1996

Current Therapy in Vascular Surgery

CURRENT THERAPY IN VASCULAR SURGERY

THIRD EDITION

Edited by

CALVIN B. ERNST, M.D.
Clinical Professor of Surgery
University of Michigan Medical School
Ann Arbor, Michigan
Head, Division of Vascular Surgery
Henry Ford Hospital
Detroit, Michigan

JAMES C. STANLEY, M.D.
Professor of Surgery
University of Michigan Medical School
Head, Section of Vascular Surgery
University Hospital
Ann Arbor, Michigan

With 784 illustrations

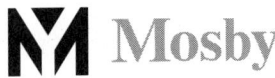

St. Louis Baltimore Boston Carlsbad Chicago Naples New York Philadelphia Portland
London Madrid Mexico City Singapore Sydney Tokyo Toronto Wiesbaden

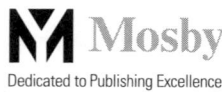
Mosby
Dedicated to Publishing Excellence

A Times Mirror Company

Publisher: Anne S. Patterson
Executive Editor: Susan M. Gay
Senior Managing Editor: Lynne Gery
Project Manager: Linda Clarke
Manufacturing Supervisor: Tim Stringham

THIRD EDITION
Copyright 1995 by Mosby–Year Book, Inc.

Previous editions copyrighted 1987, 1991

All rights reserved. No part of this publication may be reproduced, stored in a retrieval system, or transmitted, in any form or by any means, electronic, mechanical, photocopying, recording, or otherwise, without prior written permission from the publisher.

Permission to photocopy or reproduce solely for internal or personal use is permitted for libraries or other users registered with the Copyright Clearance Center, provided that the base fee of $4.00 per chapter plus $.10 per page is paid directly to the Copyright Clearance Center, 27 Congress Street, Salem, MA 01970. This consent does not extend to other kinds of copying, such as copying for general distribution, for advertising or promotional purposes, for creating new collected works, or for resale.

Printed in the United States of America.

Mosby–Year Book, Inc.
11830 Westline Industrial Drive
St. Louis, Missouri 63146

NOTICE: The authors and publisher have made every effort to ensure that the patient care recommended herein, including choice of drugs and drug dosages, is in accord with the accepted standards and practice at the time of publication. However, since research and regulation constantly change clinical standards, the reader is urged to check the product information sheet included in the package of each drug, which includes recommended doses, warnings, and contraindications. This is particularly important with new or infrequently used drugs.

ISBN 0-8151-3134-8
95 96 97 98 99 / 9 8 7 6 5 4 3 2 1

CONTRIBUTORS

WILLIAM M. ABBOTT, M.D.
Professor of Surgery, Harvard Medical School; Chief of Vascular Surgery, Massachusetts General Hospital, Boston, Massachusetts

ALI F. ABURAHMA, M.D.
Professor of Surgery, and Chief, Vascular Surgery, Robert C. Byrd Health Sciences Center of West Virginia University; Chief of Vascular Surgery, and Medical Director, Vascular Laboratory, Charleston Area Medical Center, Charleston, West Virginia

CHARLES W. ACHER, M.D.
Associate Professor of Surgery, University of Wisconsin Medical School, Madison, Wisconsin

MARK A. ADELMAN, M.D.
Assistant Professor of Surgery, New York University School of Medicine; Attending Surgeon, New York University Hospital, Bellevue Hospital, and Manhattan Veterans Administration Medical Center, New York, New York

SAMUEL S. AHN, M.D.
Associate Clinical Professor, UCLA Center for the Health Sciences, Los Angeles; Chief, Vascular Surgery, Olive View Medical Center, Sylmar, California

ERNESTO ANAYA, M.D.
Staff Surgeon, Instituto Nacional de Nutricion, Mexico City, Mexico

CHARLES A. ANDERSEN, M.D.
Clinical Professor of Surgery, Uniformed Services University of the Health Sciences, F. Edward Hébert School of Medicine, Bethesda, Maryland; Chief, Department of Surgery, Madigan Army Medical Center, Tacoma, Washington

GEORGE ANDROS, M.D.
Clinical Assistant Professor, University of Southern California School of Medicine, Los Angeles; Medical Director, Vascular Laboratory, St. Joseph Medical Center, Burbank, California

JOHN F. ANGLE, M.D.
Assistant Professor of Radiology, University of Virginia Health Sciences Center, Charlottesville, Virginia

JOSEPH P. ARCHIE, M.D., Ph.D.
Clinical Professor of Surgery, University of North Carolina School of Medicine, Chapel Hill; Adjunct Professor of Mechanical and Aerospace Engineering, North Carolina State University, Raleigh, North Carolina

ENRICO ASCER, M.D.
Professor of Surgery, State University of New York Health Science Center at Brooklyn; Director, Division of Vascular Surgery, Maimonides Medical Center, Brooklyn, New York

ALLEN W. AVERBOOK, M.D.
Staff Surgeon, Ohio Permanente Medical Group, and Staff, The Cleveland Clinic Foundation Hospital, Cleveland, Ohio

RACHEL PODRAZIK BAER, M.D.
Assistant Professor of Surgery, Wayne State University Medical School, Detroit, Michigan

AMINE BAHNINI, M.D.
Staff Surgeon, Vascular Surgery Service, Pitié-Salpêtrière University Hospital, Paris, France

J. DENNIS BAKER, M.D.
Professor of Surgery, University of California, Los Angeles, School of Medicine, Los Angeles; Chief, Vascular Surgery Section, Sepulveda Veterans Administration Medical Center, Sepulveda, California

WILLIAM H. BAKER, M.D.
Professor of Surgery, Loyola University of Chicago Stritch School of Medicine; Chief, Section of Vascular Surgery, and Director, Peripheral Vascular Laboratory, Loyola University Medical Center, Maywood, Illinois

DENNIS F. BANDYK, M.D.
Professor of Surgery, University of South Florida College of Medicine, Tampa, Florida

ROBERT W. BARNES, M.D.
Professor and Chairman, Department of Surgery, University of Arkansas for Medical Sciences; Chief of Surgery, University Hospital of Arkansas, and Attending Surgeon, McClellan Veterans Administration Medical Center, Little Rock, Arkansas

RICHARD A. BAUM, M.D.
Assistant Professor of Radiology and Surgery, University of Pennsylvania School of Medicine; Staff Interventional Radiologist, University of Pennsylvania Medical Center, Philadelphia, Pennsylvania

B. TIMOTHY BAXTER, M.D.
Assistant Professor of Surgery, Section of Vascular Surgery, University of Nebraska Medical Center; Chief of Vascular Surgery, Omaha Veterans Administration Medical Center, Omaha, Nebraska

FRITZ R. BECH, M.D.
Assistant Professor of Surgery, Dartmouth Medical School, Hanover; Staff Surgeon, Mary Hitchcock Memorial Hospital, Lebanon, New Hampshire, and Veterans Administration Medical Center, White River Junction, Vermont

HUGH G. BEEBE, M.D.
Adjunct Professor of Surgery, University of Michigan Medical School, Ann Arbor, Michigan; Director, Jobst Vascular Center, Toledo, Ohio

FOLKERT O. BELZER, M.D.
Professor and Chairman, Department of Surgery; Chairman, Division of General Surgery; Head, Section of Transplantation; and Chief of Surgery, University of Wisconsin Hospital, Madison, Wisconsin

JOHN D. BENNETT, M.D., C.M.
Assistant Professor of Diagnostic Radiology, University of Western Ontario Faculty of Medicine; London X-Ray Associates, St. Joseph's Health Centre, London, Ontario, Canada

RAMON BERGUER, M.D., Ph.D.
Professor of Surgery and Chief, Division of Vascular Surgery, Wayne State University School of Medicine; Chief, Section of Vascular Surgery, Harper Hospital, Detroit, Michigan

HENRY D. BERKOWITZ, M.D.
Associate Professor of Surgery, University of Pennsylvania School of Medicine; Chief, Division of Vascular Surgery, Presbyterian Medical Center, Philadelphia, Pennsylvania

SCOTT S. BERMAN, M.D.
Assistant Professor of Clinical Surgery, University of Arizona Health Sciences Center, Tucson, Arizona

VICTOR M. BERNHARD, M.D.
Clinical Professor of Surgery, Stanford University School of Medicine, Stanford, California

MICHAEL A. BETTMANN, M.D.
Professor of Radiology, Dartmouth Medical School, Hanover; Director, Cardiovascular and Interventional Radiology, Dartmouth-Hitchcock Medical Center, Lebanon, New Hampshire

F. WILLIAM BLAISDELL, M.D.
Professor and Chairman, Department of Surgery, University of California, Davis, School of Medicine, Davis, California

JAMES P. BOLAND, M.D.
Professor and Chairman, Department of Surgery, Robert C. Byrd Health Sciences Center of West Virginia University, Charleston, West Virginia

DAVID C. BREWSTER, M.D.
Associate Clinical Professor of Surgery, Harvard Medical School and Massachusetts General Hospital, Boston, Massachusetts

THOMAS E. BROTHERS, M.D.
Assistant Professor of Surgery, Medical University of South Carolina; Attending Surgeon, Medical University Hospital and Ralph Henry Johnson Department of Veterans Affairs Medical Center, Charleston, South Carolina

STEVEN R. BUCHMAN, M.D.
Assistant Professor, Plastic and Reconstructive Surgery, University of Michigan Medical School; Director, Craniofacial Surgery, University of Michigan Medical Center, and Chief, Pediatric Plastic Surgery, C.S. Mott Children's Hospital, Ann Arbor, Michigan

JEFFREY L. BUEHRER, M.D.
Staff Vascular Surgeon, Wilford Hall Medical Center, Lackland Air Force Base, San Antonio, Texas

RONALD W. BUSUTTIL, M.D., Ph.D.
Professor of Surgery and Dumont Chair in Transplantation Surgery, University of California, Los Angeles, School of Medicine, Los Angeles, California

MICHAEL P. BYRNE, M.D.
Chief, Section of Vascular Surgery, Brooke Army Medical Center, San Antonio, Texas

ALLAN D. CALLOW, M.D., Ph.D.

Research Professor of Surgery and Director, Vascular Biology Research Laboratory, Boston University School of Medicine; Surgeon, University Hospital and Boston City Hospital, Boston, Massachusetts

RICHARD P. CAMBRIA, M.D.

Associate Professor of Surgery, Harvard Medical School; Associate Visiting Surgeon, Massachusetts General Hospital, Boston, Massachusetts

DARRELL A. CAMPBELL, Jr., M.D.

Professor and Associate Chairman, Department of Surgery, University of Michigan Medical School; Head, Section of General Surgery, University of Michigan Hospitals, Ann Arbor, Michigan

RICHARD E. CARBALLO, M.D.

Vascular Surgery Fellow, Medical College of Wisconsin, Milwaukee, Wisconsin

JEFFREY P. CARPENTER, M.D.

Assistant Professor of Surgery, University of Pennsylvania School of Medicine; Attending Surgeon and Director, Vascular Laboratory, Hospital of the University of Pennsylvania, Philadelphia, Pennsylvania

ELLIOT L. CHAIKOF, M.D., Ph.D.

Assistant Professor of Surgery, Emory University School of Medicine; Attending, Emory University Hospital and Grady Memorial Hospital, Active Attending, Egleston Children's Hospital, and Staff Surgeon, Veterans Administration Medical Center, Atlanta, Georgia

BENJAMIN B. CHANG, M.D.

Assistant Professor of Surgery, Albany Medical College, Albany, New York

KENNETH J. CHERRY, Jr., M.D.

Associate Professor of Surgery, Mayo Medical School; Consultant, Division of Vascular Surgery, Mayo Clinic and Foundation, Rochester, Minnesota

MARC I. CHIMOWITZ, M.D.

Assistant Professor of Neurology, and Director, Cerebrovascular Program, University of Michigan Medical School, Ann Arbor, Michigan

KYUNG J. CHO, M.D.

Professor of Radiology, and Director, Division of Vascular and Interventional Radiology, University of Michigan Medical School, Ann Arbor, Michigan

TIMOTHY A. M. CHUTER, M.D.

Assistant Professor of Surgery, Columbia University College of Physicians and Surgeons; Assistant Attending Surgeon, Columbia-Presbyterian Medical Center, New York, New York

G. PATRICK CLAGETT, M.D.

Professor of Surgery and Head, Vascular Surgery Section, University of Texas Southwestern Medical Center, Dallas, Texas

ELIZABETH T. CLARK, M.D.

Research Associate and Clinical Vascular Fellow, Section of Vascular Surgery, Department of Surgery, University of Chicago Pritzker School of Medicine, Chicago, Illinois

JAMES A. COFFEY, M.D.

Clinical Assistant Professor of Surgery, Uniformed Services University of the Health Sciences, Bethesda, Maryland; Peripheral Vascular Surgeon, The Reading Hospital and Medical Center, Reading, Pennsylvania

JAY D. COFFMAN, M.D.

Professor of Medicine, Boston University School of Medicine; Chief, Vascular Medicine Section, Boston University Medical Center Hospital, Boston, Massachusetts

LISA COLLETTI, M.D.

Assistant Professor of Surgery, University of Michigan Medical School, Ann Arbor, Michigan

JOHN E. CONNOLLY, M.D.

Professor of Surgery and Chief of Vascular Surgery, University of California, Irvine, College of Medicine, Irvine, California

JOSEPH S. COSELLI, M.D.

Associate Professor of Surgery, Baylor College of Medicine; Attending Surgeon, The Methodist Hospital, Houston, Texas

ENRIQUE CRIADO, M.D.

Assistant Professor of Surgery, Division of Vascular Surgery, University of North Carolina School of Medicine, Chapel Hill, North Carolina

JACK L. CRONENWETT, M.D.

Professor of Surgery, Dartmouth Medical School; Chief, Section of Vascular Surgery, Dartmouth-Hitchcock Medical Center, Lebanon, New Hampshire

CHRISTOPHER G. CUNNINGHAM, M.D.
Assistant Professor of Vascular Surgery, Uniformed Services University for the Health Sciences; Chief, Section of Peripheral Vascular Surgery, National Naval Medical Center, Bethesda, Maryland

BRUCE S. CUTLER, M.D.
Professor of Surgery, University of Massachusetts Medical School; Chief of Vascular Surgery, University of Massachusetts Medical Center, Worcester, Massachusetts

MICHAEL D. DAKE, M.D.
Assistant Professor of Radiology and Medicine, Stanford University School of Medicine; Chief, Cardiovascular and Interventional Radiology, and Co-Director, Cath/Angio Laboratories, Stanford University Hospital, Stanford, California

HERBERT DARDIK, M.D.
Clinical Professor of Surgery, Mt. Sinai Medical Center; New York, New York; Chief, Department of Surgery, Englewood Hospital and Medical Center, Englewood, New Jersey

R. CLEMENT DARLING III, M.D.
Assistant Professor of Surgery, Albany Medical College, Albany, New York

RICHARD H. DEAN, M.D.
Professor and Chairman, Department of Surgery, Bowman Gray School of Medicine; Chief of Surgery, North Carolina Baptist Hospital, Winston-Salem, North Carolina

DAVID H. DEATON, M.D.
Assistant Clinical Professor of Surgery, University of Pennsylvania School of Medicine; Staff Surgeon, Jeanes Hospital and Presbyterian Hospital, and Associate Staff Surgeon, Fox Chase Cancer Institute, Philadelphia, Pennsylvania

ROBERT D. DeFRANG, M.D.
Assistant Professor of Surgery, Division of Vascular Surgery, University of New Mexico School of Medicine, Albuquerque, New Mexico

DOMINIC A. DeLAURENTIS, M.D.
Professor of Surgery, University of Pennsylvania School of Medicine; Chief, Section of Vascular Surgery, Pennsylvania Hospital, Philadelphia, Pennsylvania

RALPH G. DePALMA, M.D.
Professor and Vice Chairman of Surgery, and Associate Dean, University of Nevada School of Medicine; Chief of Surgery, Ionnis A. Lougaris Veterans Administration Medical Center, Reno, Nevada

JAMES A. DeWEESE, M.D.
Professor of Surgery and Chief Emeritus of Cardiothoracic and Vascular Surgery, University of Rochester Medical Center, Rochester, New York

THOMAS F. DODSON, M.D.
Associate Professor of Surgery, Emory University School of Medicine, Atlanta, Georgia

MAGRUDER C. DONALDSON, M.D.
Associate Professor of Surgery, Harvard Medical School; Surgeon, Brigham and Women's Hospital, Boston, Massachusetts

CHRISTOS D. DOSSA, M.D.
Staff Vascular Surgeon, Staten Island University Hospital, Staten Island, New York

RICHARD W. DOW, M.D.
Associate Professor of Surgery, Dartmouth Medical School, Hanover, New Hampshire; Physician and Chief of Surgical Service, Veterans Administration Medical and Regional Office Center, White River Junction, Vermont

CHRISTOPHER F. DOWD, M.D.
Assistant Professor of Radiology and Neurological Surgery, University of California, San Francisco, School of Medicine, San Francisco, California

ALLAN R. DOWNS, M.D.
Professor of Surgery, University of Manitoba Faculty of Medicine; Head, Vascular Surgery Service, Health Sciences Centre, Winnipeg, Manitoba, Canada

PAUL W. DURANCE, PH.D.
Assistant Professor of Health Services Management and Policy, University of Michigan School of Public Health, Ann Arbor, Michigan

FREDERIC E. ECKHAUSER, M.D.
Professor of Surgery and Chief, Division of Gastrointestinal Surgery, University of Michigan Medical School, Ann Arbor, Michigan

WILLIAM H. EDWARDS, M.D.
H. William Scott, Jr. Professor of Surgery and Chief, Division of Vascular Surgery, Vanderbilt University Medical Center, Nashville, Tennessee

WILLIAM K. EHRENFELD, M.D.
Professor of Surgery, University of California, San Francisco, School of Medicine, San Francisco, California

BO EKLOF, M.D., Ph.D.
   Clinical Professor of Surgery, University of Hawaii John A. Burns School of Medicine; Vascular Surgeon, Straub Clinic and Hospital, Honolulu, Hawaii

SHERIF EL-MASSRY, M.D.
   Assistant Professor, Department of General Surgery, El Mansoura University, El Mansoura, Egypt; Clinical and Research Fellow, The Hope Heart Institute, Seattle, Washington

MARTIN I. ELLENBY, M.D.
   Fellow, Division of Vascular Surgery, Henry Ford Hospital, Detroit, Michigan

JOSEPH P. ELLIOTT, Jr., M.D.
   Clinical Associate Professor of Surgery, University of Michigan Medical School, Ann Arbor; Senior Surgeon, Division of Vascular Surgery, Henry Ford Hospital, Detroit, Michigan

FRANK D. ELLIS, M.D.
   Resident, Department of Orthopaedic Surgery, Emory University Hospital, Atlanta, Georgia

ERIC D. ENDEAN, M.D.
   Associate Professor of Surgery, University of Kentucky College of Medicine; Attending Physician, Chandler Medical Center and Veterans Administration Hospital, Lexington, Kentucky

CALVIN B. ERNST, M.D.
   Clinical Professor of Surgery, University of Michigan Medical School, Ann Arbor; Head, Division of Vascular Surgery, Henry Ford Hospital, Detroit, Michigan

WILLIAM E. EVANS, M.D.
   Clinical Professor of Surgery, Ohio State University College of Medicine, Columbus, Ohio

JAMES I. FANN, M.D.
   Fellow, Cardiothoracic Surgery and Vascular Surgery, Stanford University School of Medicine, Stanford, California

MARK F. FILLINGER, M.D.
   Assistant Professor of Surgery, Dartmouth-Hitchcock Medical Center, Lebanon, New Hampshire

DANIEL F. FISHER, Jr., M.D.
   Associate Professor of Surgery, Chattanooga Unit of University of Tennessee College of Medicine; Staff Surgeon, Erlanger Medical Center, Chattanooga, Tennessee

LAMAR L. FLEMING, M.D.
   Professor and Chairman, Department of Orthopaedic Surgery, Emory University School of Medicine, Atlanta, Georgia

WILLIAM R. FLINN, M.D.
   Professor of Surgery, University of Maryland School of Medicine; Head, Section of Vascular Surgery, University of Maryland Medical Center, Baltimore, Maryland

THOMAS J. FOGARTY, M.D.
   Professor of Surgery, Stanford University School of Medicine, Stanford, California

RICHARD J. FOWL, M.D.
   Associate Professor of Surgery, University of Cincinnati Medical Center, Cincinnati, Ohio

JOSEPH E. FRANKHOUSE, M.D.
   Clinical Resident Instructor in General Surgery, University of Southern California School of Medicine, Los Angeles, California

PAUL FRIEDMANN, M.D.
   Professor of Surgery, Tufts University School of Medicine, Boston; Chairman, Department of Surgery, Baystate Medical Center, Springfield, Massachusetts

ARNOST FRONEK, M.D., Ph.D.
   Professor of Surgery and Bioengineering, University of California, San Diego, School of Medicine; Chief, Vascular Laboratory, Veterans Administration Medical Center, La Jolla, California

MAX R. GASPAR, M.D.
   Clinical Professor of Surgery Emeritus, University of Southern California School of Medicine; Consultant, Vascular Surgery, Los Angeles County/University of Southern California Medical Center, Los Angeles, California

JONATHAN P. GERTLER, M.D.
   Assistant Professor of Surgery, Harvard Medical School; Assistant Surgeon, Massachusetts General Hospital, Boston, Massachusetts

BRUCE L. GEWERTZ, M.D.
   Dallas B. Phemister Professor and Chairman, Department of Surgery, University of Chicago Pritzker School of Medicine, Chicago, Illinois

GARY W. GIBBONS, M.D.
   Associate Clinical Professor of Surgery, Harvard Medical School; Clinical Chief, Division of Vascular Surgery, New England Deaconess Hospital, Boston, Massachusetts

JOSEPH GIGLIA, M.D.
Research Fellow and Surgical Resident, Department of Surgery, University of Michigan Medical School, Ann Arbor, Michigan

ENRIQUE GINZBURG, M.D.
Department of Surgery, M.D. Jackson Memorial Hospital, University of Miami Hospital and Clinics, and Veterans Administration Hospital, Miami, Florida

JOSEPH M. GIORDANO, M.D.
Professor and Chairman, Department of Surgery, George Washington University Medical Center, Washington, DC

PETER GLOVICZKI, M.D.
Professor of Surgery, Mayo Medical School; Consultant, Division of Vascular Surgery, Mayo Clinic and Foundation, Rochester, Minnesota

MITCHELL H. GOLDMAN, M.D.
Professor of Surgery, University of Tennessee Graduate School of Medicine; Chief of Vascular and Transplant Surgery, University of Tennessee Medical Center, Knoxville, Tennessee

HARRY S. GOLDSMITH, M.D.
Professor of Surgery and Adjunct Professor of Neurosurgery, Boston University School of Medicine; Attending Surgeon, University Hospital, Boston, Massachusetts

JERRY GOLDSTONE, M.D.
Professor and Vice-Chairman, Department of Surgery, University of California, San Francisco, School of Medicine; Staff Surgeon, Department of Veterans Affairs Medical Center, San Francisco, California

DAVID GORDON, M.D.
Associate Professor of Pathology, University of Michigan Medical School, Ann Arbor, Michigan

ROBERT C. GORMAN, M.D.
Instructor of Surgery and Surgical Resident, Hospital of the University of Pennsylvania, Philadelphia, Pennsylvania

ALAN M. GRAHAM, M.D.
Associate Professor and Chief, Division of Vascular Surgery, University of Medicine and Dentistry of New Jersey–Robert Wood Johnson Medical School; Attending Staff, Robert Wood Johnson University Hospital, New Brunswick, New Jersey

LINDA M. GRAHAM, M.D.
Professor of Surgery, Case Western Reserve University School of Medicine; Chief, Vascular Surgery Section, Veterans Affairs Medical Center, Cleveland, Ohio

ROBERT A. GRAOR, M.D.
Associate Professor of Medicine and Chairman, Department of Vascular Medicine, The Cleveland Clinic Foundation, Cleveland, Ohio

JOHN L. GRAY, M.D.
Assistant Professor of Surgery, Rush Medical Center; Staff Surgeon, Section of Vascular Surgery, Cook County Hospital, Chicago, Illinois

RICHARD M. GREEN, M.D.
Associate Professor of Surgery and Chief, Section of Vascular Surgery, University of Rochester School of Medicine and Dentistry, Rochester, New York

LAZAR J. GREENFIELD, M.D.
Frederick A. Coller Professor and Chairman, Department of Surgery, University of Michigan Medical School; Surgeon-in-Chief, University of Michigan Hospitals, Ann Arbor, Michigan

ROGER M. GREENHALGH, M.D., M.CHIR.
Professor and Chairman, Department of Surgery, Charing Cross and Westminster Medical School; Director, Regional Vascular Service, Charing Cross Hospital, London, United Kingdom

ANITA K. GREGORY, M.D.
Research Fellow in Vascular Science and Surgical Resident, St. Luke's-Roosevelt Hospital Center of Columbia University, New York, New York

SUSHIL K. GUPTA, M.D.
Associate Clinical Professor of Surgery, Harvard Medical School, Boston; Chairman, Department of Surgery, MetroWest Medical Center, Framingham, Massachusetts

KEVIN A. HALL, M.D.
Chief Resident in Surgery, University of Arizona Health Sciences Center, Tucson, Arizona

JOHN W. HALLETT, JR., M.D.
Professor of Surgery, Mayo Medical School, Mayo Clinic, Rochester, Minnesota

KIMBERLEY J. HANSEN, M.D.
Associate Professor of Surgery, and Director, Clinical Vascular Laboratory, Bowman Gray School of Medicine, Winston-Salem, North Carolina

DOUGLAS W. HARRINGTON, D.O.
William Beaumont Hospital, Royal Oak, St. Johns Hospital, Detroit, and Mt. Clemens General Hospital, Mt. Clemens, Michigan

E. JOHN HARRIS, JR., M.D.
Assistant Professor of Surgery, Stanford University School of Medicine, Stanford; Staff Vascular Surgeon, Palo Alto Veterans Administration Medical Center, Palo Alto, California

ROBERT W. HARRIS, M.D.
Associate Clinical Professor of Surgery, University of Southern California School of Medicine, Los Angeles, California

TIMOTHY R. S. HARWARD, M.D.
Associate Professor of Surgery, University of Florida College of Medicine, Gainesville, Florida

ZIV J. HASKAL, M.D.
Assistant Professor of Radiology and Surgery, Hospital of the University of Pennsylvania, Philadelphia, Pennsylvania

JAMES L. HAYNES, M.D.
Professor of Surgery, University of South Carolina School of Medicine; Staff, Richland Memorial Hospital and Veterans Administration Medical Center, Columbia, South Carolina

NORMAN R. HERTZER, M.D.
Chairman, Department of Vascular Surgery, The Cleveland Clinic Foundation, Cleveland, Ohio

DAN J. HIGMAN, FRCS
Department of Surgery, Charing Cross Hospital, London, United Kingdom

ANIL P. HINGORANI, M.D.
Fellow in Vascular Science and Surgical Resident, St. Luke's-Roosevelt Hospital Center of Columbia University, New York, New York

ASHER HIRSHBERG, M.D.
Lecturer in Surgery, Sackler School of Medicine, Tel Aviv University, Tel Aviv; Attending Surgeon, Chaim Sheba Medical Center, Tel Hashomer, Israel

ROBERT W. HOBSON II, M.D.
Professor of Surgery, and Chief, Section of Vascular Surgery, University of Medicine and Dentistry of New Jersey/New Jersey Medical School, Newark, New Jersey

LARRY H. HOLLIER, M.D.
Executive Director of Clinical Affairs, Healthcare International (Scotland), Clydebank, Glasgow, Scotland

WILLIAM HOLMES, M.D.
Department of Surgery, University Hospital, Boston, Massachusetts

THOMAS S. HUBER, M.D., PH.D.
Assistant Professor of Surgery, University of Florida College of Medicine; Staff, Veterans Administration Medical Center, Gainesville, Florida

GLENN C. HUNTER, M.D.
Associate Professor of Surgery, University of Arizona Medical Center; Staff, Veterans Administration Medical Center, and Kino Community Hospital, Tucson, Arizona

GORDON L. HYDE, M.D.
Professor of Surgery, University of Kentucky College of Medicine; Chief, Vascular Surgery, University of Kentucky Hospital, Lexington, Kentucky

MARK IANNETTONI, M.D.
Assistant Professor of Surgery, University of Michigan Medical School; Staff, Veterans Administration Medical Center, Ann Arbor, Michigan

ANTHONY M. IMPARATO, M.D.
Professor of Surgery, New York University Medical Center, New York, New York

DONALD L. JACOBS, M.D., M.S.
Assistant Professor of Surgery, St. Louis University School of Medicine; Staff, St. Louis University Hospital and Veterans Administration Medical Center, St. Louis, Missouri

LLOYD A. JACOBS, M.D.
Associate Professor of Surgery, University of Michigan Medical School; Chief of Staff, Veterans Administration Medical Center, Ann Arbor, Michigan

DOUGLAS L. JICHA, M.D.
Assistant Professor of Vascular Surgery, University of Utah Health Science Center, Salt Lake City, Utah

KAJ H. JOHANSEN, M.D., PH.D.
Professor of Surgery, University of Washington School of Medicine; Director, Surgical Education, Providence Medical Center, Seattle, Washington

GEORGE JOHNSON, JR., M.D.
Roscoe B.G. Cowper Distinguished Professor and Vice Chairman, Department of Surgery, University of North Carolina School of Medicine, Chapel Hill, North Carolina

K. WAYNE JOHNSTON, M.D.
Professor and Associate Chairman, Department of Surgery, University of Toronto Faculty of Medicine; Head, Division of Vascular Surgery, The Toronto Hospital, Toronto, Ontario, Canada

JOHN W. JOYCE, M.D.
Professor of Medicine, Mayo Medical School; Consultant, Division of Internal Medicine, Cardiovascular Diseases, Mayo Clinic, Rochester, Minnesota

SAADOON KADIR, M.D.
Clinical Professor of Radiology, St. Louis University School of Medicine, St. Louis, Missouri

DOROTHY M. KAHKONEN, M.D.
Clinical Assistant Professor of Internal Medicine, University of Michigan Medical School, Ann Arbor; Senior Staff Physician, Division of Endocrinology and Metabolism, Henry Ford Hospital, Detroit, Michigan

PETER G. KALMAN, M.D.
Associate Professor of Surgery, University of Toronto Faculty of Medicine; Staff Vascular Surgeon, The Toronto Hospital, Toronto, Ontario, Canada

FREDERICK M. KARRER, M.D.
Associate Professor of Surgery and Assistant Professor of Pediatrics, University of Colorado School of Medicine; Director, Pediatric Transplantation, Children's Hospital/ University of Colorado Health Sciences Center, Denver, Colorado

DAVID J. KASTAN, M.D.
Senior Staff, Department of Radiology, Henry Ford Hospital, Detroit, Michigan

ANDRIS KAZMERS, M.D., M.P.H.
Associate Professor of Surgery, Wayne State University School of Medicine; Director, Vascular Surgery Laboratory, Harper Hospital, Detroit, Michigan

BLAIR A. KEAGY, M.D.
Professor of Surgery, University of North Carolina School of Medicine; Chief, Division of Vascular Surgery, University of North Carolina Hospitals, Chapel Hill, North Carolina

RICHARD F. KEMPCZINSKI, M.D.
Professor of Surgery and Chief, Vascular Surgery, University of Cincinnati Medical Center, Cincinnati, Ohio

ROBERT K. KERLAN, Jr., M.D.
Associate Clinical Professor of Radiology and Chief of Interventional Radiology, Mount Zion Medical Center, San Francisco, California

MORRIS D. KERSTEIN, M.D.
Deissler Professor of Surgery, Hahnemann University School of Medicine, Philadelphia, Pennsylvania, and Clinical Professor of Surgery, Uniformed Services University of the Health Sciences F. Edward Hébert School of Medicine, Bethesda, Maryland

EDOUARD KIEFFER, M.D.
Professor of Surgery, Pitié-Salpêtrière School of Medicine; Chief of Vascular Surgery, Pitié-Salpêtrière University Hospital, Paris, France

MICHAEL J. KIKTA, M.D.
Vascular Surgery Resident, University of Missouri–Columbia School of Medicine, Columbia, Missouri

LOIS A. KILLEWICH, M.D., Ph.D.
Assistant Professor of Surgery, University of Maryland School of Medicine, Baltimore, Maryland

MARVIN M. KIRSH, M.D.
Professor of Surgery, University of Michigan Medical School; Chief, Cardiothoracic Surgery, Veterans Administration Medical Center, Ann Arbor, Michigan

ROBERT L. KISTNER, M.D.
Clinical Professor of Surgery, University of Hawaii John A. Burns School of Medicine; Staff Surgeon, Straub Clinic and Hospital, Honolulu, Hawaii

JAMES A. KNOL, M.D.
Associate Professor of Surgery, University of Michigan Medical School; Staff Surgeon, University of Michigan Hospital, Ann Arbor, Michigan

TED R. KOHLER, M.D.
Associate Professor of Surgery, University of Washington School of Medicine; Chief, Vascular Surgery Section, Veterans Administration Medical Center, Seattle, Washington

FABIEN KOSKAS, M.D.
Praticien-Hospitalier, Pitié-Salpêtrière University Hospital, Paris, France

TIMOTHY F. KRESOWIK, M.D.
Associate Professor of Surgery, University of Iowa College of Medicine, Iowa City, Iowa

WILLIAM C. KRUPSKI, M.D.
Professor of Surgery, University of Colorado Health Sciences Center; Chief, Vascular Surgery Section, University Hospital, Denver, Colorado

CHRISTOPHER J. KWOLEK, M.D.
Clinical Fellow in Vascular Surgery, Massachusetts General Hospital, Boston, Massachusetts

WAYNE W. LaMORTE, M.D., Ph.D., M.P.H.
Associate Professor of Surgery, Boston University School of Medicine, Boston, Massachusetts

PATRICK J. LAMPARELLO, M.D.
Associate Professor of Surgery, New York University School of Medicine, New York, New York

GLENN M. LaMURAGLIA, M.D.
Assistant Professor of Surgery, Harvard Medical School; Assistant Surgeon, Massachusetts General Hospital, Boston, Massachusetts

RAUL A. LANDA, M.D.
General and Vascular Surgeon, MetroWest Medical Center, Framingham, Massachusetts

PETER F. LAWRENCE, M.D.
Professor and Chairman, Division of Vascular Surgery, University of Utah Health Science Center, Salt Lake City, Utah

ROBERT P. LEATHER, M.D.
Professor of Surgery, Albany Medical College; Chief, Vascular Surgery, Albany Medical Center, Albany, New York

PAVEL J. LEVY, M.D.
Clinical Fellow, Department of Vascular Medicine, The Cleveland Clinic Foundation, Cleveland, Ohio

JOHN R. LILLY, M.D.
Professor of Surgery and Pediatrics, and Chief, Section of Pediatric Surgery, University of Colorado School of Medicine; Chairman, Department of Pediatric Surgery, The Children's Hospital, Denver, Colorado

MICHAEL P. LILLY, M.D.
Associate Professor of Surgery, University of Maryland School of Medicine, Baltimore, Maryland

S. MARTIN LINDENAUER, M.D.
Professor of Surgery, University of Michigan Medical School; Assistant Chief of Staff, Ann Arbor Veterans Administration Medical Center, Ann Arbor, Michigan

JOHN P. LOFTUS, M.D.
Fellow, Division of Vascular Surgery, Department of Surgery, Mayo Graduate School of Medicine, Rochester, Minnesota

FRANK W. LoGERFO, M.D.
Professor of Surgery, Harvard Medical School; Chief, Division of Vascular Surgery, New England Deaconess Hospital, Boston, Massachusetts

HERBERT I. MACHLEDER, M.D.
Professor of Surgery, University of California, Los Angeles, School of Medicine; Attending Surgeon, Vascular Service, UCLA Medical Center, Los Angeles, California

WILLIAM C. MACKEY, M.D.
Associate Professor of Surgery, Tufts University School of Medicine; Attending Vascular Surgeon, New England Medical Center Hospitals, Boston, Massachusetts

JOHN A. MANNICK, M.D.
Moseley Distinguished Professor of Surgery, Harvard Medical School, Boston, Massachusetts

JOHN M. MAREK, M.D.
Vascular Fellow, University of Arizona Health Sciences Center, Tucson, Arizona

PHILIPPE A. MASSER, M.D.
Fellow, Division of Vascular Surgery, Oregon Health Sciences University, Portland, Oregon

ALAN H. MATSUMOTO, M.D.
Associate Professor of Radiology, Division of Angiography and Interventional Radiology, University of Virginia Health Sciences Center, Charlottesville, Virginia

MARK A. MATTOS, M.D.
Assistant Professor of Surgery, Southern Illinois University School of Medicine, Springfield, Illinois

KENNETH L. MATTOX, M.D.
Professor of Surgery, Baylor College of Medicine; Chief of Staff and Chief of Surgery, Ben Taub General Hospital, Houston, Texas

RICHARD L. McCANN, M.D.
Professor of Surgery and Chief of Vascular Surgery, Duke University Medical Center, Durham, North Carolina

WALTER J. McCARTHY, M.D.
Assistant Professor of Surgery, Northwestern University Medical School; Staff Surgeon, Northwestern Memorial Hospital, Chicago, Illinois

HOLT A. McDOWELL, JR., M.D.
Professor of Surgery and Medical Staff, University of Alabama at Birmingham; Consultant, Veterans Administration Medical Center, Birmingham, Alabama

JOSE MENA, M.D.
Assistant Professor of Surgery, Medical College of Georgia, Augusta, Georgia

JAMES O. MENZOIAN, M.D.
Professor of Surgery, Boston University School of Medicine; Chief, Section of Vascular Surgery, Boston University Medical Center, Boston, Massachusetts

ROBERT M. MERION, M.D.
Associate Professor of Surgery, University of Michigan Medical School; Chief, Division of Transplantation, University of Michigan Medical School, Ann Arbor, Michigan

CHARLES L. MESH, M.D.
Assistant Professor of Surgery, Case Western Reserve University School of Medicine; Staff Surgeon, Veterans Administration Medical Center, Cleveland, Ohio

LOUIS M. MESSINA, M.D.
Associate Professor of Surgery, University of Michigan Medical School; Staff Surgeon, University Hospital and Co-Chief, Vascular Surgery Service, Veterans Administration Medical Center, Ann Arbor, Michigan

D. CRAIG MILLER, M.D.
Professor of Cardiovascular and Thoracic Surgery, and Director, Cardiovascular Physiology Research Laboratory, Stanford University School of Medicine, Stanford, California

TIMOTHY A. MILLER, M.D.
Professor, Plastic and Reconstructive Surgery, University of California, Los Angeles, School of Medicine; Chief of Plastic Surgery, West Los Angeles Veterans Administration Medical Center, Los Angeles, California

JOSEPH L. MILLS, M.D.
Associate Professor of Surgery and Chief of Vascular Surgery, University of Arizona College of Medicine; Attending Surgeon, University Medical Center and Veterans Administration Medical Center, Tucson, Arizona

PANAYIOTIS MITSIAS, M.D.
Senior Staff Neurologist, Henry Ford Hospital, Detroit, Michigan

J. GREGORY MODRALL, M.D.
Research Fellow in Vascular Surgery, and Resident, Department of Surgery, University of Southern California School of Medicine, Los Angeles, California

ASHBY C. MONCURE, M.D.
Associate Clinical Professor of Surgery, Harvard Medical School; Visiting Surgeon, Massachusetts General Hospital, Boston, Massachusetts

GREGORY L. MONETA, M.D.
Associate Professor of Surgery, Oregon Health Sciences University; Staff Surgeon, Oregon Health Sciences University Hospital and Veterans Administration Medical Center, Portland, Oregon

SAMUEL R. MONEY, M.D.
Clinical Assistant Professor of Surgery, Tulane University School of Medicine; Staff Surgeon, Ochsner Clinic, and Director, Surgery Research Laboratory, Ochsner Medical Foundation, New Orleans, Louisiana

WESLEY S. MOORE, M.D.
Professor of Surgery, University of California, Los Angeles, School of Medicine; Chief, Section of Vascular Surgery, UCLA Medical Center, Los Angeles, California

MOHAMMED M. MOURSI, M.D.
Lecturer in Vascular Surgery, University of Michigan Medical School, Ann Arbor, Michigan

STEPHEN P. MURRAY, M.D.
Clinical Instructor in Surgery, University of California, San Francisco School of Medicine, San Francisco, California, and Assistant Clinical Professor of Surgery, Uniformed Services University of the Health Sciences, Bethesda, Maryland

MASSIMO M. NAPOLITANO, M.D.
Clinical Fellow, Division of Vascular Surgery, Henry Ford Hospital, Detroit, Michigan

EILEEN S. NATUZZI, M.D.
Surgical Resident, University of California, San Francisco, Medical Center, San Francisco, California

MARK R. NEHLER, M.D.
Resident in Vascular Surgery, Oregon Health Sciences University, Portland, Oregon

CONSTANCE NEWMAN, R.N.
Section of Cardiothoracic Surgery, Ann Arbor Veterans Administration Medical Center, Ann Arbor, Michigan

ANDREW N. NICOLAIDES, M.D.
Academic Vascular Surgery, St. Mary's Hospital, London, United Kingdom

ANDREW C. NOVICK, M.D.
Chairman, Department of Urology, The Cleveland Clinic Foundation, Cleveland, Ohio

DANIEL B. NUNN, M.D.
Clinical Professor of Surgery, University of Florida Health Science Center, Jacksonville, Florida

TIMOTHY J. NYPAVER, M.D.
Assistant Professor of Surgery, University of Kentucky Medical Center; Attending Surgeon, A.B. Chandler Medical Center and Veterans Administration Hospital, Lexington, Kentucky

THOMAS F. O'DONNELL, JR., M.D.
Professor and Chairman, Department of Surgery, Tufts University School of Medicine; Surgeon-in-Chief and Chief, Division of Vascular Surgery, New England Medical Center, Boston, Massachusetts

PATRICK J. O'HARA, M.D.
Associate Professor of Surgery, The Ohio State University College of Medicine; Staff Surgeon, Department of Vascular Surgery, The Cleveland Clinic Foundation, Cleveland, Ohio

CORNELIUS OLCOTT IV, M.D.
Professor of Surgery, Stanford University School of Medicine, Stanford, California

KIM M. OLTHOFF, M.D.
Clinical Instructor, Department of Surgery, University of California, Los Angeles, School of Medicine; Multi-Organ Transplant Fellow, Dumont–UCLA Transplant Center, Los Angeles, California

KENNETH OURIEL, M.D.
Clinical Associate Professor of Surgery, University of Rochester School of Medicine and Dentistry, Rochester, New York

FRANK T. PADBERG, JR., M.D.
Associate Professor of Surgery, University of Medicine and Dentistry of New Jersey/New Jersey Medical School, Newark; Associate Chief of Surgery, Veterans Administration Medical Center, East Orange, New Jersey

WILLIAM H. PEARCE, M.D.
Professor of Surgery, Northwestern University Medical School; Chief, Vascular Surgery Section, Veterans Administration Lakeside Medical Center, and Attending Surgeon, Northwestern Memorial Hospital, Chicago, Illinois

BRUCE A. PERLER, M.D.
Associate Professor of Surgery, The Johns Hopkins University School of Medicine; Director, Vascular Surgery Service and Noninvasive Vascular Laboratory, Johns Hopkins Hospital, Baltimore, Maryland

MALCOLM O. PERRY, M.D.
Professor and Chief of Vascular Surgery, Texas Tech University Health Sciences Center, Lubbock, Texas

MICHAEL J. PETERSEN, M.D.
Resident in Vascular Surgery, Harvard Medical School and Massachusetts General Hospital, Boston, Massachusetts

THOMAS PFAMMATTER, M.D.
Lecturer, University of Michigan Medical School; Fellow, Division of Vascular and Interventional Radiology, University of Michigan Hospitals, Ann Arbor, Michigan

JOHN R. PFEIFER, M.D.
Clinical Associate Professor of Surgery, Wayne State University School of Medicine, Detroit, and Adjunct Professor of Health Sciences, Oakland University, Rochester; Director of Surgical Research, Providence Hospital and Medical Center, Southfield, Michigan

THOMAS G. PICKERING, JR., M.D., PH.D.
Professor of Medicine, Cornell University Medical College; Attending Physician, The New York Hospital, New York, New York

LAKSHMIKUMAR PILLAI, M.D.
Assistant Professor of Vascular Surgery, State University of New York at Buffalo School of Medicine and Biomedical Sciences, Buffalo, New York

ROBERT J. PITSCH, M.D.
Instructor, Department of Surgery, Veterans Administration Medical Center and University of Utah School of Medicine, Salt Lake City, Utah

ROBERT M. POLLINA, M.D.
Fellow in Vascular Surgery, Maimonides Medical Center, Brooklyn, New York

JOHN POPOVICH, JR., M.D.
Clinical Associate Professor of Medicine, University of Michigan Medical School, Ann Arbor; Division Head, Pulmonary and Critical Care Medicine, Henry Ford Hospital, Detroit, Michigan

JOHN M. PORTER, M.D.
Professor of Surgery, and Chief, Division of Vascular Surgery, Oregon Health Sciences University, Portland, Oregon

JANET T. POWELL, Ph.D., M.D.
Reader in Cardiovascular Biology, University of London, London, United Kingdom

JOHN L. PROVAN, M.S.
Professor of Surgery and Associate Dean of Postgraduate Medical Education, University of Toronto; Consultant, Departments of Surgery, The Wellesley Hospital and The Toronto Hospital, Toronto, Ontario, Canada

JEFFREY D. PUNCH, M.D.
Assistant Professor of Surgery, University of Michigan Medical School, Ann Arbor, Michigan

WILLIAM J. QUIÑONES-BALDRICH, M.D.
Associate Professor of Surgery, University of California, Los Angeles, School of Medicine; Staff Surgeon, UCLA Medical Center, Los Angeles, California

SESHADRI RAJU, M.D.
Professor of Surgery, University of Mississippi Medical Center, Jackson, Mississippi

TAMMY K. RAMOS, M.D.
Assistant Professor of Surgery, University of California, San Francisco, School of Medicine; Staff Surgeon, Medical Center at the University of California, San Francisco, and Veterans Administration Medical Center, San Francisco, California

TIMOTHY J. RANVAL, M.D.
Assistant Professor of Surgery, Vanderbilt University School of Medicine, Nashville, Tennessee

SCOTT W. REAVIS
Clinical Director, Surgery Vascular Laboratory, Bowman Gray School of Medicine, Winston-Salem, North Carolina

DANIEL J. REDDY, M.D.
Clinical Associate Professor of Surgery, University of Michigan Medical School, Ann Arbor; Senior Staff Vascular Surgeon, Henry Ford Hospital, Detroit, Michigan

LINDA M. REILLY, M.D.
Associate Professor of Surgery, University of California, San Francisco, Medical Center, San Francisco, California

MARK REYNOLDS, M.D.
Assistant Professor of Surgery, West Virginia University School of Medicine, Morgantown, West Virginia

ROBERT Y. RHEE, M.D.
Vascular Surgery Fellow, Mayo Clinic, Rochester, Minnesota

NORMAN M. RICH, M.D.
Professor and Chairman, Department of Surgery, Uniformed Services University of the Health Sciences, Bethesda, Maryland

J. DAVID RICHARDSON, M.D.
Professor and Vice Chairman, Department of Surgery, and Chief of General Surgery, University of Louisville School of Medicine, Louisville, Kentucky

JOHN J. RICOTTA, M.D.
Professor of Surgery and Director, Division of Vascular Surgery, State University of New York at Buffalo School of Medicine and Biomedical Sciences; Chief of Surgery, Millard Fillmore Hospital, Buffalo, New York

LAYTON F. RIKKERS, M.D.
M.M. Musselman Professor and Chairman, Department of Surgery, University of Nebraska Medical Center, Omaha, Nebraska

THOMAS S. RILES, M.D.
Professor of Surgery and Director, Division of Vascular Surgery, New York University Medical Center; Attending Surgeon, Tisch Hospital, New York, New York

ERNEST J. RING, M.D.
Professor of Radiology, University of California, San Francisco, School of Medicine; Chief, Interventional Radiology, University of California, San Francisco, and Chief, Radiology Service, Mt. Zion Hospital, San Francisco, California

AGUSTIN A. RODRIGUEZ, M.D.
Vascular Surgery Fellow, Tufts-New England Medical Center, Boston, Massachusetts

MICHAEL J. ROHRER, M.D.
Assistant Professor of Surgery, University of Massachusetts Medical School; Director, Venous Clinic, University of Massachusetts Medical Center, Worcester, Massachusetts

ALEXANDER ROMASCHIN, Ph.D.
University of Toronto, Toronto, Ontario, Canada

ERNEST F. ROSATO, M.D.
Professor of Surgery, University of Pennsylvania School of Medicine; Chief, Gastrointestinal Surgery Division, Hospital of the University of Pennsylvania, Philadelphia, Pennsylvania

DAVID ROSENTHAL, M.D.
Clinical Professor of Surgery, Medical College of Georgia, Augusta; Chief of Vascular Surgery, Georgia Baptist Medical Center, Atlanta, Georgia

BRIAN G. RUBIN, M.D.
Assistant Professor of Surgery, Washington University School of Medicine; Director, Noninvasive Vascular Laboratory, Jewish Hospital, St. Louis, Missouri

GEORGE H. RUDKIN, M.D.
Resident, Department of Surgery, UCLA Medical Center, Los Angeles, California

MARK C. RUMMEL, M.D.
Vascular Fellow and Instructor in Surgery, Hahnemann University Hospital and School of Medicine, Philadelphia, Pennsylvania

CARLO RUOTOLO, M.D.
Staff Surgeon, Pitié-Salpétrière University Hospital, Paris, France

DANIEL S. RUSH, M.D.
Associate Professor of Surgery and Chief, Vascular Surgery Service, University of South Carolina School of Medicine; Chief, Vascular Surgery Service, Veterans Administration Medical Center, and Staff Surgeon, Richland Memorial Hospital, Columbia, South Carolina

ROBERT B. RUTHERFORD, M.D.
Professor of Surgery, University of Colorado Health Sciences Center; Staff Surgeon, University Hospital, Denver, Colorado

ATEF A. SALAM, M.D.
Professor of Surgery, Emory University Affiliated Hospitals, Atlanta, and Veterans Administration Medical Center, Decatur, Georgia

RAJABRATA SARKAR, M.D.
Research Fellow, Section of Vascular Surgery, University of Michigan Medical School, Ann Arbor, Michigan; Resident in General Surgery, UCLA Center for the Health Sciences, Los Angeles, California

LESTER R. SAUVAGE, M.D.
Clinical Professor of Surgery, The University of Washington School of Medicine; Medical Director, The Hope Heart Institute, Seattle, Washington

PETER A. SCHNEIDER, M.D.
Division of Cardiovascular and Thoracic Surgery, Hawaii Permanente Medical Group, Honolulu, Hawaii

JAMES J. SCHULER, M.D.
Professor of Surgery, University of Illinois College of Medicine; Chief, Division of Vascular Surgery, University of Illinois Hospital, and Attending Surgeon, Cook County Hospital, West Side Veterans Administration Medical Center, Edgewater Hospital, and Michael Reese Hospital, Chicago, Illinois

SHELDON A. SCHWARTZ, M.D.
Senior Staff Surgeon, Henry Ford Hospital, Detroit, Michigan

JAMES M. SEEGER, M.D.
Professor of Surgery and Chief, Section of Vascular Surgery, University of Florida College of Medicine, Gainesville, Florida

JOHN GRAY SEILER III, M.D.
Assistant Professor of Orthopaedic Surgery and Director of Orthopaedic Education, Emory University School of Medicine, Atlanta, Georgia

MARK E. SESTO, M.D.
Chairman, Department of General and Vascular Surgery, Cleveland Clinic Florida, Fort Lauderdale, Florida

DHIRAJ M. SHAH, M.D.
Professor of Surgery and Head, Division of General Surgery, Albany Medical College, Albany, New York

CHARLES J. SHANLEY, M.D.
Lecturer, Section of Vascular Surgery, University of Michigan Medical School, Ann Arbor, Michigan

ALEXANDER D. SHEPARD, M.D.
Clinical Associate Professor of Surgery, University of Michigan Medical School, Ann Arbor; Senior Staff Surgeon, and Medical Director, Clinical Vascular Laboratory, Henry Ford Hospital, Detroit, Michigan

P. C. SHETTY, M.D.
Division Head, Neuroradiology and Vascular Radiology, Henry Ford Hospital, Detroit, Michigan

GREGORIO A. SICARD, M.D.
Professor of Surgery, Washington University School of Medicine; Director, Vascular Service, Barnes Hospital, St. Louis, Missouri

DONALD SILVER, M.D.
W. Alton Jones Professor and Chairman, Department of Surgery, University of Missouri–Columbia School of Medicine; Surgeon and Chief, University of Missouri Health Sciences Center, Columbia, Missouri

DAVID J. SMITH, JR., M.D.
Professor of Surgery, University of Michigan Medical School; Head, Section of Plastic Surgery, University of Michigan Medical Center, Ann Arbor, Michigan

JOHN W. SMITH, M.D.
Clinical Associate Professor of Surgery, University of Nebraska College of Medicine; Vascular Surgeon, Methodist Hospital, Omaha, Nebraska

ROBERT B. SMITH III, M.D.
Professor of Surgery and Head of Vascular Surgery, Emory University School of Medicine; Director of Vascular Surgery and Associate Medical Director, Emory University Hospital, Atlanta, Georgia

KENNETH W. SNIDERMAN, M.D.
Associate Professor of Medical Imaging, University of Toronto Faculty of Medicine; Co-Director of Vascular and Interventional Radiology, The Toronto Hospital, Toronto, Ontario, Canada

MICHAEL SOBEL, M.D.
Associate Professor of Surgery, Medical College of Virginia; Chief, Vascular Surgery Service, H.H. McGuire Veterans Affairs Medical Center, Richmond, Virginia

THOMAS A. SOS, M.D.
Professor of Radiology, Cornell University Medical College; Director, Division of Cardiovascular and Interventional Radiology, The New York Hospital, New York, New York

VIKROM S. SOTTIURAI, M.D., PH.D.
Associate Professor of Surgery and Physiology, Louisiana State University Medical Center, New Orleans, Louisiana

DONALD P. SPADONE, M.D.
Assistant Professor of Surgery, University of Missouri–Columbia School of Medicine; Vascular Surgeon, University Hospital and Clinics and Harry S Truman Memorial Veterans Administration Medical Center, Columbia, Missouri

DAVID A. SPAIN, M.D.
Assistant Professor of Surgery, University of Louisville School of Medicine, Louisville, Kentucky

JAMES C. STANLEY, M.D.
Professor of Surgery, University of Michigan Medical School; Head, Section of Vascular Surgery, University Hospital, Ann Arbor, Michigan

RONALD J. STONEY, M.D.
Professor of Surgery, University of California, San Francisco, School of Medicine, San Francisco, California

D. EUGENE STRANDNESS, JR., M.D.
Professor of Surgery and Chief, Division of Vascular Surgery, University of Washington School of Medicine; Attending Vascular Surgeon, University of Washington Medical Center, Seattle, Washington

S. TIMOTHY STRING, M.D.
Clinical Professor of Surgery, University of South Alabama College of Medicine, Mobile, Alabama

WILLIAM E. STRODEL, M.D.
Professor and Associate Chairman, Department of Surgery, University of Kentucky College of Medicine, Lexington, Kentucky

WILLIAM D. SUGGS, M.D.
Assistant Professor of Surgery, Albert Einstein College of Medicine; Assistant Surgeon, Montefiore Medical Center, and Director of Vascular Surgery Services, North Central Bronx Hospital, Bronx, New York

DAVID S. SUMNER, M.D.
Distinguished Professor of Surgery and Chief, Section of Peripheral Vascular Surgery, Southern Illinois University School of Medicine, Springfield, Illinois

MARK TAGETT, M.D., PH.D.
Fellow, Vascular Surgical Service, Wayne State University Detroit Medical Center, Detroit, Michigan

ROY L. TAWES, JR., M.D.
Associate Clinical Professor of Surgery, University of California, San Francisco, School of Medicine, San Francisco, California

LLOYD M. TAYLOR, JR., M.D.
Professor of Surgery, Oregon Health Sciences University, Portland, Oregon

CHARLES J. TEGTMEYER, M.D.
Professor of Radiology and Director, Division of Angiography, Interventional Radiology and Special Procedures, University of Virginia Health Sciences Center, Charlottesville, Virginia

R. BRADLEY THOMASON III, M.D.
Clinical Instructor in Surgical Sciences/General Vascular Surgery, Bowman Gray School of Medicine; Attending Physician in Surgery, Forsyth Memorial Hospital, Winston-Salem, North Carolina

JESSE E. THOMPSON, M.D.

Clinical Professor of Surgery, University of Texas Southwestern Medical Center, Dallas, Texas

M. DAVID TILSON, M.D.

Ailsa Mellon Bruce Professor of Surgery, Columbia University College of Physicians and Surgeons; Director of Surgery, St. Luke's-Roosevelt Hospital Center, New York, New York

DAVID F. J. TOLLEFSON, M.D.

Clinical Assistant Professor of Surgery, Uniformed Services University of the Health Sciences F. Edward Hébert School of Medicine, Bethesda, Maryland; Chief, Section of Vascular Surgery, Madigan Army Medical Center, Tacoma, Washington

JONATHAN B. TOWNE, M.D.

Professor of Surgery and Chairman of Vascular Surgery, Medical College of Wisconsin, Milwaukee, Wisconsin

JEFFREY D. TRACHTENBERG, M.D.

Vascular Surgery Research Fellow and Resident, Department of Surgery, Washington University School of Medicine, St. Louis, Missouri

WILLIAM D. TURNIPSEED, M.D.

Professor of Surgery, University of Wisconsin Medical School; Chief, Vascular Surgery, University of Wisconsin Hospital, Madison, Wisconsin

JAMES G. TYBURSKI, M.D.

Assistant Professor of Surgery, Wayne State University School of Medicine, Detroit, Michigan

ARMEN VARTANY, M.D.

Chief Resident, Department of Surgery, University of California, Irvine, Medical Center, Orange, California

FRANK J. VEITH, M.D.

Professor of Surgery, Albert Einstein College of Medicine; Chief, Vascular Surgical Services, Montefiore Medical Center, Bronx, New York

HENRY C. VELDENZ, M.D.

Assistant Professor of Surgery, University of Florida Health Science Center, Jacksonville, Florida

J. LEONEL VILLAVICENCIO, M.D.

Professor of Surgery, Uniformed Services University of the Health Sciences; Director, Venous and Lymphatic Surgical Clinics, National Naval Medical Center, Bethesda, Maryland; Senior Consultant and Staff, Department of Surgery, and Director, Venous and Lymphatic Surgical Clinics, Walter Reed Army Medical Center, Washington, DC

MICHAEL J. VITTI, M.D.

Department of Surgery, University of Arkansas for Medical Sciences, Little Rock, Arkansas

ROBERT L. VOGELZANG, M.D.

Professor of Radiology, Northwestern University Medical School; Chief of Vascular and Interventional Radiology, Northwestern Memorial Hospital, Chicago, Illinois

THOMAS W. WAKEFIELD, M.D.

Associate Professor of Surgery, University of Michigan Medical School; Staff Surgeon, University Hospital, and Co-chief, Peripheral Vascular Surgery Service, Veterans Administration Medical Center, Ann Arbor, Michigan

PAUL M. WALKER, M.D., PH.D.

Surgeon-in-Chief, The Toronto Hospital, Toronto, Ontario, Canada

MATTHEW J. WALL, JR., M.D.

Assistant Professor of Surgery, Baylor College of Medicine; Chief of General Surgery and Director of Trauma Services, Ben Taub General Hospital, Houston, Texas

DANIEL B. WALSH, M.D.

Associate Professor of Surgery, Dartmouth-Hitchcock Medical Center, Lebanon, New Hampshire

HARRIS J. WATERS, M.D.

Clinical Assistant Professor of Surgery, University of Nevada School of Medicine, Las Vegas, Nevada

FRED A. WEAVER, M.D.

Associate Professor of Surgery, University of Southern California School of Medicine, Los Angeles, California

THOMAS H. WEBB III, M.D.

Assistant Professor of Surgery and Chief of Vascular Surgery, Medical College of Ohio, Toledo, Ohio

MARSHALL W. WEBSTER, M.D.

Professor and Vice Chairman, Department of Surgery, University of Pittsburgh School of Medicine; Chief, Section of Vascular Surgery and Wound Healing, University of Pittsburgh Medical Center, Pittsburgh, Pennsylvania

ALAN B. WEDER, M.D.

Associate Professor of Internal Medicine, Division of Hypertension, University of Michigan Medical School, Ann Arbor, Michigan

K. M. A. WELCH, M.D.

Professor of Neurology, Case Western Reserve University School of Medicine, Cleveland, Ohio; William T. Gossett Chair, Department of Neurology, Henry Ford Hospital, Detroit, Michigan

RICHARD E. WELLING, M.D.

Director, Surgical Residency Program, Vascular Fellowship Program, and Department of Surgery, Good Samaritan Hospital, Cincinnati, Ohio

H. BROWNELL WHEELER, M.D.

Harry M. Haidak Distinguished Professor and Chairman of Surgery, University of Massachusetts Medical School; Chief of Surgery, University of Massachusetts Medical Center, Worcester, Massachusetts

RODNEY A. WHITE, M.D.

Professor of Surgery, University of California, Los Angeles, School of Medicine, Los Angeles; Chief, Vascular Surgery, and Associate Chairman, Department of Surgery, Harbor-UCLA Medical Center, Torrance, California

THOMAS A. WHITEHILL, M.D.

Assistant Professor of Surgery, University of Colorado Health Sciences Center; Chief of Vascular Surgery, Veterans Administration Medical Center, and Staff Surgeon, University Hospital, Denver, Colorado

ANTHONY D. WHITTEMORE, M.D.

Professor of Surgery, Harvard Medical School; Chief, Division of Vascular Surgery, Brigham and Women's Hospital, Boston, Massachusetts

BERNARD R. WILCOSKY, Jr., M.D.

Associate Medical Director, Sequoia Pain Treatment Clinic, and Chairman, Department of Anesthesiology, Sequoia Hospital District, Redwood City, California

DAVID M. WILLIAMS, M.D.

Associate Professor of Radiology, University of Michigan Medical School, Ann Arbor, Michigan

G. MELVILLE WILLIAMS, M.D.

Bertram M. Bernheim Professor of Surgery, The Johns Hopkins University School of Medicine; Surgeon-in-Charge, Division of Vascular Surgery, Johns Hopkins Hospital, Baltimore, Maryland

ROBERT F. WILSON, M.D.

Professor of Surgery, Wayne State University School of Medicine; Chief of Surgery and Director of Trauma Services, Detroit Receiving Hospital, Detroit, Michigan

SAMUEL E. WILSON, M.D.

Professor of Surgery, University of California, Irvine, College of Medicine, Irvine; Chairman, Department of Surgery, University of California, Irvine, Medical Center, Orange, California

MARTIN J. WINKLER, M.D.

Clinical Assistant Professor of Surgery, University of Nebraska Medical Center, Omaha, Nebraska

JONATHAN WOODSON, M.D.

Assistant Professor of Surgery, Boston University School of Medicine; Attending Surgeon, Boston University Medical Center, Boston, Massachusetts

JAMES S. T. YAO, M.D., Ph.D.

Magerstadt Professor of Surgery, Northwestern University Medical School; Chief, Division of Vascular Surgery, Northwestern Memorial Hospital, Chicago, Illinois

ALBERT E. YELLIN, M.D.

Professor of Surgery, and Chief, Division of Vascular Surgery, University of Southern California School of Medicine, Los Angeles, California

JESS R. YOUNG, M.D.

Chairman, Department of Vascular Medicine, The Cleveland Clinic Foundation, Cleveland, Ohio

CHRISTOPHER K. ZARINS, M.D.

Chidester Professor of Surgery, Stanford University School of Medicine; Chairman, Division of Vascular Surgery, Stanford University Medical Center, Stanford, California

GERALD B. ZELENOCK, M.D.

Professor of Surgery, University of Michigan Medical School, Ann Arbor, Michigan

R. EUGENE ZIERLER, M.D.

Associate Professor of Surgery, University of Washington School of Medicine, Seattle, Washington

THOMAS N. ZWENG, M.D.

Assistant Professor of Surgery, University of Kentucky College of Medicine; Attending Surgeon, Albert B. Chandler Medical Center, Lexington, Kentucky

PREFACE

As the knowledge base of vascular disease has continued to expand so has *Current Therapy in Vascular Surgery*, from 155 chapters and 194 contributors in the first edition in 1987, to 239 chapters and 313 contributors in the second edition of 1991, to 249 chapters and 339 contributors in this, the third edition. The format for the third edition of *Current Therapy in Vascular Surgery* remains the same as previous offerings. It is a hard-hitting, no-nonsense, up-to-date, and comprehensive review of contemporary vascular disease problems encountered by practicing surgeons, physicians, and radiologists.

The essential elements of vascular surgery, arterial, venous, and lymphatic diseases are updated in this third edition of *Current Therapy in Vascular Surgery*. New information has been included in each of the major sections on cerebrovascular disease, upper extremity arterial disease, aortic aneurysms, lower extremity aneurysms, aortoiliac occlusive disease, lower extremity occlusive disease, embolic disease of the extremities, vascular trauma, amputations, mesenteric vascular disease, portal hypertension, renovascular disease, arteriovenous fistulas and malformations, angioaccess, venous disease, and lymphatic disease.

Emphasis is on management with inclusion of diagnosis and basic pathophysiology where such is important in understanding therapeutic options. All chapters are new and by different authors from the first two editions of *Current Therapy in Vascular Surgery*, reflecting contemporary clinical practice, and occasionally revealing different viewpoints from those of the first two editions. Consequently, the third edition is complementary to the previous two editions in supplementing our contemporary knowledge of vascular diseases.

The Editors are grateful to our dedicated contributors without whose efforts this text would not have come to fruition. We would be remiss if we did not recognize Barbara Humenny, personal secretary to the Senior Editor, for her dedicated efforts in facilitating the handling of manuscripts and correspondence for a volume of this magnitude. Finally, we are most appreciative of the assistance of our publisher Mosby–Year Book and associates Lynne Gery and Susan Gay who energetically assisted the Editors in helping this book come to print.

Calvin B. Ernst, M.D.
James C. Stanley, M.D.

CONTENTS

CEREBROVASCULAR DISEASE

Human Carotid Artery Atherosclerosis   1
David Gordon

Pathology of Carotid and Vertebral Arterial Fibrodysplasia   4
Elliot L. Chaikof
Robert B. Smith III

Duplex Scanning and Spectral Analysis of Carotid Artery Occlusive Disease   8
R. Eugene Zierler

Angiographic Evaluation of the Carotid Artery   13
William K. Ehrenfeld
Stephen P. Murray
Christopher F. Dowd

Transcranial Doppler Evaluation of Cerebrovascular Disease   15
Marc I. Chimowitz

Computed Tomography Evaluation of Cerebrovascular Disease   19
Ramon Berguer

Magnetic Resonance Imaging in Assessment of Cerebrovascular Disease   21
Magruder C. Donaldson

Medical Therapy for Transient Ischemic Attacks and Ischemic Stroke   24
Panayiotis Mitsias
K. M. A. Welch

Diagnosis and Surgical Management of Asymptomatic Carotid Stenosis   29
Allan D. Callow
Jeffrey D. Trachtenberg

Surgical Treatment of Evolving Stroke Secondary to Carotid Artery Atherosclerosis   34
G. Patrick Clagett

Surgical Treatment of Fixed Stroke Secondary to Carotid Artery Atherosclerosis   38
Hugh G. Beebe

Technical Aspects of Carotid Endarterectomy for Atherosclerotic Disease   40
Calvin B. Ernst

Regional and Local Anesthesia for Carotid Endarterectomy   44
William E. Evans
Enrique Ginzburg

Management of Occluded or Nearly Occluded Extracranial Carotid Arteries   45
William J. Quiñones-Baldrich

Recognition of Cerebral Ischemia During Carotid Artery Reconstruction   54
Marshall W. Webster

Role of Shunting During Carotid Endarterectomy   57
Jesse E. Thompson

Patch Graft Closure for Carotid Endarterectomy   60
Patrick J. O'Hara

Intracranial Occlusive Disease and Aneurysms: Influence on Carotid Endarterectomy Outcome   65
William C. Mackey

Cerebral Hyperperfusion Syndrome Following Carotid Endarterectomy   68
Anthony M. Imparato

Blood Pressure Instability Following Carotid Endarterectomy   71
David H. Deaton
Wesley S. Moore

Recognition and Management of Acute Stroke Following Carotid Endarterectomy ... 73
John L. Gray
William H. Baker

Recurrent Carotid Artery Stenosis Following Endarterectomy ... 76
D. Eugene Strandness, Jr.

Surgical Management of Recurrent Carotid Artery Stenosis ... 78
William C. Mackey

Surgical Treatment of Transient Ischemic Attack and Stroke Secondary to External Carotid Atherosclerosis ... 80
Jonathan P. Gertler

Vertebral Artery Reconstruction for Vertebrobasilar Insufficiency ... 84
Edouard Kieffer
Amine Bahnini
Fabien Koskas
Carlo Ruotolo

Subclavian to Carotid Transposition ... 89
William H. Edwards

Carotid-Subclavian Bypass and Other Extra-Anatomic Revascularizations for Proximal Subclavian Artery Stenosis Causing Cerebral Steal Syndrome ... 93
Thomas S. Riles
Patrick J. Lamparello

Surgical Treatment of Innominate Artery Atherosclerosis ... 96
John P. Loftus
Kenneth J. Cherry, Jr.

Management of Concomitant Carotid and Coronary Arterial Occlusive Disease ... 100
Richard P. Cambria

Extracranial Carotid Artery Aneurysm ... 105
Gerald B. Zelenock
Joseph Giglia

Carotid Artery Dissection ... 109
Tammy K. Ramos
Jerry Goldstone

Fibromuscular Disease of the Carotid Artery ... 114
Eileen S. Natuzzi
Ronald J. Stoney

Carotid Kinks and Coils ... 118
Mark Tagett
Andris Kazmers

Carotid Body Tumors ... 121
Glenn M. LaMuraglia

Surgical Treatment of Takayasu's Arteritis ... 125
Fred A. Weaver
J. Gregory Modrall
Albert E. Yellin

Giant Cell Arteritis ... 130
Jess R. Young

Radiation-Induced Arteritis ... 133
George Andros
Peter A. Schneider
Robert W. Harris

UPPER EXTREMITY ARTERIAL DISEASE

Pathology of Upper Extremity Arterial Disease ... 138
James S. T. Yao

Revascularization of the Upper Extremity ... 142
Henry Veldenz
Gordon L. Hyde

Diagnosis of Upper Extremity Vasospastic Disease ... 145
David S. Sumner

Treatment of Upper Extremity Vasospastic Disease ... 151
John W. Joyce

Buerger's Disease ... 154
Timothy F. Kresowik

Ergotism ... 159
Marshall W. Webster

Extremity Causalgia and Mimocausalgia ... 162
Cornelius Olcott IV
Bernard R. Wilcosky

Upper Extremity Sympathectomy ... 165
Ali F. AbuRahma
James P. Boland

Etiology and Anatomic Pathology of Thoracic Outlet Syndrome ... 169
Herbert I. Machleder

Diagnosis of Thoracic Outlet Syndrome 176
Lazar J. Greenfield

Nonoperative Management of Thoracic Outlet Syndrome 179
Robert D. DeFrang
Lloyd M. Taylor, Jr.
Gregory L. Moneta
John M. Porter

Transaxillary Operative Management of Thoracic Outlet Syndrome 182
Richard M. Green

Supraclavicular Operative Approach to Thoracic Outlet Syndrome 185
Lazar J. Greenfield

Subclavian and Axillary Artery Aneurysms 188
Glenn C. Hunter
Kevin A. Hall

Hypothenar Hammer Syndrome 195
Mark R. Nehler
Lloyd M. Taylor, Jr.
John M. Porter

AORTIC ANEURYSM

Genetics of Abdominal Aortic Aneurysmal Disease 198
Anita K. Gregory
Anil P. Hingorani
M. David Tilson

Pathogenesis of Aortic Aneurysms 200
Christopher K. Zarins

Pathology of Inflammatory Aortic Aneurysm 204
Mitchell H. Goldman

Pathophysiology of Aortic Dissection 206
James I. Fann
D. Craig Miller

Role of Arteriography in Assessment of Abdominal Aortic Aneurysm 210
Michael J. Petersen
David C. Brewster

Magnetic Resonance Imaging, Ultrasonography, and Computed Tomography in Assessment of Abdominal Aortic Aneurysm 214
David Rosenthal

Surgical Treatment of Nonruptured Infrarenal and Juxtarenal Aortic Aneurysms 218
Calvin B. Ernst

Surgical Treatment of Ruptured Infrarenal Aortic Aneurysm 224
Mohammed M. Moursi
James C. Stanley

Management of Small Abdominal Aortic Aneurysms 227
John W. Hallett, Jr.

Surgical Treatment of Inflammatory Abdominal Aortic Aneurysms 229
Samuel R. Money
Larry H. Hollier

Surgical Treatment of Infected Abdominal Aortic Aneurysms 232
Martin I. Ellenby
Calvin B. Ernst

Management of Concurrent Intra-Abdominal Disease and Abdominal Aortic Aneurysm 235
S. Timothy String

Retroperitoneal Approach for Elective Abdominal Aortic Aneurysmectomy 238
Robert P. Leather
R. Clement Darling III
Benjamin B. Chang
Dhiraj M. Shah

Aortic Aneurysm Repair with Coexistent Visceral and Renal Artery Disease 242
David F. J. Tollefson
Charles A. Andersen

Renal Ectopia and Renal Fusion in Patients Requiring Abdominal Aortic Operations 246
Max R. Gaspar
Harris J. Waters
Allen W. Averbook

Aortic Reconstruction in Renal Transplant Patients 250
Gary W. Gibbons
Christopher J. Kwolek

Venous Anomalies Encountered During Aortic Reconstruction 252
Joseph M. Giordano

Management of Thoracoabdominal Aortic Aneurysm 255
G. Melville Williams

Surgical Treatment of Abdominal Aortic Aneurysm–Inferior Vena Cava Fistula 261
John E. Connolly

Management of Primary Aortoenteric Fistula 262
Scott S. Berman
Victor M. Bernhard

Treatment of Abdominal Aortic Aneurysm by Endovascular Grafting 265
Tim Chuter
James A. DeWeese

Acute Limb Ischemia Following Aortic Reconstruction 271
Richard E. Carballo
Jonathan B. Towne

Intestinal Ischemia as a Complication of Abdominal Aortic Reconstruction 274
Massimo M. Napolitano
Alexander D. Shepard

Neurologic Complications of Abdominal Aortic Reconstruction 278
Elliot L. Chaikof
Atef A. Salam

Prevention of Spinal Cord Ischemia During Thoracoabdominal Aortic Reconstruction 282
Robert Y. Rhee
Peter Gloviczki

Autotransfusion in Aortic Reconstruction 287
Daniel J. Reddy

Aneurysmal Deterioration of Arterial Prostheses 289
Daniel B. Nunn

Aortic Aneurysm, Arteriomegaly, and Aneurysmosis 292
Charles L. Mesh
Linda M. Graham

Isolated Iliac Aneurysm 296
William C. Krupski

Vascular Complications of Ehlers-Danlos Syndrome and Marfan Syndrome 302
Thomas A. Whitehill

Medical Management of Acute Aortic Dissection 305
Marvin M. Kirsh
Constance A. Newman

Surgical Treatment of Acute and Chronic Thoracic Aortic Dissections 309
Joseph S. Coselli

LOWER EXTREMITY ANEURYSM

Arteriosclerotic Femoral Artery Aneurysm 315
Bruce S. Cutler

Infected Femoral Artery False Aneurysm Associated with Drug Abuse 319
Frank T. Padberg, Jr.

Obturator Foramen Bypass Grafts in Groin Sepsis 322
S. Martin Lindenauer

Popliteal Artery Aneurysm 325
Robert W. Hobson, II

AORTOILIAC OCCLUSIVE DISEASE

Anatomic Distribution and Natural History of Aortoiliac and Infrainguinal Atherosclerosis 328
Mark F. Fillinger
Jack L. Cronenwett

Smoking and Vascular Disease 333
Dan J. Higman
Janet T. Powell
Roger M. Greenhalgh

Treatment of Hyperlipidemia 336
Dorothy M. Kahkonen

Hypertension as a Risk Factor in Atherosclerotic Cardiovascular Disease 340
Alan B. Weder

Assessment and Importance of Coronary Artery Disease in Patients with Aortoiliac Occlusive Disease and Abdominal Aortic Aneurysms 345
Richard P. Cambria

Physiologic Studies to Document Severity of Aortoiliac Occlusive Disease 350
Joseph P. Archie, Jr.

Aortofemoral Bypass for Atherosclerotic Aortoiliac Occlusive Disease 355
William M. Abbott
Christopher J. Kwolek

Coarctation and Hypoplasia of the Subisthmic Thoracic and Abdominal Aorta 359
Charles J. Shanley
James C. Stanley

Endarterectomy for Atherosclerotic Aortoiliac Occlusive Disease 363
Allan R. Downs

Percutaneous Arterial Dilation for Atherosclerotic Aortoiliac Occlusive Disease 365
Kyung J. Cho
Thomas Pfammater

Management of Juxtarenal Aortic Occlusive Disease by Transabdominal Exposure of the Pararenal and Suprarenal Aorta Using Medial Visceral Rotation 373
Linda M. Reilly

Acute Aortic Occlusion 378
Alexander D. Shepard
Christos D. Dossa

Descending Thoracic Aorta to Femoral Bypass 381
Walter J. McCarthy

Axillofemoral Bypass 384
Lester R. Sauvage
Sherif El-Massry

Unilateral Retroperitoneal Iliofemoral Bypass 391
Dhiraj M. Shah
R. Clement Darling III
Benjamin B. Chang
Robert P. Leather

Femorofemoral Bypass for Aortoiliac Occlusive Disease 393
Sushil Gupta
Raul Landa
Frank Veith

Vasculogenic Impotence 397
James S. T. Yao

Diagnosis of Aortic Graft Infection 400
Thomas W. Wakefield

Treatment of Aortic Graft Infection 405
Dennis F. Bandyk

Aortic Graft–Enteric Fistula 411
John W. Smith

Management of Groin Lymphocele and Lymph Fistula 413
Mark C. Rummel
Morris D. Kerstein

Anastomotic Aneurysm 415
Calvin B. Ernst

Aortic Graft Limb Occlusion 419
David C. Brewster

Management of Chyloperitoneum and Chylothorax After Aortic Reconstruction 426
Mark A. Mattos
David S. Sumner

LOWER EXTREMITY OCCLUSIVE DISEASE

Doppler Pressure Assessment of Infrainguinal Occlusive Disease 432
J. Dennis Baker

Duplex Imaging of Infrainguinal Occlusive Disease 436
Gregory L. Moneta

Conventional Arteriographic Diagnosis of Infrainguinal Occlusive Disease 441
P. C. Shetty
David J. Kastan

Magnetic Resonance Arteriography for Assessment of Infrainguinal Occlusive Disease 447
Jeffrey P. Carpenter
Richard A. Baum

Superficial Femoral Artery Endarterectomy for Atherosclerotic Lower Extremity Occlusive Disease 453
Fritz R. Bech
Daniel B. Walsh

Profundaplasty
  Donald L. Jacobs
  Jonathan B. Towne
	457	Popliteal Vascular Entrapment Syndrome
		  William D. Turnipseed
			504

Lumbar Sympathectomy for Lower Extremity Cutaneous Ischemic Ulcers
  Timothy J. Ranval
  Robert W. Barnes
	462	Popliteal Artery Adventitial Cystic Disease
		  Lois A. Killewich
		  Michael P. Lilly
		  William R. Flinn
			509

Reversed Autogenous Vein Graft for Atherosclerotic Lower Extremity Occlusive Disease
  Philippe A. Masser
  Lloyd M. Taylor, Jr.
  Gregory L. Moneta
  John M. Porter
	465	Percutaneous Arterial Dilatation for Atherosclerotic Lower Extremity Occlusive Disease
		  K. Wayne Johnston
			512

In Situ Saphenous Vein Graft for Lower Extremity Occlusive Disease
  John A. Mannick
  Anthony D. Whittemore
  Magruder C. Donaldson
	469	Atherectomy Devices in the Management of Infrainguinal Occlusive Disease
		  Samuel S. Ahn
			517

Sequential Bypass Procedures for Atherosclerotic Lower Extremity Disease
  Paul Friedmann
  Dominic A. DeLaurentis
	473	Balloon Angioplasty in the Management of Failing Infrainguinal Bypass Grafts
		  Anthony D. Whittemore
			521

Arm Veins for Lower Extremity Revascularization
  Norman R. Hertzer
  Mark E. Sesto
	476	Angioscopy in the Management of Infrainguinal Occlusive Arterial Disease
		  Frank W. LoGerfo
		  Christopher J. Kwolek
			524

Expanded Polytetrafluoroethylene Graft for Atherosclerotic Lower Extremity Occlusive Disease
  William D. Suggs
  Frank J. Veith
	480	Intravascular Ultrasound for Imaging of Diseased Arteries
		  Rodney A. White
			527

Umbilical Vein Grafts for Atherosclerotic Lower Extremity Occlusive Disease
  Herbert Dardik
	484	Nonoperative, Nonpharmacologic Management of Lower Extremity Occlusive Disease
		  Robert A. Graor
			531

Short Vein Grafts from the Distal Superficial Femoral, Popliteal, or Infrapopliteal Arteries for Limb Salvage
  Enrico Ascer
  Robert M. Pollina
	488	Pharmacologic Treatment of Lower Extremity Arterial Occlusive Disease
		  Jay D. Coffman
			534

Surveillance of Lower Extremity Bypass Grafts
  Dennis F. Bandyk
	492	Operative Management of Acute Thrombosis of Lower Extremity Bypass Grafts
		  Lakshmikumar Pillai
		  John J. Ricotta
			537

Persistent Sciatic Artery
  Vikrom S. Sottiurai
	499	Fibrinolytic Therapy for Acutely Thrombosed Lower Extremity Arteries and Grafts
		  Bruce A. Perler
			540

		Role of Antithrombotic Drugs in Maintaining Graft Patency Ted R. Kohler	544
		Prothrombotic States and Vascular Thromboses Michael Sobel	550

Complications of Heparin Therapy 554
   Michael J. Rohrer
   H. Brownell Wheeler

Cutaneous Ulcers in the Ischemic
Diabetic Foot 558
   John M. Marek
   William C. Krupski

Treatment of Infected Vascular Grafts
in the Groin 564
   Alan M. Graham

EMBOLIC DISEASE OF THE EXTREMITIES

Spontaneous Atheroembolism 568
   Ralph G. DePalma

Anticoagulant and Lytic Therapy for Arterial
Macroembolism in the Extremities 572
   Robert J. Pitsch
   Peter F. Lawrence

Balloon Catheter Embolectomy for
Macroembolism in the Extremities 576
   Roy L. Tawes, Jr.

Percutaneous Aspiration
Thromboembolectomy 580
   Peter G. Kalman
   Kenneth W. Sniderman

Oxygen Free Radical Scavengers in Acute
Ischemia and Reperfusion Syndrome 582
   Paul M. Walker
   Alexander Romaschin

Noninvasive Methods of Diagnosing Cardiac
Sources of Macroemboli 586
   Brian G. Rubin
   Gregorio A. Sicard

Paradoxical Embolism 589
   Timothy F. Kresowik

VASCULAR TRAUMA

Nonarteriographic Assessment of Penetrating
Vascular Injuries 593
   Kaj Johansen

Role of Arteriography in Penetrating Vascular
Injuries 596
   Malcolm O. Perry

Penetrating and Blunt Extracranial Carotid
Artery Injuries 598
   Michael P. Byrne
   Richard E. Welling

Penetrating and Blunt Vertebral Artery
Trauma 604
   Thomas H. Webb III
   Bruce L. Gewertz

Penetrating Trauma to the Aortic Arch,
Innominate, and Subclavian Arteries 608
   Robert F. Wilson
   James G. Tyburski

Blunt Arterial Injuries of the Shoulder and
Elbow 614
   Eric D. Endean

Penetrating Arterial Injuries in the Extremities 617
   Norman M. Rich

Blunt and Penetrating Abdominal Vascular
Injuries 619
   Asher Hirshberg
   Kenneth L. Mattox
   Matthew J. Wall, Jr.

Iatrogenic Upper Extremity Arterial Catheter
Injury 625
   Richard J. Fowl
   Richard F. Kempczinski

Complications of the Lower Extremities After
Percutaneous Arterial Puncture 628
   Richard L. McCann

Arterial Injuries Associated with Fractures
and Extensive Soft Tissue Trauma 631
   J. David Richardson
   David A. Spain

Blunt Arterial Injuries to the Knee 634
   Allan R. Downs

Vascular Injury Secondary to Drug Abuse 637
   Albert E. Yellin
   Joseph H. Frankhouse
   Fred A. Weaver

Fasciotomy in Vascular Trauma
and Compartment Syndrome — 644
  Joseph L. Mills

Ischemia-Induced Myonecrosis,
Myoglobinuria, and Secondary Renal Failure
(Reperfusion Syndrome) — 650
  F. William Blaisdell

Concomitant Venous Repair in the
Management of Extremity Arterial Injuries — 652
  James J. Schuler

Blunt and Penetrating Renal Vascular Injuries — 657
  Gerald B. Zelenock

Iatrogenic Pediatric Vascular Injuries — 659
  Philippe A. Masser
  Lloyd M. Taylor, Jr.
  Gregory L. Moneta
  John M. Porter

Cold Injury — 663
  Rachel Podrazik Baer

AMPUTATION

Noninvasive Methods of Determining
Amputation Levels — 669
  John L. Provan

Toe and Foot Amputation — 672
  Daniel F. Fisher, Jr.

Below-the-Knee Amputation — 674
  Lloyd A. Jacobs
  Paul W. Durance

Above-the-Knee Amputation and Hip
Disarticulation — 677
  Eric D. Endean

Upper Extremity Amputation — 680
  John Gray Seiler, III
  Frank D. Ellis
  Lamar L. Fleming

MESENTERIC VASCULAR DISEASE

Duplex Scanning in the Diagnosis of
Splanchnic Artery Occlusive Disease — 686
  D. Eugene Strandness, Jr.

Percutaneous Transcatheter Therapy
of Visceral Ischemia — 689
  Charles J. Tegtmeyer
  Alan H. Matsumoto
  J. Fritz Angle

Acute Embolic and Thrombotic Mesenteric
Ischemia — 693
  Daniel S. Rush
  Pavel J. Levy
  James L. Haynes

Transaortic Splanchnic Endarterectomy
for Chronic Mesenteric Ischemia — 697
  Louis M. Messina
  Rajabrata Sarkar

Bypass Procedures for Chronic Mesenteric
Ischemia — 701
  Jose Mena
  Larry H. Hollier

Celiac Compression Syndrome — 703
  Douglas L. Jicha
  Ronald J. Stoney

Nonocclusive Mesenteric Ischemia — 706
  Elizabeth T. Clark
  Bruce L. Gewertz

Mesenteric Venous Thrombosis — 710
  Timothy R. S. Harward
  James M. Seeger

Celiac, Hepatic, and Splenic Artery
Aneurysms — 714
  Linda M. Graham
  Charles L. Mesh

Vascular Malformations of the Splanchnic
Circulation — 718
  Ashby C. Moncure

Splanchnic and Portal Arteriovenous Fistulas — 721
  Thomas E. Brothers

PORTAL HYPERTENSION

Anatomic Basis of Portal Hypertension — 725
  Frederic E. Eckhauser
  Lisa Colletti
  James A. Knol

Pharmacologic Intervention, Balloon
Tamponade, and Catheter Embolization
for Variceal Hemorrhage 732
   B. Timothy Baxter
   Layton F. Rikkers

Endoscopic Sclerotherapy and Ligation
of Esophageal Varices 735
   Thomas N. Zweng
   William E. Strodel

Operative Variceal Ligation and
Gastroesophageal Devascularization
for Variceal Hemorrhage 740
   Robert C. Gorman
   Ernest F. Rosato

Decompressive Shunts for Variceal
Hemorrhage 744
   Atef A. Salam

Budd-Chiari Syndrome 748
   Darrell A. Campbell, Jr.
   Frederic E. Eckhauser

Transjugular Portosystemic Shunts 751
   Robert K. Kerlan, Jr.
   Ziv J. Haskal
   Ernest J. Ring

Liver Transplantation in the Management
of Portal Hypertension 755
   Kim M. Olthoff
   Ronald W. Busuttil

Portal Hypertension in Children 759
   Frederick M. Karrer
   John R. Lilly

RENOVASCULAR DISEASE

Pathology of Renal Artery Occlusive Disease 764
   Rajabrata Sarkar
   Louis M. Messina

Duplex Scanning for Renal Arterial Occlusive
Disease 768
   Kimberley J. Hansen
   Scott W. Reavis
   Richard H. Dean

Functional Significance of Renal Arterial
Occlusive Disease 774
   Thomas G. Pickering, Jr.

Arteriographic Diagnosis of Renovascular
Hypertension 779
   Thomas A. Sos

Percutaneous Arterial Dilation
for Renovascular Hypertension 780
   David M. Williams
   Michael D. Dake

Aortorenal Bypass for Renovascular
Hypertension in Adults 785
   Calvin B. Ernst

Ex Vivo Arterial Repair for Renovascular
Hypertension Secondary to Fibrodysplasia 790
   Folkert O. Belzer
   Charles W. Acher

Aortorenal Endarterectomy for Treatment
of Renal Artery Atherosclerosis 793
   Thomas S. Huber
   James C. Stanley

Alternative Renal Artery Reconstructive
Techniques: Hepatorenal, Splenorenal,
and Other Bypass Procedures 799
   Andrew C. Novick

Operative Assessment of Renal and Visceral
Arterial Reconstruction Using Duplex
Sonography 804
   Kimberley J. Hansen
   R. Bradley Thomason
   Richard H. Dean

Surgical Treatment of Renovascular
Hypertension in Children 808
   Henry D. Berkowitz

Renal Artery Aneurysm 813
   James C. Stanley

Renal Artery Dissection 818
   Linda M. Reilly

Renal Artery Embolism 821
   Kenneth Ouriel

Renal Vein Thrombosis 823
   Timothy J. Nypaver

Renal Artery Occlusive Disease in Chronic
Renal Failure   827
   Richard H. Dean

Renal Arteriovenous Malformation
and Arteriovenous Fistula   830
   John D. Bennett
   Saadoon Kadir

ARTERIOVENOUS FISTULAS AND ARTERIOVENOUS MALFORMATIONS

Classification of Peripheral Congenital
Vascular Malformations   834
   Robert B. Rutherford

Evaluation of Congenital Vascular
Malformations of the Extremities
by Nonangiographic Methods   839
   William H. Pearce
   Robert L. Vogelzang

Acquired Arteriovenous Fistula   841
   S. Martin Lindenauer

Congenital Vascular Lesions in Infancy
and Childhood   846
   Steven R. Buchman
   David J. Smith, Jr.

Management of Congenital Arteriovenous
Fistulas and Malformations in Adults   850
   Thomas S. Riles
   Mark A. Adelman

ANGIOACCESS SURGERY

External Methods of Angioaccess   853
   Jeffrey D. Punch
   Robert M. Merion

Direct Arteriovenous Anastomosis
for Angioaccess   857
   Jeffrey L. Buehrer
   Blair A. Keagy

Bridge Grafts for Angioaccess   860
   Richard W. Dow
   Sheldon A. Schwartz

Surveillance of Angioaccess Graft Function   865
   Armen Vartany
   Martin J. Winkler
   Samuel E. Wilson

VENOUS DISEASE

Coagulation Cascade and Thromboembolism   868
   Thomas W. Wakefield

Pathophysiology of Venous Thrombosis   874
   Seshadri Raju

Noninvasive Methods of Diagnosing Venous
Disease   879
   Enrique Criado
   George Johnson, Jr.

Invasive Methods of Diagnosing Venous
Disease   884
   Andrew N. Nicolaides

Nonoperative Treatment of Acute Superficial
Thrombophlebitis and Deep Femoral Venous
Thrombosis   888
   Michael J. Vitti
   Robert W. Barnes

Injection Compression Sclerotherapy of
Spider Telangiectasia and Varicose Veins   894
   John R. Pfeifer

Excision of Varicose Veins   898
   Joseph P. Elliott, Jr.

Surgical Treatment of Acute Saphenous
and Deep Femoral Venous Thrombosis   904
   Robert L. Kistner
   Bo Eklöf

Deep Venous Thrombosis in Pregnancy   907
   Ali F. AbuRahma

Nonoperative Management of Chronic
Venous Insufficiency   910
   Mark C. Rummel
   Morris D. Kerstein

Surgical Management of Chronic Venous
Insufficiency   914
   Agustin A. Rodriguez
   Thomas F. O'Donnell, Jr.

Warfarin-Induced Skin Necrosis 919
Donald P. Spadone
Donald Silver

Pathogenesis of Cutaneous Venous Ulcers 922
Arnost Fronek

Nonoperative Treatment of Venous Ulcers 924
James O. Menzoian
Wayne W. LaMorte
Jonathan Woodson

Operative Treatment of Venous Ulcers 927
J. Leonel Villavicencio
James A. Coffey
Christopher Cunningham

Surgical Treatment of Acute Iliofemoral Thrombosis 932
Bo Eklof
Robert L. Kistner

Nonoperative Treatment of Acute Iliofemoral and Caval Thrombosis 936
Michael J. Kikta
Donald Silver

Nonoperative Treatment of Acute Pulmonary Embolism 940
Douglas W. Harrington
John Popovich, Jr.

Percutaneous Devices for Vena Cava Filtration 945
Daniel B. Walsh
Michael Bettmann

Operative Inferior Vena Cava Interruption 949
Holt A. McDowell, Jr.
Ernesto Anaya

Transvenous Catheter Pulmonary Embolectomy 951
E. John Harris, Jr.
Thomas J. Fogarty
Christopher K. Zarins

Surgical Treatment of Acute and Chronic Pulmonary Emboli 955
Mark Iannettoni
Marvin Kirsh

Upper Extremity Venous Occlusion 958
Herbert I. Machleder

Septic Thrombophlebitis 963
Mark Reynolds
J. David Richardson

Primary and Secondary Vena Caval Tumors 967
Thomas F. Dodson
Robert B. Smith, III

Venous Aneurysms 970
Bruce A. Perler

LYMPHATIC DISEASE

Primary Lymphedema 973
George H. Rudkin
Timothy A. Miller

Secondary Lymphedema 978
Harry S. Goldsmith
William Holmes

CEREBROVASCULAR DISEASE

HUMAN CAROTID ARTERY ATHEROSCLEROSIS

DAVID GORDON, M.D.

TOPOGRAPHY AND COMPOSITION OF ESTABLISHED PLAQUES

Atherosclerotic involvement of human carotid arteries tends to be localized principally in three regions: (1) at the origin of the common carotid artery from the aortic arch or the innominate artery, (2) at the bifurcation of the common carotid artery into internal and external branches, and (3) within the intracranial siphon region of the internal carotid artery. The plaques that form at the bifurcation of the common carotid artery are by far the most common and prominent from a clinical standpoint.

Similar to atherosclerotic plaques that develop elsewhere in the arterial tree, carotid bifurcation plaques are large, usually eccentric intimal lesions that nearly always involve the outer walls of the carotid bifurcation region.[1] The flow divider itself is relatively spared of direct atherosclerotic involvement. The atherosclerotic lesion is usually confined to the intima, although secondary erosion into the media and thinning of the media commonly occurs. As for tissue composition, the most predominant cell type is the smooth muscle cell.[2] In addition to proliferation within the intima, these cells have other properties relevant to atherosclerotic lesion development that include the accumulation of cholesterol and other lipids. This may result in the production of vacuolated cells called smooth muscle–derived foam cells that are characteristic of the atherosclerotic lesion. The other main function of these smooth muscle cells is the production of extracellular matrix, particularly collagen.

Other cell types present in human carotid plaque lesions include numerous monocyte/macrophages that also ingest lipid and become vacuolated, producing the macrophage-derived foam cells that are also characteristic of atherosclerotic lesions. Macrophages may also be an important source of growth factors that act on the surrounding smooth muscle cells to stimulate their growth and extracellular matrix production.[2] Finally, numerous T cells are present in these atherosclerotic lesions, along with a few scattered B cells. The roles played by these lymphocytes are currently not clear, although their presence in such lesions, as well as the similarities between ordinary atherosclerosis and transplant arteriosclerosis, has given rise to immune-based theories of the genesis of human atherosclerosis.[2]

Atherosclerotic plaques also have other important topographic features. Although a minority of established carotid plaques are solid, fibrous lesions, composed of the cells and extracellular matrix as just described, the vast majority have a necrotic core that usually has few if any viable cells, is composed of much loosely aggregated necrotic cellular debris, and contains numerous characteristic cholesterol crystals. This necrotic core is also rich in the potent procoagulant "tissue factor."[3] This necrotic core is separated from the lumen by a fibrous cap, a rim of solid plaque tissue composed of cells and extracellular matrix as previously described, which is of variable thickness. The integrity of this fibrous cap can be diminished by the marked influx of monocyte/macrophages and the loss of smooth muscle and collagen. It is the rupture of this fibrous cap that commonly leads to overlying thrombus formation because the blood elements now come into direct contact with the interstitial collagen and tissue factor of the underlying plaque and necrotic core. Necrotic core material and thrombus can also embolize distally.

Other common features of these advanced, complicated atherosclerotic plaques include intraplaque hemorrhage and calcification. Intraplaque hemorrhage is felt to arise from rupture of the fibrous cap with an associated infiltration of the softer plaque elements by blood under arterial pressure. The occasional finding of intraplaque hemorrhage in plaques without an overlying break in the fibrous cap has also been used to suggest that such hemorrhage can occur from rupture of one of often several thin-walled, capillary-like vessels that are prevalent in these plaques. This plaque vascularization is a common, sometimes less appreciated feature of advanced atherosclerosis, and the structurally weak walls are felt to be prone to rupture. Based on detailed studies of human coronary atherosclerosis, most of these small, penetrating vessels are derived from vasa vasora of the adventitia that secondarily penetrate through the media and arborize in the atherosclerotic intima. A few, however, can apparently arise directly from the arterial lumen.[4] Angiogenic activity has been described in atherosclerotic plaques, and these vessels also appear to have important growth-supporting roles.

Calcification commonly occurs in atherosclerotic plaques, usually in regions of necrosis. Thus, focal calcification is commonly seen in the necrotic cores, but it also frequently involves acellular, fibrous regions of the plaque as well. Calcification is usually felt to be dystrophic in nature, with dead cellular debris forming a nidus for calcium phosphate crystal formation. However, the recent demonstration of specific proteins such as osteopontin and morphogenic bone protein in such lesions suggests that the biology of plaque calcification may have parallels with early bone formation processes.[5]

HEMODYNAMIC FACTORS IN THE DEVELOPMENT OF CAROTID BIFURCATION PLAQUES

The location of early intimal thickenings and later atherosclerotic plaque development in the carotid bifurcation region is correlated with certain hemodynamic factors. In particular, regions of low shear stress and disturbed, nonlaminar flow almost uniformly occur in the carotid bulb region of the proximal internal carotid artery and away from the flow divider, which is a relatively high shear stress region. This is the same site of preferred plaque development, and it has been suggested that particulate elements in the blood such as platelets and leukocytes, can more easily interact with the arterial wall at these sites.[1] More recent studies focus on lymphocyte and monocyte adherence to arterial endothelium, which is felt to be an initial stage in the formation of the fatty streak and subsequent atherosclerosis development.[2] Specific leukocyte-endothelial adhesion molecules are felt to mediate this initial attachment, and at least one such ligand intercellular adhesion molecule-1 (ICAM-1) has been shown to be expressed in arterial endothelium in a flow-dependent manner,[6] associated with mononuclear inflammatory cell adhesion.[7] Additionally, molecular biology studies have documented a similar shear stress response element in the platelet-derived growth factor (PDGF)-B gene.[6] Elucidation of the hemodynamic controls of leukocyte adhesion to endothelium and arterial wall adaptations await further research.

GROWTH FACTORS AND CELL PROLIFERATION IN CAROTID PLAQUES

Several arterial wall growth factors have now been described.[2] Some of these, such as PDGF-A and -B isoforms and acidic and basic fibroblast growth factors, have also been demonstrated in human arterial tissues. Currently no direct data bear on the question of which of these growth factors is most responsible for smooth muscle and other cell proliferation in human atherosclerosis. Although a spatial correlation has been noted between PDGF-A chain and cell proliferation in human carotid plaques,[8] other growth-promoting activities associated with penetrating microvessels in these plaques appear to be more important with regard to proliferative activity.

As for the equally important question, What is the extent of cell proliferation in human vascular intimas? some data are beginning to come forth.[9] Studies using problematic ex vivo tritiated thymidine labeling of human arteries indicate very low levels of cell proliferation (0 to 0.09% of cells being labeled). This was found in "normal artery" samples, and qualitatively similar levels were seen in atherosclerotic plaques. There now exist antibodies against cell cycle-specific proteins that can be applied to freshly obtained human tissues without the need for prior injections. One class of such antibodies has been to the proliferating cell nuclear antigen (PCNA), an auxiliary protein to DNA polymerase delta. With such antibodies, the first look at human arteries focused on segments of normal internal mammary artery excised at the time of coronary bypass procedures, as well as the coronary arteries of the diseased hearts removed at the time of heart transplantation.[9] The internal mammary arteries revealed a 0 to 0.11% PCNA index.[9] The normal adult human coronary arteries exhibit a prominent amount of nonocclusive diffuse intimal thickening, which is universal among the epicardial arteries. The PCNA indices here in the intimae averaged 0.31% (range 0 to 1.24%) and their underlying mediae averaged 0.19% (range 0 to 0.25%). Finally, the coronary atherosclerotic intimae exhibited PCNA indices averaging 0.85% (range 0 to 4.68%), and their underlying mediae averaged 0.4% (range 0 to 3.43%). Similar levels of proliferative activity were obtained by using a different proliferation marker, Ki-67.[9] Similar levels of cell proliferation have been seen in advanced human carotid artery plaques removed at the time of carotid endarterectomy (Fig. 1). Other investigators have also found similarly low levels of proliferative activity in human atherosclerotic arterial material.

These proliferative indices are certainly low compared with the 30% to 50% maximal levels seen in the balloon catheter–induced intimal thickening in the rat carotid artery.[10] This rat model exhibits an abrupt, large increase in arterial cell proliferation over an approximate 2 day period, which is subsequently followed by a gradual decrease in proliferative index to less than 1% by 8 weeks after injury. It is nevertheless conceivable that human atherosclerosis could have such a pattern with very rare bursts of major proliferative activity. Sampling could have been all in the long subsequent latent periods. However, the relatively low levels seen in human arteries are also in concert with the levels of cell proliferation seen with hypercholesterolemia models of atherosclerosis in pigs and in rabbits, here measured by in vivo tritiated thymidine labeling.[9] In those hypercholesterolemia models in which cell proliferation has been

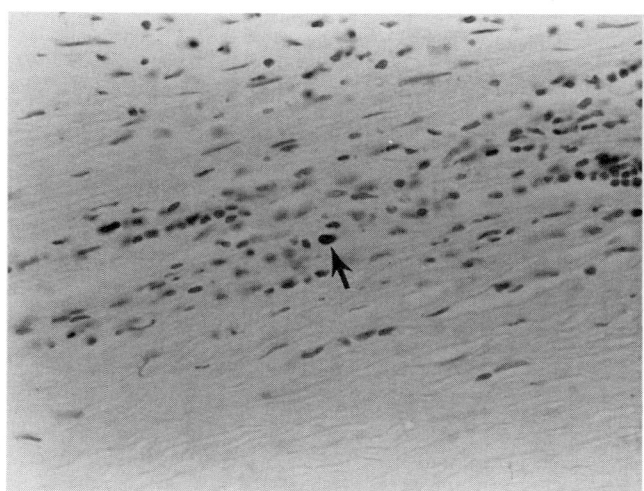 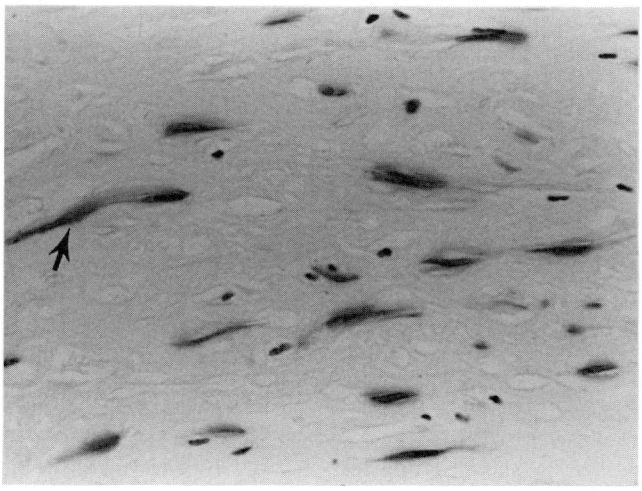

Figure 1 Human carotid atherosclerotic plaque stained with anti-PCNA antibody and showing focal cell proliferation, black nuclear reaction product *(arrow)*. (Methyl green nuclear counterstain, × 300.)

Figure 2 Human carotid plaque showing immunoreaction for type I procollagen protein in the fibrous cap region *(arrow)*. (Hematoxylin nuclear counterstain, × 300.)

measured, the time course of cell proliferation is more protracted. Although increased mitotic activity can be detected within days after the start of a cholesterol-rich diet in pigs, proliferative indices remain in the 0 to 3% range and do not exceed 5%. Thus, the hypercholesterolemia model data suggest a slow-growing, indolent proliferative response that is able to produce significant stenotic lesions over several months to years and as such may be more representative of human atherosclerosis.

In initial studies of human coronary arteries, specific antibodies were used in a double-labeling procedure to determine the cell types displaying PCNA immunoreactivity.[9] About 16% of PCNA positive cells reacted with smooth muscle–specific actin, implying smooth muscle origin. A significant number (up to 27%) of the PCNA-positive cells also reacted with macrophage markers. Many of these cells are foam cells. The conclusion may be that, in addition to smooth muscle cells, monocytes, macrophages, and possibly lymphocytes account for much of the proliferative activity seen in human atherosclerotic plaques. However, several cells displaying proliferative activity remain to be defined. Similar data have been obtained with human carotid plaques.

COLLAGEN GENE EXPRESSION IN CAROTID BIFURCATION PLAQUES

For most intima, and particularly for clinically significant atherosclerotic plaques, extracellular matrix comprises the largest volume component of the lesion. Thus, control of extracellular matrix synthesis is very important in overall intimal growth. The intimal extracellular matrix is composed of several proteoglycan species as well as several collagen types.[11] Recent studies have begun investigating collagen gene expression in the vessel wall because collagen is a very prominent protein class in the normal vessel wall and in atherosclerosis.[11] Collagen also provides much of the tensile strength of the intima, which is particularly significant because fibrous cap rupture is felt to be the immediate precursor to atherosclerosis-related arterial thrombosis. The vast majority of arterial wall collagenous protein is accounted for by types I, III, and IV.[11] These mature types have also been well demonstrated in human atherosclerosis and in intimal hyperplasia by biochemical and immunocytochemical methods.

A putative inflammatory link to collagen gene expression in human atherosclerosis recently has been highlighted.[11] Qualitatively increased collagen type I and III mRNAs was found using in situ hybridization on human arterial intima compared to media. Based on serial section immunocytochemistry, expression was suggested to be in smooth muscle cells adjacent to macrophages. Increased type I collagen mRNA and type I procollagen protein expression have been seen in carotid (Fig. 2) and coronary atherosclerotic plaques, compared with normal coronary or internal mammary arteries, but have not seen a tight spatial correlation with the presence of macrophages.[12] Rauterberg and Jaeger reported no such collagen-macrophage association in human aortic coarcts.[11] Additionally, the rat carotid artery injury model does not exhibit significant numbers of inflammatory cells but does show prominent collagen gene expression. Therefore, macrophages are clearly not required for arterial wall collagen synthesis. Additionally, prominent PDGF -A and -B expression has been seen associated with intraplaque capillaries in human carotid plaques,[3] as well as prominent perivascular type I procollagen immunostaining in human carotid and coronary plaques.[12] Finally, a negative association between plaque regions displaying type I collagen gene expression and the presence of T cells has been seen, raising the possibility that T-cell mediators such as interferon-γ may play an important regulatory role for this prominent extracellular protein.[12] This area requires further study because macrophages and T cells in the artery wall may be in various states of cell activation.

In summary, hemodynamic factors, the expression of leukocyte-endothelial adhesion molecules, and growth factors are important aspects of the development of human atherosclerosis. However, their definite roles in regard to the low levels of cell proliferation seen need further elucidation. In addition, extracellular matrix synthesis by arterial smooth muscle–derived cells represents a major growth component to these lesions and may be governed by the same or separate controlling factors. In particular, the balance between collagen synthesis and degradation may be important, both for this aspect of plaque growth and in determining the strength or weakness of the fibrous cap region, which in turn may be critical for the transition from stable to clinically unstable arterial lesions.

REFERENCES

1. Glagov S, Zarins C, Giddens DP, Ku DN. Hemodynamics and atherosclerosis: Insights and perspectives gained from studies of human arteries. Arch Pathol Lab Med 1988; 112:1018–1031.
2. Ross R. The pathogenesis of atherosclerosis: A perspective for the 1990s. Nature 1993; 362:801–809.
3. Wilcox JN. Analysis of local gene expression in human atherosclerotic plaques by in situ hybridization. Trends Cardiovasc Med 1991; 1:17–24.
4. Barger AC, Beeuwkes R, Lainey LL, Silverman KJ. Hypothesis: Vasa vasorum and neovascularization of human coronary arteries. A possible role in the pathophysiology of atherosclerosis. N Engl J Med 1984; 310:175–747.
5. Boström K, Watson KE, Horn S, et al. Bone morphogenetic protein expression in human atherosclerotic lesions. J Clin Invest 1993; 91:1800–1809.
6. Resnick N, Collins T, Atkinson W, et al. Platelet-derived growth factor B chain promoter contains a cis-acting fluid shear-stress-responsive element. Proc Natl Acad Sci U S A 1993; 90:4591–4595.
7. Walpola PL, Gotlieb AI, Langille BL. Monocyte adhesion and changes in endothelial cell number, morphology and F-actin distribution elicited by low shear stress in vivo. Am J Pathol 1993; 142:1392–1400.
8. Rekhter MD, Gordon D. Does PDGF A stimulate proliferation of arterial mesenchymal cells in human atherosclerotic plaques? Circ Res 1994; 75:410–417.
9. Gordon D, Schwartz SM. Cell proliferation in human atherosclerosis. Trends Cardiovasc Med 1991; 1:24–28.
10. Clowes AW, Reidy MA, Clowes MM. Kinetics of cellular proliferation after arterial injury: I. Smooth muscle growth in the absence of endothelium. Lab Invest 1983; 49:327–333.
11. Rauterberg J, Jaeger E. Collagen and collagen synthesis in the atherosclerotic vessel wall. In: Robenek H, Severs NJ, eds. Cell interactions in atherosclerosis. Boca Raton, Fla: CRC Press, 1992:101.
12. Rekhter MD, Jhang K, Narayanan AS, et al. Type I collagen gene expression in human atherosclerosis: Localization to specific plaque regions. Am J Pathol 1993; 143:1634–1648.

PATHOLOGY OF CAROTID AND VERTEBRAL ARTERIAL FIBRODYSPLASIA

ELLIOT L. CHAIKOF, M.D., PH.D.
ROBERT B. SMITH III, M.D.

Despite a 30-year history of case reports and collected retrospective reviews, our understanding of the pathology, pathogenesis, and natural history of extracranial arterial fibromuscular dysplasia (FMD) remains incomplete. The rarity of the process and the sole reliance on angiographic findings to diagnose and categorize FMD have limited clinical decision making. We suspect that in the coming years widespread use of ever-improving imaging modalities will present an increasing pool of such patients. The challenge will be to continue a careful examination of this nonatheromatous, noninflammatory process, for ultimately we must base our clinical recommendations on an understanding of disease progression and our ability to alter this process.

CLASSIFICATION AND DISEASE ASSOCIATIONS: EVIDENCE FOR A SYSTEMIC ARTERIOPATHY

Harrison and McCormack[1] proposed the first pathologic classification of FMD, which was revised by Stanley and associates[2] in 1975. The classification is based on the predominant site of dysplasia in the arterial wall: intimal fibroplasia, medial dysplasia, and periarterial or periadventitial fibroplasia. Lesions involving the media may be subclassified into medial fibroplasia, perimedial fibroplasia, and medial hyperplasia. Medial fibroplasia is the most common form of FMD and accounts for 70% to 95% of all fibromuscular lesions. Medial dissection used to be considered a fourth subtype of medial FMD but is in fact a complication of FMD and should be considered a distinct entity. The advantage of this classification is its excellent correlation with angiographic findings.

This classification is derived from an examination of renovascular FMD. For the most part, extracranial fibromuscular disease consists of two primary pathologic subtypes, intimal and medial fibroplasia. Intimal fibroplasia is the less common of the two and is typically associated with either an isolated web or a smooth tubular stenosis of the internal carotid artery (Fig. 1). Webs appear to be more common among older patients,

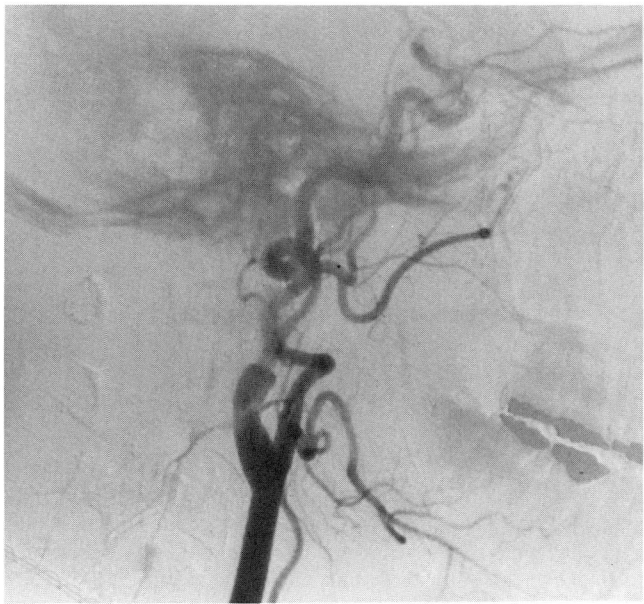

Figure 1 Tubular stenosis of the internal carotid artery is typically associated with intimal fibroplasia.

and long stenoses typically occur in the young adult. Histologically, intimal fibroplasia consists of an eccentric or circumferential accumulation of fibrous tissue in the intima, with an intact internal elastic lamina and no significant inflammatory infiltrate. Elongation, kinking, or coiling of the carotid artery may also be noted. This process appears to be predominantly a localized arteriopathy, and simultaneous lesions, whether aneurysmal or fibrodysplastic, are unusual. Several authors have suggested that a highly stenotic web may represent a lesion associated with a relatively high risk of stroke.

Medial fibroplasia has been documented in the celiac, hepatic, superior mesenteric, iliac, and profunda femoris arteries as well as within the subclavian and brachial arteries and branches of the external carotid artery. However, the most common sites remain the renal and extracranial internal carotid arteries. Morphologically, medial fibroplasia is characterized by multiple stenoses with intervening mural dilations, most often noted on nonbranching arterial segments. Histologic examination reveals disruption of the internal elastic lamina, a disordered mix of medial cellular and matrix components, and the absence of associated necrosis, calcification, and inflammation. The angiographic appearance is the classic string-of-beads stenoses (Fig. 2). Typically the beads are larger than the diameter of the proximal uninvolved artery. Medial fibroplasia of the extracranial internal carotid artery most often involves a 2 to 6 cm segment adjacent to the second and third cervical vertebrae and spares the origins and proximal portions of the carotid. The artery is often elongated, and kinking is noted in approximately 5% of patients. Reviews have documented bilateral disease in 35% to 85% of patients. Perimedial

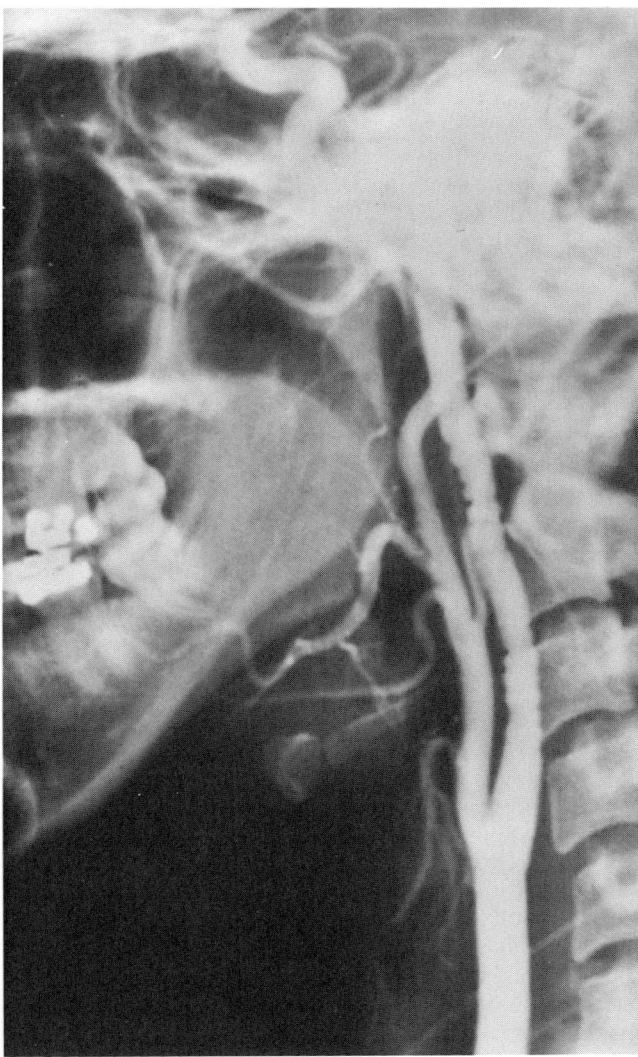

Figure 2 Angiographic demonstration of string-of-beads stenosis characteristic of carotid artery medial fibroplasia.

fibroplasia is found almost exclusively in the renal circulation and has not to our knowledge been documented in either vertebral or carotid arteries. Medial hyperplasia probably accounts for fewer than 5% of FMD cases and histologically consists of increased medial smooth muscle without associated fibrosis. It has been observed in the internal carotid, typically at the C1 to C2 level. The lesion produces a focal smooth concentric and at times tubular stenosis. In this regard it is sometimes difficult to distinguish from intimal fibroplasia. Periadventitial (periarterial) fibroplasia, the rarest form of FMD, has not been observed to affect the extracranial vessels.

Vertebral artery fibrodysplasia is a medial process but differs morphologically from the lesions observed in renal and carotid arteries. It typically presents as multiple stenoses or nonocclusive mural aneurysms in the lower portion of the vessel adjacent to the fifth cervical vertebra or more distally at the level of the second cervical vertebra.

Although most cases of medial fibroplasia occur as isolated findings, this process should be considered a systemic arteriopathy. In approximately 10% to 20% of patients who present with a carotid dissection, contralateral fibromuscular disease is present. Coexistent carotid and vertebral fibrodysplasia occurs in approximately 20% of patients. Additionally, carotid fibromuscular disease associated with intracranial and on rare occasion extracranial aneurysms has been observed. In a review of 102 ruptured intracranial aneurysms, cervical FMD was noted in 31 cases.[3] Aneurysms were saccular, frequently multiple, and within the ipsilateral intracranial portion of the internal carotid and vertebral arteries. Moreover, aneurysms may involve any intracranial site and are not necessarily contiguous with a neighboring region of fibrodysplasia. Certainly the most common site for either simultaneous or subsequent development of fibrodysplasia is the renal artery. Concomitant renovascular and extracranial fibromuscular disease has been noted in 25% to 50% of patients.

The pathogenesis of arterial fibromuscular disease is unknown, and little new information has emerged regarding postulates that first arose nearly 2 decades ago. The causative factors considered most important are hormonal, mechanical, and genetic. The predominance of fibroplasia in women of childbearing age has raised speculation about the role of estrogens. In one report cerebrovascular FMD was noted in 18% of women who presented with a cerebral ischemic event while taking oral contraceptives. Intimal hyperplasia may be induced by oral contraceptives, and alterations in the vascular media may occur during pregnancy. However, there appears to be no relationship between gravidity or parity rates and the incidence of FMD in the general population.

Sottiurai and co-workers[4] have suggested that medial fibroplasia may occur as a consequence of an impairment of adaptive repair mechanisms that normally respond to mechanically or hemodynamically induced arterial wall injury. Long vessels lacking arterial branches presumably have a paucity of vasa vasora, which creates localized regions of relative medial ischemia. In this model the extent of medial injury produced by hemodynamic factors, trauma, or repetitive stretching during extension and rotation of the head determines the pathologic type of fibrodysplasia. However, this hypothesis does not account for the large number of patients with carotid loops, kinks, and coils who fail to develop FMD. Further, it fails to explain the observation of fibromuscular disease in the superficial temporal artery and the clear association of fibroplasia with intracranial aneurysms.

Recent reports of extracranial fibromuscular disease in siblings and family clusters suggest a possible genetic component. Rushton[5] analyzed the occurrence of FMD in 20 families and suggested an autosomal dominant inheritance pattern with variable penetrance.

DIAGNOSTIC APPROACHES

Conventional arteriography remains the sole means of definitively diagnosing carotid or vertebral fibrodysplasia. The presence of FMD in any one of the extracranial vessels should prompt a thorough four-vessel cerebral angiogram, including examination of the intracranial vessels to detect possible sites of aneurysmal disease. In addition, the predilection of concomitant disease necessitates renal arteriography. The accuracy of noninvasive techniques, including magnetic resonance angiography and duplex ultrasonography, remains limited. At present they cannot be relied on in screening arteries at risk.

Recent reports of concurrent fibromuscular disease in the superficial temporal artery imply that biopsy may be helpful to confirm the diagnosis in patients who have either a carotid dissection or multiple intracranial aneurysms of the internal carotid artery and no other evidence of systemic FMD. This information has important prognostic implications and may aid in obtaining a more precise disease classification.

Although radiographic findings are pathognomonic for medial fibroplasia, a differential diagnosis should always be considered when intimal fibroplasia or medial hyperplasia is a possibility. These lesions may be confused with arteriosclerotic plaques, inflammatory processes such as Takayasu's arteritis, and vascular lesions of neurofibromatosis or Ehlers-Danlos syndrome. Arteriosclerotic lesions can usually be distinguished by their eccentric appearance and location at the level of the carotid bifurcation. In Takayasu's arteritis the aorta is usually involved and the large arteries are stenotic at their origin. The associated stigmata of Ehlers-Danlos syndrome and neurofibromatosis should aid in identifying these entities.

CLINICAL PRESENTATION AND NATURAL HISTORY

The incidence of medial fibroplasia in most carotid arteriographic studies ranges between 0.25% and 0.68%. It presents commonly in women and infrequently in blacks. Most patients with extracranial FMD are diagnosed at a later age than those with renovascular dysplasia. Notably, approximately 20% to 50% of patients may have associated atherosclerotic disease of the carotid bulb. Some 39% of the patients treated by graded intraluminal dilation in a series reported by Collins and co-workers[6] and 20% of those reported by Effeney and associates[7] also required a concomitant carotid bifurcation endarterectomy. Although there are fewer patients with intimal fibroplasia or vertebral artery involvement, the demographic profile appears similar to that of medial fibroplasia. Extracranial FMD has been documented in children, and it should be considered in the differential diagnosis of the symptomatic pediatric patient.

In reported surgical series, as in our experience, the spectrum of symptoms is similar to that of patients with atherosclerosis undergoing carotid endarterectomy: amaurosis fugax, transient ischemic attacks, nonfocal cerebral ischemia, and stroke. Suggested causes of symptoms include both impaired perfusion as a consequence of multiple stenoses and embolic debris originating from aneurysmal cul de sacs. Alternatively, symptoms may originate following dissection of the vertebral or internal carotid artery. Occipital or neck pain followed by basilar ischemic symptoms is characteristic of vertebral artery dissection. The patient with carotid dissection more often complains of facial and neck pain, blurred vision, and associated facial numbness and dysthesias. Horner's syndrome may be noted on physical examination. Headaches, vertigo, and tinnitus have also been observed in association with extracranial arterial fibroplasia. It has been suggested that headache is related to the release of vasoactive substances, such as serotonin or thromboxane A2 from aggregating platelets. In many patients, however, the angiographic finding of carotid FMD is only incidental, with no symptomatic correlation.

The assumption that patients with carotid FMD have a prognosis and natural history similar to that of patients with atherosclerosis is unproved. Repeat angiography has rarely been documented in patients with carotid FMD, and the incidence of progressive disease has not been clarified. Only 15 patients with carotid FMD undergoing serial angiography have been described in the literature. Of these, progressive FMD was observed in five and a new lesion in two. Of 8 patients followed at Emory, only one developed a new lesion of FMD in the contralateral vessel, and atherosclerotic stenosis evolved in one other. The significance of angiographic progression is uncertain, as these changes were not correlated with new clinical symptoms. Similarly, in a series of 79 patients reported by Corrin, Sandok, and Houser[8] from the Mayo Clinic, carotid FMD was an incidental finding in the majority, and only three had or developed ischemic symptoms during a mean follow-up period of 5 years. This is in direct contrast to renovascular FMD, where progression is much more common. In one report, progression of renal FMD was documented in 35% of patients after a 3-year observation period.

The presumption that recurrent symptoms and/or cerebral infarction is inevitable in the patient with symptomatic carotid FMD remains an open question. In a review from the Emory University Hospital of 35 nonoperated patients with carotid FMD, all but 7 of whom were symptomatic, none had a stroke during an average follow-up period of 91 months.[9] Only two patients had persistent symptoms of nonfocal cerebral ischemia. In our experience even patients with symptoms of focal ischemia will probably have spontaneous cessation of these symptoms on antiplatelet therapy. Similar findings have been observed by others. Wessen and Elliott[10] followed 19 patients with cerebrovascular FMD treated with antiplatelet agents. Only 2 had recurrent symptoms after a mean observation period of approximately 24 months. This is not to say that carotid FMD cannot cause cerebral infarction but rather that the incidence is probably very low. Certainly, there seems little need to intervene surgically in the asymptomatic patient with carotid or vertebral FMD.

REFERENCES

1. Harrison EG Jr, McCormack LJ. Pathologic classification of renal arterial disease in renovascular hypertension. Mayo Clin Proc 1971; 46:161–167.
2. Stanley JC, Gewertz BL, Bove EL, Sottiurai V, Fry WJ. Arterial fibrodysplasia: histopathologic character and current etiologic concepts. Arch Surg 1975; 110:561–566.
3. George B, Zerah M, Mourier KL, et al. Ruptured intracranial aneurysms: The influence of sex and fibromuscular dysplasia upon prognosis. Acta Neurochir 1989; 97:26–30.
4. Sottiurai V, Fry WJ, Stanley JC. Ultrastructural characteristics of experimental arterial medial fibrodysplasia induced by vasa vasorum occlusion. J Surg Res 1978; 24:169–177.
5. Rushton AR. The genetics of fibromuscular dysplasia. Arch Intern Med 1980; 140:233–236.
6. Collins GJ Jr, Rich NM, Clagett GP, et al. Fibromuscular dysplasia of the internal carotid arteries: Clinical experience and follow-up. Ann Surg 1981; 194:89–96.
7. Effeney DJ, Ehrenfeld WK, Stoney RJ, et al. Why operate on carotid fibromuscular dysplasia? Arch Surg 1980; 115:1261–1265.
8. Corrin LS, Sandok BA, Houser OW. Cerebral ischemic events in patients with carotid artery fibromuscular dysplasia. Arch Neurol 1981; 38:616–618.
9. Stewart MT, Moritz MW, Smith RB III, et al. The natural history of carotid fibromuscular dysplasia. J Vasc Surg 1986; 3:305–310.
10. Wessen CA, Elliott BM. Fibromuscular dysplasia of the carotid arteries. Am J Surg 1986; 151:448–451.

DUPLEX SCANNING AND SPECTRAL ANALYSIS OF CAROTID ARTERY OCCLUSIVE DISEASE

R. EUGENE ZIERLER, M.D.

The clinical importance of the carotid artery bifurcation in the pathogenesis of stroke was not generally recognized until the observations of C. Miller Fisher in 1951.[1] Even at the time of the Joint Study of Extracranial Arterial Occlusion in 1968, arteriography was the only diagnostic method of classifying the severity of carotid artery disease.[2] However, because of its invasive nature, arteriography was not suitable for screening asymptomatic patients or performing serial follow-up studies. In addition, arteriography is a strictly anatomic investigation that gives no direct information on the physiologic consequences of the observed lesions.

The risks and limitations of arteriography stimulated the development of noninvasive methods for the evaluation of cerebrovascular disease. These tests are characterized by minimal risk, absence of patient discomfort, and relatively low cost, so they can be used to document both the extent of disease at a single time and any subsequent changes. Noninvasive tests for extracranial carotid artery disease can be considered as either indirect or direct. Although indirect tests such as periorbital Doppler examination and various types of oculoplethysmography may still be of value in selected patients, the direct approach of duplex scanning is clearly the method of choice for routine diagnostic use.

THE DUPLEX CONCEPT

The early attempts to use ultrasound in the evaluation of the carotid artery bifurcation relied on B-mode imaging alone. While satisfactory images could be obtained, the resolution was not sufficient to distinguish flowing blood from noncalcified atherosclerotic plaque or thrombus. It became apparent that a method for identifying blood flow within B-mode images was needed.[3] Since Doppler ultrasound was being used to assess blood flow in arterial occlusive disease of the extremities, it seemed logical to combine these ultrasound methods into a single diagnostic test. Thus, the duplex concept of combining B-mode imaging and pulsed Doppler flow detection for the direct evaluation of arterial disease led to the construction of the first duplex scanning instruments.

Duplex scanning makes it possible to obtain anatomic and physiologic information directly from sites of vascular disease. This approach is based on the concept that arterial lesions produce disturbances in blood flow patterns that can be characterized by analysis of Doppler flow signals. In conventional duplex scanning the B-mode image is used as a guide for placement of a pulsed Doppler sample volume within the artery of interest, and the local flow pattern is assessed by spectral waveform analysis. While the B-mode image may be useful for identifying anatomic variants and arterial wall thickening or calcification, the classification of arterial disease severity is based primarily on interpretation of pulsed Doppler spectral waveforms. An important aspect of duplex scanning is the use of a pulsed Doppler, which permits evaluation of the arterial flow pattern at a discrete site within the B-mode image. The sample volume of a pulsed Doppler is the region in which flow is actually detected. Adjusting the size and position of the sample volume allows center stream flow patterns to be assessed without interference from flow disturbances near the arterial wall or flow in adjacent vessels.

B-MODE IMAGING

B-mode imaging alone has been used with varying degrees of success to assess the histologic and surface features of carotid bifurcation lesions. Although the sonographic appearance of a plaque may correlate qualitatively with its histologic composition, the clinical relevance of this information is controversial.[4] Calcified atherosclerotic plaque, which is extremely echogenic, results in bright echoes with acoustic shadows (Fig. 1). The B-mode characteristic of plaque that appears to correlate most closely with clinical outcome is het-

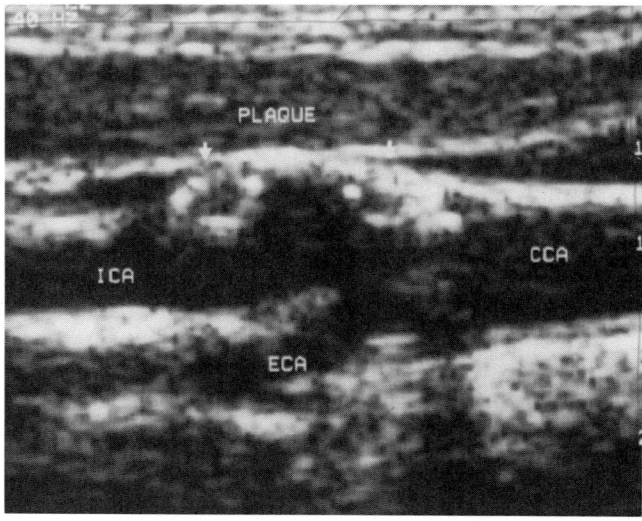

Figure 1 B-mode image of a diseased carotid bifurcation. A brightly echogenic calcified atherosclerotic plaque is present along the near wall of the carotid bulb *(arrows)* with acoustic shadowing in the distal common carotid artery (CCA). Although the arterial lumen is clearly seen, it is difficult to classify the severity of stenosis based on the image alone. ICA, internal carotid artery; ECA, external carotid artery.

erogeneity, a feature attributed to intraplaque hemorrhage. This particular feature has been observed more frequently in symptomatic than in asymptomatic patients.

Experience with B-mode imaging for the classification of carotid artery disease has generally shown that interpretation of the image is most accurate for lesions of minimal to moderate severity and least accurate for high-grade stenoses or occlusions. It is often difficult to estimate the size of the arterial lumen from a B-mode image because the interface between the arterial wall and flowing blood is not clearly seen. Furthermore, acoustic shadows from calcified plaques may prevent complete visualization of the arterial wall and lumen. These limitations are largely overcome by duplex scanning.

SPECTRAL WAVEFORM ANALYSIS AND COLOR-FLOW IMAGING

In the conventional approach to carotid duplex scanning, the B-mode image is used to locate the arteries and facilitate placement of the pulsed Doppler sample volume at the site of interest (Fig. 2). The severity of disease is then determined by spectral analysis of the Doppler signal. Spectral waveform analysis is a signal processing technique that displays the complete frequency and amplitude content of the Doppler signal. The Doppler-shifted frequency is directly proportional to blood cell velocity, and the amplitude of the signal depends on the number of blood cells moving through the pulsed Doppler sample volume. As the number of blood cells producing the Doppler frequency shift increases, the signal amplitude becomes stronger. Spectral information is usually presented graphically with frequency or velocity on the vertical axis, time on the horizontal axis, and amplitude indicated by shades of gray (Fig. 3).

The center stream flow pattern in a normal artery is uniform or laminar, and a spectral waveform taken with the pulsed Doppler sample volume in the center of the lumen shows a relatively narrow band of frequencies. Stenoses and other arterial wall abnormalities disrupt this normal pattern and produce flow disturbances that are apparent in the Doppler spectral waveform as a wider range of frequencies and amplitudes. This increase in the width of the frequency band is called spectral broadening. A localized increase in the peak systolic frequency is associated with severe stenoses that produce high-velocity jets. The end-diastolic frequency is also increased in very severe stenoses. The spectral waveform criteria for classifying the severity of internal carotid disease (Table 1, Fig. 3), have been validated by a series of comparisons with independently interpreted contrast arteriograms. These criteria can distinguish between normal and diseased internal carotid arteries with a specificity of 84% and a sensitivity of 99%. The accuracy for detecting 50% to 99% diameter stenosis or occlusion is 93%.[5]

Color-flow imaging is an alternative to spectral waveform analysis for displaying the pulsed Doppler information obtained by duplex scanning.[6] In contrast to spectral analysis, which evaluates the entire frequency and amplitude content of the signal at a single sample site, color-flow imaging provides an estimate of the Doppler-shifted frequency or flow velocity for each site within the B-mode image. The main advantage of the color-flow display is that it presents simultaneous flow information on the entire image. Spectral waveforms contain a range of frequencies and amplitudes, allowing determination of flow direction and spectral parameters such as mean, mode, peak, and bandwidth. The color assignments in the color-flow image are based on flow direction and a single mean or average frequency estimate for each site in the B-mode image plane. Consequently, the peak Doppler frequency shifts or velocities shown by spectral waveforms are generally higher than the frequencies or velocities indicated by color-flow imaging.

In a color-flow image shades of two or more distinct colors, usually red and blue, indicate the direction of flow relative to the ultrasound scan lines. The display is generally set up by the examiner to show flow in the arterial direction as red and flow in the venous direction as blue. Variations in the Doppler-shifted frequency or flow velocity are then indicated by changes in color, with lighter shades typically representing higher flow velocities. The specific features of color-flow images vary considerably among the commercially available duplex scanning instruments. However, a single-sample volume-pulsed Doppler and spectrum analyzer are always available for a detailed evaluation of flow patterns at selected arterial sites.

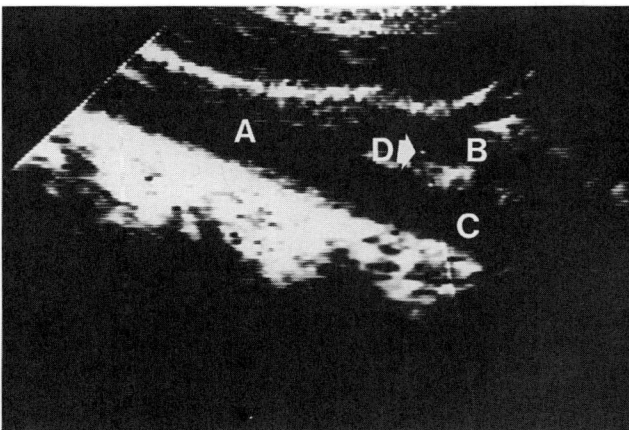

Figure 2 Conventional duplex scan image of a left carotid bifurcation. A, common carotid artery; B, external carotid artery; C, internal carotid artery. A white line indicates the position of the pulsed Doppler beam, and the sample volume is represented by a dot (D). (From Zierler RE, Strandness DE Jr. Noninvasive dynamic and real-time assessment of extracranial cerebrovasculature. In: Wood JH, ed. Cerebral blood flow: Physiologic and clinical aspects. New York: McGraw-Hill, 1987:316; with permission.)

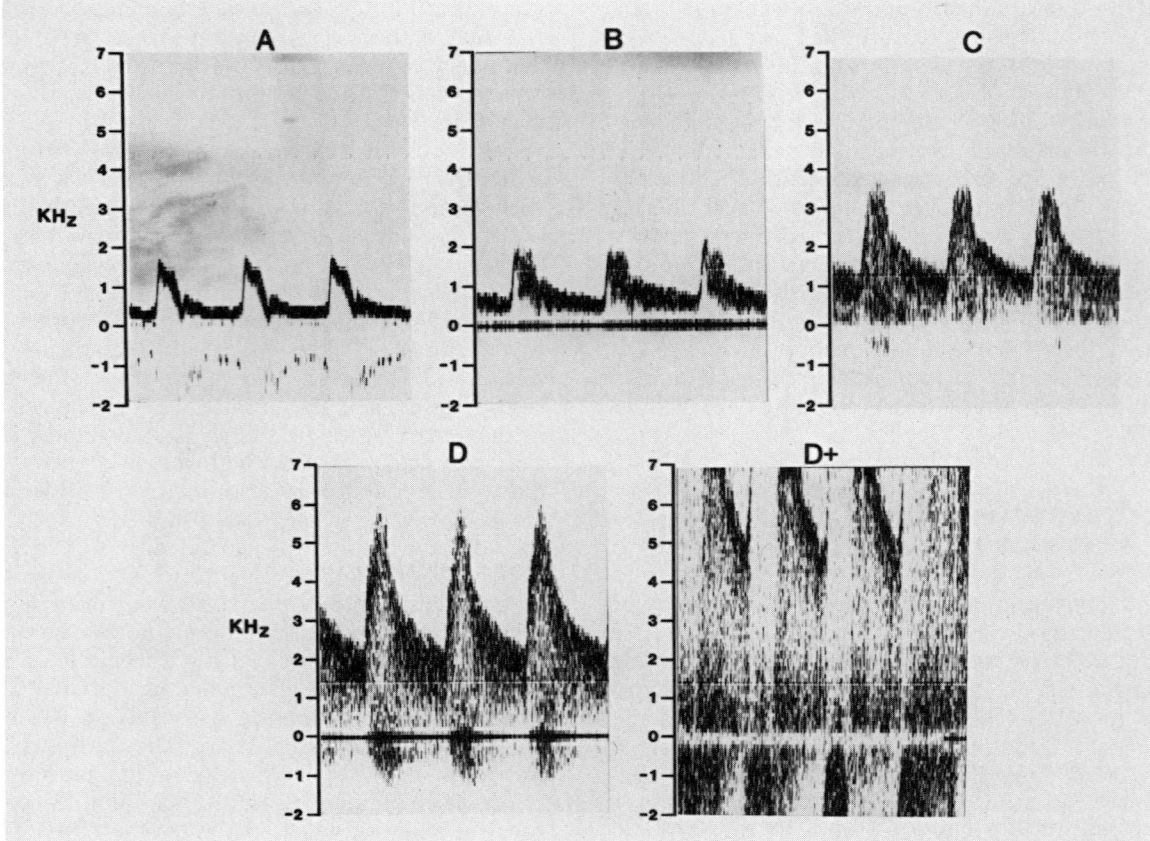

Figure 3 Examples of internal carotid spectral waveforms classified according to the criteria given in Table 1. *A*, Normal; *B*, 1 to 15 percent diameter reduction; *C*, 16 to 49 percent diameter reduction; *D*, 50 to 79 percent diameter reduction; D+, 80 to 99 percent diameter reduction. (From Zierler RE, Strandness DE Jr. Noninvasive dynamic and real-time assessment of extracranial cerebrovasculature. In: Wood JH, ed. Cerebral blood flow: Physiologic and clinical aspects. New York: McGraw-Hill, 1987:317; with permission.)

Table 1 Criteria for Classification of Internal Carotid Artery Disease by Duplex Scanning with Spectral Waveform Analysis of Pulsed Doppler Signals

Arteriographic Lesion (% Diameter Reduction)		Spectral Criteria
A.	0	Peak systolic frequency <4 kHz; no spectral broadening
B.	1–15	Peak systolic frequency <4 kHz; spectral broadening in deceleration phase of systole only
C.	16–49	Peak systolic frequency <4 kHz; spectral broadening throughout systole
D.	50–79	Peak systolic frequency ≥4 kHz; end-diastolic frequency <4.5 kHz
D+.	80–99	End-diastolic frequency ≥4.5 kHz
E.	Occlusion (100)	No internal carotid flow signal; flow to zero in common carotid artery

Criteria are based on a pulsed Doppler with a 5 MHz transmitting frequency, a sample volume that is small relative to the internal carotid artery, and a 60° beam-to-vessel angle of insonation. Approximate angle-adjusted velocity equivalents are 4 kHz = 125 cm/sec and 4.5 kHz = 140 cm/sec.

INSTRUMENTATION AND TECHNIQUE

Since the attenuation of ultrasound as it travels through tissue is directly proportional to the transmitting frequency, low frequencies can penetrate to greater depths than high frequencies. Thus, low ultrasound frequencies are required for obtaining image and Doppler information from deeply located structures such as those in the abdomen. However, because the blood vessels in the neck are relatively superficial, ultrasound transmitting frequency is generally not a major consideration in carotid duplex scanning. Transducers with frequencies in the range of 5 to 10 MHz give optimal results.

One of the principal limitations of the conventional approach to carotid duplex scanning is the small region of the arterial lumen that can be evaluated at any one time. To obtain complete information on flow patterns throughout the B-mode image, the single-pulsed Doppler sample volume must be moved serially to various sites. Even with extreme diligence on the part of the examiner, flow disturbances that are confined to a small section of the vessel may be missed. In addition, it is more difficult to appreciate the complex three-dimensional features of flow in the carotid bifurcation with the single-sample volume technique than it is with color-flow imaging.

The basic examination technique is the same for both color-flow imaging and conventional duplex scanning. First the common carotid artery is imaged low in the neck and followed distally. The common carotid bifurcation is usually at the level of the upper border of the thyroid cartilage, and the internal and external carotid arteries can be distinguished by their typical location with the internal carotid posterolaterally and the external carotid anteromedially. The carotid sinus or bulb may be seen as a dilatation of the arterial lumen at the origin of the internal carotid artery. A region of boundary layer separation is normally present along the posterior or outer wall of the bulb on the side opposite the flow divider. This region is characterized by low flow velocity with alternating forward and reverse components. Continuous forward flow is present in the bulb along the flow divider, and a more laminar flow pattern is re-established in the internal carotid artery distal to the bulb. The features of boundary layer separation in normal carotid bifurcations have been demonstrated by model studies and clinical pulsed Doppler examinations.[7] Once the internal carotid artery is identified, it should be followed as far distally as possible. Flow patterns are most easily visualized when the arteries are scanned in longitudinal section. Occasionally, transverse scans are useful for showing unusual anatomic relationships between the various carotid branches.

As the carotid branches are visualized on the B-mode image, pulsed Doppler signals are obtained at frequent intervals along the vessels. This is necessary because the flow disturbances produced by arterial lesions are propagated only for short distances downstream. Particular care is taken to completely assess the flow pattern in the carotid bulb or proximal internal carotid artery. Abnormal flow disturbances such as high-velocity jets and poststenotic turbulence are noted. Although the color-flow image may also be helpful for identifying flow disturbances, some high-velocity jets may not be apparent on the color-flow image because the colors are based on a mean Doppler frequency estimate rather than the peak systolic frequency.

The color-flow image has been particularly useful for identifying unusual anatomic features such as tortuosity and kinking, which can be difficult to recognize with conventional duplex scanning techniques. Color-flow imaging is also valuable for documenting internal carotid occlusion. With conventional duplex scanning, internal carotid occlusion is indicated by the absence of a pulsed Doppler flow signal in the imaged vessel, decreased diastolic flow velocity in the ipsilateral common carotid artery, and the presence of flow in the external carotid artery. In this situation the flow pattern in the common carotid artery on the side of occlusion resembles that found in the external carotid. The site of occlusion in the proximal internal carotid can often be visualized on the color-flow image. When there is unilateral internal carotid occlusion, flow velocities in the contralateral carotid bifurcation may be increased because of collateral flow and may result in overestimation of stenosis severity in the patent internal carotid artery.

Some variability is unavoidable with any diagnostic test. In carotid duplex scanning, the greatest variability has been noted for normal, minimal, and moderate stenosis (A, B, and C lesions in Table 1). Agreement is much better for classification of lesions that reduce arterial diameter by more than 50%. Similarly, interpretation of carotid arteriograms is subject to the most variability when the arteries are normal or minimally diseased.

CLINICAL APPLICATIONS

Although advances in technology have expanded the capabilities of duplex scanning to include detection of vascular disease in the abdomen and extremities, the identification of extracranial carotid artery disease continues to be one of the most frequent clinical applications. The main goal in the noninvasive carotid evaluation is to identify patients who are at risk for stroke. Once this is accomplished, decisions can be made regarding the need for arteriography and the potential benefits of carotid endarterectomy. The major indications for carotid duplex scanning are (1) an asymptomatic carotid bruit, (2) hemispheric cerebral or ocular transient ischemic attacks, (3) prior stroke with good neurologic recovery, (4) screening prior to major cardiac or peripheral vascular surgery, and (5) follow-up after carotid endarterectomy.

The finding of a bruit in the neck is one of the most common indications for a duplex scan of the carotid arteries. Among 100 patients with 165 asymptomatic bruits, duplex scanning showed a normal internal carotid in 12 (7%), less than 50% diameter stenosis in 83 (50%), a 50% or greater stenosis in 61 (37%), and internal carotid occlusion in 9 (6%).[5] Thus, although most neck bruits are associated with some disease of the carotid artery, only about one-third are related to severe internal carotid stenoses.

Therapeutic decisions for patients with asymptomatic carotid disease must take into account not only the severity of stenosis but also the natural history of the lesion. In a serial follow-up study of 167 patients with asymptomatic neck bruits, duplex scanning showed progression of disease in 60% of the internal carotid arteries.[8] The mean annual rate for development of ipsilateral neurologic symptoms (transient ischemic attack or stroke) was 4%. There was a strong correlation between the presence of an 80% to 99% internal carotid stenosis and the occurrence of neurologic symptoms or internal carotid occlusion. Patients with lesions of this severity had a 46% incidence of one or more of these events, and those with less severe stenoses had only a 1.5% incidence. Thus, duplex scanning can be used as a screening test to identify patients with especially severe carotid stenoses who are at increased risk for neurologic events.

The purpose of carotid screening in patients with hemispheric neurologic symptoms is to identify lesions that could reduce hemispheric blood flow or be the source of cerebral emboli. In the North American Symptomatic Carotid Endarterectomy Trial (NASCET), carotid endarterectomy was highly beneficial for patients with recent hemispheric transient ischemic attacks or mild strokes and 70% to 99% stenosis of the ipsilateral internal carotid artery. These results indicate that symptomatic patients with severe carotid stenoses should be treated by endarterectomy unless their general medical condition makes the risk of operation prohibitive. Although the specific NASCET guidelines for carotid endarterectomy in symptomatic patients require a 70% to 99% stenosis by arteriography, many stenoses in the 50% to 79% category and virtually all the stenoses in the 80% to 99% category by duplex scanning will fall into this group. Thus, the duplex scan finding of a 50% to 99% carotid stenosis in a symptomatic patient should be considered an indication for further evaluation. To be more consistent with the NASCET guidelines, a proposed modification of the duplex criteria is based on the ratio of the peak systolic velocities in the internal and common carotid arteries (ICA-CCA ratio). An ICA-CCA ratio of 4 or greater is consistent with a 70% to 99% diameter carotid stenosis.[9] Occasionally a duplex scan shows a normal or minimally diseased internal carotid artery in a patient with neurologic symptoms. Follow-up of these patients generally supports a nonoperative approach, since the incidence of subsequent neurologic events is extremely low and a noncarotid cause for symptoms may exist.

It has been difficult to define the role of screening for carotid artery disease prior to cardiac or other major surgical procedures. Such studies have not shown a consistent relationship between perioperative neurologic events and the presence asymptomatic carotid stenoses.[5] Therefore, routine carotid endarterectomy for prevention of perioperative stroke is difficult to justify. However, as noted previously, severe asymptomatic internal carotid stenoses are associated with an increased risk of neurologic symptoms and carotid occlusion. If endarterectomy is indicated for asymptomatic carotid stenosis, this may take precedence over other elective surgical procedures.

Since duplex scanning can be repeated at relatively frequent intervals, it is ideal for follow-up testing after carotid endarterectomy to document the incidence and clinical significance of recurrent carotid stenosis. Although symptomatic recurrent stenosis occurs in only about 5% of patients, when asymptomatic lesions are included, the incidence is in the range of 9% to 21%.[10] Serial duplex scanning also indicates that recurrent lesions tend to occur during the first 2 years after operation, are smoothly tapered, and may regress over time. Recurrent lesions that persist usually remain stable, and progression to internal carotid occlusion is uncommon. Since the incidence of neurologic symptoms does not appear to be significantly different in patients with and without recurrent carotid stenosis, a conservative approach to asymptomatic recurrent stenosis is justified.

Although standard contrast arteriography is still generally considered to be the definitive diagnostic test for carotid artery disease, there has been increasing interest in performing carotid endarterectomy based on the clinical evaluation and duplex scan findings alone. This trend has been stimulated by improvements in the accuracy and reliability of carotid duplex scanning, along with increasing demands to minimize both the costs and risks of medical care. Carotid endarterectomy may be indicated for high-grade stenoses in asymptomatic patients and moderate to severe stenoses in patients with hemispheric neurologic symptoms. These categories of lesions can be accurately detected by duplex scanning. While duplex scanning does not provide any direct information on lesions involving the proximal aortic arch branches or the intracranial circulation, significant lesions proximal or distal to the carotid bifurcation are uncommon and rarely have an adverse effect on the outcome of carotid endarterectomy. In addition, most stenoses in the proximal brachiocephalic vessels can be diagnosed on the basis of common carotid flow abnormalities or unequal arm blood pressures.

While the specific indications for carotid reconstruction without arteriography remain controversial, the results of arteriography rarely alter the clinical treatment plan when a technically adequate duplex scan shows an 80% to 99% stenosis in an asymptomatic patient or an ipsilateral 50% to 99% stenosis in a patient with hemispheric neurologic symptoms.[11] Arteriography is most likely to be useful when the duplex scan is nondiagnostic, for atypical lesions that appear to extend beyond the carotid bifurcation, and for less than 50% internal carotid stenoses in patients with neurologic symptoms. It is inevitable that the tendency to perform carotid endarterectomy without contrast arteriography will increase with further improvements in duplex scanning technology.

REFERENCES

1. Fisher CM. Occlusion of the internal carotid artery. Arch Neurol Psychiat 1951; 65:346-377.
2. Hass WK, Fields WS, North RR, et al. Joint study of extracranial arterial occlusion II: Arteriography, techniques, sites, and complications. JAMA 1968; 203:961-968.
3. Strandness DE Jr. Duplex scanning in vascular disorders. New York: Raven Press, 1990:1.
4. Reilly LM. Importance of carotid plaque morphology. In: Bernstein EF, ed. Vascular diagnosis, 4th ed. St. Louis: Mosby–Year Book, 1993:333.
5. Zierler RE. Carotid artery evaluation by duplex scanning. Semin Vasc Surg 1988; 1:9-16.
6. Zierler RE, Phillips DJ, Beach KW, et al. Noninvasive assessment of normal carotid bifurcation hemodynamics with color-flow ultrasound imaging. Ultrasound Med Biol 1987; 13:471-476.
7. Ku DN, Phillips DJ, Giddens DP, et al. Hemodynamics of the normal human carotid bifurcation: In vitro and in vivo studies. Ultrasound Med Biol 1985; 11:13-26.
8. Roederer GO, Langlois YE, Jager K, et al. The natural history of

carotid arterial disease in asymptomatic patients with cervical bruits. Stroke 1984; 15:605-613.
9. Moneta GL, Edwards JM, Chitwood RW, et al. Correlation of North American Symptomatic Carotid Endarterectomy Trial (NASCET) angiographic definition of 70 percent to 99 percent internal carotid artery stenosis with duplex scanning. J Vasc Surg 1993; 17:152-159.
10. Healy DA, Zierler RE, Nicholls SC, et al. Long-term follow-up and clinical outcome of carotid restenosis. J Vasc Surg 1989; 10: 662-669.
11. Dawson DL, Zierler RE, Strandness DE, Jr, et al. The role of duplex scanning and arteriograpy before carotid endarterectomy: A prospective study. J Vasc Surg 1993; 18:673-683.

ANGIOGRAPHIC EVALUATION OF THE CAROTID ARTERY

WILLIAM K. EHRENFELD, M.D.
STEPHEN P. MURRAY, M.D.
CHRISTOPHER F. DOWD, M.D.

Catheter-based intra-arterial digital subtraction angiography (IADSA) is the procedure of choice of the Division of Vascular Surgery at the University of California at San Francisco for patients selected for diagnosis and treatment of carotid artery disease. We have a long-standing interest in the importance of angiographic evaluation in the diagnosis and management of patients with extracranial cerebrovascular disease.[1] The extent of the individual arteriographic procedure varies within our group. Some request only selective injection of the carotid artery bifurcations; others request traditional arch and complete four vessel studies, including intracranial views with variations often dependent upon the patient's clinical presentation.

The evolution of safer and better invasive contrast studies began with direct arterial punctures, and progressed to catheter-based conventional cut film examinations and then to IADSA. Like many others, we had a short-lived but enthusiastic experience with intravenous digital subtraction angiography (IVDSA).[2] This experience a decade ago was reviewed retrospectively and prospectively, and we concluded that IADSA was our preferred method of study. Since then it has completely supplanted all other invasive techniques.

Increasingly in recent years many excellent centers have supplanted invasive carotid angiography with noninvasive duplex scanning as the sole study before carotid endarterectomy. A well-conceived detailed prospective study[3] supports duplex scanning before carotid endarterectomy in a large majority of patients. However, others have presented conflicting evidence and views that make this subject controversial.[4,5]

TECHNIQUES OF ANGIOGRAPHY

The angiographer should be familiar with pertinent history, both from the referring physician and from the patient, to document the necessity of the angiogram, to tailor the examination to the suspected pathology, and to elicit any history of contrast medium allergy. All of this is predicated upon an approach that includes open and free communication between the vascular surgeon and the neuroradiologist. Review of all prior radiographs, including computed tomography, magnetic resonance angiography, magnetic resonance imaging, duplex sonograms, and angiograms, is crucial to planning a proper examination. Evaluation and possibly treatment of any allergy are important. When a contrast medium allergy is ascertained, nearly all patients can be studied under drug coverage. This calls for experience and restraint as to selection of the most appropriate contrast agent and the amount of contrast necessary. Nephrotoxicity is less of a problem with the use of nonionic contrast agents.

IADSA is usually performed by way of a femoral artery puncture. Brachial, axillary, and direct carotid arterial approaches are possible when significant aortoiliac atherosclerotic disease precludes a safe transfemoral approach. The benefits of the transfemoral route include the ability to reach several carotid or vertebral arteries from the same puncture, superior control for hemostasis at the puncture site, and fewer complications, which may include hematoma, dissection, occlusion, and false aneurysm formation, than at other sites.

After proper preangiographic evaluation, the patient is placed supine on the fluoroscopy table. A puncture needle is positioned over the artery and advanced until a return of pulsatile blood occurs. A soft-tipped guide wire is run through the puncture needle into the artery, and the needle is removed. The angiography catheter is directed over the guide wire into the artery, and this guide wire–catheter combination is advanced under fluoroscopic guidance in a retrograde manner through the abdominal aorta to the aortic arch.

If disease of the proximal great vessels is suspected, an arch aortogram can be obtained. This is best done in the left anterior oblique position to visualize the origins of the great vessels optimally. Many types of catheters are used to study the common carotid bifurcations. However, in a patient population in which there may be significant bifurcation atherosclerotic disease, it is wise to choose a catheter–guide wire combination that does not require crossing the bifurcation for the angiographic study; a variety of catheters are excellent for this. This particular catheter must be reformed in the aortic arch and then positioned under fluoroscopic guidance in the common carotid artery. Flow is checked to ensure proper catheter position and avoidance of dissection. Angiographic runs are made in multiple projections using 5 to 8 ml of contrast over 1 second duration. Several projections are necessary to visualize the bifurcation in profile and enface. The appearance of the carotid siphon can easily be studied with the same injection. Additional information obtained from intracranial views includes evidence of branch occlusions from emboli and possible collateral circulation, including visualization of anterior communicating, posterior communicating, and leptomeningeal collateral arteries.

The catheter is next repositioned into the contralateral common carotid artery for a similar study. The subclavian and vertebral arteries can be studied in like fashion. This may require changes in the catheter–guide wire combination.

At the conclusion of the study the catheter is removed and hemostasis is achieved by manual compression of the femoral artery puncture site. Compression must be maintained for 15 minutes, and the patient is immobilized for the next 6 hours with the lower extremity extended, to avoid hemorrhage from the puncture site. After the procedure neurologic examination is performed along with evaluation of the peripheral pulses.

The most severe complication of carotid angiography is stroke. Risk factors include age, extensive atherosclerosis, experience of the angiographer, duration of catheterization, and the number of catheter exchanges. In an early study the overall risks at our medical center for a neurological event was 0.6% for a permanent neurological deficit and less than 0.1% for death.[6] These complication rates have remained virtually unchanged since that report. Other complications include arterial dissection, disruption, and embolization by catheter manipulation.

With the advent of digital subtraction angiography, the procedures are shorter and several views of a single vessel may be obtained rapidly. At one time the spatial resolution for digital subtraction techniques was suboptimal, but advances in technology have permitted resolution that approaches that of cut-film angiography. The digital subtraction technique consists of substituting an image intensifier for the angiographic film. This image intensifier digitally records the locations of the striking x-ray beams, and a computerized digital image of the angiogram is created.

A shortcoming of IADSA is loss of a clear relationship between the carotid bifurcation and the angle of the mandible. The subtraction method often renders bony areas ill defined or not defined. Thus, the opportunity of easily locating the most advantageous position for placement of the skin incision relative to the level of the carotid bifurcation may be lost. This is even more significant if shunts are selected during carotid cross-clamping. Another shortcoming is the relative loss of definition of surface changes such as ulceration, of intimal changes such as those associated with neointimal hyperplasia, and of the fibrous bands associated with fibromuscular dysplasia, which are best seen by conventional angiography. Angiography does not allow assessment of whether a lesion is homogeneous or heterogeneous. Fresh thrombus may be less readily identified and whether intraplaque hemorrhage is present, is rarely clear.

DUPLEX SCANNING

In the past decade there has been increasing interest in and support for duplex scanning instead of angiography in the treatment of carotid artery disease.[3,4,7,8] To varying degrees the advocates of this approach acknowledge that patients with symptomatic extracranial lesions other than those at the carotid bifurcation will not be identified by scanning techniques. Most proponents of this position purport that with proper history and physical examination these patients will be recognized and angiography will be selectively and appropriately used.[9] A recent report by Dawson and collegues[3] concluded that clinical assessment and duplex scanning were sufficiently accurate in 93% of the patients to undergo carotid endarterectomy. In an earlier study from another institution approximately two-thirds of carotid artery operations were performed with duplex scanning alone.[8] In the 1991 North American Symptomatic Carotid Endarterectomy Trial (NASCET), collaborators recommended that duplex scanning alone before operation should not be considered.[4] A strong rebuttal of these findings was recently presented by Strandness,[10] who disputes NASCET's data.

Proponents of duplex scanning come from centers of excellence in this technique. The overwhelming majority of like-minded proponents have laboratories that are known for their vast experience, technical excellence, and proven abilities to perform and correctly analyze the data. It is our belief as well as that of the proponents of duplex scanning that before any institution chooses this methodology, it is incumbent upon them to prove that their laboratory can achieve a high level of excellence. We believe that before proceeding with this approach, those who elect to use scanning instead of angiography have the responsibility to perform a prospective study of at least 100 of their own patients. Only when their data conclusively show that the sensitivity and specificity levels approach those of the published data can there be justification for a shift of the gold standard from routine IADSA to duplex scanning alone. Despite our long-standing interest and experience with both modalities, we do not yet have conclusive data to shift from our present position.

REFERENCES

1. Wylie EJ, Ehrenfeld WK. Extracranial occlusive cerebrovascular disease: Diagnosis and management. Philadelphia: WB Saunders, 1970.

2. Reilly LM, Ehrenfeld WK, Stoney RJ. Carotid digital subtraction angiography: The comparative roles of intra-arterial and intravenous imaging. Surgery 1984; 95:909–917.
3. Dawson DL, Zierler RE, Strandness DE Jr, et al. The role of duplex scanning and arteriography before carotid endarterectomy: A prospective study. J Vasc Surg 1993; 18:678–683.
4. North American Symptomatic Carotid Endarterectomy Trial Collaborators. Beneficial effect of carotid endarterectomy in symptomatic patients with high-grade carotid stenosis. N Engl J Med 1991; 325:445–463.
5. Haynes B, Thorpe W, Taylor W, et al. Poor performance of ultrasound in detecting high-grade carotid stenosis. Can J Surg 1992; 35:446 (abstract).
6. Mani R, Eisenberg RL, McDonald EJ Jr, et al. Complications of catheter cerebral angiography: Analysis of 5,000 procedures 1: Criteria and incidence. Am J Roentgenol 1978; 131:861–865.
7. Sandmann W, Hennerici M, Nullen H, et al. Carotid artery surgery without angiography: Risk or progress. In: Greenhalgh RM, Rose FC, eds. Progress in Stroke Research II. London: Pitman, 1983:447.
8. Ahn SS, Baker JD, Moore WS. Carotid endarterectomy based on duplex scanning without routine arteriography. Perspect Vasc Surg 1991; 4(1):109–118.
9. Moore WS, Ziomek S, Quinones-Baldrich WJ, et al: Can clinical evaluation and noninvasive testing substitute for arteriography in the evaluation of carotid artery disease? Ann Surg 1988; 208: 91–94.
10. Strandness DE Jr. Carotid endarterectomy: Current status and effects of clinical trials. Cardiovasc Surg 1993; 1:311–316.

TRANSCRANIAL DOPPLER EVALUATION OF CEREBROVASCULAR DISEASE

MARC I. CHIMOWITZ M.B., CH.B.

In 1982, Aaslid, Markwalder, and Nornes[1] described a noninvasive technique using transcranial Doppler ultrasound (TCD) to measure blood flow velocity in distinct cerebral arteries at the base of the brain. Subsequently TCD has become a widely used diagnostic technique for evaluating patients with a variety of cerebrovascular diseases, raised intracranial pressure, and brain death.[2] TCD is particularly useful for evaluating patients with extracranial and intracranial occlusive disease and certain other cerebrovascular disorders such as emboli, vasospasm after subarachnoid hemorrhage, and arteriovenous malformations.

TECHNIQUE AND PRINCIPLES OF SIGNAL INTERPRETATION

Whereas carotid ultrasound imaging uses continuous-wave Doppler ultrasound at a frequency of 5mHz, TCD uses pulsed-wave Doppler ultrasound at 2mHz, which can penetrate bone. The focal length of ultrasound emitted by the TCD transducer can be varied to enable insonation of vessels at different depths. The TCD transducer emits ultrasound that penetrates the temporal bone and is focused on the vessel of interest. The ultrasound is reflected to the transducer by blood flowing in the vessel. The frequency of the reflected ultrasound is shifted in direct proportion to blood flow velocity. Fourier transformation of the Doppler signal enables spectral display of the signal and measurement of systolic, diastolic, and mean blood flow velocities as well as the pulsatility index (systolic velocity minus diastolic velocity divided by mean velocity).

Choosing the appropriate skull window and varying the angle of insonation on the skull and the focal length of the ultrasound beam allows individual cerebral arteries to be identified using TCD. The internal carotid artery (ICA), middle cerebral artery (MCA), anterior cerebral artery (ACA), and posterior cerebral artery (PCA) signals can be obtained through the temporal window, and the vertebral artery and basilar artery signals can be obtained suboccipitally through the foramen magnum. Additionally, the ophthalmic artery and carotid siphon signals can be obtained through the transorbital window. In approximately 5% to 10% of patients, the ICA, MCA, ACA, and PCA signals cannot be obtained because of poor ultrasound penetration of the temporal bone.

Accurate diagnosis of intracranial vascular lesions using TCD requires a thorough analysis of the Doppler signals obtained from all the major cerebral arteries. Special attention is paid to (1) the direction of flow in the arteries, (2) characteristics of the velocity waveform such as the presence of spectral broadening or symmetrical low-frequencies suggesting stenosis, (3) comparison of blood flow velocities in each artery with normal values, (4) side-to-side comparison of blood flow velocities in the major cerebral arteries, (5) the ratios of blood flow velocities in the major ipsilateral cerebral arteries, and (6) the pulsatility index of each cerebral artery. Knowledge about the clinical presentation and the presence of extracranial carotid artery or vertebral artery disease is also essential for accurate interpretation of the intracranial Doppler signals.

The following example illustrates the diagnostic process using TCD. A 65-year-old diabetic man had several episodes of right-hand weakness, each lasting 1 to 3 minutes. Carotid ultrasound showed mild intimal thickening of both extracranial internal carotid arteries. This patient had frequent stereotypical spells involving right-hand weakness, suggesting episodic ischemia in the territory supplied by the left MCA artery. Diagnostic

Table 1 Transcranial Doppler Ultrasound Readings in a Patient with Episodes of Right Hand Weakness

Artery	Mean Blood Flow Velocity (cm/sec)		
	R	L	Normal
MCA	60	40*	50–75
ACA	65	45†	39–63
Carotid siphon	70	120	40–70

MCA, middle cerebral artery; ACA, anterior cerebral artery.
*Signal had low pulsatility; i.e., systolic velocity = 46 cm/sec; diastolic velocity = 37 cm/sec.
†Direction of flow is reversed.

possibilities included a stenotic lesion of the left extracranial carotid artery, left carotid siphon, and left MCA. Carotid ultrasound ruled out extracranial stenosis. TCD documented extremely high velocity in the left carotid siphon suggesting high-grade stenosis of this vessel (Table 1). The hemodynamic significance of the left carotid siphon lesion was evidenced by reversal of flow in the left ACA, indicating collateral flow from the right ACA through the anterior communicating artery. Ordinarily, the MCA velocity exceeds the ACA velocity but in this case the right ACA velocity exceeded the right MCA velocity because the right ACA was providing collateral flow to the left hemisphere. The low mean blood flow velocity and pulsatility of the left MCA was due to the proximal high-grade carotid siphon stenosis. Another factor that may have contributed to the low pulsatility of the left MCA was distal arteriolar vasodilation, an autoregulatory compensatory mechanism to maintain cerebral blood flow when perfusion pressure is reduced. Arteriolar vasodilatation results in a low-resistance vascular bed, higher diastolic flow velocity, and lower pulsatility.

EVALUATION OF EXTRACRANIAL CAROTID OCCLUSIVE DISEASE

TCD may serve many useful roles in the evaluation and management of patients with extracranial carotid occlusive disease. TCD is most commonly used in this setting to provide information on collateral blood flow to the brain distal to the extracranial carotid stenosis. Other clinical roles for TCD include detection of emboli in the MCA that originate in the extracranial carotid artery, determination of cerebral perfusion reserve distal to the carotid lesion, and monitoring of ipsilateral MCA blood flow velocity during carotid endarterectomy.

Collateral Cerebral Blood Flow and Carotid Stenosis

Since TCD can determine direction of flow in the major cerebral arteries and ophthalmic artery, it is a useful technique for establishing collateral flow patterns in patients with extracranial carotid occlusive disease. Collateral flow from the contralateral ACA through the anterior communicating artery is detected by finding reversed flow in the ACA ipsilateral to the carotid stenosis and high velocities in the contralateral ACA. Collateral flow from the external carotid artery–ophthalmic artery system to the supraclinoid carotid artery is recognized by reversal of flow in the ophthalmic artery. Detection of flow through the posterior communicating artery from the PCA to the supraclinoid carotid artery is also possible but technically more difficult. This pattern of collateral flow can often be inferred if markedly elevated blood flow velocities are detected in the ipsilateral PCA and vertebrobasilar circulation.

Cerebral angiography to determine the extent of carotid disease, the presence of severe coexistent intracranial disease, and collateral patterns of blood flow is performed in virtually all patients undergoing carotid endarterectomy. However, since the combination of carotid ultrasound and TCD enables these data to be documented reliably, it is possible that these safe, less expensive, nonivasive procedures will ultimately replace cerebral angiography as the method of choice for preoperative evaluation of patients with carotid stenosis.

Detection of Emboli from Extracranial Carotid Disease

Doppler ultrasound is a very sensitive technique for detecting emboli in the carotid or MCA. Recent studies have documented that in patients with atrial fibrillation or a prosthetic heart valve, spontaneous asymptomatic emboli to the MCA from the heart or from the internal carotid artery are common.[3] Simultaneous ultrasound monitoring of the carotid artery and MCA offers the potential for localizing the source of emboli to the carotid artery or to the heart. The ability to identify the extracranial carotid artery as a source of microemboli may help clarify the need for carotid endarterectomy in some patients; for example, symptomatic patients with only moderate carotid stenoses and patients with complex ulcers. Additionally, simultaneous carotid and TCD imaging may permit monitoring of the effects of surgical or medical therapy on the frequency of distal emboli.

Evaluation of Cerebral Perfusion Reserve in Patients with Carotid Disease

Studies using positron emission tomography have shown that some patients with carotid occlusive disease have high cerebral blood volume–cerebral blood flow ratios and high oxygen extraction fractions ipsilateral to the carotid lesion. These findings are consistent with maximal ipsilateral regional arteriolar vasodilation and collateral flow in response to diminished cerebral perfusion pressure; that is, a state of impaired ipsilateral cerebral perfusion reserve. Several investigators have used TCD to identify patients with carotid occlusive disease and impaired cerebral perfusion reserve by comparing side-to-side differences in MCA velocity

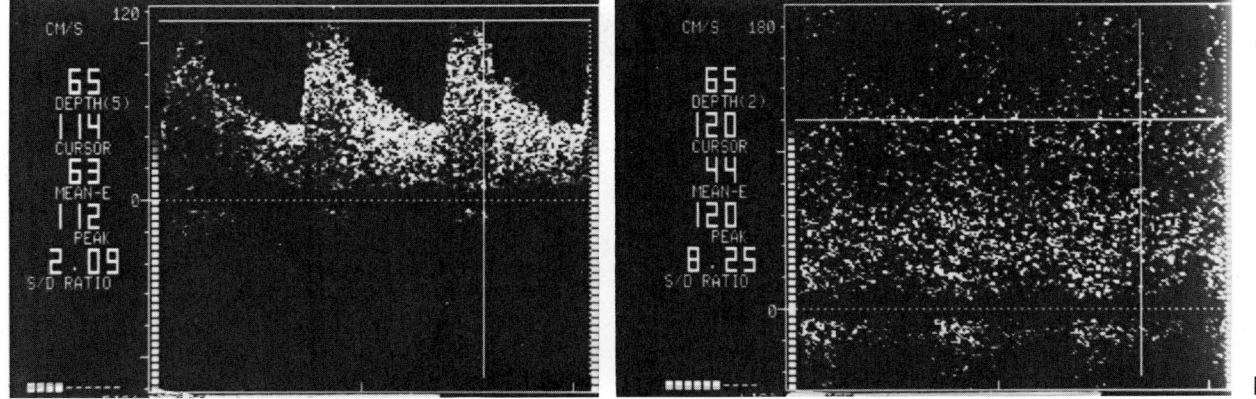

Figure 1 Patient with high-grade stenosis of the left intracranial carotid artery. A, Normal right intracranial carotid artery signal at a depth of 65 mm. The mean blood flow velocity is 71 cm/sec. B, Spectral broadening of the waveform of the left intracranial carotid artery at a depth of 65 mm. The mean blood flow velocity exceeds 140 cm/sec. These findings indicate a high-grade stenosis, confirmed at angiography.

before and after the application of a cerebral vasodilatory stimulus such as acetazolamide or hypercapnia. Patients with impaired perfusion reserve have little or no increase in MCA velocity distal to the diseased carotid artery and a marked increase in MCA velocity on the contralateral side. Moreover, a recent TCD study of patients with unilateral carotid occlusive disease documented that patients with impaired perfusion reserve had a significantly higher frequency of ipsilateral transient ischemic attack (TIA) than patients without impaired perfusion reserve.[4] This finding suggests that TCD may enable identification of a subgroup of patients with carotid occlusive disease who are at higher risk of stroke; however, this hypothesis must be tested in a large prospective study. It has been well established using TCD that cerebral perfusion reserve is usually restored in patients who have undergone carotid endarterectomy.

Monitoring of MCA Velocity During Carotid Endarterectomy

Neurovascular monitoring during carotid endarterectomy (CEA) is frequently used to help the surgeon decide on the need for a temporary intraluminal shunt after carotid cross-clamping. Monitoring techniques include measurement of carotid stump blood pressure, electroencephalography (EEG) recording, and use of local anesthesia so that the patient's level of consciousness, speech, and contralateral hand strength can be evaluated. More recently, TCD has also been used during CEA to detect diminished ipsilateral MCA velocity after carotid cross-clamping and to detect emboli throughout the procedure.

Most emboli are detected after release of the carotid clamp following endarterectomy, but a few are also detected during manipulation of the artery before clamping, during the introduction of a shunt, and after introduction of a needle to measure carotid stump blood pressure. Most of these emboli have no clinical significance. In one recent study of 123 patients undergoing endarterectomy, 75 episodes of embolization were detected in 55 patients (45%). Only one of these patients had a clinical deficit.[5]

Several studies have documented that TCD measurements of MCA blood flow velocity after carotid clamping correlate directly with carotid stump blood pressure and are higher when major collaterals are functional. Most studies, however, have not shown a predictable relationship between low MCA blood flow velocity during cross clamping and increased stroke risk. One retrospective study of 1,495 CEAs monitored with TCD showed that severe ischemia occurred in 7.2% of patients after carotid cross-clamping, but in half of these the ischemia cleared spontaneously. In instances of persisting ischemia the rate of severe stroke was very high unless shunting was performed. If ischemia did not occur after cross-clamping, the use of shunting was associated with an increased risk of stroke.[6] Large prospective studies are needed to clarify whether TCD monitoring during carotid endarterectomy will enable the surgeon to lower the risk of intraoperative stroke by adjusting the surgical technique.

EVALUATION OF INTRACRANIAL OCCLUSIVE DISEASE

TCD is commonly used to detect stenoses or occlusions of major intracranial arteries in patients with TIA or stroke. Focal stenosis of an intracranial artery is diagnosed if one of the following findings are detected at a circumscribed insonation depth: (1) mean blood flow velocity at least 85 cm/sec with dampened flow velocities more distally, (2) spectral broadening of the velocity waveform indicating turbulent flow, (3) symmetric systolic low frequencies indicating arterial wall vibrations (Fig. 1). In my experience these findings are detected only if there is at least 50% narrowing of the arterial

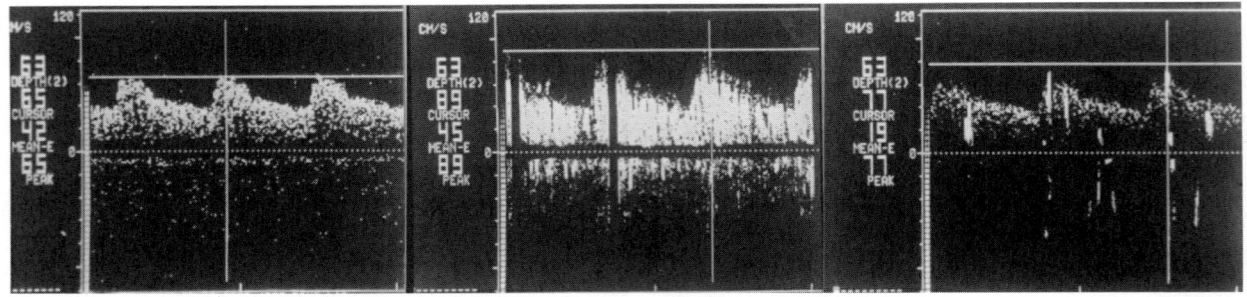

Figure 2 Air microemboli detected in the middle cerebral artery after intravenous injection of bubble contrast in a patient with multiple pulmonary arteriovenous fistulae. *A,* Normal middle cerebral artery signal before contrast injection. *B,* Multiple air microemboli initially detected in the middle cerebral artery after contrast injection. *C,* Thirty to 60 seconds later, individual air emboli detected in the middle cerebral artery. (From Chimowitz MI, Nemec J, Marwick T, et al. Transcranial Doppler ultrasound identifies patients with right to left cardiac or pulmonary shunts. Neurology 1991; 41:1902–1904; with permission.)

diameter. TCD is insensitive at detecting low-grade intracranial stenoses, nor can it detect a stenosis of a distal branch of a major intracranial artery.

Occlusion of a major intracranial artery is diagnosed when a signal from that artery cannot be obtained but the signals of neighboring arteries can be recorded through the same bone window. Intracranial stenosis or occlusion is often suggested by collateral flow patterns. For example, MCA stenosis or occlusion is associated with high ipsilateral ACA or PCA velocities because these arteries provide collaterals to the MCA through distal leptomenigeal anastomoses.

Several TCD-angiographic correlative studies have been performed in patients with intracranial occlusive disease. These studies indicate that the sensitivity of TCD for detecting high-grade stenosis or occlusion of the carotid siphon or MCA occlusive lesions is 80% to 90%, and the specificity is 95% to 98%.[7] TCD is less reliable for detecting occlusive lesions in the vertebrobasilar circulation (sensitivity 75%, specificity 97%), especially in the distal basilar region. These data suggest that TCD may not be sensitive enough to stand alone as a screening test for intracranial occlusive disease. Recent studies have shown that the combination of TCD and magnetic resonance arteriography are highly reliable for diagnosis of intracranial occlusive disease. TCD has also been established as a reliable method for documenting a subclavian steal.

DETECTION OF CEREBRAL EMBOLI

In 1969 Spencer and associates[8] showed that Doppler ultrasound could detect gas bubbles in the blood stream of divers with decompression sickness. This discovery raised the possibility that Doppler ultrasound could be used to detect emboli. In recent years several studies have shown that TCD is a highly sensitive technique for detecting emboli to the MCA. Emboli as small as 100 microns in diameter are recognized by high-amplitude spikes in the Doppler signal (Fig. 2) that are associated with a characteristic auditory chirp.

Numerous spontaneous emboli to the MCA have been detected in patients with artificial heart valves, atrial fibrillation, or carotid stenosis. Multiple emboli have also been detected during operative procedures such as coronary artery bypass and carotid endarterectomy. TCD has also been used to diagnose right-to-left cardiac or pulmonary shunts by detecting air microemboli in the MCA after intravenous injection of bubble contrast.[9] Recent experimental work suggests that TCD may be able to differentiate between embolic materials such as thrombus, platelet-rich aggregates, atheromatous material, and fat.[10] The ability to distinguish between types of embolic material may enable physicians to choose therapy according to the type of emboli detected (e.g., anticoagulation for thrombus emboli, antiplatelet agents for platelet emboli).

OTHER CLINICAL APPLICATIONS

One of the most common clinical applications of TCD is the detection of intracranial vasospasm after subarachnoid hemorrhage. Vasospasm usually involves several vessels and is diagnosed by TCD if mean blood flow velocities exceed 120 cm/sec in long segments of multiple arteries. A fixed intracranial stenosis from atherosclerosis may also be associated with a mean blood flow velocity exceeding 120 cm/sec. However, the abnormal signal in this setting is detected at a circumscribed depth of a single vessel. Recent TCD-angiographic correlative studies have shown that the specificity of TCD for detecting vasospasm approaches 100% with sensitivity of 60% to 85%.[2]

TCD is also useful for evaluating patients with intracranial arteriovenous malformations (AVMs). Arteries feeding an AVM can be identified by markedly elevated high blood flow velocities and very low pulsatility.[2] The effects of surgical or embolic therapy for AVMs can be monitored by assessing blood flow velocities and pulsatility of the feeding arteries. Successful therapy usually results in near normalization of these parameters. Recently TCD has also been used for documenting intracranial circulatory arrest in patients who fulfill the clinical criteria of brain death.[2]

Transcranial color-coded real-time ultrasonography is an exciting new development that enables rapid visual identification of the major cerebral arteries as well as identification of central nervous system parenchymal lesions, such as hemorrhages, tumors, and hydrocephalus.

REFERENCES

1. Aaslid R, Markwalder T-M, Nornes H. Noninvasive transcranial Doppler ultrasound recording of flow velocity in basal cerebral arteries. J Neurosurg 1982; 57:769–774.
2. Caplan LR, Brass LM, De Witt LD, et al. Transcranial Doppler ultrasound: Present status. Neurology 1990; 40:696–700.
3. Berger MP, Tegeler CH. Embolus detection using Doppler ultrasonography. In: Babikian VL, Wechsler LR, eds. Transcranial Doppler ultrasonography. St. Louis: Mosby–Year Book, 1993, pp 232–241.
4. Chimowitz MI, Furlan AJ, Jones SC, et al. Transcranial Doppler assessment of cerebral perfusion reserve in patients with carotid occlusive disease and no evidence of cerebral infarction. Neurology 1993; 43:353–357.
5. Jansen C, Vriens EM, Eikelboom BC, et al. Carotid endarterectomy with transcranial Doppler and electroencephalographic monitoring: A prospective study in 130 operations. Stroke 1993; 24:665–669.
6. Halsey JH Jr for the International Transcranial Doppler Collaborators. Risks and benefits of shunting in carotid endarterectomy. Stroke 1992; 23:1583–1587.
7. Ley-Pozo J, Ringelstein EB. Noninvasive detection of occlusive disease of the carotid siphon and middle cerebral artery. Ann Neurol 1990; 28:640–647.
8. Spencer MP, Campbell SD, Sealey JL, et al. Experiments on decompression bubbles in the circulation using ultrasonic and electromagnetic flowmeters. J Occup Med 1969; 11:238–244.
9. Chimowitz MI, Nemec J, Marwick T, et al. Transcranial Doppler ultrasound identifies patients with right to left cardiac or pulmonary shunts. Neurology 1991; 41:1902–1904.
10. Markus HS, Brown MM. Differentiation between different pathological cerebral embolic materials using transcranial Doppler in an in vitro model. Stroke 1993; 24:1–5.

COMPUTED TOMOGRAPHY EVALUATION OF CEREBROVASCULAR DISEASE

RAMON BERGUER, M.D., Ph.D.

MONITORING OF BRAIN INFARCTION

Although computed tomographic (CT) scan may suggest cerebral infarction a few hours after the onset of symptoms, in general the low-density signal appears 1 to 3 days after the clinical event. Cortical infarctions are the easiest to detect. In contrast, some lesions are notoriously difficult to identify on a CT scan even after 3 days. These lesions are (1) small infarcts with little edema such as those that occur in the internal capsule and (2) small infarctions in the posterior fossa and brain stem, which are difficult to resolve because of interference created by the dense petrous bone.

It has been stated that modern CT scanners can pick up about 90% of the supratentorial infarcts within 24 hours.[1] Infratentorial infarction, on the other hand, is detected by CT scan in only 31% to 44% of patients.[2,3]

The hypodense area noticed in the CT scan at the site of a brain infarct represents both necrotic brain tissue and intracellular swelling. This hypodensity is patchy at the beginning, but the pattern becomes homogeneous and develops a sharp outline in 3 to 5 days. This is also when there is maximum necrosis within and edema around an infarction. In large infarcts, however, hypodensity and evidence of brain swelling will appear much earlier, often in the first few hours. The latter is suggested by obliteration of the cortical sulci, a decrease in the size of the ipsilateral ventricle, and a shift in the midline. Brain swelling usually resolves in about 2 to 3 weeks.

Contrast enhancement is seen in most infarctions 2 or 3 weeks after the clinical event. The likelihood of enhancement of an infarction increases with the amount of iodine contrast injected.[4] Contrast enhancement has been reported variably during the first week as not occurring[4] and as being present in 62% of patients.[5] Enhancement between weeks 2 and 4 is reported in 82% to 88% of patients.[5,6] Although the breakdown of the blood-brain barrier probably takes place within a few hours, contrast enhancement is not seen early because blood flow into the infarct and peri-infarct area is severely reduced; hence there is little capillary leakage. After 7 days, as edema begins to subside and collateral flow improves, the rate of transmural leakage is sufficient to enhance contrast. The infarcts most likely to enhance are the embolic ones; the lysis of the clot usually results in reperfusion of the infarct with a damaged blood-brain barrier. Infarcts that enhance in the 3 hour–delayed CT scan after high-dose contrast infusion have poor prognosis and are likely to progress to hemorrhagic infarction.[7] Enhancement declines after the third week, although it may persist up to 7 weeks.

The mechanisms of enhancement are (1) increased vascular permeability, (2) increased vascularity (neovascularization, collaterals), and (3) luxury perfusion. Most enhancement occurs because there is contrast in the extracellular space. The damaged blood-brain barrier allows the passage of large molecules such as contrast medium, which are normally unable to filter through the tight endothelial junctions of the vessels of the brain. Usually there is little enhancement in the first week because the number of collaterals and the anterograde circulation are limited; this results in a slow delivery of contrast to the peri-infarct area. The neovascular proliferation seen around an infarct for about 1 to 2 months results in enhancement because these newly formed vessels have an incompetent blood-brain barrier.

A good reason to obtain CT scans with and without contrast is the well-known fact that contrasting, by increasing density, may obliterate a hypodense infarction that was previously seen on a noncontrast scan. Conversely, in 90% of the patients who have had a stroke and have a normal noncontrast scan, the administration of contrast will result in enhancement, and therefore identification of a new infarct. There is no general agreement on the prognostic value of enhancement.[4,6]

In embolic infarction, as opposed to atherosclerotic thrombosis, lysis of the thrombus or its partial fragmentation results in hyperfusion of the infarcted area, which has lost its autoregulation and has a damaged blood-brain barrier. Leakage through this damaged blood-brain barrier and to a lesser extent the luxury perfusion,[8] result in prominent enhancement and petechial hemorrhages.[1]

Hemorrhagic infarction is generally the result of reperfusion of brain tissue previously damaged by ischemia. It is more common in embolic than in atherosclerotic infarction, presumably because lysis and fragmentation of the embolus result in reperfusion.[9] However, hemorrhagic infarction may develop after atherothrombotic ischemic infarction in patients with coagulation disorders and in those receiving heparin sodium or fibrinolytic therapy. Hemorrhages range from diffuse petechiae to frank hemorrhage[10] and usually involve the cortex or basal ganglia.

CORRELATION BETWEEN TRADITIONAL CLINICAL CATEGORIES OF CEREBROVASCULAR DISEASE AND BRAIN CT FINDINGS

Carotid Artery Disease

Disease of the carotid artery traditionally has been rated by its end-organ clinical manifestations. Indications for treatment are different for asymptomatic lesions, for those causing transient ischemic attacks (TIAs), and for those that have caused stroke. The routine use of brain CT scan in patients with carotid disease has shown that the correlation between clinical symptoms and the finding of the CT scan is often poor.[11] Patients who are asymptomatic may show areas of infarction in the brain in the territory supplied by the carotid artery. That their infarctions occurred in clinically silent areas does not detract from the fact that the presence of these infarcts proves the virulence or instability of the carotid plaque that is likely their cause.

Patients with TIAs are implicitly assumed to have had a compensated transient disturbance. About 26% of patients with a history of a hemispheric TIA who have normal neurologic examinations show an infarction by CT scan involving the territory where the TIA originated. Conversely, a third of patients who have had clinical strokes may not show an infarction on the CT scan. These patients usually have had small infarcts in either the internal capsule or brain stem that escape detection by CT scanning.

Routine CT scanning done 2 to 4 days after carotid endarterectomy will detect evidence of brain infarction six times as frequently as neurologic examination.[11] These neurologically silent infarcts are usually small but can nevertheless be attributed to the carotid operation. In other words, the CT scan of the brain is superior to clinical examination in monitoring the technical morbidity of carotid endarterectomy.

The appearance of a silent infarct in the territory of a severe but otherwise asymptomatic plaque is partly a random event. The microembolus causing the infarct was directed by the complex patterns of the flow stream to a silent area of the hemispheres. The next bout of embolization may end up in an area with obvious somatic representation and result in a clinical deficit. A carotid plaque causing a silent infarction is by definition asymptomatic but can be called "signomatic." Such a carotid lesion should be evaluated for surgical treatment with more circumspection than an asymptomatic plaque.

Given that CT scanning of the brain detects unsuspected lesions before and after carotid endarterectomy, studies on the natural history of the disease and on randomization of treatment should take this information into account. This will permit further refinement of indications for operation.

We advocate routine use of CT scanning in patients undergoing carotid endarterectomy. Some published studies[12] have documented retrospectively that a brain CT scan would not have made any difference in indications for operation. This does not hold true in our clinical practice. The presence of a silent infarction or of an unsuspected infarction in a patient with a history of TIA may change our threshold for operability. The finding of a meningioma or large intracranial aneurysm has occasionally modified my treatment strategy. I find it useful to know preoperatively if a patient who has TIA has in fact had either an infarction or a rare episode of cortical bleeding. The latter finding is likely to result in the postponement of the operation. For patients with an old history of stroke, assessment of the size of the infarction preoperatively may modify the strategy of brain protection during the operation.

Finally, in a patient with a recent stroke the CT scan with contrast may display a pattern of contrast enhancement associated with gross damage of the blood-brain barrier, and this has occasionally resulted in a delay in surgical treatment.

Posterior Circulation

In contraposition to what is seen in the carotid territory, CT scanning is of little use in the evaluation of patients with vertebrobasilar ischemia. Most of the small infarctions of the infratentorial brain and brain stem are missed by CT scan, although large cerebellar infarctions such as those following occlusion of the posterior-inferior cerebellar artery are usually seen. I advocate the routine use of MRI rather than CT scan in the evaluation of vertebrobasilar ischemia. Rarely, a patient with multiple sclerosis, often detectable by CT scanning, may have severe anatomic lesions of the vertebral artery and symptoms suggestive of vertebrobasilar ischemia.

REFERENCES

1. Inove Y, Takemota K, Miyamoto T, et al. Sequential computed tomography scans in acute cerebral infarction. Radiology 1980; 135:655–662.
2. Campbell JK, Houser O, Stevens JC, et al. Computed tomography and radionuclide imaging in the evaluation of ischemic stroke. Radiology 1978; 126:695–702.
3. Kingsley DPE, Wradue E, Duboulay EPGH. Evaluation of computed tomography in vascular lesions of the vertebrobasilar territory. J Neurol Neurosurg Psychiatr 1980; 43:193–197.
4. Weisberg LA. Computerized tomographic enhancement patterns in cerebral infarction. Arch Neurol 1980; 37:21.
5. Lee KF, Chambers RA, Diamond C, et al. Evaluation of cerebral infarction by computed tomography with special emphasis on microinfarction. Neuroradiology 1978; 16:156–158.
6. Pullicino P, Kendall BE. Contrast enhancement in ischaemic lesions I: Relationship to prognosis. Neuroradiology 1980; 19: 235–239.
7. Hayman LA, Evans RA, Bastion FO, et al. Delayed high dose contrast CT: Identifying patients at risk of massive hemorrhagic infarction. Am J Neuroradiol 1981; 2:139–147.
8. Kohlmeyer K, Graser C. Comparative studies of computed tomography and measurements of regional cerebral blood flow in stroke patients. Neuroradiology 1978; 16:233–237.
9. Irino T, Taneda M, Minami T. Angiographic manifestations in postrecanalized cerebral infarction. Neurology 1977b; 17:471–475.
10. Adams RD, Vander Eecken HM. Vascular diseases of brain. Ann Rev Med 1953; 4:213.
11. Berguer R, Sieggreen MY, Hodakowski GT, et al. The silent brain infarct in carotid surgery. J Vasc Surg 1986; 3:442–447.
12. Martin JD, Valentine RJ, Myers SI. Is routine CT scanning necessary in the preoperative evaluation of patients undergoing carotid endarterectomy? J Vasc Surg 1991; 14:267–270.

MAGNETIC RESONANCE IMAGING IN ASSESSMENT OF CEREBROVASCULAR DISEASE

MAGRUDER C. DONALDSON, M.D.

Magnetic resonance (MR) imaging, with rapidly evolving capabilities of producing exquisitely detailed images of intracranial structures and valuable information about vascular anatomy in one sitting, is a promising means of assessing cerebrovascular disease.[1]

Most clinically available MR imaging machines use two-dimensional time-of-flight technique to capture cross sections of anatomy at intervals as small as 1.5 mm. Data acquired in this manner are reconstructed by computer for display on a screen or translucent film. Complex vascular structures such as the carotid and vertebral arteries and the circle of Willis can be routinely demonstrated by this technology. Lesions can usually be detected in the siphon and other intracranial portions of the cerebrovascular tree, and intracranial aneurysms are precisely documented. Although not yet regularly available in most hospitals, three-dimensional reconstruction allows superior resolution of vascular structures.[2] Combined MR angiography and brain imaging provide correlation of vascular pathology with intracranial findings, a screen for occult strokes and mass lesions, and a preoperative baseline for possible later comparison.

Finally, MR imaging is safe, painless, and free of the small but measurable risks of angiography and contrast-enhanced computed tomography.

With technology now in common use, resolution is generally excellent for static structures, but with excessive turbulence the signal is distorted, producing irregularity or gaps in the image. Most dramatically, with flow perpendicular to the axis of acquisition, total signal loss may occur. Tortuosity, kinks, and loops may be completely obscured by turbulence. In the typical two-dimensional technique, this phenomenon accentuates the apparent degree of vascular stenosis, leading to overestimation of the disease's severity (Fig. 1). These limitations have so far limited application of MR imaging to simple qualitative assessment of vascular patency and rough quantitative estimation of moderate and severe stenoses by the length of the typical flow gap at the site of the lesion (Fig. 2). Diagnosis of internal carotid occlusion is usually possible by MR alone, although a small incidence of false positives and false negatives requires confirmation by a second modality. Despite intensive developmental efforts, precise documentation of plaque morphology and degree of stenosis is probably beyond the capabilities of MR imaging. In addition, the accession window usually excludes the aortic arch and proximal common carotid and vertebral arteries, possibly leaving disease undetected in these areas. While calcium has no deleterious effect, clips and other metallic objects will produce artifacts. MR imaging cannot be performed in the presence of pacemakers, nerve stimulators, cochlear implants, or ferromagnetic intracranial aneurysm clips. Motion by the patient

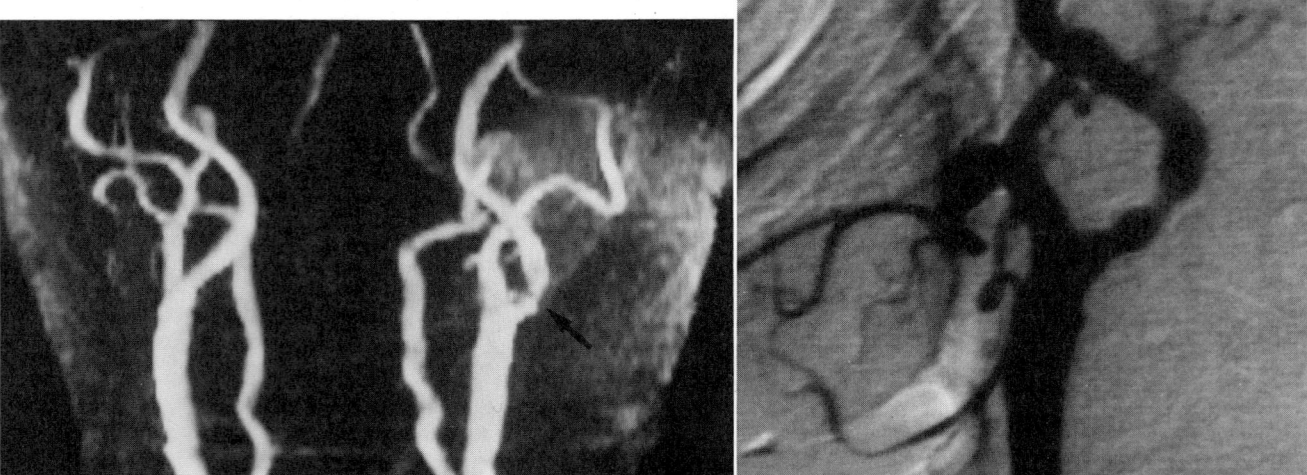

Figure 1 *A,* MR angiogram of left carotid bifurcation suggesting roughly 80% stenosis *(arrow)*. *B,* Contrast angiogram of artery demonstrating 60% stenosis.

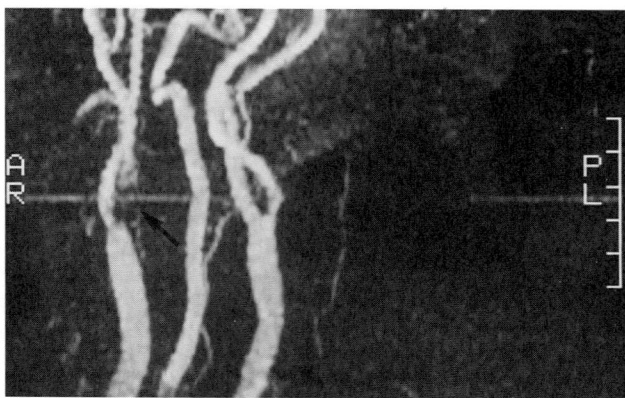

Figure 2 Typical flow gap *(arrow)* in MR image of proximal right internal carotid artery with 90% stenosis.

compromises clarity and resolution in 10% to 15% of studies, and 5% to 10% of patients are sufficiently claustrophobic that they cannot be adequately examined within the confines of the magnet. Finally, the logistics of safely scanning patients who are ventilator dependent or unstable are usually formidable.

Correlation of MR angiography with duplex ultrasound and contrast arteriography is reasonably good. When duplex and MR imaging agree, there is virtually 100% accuracy compared with arteriography,[3,4] including cases of internal carotid occlusion. However, because of the limitations mentioned, MR imaging does not often add to the accuracy of a technically satisfactory duplex ultrasound examination in evaluating the middle and distal common carotid, bifurcation, and proximal internal and external carotid arteries. Adequate evaluation of the proximal common carotid artery and aortic arch may require a second study session, and MR imaging provides insufficient anatomic detail to substitute for contrast arteriography when such detail is required.

Screening and preoperative evaluation for carotid endarterectomy should be conducted sequentially with a combination of modalities with the goal of keeping inconvenience, cost, and morbidity at a minimum without compromising diagnostic value. Although still in the process of validation, a suggested diagnostic algorithm is presented (Fig. 3). Since tandem lesions and intracranial aneurysms are rarely a concern, the diagnostic focus is upon the extracranial carotid artery. Once the noninvasive ultrasound laboratory has proven itself reliable in detecting extracranial disease and quantifying degrees of stenosis, patients with suspicious symptoms or physical findings are evaluated first with this modality. During the examination, the common carotid blood flow pattern is investigated for turbulence and abnormalities in inflow that may indirectly indicate a proximal common carotid lesion. Also, abnormalities around the carotid bulb suggesting unusual tortuosity or aneurysm and absent or equivocal internal carotid blood flow compatible with unusually distal disease or occlusion are noted. Interrogation of the vertebral arteries is performed if there is a suggestive pattern of symptoms or physical findings.

Information obtained by ultrasound is considered in light of the overall clinical picture. When ultrasound documents typical high-grade bifurcation disease with internal carotid stenosis greater than 75% in concert with a history of either no symptoms or classic ocular or cortical transient ischemic attack, no further carotid evaluation ordinarily must be pursued. When the ultrasound findings suggest unusual pathology such as proximal common carotid disease, tortuosity, aneurysm, or possible internal carotid occlusion, diagnostic confirmation by further imaging is indicated. In addition, ultrasound is occasionally frustrated by technical issues such as heavily calcified plaque obscuring the degree of stenosis. Further study is also necessary if there are atypical symptoms suggesting vertebrobasilar disease, subclavian steal, or a confusing pattern of ocular or

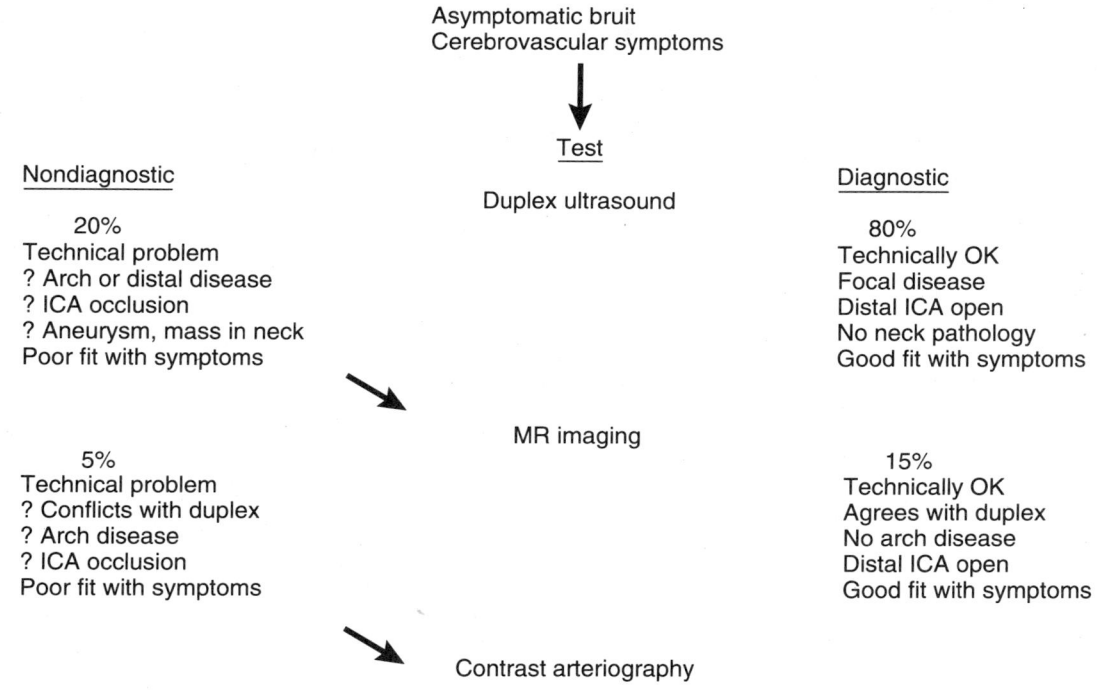

Figure 3 Diagnostic algorithm for extracranial carotid occlusive disease.

cortical transient attacks. In the presence of evolving or completed stroke, brain imaging is mandatory to establish the size and location of the intracranial lesion and the absence of hemorrhage. In other circumstances brain imaging may be useful to exclude silent stroke, tumor, and other intracranial pathology and to establish a preoperative baseline.

MR imaging is used next in the diagnostic sequence because the combination of brain scan and vascular mapping answers most of the issues unresolved by duplex. For example, the presence of intracranial mass lesions or stroke can be easily verified. When MR imaging and duplex ultrasound both detect internal carotid occlusion, the diagnostic accuracy is virtually 100% (Fig. 4).[3,4] A third modality is employed to confirm occlusion only when ultrasound and MR imaging disagree or when ongoing transient symptoms suggest persistence of a tiny, possibly operable arterial channel. The presence of extracranial aneurysm and carotid body tumor can be verified by MR, as can patency of the vertebral arteries. Although rough, findings consistent with tortuosity and extracranial or intracranial stenosis can confirm suspicions raised by ultrasound screening.

Arteriography is thus reserved for a small minority of patients in whom arch or proximal carotid artery disease is suspected, internal carotid artery occlusion remains unresolved after duplex ultrasound and MR imaging, or symptoms and extracranial vascular findings cannot be linked sufficiently strongly to clarify a possible therapeutic role for operation. Arteriography is generally used, for example, to clarify brachiocephalic anatomy in the presence of relatively nonspecific verte-

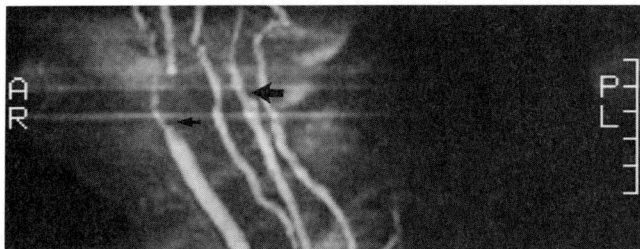

Figure 4 MR angiogram indicating occlusion of the left internal carotid artery *(large arrow)* and 95% stenosis of right internal carotid *(small arrow)*.

brobasilar symptoms or, possibly without preliminary MR imaging, to exclude ulceration or proximal or distal sources of emboli in a patient with a shallow bifurcation plaque and ongoing symptoms.

MR imaging fulfills an important role in clinical evaluation of patients suspected of having extracranial cerebrovascular disease. With a noninvasive laboratory of proven reliability and accumulating evidence that various types of intracranial vascular or mass lesions may not significantly affect surgical morbidity and long-term success, many vascular surgeons are gradually coming to rely on duplex ultrasound without further investigation. This approach is used in 60% of patients. However, with validation of the protocol described, it is likely that MR imaging will be necessary in only about 20% of patients, further reducing the need for contrast arteriography from the current level of 25% to approximately 5%. With further developments in technology and experience, noninvasive diagnostic methods will likely completely replace arteriography.

REFERENCES

1. Edelman RR, Warach S. Magnetic resonance imaging. New Eng J Med 1993; 328:708–716, 785–791.
2. Wilkerson DK, Keller I, Mezrich R, et al. The comparative evaluation of three-dimensional magnetic resonance for carotid artery disease. J Vasc Surg 1991; 14:803–811.
3. Mattle HP, Kent KC, Edelman RR, et al. Evaluation of the extracranial carotid arteries: Correlation of magnetic resonance angiography, duplex ultrasonography, and conventional angiography. J Vasc Surg 1991; 13:838–845.
4. Turnipseed WD, Kennell TW, Turski PA, et al. Combined use of duplex imaging and magnetic resonance angiography for evaluation of patients with symptomatic ipsilateral high-grade carotid stenosis. J Vasc Surg 1993; 17:832–840.

MEDICAL THERAPY FOR TRANSIENT ISCHEMIC ATTACKS AND ISCHEMIC STROKE

PANAYIOTIS MITSIAS, M.D.
K.M.A. WELCH, M.D.

Ischemic stroke is one of the leading causes of death and disability in the United States and many other industrialized nations. It is estimated that 500,000 people in the United States have a new or recurrent stroke each year, and approximately 150,000 die as a result. The annual cost of strokes, in terms of health care expenditure and loss of productivity, is estimated to be more than $18 billion.

Every year 50,000 patients in the United States suffer transient ischemic attacks (TIAs), and about one third develop a stroke. A TIA identifies a patient at substantial risk of stroke, providing a warning that allows the physician to intervene before stroke occurs.

DEFINITION

Transient ischemic attacks are temporary focal brain or anterior visual pathway deficits caused by vascular disease that clear completely in less than 24 hours. The 24 hour limit is arbitrary, selected in prospective surveys in the early 1970s. Most TIAs are much shorter, resolving within 1 hour. The median duration of carotid system TIAs is 14 minutes and that of the vertebrobasilar TIAs is 8 minutes. If a symptom is present for more than 1 hour, there is a high probability that the patient will have a cerebral infarct since only 14% of these longer TIAs resolve within 24 hours.

MECHANISMS

TIAs are symptoms and they have diverse causes. Proper diagnosis is crucial in choosing the appropriate therapy to minimize stroke. Occasionally, a transient neurological deficit from a nonvascular cause may mimic a TIA (Table 1).

TIAs may herald all types of stroke, but their frequency varies depending on etiology. TIAs are most common in patients with large-artery atherosclerosis. In stroke studies, TIAs have occurred before 25% to 50% of atherosclerotic infarcts, but before only 11% to 30% of cardioembolic infarcts and 11% to 14% of lacunar infarcts. Less common causes of TIAs include hypercoagulable states, arterial dissection, arteritis, and illicit drug use. Thus, although the occurrence of a TIA may suggest certain stroke etiologies, a TIA is not diagnostic for any specific stroke type.

Ischemic strokes and TIAs are part of a continuum of pathology caused by cerebral ischemia. Cerebral infarction is also commonly considered atherothrombotic, cardioembolic, or lacunar (Table 2). About 30% to 40% of patients with infarction cannot be easily classified clinically as having one of these types, and are best labeled as having infarction of unknown type. Atherothrombotic infarction occurs when atherosclerosis involves selected sites in the extracranial or intracranial arteries. Infarction is produced by the plaque enlarging to seriously compromise the lumen, more often with superimposed thrombus, or by artery-to-artery embolism. The basis for the clinical diagnosis of cardioembolic infarction is the documentation of a cardiac source of embolus (Table 3) and no other causes of stroke. Lacunar infarcts are small lesions resulting from involve-

Table 1 Differential Diagnosis of TIAs

Migraine and migraine equivalents
Antiphospholipid syndrome
Partial seizure
Subdural hematoma
Hypoglycemia
Metabolic encephalopathy
Cerebral neoplasm
Demyelinating disease
Dystonia, tremor, chorea or other movement disorders
Syncope/cardiac arrhythmia
Narcolepsy, cataplexy
Conversion reaction, malingering
Hyperventilation, panic attack, anxiety

Table 2 Classification of Ischemic Stroke by Mechanism

Large artery atherosclerosis
  Extracranial vessels
    Internal carotid artery origin
    Vertebral artery origin
  Intracranial vessels
    Middle cerebral artery
    Anterior cerebral artery
    Basilar artery
    Posterior cerebral artery
Cardiogenic embolism
Small vessel disease (lacunar infarction)
Watershed infarction (associated with systemic hypotension)
Others
  Nonatherosclerotic vasculopathy
  Hypercoagulable states
  Paradoxical embolism
  Migraine-related stroke

Table 3 Cardiac Lesions Associated with Embolic Stroke*

High-risk
Valvular surgery
Atrial fibrillation, atrial flutter or sick-sinus syndrome with valvular heart disease
Atrial fibrillation, atrial flutter or sick-sinus syndrome without valvular heart disease
Ventricular aneurysm by echocardiogram
Mural thrombus by echocardiogram
Cardiomyopathy or left ventricular hypokinesis by echocardiogram
Akinetic region by echocardiogram

Medium-risk
Myocardial infarction within 6 months
Valvular heart disease without atrial fibrillation, atrial flutter or sick-sinus syndrome
Congestive heart failure
Decreased left ventricular function by echocardiogram
Hypokinetic segment by echocardiogram
Mitral valve prolapse by history or echocardiogram
Mitral annular calcification by echocardiogram

*Adapted from Kittner SJ et al. Neurology 1992;42:299-302; with permission.

Table 4 Selected Etiologies of Stroke in Young Patients

Nonatherosclerotic arteropathy
  Arterial dissection
  Fibromuscular dysplasia
  Moya-moya disease
  Takayasu's arteritis
  Sickle-cell disease
  Fabry's disease
Hypercoagulable state
  Oral contraceptives, peripartum
  Deficiency of protein C, or S, or antithrombin III
  Antiphospholipid syndrome
Cardiogenic embolism
  Mitral valve prolapse
  Patent foramen ovale
Drug abuse
  Cocaine
  Infectious endocarditis from intravenous drug use
  Amphetamines
Systemic Lupus Erythematosus
Migraine-related stroke
Thrombotic thrombocytopenic purpura

ment of deep, small, penetrating arteries. Cerebral infarction in young patients is usually related to other, less frequent etiologies (Table 4).

DIAGNOSIS

Even when a careful history is taken, recognition of TIAs is sometimes difficult, and experienced observers do not always agree. The symptoms of TIAs are protean and depend on the vascular territory involved. When the carotid territory is involved, the symptoms reflect ischemia of the ipsilateral eye or cerebral hemisphere. The visual disturbance is a transient graying, fogging or blurring of vision, sometimes with a "shade" seeming to descend over the line of sight. Hemispheral ischemia usually causes weakness or numbness of the contralateral face or limbs. Language difficulties (dominant hemisphere) and cognitive and behavioral disturbances (dominant and non-dominant hemisphere) may also occur.

Vertebrobasilar TIAs often include ataxia, dizziness, vertigo, dysarthria, abnormalities of eye movements (diplopia), and unilateral or bilateral motor and sensory symptoms. Hemianopsia and bilateral loss of vision also occur. Isolated vertigo, dizziness or nausea are rarely caused by TIAs. Syncope, light-headedness, incontinence, confusion, amnesia, or seizures are also rarely due to TIAs.

PROGNOSIS

Patients who have had TIAs are at a much higher risk of stroke than the general population. Overall, the risk of stroke is 24% to 29% during the 5 years after a TIA, a sevenfold increase.[1] The risk is 4% to 8% in the 1st month and 12% to 13% during the 1st year, a 13 to 16-fold increase. Patients with hemispheric TIAs and carotid stenoses of more than 70% have a particularly ominous prognosis, with a stroke rate of more than 40% in 2 years. In contrast, isolated monocular visual symptoms have a better prognosis, and young patients with TIAs have a generally lower stroke risk.

A frequently overlooked issue is the risk of cardiac mortality in patients with typical TIAs, approaching 5% per annum, higher than the 3% to 4% annual mortality of patients with angina pectoris. This mortality is even higher in patients with atypical TIAs. Despite this, firm guidelines for evaluation of silent coronary artery disease have not been established for this group of patients.

RISK REDUCTION

Hypertension. Hypertension is the most powerful, prevalent and treatable risk factor for stroke. Both systolic and diastolic blood pressure are independently related to stroke incidence. Borderline hypertension or isolated systolic hypertension also increase the risk of stroke. Patients with hypertension can substantially reduce their risk of stroke by controlling their blood pressure. An analysis of 14 treatment trials indicates that an average reduction of diastolic blood pressure of 6mm Hg produces a 42% reduction in stroke risk.[2] In patients with acute stroke, aggressive treatment of hypertension is not recommended. Also, some patients with a high-grade arterial stenoses have a hemodynamic basis for the TIA, and blood pressure lowering could theoretically precipitate symptoms. Thus, although aggressive therapy of hypertension is important in the followup care of patients with TIA or stroke, it might be advisable to delay it until after the acute phase of stroke or TIA.

Cigarette smoking. Most studies document that cigarette smoking can double the risk of stroke. Data from the Framingham study[3] documented that smoking cessation can promptly reduce the risk of stroke, and that after only 5 years of not smoking, the risk of stroke is no different from that of people who have never smoked.

Oral contraceptive use. Women who take oral contraceptives have an approximately five-fold increase in the risk of stroke. The increased risk occurs primarily in women over age 35 and in those who smoke or have other cardiovascular risk factors. Women who discontinue the oral contraceptives have risk of stroke no higher than those who never used them.

Alcohol consumption. Heavy alcohol use, either daily or in binges, is related to excess stroke risk. Light or moderate alcohol consumption raises the high-density lipoproteins, lowers the risk of coronary artery disease, and has no effect or a mild protective effect against the risk of stroke.

Blood lipids. Increased levels of serum cholesterol and triglycerides are independently related to the development of coronary artery disease. Their relation to stroke is less clear, although serum lipid levels have been related to carotid artery atherosclerosis in ultrasonographic and arteriographic studies. No prospective trials have suggested that therapy to reduce excessive lipid levels can reduce the risk of stroke. However, medications for hyperlipidemia reduce the risk of coronary artery disease, and cholesterol lowering may be recommended for these patients.

Diabetes mellitus. Diabetes is an independent risk factor for ischemic stroke, but whether strict control of blood glucose in diabetic patients reduces their risk for stroke is unknown.

Physical activity. No prospective trials have addressed the relation between physical activity and stroke risk. Exercise may exert a beneficial effect on risk factors for atherosclerotic disease, and it is possible that increased physical activity by sedentary people will reduce stroke risk.

ANTITHROMBOTIC THERAPY FOR TIA AND ISCHEMIC STROKE (TABLE 5)

Antiplatelet Agents

It has been reliably established that in patients with unstable angina, suspected acute myocardial infarction, or a history of myocardial infarction, stroke or a transient ischemic attack,[4] antiplatelet therapy reduces the risk of vascular death by about one-sixth and the risk of nonfatal myocardial infarction and stroke by one-third.

Aspirin

Aspirin is the standard medical therapy for prevention in patients at risk for stroke. Aspirin inhibits platelet function by blocking cyclooxygenase. At least ten clinical trial studies of aspirin for patients with TIAs and minor stroke have been reported, and in all but two, a statistically significant benefit from aspirin was documented. In aggregate, the studies overwhelmingly establish the beneficial effect of aspirin for reducing stroke and death in these patients.[4] Despite this evidence, several issues are still debated. Among these are the ideal dose, gender differences, and the risk: benefit ratio as compared to ticlopidine.

Most clinical trials documenting a beneficial effect of aspirin for patients with cerebrovascular disease used

Table 5 Guidelines for Antithrombotic Therapy*

Clinical Situation	Recommended Therapy	Alternative Options
TIA or minor stroke†	Aspirin 975-1300 mg/day	Low dose aspirin 75 to 325 mg/day Ticlopidine 250 mg twice daily
TIA or minor stroke and aspirin intolerance	Ticlopidine 250 mg twice daily	Warfarin - INR 2.0-3.0
Crescendo TIA or stroke-in-evolution		IV Heparin (PTT: 1.5-2 times control) or aspirin 325 to 1,300 mg/day
Acute cardiogenic embolism		
TIA or small infarct	IV Heparin (after CT negative for hemorrhage) followed by Warfarin (INR: 2-3)	Warfarin, delayed anticoagulation, aspirin 325 to 1300 mg/day
Large infarct	Delayed anticoagulation 5-14 days	Aspirin, no treatment

*Adapted from Sherman et al. Chest 1992;102(suppl):529S-537S
†No evidence of cardiogenic embolism or high-grade (70-99%) stenosis of the internal carotid artery in patients with hemispheric or ocular ischemia.

doses of 975 to 1,300 mg/day. It is unclear whether lower doses are equally effective. The antiplatelet trialists stated that there appears no good reason to use a dose higher than 300 to 325 mg/day based on the assumption that patients with coronary artery disease and cerebrovascular disease would respond similarly to the same dose of aspirin. The Swedish Aspirin Low-dose Trial documented that 75 mg/day was significantly better than placebo[5] and the Dutch TIA Trial documented equal effectiveness between low-dose (283 mg/day) and very low dose (30 mg/day) aspirin.[6] However, no conclusions can be reached regarding whether the low dose is as effective as the higher doses.

Early aspirin trials suggested either no or minimal effect in women. However, in TIA studies where stroke and death rates were documented, women with TIA had a much lower event rate than men, so that a true effect could not be found during the few years of follow-up. In the European Stroke Prevention Study[7] and the French AICLA[8] study a beneficial effect was seen for both women and men.

It is difficult to know how long antiplatelet therapy should be continued, as no large directly randomized comparisons between different durations of treatment have been reported. There is a suggestion from trials conducted so far that the effects of antiplatelet therapy diminish over time.

Dipyridamole

Although a combination of aspirin and dipyridamole offers a theoretical advantage, four clinical trials (French Toulouse Study, French AICLA Study, American-Canadian Cooperative Study and European Stroke Prevention Study) documented that dipyridamole added no benefit.

Ticlopidine

Ticlopidine hydrochloride is a novel antiplatelet agent recently approved in the United States for prevention of stroke in patients with TIA or minor stroke. The antiplatelet action is not completely understood, but it appears to inhibit adenosine diphosphate in the platelet membrane. Ticlopidine exerts this effect within 24 to 48 hours after administration and it lasts for the lifetime of the platelet. Two recent large, multicenter, randomized trials have evaluated the efficacy of ticlopidine in patients with cerebrovascular disease.[9,10] The Canadian American Ticlopidine Study (CATS)[9] evaluated the efficacy of ticlopidine in patients with a recent moderate to severe atherothrombotic or lacunar strokes. The relative risk reduction for the cluster of vascular events, including recurrent nonfatal stroke, nonfatal myocardial infarction, and vascular mortality, was 23.3%. The other study, Ticlopidine Aspirin Stroke Study (TASS),[10] compared the efficacy of ticlopidine with 1,300 mg/day aspirin in reducing the incidence of stroke and death from all causes in patients with a recent TIA or minor stroke. Even in 3 years the risk reduction for fatal and nonfatal stroke was 21% better than aspirin. The effect was present in both men and women. The relative risk reduction was greatest in the first year after entry into the study.

Diarrhea was the most frequent side effect in the drug trials, occurring in 12.5% of patients. Neutropenia developed in 2.4% of patients, and was severe in 0.8%. Severe neutropenia occurred within 90 days of starting therapy, but was reversible. Because of this, a complete blood count and differential must be obtained every 2 weeks during the first 3 months of therapy.

Considering the minor additional benefit of ticlopidine in light of its cost and side effects, many clinicians may choose to start antiplatelet therapy with aspirin and reserve ticlopidine for patients who are intolerant of or fail aspirin treatment.

Anticoagulants

Heparin Sodium

Heparin sodium is often considered in the management of patients with TIAs, cardioembolic stroke, or stroke-in-evolution. Patients with uncontrolled arterial hypertension, hemorrhagic diatheses, peptic ulcer disease, or intracranial hemorrhage must be excluded from treatment. A complete blood count, including platelet count, prothrombin, time, and partial thromboplastin time should be obtained prior to treatment.

Immediate anticoagulation with heparin sodium should be considered in patients with crescendo TIAs, and in those with a high risk of recurrent cardiogenic emboli who suffer TIAs or small-volume ischemic strokes. Following a cardioembolic stroke, the optimal time to initiate anticoagulation with heparin sodium is controversial. The dilemma balances the potential reduction in early recurrent embolism against the risk of potentiating secondary brain hemorrhage because cardioembolic strokes appear to have a special, but not exclusive, propensity for delayed hemorrhagic transformation. Approximately 12% of patients with cardioembolic strokes will experience a second embolic stroke within 2 weeks (range 0% to 21%). The only exception is patients with nonrheumatic atrial fibrillation, who have a lower risk of early stroke recurrence. The frequency of clinical worsening due to hemorrhagic conversion of the ischemic infarct after immediate anticoagulation ranges from 1.4% to 24%. By 48 hours about 75% of the infarctions undergoing spontaneous hemorrhagic conversion will be visible on computed tomography (CT). As a result it is recommended that heparin sodium followed by sodium warfarin therapy be instituted in normotensive patients with small- to moderate-sized embolic infarcts, in whom CT scans performed at approximately 48 hours document no evidence of spontaneous hemorrhagic conversion. Anticoagulation should be postponed for 5 to 14 days in patients with large embolic infarcts occupying more than 30% of one cortical lobe, especially if they occur in elderly patients or in the setting of uncontrolled hypertension.

Approximately 15% of ischemic infarcts progress, usually in the first 7 to 10 days. The cause of progression is usually unknown, but may be due to clot propagation. Although early trials suggested a benefit of anticoagulation, recent evidence does not support this. Overall, heparin anticoagulation for 3 to 5 days appears most reasonable, especially for progressing ischemic stroke in the vertebrobasilar circulation.

Sodium Warfarin

Oral anticoagulants have been used for decades to prevent stroke, but there are no conclusive data to support their routine use in patients with cerebral ischemia due to atherothrombotic disease of the extracranial or intracranial arteries. Sodium warfarin is considered only when other modes of therapy have failed, are contraindicated, or if TIAs have a cardiac course.

In patients with cardioembolic stroke, long-term treatment with oral anticoagulants is the treatment of choice. The range of prothrombin time prolongation that optimally balances antithrombotic effect and bleeding complications has not been established by adequate clinical trials for most cardioembolic sources. Pending further clinical data, anticoagulation to an international normalized ratio of 2.0 to 3.0 would appear satisfactory for embolism prophylaxis for many types of heart disease with the possible exception of mechanical prosthetic heart valves in which a higher intensity of anticoagulation is required.

Sodium warfarin is indicated for the prevention of stroke in patients with non-valvular atrial fibrillation, although aspirin may be preferred to sodium warfarin in patients at lower risk for embolic stroke because of the hemorrhagic side effects of the latter, particularly in the very elderly. High risk factors for stroke in this condition include age over 75, hypertension, congestive heart failure, and previous thromboembolism.

Thrombolytic Therapy

There is currently no proven therapy for acute ischemic stroke. There is, however, preliminary optimism concerning therapies designed to reduce neurologic deficits and infarct size by: restoring or increasing perfusion to ischemic regions by thrombolytic agents; or attempting to improve the cellular, metabolic, and biochemical consequences of ischemia by neuroprotective agents.

Reestablishing blood flow can be attempted by medical or surgical intervention. The presence of an intravascular clot suggests that thrombolytic therapy is a viable approach in the treatment of acute ischemic stroke, provided that it is not associated with an unacceptably high hemorrhagic risk. Patients with arteriographically documented cerebrovascular occlusions were treated with escalating tissue plasminogen activator (tPA) doses within 8 hours of stroke onset. Partial or complete arterial recanalization was documented in 34% of patients.[11] Parenchymatous hemorrhage associated with clinical deterioration was observed in 5.8% of patients. The risk for intracranial hemorrhage was significantly higher in patients treated more than 6 hours after stroke onset. In another dose escalation trial, tPA was administered within 90 minutes of stroke onset, but without prior arteriography.[12] Only 2 of 74 patients suffered an intracranial hemorrhage in the region of presumed infarction and 1 other hematoma was observed in an unassociated region, for a 4% hemorrhagic rate. At least four multicenter randomized trials of thrombolytic agents are now under way to determine the clinical efficacy of this treatment.

GENERAL THERAPEUTIC MEASURES IN ACUTE ISCHEMIC STROKE

In addition to pharmacologic therapies, some general considerations apply to all patients, independent of stroke mechanism. Overzealous therapy of hypertension should be avoided. Hyperglycemia and fever should be treated promptly, as they may result in increased infarct size. An optimal fluid balance should be maintained. Patients in coma or at risk for aspiration, especially those with brainstem strokes, should be admitted to an intensive care unit and considered for elective intubation.

Endotracheal intubation, elevation of head of bed, hyperventilation, and intravenous mannitol should be considered in patients with brain edema and increased intracranial pressure. Such interventions offer only short-term benefit, but may influence survival.

REFERENCES

1. Dennis M, Bamford J, Sandercock P, Warlow C. Prognosis of transient ischemic attacks in the Oxfordshire Community Stroke Project. Stroke 1990;21:848–853.
2. Collins R, Peto R, MacMahon S, et al. Blood pressure, stroke, and coronary heart disease, II: short-term reductions in blood pressure: overview of randomized drug trials in their epidemiological context. Lancet 1990;335:827–838.
3. Wolf P, D'Agostino RB, Kannel WB, et al. Cigarette smoking as a risk factor for stroke: the Framingham Study. JAMA 1988;259:1025–1029.
4. Antiplatelet Trialists' Collaboration. Collaborative overview of randomized trials of antiplatelet therapy-I: Prevention of death, myocardial infarction, and stroke by prolonged antiplatelet therapy in various categories of patients. BMJ 1994;308:81–106.
5. The SALT Collaborative Group. Swedish Aspirin Low-dose Trial (SALT) of 75mg aspirin as secondary prophylaxis after cerebrovascular ischemic events. Lancet 1991;338:1345–1349.
6. The Dutch TIA Trial Study Group. A comparison of two doses of aspirin (30mg vs 283mg a day) in patients after a transient ischemic attack or minor ischemic stroke. N Engl J Med 1991;325:1261–1266.
7. European Stroke Prevention Study Group. ESPS: principal end points. Lancet 1987;2:1351-1354.
8. Bousser MG, Eschwege E, Haguenan B, et al. A.I.C.L.A.: Controlled trial of aspirin and dipyridamole in the secondary prevention of atherothrombotic cerebral ischemia. Stroke 1983;14:5-14.
9. Gent M, Easton JD, Hachinski VC, et al. The Canadian American Ticlopidine Study. Lancet 1989;1:1215–1220.

10. Hass WK, Easton JD, Adams HP, et al. A randomized trial comparing ticlopidine hydrochloride with aspirin for the prevention of stroke in high-risk patients. N Engl J Med 1989;321: 501–507.
11. The rt-PA/Acute Stroke Study Group. An open safety/efficacy trial of rt-PA in acute thromboembolic stroke (abstract). Stroke 1991;22:153
12. Brott T, Halet C, Levy D, et al. Safety and potential efficacy of tissue plasminogen activator for stroke. Stroke 1990;21:181

DIAGNOSIS AND SURGICAL MANAGEMENT OF ASYMPTOMATIC CAROTID STENOSIS

ALLAN D. CALLOW, M.D., PH.D.
JEFFREY D. TRACHTENBERG, M.D.

Stroke remains the third leading cause of death in the United States. Equally important, however, are the survivors who are left with permanent deficits, robbed of their independence and unable to care for themselves. In the current climate of cost containment, the treatment of these patients—not only during the acute phase but also during their subsequent rehabilitation—exacts a staggering toll on the health care system. Prevention, therefore, is paramount, and therein lies the problem of asymptomatic carotid stenoses.

Somewhat less than one-third of ischemic strokes are due to identifiable arteriosclerotic lesions of major vessels. Cardiac-origin emboli account for about the same number. Lacunar infarctions, the consequence of small artery and arteriolar occlusions, account for about one-fourth, and the remainder are due to a host of disorders, including fibromuscular dysplasia, coagulation disorders, and aorta-based emboli. All these possibilities complicate the problem of interpretation of the asymptomatic carotid lesion. An individual with such a lesion may, indeed, suffer a stroke in the course of long-term surveillance, but it may not be due to the carotid lesion. This distinction, allocation of cause, has plagued the analysis and obfuscated the role of treatment of the asymptomatic carotid lesion.

PREVALENCE OF ASYMPTOMATIC CAROTID ARTERY DISEASE

The prevalence of asymptomatic carotid occlusive disease is not known. Most studies are of small groups, often with coexisting cardiac or peripheral vascular disease. The small sample size and the narrow demographics are major limitations.

By a variety of noninvasive techniques, asymptomatic disease among unselected patients, chosen at random in that a carotid bruit was not a selection criterion, was found in 54% of individuals over 65 years. Lesions greater than 50% were found in only 4.6%, and less than 1% had lesions greater than 80%. There is a clear correlation with age. In patients younger than 60 years, there is a 4% prevalence that increases to 11% after the seventh decade. From these very limited studies, it appears that carotid disease is common in unselected populations but very few have threatening lesions.

Among patients with carotid bruits, common in elderly people, Chambers and Norris found 52% of 500 individuals with lesions greater than 30% stenosis; 23% had lesions greater than 75%.[1]

In another risk category, patients undergoing cardiac or peripheral vascular operations, the prevalence of lesions with greater than 50% stenosis ranged from a low of 3.8% to a high of 25%, not very helpful data. Arteriographic evaluation of patients identified as peripheral vascular surgical candidates with carotid bruits, however, documented a prevalence rate of 66% for greater than 50% stenosis and 33% for lesions greater than 75% to 80%. This is the largest reported prevalence rate. By contrast, Berens and colleagues[2] reviewed 4,047 cardiac surgery candidates and found only 3.8% with lesions greater than 50% stenosis.

In summary, in an unselected population, 5% of individuals may be expected to have a carotid lesion of greater than 50% stenosis, and less than 1% have a lesion with greater than 75% stenosis. Among individuals with bruits alone, 10% to 20% have lesions with greater than 50% stenosis, and only 5% show lesions greater than 75%. For patients selected for cardiac or peripheral vascular operations, 40 to 50% have lesions of greater than 50% stenosis, and 10 to 20% have greater than 75% stenosis (Table 1). At this time screening for asymptom-

Table 1 Estimated Prevalence of Asymptomatic Carotid Artery Disease in Various Groups of People

		Prevalence	
	Disease	Stenosis >50%	Stenosis >75%
Unselected population	10–50%	5%	<1%
Cardiac or vascular patients	—	10–20%	5%
Patients with bruits	—	40–50%	10–20%

atic carotid disease in an unselected population can be justified only for epidemiologic reasons. It is important information, but it is research and not patient care. By contrast, in especially high-risk groups, such as those undergoing cardiac or peripheral vascular operations, screening seems justified.

NATURAL HISTORY OF ASYMPTOMATIC CAROTID ARTERY DISEASE

For many years a bias persisted among many neurologists that the asymptomatic stenotic carotid lesion is benign. This misconception appears to have had its origin in two reports, one from Evans County, Georgia,[3] and the second from Framingham, Massachusetts.[4] These studies reported the stroke risk of an asymptomatic bruit to be approximately 2% per year. Both studies were flawed because of failure to define the underlying lesion in patients with carotid bruits. We now know that many patients with carotid bruit may have minimal lesions. In fact, the incidence of high-grade carotid artery stenosis in a patient population with carotid bruit is only about 20%. It is of interest and often overlooked by critics of prophylactic carotid endarterectomy (CEA) that in the Framingham study the presence of a carotid bruit correlated much better with fatal myocardial infarction than it did with subsequent stroke. Subsequent studies have corroborated this, documenting the likelihood of cardiac ischemia and vascular death in individuals with greater than 75% carotid artery stenosis to be 9.9% per year.

Further, with the report of Roederer and associates[5] utilizing duplex scanning, it was realized that approximately 30% of individuals with minimal lesions at the time of evaluation progress to more than 50% stenosis within 3 years of surveillance. Disease progression to more than 80% stenosis was associated with transient ischemic attacks (TIAs) or stroke in 89% of their patients. Progression to greater than 80% stenosis carried a 35% risk of neurologic symptoms or occlusion of that carotid artery within 6 months of the observed progression plus a 46% risk of adverse events within 12 months of observation. The progression to occlusion of an asymptomatic lesion is not a benign event, for patients with an occluded carotid artery are at risk for stroke at the rate of 5 to 10% per year. At this end point of arterial disease, endarterectomy is impossible.

Chambers and Norris[1] identified two critical predictors of neurologic events in their noninvasive follow-up examination of 500 asymptomatic patients every 6 months: (1) stenosis greater than 75% or evidence of disease progression between two examinations, and (2) failure of daily prophylactic administration of aspirin to influence outcome. For patients with greater than 75% stenosis the 1 year TIA and stroke rate was 18%. The 1 year stroke rate was 5%. Even though half of these patients were taking aspirin, the neurologic event rate of the two groups was identical.[1] A more recent report by this group documented a low annual stroke rate of 1.3% among individuals with carotid stenoses of less than 75%. This stroke rate increases to 3.3% for patients with greater than 75% stenoses. The combined stroke and TIA rate for patients with greater than 75% stenoses was 10.5% per year, with 75% of events ipsilateral to the stenosed artery.[6]

These studies highlight the importance of critical, i.e., greater than 75% stenosis plus progression of disease, as markers for subsequent neurologic events. Recent studies have also identified plaque morphology as a risk factor. An echolucent lesion is probably more dangerous than an echogenic one, as the lucency reflects cholesterol deposition or hemorrhage. Such plaque may be unstable and more likely to ulcerate. Other factors that may also correlate with an increased incidence of neurologic sequelae are imperfections in the circle of Willis and the presence of hypodense lesions on computed tomography (CT).

SURGICAL RESULTS OF CAROTID ENDARTERECTOMY FOR ASYMPTOMATIC LESIONS

For CEA to be a valid therapeutic option, the combination of the perioperative and postoperative morbidity and mortality must be less than in patients treated with medical therapy alone. In this regard, beneficial effects have been suggested in the clinical setting.[7] In the discussions currently underway concerning health care reform, treatment outcome will be carefully scrutinized. In this regard, the Stroke Council of the American Heart Association has recommended that the combined operative morbidity and mortality due to stroke for patients with asymptomatic carotid stenosis must be below 3%. In centers of excellence, CEA can be performed successfully with exemplary results, not only with low perioperative morbidity and mortality and immediate benefit but also with continuation of protection against stroke over the long term.

A review by Colburn and Moore of studies published since 1971 of the risk of CEA in asymptomatic patients documented a perioperative stroke rate of 1.5% and an operative mortality of 0.8% in a total of 2,316 patients.[8] The same report documented the incidence of TIAs to range from 0 to 6% and the incidence of stroke from 0 to 11.8% after 2 to 5 years. Comparisons between reports are difficult because of varying lengths of follow-up, the criteria for surgical intervention, and the methods used for reporting neurologic events.

In a study by Freischlag and co-workers[9] of asymptomatic CEA, the perioperative mortality was 0. The perioperative stroke rate was 1.6%. Using life table analysis in a follow-up of 10 years, the ipsilateral TIA rate was 2% or 0.2% per year. Including all neurologic events in all arterial territories during this decade, overall TIA rate was 6%, or 0.6% per year. The overall stroke rate was 7% or 0.7% per year, an experience substantially lower than the 18% per year event rate and the 5% stroke rate reported by Chambers and Norris.

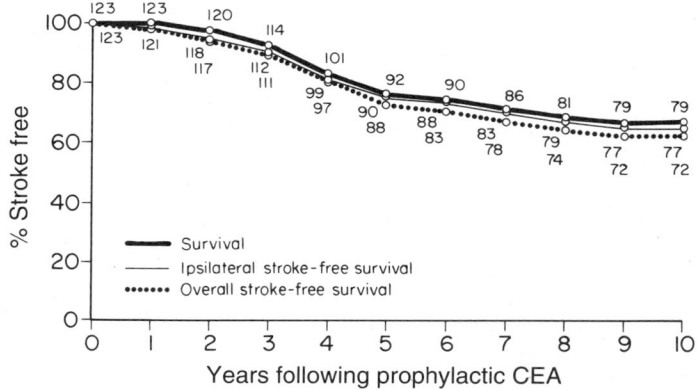

Figure 1 Life table analysis revealing stroke-free survival rates of 90%, 72%, and 62% at 3, 4, and 10 years, respectively, after carotid endarterectomy (CEA). Ipsilateral stroke-free survival rates were 90%, 75%, and 65% at 3, 5, and 10 years, respectively. Overall survival rate was 92.4% at 3 years, 76% at 5 years, and 66.5% at 10 years. (From Freischlag JA, Hanna D, Moore WS. Improved prognosis for asymptomatic carotid stenosis with prophylactic carotid endarterectomy. Stroke 1992; 23:479–482; with permission.)

The somewhat nettlesome allegation that coexisting coronary artery occlusive disease precludes meaningful realization of benefits that might be conferred by prophylactic CEA is denied in this same series. Survival at 3 years was 92%, at 5 years 76%, and at 10 years 66%. Comparison of stroke-free survival curves reveals a nearly identical experience; i.e., surviving patients do so without suffering a stroke (Fig. 1). The 3.4% mortality per year is striking evidence that patients live long enough to benefit from operation for asymptomatic lesions.

Our personal experience lends strong support. Of 179 CEAs for asymptomatic stenosis, the 30 day perioperative stroke rate was 1.1% and the death rate was 0.56%, for a combined rate of 1.7%. The operation-specific 30 day stroke rate was 1.6%, and the operation-specific death rate was 0.62%. Life table stroke-free survival was 98% at 1 year, 93% at 5 years, and 87% at 10 years.[10]

These reports of superior experience originate for the most part from centers of established excellence. Whether "occasional vascular surgeons," in the words of Eastcott, can duplicate these results rests upon them. There is an understandable concern that results equal to those of specialized centers cannot be duplicated countrywide. We doubt this, given the strong motivation for excellent patient care that we have witnessed for decades and that exists throughout the vascular surgery fraternity. However, continuing audit of individual surgeons and institutions is in the best interest of all.

RANDOMIZED PROSPECTIVE CONTROLLED TRIALS FOR ASYMPTOMATIC LESIONS

Four multicenter prospective trials of asymptomatic carotid lesions deserve mention. Two can be dismissed promptly: the Mayo Clinic trial[11] comparing aspirin therapy with endarterectomy and the Carotid Artery Stenosis with Asymptomatic Narrowing Trial, Operation versus Aspirin (CASANOVA) trial.[12] The Mayo Clinic trial was a single-center study that was terminated early because of an excess of myocardial infarction in the surgical group.

The CASANOVA trial, performed in Europe, enrolled patients with asymptomatic stenoses ranging from 50% to 90%. Patients with greater than 90% stenoses were excluded. Patients were randomized to receive either CEA and antiplatelet agents or antiplatelet agents alone. No difference between the surgical and medical groups could be documented, and the authors erroneously concluded that operation should not be recommended to patients with carotid stenoses of less than 90%. This study was severely flawed. First, exclusion of patients with greater than 90% stenoses missed the opportunity to study the effects of operation in this very high-risk group. These patients all underwent CEA. Also, 118 of 206 patients in the medical group actually underwent CEA, including patients who became symptomatic (i.e., developed TIAs), patients with lesion progression beyond 90%, and patients who developed bilateral stenoses with one side greater than 50%. In addition, if a patient was randomized to medical therapy and had bilateral stenoses, the carotid with the greater lesion underwent CEA and the other was followed. Nevertheless, all these patients were considered to have been treated medically, using the intent-to-treat method of statistical analysis.

The third trial, the Asymptomatic Carotid Stenosis Veterans Administration Study was the first multicenter randomized prospective controlled trial in the United States.[13] Entrants had greater than 50% stenosis by arteriography and were allocated to one of two groups: best medical therapy or best medical therapy with carotid endarterectomy. The study documented that the combined incidence of ipsilateral neurologic events (TIA plus stroke) was reduced in the surgically treated patients, 8% versus 20.6% (p less than 0.001). Unfortunately, the study size was not sufficient to show a significant difference for stroke alone, although there was a trend toward decreased stroke in the surgical group, i.e., 4.7% versus 9.4%. When perioperative mortality was added to the surgical stroke rate, there was no statistical difference between the two groups. In addition, no worse prognosis was found in the medically managed group for those with lesser degrees of stenosis, ranging from 50 to 75%. The major problem with this study is the lack of statistical power due to small sample size. A second major criticism involves the lumping together of patients with stroke, transient cerebral ischemia, and transient monocular blindness as a single neurologic event. These are not equivalent events and do not exert equivalent negative impacts on patient quality of life.

The fourth trial, the Asymptomatic Carotid Artery Study (ACAS), is the largest study to date.[14] It is designed to answer the question of whether CEA, when added to aspirin and risk factor modification, will reduce the incidence of neurologic events in patients with hemodynamically significant asymptomatic carotid stenoses. Debate continues as to the end points, but given the results of the recent trials in symptomatic patients,[15] TIA becomes a clear end point. Thus, patients treated medically can undergo CEA.

THE CONTROVERSY

The controversy of whether asymptomatic patients with carotid stenoses should undergo prophylactic CEA has focused on three specific points:

1. The long-term natural history of asymptomatic carotid stenosis is not known.
2. There is substantial variation in perioperative morbidity and mortality in reported results from community and larger institutions.
3. The benefit of CEA in terms of reduction in stroke rate and incidence of TIA in asymptomatic patients has not yet been undeniably established in a prospective randomized clinical trial.

Barnett and Haines state that "on the basis of evidence to date (Jan 1993) we are forced to conclude that endarterectomy is of as yet unproven benefit for any group of patients with asymptomatic arteriosclerotic stenosis of the carotid artery."[16] In this opinion they include patients we would consider in need of operation, those with the most marked stenosis, those for whom other major surgical procedures are planned, and those with stenosis in the presence of asymptomatic lesions ascribed to ischemia by CT.

Critics of prophylactic CEA recommend waiting for symptoms to develop. Although there are reports of almost all strokes being heralded by a TIA, this is not reliable, for as many as two-thirds of all strokes may occur in the absence of any warning. In addition, the prevention of TIAs may have an as yet unrecognized benefit. Awad and colleagues have identified cerebral abnormalities in 32% of patients with TIAs by CT imaging, and, with magnetic resonance imaging (MRI), focal cerebral abnormalities have been detected in 77% of such patients.[17] Hobson and associates noted that half of all neurologic events in the VA Cooperative trial were strokes without antecedent or warning TIA.[13] Consequently, the implied recommendation of waiting for a TIA before intervening surgically may not constitute an optimal management program for many patients.

CURRENT MANAGEMENT RECOMMENDATIONS

Ideally, management of the patient with asymptomatic carotid artery stenosis should be based on a thorough understanding of the natural history of the asymptomatic lesion, the surgical risk, and the expected long-term benefit. Conflicting information makes generalizations regarding treatment difficult to substantiate. Because the greatest risk to patients with asymptomatic carotid disease is related to cardiac morbidity and not stroke, an aggressive approach to risk factor modulation should be encouraged. Based on the available evidence, we would add aspirin to this regimen. Clearly, however, there are patients who would benefit from operation. In centers where the operation can be performed with acceptably low morbidity and mortality, such a course is warranted. It must be remembered, however, that this is a prophylactic operation, and the operative risks of stroke are the very events the operation is designed to prevent. A policy of individualization is prudent, and patients should be selected for operation based on their individual stroke risk and long-term survivability.

Patients with asymptomatic carotid disease most often present in a number of defined clinical situations. First, a patient is referred to a vascular physician for evaluation of an asymptomatic cervical bruit. Second, an asymptomatic lesion contralateral to a symptomatic lesion requires treatment. Finally, an asymptomatic lesion is identified in a patient who is screened prior to undergoing a major cardiovascular or peripheral vascular procedure. An algorithm for managing these patients is suggested (Fig. 2).

Patients with asymptomatic bruits should undergo duplex screening for documentation of lesion severity. Patients with stenoses of less than 75% are routinely followed every 3 to 6 months, and no intervention is recommended unless there is significant progression of the lesion or the appearance of symptoms. In general, in centers of excellence in which the perioperative stroke and death rates have been documented to be less than 3%, we advocate an aggressive approach to the treatment of patients with asymptomatic disease and high-grade (greater than 75%) carotid stenoses who have no other life-threatening illnesses and are acceptable operative risk. Although results of the VA Cooperative trial

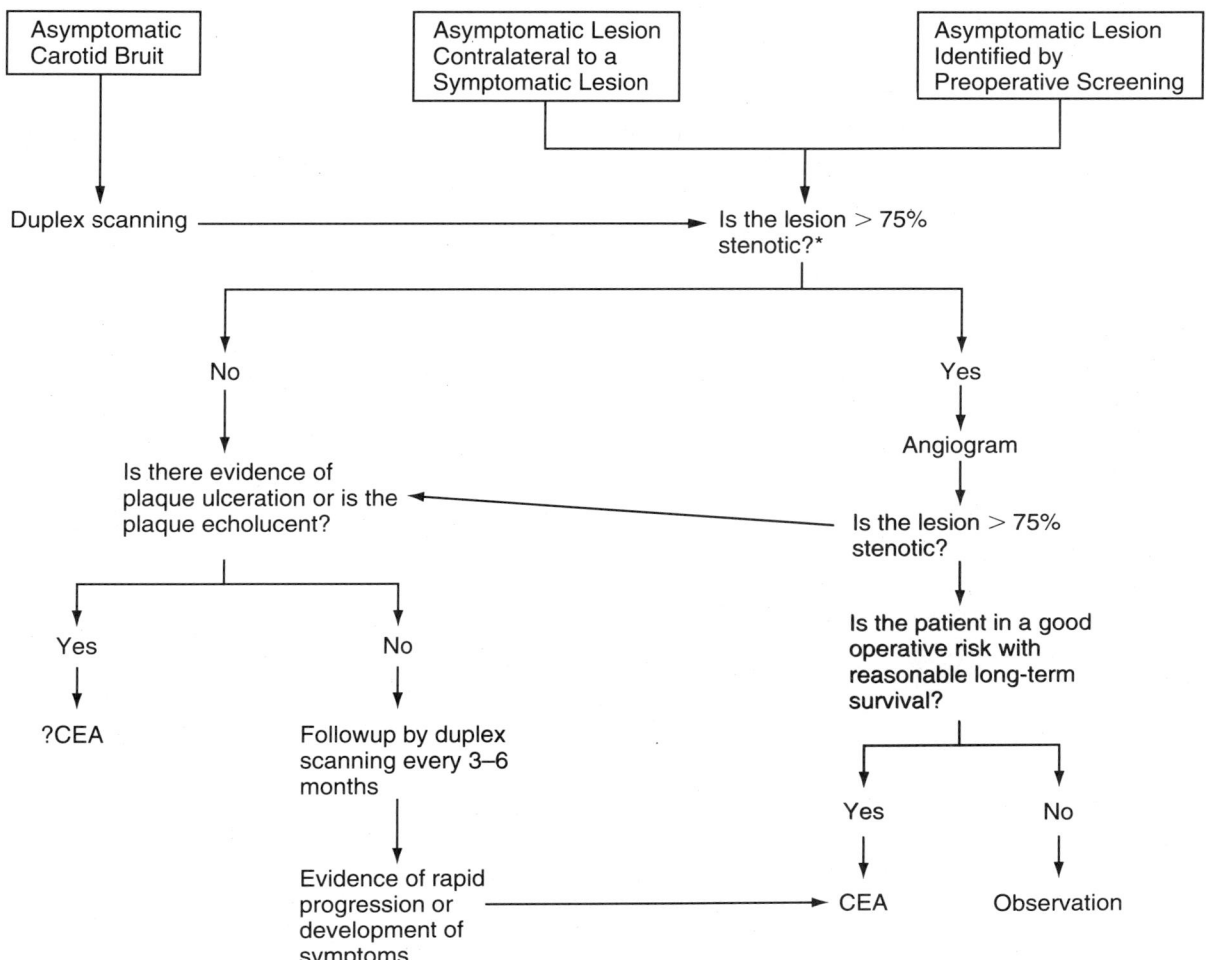

Figure 2 Algorithm for management of asymptomatic atherosclerotic carotid occlusive disease. *Patients with asymptomatic lesions detected on preoperative screening with bilateral stenosis greater than 50% or greater than 50% stenosis contralateral to an occluded carotid artery may also be candidates for prophylactic CEA.

are promising, given the small sample size further validation will have to wait until the ACAS trial is completed. Although we do not advocate operation for a stenosis of less than 50%, this is not a hard-and-fast rule. In those patients who demonstrate rapid plaque progression or have an ulcerated, unstable plaque, operative intervention may be warranted.

For patients with a lesion contralateral to a symptomatic operated carotid artery, available data suggest that the same criteria be employed for the evaluation of this vessel as for the patient with unilateral disease; that is, an artery with greater than 75% stenosis should be operated upon, and those with lesser stenosis are watched. Much of the uncertainty relates to the fact that the natural history of an asymptomatic lesion contralateral to an operated carotid artery may not be the same as an asymptomatic lesion in a patient with a nonoperated contralateral carotid artery.

For patients with carotid bifurcation disease identified prior to a major surgical procedure, current data suggest that the risk of perioperative stroke is the same for those undergoing CEA and those who do not. The difference appears to be that in patients undergoing prophylactic CEA there appears to be a reduced rate of late neurologic events. The presence of extracranial carotid disease, however, is a risk factor for increased perioperative cardiac morbidity and mortality. We recommend that these patients be treated the same as patients who are not undergoing a major operation. If a patient does have a high-grade stenosis, then the decision as to whether CEA be performed concomitantly or in staged fashion can be based on the bias of the operating surgeon and the individual patient's risk factors. There are two caveats in this group of patients: those with bilateral disease in which each side has greater than 50% stenosis, and those patients with at least 50% stenosis opposite an occluded carotid artery. Although we recommend CEA under these circumstances, confirmation by prospective trials is needed.

REFERENCES

1. Chambers RB, Norris JW. Outcome in patients with asymptomatic neck bruits. N Engl J Med, 1986; 315:860–865.
2. Berens ES, Kouchoukos NT, Murphy SF, Wareing THE. Preoperative carotid artery screening in elderly patients undergoing cardiac surgery. J Vasc Surg 1992; 15:313–323.
3. Heyman A, Wilkinson WE, Heyden S, et al. Risk of stroke in asymptomatic persons with cervical arterial bruits. A population study in Evans County, Georgia. N Engl J Med 1980; 302:838–841.
4. Wolf PA, Kannel WB, Sorlie P, McNamara P. Asymptomatic bruit and risk of stroke: The Framingham Study. JAMA 1981; 245:1442–1445.
5. Roederer GO, Langlois YE, Jager KA, et al. The natural history of carotid artery disease in asymptomatic patients with cervical bruits. Stroke 1984; 15:605–613.
6. Norris JW, Zhu CZ, Bornstein NM, Chambers BR. Vascular risks of asymptomatic carotid stenosis. Stroke 1991; 22:1485–1490.
7. Hobson RW, Krupski WC, Weiss DG, and the VA Cooperative Study on Asymptomatic Carotid Stenosis. Influence of aspirin in the management of asymptomatic carotid stenosis. J Vasc Surg 1993; 17:257–263.
8. Colburn MD, Moore WS. The risk of carotid endarterectomy in asymptomatic patients. In: Bernstein EF, Callow AD, Nicolaides AN, Shifrin EG, eds. Cerebral revascularization. London: Med-Orion, 1993:523.
9. Freischlag JA, Hanna D, Moore WS. Improved prognosis for asymptomatic carotid stenosis with prophylactic carotid endarterectomy. Stroke 1992; 23:479–482.
10. Callow AD, Mackey WC. Long-term followup of surgically managed carotid bifurcation atherosclerosis. Justification for an aggressive approach. Ann Surg 1989; 210:308–315.
11. Mayo Asymptomatic Carotid Endarterectomy Study Group. Results of a randomized controlled trial of carotid endarterectomy for asymptomatic carotid stenosis. Mayo Clin Proc 1992; 67:513–518.
12. The CASANOVA Study Group. Carotid surgery versus medical therapy in asymptomatic carotid stenosis. Stroke 1991; 22:1229–1235.
13. Hobson RW II, Weiss DG, Fields WS, et al. Efficacy of carotid endarterectomy for asymptomatic carotid stenosis. N Engl J Med 1993; 328:221–227.
14. The Asymptomatic Carotid Artery Stenosis Group. Study design for randomized prospective trial of carotid endarterectomy for asymptomatic atherosclerosis. Stroke 1989; 20:844–849.
15. North American Symptomatic Carotid Endarterectomy Trial Collaborators. Beneficial effect of carotid endarterectomy in symptomatic patients with high-grade carotid stenosis. N Engl J Med 1991; 325:445–453.
16. Barnett HJM, Haines SJ. Carotid endarterectomy for asymptomatic carotid stenosis. N End J Med 1993; 328:276–279.
17. Awad I, Modic M, Little JR, et al. Focal parenchymal lesions in transient ischemic attacks: correlation of computed tomography and magnetic resonance imaging. Stroke 1986; 17:399–403.

SURGICAL TREATMENT OF EVOLVING STROKE SECONDARY TO CAROTID ARTERY ATHEROSCLEROSIS

G. PATRICK CLAGETT, M.D.

Evolving stroke is an imprecise term that may include three clinical syndromes characterized by neurologic instability stemming from acute thrombus formation on a carotid bifurcation atherosclerotic plaque. First is stroke in evolution associated with advanced carotid stenosis that is manifested by an acute neurologic deficit that progresses in greater severity over hours to days with waxing and waning of signs but without complete resolution of the deficit. Second is an acute neurologic deficit from thrombotic occlusion of the internal carotid artery (ICA) that occurs at the time of, or shortly after, angiography. Finally, there are crescendo transient ischemic attacks (TIAs) that have been defined as recurrent cerebral ischemia in the distribution of the carotid artery, characterized by a definite change in pattern to include increased frequency with multiple TIAs occurring singly or in a cluster in a single day or over 2 or 3 days; and/or increased duration of TIAs with episodes lasting longer than the initial event, or lasting several hours; and/or increased severity of TIAs with expansion in the distribution of ischemia with more extensive or new motor, sensory, speech, or visual deficits.[1] All of these conditions require emergency evaluation and treatment because of the underlying pathologic condition, a severely stenotic atherosclerotic plaque associated with thrombus formation that will inexorably lead to occlusion of the ICA if it has not already occurred at the time of presentation.

The natural history of evolving stroke syndromes associated with severe carotid stenosis and thrombosis is grim. Recent reviews document that, without treatment, good recovery occurs in only 2% to 12% of patients; another 40% to 69% survive with a major neurologic deficit, and 16% to 55% die.[2] Anticoagulation with heparin sodium has been recommended as treatment for patients presenting with progressing stroke,[3] but critical review of randomized trials suggests no benefit of heparin sodium over placebo or aspirin in halting progression to completed stroke.[4,5] Despite these negative trial results, we recommend heparin sodium anticoagulation as initial therapy because it may slow the thrombotic process and buy time, during which intervention can be planned and carried out. We have noted resolution of crescendo TIAs and stabilization of waxing and waning neurologic symptoms with prompt heparin sodium administration.

Carotid endarterectomy (CEA) is being increasingly and successfully used in patients with evolving stroke syndromes. Because of the stunning success of the North American Carotid Endarterectomy Trial (NASCET) and other trials in documenting the benefit of CEA in patients with advanced carotid stenosis who present with stable TIA or small strokes and because of the malignant prognosis with medical treatment,[6] more neurologically unstable patients with severe carotid stenoses are being referred for endarterectomy. Although the results cannot be directly extrapolated, vascular surgeons can expect to be confronted with increasing numbers of these difficult cases. Since publication of NASCET results, we have found ourselves in the surprising and paradoxic position of arguing with some formerly conservative colleagues against CEA in some hopeless patients dying from completed stroke.

The early results of CEA for acute stroke and ICA occlusion were dismal.[7,8] Underlying these poor results was the fear of turning a bland infarct into a hemorrhagic infarct and the high rate of reocclusion with worsening of the neurologic deficit. However, improvements in patient selection based on modern brain imaging and angiographic methods, as well as refinements in anesthetic and perioperative care, especially control of hypertension, have led to successful surgical results in patients with evolving stroke syndromes. The collective experience of several contemporary studies indicates successful results, with improvement in neurologic deficit in about 80%, unsatisfactory results with deterioration in 10% to 15%, and death in 5% to 10%.[2,9] Although these results would be unacceptable for neurologically stable patients undergoing CEA, they are a dramatic improvement compared to the natural history or results with medical treatment alone. In a recent report of 70 neurologically unstable patients undergoing CEA, 93% had improvement or resolution of neurologic deficits, 4.3% deteriorated, and 2.9% died.[9]

Thrombolytic therapy with urokinase and recombinant tissue plasminogen activator is receiving increasing interest in the management of patients with evolving stroke syndromes.[10,11] The rationale behind both thrombolytic therapy and early CEA involves the concept of the "ischemic penumbra" that is now reasonably well established by electrophysiologic work in animals,[12] as well as positron emission tomography. After acute interruption of blood supply, some brain tissue suffers irreparable damage within minutes, but a surrounding penumbra of dysfunctional but viable brain tissue remains salvageable for several hours.[12,13] This provides a window of opportunity during which thrombolytic therapy can be initiated. The early results of thrombolytic therapy for acute stroke are encouraging, and several trials are underway.

Three features make thrombolytic therapy especially attractive as the initial intervention before consideration of CEA in patients with evolving stroke. First, therapy can be started at the time of angiographic diagnosis, and the time to re-establish perfusion is faster than with CEA after angiography. Second, selective thrombolytic therapy can clear thrombus from the middle cerebral artery (Figs. 1 and 2). In one series, the presence of a middle cerebral artery (MCA) embolus was a predictor of a poor neurologic outcome following otherwise successful endarterectomy for acute ICA occlusion.[2] Finally, thrombolytic therapy may clear ICA partially occlusive thrombus or so-called free-floating thrombus (Fig. 3). The presence of ICA thrombus noted on preoperative angiograms is an important risk factor for stroke morbidity with CEA.[9] Despite excellent overall surgical results, this subgroup sustained a 22% perioperative stroke rate in the NASCET study.[6] Re-

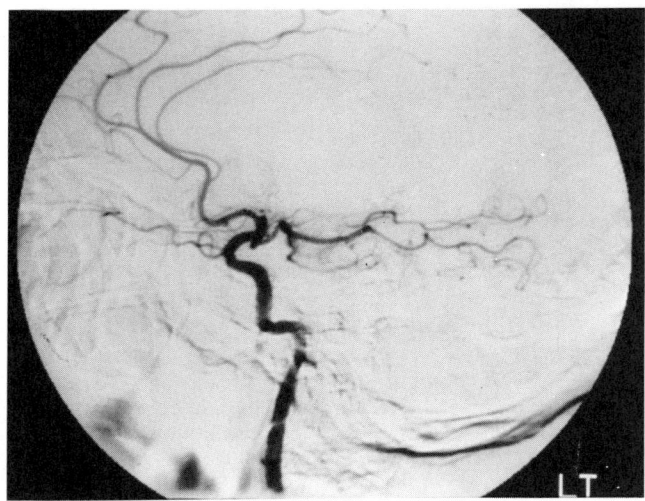

Figure 1 Selective injection of the left internal carotid artery demonstrates embolic occlusion of the left middle cerebral artery.

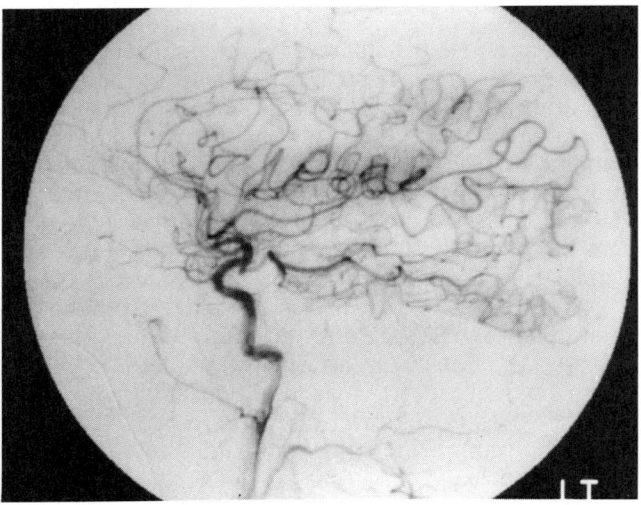

Figure 2 Repeat injection following urokinase infusion demonstrates successful thrombolysis with good filling of the middle cerebral artery. The patient improved and was left with a mild deficit.

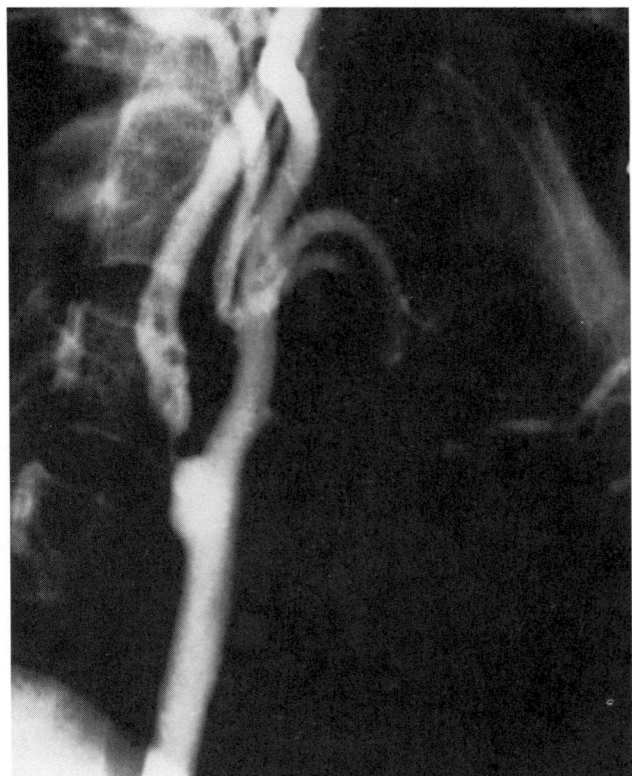

Figure 3 This patient presented with crescendo TIAs, and an arteriogram disclosed intraluminal filling defects that proved to be fresh thrombus distal to an advanced stenosis at the origin of the right internal carotid artery.

moval of this risk factor with thrombolytic therapy before endarterectomy is an attractive concept, but as yet an unproven one.

Based on these considerations, a multidisciplinary approach has been developed to patients with evolving stroke syndromes from severe carotid stenosis. Anticoagulation with heparin sodium is begun at the time of presentation and carried through the period of diagnostic evaluation and intervention. A head computed tomography (CT) scan or magnetic resonance imaging study is performed to rule out intracranial hemorrhage, subdural hematoma, or intracranial pathologies other than acute cerebral ischemia. Immediately after CT, diagnostic arteriography is performed and, if acute occlusion of the ICA or intraluminal thrombus is identified, selective carotid infusion of urokinase is started. The technical aspects of catheter-delivered thrombolytic therapy for carotid occlusion are evolving, but the goal is to clear proximal thrombus before advancing small catheters intracranially into the MCA and its branches.

After complete thrombolysis, CEA for the underlying atherosclerotic plaque is carried out at variable times later, depending on the severity of the underlying stenosis and the clinical condition of the patient. Preference is to allow the patient to stabilize and the

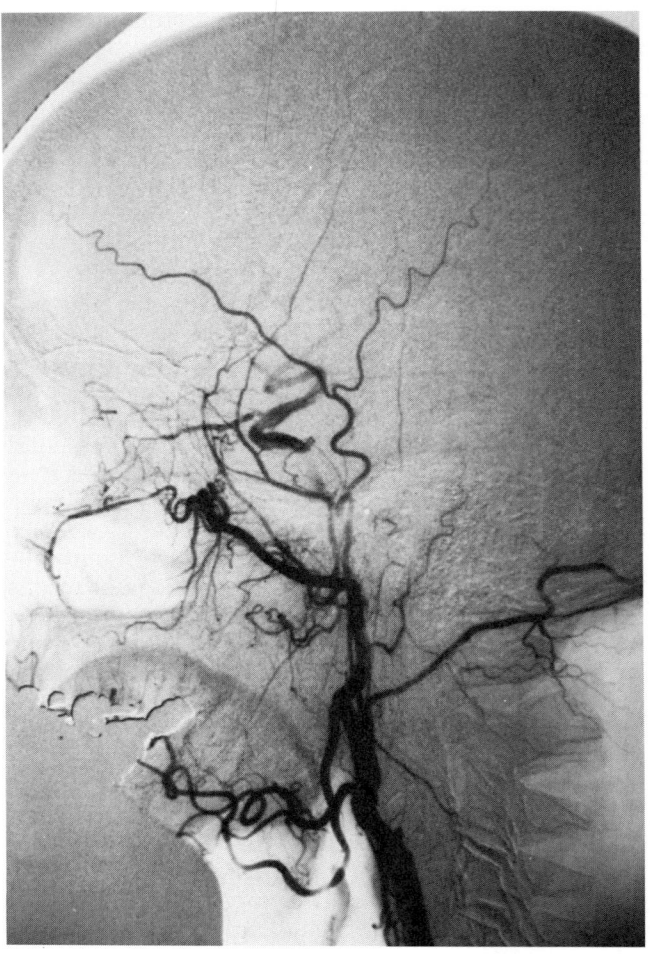

Figure 4 This patient had a known advanced left carotid stenosis and developed crescendo TIAs followed by a nondisabling left hemispheric stroke over 48 hours shortly after an inguinal hernia repair. Emergency arteriography disclosed occlusion of the proximal left internal carotid artery with retrograde filling via collaterals of most of the intracranial internal carotid artery.

neurologic deficit to plateau before undertaking CEA. We have waited days to weeks while maintaining anticoagulant therapy with equivalent good results. However, early operation is preferred because of the safety of early CEA after nondisabling stroke and the risk of recurrent stroke from severe carotid stenosis, even while the patient is on anticoagulant therapy.[14]

When thrombolytic therapy is unavailable or unsuccessful, emergency CEA should be performed immediately after angiography. Prograde flow of tiny amounts of contrast medium seen on late phase films ("ghost" carotid or a "string" sign) or retrograde filling of the carotid siphon from collateral sources appear to be good predictors of a patent ICA with the anticipation of an excellent result following CEA. In the latter case the ICA appears angiographically "nonpatent" with a column of nonopacified blood distal to a short segment occlusion (Fig. 4, 5, and 6).

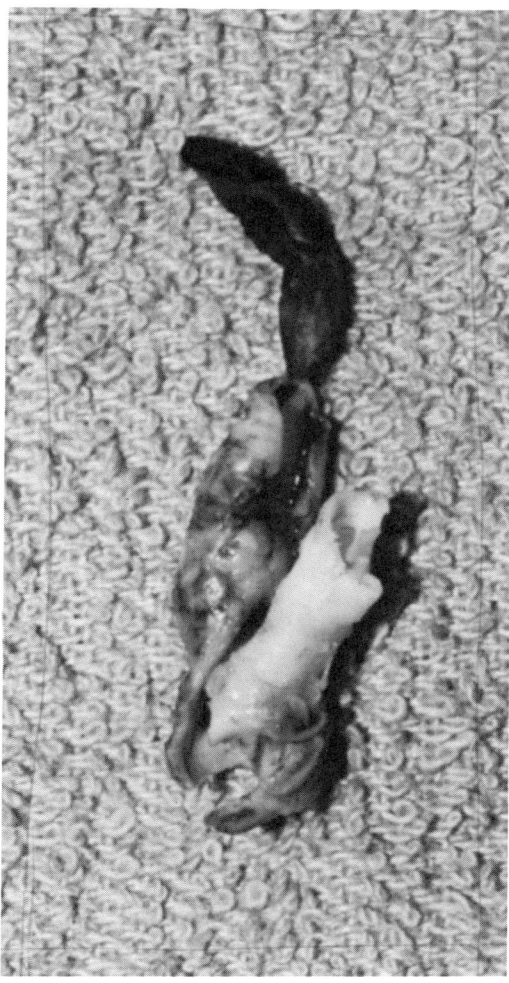

Figure 5 Operative specimen after emergency carotid endarterectomy in patient whose angiogram is shown in Figure 4. A small amount of occluding thrombus was present at the distal portion of the severely stenotic plaque. The internal carotid artery was patent distally.

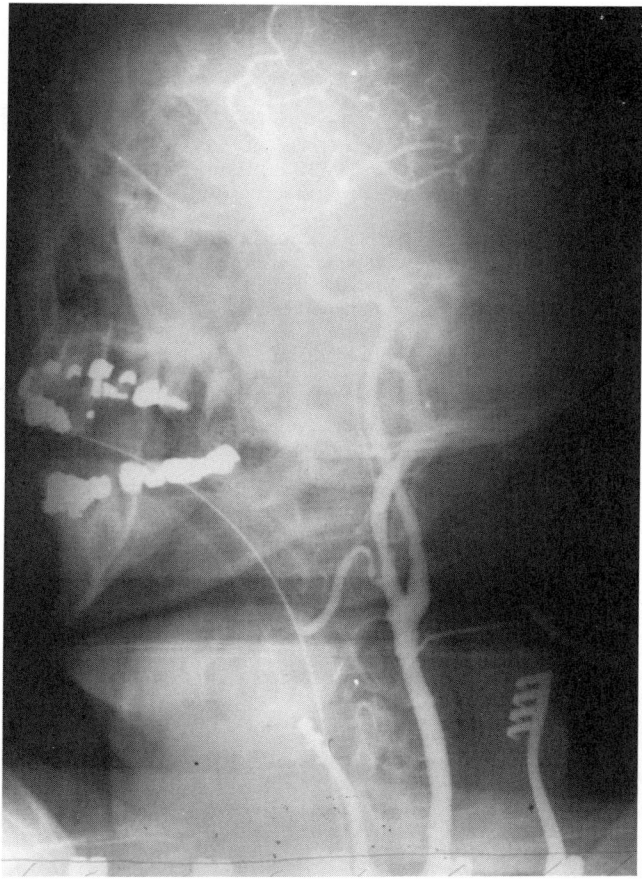

Figure 6 Operative arteriogram in the patient presented in Figures 4 and 5. Complete patency of the left internal carotid artery was restored, and the patient made an excellent recovery with no permanent neurologic deficit.

There are several important technical considerations in performing CEA under these circumstances. First, heparin sodium anticoagulation is maintained throughout. Second, the utmost care must be taken during dissection not to embolize loose thrombus in the ICA. The ICA is not cross-clamped initially for fear of fragmenting thrombus. Clamps are applied to the common and external carotid arteries, and an arteriotomy is begun distally on the ICA just beyond the bifurcation plaque. Most often, a small amount of thrombus is extruded through the arteriotomy by backbleeding. On occasion, teasing thrombus free with the help of a 3 Fr embolectomy catheter carefully placed up the ICA may be necessary. If thrombus is adherent and backbleeding cannot be obtained, the ICA should be ligated. If significant stenosis of the external carotid artery is present, consideration for CEA and reconstruction of this vessel is warranted. If good backbleeding of the ICA is obtained, the vessel may then be cross-clamped, the arteriotomy extended down into the common carotid artery, and a small, straight 10 Fr shunt inserted. Because minutes may be important in reversing and salvaging the ischemic penumbra, a shunt is important. Finally, at the conclusion of endarterectomy, an operative arteriogram is obtained to ensure patency of the distal ICA. An operative arteriogram is usually inadequate to fully assess the MCA. However, visualization of this vessel is not needed if the patient awakens neurologically intact. In the event that the patient awakens with no improvement or worsening of the deficit, consideration should be given to repeat formal angiography to assess the MCA. If an embolus is present in this vessel, selective thrombolytic therapy with small catheters would be feasible.

REFERENCES

1. Mayberg MR, Wilson SE, Yatsu F, et al. Carotid endarterectomy and prevention of cerebral ischemia in symptomatic carotid

stenosis. Veterans Affairs Cooperative Studies Program 309 Trialist Group. JAMA 1991; 266:3289–3294.
2. Meyer FB, Sundt TM Jr, Piepgras DG, et al. Emergency carotid endarterectomy for patients with acute carotid occlusion and profound neurological deficits. Ann Surg 1986; 203:82–89.
3. Sherman DG, Dyken ML Jr, Fisher M, et al. Antithrombotic therapy for cerebrovascular disorders. Chest 1992; 102:529S–537S.
4. Duke RJ, Bloch RF, Turpie AGG, et al. Intravenous heparin for the prevention of stroke progression in acute partial stable stroke: randomized controlled trial. Ann Intern Med 1986; 105:825–828.
5. Biller J, Bruno A, Adams HP Jr, et al. A randomized trial of aspirin or heparin in hospitalized patients with recent transient ischemic attacks. A pilot study. Stroke 1989; 20:441–447.
6. North American Symptomatic Carotid Endarterectomy Trial Collaborators. Beneficial effect of carotid endarterectomy in symptomatic patients with high-grade carotid stenosis. N Engl J Med 1991; 325:445–453.
7. Blaisdell WF, Clauss RH, Galbraith JG, et al. Joint study of extracranial arterial occlusion. IV. A review of surgical considerations. JAMA 1969; 209:1889–1895.
8. Wylie EJ, Hein M, Adams JE. Intracranial hemorrhage following surgical revascularization for treatment of acute strokes. J Neurosurg 1964; 21:212–215.
9. Gertler JP, Blankensteijn JD, Brewster DC, et al. Carotid endarterectomy in neurologically unstable patients: Do results justify an aggressive approach? J Vasc Surg 1994;19:32-42.
10. Wardlaw JM, Warlow CP. Thrombolysis in acute ischemic stroke: Does it work? Stroke 1992; 23:1826–1839.
11. Brott TG, Haley EC Jr, Levy DE, et al. Urgent therapy for stroke. Part I. Pilot study of tissue plasminogen activator administered within 90 minutes. Stroke 1992; 23:632–640.
12. Astrup J, Siesjo BK, Symon L. Thresholds in cerebral ischemia: The ischemic penumbra. Stroke 1981; 12:723–725.
13. Jones TH, Morawetz RB, Crowell RM, et al. Thresholds of focal cerebral ischemia in awake monkeys. J Neurosurg 1981; 54: 773–782.
14. Gasecki AP, Eliasziw M, Ferguson GG, et al. The importance of early endarterectomy for severe carotid stenosis after a nondisabling stroke: Results from NASCET. J Vasc Surg (in press).

SURGICAL TREATMENT OF FIXED STROKE SECONDARY TO CAROTID ARTERY ATHEROSCLEROSIS

HUGH G. BEEBE, M.D.

The fundamental rationale for carotid endarterectomy after stroke has occurred is protection from greater neurologic damage. Carotid endarterectomy (CEA) following stroke can be considered in patients meeting three criteria: (1) a patent carotid artery ipsilateral to the hemisphere affected, (2) a degree of stenosis and/or ulceration in that artery consistent with current standards of severity that qualify for surgical intervention, and (3) enough recovery from stroke to afford reasonable function. Examination of the results of best medical management with or without CEA should disclose whether such surgical therapy is worthwhile.

One recent report on this subject documented recurrent ischemic stroke in patients with carotid bulb atherosclerosis to be essentially the same whether treated surgically or not.[1] Although this report suggested a significant benefit to surgical therapy, the number of patients in each cohort beyond the 6 year interval (23 surgical versus 17 nonsurgical) makes statistical interpretation difficult. Hertzer and Arison documented a cumulative stroke rate of 25% in 80 patients followed for at least 10 years after CEA for prior stroke, but the large majority of these also occurred during the first 5 years.[2]

In the opinion of some thoughtful physicians, little benefit can be derived from CEA in patients who have suffered an ischemic stroke because of the high rate of mortality, principally from cardiac cause, that runs about 6% to 10% per year. However, many patients fear stroke more than death. Recurrent stroke is common, with estimates as high as 5% to 10% per year. It is usually increased by diabetes. However, these data include little that serves as an adequate comparison for evaluating surgical therapy because they lack information about the degree of carotid atherosclerosis.

Bernstein and colleagues analyzed late outcome following CEA in 127 patients who sustained a preoperative stroke and found that CEA may not be superior to nonoperative treatment.[3] In the stroke patients, compared to a consecutive series of 456 operations for all indications, operative mortality was higher (3.1% versus 0.9%), as was postoperative permanent neurologic deficit (3.9% versus 2.1%). Five years postoperatively, 24% of the preoperative stroke cohort had suffered serious morbidity or death. Rubin and colleagues reported that 95 patients had a 96.8% cumulative stroke-free survival for 5 years after CEA done for history of prior stroke with a combined operative morbidity and mortality of 2.7%.[4]

A report of the Ad Hoc Committee of the Joint Council of the Society for Vascular Surgery and the North American Chapter of the International Society for Cardiovascular Surgery noted[5]: "Carotid endarterectomy has been used effectively to reduce the risk of recurrent stroke in patients with cerebral infarction as a result of carotid bifurcation disease. The operation carries an increased risk, and the recommendation of the Stroke Council of the American Heart Association has been that operation should be undertaken only by those who can achieve an operative morbidity and mortality rate of less than 7% for this group of patients.[6] Ideally, the rate should be less than 5%."

Another matter is the growing recognition that many patients who are categorized as having had a transient ischemic attack (TIA) or who are asymptomatic have computed tomography (CT) evidence of cerebral infarction. Ricotta and colleagues have documented positive CT scans from 21% in asymptomatic patients with carotid bifurcation disease to nearly 33% of those with symptoms of TIA.[7,8] If such patients can be thought of as having an "asymptomatic stroke," what is the correct assignment of their operative risk and expected result? Should they be categorized together with those whose stroke is clinically apparent?

Two recently completed randomized prospective trials of CEA included patients with prior stroke. In the North American Symptomatic Carotid Endarterectomy Trial (NASCET), the cumulative risk of ipsilateral stroke at 2 years was 26% in 331 medical patients and 9% in 328 surgical patients.[9] It was concluded that CEA is highly beneficial to patients with nondisabling strokes and ipsilateral high-grade stenosis of the internal carotid artery.

The Veterans Administration Cooperative Trial documented benefit in a group of 193 patients randomly assigned carotid endarterectomy, of whom slightly more than one-third had prior stroke.[10] At a mean follow-up of less than 1 year, there was a significant reduction in stroke or crescendo TIA in patients who underwent CEA (7.7%) compared to nonsurgical patients (19.4%).

TIMING OF OPERATION

Several recent trends make it increasingly difficult to determine the timing of operation following stroke. For one thing, the definition of what constitutes a "completed stroke" appears to be blurred because of the information gathered from brain CT studies. The category of a reversible ischemic neurologic deficit (RIND), a neurologic deficit lasting more than 24 hours but resolving within 3 weeks, seems less useful than in the past. The tendency in recent years is to group these patients together as simply having had a stroke with good early recovery. There is also the difficulty of how to classify patients whose symptoms are characteristic of TIA with evidence of cerebral infarction on CT scan. Furthermore, patients with relatively minor fixed neurologic deficits who do not have CT scan abnormalities are not clearly different from those with similar symptoms whose CT scans are positive.

More than 25 years ago, high mortality rates were associated with CEA following acute stroke. This was well documented in reports of the classic joint study of extracranial arterial occlusion. Whittemore and associates reported that half of 28 patients with hemodynamically significant carotid lesions and small, fixed strokes were operated upon within 7 days of the onset of symptoms, and none sustained a new postoperative deficit.[11] However, Ricotta and co-workers identified a 40% increase in neurologic morbidity and 10% mortality in operating acutely upon patients with a positive CT scan.[7]

More recently, Piotrowski and colleagues questioned the traditional delay of at least 6 weeks before performing CEA after acute stroke.[12] They examined the outcomes after CEA in 140 patients whose operations occurred at variable intervals after stroke. Although this group included a variety of subsets of patients, no significant difference was found in the incidence of postoperative cerebrovascular complications with respect to the timing of CEA. They concluded that the operation could be done safely after acute stroke so long as neurologic recovery had reached a plateau.

The traditional interval of 4 to 6 weeks between the onset of a fixed neurologic deficit and subsequent CEA has become dogma largely on the basis of anecdotal evidence. Still, because the consequences of hemorrhage into areas of brain infarction are so severe, the onus for proof of safety rests upon those who would operate earlier. There is little documentation of the incidence of recurrent stroke during the first 6 weeks in unoperated patients in whom the cause of stroke was a carotid bifurcation lesion.

The Ad Hoc Committee for carotid endarterectomy guidelines of the Joint Council of the two major vascular societies also commented upon timing issues: "The timing of intervention has never been agreed on, and there are recommendations that range from a specifically defined interval of 6 weeks to 3 months to an interval that varies depending on the clinical condition of the patient."[5] The timing of operation in patients who have sustained a stroke is important. Although serial CT scanning offers a theoretical basis for selective timing of operation, the reported experience with this modality is neither extensive nor prospective. Thus, a cautious approach that takes into account the angiographic appearance of the carotid lesion in question would seem appropriate at present. The combination of appropriately timed serial CT scans showing no evidence of extensive infarction or surrounding hyperemia, an interval of neurologic stability, and the suggestion of an unstable or preocclusive lesion by duplex scan or arteriography would favor early operation.

TECHNIQUE OF OPERATION

Carotid endarterectomy after stroke should be conducted in the same way that endarterectomy is performed for other indications with two differences. The first is recognition that the range of patient tolerance for any physiologic aberration is smaller than in patients who have not sustained a preoperative neurologic deficit. Thus, defining blood pressure limits during and after operation within a narrow range and accepting the expense of premixing vasoactive drugs for immediate intravenous use in advance of actual need are useful. The second difference is in consideration of methods to ensure cerebral protection during the operation. Routine shunting in all such patients has the theoretical benefit of protecting brain tissue that may be marginally perfused. Some patients who have sustained a cerebral infarction can be presumed to have an area of adjacent brain tissue that is marginally perfused, and thus may develop an ischemic penumbra when the carotid artery is clamped during operation. Not all brain effects from transient, barely inadequate blood flow are immediately noticed, no matter whether the operation is done using regional or general anesthesia and with electroencephalographic (EEG) or carotid stump blood pressure monitoring. Indeed, monitoring techniques such as EEG or carotid stump blood pressures after clamping may not be reliable in patients having sustained a preoperative stroke. Stroke patients are frequently observed to have lower carotid stump blood pressures than those without neurologic deficit, and this blood pressure may be variable during the procedure.

Some surgeons who are opposed to shunting have shown acceptable morbidity rates in poststroke patients. Conversely, other surgeons have evidence that patients with a stroke history more often need shunt protection than those with transient or asymptomatic carotid disease. For example, Whittemore and associates employed selective shunting based on intraoperative EEG monitoring and found that 40% of their patients demonstrated the need for a shunt.[11] Either routine shunting or effective monitoring for shunt need, probably best accomplished by interrogating a regionally anesthetized patient during operation, ought to be standards of care.

REFERENCES

1. Rosenthal D, Borrero E, Clark MD, et al. Carotid endarterectomy after reversible ischemic neurologic deficit or stroke: Is it of value? J Vasc Surg 8:527-534, 1988.
2. Hertzer NR, Arison R. Cumulative stroke and survival ten years after carotid endarterectomy. J Vasc Surg 2:661-668, 1985.
3. Bernstein EF, Humber PB, Collins GM, et al. Life expectancy and late stroke following carotid endarterectomy. Ann Surg 198:80-86, 1983.
4. Rubin JR, Goldstone J, McIntyre KE Jr, et al. The value of carotid endarterectomy in reducing the morbidity and mortality of recurrent stroke. J Vasc Surg 4:443-449, 1986.
5. Moore WS, Mohr JP, Najafi H, et al. Carotid endarterectomy: Practice guidelines. Report of the Ad Hoc Committee to the Joint Council of the Society for Vascular Surgery and the North American Chapter of the International Society for Cardiovascular Surgery. J Vasc Surg 15:469-479, 1992.
6. Beebe HG, Clagett GP, DeWeese JA, et al. Assessing risk associated with carotid endarterectomy. Stroke 20:314–315, 1989.
7. Ricotta JJ, Ouriel K, Green RM, DeWeese JA. Use of computerized cerebral tomography in selection of patients for elective and urgent carotid endarterectomy. Ann Surg 202:783-787, 1985.
8. Street DL, O'Brien MS, Ricotta JJ, et al. Observations on cerebral computed tomography in patients having carotid endarterectomy. J Vasc Surg 7:798-801, 1988.
9. North American Symptomatic Carotid Endarterectomy Trial Collaborators. Beneficial effect of carotid endarterectomy in symptomatic patients with high-grade carotid stenosis. N Engl J Med 325:445-453, 1991.
10. Mayberg MR, Wilson SE, Yatsu F, et al. Carotid endarterectomy and prevention of cerebral ischemia in symptomatic carotid stenosis. JAMA 266:3289-3294, 1991.
11. Whittemore AD, Ruby ST, Couch NP, Mannick JA: Early carotid endarterectomy in patients with small, fixed neurologic deficits. J Vasc Surg 1:795-799, 1984.
12. Piotrowski JJ, Bernhard VM, Rubin JR, et al. Timing of carotid endarterectomy after acute stroke. J Vasc Surg 11:45-52, 1990.

TECHNICAL ASPECTS OF CAROTID ENDARTERECTOMY FOR ATHEROSCLEROTIC DISEASE

CALVIN B. ERNST, M.D.

There is almost universal agreement that carotid endarterectomy (CEA) is indicated for symptomatic atherosclerotic lesions of the carotid bifurcation. Reports of recent randomized clinical trials have confirmed what vascular surgeons have suspected for many years.[1,2] Since the first successful CEA, millions of patients have benefited from this conceptually straightforward operation. Over the subsequent four decades, the technical aspects of CEA have been refined and become standardized. Yet in the hands of an inexperienced surgeon, this established procedure may prove disastrous. Few vascular operations are as unforgiving as a technically inadequate CEA. Consequently, strict attention to operative technical details is mandatory for success. The procedure must be flawless. To this end, it has been suggested that only experienced surgeons, those with a combined operative mortality and stroke rate of less than 5%, should perform CEAs.[3] Controversy remains, however, over appropriate management of the asymptomatic carotid bifurcation lesion. Some surgeons recommend operation for high-grade asymptomatic lesions, whereas others remain circumspect and await the results of randomized clinical trials addressing the asymptomatic lesion.[4]

After thorough preoperative preparation, many patients are admitted to the hospital the morning of operation. Those with complicating comorbidities are admitted the day before.

All preoperative medications are continued, including aspirin. The nuisance of wound oozing secondary to aspirin effect is offset by the platelet antiaggregating effect and potential to prevent platelet thrombus formation at the endarterectomy site. Antibiotics are not routinely given.

ANESTHESIA AND MONITORING

A radial artery cannula is inserted prior to induction of anesthesia in all patients to monitor blood pressure and for arterial blood gas sampling. Pulmonary artery catheters are rarely used.

General endotracheal anesthesia is preferred unless the patient is very cooperative and desires regional block anesthesia. General endotracheal anesthesia assures a relaxed, stable milieu for both patient and surgeon, which is particularly helpful in a teaching hospital environment. When regional block anesthesia is employed, local tissue infiltration with 1% lidocaine without epinephrine is often required. It is important that supplemental sedation be used judiciously so that the patient remains responsive enough to permit evaluation of the neurologic status during carotid clamping.

After induction of anesthesia, the patient's head is turned slightly to the opposite side and the neck slightly extended. The table is placed in approximately 15° reversed Trendelenburg to minimize venous bleeding. When regional block anesthesia is used, draping must assure patient comfort by tenting the drape over the face. The anesthesiologist must have ready access to the airway in the event endotracheal intubation is required.

EXPOSURE OF THE CAROTID VESSELS

If the atherosclerotic lesion appears complex and extends into the mid to distal one-third of the internal carotid artery, which occurs in approximately 3% of patients, ipsilateral temporary mandibular subluxation has proven useful in exposing the internal carotid artery to within 1 to 2 cm of the base of the skull.[5] Such distal exposure assures precise and complete removal of the offending plaque, which, under the unusual circumstances of extensive distal disease, may not be possible with standard exposure. Temporary mandibular subluxation requires nasotracheal intubation and general anesthesia. Such subluxation maneuvers are performed in cooperation with an oral surgeon. It is important only to sublux the ipsilateral mandible and avoid dislocation, which may damage the temporomandibular joint cartilage. In dentate patients the subluxation position is held by Ivy loop interdental diagonal wiring of an ipsilateral mandibular cuspid or bicuspid tooth to a contralateral maxillary bicuspid or cuspid tooth with 25 gauge stainless-steel wire. In edentulous patients, stabilization is maintained by intermaxillary-mandibular wiring around two 3/32 inch Steinmann pins drilled intraorally at the gingival margins into the ipsilateral mandible and the contralateral maxilla. After the endarterectomy, the fixation wires are removed, and the subluxation is reduced.

A 10 cm skin incision is made along the anterior border of the sternocleidomastoid muscle and extended through the platysma muscle and superficial layer of the deep cervical fascia. Hemostasis is obtained with fine silk ties and electrocautery. If distal exposure is required, the skin incision is extended cephalad behind the parotid gland, often to the retroauricular area.

The anterior facial vein, under which the carotid bifurcation lies, is divided between silk ties after the fascia along the anterior border of the sternocleidomastoid muscle is incised. After the sternocleidomastoid muscle is mobilized and retracted posteriorly, the carotid sheath is incised and the distal common carotid artery is mobilized and encircled with a suitable loop. A short length of PE-90 polyethylene tubing serves well because by lifting it carotid dissection is facilitated by the no-touch technique. The vagus nerve is identified lying between the internal jugular vein and the common carotid artery. Two Wietlaner retractors are placed, and dissection proceeds cephalad on the common carotid artery to its bifurcation. The self-retaining retractors must be placed with care so as not to impale and injure the vagus nerve. The superior thyroid artery, which branches from the most distal common carotid artery or most proximal external carotid, is ligated and divided flush with its origin to avoid injury to the superior laryngeal nerve.

The interval between the internal and external carotid vessels is incised, and the proximal external carotid artery is encircled with PE-90 polyethylene tubing, which is threaded through an 8 cm segment of an 18 Fr catheter. This will later serve for external carotid snare occlusion. The carotid sinus nerve is preserved insofar as possible. If, during dissection of the carotid bifurcation, hypotension or bradycardia develops, 1 to 2 ml of 1% lidocaine is injected into the carotid sinus area between the internal and external carotid vessels to block the baroreceptor mechanism. This is rarely required. Traction on both polyethylene catheters allows gentle, atraumatic, no-touch dissection of the carotid bifurcation and proximal internal carotid artery. As dissection proceeds cephalad, the hypoglossal nerve is identified as it crosses the external carotid artery. Ligating the sternocleidomastoid branch of the external carotid artery, which passes over and tethers the hypoglossal nerve, facilitates mobilization of the nerve during distal dissection. Also, the descending branch of the hypoglossal nerve serves as a marker to the hypoglossal nerve by tracing it cephalad. If in the way, the descending branch can be divided 0.5 cm from the main trunk.

The internal carotid artery is dissected approximately 2 cm beyond the lesion. Occasionally, the posterior belly of the digastric muscle must be divided to gain adequate exposure of the internal carotid artery beyond the plaque. Additional exposure may be obtained by dividing the styloglossus, the stylopharyngeus, and the stylohyoid muscles. If necessary, the styloid process can be excised. It must be kept in mind that the spinal accessory nerve is vulnerable when the mastoid insertion of the sternocleidomastoid muscle is mobilized to excise the styloid process. During dissection of the mid to distal internal carotid artery, delicate overlying veins must be carefully ligated. Use of the electrocautery is discouraged lest injury to the hypoglossal, vagus, or glossopharyngeal nerves occur during such high dissections. In addition, the occipital artery that courses posteriorly and overlies the internal carotid may require ligation and division. Most plaques extend only 1 to 2 cm into the internal carotid artery, and the extensive distal dissection described is usually not required.

Electroencephalographic (EEG) monitoring is preferred in the anesthetized patient. A standard 18 lead EEG is employed. During carotid clamping an EEG technologist monitors the recording. In the event cortical ischemia develops after 2 minutes of test occlusion of the common and external carotid vessels, which is manifested by diminished wave amplitudes and frequencies, a long Sundt shunt is placed. If a pulse is felt in the internal carotid artery after clamping the common carotid and tightening the PE-90 snare on the external carotid, it is almost never necessary to use a shunt. When performing the endarterectomy without a shunt, it is important that the anesthesiologist maintain the patient's systolic blood pressure at a level to maintain normal EEG tracings.

It has been suggested that patients with contralateral internal carotid occlusions or previous ipsilateral hemispheric strokes routinely require a shunt. In my experience this has not been true, especially when employing EEG monitoring or operating upon the awake patient. When using cervical block anesthesia supplemented with local anesthesia injection, the patient's continued conversation with the anesthesiologist or surgeon in addition to the patient squeezing a squeaker device with the contralateral hand documents adequate cerebral perfusion.

Routine shunting obviates need for monitoring cerebral perfusion, but working around a shunt adds some technical complexity to the endarterectomy. In the event cerebral perfusion deteriorates after carotid clamping or during the endarterectomy, the Sundt shunt is expeditiously inserted and secured by Javid shunt clamps. The shunt is inserted into the internal carotid artery first, backbled to flush air, and then inserted into the common carotid artery. It is important to backbleed the shunt and fill the cul-de-sac at the proximal end of the arteriotomy to remove any trapped air. The shunt is temporarily clamped while it is inserted and secured in the common carotid artery. The shunt clamp is then removed, and the blood flow stream in the shunt is scrutinized for any bits of debris or air. If such material is seen, the shunt is reclamped, extracted from the common carotid artery, backbled once again, and then reinserted. The properly placed shunt assumes a loop configuration. Because a shunt complicates the endarterectomy, particularly at the distal extent, a shunt is not used routinely but only when necessary, in about 10% of patients.

CAROTID ENDARTERECTOMY

After complete mobilization of the common, internal, and proximal external carotid arteries, 50 to 100 units/kg of heparin sodium are given intravenously and monitored by the activated clotting time. After 2 to 3 minutes, the external carotid artery snare is tightened and the common carotid artery is clamped while the EEG technician monitors the tracing. The internal carotid artery pulse is palpated and if there are no EEG tracing abnormalities, the internal carotid is clamped with a low-tension serrefine clamp. An arteriotomy is made in the common carotid artery extending anterolaterally through the plaque into the internal carotid artery beyond the distal extension of the plaque. Straying too far medially along the bifurcation into the internal carotid artery complicates subsequent arteriotomy closure.

If the EEG tracing remains normal, the appropriate plane in the deep layer of the media is entered with a Freer elevator, and the endarterectomy proceeds from the common carotid artery cephalad. The intimomedial layer is dissected circumferentially in the common carotid and transected, providing a sharp transition at the proximal end of the specimen. The specimen is further dissected, pushing the plaque away from the artery up to the external carotid artery ostium. The external carotid artery snare is released, and an eversion endarterectomy of the proximal external carotid is performed, transecting the plaque sharply in the external carotid. After assuring a smooth external carotid plaque transition by direct inspection, the snare is retightened. The endarterectomy proceeds into the internal carotid artery. With gentle caudad traction on the specimen, it usually feathers out into a smooth transition from the endarterectomized segment to normal appearing intima. Occasionally, however, the distal portion of the specimen must be sharply divided because a smooth, feathered transition cannot be obtained. Under these circumstances, if the distal intima is not firmly attached, one or two 7-0 double-armed polypropylene tacking sutures are placed to secure the distal intima to prevent intimal flap development.

After excision of the specimen, loose strands of media are meticulously removed from the endarterectomized segment. Fine-tipped ringed forceps facilitate such fragment removal. The endarterectomized segment is vigorously irrigated with heparin sodium–saline solution using a bulb syringe and an 18 gauge blunt-tipped needle. Removing loose fragments of retained media is one of the most important parts of the operation because overlooked and retained bits of medial debris may embolize and cause a neurologic deficit after restoration of blood flow.

The arteriotomy is closed without a patch unless the internal carotid is less than 3 mm in diameter or unless it is a redo operation. Arteriotomy closure begins distally by using a continuous 7-0 double-armed polypropylene suture to place the first suture from inside out at the arteriotomy apex. This is continued proximally to the level of the bifurcation, and then a second 6-0 double-armed polypropylene suture is used, closing the proximal portion of the arteriotomy. It is important to place the most distal 7-0 suture and most proximal 6-0 suture precisely to avoid constricting the lumen. Before the final three to four sutures are placed, the vessels are flushed first by temporarily releasing the external carotid snare, then the internal carotid clamp, and finally the common carotid clamp. After each flush, the endarterectomized lumen is irrigated with heparin sodium–saline solution.

After the flushing and irrigation maneuvers, approximately 10 to 20 ml of low-molecular-weight dextran is instilled into the lumen, the arteriotomy closure is completed, and the two sutures are tied to each other. After removing the external carotid artery snare and the common carotid artery clamp and while temporarily pinching the internal carotid artery at its origin with forceps, several pulses of blood are allowed into the external carotid artery circulation. Finally, the internal carotid artery is released, restoring pulsatile flow.

If a shunt was required, it is removed prior to placing the final four or five sutures, and the flushing sequence follows. There is no need for haste because shunt removal and arteriorrhaphy completion can almost always be accomplished in a few minutes.

If it appears that closure of the arteriotomy will compromise the lumen, patch angioplasty closure is performed using autogenous saphenous vein harvested from the groin. Using meticulous suturing technique with double-armed 7-0 and 6-0 polypropylene suture as described for the primary closure, the patching maneuver is completed. It is important to limit the diameter of the patch to about 5 mm so as not to create an aneurysmal configuration at the site of closure.

Following restoration of blood flow and assuring that the suture line is secure and hemostasis is complete, the heparin sodium effect is reversed by using protamine sulfate. The appropriate dose is calculated, depending upon the activated clotting time, duration, and amount of heparin sodium given. For example, for 5,000 units of heparin sodium and a 30 minute clamp time, approximately 25 mg of protamine sulfate is required to reverse the heparin sodium effect.

A sterile, continuous-wave Doppler pencil-tipped probe is placed over the internal, external, and common carotid vessels to assure normal sounding pulsatile flow, following which the wound is closed without a drain. The platysma is closed with 4-0 absorbable sutures and the skin with clips. The patient is awakened in the operating room and, after an unchanged neurologic examination is documented, moved to the recovery room.

Although endarterectomy techniques may vary slightly from surgeon to surgeon, the one described works well in my hands. The critical elements common to all flawless carotid endarterectomies include adequate mobilization of the internal carotid artery beyond the plaque, precise placement of the arteriotomy, meticulous debridement of all loose fragments from the endarterectomized segment, and meticulous arteriotomy closure to prevent a proximal constrictive shelf forming at the transition point or distal intimal flap development.

REFERENCES

1. NASCET Collaborators. Beneficial effect of carotid endarterectomy in symptomatic patients with high-grade carotid stenosis. N Engl J Med 1991; 325:445–453.
2. European Carotid Surgery Trialists' (ECST) Collaborative Group. MRC European carotid surgery interim results for symptomatic patients with severe (70–99%) or mild (0–29%) carotid stenosis. Lancet 1991; 337:1235–1243.
3. Moore WS, Mohr JP, Jr., Najafi H, et al. Carotid endarterectomy: Practice guidelines. Report of the Ad Hoc Committee to the Joint Council of the Society for Vascular Surgery and the North American Chapter of the International Society for Cardiovascular Surgery. J Vasc Surg 1992; 15:469–479.
4. The Asymptomatic Carotid Atherosclerosis Study Group: Study for design for randomized prospective trial of carotid endarterectomy for asymptomatic atherosclerosis. Stroke 1989; 20:844–849.
5. Dossa C, Shepard AD, Wolford DG, et al. Distal internal carotid exposure: A simplified technique for temporary mandibular subluxation. J Vasc Surg 1990; 12:319–325.

REGIONAL AND LOCAL ANESTHESIA FOR CAROTID ENDARTERECTOMY

WILLIAM E. EVANS, M.D.
ENRIQUE GINZBURG, M.D.

Many and varied methods of cerebral protection have been used in the attempt to increase the safety of carotid artery reconstruction. For many years, our carotid artery operations were done under general anesthesia, with selective shunting determined by findings of electroencephalography (EEG) and/or carotid artery stump blood pressure. Unfortunately, criteria employed tended to vary not only from surgeon to surgeon but also from time to time with individual surgeons. In 1983, a review of our carotid artery operations showed a permanent stroke rate for elective endarterectomy of slightly over 3%. These results were considered unacceptable, leading to a re-evaluation of our approach to carotid endarterectomy (CEA). Technical features were discussed in detail, videotapes of own procedures as well as those of others were critiqued, and respected colleagues were consulted. From this review it was concluded that our surgical techniques were standard and safe and probably did not need to be altered.

Next, we reassessed our method of intraoperative monitoring. Although others had obtained excellent results using EEG and carotid stump blood pressure monitoring, we decided to seek a different approach. We evaluated various methods. Some we felt to be unproved. Others appeared cumbersome. A few necessitated expensive equipment, and the most popular, routine shunting, appeared to have risks inherent to the protective method itself. We were aware of the studies of Imparato and colleagues, as well as those of Hafner, where CEA was being done using local or regional anesthesia, thus allowing direct assessment of neurologic status.[1,2] It was felt that direct assessment might have distinct advantages over the more traditional indirect methods, and the reported results convinced us to evaluate regional and/or local anesthesia as our standard anesthesia approach. We agreed that a shunt would be inserted only as a response to neurologic change. The EEGs and carotid stump blood pressures were routinely recorded, but this information was not available to influence the decision for or against shunt insertion. It was used retrospectively to help interpret results. The initial group of 134 operations was reported in 1985, followed by a combined study with Hafner of more than 1,200 carotid artery operations in 1988.[3,4] As expected, changes in the EEG or carotid stump blood pressure either predicted the onset of neurologic events or occurred simultaneously with the onset of the events in most, but unfortunately not all, patients. We concluded that monitoring awake neurologic status was at least as reliable as other methods, and in a small but significant minority probably better, because a few patients had neurologic events without the EEG or carotid stump blood pressure predicting such an event.

In these series, about 10% of patients developed deficits and thereby required a shunt. This rate for shunt insertion was much lower than would have been predicted if a carotid stump blood pressure of 50 mm Hg or even a pressure of 25 mm Hg had been used to determine the need for shunting. We were particularly gratified to find that the permanent stroke rate was less than 1%. The mortality rate was also under 1%, even though it appeared that more patients with severe medical problems had been included.

Although our initial approach was to use local anesthesia by layer-to-layer infiltration of local agents, regional cervical block supplemented by local infiltration is now our preferred method. The service of an experienced anesthesiologist is recommended, although results still are somewhat unpredictable, reflecting regional neuroanatomy, which appears obscure at best. This factor is reflected in the results of regional block. Approximately 40% to 50% of patients obtained a satisfactory block. The rest had an anesthetic response ranging from good to poor, requiring additional local infiltration. Even though the regional block is not always optimal, it is worth the attempt because a successful block provides a superior level of patient comfort. Pain, when it occurs in the surgical wound, is usually easily controlled with local infiltration. Occasional patients complain of severe pain referred to the ipsilateral teeth and external ear canal. The pain usually begins at the time of carotid artery clamping and can be controlled with infiltration of the adventitia.

Local and/or regional anesthesia is supplemented by sedation and analgesia, although in most patients intravenous midazolam hydrochloride (Versed) is adequate. The goal with the use of local and parenteral agents is a patient who is comfortable, quiet, and responsive because cooperation is vital for monitoring neurologic status.

Test clamping is routinely carried out for 2 to 3 minutes. Developing neurologic deficits prompts immediate restoration of carotid blood flow. Blood pressure should also be assessed because decreased consciousness occasionally results from hypotension. Restoration of normal blood pressure in such cases often allows subsequent successful carotid artery clamping. When not related to low blood pressure, unclamping the carotid artery restores perfusion and allows time to reassess the situation and to prepare for shunt insertion.

The operation is more difficult using local anesthesia than it is using general anesthesia. First, the neck can seldom be extended optimally, creating a slightly deeper field of dissection. With experience, this becomes less troublesome. Second, dissection must proceed more slowly and gently, particularly when the cervical block has not rendered the patient completely pain-free. It is vital to tend to the patient's comfort, thus allaying fear, anxiety, and agitation. This is particularly important when local and/or regional anesthesia has been chosen based on concerns about coronary disease and possible cardiac decompensation. Third, the patient, even under ideal conditions, is more mobile than if unconscious, which on occasion tries the patience of even the most imperturbable surgeon. Proper attention by anesthesiologist and surgeon can greatly attenuate this potential problem. Fourth, especially during a surgeon's early experience operating upon awake patients, the sudden onset of aphasia, hemiparesis, or changing mental status tends to test the surgeon's mettle. However, the knowledge that the episode clearly identifies a deficit of cerebral blood flow and that rapid shunt insertion restores neurologic function eventually results in an enhanced comfort level for the surgeon.

Patient selection is important, but one must be diligent lest the cause for exclusion be surgeon timidity rather than patient need. Occasional patients have general or local problems that make awake operations hazardous. For example, a patient with a rapid tic involving the head and neck was relegated to general anesthesia. Some patients simply refuse to be operated upon while awake, although it is of interest that most patients requiring a later contralateral endarterectomy, the first side having been done under regional, seldom request general anesthesia for the second side. Occasional patients present who are not emotionally stable or who are uncooperative. In these patients general anesthesia is usually a better choice. Patients operated upon for recurrent carotid artery problems are also best handled under general anesthesia. Scar tends to decrease the effectiveness of the blocks and of local infiltration. In addition, these operations are usually more tedious, requiring a well-controlled patient. The operations can be prolonged, which would unduly add to patient discomfort if done awake.

In addition to patient selection, surgeon temperament and abilities should be taken into consideration in anesthetic choice. If one's approach to carotid artery reconstruction is one of excessive tedium or if one's psyche is more attuned to the placid and the unmarred, general anesthesia is probably a better choice. Although I agree with Riles[3] that awake CEA is appropriate for trainees, the guidance of appropriate surgical staff is mandatory in order to proceed safely and quickly. In the main I remain convinced that CEA should be the purview of the facile, the intrepid, and the perspicacious. Nowhere is this more germane than in the patient operated upon while awake.

REFERENCES

1. Imparato AM, Ramirez A, Riles T, Mintzer R. Cerebral protection in carotid surgery. Arch Surg 1982; 117:1073–1078.
2. Hafner CD. Minimizing the risks of carotid endarterectomy. J Vasc Surg 1984; 1:392–397.
3. Hafner CD, Evans WE. Carotid endarterectomy with local anesthesia: Results and advantages. J Vasc Surg 1988; 7:232–239.
4. Evans WE, Hayes JP, Waltke EA, Vermilion BD. Optimal cerebral monitoring during carotid endarterectomy: Neurologic response under local anesthesia. J Vasc Surg 1985; 2:775–777.

MANAGEMENT OF OCCLUDED OR NEARLY OCCLUDED EXTRACRANIAL CAROTID ARTERIES

WILLIAM J. QUIÑONES-BALDRICH, M.D.

Management of patients with extracranial carotid artery occlusion depends on the etiology of the process, presence or absence of symptoms, and the responsible mechanism. Specific recommendations for management require delineation of the vascular anatomy in a particular patient. An understanding of the process responsible for the patient's symptoms must be sought in order to select an intervention with the most likelihood of success.

ETIOLOGY AND NATURAL HISTORY

The most common cause of extracranial carotid artery occlusion is atherosclerosis, either at the level of the carotid bulb and internal carotid artery, or at the origin of the common carotid artery. Progression of disease leads to thrombosis of the internal or common carotid artery, respectively. Three specific mechanisms may be responsible for symptoms in these patients. Occlusion of the internal carotid artery may lead to hypoperfusion of the ipsilateral hemisphere when collateral blood flow through the circle of Willis is inadequate. It is estimated that only 15% to 45% of patients have a complete circle of Willis. Then again, the process of atherosclerotic occlusion at the origin of the internal carotid artery may allow sufficient time for collateral circulation to develop, so that acute occlusion is often asymptomatic. As the artery thromboses, however, propagation of clot may occur to the intracranial portion of the carotid artery, with embolization to the middle or anterior cerebral artery occurring as collateral flow may wash out the distal end of this thrombus. Thus, although symptoms may not occur at the outset of the thrombosis, they may be manifested days or weeks later by this mechanism. Once a chronic occlusion has been established, symptoms may occur secondary to embolization through the external carotid artery either from the cul-de-sac formed by the internal carotid artery thrombosis or from a stenotic external carotid artery lesion that, in addition, may lead to hypoperfusion of the ipsilateral hemisphere. There are well-established communications between the external carotid and the internal carotid systems that acquire importance in patients with internal carotid artery occlusion (Fig. 1).

Certainly, recommended intervention must take into account the mechanism of the patient's symptoms. The presence of contralateral carotid artery disease also influences the choice of operation. Precise angiographic delineation of the perfusion of the cerebral hemispheres, with specific attention to the vascular supply of the symptomatic territory, will dictate the best intervention in such a patient. A patient with an internal carotid artery occlusion and significant contralateral carotid artery disease will benefit from contralateral endarterectomy, if the hemisphere ipsilateral to the occlusion is perfused by the patent stenotic contralateral system. If significant external carotid to internal carotid collaterals can be demonstrated with perfusion of the symptomatic hemisphere by the external system, however, a better choice of operation may be addressing an embolic source or stenotic lesion in the ipsilateral external carotid artery.

An additional cause of internal carotid artery thrombosis secondary to atherosclerosis is a stenosis in the intracranial carotid siphon, progressing to occlusion and leading to retrograde thrombosis of the internal carotid artery. The exact incidence of this process is not known. Based on studies done with transcranial Doppler, however, most patients with carotid artery thrombosis do not have significant siphon stenosis, and this is a relatively rare cause of internal carotid artery occlusion. The presence of a contralateral siphon stenosis or of significant intracranial arterial occlusive disease

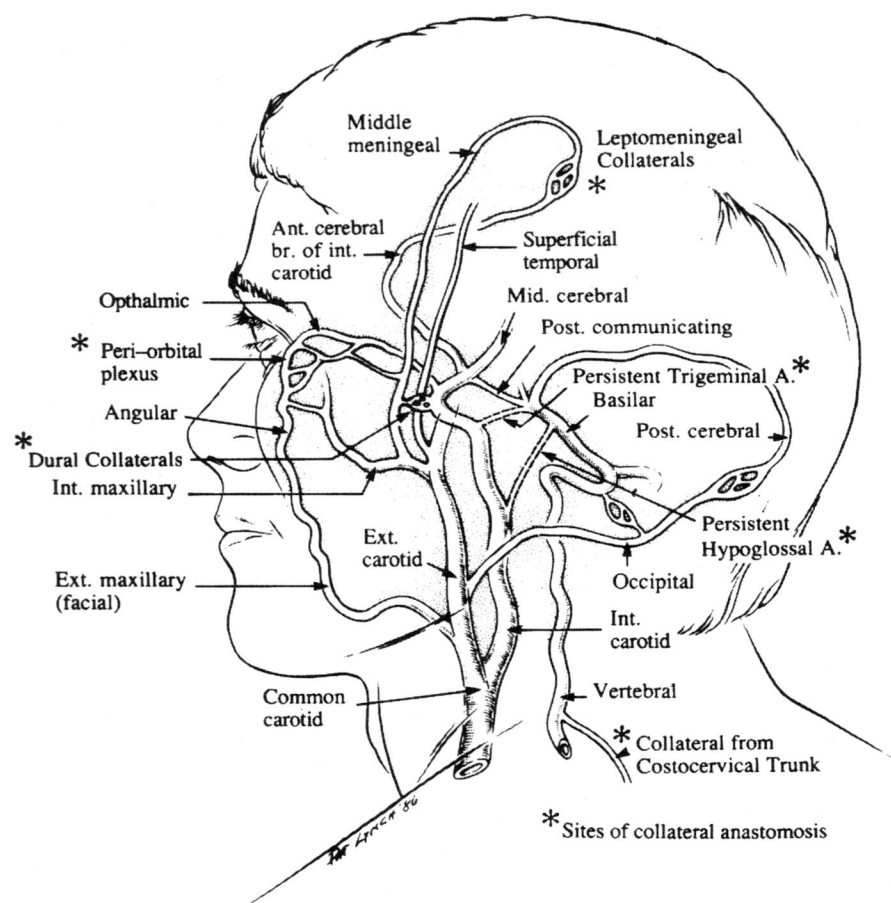

Figure 1 Collateral pathways that may acquire clinical importance in the presence of internal carotid artery occlusion. Note those collaterals denoted by the asterisk are specifically between the external carotid system and the internal carotid artery. These can provide perfusion through the external carotid artery to the internal system but may also serve as pathways for emboli originating at the origin of the external carotid artery. (From Gertler JP, Cambria RP. The role of external carotid endarterectomy in the treatment of ipsilateral internal carotid occlusion: Collective review. J Vasc Surg 1987; 6:158–167; with permission.)

documented by angiography should raise the suspicion of this process in specific patients. Intracranial disease is more common in diabetics, and the presence of this risk factor, especially with appropriate findings on angiography, would support this diagnosis. Certainly, the presence of a siphon stenosis leading to thrombosis of the internal carotid artery would be a contraindication for extracranial attempts at re-establishing patency. Conversely, other mechanisms responsible for symptoms (e.g., presence of a cul-de-sac with embolization through the external carotid or hypoperfusion through the external collaterals) can be managed similar to internal carotid artery occlusion secondary to other processes.

The natural history of patients with internal carotid artery occlusion secondary to atherosclerosis is mostly influenced by the occurrence of a stroke around the time of occlusion. Based on reports in the literature, patients with cerebral infarcts secondary to carotid thrombosis have a subsequent stroke risk of 8% to 12% per year. However, the long-term outcome of a patient with asymptomatic internal or common carotid artery thrombosis was no worse and, in fact, perhaps better than that of a patient with stenotic lesions. Thus, in the asymptomatic patient with a chronic occlusion, the benefit of revascularization is questionable. Conversely, symptomatic patients with carotid artery occlusion remain at a significant risk of future stroke and should be considered candidates for intervention, provided that specific anatomic delineation of the mechanisms of their symptoms can be established and proper intervention planned. Timing of the operation, as discussed later, is critical in patient selection. Results previously reported in the literature would suggest that patients with acute occlusion of the carotid artery should not undergo an operation if they are unstable or have a dense neurologic deficit or loss of consciousness. The natural history of a bland ischemic infarct is hemorrhagic conversion in approximately 20% of patients. This acute group of patients is at a significant potential risk of a hemorrhagic infarct when a thrombotic occlusion is surgically removed during the early critical period following a cerebral infarct.

DIAGNOSIS

Pseudo-occlusion of the internal carotid artery is one of several terms used to describe angiographically occluded, but anatomically patent, carotid arteries. Management of patients with documented patency of the internal carotid arteries distal to a severe stenosis is relatively straightforward, as standard carotid endarterectomy produces excellent results in this group of patients.[1] Symptomatic patients in this group are clearly candidates for operation, and a strong argument can be made to avoid progression to occlusion by prophylactic intervention in asymptomatic patients. Confirmation of internal carotid artery patency, however, remains difficult at times. Even with selective angiography, patency of the internal carotid artery may not be established preoperatively. Rapid-sequence computed tomographic (CT) scanning has been advocated in these instances, with the injection of contrast material delineating a patent internal carotid artery that otherwise was not visualized on angiography.[2] Duplex imaging cannot reliably distinguish pseudo-occlusion from occlusion of the internal carotid artery.[3] As the degree of stenosis increases, erythrocyte velocity through the point of maximal stenosis increases up to a point where extreme degrees of stenosis decrease the velocity of the erythrocytes. Filtration of the Doppler signal, necessary in these instruments, does not allow detection of blood flows that occur with extreme degrees of stenosis; an occlusion is suggested when, in reality, the vessel remains patent. O'Leary and colleagues suggested that pseudo-occlusion should be suspected when criteria for occlusion are present on the duplex scan and symptoms appropriate to that territory have occurred within the month preceding the noninvasive studies.[4] When pseudo-occlusion was suspected, they recommended selective catheterization of the common carotid artery with prolonged injection of contrast medium; filming in the lateral projection with coning to include both the carotid bifurcation and the supraclinoid carotid artery for at least 14 seconds using subtraction techniques. Alternatively, selective catheterization of the common carotid artery, with digital subtraction angiography with delayed views, may be used. Thus, the diagnosis of pseudo-occlusion was based on both thorough angiography and clinical presentation. Emerging new technology, such as magnetic resonance imaging, may improve the ability to establish vessel patency in these patients prior to exploration. Early experience with magnetic resonance angiography, however, has been limited and inconclusive.

From a practical standpoint, patients presenting with symptoms ipsilateral to a suspected carotid occlusion should be studied with selective angiography. If occlusion is diagnosed, carotid exploration may be recommended in symptomatic stable patients, as it may disclose an anatomically patent artery. If the internal carotid artery is found to be chronically occluded, external carotid artery endarterectomy and/or patch angioplasty with elimination of the cul-de-sac from the occluded internal carotid artery is of benefit in most instances. Thus, the combination of clinical and angiographic criteria may help select patients for intervention in the presence of suspected carotid artery occlusion or pseudo-occlusion. An additional angiographic criterion suggestive of pseudo-occlusion is the presence of a long, tapered, proximal internal carotid artery stump, as opposed to the short, blunt stump of true occlusion. In our experience, retrograde filling of the intracranial portion of the internal carotid artery through collaterals from the external carotid artery supports the diagnosis of pseudo-occlusion (Fig. 2). The well-described string sign, seen as a thin line of opacification in the area of the internal carotid artery, is highly suggestive of persistent patency of the internal carotid artery. Differential diagnosis of the string sign includes dissection of the internal carotid artery, radiation-associated carotid ar-

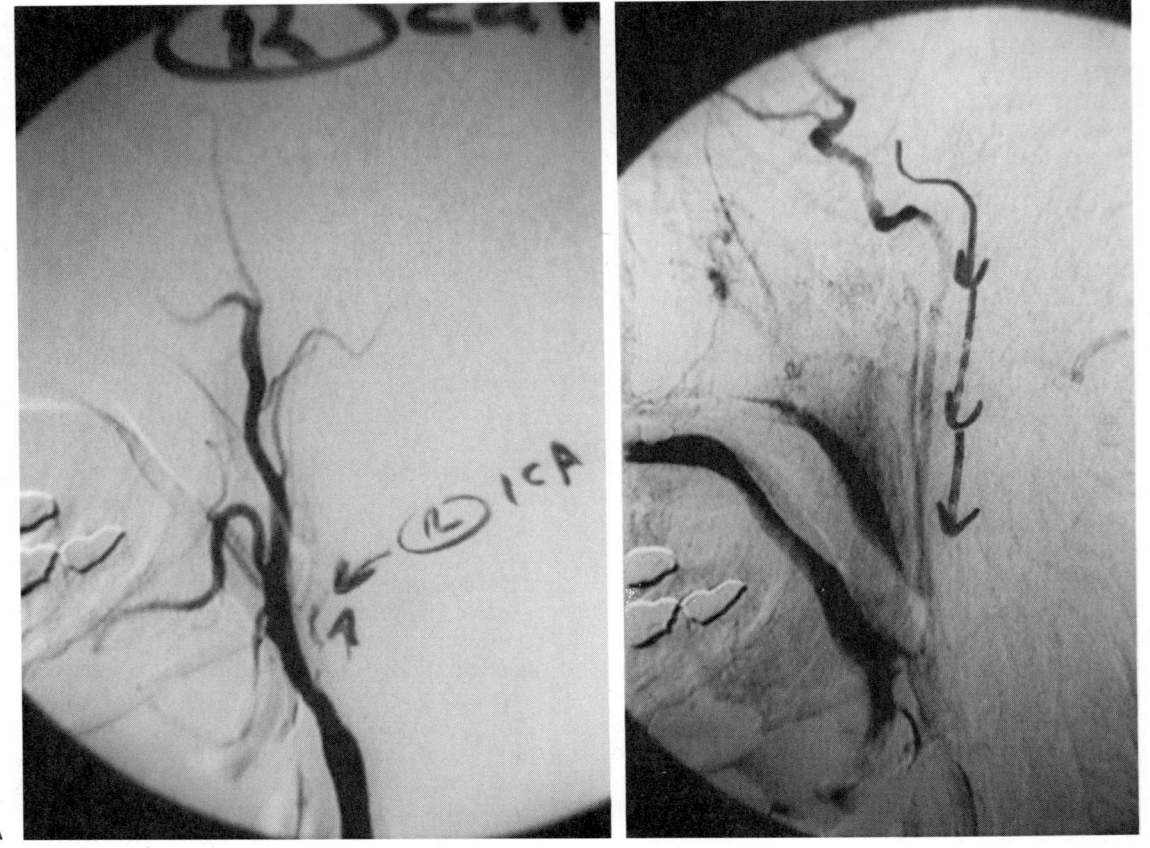

Figure 2 Patient presenting 6 weeks following a right hemispheric stroke, now with recurrent transient ischemic attacks referable to the right hemisphere. Angiography shows *(A)* apparent occlusion of the internal carotid artery. On delayed views *(B)*, there is retrograde filling of the internal carotid artery suggesting pseudo-occlusion of the internal carotid artery. The patient underwent carotid endarterectomy with complete resolution of transient ischemic attacks.

tery disease, preocclusive atherosclerosis at the carotid bifurcation, subacute partial thrombosis of the carotid artery, and chronic subtotal thrombosis of the internal carotid artery.[5]

On occasion, a patient presenting with hemispheric symptoms is found on duplex scan to have a patent internal carotid artery supplied by the external carotid artery, with a chronic occlusion of the common carotid artery. Thrombectomy of the common carotid artery usually re-establishes flow to a normal system (Fig. 3). In approximately 50% of these instances, however, one can expect the causative lesion to be at the arch level, and the surgeon must be prepared for alternative inflow sites, most commonly the subclavian artery.

Patients with common carotid artery thrombosis seldom have their distal internal-external carotid artery visualized on angiography. Riles and co-workers explored 24 patients with common carotid artery occlusion.[2] On angiography, only four patients had visualization of a patent external or internal carotid artery. On exploration, the internal carotid artery was found to be patent in 46% of patients, and the external carotid artery in 62%. Even in patients in whom the internal carotid artery was occluded, external carotid endarterectomy and common carotid artery thrombectomy were possible.

MANAGEMENT

Medical management is indicated in patients with carotid artery occlusion who are asymptomatic or who have acute, severe neurologic deficits including dense hemiplegia, aphasia, and loss of consciousness. Surgical intervention in the latter group is associated with high morbidity and mortality.

Anticoagulation is indicated in patients without evidence of intracranial hemorrhage, as documented by CT scan. Anticoagulation is aimed at preventing distal embolization into the middle cerebral artery from the most distal portion of the occluded internal carotid artery. The duration of chronic anticoagulation has varied from a few weeks to several months, with 3 months a reasonable period.

Control of hypertension is essential in the management of patients with symptomatic carotid artery occlusion. The contribution of hypertension to cerebral hemorrhage following a bland infarct is well recog-

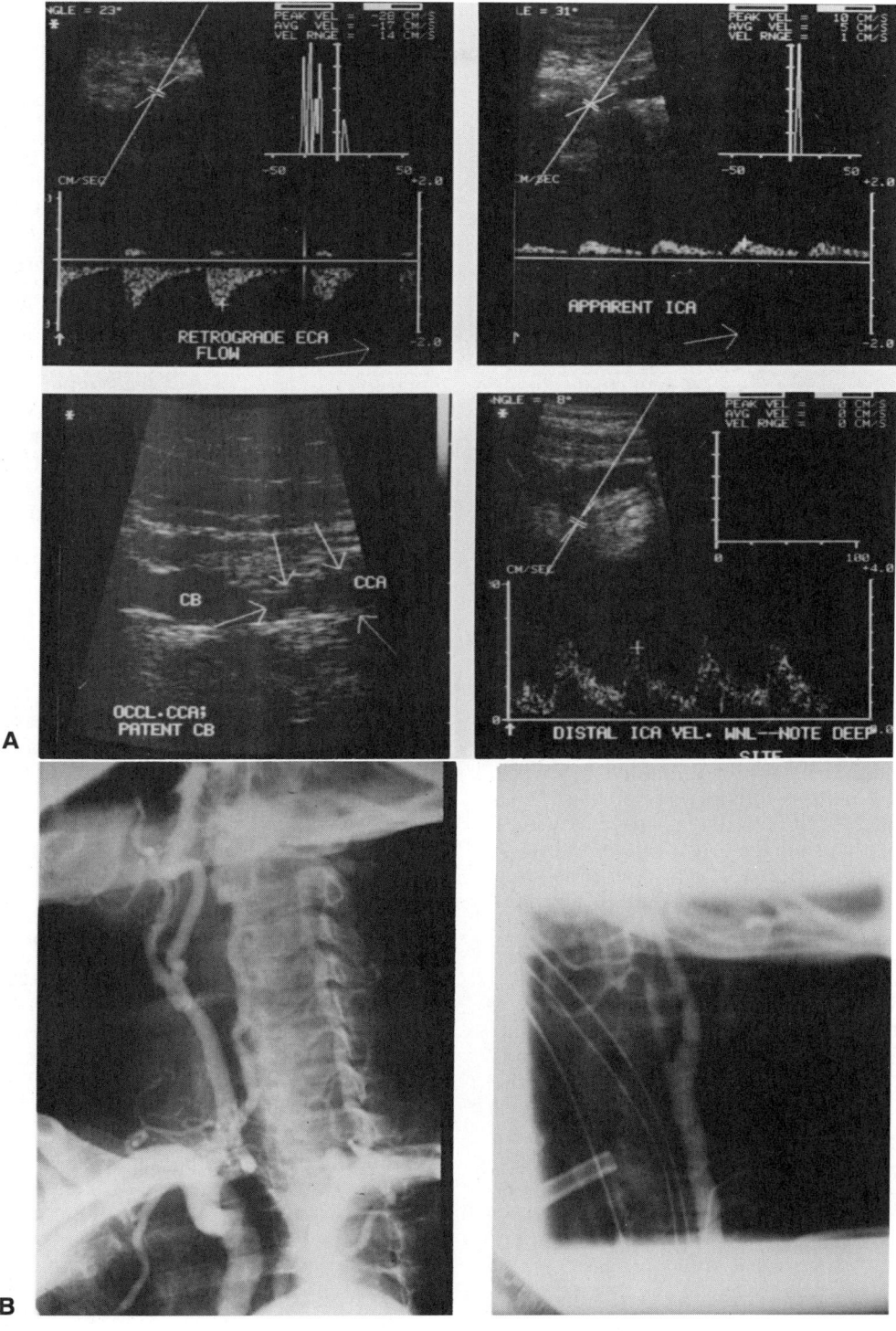

Figure 3 *A,* Duplex scan of patient presenting with transient ischemic attacks referable to the left hemisphere. *Upper left:* Retrograde external carotid artery flow demonstrated by duplex scan. *Upper right:* Apparent internal carotid artery flow with low velocity. *Lower left:* Occlusion of common carotid artery demonstrating patent carotid bulb with external to internal carotid artery flow. *Lower right:* Internal carotid artery duplex scan following common carotid artery thrombectomy. *B, Left:* Angiogram of patient with common carotid artery thrombosis. Note that patent carotid bulb was not visualized on angiography but was patent by duplex scan. *Right:* Completion arteriography after common carotid thrombectomy.

nized, especially in patients treated with anticoagulation.

Surgical intervention in asymptomatic patients should be limited to those in whom the occlusion occurs under medical supervision. This represents a small group of patients in whom the physician observes the disappearance of a bruit and/or change in noninvasive studies done within a short time of each other. These are usually patients who are known to have severe carotid stenosis, and one is likely to re-establish patency of the internal carotid with a bifurcation endarterectomy. Asymptomatic patients with a diagnosis of pseudo-occlusion are also candidates for prophylactic carotid endarterectomy (CEA).

Symptomatic patients with carotid artery thrombosis may be selected for intervention, depending on clinical circumstances. In the presence of an acute neurologic deficit, proper timing of the intervention is essential. The presence of a profound neurologic deficit, defined as dense hemiplegia, aphasia, and/or loss of consciousness, constitutes a contraindication to emergency surgical intervention. Emergency CEA should be limited to stroke patients who can undergo operation within the first 1 to 2 hours after the acute event, and to symptomatic patients who have fluctuating symptoms consistent with stroke in evolution. In the latter group, exclusion of a hemorrhagic component to the infarct must be established by preoperative CT scan; otherwise, intracerebral hemorrhage may follow operation.

Preferably, intervention for acute stroke should be delayed until the patient has reached a plateau in recovery. Some authors have recommended a 6 week interval between the acute event and intervention.[6] With this approach, up to 21% of patients may have recurrent symptoms or stroke during the observation interval.[7] Many surgeons prefer to proceed with operation once neurologic recovery has reached its maximum. This may occur after a few days or several weeks, depending on the individual patient.

Elective operation for carotid occlusion should be considered in patients with prior stroke who are currently symptomatic and patients presenting with transient ischemic attacks. The choice of operation depends on the preoperative evaluation aimed to establish the mechanism of the symptoms and the anatomic pattern of the occlusion. Operation is aimed at correcting the causative process, and the choice depends on appropriate clinical and angiographic preoperative evaluation.

Careful postoperative management is crucial in assuring good results following surgical intervention. Management of hypertension should be aggressive to decrease the risk of intracerebral hemorrhage. In addition, some patients may develop hyperperfusion syndrome manifested by a severe headache, usually ipsilateral to the reconstructed artery.[8] This may progress to seizures, and aggressive management is recommended. Patients with this syndrome should be observed in the hospital, their blood pressure controlled, and anticoagulation avoided.

Anticoagulation following surgical intervention for thrombosis of the carotid artery should be individualized. In patients shortly after a stroke, concern about intracerebral hemorrhage would argue against full anticoagulation. In patients presenting with transient ischemic attacks or stroke in the remote past, anticoagulation to protect against rethrombosis carries a lower risk and should be considered.

CHOICE OF OPERATION

Contralateral Carotid Endarterectomy

Contralateral CEA is indicated in patients with internal carotid artery occlusion who have a significant contralateral stenosis and can be documented by angiography to have filling of the symptomatic hemisphere from the diseased, but patent, artery. When the indication is a stroke, whether in the hemisphere ipsilateral or contralateral to the stenosis, a shunt should be used during CEA to protect from hypoperfusion. In this setting, the hemisphere contralateral to the stenosis is in a watershed area of perfusion.

Many reports in the literature have documented the safety and efficacy of CEA contralateral to an internal carotid artery occlusion. A statistically significant benefit, with reduced incidence of late strokes following operation compared to nonoperated cohorts, was reported by Hertzer and co-workers.[9] In asymptomatic patients with an internal carotid artery occlusion, prophylactic CEA of the contralateral stenotic artery may be considered for lesions greater than 50% to 60% diameter stenosis. The latter recommendation, however, is not universally accepted and may be supported or modified following the results of ongoing randomized trials.

Thrombectomy of the Carotid Artery

Thrombectomy of the occluded carotid artery is indicated in symptomatic patients with common carotid artery thrombosis and patency of either the external or the external-internal carotid vessels and in highly selected patients with internal carotid artery occlusion who are identified very early after the event and in the absence of a dense neurologic deficit or loss of consciousness. Unstable patients are not candidates for acute intervention. Because of the associated increased risks of this intervention, asymptomatic patients are not candidates for carotid thrombectomy, unless the diagnosis of pseudo-occlusion is established preoperatively, in which case standard endarterectomy is the procedure of choice, or unless the occlusion has occurred under medical supervision, as mentioned previously.

Several important points must be made regarding the technical aspects of both acute and chronic carotid artery thrombectomy. In patients operated upon acutely, re-establishment of blood flow through the system as soon as possible is a priority. Although brisk backbleeding after thrombectomy is a good sign of potential success, arteriography of the distal system is recommended prior to establishment of flow. Operative arteriography can identify small filling defects that may require retrieval either by allowing backbleeding or repassage of the embolectomy catheter prior to restoration of blood flow. The operative arteriogram, however, should not be performed with the usual flush technique, as one may embolize material beyond retrieval. It is best just simply to fill the system under fluoroscopy by using the distal end of the carotid shunt and then allowing the contrast material to exit in a retrograde fashion. Once this has confirmed patency and the completeness of the thrombectomy, shunt placement follows, restoring blood flow.

Findings at operation are critical in deciding the best way to proceed, from both a technical and a management standpoint. If a chronically occluded internal carotid artery is encountered where the artery beyond the bulb is contracted and fibrotic, the best alternative is to ligate the internal carotid artery and eliminate the cul-de-sac formed by the stump of the occluded vessel. This is best accomplished by resection of the origin of the internal carotid artery, using the bulb to tailor the transition from the common to the external carotid artery. Attempts at thrombectomy of chronically occluded contracted internal carotid arteries are not only contraindicated but also hazardous. Short- or long-term patency in these instances is dismal with considerable risk of neurologic morbidity. When the occlusion has been recent, the nature of the occluding thrombus allows easy separation once the carotid bulb has been opened. The decision to proceed with chronic thrombectomy, as opposed to ligation, requires considerable judgment. If there is any question about the feasibility of chronic thrombectomy, it is best not to make any forceful attempts at reestablishing patency but rather to proceed with stumpectomy and external carotid artery repair. When patency of the distal internal carotid artery has been documented preoperatively, chronic thrombectomy is often possible.

Passage of the Fogarty catheter during chronic thrombectomy is best done at several points along the plane between the thrombus and the endothelium. In acute occlusions, it is common to find thrombus at the origin of the internal carotid artery, with a tail of fresh clot in its distal portion. Retrieval by maintaining its continuity is possible, avoiding passage of embolectomy catheters altogether. During internal carotid thrombectomy, use of fluoroscopy while passing the Fogarty catheter helps identify when the catheter has reached the intracranial portion of the carotid system. Filling the balloon with contrast helps visualization. Fluoroscopy also assists in recognizing when there is difficulty in traversing the occlusion. In these instances, the tip of the catheter can be seen bending against resistance. Passage beyond the carotid siphon is unnecessary and hazardous. Extraction of the catheter during internal carotid thrombectomy must be done with great caution. It should be recognized that the two mechanisms responsible for the development of carotid cavernous sinus fistula are forceful passage of the Fogarty catheter and overinflation and forceful retrieval, causing a traction injury of the vessel adjacent to the carotid siphon. Completion angiography is highly recommended.

When the indication for operation has been a string sign or the artery is seen in spasm (contracted but without thrombus within its lumen) on completion angiography, it is advisable to gently dilate the artery with dilators. This must be done with great caution to avoid disruption of the intima. The process of dilation should be gradual, in half-millimeter increments, and not exceed 4 mm. Adventitial instillation of papaverine has been of anecdotal benefit.

During proximal common carotid artery thrombectomy, the same principles apply. We have found, however, that angioscopy is helpful in the evaluation of the completeness of the thrombectomy. Proximal inflow control can be obtained by a balloon catheter with passage of the angioscope in a retrograde fashion. Flexible biopsy forceps may allow one to retrieve small flaps that remain after common carotid artery thrombectomy. During internal carotid artery thrombectomy, use of angioscopy is less attractive as one must be concerned about the irrigation causing embolization of thrombotic material.

The cause of common carotid artery thrombosis may be either an embolus to the carotid artery bifurcation with retrograde thrombosis, a high-grade stenosis of the internal carotid artery leading to thrombosis of the entire system, or an origin lesion at the arch, which causes prograde thrombosis. In the first two instances, retrograde thrombectomy of the common carotid artery and standard carotid endarterectomy of the carotid bulb usually suffice. When thrombosis is secondary to an arch lesion, however, the thrombus may end at the distal common carotid artery with a patent internal carotid artery through retrograde flow from the external carotid artery. When common carotid artery thrombosis is present, the surgeon must be prepared to use alternative inflow sites, most commonly the subclavian artery. The need for such alternative sites is recognized by failure to establish adequate inflow during common carotid thrombectomy or after completion angiography or angioscopy following thrombectomy.

The goal of common carotid thrombectomy is, at the least, establishment of flow into the external carotid artery. When the external and the internal carotid arteries are open, restitution of a completely normal system should be the goal of operation. On occasion, a pseudo-occlusion is identified, which also allows restoration to a normal carotid system.

When patients are properly selected, the results of operation for internal carotid artery occlusion appear to be beneficial. In a retrospective review over a 10 year period, 47 thromboendarterectomies were performed for recent occlusion of the internal carotid artery by Hafner and Tew.[10] Of these, 32% were considered immediate surgical failures, as suggested by no backbleeding or minimal backbleeding, leading to ligation of the artery. In 68%, however, they were able to establish patency of the internal carotid artery, which was documented by postoperative angiography or noninvasive studies in most patients. Postoperative patency correlated with the duration of the occlusion. Whereas occlusions suspected for less than 48 hours had 100% postoperative patency, occlusions older than 1 month had a 68% long-term patency. Of the 32 patients who were considered surgical successes, there were no recurrent cerebral infarctions or transient ischemic attacks with follow-up as long as 8½ years. There were no operative deaths or morbidity. Patient selection was clearly a factor in these excellent results.

When urgent operation is performed for acute symptoms, the morbidity of the procedure increases. In Meyer and colleagues' series of 34 patients undergoing emergency endarterectomy for acute internal carotid artery occlusion, there was a 94% success rate in restoring patency.[11] During follow-up, however, only 26% of patients were normal and 11% had minimal deficit. Mortality was 20% in this series. The authors felt, however, that these results compared favorably to the natural history of acute carotid occlusion in symptomatic patients. Overall, the results of carotid artery thrombectomy for internal carotid artery occlusion can be expected to have a higher risk and should be limited to patients whose natural history would favor intervention.

External Carotid Thromboendarterectomy

External carotid artery reconstruction is indicated in symptomatic patients with internal carotid artery thrombosis who have symptoms secondary to hypoperfusion of external to internal carotid artery collaterals, as documented by angiography, and a high-grade stenosis of the external carotid artery (Fig. 4). External carotid artery reconstruction is also indicated in patients with a large stump formed by the occluded internal carotid artery, which serves as an embolic source through external-internal carotid collaterals, in patients with severe stenosis of the external carotid artery, which may produce symptoms as a source of emboli; or, alternatively, in patients with an occluded external carotid artery, where the stump may serve as an embolic source through the normal internal carotid artery. The last is a rare cause of symptoms.[12] It may be manifested shortly after standard carotid endarterectomy secondary to a technical error leading to external carotid artery thrombosis, or in late follow-up secondary to progression of an external carotid lesion.

External carotid artery reconstruction is best accomplished by removal of the stump of the internal carotid artery and creation of a smooth transition between the common and external carotid arteries. When a stenotic

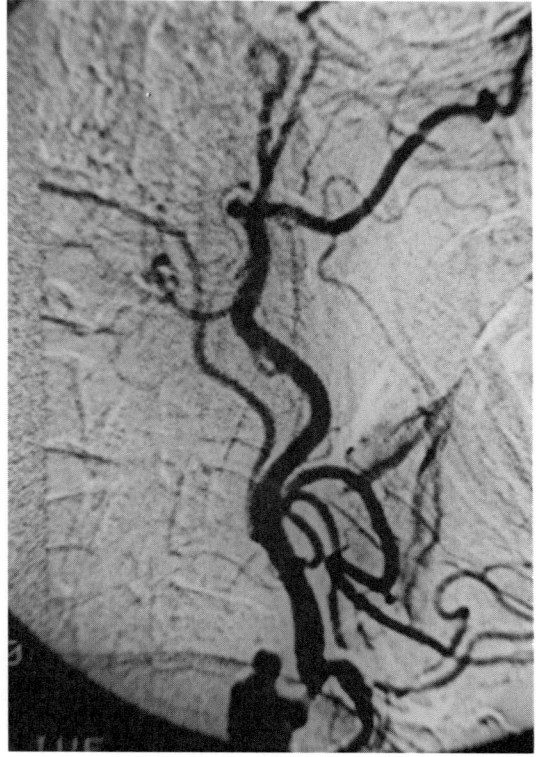 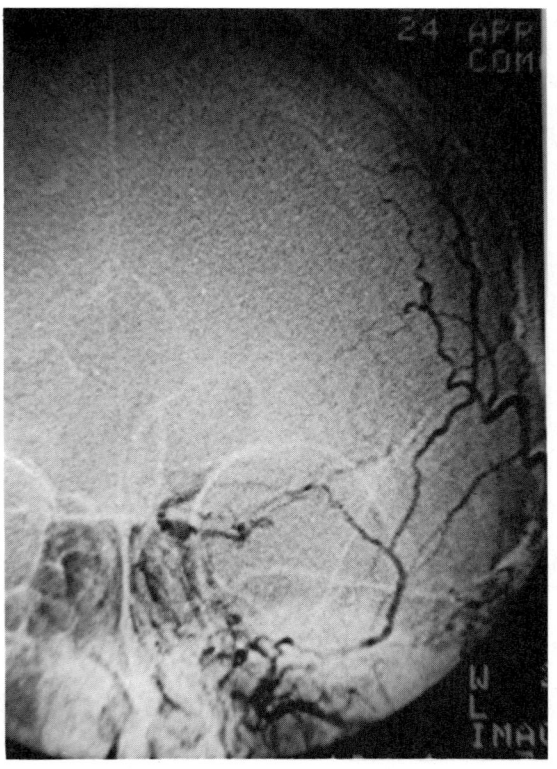

Figure 4 Patient presenting with left amaurosis fugax. *A,* Angiogram demonstrating internal carotid artery thrombosis with large cul-de-sac and external carotid origin stenosis. *B,* Delayed views demonstrating external carotid to internal carotid artery collaterals reconstituting internal carotid siphon. An external carotid endarterectomy with stumpectomy was performed. No recurrent symptoms have occurred during 29 months of follow-up.

lesion is present in the external carotid artery, local endarterectomy and patch angioplasty is indicated. When performing endarterectomy of the external carotid artery, the surgeon has to control its branches so that exposure beyond the area of endarterectomy can be accomplished. This assures a smooth end point with patch closure and avoids narrowing its origin. When the indication for reconstruction is external carotid artery occlusion, it is probably best to detach the external carotid artery origin and 'close the carotid bulb with a patch rather than reconstruct the external carotid artery and risk rethrombosis. Completion arteriography to document the end result is highly recommended.

In a collective review of external CEA for the treatment of ipsilateral internal carotid artery occlusion, Gertler and Cambria summarized 23 reports describing 218 patients. Resolution of symptoms was seen in 83% of patients, with an additional 7% showing improvement. The perioperative mortality was 3% with the overall neurologic complication rate of 5%. A diseased contralateral carotid artery was associated with higher neurologic morbidity, whereas disease in the vertebral arteries had no impact on outcome. The best results were obtained when operation was performed to relieve specific hemispheric or retinal symptoms as opposed to nonspecific neurologic complaints or previous strokes.[13] Others have suggested that the complications of external carotid artery reconstruction are increased when additional procedures are performed at the same time, such as external carotid–internal carotid bypass or bypass grafts from the subclavian artery.[14]

Extracranial-Intracranial Bypass

In an attempt to increase blood flow to the cerebral hemisphere, extracranial-intracranial bypass, using branches of the external carotid artery directly anastomosed to the middle cerebral artery branch, was performed with increasing frequency in the late 1970s. However, a randomized prospective trial documented that patients operated upon did no better than patients treated medically.[15] However, the high patency rate of such reconstructions was remarkable. In spite of the results of the randomized study, extracranial-intracranial bypass remains an alternative for selected patients with symptoms related to hypoperfusion of the hemisphere ipsilateral to an internal carotid artery occlusion when no other alternative method to increase cerebral blood flow by extracranial reconstruction is available.

REFERENCES

1. Archie JP Jr. Carotid endarterectomy when the distal internal carotid artery is small or poorly visualized. J Vasc Surg 1993; 19:23–31.
2. Riles TS, Imparato AM, Posner MP, Eikelboom BC. Common carotid occlusion. Assessment of the distal vessels. Ann Surg 1984; 199:363–366.
3. O'Leary DH, Gibbons GW, Pinel DF. Limitations of noninvasive testing in assessing the "occluded" carotid artery. AJNR 1983; 4:759–763.
4. O'Leary DH, Mattle H, Potter JE. Atheromatous pseudo-occlusion of the internal carotid artery. Stroke 1989; 20:1168–1173.
5. Mehigan JT, Olcott C. The carotid "string" sign: Differential diagnosis and management. Am J Surg 1980; 140:137–143.
6. Giordano JM, Trout HH III, Kosloff L, DePalma RG. Timing of carotid artery endarterectomy after stroke. J Vasc Surg 1985; 2:250–255.
7. Dosick SM, Whalen RC, Gale SS, Brown OW. Carotid endarterectomy in the stroke patient: Computerized axial tomography to determine timing. J Vasc Surg 1985; 2:214–219.
8. Reigel MM, Hollier LH, Sundt TM Jr, et al. Cerebral hyperperfusion syndrome: A cause of neurolgic dysfunction after carotid endarterectomy. J Vasc Surg 1987; 5:628–634.
9. Hertzer NR, Flanagan RA Jr, Beven EG, O'Hara PJ. Surgical versus nonoperative treatment of symptomatic carotid stenosis. Surgery 1986; 204:154–162.
10. Hafner CD, Tew JM. Surgical management of the totally occluded internal carotid artery: A ten-year study. Surgery 1981; 89:710–717.
11. Meyer FB, Piepgras DG, Sandok BA, et al. Emergency carotid endarterectomy for patients with acute carotid occlusion and profound neurological deficits. Ann Surg 1986; 203:82–88.
12. Moore WS, Martello JY, Quiñones-Baldrich WJ, Ahn SS: Etiologic importance of the intimal flap of the external carotid artery in the development of postcarotid endarterectomy stroke. Stroke 1990; 21:1497–1502.
13. Gertler JP, Cambria RP. The role of external carotid endarterectomy in the treatment of ipsilateral internal carotid occlusion: Collective review. J Vasc Surg 1987; 6:158–167.
14. O'Hara PJ, Hertzer NR, Beven EG. External carotid revascularization: Review of a ten-year experience. J Vasc Surg 1985; 2:709–714.
15. Barnett WJM. EC-IC Bypass Study Group. Failure of extracranial-intracranial arterial bypass to reduce the risk of ischemic stroke. N Engl J Med 1985; 313:1191–1200.

RECOGNITION OF CEREBRAL ISCHEMIA DURING CAROTID ARTERY RECONSTRUCTION

MARSHALL W. WEBSTER, M.D.

Although most neurologic deficits occurring intraoperatively or after carotid endarterectomy (CEA) probably have a thromboembolic etiology, there are undeniably some patients (5% to 10%) who have severely impaired cerebral blood flow during temporary carotid artery occlusion and who are at risk for cerebral infarction on a low-flow basis during that period.

Cerebral blood flow below 15 to 20 ml/100 g of brain tissue/minute may lead to irreversible ischemia, especially in the watershed or boundary areas, and the lower the flow, the shorter the time required for cerebral infarction. Because shunting is accompanied by its own risks and expense, and the presence of a shunt makes CEA technically more difficult, most surgeons believe it is important to monitor cerebral function or blood flow intraoperatively. Even if shunting is used routinely, the shunt may not be functioning adequately, and without monitoring ischemia may go unrecognized. Further, by monitoring, neurologic deficits secondary to intraoperative thromboembolic events may be detected and successfully treated on the operating table. Some form of monitoring is therefore considered a standard of care to permit recognition of cerebral ischemia during carotid artery reconstruction.[1,2]

Many techniques have been proposed to determine if temporary carotid occlusion results in critically low cerebral perfusion. Each has advantages and disadvantages; none is perfect (Table 1). They can be divided into techniques that monitor blood flow (or a derivative) and those that monitor neurologic function. They can be further divided into techniques used preoperatively and those employed intraoperatively. All monitoring may detect changes sensitive to perfusion pressure. Cerebral blood flow may be critically low at a low systemic arterial blood pressure, but flow may be sufficient at a higher systemic blood pressure. Maintenance of an adequate cerebral perfusion pressure may be as critical in some patients as the placement of an indwelling shunt, although inducing significant hypertension carries its own risks and is not recommended.

The pattern of carotid and vertebral obstruction on preoperative arteriograms and the apparent cerebral perfusion observed from contrast flow (e.g., cross-filling) are notoriously unreliable in predicting the ability of the brain to tolerate carotid cross-clamping, not withstanding some claims to the contrary. Even the presence of contralateral carotid occlusion is not a good indicator of the hemodynamic effects to be anticipated from ipsilateral carotid occlusion, although clearly such patients are more likely to become ischemic.

TRIAL CAROTID ARTERY BALLOON OCCLUSION

The ability of the brain to tolerate temporary or permanent carotid occlusion can be determined preoperatively by percutaneous insertion of an arterial catheter and temporary balloon occlusion of the common or internal carotid artery.[3] At the time of carotid balloon occlusion, internal carotid artery back blood pressure (stump pressure) may be measured just beyond the occluding balloon, cerebral function may be assessed by clinical neurologic examination if the patient is awake, and cerebral blood flow may be measured by, for example, the stable (nonradioactive) xenon–computed tomography (CT) technique. The balloon may be deflated immediately if a deficit occurs. Temporary balloon occlusion of the carotid preoperatively in the angiography suite has been most useful when it is anticipated that carotid artery resection might be required or there would be an inability to place a shunt temporarily during carotid clamping. This has been especially helpful with skull base tumor surgery or with resection of a large carotid body tumor. Preoperative trial carotid artery occlusion has little applicability for standard CEA and carries its own risk of arterial injury or embolization, especially in the atherosclerotic patient.

LOCAL OR REGIONAL BLOCK ANESTHESIA

The simplest and most widely employed monitoring technique in the past has been the continuous clinical neurologic assessment of the awake patient while the operation is performed under local or regional cervical block anesthesia. The patient's speech, motor function, and level of consciousness can be easily assessed by the surgeon or anesthesiologist. The patient may be asked to count backwards or use a hand-held "clicker." Cerebral ischemia may be manifest within 30 to 60 seconds after carotid occlusion, although evidence may appear much

Table 1 Methods to Detect the Adequacy of Cerebral Blood Flow During Temporary Carotid Occlusion

Preoperative
    Trial carotid balloon occlusion
        Clinical neurologic function
        Carotid "stump" blood pressure
        Cerebral blood flow
Intraoperative
    Hemodynamic parameters
        Carotid stump blood pressure
        Transcranial Doppler flow
        Cerebral blood flow
    Neurologic function
        Clinical neurologic function in awake patient
        Electroencephalogram
        Somatosensory evoked potentials

later. This has been a reliable means of detecting cerebral ischemia during carotid clamping and is acceptable today. Our institution discontinued this approach in the early 1980s, although it is still the preference of many surgeons. In our experience, approximately 5% of patients required intraoperative shunting when operation was performed under regional anesthesia.

CAROTID STUMP BLOOD PRESSURE

When carotid artery reconstruction is performed under general anesthesia, indirect evidence of neurologic function or a direct or indirect measurement of cerebral blood flow must be chosen. The most easily obtained hemodynamic information is the measurement of internal carotid artery stump blood pressure. After occlusion of the external and common carotid arteries, a needle is inserted into the carotid bulb and blood pressure measured through a catheter connected to an off-table arterial transducer. In some instances the internal carotid artery even remains pulsatile with proximal clamp occlusion. More commonly a reduced systolic or mean arterial pressure is noted. The minimal acceptable arterial back pressure is uncertain. A level of 50 mm Hg systolic pressure or greater has been suggested as indicating that collateral blood flow is adequate. Unfortunately, the stump blood pressure is a crude measure of mean global cerebral blood flow and may not detect critical regional variances in patients with relatively isolated vascular territories secondary to intracranial vascular abnormalities or stenosis. Further, there is the risk of distal embolization by puncture and manipulation of the carotid artery. For these reasons the measurement of stump blood pressure has lost favor with many surgeons as a reliable monitoring technique. Monitoring of conjunctival PO_2 or internal jugular vein oxygen saturation is mainly of historical interest.

TRANSCRANIAL DOPPLER

A potentially more reliable and less invasive method of monitoring intracranial blood flow is the transcranial Doppler (TCD).[4,5] It has the advantage of allowing monitoring of both hemodynamic and embolic events, primarily in the middle cerebral artery (MCA) distribution. The MCA cannot be insonated in 5% to 15% of patients, most commonly because of the lack of a "window" for Doppler signal penetration of the skull. Severe ischemia is considered present in the first minute after carotid occlusion if the MCA mean velocity (MV) decreases to 15% of baseline or lower, mild ischemia if 15% to 40%, and adequate perfusion if greater than 40% of baseline.[6] Following insertion of a shunt or upon declamping, a brisk recovery in velocity should be seen, usually greater than 80%. Absolute MV of 15 cm/second or even 30 cm/second have been alternately suggested. An MCA MV of 30cm/second has correlated roughly with a carotid artery stump blood pressure of 50 mm Hg.

There has been the belief by some that TCD detects critically low flow that results in neurologic deficit even in the absence of electroencephalogram (EEG) changes. The converse is also true; a pronounced drop in MV has been observed in conjunction with a normal EEG and no resultant cerebral infarction, the cortex surviving from the other cerebral and leptomeningeal vessels.

There may be a significant role for TCD monitoring in the postoperative period to detect early thrombosis of the carotid artery, continued embolization, or the hyperperfusion syndrome. A markedly increased MV (150% of baseline) may herald an intracranial hemorrhage. The TCD appears to have increasing acceptance as a monitoring technique. The use of TCD monitoring has even led some surgeons to modify their operative technique based on hearing a distressing frequency of emboli while operating with the continuously audible TCD.

CEREBRAL BLOOD FLOW MEASUREMENTS

Actual cerebral blood flow, both global and regional, may be directly measured intraoperatively. The techniques that have been used include the intravascular injection of a radioactive tracer (Fick-Kety principle), the intravascular injection of radioactive xenon with extracranial scintillation counters, or the stable (nonradioactive) xenon-CT mapping system. The use of these techniques intraoperatively is cumbersome, expensive, and time-consuming. The xenon-CT technique, for example, requires a CT scanner in the operating room. These techniques are not useful for detecting rapid changes in cerebral blood flow, but historically they have provided important data about the effects of carotid occlusion and critical flow levels.

EEG AND SEP

The most accepted monitoring technique at present is indirectly confirming neurologic function through normal electrical activity.[7] This is done most commonly by continuously following either the EEG or somatosensory evoked potentials (SEP). These techniques accurately and rapidly detect cerebral ischemia, but they tend to "over-read" the ischemia. The reported experience of many surgeons would suggest that irreversible ischemia may not occur even if a shunt is not used when EEG or SEP changes occur, in part because of the relatively short period of ischemia before blood flow is restored and because neuronal electrical activity ceases at blood flow levels that will still support cell survival. Unfortunately, there is no reliable means of distinguishing those patients who will tolerate the ischemia and those who will not by the pattern of EEG or SEP change. Both EEG and SEP monitoring require sophisticated equipment and an experienced technologist. The EEG can be altered by general anesthetics and certain drugs, for example, barbiturates, which make interpretation more complex and subjective or even impossible. Derivatives of the EEG, which use compressed spectral array of the hemispheric EEG signals from a standard 12 (or fewer) lead EEG, may simplify monitoring and obviate the need for an EEG technologist in the operating room. Whether these processed EEGs are as sensitive as the full-lead EEG is uncertain, and they require that the anesthesiologist have special training and confidence in the data. Up to 25% of patients may require shunting based on change in EEG with carotid clamping, although in our experience it has been 10% to 15%. When significant change is seen in the EEG, it is usually apparent within 15 to 60 seconds following carotid clamping. Slowing and dampening of the electrical activity may be seen, either regional, hemispheric, or global. At very low blood flows, the EEG may become isoelectric. These changes, when present, revert quickly with shunt insertion. In patients who have had a previous significant infarction, EEG changes may be difficult to interpret and may not reflect significant ischemia. For this reason there is some preference for routinely shunting patients with previous cerebral infarction regardless of EEG abnormalities because surrounding tissue may be particularly vulnerable to marginal perfusion.

There have been postoperative neurologic deficits reported despite EEG monitoring, but whether this is a failure of the EEG to detect areas of ischemia or whether these neurologic events are secondary to embolic episodes that occurred following the period of carotid artery cross-clamping is uncertain. The EEG may be less reliable at detecting brain stem ischemia than cortical hypoperfusion. There may be a role for combined TCD and EEG monitoring, as proposed by Jansen and associates,[8] because of their complementary information.

The monitoring of SEP as an indication of central nervous system ischemia, as opposed to SEP monitoring for spinal cord ischemia, is favored by some surgeons but is even more dependent on specialized equipment and expertise and is used primarily in institutions with a large neurosurgical unit and an active neurophysiology diagnostic service.[9] Although the SEP may be less influenced by anesthetics and drugs and may better detect deep brain ischemia, in a comparison study of SEP versus EEG, Kearse and colleagues found the EEG to be a more reliable indicator than SEP of cerebral ischemia.[10]

The ability to recognize cerebral ischemia during CEA is now viewed by most surgeons as an essential part of carotid artery reconstructive operations. Neurologic evaluation of the awake patient, TCD, EEG, and possibly SEP are all acceptable monitoring techniques at present. A combination of TCD and EEG may hold promise for optimizing monitoring at this time. The team of surgeon and anesthesiologist must choose what they are comfortable with, depending on the resources available to them. If we are to reduce the incidence of neurologic complications during carotid operations to a level approaching zero, which is unfortunately not yet obtainable, we must at least attempt to minimize those neurologic deficits that occur because of operative ischemia, which we are able to avert through appropriate action that is possible only by recognition of its presence.

REFERENCES

1. Sundt TM Jr. The ischemic tolerance of neural tissue and the need for monitoring and selective shunting during carotid endarterectomy. Stroke 1983; 14:93–98.
2. Naylor AR, Bell PRF, Ruckley CV. Monitoring and cerebral protection during carotid endarterectomy. Br J Surg 1992; 79:735–741.
3. Steed DL, Webster MW, DeVries EJ, et al. Clinical observations on the effect of carotid artery occlusion on cerebral blood flow mapped by xenon computed tomography and its correlation with carotid artery back pressure. J Vasc Surg 1990; 11:38–44.
4. Chiesa R, Minicucci F, Mellissano G, et al. The role of transcranial Doppler in carotid artery surgery. Eur J Vasc Surg 1992; 6:211–216.
5. Jergensen LG, Schroeder TV. Transcranial Doppler for detection of cerebral ischaemia during carotid endarterectomy. Eur J Vasc Surg 1992; 6:142–147.
6. Halsey JH Jr. Risks and benefits of shunting in carotid endarterectomy. Stroke 1992; 23:1583–1587.
7. Messick JM Jr, Casement B, Sharbrough FW, et al. Correlation of regional cerebral blood flow (rCBF) with EEG changes during isoflurane anesthesia for carotid endarterectomy: Critical rCBF. Anesthesiology 1987; 66:344–349.
8. Jansen C, Moll FL, Vermeulen FEE, et al. Continuous transcranial Doppler ultrasonography and electroencephalography during carotid endarterectomy: A multimodal monitoring system to detect intraoperative ischemia. Ann Vasc Surg 1993; 7:95–101.
9. Tiberio G, Floriani M, Giulini SM, et al. Monitoring of somatosensory evoked potentials during carotid endarterectomy: Relationship with different hemodynamic parameters and clinical outcome. Eur J Vasc Surg 1991; 5:647–653.
10. Kearse LA Jr, Brown EN, McPeak K. Somatosensory evoked potentials sensitivity relative to electroencephalography for cerebral ischemia during carotid endarterectomy. Stroke 1992; 23: 498–505.

ROLE OF SHUNTING DURING CAROTID ENDARTERECTOMY

JESSE E. THOMPSON, M.D.

The most serious complication of carotid endarterectomy (CEA) is the occurrence or aggravation of a neurologic deficit.[1] Many of these episodes are transient weakness lasting only a few hours or a few days with complete clearing; others remain as permanent deficits, either mild or severe. A common cause of such deficits is cerebral embolization of platelet aggregations or debris from necrotic atherosclerotic plaques. Embolization is avoided by gentleness in dissection of the artery, proper insertion of a shunt, and proper flushing of the vessels following closure of the arteriotomy.

The second cause of operative induced deficits is cerebral ischemia. Although many patients can tolerate temporary clamping without deleterious effects, some require cerebral protection if neurologic deficits are to be avoided. Patients with severe vascular disease and multiple large vessel occlusions and those with intracranial occlusions and stenoses are least tolerant of carotid clamping. Cerebral ischemia may also result from hypotension, arterial thrombosis of intracerebral vessels, or inadequate cerebral protection.

Hypotension may be caused by manipulation of the carotid sinus area or inappropriate anesthesia. Infiltration of the carotid bifurcation region with 1% lidocaine prevents the reflex effects of carotid sinus stimulation. Blood pressure should be maintained at or slightly above normal levels for the individual patient by intravenous administration of lactated Ringer's solution or small amounts of vasopressors.

The critical threshold value for regional cerebral blood flow (rCBF) with halothane anesthesia and a $Paco_2$ of 30 to 40 mm Hg is 18 to 23 ml/100 g/minute. When rCBF falls below this level, cerebral circulation becomes insufficient to support cerebral metabolic activity, physiologic paralysis ensues, and changes occur in the electroencephalogram (EEG). Clamping of the internal carotid artery (ICA) results in reduction of rCBF, which can be restored to preocclusive levels by insertion of a shunt. The ICA stump blood pressure correlates closely with rCBF and the EEG. The critical mean stump blood pressure has been found to be 50 to 55 mm Hg, below which EEG changes occur and rCBF drops below the threshold level of 18 to 23 ml/100 g/minute.[1,2]

Methods now available to determine the adequacy of cerebral collateral blood flow during carotid clamping include determination of rCBF,[2] temporary ICA occlusion under local anesthesia while the neurologic status is being checked,[3] determination of mean stump blood pressure in the occluded distal ICA,[4,5] EEG monitoring,[2,6] transcranial Doppler (TCD) monitoring,[7,8] and somatosensory evoked potential (SEP) monitoring.[9]

Techniques designed to enhance cerebral protection during CEA when collateral circulation is inadequate include general anesthesia and the use of a temporary intraluminal bypass shunt.[1] General anesthesia is indeed helpful by increasing the tolerance of the brain to ischemia and reducing cerebral metabolic demands for oxygen.

The use of a temporary inlying bypass shunt remains the most reliable method for cerebral support. Extensive discussion has centered on the necessity for its routine use. Some surgeons employ it routinely in all partially occlusive lesions,[1,10] some use it selectively based on assessment of cerebral collateral circulation, and a few state they rarely or never use it.[4] That an inlying shunt is a satisfactory method of cerebral protection is based on both clinical and laboratory data. Its insertion promptly restores depressed rCBF to preocclusive values and reverses changes in the EEG and those seen during TCD and SEP monitoring. The ICA blood flow studies with a shunt in place are within the normal range.[1]

Those who advocate selective shunting base its use on the inadequacy of cerebral collateral circulation. Although actual determination of rCBF by the xenon-133 method would be ideal, the technique is rarely available. However, Sundt and colleagues at the Mayo Clinic have used it extensively in conjunction with EEG monitoring in 1,145 patients.[2] They used a shunt if rCBF was less than 18 to 20 ml/100 g/minute, which occurred in 44.6% of patients. With this technique the operative mortality was 1.5%, major stroke mortality 1%, major stroke morbidity 1%, minor stroke morbidity 1%, and transient neurologic dysfunction 2%. Callow and Mackey have used the EEG extensively for many years and in a recent important study reported an operative mortality of 0.7% and a perioperative stroke rate of 2.7% while using this monitoring technique.[6]

Another method to determine adequacy of collateral blood flow is the use of temporary occlusion of the ICA with the patient under local anesthesia while the neurologic status is being checked. A shunt is inserted if the patient begins to show signs of neurologic dysfunction.[3]

Stump blood pressure in the occluded distal ICA has commonly been used to determine the adequacy of collateral blood flow.[4,5] Mean stump blood pressures of 50 mm Hg or above have been considered to reflect adequate cerebral collateral circulation. Archie, following Moore's recommendation, has reported that a mean stump blood pressure of 25 mm Hg or higher and a cerebral perfusion pressure greater than 18 mm Hg indicate adequate cerebral circulation.[5] In a study of 665 CEAs using this technique, his operative mortality was 1.5% and his permanent stroke rate 0.6%.

A relatively new method for monitoring patients during carotid clamping under general anesthesia is the TCD technique, which measures blood flow velocity, not volume flow, in the middle cerebral artery (MCA).

Ruckley and Naylor have used this technique in more than 100 operations.[8] They observed an overall correlation between MCA velocity, stump blood pressure, and ICA back flow. When the ICA is clamped, MCA velocity falls. They found that insertion of a shunt restored blood flow velocity to preclamp levels. A carotid stump systolic blood pressure of 50 mm Hg correlated with an MCA systolic velocity of 40 cm/second and a mean MCA velocity of 30 cm/second. With velocities above 40 cm/second they had no neurologic deficits of hemodynamic origin.

Halsey has reported a retrospective study of 1,495 CEAs using TCD monitoring in patients operated upon with and without a shunt.[7] In patients showing severe ischemia by TCD during operation without a shunt, the perioperative stroke rate was 46%, whereas in similar patients with severe ischemia by TCD in which a shunt was used during carotid clamping there were no strokes. This study documented clearly that certain patients with severe degrees of cerebral ischemia require cerebral protection, if neurologic deficits are to be avoided. Further studies with TCD monitoring are needed to establish appropriate guidelines for its use during carotid artery reconstruction.

Another method of determining the adequacy of cerebral collateral when the carotid artery is clamped during endarterectomy is SEP monitoring, which is founded on the relationship between CBF, brain metabolism, and the electrical responses of the nervous system to sensory stimulation, in this case, of the median nerve at the wrist. Panetta and co-workers have reported that cortical SEPs progressively attenuate as rCBF falls below 18 ml/100 g/minute and actually disappear at about 15 ml/100 g/minute or below.[9] In a study of 50 patients undergoing CEA, they found major changes in the SEPs in 10% of the patients. They state that the SEP correlates fairly well with carotid stump blood pressures. Additional studies are necessary to determine the appropriate criteria for the use of SEP during CEA.

From data in the literature on operative mortality and morbidity associated with CEA, it is clear that an assessment of collateral circulation is necessary in all patients and that provision for cerebral protection must be made for those with inadequate flow.

Baker and associates have advocated CEA without the use of a shunt and reported on 783 patients using carotid stump systolic blood pressure monitoring.[4] Operative mortality in the entire group of patients was 0.5%. They found that with carotid stump systolic blood pressures of less than 50 mm Hg the incidence of permanent deficits was 4.7%; when such pressures were 50 mm Hg or higher, permanent deficits occurred in 1.1% of patients. They also found that when the contralateral carotid artery was occluded and no shunt was used in the operated artery, the incidence of stroke was 9.3%; when the contralateral artery was patent, the incidence of stroke was 1.5%. In patients in whom the carotid stump systolic blood pressure was less than 50 mm Hg and the contralateral carotid was occluded, the incidence of permanent deficits was 11%. This study, like that of Halsey, again points out that in certain patients cerebral protection, as with a temporary shunt, is mandatory if neurologic deficits are to be avoided. As a result of this study, Baker and associates have changed their policy to include the use of a shunt when carotid stump systolic blood pressure is below 50 mm Hg, the contralateral artery is occluded, or both factors are present.

Sandmann and colleagues have reported a randomized study of 250 CEAs performed with a shunt and 253 CEAs done without a shunt.[11] Overall operative mortality was 1.8%, and the overall stroke rate was 4%. The operative mortality in the shunted patients was 0.9%; in the nonshunted group it was 2.5%. The perioperative stroke rate in the shunted patients was 4.2%, and that in the nonshunted patients was 3.3%. However, 10 patients in the original nonshunted group, because of EEG or SEP changes during operation, crossed over and were shunted for ethical reasons. Assuming that all of these would have had strokes if shunts had not been used, Sandmann and colleagues state that the stroke rate would have been 7.1% in the nonshunted patients, thus favoring the trend toward the use of a shunt in these particular individuals. In patients with severe changes in neuromonitoring status during operation, the stroke rate was 42%; in those without neuromonitoring changes, the stroke rate was 1.2%. This group found high stroke rates in patients with preoperative positive computed tomography (CT) scans, those with prior strokes, and those with contralateral carotid occlusions. They advocate the use of a shunt routinely in these particular patients and use EEG-SEP monitoring techniques to determine the indication for selective shunting in the others.

The duration of carotid clamping must also be considered. Monitoring methods that may indicate safety for short periods of occlusion may not be adequate for unexpected long periods of occlusion. This is not the case when a shunt is in place.

Jensen and Becker have reported on 1,781 CEAs using general anesthesia and routine shunting without other cerebral monitoring.[10] They make the point that general anesthesia reduces the cerebral metabolic rate and thus reduces the cerebral metabolic requirements for oxygen. With routine shunting, their operative mortality was 1.1%, transient deficits 1.4%, and persisting deficits 0.6%.

For many years my associates and I have used a shunt routinely during the performance of CEA for all partially occlusive lesions.[1] Proper technique of insertion of a shunt is necessary in order to avoid damage to the artery wall and to prevent embolization of debris into the brain (Fig. 1). To this end the occluding plaque is cut completely across at both its proximal and distal ends so that normal artery can be visualized. The shunt is first inserted into the distal ICA, and blood is allowed to back flow. The proximal end of the shunt is then placed into the common carotid lumen, and the umbilical tapes with rubber tourniquets are made snug. Cerebral blood flow is thus restored through the shunt, a step requiring approximately 60 seconds. The average size shunt that

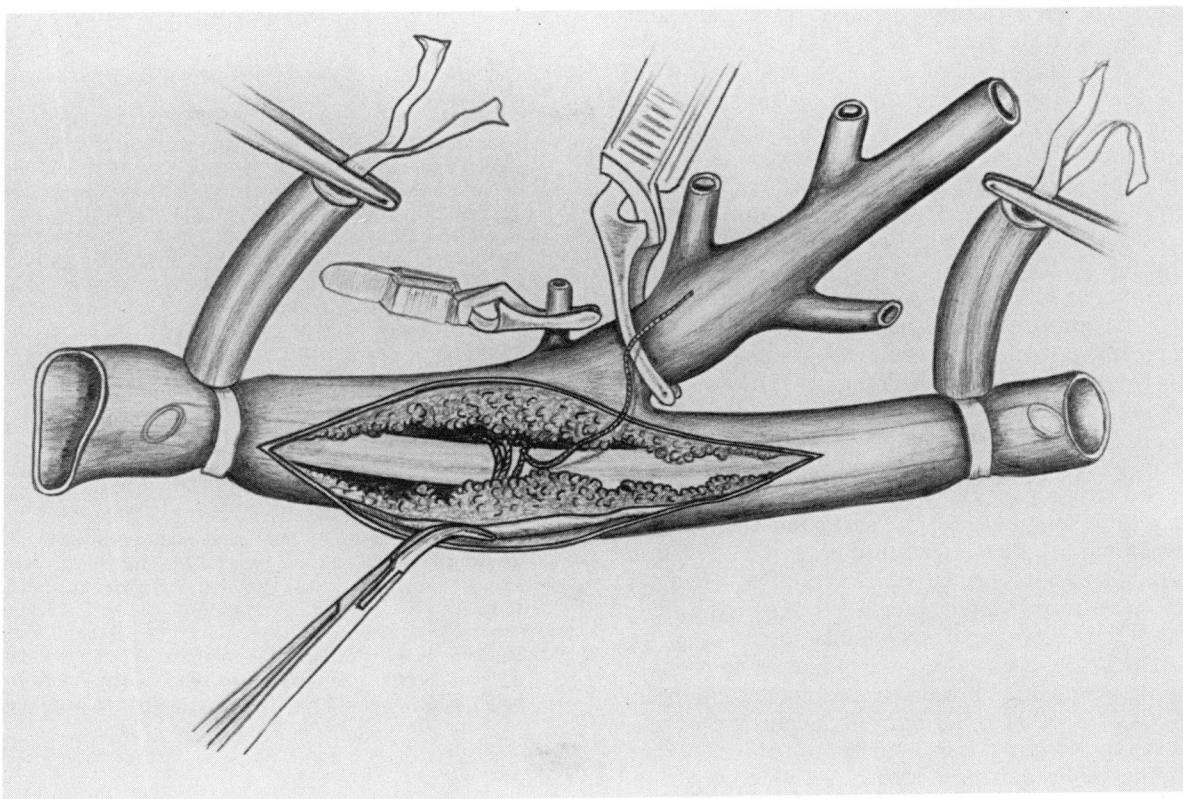

Figure 1 Technique of carotid endarterectomy with routine use of a temporary inlying shunt. (From Thompson JE. Carotid endarterectomy with shunt. In: Nyhus LM, Baker RJ, eds. Mastery of surgery, 2nd ed. Boston: Little, Brown, 1992:1641–1647; with permission.)

we use that fits the distal ICA is a simple 10 Fr plastic catheter about 9 cm in length. An 8 or 12 Fr catheter is used if the artery is smaller or larger than usual. The internal diameter (ID) of the 10 Fr catheter is 2.5 mm, which is greater than the ID of the 10 Fr Pruitt-Inahara shunt or the distal end of the Javid shunt. With normal levels of blood pressure, this shunt carries 125 ml or more of blood per minute. Experience has shown that this flow is adequate during the period required for endarterectomy.

The external carotid artery (ECA) is an important source of intracranial collateral circulation in the presence of a stenosed or occluded ICA. With symptomatic chronic ICA occlusion and coexisting ECA stenosis, removal of ECA plaques may be followed by improvement in the symptoms of transient ischemic attack and amaurosis fugax. For many years we have operated on selected lesions by using the shunt in the ECA to protect the collateral circulation to the eye. A shunt is important in these patients, as we have seen permanent blindness occur when a shunt was not used as a result of clamping the ECA when the ICA is occluded. The shunt technique used in the ICA is easily adapted for use in the ECA.

With my CEA technique, using general anesthesia and routine shunting, in a personal series of 707 patients the operative mortality was 0.42%. The incidence of severe deficits was 0.56%, and that of mild deficits 1%, for a total operation-related stroke morbidity of 1.56%. No other monitoring techniques were used.

A strenuous test for any method of cerebral protection is its efficacy in a patient undergoing operation for ipsilateral carotid stenosis in the presence of a contralateral carotid artery occlusion. That a shunt is necessary under this circumstance is corroborated by Baker and associates, who had a 9.3% incidence of stroke when the contralateral artery was occluded and no shunt was used.[4] In my series of more than 200 carotid operations on patients with unilateral stenoses and contralateral occlusions in whom a shunt was used routinely, operative mortality has been less than 1% and the incidence of neurologic deficits likewise less than 1%.

From data in the literature it would appear that shunting is mandatory in patients who have had prior strokes, in those whose contralateral ICA is occluded, in those showing changes during intraoperative monitoring, and perhaps also in patients with positive CT scans.[11] An assessment of collateral circulation is clearly necessary in all patients, if best results are to be obtained. Provision for cerebral protection must be made for those with inadequate cerebral blood flow. A number of satisfactory intraoperative monitoring methods are now in use so that selective shunting may be employed if the surgeon so desires.

Those who advocate selective shunting cite the

disadvantages of having a shunt in the operative field and mention complications related to the shunt. This is not a hindrance once the surgeon becomes accustomed to its use. With routine use, complications of the shunt are practically negligible. In more than 3,000 patients, we have had only one documented instance of shunt occlusion. Operation-related strokes can occur, however, even with a shunt, from emboli or intracranial thrombosis. In addition to providing constant ICA flow during the operation, the shunt is simple, reliable, inexpensive, and reuseable. It allows for an unhurried operation in patients with complicated lesions and is useful as a stent for closure of the arteriotomy without a patch graft. It is particularly advantageous in teaching institutions where residents and fellows are being trained in vascular surgery. Thus, Sandmann and co-workers found a higher incidence of complications when trainees and less experienced surgeons were performing carotid endarterectomy (5% versus 0.5%).[11] Sandmann states, "We probably should use the shunt routinely if the operation is performed by a vascular surgeon in training." The use of a shunt also obviates the need for expensive, cumbersome, and perhaps unavailable monitoring apparatus. The shunt can be used in any operating room in any hospital at any time. For these reasons I recommend routine use of a shunt in all partially occlusive lesions. My results and those of others bear out the efficacy of the shunt. In the hands of experienced surgeons, comparable results may be obtained using selective shunting, as necessitated by one of the monitoring methods previously described.

REFERENCES

1. Thompson JE. Complications of carotid endarterectomy and their prevention. World J Surg 1979; 3:155–165.
2. Sundt TM, Sharbrough FW, Piepgras DG, et al. Correlation of cerebral blood flow and electroencephalographic changes during carotid endarterectomy. Mayo Clinic Proc 1981; 56:533–543.
3. Imparato AM, Ramirez A, Riles T, Mintzer R. Cerebral protection in carotid surgery. Arch Surg 1982; 117:1073–1078.
4. Baker WH, Littooy FN, Hayes AC, et al. Carotid endarterectomy without a shunt. The control series. J Vasc Surg 1984; 1:50–56.
5. Archie JP Jr. Technique and clinical results of carotid stump back-pressure to determine selective shunting during carotid endarterectomy. J Vasc Surg 1991; 13:319–327.
6. Callow AD, Mackey WC. Long-term follow-up of surgically managed carotid bifurcation atherosclerosis. Ann Surg 1989; 210:308–316.
7. Halsey JH Jr. Risks and benefits of shunting in carotid endarterectomy. Stroke 1992; 23:1583–1587.
8. Ruckley CV, Naylor AR. Perioperative transcranial Doppler monitoring. In: Greenhalgh RM, Hollier LH, eds. Surgery for stroke. London: WB Saunders, 1993:263–272.
9. Panetta TF, Legatt AD, Veith FJ. Somatosensory evoked potential monitoring during carotid surgery. In: Greenhalgh RM, Hollier LH, eds. Surgery for stroke. London: WB Saunders, 1993:273–285.
10. Jensen U, Becker HM. Prevention of cerebral ischaemia under general anesthesia. Eur J Vasc Surg 1993; 7(suppl A):8–12.
11. Sandmann W, Willeke F, Kolvenbach R, et al. Shunting and neuromonitoring: A prospective randomized study. In: Greenhalgh RM, Hollier LH, eds. Surgery for stroke. London: WB Saunders, 1993:287–296.

PATCH GRAFT CLOSURE FOR CAROTID ENDARTERECTOMY

PATRICK J. O'HARA, M.D.

The effectiveness of carotid endarterectomy (CEA) has been established,[1] but good results may be compromised by certain complications of operation. Technical problems leading to early postoperative thrombosis of the reconstruction or early microembolization from a stenotic or roughened endarterectomy site may contribute to an unacceptably high rate of postoperative neurologic complications that may negate the benefit of operation. Late restenosis of the internal carotid artery following CEA may occur in 30% to 40% of patients, depending upon how the recurrent stenosis is defined and identified.[2] There is consensus, nevertheless, that only about 3% of the recurrent stenoses identified are severe enough to require reoperation.[2,3] Internal carotid artery restenosis that occurs within the first 2 years after CEA is usually caused by myointimal hyperplasia, whereas late restenosis is more often the result of recurrent atherosclerosis.[4] However, some authors have speculated that some of the restenoses detected postoperatively may actually be residual stenoses in contradistinction to truly recurrent disease.[3-7]

Although the technique of CEA is not standardized, excellent results have been reported by surgeons utilizing a variety of methods to perform the operation. Much of the controversy regarding the optimal CEA surgical technique has focused upon the use of intraluminal shunts, distal intimal tacking sutures, the use of eversion or transposition methods, and the use of adjunctive anticoagulants such as low-molecular-weight dextran.

Recent interest has centered upon the method of arteriotomy closure. For years, primary closure has been the most commonly used method and has been associated with consistently good results in experienced hands. However, as more accurate methods of noninvasive imaging have provided closer postoperative scrutiny of the endarterectomy site, patch angioplasty has been advocated by some in a continuing effort to improve the early and late results of CEA. Good results utilizing both autogenous and synthetic patch materials for carotid arteriotomy closure have been reported.[3,4,6,7] Advocates of autogenous patch material, such as saphenous vein, arterial segments, or other veins including the internal jugular and lesser saphenous veins, cite ease of handling, resistance to infection, diminished bleeding, and a ready source of endothelial cells for lining the endarterectomy site as advantages of this material. Alternatively, synthetic patch advocates have usually employed knitted Dacron or polytetrafluorethylene (PTFE) as graft material. Ready availability, superior tensile strength, and the ability to conserve autogenous vein as a resource for more critical uses are cited as advantages of this approach.

THE ARGUMENT FOR PATCH ANGIOPLASTY

Proponents of routine patch angioplasty closure following CEA have argued that the procedure may be technically easier than primary closure of the arteriotomy, especially if the artery is small or unusually thin. Furthermore, patch closure may be associated with a hemodynamic advantage over primary closure if the patch diameter is appropriate. Fietsam and colleagues compared the hemodynamic changes associated with PTFE patch angioplasty to primary closure of the canine carotid artery.[8] They documented that primary vessel closure created a mild local stenosis with nonturbulent flow acceleration. Although no significant hemodynamic disturbances were caused by closure with moderately sized patches, the use of patches that were large relative to the native vessel dimensions created a marked flow disturbance throughout the cardiac cycle. Their data suggested that, from a hemodynamic point of view, a 5 mm patch was superior to primary closure. However, because unusual turbulence may predispose to late restenosis, care should be taken to avoid the use of larger patches for arteriotomy closure after CEA.

Some authors have reported a decrease in the perioperative stroke risk from early postoperative occlusion or early residual postoperative stenosis by the use of patch angioplasty closure after CEA. Archie reported a series of 200 CEAs performed over a 30 month period, half of which utilized saphenous vein patch angioplasty. Most patients were followed up to 1 year. The combined incidence of morbidity, mortality, restenosis, or occlusion was 10% in the nonpatched group and 0 in patched arteries ($p < 0.01$). Restenosis or occlusion alone occurred in 9% of the nonpatched arteries and 0 in patched arteries ($p < 0.01$). Based upon these results, the author recommended saphenous vein patch angioplasty after CEA to protect against early restenosis or occlusion.[3] Lord and associates reported a series of 140 CEAs randomized to primary closure, saphenous vein patch closure, and PTFE patch closure.[7] Considering both transient and permanent neurologic deficits, these early postoperative complications were more frequent in the nonpatched group (10%) than in either the saphenous vein patched group (2.4%) or the PTFE patched group (2.1%). On the basis of intravenous digital subtraction arteriograms, 17% of the CEAs in the nonpatched group were narrowed by 30% to 50% diameter stenosis, whereas none of the patched arteries had more than a 30% stenosis ($p < 0.005$). The authors concluded that patch closure after CEA was less likely to cause stenosis in the perioperative period. They also concluded that PTFE patches resisted dilation better than did saphenous vein patches and were less likely to become aneurysmal.[7]

In a study of 801 consecutive patients who underwent 917 primary CEAs from 1983 to 1985 at the Cleveland Clinic, standard primary closure was performed in 483 operations, and saphenous vein patch angioplasty was employed in the remaining 434 procedures. The operative mortality rate was the same for both the patched and the nonpatched groups. However, the saphenous vein patch group had a significantly lower incidence of perioperative stroke, early thrombosis of the internal carotid artery, and late recurrent stenosis of 30% or more. The late stroke incidence, however, was not altered by the use of vein patch angioplasty (Table 1). This prospective but not randomized study suggested that vein patching improved the safety and durability of CEAs.[6] Because of these beneficial results, our preference for vein patch closure has progressively increased from 1983 through 1990 (Fig. 1). In 1983, the first year of our prospective investigation of patch angioplasty, just one-third were patched and approximately two-thirds of all carotid arteriotomies were closed primarily. However, by the time our initial results were published in 1987, patch closure was used during 86% of CEAs on the vascular surgical service at the Cleveland Clinic; by September 1990, fully 96.5% of our arteriotomies were closed with patch angioplasty.[9] Considering data from our departmental vascular registry regarding our most recent experience, saphenous vein patches were used in 78% of CEA operations performed from January to September 1993. Over the same time period, prosthetic material was used in 16% and primary closure in 6% of

Table 1 Mortality and Morbidity for the Complete Series of 917 Carotid Endarterectomies

Complication	Patch Group (%)	No Patch Group (%)	p Value
Early mortality	0.5	0.5	NS
Early stroke	0.7	3.1	0.0084
Early thrombosis	0.5	3.1	0.0027
Late recurrent stenosis, 30% or greater	4.8	14	0.0137
Late ipsilateral stroke	2.0	2.7	NS
Cervical hematoma	1.6	1.4	NS

NS = not significant.
Adapted from Hertzer NR, Beven EG, O'Hara PJ, Krajewski LP. A prospective study of vein patch angioplasty during carotid endarterectomy: Three-year results for 801 patients and 917 operations. Ann Surg 1987; 206: 628–635; with permission.

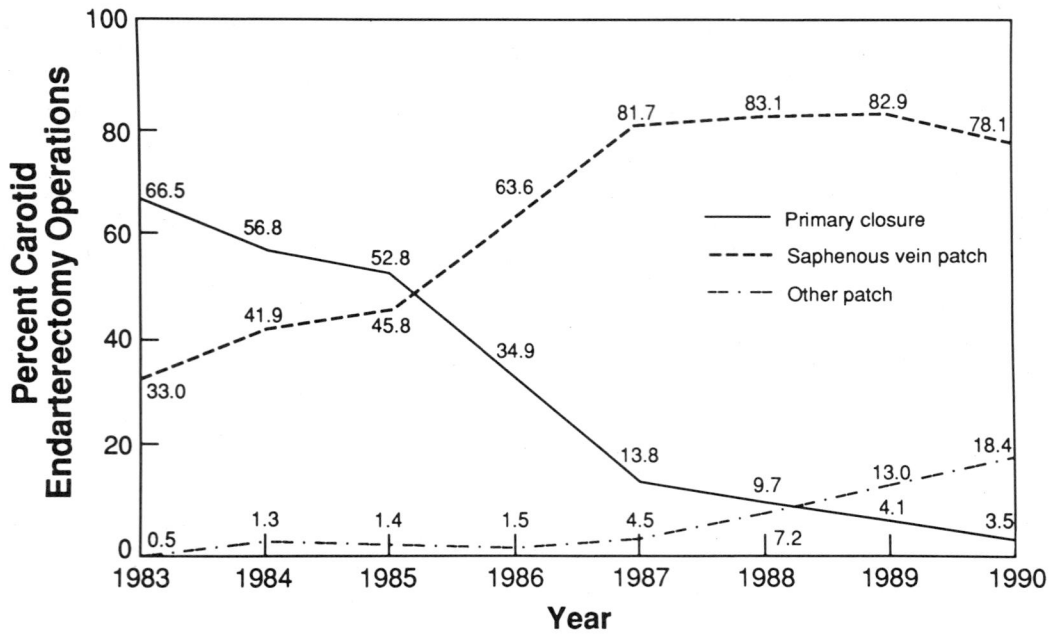

Figure 1 Method of arteriotomy closure and type of patch material used in 2,731 carotid endarterectomies from January 1983 to September 1990. (From O'Hara PJ, Hertzer NR, Krajewski LP, Beven EG. Saphenous vein patch rupture after carotid endarterectomy. J Vasc Surg 1992; 15:504–509, with permission.)

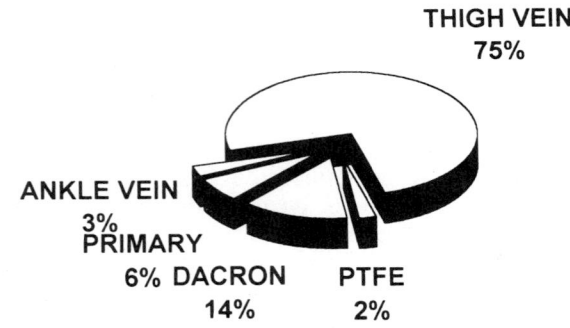

Figure 2 Type of closure and patch material used during 207 consecutive carotid endarterectomies from January to September 1993.

carotid arteriotomy closures, reflecting our current reluctance to accept a substandard saphenous vein for patching purposes (Fig. 2).

Although definitive data supporting the use of routine patch angioplasty closure for CEA for the prevention of late recurrence is not yet available, some reports, with intermediate postoperative follow-up data, suggest that a late benefit may be likely. Eickelboom and colleagues reported a prospectively randomized study of 129 CEAs followed by serial duplex scanning at 3, 6, and 12 months after operation. One year follow-up was obtained in 105 patients and revealed a significantly ($p = 0.006$) higher incidence of a 50% or greater recurrent stenosis among arteries with primary closure (21%) than those with patch closure (3.5%). The authors concluded that the rate of recurrent carotid stenosis was reduced, especially in women, by patching and suggested that it may be further reduced by intraoperative detection and correction of technical imperfections.[5] Schultz and associates, in a study of 36 Dacron patch angioplasties performed over a 10 year period, reported no perioperative deaths, strokes, or ipsilateral transient ischemic attacks. Late follow-up for 27 patients with a mean follow-up of 44 months revealed no late postoperative infections, occlusions, emboli, strokes, or pseudoaneurysms. Twenty-four of these 27 patients had late B-mode imaging and spectral analysis studies that revealed no sign of hemodynamically significant recurrent stenoses.[4]

DISADVANTAGES OF PATCH ANGIOPLASTY

Despite these favorable reports, the use of carotid patch angioplasty remains controversial. Some reservations focus upon the concept of patch angioplasty closure itself, whereas others are centered upon real or perceived limitations of the patch material utilized.

All patches require a longer suture line, which may require additional operating time and, in theory, may increase the risk of suture line disruption on the basis of length alone. This is probably not a practical concern because patching allows the use of large suture bites with impunity. Wall tension may be increased, if the patch is too large. The geometric configuration of the carotid bulb following an overly large patch angioplasty may increase turbulent flow as documented by Fietsam and colleagues.[8] Disturbed flow patterns could, theoretically, predispose to endothelial injury, platelet aggregation with embolization, or perhaps late restenosis. Limiting the patch diameter to 5 mm should obviate these problems.

Established infection in a prosthetic graft usually mandates its removal. Fortunately, this complication is rare in the cervical carotid artery, and the situation may be salvaged by replacement with an autogenous patch. Although compliance mismatch at the synthetic-carotid interface may theoretically predispose to myointimal hyperplasia affecting the durability of the carotid artery reconstruction, this has yet to be convincingly demonstrated.

Autogenous patches are a source for endothelial cells and offer the apparent advantages of ease of handling and relative resistance to infection. Nonetheless, some patients who have required multiple lower-extremity revascularization procedures or myocardial revascularization may not have sufficient autogenous vein available for carotid patch angioplasty. Furthermore, whenever vein is harvested from the leg, the potential exists for wound complications involving the harvest incision. More important, some surgeons may have avoided the routine use of autogenous vein patching because of reservations regarding the potential for bleeding from ligated branches in the patch or rupture of the patch itself.

Whereas all of these considerations have merit, and most can be managed by careful attention to surgical technique, the most dreaded complication is rupture of the saphenous vein patch.

Saphenous Vein Patch Rupture

Because of the encouraging results that we reported in 1987 with the use of saphenous vein patch angioplasty for arteriotomy closure following CEA, we began to use saphenous vein patch angioplasty as the routine method of closure at the Cleveland Clinic. We also reported at that time that acute false aneurysms required urgent reoperation in 3 patients (0.7%) in our original 434 saphenous vein patch closure group in the early postoperative period. Two of these were caused by anastomotic suture line disruptions, but the remaining patient had an inexplicable rupture of the central saphenous vein patch.[6] Riles and coauthors reported central vein patch ruptures in 4% of patients in whom ankle vein was used, but never encountered this complication in more than 600 veins harvested from the groin.[10] Eickelboom and associates also described a single incident of this complication (1.5%) among 67 CEAs closed with saphenous vein obtained from the ankle.[5] Similarly, Tawes and Treiman reported the collective experience of 48 surgeons in the Western Vascular Society consisting of 23,873 carotid operations.[11] A vein patch was used in 1,760 operations (7.4%), and rupture of the patch occurred in 13 patients (0.7%). Saphenous vein was used for all patches and was harvested from the ankle in 12 patients and from the groin in 1 patient. In this series, all but one rupture occurred within the eighth postoperative day. Four of the 13 patients died, 3 of the survivors had a stroke, and 1 had a retinal embolus. Consequently, in this series, the mortality and morbidity rates were each 31%.[11]

As a consequence of these observations and because other patch ruptures eventually occurred in our own practice, we reviewed our experience with saphenous vein patch rupture after CEA in a series of 2,731 CEAs performed from January 1983 through September 1990 at the Cleveland Clinic.[9] Sixty-two percent (1,691) of these operations utilized autogenous saphenous vein angioplasty for arteriotomy closure. Eight postoperative ruptures (0.5%) of the central portion of the patch were observed in seven patients. The complication occurred in three men and four women (mean age 69 years) all of whom were hypertensive, and all but one of whom were smokers. In each case of patch rupture, the saphenous vein had been harvested from the leg distal to the knee, a finding consistent with the report by Tawes and Treiman.[11] Although the harvest site could not be determined retrospectively for every patient, no patch ruptures were encountered among 370 procedures in saphenous veins obtained from the groin. All ruptures occurred within 5 days of the primary operation, and four occurred during the first 24 hours. The ruptures were urgently corrected by primary closure of the original arteriotomy in two patients and by replacement of the ruptured patch in the remaining six. Two (29%) of the seven patients either died or sustained a permanent neurologic deficit, comprising 25% (two of eight) of the patch ruptures.[9]

The cause of patch rupture is unclear, but it may be related to the geometry of the patch, the diameter of the saphenous vein, and possibly unknown variations in the wall strength of ankle and groin veins. It seems likely that uncontrolled hypertension increases the risk of rupture in some patches by increasing the wall stress.[9,12] Others have documented that hypertension, age, diabetes, and gender may adversely influence the tensile strength of distal saphenous vein.[13] Archie and Green documented a positive linear correlation between the diameter of intact veins and rupture pressures in vitro, but the similarity of the biomechanical properties of intact cylindrical veins to those of the opened patch remains speculative. Nonetheless, this finding may help explain the apparent difference in vein patch strength between proximal and distal saphenous veins.[12] Furthermore, they also documented that the location of the vein patch most likely to rupture is the area where the radius of curvature is greatest and, consequently, the circumferential wall stress is maximal.[12] This finding is consistent with our clinical observations[9] and suggests that a narrow vein patch may be less susceptible to early rupture, as well as more durable, as suggested by others.[8]

CURRENT RECOMMENDATIONS

The ideal patch material for closure of the arteriotomy after CEA should be strong and durable, as well as readily available. It should be relatively resistant to infection and ideally should supply a source of endothelial cells to allow rapid lining of the endarterectomy site. These properties should reasonably be expected to lessen the risk of early embolization or thrombosis, as well as late recurrent stenosis. Although no ideal patch material exists, the autogenous saphenous vein appears to fulfill most of these requirements.

We are convinced that vein patch closure enhances the outcome of CEA by minimizing the risk for postoperative thrombosis, stroke, and early recurrent stenosis. Although saphenous vein patches were harvested preferentially from the ankle from 1983 through 1985, recently we have preferred proximal saphenous veins (Fig. 3). Although the preferred patch material is proximal thigh saphenous vein, the occasional, selective use of distal saphenous vein may be appropriate, usually in men with large veins, as reflected in our 7% use of ankle veins since 1989. In our current practice, within the last year, the ankle vein utilization rate has decreased to 3% (Fig. 2). Using this approach, we have not observed a central patch rupture since 1988.

To minimize wall tension, the vein should be trimmed to provide a maximum expanded patch diameter of 5 mm after the re-establishment of flow. If the thigh saphenous vein is inadequate or unavailable because of previous harvesting for other procedures, primary arteriotomy closure may still be appropriate in men with large arteries and smooth endarterectomy planes. However, in the absence of adequate proximal vein, a synthetic patch is probably preferable when the artery is small, such as often found in women, or when reoperation is required for recurrent carotid artery stenosis.[9]

REFERENCES

1. North American Symptomatic Carotid Endarterectomy Trial Collaborators. Beneficial effect of carotid endarterectomy in symptomatic patients with high-grade carotid stenosis. N Engl J Med 1991; 325:445.
2. Civil ID, O'Hara PJ, Hertzer NR, et al. Late patency of the carotid artery after endarterectomy: Problems of definition, follow-up methodology, and data analysis. J Vasc Surg 1988; 8:79–85.
3. Archie JP. Prevention of early restenosis and thrombosis-occlusion after carotid endarterectomy by saphenous vein patch angioplasty. Stroke 1986; 17:901–905.
4. Schultz GA, Zammit M, Sauvage LR, et al. Carotid artery Dacron patch angioplasty: A ten-year experience. J Vasc Surg 1987; 5:475–478.
5. Eickelboom BC, Ackerstaff RGA, Hoeneveld H, et al. Benefits of carotid patching: A randomized study. J Vasc Surg 1988; 7:240–247.
6. Hertzer NR, Beven, EG, O'Hara PJ, Krajewski LP. A prospective study of vein patch angioplasty during carotid endarterectomy. Three year results for 801 patients and 917 operations. Ann Surg 1987; 206:628–635.
7. Lord RSA, Raj B, Stary DL, et al. Comparison of saphenous vein patch, polytetrafluoroethylene patch and direct arteriotomy closure after carotid endarterectomy. Part I. Perioperative results. J Vasc Surg 1989; 9:521–529.
8. Fietsam R, Ranval T, Cohn S, et al. Hemodynamic effects of primary closure versus patch angioplasty of the carotid artery. Ann Vasc Surg 1992; 6:443–449.
9. O'Hara PJ, Hertzer NR, Krajewski LP, Beven EG. Saphenous vein patch rupture after carotid endarterectomy. J Vasc Surg 1992; 15:504–509.
10. Riles TS, Lamparello PJ, Giangola G, Imparato AM. Rupture of the vein patch: A rare complication of carotid endarterectomy. Surgery 1990; 107:10–12.
11. Tawes RL, Treiman RL. Vein patch rupture after carotid endarterectomy. A survey of the Western Vascular Society members. Ann Vasc Surg 1991; 5:71–73.
12. Archie JP, Green JJ. Saphenous vein rupture pressure, rupture stress, and carotid endarterectomy vein patch reconstruction. Surgery 1990; 107:389–396.
13. Donovan DL, Schmidt SP, Townshend SP, et al. Material and structural characterization of human saphenous vein. J Vasc Surg 1990; 12:531–537.

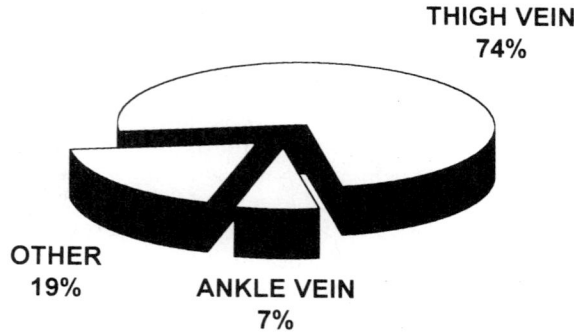

Figure 3 Type of patch material used in the closure of 1,401 consecutive carotid endarterectomies from January 1989 to September 1993.

INTRACRANIAL OCCLUSIVE DISEASE AND ANEURYSMS: INFLUENCE ON CAROTID ENDARTERECTOMY OUTCOME

WILLIAM C. MACKEY, M.D.

Carotid endarterectomy (CEA) has proven beneficial in selected patients with extracranial cerebrovascular occlusive disease. Do intracranial occlusive lesions or aneurysms alter the risk-benefit equation in these patients by increasing the risk of perioperative stroke or by decreasing the long-term benefit, reducing the risk of stroke? Should the presence of significant intracranial stenoses or aneurysms influence the decision to offer or withold CEA?

INTRACRANIAL OCCLUSIVE DISEASE

Intracranial occlusive lesions are found in approximately 20% to 40% of patients undergoing arteriography in preparation for CEA. The carotid siphon is the most frequent site of recognized occlusive disease. Mattos and colleagues[1] identified siphon stenoses of more than 20% in 84 of 393 (21.4%) carotid arteries subjected to endarterectomy. The siphon stenosis exceeded 50% in only 19 of 393 (4.8%) arteries. Similarly, in our study, intracranial lesions were identified in 134 of 597 (22.4%) patients undergoing CEA.[2] Carotid siphon occlusive disease was present in 90 patients (15.1%) but high-grade (more than 80%) siphon lesions were present in only 11 (1.8%). Schuler and co-workers[3] identified siphon lesions of at least 20% in 44 of 91 (48%) carotid arteriograms, and in 14 of 91 (15.4%) the stenosis exceeded 50%. Keagy and associates[4] and Roederer and colleagues[5], identified more than 50% siphon stenosis in 17% and 9% of arteriographically visualized carotids, respectively. Carotid siphon disease and other intracranial occlusive lesions are frequently found in patients undergoing evaluation for CEA. Most siphon lesions, however, are mild to moderate stenoses. High-grade stenoses of the siphon are unusual.

Occlusive lesions involving other intracranial vessels are less frequently reported. Lesions of the anterior and posterior communicating arteries, the middle cerebral stem, middle cerebral branches, and basilar artery, may cause symptoms or influence the risk of surgical intervention.

Perioperative stroke and death rates are not statistically significantly increased in CEA patients with intracranial occlusive lesions. Perioperative (30 day) mortality and stroke rates from recent reports comparing outcome in patients with and without intracranial occlusive lesions are shown in Table 1. In a subgroup of

Table 1 Perioperative Mortality and Stroke Risk

	Intracranial Stenosis	
	Present	Absent
Mortality	0.0%[1]	0.6%[1]
	0.5[2]	0.7[2]
Stroke	3.6[1]	2.3[1]
	1.9[2]	1.8[2]

Table 2 Life Table Stroke-Free Rates

	Intracranial Stenosis	
Interval	Present	Absent
	Stroke Free (%)	
1 year	96.2[1]	97.2[1]
	96.2[2]	95.8[2]
5 years	88.5[1]	94.9[1]
	86.7[2]	90.4[2]
8 years	83.4[1]	94.9[1]
	81.9[2]	86.2[2]
10 years	78.6[2]	84.9[2]

patients with more than 50% siphon stenosis, Mattos and co-workers found a perioperative stroke rate of 1 in 19 (5.3%), but it was not statistically significantly different from the stroke rate noted in patients without siphon disease or with mild (20% to 49%) siphon lesions. This is similar to the findings of Schuler and associates[3] of a perioperative stroke rate of 7.1% in patients with more than 50% ipsilateral siphon stenosis. In addition, they found a stroke rate of 2 in 18 (11.1%) in patients undergoing endarterectomy in whom the siphon stenosis exceeded the bifurcation stenosis. While this was greater than the perioperative stroke risk (4.1%) noted in patients with normal or less severely diseased siphons, the difference was not statistically significant. Perioperative stroke risk, then, may be slightly but not significantly increased in patients with intracranial occlusive lesions, especially in those unusual patients with more than 50% siphon lesions.

The long-term stroke prevention afforded patients by CEA is only slightly diminished by the presence of intracranial occlusive lesions. Postendarterectomy life table stroke-free rates for patients with and without intracranial occlusive disease are shown in Table 2. In neither the Mattos and associates[1] nor the Mackey, O'Donnell, and Callow[2] study did the differences in late stroke-free rates approach statistical significance. Similarly, Roederer and colleagues[5] found no correlation between the likelihood of symptoms recurring and the presence or severity of siphon disease in carotid endarterectomy patients.

The influence of intracranial occlusive disease on long-term survival after CEA remains unclear. Mattos and colleagues[1] found a statistically significant stroke-free survival disadvantage (49.1% versus 75.3% at 7 years; p = .04) in patients with siphon lesions. In the Mackey, O'Donnell, and Callow[2] study, life table stroke-free survival was not different in patients with and without siphon stenosis (p = .75). Review of the demographic and risk factor data from these two studies reveals no explanation for this apparent conflict. Most of the excess mortality in Mattos's patients with siphon disease occurred more than 5 years after CEA, and that study has relatively small numbers of patients followed beyond 5 years. These factors raise the possibility that the apparent increase in late mortality in Mattos's siphon stenosis patients is artifactual. In all studies the most frequent cause of death in patients with and without intracranial lesions was myocardial infarction, not stroke.

Intracranial occlusive lesions, then, appear to have little influence on perioperative mortality and stroke morbidity or on long-term stroke-free rates in CEA patients. Most intracranial lesions found in CEA candidates are in the carotid siphon and are less than 50% stenoses. Their lack of influence on late stroke morbidity suggests that these lesions remain stable. The benign natural history of carotid siphon lesions may be related to their morphologic characteristics. Unlike plaques at the carotid bifurcation, which calcify as they degenerate, siphon plaques may calcify early in their progression. This early calcification involves only the media and elastic lamina, is not accompanied by other morphologic characteristics of progressive atherosclerosis, and does not appear to correlate with the presence or severity of atherosclerosis elsewhere. Fisher and co-workers[6] postulated that diffuse calcification of the media and elastic lamina of the carotid siphon may actually retard local progression of more typical obstructive atherosclerosis. Many if not most of the nonstenosing plaques noted in studies of intracranial occlusive lesions may be related to diffuse medial calcification and may, therefore, be more stable than the typical atherosclerotic plaque.

Since intracranial occlusive lesions have little effect on perioperative mortality or stroke risk or on long-term stroke-free rates, most patients with appropriate carotid bifurcation pathology and intracranial occlusive lesions should be deemed acceptable candidates for CEA. An arteriogram of a symptomatic patient with a compelling bifurcation lesion and an irregular, possibly ulcerated siphon lesion is shown in Figure 1. This arteriogram documents typical tandem lesions. CEA is clearly indicated in this setting. Rarely, patients with typical carotid symptoms will be found to have intracranial lesions that make CEA inappropriate (Fig. 2).

In most symptomatic patients with carotid bifurcation and intracranial occlusive disease, the bifurcation lesion is more significant and much more likely to be the source of symptoms. The presence of intracranial occlusive disease in this setting should not influence the decision to perform CEA. For asymptomatic patients with tandem lesions and for symptomatic patients in whom the intracranial disease is more severe or deemed more likely to be the source of symptoms than the cervical lesion, surgical decision making must be individualized. CEA should rarely be denied to otherwise appropriate candidates because they have intracranial occlusive lesions.

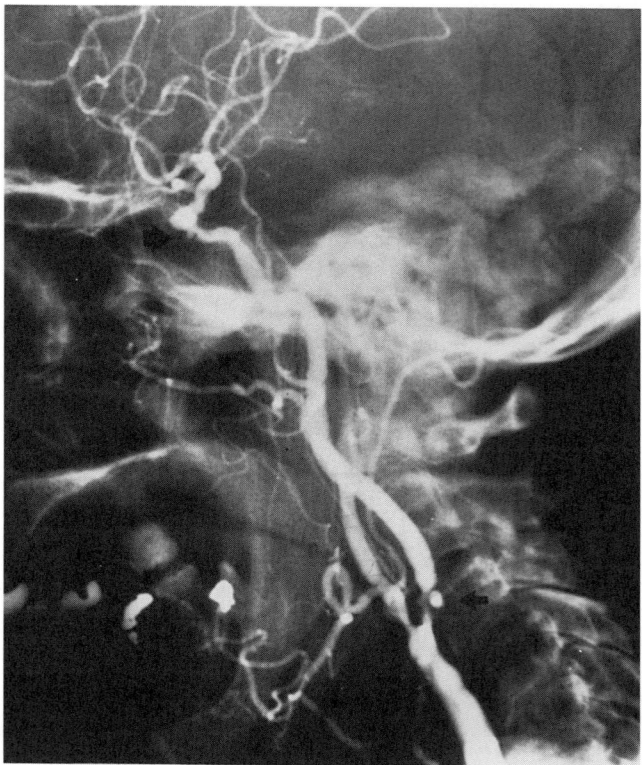

Figure 1 Severe ulcerative and stenotic carotid bifurcation plaque in association with moderate carotid siphon disease. In this patient with tandem lesion and typical carotid territory symptoms, carotid endarterectomy is appropriate.

INTRACRANIAL ANEURYSMS

Incidental intracranial aneurysms are found in approximately 5% of patients undergoing angiographic evaluation for extracranial carotid occlusive disease. Most of these are medial defect berry aneurysms involving the middle or anterior cerebral arteries, communicating arteries of the circle of Willis, or less commonly, the cavernous carotid or posterior circulation branch. Asymptomatic intracranial aneurysms have a 5 year risk of hemorrhage of 10% to 20% that will result in significant mortality and neurologic morbidity.

There are no documented cases in which CEA precipitated rupture of a previously asymptomatic intracranial aneurysm in the perioperative period. In the three largest series of combined carotid occlusive disease and intracranial aneurysms, aneurysm rupture occurred in the perioperative period in a single patient who had subarachnoid hemorrhage and severe but asymptomatic carotid disease.[7-9] Incidentally discovered intracranial aneurysms do not increase perioperative risk for CEA.

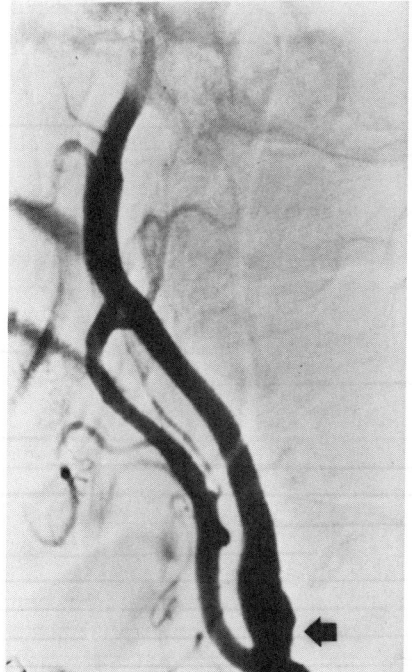

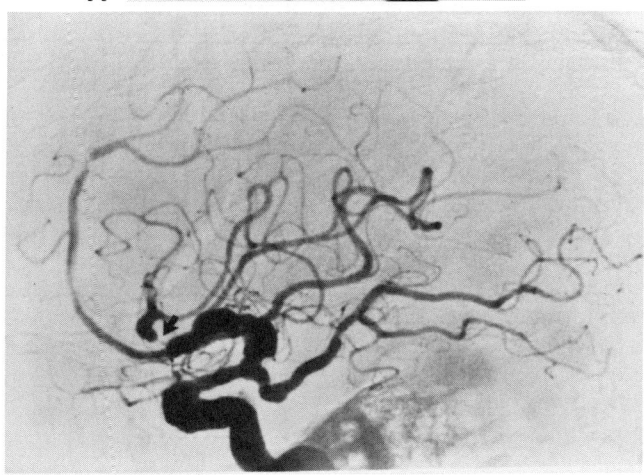

Figure 2 *A*, Mild left carotid bifurcation stenosis and possible ulceration in a patient with repeated episodes of aphasia. *B*, Severe intracranial occlusive disease with critical stenosis of an anterior branch of the middle cerebral artery. Here the intracranial disease explains the patient's symptoms. Carotid endarterectomy is inappropriate.

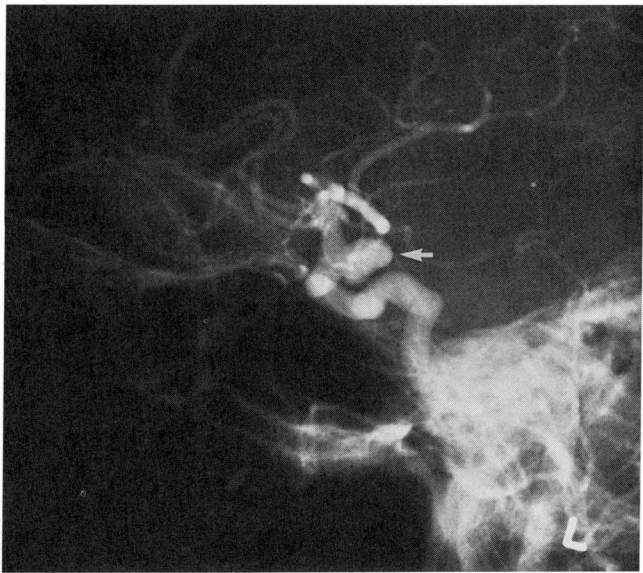

Figure 3 An incidentally discovered moderate-sized medial defect aneurysm of the left posterior communicating artery in a patient with 99% symptomatic stenosis of the right internal carotid origin.

CEA has no apparent influence on long-term enlargement and rupture rates of intracranial aneurysms. Ladowski and associates[7] reported 19 patients who underwent 20 CEAs for symptomatic carotid occlusive disease in the presence of incidentally discovered intracranial aneurysms. There were no instances of subsequent aneurysm rupture, and only 3 patients underwent elective aneurysm clipping in follow-up to 10 years. Stern and Whelan[8] obtained follow-up arteriograms in 5 of 15 patients undergoing CEA and could document no evidence of aneurysm enlargement. In these 15 patients there were no episodes of subarachnoid hemorrhage and only one elective clipping in 6 months to 8 years of follow-up. Orecchia and colleagues[9] reported a death secondary to rupture of a 10 mm right superior cerebellar aneurysm 3 months after redo right CEA. In the other 9 patients in this study there were no aneurysm ruptures and three elective aneurysm clippings. Of the 44 patients in these three reports, only 1 (2.3%) had rupture of an intracranial aneurysm, and this large aneurysm was in the posterior circulation. In addition, Adams[10] in 1977 reported a single case of fatal subarachnoid hemorrhage 7 months after carotid endarterectomy. While rupture of intracranial aneurysms can occur at any time, the relationship of intracranial aneurysm rupture and prior CEA remains unproven.

A clinical scenario with an incidentally discovered left posterior communicating artery aneurysm in a healthy 70 year old woman with recurrent episodes of transient monocular blindness related to a 99% right internal carotid stenosis is typical of this subject (Fig. 3). In this setting, CEA was not only appropriate but crucial and was carried out without delay. Later the patient and her neurosurgeon decided that elective aneurysm clipping was appropriate, and this was performed uneventfully.

Since there is no added perioperative risk and no clear relationship to late postoperative aneurysm enlargement or rupture, CEA should not be denied to appropriate candidates because of the incidental finding of an asymptomatic intracranial aneurysm. After CEA, management of the intracranial aneurysm will depend upon the size and location of the aneurysm and the age and overall medical condition of the patient.

REFERENCES

1. Mattos MA, van Bemmelen PS, Hodgson KJ, et al. The influence of carotid siphon stenosis on short- and long-Term outcome after carotid endarterectomy. J Vasc Surg 1993; 17:902–911.
2. Mackey WC, O'Donnell TF, Callow AD. Carotid endarterectomy in patients with intracranial vascular disease: Short-term risk and long-term outcome. J Vasc Surg 1989; 10:432–438.
3. Schuler JJ, Flanigan DP, Lim LT, et al. The effect of carotid siphon stenosis on stroke rate, death, and relief of symptoms following elective carotid endarterectomy. Surgery 1982; 92:1058–1067.
4. Keagy BA, Poole MA, Burnham SJ, et al. Frequency, severity, and physiologic importance of carotid siphon lesions. J Vasc Surg 1986; 3:511–515.
5. Roederer GO, Langlois YE, Chan ARW, et al. Is siphon disease important in predicting outcome of carotid endarterectomy? Arch Surg 1983; 118:1177–1181.
6. Fisher CM, Gore I, Okabe N, et al. Calcification of the carotid siphon. Circulation 1965; 32:538–548.
7. Ladowski JS, Webster MW, Yonas HO, et al. Carotid endarterectomy in patients with asymptomatic intracranial aneurysm. Ann Surg 1984; 200:70–73.
8. Stern J, Whelan M. Management of extracranial carotid stenosis and intracranial aneurysm. J Neurosurg 1979; 51:147–150.
9. Orecchia PM, Clagett GP, Youkey JR, et al. Management of patients with symptomatic extracranial carotid artery disease and incidental intracranial berry aneurysm. J Vasc Surg 1985; 1:158–164.
10. Adams HP Jr. Carotid stenosis and coexisting ipsilateral intracranial aneurysm: A problem in management. Arch Neurol 1977; 34:515–516.

CEREBRAL HYPERPERFUSION SYNDROME FOLLOWING CAROTID ENDARTERECTOMY

ANTHONY M. IMPARATO, M.D.

No outcome of carotid endarterectomy (CEA) is more distressing than death from cerebral hemorrhage several days after successful operation to correct a severe carotid artery stenosis in a neurologically intact individual whose preoperative evaluation indicated an almost certainly favorable outcome. Death from post-CEA cerebral hemorrhage when described by Wylie and co-workers[1] in 1963 was said to follow a sequence of events wherein extracranial arterial occlusive disease led to a critical degree of cerebral ischemia, which in turn led to a locally successful operation for revascularization and then days later to death, with autopsy findings of intracranial hemorrhage superimposed on cerebral infarction. The emphasis was on infarction, hypertension, and anticoagulants as causative factors.

Since then the concepts regarding the pathogenesis of this syndrome have broadened and additional clinical manifestations have been recognized, due in large measure to the work of Spetzler and colleagues,[2] who in 1978 coined the term "normal perfusion pressure break-through" (relative hyperperfusion) to characterize the malignant edema and hemorrhage that sometimes occur in a cerebral hemisphere after resection of a cerebral arteriovenous malformation.

The syndrome as now recognized is described by Bernstein and associates[3] with a typical case history:

A 56-year-old normotensive man, found to have bilateral carotid bruits but no symptoms or abnormal neurologic physical findings, underwent left CEA for angiographically documented extremely high grade carotid stenosis under general anesthesia without shunt, receiving 7,000 units of heparin sodium before arterial clamping, not subsequently neutralized. He developed unilateral severe pounding left orbital frontal and temporal headache, ipsilateral to the endarterectomy site, 24 hours postoperatively. Then 36 hours postoperatively he suffered two grand mal seizures with full neurologic recovery. Head pain, however, continued until the sixth postoperative day, when though still normotensive, he vomited and developed right hemiplegia followed by coma and bilateral dilated fixed pupils. Computed tomographic (CT) scan confirmed massive left cerebral hemorrhage, and the patient died 12 hours later. At autopsy the operative site was patent and free of thrombus, and a massive left hemispheric hematoma was found to have caused herniation of the left hypocampal gyrus. Microscopically the small arteries of the involved hemisphere showed changes reminiscent of malignant hypertension; no such changes were found in the right hemisphere.

The triad of unilateral head, eye, and face pain and seizures, sometimes followed by intracerebral hemorrhage that often proves fatal, has come to be known as cerebral hyperperfusion syndrome and is ascribed to loss of cerebral vascular autoregularity function.

PATHOGENESIS

Cerebral hyperperfusion, a state in which cerebral blood flow (CBF) exceeds the metabolic needs of the brain, may cause cerebral edema and hemorrhage, which may follow one of a number of conditions including CEA, embolic stroke, severe head injuries, and excision of large cerebral arteriovenous malformations. Clinically manifest by head pain, seizures, coma, and death, it sometimes also produces acute increases in blood pressure.[5,6] The features of the syndrome suggest common pathogenetic mechanisms, perhaps shared as well by the reperfusion injuries of ischemic limbs and other tissue including heart, skeletal muscle, intestine, and liver.

The common denominator in all appears to be reactive hyperemia. Reactive hyperemia in general has been thought to arise from the release of vasoactive substances at the sites of injury, resulting in vasodilatation through relaxation of vascular smooth muscle, generation of oxygen free radicals, disturbances in intracellular and extracellular calcium and potassium balances, abnormalities of biologic iron complexes and their participation in radical reactions, platelet activating factor–induced microvascular dysfunction, leucocyte adherence, failure of ATP syntheses, histamine release, and failure of prostaglandin protective effect. All have been cited as contributory to hyperperfusion reperfusion injury in one or more organs. On the other hand, there may be organ-specific mechanisms, an important consideration for planning prophylactic and therapeutic strategies, especially since the blood-brain barrier is unique among various vascular-organ interphases.[7]

CLINICAL MANIFESTATIONS

Neurologic deficits that develop during CEA in conscious patients or that become apparent upon awakening in those who undergo CEA under general anesthesia are due to clamping ischemia, arterioarterial cerebral embolization, or thrombosis at the endarterectomy site. Neurologic deficits that develop after the first 24 to 48 hours may be due to embolization or operative site thrombosis. An additional cause, cerebral hyperperfusion, in its most severe form results in intracerebral hemorrhage and death from herniation of the brain stem into the foramen magnum. This mechanism must be recognized to plan therapy. Varying degrees of severity of the hyperperfusion syndrome are reported. Reigel and associates[8] reported two phases of the syndrome. In the milder form, which developed in 0.04% of 2,439 patients operated upon between 1972 and 1985, each patient had very high grade carotid stenosis that was corrected, a history of long-standing chronic cerebral ischemia, and intraoperatively determined xenon-labeled CBFs as much as three to four times baseline levels. Postoperatively they did well for several days until unilateral headache on the side of operation appeared and was followed by seizures. Electroencephalography (EEG) uniformly showed periodic lateralizing epileptiform discharges ipsilateral to CEA. All patients in this group recovered fully. In a second report an additional 14 patients developed intracerebral hemorrhage after operation to relieve severe carotid stenoses associated with transient episodes of cerebral ischemia, which led to relatively abrupt appearances of contralateral neurologic deficits during the first 14 postoperative days. One death resulted, and there were only two complete recoveries. The common denominator in all these cases was preocclusive carotid stenosis and at least a 100% increase in intraoperative CBF.

Similarly, Pomposelli and colleagues[9] reported a 0.7% incidence of intracranial hemorrhage with 36% mortality in a series of 1,500 CEAs. There were only two full recoveries among the 11 patients affected.[9] The common denominator was operation for very severe carotid stenoses in the absence of obvious cerebral infarction with neurologic deficit developing within the first 10 postoperative days. Although hypertension was not thought to contribute to the development of hemorrhage, all but one patient had systolic blood pressure above 180/mm Hg intraoperatively (range 180 to 230), and none had blood pressure over 160 systolic (range 120 to 160) on admission to the hospital.

That CEA is almost immediately followed by cerebral hyperperfusion has been documented by a variety of techniques besides radioactive xenon CBF studies. Schroeder and co-workers,[6] on the basis of serial CBF studies performed in 56 patients before and as many as four times after uncomplicated CEA, found that related to the ratio between internal carotid artery (ICA) and common carotid artery (CCA) mean pressures, CBF increased 37% in the ipsilateral and 33% in the contralateral hemisphere. This was most pronounced 2 to 4 days after reconstruction, then gradually returned to normal. These changes were interpreted as signifying impairment of cerebral vascular autoregulation, possibly accentuated by postoperative hypertension, which may lead to cerebral edema or hemorrhage.

Similar defects in autoregulation were reported by Powers and Smith[10] on the basis of transcranial Doppler ultrasonography performed in two patients. These patients exhibited the first stages of hyperperfusion syndrome, i.e., unilateral headaches and nausea associated with middle cerebral artery (MCA) flow velocities that rose from 28/cm/sec preoperatively to 70/cm/sec intraoperatively and 106/cm/sec postoperatively. Systemic arterial blood pressures remained at 120/60 to 120/70 mmHg. Resolution and then return of symptoms correlated with MCA velocity that decreased to 64/cm/sec before final return to normal and disappearance of symptoms.

DIAGNOSIS

The diagnosis of cerebral hyperperfusion requires an awareness that its clinical manifestations vary in part according to the severity of the circulatory abnormality and in part according to unknown factors that predispose to fatal hemorrhage, a stage beyond mere hyperemia with or without cerebral edema. One cannot conclude with certainty that the spectrum of symptoms ascribed to hyperperfusion—beginning with headache and progressing to seizures, then hemiplegia, coma, and death from herniation of the brain stem through the foramen magnum—are due to postischemic hyperemia alone. Some asymptomatic patients with neither clinical nor laboratory evidence of cerebral ischemia, who have been relieved of very severe carotid stenoses, have abruptly and without manifesting any symptoms of early hyperperfusion become hemiplegic, comatose, and have died shortly after CEA. By contrast, relatively large series of patients operated upon for acute strokes with radiographic evidence of fresh cerebral infarcts have undergone uncomplicated CEAs with uneventful recoveries.

Nevertheless, the hallmarks of patients at risk for developing either transient postoperative symptoms or fatal cerebral hemorrhage include the following:

Cerebral infarcts larger than 1 cm on CT scan
Systemic arterial hypertension over 160 to 180/mm Hg
ICA-CCA mean blood pressure ratios less than 0.7
Transcranial Doppler MCA velocity blood flows over 100/cm/sec
Ocular pneumoplethysmography showing unilateral ocular hyperperfusion[11]

Factors that may contribute to development of the syndrome include the use of anticoagulants, antiplatelet agents, and perhaps intraoperative vasopressors, failure to treat hypertension adequately, perhaps carotid clamping ischemia, and intraoperative or postoperative microembolization, since the incidence of spontaneous intracerebral hemorrhage is greater after cerebral infarction resulting from emboli than from arterial thromboses.

Although many patients develop headaches after CEA, the characteristic headache of significant hyperperfusion is unilateral to the side of operation, is localized to the frontoparietal area and the orbit, appears any time during the postoperative course, and may be followed by focal seizures progressing to generalized. Confirmation may be obtained by EEG, which may document seizure disorder, and by CT brain scan, which may document local areas of diminished density without hemorrhage. Systemic arterial hypertension may or may not be present.

The abrupt appearance of a focal neurologic deficit appropriate to the side of operation requires differential diagnosis of three possible causes, embolization from the operative site, thrombosis, and intracerebral hemorrhage. In the absence of premonitory symptoms (headache, seizures), CT brain scan may be required to discover hemorrhage. In the absence of confirmation of cerebral hemorrhage, operative site thrombosis and embolization should be searched for.

TREATMENT

There is general agreement that predisposing factors to the development of cerebral hyperperfusion syndromes are systemic arterial hypertension, old and recent cerebral infarcts, and the postoperative use of anticoagulants. Therefore, prophylaxis must be directed at these factors even though normotensive patients have developed fatal cerebral hemorrhages, called normal perfusion pressure breakthrough. It is important not to exert too vigorous and abrupt blood pressure control during carotid clamping, when compensatory blood pressure elevations may occur and when a decrease in blood pressure to below levels recorded preoperatively may precipitate cerebral ischemia, a phenomenon observed in conscious patients. Although it is not possible to be arbitrary, my experience suggests that systemic blood pressure above 160/mm Hg may be deleterious in the postoperative period.

The most difficult aspect of prophylaxis deals with anticoagulants and antiplatelet agents, whose administration has made possible precise, unhurried operations with minimal technical faults, not possible if time restrictions are necessary to avoid thrombosis. Heparin sodium dosage routinely is 3,000 units IV, monitored by activated clotting times, 5,000 units if a shunt is to be used and not neutralized. Antiplatelet agents continue to be administered at 360/mg daily.

Although there is considerable controversy about the mechanism of post-CEA hypertension, ranging from abnormal carotid baroreceptor hypoactivity to loss of autoregulatory control, it has been my practice for the past 3 decades to avoid extensive dissection between the origins of the external and internal carotid arteries, thereby preserving the baroreceptor nerves. In my patients postoperative hypotension requiring easily maintained blood pressure support is more common than hypertension. An added dividend of this approach is that annoying bleeding from the ascending pharyngeal artery is avoided.

Recognizable early hyperperfusion syndrome requires treatment with anticonvulsants and if hypertension is present, with antihypertensives. Anticoagulants and antiplatelet agents should be discontinued and coagulation parameters checked at once so that obvious abnormalities can be corrected. Neurologic consultation to discuss the use of antiedema measures, diuretics, and anti-inflammatory agents is suggested.

When cerebral hemorrhage is detected, the additional modality to be investigated is whether decompressive craniotomy should be performed. This procedure may be life saving but not clearly effective in restoring function. The neurosurgical staff at this center has performed these procedures when clinical deterioration was progressive.

A number of therapeutic modalities are being investigated experimentally. They include iron depletion by chelation, topical application of capsaicen, blockade of receptors (Serotonin-like drugs), blockade of neurogenic inflammation by u-opioids, and blockade of neuropeptide vascular receptors, which may be the most attractive approach to pharmacologic control.[5]

REFERENCES

1. Wylie EJ, Hein MF, Adanes JE. Intracranial hemorrhage following surgical revascularization for treatment of acute strokes. J Neurosurg 1964; 21:212–215.
2. Spetzler RF, Wilson CB, Weinstein P, et al. Normal perfusion breakthrough theory. Clin Neurosurg 1978; 25:651–672.
3. Bernstein M, Fleming JFR, Deck JHN. Cerebral hyperperfusion after carotid endarterectomy: A cause of cerebral hemorrhage. Neurosurgery 1984; 15:50–56.

4. Araki CT, Babikian VL, Cantelmo NL, et al. Cerebrovascular hemodynamic changes associated with carotid endarterectomy. J Vasc Surg 1991; 13:854–860.
5. McFarlane R, Moskowitz MA, Sakas DE, et al. The role of neuroeffector mechanisms in cerebral hyperperfusion syndromes. J Neurosurg 1991; 75:845–855.
6. Schroeder, T, Silesen, H, Sorensen, O. Cerebral hyperperfusion following carotid endarterectomy. J Neurosurg 1987; 66:824–829.
7. Greenwood AJ. Mechanisms of blood-brain barrier breakdown. Neuroradiology 1991; 33:95–100.
8. Reigel MM, Hollier LH, Sundt TM, et al. Cerebral hyperperfusion syndrome: A cause of neurologic dysfunction after carotid endarterectomy. J Vasc Surg 1987; 5:628–634.
9. Pomposelli FB, Lamparello PJ, Riles TS, et al: Intracerebral hemorrhage after carotid endarterectomy. J Vasc Surg 1988; 7:248–255.
10. Powers AD, Smith RR. Hyperperfusion syndrome after carotid endarterectomy: A transcranial Doppler evaluation. Neurosurgery 1990; 26:56–60.
11. Nicholas GG, Hashemi HH, Gee W, et al. The cerebral hyperperfusion syndrome: Diagnostic value of ocular pneumoplethysmography. J Vasc Surg 1993; 17:690–695.

BLOOD PRESSURE INSTABILITY FOLLOWING CAROTID ENDARTERECTOMY

DAVID H. DEATON, M.D.
WESLEY S. MOORE, M.D.

The efficacy of carotid endarterectomy (CEA) as a prophylactic surgical intervention depends on a minimally morbid operative procedure. The patient population is typically elderly and has a variety of comorbid conditions including hypertension, coronary occlusive disease, diabetes, and occasionally previous cerebral infarction. The maintenance of the patient's normal blood pressure is important from the immediate preoperative period throughout the operation and for several weeks afterward. While most patients can be operated upon without untoward fluctuations in blood pressure, others will exhibit hypertension or hypotension that increases the risk of perioperative neurologic and cardiovascular events. Some of these patients can be identified as at high risk preoperatively. Others will develop unstable blood pressure without known risk factors during their surgical care.

The most devastating complication of postoperative hypertension after CEA is intracerebral hemorrhage (IH). The development of postoperative hypertension is usually unrelated to cerebral hyperperfusion, but most patients with this condition have postoperative hypertension. Patients with cerebral hyperperfusion are those with carotid stenosis above 90%, relative hemispheric hypoperfusion, and preoperative hypertension. Reperfusion after CEA in these patients is associated with severe hyperperfusion of the ipsilateral hemisphere and risk of IH. The accurate preoperative assessment of risk for this group of patients is an area of active research.

Hypotension associated with CEA also increases the incidence of associated morbid events, including neurologic changes and myocardial ischemia. Many patients undergoing CEA are chronically dehydrated as a result of diuretic therapy and acutely dehydrated in preparation for anesthesia. Hypotension on the induction of anesthesia is a significant risk in these patients and is particularly dangerous in patients with severe carotid stenosis and/or a history of coronary occlusive disease.

The cause of hypertension following CEA is undetermined. Denervation of the carotid sinus has been shown to have no effect on the incidence of this problem.[1] The loss of baroreceptor function with age and progression of atherosclerotic disease has been proposed but not substantiated. Another study has proposed an intracranial mechanism after noting increased norepinephrine levels both cranially and peripherally in patients with significant postoperative hypertension.[2] Severe carotid stenosis is most often associated with postoperative hypertension.

INCIDENCE

The incidence of postoperative hypertension varies from 20% to 58%, depending on the blood pressure limits used to define it. The most widely accepted definition is systolic blood pressure above 200 mm Hg. This degree of hypertension is seen in approximately 35% of patients. Some reports describe an identical incidence but a shorter duration of hypertension when local anesthesia was employed. Hypotensive episodes are less well documented and are almost uniformly related to hypovolemia, manipulation of the carotid sinus during operation, or cardiac dysfunction.

RISK FACTORS

The risk factors for hypertension following CEA are primarily preoperative hypertension and carotid stenosis greater than 90%. Preoperative hypertension is particularly important if it is severe and not well controlled.[3] The need for intraoperative shunting, indicating insufficient collateral cerebral circulation and relative hypoperfusion, has also been described as a risk factor for postoperative hypertension.[3] Identification of the group at risk for cerebral hyperperfusion and possible IH is particularly important. Sbarigia and colleagues[4] have described a technique using the transcranial Doppler and an acetazolamide challenge to determine which patients would develop cerebral hyperperfusion after CEA. The basis of the test is the expected increase in middle cerebral artery (MCA) blood flow following the vasodilating effect of acetazolamide as assessed by transcranial Doppler. Three of 36 patients had no increase in MCA flow after acetazolamide administration. This suggests a loss of reserve capacity and cerebral autoregulation. All three of these patients had a carotid stenosis above 90% and significant preoperative hypertension. They all developed the objective and subjective findings of cerebral hyperperfusion after CEA.[4] Others have used the ratio of internal carotid pressure (ICA) to common carotid pressure (CCA) as an indication of relative hemispheric hypoperfusion and insufficient collateralization. The group with an ICA-CCA ratio of 0.7 or less was at high risk for development of cerebral hyperperfusion and its attendant morbidity.[5] The control of hypertension in patients with evidence of postoperative cerebral hyperperfusion should be carefully maintained for at least 2 weeks. A variety of studies indicate that the neurologic events in these patients occur within that period and are related to the control of hypertension.[5-7]

MANIFESTATIONS AND PROGNOSIS

Hypotension

Hypotension most commonly manifests during operation or early in the postoperative period. Hypotension during the induction of anesthesia is most often the result of anesthesia-induced vasodilation in a relatively hypovolemic patient. This common event with the induction of anesthesia deserves special attention and a prompt remedy for the patient population with severe carotid stenosis and a high incidence of coronary occlusive disease. Delay in promptly restoring adequate perfusion pressure can initiate a cerebral or myocardial infarct. The manipulation of the carotid sinus during the intraoperative dissection may induce bradycardia and resultant hypotension as well. This is easily remedied by injection of the carotid bulb with a local anesthetic, usually 1% lidocaine. Postoperative hypotension is most often due to hypovolemia, but myocardial dysfunction and ischemia must be ruled out if there are symptoms or if a prompt response to volume infusion is not realized.

Hypertension

As an isolated finding, hypertension following CEA is usually manifested only by elevated blood pressure. The level of blood pressure that constitutes postoperative hypertension has been widely debated. There is no firm number, as the degree of hypertension is relative to the patient's normal mean blood pressure. For practical purposes most clinicians consider systolic pressure above 200 mm Hg or an increase in the mean blood pressure of 35 mm Hg over the preoperative value to be an indication for intervention. The duration of postoperative hypertension is most often less than 24 hours in patients without evidence of cerebral hyperperfusion. Some studies indicate that the use of local instead of general anesthesia will lessen the duration of any postoperative hypertension from an average of 19 hours to less than 2 hours.[8] The administration of antiplatelet drugs (such as aspirin and ticlopidine) increases the risk of wound hematoma formation in all patients, particularly those with hypertensive episodes in the immediate postoperative period. Hematoma formation poses its greatest risk by impairing the airway. Prompt recognition and evacuation along with timely control of the airway are of paramount importance in this setting.

Headache, seizures, facial swelling, or other symptoms in concert with postoperative hypertension raise the possibility of cerebral hyperperfusion and its attendant risks of IH. Ipsilateral cerebral blood flow can increase threefold to fourfold in these patients when assessed by xenon-labeled postocclusion cerebral blood flow.[9] These patients are usually asymptomatic for an interval in the postoperative period before developing symptoms. Vigorous maintenance of normal or slightly lower than normal blood pressure for at least 2 weeks is of paramount importance in these patients. Patients who have seizures postoperatively without computed tomographic (CT) evidence of a neurologic event usually return to normal. The fate of those developing IH is considerably grimmer, with mortality rates anywhere from 36% to 100%.[7,10]

Several mechanisms may contribute to the development of IH, but all have loss of cerebral autoregulation and resultant hyperperfusion as a basis. Intraoperative and early postoperative events are usually related to embolic phenomena. Patients who have a normal neurologic examination in the early postoperative period and then develop neurologic symptoms and/or severe hypertension must be treated aggressively with antihypertensive medication. Some patients develop IH without any evidence of an antecedent ischemic event. This is thought to be the result of massively increased blood flow in association with hypertension resulting in the rupture of an intracerebral vessel. Other patients have pathologic or CT evidence of an ischemic event in the early postoperative period followed by the development of IH. These patients presumably have an ischemic area that converts to an area of hemorrhagic infarction in the setting of cerebral hyperperfusion.

TREATMENT

The therapy of patients with hypotension either during operation or postoperatively is largely directed at volume resuscitation and correction of cardiac dysfunction. Postoperative hypertension is treated most commonly with vasodilating agents. For acute control an intravenous infusion of sodium nitroprusside has the advantages of rapid blood pressure reduction and easy titration. It does require invasive arterial monitoring and frequent adjustment of the infusion rate by the nursing staff. In patients with significant pulmonary disease it can also induce significant hypoxemia as a result of intrapulmonary shunting.

A recent study compared the effect of nitroprusside with that of the beta-blocker labetalol for the control of hypertension following CEA. The researchers found that labetalol was just as effective and concluded that it offered many of the advantages of nitroprusside without some of the disadvantages.[11] Theoretically, the use of beta-blockers is most appealing in patients at risk for intracerebral hemorrhage. The action of beta-blockers reduces the dp-dt of the cardiac cycle and has been advocated in the acute therapy of aortic dissections and the chronic therapy of aortic aneurysms. Esmolol, a short-acting beta-blocker, should be considered in the patient who has only relative contraindications to beta-blocker therapy as a trial therapy before administering a longer-acting beta-blocker.

The assessment of neurologic status coincident with any significant change in hemodynamics is of prime importance. Acute changes in blood pressure can herald new neurologic symptoms or be the result of an intracranial event. The evaluation of any change in neurologic status coincident with changes in blood pressure should be the highest priority as control of appropriate blood pressure is regained.

REFERENCES

1. Towne JB, Bernhard VM. The relationship of postoperative hypertension to complications following carotid endarterectomy. Surgery 1980; 88: 575–580.
2. Ahn SS, Marcus DR, Moore WS. Postcarotid endarterectomy hypertension: Association with elevated cranial norepinephrine. J Vasc Surg 1989; 9: 351–360.
3. Benzel EC, Hoppens KD. Factors associated with postoperative hypertension complicating carotid endarterectomy. Acta Neurochir 1991; 112(1–2): 8–12.
4. Sbarigia E, Speziale F, Giannoni MF, et al. Post-carotid endarterectomy hyperperfusion syndrome: Preliminary observations for identifying at risk patients by transcranial Doppler sonography and the acetazolamide test. Eur J Vasc Surg 1993; 7: 252–256.
5. Schroeder T, Sillesen H, Boesen J, et al. Intracerebral haemorrhage after carotid endarterectomy. Eur J Vasc Surg 1987; 1: 51–60.
6. Pomposelli FB, Lamparello PJ, Riles TS, et al. Intracranial hemorrhage after carotid endarterectomy. J Vasc Surg 1988; 7:248–255.
7. Piepgras DG, Morgan MK, Sundt T Jr, et al. Intracerebral hemorrhage after carotid endarterectomy. J Neurosurg 1988; 68: 532–536.
8. Corson JD, Chang BB, Leopold PW, et al. Perioperative hypertension in patients undergoing carotid endarterectomy: Shorter duration under regional block anesthesia. Circulation 1986; 74(3 Pt 2): I1–4.
9. Reigel MM, Hollier LH, Sundt TM Jr., et al. Cerebral hyperperfusion syndrome: A cause of neurologic dysfunction after carotid endarterectomy. J Vasc Surg 1987; 5: 628–634.
10. Hafner DH, Smith RB, King OW, et al. Massive intracerebral hemorrhage following carotid endarterectomy. Arch Surg 1987; 122: 305–7.
11. Geniton DJ. A comparison of the hemodynamic effects of labetalol and sodium nitroprusside in patients undergoing carotid endarterectomy. Aana J 1990; 58:281–287.

RECOGNITION AND MANAGEMENT OF ACUTE STROKE FOLLOWING CAROTID ENDARTERECTOMY

JOHN L. GRAY, M.D.
WILLIAM H. BAKER, M.D.

The purpose of carotid endarterectomy (CEA) is to prevent stroke. Unfortunately, the operation itself carries a risk of stroke that ideally should be less than 5%. Although it is infrequent, when a perioperative stroke occurs, the surgeon must have a plan to deal with this complication (Fig. 1).

There are three general causes of strokes immediately following CEA: an occlusion of the internal carotid artery (ICA), an embolus from the operated ICA, and intraoperative ischemia. Intraoperative ischemia and embolization to the brain are completed events. Only surgical correction of the ICA occlusion will improve flow to the endangered brain. Therefore, the surgeon must rapidly diagnose and treat postoperative ICA occlusion.

Of the other causes of stroke, neither intracranial edema nor hemorrhage usually occurs during the first few hours after operation but will become apparent days later. Causes of stroke that are unrelated to operation, such as intracranial aneurysm, arteriovenous malformation, and embolization from the heart, are not generally considered in the perioperative period.

The best treatment for occlusion is prevention. Suffice it to say that technical perfection is the hallmark of success of this operation. To assure technical success many surgeons rely upon intraoperative angiography, angioscopy, Doppler interrogation, or duplex scanning.

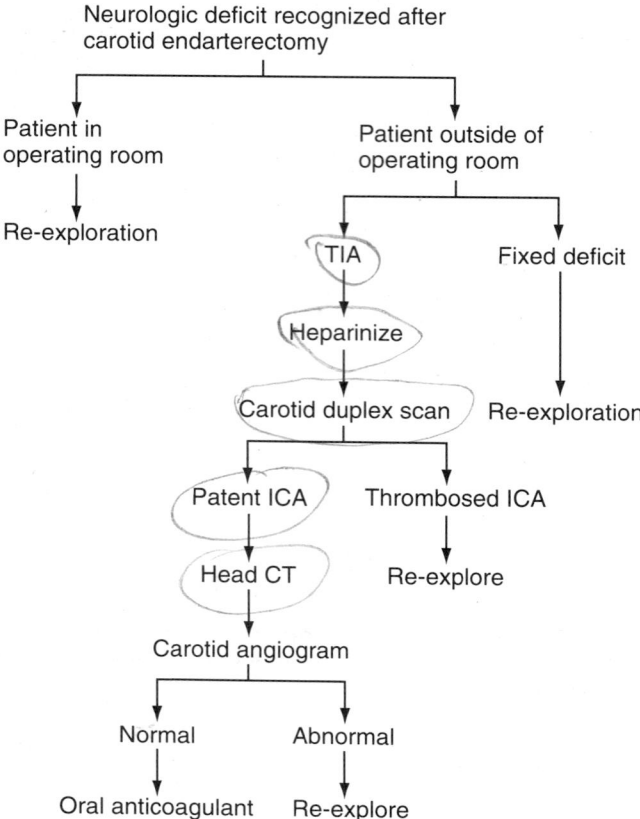

Figure 1 Algorithm for the management of neurologic deficit following carotid endarterectomy. CT = computed tomography; ICA = internal carotid artery; TIA = Transient ischemic attack.

The latter technique has been used since 1986 in our institution. Using this technique, we have detected obvious technical defects in several patients that led us to reopen the carotid artery and correct the defect.[1] In 7 years only two patients whose intraoperative duplex scans were deemed normal had immediate postoperative carotid occlusion. Although we have developed great confidence in intraoperative duplex scanning, these two instances underscore that this test, like most tests, is imperfect.

DIAGNOSIS OF PERIOPERATIVE STROKE

Detection of postoperative neurologic deficits requires that every patient receive a careful preoperative neurologic examination. Many patients who think they have completely recovered from transient ischemic attacks are mistaken. Subtle neurologic deficits may persist. They may have decreased ability to perform fine movements or may demonstrate hyperreflexia or arm drift. These subtle preoperative findings are important because neurologic function in these patients may temporarily worsen after general anesthesia. The finding of a worsened but still mild upper extremity paresis in a patient who had a subtle finding preoperatively is not nearly so unsettling as the finding of a similar deficit in a patient who was perfectly normal preoperatively. Similarly, the patient's preoperative brain scan should be immediately available to the postoperative examiner. Patients who have a preoperative brain scan deficit may have an increased neurologic deficit as a result of general anesthesia, not as the result of a technical misadventure. Most of the neurologic events that are blamed upon anesthetic depression of a damaged brain usually show rapid improvement if not total reversal within an hour.

STROKE RECOGNIZED IN THE OPERATING ROOM

It is especially helpful to the vascular surgeon that the patient awaken promptly from anesthesia. Ideally, all patients should awaken in the operating room and be capable of being tested neurologically. From a practical point of view this does not always happen after general anesthesia. Yet when the patient does awaken with a neurologic deficit, the surgeon's decision is either to continue to the recovery room or to re-explore the artery. Under almost all circumstances re-exploration is recommended. In 10 to 15 minutes the neck can be reprepped and draped, the incision opened, and a diagnosis of ICA occlusion or patency established. The odds of making a patient worse with this plan of action are negligible. If indeed the ICA is occluded, the odds of improving the patient are maximized.

Some patients have complicated perioperative courses that may muddle the surgeon's algorithm. Consider the patient with a preoperative neurologic deficit who has prolonged intraoperative ischemia because of technical problems during the endarterectomy. If the operative duplex scan is perfect yet the patient awakens with a neurologic deficit, the surgeon must decide whether the neurologic deficit is due to the prolonged intraoperative ischemia or internal carotid artery occlusion. Under such circumstances the former diagnosis is not unreasonable.

STROKE IN THE RECOVERY ROOM

The patient who arrives in the recovery room awake and talking and who later, while still in the recovery room, develops an obvious neurologic deficit appropriate to the side of the CEA is less controversial. If indeed this deficit has developed because of an ICA occlusion, this patient is best served by rapid restoration of blood flow. Expeditious return of the patient to the operating room before the brain becomes permanently damaged is recommended. Most authors report their best results when blood flow is restored within 1 or at most 2 hours.[2,3,4]

Once the diagnosis of perioperative stroke has been made by a physical examination, little else must be done. During the middle of the day, while the operating rooms are busy and the noninvasive laboratory is readily available, a rapid duplex scan that can be obtained within 15 or 20 minutes is appropriate. However, the return to the operating room should not be delayed just to obtain a scan. Although duplex scanning may be done with ease in some patients, in other patients with thick necks, postoperative swelling, or extreme tenderness, these scans are difficult.

The performance of a cerebral angiogram under ideal circumstances at our institution requires 90 minutes. If the surgeon is to restore blood flow to the ischemic brain within 1 to 2 hours, arteriography must be eliminated from the algorithm.

Therefore, in almost all circumstances the patient is returned to the operating room for re-exploration. In the operating room the wound is reopened and the carotid is gingerly palpated. If there appears to be flow in the ICA, the common, internal, and external carotid arteries are carefully controlled as before. The patient is anticoagulated, clamps are applied, and the arteriotomy opened. We do not perform either an arteriogram or duplex scan prior to this event. Even if the scan and arteriogram do not appear to be markedly abnormal, we do not rule out a small excrescence or thrombus that may be the source of a cerebral embolus. The arteriotomy is opened and the lumen explored. In patients who have had a thrombosed ICA, the thrombus is removed. Only on rare occasions will use of a Fogarty balloon catheter be necessary to clear the distal thrombus. The distal intimal end point should be carefully inspected to ensure that it is well attached. Regardless of the carotid back blood pressure or EEG, patients with neurologic deficits have demonstrated that they cannot tolerate an occluded ICA, and so blood flow must be established expeditiously by placement of a shunt. In patients who have a patent ICA a shunt is usually reinserted after inspection of the artery. The artery is reclosed with a patch. Remember, these patients now have a second downstream occlusion of a cerebral artery, presumably from an embolus, to explain their neuroloic deficit.

POSTOPERATIVE TRANSIENT ISCHEMIC ATTACK

A third decision must be made about patients who awaken without neurologic deficit and either in the recovery room or while awaiting hospital discharge have a transient ischemic attack. It has been our policy with these patients immediately to give heparin sodium and obtain an expeditious duplex scan. If the scan shows that the artery is occluded, the problem is what to do next. In patients who had excellent carotid back blood pressure at the original operation and who are neurologically intact, reoperation may not be recommended. These patients should undergo expeditious computed tomographic (CT) examination of the head to exclude intracranial hemorrhage, and heparin sodium therapy continued and converted to warfarin for 1 to 2 months. The object of the anticoagulation is to prevent distal extension or propagation of the ICA thrombus. Reoperation has the advantage of restoring blood flow into the ICA and the disadvantage of subjecting the patient to the risk of stroke during operative manipulation.

In patients who have had a postoperative transient ischemic attack and who have a patent ICA by duplex scanning, heparin sodium is continued after an expeditious head CT documents the absence of intracranial bleeding. Then an arteriogram is obtained. In the presence of a normal arteriogram we discontinue the heparin sodium therapy and maintain the patient on aspirin. The rationale for the choice between aspirin and warfarin is not based on any data. Patients with arteriographic abnormalities are reoperated upon to correct the defect.

The evidence that these algorithms are worthwhile is scanty. Edwards and co-workers have followed this protocol.[5] They reported reexploring 20 patients of whom 12 had a thrombectomy and revision, but 8 were found to have no thrombus. Three of the patients with thrombus recovered without neurologic deficit, and 9 had some neurologic deficit.[6] Of patients without thrombus, 3 recovered with no neurologic deficit and 5 continued to have some type of neurologic deficit.

Courbier and Ferdani[7] reported their experience with postoperative carotid thrombosis: 12 patients were re-explored, and 3 of them died. Three recovered completely, although 1 had a late new stroke. Three had mild residual deficits, and 3 had severe deficits. Of the 8 patients who were observed, 1 died, 1 had complete recovery, 4 had a mild deficit after recovery, and 1 had a severe deficit. One of these patients had a contralateral deficit. Thus, in this series the difference between patients reoperated upon and those observed was not significant.

If the evidence for successful re-exploration is not compelling, why do it? Most of us have experience with the occasional patient who seems to recover quickly after restoration of blood flow. These few successes compel us to recommend early reoperation. Since few series detail management of large numbers of postoperative carotid strokes in the literature, and in none was treatment randomized, decisions will continue to be based on these rare successes or failures.

REFERENCES

1. Baker WH, Koustas G, Burke K, et al. Intraoperative duplex scanning and late carotid stenosis. J Vasc Surg 1994; 19:829–833.
2. Kwaan JH, Connolly JE, Sharefkin JB. Successful management of early stroke after carotid endarterectomy. Ann Surg 1979; 190: 676–678.
3. Perdue GD. Management of postendarterectomy neurologic deficits. Arch Surg 1982; 117:1079–1081.
4. Treiman RL, Cossman DV, Cohen JL, et al. Management of postoperative stroke after carotid endarterectomy. Am J Surg 1981; 142:236–238.
5. Edwards WH Jr, Jenkins JM, Edwards WH Sr, Mulherin JL Jr. Prevention of stroke during carotid endarterectomy. Am Surg 1988; 54:125–128.
6. Edwards WH Sr. Personal communications, August 1988.
7. Courbier R, Ferdani M. Criteria for immediate reoperation following carotid surgery. In: Bergen JJ, Yao JST, eds. Reoperative arterial surgery. Orlando: Grune & Stratton, 1986:495.

RECURRENT CAROTID ARTERY STENOSIS FOLLOWING ENDARTERECTOMY

D. EUGENE STRANDNESS Jr. M.D.

The symptomatic patient who undergoes carotid endarterectomy (CEA) has an excellent prognosis compared with those patients who are treated by medical means. The results of the North American Symptomatic Carotid Endarterectomy Trial (NASCET) clearly documented that for up to 2 years of follow-up, CEA was clearly superior to conventional medical therapy for those lesions that narrowed the carotid artery by 70% or more in diameter reduction.[1]

There are basically two late postoperative problems that can develop, both of which occur within well-known time frames. The first is myointimal hyperplasia, and the second is recurrent atherosclerosis. Myointimal hyperplasia tends to develop within the first several months after the procedure and is usually stable by the end of the first year. Atherosclerosis, when it develops, is within the area of plaque removal and does not usually develop before two years after operation.

Myointimal hyperplasia occurs at sites where the arterial wall is injured. The lesion that forms is smooth, white, and tough and rarely ulcerates. This is in contrast to recurrent atherosclerotic lesions, which are indistinguishable from those commonly seen at the time of initial operation.

PREVALENCE

Before dealing with the issue of prevalence, it is important to review the categories of stenosis that have been developed and comment on their relevance to clinical outcome. Specific categories of stenosis severity were defined with the development of duplex scanning. Because this method was developed to detect carotid lesions, it became important to develop criteria that could be used for classification of the degree of narrowing. Although there are different algorithms for assessing the degree of stenosis, those developed and used by our group will serve as the basis for discussion. The following categories of stenosis have relevance to possible outcome both for the myointimal lesions and recurrent atherosclerotic plaques.

1. Normal. The carotid bulb is entirely free of disease.
2. 1% to 15% stenosis. The classification scheme has been modified since it was introduced in the late 1970s. At present, this category is reserved for patients whose carotid bulb is filled with an atheroma that has not yet extended to impinge on the blood flow stream feeding the internal carotid artery.
3. 16% to 49% narrowing. The atheroma is beginning to impinge on the blood flow into the internal carotid artery. This is not considered to be a pressure or flow-reducing lesion and is generally benign.
4. 50% to 79% stenosis. This lesion is generally referred to as hemodynamically significant because it may be associated with a decrease in blood pressure and blood flow across the lesion itself.
5. 80% to 99% narrowing. These are preocclusive or prethrombotic lesions. If not removed, they frequently progress to a occlusion of the internal carotid artery.
6. Occlusion.

Our own studies of this problem have extended over more than 10 years with the first report appearing in 1982.[2] Validation studies comparing duplex scanning with arteriography were done in patients with suspected carotid disease and in those who had undergone CEA.[3] The sensitivity has been in the range of 98% with a specificity of 94%. Arteriography (Table 1) after CEA was performed in 36 patients (44 segments) with a mean follow-up of 29 months (range 1 week to 10 years). Arteriography was performed for clinical indications, not simply to document the status of the operated segment of carotid artery.

The extent of agreement with arteriography in this group of patients is as follows:

1. One normal artery was classified as 16% to 49% stenosis.
2. Two of the 5 arteries in the 1% to 15% group were classified in the 16% to 49% category.
3. In the 16% to 49% stenosis group, in the 21 sides, 1 was classified as less severe, with the remaining 5 placed into a higher category of narrowing.
4. Of the 15 in the 50% to 99% group, 14 were properly classified with 1 in the 16% to 49% group.
5. The 2 occlusions were correctly identified.

If we consider only the high-grade lesions (50% to 99%), the overall accuracy of duplex scanning is 94%.

Table 1 Distribution of Lesions in 36 Patients (44 Segments) Who Have Undergone Endarterectomy

Diameter Reduction (%)	Number of Sides	Percent
Normal	1	2.3
1–15	5	11.4
16–49	21	47.7
50–99	15	34.1
Occlusion	2	4.5

PROSPECTIVE STUDY POPULATIONS

Our studies in this area have covered different time periods and dealt with some slightly different issues. In our first publication (1982), we were able to study prospectively 76 patients (89 operations), all of whom had operative arteriograms to document the status of the endarterectomized segment.[2] The follow-up studies for this group showed that the prevalence of a 50% to 99% stenosis was 36%. However, in nine of these arteries, the lesions appeared to regress, giving an overall restenosis rate of 19%. Only one artery developed occlusion. Of the entire group, eight patients developed recurrent neurologic symptoms appropriate to the operated segment. In one-half of the symptomatic patients, less than 50% stenosis was found, with the remainder falling into the greater than 50% category.

In a subsequent prospective study published in 1985, we evaluated 107 men and 27 women (145 sides) with a follow-up period that extended to 4 years.[4] There were 9 deaths, of which 2 were stroke related. Focal symptoms developed in 12 patients relative to the operated segment, 6 of which were strokes (one lacunar). Transient ischemic attacks occurred in 7 patients, but in only 2 were these related to a greater than 50% diameter reducing stenosis. The persistent recurrent stenosis rate was found to be 17% (greater than 50% diameter reduction). In this study, the restenosis appeared early and was stable by 24 months.

Our final study of this problem concluded in 1989. In the course of evaluating the outcome of 301 patients, the overall restenosis rate at 7 years was 31%.[5] Regression of the lesion appeared to occur in 10%, leaving a persistent restenosis rate of 21%. Transient ischemic attacks developed in 12%, with stroke in 3%. However, it became clear that the cumulative prevalence of symptoms was no higher in those with restenosis as compared to those without.

One very important question relates to the likelihood that a myointimal hyperplastic lesion might progress to occlusion of the internal carotid artery. Healy and colleagues investigated this in 200 consecutive patients who had been followed by serial duplex scans for a mean follow-up period of 31 months.[6] In this group, there were five occlusions: one perioperative and four during follow-up. In three of the four, a stroke occurred at the time of the occlusion. It is not clear what relationship the occlusions had to either myointimal hyperplasia or recurrent atherosclerosis.

DISCUSSION

Our knowledge of the development of myointimal hyperplasia has evolved over the years, but most of the information is observational in that we do not understand its pathogenesis or methods of prevention. The facts that have emerged are as follows:

1. The process can develop very early (weeks) but appears to be complete within the first 2 years.
2. The lesions themselves are uniform in composition and appear to be primarily smooth muscle cells.
3. The surface of the lesion appears to be smooth and, as far as is known, does not appear to ulcerate regularly.
4. Although not absolutely proven, some of these lesions appear to regress to a lesser degree of narrowing.
5. Although there appears to be no doubt that some lesions may be responsible for the development of ischemic events, this association is not as well established. In fact, when the patient becomes symptomatic, the diagnosis appears to be one of exclusion.
6. After 2 years, it is generally agreed that recurrent stenoses should be considered likely to be secondary to atherosclerosis. It is not certain but likely that all of the factors that pertain to those lesions that occur de novo also pertain here.

It is difficult to develop firm management guidelines when the prevalence of symptoms is so low. However, for myointimal lesions that are less than 80% diameter reduction, operation is not indicated in the absence of symptoms. There is no evidence that recurrent operation will have any benefit for the prevention of subsequent events. The one category where uncertainty remains is very high-grade (greater than 80%) lesions and their potential for progressing to occlusion. These patients should be given consideration for operation because progression to occlusion carries a 25% chance of a completed stroke. With regard to the issue of progression to occlusion, some data may be relevant to this issue. As noted, the study by Healy and co-workers suggests that some lesions in the long-term can progress to occlusion and then lead to the development of a completed stroke.[6]

The surgical procedures designed to correct recurrent carotid stenosis depend upon the extent of involvement, the degree of narrowing, the material itself, ability to repeat the endarterectomy, and the size of the artery. In 1988 we reported the results of reoperation in 14 patients.[7] The indications for operation were recurrent transient ischemic attacks in 8 patients, 2 with a stroke, and 4 with veterbrobasilar insufficiency. These 14 represented 1.3% of the patients who had undergone CEA from 1979 to 1986. In all but 2, the area of restensois was in the proximal internal carotid artery and within 2 cm of the bifurcation. In the remaining 2 patients, the area of recurrence was in the common carotid artery.

The material found at the time of operation was myointimal hyperplasia alone in two, with the remaining patients having lesions that appeared to be mainly atherosclerosis with some remnants of myointimal hyperplasia. The surgical therapy depended upon the findings at operation. Eleven underwent repeat CEA with patch angioplasty, two had patch angioplasty alone, and one needed arterial replacement with a vein graft. Thus, the local treatment of the lesion varied, but in nearly all patients it is felt that a patch is needed. There were no ischemic complications, but two patients had injury to the cranial nerves.

REFERENCES

1. North American Symptomatic Carotid Endarterectomy Trial Collaborators (NASCET). Beneficial effect of carotid endarterectomy in symptomatic patients with high grade carotid stenosis. N Engl J Med 1991; 325:445-463.
2. Zierler RE, Bandyk DF, Thiele BL, et al. Carotid artery stenosis following carotid endarterectomy. Arch Surg 1982; 117:1408-1415.
3. Roederer GO, Langlois Y, Chan ATW, et al. Postendarterectomy carotid ultrasonic duplex scanning concordance with arteriography. Ultrasound Med Biol 1983; 9:73-78.
4. Nicholls SC, Phillips DJ, Bergelin RO, et al. Carotid endarterectomy: Relationship of outcome to early restenosis. J Vasc Surg 1985; 2:375-381.
5. Healy DA, Zierler RE, Nicholls SC, et al. Long-term follow-up and clinical outcome of carotid restenosis. J Vasc Surg 1989; 10: 662-669.
6. Healy D, Clowes AW, Zierler RR, et al. Immediate and long-term results of carotid endarterectomy. Stroke 1989; 20:1138-1142.
7. Kazmers A, Zierler RE, Huang TW, Pulliam CW. Reoperative carotid surgery. Am J Surg 1988; 156:346-352.

SURGICAL MANAGEMENT OF RECURRENT CAROTID ARTERY STENOSIS

WILLIAM C. MACKEY, M.D.

The natural history of untreated recurrent carotid stenosis has not been described in detail. Recurrent carotid stenoses, exceeding 50% reduction in diameter, occur in 16% to 22% of patients after carotid endarterectomy (CEA).[1-3] Despite the frequency with which significant recurrence is found, transient cerebral ischemic events or strokes related to recurrent stenoses are unusual, occurring in only 3% to 4% of all patients.

Even in patients with documented recurrent stenoses, neurologic symptoms and especially strokes are unusual. More than half of patients with significant restenosis remained asymptomatic without intervention and did not progress to carotid occlusion over a mean follow-up period of 52.6 months (Table 1).[1] The 5 year life table stroke-free rate in patients with 50% or more carotid restenosis was 96%, which was not significantly different from the 97% 5 year life table stroke-free rate in patients without recurrent stenosis.[1] Recurrent carotid stenosis, then, although frequently discovered on follow-up duplex ultrasound, most often remains asymptomatic or results in transient symptoms that prompt further evaluation and therapy. Unheralded stroke related to recurrent carotid stenosis is unusual.

Using our carotid follow-up registry, we evaluated all patients who suffered a stroke more than 30 days

Table 1 Clinical Outcome in Patients with 50% or Greater Recurrent Stenosis

Patient Status	Number	Percent
Asymptomatic, no occlusion, no reoperation	29/55	52.8%
Occlusion with no neurologic residua	8/55	14.5%
Reoperation for transient ischemic attacks	8/55	14.5%
Reoperation for asymptomatic restenosis	8/55	14.5%
Unheralded stroke	2/55	5.5%

after CEA.[4] In this group the incidence of late stroke was 35 of 688 (5.1%). Of these 35 late strokes, only 11 (31.4%) were clearly related to recurrent stenosis. Only 3 of 20 (15%) strokes occurring within 36 months of CEA were related to recurrent stenosis, but 8 of 15 (53.3%) occurring after 36 months were related to restenosis. It is likely, therefore, that early restenoses related to neointimal fibrous hyperplasia are less likely to result in stroke than later restenoses related to atherosclerotic degeneration of the endarterectomized segment. Neointimal hyperplastic lesions are of smooth, uniform, fibrous consistency, whereas recurrent atherosclerotic lesions are more likely to have irregular, ulcerated surfaces lined by thrombus and pultaceous debris. This difference in plaque morphology may explain the possible difference in clinical behavior of the early and late restenoses.[5]

INDICATIONS FOR REOPERATION

Because stroke related to recurrent stenosis is uncommon and because the risks of reoperation may be high, the indications for redo CEA must be carefully evaluated. Most neurologists and vascular surgeons agree that patients with symptoms related to a high-grade recurrent stenosis should undergo another CEA, although no compelling data exist to support this approach. Less certain is the role of redo endarterectomy for asymptomatic lesions. In considering the role of redo endarterectomy in asymptomatic restenosis, it must be kept in mind that the role of CEA for asymptomatic primary lesions is unclear. Because the risks of redo endarterectomy, especially local anatomic complications such as cranial nerve injury, are higher than the risks of primary endarterectomy, a risk-benefit analysis of redo endarterectomy for asymptomatic restenosis may favor a conservative approach. Only patients deemed to be at highest risk from asymptomatic restenoses and at lowest risk for operation should be considered candidates for reoperation.

Based on our experience with early (up to 36 months) restenosis, we recommend a nonoperative approach. Only symptomatic patients or good-risk asymptomatic patients with progressive or preocclusive (greater than 90%) early restenoses are considered for operation. All other patients with early restenoses are followed. In some patients these lesions have been noted to regress slightly.

Patients with late (after 36 months) restenoses are offered operation if they are symptomatic or if they are good risk and have a high-grade (greater than 75%) lesion or a shaggy, ulcerated plaque. Many patients with late restenoses are followed because of advanced age or significant comorbidities.

SURGICAL TECHNIQUE

Meticulous dissection of the artery with adequate proximal and distal exposure is essential for safe redo endarterectomy. Cranial nerve injury is the most frequently reported complication of redo endarterectomy in that it occurs in over 15% of patients.[6] The frequency and potential morbidity of this complication underscore the importance of care during arterial exposure. Ideally, proximal and distal exposure should extend beyond the limits of the exposure for the primary operation in order to ensure that complete endarterectomy is possible. Some surgeons have advocated dissection outside the scar from the prior operation until proximal and distal control are achieved in order to lessen the likelihood of embolization from arterial manipulation. Dissecting in this manner may be especially important in patients with friable, ulcerated lesions, characteristic of late recurrent stenoses. Mandibular subluxation may be an appropriate adjunct in patients where the need for very high exposure is anticipated.

Cerebral monitoring and protection techniques are no different than for primary CEA. Routine shunting and selective shunting based on electroencephalography or carotid stump blood pressure measurements are acceptable alternatives in redo endarterectomy. Because of the technical difficulty of many reoperations, regional anesthesia with neurologic monitoring by direct patient observation is not applicable.

In instances of early recurrent stenosis due to neointimal fibrous hyperplasia, CEA may be very difficult. Persistent attempts to achieve an endarterectomy plane where none exists may result in disruption of the artery and need for vein interposition. Nevertheless, the hyperplastic lesion can usually be shaved from the underlying arterial wall by using a fine blade and gentle blunt technique. Once an adequate flow surface has been achieved, a patch of saphenous vein harvested from the thigh or groin or a synthetic patch should be used to enlarge the luminal diameter to prevent a secondary recurrence.

Recurrent stenosis occurring late and related to atherosclerotic degeneration is usually amenable to standard endarterectomy. An appropriate endarterectomy plane is often achieved without difficulty. Again, patch closure is almost always performed unless the artery is large and the lesion confined to the common carotid and proximal bulb.

RESULTS

With these criteria for patient selection and guidelines for surgical technique, satisfactory results have been reported in patients requiring reoperation.[6] Our perioperative stroke rate was 3.5% and there were no perioperative deaths. Postoperative cranial nerve palsies were noted in 17.2% of patients, but all have been transient. Life table stroke-free rates (92% 1 year and 83.3% 5 year) following redo endarterectomies are acceptable and only slightly lower than those following primary operation (96.7% 1 year and 90.9% 5 year).[6,7]

Comparison of stroke-free rates from the time of primary operation in patients who were and were not operated upon for recurrent stenoses documented no statistically significant differences.[6] However, patients with recurrent stenoses, regardless of whether they underwent reoperation, in aggregate do not appear to fare differently than patients without recurrent stenoses in stroke-free rates. Because the incidence of stroke related to recurrent stenosis is so low, it is difficult to prove that operation for recurrent stenosis reduces stroke risk. Nevertheless, experience suggests that selected patients with recurrent stenoses deemed to be at high risk for stroke can be managed surgically with acceptable perioperative morbidity and mortality rates and with long-term benefit similar to that following primary operations.[6] Careful patient selection and conduct of the reoperation in a center with sufficient experience in reoperative carotid procedures are necessary to ensure that benefit exceeds risk in these patients.

REFERENCES

1. Mackey WC, Belkin M, Sindhi R, et al. Routine postendarterectomy duplex surveillance: Does it prevent late stroke? J Vasc Surg 1992; 16:934–940.
2. Cook JM, Thompson BW, Barnes RW. Is routine duplex examination after carotid endarterectomy justified? J Vasc Surg 1990; 12:334–339.
3. Nichols SC, Phillips DJ, Bergelin RO, et al. Carotid endarterectomy: Relationship of outcome to early restenosis. J Vasc Surg 1985; 2:375–381.
4. Washburn WK, Mackey WC, Belkin M, O'Donnell TF. Late stroke after carotid endarterectomy: The role of recurrent stenosis. J Vasc Surg 1992; 15:1032–1037.
5. O'Donnell TF, Callow AD, Scott G, et al. Ultrasound characteristics of recurrent carotid disease: Hypothesis explaining the low incidence of symptomatic recurrence. J Vasc Surg 1985; 2:26–41.
6. Nitzberg RS, Mackey WC, Prendiville E, et al. Long-term follow-up of patients operated on for recurrent carotid stenosis. J Vasc Surg 1991; 13:121–127.
7. Callow AD, Mackey WC. Long-term follow-up of surgically managed carotid bifurcation atherosclerosis: Justification for an aggressive approach. Ann Surg 1989; 210:308–316.

SURGICAL TREATMENT OF TRANSIENT ISCHEMIC ATTACK AND STROKE SECONDARY TO EXTERNAL CAROTID ATHEROSCLEROSIS

JONATHAN P. GERTLER, M.D.

Internal carotid artery (ICA) occlusion carries a poor prognosis despite what is frequently an asymptomatic presentation. It is difficult to estimate the number of patients in whom an ICA occlusion will manifest initially with either transient ischemic attack or frank stroke. However, prospective studies of patients with known ICA occlusions suggest a delayed stroke rate approaching 25% within 2 to 3 years.[1]

The mechanism of acute stroke after ICA occlusion is typically embolism to the middle cerebral artery distribution, thrombus extension past the ophthalmic artery into the circle of Willis, or hemodynamic insufficiency in association with either an isolated hemisphere or diffuse extracranial cerebral vascular disease. Stroke at an interval following ICA occlusion may be due to similar mechanisms but may also arise from a diseased external carotid artery (ECA) or a remnant ICA cul-de-sac containing thrombus and/or platelet or fibrin debris. In either case turbulent flow at the carotid bifurcation may sweep atheroembolic material into the intracranial vasculature via external carotid collaterals. Occasionally the ECA is the major cerebral collateral in the setting of ICA occlusion, and a proximal ECA stenosis may have a hemodynamic impact on cerebral perfusion.

ANATOMY OF CEREBRAL COLLATERAL CIRCULATION

Although cerebral collateral blood flow may depend on contralateral intracranial supply and/or basilar artery blood flow from either or both vertebral arteries, it is important to recognize that the circle of Willis is incomplete in as many as 60% of patients.[2] The ECA may also provide significant ipsilateral collateralization and at the very least may be a source of significant-sized collaterals through which atherosclerotic debris may reach the intracranial vessels.[3]

Adult cerebral collateral arterial branches have been categorized by Alksne[4] into large interarterial connections, intracranial-extracranial connections, and small interarterial anastomoses. Other rarer collateral vessels are based on persistent trigeminal and hypoglossal arteries, which provide carotid basilar connections.

The ECA serves as a major extracranial arterial collateral primarily through periorbital branches. Periophthalmic channels depend on the superficial temporal, angular, middle meningeal, and infraorbital arteries. Vertebral collateral is provided through the occipital branch of the ECA as well as the costocervical trunk and the contralateral vertebral artery, which communicates at the level of the intervertebral foramen. Perimeningeal, stylomastoid, and anterior tympanic branches of the ECA may all provide collateral channels of varying degrees of significance (Fig. 1).

EVALUATION OF THE PATIENT WITH SYMPTOMATIC ICA OCCLUSION

Although metabolic testing for patients with ICA occlusion is accelerating on an experimental basis and transcranial Doppler determination of existing cerebral collaterals has been developed from a technical viewpoint, decision making for ECA endarterectomy remains

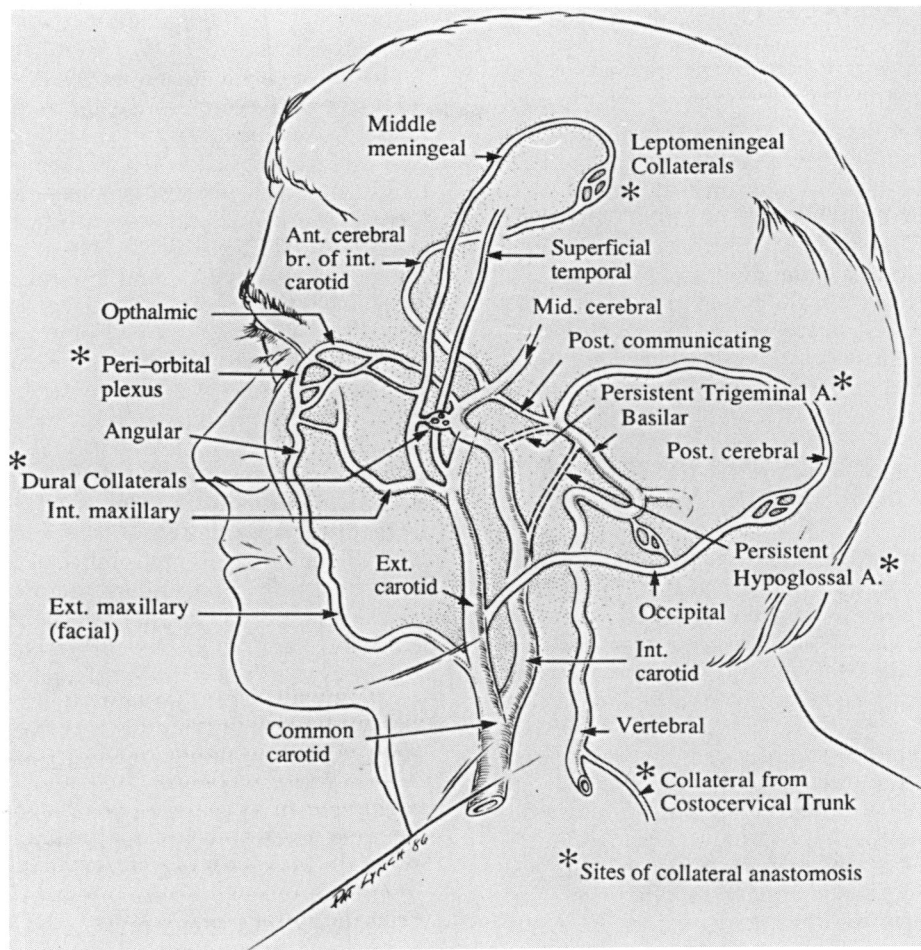

Figure 1 Extracranial collateral pathways.

primarily clinical. To this end, thorough extracranial vascular examination, with special attention to evidence of subclavian stenoses and complete evaluation of the palpable branches of the ECA, remains the basis of all other testing. The patient's history is equally important. It is important to differentiate vague neurologic complaints from specific hemispheric and ocular findings. Ophthalmologic examination to corroborate suspected retinal embolic events is recommended. Although global cerebral hypoperfusion manifest as vertebral basilar insufficiency and/or focal watershed hemodynamic problems may be correctable by ECA endarterectomy, it is the specific hemispheric event ipsilateral to an appropriately occluded ICA and diseased ECA that is most confidently treated.

A battery of evaluations can provide supplemental data and provide an important postoperative means of assessing the results of any ECA intervention. Baseline computed tomography or magnetic resonance imaging (MRI) should be performed to document existing cerebral tissue loss as well as any unsuspected lesions in the distribution of the occluded ICA. Carotid duplex examination will add hemodynamic data about the degree of ECA stenosis and identify turbulent areas around an ICA cul-de-sac. Transcranial Doppler along with the noninvasive examination can identify cerebral collateral pathways as either contributory or not, and considered with subsequent arteriography, may provide corroborative data to ignore or repair a significant ECA stenosis.[5] It has been suggested that cerebral compensation for carotid occlusion is primarily hemodynamic rather than metabolic.[6] Given that the ECA does not always develop as an important hemodynamic collateral pathway, in the absence of clear embolic events related to a diseased ECA or occluded ICA, hemodynamic assessment of the collateral blood supply will increase the accuracy of the decision-making process.

Alternative testing such as magnetic resonance angiography of the distal ICA[7] and assorted metabolic tests of the brain such as position emission tomography (PET) scanning,[6] MRI variants, CO_2 reactivity, and calculations of regional blood flows[5] are not sufficiently well developed or widespread to justify their inclusion in the routine preoperative evaluation. Nonetheless, for a true sense of how ECA endarterectomy is to be applied in the setting of global hypoperfusion, these types of evaluation will be critically important.

There is an absolute necessity for four-vessel angiography in any patient with noninvasively proven diffuse cerebral vascular disease being evaluated for recurrent or new-onset symptoms in the presence of ICA occlusion. Arteriography should include aortic arch views to exclude proximal sources of emboli from the great vessels as well as subclavian stenoses, which may compromise the posterior circulation. Precise definition of the status of the vertebral arteries as well as both carotid bifurcations is necessary, as is a thorough delineation of the intracranial vasculature and their collateral (cross-filling) relationships.

CURRENT INDICATIONS AND RESULTS OF SURGICAL TREATMENT

Patients with either an ICA occlusion and an ECA stenosis or a prominent ICA cul-de-sac and appropriate ipsilateral symptoms are well treated by ECA endarterectomy and ICA cul-de-sac obliteration (Fig. 2). In individuals with either contralateral hemispheric complaints or evidence of global hypoperfusion in the absence of other correctable extracranial pathology (i.e., contralateral carotid stenosis or vertebral disease of hemodynamic significance) and with evidence of ECA collaterals on arteriographic and noninvasive evaluation, symptomatic improvement after ECA endarterectomy may be anticipated. However, this less precise indication does not appear to offer the same security of neurologic improvement as does ECA endarterectomy in the patient with more specific hemispheric complaints.

In a collective review of ECA endarterectomy in 1987[8] and in several publications since that time,[9,10] these personal observations have been confirmed. Most ECA endarterectomies are performed for either amaurosis fugax or transient hemispheric ischemic attacks. In the 1987 review of patients with transient ischemic attack (TIA) or amaurosis in whom outcome data were available, 92% resolved and 8% improved. Other interesting indications included patients who were being prepared for the now rarely performed temporal artery–middle cerebral artery bypass by having ECA reconstruction as a preliminary step. All of these had resolution of symptoms without the intracranial procedure. The problem that continues to vex students of ECA reconstruction is that these reports are anecdotal and provide little justification for the procedure beyond the theoretic appeal. Earlier work using xenon perfusion scans documented the feasibility of increasing cerebral blood flow with ECA endarterectomy, but far-reaching clinical data are not available. Therefore, although the decision to perform ECA endarterectomy remains clinical, any available cerebral perfusion studies and careful preoperative and postoperative neurologic examinations should be obtained. This is especially true for patients in whom the indications for operation are inexact.

TECHNIQUE OF EXTERNAL CAROTID ENDARTERECTOMY

Exposure of the carotid bifurcation is carried out in routine fashion. Continuous EEG monitoring is desirable, since shunting through the ECA during the procedure is feasible and can be a highly effective means of increasing intracranial perfusion intraoperatively. The ICA is excised flush with the carotid bulb and oversewn with fine polypropylene suture even in the absence of an ICA cul-de-sac (Fig. 3). Mere ligation of the ICA origin may extrude atherosclerotic debris or thrombus into the ECA reconstruction, undermining the procedure. A longitudinal arteriotomy is made into the ECA, which should be dissected well up into the neck and its branches controlled. Precise excision of the ECA plaque with eversion endarterectomy of branch vessels is recommended, avoiding tacking sutures if a clean intimal end point can be obtained. A saphenous vein patch, or alternative if no vein is available, is placed over the ECA in standard fashion (Fig. 3).

RECOMMENDATIONS

External carotid endarterectomy may be useful in the unusual patient with ongoing hemispheric symptoms ipsilateral to an ICA occlusion (Table 1). Although theoretically appealing for improving cerebral perfusion in the setting of diffuse extracranial vascular disease, this indication is less common and less clearly effective.

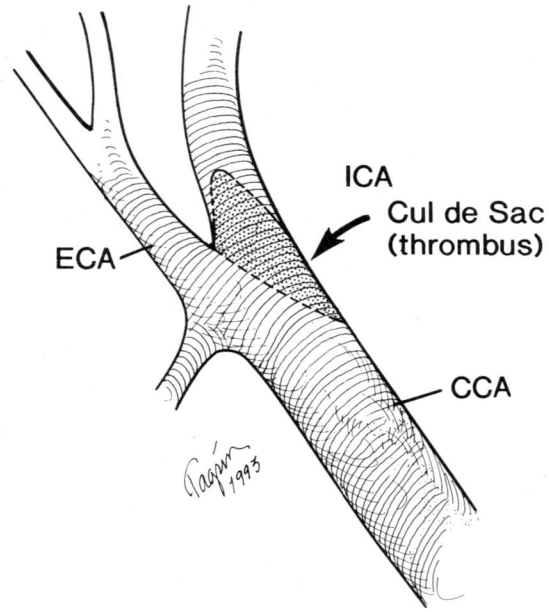

Figure 2 Internal carotid artery cul-de-sac, a potential source of cerebral emboli via the external carotid collaterals.

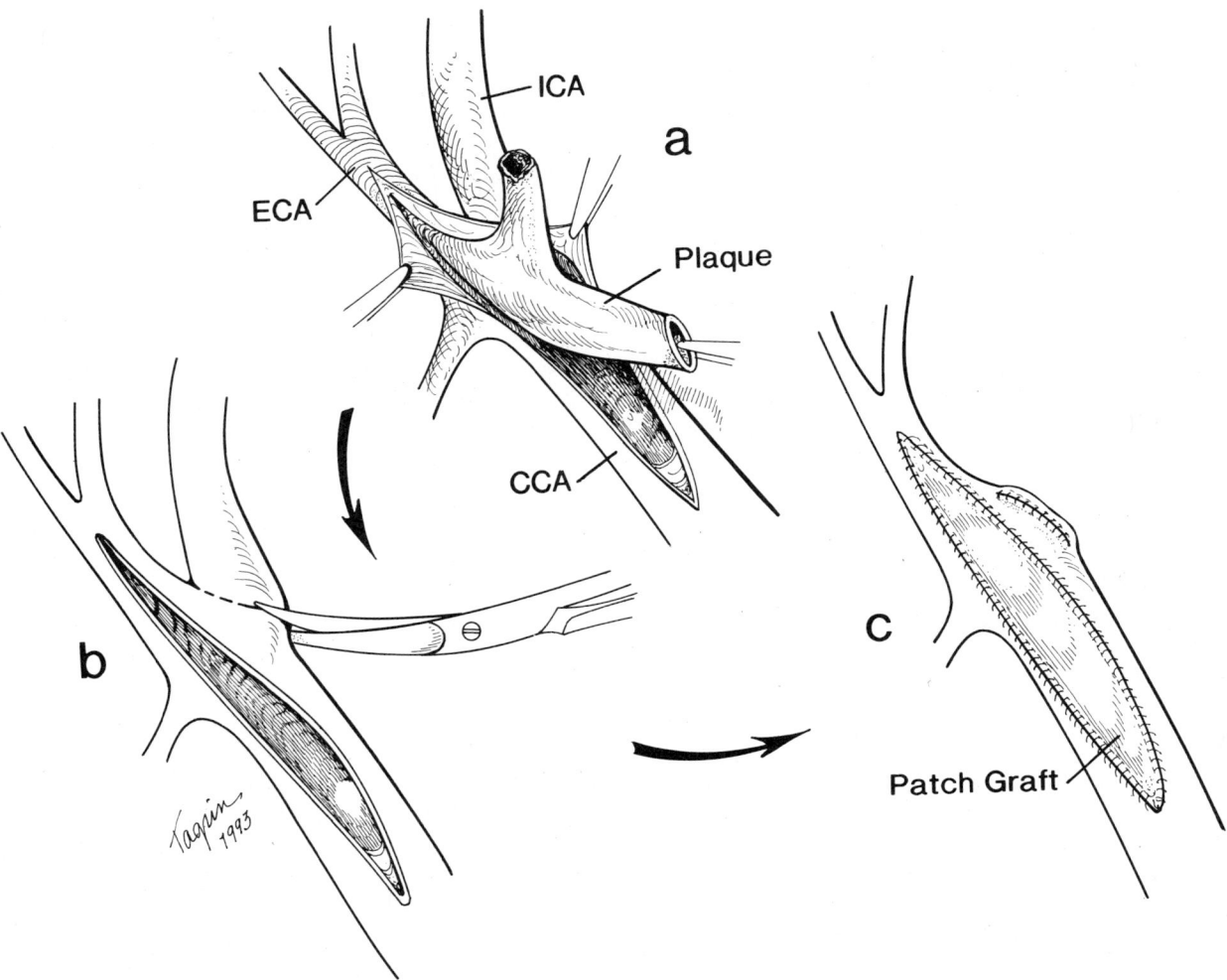

Figure 3 Technique of external carotid endarterectomy. *A*, Arteriotomy is extended onto the external carotid artery past the end point of the plaque. *B*, The internal carotid artery is divided sharply several millimeters beyond its origin and disease removed by eversion endarterectomy. *C*, A patch graft is placed on the external carotid artery and the internal carotid orifice is oversewn.

Table 1 Outcome of ECA Revascularization (Endarterectomy or Bypass) vs. Indication for Operation (Updated October 1993)

Indication	Resolved	Improved	Unchanged	Worsened	Death	Unspecified
Amaurosis fugax	38	11	0	0	0	22
Hemispheric TIA	38	2	0	0	0	8
Crescendo TIA	2	0	0	0	0	2
Previous CVA	9	1	5	0	0	3
Vague Neuro SX's	11	8	0	0	0	
Pre–EC-IC bypass	7	0	0	0	0	
Unspecified	76	0	2	6	6	
	181(70%)	22(8.5%)	7(3%)	6(2.5%)	6(2.5%)	35(13.5%)

Thorough noninvasive and arteriographic evaluation, thorough neurologic examinations, and evaluation of preoperative and postoperative cerebral perfusion status, if available, offer the best chance for selecting the appropriate patient for operation. The technique of ECA endarterectomy is similar to internal carotid endarterectomy with the additions of ECA shunting as an option, careful obliteration of the ICA cul-de-sac, and routine saphenous vein patching of the endarterectomy site.

REFERENCES

1. Cote R, Barnett HJM, Taylor DW. Internal carotid occlusion: A prospective study. Stroke 1983; 14:898–906.
2. Callow AD. An overview of the stroke: Problem in the carotid territory. AM J Surg 1980; 140:181–191.
3. Barnett HJM, Peerless SJ, Kaufman JGE. Stump of internal carotid artery: A source for further cerebral embolic ischemia. Stroke 1978; 9:448–456.
4. Alksne JF. Collateral circulation. In: Strandness DE, ed. Collateral circulation in clinical surgery. Philadelphia: WB Saunders, 1969:595.
5. Norris JW, Krajewski A, Bornstein NM. The clinical role of the cerebral collateral circulation in carotid occlusion. J Vasc Surg 1990; 8:113–118.
6. Kuwert T, Hennerici M, Langen KJ, et al. Compensatory mechanisms in patients with asymptomatic carotid artery occlusion. Neurol Res 1990; 6:89–93.
7. Provinciali L, Minciotti P, Ceravolo MG, et al. Haemodynamic changes following carotid occlusion: MRI angiography and transcranial Doppler patterns. Neurol Res 1992; 14:208–210.
8. Gertler JP, Cambria RP. The role of external carotid endarterectomy in the treatment of ipsilateral internal carotid occlusion: Collective review. J Vasc Surg 1987; 8:158–167.
9. Nicholls SC, Kohler TR, Bergelin RO, Strandness DE, Jr. Management of internal carotid artery occlusion. J Cardiovasc Surg 1989; 8(9):547–552.
10. Sterpetti AV, Feldhaus RJ, Schultz RD, Farina C. Operative strategies in patients with symptomatic internal carotid artery occlusion. Surg 1989; 5:632–637.

VERTEBRAL ARTERY RECONSTRUCTION FOR VERTEBROBASILAR INSUFFICIENCY

EDOUARD KIEFFER, M.D.
AMINE BAHNINI, M.D.
FABIEN KOSKAS, M.D.
CARLO RUOTOLO, M.D.

Surgical reconstruction of the vertebral artery (VA) is gaining wider acceptance among the medical community, although operative indications are still controversial. During the last decade vertebrobasilar insufficiency (VBI) has been recognized as a specific entity with different mechanisms. Refinements in diagnostic techniques including positional arteriography, magnetic resonance imaging, and evoked potentials have allowed more objective assessment of patients presenting with symptoms suggesting brain stem ischemia. All segments of the VA have become accessible to surgical reconstruction using transposition or bypass grafting techniques. Finally, large series of patients with sufficient follow-up have now been accumulated.

PATHOPHYSIOLOGY OF VERTEBROBASILAR INSUFFICIENCY

Knowledge of the pathophysiology of VBI in each individual patient is of utmost importance in discussing the indications for VA reconstruction. Postmortem studies and clinical evaluation of patients with VBI have identified two different pathologic mechanisms, thromboembolism and hemodynamic compromise.[1,2] Although these two mechanisms may coexist in a few patients, they are usually caused by different anatomic lesions, account for different clinical manifestations (Table 1), and have different prognostic and therapeutic implications.

Thromboembolic Vertebrobasilar Insufficiency

Although it is the least frequent involvement, thromboembolism may occur in the vertebrobasilar territory much in the same way as it occurs in the carotid territory. Atherosclerosis does not play a major role in this mechanism because of the usually smooth nature of the atherosclerotic plaques of the VA. Nonatherosclerotic lesions, especially traumatic and spontaneous aneurysms or dissections, are the most frequent etiologies, because of the intimal disease and the possibility of mural thrombus formation in such lesions.

Most large emboli lodge at the end of the basilar artery or in one or both of the posterior cerebral arteries. The smallest emboli may produce transient ischemic attacks (TIAs) that usually last several hours or reversible ischemic neurologic deficits (RINDs), in which neurologic symptoms may last several days or a few weeks.

Segmental occlusions of the VA are frequent. In the most surgically favorable cases, reconstitution of the VA occurs at the C1–C2 level through ipsilateral collateral circulation from the external carotid artery or branches of the subclavian artery.[3] Occlusion may also extend intracranially up to the origin of the posteroinferior cerebellar artery (PICA) that remains patent through the opposite VA. Such segmental VA occlusions are compatible with absent or minimal neurologic complications. In more extensive occlusions that involve the origin of the PICA or the basilar artery itself, neurologic complications are usually severe, ranging from limited lateromedullary or cerebellar infarcts to massive infarctions of the brain stem.

Although complete or near complete clinical recovery occurs in about 50% of patients with vertebrobasilar strokes, early mortality remains as high as 20% to 30%, which is significantly more than for carotid strokes. The prognosis for thromboembolic vertebrobasilar TIAs is

Table 1 Comparison of Timing, Circumstances, Responsiveness to Medical Therapy, and Spontaneous Course of Thromboembolic and Hemodynamic Vertebrobasilar Transient Ischemic Attacks

Thromboembolic	Hemodynamic
Long, minutes to several hours (up to 24 hours)	Brief, seconds to minutes (up to 30 minutes)
Varied, polymorphic	Stereotyped, monomorphic
Low recurrence rate, can be numbered; no periodic clusters of symptoms during follow-up	High recurrence rate, often innumerable; periodic clusters of symptoms during follow-up
Independent of body and neck position; not relieved by lying down	Triggered by erect body and specific neck positions; relieved by lying down
Nonreproducible by VA compression	Reproducible by VA compression
Responsive to antiplatelet and anticoagulant therapy	Responsive to alpha-blockers
Prognosis: infarcts during follow-up; life-threatening risk; risk of permanent sequelae	Prognosis: no infarcts during long-term follow-up; trauma from falls; functional disability

From Rancurel G, Kieffer E, Arzimanoglou A, et al. Hemodynamic vertebrobasilar ischemia: Differentiation of hemodynamic and thromboembolic mechanisms. In: Berguer R, Caplan LR, eds. Vertebrobasilar Arterial Disease. St Louis: Quality Medical Publishing, 1992:40; with permission.

Table 2 Factors Contributing to Hemodynamic Vertebrobasilar Insufficiency and Their Management

Level	Contributing Factors	Management
Hindbrain	Watershed ischemia, autoregulation disturbances	Carotid artery reconstruction Alpha-blockers
Vertebral arteries	Obstruction (permanent or transient)	Vertebral artery reconstruction
Blood	Anemia, hypoxemia, thrombocytosis, polycythemia	Medical treatment
Systemic pressure	Orthostatic hypotension	Medical treatment
Heart	Cardiac failure, rhythmic disturbances, atrioventricular conduction defects	Medical treatment Pacemaker implantation

From Kieffer E, Bahnini A, Rancurel G. Surgery of vertebral artery insufficiency. In: Bergan JJ, Yao JST, eds. Arterial surgery: New diagnostic and operative techniques. New York: Grune & Stratton, 1988:187; with permission.

probably not as good as usually believed. Recent studies using strict criteria for thromboembolic vertebrobasilar TIAs have shown a 22% to 35% 5-year stroke rate, very similar to that of carotid TIAs.

Hemodynamic Vertebrobasilar Insufficiency

Hemodynamic compromise of the posterior circulation is the primary cause of VBI. A variety of contributing factors should be considered in the discussion and management of hemodynamic VBI (Table 2).

The anatomic configuration of the vertebrobasilar arterial system and circle of Willis is unique in the human anatomy. Due to the contribution of both VAs to the formation of the basilar artery, one patent VA of sufficient diameter is usually enough to ensure satisfactory blood flow to the basilar artery. The anatomic requisites for hemodynamic VBI are, thus, either bilateral VA disease or unilateral VA disease with contralateral absent or hypoplastic VA or a small contralateral VA ending in the PICA without participating in the formation of the basilar artery. These anatomic situations logically constitute the only justified indications for VA reconstructions in hemodynamic VBI. Furthermore, the normal basilar artery is in continuity with the anterior circulation through both posterior communicating arteries. Two anatomic factors may, therefore, increase the potential for hemodynamic VBI: (1) associated carotid artery disease, a finding that is particularly frequent in atherosclerotic patients; and (2) congenital absence or hypoplasia of one or both posterior communicating arteries, a finding that is present in approximately 30% of normal individuals. These factors may be absent in some of the most severe and indisputable hemodynamic VBIs and should therefore not be considered indispensable to a justified indication for operation for hemodynamic VBI.

The susceptibility of the hindbrain to ischemia is another contributing factor. In the basilar artery there is a competition between flow coming from the vertebral arteries and that coming from the carotid arteries. This "dead point" located somewhere in the midportion of the basilar artery varies according to local factors affecting vertebrobasilar flow. Extrinsic, positional compressions of the VA (Table 3), the importance of which has been recognized only recently,[4] may be responsible for rapid variations in hindbrain perfusion, a fact that accounts for the apparently paradoxic patency of both carotid and posterior communicating arteries in a significant number of patients. The branches of the basilar artery that perfuse the hindbrain are small, terminal vessels, a situation that favors the appearance of watershed ischemia. The vestibular nucleus, which is fed by very long, small, terminal arteries, is indeed one of the most frequently ischemic structures in patients with hemodynamic VBI. Finally, elderly people, especially if hypertensive or diabetic, tend to have poor

Table 3 Extrinsic Compressions of the Extracranial Vertebral Artery That May Cause Hemodynamic Vertebrobasilar Insufficiency

VA Level	Cause
V1	Stellate ganglion
	Fibrous band
	Anterior scalene muscle
V1–V2 junction	Insertion of longus colli and anterior scalene muscle on C6
	Abnormal entrance of vertebral artery into the bony canal
V2	Cervical spondylosis
	Cervical spine trauma
	Neural or bony tumor
V3	Extraosseous course of vertebral artery
	Anterior branch of C2 nerve
	Hypermotility of C1–C2 joint
	Bony canal of the upper aspect of C1
V3–V4 junction	Foramen of the atlantooccipital membrane
	Bony abnormalities of the atlantooccipital joint

From Kieffer E, Bahnini A, Rancurel G. Surgery of vertebral artery insufficiency. In: Bergan JJ, Yao JST, eds. Arterial surgery: New diagnostic and operative techniques. New York: Grune & Stratton, 1988:187; with permission.

cerebral autoregulation, a fact that may account for failure of local compensatory mechanisms.

Cardiac function is also an important factor in hemodynamic VBI. Low cardiac output due to coronary artery insufficiency, rhythm disturbances, or atrioventricular conduction defects may lower total cerebral blood flow. Similarly, patients with orthostatic hypotension, either spontaneous or due to medication, also have the potential for decreased cerebral blood flow.

Finally, rheologic factors such as anemia, hypoxemia, thrombocytosis, or polycythemia may also contribute to tissue ischemia and aggravate hemodynamic VBI.

Although any one of the aforenoted factors may predominate in an individual patient, they usually combine in different manners to cause hemodynamic VBI. In these patients, symptoms are of short duration and repetitive. They affect mainly the territories that are fed by long terminal arteries. The nearly constant vestibular symptoms in hemodynamic VBI are due to the fact that vestibulolabyrinthine arteries are long, terminal branches arising in the midportion of the basilar artery in the vicinity of the hemodynamic dead point. Other symptoms related to brain stem or cerebellar ischemia are due to hypoperfusion in watershed areas of the cerebellum, brain stem nuclei, reticulate substance, long motor or sensory tracts of the brain stem, or upper part of the medulla. Ischemia of the occipital lobe is frequent when posterior cerebral arteries act as terminal vessels in the absence of functioning posterior communicating arteries.

The prognosis of hemodynamic VBI seems to be relatively good. Although the daily repetition of TIAs may become a functional and social handicap and cause trauma from falls, vertebrobasilar strokes are rather rare in this setting. However, the repetition of TIAs and the presence of symptoms related to ischemia of the long tracts of the brain stem should be considered ominous manifestations and harbingers of vertebrobasilar strokes.

INDICATIONS FOR OPERATION

The rationale for operation is different in thromboembolic and hemodynamic VBI.[1,5]

Thromboembolic Vertebrobasilar Ischemia

Operation for thromboembolic VBI should be considered only in patients with TIAs or a small residual deficit. It is aimed at the prevention of further thromboembolic events. Even though the contralateral VA may be widely patent, the presence of an embolic source is a logical indication to surgical treatment using either a direct reconstruction or a distal bypass excluding the lesion. Occlusion of the VA is an indication for operation only in patients with limited distal extension leaving the V3 segment accessible for bypass. In patients with more extensive occlusions, operation may be indicated in order to reconstruct a large contralateral stenotic VA and, therefore, to avoid bilateral occlusion with its attending risk of stroke.

Hemodynamic Vertebrobasilar Ischemia

The indications for operation in hemodynamic VBI are quite different (Fig. 1). The patient is fully evaluated for associated medical problems and the presence of significant carotid artery disease. Maximal treatment of medical problems is undertaken, and a specific medical treatment of VBI, including antiplatelet and alpha-adrenergic blocking drugs, is prescribed. Medical management is successful in a good number of patients. Four-vessel arteriography is indicated only in suitable surgical candidates in the presence of significant carotid artery disease, with or without symptoms, or if medical treatment of incapacitating VBI has been unsuccessful in patients with or without significant carotid artery disease. Four situations may arise according to the degree of VA disease, the association of carotid artery disease, and the possibility for reconstruction of the diseased carotid and vertebral arteries.

First, patients with significant, reconstructible carotid artery and VA disease have usually been treated by isolated carotid reconstruction. A few months later, VA reconstruction was performed, if symptoms of VBI persisted. Although many attempts have been made at predicting the clinical results of isolated carotid operations, this usually has not been possible. Failure to cure the symptoms of VBI has been noted in 30% to 50% of patients. It is our strong belief that associated carotid-vertebral reconstructions in the same operative session solve the problem without added operative risk and should therefore be performed routinely.[6]

Second, patients with VBI and significant carotid

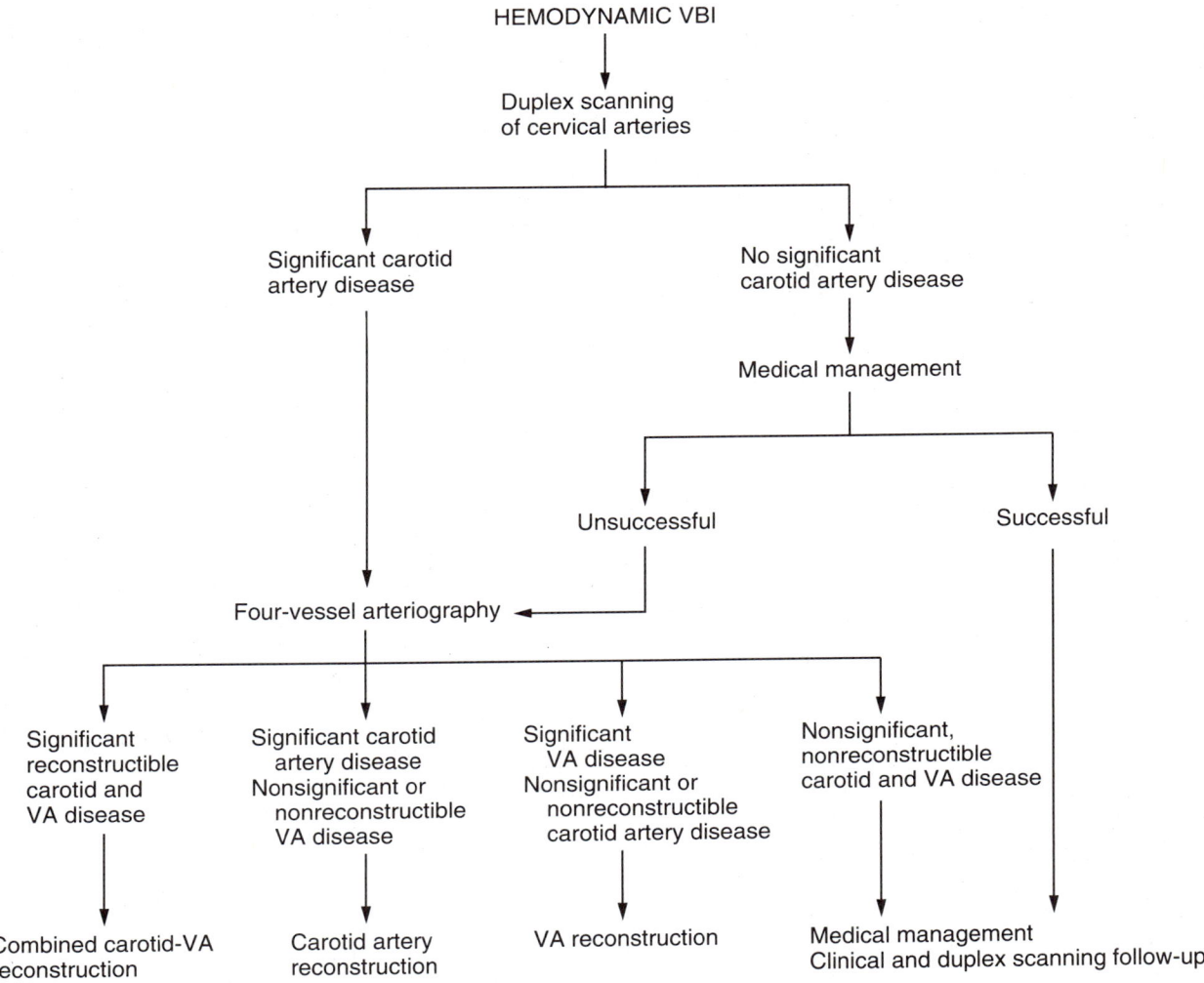

Figure 1 Algorithm for the management of hemodynamic vertebrobasilar insufficiency. VA, Vertebral artery; VBI, vertebrobasilar insufficiency.

artery disease and nonsignificant or nonreconstructible VA disease should undergo carotid reconstruction whether or not they have carotid symptoms. This situation may arise in the rare patient with diffuse nonreconstructible VA occlusions or, more frequently, in patients with bilateral, small hypoplastic VA, characteristic of hypoplasia of the vertebrobasilar arterial system.

Third, patients with VBI, significant VA lesions, and nonsignificant or nonreconstructible carotid artery lesions should have isolated VA reconstruction. The presence of nonreconstructible carotid artery disease, such as extensive common and internal carotid artery occlusion or tight stenosis of the carotid siphon, may require unusual techniques of reconstruction, such as bypass with the proximal anastomosis in the subclavian or external carotid arteries.

Finally, in the rare patient with nonsignificant or nonreconstructible lesions of both the vertebral and carotid arteries, maximal medical management is the only available therapeutic modality.

In each of these instances of hemodynamic VBI, VA reconstruction should be limited to the large, dominant VA. Very few patients, if any, need bilateral reconstructions. It should also be recognized that one or both of the VA occlusive lesions may not be evident on standard arteriograms because of variations in their anatomic position. The relationship between clinical symptoms and certain positions of the head and neck should lead to the performance of positional arteriograms under local anesthesia with the patient in the sitting position.

RECONSTRUCTIVE TECHNIQUES

Reconstruction of the VA is possible at any level of its four segments.[3,7]

V1 Segment

The approach is either through a transverse supraclavicular incision with dissociation of both heads of the sternomastoid muscle or through a presternomastoid incision in patients with short necks who require combined carotid and VA reconstruction. The VA is approached between the common carotid artery and the internal jugular vein with the vagus nerve being left adjacent to the vein. Lymphatic elements, including the thoracic duct on the left side, and the vertebral vein are carefully ligated and cut in order to avoid postoperative lymphatic drainage. The VA is then exposed along with the sympathetic chain and the stellate ganglion that should be preserved in order to avoid postoperative Horner's syndrome.

Atherosclerotic lesions at the origin of the VA have been treated using a closed transsubclavian or open endarterectomy with good results. We seldom use this technique because it needs complete exposure of the proximal subclavian artery and its branches, it may necessitate an extensive endarterectomy of the subclavian artery, it does not take into account the frequent excess in length of the V1 segment that may lead to postoperative kinking of the VA, and it entails the risk of a distal intimal flap in the VA that may be the cause of postoperative stenosis or occlusion.

Similarly, transposition into and venous bypass from the distal subclavian artery are rather complicated procedures that necessitate complete dissection of the subclavian artery. Moreover, late results may be compromised by progression of atherosclerotic disease in the subclavian artery itself. In our opinion, these two techniques should be considered only when the ipsilateral common carotid artery is not usable because of occlusion or advanced mural atherosclerosis, severe siphon stenosis, or advanced contralateral carotid occlusive disease, making clamping impossible or potentially dangerous.

The technique of choice for reconstruction of the VA in its first segment is transposition of the VA into the common carotid artery. It is a simple procedure that necessitates only limited exposure of the proximal VA and adjacent common carotid artery. It has the advantage of avoiding lesions of the subclavian artery. It allows for simultaneous management of excessive length of the VA. Finally, progression of atherosclerotic disease is seldom encountered on the common carotid artery in late follow-up. Requirements for this technique are normal common carotid and intracranial internal carotid arteries. Atherosclerotic lesions of the carotid bifurcation should be treated simultaneously, using the same presternomastoid incision. Clamping of the normal common carotid artery does not entail an added risk of cerebral ischemia because antegrade perfusion of the internal carotid artery is maintained during clamping through collaterals originating from the ipsilateral external carotid artery.

V2 Segment

Although tedious and potentially difficult, a direct approach to the VA in the V2 segment is feasible by unroofing the artery in the bony canal of the transverse processes. This segment of the VA is surrounded by a venous plexus that has to be coagulated and transsected and may constitute an operative difficulty.

Although this approach has been used extensively for direct decompression of the VA in patients with cervical spondylosis, a much simpler distal bypass from the carotid or subclavian to the V3 segment is usually preferred. In our opinion the only remaining indication to a direct approach of the V2 segment is penetrating trauma to the artery or combined neurologic and arterial compression in patients with cervical spondylosis or tumors.

V3 Segment

The introduction of a direct approach to the distal cervical VA has been a major advance in the management of VA disease.[8,9] The VA is usually approached in the C1–C2 interspace with a high presternomastoid incision. The internal jugular vein remains in the anterior part of the surgical field. The spinal accessory nerve is identified and preserved. The C1 transverse process leads to the underlying C1–C2 interspace that is exposed by resecting the muscles inserting in the lower aspect of C1. The VA is then dissected from the anterior branch of the C2 nerve and freed from the surrounding venous plexus. Approximately 2 to 3 cm of normal VA are available for the distal implantation of a saphenous bypass originating from the common carotid artery or, much less frequently, from the external carotid, internal carotid, or subclavian arteries.

Alternative techniques include transposition of the distal VA into the internal carotid artery, transposition of the occipital artery into the VA, or the use of arterial autograft obtained from the proximal V1 segment or from an endarterectomized internal carotid artery. These techniques have the advantage of bypassing all the lesions of the V2 segment with a distal anastomosis or implantation in a usually normal portion of the VA.

Rarely, a more distal approach to the VA is needed above C1. It may be obtained through a posterior extension of the previous incision or through a posterior midline incision with a lateral extension. In both cases, resection of the posterior arch of C1 allows a relatively easy approach to the VA that can be dissected up to the atlantooccipital membrane.

V4 Segment

Direct approach to the V4 segment in the posterior fossa is feasible. Successful segmental endarterectomy of the intracranial VA has been reported. However, the usual technique has been extracranial-intracranial revascularization using occipital artery-to-PICA anastomosis or venous graft from the external carotid artery to the posterior cerebral artery.

RESULTS

Generally, VA reconstructions have been gratifying. In the collective review of Kline and Berguer,[10] the early postoperative (30 days) stroke rate was less than 1%, cure of symptoms was achieved in 85% of patients while 7% were improved, and the expected 10-year survival rate was 71%, not significantly different from that of the normal population. Proximal and distal VA reconstructions had slightly different results, with a tendency for distal reconstructions to have a higher mortality rate (3.3% versus 0.5%) and lower patency rate (85% versus 93%) but better clinical results (85% versus 62% VBI-free patients at late follow-up). Combined carotid-VA reconstructions had the worst prognosis, with a 5% combined postoperative morbidity and mortality rate, and with survival, freedom from stroke, and freedom from VBI at 10 years being 69%, 79%, and 88%, respectively.

REFERENCES

1. Kieffer E, Bahnini A, Rancurel G. Surgery of vertebral artery insufficiency. In: Bergan JJ, Yao JST, eds. Arterial surgery: New diagnostic and operative techniques. New York, Grune & Stratton, 1988:187.
2. Rancurel G, Kieffer E, Arzimanoglou A, et al. Hemodynamic vertebrobasilar ischemia: Differentiation of hemodynamic and thromboembolic mechanisms. In: Berguer R, Caplan LR, eds. Vertebrobasilar arterial disease. St Louis, Quality Medical Publishing, 1992:40.
3. Berguer R. Distal vertebral artery bypass: Technique, the "occipital connection," and potential uses. J Vasc Surg 1985; 2:621–626.
4. Kieffer E. Nonatherosclerotic disease of the vertebral artery. In: Berguer R, Caplan LR, eds. Vertebrobasilar arterial disease. St Louis, Quality Medical Publishing, 1992:29.
5. Berguer R, Kieffer E. Surgery of arteries to the head. New York, Springer Verlag, 1992:138.
6. Bahnini A, Koskas F, Kieffer E. Combined carotid and vertebral artery surgery. In: Berguer R, Caplan LR, eds. Vertebrobasilar arterial disease. St Louis, Quality Medical Publishing, 1992:248.
7. Kieffer E. Chirurgie de l'artère vertébrale. Encyclopédie Médico-Chirurgicale. Techniques Chirurgicales. Chirurgie Vasculaire (in press).
8. Kieffer E, Rancurel G, Richard T. Reconstruction of the distal cervical vertebral artery. In: Berguer R, Bauer RB, eds. Vertebrobasilar arterial occlusive disease. New York, Raven Press, 1984:265.
9. Kieffer E, Koskas F, Rancurel G, et al. Reconstruction of the distal cervical vertebral artery. In Berguer R, Caplan LR, eds. Vertebrobasilar arterial disease. St Louis, Quality Medical Publishing, 1992:278.
10. Kline RA, Berguer R. Basic data underlying clinical decision making: Vertebral artery reconstruction. Ann Vasc Surg 1993; 7:497–501.

SUBCLAVIAN TO CAROTID TRANSPOSITION

WILLIAM H. EDWARDS, M.D.

Atherosclerotic lesions of the proximal subclavian artery occur with less frequency than those of the common or internal carotid arteries, but can produce brain stem or arm symptoms. Stenotic lesions of the proximal vertebral artery may occur as isolated lesions or in combination with the atherosclerotic process present also in the subclavian artery.

HEMODYNAMIC CONDITIONS

The left subclavian artery, arising from the distal aortic arch, is more prone to plaque formation and stenosis than its counterpart on the right (Fig. 1). In addition, lesions of the left subclavian artery occur more frequently than those of the innominate artery. The vertebral artery arising as the first major branch of the subclavian along its superior-posterior portion as it arches from the thoracic outlet makes the proximal vertebral prone to the same plaque formation. Thus, formation of atherosclerotic stenotic or ulcerated lesions of the subclavian and vertebral arteries may lead to symptoms on the basis of hypoperfusion or embolic events (Fig. 2).

HISTORICAL PERSPECTIVES

In 1957, Hutchinson and Yates described the vertebral and subclavian arteries in their entirety.[1] They concluded that atherosclerotic lesions contributed to infarcts found in the cerebellum and brain stem and were the cause of transient ischemic events.

Also in 1957 Cate and Scott first performed a subclavian-vertebral arterial endarterectomy to relieve symptoms of combined subclavian and vertebral stenosis.[2] With that beginning, symptomatic stenoses of the subclavian artery were found to be amenable to surgical reconstruction.

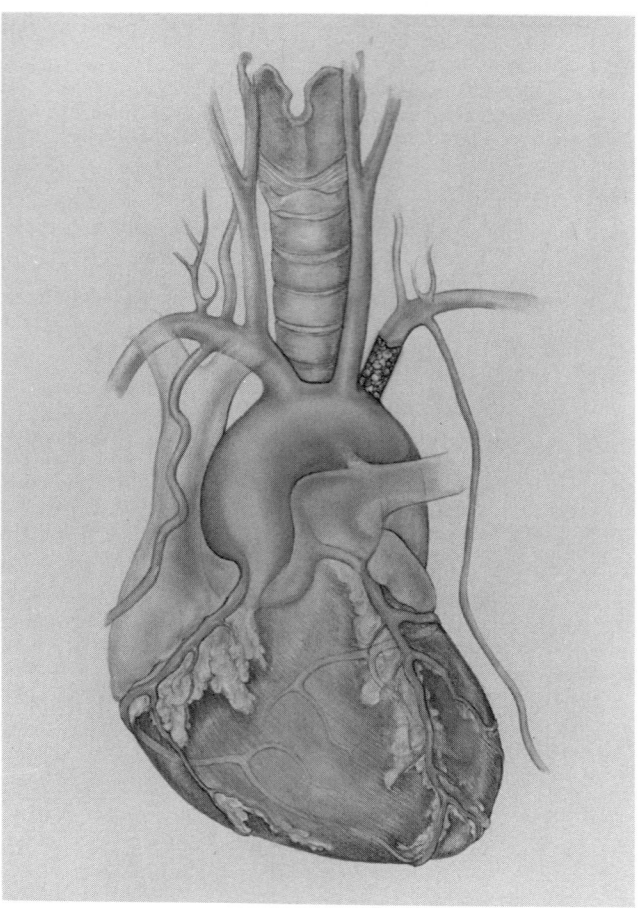

Figure 1 Proximal subclavian atherosclerotic lesion.

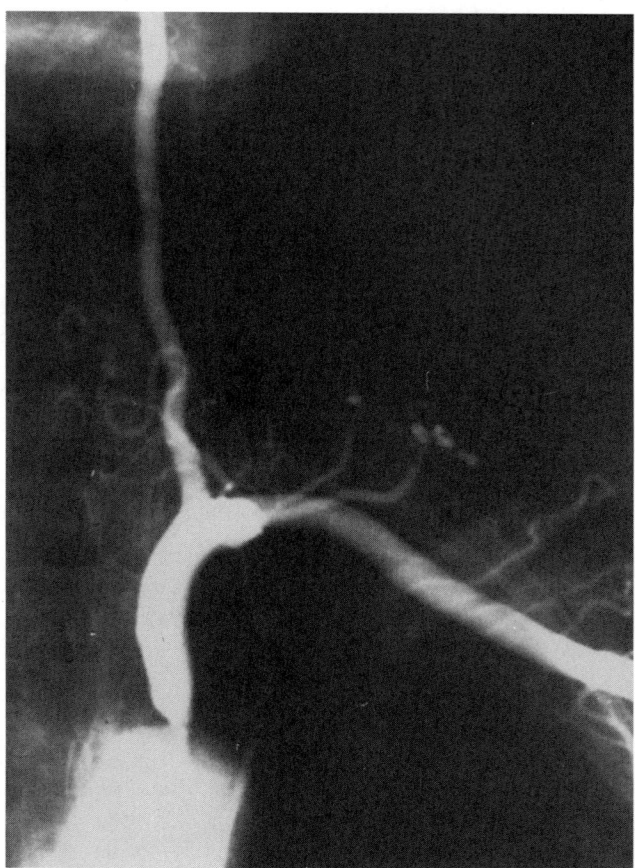

Figure 2 Typical stenotic arteriosclerotic lesion of the proximal left subclavian artery.

In a 1961 editorial in the *New England Journal of Medicine,* Fisher coined the term subclavian steal for retrograde vertebral blood flow that is associated with proximal subclavian stenosis or occlusion.[3] This phenomenon has been widely discussed since that time.

DIAGNOSTIC STUDIES

Duplex scanning and spectral analysis of extracranial circulation continue to improve and can document the blood flow and the degree of stenosis not only in the carotid arterial system but in the subclavian-vertebral system as well.

Blood flow patterns can be recorded with color imaging for identification of the arteries and veins to allow for immediate assessment. A competent technologist with state-of-the-art equipment in most situations can document the presence or absence of a proximal subclavian stenosis, as well as retrograde vertebral flow, if present.

Arch aortography is the technique most frequently employed, but unless the interventional radiologist is aware of the need for visualization of the proximal vertebral arteries, these vessels are sometimes poorly documented. Stenotic lesions of the proximal subclavian artery are more easily visualized.

An alternative to an arch aortogram is a retrograde brachial injection by means of a needle puncture of the brachial artery. This technique is safe and easily performed and provides excellent radiographs that allow the surgeon to decide on the proper treatment.

SURGICAL MANAGEMENT

In symptomatic patients, the proximal subclavian artery may be approached by the transthoracic or extrathoracic route.[4] The latter technique is generally preferred; sternotomy or thoracotomy is not necessary. The three operations of endarterectomy, bypass grafting, and transposition of the subclavian artery to carotid artery are all suitable for stenotic lesions. Subclavian-carotid transposition offers the advantage of avoidance of synthetic material with excellent compliance of the anastomosed arteries and good long-term results.[5] It must be remembered that the portion of the subclavian artery to be transected and transposed is quite delicate, and adventitial tears can easily occur. This will some-

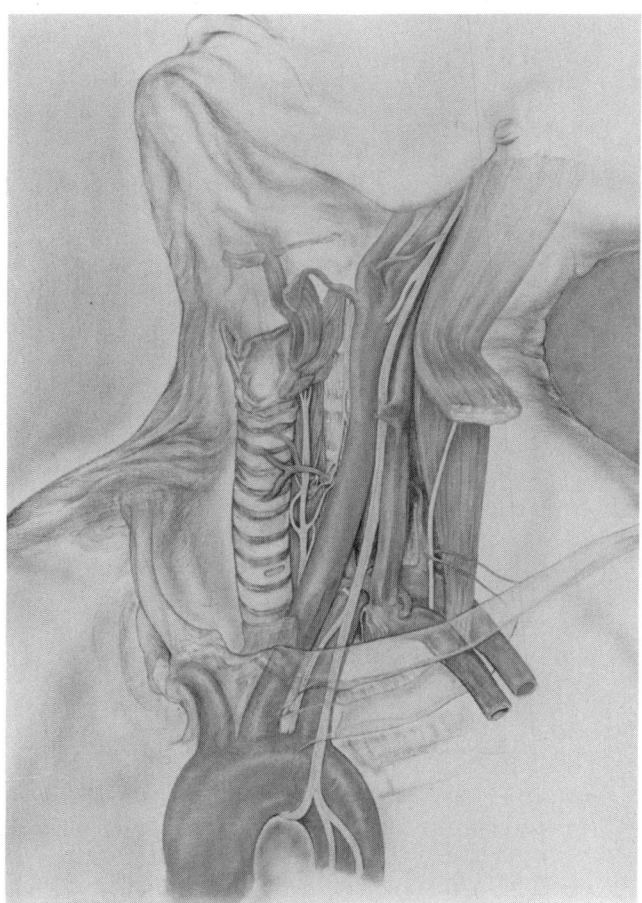

Figure 3 Proximity of subclavian and carotid artery can be appreciated from the drawing.

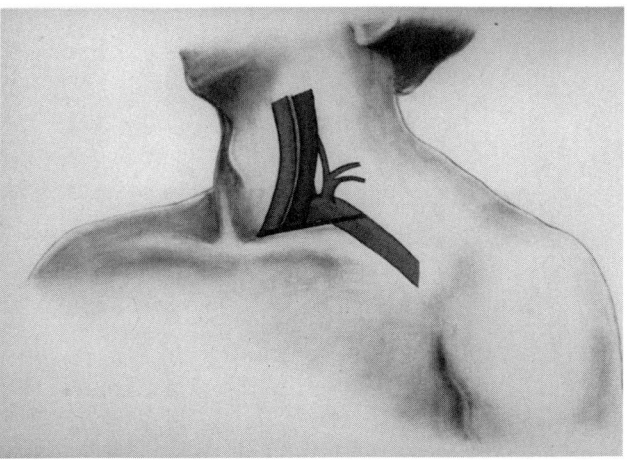

Figure 4 Supraclavicular incision extends from the suprasternal notch over a length of 6 to 8 cm.

times create an artery that is of insufficient length for a transposition.

The origin of the subclavian artery, especially on the left side, can be located deep in the thorax (Fig. 3). Its level can usually be determined preoperatively by the extent to which the subclavian arches out of the thorax through the thoracic outlet prior to dipping under the scalenus anticus to descend to the arm. With proper attention to delicate dissection, the operation can be safely performed.

An incision is placed just above the clavicle on the appropriate side, extending 5 to 6 cm from the suprasternal notch laterally (Fig. 4). The platysma and sternocleidomastoid muscles are divided to expose the common carotid artery and the internal jugular vein. The vagus nerve lies deep between these two vessels. Cephalad and caudad dissection along the course of the jugular vein and the carotid artery facilitates the deeper dissection that follows. This, in addition, isolates a portion of the carotid artery for the subsequent anastomosis. The vagus nerve can be mobilized adequately and excluded from the dissection. The jugular vein and the vagus nerve are retracted laterally, and the common carotid artery is displaced medially. The exposure from this point is through the deep fascia approaching the subclavian artery. If the surgeon sees the scalenus anticus muscle, then the dissection has been developed too far laterally and needs to move more medially. The ansa subclavia nerve is usually visualized as it crosses the subclavian artery.

We make a specific point to identify, ligate, and divide the thoracic duct. We feel that by dividing the duct the likelihood of a fistula is minimized. We have had no problems from ligating the duct.

It is generally not necessary to mobilize the internal mammary artery or the thyrocervical trunk. Adequate distal control of the subclavian artery for clamping can be achieved proximal to both these arteries. Because the vertebral artery is the first branch of the subclavian artery, it is necessary to ligate the vertebral vein and to dissect the proximal portion of the vertebral artery. The dissection is then developed toward the proximal subclavian artery as it comes through the thoracic outlet. The depth of dissection depends, to some extent, on the degree of disease and site of obstruction in the subclavian artery. However, in order to obtain an adequate length of distal subclavian artery for the transposition and for a safe closure of the proximal subclavian, we do not hesitate to dissect deeply along the course of the subclavian artery, realizing that we may place a properly angled clamp well down on the proximal artery to allow sufficient length once it is transected.

Following adequate exposure, we administer 5,000 units of intravenous heparin sodium, apply proximal and distal occlusive clamps, and transect the subclavian artery at the appropriate level. The proximal stump is oversewn with 5-0 monofilament suture, and on completion of this closure the proximal clamp is removed. Following this, the distal subclavian artery is then tailored to complete an end-to-side anastomosis between the common carotid and the subclavian arteries. An incision is made along the lateral wall of the common carotid artery and, utilizing a Goosen punch, we remove

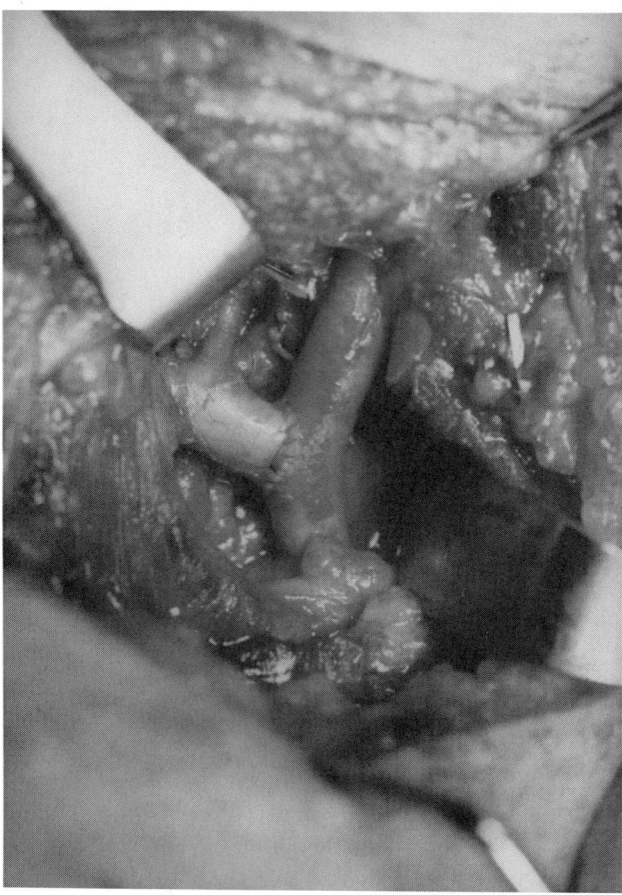

Figure 5 Completed right subclavian-to-carotid transposition. The vertebral artery is seen on the superior wall of the subclavian.

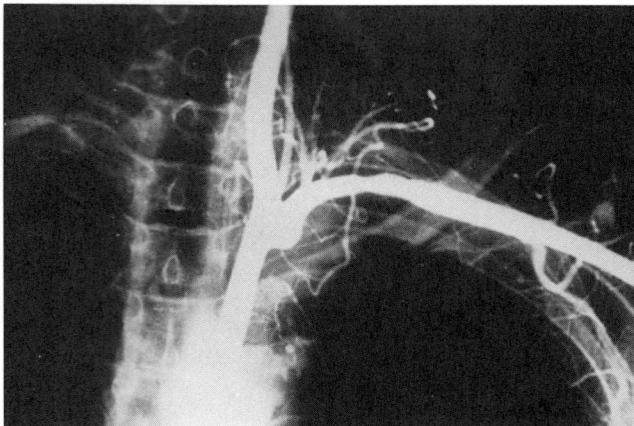

Figure 6 Arteriogram showing left subclavian-to-carotid transposition, 15 years postoperatively.

a portion of the common carotid artery for the subclavian artery transposition. We do not use an internal shunt but confirm that there is no distal internal carotid stenosis and that the contralateral internal carotid artery is widely patent on the arteriograms. The anastomosis is performed with a 6-0 monofilament suture on a special curved needle designed to facilitate the anastomosis in the small arteries (Fig. 5). Loop magnification is, in our opinion, necessary.

After completion of the anastomosis, the incision is closed in layers with no drains. Total operative time is about 1 hour and 15 minutes; unless complications develop, the patient is ready for discharge on the first or second postoperative day.

SPECIAL SITUATIONS

In patients with multiple arterial involvement in the extracranial circulation, innovative combinations of operations may be necessary. One possibility is a combined subclavian-to-carotid transposition with an internal carotid endarterectomy, in which case an internal shunt is used in the carotid system.

RESULTS

Over the last quarter century, we have undertaken 190 operations for lesions of the proximal subclavian artery in 185 patients.[5] In the early years of practice, the most common procedure was subclavian endarterectomy and/or intrathoracic to extrathoracic bypass. Beginning in 1969, however, we performed the first side-to-side, subclavian-to-carotid transposition and have since that time switched to an end-to-side transposition that we found to be quite satisfactory (Fig. 6).

Follow-up in over 80% of these patients has revealed only one occlusion of a subclavian-carotid transposition. In contrast, there is a follow-up of carotid-subclavian bypasses in which 40% of the bypasses have occluded during the period of follow-up.

Not only has the operation proven to be effective in long-term patency but also patients have been relieved of their vertebral basilar or arm symptoms.

REFERENCES

1. Hutchinson EC, Yates PO. Carotid-vertebral stenosis. Lancet 1957; 1:2–8.
2. Cate WR, Scott HW. Cerebral ischemia of central origin: relief by subclavian vertebral artery thromboendarterectomy. Surgery 1959; 45:19–31.
3. Fisher CM. A new vascular syndrome: The subclavian steal. N Engl J Med 1961; 265:912–913.
4. Crawford ES, DeBakey ME, Morris GC, Cooley DA. Thromboobliterative disease of the greater vessels arising from the aortic arch. J Thorac Cardiovasc Surg 1962; 43:38.
5. Edwards WH Jr, Tapper SS, Edwards WH Sr, et al. Subclavian revascularization: A quarter century experience. Ann Surg 1994; 219:673–678.

CAROTID-SUBCLAVIAN BYPASS AND OTHER EXTRA-ANATOMIC REVASCULARIZATIONS FOR PROXIMAL SUBCLAVIAN ARTERY STENOSIS CAUSING CEREBRAL STEAL SYNDROME

THOMAS S. RILES, M.D.
PATRICK J. LAMPARELLO, M.D.

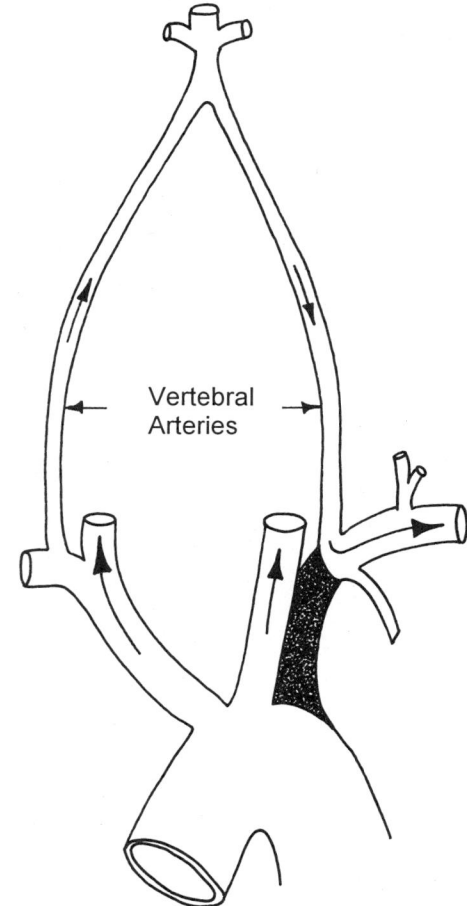

Figure 1 The subclavian steal.

Of arteriograms performed for the diagnosis of extracranial vascular disease, 8% to 12% will have evidence of stenosis or occlusion of one or both proximal subclavian arteries. Presumably because of the difference in anatomy between the two sides, the lesions are more commonly found on the left. In our experience the left-sided lesions are predominant by a ratio of 4:1. The plaque typically begins near the origin of the subclavian artery and ends just proximal to the origin of the vertebral artery. The vast majority of these lesions are atherosclerotic. However, the differential diagnosis should include Takayasu's arteritis, other types of arteritis, aneurysmal disease, embolism, and dissection.

Most patients with a subclavian artery stenosis are asymptomatic. It is not uncommon for the patient to be totally unaware of the condition until an astute clinician notes a differential in the blood pressure between the two arms.

The paucity of arm symptoms with a proximal subclavian artery occlusion is explained by the excellent collateral circulation provided by the vertebral arteries. The anatomy of these vessels is such that once the subclavian artery reduces the pressure distal to the plaque, the blood flow in the ipsilateral vertebral artery reverses, compensating for the subclavian lesion (Fig. 1). If the contralateral vertebral artery is sufficiently large to supply both the arm and the posterior circulation, the patient remains asymptomatic.

Besides the decreased blood pressure and diminished pulse on the affected side, an interesting physical finding that confirms the diagnosis of a proximal subclavian artery occlusion is the pulse lag. Assuming the patient has pulses bilaterally, simultaneous palpation of the radial arteries will often demonstrate a delayed peak of the pulse wave on the affected side. This is due to the longer transit time of the pulse wave to that side, which has to course through both vertebral arteries. With a subclavian stenosis, a bruit may be heard above or below the clavicle. If the subclavian artery is occluded, there often is no bruit.

Symptoms of a subclavian artery stenosis may be related to either the ipsilateral arm or the central nervous system. Arm symptoms are typically effort related, analogous to claudication in the lower extremity. Occasionally the ischemia is severe, especially with an acute arterial occlusion. Also, distal embolization may cause ischemia of one or more fingers on the hand.

Neurologic symptoms, usually of posterior cerebral insufficiency, include dizziness, vertigo, dyplopia, ataxia, bilateral sensory or motor deficits, dysarthria, and drop attacks. The classic description of a patient with the subclavian steal syndrome is one who develops one or more of these neurologic symptoms on exercising the arm on the affected side. Presumably the exercise increases the retrograde blood flow through the ipsilateral vertebral artery. As a result, flow to the basilar artery is either decreased or reversed, stealing blood from the posterior brain. In our experience this is the exception. Episodic symptoms more commonly occur with changes in the blood pressure or cardiac output. Symptoms may also occur with head rotation or extension, which may temporarily occlude the remaining vertebral artery, further decreasing the posterior circulation. The effects of a subclavian artery occlusion may be accentuated by concomitant carotid artery disease. These varying mechanisms of posterior circulatory insufficiency must be considered when evaluating a patient with a subclavian steal syndrome.

INDICATIONS FOR OPERATION

Once it is established that a patient has an insufficiency of the posterior circulation and a subclavian steal, a decision must be made as to how the patient can best be managed. If the patient has a severe stenosis of the carotid artery, particularly if there is bilateral disease, we have often corrected the carotid lesion first and found that this alone will improve the posterior circulation through the posterior communicating arteries, eliminating need to correct the subclavian steal. If there are no lesions restricting carotid blood flow or if the carotids are inoperable, perhaps because of an internal carotid occlusion, the operation must include some means of increasing the blood pressure to the subclavian artery to restore antegrade blood flow to the vertebral artery.

SURGICAL TECHNIQUE

Among the many described techniques for repairing a subclavian steal, the three most common are the carotid-subclavian bypass, the axilloaxillary bypass, and the reimplantation of the subclavian artery into the carotid artery. The last will be described in a separate chapter.

Of the two bypass procedures, the carotid subclavian bypass, first described in 1957,[1] is more common.[2] This bypass is usually performed between the proximal portion of the common carotid artery and the second or third portion of the subclavian artery. Our approach is through transverse supraclavicular incision dividing the clavicular head of the sternocleidomastoid muscle. Dissection is performed lateral to the jugular vein. The scalene fat pad is freed along its medial and inferior border, exposing the anterior scalene muscle. The phrenic nerve is identified and carefully mobilized medially off the anterior scalene. The brachial plexus is identified laterally along with the distal subclavian artery. Usually the anterior scalene muscle is divided to provide access to the proximal subclavian artery. The site for anastomosis, usually distal to the thyrocervical trunk, is chosen.

The graft material we prefer for this bypass is 8 mm Dacron or expanded polytetrefluoroethylene (PTFE). In earlier years we routinely used saphenous vein but have found no particular advantage to the use of autologous tissue for this operation. Also, the saphenous vein often was of insufficient caliber for this reconstruction. Long-term results may also be better with prosthetic grafts.[3]

Once the vessels are prepared, the patient is given heparin sodium. We perform the carotid anastomosis first, sewing the graft to the side of the carotid artery in a T configuration (Fig. 2). Cerebral ischemia during the carotid clamping is rare if the contralateral carotid artery is patent (4%), but it may occur in up to 25% of patients

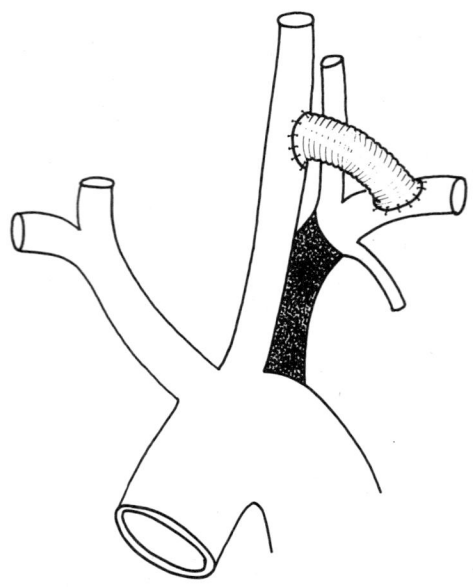

Figure 2 The carotid-subclavian bypass.

if the contralateral carotid is occluded. Since the shunt is awkward to use in this portion of the carotid artery, we generally test-clamp the carotid artery under cervical block anesthesia to determine whether a shunt is required. Others prefer EEG monitoring for selective shunting. A number of techniques may facilitate the placement and removal of a shunt, including a long arteriotomy with an oblique anastomosis and an extension of the dissection to the carotid bifurcation. The latter requires an extension of the incision along the anterior border of the sternocleidomastoid muscle.

After completing this end-to-side anastomosis the graft is tunneled under the jugular vein into the proximity of the subclavian artery. An end-to-side subclavian artery anastomosis is constructed. If the procedure is to prevent microembolization from the subclavian plaque, it is necessary to ligate the subclavian artery proximal to the vertebral artery origin.

If the patient has a severe stenosis at the carotid bifurcation, the procedure may have to include a carotid endarterectomy. The incision is curvilinear from the superior border of the clavicle artery to the medial head of the sternocleidomastoid muscle, then along the anterior border of the muscle. Some surgeons perform the carotid side of the bypass from the carotid bifurcation, constructing the end of the graft as an onlay patch. We prefer to perform the anastomosis lower on the carotid artery and to manage the bifurcation stenosis through a separate arteriotomy.

Occasionally carotid subclavian bypass is not technically feasible. The main reason for this is severe atherosclerotic stenosis of the donor carotid artery, particularly if there is a proximal common carotid plaque. Our preference in this situation is the axilloaxillary bypass (Fig. 3). This procedure is safe, since it does not require clamping any blood flow to the brain.

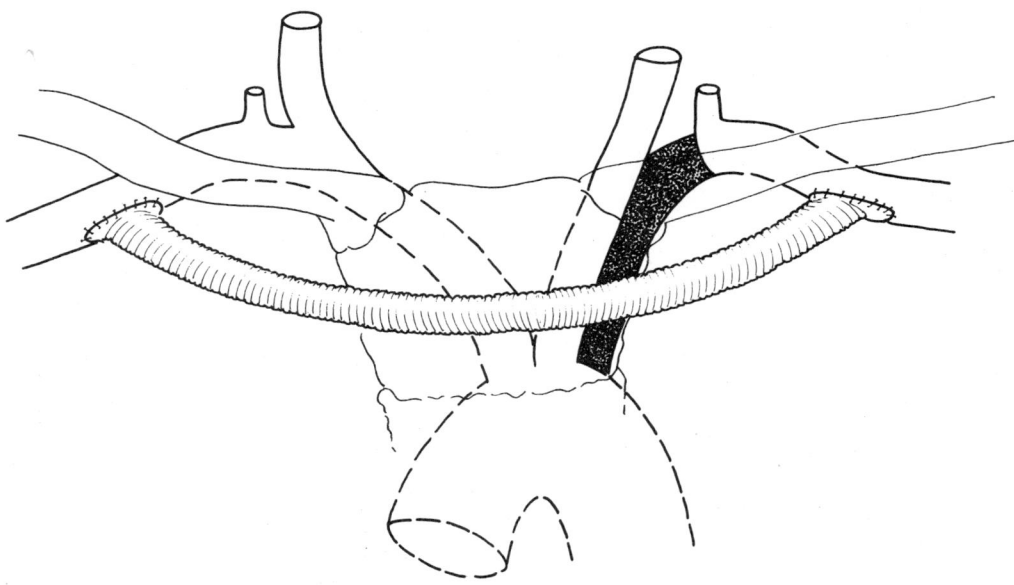

Figure 3 The axilloaxillary bypass.

With the patient under general anesthesia, bilateral infraclavicular incisions are made. The pectoralis major muscle is split transversely. The pectoralis minor muscle is identified. Our preference is to dissect and perform the anastomosis at the most proximal portion of the axillary artery, medial to the insertion of the pectoralis minor muscle. In some individuals this is not technically feasible and division of the pectoralis minor muscle is required. A subcutaneous tunnel is made between the two incisions. The Dacron or PTFE graft is passed over the manubrium below the sternal notch. Standard end-to-side anastomoses are performed. The operative morbidity for the axilloaxillary bypass is very low, and the long-term results are excellent.[4]

In properly selected patients, the operative mortality for either extraanatomic repair for subclavian steal is low, ranging from 0 to 2%.[5] The major complications are myocardial infarction and stroke, but these are relatively infrequent (1% to 3%). Other possible problems include postoperative bleeding, graft thrombosis, and infection. The subclavian carotid bypass may also include the risk of phrenic nerve injury or lymphocele if there is an unrecognized injury to the thoracic duct. Long-term results are generally excellent, with 5 year patency rates of 85% being reported.[6]

REFERENCES

1. Lyons C, Gaillraiter G. Surgical treatment of atherosclerotic occlusion of the internal carotid artery. Ann Surg 1957; 146: 487–494.
2. Crawford ES, Stowe CL, Dwers RW Jr. Occlusion of the innominate, common carotid, and subclavian artery: Long term results of surgical treatment. Surgery 1983; 94:781–791.
3. Ziomek S, Quinones-Baldrich WJ, Busuttil RW, et al. The superiority of synthetic arterial grafts over autologous veins in carotid-subclavian bypass. J Vasc Surg 1986; 3:140–145.
4. Posner MP, Riles TS, Ramirez AA, et al. Axillo-axillary bypass for symptomatic stenosis of the subclavian artery. Am J Surg 1983; 145: 644–646.
5. Zelenock GB, Cronenewitt, JL, Graham LM, et al. Brachiocephalic arterial occlusions and stenosis: Manifestations and management of complex lesions. Arch Surg 1985; 120:370–376.
6. Vogt DP, Mertzer NR, O'Hara PJ, et al. Brachiocephalic arterial reconstruction. Ann Surg 1992; 196–541.

SURGICAL TREATMENT OF INNOMINATE ARTERY ATHEROSCLEROSIS

JOHN P. LOFTUS, M.D.
KENNETH J. CHERRY Jr., M.D.

Seventeen percent of patients undergoing arteriographic evaluation of extracranial arterial occlusive disease (AOD) have atherosclerotic lesions of the subclavian or innominate artery.[1] However, only a small percentage of these patients undergo operation. The actual number of affected patients is unknown. Thus, the natural history of innominate artery occlusive disease remains poorly defined. Because of the rarity of patients undergoing surgical reconstruction for innominate artery stenosis or occlusion, surgical management strategies must be gleaned from large retrospective studies from referral centers.[2-10] Published reports from these institutions form the basis of this chapter, which focuses on patient characteristics and their presenting signs and symptoms, diagnostic evaluation, operative indications, techniques, and long-term results.

PATIENT PRESENTATION

Innominate artery atherosclerosis manifests itself in patients who are relatively younger than those with AOD in other regions. Patients are most commonly in their fifth or sixth decades. Men and women are nearly equally affected, although there may be a slight male predominance. Risk factors are similar to those found in other patients with vascular disease and include smoking (78% to 100% of patients), coronary artery disease (25% to 65%), hypertension (50%), diabetes (23%), and hyperlipidemia (19%).[3,6,8]

Innominate artery lesions may become symptomatic from hemodynamic compromise or atheroembolism to the central nervous system and/or to the right upper extremity. Neurologic symptoms may be referable to either the anterior cerebral circulation or the posterior cerebral circulation. In the reports from the Mayo Clinic and the Texas Heart Institute, approximately three-quarters of patients manifested neurologic symptoms.[3,5] In the Mayo Clinic study, 50% of patients had anterior circulation symptoms, 40% had posterior circulation symptoms, and 10% had global ischemia. Right upper extremity symptoms are less common than neurologic symptoms, occurring in a range of 14% to 54%.[3,5] The upper extremity symptoms include exercise ischemia (63%) and microembolization (37%).[3] For patients with combined neurologic and extremity complaints, most have upper extremity exercise ischemia, usually resulting from a high-grade stenosis rather than an ulcerated lesion, which more commonly results in microembolization. Patients with upper extremity symptoms alone tend to have microembolization associated with ulcerative plaques.[3]

DIAGNOSIS

The examiner should focus on palpation and auscultation of proximal and mid-cervical carotid and subclavian artery pulses. The presence of bruits or thrills over these vessels suggests innominate artery or other great vessel stenosis. Absent proximal, cervical, or subclavian pulses indicate occlusion. Palpation of superficial temporal, brachial, radial, and ulnar artery pulses is also performed, and asymmetry noted. Digital artery patency can be assessed with Allen's test or its variations. Bilateral upper extremity blood pressure measurements are taken; they assist in localizing these stenotic lesions. In the presence of bilateral upper extremity occlusive disease, comparison with lower extremity blood pressures should be performed. Microembolization from ulcerative lesions presents as painful bluish discoloration of the fingertips, subungual splinter hemorrhages, or livedo reticularis. These findings can occur in both the presence and the absence of wrist pulses. The presence of pulses with atheroembolization strongly suggests ulcerative, nonstenotic lesions.

Although duplex ultrasonography has become an accurate screening technique for evaluation of extracranial AOD, examination of the innominate artery is not usually possible with this modality. Indirect evidence, however, may be attained by waveform analysis of the carotid and upper extremity circulations. The diagnosis can be confirmed, however, only with arch aortography, including runoff views of the carotid, subclavian, and vertebral artery circulations. Aortography not only provides the means to confirm the diagnosis but also localizes the lesions, determines the etiology, and allows planning of operative therapy. The need for complete aortography is underscored by the 60% to 70% incidence of multiple arch lesions and the 10% incidence of concomitant vertebral or carotid bifurcation lesions.[3,5] Finally, aortography provides important anatomic information concerning the feasibility of endarterectomy versus prosthetic graft reconstruction.

SURGICAL MANAGEMENT

Atherosclerotic lesions of the innominate artery can be managed directly through a median sternotomy or by extrathoracic bypass procedures. Although early experience with direct transthoracic repair yielded good results, the early morbidity and mortality rates were high. Later attempts at reducing surgical morbidity and mortality by using extra-anatomic bypass, and thus avoiding median sternotomy, resulted in lower patency rates.[8,9] The experience with coronary artery bypass grafting over the years has proven that median sternotomy is a safe approach, with acceptable morbidity and mortality, and there has been a trend back to direct repair of innominate artery lesions. Other arguments against extra-anatomic reconstruction, in addition to the lower patency rates, include the obligatory retrograde blood flow through the graft that may contribute to lower patency rates, the failure to remove the source of atheroembolism from the circulation, and the potential for using another diseased great vessel as the inflow source in the case of multiple arch lesions. Presently, most surgeons who have experience in treating innominate artery occlusive disease favor direct transthoracic approach.

Innominate artery endarterectomy and ascending aortic origin grafting are the principle means of reconstruction. Endarterectomy is performed infrequently because fewer lesions are anatomically amenable to this procedure, and it is technically more demanding. There is no difference, however, in the outcome of properly selected patients having endarterectomy versus graft reconstruction.[3,5,10] Patients amenable to innominate artery endarterectomy are those with minimal associated aortic disease at the base of the innominate artery and those in whom the left common carotid artery is far enough away from the innominate artery to allow safe clamp placement. Multiple arch lesions requiring repair are best treated with graft reconstruction. Graft reconstruction of the innominate artery utilizes the ascending aorta, which is normally soft, as the inflow source. The intrapericardial ascending aorta is almost always free of atherosclerotic disease. Reconstruction can be accomplished by using either a single 8 or 10 mm Dacron graft, sewing side arms to this as needed or alternatively using a bifurcated graft. Proponents of the former find the minimal graft material within the mediastinum appealing, as some failures have been attributed both to the bulk of graft material in the mediastinum and to turbulence within the proximal segment of graft trunk. If a bifurcated graft is used, the trunk should be longer than is the case with infrarenal aortic repair to minimize turbulence of the bifurcation. The Texas Heart Institute has had excellent results with bifurcated grafts used in this manner.[5]

Because of the high incidence of associated lesions occurring in the presence of innominate artery stenosis or occlusion, there are varying opinions regarding the extent of reconstruction that should be performed. Reul and colleagues advocate bypass of all diseased vessels, which results in placement of multiple grafts.[5] They have published excellent results. Others reconstruct only symptomatic lesions and those that by virtue of their anatomy require repair.[3] Such would be the case with a left common carotid artery arising from a common brachiocephalic trunk. High-grade carotid bifurcation stenoses generally would also be repaired concurrently. The point of contention is the concomitant left subclavian artery stenosis or occlusion. In the Mayo Clinic experience,[3] relief of left upper extremity exercise ischemia was often obtained without direct reconstruction of the subclavian artery. Subsequent carotid-subclavian artery bypass, if needed, may be easier to perform than ascending aorta to left subclavian artery grafting, as the left subclavian artery lies far posterior in the mediastinum. Both approaches have yielded comparable results.[3,5]

OPERATIVE TECHNIQUE

Utilizing general anesthesia, the patient is placed supine with a rolled towel placed vertically along the spine allowing the shoulders to roll posteriorly. The neck is extended and turned to the left. Excessive hyperextension is avoided. The chest and both sides of the neck are prepped into the operative field. Both arms are tucked at the sides. Monitoring intravascular catheters are utilized as needed. Communication between surgeon and anesthesiologist is important as use of the left internal jugular or subclavian veins should be avoided because of the need for extensive mobilization or ligation of the innominate vein. Monitoring of cerebral perfusion is accomplished by the same means the surgeon prefers during carotid endarterectomy. The authors typically employ intraoperative electroencephalographic monitoring, although shunting is rarely required owing to the proximal clamp placement and rich collateral circulation in these areas.

Median sternotomy is performed with extension of the incision to the right side of the neck along the anterior border of the sternocleidomastoid. The sternal muscular attachments are divided. The innominate vein is mobilized and divided if needed. Division of this vessel results in minimal morbidity.[10] The innominate artery is dissected from its origin on the aortic arch to its bifurcation into the right common carotid and right subclavian arteries. The vagus nerve should be identified, as well as the recurrent laryngeal nerve as it courses around the subclavian artery. The left common carotid artery is isolated at its origin from the aortic arch. If the lesion is located in the mid to distal third of the innominate artery, if the dome of the aorta is spared from significant disease, and if the origin of the left common carotid artery is sufficiently distant to allow safe clamp placement, endarterectomy may be performed (Fig. 1). The right subclavian and common carotid arteries are clamped prior to placement of a Wylie J-clamp at the base of the innominate artery partially occluding the aorta. Prior to the innominate arteriotomy and the initiation of endarterectomy, the clamp should be placed for at least 1 minute to determine the adequacy of cerebral perfusion. If perfusion is deemed inadequate, endarterectomy should be abandoned and graft reconstruction performed; otherwise, one proceeds with endarterectomy. A longitudinal arteriotomy is made in the innominate artery. The plaque tends to course along the lateral aspect of the innominate artery and preferentially into the right subclavian artery. As such, if needed, the arteriotomy can be extended beyond the bifurcation and onto the right subclavian artery or, more

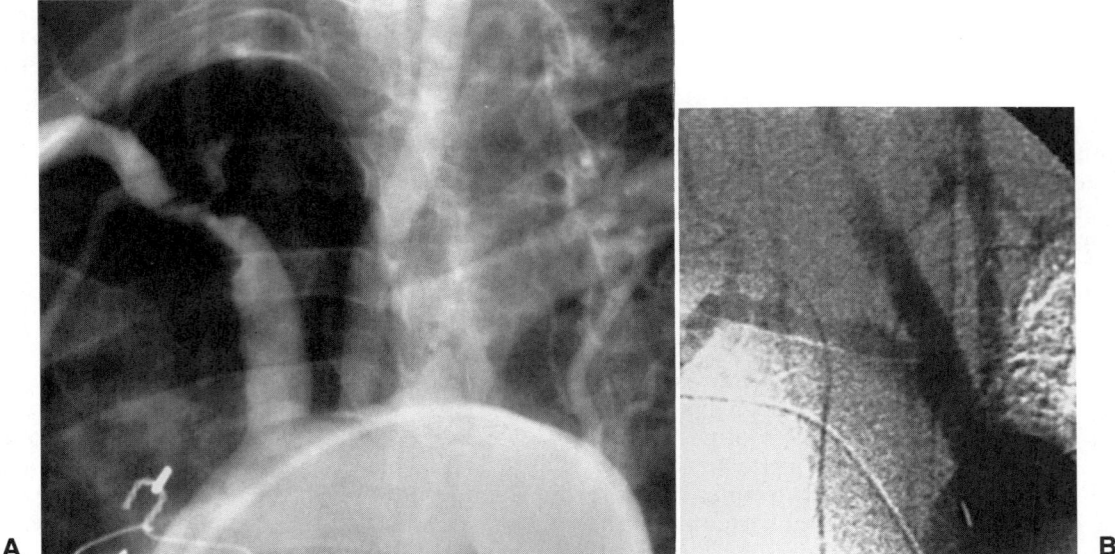

Figure 1 *A,* Arch aortogram of 45-year-old woman demonstrating high-grade stenosis of distal innominate artery. *B,* Digital subtraction angiogram following innominate artery endarterectomy.

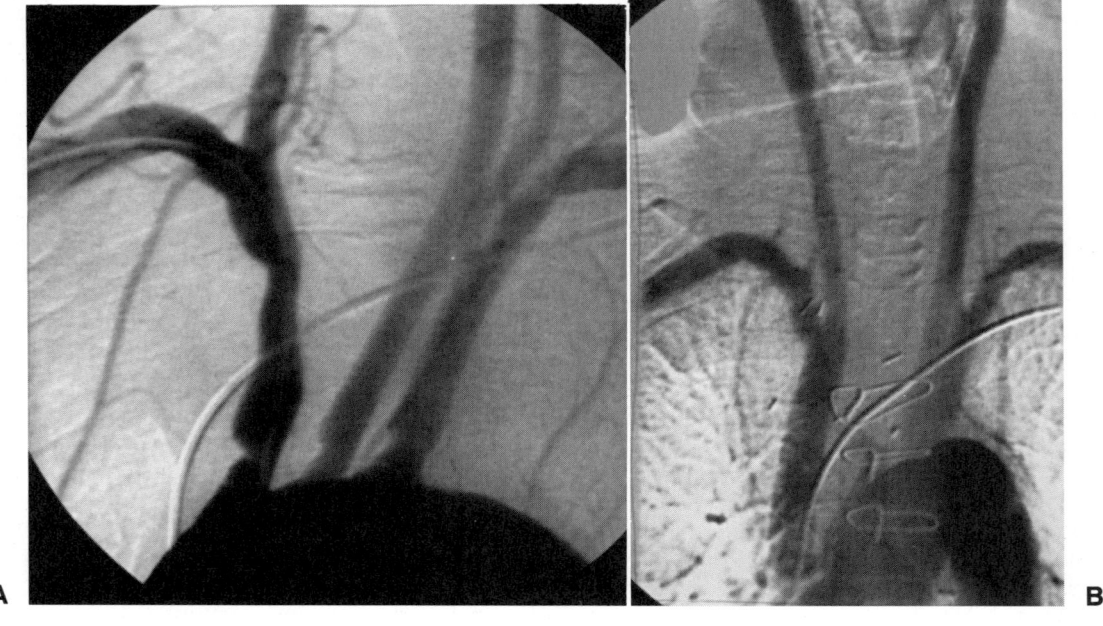

Figure 2 *A,* Arch aortogram of 56-year-old man with atherosclerotic disease of innominate artery. *B,* Digital subtraction angiogram following aortoinnominate graft reconstruction.

rarely, the right common carotid artery. Once endarterectomy is completed, the artery is closed with running fine polypropylene suture. Prosthetic patching is rarely necessary.

For graft reconstruction, the intrapericardial portion of the ascending aorta must be exposed. A partial occluding clamp is placed on the ascending aorta and an 8 or 10 mm woven or collagen-impregnated knitted Dacron graft is chosen. After making the aortotomy, the graft is trimmed and sewn end to side with running 3-0 or 4-0 polypropylene or Dacron suture. Upon completion and hemostasis of this anastomosis, the aortic clamp

Table 1 Morbidity and Mortality in Published Series of Direct Reconstruction for Innominate Artery Stenosis or Occlusion

Institution	No. of Patients	Perioperative Transient Ischemic Attack or Stroke (%)	Mortality (%)	Relief of Symptoms (%)
University of California, San Francisco, 1977	37	2.9	6	94
Cleveland Clinic, 1982	34	0	14.7	82
Baylor, 1983	43	5.5	4.7	94
University of Michigan, 1985	17	5.9	0	100
Massachusetts General Hospital, 1985 (intrathoracic approach)	29	6.9	3.4	88
Ohio State University, St. Anthony, 1988	26	7.6	7.6	96
Mayo Clinic, 1989	26	0	3.8	96
Texas Heart Institute, 1991	38	2.7	0	92

Adapted from Cherry KJ, McCullough JL, Hallett JW Jr, et al. Technical principles of direct innominate artery revascularization: A comparison of endarterectomy and bypass grafts. J Vasc Surg 1989; 9:718–724; with permission.

is removed and the graft clamped just beyond the anastomosis. The patient is then systemically heparinized and control obtained of the right subclavian, right common carotid, and innominate arteries. The innominate artery is divided just below its bifurcation, and the graft is sewn end to end with running suture. After appropriate back and fore bleeding, flow is restored first to the subclavian artery and then to the carotid artery. The proximal portion of the innominate artery is excised and the stump oversewn, utilizing a double suture line of a running horizontal mattress and over-and-over permanent suture. Division of the innominate vein and lateral placement of the graft, in addition to excision of the diseased innominate artery, may help decompress the anterior mediastinum and prevent graft occlusion (Fig. 2).

If additional vessels are to be reconstructed as a planned part of the operation, side arms to the first graft are sewn end to side before the graft–innominate artery anastomosis is performed. In this manner, cerebral hypoperfusion time is minimized. Concomitant carotid bifurcation endarterectomy can be performed by extending the incision on the right higher along the anterior border of the sternocleidomastoid and on the left by making a standard carotid incision. Once hemostasis is secured, one or two mediastinal chest tubes are placed through separate stab wounds, previously transected muscles are reapproximated, and the sternum is closed with sternal wires and standard technique.

RESULTS

The long-term results of direct innominate revascularization are excellent with relief of symptoms noted in 87% to 90% of patients (Table 1). Perioperative neurologic events and mortality range from 0 to 7, and 0.6%,[2,3,5-8] although the Cleveland Clinic reported a mortality of 14.7%.[4] Patients in this report had a notably high percentage of coronary artery and valvular heart disease. In addition, the deaths in the University of California and in the Mayo Clinic studies were all cardiac in nature, underscoring the need for preoperative cardiac evaluation.[2,3] Concomitant brachiocephalic and coronary artery revascularization has been performed successfully and is probably preferable to staged operations that require repeat sternotomy.[3]

REFERENCES

1. Fields WS, Lernak NA. Joint study of extracranial arterial occlusion: VII. Subclavian steal: A review of 168 cases. JAMA 1972; 222:1139–1143.
2. Carlson RE, Ehrenfeld WK, Stoney RJ, et al. Innominate artery endarterectomy: A 16-year experience. Arch Surg 1977; 112:1389–1393.
3. Cherry KJ, McCullough JL, Hallett JW Jr, et al. Technical principles of direct innominate artery revascularization: A comparison of endarterectomy and bypass grafts. J Vasc Surg 1989; 9:718–724.
4. Vogt DP, Hertzer NR, O'Hara PJ, Beren EG. Brachiocephalic arterial reconstruction. Ann Surg 1982; 196:541–552.
5. Reul GJ, Jacobs MJ, Gregoric ID, et al. Innominate artery occlusive disease: Surgical approach and long-term results. J Vasc Surg 1991; 14:405–412.
6. Crawford ES, Stone CL, Powers RW Jr. Occlusion of the innominate, common carotid, and subclavian arteries: Long-term results of surgical treatment. Surgery 1983; 94:781–791.
7. Zelenock GB, Cronenwett JL, Graham LM, et al. Brachiocephalic arterial occlusions and stenoses: Manifestations and management of complex lesions. Arch Surg 1985; 120:370–376.
8. Brewster DC, Moncure AC, Dorling RC, et al. Innominate artery lesions: Problems encountered and lessons learned. J Vasc Surg 1985; 2:99–112.
9. Criado FJ. Extrathoracic management of aortic arch syndrome. Br J Surg 1982; 69(Suppl):45–51.
10. Kieffer E, Sabatien J, Koskas F, et al. Atherosclerotic innominate artery occlusive disease: Early and long-term results of surgical reconstruction (submitted).

MANAGEMENT OF CONCOMITANT CAROTID AND CORONARY ARTERIAL OCCLUSIVE DISEASE

RICHARD P. CAMBRIA, M.D.

Any discussion of the management of the patient with coexistent carotid and coronary artery disease must begin with an acknowledgment that such patients present for treatment in a number of clinically distinct subsets. The circumstances of the initial clinical presentation guide the subsequent management. The preoperative evaluation and management of a patient with clearly symptomatic carotid artery disease and even active coronary artery disease (CAD) differ from that applied to a patient who is scheduled to undergo intervention for CAD and in whom significant, often asymptomatic, carotid disease is discovered. Most would agree that symptomatic carotid atherosclerosis requires prompt and, in some cases, even urgent surgical correction, and in such patients concurrent CAD would ordinarily be managed by maximizing medical therapy in the perioperative period. A more controversial issue is the appropriate management of the patient who requires coronary artery bypass grafting (CABG) and in whom significant carotid artery occlusive disease is found. The management of these latter patients varies widely across the country. A recently convened expert panel consensus report by the Rand Corporation considered the simultaneous performance of carotid endarterectomy and CABG of "uncertain" appropriateness, and a companion conference of vascular surgeons and neurosurgeons from 13 leading U.S. medical centers agreed with this designation. Furthermore, an ad hoc committee of the Society for Vascular Surgery and the National Institutes of Health's Asymptomatic Carotid Atherosclerosis study group have identified the issue of surgical staging in patients with coexistent carotid and coronary artery disease as among the unanswered questions in the management of carotid artery disease. Thus, it is not surprising that there is no consensus approach to these patients across the country, and no single approach will suffice for the various clinical subsets that constitute the spectrum of patients with coexistent coronary and carotid artery disease.

From a practical standpoint, two management scenarios constitute the bulk of clinical decision-making issues in these patients. First is the extent to which the patient who is a potential candidate for carotid endarterectomy ought to be investigated for the presence of occult CAD and what effect such data should have on the decision of whether to proceed with carotid endarterectomy. The second and more controversial circumstance is that of the patient who requires CABG and in whom carotid artery disease, which is often asymptomatic, is discovered.

CARDIAC RISK STRATIFICATION PRIOR TO CAROTID ENDARTERECTOMY

An assessment of CAD prior to vascular reconstruction has a dual purpose. First is the prevention of perioperative cardiac ischemic complications, and second is some assessment of the patient's long-term prognosis, which is usually dominated by the presence and severity of associated CAD. With respect to carotid endarterectomy, the latter consideration is, in fact, more important because all carotid operations are prophylactic in nature and rational only if the patient is likely to live long enough to derive benefit from such a prophylactic operation. This is particularly true in patients with asymptomatic carotid artery stenoses.

In deciding the wisdom of investigation for potential CAD in patients with carotid disease, a summary of pertinent data is appropriate.

First, the prevalence of significant CAD in patients with carotid artery bifurcation atherosclerosis is astounding, with some studies indicating a linear relationship between the severity of the carotid artery stenosis and the extent of coronary artery disease. Hertzer and colleagues from the Cleveland Clinic documented severe CAD in one-third of patients presenting for carotid endarterectomy and Urbinati and associates noted clinically silent CAD in 25% of carotid endarterectomy patients.[1,2]

Second, cardiac complications rather than stroke are the more common source of morbidity and mortality after carotid endarterectomy. In our unit, 294 carotid endarterectomies were performed during 1990 and 1991. Whereas permanent stroke and death rates were both in the 1% range, cardiac complications both major and minor occurred in nearly 6% of these patients. The reported incidence of myocardial infarction complicating carotid endarterectomy ranges from 1.5% to 5%.[3]

Third, studies that detail long-term follow-up after carotid endarterectomy implicate CAD as the principal source of late mortality after carotid endarterectomy.

Fourth, natural history studies of patients followed with asymptomatic carotid stenosis implicate CAD as the more frequent source of morbidity and mortality. Norris and co-workers noted an annual cardiac death rate of 6.5% in patients with severe yet asymptomatic carotid stenosis.[4] Alternatively, natural history studies of asymptomatic carotid stenosis indicate that the risk of "de novo" stroke in such patients is in the 3% to 5%/year range.

Thus, the patient being considered for carotid endarterectomy is likely to have some degree of CAD, which is the most important factor in predicting longevity irrespective of protection from stroke that may be afforded by carotid endarterectomy. It is also true that in current practice carotid endarterectomy is quite safe, and many patients even with anatomically threatening

CAD can be safely carried through carotid endarterectomy with appropriate medical management of the coincident CAD. When considering carotid endarterectomy, preoperative cardiac risk stratification is typically more valuable in making an appropriate judgment as to the wisdom of endarterectomy in asymptomatic patients than it is for considerations of perioperative safety. Therefore, the desirability of cardiac testing prior to carotid endarterectomy is largely a function of the urgency of the carotid operation (Fig. 1).

In clinical circumstances such as crescendo or multiple transient ischemic attacks (TIAs), recent strokes, carotid string sign, or a carotid anatomy that is imminently threatening as with occlusion with contralateral severe stenosis or bilateral preocclusive lesions, delay of operation for cardiac evaluation would be inappropriate even in patients with clinically evident CAD. At the other extreme are patients with unilateral asymptomatic carotid lesions being considered for endarterectomy. Because the annual risk of stroke in such patients is low and the mere presence of the carotid stenosis is a marker of CAD, we recommend a low threshold for cardiac risk stratification prior to operation for asymptomatic carotid stenosis. Our approach to cardiac risk stratification begins with the elemental question of whether further knowledge of the patient's coronary anatomy would influence patient management. It is clear that in decision making as to the wisdom of operation for asymptomatic carotid disease, further knowledge of the patient's CAD would indeed influence management, and cardiac investigation prior to carotid endarterectomy may be entirely appropriate. Recently available data from the Veteran's Administration Cooperative Study that documented efficacy for carotid endarterectomy in asymptomatic patients have not altered this position because late mortality from CAD in the VA study was at least as impressive as protection from stroke afforded by carotid endarterectomy. Indeed, Hobson and colleagues recommended consideration of carotid endarterectomy in asymptomatic patients only in

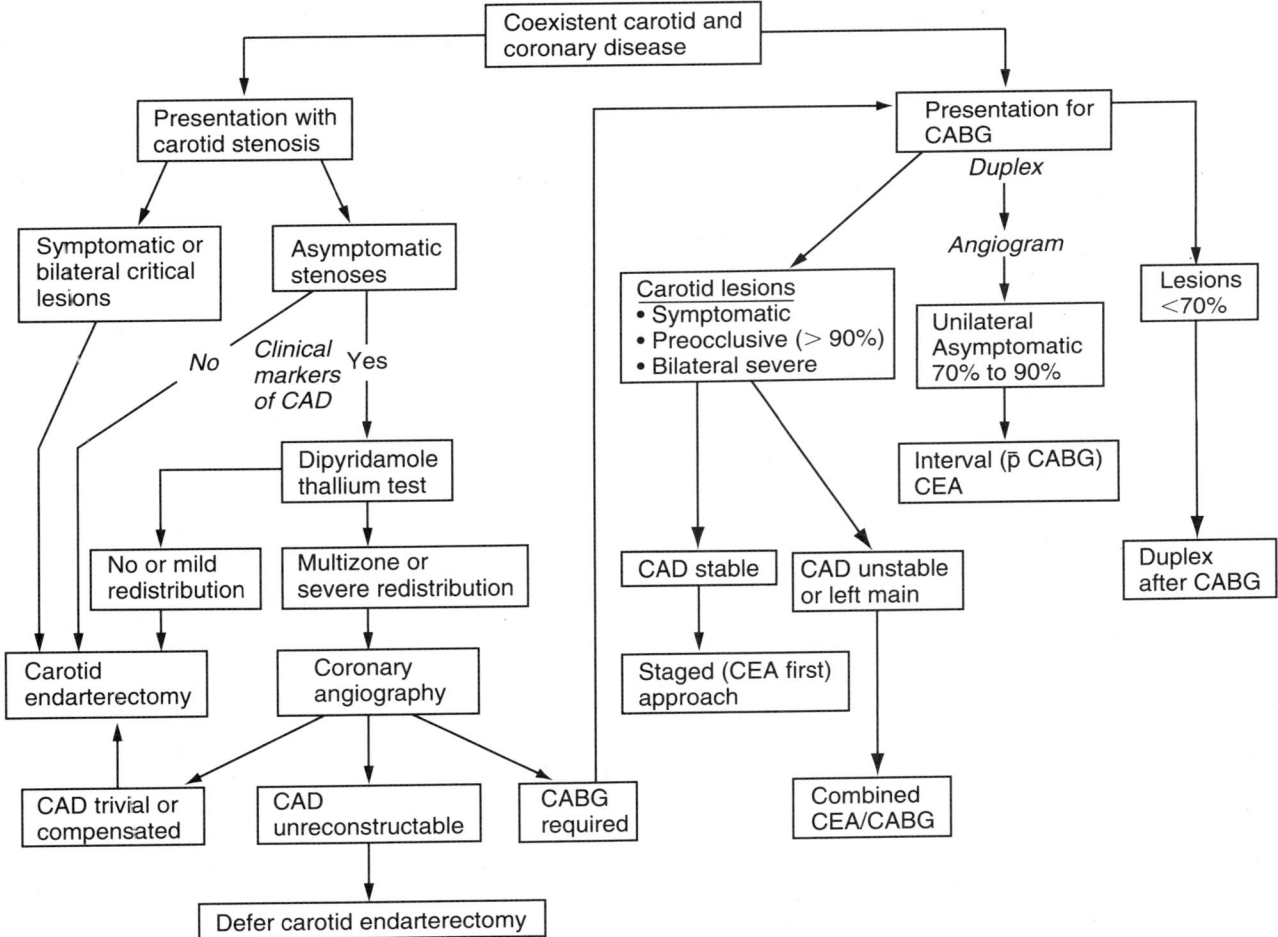

Figure 1 Suggested algorithm for management of patients with carotid and coronary artery disease. Clinical markers of CAD are age older than 70 years, diabetes, history of angina, myocardial infarction, heart failure, and ventricular arrhythmias. The term preocclusive refers to a carotid lesion greater than 90% diameter stenosis or when the residual carotid lumen is 1 mm or less. CAD, Coronary artery disease; CABG, coronary artery bypass graft.

the context of the severity of and limitations on longevity imposed by associated CAD.[5]

In our practice, candidates for endarterectomy for asymptomatic carotid artery stenosis are further evaluated with dipyridamole-thallium (D-THAL) myocardial scans based on the presence or absence of readily apparent clinical markers of CAD. A series of studies with routine performance of D-THAL scans and prospective recording of data referrable to antecedent CAD has defined the following clinical markers as useful in the selective application of cardiac testing: (1) diabetes, (2) age older than 70 years, (3) prior angina, (4) Q waves on electrocardiogram or prior myocardial infarction, and (5) history of congestive heart failure or ventricular arrhythmias. The presence of any of these factors engenders a recommendation for D-THAL. If such testing documents severe CAD, the patient is considered for coronary arteriography, and decisions referrable to treatment of CAD become the first priority (Fig. 1). Even in those patients who undergo carotid endarterectomy without initial cardiac testing, interval thallium scintigraphy should be considered for its potential benefit on long-term cardiac prognosis. Urbinati and associates found that the 7 year survival free from coronary events was a mere 51% in patients with "silent" CAD who underwent carotid endarterectomy.[2]

CAROTID DISEASE IN PATIENTS REQUIRING CORONARY REVASCULARIZATION

The proper role of preliminary or concomitant carotid endarterectomy in the patient who requires a CABG remains controversial. Those who have advocated what could be considered an intuitive approach have favored either preliminary or simultaneous correction of significant carotid stenosis to afford protection from stroke during cardiopulmonary bypass and from potential instability in a critical carotid lesion in the immediate perioperative period following CABG. This approach has been refuted by those who have suggested that asymptomatic carotid artery stenosis, in particular, can safely be ignored during CABG. The interrelated issues that bear on the management of such patients include the prevalence of hemodynamically significant carotid artery disease in patients who require CABG, the frequency of perioperative stroke associated with CABG in contemporary practice, and the importance of uncorrected carotid artery disease in the etiology of stroke during cardiopulmonary bypass grafting. Finally, how safe is the combined carotid endarterectomy–CABG procedure in current practice? Much of the objection to it in the past has focused on unacceptable complication rates that appeared to negate any potential benefit from preliminary cerebral revascularization.

As noted before, the incidence of coexistent CAD in patients presenting for treatment of carotid artery disease is significant. However, the converse is not true. The incidence of hemodynamically significant carotid artery stenosis in screening studies of patients presenting for CABG is generally quoted as less than 5%.[6] Even if such screening is restricted to CABG patients older than 60 years of age, the figure has been no higher than the 11% range.[7] Thus, it is clear that, from the perspective of the cardiac surgeon, complicating carotid artery stenosis is not a common problem, and routine screening for carotid disease is ill advised. Most authors reporting experience with combined carotid endarterectomy–CABG note it constitutes but a small fraction of their overall coronary surgical practice. In our unit this figure is less than 2% of CABG procedures in an environment where a relatively aggressive approach to the combined procedure has been embraced. Despite the modest incidence of hemodynamically significant carotid disease in CABG patients, an important distinction in this clinical subset is that the severity of the cardiac disease in these patients is advanced when compared to a "control" CABG population without such carotid disease. We and others have documented that patients who require CABG and have significant coexistent carotid disease have more left main CAD, significantly more left ventricular dysfunction, and advanced age. Such factors become important when one attempts to compare surgical risks of the combined operation versus CABG alone. Simply stated, such comparisons are not valid because the cardiac risk factors are not equivalent.

The initial rationale for the combined carotid endarterectomy–CABG operation was the prevention of stroke during cardiopulmonary bypass. This intuitive approach was based more on empiricism than on data. There seems little doubt that the improvement in neurologic complications attending cardiopulmonary bypass over the past two decades relates more to technical improvements, blood filtration, and surgical techniques than to any attempt to address coexistent carotid disease. Furthermore, the etiology of stroke during cardiopulmonary bypass is multifactorial, and potentially important contributing factors include significant atherosclerotic disease in the ascending aorta as a source of atheromatous emboli, increased patient age, prolonged duration of cardiopulmonary bypass, and a history of stroke. The low incidence of stroke complicating CABG in general and the modest incidence of significant carotid artery disease in these patients lead to the conclusion that carotid artery stenosis is but a small component in the overall problem of stroke during cardiopulmonary bypass.

The more relevant question for the vascular surgeon is the importance of carotid artery disease in that small subset of CABG patients who harbor it. In this regard the available data suggest that major carotid artery stenosis significantly increases the risk of stroke during CABG. Brenner and associates noted a 9.2% incidence of stroke and/or TIA during CABG in patients with significant carotid artery disease as compared to a 1.9% risk in those without such disease.[6] Reed and colleagues noted that the presence of carotid artery bruit was accompanied by a fourfold increase in the risk of stroke during CABG.[8] Data reported from the Cleveland Clinic documented a stroke rate of 8.9% in a series of 275

CABG patients with arteriographically documented critical carotid artery stenoses as compared to an institutional stroke rate of 1.3% for CABG in general.[9]

Two considerations relative to the pathophysiology of stroke from carotid artery disease are worthy of mention. First, watershed infarctions from cerebral hypoperfusion clearly do occur, as evidenced by the extraordinary stroke risk of 14% reported by Brenner and co-workers in the setting of internal carotid artery occlusion.[6] Indeed, the highest-risk situation is in those cerebral hemispheres subtended by a chronic internal carotid artery occlusion. Obviously, the vascular surgeon can only improve this circumstance by contralateral carotid endarterectomy with resultant increase in the collateral circulation to the hemisphere ipsilateral to a carotid occlusion. A second mechanism of stroke from carotid artery disease relates to instability and/or thrombosis on a pre-existent critical carotid artery stenosis in the immediate perioperative period, possibly related to "rebound" from large doses of intraoperative heparin sodium used during cardiopulmonary bypass and/or increased thrombogenicity in the immediate postoperative period. In this regard, concern is focused on the "preocclusive" stenoses, lesions with greater than 90% diameter stenosis or a residual lumen diameter of 1 mm or less. Thus, in formulating a rationale for the combined carotid endarterectomy–CABG operation, several components can be cited: (1) prevention of stroke during cardiopulmonary bypass, which likely relates to flow-related phenomenon; (2) stroke prevention in the immediate perioperative CABG period, referable to embolization or thrombosis of an antecedent critical carotid lesion; and (3) long-term stroke prevention. With respect to the last consideration, even opponents of the combined operation have emphasized the genuine risk of late stroke in CABG patients with unrepaired carotid lesions, and these data are consistent with the available natural history studies of critical carotid stenosis.[10] Of course, the consideration of late stroke prevention could be addressed with interval carotid endarterectomy weeks or months after CABG, but the efficiency and economy of a combined procedure have appeal, if it can be performed safely.

The final component relating to the combined carotid endarterectomy–CABG procedure is the safety of the operation. Many authors have cited undue operative risk as a prime argument against the combined operation, and frequently the standard of comparison is a concurrent series of isolated CABG procedures. Yet, as previously noted, patients with simultaneous carotid and coronary lesions generally have more advanced CAD, and this is reflected in the reported results of the combined operation. Schultz and associates documented that patients undergoing isolated CABG operation with uncorrected carotid lesions had an operative mortality of 7.2% when their cardiac status was matched for a concurrent series of combined carotid endarterectomy-–CABG operations.[11] Similar findings of increased operative mortality (more than 5%) for CABG in patients with diffuse vascular disease have been reported.[9] In a previous report, we noted an acceptable 2% rate of both perioperative mortality and stroke after the combined carotid endarterectomy–CABG operation.[12] In a review of the English literature, the author found 19 reports of the carotid endarterectomy–CABG operation with 25 or more cases reported since 1981. Experience with 1,638 patients is represented in these series; the mean operative mortality for the operation was 4.7% (range 0 to 11%), and the stroke (permanent deficit) rate was 2.4% (range 0 to 6.5%). These figures represent an acceptable operative morbidity for the combined operation, given the advanced CAD typically found in such patients. The notion that the combined carotid endarterectomy–CABG operation is inherently dangerous is born of multiple reports that "match" carotid endarterectomy–CABG patients with companion series of isolated CABG operations that, in fact, are inappropriate comparisons. Although the indications for the combined operation remain ill defined, the safety of this approach has been amply documented. In a personal series of 60 such operations carried out over the past 6 years, there has been no mortality and a single stroke related to bilateral atheromatous microemboli.

What practical guidelines can be given in selecting patients for the combined carotid endarterectomy–CABG operation? Focusing for the moment on those patients whose primary clinical presentation is for correction of coronary disease, the same factors that influence decision making in all carotid artery operations, that is, severity and symptomatic status of the carotid lesion, and the stability of the CAD are addressed. Discussion about a potential combined operation is entertained regarding patients whose carotid lesions would be repaired on their own merits. However, there are enough practical and logistical disadvantages to a combined operation to temper enthusiasm about extending this approach to all patients whose carotid lesions would ordinarily be repaired. These limitations include the obvious prolongation of an already major procedure, disparate blood pressure requirements for the coronary versus the carotid operation, and an anesthetic technique for cardiopulmonary bypass that necessitates a deeply anesthetized patient and disallows an immediate postoperative neurologic assessment. Other practical limitations include a premium on an expeditious carotid artery operation, making such procedures inappropriate for resident teaching, and that EEG monitoring becomes cumbersome or not feasible with the hypothermia and low perfusion pressures used in cardiac anesthesia. The carotid artery operation is done while vein harvest is proceeding in the leg, but prior to the induction of cardiopulmonary bypass. Some prefer to institute cardiopulmonary bypass and systemic hypothermia prior to the carotid operation, citing the theoretic cerebral protection of this method.[7] However, this approach negates the benefit of a widely patent carotid artery prior to the lowered perfusion pressures used with cardiopulmonary bypass.

The combined operation clearly adds a degree of complexity not evident if the carotid lesion is ignored.

Therefore, despite the demonstrated safety of the combined operation, its use is restricted to patients whose carotid lesions appear to present a genuine threat in the perioperative CABG period (Fig. 1). These include symptomatic high-grade lesions, irrespective of contralateral carotid anatomy, and patients whose anatomy is precarious for hemodynamic or low-flow mediated injury, e.g., carotid occlusion with contralateral stenosis or bilateral high-grade stenosis, in which case the lesion referable to the dominant hemisphere is repaired. It is important to emphasize that in selection of patients for the combined operation, particularly those with asymptomatic lesions, "high-grade" stenoses refers to a 90% lesion or one with a residual lumen of 1 mm or less. This implies that contrast carotid arteriography is mandatory in these patients and, if the overall clinical situation does not permit it, the carotid lesion should be ignored. Unless clear-cut symptoms are referable to the carotid artery lesions, the precise determination of the severity of the stenosis is an important piece of data that cannot be reliably ascertained short of contrast arteriography. Other factors potentially important in selecting patients for the combined operation include patient age, history of prior stroke, and anticipated length of cardiopulmonary bypass run, which is known to increase the risk of stroke during CABG.

Of the various staging schemes applicable to patients with coexistent carotid and coronary disease, each has its merits and disadvantages. Initial carotid endarterectomy followed by interval CABG is frequently applied to patients who present with symptomatic carotid lesions and/or those with clinically stable CAD. The combined operation is preferred for patients with critical carotid lesions whose CAD does not permit an initial carotid artery operation. Finally, the so-called reversed staged procedure or CABG followed by interval carotid endarterectomy is utilized in patients whose carotid artery stenoses are not repaired during CABG, typically because of emergent circumstances of the latter or lesions of less than critical diameter. In this situation, Hertzer and associates[9] have emphasized the increased morbidity of performing carotid endarterectomy in the immediate post-CABG period; therefore, the carotid artery procedure should be deferred to a subsequent admission. In practice, the most important factor in choosing among the various staging schemes is the stability of the CAD. Patients with left main CAD or unstable angina or those requiring intravenous nitroglycerin or intra-aortic balloon counterpulsation are too tenuous to be managed with initial staged carotid endarterectomy. However, with current surgical and anesthetic techniques, it is obvious that many patients with both overt and occult CAD can be safely managed through a carotid artery operation, and this is generally the route taken when the carotid lesion is the mode of clinical presentation.

REFERENCES

1. Hertzer NR, Beven EG, Young JR, et al. Coronary artery disease in peripheral vascular patients. A classification of 1,000 coronary angiograms and results of surgical management. Ann Surg 1984; 199:223–233.
2. Urbinati, S, DiPasquale G, Andreoli A, et al. Frequency and prognostic significance of silent coronary artery disease in patients with cerebral ischemia undergoing carotid endarterectomy. Am J Cardiol 1992; 69:1166–1170.
3. Yeager R, Moneta R. Assessing cardiac risk in vascular surgical patients. Current status. Perspect Vasc Surg 1989; 2:18–36.
4. Norris JW, Zhn CZ, Bornstein NM, Chambers BR. Vascular risks of asymptomatic carotid stenosis. Stroke 1991; 22:1485.
5. Hobson RW, Weiss DG, Fields WS, et al. Efficacy of carotid endarterectomy for asymptomatic carotid stenosis. N Engl J Med 1993; 328:221.
6. Brener B, Brief D, Alpert J, et al. The risk of stroke in patients with asymptomatic carotid stenosis undergoing cardiac surgery: A follow-up study. J Vasc Surg 1987; 5:269–279.
7. Berens E, Kouchoukos N, Murphy S, Wareing T. Preoperative carotid artery screening in elderly patients undergoing cardiac surgery. J Vasc Surg 1992; 15:313–323.
8. Reed G, Singer D, Picard D, DeSanctis R. Stroke following coronary artery bypass surgery. N Engl J Med 1988; 10:1246–1250.
9. Hertzer N, Loop F, Beven E, et al. Surgical staging for simultaneous coronary and carotid disease: A study including prospective randomization. J Vasc Surg 1989; 9:455–463.
10. Barnes R, Nix M, Sansonetti D. Late outcome of untreated asymptomatic carotid disease following cardiovascular operations. J Vasc Surg 1985; 2:843–849.
11. Schultz JW, Sterpetti A, Feldhaus R. Early and late results in patients with carotid disease undergoing myocardial revascularization. Ann Thorac Surg 1988; 45:603–609.
12. Cambria RP, Ivarsson BL, Akins CW, et al. Simultaneous carotid and coronary disease: Safety of the combined approach. J Vasc Surg 1989; 9:56–64.

EXTRACRANIAL CAROTID ARTERY ANEURYSM

GERALD B. ZELENOCK, M.D.
JOSEPH GIGLIA, M.D.

Extracranial carotid artery aneurysms (ECAAs) are rare vascular lesions.[1-8] Clinical series reporting 20 or more patients are distinctly uncommon. One clinical series reports that during a period in which 1,500 carotid endarterectomies were performed, only 6 such aneurysms were encountered.[2] The clinical importance of such lesions lies in the fact that they may cause transient ischemic attacks or stroke and can be encountered in the differential diagnosis of cervical, pharyngeal, and tonsillar masses.

The clinical classification of these aneurysms recognizes several distinct pathophysiologic entities (Table 1). Atherosclerotic aneurysms represent approximately half of the cases of ECAA (Figs. 1 and 2).[1-3,7] In most series, fibrodysplastic lesions, traumatic aneurysms secondary to blunt or penetrating trauma (Figs. 3 and 4), and postendarterectomy pseudoaneurysms are equally likely to be reported (Fig. 5). Mycotic aneurysms are less commonly a cause of ECAA. An occasional association between ECAA and intracranial aneurysms has been reported.[6] However, given the common occurrence of the latter, this seems likely to be on the basis of chance alone. Two reports from Japan note an association between carotid aneurysms and visceral aneurysms that is likely the result of a systemic inflammatory vasculopathy.

CLINICAL PRESENTATION

Recent reports have emphasized the diversity of symptoms that may accompany a carotid aneurysm. Clearly, most worrisome are transient ischemic attacks or a completed stroke. When clear-cut, these symptoms are likely to proceed to an expeditious diagnosis, as noninvasive testing or arteriography should readily identify the aneurysm. Patients complaining of tinnitus or a cervical bruit are likewise readily evaluated, and the diagnosis rapidly confirmed. Other presentations such as a mass in the neck or the posterior pharynx can be quite subtle and are deceptive, particularly if the pulsatile component to the aneurysm is not appreciated. The otolaryngologic and dental literature describe multiple cases where inadvertent biopsy of a neck mass or incision and drainage of a suspected tonsillar abscess has resulted in significant hemorrhage. Spontaneous hematemesis has also been reported as a result of a carotid aneurysm, as have cranial nerve palsies involving the hypoglossal nerve, the recurrent branch of the vagus, and other branches of cranial nerves IX to XII. A partial Horner's syndrome is common. In the case of trauma-related aneurysms, diagnosis can be significantly delayed, often weeks or months following the initial injury. Carotid artery dissections, whether traumatic or spontaneous, are felt to predispose to pseudoaneurysm formation.[7] In more recent reports, the number of asymptomatic patients detected at the time of screening for other diseases has increased substantially.

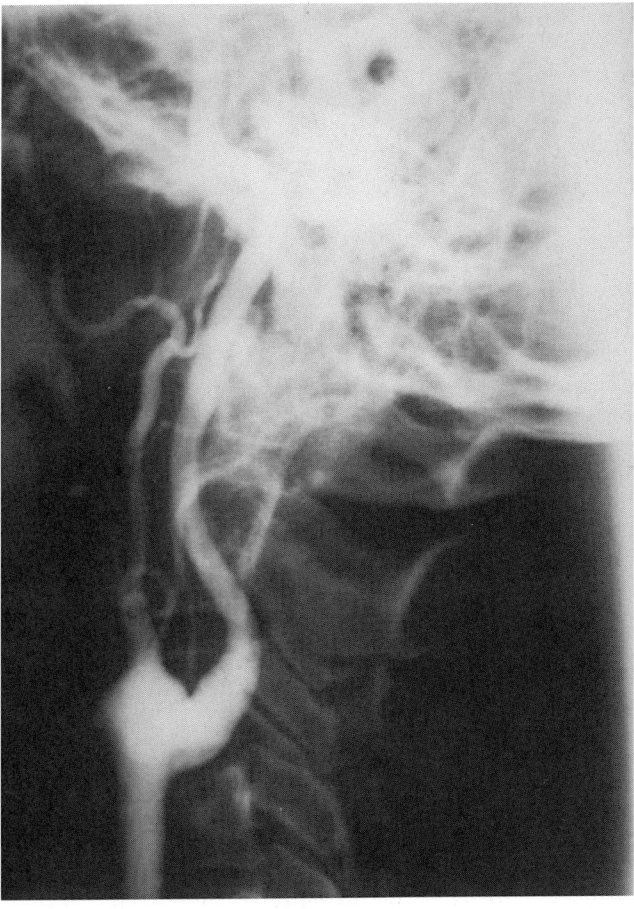

Figure 1 Atherosclerotic aneurysm of the carotid artery. Both the internal and external carotid arteries are involved in the degenerative process.

Table 1 Clinical Classification of Extracranial Carotid Aneurysm

Atherosclerotic
Fibromuscular dysplasia
Postendarterectomy pseudoaneurysms
Trauma-associated pseudoaneurysms
   Blunt
   Penetrating
Mycotic/infectious
   Tuberculosis
   Otitis media/tonsillar abscess
Congenital
Associated with intracranial aneurysms
Associated with visceral artery aneurysms

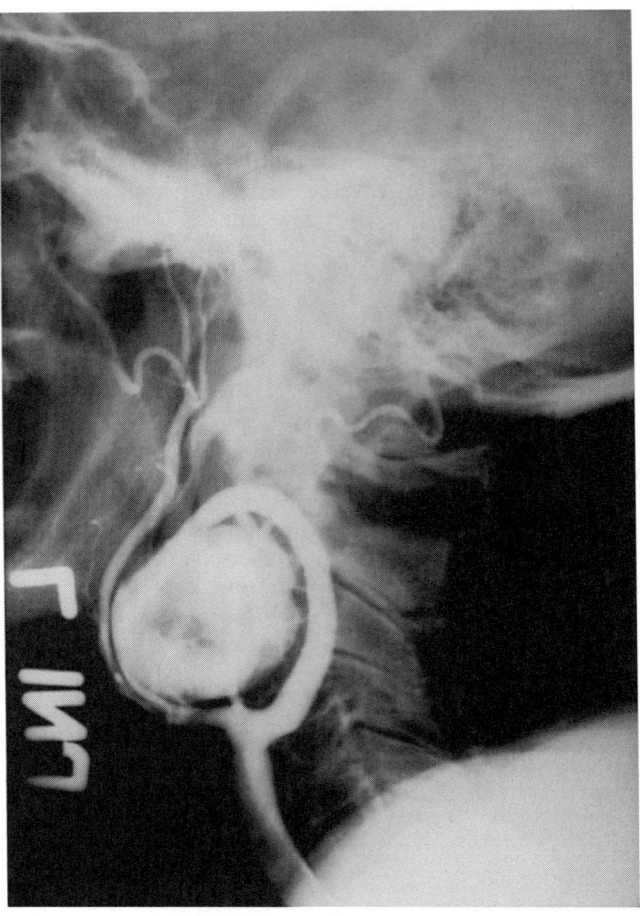

Figure 2 Large saccular atherosclerotic internal carotid artery aneurysm. (From Zwolak RM, Whitehouse Wm Jr, Knake JE, et al. Atherosclerotic extracranial carotid artery aneurysms. J Vasc Surg 1984; 1:415–422.)

Once the diagnosis is suspected, a number of imaging modalities are utilized to confirm the clinical impression. Duplex scanning of carotid aneurysms should be relatively reliable for lesions at the carotid bifurcation or in the proximal internal carotid artery (ICA). However, lesions very high in the ICA at the skull base may not be accessible for operative treatment. At present, in most instances, confirmation of the diagnosis of ECAA rests with arteriography, either conventional or with intravenous digital subtraction techniques (Figs. 2 and 3). Detailed arteriography allows precise delineation of the carotid aneurysm, as well as localization and assessment of the adequacy of the collateral circulation. The enormous technical advances in magnetic resonance angiography (MRA) have allowed enhanced resolution and detail, and it has begun to be utilized to detect such lesions. It has the obvious advantages of not requiring ionizing radiation or nephrotoxic contrast media. In addition, iatrogenic embolization of aneurysm contents is avoided, as there is no need for intra-arterial catheters or intracarotid injections. Although not yet widely available, this technique seems certain to become the imaging modality of choice in the near future. Computed tomography (CT) scanning is frequently employed in patients with cranial-cervical complaints. It has allowed diagnosis, but generally these were incidental findings on a scan ordered to investigate cranial-cervical trauma or a neck mass. Computed tomography scanning does not provide enough anatomic detail for appropriate therapeutic planning but often excludes other important diagnostic possibilities. The variability of the initial clinical presentation means that the potential differential diagnosis is initially large; however, the algorithms to reach certain key decision points are straightforward and allow an efficient elimination of alternative diagnoses.

TREATMENT

Management decisions must be highly individualized. There have been no randomized prospective clinical trials comparing different treatments, and there are no absolute guidelines applicable to all patients and all clinical settings. The type of aneurysm, its anatomic location, the adequacy of the collateral circulation, and the presence or absence of symptoms are all appropriate determinants of therapy in a specific patient. Some physicians favor a conservative approach involving expectant treatment. Others use antiplatelet agents or anticoagulation with heparin sodium and warfarin to reduce the thromboembolic risk. Direct cervical repair with or without ancillary or adjunctive techniques to maintain cerebral blood flow has been described. These are often suitable for low-lying and midrange aneurysms and are similar to standard carotid reconstruction techniques.

Although standard carotid endarterectomy is usually performed under regional anesthesia at our institution, carotid aneurysm repair requires general anesthesia and full cardiovascular monitoring. Exposure of the carotid proceeds in normal fashion until the carotid sheath is encountered. Proximal and distal control remote from the aneurysm itself is achieved. Under full anticoagulation, the aneurysm is dissected and opened. Aneurysm contents are extracted, and the normal proximal and distal arteries identified. Either primary end-to-end or, more commonly, a short interposition graft is placed to restore arterial continuity. In favorable circumstances, a simple aneurysmorrhaphy with patch angioplasty suffices.

Aneurysms at the base of the skull require extensive exposure. Exposure of the distal carotid artery can be facilitated by using a number of techniques. Routine transection of the digastric muscle and mobilization of the XII nerve allow excellent distal exposure. Full mobilization may require division of the ansa hypoglossus branch. Foward displacement of the mandible, using arch bar retraction and selective styloid process resection, allows exposure of the distal extracranial ICA. Rarely, more distal exposure may require mastoid resection to mobilize the first portion of the intraosseous carotid artery. At our institution, this latter procedure is

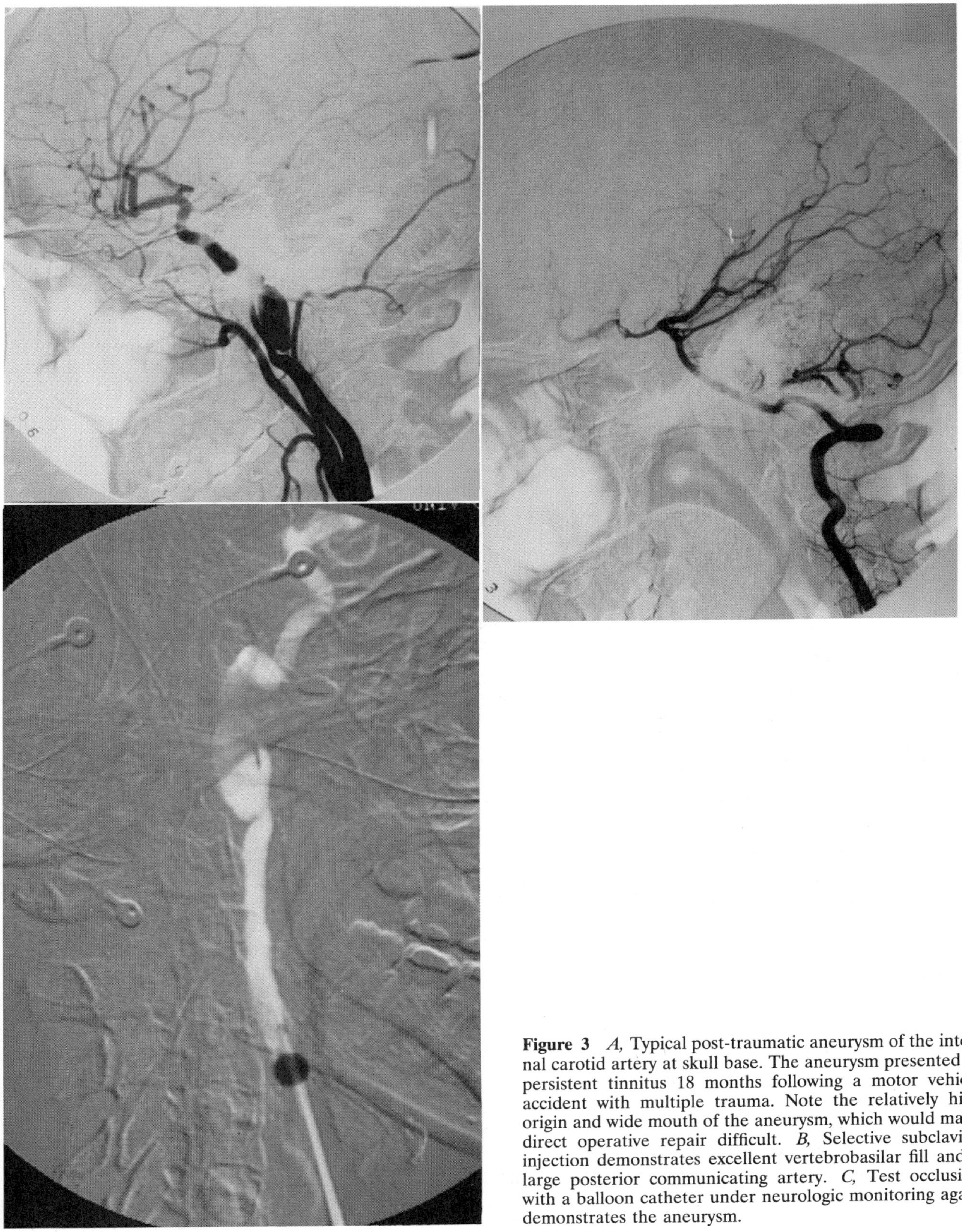

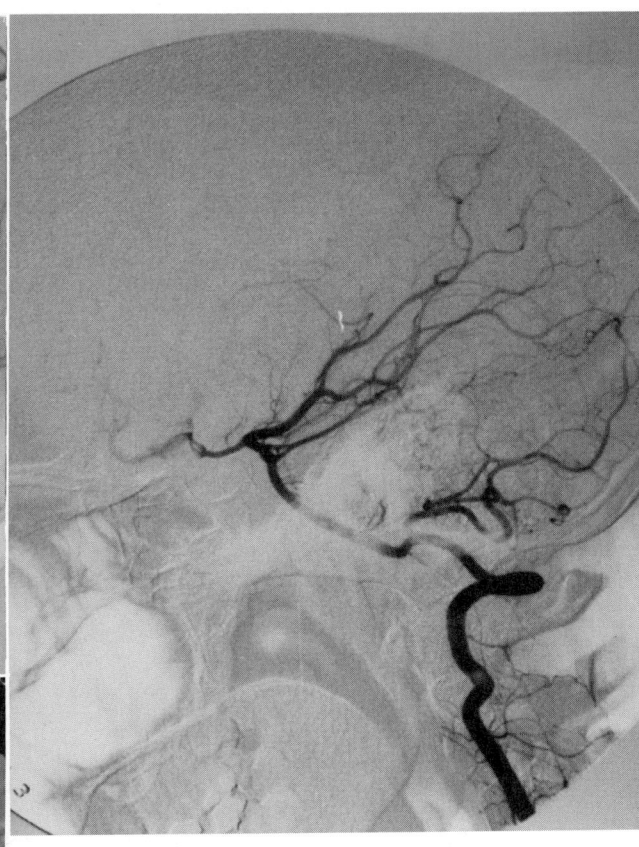

Figure 3 *A,* Typical post-traumatic aneurysm of the internal carotid artery at skull base. The aneurysm presented as persistent tinnitus 18 months following a motor vehicle accident with multiple trauma. Note the relatively high origin and wide mouth of the aneurysm, which would make direct operative repair difficult. *B,* Selective subclavian injection demonstrates excellent vertebrobasilar fill and a large posterior communicating artery. *C,* Test occlusion with a balloon catheter under neurologic monitoring again demonstrates the aneurysm.

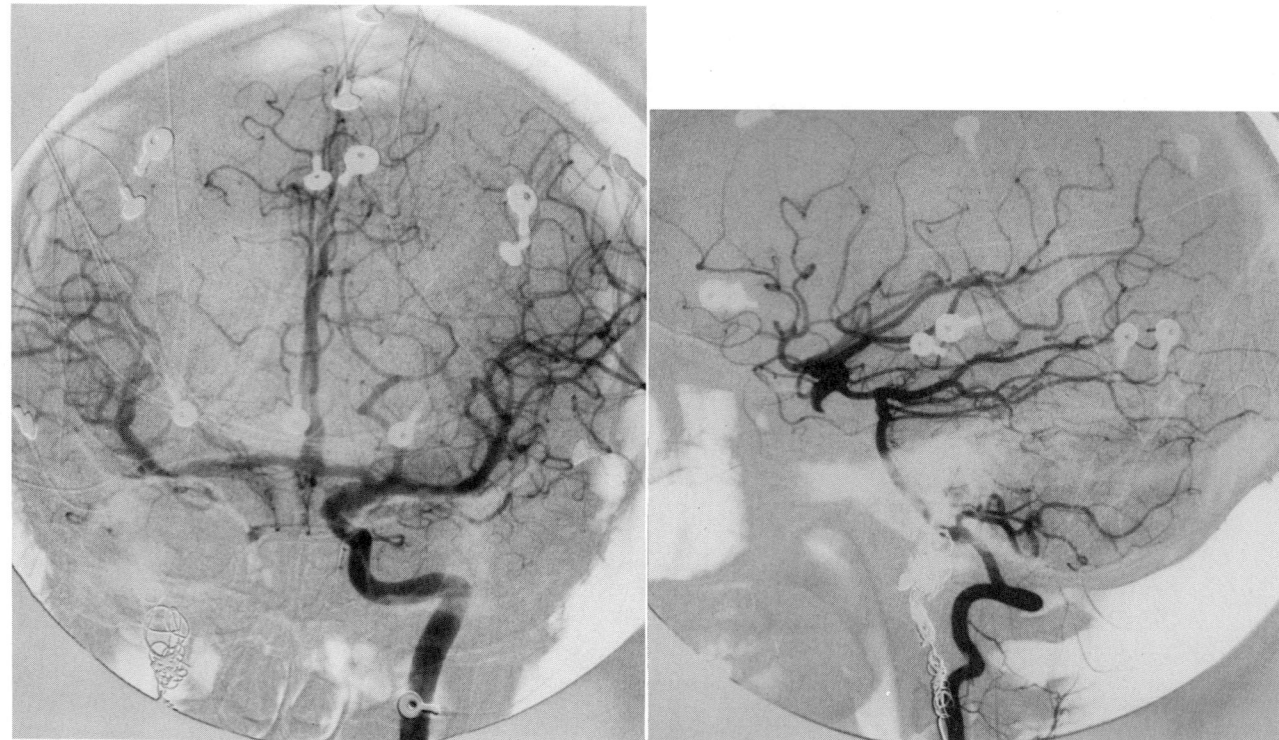

Figure 4 *A,* Permanent occlusion of the right internal carotid artery has been accomplished. (Note the metallic wire occluding the right carotid artery.) There is excellent left-to-right flow through the fully competent anterior communicating artery. *B,* A lateral view following subclavian artery injection demonstrates excellent posterior-to-anterior flow via the posterior communicating artery and the superimposed carotid occlusion.

done in conjunction with the neurologist and utilizes somatosensory monitoring of cranial nerve VII in addition to routine cardiovascular and cerebral support.

In general, arterial reconstruction involves aneurysm resection and end-to-end spatulated anastomoses. Reasonable alternatives include (1) resection of the aneurysm and patch angioplasty using either autogenous vein or a prosthetic patch or (2) resection and bypass grafting. For some very high-lying aneurysms, an extracranial to intracranial bypass procedure with ligation of the ICA has been utilized when direct reconstruction is not possible. In some circumstances, carotid ligation without reconstruction, to eliminate a potential embolic source, is the most appropriate treatment. Clearly, prior to permanent ligation, test occlusion of the carotid artery should be performed to ensure the adequacy of collateral flow. Because many of the carotid reconstructive procedures are more complex than standard carotid endarterectomy, they are typically performed under general anesthesia and may require use of an indwelling shunt.

Aggressive interventional neuroradiology support may allow a therapeutic approach in selected patients at risk for thromboembolic strokes but not amenable to direct reconstruction. Balloon occlusion techniques for either the carotid aneurysm or the ICA have been described. The technique for the latter clearly requires documentation of adequate collateral flow and does carry a small but real risk of cerebral ischemia (1% to 5%) due to embolism or low flow. Although a simple test occlusion and clinical observation are standard practice, position emission tomography (PET) scanning during arterial occlusion allows a more precise definition of the metabolic end organ effects of interrupting carotid artery blood flow. Permanent carotid occlusion utilizes a variety of coils, loops, wires, and thrombotic matrices to assure complete luminal obliteration with minimal embolic potential (Fig. 4).

RESULTS

Summating all patients with a variety of etiologies and means of therapy together, the overall mortality in reported series ranges from 0 to 16%, but it must be re-emphasized that these represent very small numbers of patients from any single institution. The overall complication rate is in the 15% to 20% range and includes strokes and cranial nerve injury. The latter typically involves nerves X and XII; with high or more extensive exposures, potential injury to IX, XI, and VII becomes more likely. The multiplicity of potential

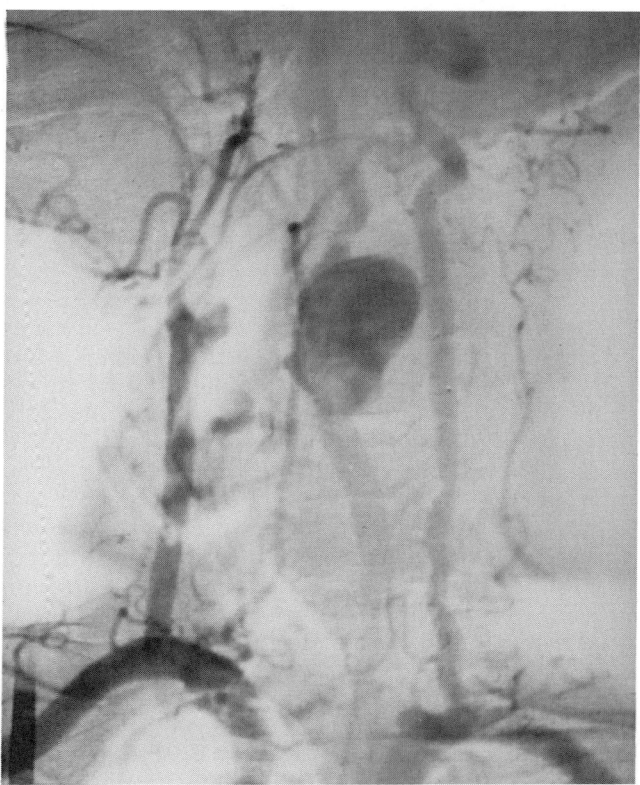

Figure 5 A postendarterectomy pseudoaneurysm appearing 38 months after carotid endarterectomy.

treatments indicates that patient management decisions must be individualized but also implies a variety of outcomes. Because the patients vary markedly in presentation, the lesions are anatomically quite dissimilar, the adequacy of the collateral circulation highly variable, and the numbers of patients reported by any single institution so small, prediction of anticipated outcome for a specific treatment plan is problematic.

REFERENCES

1. McCollum CH, Wheeler WG, Noon GP, DeBakey ME. Aneurysms of the extracranial carotid artery. Twenty-one years' experience. Am J Surg 1979; 137:196–200.
2. Painter TA, Hertzer NR, Beven EG, O'Hara PJ. Extracranial carotid aneurysms: Report of six cases and review of the literature. J Vasc Surg 1985; 2:312–18.
3. Rhodes EL, Stanley JC, Hoffman GL, et al. Aneurysms of extracranial carotid arteries. Arch Surg 1976; 111:339–343.
4. Sahlman A, Salo J, Kostiainen S, et al. Extracranial carotid artery aneurysms. Vasa 1991; 20:369–373.
5. Sharma S, Rajani M, Mishra N, et al. Extracranial carotid artery aneurysms following accidental injury: Ten years experience. Clin Radiol 1991; 43:162–165.
6. Tokimura H, Todoroki K, Asakura T, et al. Coexistence of extracranial internal carotid artery aneurysm and multiple intracranial aneurysms: Case report. Neurol Med Chir (Tokyo) 1992; 32:292–295.
7. Zelenock GB, Kazmers A, Whitehouse WM Jr, et al. Extracranial internal carotid artery dissections: Noniatrogenic traumatic lesions. Arch Surg 1982; 117:425–432.
8. Zwolak RM, Whitehouse WM Jr, Knake JE, et al. Atherosclerotic extracranial carotid artery aneurysms. J Vasc Surg 1984; 415–422.

CAROTID ARTERY DISSECTION

TAMMY K. RAMOS, M.D.
JERRY GOLDSTONE, M.D.

Carotid artery dissection is the result of hemorrhage into the tunica media of the arterial wall. The hemorrhage may result from a tear in the intima or from ruptured vasa vasora. Progression of the dissecting hematoma leads to enlargement of the vessel wall, both compressing the true lumen and causing an overall increase in vessel diameter. When the dissection is subintimal, occlusion of the true lumen may result. Alternatively, when the dissection is subadventitial, aneurysmal dilation of the artery wall is more likely to occur. Carotid artery dissections may be secondary to trauma, or they may occur spontaneously. This discussion is limited to spontaneous carotid dissections, which most frequently involve the extracranial internal carotid artery but may also occur in the common carotid and in the intracranial internal carotid arteries.

The etiology of spontaneous carotid artery dissection is unknown. By definition such is not associated with a history of antecedent trauma, but minor unrecognized trauma such as sneezing, coughing, or exaggerated neck movements may play a role. In certain patients underlying arterial wall pathology seems to predispose to dissection. Fifteen percent of extracranial internal carotid artery dissections are associated with fibromuscular dysplasia, and this number increases to 50% in the quarter of patients who present with bilateral dissections. Many early reports implicated cystic medial necrosis as a predisposing factor to dissection, but this finding and its relationship to spontaneous carotid artery dissection are less well characterized. Interestingly, Schievink and colleagues reported an increased frequency of saccular intracranial aneurysms in patients with spontaneous cervical carotid and vertebral artery dissections.[1] The preponderance of these aneurysms in the supraclinoid internal carotid artery, where they also commonly occur in patients with connective tissue disorders, supports the possibility that underlying arterial wall pathology may predispose to both of these abnormalities. Reported risk factors for carotid artery dissection including hypertension, migraine headaches, smoking, and the use of oral contraceptives have been identified in a variable number of patients.

PRESENTATION

Carotid artery dissection is a recognized cause of focal cerebral ischemic symptoms, especially in younger patients. Lanzino and associates identified internal carotid artery dissection as the etiology of transient ischemic attack or stroke in 4.5% of patients between the ages of 16 and 45 years.[2] A population-based survey of Rochester, Minnesota, defined the average annual incidence rate of cervical internal carotid artery dissection as 2.6 per 100,000 for patients of all ages, and the mean age at presentation was 44 years.[3] According to a recent review, 76% of patients with extracranial internal carotid artery dissection present with symptoms of focal cerebral ischemia.[4] Mokri found that more than half of such patients treated at the Mayo Clinic presented with one of three distinct syndromes: (1) hemicrania and oculosympathetic palsy; (2) hemicrania and delayed focal cerebral ischemic events; or (3) hemicrania, oculosympathetic palsy, and focal cerebral ischemic symptoms.[5] Over the last several years the use of noninvasive testing has led to the diagnosis of carotid artery dissection in patients with more subtle and unusual symptoms and signs, such as unilateral head, face, or neck pain associated with ipsilateral oculomotor or lower cranial nerve palsies.[6,7] Occasionally, asymptomatic carotid artery dissections are incidentally diagnosed by arteriography done for another reason.

Cerebral ischemic symptoms may be hemodynamic in origin, resulting from compression of the true lumen by the enlarging hematoma in the false lumen. More commonly they are thought to be due to distal embolization of thrombus that has developed at the site of the intimal tear or within an aneurysmal dilation. Involvement of the postganglionic sympathetic fibers traveling with the internal carotid artery by the dissection results in the characteristic incomplete Horner's syndrome with ptosis and miosis. Facial sweating remains normal because the postganglionic sympathetic fibers traveling with the external carotid artery are spared. Both nerve compression by the expanding intramural hematoma and transient ischemia have been postulated as the etiology of ipsilateral cranial nerve palsies.[6,7] Referred pain to the ipsilateral head, face, or neck is the most common symptom of carotid artery dissection, and its presence, especially in association with any of the other symptoms or signs already mentioned, should alert one to this diagnosis.

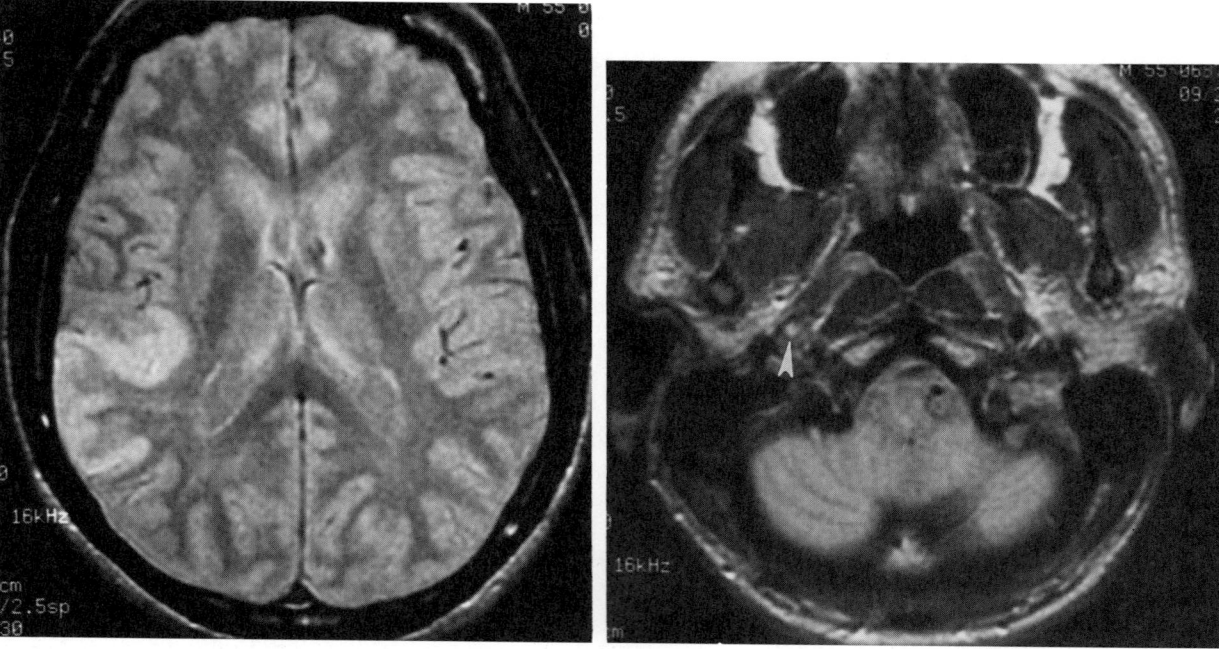

Figure 1 Imaging studies performed in a 55-year-old patient who presented with a 3 day history of severe generalized headache and new-onset confusion with mild sensory neglect of left side. *A,* Transaxial proton-density magnetic resonance imaging (MRI) section at the level of the lateral ventricles shows a right parietal infarct in the distribution of the posterior division of the middle cerebral artery. *B,* Transaxial proton-density MRI section at the cervicopetrous carotid junction reveals a hyperintense signal filling the right carotid lumen *(arrowhead).* Note the normal flow void in the left carotid artery.

DIAGNOSIS

Traditionally, the diagnosis of carotid artery dissection has been made by arteriography, although the pathognomonic finding of a double lumen is rarely present. The most common arteriographic finding is an irregular, tapered narrowing of the internal carotid artery beginning 2 to 3 cm distal to the bifurcation and extending rostrally to the base of the skull, where the artery usually regains its normal diameter. Less commonly, there is gradual tapering of the true lumen to occlusion resembling a dunce cap or flame (Fig. 1D). Occasionally, digital subtraction techniques and delayed filming can document a string sign or antegrade flow in what was initially thought to be an occluded vessel. Other arteriographic findings include aneurysms, intimal flaps, and occlusion of the middle cerebral artery or its branches.

Over the past few years, we have employed magnetic resonance imaging (MRI) early in the evaluation of patients with suspected carotid artery dissection. More recently, we have combined this study with magnetic resonance angiography (MRA) that can be performed at the same time. The brain can be imaged for evidence of infarction or hemorrhage while considerable information can be obtained about the arterial system (Fig. 1A, B, and C). In the axial plane, MRI can document the vessel lumen as well as intramural changes in the vessel wall that frequently cannot be appreciated by arteriography. The mural hematoma is best appreciated on fat-saturated T1-weighted images and proton-density T2-weighted images in which the surrounding adipose tissue gives a hypointense signal, allowing better definition of the intramural hemorrhage. Such images identify the typical hyperintense, crescent-shaped hematoma in the wall of the internal carotid artery (Fig. 2A). If the normal flow void is present, luminal narrowing can be readily appreciated by comparing the affected artery to the contralateral side. In contrast, if a hyperintense signal replaces the flow void, it is not always possible to distinguish mural hematoma from luminal thrombosis or slow flow (Fig. 1B). Sometimes MRA is helpful in this situation (Fig. 1C). If uncertainty exists, we proceed to digital subtraction angiography (DSA) to acquire further

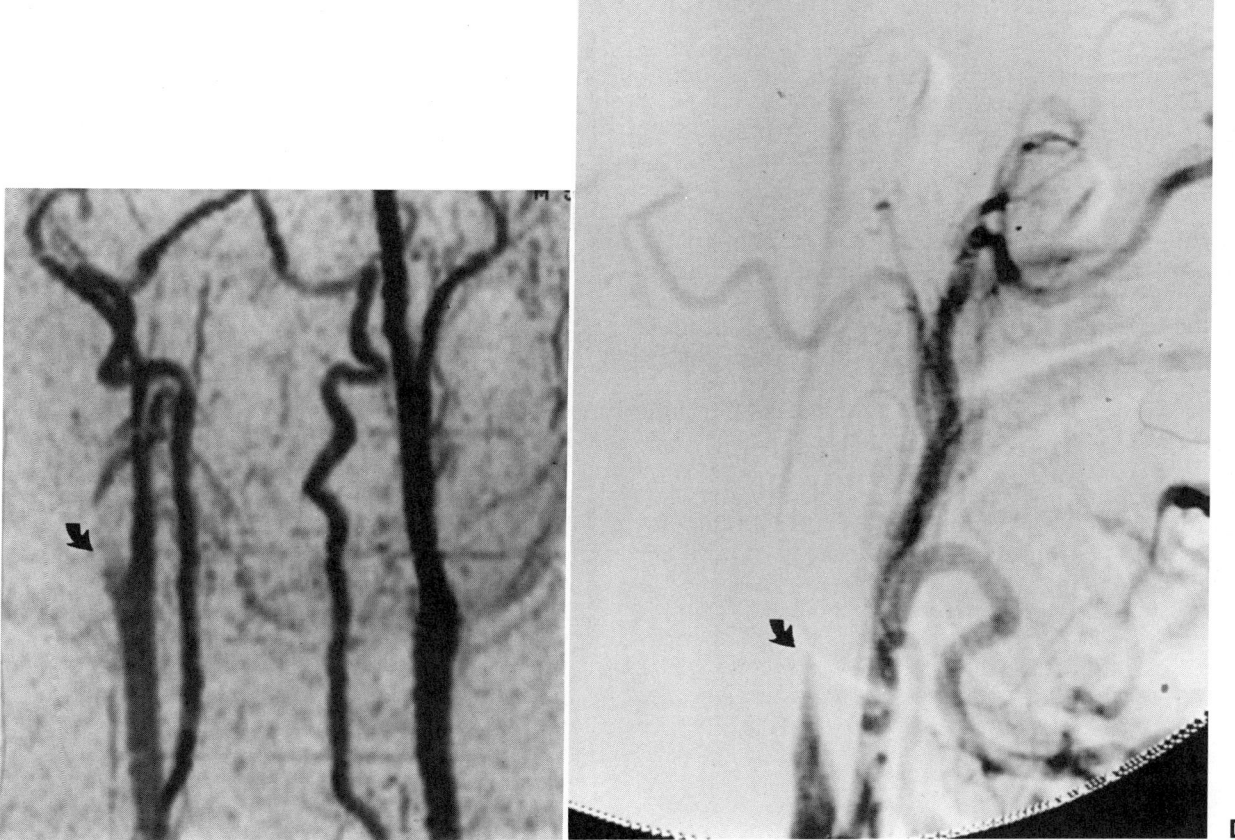

Figure 1 cont'd C, Magnetic resonance angiogram (MRA), right anterior oblique projection, shows occlusion of the right internal carotid artery at its origin *(arrow)*. D, Right common carotid digital subtraction angiogram (DSA), lateral projection, confirms internal carotid artery occlusion *(arrow)* and demonstrates the typical dunce cap or flame appearance of arterial occlusion secondary to dissection.

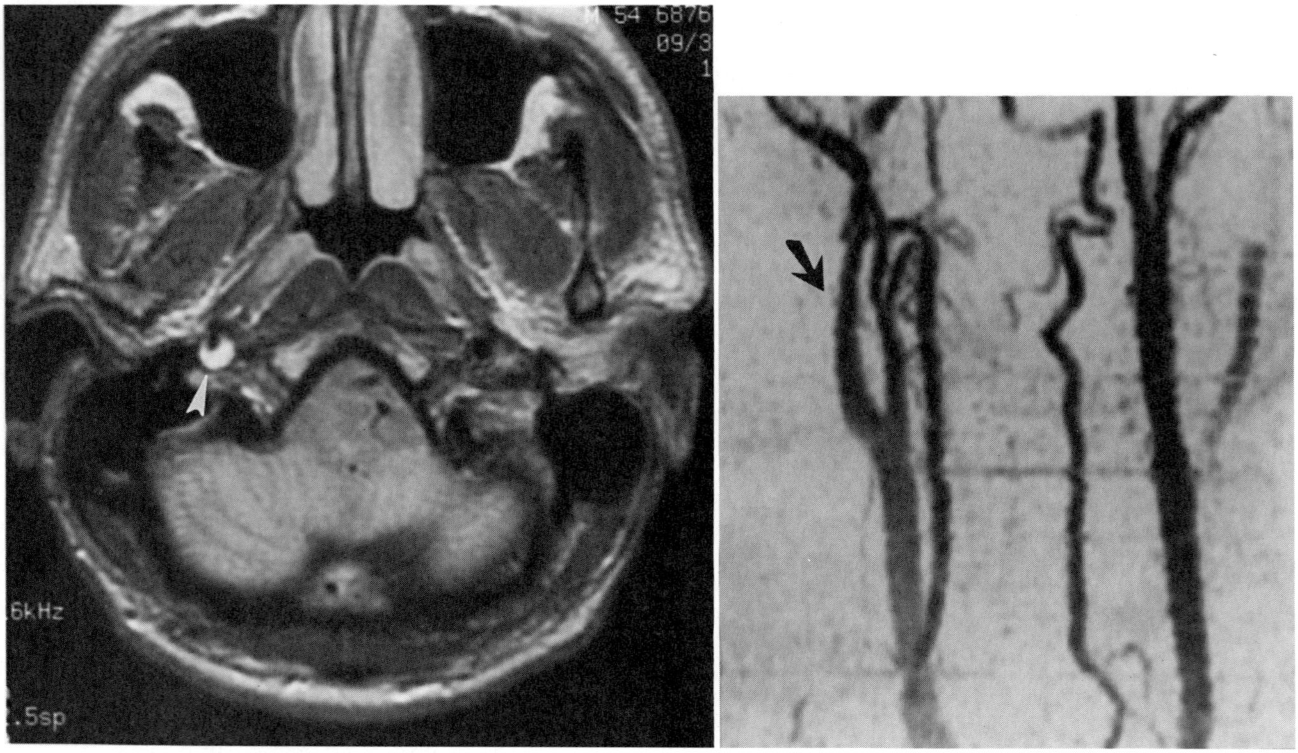

Figure 2 Imaging studies in the same patient performed 1 week after those shown in Figure 1. *A,* Transaxial proton-density MRI section shows recanalization of right internal carotid artery, indicated by the appearance of a flow void within the arterial lumen. Note the crescent-shaped hyperintense mural hematoma posteriorly *(arrowhead),* representing the classic appearance of a dissection. *B,* Two-dimension time of flight MRA, right anterior oblique projection, demonstrates recanalization of the right internal carotid artery *(arrow).*

information about vessel patency and to confirm the diagnosis (Fig. 1D). However, as we gain experience with MRI and with improvement in the techniques for MRA, we anticipate that contrast arteriography will be used less frequently to diagnose carotid artery dissection.

Other noninvasive tests that have been used to confirm the diagnosis of carotid artery dissection include duplex scanning, transcranial Doppler, and ocular pneumoplethysmography. Of these three studies we have found duplex scanning the most helpful. Rarely, when the proximal internal carotid artery or the common carotid artery is involved, duplex scanning can identify a double lumen, intimal flap, or tapered occlusion, all direct signs of dissection.[8] However, the usual finding is a patent, normal-appearing carotid bulb and proximal internal carotid artery without a flow signal or with a high-resistance flow pattern suggesting dissection.

TREATMENT

Over the last 40 years, much has been learned about the treatment of extracranial carotid artery dissections, but little knowledge has been gained about the natural history of this disease because most patients have received some form of therapy. In the early experience at the University of California, San Francisco, more than 80% of patients with cervical carotid artery dissections presented with acute focal cerebral ischemic symptoms, and more than a quarter of these patients presented with a completed stroke.

Extrapolating from experience with atherosclerotic extracranial cerebral vascular disease, we emphasized surgical treatment for carotid artery dissections, especially in those patients presenting with transient ischemic attacks. However, this initial experience with surgical interventions including segmental resection and saphenous vein grafting, intraluminal dilation, balloon catheter thrombectomy and intimectomy, and internal carotid artery ligation was disappointing. Fewer than 30% of the vessels remained patent after operation, and the perioperative stroke rate was 15%. In contrast, patients treated with only systemic anticoagulation seemed to do better. They suffered no additional neurologic symptoms and in patients who had repeat arteriograms the carotid lumen had become normal in 90%.

As a result of this experience and similar experiences reported by others, we currently treat patients with cervical carotid artery dissections with systemic anticoagulation to decrease the risk of distal embolization and vessel thrombosis. It may not be necessary to treat all patients with systemic anticoagulation, but it is difficult to know what the appropriate treatment is from one situation to another without prospective randomized trials upon which to base decision making. Some authors recommend only observation or antiplatelet therapy for patients presenting with local symptoms and reserve the use of systemic anticoagulation for patients who present with focal cerebral ischemic symptoms. In our experience many patients with acute carotid artery dissection have significant narrowing of the vessel lumen, even when they present with local symptoms. However, if the lumen is not compromised, suggesting that the local symptoms are the result of nerve compression from aneurysmal dilation, an antiplatelet agent may be all that is necessary. With experience, MRI may guide therapeutic decision making because it allows one to relate the symptoms at presentation directly to the size and location of the intramural hematoma and its relationship to the arterial lumen and surrounding structures. But for now, we anticoagulate acutely with heparin sodium and then chronically with sodium warfarin (Coumadin) for 3 months. When contraindications to systemic anticoagulation are present and if it is reasonable, an antiplatelet agent such as aspirin is used as an alternative. If heparin sensitivity is a concern, a rheologic agent such as low-molecular-weight dextran (Rheomacrodex) is substituted for the acute therapy. When patients present with a hemorrhagic or massive cerebral infarction, they are treated initially with supportive measures to assure adequate volume resuscitation and blood pressure control. Institution of delayed anticoagulation or antiplatelet therapy is determined by their clinical course and early follow-up studies.

All patients recieve a follow-up arteriogram at 3 months to guide further anticoagulation therapy. When high-resolution MRI and MRA have accurately defined the acute dissection, we use these studies for follow-up instead of contrast arteriography. Resolution of the dissection can be documented by changes in signal intensity of the intramural hematoma on sequential MRI studies. When MRI is complimented by MRA, normalization of the vessel lumen as well as residual aneurysmal changes in the vessel wall can be determined (Figs. 1B, 1C, 2A, and 3).

Instituting anticoagulation therapy, even when the vessel appears occluded by the dissection, may result in a normal vessel, a phenomenon that has been documented even in the absence of specific therapy. If follow-up studies document a normally healed vessel, then anticoagulation therapy is discontinued. However, if there is residual intramural hematoma or persistent luminal narrowing, anticoagulation is continued for a total of 6 months. Follow-up studies are obtained to document the status of the vessel and when anticoagulation therapy is to be discontinued. It has been our experience and that of others that if resolution of the dissection is going to occur, it does so within this interval.[9] When follow-up studies reveal a residual aneursym, repeat examinations are performed every 3

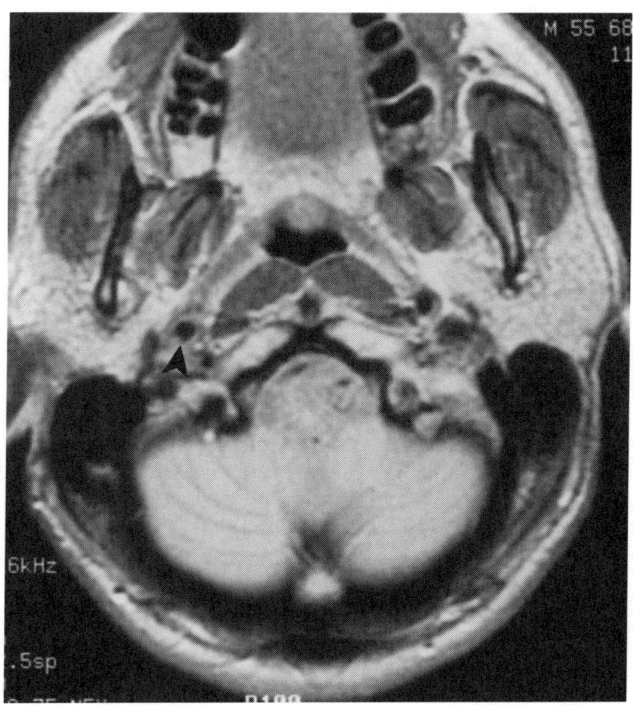

Figure 3 Follow-up transaxial proton-density MRI 6 weeks after the initial presentation of the patient in Figure 1 shows disappearance of the hyperintense mural hematoma and a normal right internal carotid artery flow void *(arrowhead)*, indicative of resolution of the dissection.

months for the first year and then biannually to monitor for enlargement.

Surgical treatment of carotid artery dissection is indicated in patients who develop recurrent neurologic symptoms despite adequate systemic anticoagulation. The acutely dissected artery is recognized by its dilation and bluish hue. It is extremely friable, making surgical manipulation hazardous, especially considering the very high exposure required for treatment of most dissections. When the dissection is limited and can be easily exposed, resection with interposition grafting is the preferred treatment for symptoms of both distal embolization and hypoperfusion. However, when the dissection extends to the base of the skull, ligation is the preferred and safest treatment for symptoms of distal embolization, if the systolic carotid stump blood pressure is greater than 70 mm Hg. If the carotid stump blood pressure is less than 70 mm Hg, the risk of perioperative stroke is increased following ligation; therefore, ligation should be combined with extracranial-intracranial (EC-IC) bypass grafting. For patients who fail systemic anticoagulation because of low-flow symptoms, EC-IC bypass grafting is also recommended. Another indication for surgical treatment of carotid artery dissection is enlargement of a residual aneurysm to 2 cm or greater in diameter. Resection with interposition grafting is the procedure of choice. Because most of these aneurysms are located at the base of the skull, however, ligation with or without EC-IC bypass grafting, as determined by the carotid stump blood pressure, is frequently necessary.

The outcomes of patients with cervical carotid artery dissections can be related more to symptoms at presentation than to the type of treatment. In a recent study of 30 patients presenting with acute stroke and carotid artery dissection with occlusion, the mortality was nearly 25%, and among the survivors almost half were severely disabled and unable to return to their previous activities.[9] In contrast, of the 70 patients with spontaneous carotid artery dissection, that Mokri reviewed, just over 25% presented with acute stroke and at follow-up 76% were asymtomatic. There were no deaths, and fewer than 1% of the patients were left with a marked or moderate deficit that interfered with their lifestyle. The patients in these two studies were treated in a variety ways. Nevertheless, patients who present with stroke fare more poorly than patients who present with transient ischemic attacks or local symptoms. Generally, similar to the resolution of arteriographic abnormalities, most symptoms resolve within 6 months, and there is little improvement in residual symptoms past this time. The relationship between residual abnormalities on arteriography and persistent symptoms is not always clear. Hopefully, sequential MRI will elucidate this relationship as well as provide new information about the healing response of the artery wall that will guide therapy.

Recurrent spontaneous carotid artery dissections, although uncommon, are not rare and are therefore, worth mentioning. They are more likely to occur in young patients, usually a year or more after the initial event, and they almost always involve a different vessel than the original dissection.[10] Determinants of outcome for recurrent dissections are similar to those for first-time dissections.

REFERENCES

1. Schievink WI, Mokri B, Peipgras DG. Angiographic frequency of saccular intracranial aneurysms in patients with spontaneous cervical artery dissection. J Neurosurg 1992; 76:62–66.
2. Lanzino G, Andreoli A, Di Pasquale G, et al. Etiopathogenesis and prognosis of cerebral ischemia in young adults. A survey of 155 treated patients. Acta Neurol Scand 1991; 84:321–325.
3. Schievink WI, Mokri B, Whisnant JP. Internal carotid artery dissection in a community: Rochester, Minnesota, 1987–1992. Stroke 1993; 24:1678–1680.
4. Anson J, Crowell RM. Cervicocranial arterial dissection. Neurosurgery 1991; 29:89–96.
5. Mokri B. Traumatic and spontaneous extracranial internal carotid artery dissections. J Neurol 1990; 237:356–361.
6. Schievink WI, Mokri B, Garrity JA, et al. Ocular motor nerve palsies in spontaneous dissections of the cervical internal carotid artery. Neurology 1993; 43:1938–1941.
7. Sturzenegger M, Huber P. Cranial nerve palsies in spontaneous carotid artery dissection. J Neurol Neurosurg Psychiatry 1993; 56:1191–1199.
8. Sturzenegger M. Ultrasound findings in spontaneous carotid artery dissection: The value of duplex sonography. Arch Neurol 1991; 48:1057–1063.
9. Bogousslavsky J, Despland P-A, Regli F. Spontaneous carotid dissection with acute stroke. Arch Neurol 1987; 44:137–140.
10. Schievink WI, Mokri B, O'Fallon WM. Recurrent spontaneous cervical artery dissection. N Engl J Med 1994; 330:393–397.

FIBROMUSCULAR DISEASE OF THE CAROTID ARTERY

EILEEN S. NATUZZI, M.D.
RONALD J. STONEY, M.D.

The first case of extrarenal fibromuscular dysplasia (FMD) was reported in 1964. It described a young female with intestinal angina and celiac artery stenosis due to fibromuscular hyperplasia.[1] A year later the first report of FMD involving the internal carotid artery was published.[2] Although FMD most commonly involves the renal arteries, it also affects vessels such as the vertebral, subclavian, mesenteric, hepatic, splenic, and iliac arteries. Of patients undergoing carotid angiography for cerebrovascular disease, as many as 2.5% are found to have angiographic evidence of carotid FMD.[3,4]

EPIDEMIOLOGY

Carotid FMD affects females more frequently than males. Young white women in their childbearing years are most often affected, suggesting there may be a link between hormones and the development of the lesions. This hypothesis, however, has not been supported by an increased incidence of the disease in multiparous women or by worsening of pre-existing disease during pregnancy. Reports of a link between FMD and oral contraceptive use have yielded conflicting and inconclusive results.

Other hypothetical causes of the disease include mechanical and ischemic vessel wall damage. Vessels most commonly affected by FMD, such as the right renal artery and the extracranial carotid artery, tend to have longer nonbranched segments, making them more dependent upon their vasa vasora for blood supply. Occlusion or decreased numbers of these small nutrient vessels may cause ischemia and subsequent deposition of connective tissue and myofibroblasts in the arterial wall.

In addition, the extracranial carotid artery may undergo stress injury due to stretching secondary to hyperextension and rotation of the neck. The combination of the mechanisms of injury, mechanical stress, and ischemia may make some vessels particularly vulnerable to mural damage. Finally, familial clustering of FMD has been reported. There appears to be evidence of an autosomal dominant trait with variable penetrance in 60% of patients.[5]

CLINICAL PRESENTATION

Patients with carotid FMD are often symptomatic; however, many lesions are found in patients undergoing angiography for other reasons. In one of the largest series of patients with carotid FMD, presenting symptoms were reported in 101 patients with angiographically proven FMD.[6] Patients with FMD present with a variety of symptoms and physical findings (Tables 1 and 2). The most disturbing and significant initial presentation is that of a completed stroke, seen in 22% of the patients. Nearly one-half of these patients are left with residual neurologic deficits. Pulsatile tinnitus heard by the patient is more commonly associated with FMD than with atherosclerotic disease and may be due to the close proximity of the flow-distorting carotid lesion to the middle ear.

Aneurysms or dissections that encroach upon neighboring neurologic structures may cause Horner's syndrome, headache, neck pain, and cranial nerve paralysis. The onset of such symptoms in patients with dissections and aneurysms may be preceded by cervical trauma or physical exercise.

Studies and reports describing surgical intervention for FMD tend to focus on symptomatic patients. Most of these reports do not define the incidence and natural history of asymptomatic FMD. Stewart and colleagues reviewed angiographically proven diagnoses of FMD and found 22% to be asymptomatic.[7] This report included a total of 49 patients, 11 of whom were asymptomatic. Thirty-five of these patients did not undergo operative intervention for a number of reasons. Their course may represent the natural history of the disease. Of them, one-fifth were asymptomatic, and the remainder had symptoms. In an 8 year follow-up period three (8%) patients died of nonneurologic causes, and three patients underwent operation due to persistent symptoms of cerebral ischemia. There were no instances of spontaneous dissection or aneurysmal rupture. These observations, although derived from a small number of patients, suggest that FMD, without associated atherosclerosis, may be a more benign disease than was initially thought. It is our belief, however, that when symptoms appear, the disease requires surgical intervention. This approach is supported by a 22% incidence of completed stroke as the presenting symptom in our series.

CAUSES OF SYMPTOMS IN FMD

The pathophysiology of symptom production in patients with FMD is unknown. A number of hypotheses have been advanced, including thromboembolic events, hypoperfusion caused by a solitary critical stenosis, serial subcritical stenoses, or multiple vessel disease. Uncontrolled hypertension may lead to lacunar infarcts and may also weaken already compromised blood vessel walls. The classic "string of beads" lesion seen in medial fibroplasia may cause turbulence and formation of mural thrombi between the stenotic fibromuscular thickenings, which later may embolize. Intracranial aneurysms may also be a source of embolized thrombotic material. When aneurysms rupture, subarachnoid or intracranial hemorrhages result.

Occlusion of the internal carotid artery and subsequent stroke may be due to spontaneous carotid dissections. Rarely, dissections result in carotid–cavernous sinus fistulas. In one atypical FMD lesion, intimal disruption resulted in a subintimal hematoma. This lesion was believed to be the source of emboli in a patient with multiple hemispheric transient ischemic attacks (TIAs).[8] Whatever the cause of neurologic symptoms may be, it seems clear that surgical intervention is indicated for symptomatic patients.

DIAGNOSIS

The diagnostic gold standard for FMD is carotid arteriography. Noninvasive studies such as duplex scans or B-mode real-time ultrasound imaging may show flow changes at narrowings in the extracranial carotid vessel. However, these studies do not identify the site of disease or the intracranial vessels that frequently contain aneurysms. In addition, ultrasound may not detect intimal flaps or dissections as readily as angiography or magnetic resonance angiography, a modality that

Table 1 Symptoms at Presentation

Symptom	Patients (%)
Transient ischemic attacks	41
Nonlocalizing neurologic signs	31
Bruits audible by patient	23
Amaurosis fugax	23
Completed strokes	22
Asymptomatic bruits	8
Prolonged ischemic attack	2
Other	6

Table 2 Physical Findings at Presentation

Finding	Patients (%)
Carotid bruit	77
Hypertension	37
Neurologic deficits	9
Electrocardiogram abnormalities	17

appears to be most sensitive for detecting internal carotid dissection.

There are a number of typical appearances of FMD on angiography. Most common is the string of beads appearance in a vessel with medial involvement (Fig. 1). This is due to multifocal thickening and alternating areas of thinned dilated wall. Lesions may also appear as tubular and localized luminal defects. The mid to distal one-third of the cervical internal carotid artery is the most common site of involvement. The high incidence of bilateral disease and concomitant atherosclerosis dictates that both carotids should be fully examined. Intracranial vessels should also be visualized for the presence of aneurysms. Saccular aneurysms, both solitary and multiple, are the most common type seen, whereas fusiform wall changes are quite rare. Spontaneous dissections are recognizable by the creation of a string sign (Fig. 2). If this long, irregular filling defect is found, it should prompt a search for evidence of FMD in other vessels.

Arteriographic studies of patients suspected of having FMD should be modified to include an aortic arch study with selected carotid injections, intracranial artery views, and visualization of the renal and external iliac arteries.

TREATMENT

The area of greatest debate in the treatment of FMD is not necessarily what operation or procedure to perform once the disease has been diagnosed but rather when is operation indicated. Stewart and colleagues emphasized the benign natural history of the disease, and therefore recommended operation for persistently symptomatic patients only.[7] Asymptomatic patients should be followed closely and at regular intervals.

Management of patients with a single minor neurologic event and angiographically proven disease is more controversial. Some patients have been treated with antiplatelet therapy (aspirin, dipyridamole), which may prevent recurrent symptoms. However, we favor surgical intervention for all symptomatic patients.

The technique for the repair of internal carotid FMD depends upon the location of the lesion and its surgical accessibility. Proximal carotid lesions with a

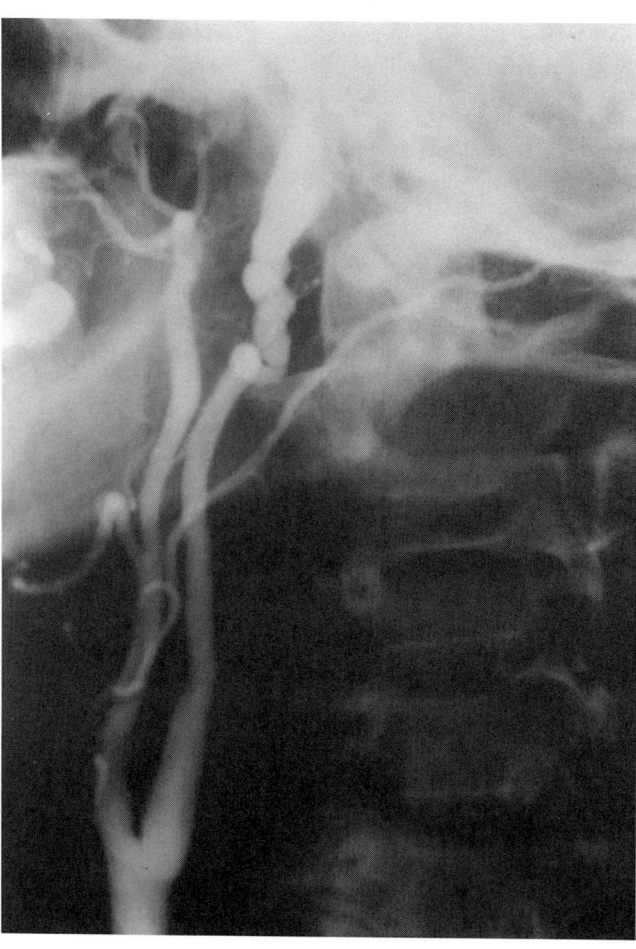

Figure 1 Carotid angiography demonstrating the classic string of beads appearance of FMD.

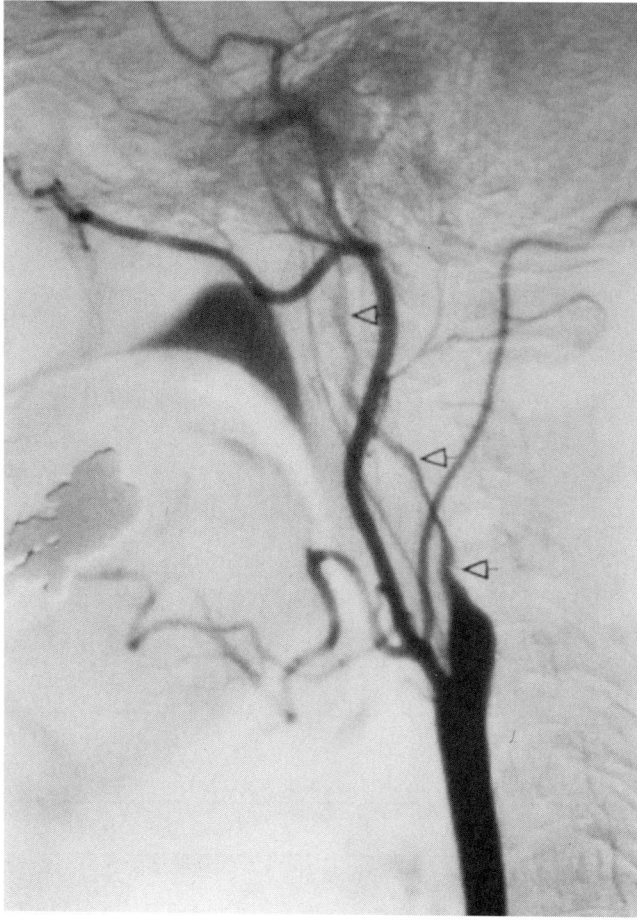

Figure 2 Spontaneous dissection of the carotid artery, creating a string sign.

redundant distal artery can be resected and reanastomosed or repaired by an interposition graft. Lesions located in the middle and distal portions of the internal carotid artery are exposed by division of the occipital artery as well as the stylohyoid and posterior belly of the digastric muscles. Occasionally, anterior subluxation of the mandible allows enlargement of the retromandibular space and extra exposure of the distal portion of the artery. If this approach is undertaken, the patient should have nasal-tracheal intubation. When significant atherosclerotic disease involves the carotid artery bifurcation, endarterectomy is performed in addition to treatment of the FMD lesion.

The vast majority of FMD lesions are not amenable to resection and repair because of the distal location in the extracranial internal carotid artery. Since 1970 we have been using graduated intraluminal dilation (GID) under direct visualization to treat these lesions. The entire length of the internal carotid artery is mobilized free of its investing fascia up to the level of the styloid process or skull base, if necessary. The carotid sinus nerve is divided in order to facilitate caudal retraction of the internal carotid artery. Patients are routinely anticoagulated with heparin sodium prior to the longitudinal arteriotomy in the carotid bulb. Rubber tubing is used to retract and straighten the internal carotid artery during dilation. The key to minimal complications following GID is to thoroughly straighten the artery prior to intraluminal dilation by caudal traction. Starting with a 1.5 or 2 mm dilator, the instrument is passed gently into the artery until resistance is encountered. The dilator is advanced slowly through this resistance (Fig. 3). Increasingly larger-diameter instruments are passed into the artery, thereby gradually dilating it. Small vessels should not be dilated beyond 3.5 mm and larger vessels not beyond 4 mm. At the completion of the dilation, the artery should be allowed to backbleed vigorously in order to flush out intimal particles and thrombi that may be dislodged during the procedure. The arteriotomy is closed with a continuous 6-0 suture. An intraoperative angiogram or, preferably, intraoperative duplex ultrasound is performed to assess the postdilation appearance of the artery.

Lord and associates have reported the use of intraoperative balloon dilation to accomplish the same goals as GID.[9] Under fluoroscopic visualization a 4.0 Gruntzig balloon dilating catheter is passed through an arteriotomy and positioned within the stenotic segment. The balloon is inflated for 4 minutes. At our institution this technique has not been used because of concerns about creating aneurysms or dissections by vigorous balloon dilation. We have found that balloon dilation

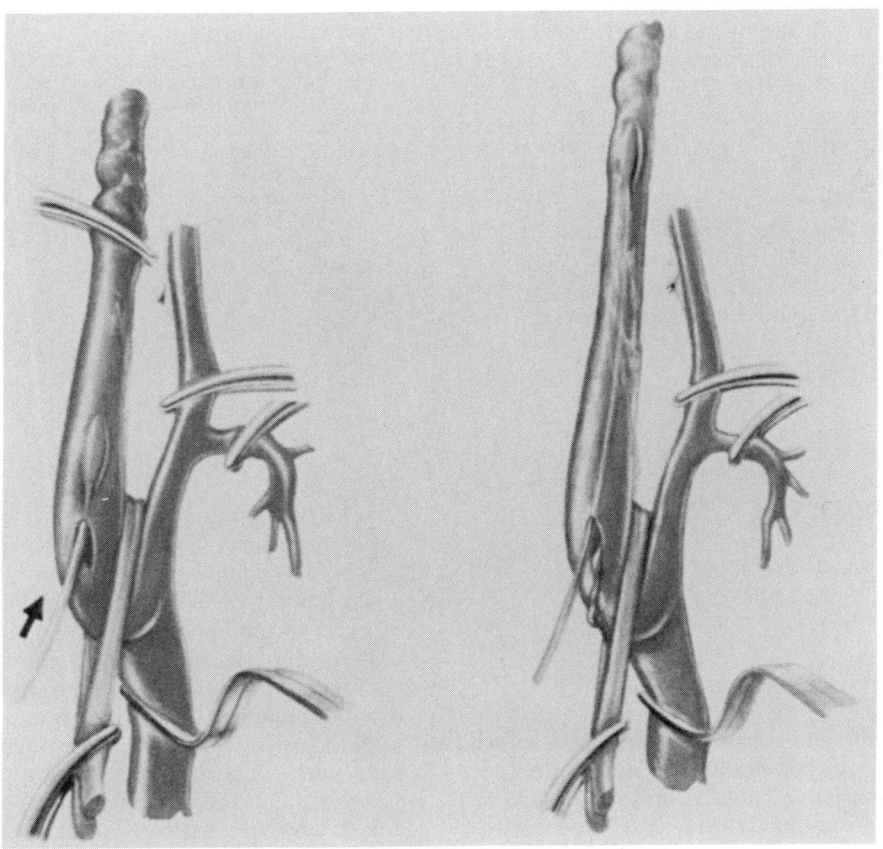

Figure 3 Technique demonstrating caudal retraction and straightening of the distal internal carotid artery prior to gradual intraluminal dilation.

does not appear to offer any advantages over rigid dilation.

There have been some reports of successful treatment of carotid FMD by percutaneous transluminal angioplasty (PTA).[10,11] Tsai and associates published a series of 27 patients who underwent carotid artery angioplasty, 5 of whom had FMD.[10] Stenotic lesions were successfully dilated without neurologic complications. Despite this safe and successful treatment in a small number of patients, concern remains about emboli from the traumatized dilation site. During PTA the cerebral blood flow remains antegrade, in contrast to GID, where blood flow is reversed and embolic debris is flushed out through the arteriotomy site. Treatment of patients with anticoagulants prior to PTA has been recommended to avoid dislodging thrombi. The development of triple coaxial catheters that have an occlusive balloon that is inflated distal to the dilating balloon and a suction port between the two balloons in order to remove dislodged debris may eliminate these concerns.

OUTCOME OF SURGICAL TREATMENT

A number of criteria are used in evaluating patients who have undergone GID at our institution. These include surgical accessibility of the lesion, safety of the procedure performed, and durability of the result.

Despite the distal location of the majority of carotid FMD lesions, access to the diseased segment has been achieved consistently using GID. This technique allows visualization of the arterial segment to be dilated during straightening and sequential dilation as far distally as the skull base.

Our results enable us to conclude that this operative approach is safe in the symptomatic patient. In 150 dilations performed in 101 patients, there were no deaths, 3 early postoperative strokes, and 9 patients with early postoperative TIAs. There was one instance of an arterial perforation early in our experience. Judicious complete mobilization and straightening of the internal carotid artery has prevented recurrence of this problem. Non-neurologic surgical complications did not differ from those seen in patients undergoing carotid endarterectomy.

Arterial patency and durability of GID were confirmed during follow-up visits. In a 17 year period, two patients required reoperation, one of whom developed reocclusion at a previously dilated site. Two patients had strokes, and two suffered subarachnoid hemorrhages from rupture of associated intracranial aneurysms. Three patients continued to have persistent generalized neurologic symptoms and probably represented inappropriate patient selection.

REFERENCES

1. Palubinskas AJ, Ripley HR. Fibromuscular hyperplasia in extrarenal arteries. Radiology 1964; 82:451–455.
2. Connett MC, Lansche JM. Fibromuscular hyperplasia of the internal carotid artery. Ann Surg 1965; 162:59–62.
3. Corrin LS, Sandok BA, Houser OW. Cerebral ischemic events in patients with carotid artery FMD. Arch Neurol 1981; 38:616–618.
4. Osborn AG, Anderson RE. Angiographic spectrum of cervical and intracranial FMD. Stroke 1977; 8:617–626.
5. Luscher TF, Lie JT, Stanson AW, et al. Arterial fibromuscular dysplasia. Mayo Clin Proc 1987; 62:931–952.
6. Effeney DJ, Fibromuscular dysplasia of the carotid artery. Aust N Z J Surg 1983; 53:527–531.
7. Stewart MT, Moritz M, Smith RB III, et al. Natural history of carotid fibromuscular dysplasia. J Vasc Surg 1986; 3:305–310.
8. Gee W, Burton R, Stoney RJ. Atypical fibromuscular hyperplasia involving the carotid artery. Ann Surg 1974; 180:136–138.
9. Lord RS, Graham AR, Benn IV. Radiologic control of operative carotid dilation. Aneurysm formation following balloon dilation. J Cardiovasc Surg 1986; 27:158–161.
10. Tsai FY, Matovich V, Hieshima G, et al. Percutaneous transluminal angioplasty of the carotid artery. AJNR, 1986; 7:349–358.
11. Brown MM. Balloon angioplasty for cerebrovascular disease. Neurol Res 1992; 14:159–163.

CAROTID KINKS AND COILS

MARK TAGETT, M.D., PH.D.
ANDRIS KAZMERS, M.D., M.S.P.H.

The clinical significance of carotid kinks and coils is controversial because sufficient data are not available to define clearly either their incidence or natural history. Information available about carotid kinks and coils is primarily anecdotal. Nevertheless, such carotid artery abnormalities may be responsible for cerebrovascular symptoms and stroke.

Not until the 1950s were carotid artery kinks or coils thought to have potential cerebrovascular pathophysiologic significance. Riser and colleagues in 1951 described a patient with vertebrobasilar insufficiency that was attributed to kinking of the carotid artery.[1] By the end of that decade Quattlebaum and associates had performed resection and reanastomosis of the common carotid artery (CCA) in three patients with carotid kinks.[2] In two of these patients, the kinks were associated with synchronous carotid atherosclerotic lesions.

Although the incidence of carotid kinks and coils in the general population is not known, excessive length leading to potential kinking of the carotid system is observed in 43% of children and 20% of adults undergoing cerebral arteriography.[3] The reported incidence of actual kinking or coiling is lower. In a review of nearly 1,500 consecutive carotid arteriograms, Weibel and Fields found tortuosity in 31%, coiling in 7%, and kinking in 5%.[4] The incidence of bilaterality has been variable. A 16% incidence of internal carotid artery (ICA) kinking and coiling was observed by Metz and co-workers on a review of 1,000 arteriograms.[5]

A useful although not universally accepted classification of carotid artery tortuosity was offered by Weibel and Fields in 1965.[4] The myriad descriptive names used to classify the different expressions of carotid redundancy has caused confusion. Among the descriptive terms worth retaining are tortuosity, coil, and kink. According to Weibel and Fields, (1) tortuosity is as any C- or S-shaped elongation of the carotid artery; (2) a coil is a circular configuration or an exaggerated S-shape; and (3) a kink is an abrupt angle in the carotid artery associated with a stenosis.[4]

PATHOPHYSIOLOGY

The cause of extracranial carotid system elongation is uncertain. Kinking or coiling of the carotid artery has been noted in all age groups. That coils are observed in children supports the theory that these coils may be congenital. The carotid system can be tortuous in utero. It is thought that as the fetal heart and great vessels descend into the mediastinum during embryogenesis, the carotid arteries become uncoiled. If the descent of the heart and great vessels is incomplete, it is theorized, bilateral carotid tortuosity can result.

Although the possibility of crossing fibrotic, nervous, or muscular adhesions leading to carotid kinks has been proposed, it is more likely that such adhesions are casual, not causal. The absence of kinking or redundancy in the external carotid artery (ECA) may be due to the presence of the many branches of the ECA that fix the vessel in place. Such branching is not present in the extracranial ICA or in the CCA proximal to the carotid bifurcation, and kinking has been reported in both these latter locations. When the ICA is involved, the kink or coil can occur 2 to 3 cm or more distal to the carotid bifurcation and can be found up to the base of the skull.

An additional etiology is that carotid kinks can result from other associated carotid artery lesions. Atherosclerotic disease, carotid aneurysms, and fibromuscular dysplasia have all been associated with carotid kinks. Whether such associated carotid lesions are involved with the pathogenesis of carotid kinking is unclear. The presence of these synchronous carotid lesions complicates surgical management of carotid kinks and coils. Treatment of these associated carotid lesions may accentuate any carotid kinking that may be present. Carotid kinks, however, may occur in the absence of any concomitant carotid lesions. It has been suggested that, unlike carotid coils, carotid kinks typically are acquired lesions that may be more likely to cause neurologic symptoms such as transient ischemic accidents (TIAs), positional cerebral ischemia, or cerebral infarction.

When kinks are not associated with other carotid lesions, ischemic or embolic neurologic symptoms may be attributed to the carotid kink. It is difficult to implicate a carotid kink or coil as being responsible for neurologic symptoms in the presence of associated carotid artery bifurcation atherosclerosis, fibromuscular disease, carotid artery aneurysms, valvular heart disease, inflammatory vascular disorders such as giant cell arteritis, or primary neurologic disorders. Before attributing neurologic symptoms to a carotid kink, it is also necessary to exclude disorders of heart rate and rhythm and central nervous system neoplasms. Occasionally, it is not possible to identify definitively the source of neurologic symptoms or complications. In the absence of associated lesions, cerebrovascular symptoms can be assumed to be due to a carotid kink after thorough evaluation including Holter monitoring, echocardiography, magnetic resonance imaging or computed tomography of the head, and four-vessel cerebral and arch arteriography.

In decreasing frequency, atherosclerosis, carotid aneurysms, and fibrodysplastic disease accompany carotid kinks in up to 80% of patients with such kinks. This confounds the issue as to which lesion may be responsible for TIAs or stroke. Isolated carotid kinks have been reported to result in TIAs or stroke, whereas carotid coils are typically clinically silent.

Although the embologenic nature of an ulcerated plaque is not to be disregarded, a kink may result in reduction of cerebral perfusion. A carotid kink in the presence of contralateral carotid artery disease or an incomplete circle of Willis could explain the presence of global cerebral ischemic symptoms in some individuals with significant carotid kinks.

CLINICAL MANIFESTATIONS AND DIAGNOSIS

Few clinical signs result from carotid tortuosity. Prominent pulsations in the neck or oropharynx may be the presenting sign of a carotid kink or coil. There may be a cervical bruit or thrill. Although it is likely that most patients with redundant carotid vessels are asymptomatic, cerebral thromboembolism or global cerebral ischemia may result in symptoms such as TIAs, vertebrobasilar insufficiency, or stroke. One classic manifestation of carotid kinks is the potentiation of cerebrovascular symptoms on abrupt rotation, flexion, or hyperextension of the head and neck. In children, neurologic insult resulting from carotid redundancy may be more severe, with seizures or ischemic hemiplegia being common presenting symptoms.[6]

Most diagnoses of carotid tortuosity or kinking are made following arteriographs. A high index of suspicion would be necessary to anticipate their presence before arteriography. Given the probability that cerebrovascular symptoms most likely result from extracranial atherosclerosis, it is not apparent that making the diagnosis of symptomatic carotid tortuosity before arteriography would be feasible, likely, or advantageous. Most carotid kinks or coils reported in the literature were diagnosed after cerebral arteriography. Duplex scanning can detect carotid redundancy, coils, or kinks, but these lesions may not all be routinely imaged by duplex because they can be distal to the carotid bifurcation. Lesions at the skull base may be difficult to image by duplex.

When arteriography documents a kink and all other causes for the symptoms have been excluded, it is possible that the kink is responsible. If the kink is present in addition to carotid bifurcation atherosclerotic disease, it is less likely, but possible, that the kink is the cause of symptoms. In this circumstance, both carotid lesions should be corrected at operation.

SURGICAL MANAGEMENT

Operation is appropriate for symptomatic carotid kinks or kinks associated with surgically significant atherosclerotic carotid lesions. The benefit of surgical management for asymptomatic carotid kinks or coils remains to be proven. Patients with asymptomatic kinks, once diagnosed, should be followed. Although the risk of stroke is not known, such asymptomatic lesions might become symptomatic. The kink or coil should be corrected in the symptomatic patient in which all other etiologies responsible for the neurologic symptoms have been excluded. Patients with atherosclerotic lesions of the carotid bifurcation often develop distal ICA redundancy. Dissection and mobilization of the ICA for endarterectomy increase the likelihood and severity of a kink. In patients undergoing endarterectomy, the plaque may serve as a stent for the carotid artery, and removal may aggravate a carotid kink. Because of these considerations, the kink as well as the atherosclerotic carotid lesion both need to be addressed, or subsequent worsening of the kink may cause perioperative carotid artery thrombosis and stroke.[7] One must be alert to the fact that the area adjacent to the kink may be exceptionally fragile, even in the absence of substantial poststenotic dilation, and it may not hold sutures well.

The many technical options that have been described to correct carotid artery kinks or coils include (1) patch angioplasty, with or without concomitant carotid endarterectomy; (2) resection and bypass; and (3) excision of the ICA or CCA, with or without eversion endarterectomy, and proximal reanastomosis. Kinking of the ICA is often suitably managed by a patch angioplasty, particularly if carotid endarterectomy is also performed. This straightens the vessel that could otherwise kink at

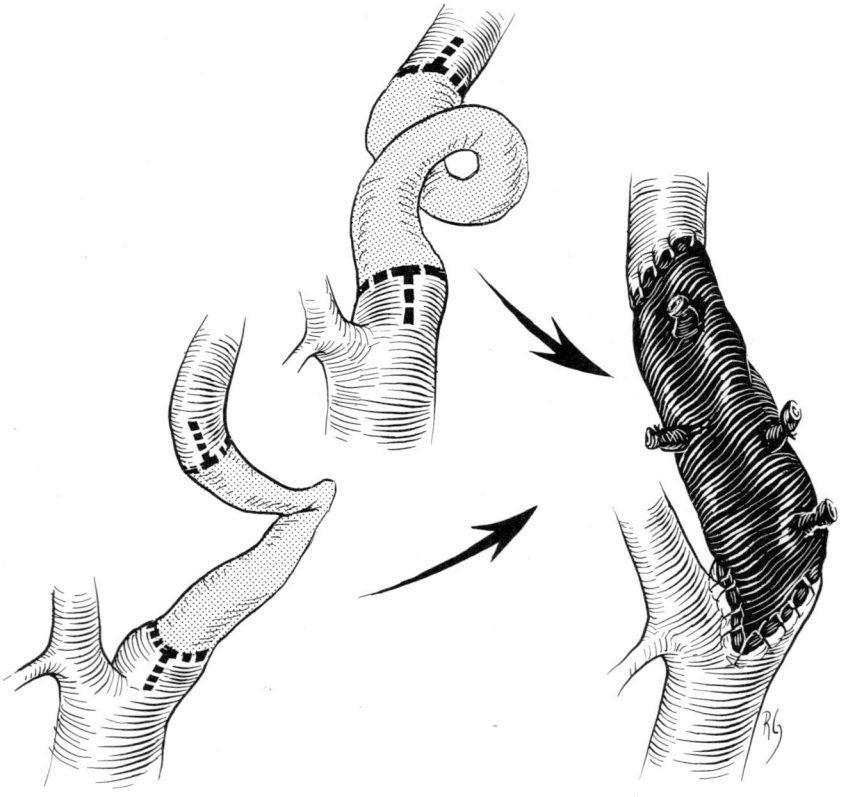

Figure 1 Resection with bypass is a useful technique for management of symptomatic carotid kinks or coils. The artery is spatulated proximally and distally after excision of the responsible lesion. Direct intraluminal inspection of the carotid bifurcation should be performed. When endarterectomy is necessary, the arteriotomy in the common carotid artery can be extended. The vein graft is also spatulated appropriately in order to prevent anastomotic narrowing. A completion angiogram is recommended to assess the technical results of carotid artery reconstruction.

or distal to the endarterectomy end point unless the patch is extended past the kink. This approach often requires an extensive patch because of the distal location of most carotid kinks. One must be prepared to expose the ICA up to the skull base in patients who require repair of a carotid kink or coil.

If the kink is extensive or associated with extreme fragility or poststenotic dilation, the lesion and abnormal artery can be excised and replaced with a reversed segment of saphenous vein. Such resection and grafting are preferred by the senior author for management of symptomatic isolated carotid kinks. The same approach is preferred for management of symptomatic carotid coils, whether or not there is associated atherosclerosis or carotid dissection (Fig. 1). Resection and grafting avoid the potential of transforming a coil into a kink when using proximal reimplantation techniques. When it appears that one is dealing with a symptomatic kink, it is recommended that the carotid bifurcation be directly inspected to rule out the presence of associated carotid atherosclerosis.[8]

Alternative techniques to correct redundancy are segmental resection and primary anastomosis of either the CCA or ICA. Another method for a redundant ICA is partial excision of the carotid bulb and reimplantation angioplasty. This can be combined with eversion endarterectomy. An alternative is transposition of the ICA to a more proximal arteriotomy in the CCA. This may also be accompanied by an eversion endarterectomy.

The technique used extensively by Quattelbaum and associates involved resection of the carotid bifurcation and sacrifice of the external carotid artery.[2] Although this has been successful, it would be preferable to maintain ECA flow and use the alternative approaches described here.

Satisfactory results have been obtained by using plication and patching of the redundant area along with a standard carotid endarterectomy. The back wall of the artery can be plicated (or resected) and then subsequently patched anteriorly with saphenous vein or synthetic material. A simple extended patch angioplasty without plication might be preferable. Regardless of the surgical technique employed, completion arteriography is necessary to assess the results.

Clearly, there are many successful alternatives for surgical treatment of carotid kinking and coiling. Definitive information is not available, however, to define which of these is the best or when such treatment is unequivocally justified because the natural history of these lesions is unclear. It would be most prudent to reserve surgical treatment for the following situations: (1) when a coil or kink is symptomatic and there is no other apparent cause for the symptoms and (2) when a kink is associated with another surgically important carotid lesion.

REFERENCES

1. Riser MM, Geraud J, Ducoudray J, Ribaut L. Dolicho-carotide interne avec syndrome vertigineux. Rev Neurol 1951; 85:10–12.
2. Quattelbaum JK Jr, Upson ET, Neville RL. Strokes associated with elongation and kinking of the internal carotid artery. Ann Surg 1959; 150:824–832.
3. Perdue GD, Barreca JP, Smith RB III, King OW. The significance of elongation and angulation of the carotid artery: A negative view. Surgery 1975; 77:45–52.
4. Weible T, Fields WS. Tortuosity, coiling and kinking of the internal carotid artery. Neurology 1965; 15:7–11.
5. Metz H, Muray-Leslie RM, Bonnister RG, et al. Kinking of the internal carotid artery in relation to cerebrovascular disease. Lancet 1961; 1:424–426.
6. Sarkari NBS, Macdonald-Holmes J, Bickerstaff ER. Neurological manifestations associated with internal carotid loops and kinks in children. J Neurol Neurosurg Psychiatry 1970; 33:194–200.
7. Mukherjee D, Inahara T. Management of the tortuous internal carotid artery. Am J Surg 1985; 149:651–655.
8. Vollmar J, Nadjafi AS, Stalker CG. Surgical treatment of kinked internal carotid arteries. Br J Surg 1976; 63:847–850.

CAROTID BODY TUMORS

GLENN M. LaMURAGLIA, M.D.

Carotid body tumors are uncommon neoplasms of neuroectoderm paraganglion cells of the carotid body; hence, they have been called paragangliomas of the carotid artery. They arise from the afferent ganglion of the glossopharyngeal nerve, which is primarily responsive to hypoxia but also to hypercapnia and acidosis. Carotid body tumors are usually well encapsulated and, as they grow, splay the bifurcation of the carotid artery and develop an intimate adherence to the adventitial surface of the artery. These tumors are highly vascular and take their blood supply from the external carotid and ascending cervical artery branches and the vasa vasora of the adjacent carotid arteries. These tumors are rarely malignant in their behavior, but metastatic spread is thought to occur in approximately 5%.[1,2]

The classification described by Shamblin and associates[1] divides carotid body tumors into three groups. Type I tumors are small and readily resected. Type II are larger tumors densely adherent to the carotid arteries; however, they do not encase the carotid artery or adjacent nerves, as do type III tumors.

PRESENTATION

Carotid body tumors are rare and usually present as an asymptomatic mass. They are usually located below the angle of the jaw with a characteristic anterior and posterior mobility, but are relatively fixed in the vertical axis. Carotid body tumors are very slow growing, can be pulsatile, and are rarely associated with a bruit. When they become large, carotid body tumors may present with cranial nerve dysfunction or airway compression.[1,2]

There is a 5% incidence of bilateral carotid body tumors, and familial aggregation exists.[3] People exposed to chronic hypoxia, such as those with severe lung disease or living at elevated altitudes, have been noted to have a higher incidence of this disease.[2]

Other causes of neck masses can be confused with carotid body tumors. These include metastatic cancer to the cervical nodes, glomus tumor, branchial cleft cyst, and low parotid tumors. It is therefore imperative to perform a careful head and neck examination and a radiologic assessment prior to biopsy of these lesions, in that their vascularity can precipitate significant bleeding.

DIAGNOSIS

Color flow ultrasound can suggest the diagnosis of a carotid body tumor. However, a carotid body tumor can be best confirmed noninvasively by computed tomography with intravenous contrast. The administration of contrast defines the splaying of the carotid arteries by the tumor and the presence of a homogeneous, highly vascularized mass between the carotid arteries (Fig. 1). Magnetic resonance imaging may also be diagnostic, but at a higher cost. It does not provide additional useful information over computed tomography. Once the diagnosis is made, the need for carotid arteriography and possible embolization must be assessed prior to any surgical approach. Carotid angiograms are helpful in confirming the diagnosis and planning the surgical approach by elucidating the major blood supply of the carotid body tumor (Fig. 2).

PREOPERATIVE EMBOLIZATION

There have been multiple reports of successful preoperative embolization of carotid body tumors.[4,5] This procedure helps diminish the highly vascular nature of these tumors and thereby facilitates surgical removal (Figs. 2 and 3). Tumors that are smaller than 3 cm in diameter (Shamblin I) do not pose a major surgical challenge. Therefore, preoperative embolization of feeding branches of these small tumors may not be worth the risk or expense. Patients with carotid body tumors larger than 3 cm, however, may benefit from preoperative embolization to decrease the otherwise large intraoperative blood loss, facilitate the operation, and potentially diminish the morbidity. It must be emphasized, however, that embolization is a difficult and potentially hazardous procedure that should be undertaken only by highly qualified personnel.

The technique of carotid body tumor embolization involves the use of highly selective catheter cannulation of the arteries feeding the tumor. This includes many ascending cervical and external carotid artery branches with occasional branches of the common carotid artery itself. Before injecting embolic material, each branch must first be checked angiographically for anastomoses to the vertebral or internal carotid artery circulation.

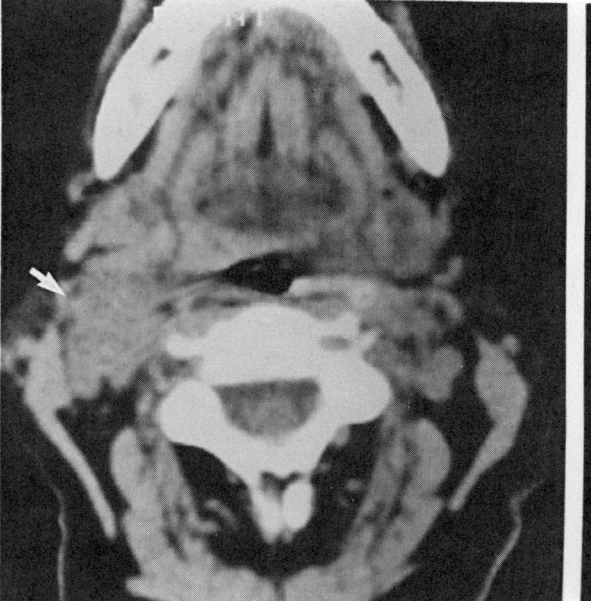 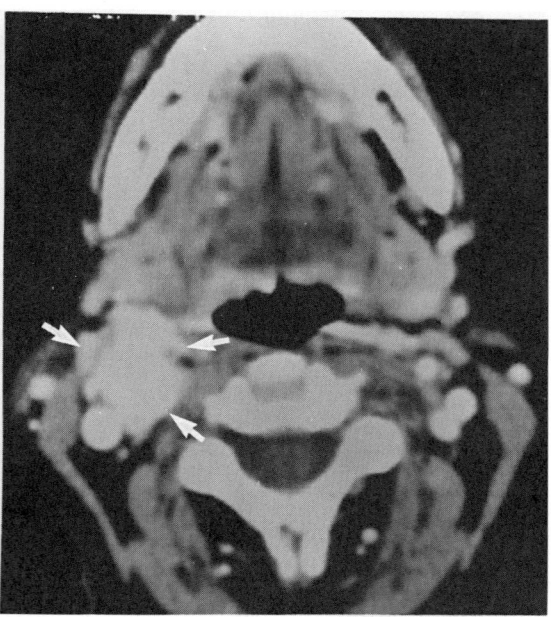

Figure 1 Computed tomography without (A), and with (B), intravenous contrast of a carotid body tumor. A, The poorly defined mass in the right neck is demonstrated (arrow). B, The mass is shown to be a homogeneous, highly vascularized mass (arrows) splaying the carotid bifurcation. This can be compared to the contralateral carotid arteries.

These dangerous anastomoses are carefully identified and not embolized (Fig. 4). Inadvertent embolization of vessels that perfuse cranial nerves are also avoided by initially injecting opacified lidocaine into the arteries while performing neurologic examinations to try to elicit nerve dysfunction. Embolization is performed by slowly injecting 150 to 300 μm polyvinyl alcohol beads (Ivalon) into the microvasculature of the tumor. Once blood flow in the feeder vessel is negligible, absorbable gelatin sponge (Gelfoam) is injected at its origin to induce thrombosis. To avoid encountering complications of tissue edema or necrosis at the time of operation, preoperative embolization should be performed on the day before operation.

During angiography, temporary balloon occlusion of the internal carotid artery can also be performed. This technique attempts to elicit symptoms of ipsilateral cerebral ischemia and provide preoperative assessment of the adequacy of collateral cerebral circulation. It, therefore, alerts the surgeon to the safety of intraoperative internal carotid artery clamping or the need for temporary intraluminal shunting, if carotid bypass should be indicated.

THERAPY

Surgical resection of the carotid body tumor is the only proper treatment. Historically, operation upon these highly vascular and densely adherent tumors to the carotid bifurcation has resulted in high morbidity and mortality.[6,7] In fact, the mortality of resection had been reported as high as 29% with a complication rate of approximately 40%. However, attempts to treat carotid body tumors with conservative management or radiation therapy have proven unsatisfactory.[8]

With advances in surgical and anesthetic techniques, perioperative mortality for carotid body tumor resection has become negligible.[4,6] Morbidity, especially with cranial nerve dysfunction, has remained high. The highly

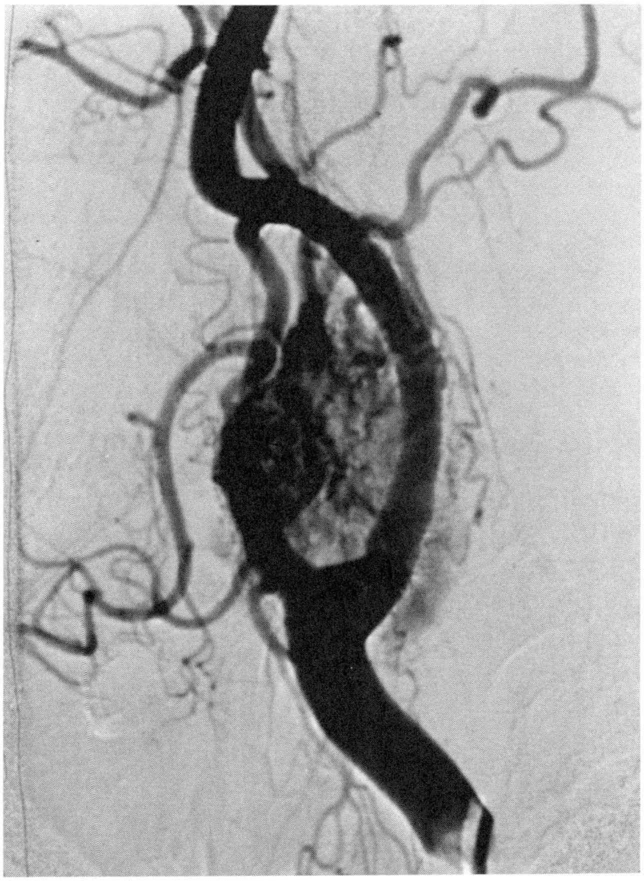

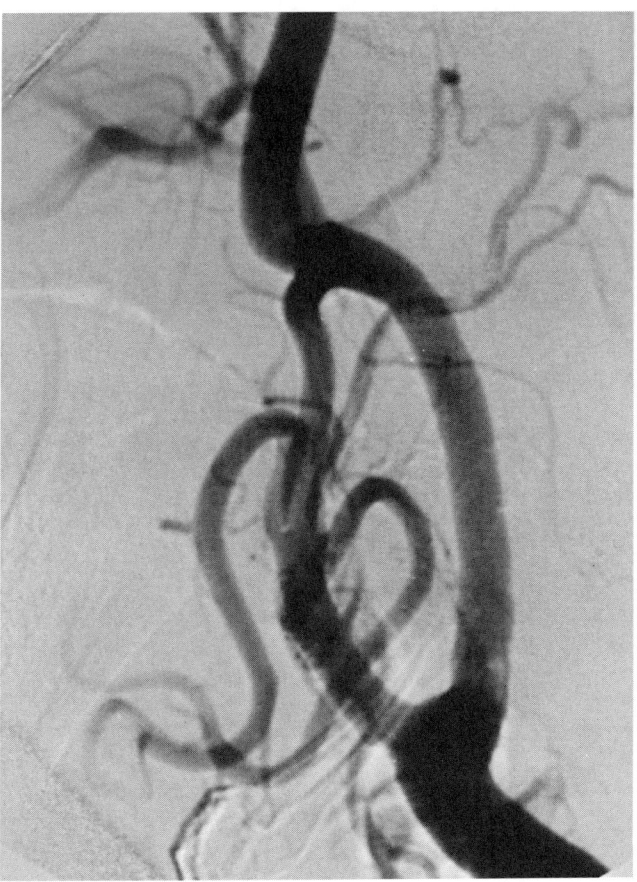

Figure 2 Digital subtraction angiogram of a carotid body tumor before embolization. It reveals a large, very vascular mass splaying the carotid bifurcation. Note the overhanging nature of the mass around the arteries. (From LaMuraglia GM, Fabian RL, Brewster DC, et al. The current surgical management of carotid body paragangliomas. J Vasc Surg 1992; 15:1038–1045; with permission.)

Figure 3 Digital subtraction angiogram of carotid body tumor after complete embolization of the tumor and afferent arteries. Note the decrease in size and the absence of the tumor blush noted in Figure 2. (From LaMuraglia GM, Fabian RL, Brewster DC, et al. The current surgical management of carotid body paragangliomas. J Vasc Surg 1992; 15:1038–1045; with permission.)

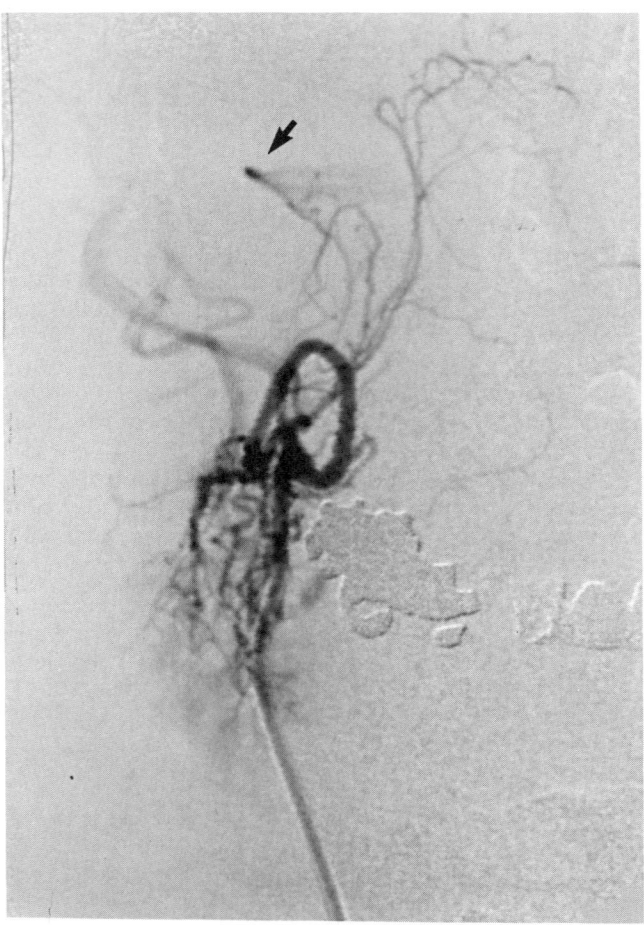

Figure 4 Digital subtraction, superselective angiogram in the ascending pharyngeal artery, which is an afferent feeding artery into the carotid body tumor. Note the dangerous anastomosis *(arrow)* of an arterial collateral from the feeder vessel into the vertebral artery. (From LaMuraglia GM, Fabian RL, Brewster DC, et al. The current surgical management of carotid body paragangliomas. J Vasc Surg 1992; 15:1038–1045; with permission.)

vascular nature of these lesions and the close proximity and adherence of large tumors to the cranial nerves provide the basis for the problems associated with this type of operation. With advances in surgical techniques and by providing significantly less bleeding in the operative field with preoperative embolization, the historically high incidence of stroke and cranial nerve injury has also diminished and become acceptable.

SURGICAL TECHNIQUE

The incision for carotid body tumor resection should be the standard incision utilized for carotid endarterectomy. However, for very large tumors requiring higher cephalad exposure, a **Y** incision can be used and centered on the inferior aspect of the tumor. Elevation of the superior flap with this incision can provide additional exposure. Nasal tracheal intubation and anterior subluxation of the jaw may improve access to the tumor, if it extends high under the mandible. It is usually at the most cephalad and posterior dissection where the hypoglossal nerve, superior laryngeal nerve, vagus nerve, or the mandibular branch of the facial nerve can be injured. If cranial nerves are involved in the capsule and adherent to the tumor, but not frankly invaded, it is important to identify the nerves prior to their course near the tumor and to dissect them free. However, should the nerves be encased in the tumor and nonfunctional preoperatively, there has been no evidence that laborious dissection from the tumor can restore their function.

Prior to dissecting the carotid body tumor off the artery, proximal control of the common carotid artery should be obtained. Careful periadventitial carotid dissection is important to avoid injury to the arterial wall. Bleeding from arterial injury can be repaired by a stitch or patch reconstruction. It should be noted that in large carotid body tumors that significantly splay and stretch the carotid bifurcation, the adventitial surface of the arteries may be attenuated. This is in contrast to patients with arteriosclerotic disease or metastatic disease in the neck when the carotid artery may be fibrotic. Therefore, extra care needs to be taken in dissecting the carotid body tumor from the artery surface. During the dissection of the carotid body tumor off the artery wall, some have suggested early clamping of the common carotid artery with insertion of a temporary intraluminal shunt to minimize blood loss. Although temporary clamping of the carotid artery may be necessary for repair of the adventitia, routine clamping of the carotid should be avoided. It decreases the pressure in the artery wall, making the vessel soft and obscuring the proper dissection planes between the artery and the tumor. Prolonged carotid artery clamping and shunting would also require systemic heparin sodium anticoagulation. It also does not diminish the substantial retrograde perfusion to the carotid body tumor from its other arterial blood supply when preoperative embolization has not been undertaken.

Resection of the external carotid artery is useful when large tumors are present. This facilitates the medial and posterior dissection of the carotid vessels, especially at the posterior portion of the bifurcation where carotid body tumors are usually most intimately adherent to the artery wall. Division of the external carotid artery also facilitates the identification of the vagus nerve. Once the medial dissection and posterior rotation of the carotid body tumor is completed, there is improved exposure of the superior laryngeal and hypoglossal nerves.

There are two indications for carotid artery reconstruction. They are tumor encasement of the internal carotid artery and invasion of the artery wall precluding its dissection. Often this cannot be predicted preoperatively; therefore, the surgeon should be ready to harvest greater saphenous vein, should it become necessary for the bypass.

When available, electroencephalographic (EEG) monitoring may be useful for intraoperative management. It can help determine the indication for temporary intraluminal shunting, should carotid reconstruction be needed. Should temporary clamping of the carotid artery be necessary, it can provide information regarding ipsilateral cerebral ischemia. Unsuspected carotid artery thrombosis secondary to manipulation or retraction of the artery can occur and be heralded by EEG changes.

Other surgical maneuvers have been found useful for this operation. Bipolar forceps are useful for coagulating small adventitial vasa vasora that may be providing significant blood supply to the tumor. Their use during the procedure also minimizes the thermal injury to the artery and adjacent cranial nerves. Topical papaverine or nitroglycerin can successfully reverse arterial spasm of the internal carotid artery secondary to periadventitial dissection and manipulation. Hemostatic pads soaked in thrombin can be used locally to retract the dissected surface of carotid body tumors to help minimize bleeding from the dissected surface.

Careful, meticulous dissection is the most important part of the surgical resection of carotid body tumors. Cranial nerve injury remains the highest reported morbidity of this operation, and the anatomy of these nerves must be carefully identified and these structures preserved.[6] For surgeons not familiar with the distorted anatomic relationships of these cranial nerves or not familiar with carotid and arterial reconstruction, a multidisciplinary approach involving a vascular and head and neck surgeon can be advantageous.

REFERENCES

1. Shamblin WR, ReMine WH, Sheps SG, Harrison EG. Carotid body tumor (chemodectoma). Clinicopathology analysis of ninety cases. Am J Surg 1971; 122:735–739.
2. Farr HW. Carotid body tumors: A 40-year study. CA 1980; 30:260–265.
3. Ridge BA, Brewster DC, Darling RC, et al. Familial carotid body tumors: Incidence and implications. Ann Vasc Surg 1993; 7:190-94.
4. LaMuraglia GM, Fabian RL, Brewster DC, et al. The current surgical management of carotid body paragangliomas. J Vasc Surg 1992; 15:1038–1045.
5. Smith RF, Shetty PC, Reddy DJ. Surgical treatment of carotid paragangliomas presenting unusual technical difficulties. The value of preoperative embolization. J Vasc Surg 1988; 7:631–637.
6. Hallett JW, Nora JD, Hollier LH, et al. Trends in neurovascular complications of surgical management for carotid body and cervical paragangliomas: A fifty-year experience with 153 tumors. J Vasc Surg 1988; 7:284–291.
7. Krupski WC, Effeney DJ, Ehrenfeld WK, Stoney RJ. Cervical chemodectoma: Technical considerations and management options. Am J Surg 1982; 144:215–220.
8. Mitchell DC, Clyne CAC. Chemodectomas of the neck: The response to radiotherapy. Br J Surg 1985; 72:903–905.

SURGICAL TREATMENT OF TAKAYASU'S ARTERITIS

FRED A. WEAVER, M.D.
J. GREGORY MODRALL, M.D.
ALBERT E. YELLIN, M.D.

In 1908, Takayasu, a Japanese ophthalmologist, reported retinal arteriovenous shunts in a "wreathlike" distribution around the optic disc and microaneurysms of the retinal vessels in a 19-year-old Japanese woman.[1] In an ensuing discussion, Onishi related similar findings in a patient with pulseless, cool upper extremities. The etiology of the described ocular and vascular findings was at that time obscure but has since become known as Takayasu's arteritis (TA). Other common synonyms for this entity include Onishi's disease, aortic arch syndrome, female arteritis, Martorell syndrome, and pulseless disease.

It is now recognized that, although the arterial involvement may be confined to the aortic arch as in Takayasu's original patient, involvement of multiple aortic segments or the entire aorta, its major branches, and the pulmonary artery can occur. Arterial pathology varies from a fulminant acute inflammatory process to extensive postinflammatory mural fibrosis. Infectious, hereditary, and autoimmune etiologies have all been suggested, yet a definitive demonstration of a causal relationship has been elusive.

The inflammatory process results in segmental stenoses, occlusions, and aneurysmal degeneration of the aorta and proximal arterial tree. This results in a variety of clinical presentations that may include renovascular hypertension, renal failure, stroke, ocular ischemia, mesenteric ischemia, extremity ischemia, aortic insufficiency, or aortic aneurysm formation. The benefits of revascularization for these conditions are well recognized, but the unique pathogenesis and uncertain natural history of TA have tempered enthusiasm for a surgical approach to this entity. Thus, surgical therapy has been traditionally reserved for severe symptomatic manifestations of arterial occlusive disease refractory to high-dose corticosteroids or other medicinal therapies.

At the University of Southern California (USC), the clinical experience with this disease began in 1973 and now includes 28 patients, 18 of whom have required 26 reconstructive procedures for the treatment of symptomatic arterial occlusive disease or aneurysm formation.[2,3] Extended follow-up of these patients has accrued, and information regarding the durability of arterial reconstruction, incidence of graft occlusion, and patient survival is available.

CLINICAL FEATURES

Relatively large series of patients with this arteriopathy have now been reported from Japan, Korea, Thailand, China, India, and Mexico, and the natural history and pattern of arterial involvement are well defined.[4,5] The clinical course of TA may include a prodromal "prepulseless phase," which is manifested by a variety of constitutional symptoms including pyrexia, weight loss, anorexia, night sweats, malaise, arthralgias, and myalgias. Because these symptoms are nonspecific and protean, they are often not recognized as indicative of acute arteritis. Unlike the large studies reported from Japan and Mexico, patients evaluated at our institution rarely manifest the constitutional symptoms of an acute arteritis. Rather, patients seek medical attention for the secondary complications of arterial insufficiency or aneurysm formation. Invariably, the clinical picture is one of a "burned-out" arteritis with a progressive deterioration in overall well-being that climaxes in a life- or limb-threatening event. On being questioned, a minority of patients report a prodromal symptom complex of malaise, fever, weight loss, anorexia, myalgias, or arthralgias antedating the clinical symptoms by 1 to 12 years.

The clinical manifestations of the patients seen at USC with a diagnosis of TA were varied (Table 1). The most impressive constellation of symptoms has been severe systemic hypertension associated with renal failure or varying degrees of cardiac failure. Hypertension has been present in 18 patients and associated with overt cardiac failure in 7 and dialysis-dependent renal failure in 2. This preponderance of hypertension is quite similar to recent reports from many Asian countries.[4]

The anatomic distribution of disease is most commonly combined aortic arch, thoracic, and abdominal aortic disease, so-called type III of Ueno's classification[6] (Fig. 1). In our experience, patients with pulmonary artery involvement, type IV (named after the pathologist Oota who first described the pulmonary findings), have been rare, although Lupi and associates reported pulmonary involvement in 50% of patients evaluated at his institution in Mexico City.[7]

All patients suspected of TA should undergo ab-

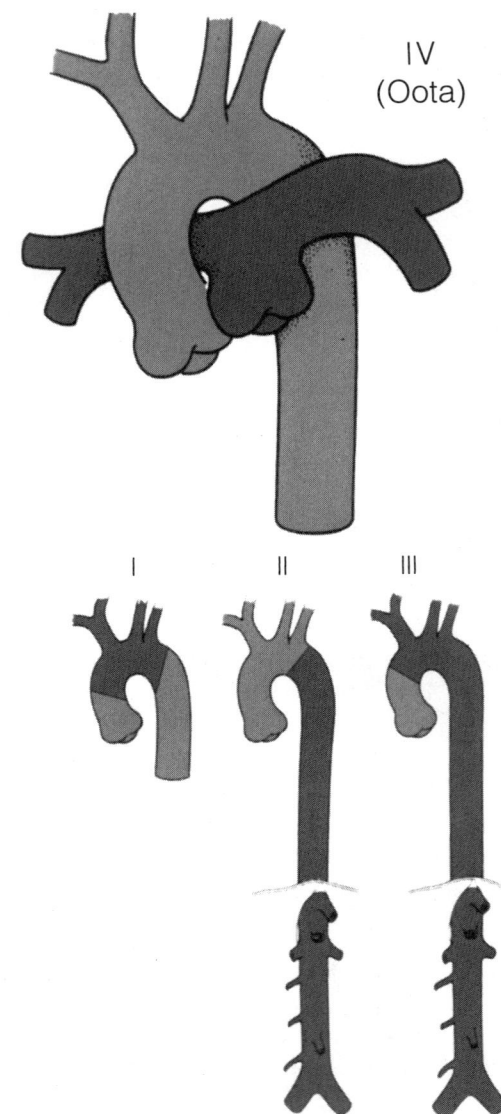

Figure 1 Ueno's[6] anatomic classification of Takayasu's arteritis as modified by Lupi.[7] Darkly shaded area indicates involvement by Takayasu's arteritis. Type IV is type I, II, or III in combination with pulmonary involvement.

Table 1 Clinical Manifestations of 28 Patients with Takayasu Arteritis at University of Southern California (1973–1993)

Clinical Manifestation	n	(%)
Age at diagnosis ≤ 40 years	27	96
Female	27	96
Hypertension	18	64
Extremity ischemia		
Upper (12)	16	57
Lower (8)		
Congestive heart failure	9	32
Transient ischemic attack	5	18
Stroke	3	11
Ocular ischemia	3	11
Renal failure	2	7
Aortic aneurysm	1	4
Pulse deficits	26	93
Cervical, abdominal bruits	19	68
Elevated erythrocyte sedimentation rate	19	68

dominal and thoracic angiography. The thoracoabdominal aorta and renal arteries are carefully evaluated. This frequently documents renovascular occlusive disease or a thoracoabdominal aortic coarctation (Fig. 2). In addition to the standard anteroposterior views, lateral and oblique views of the renal and mesenteric vessels are also important. For patients with a thoracoabdominal aortic coarctation, intra-arterial blood pressures above and below the stenosis are helpful to document a blood pressure differential and plan an operative strategy. Arteriographic findings are characteristically tubular, long-segment stenoses or occlusions usually involving the origins of major aortic branches, aortic arch, distal descending thoracic aorta, and suprarenal abdominal aorta. Such a pattern of arterial involvement in a woman younger than 40 years with an elevated ergthrocyte sedimentation rate (ESR) provides a clinical diagnosis of TA. Although TA can occur in males, it is rare.

Although an elevated ESR is helpful in establishing a diagnosis, it is a poor indicator of disease activity. Despite an elevated ESR in most patients with TA, very few have findings consistent with acute arteritis in arterial specimens obtained at time of operation. Furthermore, we have noted little difference in the clinical course of patients with an elevated ESR as compared to those whose ESR is normal.

Other specific diagnostic tests should be tailored to specific organ system dysfunction. In patients with renovascular hypertension or renal failure, renal perfusion and function are assessed by isotopic renography. Renal color-flow duplex imaging is used to assess renal parenchymal size, cortical thickness, vascular resistance, and blood flow velocity. Severe cardiac dysfunction is assessed by echocardiography because both mitral and aortic valvular insufficiency can occur. Cardiac catheterization is indicated if significant valvular dysfunction is documented or there is suspicion of coronary or pulmonary artery involvement. Right-sided heart failure, dyspnea, or hypoxemia should raise a suspicion of pulmonary involvement. Cerebrovascular symptoms are evaluated with computed tomography or magnetic resonance imaging. Information concerning the hemodynamics of the cerebral circulation can be provided by carotid duplex and transcranial Doppler studies.

TREATMENT

Medical

Corticosteroids are usually the initial treatment offered for symptomatic TA because dramatic symptomatic improvement and restoration of absent pulses have been reported to follow its use.[8] Cyclophosphamide and methotrexate have also been used alone or in combination with corticosteroids.[9] However, the efficacy of corticosteroids and medical therapy, in general, for TA has not been universally acknowledged, and in many centers, including our own, medical therapy has fallen into disfavor. Most patients with symptomatic arterial insufficiency have entered the chronic burned-out phase and do not manifest a dramatic clinical response to medical intervention. The contention that medical therapy provides the additional benefit of arresting disease progression is also suspect because serial arteriographic follow-up of surgical patients has not documented disease progression despite the absence of medical treatment. Conversely, prolonged attempts at steroid therapy can be deleterious in that an unwarranted delay in definitive surgical therapy causes further deterioration in organ function. Therefore, as experience with TA has increased, surgical revascularization has evolved to become the primary intervention for most patients with symptomatic arterial insufficiency.

Transluminal Angioplasty

Conceptually, transluminal angioplasty should have a limited role in the patient with TA. Although anecdotal reports and a few large series have reported favorable results, the fibrous nature of the arterial obliteration mitigates against a durable, long-term benefit.[2] Thus, the use of percutaneous transluminal angioplasty is a temporizing strategy to provide short-term symptomatic relief when more urgent medical problems exist. At USC, transluminal angioplasty has been used selectively in five patients. Arterial segments dilated have included five renal arteries, two infrarenal aortas, and two common iliac arteries. All dilations, with one exception, have restenosed within 6 months. The one angioplasty that remains patent was of the common iliac artery and

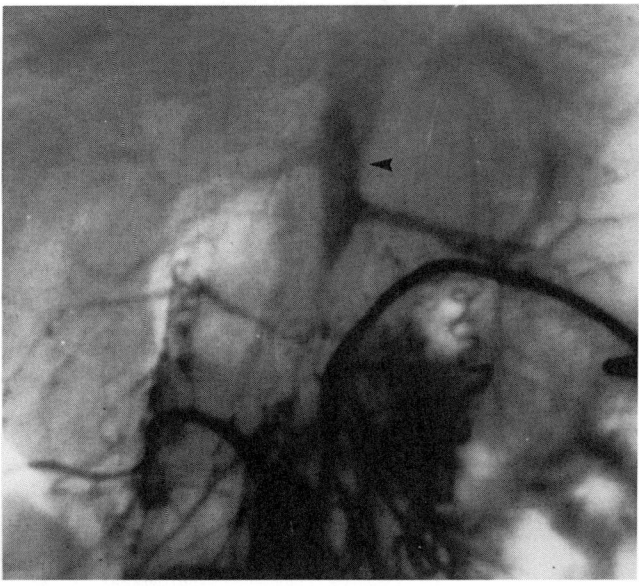

Figure 2 Arteriogram of patient with occlusion of distal descending thoracic aorta (not seen) and reconstitution of suprarenal aorta and renal arteries *(arrow)*. Infrarenal aorta also occluded with reconstitution at large inferior mesenteric artery, which supplies occluded celiac and superior mesenteric arteries.

employed an intravascular stent. Follow-up of this patient is now almost 1 year, and symptomatic improvement remains. Whether a more liberal use of stents will improve angioplasty results in TA remains to be seen.

Arterial Reconstruction

Indications for arterial reconstruction parallel those for the patient with atherosclerosis. However, unlike the atherosclerotic patient, we have not found TA lesions to be necessarily progressive or documented new lesions in previously arteriographically normal segments. Eight patients at our institution have undergone serial arteriographic studies over a 132 month period. Progressive obstruction of native distal segments or new involvement of adjacent arterial segments has not been identified. Given these findings, one would anticipate that the long-term patency of bypass procedures performed for TA would be excellent.

Arterial reconstruction requires a flexible and creative approach and relies on the exclusive use of bypass or interposition grafts tailored to the existing anatomy. We have used a variety of graft materials including Dacron, polytetrafluoroethylene, saphenous vein, and hypogastric artery. Prosthetic grafts are used for major aortic reconstructions, with the autogenous conduits reserved for extremity or isolated renal or mesenteric revascularization. In adolescents, hypogastric artery is preferred for renal revascularization because of the known propensity for saphenous vein to undergo aneurysmal degeneration.

The basic tenets of vascular surgery must be adhered to, if one is to perform procedures that result in long-term benefit. Graft inflow should originate from proximal uninvolved aorta or, in the case of upper extremity revascularizations, uninvolved carotid artery. Of critical importance is that the distal anastomosis is performed in an arterial segment entirely free of and distal to the inflammatory involvement.[2,10] Failure to follow this principle will result in early graft failure. On occasion, locating distal segments free of arteritic involvement may require a complex distal dissection. However, the typical pattern of TA with its involvement limited primarily to the aorta and proximal portion of major aortic branches provides a satisfactory distal vessel in almost all patients.

With hypertension a frequent finding in patients with TA, it is not surprising that renovascular procedures are common. At USC, it is the most frequent indication for operative intervention (Table 2). Most patients requiring renal revascularization have severe hypertension that is refractory to medical management. Congestive heart failure and aortic or mitral valvular insufficiency or renal failure may be present. Aorta-aorta bypass for thoracoabdominal coarctation and/or aorta-renal bypass are the most common procedures performed. Nephrectomy is rarely required. Aortic inflow for aorta-renal bypass may originate from supraceliac or infrarenal aorta, depending on the extent of aortic involvement. Hepatic- and splenic-renal bypass are usually poor options because occlusive visceral artery disease is frequent.

Table 2 Surgical Procedures for Takayasu's Arteritis at University of Southern California (1973–1993)

Indication	Procedure	n
Renovascular hypertension	Aorta-renal bypass	8
	Aorta-aorta bypass	2
	Nephrectomy	1
Cerebrovascular insufficiency	Ascending aorta-carotid and/or subclavian bypass	3
	Subclavian-carotid bypass	2
Extremity ischemia	Carotid-axiliary and/or brachial bypass	4
	Iliac-femoral bypass	1
	Aorta-femoral bypass	1
Aortic aneurysm	Aortic replacement	2
Cardiac failure	Aortic valve replacement	1
	Aortic valve and ascending aorta replacement	1

Upper or lower extremity ischemia accounts for another major group of patients who require revascularization. Severe debilitating claudication is the most common indication. Bypasses for upper extremity ischemia can usually be performed via an extrathoracic approach by utilizing ipsilateral cervical common carotid artery for proximal inflow with the distal anastomosis in the subclavian, axillary, or brachial arteries. A variety of procedures including aorta-femoral bypass and unilateral iliac-femoral bypass are used for correcting lower extremity ischemia. In general, occlusive involvement of the lower extremities is confined to the distal aorta and proximal iliac vessels, although we have seen two patients with superficial femoral artery involvement. Proximal aorta-iliac revascularization in both patients restored palpable pedal pulses due to generous profunda femoris collaterals.

Despite the frequent arteriographic presence of brachiocephalic occlusive disease, cerebrovascular insufficiency, although reported to be a common indication for revascularization, is a relatively rare indication in our experience (Fig. 3). When required, the diffuse involvement of all branches of the aortic arch requires that inflow originates from the ascending aorta. Usually the most distal extent of carotid involvement is the middle third of the common carotid, leaving the distal third or internal carotid as a satisfactory vessel. Revascularization is best in patients with occlusion of all arch branches by constructing a bypass to both carotids or a carotid and subclavian with a bifurcated 12 by 6 mm graft.

Other procedures that are occasionally required include aortic or mitral valve replacement, aortic aneurysm resection, and mesenteric revascularization. The need for coronary revascularization is rare and has not been necessary at our institution.

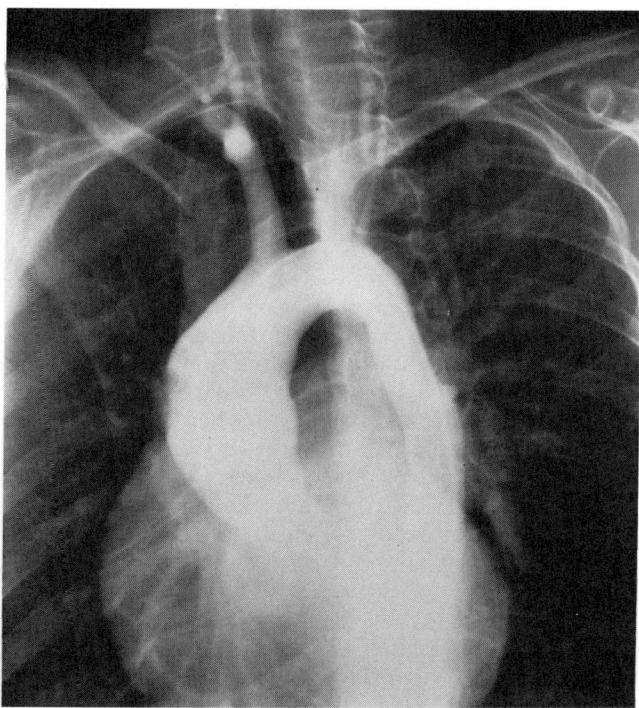

Figure 3 Enlarged cardiac silhouette and ascending aorta due to aortic valve insufficiency. Asymptomatic occlusion of left subclavian and carotid arteries is present.

SURGICAL RESULTS

A surgical approach is well tolerated because of the relatively young age of patients with TA. Preoperative medical morbidity such as cardiac or renal failure poses the greatest perioperative risk, but a successful operation, particularly in patients undergoing renovascular procedures, can rapidly improve the overall well-being of the patient with TA. Postoperative complications are few, and early graft occlusion is rare. No mortality has occurred in our series, and in another report it is less than 5%.[10]

For the 18 patients who have undergone procedures at our institution, a follow-up of 3 to 190 months (mean 75 months) is available. Two patients have been lost to follow-up, and the remaining 16 are alive and well. Corticosteroids, if administered perioperatively, have been tapered and discontinued. Late graft complications include three graft occlusions and four distal anastomotic stenoses. Two grafts occluded early because of placement of the distal anastomosis in a patent but thickened artery. The third occlusion was due to severe graft calcification and fibrosis that developed in a graft placed 10 years earlier. Of the four distal anastomotic stenoses, two have been successfully revised and two successfully managed by transluminal angioplasty.

Pathologic material from operative revisions has documented intimal hyperplasia as the cause of the anastomotic narrowing. Pathologic findings of acute or chronic arteritis have not been found.

Of the patients who have undergone operations for renovascular hypertension, eight are normotensive, one is normotensive but receiving two antihypertensive agents, one is normotensive but with parenchymal-based renal failure of unknown etiology, and one continues to have significant hypertension despite intensive medical therapy. Of significance, cardiac function has markedly improved in all patients with preoperative congestive heart failure. This underscores the influence surgical correction of renovascular hypertension can have on cardiac morbidity, a major cause of death in this patient population.

Other reconstructive procedures have provided significant symptomatic benefit with the exception of a cerebrovascular reconstruction in a patient with occlusive disease of the aortic arch. This patient remains neurologically intact with the exception of severe ocular ischemia that has resulted in near-blindness.

The surgical experience with Takayasu's arteritis suggests that patients with long-standing symptomatic arterial disease are poorly managed by medicinal therapy alone. Thus, most patients with symptomatic arterial disease require surgical revascularization that uses standard techniques of arterial reconstruction. Over an extended period, our experience documents that such an approach has relatively few long-term graft complications, effectively relieves symptoms, and limits the potential for irreversible end-organ ischemic injury in the patient with Takayasu's arteritis.

REFERENCES

1. Takayasu M. A case of peculiar changes of the central retinal vessels. Acta Soc Ophth Jap 1908; 12:554.
2. Weaver FA, Yellin AE, Campen DH, et al. Surgical procedures in the management of Takayasu's arteritis. J Vasc Surg 1990; 12:429–439.
3. Weaver FA, Yellin AE. Surgical treatment of Takayasu arteritis. Heart Vessels 1992; 7 (suppl):154–158.
4. Numano F, Kyu TL, Chang YH. Takayasu arteritis. Heart Vessels 1992; 7 (suppl):1–178.
5. Herrera EL, Torres GS, Marcushamer J, et al. Takayasu's arteritis: Clinical study of 107 cases. Am Heart J 1977; 93:94–103.
6. Ueno A, Awane Y, Wakabayashi A, Shimizu K. Successfully operated obliterative brachiocephalic arteritis (Takayasu) associated with the elongated coarctation. Jpn Heart J 1967; 8:538–544.
7. Lupi HE, Sanchez GT, Horwitz S, Gutierrez EF. Pulmonary artery involvement in Takayasu's arteritis. Chest 1975; 67:69–74.
8. Fraga A, Mintz G, Valle L, Izquierdo GF. Takayasu's arteritis: Frequency of systemic manifestations (study of 22 patients) and favorable response to maintenance steroid therapy with adenocorticosteroids (12 patients). Arthritis Rheum 1972; 15:617–624.
9. Shelhamer JH, Volkman DJ, Parrillo JE, et al. Takayasu's arteritis and its therapy. Ann Intern Med 1985; 103:121–126.
10. Lagneau P, Michel JB, Vuong PN. Surgical treatment of Takayasu's disease. Ann Surg 1987; 205:157–166.

GIANT CELL ARTERITIS

JESS R. YOUNG, M.D.

Giant cell arteritis (GCA), also known as temporal arteritis or cranial arteritis, is a systemic vasculitis of unknown cause occurring almost exclusively in individuals over the age of 50 years. Its variable features and multiple presentations may make recognition difficult. However, it is one of the most satisfying of conditions for physicians to diagnose and treat because the unpleasant effects and serious consequences of this condition can be almost entirely prevented or improved by steroid therapy. Although the terms temporal arteritis and giant cell arteritis are often used interchangeably, giant cell arteritis is preferred because the disease affects more than just the temporal arteries.

PATHOPHYSIOLOGY

The pathogenesis of GCA remains unknown, but autoimmune, genetic, and environmental mechanisms have been implicated. The immunologic mechanism is favored, and the role of elastin as a possible antigen has been documented.[1]

Giant cell arteritis is a systemic disease that can affect any of the large or medium-sized arteries, including the aortic arch and its branches, the abdominal aorta, and the intracranial, mesenteric, femoral, and coronary arteries.

Mononuclear cells infiltrate the media, particularly in the region of the internal elastic lamina. The infiltrates can be extensive and enter the adventitia, particularly in those vessels that contain abundant elastin. Often present are granulomas that contain multinucleated giant cells, histiocytes, and lymphocytes.

The occurrence of intermittent "skip lesions" has long been recognized and poses a problem for the clinician treating a patient with negative biopsy findings but otherwise typical clinical presentations. Sampling inadequacy and skip lesions may be two of the reasons for the negative biopsy findings in the presence of obvious GCA.

Blindness results from arteritic involvement in several vessels that feed the eye, but mainly the posterior ciliary artery. Involvement of the central retinal artery is less frequent. Giant cell arteritis is also one of the arterial lesions that can result in aortic dissection.

Anticardiolipin antibodies are prevalent with patients in GCA and may play an important role in the pathogenesis of the vasculopathy observed in this disease.

CLINICAL PRESENTATION

Giant cell arteritis rarely affects patients under age 50. The mean age of onset is about 70 years. About 70% of patients affected are women. The condition is more common in people of central and northern European origin, less common in people from the Mediterranean area, and uncommon in people of Asian or African heritage.

About 50% of patients with GCA have the associated condition polymyalgia rheumatica (PMR), an illness characterized by pain and stiffness of the pectoral and pelvic girdles and by systemic features that often include fatigue and a low-grade fever. Most laboratory studies are normal except for a marked increase in the erythrocyte sedimentation rate (ESR) and often a normocytic, normochromic anemia. A dramatic response to 10 to 15 mg of prednisone daily is considered a prominent feature of this disease. The patient often feels remarkably better within hours of starting treatment.

In addition to symptoms of PMR, other possible clinical features of GCA are numerous and include headache, weight loss, fever, jaw "claudication," carpal tunnel syndrome, radiculopathy, psychosis, breast mass, pulseless disease due to brachiocephalic arteritis, transient ischemic attacks, strokes, vision loss, hearing loss, intermittent claudication, and dissecting aortic aneurysm.

Vision loss is the most serious complication of GCA. Fortunately, blindness usually, but not always, tends to follow other ocular or systemic symptoms by weeks or months, and thus may be a late, preventable complication. Once blindness occurs in one eye, the other eye may become blind within a few weeks in the absence of appropriate treatment. It is unusual for visual loss to occur once high-dose steroid therapy has been started.

Giant cell arteritis commonly affects the subclavian and axillary arteries and should be considered in patients, especially elderly women, with occlusive disease of the upper extremities.[2] Raynaud's phenomenon, intermittent exercise ischemia, and even rest pain can occur. Arm exercise ischemia or severe ischemia may at times be the only manifestation of GCA. In a review of 26 patients in whom arm ischemia was the only finding, 21 patients had a positive temporal artery biopsy, and steroid therapy improved 24 of the 26 patients.[3] Arteritic involvement of the iliac, femoral, and calf arteries can also occur but is much less common than upper extremity involvement.

Death from GCA is unusual, although a dissecting aneurysm can occur and be fatal. Occasionally coronary arteritis or strokes can result in death.

DIAGNOSIS

The American College of Rheumatology 1990 criteria for the diagnosis of GCA are (1) age equal to or greater than 50 years at disease onset, (2) new onset of localized headache, (3) temporal artery tenderness or decreased temporal artery pulse, (4) elevated Westergren ESR equal to or greater than 50 mm/hour, and (5) biopsy evidence of GCA.[4] The presence of three or more of these five criteria was associated with a sensitivity of 93.5% and a specificity of 91.2% in making the correct diagnosis.

Laboratory Findings

The Westergren ESR averages 70 to 80 mm/hour in GCA but may reach 120 to 140 mm/hour. However, in 1% to 2% of patients, the ESR is normal or only minimally elevated. Mild to moderate liver function abnormalities occur in 20% to 35% of patients with GCA.

One report noted an increase in anticardiolipin antibodies in 16 of 20 (80%) patients with GCA.[5] Six of these 20 patients had vascular complications including strokes, myocardial infarctions, blindness, diplopia, and transient ischemic attacks. Of seven patients with IgG and IgM antibodies, five had vascular complications. These results suggest that high titers of anticardiolipin antibodies may help to predict which patients with GCA are at greater risk for arterial thrombosis. Higher doses of corticosteroids and intravenous heparin sodium could be considered for that group of patients.

Temporal Artery Biopsy

The need for doing a temporal artery biopsy even when clinical suspicion is high for GCA continues to be debated. Some still favor a routine biopsy because of the risk of unnecessary long-term corticosteroid treatment. A biopsy is most helpful when PMR and GCA cannot be differentiated on the basis of clinical information. A biopsy should be done whenever any doubt about the correct diagnosis exists.

If the artery is clearly abnormal, with a tender, inflamed, thickened segment, only a 2 cm segment is needed for histologic diagnosis. If the artery is not distinctly abnormal, however, a longer, 4 cm to 6 cm segment is needed because of the intermittent, skipped distribution of lesions.

If the clinical picture suggests GCA but the temporal artery biopsy is negative, performing a second biopsy on the contralateral temporal artery increases the diagnostic yield by about 15%. Sometimes both biopsies are negative, yet the physician still suspects GCA. In these situations, the patients should be treated as if they had GCA, but the physician must remain constantly alert for other diseases that could cause a similar clinical picture, such as rheumatoid arthritis, polymyositis, or systemic lupus erythematosus.

If the biopsy results are not available for several days, treatment for GCA should be started immediately. If the patient has had a transitory loss of vision or other problems suggesting a vascular complication, treatment should also be started immediately, and even the parenteral administration of steroids and heparin sodium should be considered.

Angiography

Angiography should be considered in all patients with extracranial vascular manifestations of GCA. Ar-

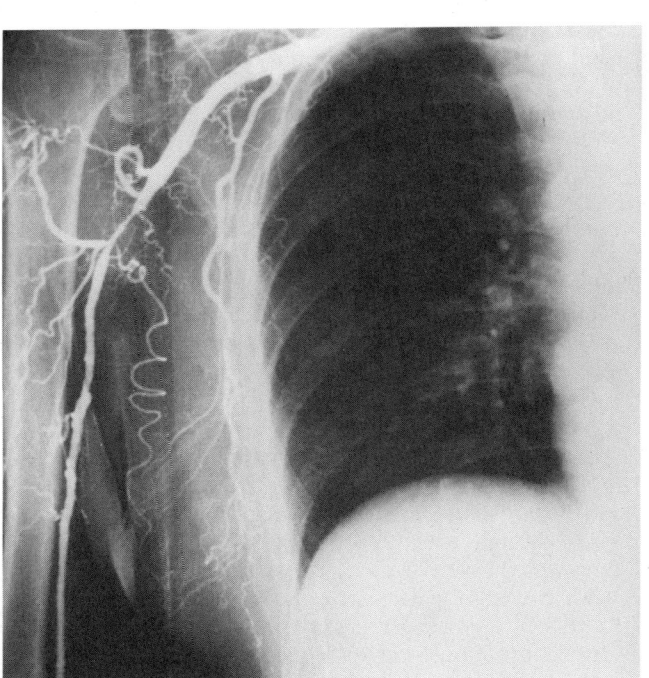
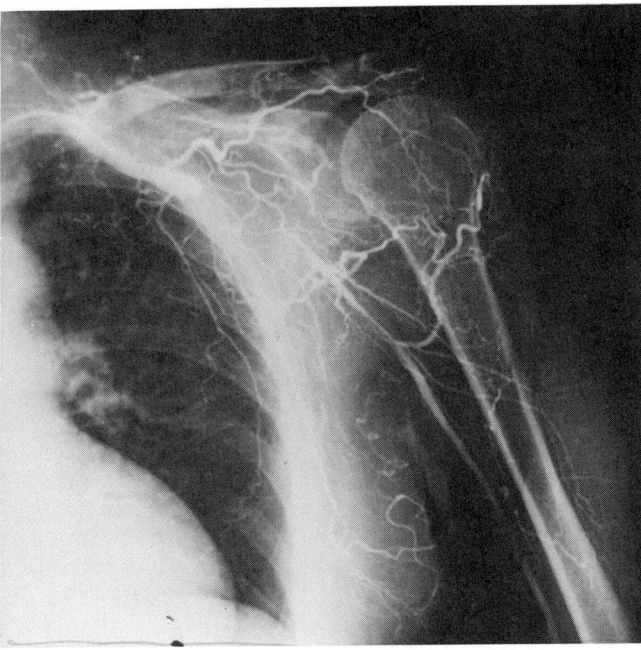

Figure 1 Bilateral subclavian arteriograms in a 68-year-old woman with rest pain in her left hand. Note the typical long, smooth, narrowed arteries.

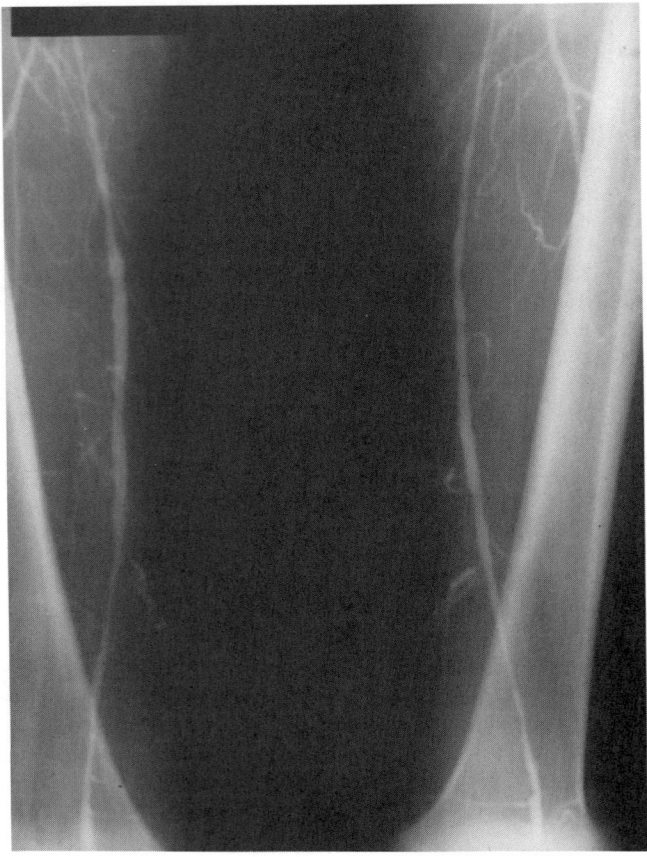

Figure 2 Bilateral femoral arteriograms in a 72-year-old woman who had intermittent claudication in both calves at 50 yards.

teriography may be helpful in making or confirming a diagnosis even when a temporal artery biopsy is negative, or it may suggest an alternative diagnosis. Typical GCA lesions are multiple, long, smooth, and tapered and are accompanied by some occlusions and collateral vessel formation (Figs. 1 and 2). The diagnosis may be aided by ultrasonography and magnetic resonance angiography. Neither method has replaced arteriography as the gold standard for diagnosis, but both measures may help monitor the response to therapy.

TREATMENT

Glucocorticosteroids are the only generally accepted treatment for GCA. The aim is to relieve troublesome symptoms and to prevent ischemic catastrophes. The main controversies today are the initial dose of steroids, the rate at which the dose is tapered to a maintenance level, and the duration of treatment.

Prednisone is usually started at a dosage of 60 mg/day and kept at that level for about 2 weeks if the clinical response is good. Other recommended starting doses have included 40 mg/day, 80 mg/day, and 1 mg/kg/day. In the rare patient whose clinical response to the initial starting dose is not good, the dose can be increased.

After 2 to 4 weeks, if the clinical response is good and the sedimentation rate is falling, the dose is tapered. There are no hard-and-fast rules for tapering. Some physicians decrease the dose by 5 mg every 1 to 2 weeks, and others decrease the dose by 10% every 2 to 4 weeks. When the dose has been tapered to 20 mg/day, the patient continues to do well, and the ESR is falling, slower tapering is suggested. One method is to decrease the dosage by 2.5 mg/week as long as the patient remains comfortable and the ESR is normal.

Traditionally, the ESR is used to guide therapy reductions. However, this cannot be used as the sole criterion for adjusting the dose of steroids. Some patients undergo a dramatic improvement in symptoms despite little or no fall in ESR. In addition, the ESR can be increased secondary to other concurrent illnesses. An occasional patient can show evidence of progressive arterial worsening in spite of a normal ESR.

If the signs, symptoms, or ESR do not greatly improve after 4 to 6 weeks of steroid treatment, a cytotoxic drug should be considered. Azathioprine (Imuran), intravenous cyclophosphamide (Cytoxan), and methotrexate have all been reported as useful in some instances. However, controlled studies are necessary to establish efficacy because GCA tends to subside gradually on its own. The choice of a drug is a personal one, given the lack of studies on the subject.

Corticosteroid therapy is usually continued for 18 to 24 months. Although most patients can be weaned within 24 months, a small minority may require more prolonged treatment.

If the patient has amaurosis fugax when originally seen or has evidence of retinal or optic nerve ischemia, higher doses of oral prednisone such as 100 mg a day or intravenous corticosteroid such as a bolus of 500 mg of methylprednisolone and methylprednisolone 1,000 mg every 12 hours for 5 days, can be given.

A prolonged corticosteroid regimen carries considerable risk of osteoporosis, especially when the patient is a postmenopausal white woman. Possible preventive measures against osteoporosis should be considered, such as estrogen and possibly cyclic progesterone, as well as calcium and vitamin D. The usefulness of drugs such as calcitonin and etidronate is yet to be determined.

SURGICAL TREATMENT

Reconstructive vascular surgery is rarely necessary, even though arteriography after stabilization usually does not show revascularization of the occluded vessels. With the administration of steroid therapy, upper and lower limb vascular symptoms may recede rapidly. Operation should be restricted to patients with severe persistent ischemia and should be performed after the inflammatory process has receded to prevent early thrombosis of the bypass graft.

PROGNOSIS

Giant cell arteritis tends to run a self-limited course of 1 to 2 years. Some patients, however, require low-dose prednisone (1 to 10 mg) for many years to control musculoskeletal symptoms. Fatal or serious complications other than blindness, stroke, or dissecting aneurysm are rare. Relapses are uncommon after 2 years, and most patients have a normal life span.

REFERENCES

1. Shiki H, Shimokoma T, Watanabe T. Temporal arteritis: Cell composition and the possible pathogenetic role of cell-mediated immunity. Hum Pathol 1989; 20:1057–1064.
2. Walz-Leblanc BA, Ameli FM, Keystone EC. Giant cell arteritis presenting as limb claudication. Report and review of the literature. J Rheumatol 1991; 18:470–472.
3. Minet JP, Bachet P, Dumontet CM, et al. Subclavian and axillary involvement in temporal arteritis and polymyalgia rheumatica. Am J Med 1990; 88:13–20.
4. Hunder GG, Block DA, Michel BA, et al. The American College of Rheumatology 1990 criteria for the classification of giant cell arteritis. Arthritis Rheum 1990; 33:1122–1128.
5. Espinoza LR, Jara LJ, Silveira LH, et al. Anticardiolipin antibodies in polymyalgia rheumatica–giant cell arteritis: Association with severe vascular complications. Am J Med 1991; 90:474–478.

RADIATION-INDUCED ARTERITIS

GEORGE ANDROS, M.D.
PETER A. SCHNEIDER, M.D.
ROBERT W. HARRIS, M.D.

With the expanded application of the radiation therapy of malignancies has come the increased recognition of radiation-induced arteritis. Because ensuing vascular complications often develop insidiously into chronic ischemic syndromes, the role of radiation is frequently overlooked.

Radiation-associated arteriopathy is often misconstrued to be the more widely prevalent lesion of arteriosclerosis. Both are diseases of the elderly and are seen most often in technologically advanced societies, arteriosclerosis with its multiple risk factors and postirradiation arterial degenerative lesions many years after the treatment of neoplasms. A synergistic effect with arteriosclerosis is suggested because the predisposing factors of arteriosclerosis appear to potentiate the injurious effects of radiation therapy on major arteries.

Based on our experience with the management of 28 patients with radiation-induced arterial lesions, our objectives here are to describe the similarities and diversities of these lesions; to present current concepts of the pathophysiology of the vascular lesions; to provide an understanding of the various clinical syndromes seen in different segments of the arterial system; to recommend therapeutic interventions that are safe, effective, and durable; and to discuss the role of arterial surveillance and possible techniques for prevention.[1]

COMPARISON TO ARTERIOSCLEROSIS

Radiation-associated arterial lesions and arteriosclerosis are both segmental in nature, although the latter can be diffuse. It is axiomatic that the vessels affected by radiation lie within the field of treatment. Concordantly, vessels outside the irradiated field are essentially disease-free. We and others have observed associated injuries to adjacent tissue such as skin, muscle, lung, rectum, bladder, and other tissues. However, venous injury is rare, and we have not observed clinically relevant damage to nerves adjacent to radiation-injured arteries.

Compared to the segmental distribution of arteriosclerotic lesions, the sites of radiation arteritis are atypical. In the cerebrovascular circulation, one or both common carotid arteries may be affected while the bifurcation is spared. Subjacent vertebral arteries often are narrowed not at their origins, but distally, corresponding to the radiation portal. When carotid bifurcation disease is identified by a bruit, there may be an external carotid stenosis rather than the more prevalent bifurcation and internal carotid involvement. Clinically important upper extremity ischemia following radiation therapy for breast carcinoma results from poorly collateralized, often ulcerated occlusive lesions near the subclavian-axillary junction. In contrast, arteriosclerosis usually arises proximally at the subclavian artery origin, not infrequently with an associated steal syndrome. Additional sites of atypical arterial stenoses include isolated renal artery lesions after abdominal irradiation for Hodgkin's disease, external iliac artery lesions after uterine or prostate cancer treatment, superficial femoral artery occlusion many years after successful radiation of lower extremity sarcoma, and midaortic and visceral artery stenoses decades after external irradiation to the midabdomen for benign and malignant lesions.

The clinical syndromes of radiation arteritis tend to present at a younger age by 10 to 15 years than those of arteriosclerotic patients.[2] This relative prematurity has been observed for both carotid and subclavian-axillary occlusions. The coexistence of risk factors for arteriosclerosis, such as hyperlipidemia, male gender, smoking, and hypertension, also predisposes to radiation arteritis. For example, 26 of the 28 patients in our study were smokers. The microscopic similarity of arteriosclerosis and radiation-induced lesions suggests possible shared mechanisms of pathogenesis. Superimposed arteriosclerosis may accelerate the development of stenosing or aneurysmal lesions initiated by irradiation.

PATHOPHYSIOLOGY

The early and late sequelae of arterial irradiation have been characterized clinically and histopathologically. The severity of arterial injury is related to radiation dose; smaller doses provide lesser degrees of cellular damage, whereas larger doses may be acutely or subacutely necrotizing. Macroscopic radiation effects include arterial spasm and epithelial denudation. Within 24 hours, intimal disruption, subintimal edema, and internal elastic membrane fragmentation are widespread. They are followed by collagen and smooth muscle degeneration. Subsequently, adventitial fibrosis, hemorrhage, and lymphocytic infiltration develop. The sensitivity of elastic tissue to irradiation damage, in particular, may partially account for the preferential occurrence of rupture in elastic arteries.

Signs of healing tend to occur along with myointimal fibrous proliferation and intimal resurfacing with nonendothelial cells. The resultant artery, with its altered architecture, can subsequently undergo arteriosclerotic degeneration with foam cell deposition and plaque formation. Diminished fibrinolytic activity, endothelium-derived plasminogen activator activity, and prostacylin synthesis have been reported.[3]

With early lesions (less than 5 years), mural thrombosis predominates. The findings in intermediate lesions (5 to 10 years) include panmural fibrosis, occlusions, and a relative paucity of collaterals. Late lesions (mean 26 years) had periarterial fibrosis incorporating a pronounced arteriosclerosis.[4]

CLINICAL MANIFESTATIONS

The lengthy interval between irradiation and the appearance of the arterial lesion requires either cure of the underlying malignancy or a very long disease-free interval. None of our 28 patients with symptomatic arterial lesions had recurrent or residual cancer. Because of this latency and the mortality from cancer, the true incidence of arterial lesions is unknown. Not to be overlooked are the important lesions of the aorta in children and symptomatic coronary artery stenoses.[5,6]

Axillary-Subclavian Lesions

Axillary-subclavian arterial lesions presented with upper extremity effort fatigue, coldness, discoloration, and/or painful ulceration of the fingertip(s) on average 6 to 7 years after irradiation for carcinoma of the breast. Stenosis, arterial ulceration, or occlusion with a paucity of collaterals was seen on arteriograms (Fig. 1).

Extracranial Cervical Lesions

Squamous cell carcinoma of the oropharynx was the most common indication for cervical radiation in our study. Six of nine patients presented with transient ishemic attack or stroke 1 to 13 years after treatment (mean 9.4 years). Atypical locations of lesions included the mid-common carotid artery, the external carotid artery, and vertebral arteries (Fig. 2). Arteriography documented intraluminal thrombus in two of nine patients.

Abdominal Aorta and Its Branches

The abdominal aorta and its branches were affected in 10 patients 5 to 44 years (mean 14.9 years) after irradiation. Included were five patients with limb-threatening ischemia and three with disabling claudication (Fig. 3). Two patients had evidence of visceral artery occlusive disease. One had hypertension due to unilateral renal artery stenosis following treatment for Hodgkin's disease (Fig. 4). The other developed midaortic stenosis and multiple visceral arterial lesions resulting from gastric irradiation for benign peptic ulcer disease. Unusual sites and patterns of radiation arteritis also characterized this group of patients.

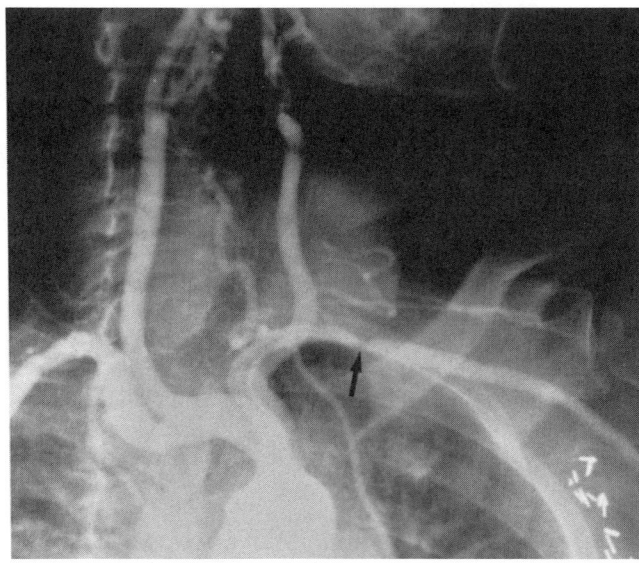

Figure 1 Subclavian-axillary stenosis (*arrow*) in a 71-year-old woman, 16 years after radiotherapy of breast carcinoma.

MANAGEMENT

Indications for revascularization were the same as for patients with arteriosclerotic occlusive disease. There were no instances of false aneurysm or cutaneous fistulas and hemorrhage. Although it is not essential to clinical management of the arterial lesion, a comprehensive record of past radiation therapy ought to be an integral part of the patient's record at the time of revascularization. Pertinent information should include at least the type and grade of neoplasm, treating physicians, place and date of radiation therapy, details of treatment (e.g., dose, number of treatments, radiation source), and any untoward events associated with treatment.

Carotid Lesions

Extracranial carotid lesions were treated with endarterectomy. We routinely augment the repair with greater saphenous vein patch angioplasty. If the endarterectomized vessel appears too friable for vein patch angioplasty, an interposition graft of reversed greater saphenous vein is inserted over an indwelling shunt. Often, common carotid artery occlusions, because they are proximal to the bifurcation, are not amenable to carotid endarterectomy. A bypass graft around mid-carotid artery lesions are terminated at or near the carotid bifurcation. Inflow can be obtained from the proximal contralateral carotid artery by tunneling either in front of or behind the trachea. Alternatively, either subclavian artery can be used for inflow sites with the graft tunneled adjacent to the carotid artery. Synthetic bypasses are to be avoided whenever possible because of the risk of graft nonincorporation by irradiation-damaged tissue. Compromised healing of wounds in the irradiated tissues may necessitate graft coverage with myofascial flaps.

Subclavian-Axillary Lesions

Bypass grafting has been our sole means of treating subclavian-axillary lesions. Endarterectomy and patch angioplasty, with potential for damage to the adjacent brachial plexus, are hazardous. Orthotopic tunnels under the clavicle and adjacent to the native artery are preferred when either the common carotid artery or supraclavicular subclavian artery is used as an inflow site. Occasionally, inflow may be taken from the proximal axillary artery, and dissection is promoted by dividing the pectoralis minor muscle. Prosthetic graft material is to be avoided.

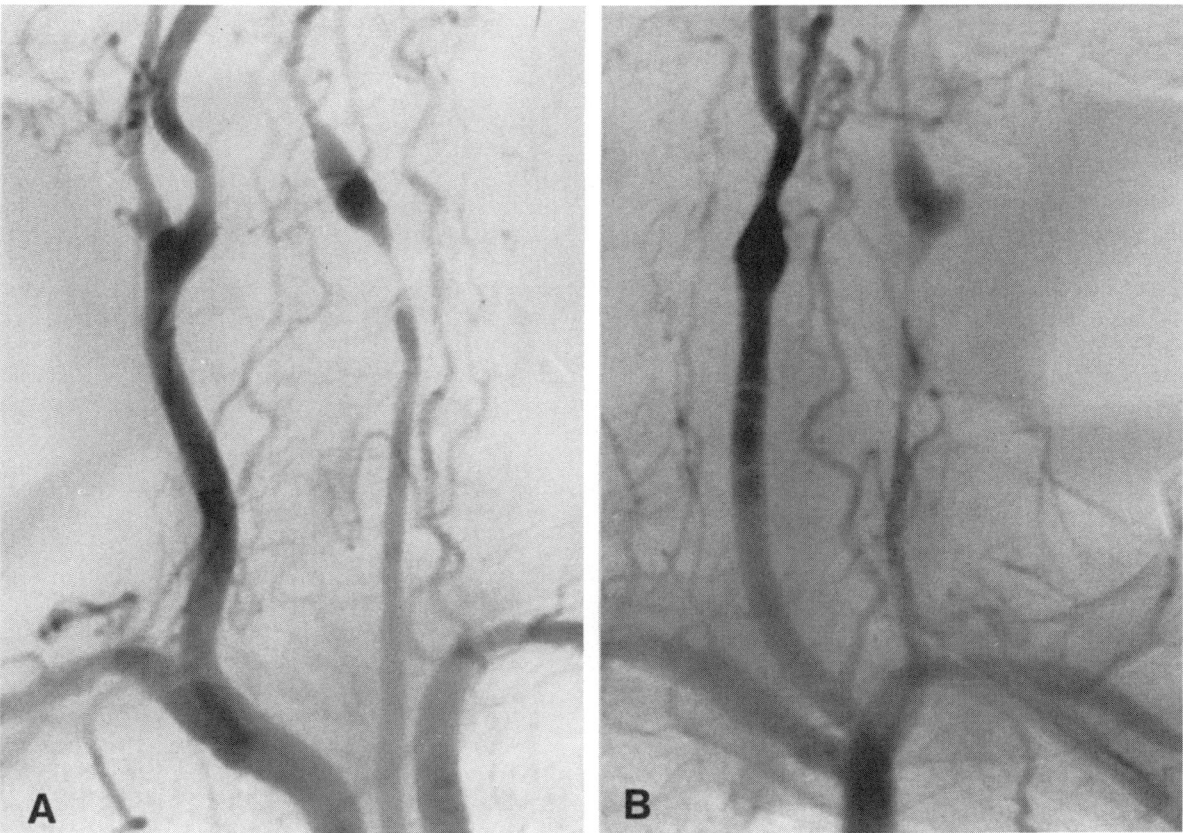

Figure 2 *A*, Left common carotid artery stenosis in 75-year-old woman 6 years after treatment of squamous cell carcinoma of the epiglottis. *B*, The right vertebral and left external carotid arteries are occluded.

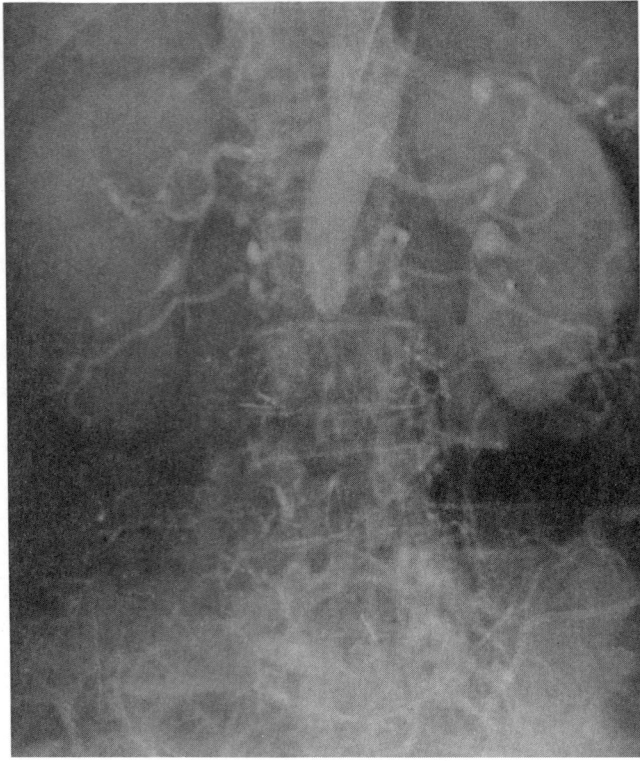

Figure 3 Aortic occlusion 5 months after irradiation for uterine cancer. Note paucity of collaterals. Common femoral arteries were found to be patent bilaterally.

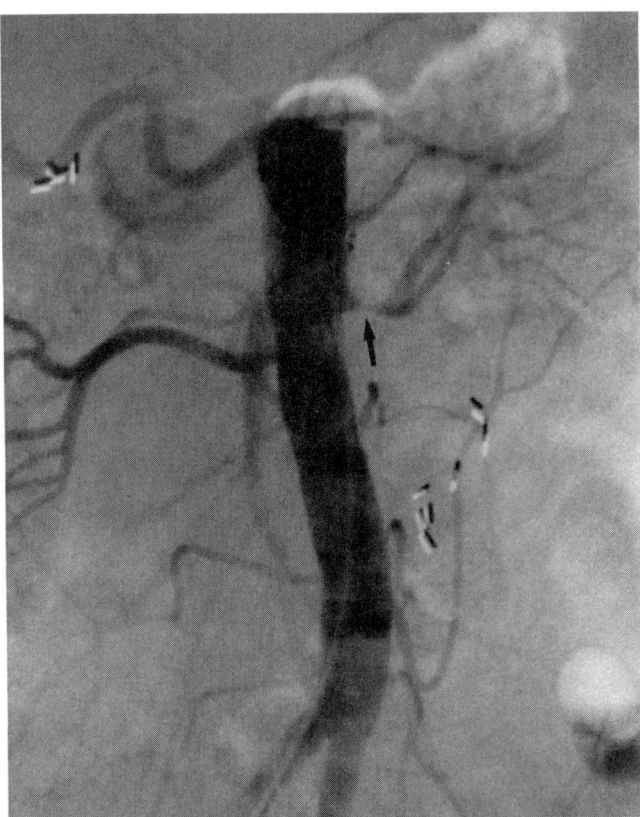

Figure 4 Left renal arterial stenosis in hypertensive male 17 years after external irradiation for lymphoma. Other arteriosclerotic disease is not observed.

Lesions of the Abdominal Aorta and Its Branches

Standard bypass techniques are usually applicable for treating aortic and branch lesions. Mid-abdominal aortic lesions are treated with aortoaortic bypass. Associated visceral occlusions are bypassed with side arm grafts to affected vessels. Celiac and superior mesenteric arterial lesions may be treated with bifurcated grafts originating from the supraceliac aorta. An isolated renal artery stenosis is well suited to hepatorenal or splenorenal vein bypass grafting. If lesions are focal, balloon angioplasty with or without stenting has proven to be effective and durable in some patients.[7]

Aortoiliac lesions are treated with Dacron aortofemoral bypasses. External iliac arterial occlusions that follow pelvic irradiation are amenable to iliofemoral bypass grafting using the retroperitoneal approach. Preoperative placement of ureteral catheters is recommended to aid in ureteral identification and protection within the scarred retroperitoneum. Whether to use orthotopic tunnels adjacent to the native arteries remains controversial. Placing the graft in this position may disturb or disrupt periarterial nerves and veins.

In the postoperative period, grafts, particularly synthetic ones, may fail to incorporate because they traverse irradiated tissue and are more susceptible to infection. Many months or years after implantation, graft nonincorporation has been observed with subsequent thrombosis. In our experience we have had no instances of graft nonincorporation while using orthotopic tunnels; therefore, we have not felt the need to use axillofemoral bypass grafting except in the presence of intra-abdominal sepsis or hostile abdomen. For infrainguinal bypasses, we use ipsilateral greater saphenous vein as our first choice and contralateral saphenous vein or arm veins as second and third choices, respectively.

SURVEILLANCE AND PREVENTION

Multiple factors affect the number of instances of irradiation arteritis seen in clinical practice. Improved techniques using supervoltage equipment with tangential portals should produce focused treatment and reduce the risk of radiation damage to skin, muscle, and vascular structures. Then again, increased numbers of patients will be selected for radiation therapy because of its improved safety and efficacy. Retrospective and prospective studies of carotid stenosis after cervical irradiation for a variety of head and neck cancers have documented an increase in the occurrence of significant carotid lesions. These findings have led to the recommendation of routine postirradiation duplex surveillance of the extracranial circulation after high-dose irradiation.[8] Likewise, the greater use of partial mastectomy and radiotherapy as the preferred treatment strategy for many breast tumors has lead some to advise noninvasive monitoring of the upper extremity circulation following irradiation.[9,10]

REFERENCES

1. Andros G, Schneider PA, Harris RW, et al. Management of arterial occlusive disease following radiation therapy (in press).
2. Silverberg GD, Britt RH, Goffinet DR. Radiation-induced carotid artery disease. Cancer 1978; 41:130–137.
3. Astedt B, Bergentz S-E, Svanberg L. Effect of irradiation on the plasminogen activator content in rat vessels. Experientia 1974; 30:1466–1467.
4. Butler MJ, Lane RHS, Webster JHH. Irradiation injury to large arteries. Br J Surg 1980; 67:341–343.
5. Colquhoun J. Hypoplasia of the abdominal aorta following therapeutic irradiation in infancy. Radiology 1966; 86:454–456.
6. Huff H, Sanders EM. Coronary-artery occlusion after radiation. N Engl J Med 1972; 286:780.
7. Guthaner DF, Schmitz L. Percutaneous transluminal angioplasty of radiation-induced arterial stenoses. Radiology 1982; 144:77–78.
8. Moritz MW, Higgins RF, Jacobs JR. Duplex imaging and incidence of carotid radiation injury after high-dose radiotherapy for tumors of the head and neck. Arch Surg 1990; 125:1181–1183.
9. Kretschmer G, Niederle B, Polteraurer P, Waneck R. Irradiation-induced changes in the subclavian and axillary arteries after radiotherapy for carcinoma of the breast. Surgery 1986; 99:658–663.
10. Berqvist D, Jonsson K, Nilsson M, Takolander R. Treatment of arterial lesions after radiation therapy. Surg Gynecol Obstet 1987; 165:116–120.

UPPER EXTREMITY ARTERIAL DISEASE

PATHOLOGY OF UPPER EXTREMITY ARTERIAL DISEASE

JAMES S. T. YAO, M.D., PH.D.

Upper extremity arterial pathology is distinctly different from that of the lower extremity in which atherosclerosis dominates the clinical problems. In the upper extremity, the disease categories are diversified and the patient population is much younger. Also, occupational injury due to chronic repetitive arterial trauma appears to be a rather common pathologic condition.

THORACIC OUTLET COMPRESSION SYNDROME

This syndrome is commonly seen in young adults with a history of using their shoulders in exaggerated motions, either from their occupations or athletic activities. Individuals commonly affected are mechanics, carpenters, musicians, and professional or competitive athletes, especially baseball pitchers. These patients present with symptoms of forearm fatigue, Raynaud's phenomenon, intolerance to cold, and, in late stages, embolization to the digital arteries causing tissue loss of the fingertips.

Four locations in the thoracic outlet may cause compression of the subclavian-axillary artery and its major branches: (1) the anterior scalene muscle, (2) the interspace between the clavicle and first rib, (3) the pectoralis minor tendon, and (4) the humerus head. Patients with a bony anomaly such as cervical rib, anomalous first rib, or healed fracture of the clavicle have the subclavian artery predisposed to compression because of the limited space within the outlet. Shoulder motions, especially in an exaggerated position, subject the artery to repetitive trauma. Although a bony anomaly causes compression, it is recognized that hypertrophy of soft tissue as a result of shoulder activity may also contribute to compression of the subclavian or axillary artery. This is especially found in baseball pitchers. Hypertrophy of the anterior scalene muscle or the pectoris minor muscle can compress the artery leading to thrombosis of the artery. Recently, the humerus head has been found to cause repetitive compression to the axillary artery and thus thrombosis of the artery. Not only the main artery is compressed; major branches such as the suprascapular artery, subscapular artery, and, in particular, the anterior or posterior circumflex humeral arteries have been found subject to compression.

As a result of repetitive trauma, the subclavian artery may develop the following injury patterns: (1) intimal disruption with ulceration in the inferior surface of the artery where the artery crosses over the cervical rib, (2) aneurysm formation, and (3) poststenotic dilatation. All of these lesions, if unrecognized, may progress to thrombosis. Both intimal disruption and aneurysm formation serve as the source of embolization. In our recent review, embolization to a digital artery is common and occurs in 80% of patients. Of interest is the development of an aneurysm of the posterior or anterior circumflex humeral arteries as a result of humerus head compression. Once the aneurysm has developed, the exaggerated shoulder activity forces thrombotic debris out of the aneurysm into the main artery. The ensuing event is multiple embolization to the digital artery. Aneurysm of the circumflex humeral artery has been reported in baseball pitchers, fist-ball players, and volleyball players. All of these athletes use violent shoulder motions in their athletic activities.[1]

Diagnosis of thoracic outlet compression is established by physical examination of the thoracic outlet and pulse examination in neutral and in abduction, external rotation positions. Arteriography is needed to determine the exact site of compression. The arteriogram must include the innominate artery on the right and the subclavian artery on the left. Examination is not complete unless positional exposure is obtained with the arm placed in functional position (pitching position or hyperabduction with external rotation). Treatment consists of the removal of the offending structure and repair of the damaged artery. In the case of humerus head compression, treatment is difficult because removal of the humerus head is not possible. Treatment in this condition is to repair damage to the artery, if it has occurred. Branch aneurysms must be excluded from the circulation to prevent embolization.

OCCUPATIONAL INJURY

There are two common forms of occupational injury to the hand, the "hypothenar hammer syndrome" and the "vibratory white finger." Both are due to repetitive trauma from excessive use of the hand. This injury is frequently seen in auto mechanics, electricians, or carpenters.

In hypothenar hammer syndrome, the predisposing factor in the development of injury of the ulnar artery is the repetitive use of the palm of the hand in activity that involves pushing, pounding, or twisting. The anatomic location of the ulnar artery in the area of the hypothenar eminence places it in a vulnerable position. The terminal branches of the ulnar artery (deep palmar branch and superficial arch) arise in a groove called Guyon's tunnel, bounded medially by the pisiform bone and the hook of the hamate bone and dorsally by the transverse carpal ligament. Over a distance of 2 cm, the ulnar artery lies quite superficially in the palm, covered only by the skin, subcutaneous tissue, and the palmaris brevis muscle. When this area is repeatedly traumatized, ulnar or digital arterial spasm, aneurysm formation, occlusion, or a combination of these lesions can result. Embolization from an aneurysm may cause multiple digital artery occlusions. Clinically, the patient presents with symptoms of ulnar artery occlusion, namely, numbness, paresthesias, stiffness, coldness, and blanching of one or more digits.

Vibratory white finger occurs in workers who use vibrating tools. On exposure to vibration or cold, patients experience blanching, numbness, and pain in the finger due to exaggerated vasoconstriction. The tools associated with this disorder include power hammers, chisels, chain saws, sanders, grinders, riveters, shapers, and drills. The severity and frequency of symptoms increase with extended duration and higher intensity of vibration exposure. The mechanism of vibratory white finger may be due to central sympathetic hyperreactivity or local vasoactive factors.[2] In addition, endothelial damage caused directly by vibration may lead to platelet adherence, aggregation, and release of mitogenic mediators. One such mediator is platelet-derived growth factor that may account for proliferation of smooth muscle cells. In advanced cases, hypertrophy of vascular smooth muscle cells causes arterial occlusion and ulceration. Vibratory white finger is usually reversible if identified early and if exposure to vibration is reduced.

CONNECTIVE TISSUE DISORDERS

Connective tissue disorders refer to (1) systemic lupus erythematosus, (2) scleroderma, and (3) rheumatoid arthritis. All have systemic symptoms, with Raynaud's phenomenon as one of the vascular manifestations.

Systemic Lupus Erythematosus (SLE). Many of the clinical manifestations of SLE are a consequence of tissue damage from vasculopathy mediated by immune complexes.[3] Polyarthritis and dermatitis are the most common clinical manifestations. Raynaud's phenomenon is often bilateral and in advanced cases may be accompanied by painful, violaceous, and atrophic finger pads. Arterial involvement is often in small arteries such as digital arteries, and it is often multiple. The diagnosis is established by the presence of antinuclear antibodies. Antibodies to native or double-stranded DNA and to Sm, a ribonuclear protein antigen, are more specific than other antinuclear antibodies for the diagnosis of SLE.[3] Approximately 30% of patients with SLE have positive antiphospholipid antibodies, and antiphospholipid syndrome is known to cause thromboembolic symptoms.

Scleroderma. This is a progressive, generalized disorder of the connective tissue of the skin, muscles, fascia, visceral organs, and blood vessels. Digital arteries are often affected with the clinical manifestation of Raynaud's phenomenon in the initial stage, slowly progressing to tissue loss or gangrene changes of the fingertips. Histologic investigation of digital arteries documents intimal thickening secondary to fibrous deposition in the blood vessel wall. Characteristic arteriographic findings are multiple focal stenoses and occlusions, as well as generalized arterial narrowing. The proper digital artery is usually most severely involved, generally in the mid or distal portion of the vessel. The third and fourth digits are affected in 80% to 90% of patients, the second digit in 75%, and the fifth digit in 20%. In addition to multiple occlusive lesions in the proper digital arteries, involvement of the ulnar artery occurs in about 50% of patients. Interestingly, the radial artery is almost always normal.

Rheumatoid Arthritis. This is the most common connective tissue disorder, but involvement of arteries causing arteritis is uncommon. Two major types of arterial abnormalities are seen: (1) occlusive and (2) hyperemic. Occlusive digital artery lesions are most commonly seen with accompanying destructive and erosive osseous changes. Hyperemic abnormalities are more common in the absence of destructive bone changes. Hypervascularity is often seen in the distal tufts of the fingers and is thought to be related to an increase of collateral circulation. Arteriography of the hands documents diagnostic features such as corkscrew formation, withering, and hypervascularity with early capillary filling. In addition to involvement of the digital arteries, the subclavian or axillary arteries may also have changes in patients with rheumatoid arteritis. Long tapering of the subclavian-axillary artery is often a common arteriographic finding. As a result of major arterial occlusion, forearm fatigue is often the presenting symptom.

ATHEROSCLEROSIS

Unlike lower extremity occlusive disease, upper extremity ischemia due to atherosclerosis is uncommon. When it occurs, the subclavian artery is the most common site of involvement. Occlusion of the subclavian artery may be associated with cerebrovascular ischemic symptoms and is often referred to as "subclavian steal syndrome." In addition to forearm fatigue, ischemic symptoms such as digital embolization may occur if there is an ulcerating plaque at the subclavian or the innominate artery. This ulcerating lesion bears a resemblance to plaque seen in the carotid artery. Not infrequently, distal embolization may also occur from atherosclerotic aneurysm of the subclavian or innominate artery.

BUERGER'S DISEASE

Thromboangiitis obliterans, or Buerger's disease, is a poorly understood disease, and some authors have questioned whether it is indeed a clinical entity. Characteristically, the patient is a habitual heavy smoker. Although the disease, if it exists, is more common in the lower extremity, it may occur in the upper extremity. As arteriography became more frequent, patients suspected of having Buerger's disease were found to have atherosclerosis. The diagnosis is made by exclusion of other diseases and depends on histologic examination, with involvement not only of arteries but of veins as well. Venous manifestation includes migrating phlebitis. An arteriogram may document diagnostic features such as multiple small artery occlusions with abundant collaterals. A characteristic corrugated appearance of the artery proximal to an occlusion is often seen, and this finding has been cited as one of the diagnostic findings in Buerger's disease. However, the corrugated artery may also be seen in other conditions.

RADIATION INJURY

Injury to arteries supplying the upper limb following, radiation treatment for breast carcinoma or Hodgkin disease is well known. The most commonly affected artery is the subclavian artery, followed by the axillary artery. The pathogenesis consists of three processes: endothelial injury and disruption of the internal elastic lamina followed by intimal fibrosis and plaque formation; occlusion of the vasa vasora by proliferation and hyaline thickening of the intima, which in turn causes fibrosis of the media; and, finally, periarterial fibrosis, which causes extrinsic constriction of the artery.

Clinically, there are four patterns of manifestation of the disease process.[4] First, fatal hemorrhage occurs from acute rupture due to necrosis of the arterial wall. Second, mural thrombosis in the arterial segment at the site of irradiation usually presents thromboembolic phenomena within 5 years of the exposure. In the third, fibrotic occlusion may lead to delayed ischemia symptoms within 10 years of radiation. The fourth group manifests itself more than 20 years after radiotherapy with symptoms initiated by periarterial fibrosis and "accelerated atherosclerosis." The diagnosis is established by a history of radiation exposure and the characteristic arteriographic finding of diffuse, long narrowing of the artery.

FIBROMUSCULAR DYSPLASIA

This is probably the rarest form of arterial occlusive disease of the upper extremity. The commonly affected artery in the upper extremity is the brachial artery. Only a handful of cases have been reported, and females appear more likely to be affected.[5] Fibromuscular dysplasia is a nonatherosclerotic and noninflammatory vascular disease of unknown cause that affects primary medium-sized and small arteries. Three predominant types of fibromuscular dysplasia have been identified. Of reported cases of brachial artery involvement, intimal fibroplasia appears to be the most common.

ARTERITIS

Arteritis, collectively known as vasculitis syndromes, has recently been further classified by the American College of Rheumatology to encompass seven distinct clinical entities:[6] polyarteritis nodosa, Churg-Strauss syndrome, Wegener's granulomatosis, hypersensitivity vasculitis, Henoch-Schönlein purpura, giant cell (temporal) arteritis, and Takayasu arteritis. Of these, only polyarteritis nodosa, Takayasu arteritis, and giant cell arteritis are of surgical significance.

Takayasu Arteritis. Takayasu arteritis is a chronic inflammatory disease of unknown etiology that primarily involves the aorta and its major branches. Fatigue of the forearm is one of the manifestations of the the disease process. According to the American College of Rheumatology, there are six inclusion criteria for the diagnosis: onset before age 40 years, exercise fatigue of an extremity, decreased brachial artery pulse, less than 10 mm Hg difference in systolic blood pressure between arms, a bruit over the subclavian arteries or the aorta, and arteriographic evidence of narrowing or occlusion of the entire aorta, its primary branches, or large arteries in the proximal upper or lower extremities. The presence of three or more of these criteria had a sensitivity of 90.5% and a specificity of 97.8% for the diagnosis.

The diagnosis of Takayasu arteritis often is delayed for months to years because many patients manifest nonspecific symptoms of fever, myalgias, arthralgias, weight loss, and anemia. Unless the clinician is aware of the disease, misdiagnosis is common. The pathology in the aorta and branches during this early stage consists of granulomatous changes in the media and adventitia. This disease progresses at variable rates to a sclerotic stage, with intimal hyperplasia, medial degeneration, and adventitial fibrosis. The aorta and involved arteries develop segmental narrowings leading to the condition known as pulseless disease. Arteriographic findings include the extensive involvement of major branches of the aortic arch vessels with characteristic segmental narrowing. Elevated erythrocyte sedimentation rate, anemia, and hypergammaglobulinemia are important supportive laboratory findings. For purposes of diagnosis, all patients with suspected Takayasu arteritis should undergo a complete arteriographic study.

Giant Cell (Temporal) Arteritis. Criteria for the classification of giant cell (temporal) arteritis are age 50 years or older at disease onset, onset of localized headache, temporal artery tenderness or decreased temporal artery pulse, elevated erythrocyte sedimentation rate (Westergren) greater than 50 mm per hour, and a biopsy sample including an artery documenting necrotizing arteritis, characterized by a predominance of mononuclear cell infiltrates or a granulomatous process with multinucleated giant cells. The presence of three or more of these five criteria was associated with a sensitivity of 93.5% and a specificity of 91.2% for the diagnosis.[6]

The etiology of giant cell arteritis is unknown. The disease is common in whites, and an association with HLA-DR4 suggests a genetic predisposition. The increasing incidence after age 50 and the predominance in women suggest a relationship to aging and, perhaps, hormonal changes.

Symptoms are often nonspecific, and these include fatigue, fever, headache, jaw fatigue, loss of vision, scalp tenderness, and polymyalgia rheumatica. The sedimentation rate is often elevated.

The subclavian or axillary artery is often the site of involvement. The arteriographic findings are long tapering of the artery with segmental stenosis. The inflammatory lesions are usually scattered irregularly along the courses of involved vessels, but longer segments may be affected in a continous manner. Histologically, a granulomatous inflammatory process is seen that is usually focused along the internal elastic lamina. This often leads to occlusion of the arterial lumen or weakening of the arterial wall and subsequent rupture. Biopsy specimens often document predominance of mononuclear cell infiltration or granulomatous inflammation, usually with multinucleated giant cells.

Polyarteritis Nodosa. Necrotizing angitis is the basic pathologic change in this disorder. This form of arteritis is uncommon; when present, it may involve visceral or digital arteries of the hand. Arteriographic findings include multiple stenoses and occlusions of the proper and common digital arteries, as well as discrete aneurysm formation, similar to that in the renal and mesenteric arteries. The aneurysms represent end results of the underlying pathologic process of necrotizing angitis and are often small and multiple.

AZOTEMIC ARTERIOPATHY

This arteriopathy is often seen in patients who are diabetics with chronic renal failure. The characteristic presentation is gangrene of the fingertip due to diffuse calcification of the digital arteries. Calciphylaxis has been proposed as a possible mechanism in the pathogenesis of soft tissue and vascular calcification in chronic renal disease, and once calcification occurs, it seldom regresses. Arterial calcification usually is localized in the media, resulting in a pipestem pattern, such as is seen in Mönckeberg's arteriosclerosis. Fibrous response to the media may result in obliteration of the lumen, causing gangrene of the digits or tissue loss in the muscles. The characteristic radiologic findings are diffuse calcification in the hand and digital arteries. In patients with gangrenous changes, occlusion of the digital arteries is a common arteriographic feature.

CONGENITAL ARTERIAL WALL DEFECTS

Pseudoxanthoma elasticum and the Ehlers-Danlos syndrome may cause spontaneous rupture of the artery and hence result in occlusion with ischemia of the upper extremity. Pseudoxanthoma elasticum is a genetically determined, probably autosomal-recessive disorder of the elastic tissue with cutaneous, ocular, vascular, and gastrointestinal manifestations. It is an extremely rare disorder, and diagnosis often is made by skin biopsy or by fluorescein angiography of the ocular findings. Ehlers-Danlos syndrome is a disorder of connective tissue involving joints, tendons, ligaments, blood vessels, and dermis. Hyperextension of the joints is common. The combination of weakness of the arterial wall and hyperextension of the joints contributes to damage to the brachial artery.

REFERENCES

1. McCarthy WJ, Yao JST, Schafer MF, et al. Upper extremity arterial injury in athletes. J Vasc Surg 1989; 9:317–327.
2. Palmer RA, Collin J. Vibratory white finger. Br J Surg 1993; 80:705–709.
3. Mills JA. Sytemic lupus erythematosus. N Engl J Med 1994; 330:1871–1879.
4. Butler MS, Lane RHS, Webster JHH. Irradiation injury to large arteries. Br J Surg 1980; 67:341–343.
5. Lin WW, McGee GS, Patterson BK, et al. Fibromuscular dysplasia of the brachial artery: Case report and review of the literature. J Vasc Surg 1992; 16:66–70.
6. Lie JT. Illustrated histopathologic classification criteria for selected vasculitis syndromes. Arthritis Rheum 1990; 33:1074–1087.

REVASCULARIZATION OF THE UPPER EXTREMITY

HENRY VELDENZ, M.D.
GORDON L. HYDE, M.D.

Upper extremity ischemia is both rare and variable in presentation. A flexible and thorough approach to the evaluation and treatment of patients with this condition is essential.

ETIOLOGY

The causes of upper extremity ischemia are more diverse than the causes of ischemia in the leg. (Table 1).[1] Upper extremity ischemia may be due to disease of the arterial wall, such as atherosclerosis, Takayasu's arteritis, thromboangiitis obliterans, and giant cell arteritis. More distal ischemia may occur as a result of connective tissue disorders such as lupus erythematosus and scleroderma. Emboli, if they are large, are usually the result of ischemic cardiac disease or rhythm disturbances.

Traumatic causes of upper extremity ischemia are common and numerous. Blunt injury to the thoracic outlet can damage the axillosubclavian system and lead to either acute or chronic ischemia resulting from traumatic pseudoaneurysm formation. Compression of the subclavian and axillary arteries by soft tissue or bony structures may cause acute or chronic ischemia from thrombosis or pseudoaneurysm. Repeated low-level trauma, as is caused by the use of power tools or due to the stress placed on the hypothenar eminence while hammering, can eventually injure the vessel affected.[2] Blunt arm injury, such as a fracture or dislocation at the elbow, can cause ischemia in the hand.[3] Compartment injuries, that result from a fracture or a crush injury, can also cause hand ischemia.

Iatrogenic injury, which usually manifests acutely, is dealt with elsewhere in this text. However, delayed recognition of these conditions can lead to chronic ischemia. In addition, some patients experience upper extremity ischemia when an artery provides access for dialysis or when the axillary artery is used as inflow for lower extremity bypass.[4]

Spontaneous thrombosis of upper extremity vessels can produce ischemia that is both acute and profound. Patients with this condition represent a diagnostic and therapeutic challenge. Some have a history of thrombotic episodes. Evaluating these particular patients for a hypercoagulable state occasionally is rewarding. Diagnosing the condition in other patients may be possible only when an identifiable clotting factor deficiency or an antibody is uncovered.

DIAGNOSIS

Clinical presentations of upper extremity ischemia range from symptomatic exertional pain to digital gangrene. However, major tissue loss is an uncommon presenting complaint. A careful history provides insight into the precipitating cause. The mechanism and timing of trauma give clues to the cause. Dialysis patients may have early or late ischemic complications resulting from access procedures. Patients with cardiac disease may have classic embolic causes. Arterial damage from radiotherapy may be suggested by treatment history. Ischemia resulting from the sequelae of thoracic outlet syndromes can be challenging to discern from the history. Spontaneous thrombosis resulting from primary hypercoagulable states is also difficult to diagnose according to history; often the diagnosis must be based on the exclusion of other causes.

Complete physical examination of the upper extremity is important in determining the cause of ischemia to the hand or arm. All axillary, brachial, radial, and ulnar pulses should be noted; they should be compared with the patient's lower extremity pulses. Brachial blood pressures should be checked bilaterally, as this may indicate a subclavian lesion. In addition, palpation and auscultation for subclavian bruits and pulse changes upon arm positioning may identify a source of ischemia at the thoracic outlet. Allen's test is used to evaluate palmar arch patency. Notation and localization of ulcers, splinter hemorrhages, and tissue loss should be accurate and thorough. Likewise, cardiac rhythm should be noted.

Noninvasive vascular laboratory evaluation complements history and physical examination. Segmental

Table 1 Causes of Upper Extremity Ischemia

Intrinsic arterial diseases
  Atherosclerosis
  Systemic disorders
    Takayasu's arteritis
    Thromboarteritis obliterans
    Lupus erythematosus
Emboli
  Cardiac origin
    Mural thrombi
    Valvular
  Proximal aneurysmal disease
  Proximal pseudoaneurysmal disease
Trauma
  Blunt
    Fracture
    Dislocation
    Crush injury
  Penetrating
Iatrogenic
  Cardiac catheterization
  Angiography access
  Dialysis access
  Arterial puncture
Thoracic outlet sequelae
  Direct compression
  Poststenotic aneurysmal change
Hypercoagulable states

pressure and waveform analysis can detect subclinical stenoses proximally and distally in upper extremities. Digital blood pressures and plethysmography can localize occlusive disease distally when the proximal arterial tree is normal. Duplex examination, not yet extensively applied to the upper extremity, may aid a difficult evaluation. An important adjunct on the evaluation of upper extremity ischemia is the assessment of suspected hypercoagulable states. An initial screen should include at minimum prothrombin time, partial thromboplastin time, serum immunoelectrophoresis, protein C, protein S, antithrombin III levels, and assays to determine the presence of anticardiolipin, antiphospholipid, and lupus inhibitor antibodies.

In difficult cases arteriography may confirm strong clinical suspicion for Buerger's disease or aid in the diagnosis of occult diseases. Otherwise arteriography is usually used to plan therapy. A complete angiographic evaluation must include a patient's aortic arch through the digits. An examination of the origins of the innominate or subclavian arteries may detect stenosis, occlusion, or aneurysmal changes. Multiple views of the axillary artery with different arm position changes can document the location of rib impingement. The brachial artery and its bifurcation must be clearly delineated, as the radial and ulnar arteries may have high or anomalous origins. Additional information about the interosseus and deep brachial collateral systems is also useful.

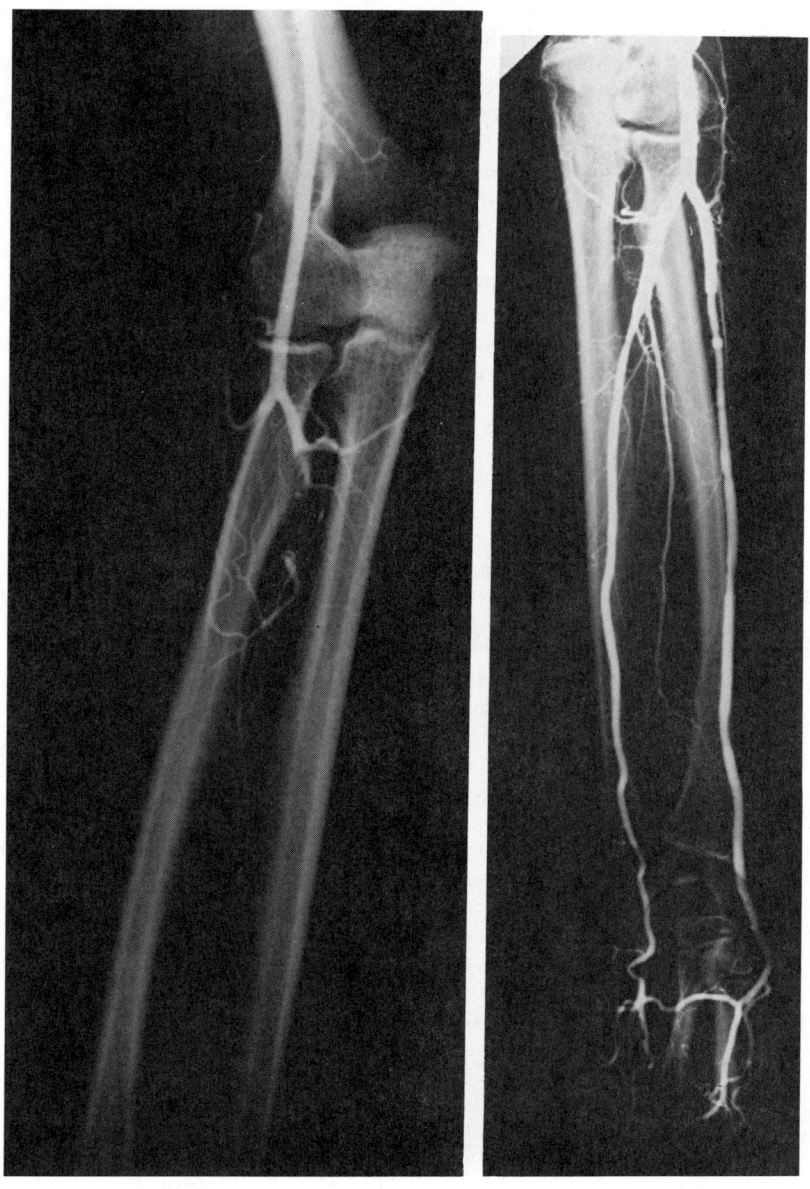

Figure 1 *A*, Thrombosis of forearm vessels in a patient with antithrombin III deficiency. *B*, Response to lytic therapy with clearing of all vasculature to the hand.

Finally, the status of the distal digital outflow must be determined.[5]

Angiography, which can be helpful even when bypass is not appropriate, is essential in evaluating the completeness of an embolectomy, especially if normal perfusion is not restored. Angiography may also provide arterial access for selective thrombolytic therapy, which may be useful when no mechanical lesion has been identified as the cause of the ischemic episode (Fig. 1).

THERAPY

Selection for Operation

Surgical treatment is offered when warranted by the patient's symptoms and the cause of the ischemia. An asymptomatic subclavian artery occlusion, often detected by blood pressure differential, usually does not need surgical intervention. However, active patients with exertional arm or hand ischemia may benefit from reconstruction. Patients with tissue loss or severe ischemic pain certainly should have reconstruction attempted.

Numerous options to treat acute ischemia are available. Simple embolectomy can remove an embolic occlusion of the brachial artery. If performed with local anesthesia, this procedure can be appropriate even for gravely ill cardiac patients. Direct repair, patch angioplasty, and bypass are all useful in treating traumatic ischemia. Occasionally, an endarterectomy may be appropriate for a localized occlusive process. Volar fasciotomy should be performed for patients with prolonged ischemia or severe crush injuries.

Bypass procedures at almost any level can be used successfully to treat chronic upper extremity ischemia.[6-8] The importance of arteriography in planning such procedures cannot be overemphasized. Subclavian occlusion is amenable to distal bypass. An aneurysm exclusion bypass can prevent further embolization. Unusual configurations of distal bypass to the brachial, radial, ulnar, or interosseous arteries are possible.[9] Even if ischemia necessitates bypass into the palm, a successful revascularization can eliminate the need to amputate the hand.

Bypass operations on the upper extremity must exclude the diseased segment. To keep the graft as short as possible, the most distal nondiseased artery is used as inflow to the most proximal nondiseased outflow vessel. Inflow sources from the carotid, subclavian, axillary, and brachial arteries are isolated with standard dissections.[9] Reversed saphenous vein grafts are the most common and useful bypass graft material. The nonreversed saphenous vein can also be used with valve lysis if size match considerations are important. Cephalic and basilic arm veins are another source of bypass material. Although usually not a preferred conduit, expanded polytetrafluenethylene is an acceptable option when no autologous material is available. The conduit for any bypass is best placed in its respective anatomic location.

One difference between upper and lower extremity revascularization is the relatively high vasoreactivity of the upper extremity arteries compared with the lower extremities. Use of topical and intra-arterial vasodilators is essential, as brachial, radial, or ulnar spasm may lead to occlusion of a reconstruction. According to experience from our own and other centers, papaverine, administered topically or intra-arterially with 60 mg in 100 ml of heparinized saline, seems to be the most useful adjunct for control of spasm.[9] Occasionally, gentle mechanical dilation must be used to relieve an episode of spasm. Maintenance of normothermia is also frequently overlooked in spasm control.

Objective assessment of the success of revascularization in the operating room is essential. Completion arteriography delineates the results of a bypass and assesses the completeness of thromboembolectomy. Even though a hand appears well perfused clinically, retained thrombus may alter the late outcome if not specifically detected and treated. Angioscopy and intraoperative duplex examination are possible alternatives, but their usefulness in assessing upper extremity revascularization has yet to be established.

Exposure

Although inflow and outflow sites in both the upper and lower extremities can be approached through anatomic longitudinal incisions, important differences exist. Dissection of vessels for upper extremity revascularization is generally closer to important peripheral nerves. Axillary artery exposure from below the clavicle can be expanded by division of the tendon of the pectoralis minor muscle. Distally, the biceps brachialis tendon can be divided at its aponeurosis to facilitate exposure. At the brachial bifurcation, a transverse incision just below the elbow, such as that used in dialysis access, also allows good exposure. Because crossing the antecubital crease longitudinally should be avoided, an S- or J-shaped incision is preferred.

Nonsurgical Therapy

Some patients with extensive distal thrombosis in the radial, ulnar, and digital arteries have no outflow and no definable mechanical source for the occlusions. In these patients with primary hypercoagulable states and thromboses, intra-arterial selective thrombolysis is useful. The distal radial, ulnar, and digital circulations do not lend themselves to adequate clearance by thrombectomy catheters. At the University of Kentucky good outcomes have been achieved with thrombolysis in some patients with defined hypercoagulable states (Fig. 1).

Thrombolytic therapy is also an important adjunct to surgical treatment. Intraoperative thrombolysis is especially useful after thromboembolectomy, when the digital circulation remains thrombosed. Isolated perfusion techniques can be used effectively during vein graft bypasses to close the small vessels. Moreover, patients with emboli and hypercoagulable states require long-term anticoagulation.

OUTCOME

The results of upper extremity revascularization vary with cause and treatment. Bypass patency depends on site distal the anastomoses. Anastomoses proximal to the brachial bifurcation fare better, with up to 83% 2-year patency compared with 53% when more distal.[10] A follow-up analysis of upper extremity bypass at Northwestern University documented durable 5-year patency rates of 62% with use of autologous conduit and 52% overall.[11] In general, limb loss is rare, even after late bypass failure. However, most patients can achieve normalization of hand perfusion and resolution of symptoms with appropriate revascularization.[6,7]

REFERENCES

1. McNamara MF, Takkai H, Yao JST, et al. A systematic approach to severe hand ischemia. Surgery 1978; 83:1–11.
2. Sachatello CR, Ernst CB, Griffen WO Jr. The acutely ischemic upper extremity: Selective management. Surgery 1974; 76:1002–1009.
3. Endean ED, Veldenz HC, Schwarcz TH, et al. Recognition of arterial injury in elbow dislocation. J Vasc Surg 1992; 16:402–409.
4. Rapp JH, Reilly LM, Goldstone J, et al. Ischemia of the upper extremity: Significance of proximal arterial disease. Am J Surg 1986; 152:122–126.
5. Erlandson EE, Forrest ME, Shields JJ, et al. Discriminant arteriographic criteria in the management of forearm and hand ischemia. Surgery 1981; 90:1025–1036.
6. Garrett HE, Morris GC, Howell JF, et al. Revascularization of the upper extremity with autologous vein bypass graft. Arch Surg 1965; 92:751–757.
7. Gross WS, Flanigan DP, Kraft RO, et al. Chronic upper extremity arterial insufficiency: Etiology, manifestations, and operative management. Arch Surg 1978; 113:419–423.
8. Wood PB. Vein-graft bypass in axillary and brachial artery occlusions causing claudication. Br J Surg 1973; 60:29–30.
9. McCarthy WJ. Revascularization of the upper extremity. In: Ernst CB and Stanley JC, eds. Current therapy in vascular surgery, 2nd ed. Philadelphia: BC Decker, 1991:182.
10. McCarthy WJ, Flinn WR, Yao JST, et al. Result of bypass grafting for upper limb ischemia. J Vasc Surg 1986; 3:741–746.
11. Mesh CL, Yao JST. Upper extremity bypass: Five-year follow-up. In: Yao JST and Pearch WH, eds. Long-term results in vascular surgery. Norwalk, CT: Appleton & Lange, 1993:353.

DIAGNOSIS OF UPPER EXTREMITY VASOSPASTIC DISEASE

DAVID S. SUMNER, M.D.

Episodic ischemia of the fingers in response to cold or emotional stimuli (Raynaud's phenomenon) is a frequent complaint of patients referred to the vascular laboratory. Estimates of the prevalence of this condition in the general population vary from less than 1% to 20%, with the higher figures being reported from regions where the climate is cold and damp. A survey of randomly selected subjects from South Carolina revealed a 10% prevalence of cold sensitivity, but only 5% of the population reported color changes, and only 3% sought medical attention.[1]

Classically, Raynaud's phenomenon consists of a triphasic color change: an ischemic phase, in which the involved fingers are white, followed by a period of sluggish blood flow, during which the fingers are cyanotic, and a final hyperemic stage, in which the fingers turn red as they rewarm. All three phases may be present simultaneously in the same finger, or different stages may occur at the same time in different fingers. Many patients note only pallor or cyanosis and never experience hyperemia with rewarming.

PATHOPHYSIOLOGY

Despite many years of research, the cause of Raynaud's phenomenon is incompletely understood. It is useful, however, from a prognostic and therapeutic point of view to classify Raynaud's phenomenon into two broad categories based on generally accepted assumptions regarding the underlying pathophysiology. Primary Raynaud's disease is the condition in which the digital arteries are morphologically normal but are hypersensitive to local cold, constricting markedly or closing completely in response to temperatures that have little effect on normal arteries. Secondary Raynaud's phenomenon designates a host of conditions in which the digital or more proximal arteries of the upper extremity are diseased, stenotic, or occluded, and therefore impede blood flow to the fingers even when they are warm. Superimposed on both conditions is the normal vasoconstrictive response to cold of the terminal arterioles, which is mediated in part through the sympathetic nervous system. The combination, therefore, of normal arteriolar vasoconstriction and digital arterial obstruction (either due to vasospasm or to fixed lesions) is responsible for Raynaud's phenomenon (Fig. 1). Unfortunately, this simple classification is somewhat arbitrary, since patients in one category sometimes show responses

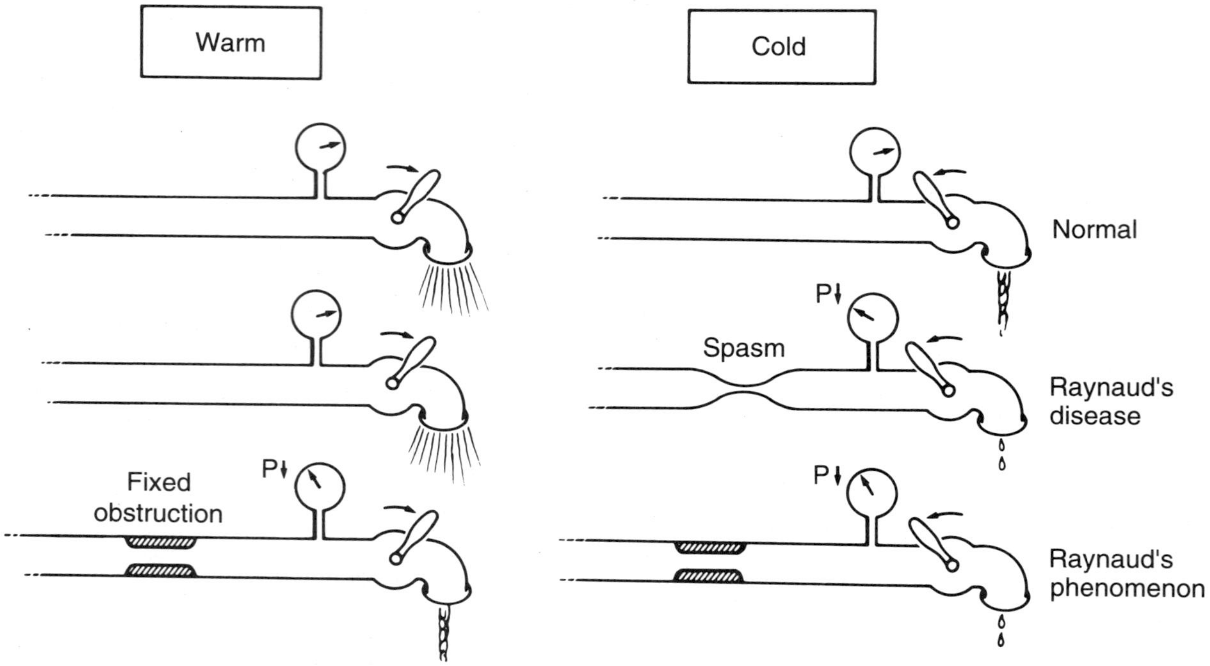

Figure 1 Effect of cold on normal fingers, fingers with primary Raynaud's disease, and fingers with Raynaud's phenomenon secondary to fixed arterial obstruction. Faucets represent arteriolar sphincters, which are dilated when the handle is turned to the right and constricted when the handle is turned to the left. Gauges represent digital arterial pressure, with increasing pressure indicated by clockwise rotation of the pointer. Digital blood flow is represented by the output from the faucets. (From Sumner DS. Evaluation of acute and chronic ischemia of the upper extremity. In: Rutherford RB, ed. Vascular surgery, 3rd ed. Philadelphia: WB Saunders, 1989: 806; with permission.)

consistent with the other. Moreover, with time, some patients originally thought to have primary Raynaud's disease will ultimately be found to have an underlying disease process. For this reason the nomenclature proposed by Edwards and Porter[2] has considerable merit. In their system, which makes no assumptions regarding the presence or absence of an associated disease, patients without laboratory evidence of arterial obstruction are said to have vasospastic Raynaud's syndrome and those in whom arterial obstruction has been demonstrated are said to have obstructive Raynaud's syndrome.

A vast array of diseases have been implicated in secondary Raynaud's phenomenon (Table 1). In fact, any pathologic entity that affects the arterial wall may be responsible for cold sensitivity under the proper circumstances. The most common offenders are the autoimmune connective tissue diseases, such as scleroderma.

CLINICAL PRESENTATION

The classic criteria for the diagnosis of primary Raynaud's disease in patients in whom exposure to moderate cold or emotional stimuli causes pallor or cyanosis of the fingers include (1) bilaterality of the phenomenon, (2) absence of ischemic lesions, and (3) failure to detect a disease that may be responsible after

Table 1 Conditions Associated with Raynaud's Phenomenon

Autoimmune Connective Tissue Diseases	Arteriosclerosis
Scleroderma (CREST syndrome)	Buerger's disease
Rheumatoid arthritis	Peripheral Emboli
Systemic lupus erythematosus	Aneurysms
Polyarteritis nodosa	Thoracic outlet syndrome
Reiter's syndrome	Trauma
Mixed connective tissue disease	Vibration
Hypersensitivity Angiitis	Percussive
Myeloproliferative disorders	Frostbite
Leukemia	Drug Induced
Myeloid metaplasia	Vasculitis
Polycythemia	Ergot derivatives
Thrombocytosis	Beta-blockers
Hypercoagulability	Cytotoxic drugs
Circulating Globulins	Oral contraceptives
Cold agglutinins	Chronic Renal Failure
Cryoglobulinemia	Occupational Chemical Exposure
Malignancy	Hypothyroidism

the condition has been present for 2 or more years. During an attack the fingers typically feel numb, but pain is rare. Although these criteria are fairly reliable, patients with secondary Raynaud's phenomenon may also have bilateral symptoms, and scleroderma or some other cause may not become evident for as long as 20

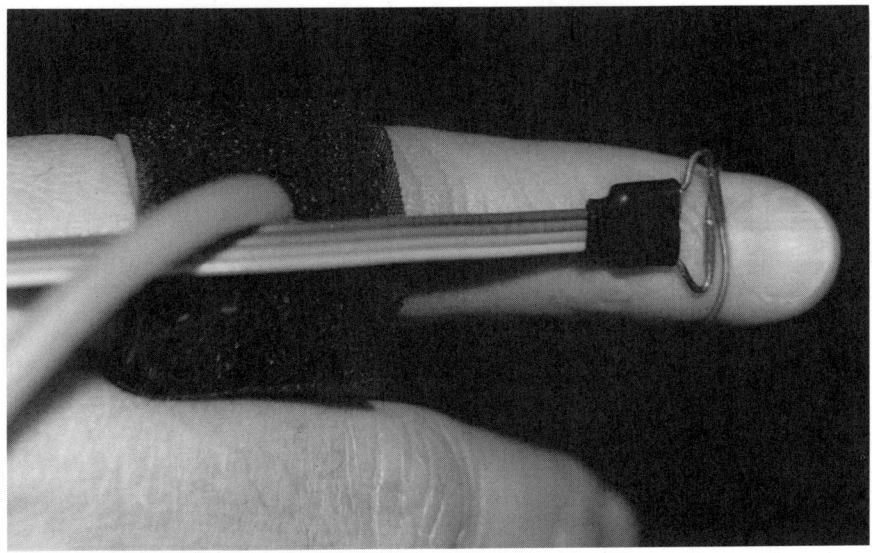

Figure 2 Apparatus for measuring finger blood pressure. A photoplethysmograph may be substituted for the mercury strain gauge shown in the figure. (From Sumner DS. Objective diagnostic techniques: Role of the vascular laboratory. In: Rutherford RB, ed. Vascular surgery, 3rd ed. Philadelphia: WB Saunders, 1989: 41; with permission.)

years. There is a marked female to male predominance, and in three-quarters of the patients the initial symptoms appear before the age of 40.

Trophic changes of the fingers or ulcers or gangrene of one or more fingertips are hallmarks of secondary Raynaud's phenomenon. These lesions are often tender and quite painful. Sclerodactyly, puffy fingers, digital pitting scars, and telangiectasias suggest a connective tissue disease. Migratory superficial phlebitis and lower extremity involvement suggest Buerger's disease. When arterial lesions are proximal to the wrist, the radial or ulnar pulses will be diminished or absent. The physical examination may also disclose bruits or pulse changes compatible with the thoracic outlet syndrome, subclavian stenosis, or subclavian aneurysms, all of which can serve as a nidus for microemboli. Valuable clues are often gleaned from the history. Vibrating tools (jackhammers, chain saws), percussive hand trauma (hypothenar hammer syndrome), and certain sports (baseball, handball) are known to cause obstruction of the digital and palmar arteries. The patient should be questioned about the use of vasospastic drugs (ergot derivatives) and exposure to chemicals toxic to arteries. Patients with connective tissue disease may complain of swallowing difficulties or arthritis.

ROLE OF THE VASCULAR LABORATORY

Noninvasive studies are designed to answer the following questions: (1) Is there fixed arterial obstruction, and if so, what is its location and how severe is the hemodynamic impairment? (2) Is there cold-induced vasospasm? (3) Do the terminal arterioles retain the ability to dilate? (4) Is sympathetic activity present? Answers to the first two questions help differentiate primary Raynaud's disease (vasospastic Raynaud's syndrome) from secondary Raynaud's phenomenon (obstructive Raynaud's syndrome). Answers to the last two questions may help determine a therapeutic approach.

Pressure Measurements

Segmental arterial blood pressure at the brachial, upper forearm, wrist, and proximal digital levels can be measured in the usual way with pneumatic cuffs and a Doppler flow sensor. In most patients with normal arteries, pressures in the two arms at each of these levels differ by only 5 to 8 mm Hg. A pressure difference that exceeds 20 mm Hg indicates a hemodynamically significant arterial obstruction proximal to the site of measurement in the arm with the lower pressure.[3]

Finger blood pressures are measured similarly. Pneumatic cuffs with a width 20% greater than the diameter of the finger are placed around the proximal phalanx (Fig. 2). Return of blood flow as the cuff is deflated can be documented with a Doppler probe placed over a volar digital artery at an interphalangeal joint distal to the cuff or with a mercury strain gauge or photoplethysmograph (PPG) placed on the terminal phalanx. Of these methods, the PPG is the most generally applicable and the easiest to use. To avoid vasoconstriction, measurements must be made in a warm (25°C, 77°F), draft-free room. It may be necessary to warm the hands by immersion in 40°C (104°F) water.

Because finger blood pressures are reduced in proportion to any reduction in brachial, forearm, or wrist blood pressure, it is helpful to calculate a finger-

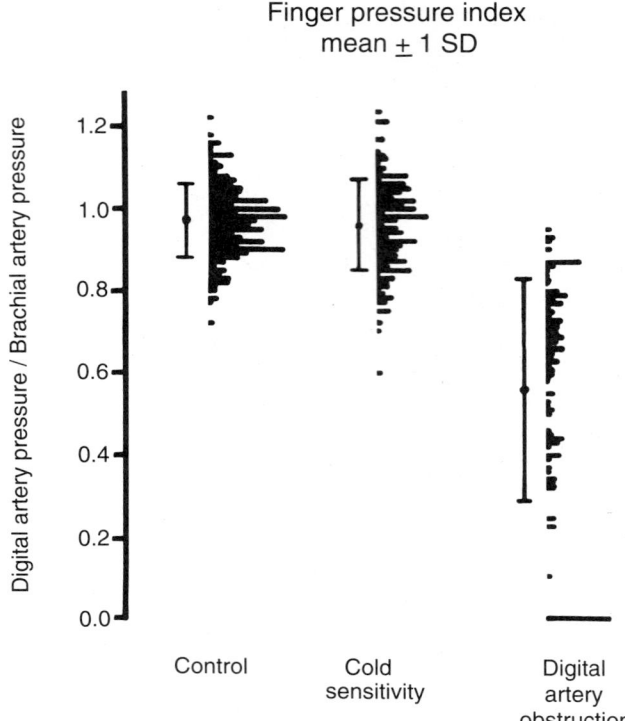

Figure 3 Finger pressure indices (mean ± 1 SD). Cold sensitivity indicates data derived from patients with primary Raynaud's disease. Digital artery obstruction indicates data from patients with fixed arterial disease who did or did not complain of cold sensitivity. (From Sumner DS, Lambeth A, Russell JB: Diagnosis of upper extremity obstructive and vasospastic syndromes by Doppler ultrasound, plethysmography, and temperature profiles. In: Puel P, Boccalon H, Enjalbert A, eds. Hemodynamics of the limbs 1. Toulouse, France: G.E.P.S.C., 1979: 365; with permission.)

brachial pressure index (FBI) by dividing the finger pressure by the ipsilateral brachial pressure. In normal subjects the FBI averages 0.97 ± 0.09 and is rarely less than 0.8 (Fig. 3).[3] Patients with vasospastic Raynaud's syndrome have FBI in the normal range provided the fingers are comfortably warm. Most patients with digital artery obstruction have FBI less than 0.8 and some have FBI of 0.

Digital Plethysmography

Pulse volumes recorded from the fingertips with a mercury strain gauge or PPG may provide additional diagnostic information (Fig. 4). Normal plethysmographic pulses have a rapid upslope, a sharp systolic peak, and a downslope that bows toward the baseline. A dicrotic notch is usually present on the downslope. Pulses recorded from fingers distal to a hemodynamically significant stenosis have a delayed upslope, a rounded peak, and a downslope with no dicrotic notch that bows away from the baseline. Obstructive pulses are useful for identifying arterial disease isolated to the

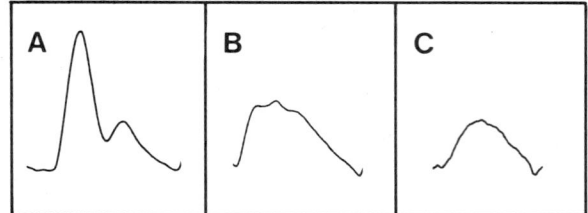

Figure 4 Finger plethysmographic pulse contours. *A*, Normal. *B*, Peaked. *C*, Obstructive. (From Sumner DS. Noninvasive assessment of upper extremity ischemia. In: Bergan JJ, Yao JST, eds. Evaluation and treatment of upper and lower extremity circulatory disorders. Orlando: Grune & Stratton, 1984: 75; with permission.)

terminal phalanges in fingers with normal FBI. An intermediate form, the peaked pulse, has an anacrotic notch or an abrupt bend that terminates in a systolic peak, followed by a dicrotic notch high on the downslope.[4] Peaked pulses have been observed in patients with autoimmune connective tissue disease in the absence of other objective evidence of arterial disease. They may also be associated with arteriolar or digital arterial vasospasm. Because vasoconstriction may alter pulse contours, it is important that plethysmographic studies be obtained when the fingers are warm.

The ability of the peripheral arterioles to dilate can be estimated by monitoring the response of the pulse amplitude to a short period of ischemia (reactive hyperemia test).[3] A pneumatic cuff placed around the forearm is inflated to supersystolic pressures for 5 minutes and then suddenly deflated. In normal subjects and in patients with vasospastic Raynaud's syndrome, plethysmographic pulses return promptly on release of cuff pressure, and the pulse amplitude rapidly increases to double that recorded prior to cuff inflation. However, when the peripheral arterioles are dilated to compensate for an increased proximal resistance or when they are stiffened by autoimmune disease, pulses return slowly and there is little or no increase in pulse amplitude.

When the sympathetic nerves are intact, digit pulse amplitude and fingertip volume decrease in response to a deep breath, to mental arithmetic, and to the application of ice placed on the chest or forehead.[3,5] A diminished or absent response, often observed in patients with connective tissue diseases, implies impaired sympathetic activity.

Duplex and Doppler Examinations

Obstructions involving axillary, brachial, and forearm arteries can be localized and their extent evaluated with conventional duplex or color-flow scanning. Surveys with a hand-held Doppler may be sufficient. Although it is difficult to image stenoses of the subclavian arteries, disturbances of the Doppler flow spectrum will usually establish the diagnosis. Aneurysms, which may give rise to emboli, are easily imaged. Patency of the distal radial or ulnar arteries and the palmar arch can be determined by noting the effect of sequential compression of the radial and ulnar arteries on the midpalmar Doppler flow signal.[3] This test is more easily interpreted than the classic Allen's test, which relies on visual evidence of return of blood flow to the hand after release of arterial compression at the wrist, the hand having first been depleted of blood by opening and closing the fist during arterial inflow compression.

Occlusions of the proper digital arteries can be detected by examining Doppler flow patterns on both sides of the fingers at the volar interphalangeal creases. Signals are occasionally detected at the distal interphalangeal joint in the absence of signals at the proximal interphalangeal joint on the same side of the finger. In this event, compression of the proximal digital artery on the other side of the finger will often obliterate the signal, confirming the presence of a cross-over collateral. A loud signal obtained from the volar surface of the fingertip indicates good perfusion and is typical of the hyperemic phase of vasospastic Raynaud's syndrome. Again, to avoid the confounding effects of vasoconstriction, Doppler surveys of the fingers must be performed when the hand is warm.

Tests for Vasospasm

A clear description of Raynaud's phenomenon may be sufficient to establish the diagnosis of episodic vasospasm in a reliable patient. However, in some instances, especially those involving industrial injury or compensation, a more objective method is desirable. Although simply shaking the cold clammy hands of a victim of this malady suggests the diagnosis, attempts to induce the typical triphasic color changes in the laboratory environment may be frustrating.

Porter and associates[6] described a simple test that involves measurement of fingertip temperature with thermistors before and after immersion of the hand in ice water for 20 seconds. Immediately after exposure to cold, fingertip temperatures in all subjects are depressed to similar levels, but the temperature returns to pre-exposure levels much more rapidly in normal subjects than it does in patients with vasospasm. When a 10-minute recovery time is used to divide normal from abnormal responses, this test is about 90% sensitive and 80% specific for detecting or ruling out cold-induced vasospasm.[3]

A more elaborate test devised by Nielsen and Lassen[7] measures digital arterial pressures at progressively decreasing finger temperatures. A cuff placed around the proximal phalanx is inflated to supersystolic pressures and perfused for 5 minutes with water at temperatures ranging from 30°C (86°F) to 10°C (50°F). The cuff is then gradually deflated until return of blood flow is sensed by a mercury strain gauge applied to the fingertip. Whereas digital arterial pressures in normal subjects decrease by only $16 \pm 3\%$ at a perfusion temperature of 10°C, the blood pressure in patients with vasospasm falls rapidly with decreasing temperature and then precipitously to 0 as a trigger point is reached. The trigger point varies from 10° to 20°C (68°F) depending on the individual patient. Unfortunately, this test is time consuming, requires expensive equipment not available in most laboratories, and is not clearly superior to the cold immersion test described above.[8]

Another less complicated method is to measure finger blood pressures while the entire hand is immersed in water at decreasing temperatures. In the absence of cold-induced vasospasm, there is little change in blood pressure at 10°C; but blood pressures in vasospastic fingers are markedly reduced, averaging 13 ± 38 mm Hg in one study.[9] Many patients with Raynaud's syndrome have reduced finger blood pressures and digit plethysmographic pulses even when they are in a warm laboratory. If the abnormal findings are due to vasospasm rather than to fixed arterial obstruction, finger blood pressures and digit pulses become normal when the hand is warmed by immersion in 40°C (104°F) water.

APPLICATION OF NONINVASIVE TESTS

The history and physical examination will usually determine which noninvasive tests are likely to be most informative. Arterial obstruction proximal to the hand is easily confirmed or ruled out by blood pressure measurements, Doppler surveys, or duplex imaging (Fig. 5). If proximal obstruction is documented, further tests are seldom necessary unless emboli to the hand are suspected.

If the inflow vessels are normal, the next step is to examine the palmar arch and finger circulation. An incomplete palmar arch may represent a congenital variant, in which case digital blood pressures and plethysmographic waveforms will be normal. An incomplete palmar arch coupled with decreased blood pressures and abnormal plethysmographic waveforms in the fourth and fifth fingers of a patient with a history of percussive trauma to the hand suggests a hypothenar hammer syndrome. In these patients compression of the radial artery will obliterate the palmar arch signal and further reduce blood pressures in the involved fingers, but compression of the ulnar artery will have no effect.

All fingers of both hands should be studied even when the patient's symptoms are confined to a single digit, since a complete examination may disclose widespread subclinical lesions in one or both hands. If only one finger is involved or if multiple fingers are affected but positive findings are restricted to one hand, localized trauma or microemboli should be considered. Such patients may give a history of using vibrating tools (jackhammers or chain saws) or may have symptoms suggesting a thoracic outlet syndrome. A poststenotic dilation or a subclavian aneurysm may be discovered by duplex examination. Patients with connective tissue (autoimmune) diseases usually have diffuse involvement of the fingers of both hands. When the disease process is confined to the terminal digital vessels, abnormal plethysmographic pulses may be the only positive finding.

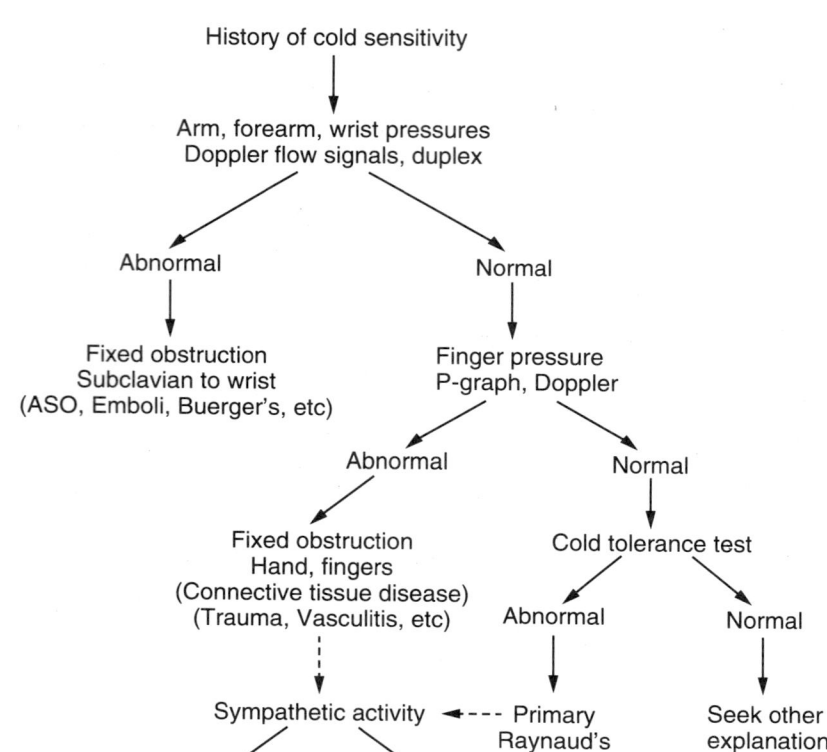

Figure 5 Algorithm depicting an approach to the diagnosis of upper extremity vasospastic disease.

If a thorough noninvasive examination documents no abnormalities when the hands are warm, it is likely that the patient has primary Raynaud's disease (vasospastic Raynaud's syndrome), provided that cold sensitivity can be documented by history, direct observation, or cold tolerance tests (see Fig. 5). When the history is in doubt and vasospasm cannot be elicited, another explanation for the patient's symptoms should be sought.

Reactive hyperemia tests and tests for sympathetic activity may be performed in a effort to predict which patients with cold sensitivity are likely to benefit from vasodilator therapy. Most patients with primary Raynaud's disease show active responses to these tests, but many patients with secondary Raynaud's phenomenon do not.

OTHER INVESTIGATIONS

Arteriography is required only when aneurysms or other sources for emboli are suspected or when operative therapy is contemplated. Selected laboratory tests for hypercoagulability, connective tissue diseases, and other associated problems may be indicated when noninvasive evaluation confirms or suggests obstructive Raynaud's syndrome and a traumatic cause has been excluded. In addition to the usual laboratory panel, routine measurement of the erythrocyte sedimentation rate, rheumatoid factor, and anti–nuclear antibody levels has been advocated. More sophisticated tests are reserved for specific indications. Blood tests are seldom positive in patients with normal noninvasive findings who fit the profile of vasospastic Raynaud's syndrome. In the vast majority, perhaps 95% of these patients, cold sensitivity is a benign condition, little more than a nuisance. Although a few patients in this category may ultimately develop a connective tissue disease, this outcome is most likely in patients with positive or equivocal noninvasive tests or in those with suggestive clinical signs or serologic abnormalities.[2] Microscopic examination of nailfold capillaries is reported to have prognostic value.[10] Patients in whom capillary loops are enlarged, dilated, and distorted with areas of nailfold avascularity are more likely to develop connective tissue diseases than those with uniformly distributed normal appearing capillaries.

REFERENCES

1. Maricq HR, Weinrich MC, Keil JE, LeRoy EC. Prevalence of Raynaud's phenomenon in the general population: A preliminary study by questionnaire. J Chron Dis 1986; 39:423–427.
2. Edwards JM, Porter JM. Long-term outcome of Raynaud's syndrome. In: Yao JST, Pearce WH, eds. Long-term results in vascular surgery. Norwalk, Conn: Appleton & Lange, 1993: 345.
3. Sumner DS. Evaluation of acute and chronic ischemia of the upper extremity. In: Rutherford RB, ed. Vascular surgery, 3rd ed. Philadelphia: WB Saunders, 1989: 806.

4. Sumner DS, Strandness DE Jr. An abnormal finger pulse associated with cold sensitivity. Ann Surg 1972; 175:294–298.
5. Delius W, Kellerova E. Reactions of arterial and venous vessels in the human forearm and hand to deep breath or mental strain. Clin Sci 1971; 40:271–282.
6. Porter JM, Snider RL, Bardana EJ, et al. The diagnosis and treatment of Raynaud's phenomenon. Surgery 1975; 77:11–23.
7. Nielsen SL, Lassen NA. Measurement of digital blood pressure after local cooling. J Appl Physiol 1977; 43:907–910.
8. Carter SA, Dean E, Kroeger EA. Apparent finger systolic pressures during cooling in patients with Raynaud's syndrome. Circulation 1988; 77:988–996.
9. DiGiacomo RA, Kremer JM, Shah DM. Fish-oil dietary supplementation in patients with Raynaud's phenomenon: A double-blind, controlled, prospective study. Am J Med 1989; 86:158–164.
10. Fitzgerald O, O'Connor GT, Spencer-Green G. Prospective study of the evolution of Raynaud's phenomenon. Am J Med 1988; 84:718–726.

TREATMENT OF UPPER EXTREMITY VASOSPASTIC DISEASE

JOHN W. JOYCE, M.D.

Raynaud's phenomenon, livedo reticularis, and acrocyanosis are well-defined entities classified as the vasospastic disorders. They are characterized by color changes of the skin induced or intensified by stimuli increasing vasomotor tone, usually reduced environmental temperature, and less frequently, emotion or drugs. Each is usually mild, and no specific therapy is required. All three, however, can cause significant symptoms, induce tissue loss, and secondary mechanisms that warrant diagnosis and treatment. These observations apply to a significant number of those with Raynaud's phenomenon and only occasionally to patients with livedo reticularis or acrocyanosis. Color and temperature changes, edema, and varying degrees of discomfort attributable to vasomotor activity are also seen with reflex sympathetic dystrophy and causalgia and various neurogenic and disuse syndromes of the limbs.

RAYNAUD'S PHENOMENON

Raynaud's phenomenon is characterized by episodes of color changes in the distal phalanges of the fingers, less frequently the toes, and rarely the nose or ears. Most common is a white or waxy blanching during the acute phase, less common cyanosis with or without blanching, followed by red or violaceous red during the recovery phase of reactive hyperemia in most. A few patients note all three colors but a history of triphasic color change is not essential for the diagnosis. The involved area is cool during the acute phase, and patients describe a numb or "dead" sensation but rarely pain. Varying degrees of distress, from burning dysesthesia to throbbing pain, are common during the hyperemic recovery phase. Attacks last as long as the exposure, and recovery takes a few minutes of rewarming. Depending on the severity of the disease, episodes may be triggered only by extreme cold or by modest temperature shifts induced by air conditioning, drafts, cool water, or handling cold objects. With progression of the syndrome, particularly when an obstructive component is present, additional digits and proximal phalanges are involved, symptoms are increased, and recovery is prolonged. The thumb is often spared. Digital infarction or ulceration is almost always indicative of secondary Raynaud's phenomenon and obstructive disease.

Both the treatment and prognosis of Raynaud's phenomenon depend upon establishing whether the pathophysiologic mechanism is primarily spasm or spasm with underlying arterial occlusive disease. The Allen and Brown[1] criteria state that if the patient has bilateral symmetrical Raynaud's phenomenon with no local, systemic, or laboratory abnormalities for 2 or more years, the process will usually remain local and benign. Such patients have been classified as having Raynaud's disease, primary Raynaud's phenomenon, idiopathic Raynaud's syndrome, and Raynaud's phenomenon, cause unknown. A modest number of such patients develop connective tissue disease, predominantly scleroderma, in later years.

Disease mechanisms associated with Raynaud's phenomenon are extensive and diverse (Table 1). Secondary causes are reported in 30% to 60% or more of patients seeking care. Such studies often reflect the type of practice reporting their experience, and the true prevalence of secondary cause is probably less, as many patients with the uncomplicated vasospastic form do not seek care. The term Raynaud's phenomenon is reserved for the event. Cases are then classified tentatively as primary (presumed spasm, no detectable secondary cause) and secondary (spasm, with demonstrable secondary cause that is usually obstructive). Periodic follow-up of patients with primary Raynaud's phenomenon is advised to detect those who later develop secondary mechanisms.

A historical and physical assessment of the patient, with selected laboratory testing, can establish a diagnosis, define secondary mechanisms, and guide initial prognosis and therapy (Table 1). Coffman[2] and Cooke and co-workers[3] provide excellent contemporary monographs for detailed documentation of the history, patho-

Table 1 Causes of Secondary Raynaud's Phenomenon

Arterial disease	Drugs
Proximal plaque, emboli	Ergot
Proximal aneurysm, emboli	Methysergide
Prior cardiac emboli	Phenylpropanolamine
Thoracic outlet, emboli	Beta-blockade
Thromboangiitis obliterans	Bleomycin/vincristin
	Bromocriptine
Connective tissue disorder	
Scleroderma	**Occupational**
Mixed collagen disease	Vibrating tools
Periarteritis nodosa	Hypothenar hammer
Polymyositis	syndrome
Rheumatoid arthritis	Vinyl chloride disease
Sjogrens syndrome	Cold injury
Systemic lupus erythematosus	
	Metabolic disorders
Hematologic disorders	Myxedema
Polycythemia vera	Pheochromocytoma
Thrombocytosis	
Cryoglobulinemia	**Neurogenic**
Macroglobulinemia	Carpal tunnel syndrome
Cold agglutinens	Thoracic outlet (neurogenic)
Hepatitis B, C antigenemia	Nerve injury
	Cord injury
Miscellaneous	
Malignancy	
Primary pulmonary hypertension	

physiology, epidemiology, pharmacologic data, and care of Raynaud's phenomenon.

TREATMENT

General Measures

Time spent explaining the normal vasoreactivity of the skin, the exaggerated response of Raynaud's phenomenon, and an insight into the natural history of the syndrome of the particular patient is well invested. As in all medical encounters, such information enhances patient compliance and removes both false fears and expectations. Complete abstinence from tobacco is advised because of both its long-term adverse effect on the respiratory and cardiovascular systems and its potential for additional vasospastic impact on the disease. A few patients report the induction of episodes with smoking, and a small number note a decrease in attacks when tobacco use is stopped. The drugs listed in Table 1 are stopped if their use parallels the onset of the syndrome. In patients with established disease, these agents can be initiated when indicated, then discontinued if episodes are potentiated. The evidence that anovulatory agents can induce Raynaud's phenomenon is negligible, but a period of observation off the drug should be considered in a patient with significant symptoms, after which a decision can be made regarding the drug's role.

It is important that the patient understand that warmth of the whole body, rather than just the hands, can significantly reduce the frequency and severity of episodes. Head wear and clothing for the neck, trunk, and limbs need emphasis equal to that of double-layered mittens. Gloves left near the deep freeze or at the door for quick outdoor errands are also suggested. Few patients benefit from a move to warmer climates, as episodes are still induced by dropping evening temperatures, air conditioning, and exposure to cool water or objects. However, some patients who work in cold environments such as the food industry or in garages and warehouses have such bothersome symptoms that a change in work should be encouraged and supported. Electric and battery-powered hand warmers and gloves help enough that their cost and inconveniences are warranted for some patients.

Drug Therapy

The great majority of patients can remain productive at home and work if they follow the measures outlined. However, some cannot change their work environment and are handicapped by insensitive, cold, or stiff hands. For these patients and those with ischemic ulcerations, a trial of pharmacologic agents is worthwhile. No single agent consistently improves Raynaud's phenomenon or clears it completely. Response can be expected in half or less of any group of patients using any agent, and with all, side effects must be weighed against any gain in symptom control. Over the decades many sympatholytic, direct-dilating, and adrenoreceptor blocking agents have been used with partial success. Each can have bothersome side effects. A partial list includes reserpine, guanethidine, phenoxybenzamine, papaverine, niacin, hydralazine, and methyldopa. Significant postural hypotension, disturbed intestinal function, edema, male impotence, fatigue, and mood alteration to the point of depression are some of the symptoms limiting their use. However, each is worthy of trial if contemporary agents fail.

Nifedipine is the most satisfactory of all agents, reducing symptoms in about half of those using it. It is the most potent peripheral dilator of all calcium channel blocking agents, and side effects of orthostatism, nausea, and headache usually clear during the first 2 weeks of use. Modest edema, which is not infrequent, can be controlled by diuretics. The initial dose is 10 mg three times daily, and it may be increased to 20 mg three or four times daily. Prazosin, 2 to 5 mg daily has also benefited a few patients. Another alpha-adrenoreceptor blocker, doxazosin meslate, 8 mg three times daily, has anecdotally been a significant help to a patient with advanced scleroderma. Clearly, a period of observed titration with several drugs in sequence or combination is often required when treating Raynaud's phenomenon.

As the understanding of endothelial biology and circulatory regulatory mechanisms has increased in the past 2 decades, new classes of agents have undergone trial. These include the angiotension-converting enzyme inhibitor Captopril; ketanserin, a serotonin antagonist;

the alpha-adrenergic blocking agent thymoxamine; and iloprost, a prostoglandin analog. All have been shown to reduce Raynaud's episodes in a modest percentage of patients treated, and iloprost has enhanced healing of ischemic digits in some patients.[4] It must be given intravenously over several days. These additional agents all warrant consideration when nifedipine, prazosin, and guanethidine fail.

Sympathectomy

That adrenergic stimuli can constrict small arteries and arterioles has long been appreciated, and sympathectomy has been documented to minimize or eliminate episodes of vasospastic Raynaud's phenomenon. Because this effect commonly dissipates within 2 years, sympathectomy is not advocated for these patients. Some advise sympathectomy for ischemic necrosis secondary to proximal occlusive disease, but I side with those who believe equal results are obtained with local wound care and selective amputation when indicated. On rare occasion cervical or lumbar sympathectomy have been recommended to manage pain in patients with thromboangiitis obliterans when a preliminary sympathetic block has given significant relief.

Reconditioning

Some success in reducing the frequency of Raynaud's episodes has been demonstrated both by biofeedback techniques and Pavlovian conditioning.[5,6] Either modality is worthy of trial if trained personnel are available.

Treating Associated Disease

Vasospastic Raynaud's phenomenon induced by drugs clears as the agent is eliminated from the body, and it also clears when myxedema and pheochromocytoma are effectively treated. Raynaud's phenomenon induced by vibrating tools will disappear if the activity is stopped before the process induces fixed arterial wall changes, a phenomenon that occurs after a few years of symptoms. Patients with a cardiac source of emboli are treated with anticoagulants. Those with proximal arterial plaque, aneurysm, or thoracic outlet lesions that embolize require arterial reconstruction to prevent further episodes. Surgical relief of nerve compression at the thoracic outlet or carpal tunnel can eliminate the syndrome. Further arterial damage can be prevented in patients with periarteritis nodosa, systemic lupus, and mixed collagen disease by treating with steroids and/or cytotoxic agents or anticoagulation when a circulating anticoagulant or anticardiolipin antibody accompanies these disorders. Further thrombotic episodes can also be prevented in polycythemia vera and thrombocytosis with appropriate medical control. Plasmapheresis has been reported to reduce occlusive events in some patients with cryoglobulinemia, hepatitis B and C antigenemia, and certain severe cases of Raynaud's syndrome with digital ulceration and uncertain etiology. Many patients who sustain occlusive Raynaud's phenomenon from an acute medical or surgical thrombotic source will show gradual improvement or clearing of the phenomenon as years pass if the primary process is treated and no new events occur. Ulceration occurs over areas of calcinosis in some patients with scleroderma. Gentle surgical debridement of deposits near the elbow, sacrum, and phalangeal pads accelerates healing and pain control.

LIVEDO RETICULARIS

Livedo reticularis, the most common vasospastic disorder, is often accepted as a normal skin variant or not even noted by patient or physician. It is seen predominantly in postpubescent women and some fair-skinned males. It is a diffuse, symmetric meshlike pattern varying from pink to pale blue to violaceous. It is seen on all four limbs and sometimes the trunk and is most prominent distally and in the legs. Cold enhances and heat and exercise decrease its intensity. Skin temperature is usually normal, but many patients get cold hands and feet more easily than normal. A modest number will also have Raynaud's phenomenon, and a few will have acrocyanosis. Spasm of the vertical dermal arterioles with dilation of distal capillaries and venules is the pathophysiologic mechanism. The color is produced by an increase in reduced oxyhemoglobin secondary to slowed blood flow. No treatment is required.

Primary livedo reticularis in a few instances will be complicated in later decades by sclerosis and/or occlusion of the feeding arterioles and by hemosiderin deposition in the mesh, chiefly in the feet, ankles, and lower legs. Small superficial and painful ulcerations occur in these areas at points of pressure or trauma and heal very slowly with bed rest and topical soaks. Many drugs, including antiplatelet agents, steroids, cyclophosphamide, methotrexate, penoxyfylline, and beta-adrenoceptor antagonists, have been tried with minimal or unpredictable results. Nifedipine 10 to 20 mg three times daily is prescribed but the drug is continued only if pain is reduced with a week's trial. Anecdotal experience suggests that lumbar sympathectomy on occasion can lessen pain, accelerate healing, and minimize recurrences. The operation is considered if a sympathetic block significantly reduces pain for 24 or more hours. Knee-length elastic support hosiery is also empirically prescribed because of the venous component and the mild edema often noted.

Secondary livedo reticularis is seen with several disease states (Table 2). The lesions caused by vasculitis and atheroembolism are often patchy, random, and asymmetric, may be inflamed and elevated, and later may infarct or ulcerate. The embolic source of atheroemboli is surgically treated when feasible. Chemotherapy of the myeloproliferative disorders and treatment of vasculitis with steroids and cytotoxic agents can prevent further episodes. Livedo reticularis associated

Table 2 Causes of Secondary Livedo Reticularis

Atherothrombotic microembolism
Systemic lupus erythematosus
Periarteritis nodosa
Cutaneous vasculitis
Polycythemia vera
Thrombocytosis
Dysproteinemia
Amantadine therapy
Prior cold injury
Neurolgenic disuse syndromes

with cold injury, neurogenic disuse syndromes, and amatadine therapy is benign.

ACROCYANOSIS

This is the least common vasospastic disorder; only 3 to 5 patients are seen yearly in this vascular center. It is characterized by a constant rather than episodic uniform cyanosis of the nails, digits, hands, feet, and sometimes forearms, with decreased skin temperature of the involved areas attributed to an increase in vasomotor tone. The findings are intensified by cold and emotion and ameliorated by warmth and exercise. Modest edema of the phalanges and some hyperhidrosis are noted by many patients. Livedo reticularis also is often present, but episodes of Raynaud's phenomenon are uncommon. Acrocyanosis is not complicated with ulceration or infarction in its primary form and is usually a cosmetic or social nuisance. Encouragingly, most patients improve with nifedipine 10 mg or prazosin 2 to 5 mg, each taken three times daily. The majority of patients are not bothered enough to require treatment. They benefit from an understanding of the benign pathophysiology.

Hyperhidrosis on rare occasions becomes a handicap. Aluminum chloride hexahydrate in alcohol solution applied to the involved skin overnight, initially daily and later every 5 to 10 days, can effectively reduce perspiration. Bilateral cervical sympathectomy, as described by Greenhalgh,[7] is reserved for very problematic symptoms.

Acrocyanosis is associated with scleroderma on occasion. It is also observed with polycythemia vera and primary thrombocytosis, sometimes with a paradoxic bipolar oversensitivity to warmth inducing erythromelalgia. Treatment of the hematologic disorder clears both the acrocyanosis and erythromelalgia. Intense acrocyanosis of the hands and feet has been noted in several patients on chronic propranolol therapy. Two such patients had periungual ulcers of the toes in winter, similar to pernio. The syndrome clears on stopping the drug.

REFERENCES

1. Allen EV, Brown GE. Raynaud's disease: A critical review of minimal requisites for diagnosis. Am J Med Sci 1932; 193:187–200.
2. Coffman JD. Raynaud's phenomenon. New York: Oxford University Press, 1989:186.
3. Cooke ED, Nicolaides AN, Porter JM. Raynaud's syndrome. London: Med-Orion, 1991:215.
4. Wigley FM, Wise RA, Seibold JR, et al. Intravenous iloprost in patients with Raynaud's phenomenon secondary to systemic sclerosis: A multicenter, placebo-controlled, double-blind study. Ann Intern Med 1994; 120:199–206.
5. Jobe JB, Sampson JB, Roberts DE, Beethan WP Jr. Induced vasodilation as treatment for Raynaud's disease. Ann Intern Med 1982; 97:706–710.
6. Freedman RR, Ianni P, Wenig P. Behavioral treatment of Raynaud's disease. J Consult Clin Psychol, 1983; 51:539–544.
7. Greenhalgh RM. The management of hyperhidrosis. In: Bergan JJ, Yao JST, eds. Evaluation and treatment of upper and lower extremity circulatory disorders. New York: Grune & Stratton, 1984:509.

BUERGER'S DISEASE

TIMOTHY F. KRESOWIK, M.D.

Buerger's disease was probably first described by Winiwarter in a case report in 1879,[1] but it was Buerger[2] in 1908 who coined the term thromboangiitis obliterans in a pathologic study of amputated limbs. The very existence of Buerger's disease as an entity distinct from atherosclerosis was questioned in the late 1950s and early 1960s, but the distinguishing features of this disease were well outlined in a report by McKusick and co-workers[3] in 1962. At present Buerger's disease is considered a relatively rare but well-accepted cause of limb-threatening ischemia in young adults. Patients with it are generally not greeted with enthusiasm by the vascular surgeon because of the often limited reconstructive options and recalcitrant smoking behavior of the patients. Emphasis on distinguishing this disease from atherosclerosis is probably misplaced, because although there may be differences in prognosis between Buerger's disease and atherosclerosis, there is no proven specific therapy for Buerger's disease. Buerger's disease in itself does not appear to have the same implications for associated coronary artery disease and poor long-term survival that is associated with extremity atherosclerotic disease.[4] The multitude of therapeutic options is testimony to the lack of clear-cut efficacy of many of them.

ETIOLOGY

Although the absolute importance of smoking in the initiation and progression of this disease has been questioned,[4] most reports have considered smoking to be an essential feature of the disease.[5,6] The mechanism through which smoking promotes the disease is unknown but may be immune related. The activation of both the cellular and humoral immune systems seen in Buerger's disease patients and the inflammatory vascular pathologic findings suggest immune-related mechanisms.[7] Genetic predisposition also appears to play a role, which is illustrated by racial differences in incidence (much higher in Asia than North America) and by the higher frequency of certain HLA patterns seen in patients with Buerger's disease.[3,7] Smoking correlates well with progression of disease.[5,6,8] It is important to recognize that self-reported smoking behavior is unreliable. Thus, reliance on self-reporting may account for reports of disease progression in the absence of smoking.[8] Passive exposure to smoke may also explain some cases of disease progression after the patient has quit smoking. The virulence of the smoking addiction in many patients with Buerger's disease is well known. It is hard to understand how otherwise healthy young adults can continue to smoke after loss of one or more limbs and a seemingly firm understanding of the relationship between smoking and the disease. The severity of the addiction leads to speculation that the mechanisms underlying the disease process also heighten some of the pleasurable effects of smoking.

DIAGNOSIS

The diagnosis of Buerger's disease rests on clinical criteria. Smoking should probably be considered an essential feature. The predilection for distal vessel involvement is characteristic (Fig. 1). In the lower extremities severe obstructive changes occur in the digital, pedal, and crural arteries, often with sparing of the popliteal and more proximal vessels, although the proximal vessels can become involved in late stages of the disease (Fig. 2). Premature atherosclerosis is a more likely diagnosis when there is early or predominant proximal involvement. Upper extremity disease is present in more than 50% of patients.[5,6] Like those of the lower extremities, the digital, palmar, and forearm vessels are usually involved, with sparing of the brachial and subclavian arteries. Because of the distal obstructive predominance, the patients often have tissue loss and concomitant ischemic rest pain as their initial complaint. Occasionally foot or hand claudication will be the presenting complaint. Raynaud's phenomenon may be present. In patients with Buerger's disease Raynaud's phenomenon is due to cold-induced collateral vasoconstriction superimposed on fixed vascular occlusions rather than an abnormal vasospastic response to cold. One-third or more of patients have a history of venous involvement, with migratory superficial phlebitis being

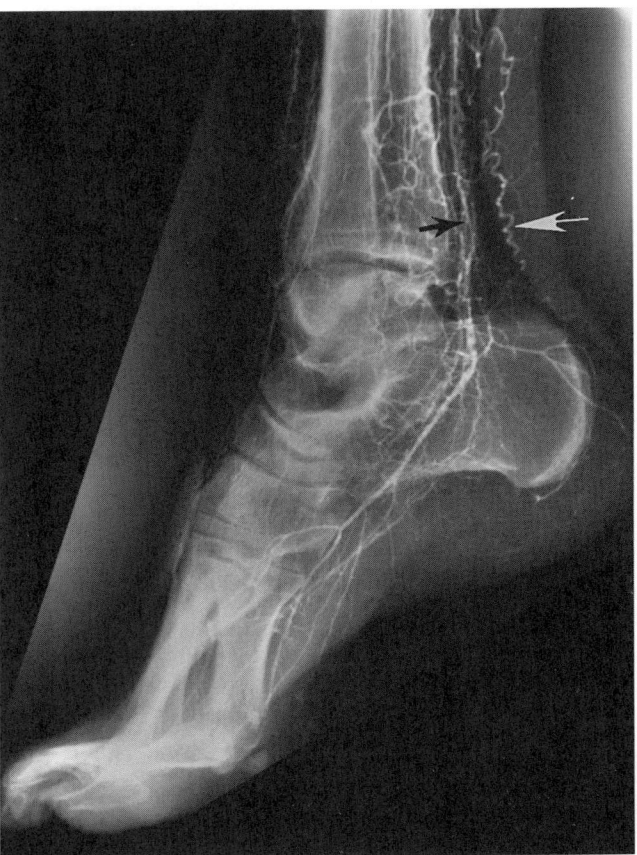

Figure 1 Arteriogram in a 31-year-old man with Buerger's disease who presented with ischemic rest pain and a nonhealing foot ulcer. The distal occlusive pattern is well demonstrated. Tree-root collaterals (*black arrow*); Corkscrew collaterals (*white arrow*).

the most common venous manifestation.[5,6] Like the arterial component, the superficial veins of the hand or foot are more commonly involved than the major saphenous or brachiocephalic trunk. The migratory superficial phlebitis may be manifest by a history of recurrent painful red nodules on the distal extremities.

Buerger's disease is a disease of young adults with an onset between ages 20 and 40 years. Individuals with onset later in life may have Buerger's disease, but the overlap with atherosclerosis makes a clear distinction more difficult. At one time Buerger's disease appeared to occur almost exclusively in men. In recent reports women account for approximately 20% of patients,[5,6] perhaps because more women smoke.

To some degree the diagnosis of Buerger's disease is made by exclusion. Patients with diabetes are excluded because a similar pattern of lower extremity arterial disease occurs in diabetic patients. Patients who have risk factors besides smoking for atherosclerosis with involvement of proximal and nonextremity vessels are usually not categorized as having Buerger's disease. Probably the inclusion of patients with premature

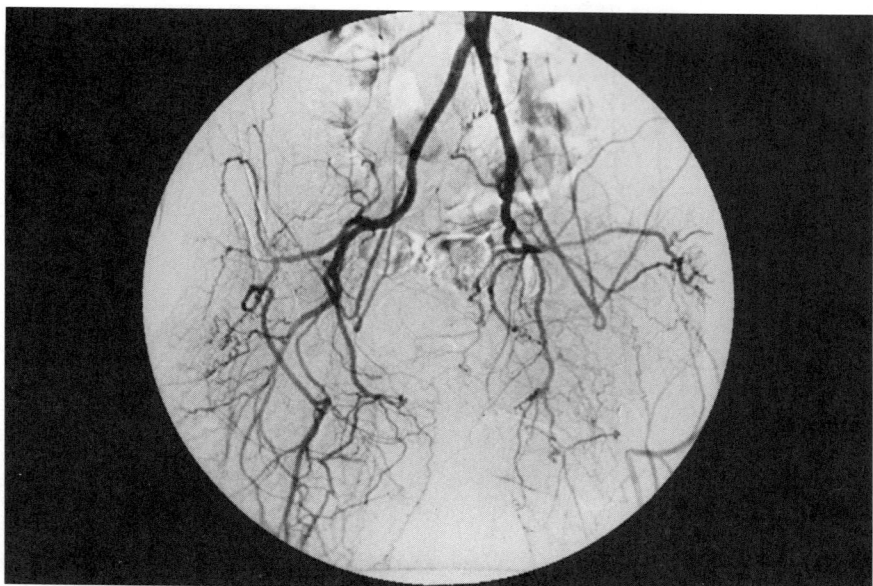

Figure 2 Pelvic arteriogram demonstrating late proximal occlusive disease in a 39-year-old man with a 10 year history of Buerger's disease who continued to smoke despite bilateral below-knee amputations and multiple bilateral finger amputations. The patient presented with a nonhealing right below-knee stump ischemic ulcer and was treated with a polytetrafluoroethylene iliac to deep femoral bypass. The patient has been maintained on both coumadin and aspirin with continued patency of the bypass at 1 year and healing of the stump ulcer.

atherosclerosis in some reports of so-called Buerger's disease has led to some of the confusion in the literature about this disease. Other forms of arteritis should be excluded before making the diagnosis of Buerger's disease. If a connective tissue disease is suggested by the history, studies such as erythrocyte sedimentation rate, anti–nuclear antigens and rheumatoid factor should be obtained. Embolic disease or local small vessel vascular trauma as is seen in the hands of patients who operate vibrating tools should also be considered in the differential diagnosis. Although hypercoagulability may play a role in the pathophysiology of Buerger's disease, patients with documented hypercoaguable states are usually excluded.

Noninvasive laboratory studies are useful in supplementing clinical findings. Extremity blood pressures may confirm the distal versus proximal obstructive pattern. Digital blood pressures measured with a small pneumatic cuff and a photoplethysmography transducer to detect the pulsatile signal are probably the most useful. Digital blood pressures less than 80% of brachial pressure are considered abnormal. In addition to having some prognostic value in predicting healing, measurement of digital blood pressure may document the presence of disease in asymptomatic limbs. The documentation of asymptomatic upper extremity small vessel involvement may help establish the diagnosis of Buerger's disease.

Arteriography may not be necessary to make the diagnosis if conservative treatment or minor amputation is planned. Arteriography should always be performed prior to consideration of a major amputation to exclude the possibility of a situation amenable to vascular reconstruction. The typical arteriographic pattern is that of distal involvement with normal-appearing proximal vessels. Abrupt occlusions and skip lesions with seemingly normal vessels in between are common findings. Corkscrew or tree-root collaterals are not specific to Buerger's disease but rather reflect the distal vessel occlusive pattern.

Arterial biopsy should not be performed solely to establish the diagnosis of Buerger's disease. Examination of amputation specimens may reveal a typical histologic picture, but the late stage of disease may be indistinguishable from other causes of small vessel occlusion. Typical histologic features of Buerger's disease[3,5] include inflammatory cells seen throughout the vessel wall without the destruction of the wall architecture that is seen in typical arteritis. Thrombus in the lumen of the vessel will also contain inflammatory cells, often clumps of polymorphonuclear leukocytes described as microabscesses. Multinucleated giant cells within the thrombus are another typical feature. In late stages there will be organization and partial recanalization of the thrombus along with perivascular fibrotic changes sometimes involving the veins and nerve in the neurovascular bundle (Fig. 3).

TREATMENT

By far the most important and perhaps the only intervention with proven benefit is helping the patient to quit smoking. Large series suggest that progression of

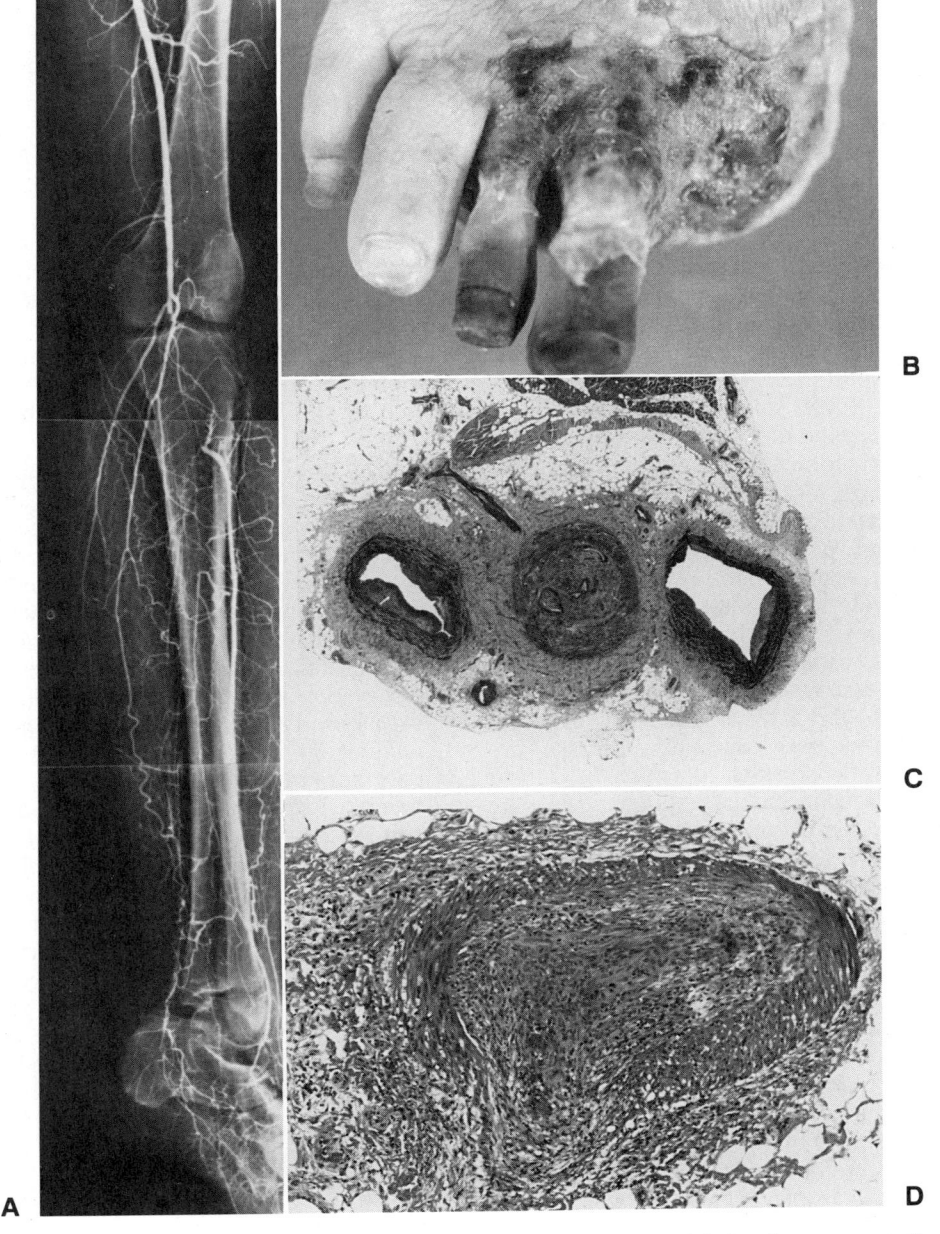

Figure 3 A 25-year-old woman with Buerger's disease who had already required a left below-knee amputation and a right great toe amputation who continued to smoke and presented with a nonhealing right toe amputation site and second and third toe gangrene. *A*, Arteriogram demonstrating popliteal, tibial, and pedal occlusive disease with segmental reconstitution of the anterior tibial artery. The patient underwent a superficial femoral to anterior tibial bypass with vein and a transmetatarsal amputation with a delayed primary closure. *B*, Photograph of amputation specimen. *C*, Microscopic (Elastichrome stain, original magnification 4X) view showing an artery in the center with occlusion of the lumen by reacanalized thrombotic material. The basic structure of the arterial wall is intact. Adventitial fibrosis surrounds both the artery and adjacent veins, which also exhibit some degree of phlebosclerosis. *D*, Higher power (H&E, original magnification 10X) view of a different artery in the same specimen demonstrating an early active lesion with acute inflammation associated with a fibrin thrombus.

disease is rare if the patient stops smoking.[5,6] Since the important component of tobacco smoke in promoting the disease is unknown and Buerger's disease has been reported with use of smokeless tobacco alone,[6] all tobacco products should be avoided. Whether or not transdermal nicotine supplements have deleterious effects on disease progression is unknown. Since nicotine supplements may be useful in helping the patient quit smoking, they should not be considered contraindicated. Chronic use of nicotine supplements should be avoided.

The addiction to tobacco is strong in the majority of these patients, but rates of smoking discontinuation approach 50% in some studies.[5] If cessation of smoking does halt the disease process, the seeming hopelessness that has been expressed about antismoking counseling in these patients may be more apparent than real. The patients who return with further problems are unable to stop smoking, and these make up the majority of the experience of the individual vascular surgeon.

A conservative approach to minor tissue loss is warranted in treating patients with Buerger's disease. If focal distal digital gangrene is present without infection, watchful waiting for autoamputation may be the most prudent course. Ischemic ulceration responds better to a moist wound environment than dry or wet-to-dry dressings. Silver sulfadiazine or antibiotic ointment is used to keep the ulcer moist and discourage bacterial growth. In addition to possibly improving the rate of healing, this type of dressing seems to be less painful for the patient. If more extensive gangrene is present, digital blood pressures may be useful in predicting healing of a minor amputation. Pressures greater than 40 mm Hg suggest a reasonable healing potential. Arteriography should be performed prior to amputation in patients with digital blood pressures less than 20 mm Hg to assess the possibility of vascular reconstruction. Although patency rates of bypasses performed for patients with Buerger's disease are markedly inferior to the results in other causes of vascular obstruction,[6] reconstruction should always be considered prior to a major amputation. Patients with multiple levels of obstruction may have enough improvement of perfusion, even with a bypass to an isolated crural artery segment, to allow healing of ulceration or a minor amputation. Since poor runoff is the rule and Buerger's disease patients may be relatively hypercoaguable, a more aggressive approach to postbypass antithrombotic therapy, e.g., warfarin and aspirin in combination, may be appropriate.

Although noninvasive measurements such as digital blood pressures are somewhat predictive of healing, even low or absent digital blood pressures should not preclude an attempt at minor amputation prior to a major amputation if vascular reconstruction is not possible or has failed. A delayed primary closure amputation technique may be helpful in patients with very marginal vascularity or in the presence of infection. In performing forefoot amputations with this technique, all gangrenous tissue is debrided, preserving viable skin for closure without adherence to standard plantar amputation flaps, if necessary. Lateral, medial, or even dorsal-based skin flaps are used for coverage. A power microsagittal saw is used to divide the metatarsal or tarsal bones far enough back to allow eventual skin closure. Divided cancellous bone is preferred to exposed cartilaginous surfaces. Exposed tissues are covered with gauze that has been generously coated with antibiotic ointment, which prevents desiccation of the tissue while the wound is left undisturbed prior to closure. Simple skin closure is performed 4 to 6 days later.

The numerous modalities used in the treatment of Buerger's disease include aspirin, anticoagulants, steroids, pentoxifylline, vasodilators, thrombolytic agents, prostacyclin analogs, hyperbaric oxygen treatments, and surgical sympathectomy. None of these measures has a proven benefit, and none have been shown to be of no benefit. A decision to employ a treatment modality with no proven benefit should be balanced against any risks associated with that modality. Surgical sympathectomy is not recommended for Buerger's disease. The sympathetic nervous system does not appear to play a role in the pathophysiology of Buerger's disease, and thus, any benefit of sympathectomy would be because of the theoretic improvement of perfusion secondary to the elimination of sympathetically mediated vasoconstriction. Alternatively, although the benefits of using systemic vasodilators such as calcium channel blockers and transdermal clonidine are equally unproven, these agents are usually well tolerated, and a surgical procedure is avoided. Pentoxifylline has few harmful side effects other than its cost. The usefulness of hyperbaric oxygen therapy may be similarly debated on a financial risk versus medical benefit basis. Steroids are intuitively attractive because of the apparent role of the inflammatory and/or the immune system in the pathophysiology of Buerger's disease. However, the risks associated with chronic steroid use, including effects on wound healing and combating infection, preclude a recommendation for steroid treatment in the absence of confirmed benefit. Intravascular thrombosis does appear to play a role in the pathophysiology of Buerger's disease. Thus, the use of aspirin as an antiplatelet agent seems appropriate. A benefit of intravenous iloprost over aspirin therapy in achieving would healing in patients with Buerger's disease was reported in a prospective randomized European trial.[9] A general recommendation for the use of iloprost awaits confirmation of these findings along with documentation of a positive effect on long-term limb salvage. Heparin sodium may be useful in the treatment of an acute exacerbation of disease, but warfarin is generally reserved for attempts to maintain bypass graft patency or in treating concomitant deep venous thrombosis. A benefit of thrombolytic therapy has been reported.[10] A trial of intra-arterial thrombolytic therapy may be appropriate in the setting of clearly limb-threatening ischemia and an acute or subacute presentation.

REFERENCES

1. Lie JT, Mann RJ, Ludwig J. The brothers von Winiwarter, Alexander (1848-1917) and Felix (1852-1931), and thromboangiitis obliterans. Mayo Clin Proc 1979; 54:802–807.
2. Buerger L. Thromboangiitis obliterans: a study of the vascular lesions leading to presenile spontaneous gangrene. Am J Med Sci 1908; 136:567–580.
3. McKusick VA, Harris WS, Ottesen OE, et al. Buerger's disease: A distinct clinical and pathologic entity. JAMA 1962; 181:93–100.
4. Ohta T, Shionoya S. Fate of the ischaemic limb in Buerger's disease. Br J Surg 1988; 75:259–262.

5. Olin JW, Young JR, Graor RA, et al. The changing clinical spectrum of thromboangiitis obliterans (Buerger's disease). Circulation 1990; 82 (suppl 4):IV3–IV8.
6. Mills JL, Taylor LM Jr, Porter JM. Buerger's disease in the modern era. Am J Surg 1987; 154:123–129.
7. Papa M, Bass A, Adar R, et al. Autoimmune mechanisms in thromboangiitis obliterans (Buerger's disease): The role of tobacco antigen and the major histocompatibility complex. Surgery 1992; 111:527–531.
8. Matsushita M, Shionoya S, Matsumoto T. Urinary cotine measurement in patients with Buerger's disease: Effects of active and passive smoking on the disease process. J Vasc Surg 1991; 14:53–58.
9. Fiessinger JN, Schafer M, for the TAO Study. Trial of iloprost versus aspirin treatment for critical limb ischaemia of thromboangiitis obliterans. Lancet 1990; 335:555–557.
10. Hussein EA, El Dorri A. Intra-arterial streptokinase as adjuvant therapy for complicated Buerger's disease: Early trials. Int Surg 1993; 78:54–58.

ERGOTISM

MARSHALL W. WEBSTER, M.D.

Ergotism comprises a variety of disorders produced by the toxic effects of a therapeutic excess or idiosyncratic reaction to ergot alkaloids or to their ingestion in contaminated food.

The symptoms of ergotism have probably been recognized for over 2500 years, but the causal relationship between ergot of rye and disease has been appreciated only since the seventeenth century.[1]

Ancient and medieval epidemics of ergotism were caused by the ingestion of bread or cereal made from rye contaminated by the fungus *Claviceps purpurea*, or ergot. Historically a gangrenous and a convulsive variety of ergotism were recognized. The term St. Anthony's fire was used to describe the gangrenous extremities, which were blackened like charcoal and said to be consumed by the "holy fire," with relief obtained at the shrine of St. Anthony. The relief may have been real, because of the dietary change imposed by travel to the shrine. These epidemics subsided in the nineteenth century, but cases have been reported in Russia in 1926, Ireland in 1929, and in France in 1953, when a baker tried to circumvent a grain tax by using contaminated flour. The last major epidemic was reported in Ethiopia in 1977 and 1978. Although ergotism from contaminated food is rare in humans today, it is still a relatively common problem in livestock feeding on contaminated grasses or silage.

PHARMACOPATHOLOGY

Thompson in 1884 recommended the fluid extract of ergot for relief of periodic headaches. In 1906, Dale gave a thorough description of the pharmacology of the ergot alkaloids, which are all derivatives of lysergic acid. Ergotamine was isolated in 1920. Lysergic acid diethylamide (LSD), an ergot alkaloid, is well known to the drug culture.

The ergot alkaloids are used pharmacologically for the treatment of migraine headaches, as oxytocics for the contraction of atonic uterine muscle in postpartum hemorrhage, and as pressor agents for patients with disturbed vasomotor control such as postural hypotension. The ergot alkaloids constitute a family of substances with diverse and even opposing effects, but the commonest form used clinically is ergotamine, an ergopeptide. Dihydroergotamine, a hydrogenated derivative of ergotamine, has been combined with heparin sodium for prophylaxis of thromboembolism.[2]

Ergotamine is an alpha-adrenergic blocking agent with a direct stimulating effect on smooth muscle of peripheral and cranial blood vessels. Ergotamine also depresses central vasomotor centers and additionally is a 5-hydroxytryptamine agonist.

Pure ergotamine (Ergost, Ergomar) or the combination of ergotamine tartrate and caffeine (Cafergot, Wigraine) has been widely prescribed for the prevention and treatment of migraine headaches. Toxicity from these medications is very uncommon, but for that reason iatrogenic ergotism with arterial insufficiency may not be recognized until irreversible gangrene is present.

CLINICAL PRESENTATION

Ergotism may appear with neurologic, gastrointestinal, or vascular symptoms. Iatrogenic ergotism occurs most commonly in young women, average age 38 years, under treatment for migraine headaches. Arterial insufficiency from ergotamine has been reported as an idiosyncratic reaction to doses as low as 2 mg as well as from long-term or excessive use. Gastrointestinal symptoms, the most common side effects of ergotamine, include nausea, vomiting, diarrhea, and cramping abdominal pain. Uterine cramping and abortions have also been noted. Neurologic symptoms include lassitude, impaired mental function, headaches, vertigo, psychoses, convulsions, and coma. It has been suggested that symptoms of bewitchment in the 1692 Salem witchcraft trials were the result of convulsive ergotism from contaminated rye.

Vascular insufficiency from ergotism appears as ischemia of the extremities, most often the legs, with pallor, coolness, numbness, and intermittent claudication progressing to pain at rest and gangrene. Anal suppositories may be more likely to cause toxic effects than the oral drug because of greater absorption.

The pulses are diminished or absent. Anterior compartment syndrome with foot drop has also been reported after an ergotamine overdose. Involvement of the aorta, carotid, digital, mesenteric (ischemic colitis, intestinal infarction), retinal (blindness), facial (tongue gangrene), and coronary arteries (angina pectoris, myocardial infarction, sudden death) have been reported from ergotism.[3] Retroperitoneal, mediastinal, pericardial, and cardiac valvular fibrosis have been reported with ergot alkaloids. Ergotamine-induced venous thrombosis, affecting the portal and splenic veins, may result primarily from severe arterial ischemia with slowing of venous blood flow and endothelial damage.

ARTERIOGRAPHIC FINDINGS

Arteriographic findings of ergotism include vascular spasm, collateral formation, and intravascular thrombi. The arterial spasm is often diffuse and frequently bilateral and symmetric but may be segmental, with long, smooth areas of narrowing (Figs. 1 and 2). Spasm most commonly begins in the superficial femoral arteries and becomes more severe distally, with threadlike narrowing and distal occlusions. Areas of spasm may mimic atherosclerosis. Intravascular filling defects believed to be thrombi result from stasis distal to arterial spasm and a direct toxic effect on the endothelium. Spasm affecting the renal and external iliac arteries can produce a roentgenographic picture indistinguishable from fibromuscular dysplasia.

Noninvasive vascular testing of the patient with ergotism documents markedly diminished or absent distal blood pressures and dampened pulse volume recordings. Exercise tolerance is also below normal. These abnormalities usually revert to normal once ergot medications are discontinued.

PATHOPHYSIOLOGY

Ergotamine acts directly via the alpha-adrenergic receptors of smooth muscle, causing vasoconstriction.

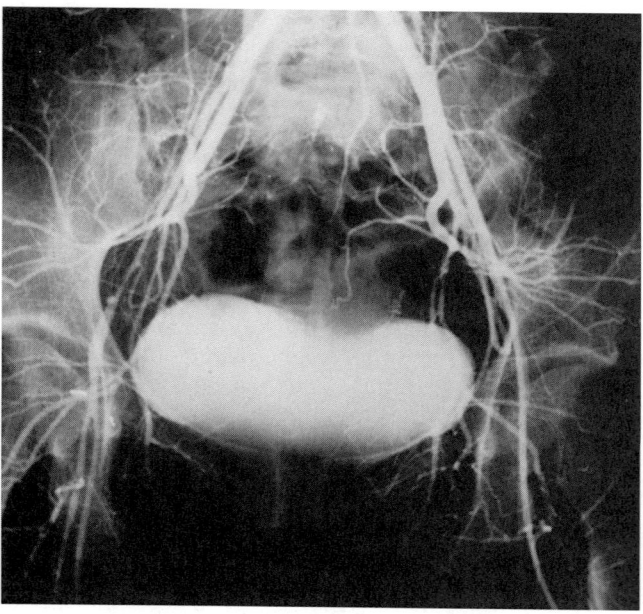

Figure 1 Aortofemoral arteriogram showing diffuse spasm, especially in the right external iliac artery.

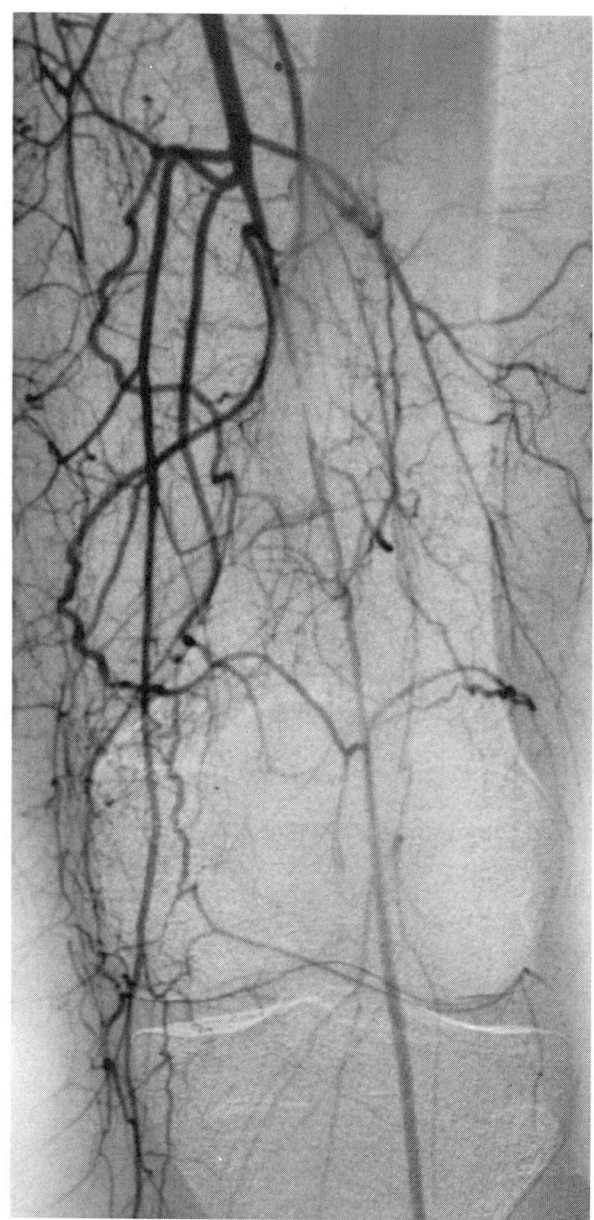

Figure 2 Localized spasm with nearly complete occlusion in the proximal popliteal artery.

Ergotamine has a direct venoconstrictor effect after local infusion in human superficial veins. This effect can be abolished by prior administration of the alpha-adrenergic blocking drug phenoxybenzamine. The peripheral venoconstrictor activity of ergotamine may also be mediated partially through enhanced formation of prostaglandin E–like substances. The potent vasoconstrictive action of ergotamine depends on the unhindered influx of extracellular calcium. Calcium is essential for the activation of vascular smooth muscle, and nifedipine has been reported to be useful in the treatment of ischemia from ergotamine.[4]

The toxic effects of ergotamine on capillary endothelium are poorly understood. Local vasoconstriction may impair perfusion through the vasa vasora, resulting in mural ischemia and necrosis leading to hyaline degeneration.

Ergotamine reduces the vasodilation and excessive pulsations of cranial arteries, especially the branches of the external carotid artery, that cause migraine headaches. A fall in plasma serotonin, a powerful vasoconstrictor of cranial vascular beds, characterizes the migraine syndrome, and ergotamine may also stimulate serotonin receptors, causing vasoconstriction.

Ergotamine is metabolized principally by the liver, and with oral administration there is a large first-pass loss with an increased proportion of metabolites. This leads to decreased systemic drug concentration compared with parenteral administration. Poorly and sporadically absorbed from the gastrointestinal tract, the effective oral dose therefore is 8 to 10 times the intramuscular dose. Absorption studies have documented an enhanced effect of ergot alkaloids when administered with a xanthine derivative such as caffeine or theophylline, probably as a result of improved intestinal absorption. Caffeine, also a cranial vasoconstrictor, is combined with ergotamine to enhance the vascular effects without increasing the dose and toxicity of ergotamine. The usual dose of ergotamine tartrate is 1 mg orally or 2 mg rectally, combined with 100 mg caffeine. The total weekly dose should not exceed 10 mg. Drugs depressing liver function can potentiate the action of ergotamine by leading to accumulation. Contraindications to the use of ergotamine include preexisting hepatic or renal disease, peripheral vascular disease, thrombophlebitis, hyperthyroidism, Raynaud's or Buerger's disease, and pregnancy. Ergotamine may sequester in tissues, producing a prolonged pharmacologic effect despite a short plasma half-life of about 2 hours.

Ergotamine produces a slow onset of vasoconstriction that is well sustained for 24 hours. It should be given no more often than every 48 hours to avoid a constant state of vasoconstriction. No cumulative effect has been observed, and hypersensitivity and tolerance to ergotamine tartrate do not occur in previous ergotamine abusers. In the prodrome of classic migraine there is a decrease in cerebral blood flow. Ergotamine may exaggerate this prodromal ischemia and should be used with caution to prevent severe, long-lasting neurologic effects.

Although ergotamine has been the drug of choice to relieve migraine headache since the first half of this century, propranolol has recently been advocated. However, ergotamine and propranolol may be synergistic for ischemia-causing severe vasospasm. There is a reported synergistic effect between cigarette smoking and ergotamine, since nicotine stimulates the sympathetic ganglia, causing vasoconstriction. A synergism with erythromycin has been reported.[5]

TREATMENT

The treatment of the ischemic effects of ergotism has been empiric, with varying results reported. It is universally recommended that the ergot alkaloid and all other vasoconstrictors, including nicotine and caffeine, be discontinued. Other treatments include the use of anticoagulants such as heparin sodium, low-molecular-weight dextran, streptokinase, and intravascular volume expansion. Various vasodilating methods such as intravenous and intraarterial nitroprusside, papaverine hydrochloride, tolazoline, procainamide, sympathetic blockade by surgical sympathectomy, epidural or spinal anesthetics, periarterial stripping, hyperbaric oxygen, and intra-arterial balloon dilation have been proposed treatments.

Heparin sodium and low-molecular-weight dextran counteract the vascular stasis and formation of thrombus. Low-molecular-weight dextran decreases the viscosity and sludging of blood in small vessels and may be helpful, since the constriction in small vessels is believed to persist for several days after spasm in large vessels has been controlled. Heparin sodium may reduce thrombus formation where necrosis has occurred and may prevent endothelial changes.

Streptokinase has a strong microvascular thrombolytic effect and may be used to dissolve thrombus in patients with impending gangrene.

Nitroprusside, a potent direct smooth muscle vasodilator, is the drug of choice in the management of severe ergotamine-induced peripheral ischemia. Nitroprusside infused either via the femoral artery or aorta or intravenously has been reported to be successful for peripheral ischemia from ergotamine. The optimal infusion rate, duration of therapy, and route of administration have not been well established. The infusion rate should be titrated to obtain the maximal clinical improvement while maintaining adequate blood pressure and urine output. Nitroglycerin also relieves ergotamine-induced arterial spasm, but the effects of ergotamine have been noted to return on withdrawal of nitroglycerin. These vasodilators are not an antidote for ergotism but only a symptomatic treatment.

Prazosin hydrochloride reduces peripheral vascular resistance by alpha-adrenergic blockade and the reduction of arterial and venous vascular tone is similar to that of the direct-acting vasodilator nitroprusside. Prazosin has the advantage of being an oral agent and does not require constant arterial blood pressure monitoring. It is not associated with serious side effects with long-term use. Therefore, it is a reasonable alternative to nitroprusside when impending gangrene is not present or when venous access is difficult. The use of alcohol, tolazoline, procainamide, magnesium sulfate, reserpine, and phenoxybenzamine have had varying effects, and the benefit of these drugs is doubtful. Infusion of prostaglandin E_1 has been reported to be effective.[6,7]

Various procedures to interrupt sympathetic tone have been advocated. These include surgical sympathectomy, epidural and spinal anesthetics, and periarterial stripping. Sympathetic block produced by epidural anesthesia inhibits the sympathetic nervous system but does not reverse the vasoconstriction produced by a drug that acts directly on the vascular smooth muscle.

The use of mechanical intra-arterial balloon dilation has been reported[8] and used in one of our patients.[9] The mechanism of relief of the arterial spasm with intraluminal balloon angioplasty is thought to be by damage to the smooth muscle of the media, which renders the artery noncontractile in response to the vasoconstrictive stimuli of ergotamine. However, rapid restenosis may occur if the ergot has not been withdrawn. The disadvantage of this technique is the risk of intimal disruption. Balloon dilatation is recommended only when more conservative treatment fails and there is danger of gangrene.

REFERENCES

1. Tanner JR. St. Anthony's fire, then and now: A case report and historical review. Can J Surg 1987; 30:291–293.
2. Kunkel DB, Jallo DS. Ergot. In: Haddad LM, Winchester JF, eds. Clinical management of poisoning and drug overdose. Philadelphia: WB Saunders, 1990:1401–1406.
3. Barinagarrementeria F, Cantu C, Balderrama J. Postpartum cerebral angiopathy with cerebral infarction due to ergonovine use. Stroke 1992; 23:1364–1366.
4. Dagher FJ, Pais SO, Richards W, Queral LA. Severe unilateral ischemia of the lower extremity caused by ergotamine: Treatment with nifedipine. Surgery 1985; 97:369–373.
5. Ghali R, De Lean J, Douville Y, et al. Erythromycin-associated ergotamine intoxication: Arteriographic and electrophysiologic analysis of a rare cause of severe ischemia of the lower extremities and associated ischemic neuropathy. Ann Vasc Surg 1993; 7:291–296.
6. Sintenie JB, Tuinebreijer WE, Kreis RW, Breederveld RS. Misleading cause of acute arterial insufficiency: Ergotamine intoxication. Eur J Surg 1992; 158:189–190.
7. Edwards RJ, Fulde GWO, McGrath MA. Successful limb salvage and prostaglandin infusion: A review of ergotamine toxicity. Med J Aust 1991; 155:825–826.
8. Baader W, Herman C, Johansen K. St. Anthony's fire: Successful reversal of ergotamine-induced peripheral vasospasm by hydrostatic dilation. Ann Vasc Surg 1990; 4:597–599.
9. Wells KE, Steed DL, Zajko AB, Webster MW. Recognition and treatment of arterial insufficiency from Cafergot. J Vasc Surg 1986; 4:8–15.

EXTREMITY CAUSALGIA AND MIMOCAUSALGIA

CORNELIUS OLCOTT IV, M.D.
BERNARD R. WILCOSKY, M.D.

Causalgia and mimocausalgia are pain syndromes mediated by the sympathetic nervous system that follow extremity trauma. Classically, causalgia describes patients in whom there is injury to a major peripheral nerve. Mimocausalgia designates cases not involving direct nerve injury. More recently, all such cases have been lumped together under the term reflex sympathetic dystrophy (RSD), or sympathetically mediated pain syndromes. These syndromes are characterized by burning pain, temperature changes, muscle and/or skin atrophy, edema, vasomotor changes, and hyperhidrosis affecting the injured extremity. These symptoms may occur after trauma of any magnitude, including very minor injuries.

There are several reasons for vascular surgeons to be familiar with RSD. First, these patients typically seek treatment for pain, cyanosis, temperature changes, and edema of the extremity, symptoms that mimic arterial or venous occlusive disease. Second, RSD may occur as a complication of vascular reconstructive procedures on the aortoiliac system or the lower extremity arterial tree or may follow prolonged nerve ischemia.[1,2] Third, surgical management of RSD requires sympathectomy, a procedure with which the vascular surgeon is most familiar.

CLASSIFICATION AND NATURAL HISTORY

The natural history of these post-traumatic pain syndromes has been classified into three stages by Druker and co-workers.[3] Stage 1 is the acute stage. It occurs during the first 1 to 3 months following injury and is characterized by burning pain, erythema, hyperthermia, edema, hyperalgesia, hyperhidrosis, and patchy osteoporosis. Chemical sympathectomy is usually successful during this period, and the effects may last beyond the usual duration of the block. Spontaneous resolution may occur during this stage. Stage 2, the dystrophic stage, occurs 3 to 6 months after injury. During this stage patients have a fixed response to sympathetic block and rarely experience spontaneous resolution. Patients typically display coolness, mottling, cyanosis, indurated edema, continuous pain, and osteoporosis of the involved extremity. Stage 3 is the atrophic phase, during which the pain may extend beyond the site of original injury. Extensive atrophy of the skin and muscles and contractures of the joints are typical. These stages, though somewhat arbitrary, may be helpful in predicting outcome. Patients in stages 1 and 2, if treated early, should expect good results. Patients in stage 3 may not respond to any form of therapy, conservative or surgical.

CLINICAL MANIFESTATIONS

Post-traumatic pain is the hallmark of RSD. Typically the pain begins immediately after injury. However, the presence of RSD may not be appreciated until the prolongation of the pain is apparent and associated signs and symptoms develop. Classically the pain is described as burning and is localized to the area of injury. However, in late stages the pain may spread beyond the site of injury. Symptoms and associated physical findings include temperature changes, atrophy of muscle and/or skin, edema, vasomotor color changes, hyperhidrosis, and osteoporosis. Typically the patient guards the involved extremity and is fearful of even minor contact. Many of these patients are emotionally labile. Women are more frequently affected than men, 83% versus 17% in our study.[4] The extent of the injury may be significant, involving a major nerve, e.g., the brachial plexus, or it may be very minor, e.g., following an intravenous needle placement. The extent of injury does not necessarily correlate with the severity of symptoms.

Although the clinical picture may be suggestive, the definitive diagnosis of RSD requires a positive response to sympathetic blockade. Ideally, the sympathetic block should be performed by a physician familiar with pain syndromes and RSD. The success of the sympathetic block should be documented by temperature change in the extremity and relief of pain. Needle placement may be documented by fluoroscopy. If necessary, several sympathetic blocks, including placebo blocks, may be performed. It is important to obtain and document an accurate block, as all future treatment depends upon it.

TREATMENT

Nonoperative

We believe that the treatment of patients with RSD is best coordinated with a multidisciplinary team approach. All of our patients are initially evaluated by a member of the Pain Service. If RSD is suspected on the basis of the clinical history and physical examination, a diagnostic sympathetic block is performed. If a documented effective block is reflected by a rise in temperature of the extremity and a decrease in pain, a diagnosis of RSD is made. Once the diagnosis is confirmed, the patient is started on a conservative regimen. There is pronounced variability in the response of RSD patients to various pharmacologic agents. Corticosteroids seem effective in early stages, but in later stages results are disappointing. Antidepressants, especially tricyclics, have universal applicability throughout the course of the disease and should be used early. Low doses, 50 to 100 mg or less, of amitriptyline or the equivalent are particularly effective for the burning component of pain and the hypersensitivity. Higher doses may treat the accompanying depression. Trials of alternative tricyclics are often required to circumvent adverse side effects. If episodic lancinating pain is pronounced, anticonvulsants of which carbamazepine is the prototype should be tried. Vasoactive drugs may be helpful. Unfortunately, guanethidine is no longer available. Research suggests that the alpha-2 agonist clonidine, given orally and transdermally, may be effective, but early results are inconclusive. Some impressive success has been reported with intravenous lidocaine and with the oral analog mexilitine. Systemic lidocaine is an effective analgesic whose application has been limited by lack of an oral analog. Mexilitine now fills that void.

In our experience, approximately 50% to 70% of patients will respond to a conservative regimen. The proportion responding is a function of duration of symptoms and patient motivation. Poorer results are seen in those with long-standing symptoms (stage 3) or with potential for secondary gain.

Operative

Patients who have a positive response to sympathetic blocks but fail to respond to a good conservative regimen are referred for surgical therapy. Patients with upper extremity RSD are treated by cervical sympathectomy. At first we performed this procedure using a supraclavicular approach. However, experience has documented that many patients managed in this fashion will develop recurrence of symptoms. Our experience has also convinced us that most such patients failed to obtain relief because of an incomplete sympathectomy. We now perform all upper extremity sympathectomies for RSD through a thoracotomy. We remove all the stellate ganglion and all ganglia down to and including T6 or T7. To date these procedures have been performed through an open thoracotomy. However, we now are exploring a thoracoscopic approach. Whether we can perform as complete a sympathectomy with the thoracoscope has yet to be determined. Patients with lower extremity RSD who require a surgical approach are managed by lumbar sympathectomy. In these patients, we remove L2 through L4 via a retroperitoneal approach.

Management of Nonresponders

One of the most difficult aspects of managing this disease is how to deal with the patient who fails to respond satisfactorily to both conservative and surgical therapy. Several considerations must kept in mind. First, the diagnosis may be incorrect. It is important to be as sure as possible of the diagnosis before beginning therapy. Second, the patient may have had an incomplete sympathectomy, particularly if the procedure was performed by someone not familiar with RSD. Third, the patient may have persistent sympathetic innervation from another source, typically the contralateral side. Should symptoms persist in a patient who one is convinced has RSD, appropriate diagnostic sympathetic blocks can help determine the site of remaining sympathetic tissue. For example, both ipsilateral and contralateral blocks can be used to document the presence and location of other contributing sympathetic pathways. Our experience is that persistent sympathetic innervation may occur from either the ipsilateral side as a result of incomplete sympathectomy or from the contralateral side.

New developments have allowed effective treatment of heretofore refractory cases of RSD. Percutaneous placement of epidural spinal cord stimulation devices holds promise. Early results suggest a 50% to 70% favorable success rate. The use of spinal opiates, with or without local anesthetics, may be delivered by implantable pumps in selected patients. Long-term results for this modality are lacking, but our experience suggests efficacy for up to 3 years in some patients. Our protocol recommends a trial of spinal cord stimulation initially, since side effects are limited and no drugs are required. Only if spinal cord stimulation fails are patients considered for a trial of spinal opiates. Both of these therapies should be considered palliative therapy for truly end-stage RSD.

Regardless of the management approach, the goal of therapy is relief of pain and restoration of extremity function. The initial emphasis should be on pain relief, as it is not usually possible to involve the patient in proper physical therapy as long as the extremity is painful. Once the pain is relieved, by either a conservative approach or operation physical therapy and rehabilitation must be emphasized so that useful extremity function may be restored.

RESULTS

In 1991 we reported the results of an analysis of 35 patients who underwent sympathectomy for RSD.[4] Follow-up in this group ranged from 1 to 40 months and averaged 14 months. Further follow-up of these patients and experience with subsequent patients has provided results similar to those of the original report. We classified results as excellent if the patient was relieved of preoperative dystrophic symptoms and required only occasional nonnarcotic medication for pain relief. Some 74% of the patients were in this group. All of these patients were rehabilitated with good function of the involved extremity and return to employment or usual activity. Patients with good results (17%) had greater than 50% relief of pain and satisfactory but not complete return of extremity function. Three of the six patients in this group returned to their usual employment. Patients who had less than 50% relief of dystrophic pain or had no improvement in extremity function were considered poor results (9%). In our experience, poor results most commonly occur in patients who have some but not complete relief of pain from sympathetic blockade and have a complex pain syndrome in which RSD is only a part of the total pain picture. Patients with excellent results tend to have less severe symptoms for a shorter period.

All patients who underwent cervical sympathectomy developed a Horner's syndrome, as we remove the entire stellate ganglion. We believe this is necessary for complete and lasting pain relief. None of these patients complained of Horner's syndrome, as they considered it a fair trade for pain relief. Some degree of postsympathectomy neuralgia occurred in 23% of the upper extremities and in 67% of the lower extremities. In all instances the neuralgia resolved spontaneously. Three patients with upper extremity RSD had had a previous cervical sympathectomy, one transaxillary and two supraclavicular, before being referred to our service. In each patient there was histologic confirmation of the sympathectomy, but in each a repeat ipsilateral sympathetic block produced relief of symptoms and a repeat sympathectomy by the transthoracic route was successful. RSD developed in a second extremity in two of our patients during follow-up, raising the question of a systemic component to this syndrome. Both of these patients responded to conservative therapy. One patient had a left lumbar sympathectomy for RSD involving her left leg that failed to provide complete relief. A block of her right sympathetic system produced relief, and she subsequently underwent a right lumbar sympathectomy with alleviation of her symptoms.

Our results[5] are similar to those of others. Mockus and associates[5] noted significant improvement in 94% of patients. Patman and colleagues[6] reported excellent results in 84% of patients, good results in 8.9%, and poor results in 7.1%. Hence, it seems reasonable to expect significant improvement with good pain relief and significant return of extremity function in 90% to 95% of patients who require sympathectomy. The important factor in obtaining good results appears to be patient selection. The importance of a good diagnostic sympathetic block and proper preoperative evaluation cannot be overemphasized. Also, the duration of symptoms is important. Best results follow prompt diagnosis and institution of therapy. In this regard it is also important not to pursue a conservative approach unless significant progress is noted. Prolonged delay may result in an unsuccessful surgical approach. As we gained experience in the surgical management of RSD, it became apparent that better results are obtained when an extensive sympathectomy is performed. This is particularly apparent in patients undergoing a repeat sympathectomy. The single ganglion sympathectomy does not produce satisfactory pain relief.

REFERENCES

1. Churcher MD. Algodystrophy after aortic bifurcation surgery. Lancet 1984; 2:131–133.
2. Priollet P, Fichelle JM, Vayssairat M, et al. Algodystrophy after vascular surgery. Lancet 1984; 2:923–924.
3. Druker WR, Hubay CA, Holden WD, et al. Pathogenesis of post-traumatic sympathetic dystrophy. Am J Surg 1959; 97:454–465.
4. Olcott C, Eltherington LG, Wilcosky BR, et al. Reflex sympathetic dystrophy: The surgeon's role in management. J Vasc Surg 1991; 14:488–495.
5. Mockus MB, Rutherford RB, Rosales C, Pearce WH. Sympathectomy for causalgia. Arch Surg 1987; 122:668–672.
6. Patman RD, Thompson JE, Persson AV. Management of post-traumatic pain syndromes: Report of 113 cases. Ann Surg 1973; 177:780–787.

UPPER EXTREMITY SYMPATHECTOMY

ALI F. ABURAHMA, M.D.
JAMES P. BOLAND, M.D.

Sympathectomy was introduced in North America by Adson and Brown[1] in 1925 for the management of vasospasm. Sympathectomy was the only alternative to amputation for chronic limb-threatening ischemia before the advent of arterial reconstruction. A better understanding of the extremity pain syndromes and progress in direct arterial reconstruction has minimized the role of sympathectomy in the last 20 years.

ANATOMIC AND PHYSIOLOGIC CONSIDERATIONS

The cervical part of the sympathetic trunk contains three ganglia, superior, middle, and lower. The lower ganglion is usually fused with the first thoracic ganglion to form the stellate ganglion. Preganglionic neurons supplying the face, neck, and upper extremity originate at the spinal cord levels of C7 through T5. Efferent fibers from these levels form multiple synapses in the stellate and thoracic ganglia. A direct fiber tract (the nerve of Kuntz) from T2 sympathetic ganglion to the brachial plexus can be identified in most patients as a frequent variation in the relay chain between the spinal cord and the upper extremity. Upper extremity sympathetic denervation has ranged from extensive resection (stellate ganglion to T5) to conservative resection (T2 ganglion and Kuntz's nerve). Most authorities advocate resection of T2 and T3 ganglia as well as the nerve of Kuntz and other rami contributing to the brachial plexus at these levels. Although providing less than 15% of upper extremity innervation, the T1 and inferior portion of the stellate ganglia make a significant contribution to the eye; therefore, complete resection of these ganglia increases the risk of permanent Horner's syndrome. To eliminate this problem, others resect only the lower third of the stellate ganglion.

The dominant effect of sympathetic denervation is vasodilation, particularly of the skin. Although some investigators question whether any increase in nutritional blood flow to the skin actually occurs, the healing of ischemic ulcers, the growth of toenails, and the increase in blood flow by xenon washout studies all suggest that some improvement in nutrient circulation follows sympathectomy. Most of the experimental studies designed to evaluate the effects of sympathectomy on blood flow have as their basis measurements of blood pressure, distribution of microspheres, clearance of injected isotopes, or measurements of the delivery of oxygen. The return of cutaneous blood flow toward normal after sympathectomy is probably the result of re-establishment of intrinsic cutaneous vasomotor tone or the increased sensitivity of blood vessels to circulating catecholamines. Sympathectomy results in ablation of sweat gland function that is usually permanent. The loss of sweating results in the dry skin that typically follows sympathectomy.

Although objective assessment of pain relief after sympathectomy in both neuropathic and ischemic extremities is difficult, aversive stimuli studies in cats have documented that sympathectomy enhances tolerance of painful stimuli. This increased pain tolerance lasts longer than the vasomotor effects of sympathectomy and may explain clinical observations of relief of rest pain and even improved exercise performance in sympathectomized extremities that have no objective increases in blood flow. Theories concerning this effect on pain thresholds suggests that sympathetic denervation decreases noxious stimulus perception both by decreasing tissue concentrations of norepinephrine and by reducing spinal augmentation of pain stimulus transmission to cerebral centers.

Despite an imposing number of clinical studies, there is no unanimity of opinion about the effectiveness of sympathectomy in the treatment of arterial occlusive diseases. Most investigators agree that mild ischemic pain and shallow ulcers can be favorably influenced by sympathectomy. The mechanism of relief of pain is believed to be a result of increased blood flow to the skin and subcutaneous tissues. Dale and Lewis[2] reported beneficial results from upper extremity sympathectomy in patients with scattered arterial occlusions in the arm and hand. However, Porter[3] could not confirm this finding.

STELLATE GANGLION BLOCK TECHNIQUE

The patient is placed supine with the head slightly raised and extended backward on a pillow. A finger inserted between the sternocleidomastoid muscle and the trachea seeks the most easily palpated transverse process (6th). Using the two-finger technique, one finger should palpate the transverse process and at the same time allow the insertion of a fine-gauge needle 5 to 8 cm long toward this transverse process until it makes contact with it. When the needle rests upon the transverse process, the tip of the needle is withdrawn a few millimeters and fixed. After aspiration, 15 ml of 0.25% bupivacaine (Marcaine) is injected to bathe the stellate ganglion, which lies at the level of C7 to D1.

It is often difficult to judge whether or not a complete sympathetic block has been obtained, especially when vascular disease is present. A significant increase in warmth, whether subjective or objective, cannot always be recognized. Increased filling of the veins is a sign of sympathetic block, which is helpful. Horner's syndrome following stellate ganglion block is not an indication of a complete sympathetic block of the upper extremity. It merely documents that the sympathetic chain in the neck has been blocked. Objective signs of a complete sympathetic block are an increased skin temperature compared with the side not blocked, an increase in arterial pulsations demonstrated by oscillometry or plethysmography, and abolished sweating in the hand. The presence of sympathetic vasomotor tone may be assessed by noting the response of the digit pulse amplitude to a deep breath. Normally the pulse amplitude is attenuated with such a maneuver, whereas patients with autosympathectomy (diabetes mellitus), surgical sympathectomy, or advanced ischemia may lose such a vasoconstrictive reflex. The ability of the digit circulation to increase in response to ischemia (reactive hyperemia) may be assessed by noting the pulse waveform response to temporary arterial occlusion induced by a pneumatic cuff on the proximal digit. Normally the digit pulse amplitude should at least double after 3 minutes of digit ischemia.[4] Digits with advanced occlusive disease may not have the capacity to vasodilate further. Such patients are unlikely to benefit from sympathectomy.

INDICATIONS FOR UPPER EXTREMITY CERVICODORSAL SURGICAL SYMPATHECTOMY

The best results of upper extremity surgical sympathectomy are achieved in patients with hyperhidrosis, reflex sympathetic dystrophy (causalgia), and vasospastic disorders complicated by digital ulceration (Table 1). Improved medical management of patients with Raynaud's disease has largely replaced cervicodorsal surgical sympathectomy for disabling digital vasospasm.

The most successful indication for upper extremity sympathectomy is hyperhidrosis. T2 and T3 ganglionectomy is sufficient. No short- or long-term failures have been reported, with maximal follow-up of 7 years in one series.[5]

Table 1 Indications for Cervico-Dorsal Sympathectomy and Clinical Outcome

Outcome	Indications	Number of Patients in Our Series (12 years)
Excellent	Hyperhidrosis	3
	Reflex sympathetic dystrophy (causalgia and mimocausalgia)	7
	Vasospastic disorders complicated by digital ulceration (frost bite sequelae or occlusive Raynaud's disease secondary to distal emboli or trauma)	4
Good to fair	Buerger's disease	2
	Distal arterial occlusion or atherosclerosis	2
Poor	Simple nonocclusive Raynaud's disease	0

Approximately 60% of the post-traumatic pain syndromes causalgia and mimocausalgia can be managed with physical therapy, mild narcotics, tricyclic antidepressants, and anticonvulsants. Cervicodorsal sympathectomy is indicated for selected patients in whom medical treatment fails.[6]

Among a small number of patients with occlusive Raynaud's syndrome complicated by digital ulceration, healing followed sympathectomy in over 75% of these lesions and prevented recurrent tissue loss even though cold-induced digital ischemia reappeared.[5] Sympathectomy does not prevent recurrent symptoms because denervation does not affect the cause and natural course of the underlying vascular disease. Occlusive Raynaud's syndrome due to embolism, trauma, or chronic occupational trauma has a more favorable and lasting response to sympathectomy.[7]

Raynaud's disease resulting from abnormal digital vasoconstriction without obstructing lesions has a more benign course than the occlusive variety. Although up to one-third of patients initially thought to be free of underlying disease may ultimately manifest signs of autoimmune vasculitis, true vasoconstrictive Raynaud's disease does not tend to be recurrent or associated with digital ulceration.[8] Treatment of primary Raynaud's disease with alpha-adrenergic antagonists or calcium channel blocking agents relieves symptoms during the acute phase. Surgical sympathectomy is, therefore, not indicated because medical management is sufficient.

Experience with upper extremity sympathectomy in the treatment of atherosclerotic disease is limited. Increased digital blood flow in response to intravenous injections of tolazoline hydrochloride (Priscoline) or other methods of sympathetic blockade helps to identify patients likely to respond to a surgical sympathectomy.

Although initial symptom relief or healing of ischemic ulcers is obtained in 50% of the patients, lasting improvement should not be expected because of the diffuse distribution of the upper extremity atherosclerotic lesions.[5] The best results are usually obtained in patients who have distal occlusive disease.

PATIENT SELECTION CRITERIA

A thorough history and examination should be done to identify concomitant peripheral vascular disease, collagen vascular disease, and antecedent trauma. Further testing may include serologic tests or tissue biopsy to identify collagen vascular disease as well as upper extremity digital blood pressures and plethysmography to define the extent, severity, and level of any occlusive disease. Arteriography may be indicated to characterize both proximal and distal occlusive disease detected by segmental limb blood pressure measurements among patients in whom therapeutic intervention is clearly needed. A trial of conservative treatment is indicated for all patients. If medical measures such as calcium channel blockers and cessation of smoking fail, proper patient selection for sympathectomy is improved by temporary stellate ganglion blockade to document the effectiveness of sympathetic denervation. For causalgia, vasospastic disorders, and digital occlusive disease, injections with local anesthetic and saline placebo are indicated to observe both the subjective response and objective improvement. Among patients with vasospastic disease, abolition of cold-induced digital ischemia, as monitored by digital pressures and plethysmography, must be documented prior to surgical sympathectomy. Ideally, a minimum of three sympathetic blocks should be done at regular intervals. Results indicating favorable outcome after sympathectomy include subjective relief of symptoms for a period equal to or longer than the duration of action of local anesthetic used for ganglion block, no symptomatic response to saline placebo, greater than 50% increase in the amplitude of the digital plethysmographic tracing as compared to baseline, and abolition of the abnormally prolonged decline in the amplitude of digital plethysmographic tracings following ice water immersion.

OPERATIVE TECHNIQUE AND COMPLICATIONS

Several techniques have been described to gain exposure to the upper dorsal sympathetic ganglia. A review of reported series using each technique indicates that the axillary, transthoracic, and extrapleural axillary approaches to the stellate and upper thoracic ganglia have the lowest complication rates. Both techniques involve exposure of the posterior superior mediastinum through a transverse axillary incision. First rib resection has been recommended to facilitate extrapleural retraction of the upper lung and identification of the sympathetic connections between the brachial plexus and higher ganglia. Similar exposure is obtained with a transthoracic approach by entering the chest through the third intercostal space. Transaxillary approaches are preferred because less dissection is required to visualize the ganglia fully, and the incision is cosmetically acceptable. The major disadvantages of the transthoracic approach are the pain of a rib-spreading incision and common need for tube thoracostomy.

The supraclavicular approach poses the greatest risk of injury to adjacent structures, e.g., the phrenic nerve, brachial plexus, subclavian artery, and cupola of the lung. It also carries a higher risk of Horner's syndrome and presents difficulty in getting to the lower ganglia (T3 and T4). The most painful approach is the posterior paravertebral approach because extensive paraspinal muscle division and rib resection are required.

Transaxillary Thoracic Dorsal Sympathectomy

With the patient in lateral decubitus position, transverse skin incision is made at the inferior margin of the axillary hair and extends from the lateral border of the pectoralis major muscle to the anterior border of the latissimus dorsi muscle (Fig. 1). The anterior thoracic nerve anteriorly and the thoracodorsal nerve posteriorly should be preserved. The incision is usually 4 inches long. The lateral cutaneous branch of the second thoracic nerve is preserved. This nerve is retracted anteriorly. Next an incision is made in the anterior serratus muscle. The incision is carried down to the third rib, and dissection is carried upward on the surface of the thoracic cage to the second interspace, through which the pleural space is entered. A small rib spreader is used to open the chest, and the dome of the lung is retracted with a malleable retractor. The stellate ganglion and upper dorsal chain can then be identified through the pleura, which is incised. The cut margins of the posterior parietal pleura are retracted. The dorsal sympathetic chain is transected with metal clips just distal to the fourth ganglion and is mobilized upward by sharp dissection. Separation of the ganglia from adjacent intercostal vessels can be facilitated by gentle traction of the chain with right angle clamp or nerve hook. T4, T3, T2, and the lower third of the stellate ganglion are resected. The pleural space is drained with a chest tube placed anteriorly. Closure is achieved by two or three paracostal sutures and running suture for the muscle and subcutaneous tissue.

Anterior Transthoracic Dorsal Sympathectomy

The patient is placed in supine position with the arm elevated and supported above the head. The incision is made in the third intercostal space extending from the sternum laterally to the anterior axillary line. The pectoralis major muscle is split along its fibers. The intercostal muscles are then incised and the pleura is opened. After a rib spreader is inserted, the lung is retracted inferiorly with Harrington retractors. The

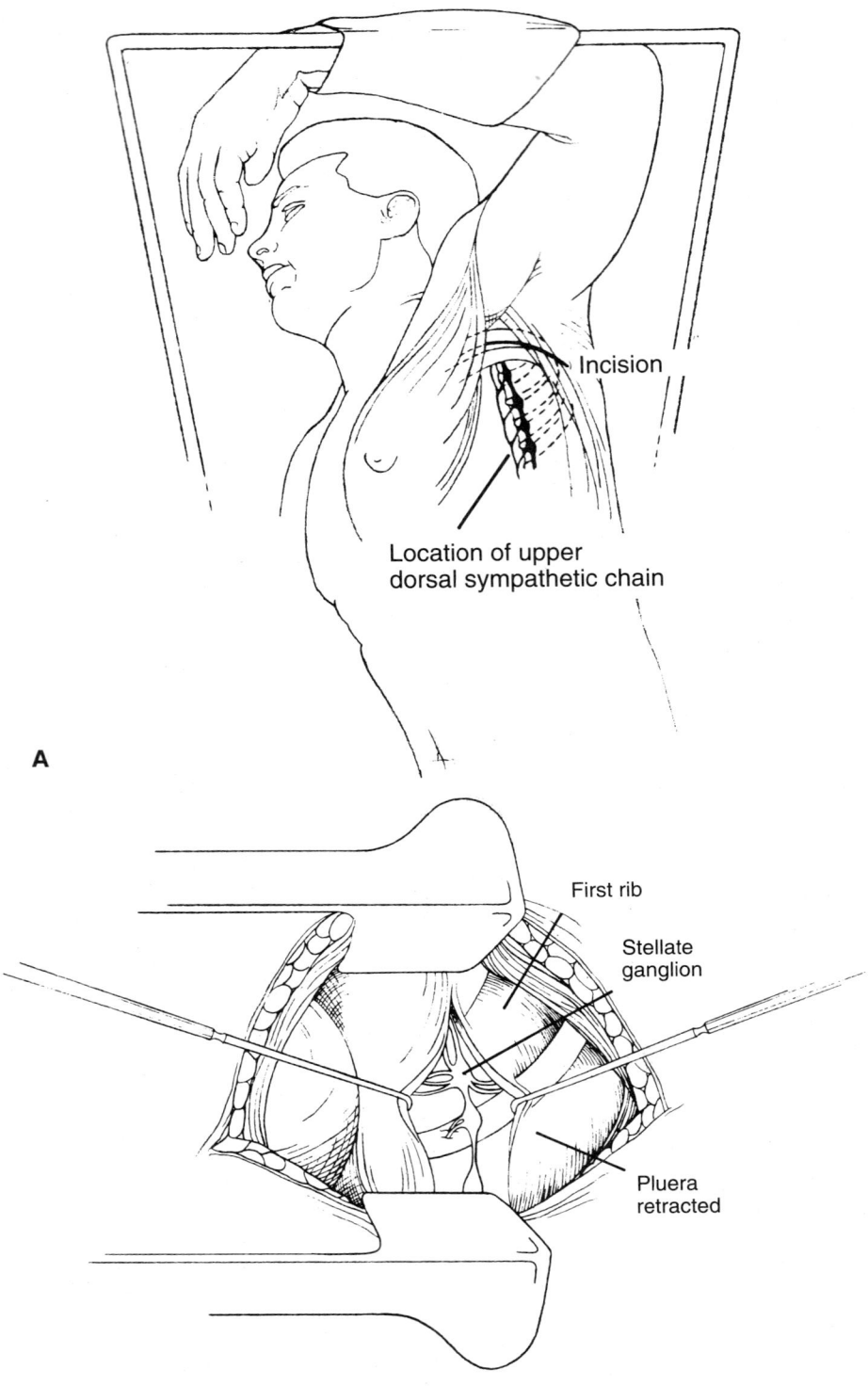

Figure 1 *A*, Axillary transpleural thoracic dorsal sympathectomy: patient positioning and incision site. *B*, Axillary transpleural thoracic dorsal sympathectomy: minithoracotomy through second or third interspace showing stellate ganglion and upper dorsal sympathetic ganglia.

superior vena cava and the phrenic nerve appear on the right side and the aorta and the subclavian artery on the left side. The upper dorsal sympathetic chain can be identified and the pleura is opened over the chain. The ganglia are excised as previously described. Upon completion of the procedure, a chest tube is inserted anteriorly and the ribs approximated using several pericostal sutures. The pectoral fascia and subcutaneous tissue can be closed with continuous suture.

Horner's syndrome, the major complication of sympathetic denervation, varies with the extent of stellate ganglion resection. When the lower half is resected, 3% to 36% of patients experience temporary ptosis and miosis with 3% to 10% incidence of permanent Horner's syndrome.[5] Significant postsympathectomy neuralgia in the face, shoulder, or chest may occur in 20% to 40% of patients.[6] The discomfort is temporary, usually lasting about 6 weeks, and requires only mild analgesics for relief.

Thoracoscopic Dorsal Sympathectomy

While it is possible to perform a thoracic sympathectomy with a one-trocar approach,[9] the current trend is to use single-lung ventilation, three or four access ports, and video imaging.[10] The first port is placed in the fifth or sixth intercostal space in the mid to posterior axillary line for the video endoscope and subsequently serves as the chest tube exit site. A reasonable strategy is to place an anterior and posterior access port along the line of the usual transaxillary incision with the option to complete the incision if thoracoscopic exposure is unsatisfactory. A hook is inserted in one port, and the other port is used for scissor, cautery, and/or clip applier. If conversion to an open procedure is necessary, the continued use of the video endoscope (a video-assisted axillary thoracotomy) will require less intercostal spreading, and therefore produce less postoperative discomfort. Radio frequency cautery can usually be used, especially anteriorly and posteriorly to the main sympathetic trunk, to assist in interrupting accessory fibers. Such cautery should be used cautiously if at all, when resecting the stellate ganglion in its lower third. The ganglion should be clipped and cut instead. This should reduce the chance of producing a Horner's syndrome. Our experience is limited to two patients, who had percutaneous transthoracic endoscopic sympathectomy with no complications and good results.

REFERENCES

1. Adson AW, Brown GE. Treatment of Raynaud's disease by lumbar ramisection and ganglionectomy and perivascular neurectomy of the common iliacs. JAMA 1925; 84:1908–1910.
2. Dale WA, Lewis MR. Management of ischemia of the hand and fingers. Surgery 1970; 67:62–79.
3. Porter JM. Upper extremity ischemia: Role of the vascular surgeon in Raynaud's syndrome and finger gangrene. In: Veith EJ, ed. Critical problems in vascular surgery. New York: Appleton-Century-Crofts, 1982: 277.
4. Barnes RW. Role of lumbar sympathectomy. In: Brewster, DC, ed. Common problems in vascular surgery. Chicago: Year Book Medical Publishers, 1989:404.
5. Welch E, Geary J. Current status of thoracic dorsal sympathectomy. J Vasc Surg 1984; 1:202–214.
6. Mockus M, Rutherford RB, Rosales C. Sympathectomy for causalgia: Patient selection and long-term results. Arch Surg 1987; 122:668–672.
7. Conn J Jr, Bergan JJ, Bell JL. Hypothenar hammer syndrome: Post-traumatic digital ischemia. Surgery 1970; 68:1122–1127.
8. Porter JM. Raynaud's syndrome and associated vasospastic conditions of the extremities. In: Rutherford RB, ed. Vascular surgery. Philadelphia: WB Saunders, 1984:697.
9. Kux M. Thoracic endoscopic sympathectomy in palmar and axillary hyperhidrosis. Arch Surg 1978; 113:264–266.
10. Landreneau RJ, Mack MJ, Hazelrigg SR, et al. Video assisted thoracic surgery: Basic technic concepts and intercostal approach strategies. Ann Thorac Surg 1992; 54:800–807.

ETIOLOGY AND ANATOMIC PATHOLOGY OF THORACIC OUTLET SYNDROME

HERBERT I. MACHLEDER, M.D.

The preponderance of evidence suggests that neurovascular compression in the region of the thoracic outlet derives from a combination of factors. These factors include predisposing morphologic variations, structural modifications conditioned by functional requirements, and changes in scalene muscle fiber type as a consequence of trauma.[1]

In their most obvious manifestations, the congenital and acquired abnormalities associated with thoracic outlet compression are considered discrete anomalies (e.g., cervical rib, supernumerary scalene muscle). The most useful classification places these discrete anomalies within a continuum of developmental variation. With the addition of increased functional requirements or post-traumatic change in muscle fiber type, the particular developmental abnormality may be a significant predisposing element in the clinical expression of the compression syndrome.

Coincident with the range and continuum of developmental abnormalities is a range and continuum of compressive forces on the normal structures that traverse the thoracic outlet. Symptoms associated with the extremes of the compressive abnormalities are easy to distinguish, as they represent the "classic" cases: (1)

Paget-Schroetter axillosubclavian vein occlusion, (2) hand ischemia from thrombosis or embolization from the compressed or aneurysmal subclavian artery, and (3) the "wasted hand" of cervical band compression of the brachial plexus.

Nevertheless, lesser degrees of symptoms may be disabling in settings of specific physical or occupational requirements. Greater resilience of the arterial and venous system seems to result in relatively innocuous symptoms until compression reaches levels of hemodynamic significance or structural damage. It is evident from the clinical pattern that the threshold for neurogenic symptoms from the brachial plexus is lower than that from the vascular system.

Although several unique anatomic and clinical relationships such as in Paget-Schroetter syndrome have been identified, the clinical manifestation of any particular compressive abnormality depends more on the variable tolerance of the three different systems, arterial, venous, and neural, than on the specific nature of the anatomic anomaly.

DEVELOPMENTAL VARIATION

Anatomic variation at the region of the thoracic outlet has intrigued surgical anatomists from early descriptions of supernumerary ribs to modern studies of ultrastructural changes in the scalene muscles.[2,3] A spectrum of configurations can be encountered during transaxillary exploration of the thoracic outlet for arterial, venous, or brachial plexus compression. These represent intermediate anatomic configurations occurring in addition to the discrete abnormalities previously described, e.g., cervical ribs, cervical fibrocartilagenous bands, and supernumerary scalene muscles.[4] The relationship of various congenital abnormalities is more easily appreciated when considered in a developmental context.

Anomalies of the thoracic outlet structures rarely exist in isolation, as there is interaction in development of the different elements. The anatomist White and his colleagues elaborated on this concept when they described cervical ribs and congenital malformations of first thoracic ribs as linked to errors of bodily segmentation in early embryonic development.[5] These rib malformations result from variation in the formation of the brachial plexus before skeletal development. Cervical rib development, for example, is determined by the formation of the spinal nerve roots. The regression of the C5 through C7 ribs is occasioned by the rapid development of the enlarging roots of the brachial plexus in the region of the limb bud. In cases of a cervical C7 rib, there is generally a prefixed plexus with only a small neural contribution from the T1 nerve root. The inhibition to rib development at that level is lost or reduced, and the size of the cervical rib is then related to the extent of contribution of this T1 root to the brachial plexus. As a corollary, in the postfixed plexus, where there is a contribution of the T2 root to the brachial plexus, the first thoracic rib is often rudimentary, having been inhibited in its development by the unusual nerve growth. This embryologically determined morphologic interdependence is evident with other structural relationships at the thoracic outlet.

Anomalies regularly encountered during thoracic outlet decompression can be categorized as (1) anomalies of the first thoracic rib or cervical rib, including the residual fibrous band from an incomplete cervical rib, (2) anomalies of scalene muscle development or insertion, including enlargement of the scalenus anticus or scalenus medius, unusual insertion of these muscles such as overlapping and enlargement of the insertion tubercle; (3) scalenus minimus muscle or its fibrous remnant; (4) anomaly of subclavius tendon, or tubercle of insertion; and (5) an anomaly not clearly identifiable as a developmental variation, often a consequence of trauma.

CLINICAL CHARACTERISTICS

In a group of 200 consecutive patients undergoing thoracic outlet operations at UCLA, 80% were women with an average age of 39 years and 20% were men with an average age of 31 years. Some 20% of these patients had problems related to venous obstruction or arterial insufficiency and embolization. Of this vascular subgroup, 65% had additional neurogenic symptoms associated with abnormal sensory evoked responses in the affected extremity. In the entire group of 200 patients with symptomatic extremities, 76.5% exhibited signs of arterial compression in stress positions, either on clinical examination or with digital photoplethysmography. The right side was operated upon 58% of the time and the left, 42% of the time. The dominant arm was corrected preferentially in cases of bilateral symptoms. In 44% of patients with neurogenic compression there was a clear history of trauma.

DISTRIBUTION OF DEVELOPMENTAL ANOMALIES

Seventeen patients (8.5%) had a cervical rib articulating with the first thoracic rib, directly or by fibrocartilaginous extension. This group included patients with associated anomalies of the first rib. Twenty (10%) had a scalenus minimus abnormality inserting either on the first rib or on Sibson's fascia, and 39 (19.5%) had an anomaly of the subclavius tendon or its insertion. In 15 patients (7.5%) there were other categories of anomalies that could not be related to specific developmental characteristics. These unique anomalies included ligamentous or fibrous structures that did not correspond to regression residua of recognized embryologic structures. More than one abnormality was recognized in 22.5% of the patients, and 32% of 25 patients undergoing bilateral procedures had similar anomalies on both sides. In 34% of patients no developmental anomaly could be identified from the transaxillary exposure.

In review, one clinical setting could be consistently correlated with characteristic anatomic abnormalities. Of 33 patients with spontaneous axillosubclavian vein thrombosis, or Paget-Schroetter syndrome, 18 (55%) had hypertrophy of the subclavius tendon associated with enlargement of the insertion tubercle. Among male patients with Paget-Schroetter syndrome 14 (70%) had this anomaly.[6]

DESCRIPTION OF SPECIFIC ANOMALIES

Anomalies of the First Rib or Cervical Rib

During development the C7 rib forms, then regresses to the C7 transverse process. Various stages in this evolution range from a complete C7 rib to rudimentary forms associated with a fibrocartilagenous band. The only radiologic indication of this residual band may be an enlarged C7 transverse process.

Cervical ribs occur in 0.17% to 0.74% of different populations. In all reporting countries there is a decided female predominance of this anomaly, with about 75% of cervical ribs occurring in women. In a large series of anatomic dissections, the German anatomist Johannes Lang found that 67% of cervical ribs were bilateral. He recognized that when the cervical rib measured 5.6 cm or greater, the subclavian artery passed over the cervical rib. If the rib measured less than 5.1 cm, the artery crossed over the first rib. This observation has helped to clarify from the screening x-ray film the likelihood of arterial injury in cases of symptomatic cervical rib and provides guidance for the decision to proceed with arteriography. When the C7 rib is incomplete, there is often a rudimentary band in place of the regressed portion of the rib (Figs. 1 and 2).

In a comparison between representative studies in the literature and our own operative observations, first rib and cervical rib abnormalities occur with a significantly higher incidence in patients with thoracic outlet syndrome (TOS) than in the general population. These variations clearly represent one of the predisposing abnormalities for development of the clinical neurovascular compressive syndromes. The considerably higher incidence of these recognized congenital abnormalities in women than in men is very likely reflected in the higher incidence of nerve compression symptoms in women.

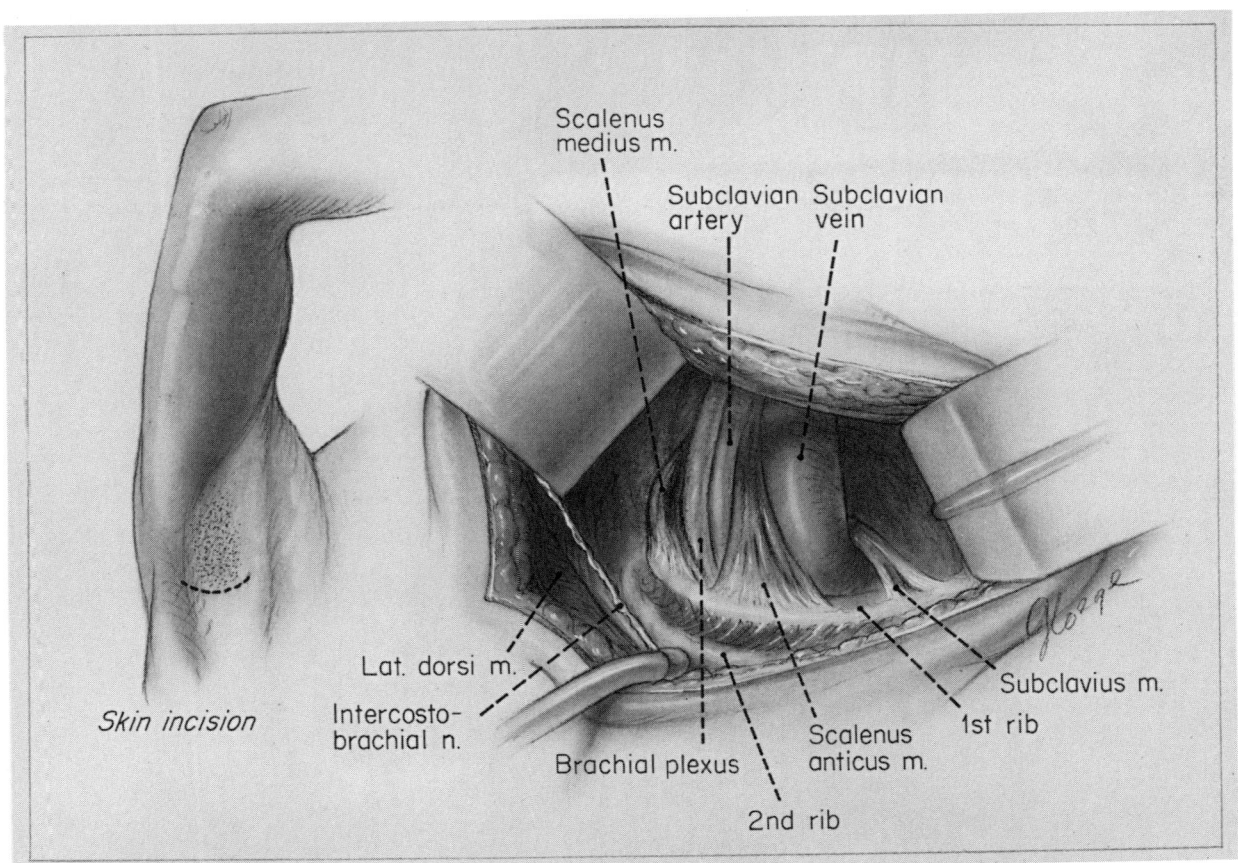

Figure 1 Anatomic relationships at the thoracic outlet as seen from the transaxillary surgical approach. (From Machleder HI. Vascular disorders of the upper extremity, 2nd ed. Mt Kisko, NY: Futura Press, 1989; with permission.)

Fibrocartilaginous Bands

Anomalous fibrous bands from rudimentary cervical ribs have been described by many anatomists investigating structures in the thoracic outlet. These bands, which extend from the ends of incompletely formed cervical ribs, are best thought of as an anomaly of cervical rib formation (Fig. 3). In his descriptive terminology Roos has referred to them as type 1 and type 2 bands.[4] Fibrous bands from the C3, C4, or C5 transverse processes that insert on the first rib or on Sibson's fascia occur when a scalenous minimus muscle has regressed. Roos[4] has described these bands in his numeric system, and Makhoul[1] has placed them in the context of embryologic development. Gilliatt provided the classic description of the clinical neurogenic consequences of these bands as they impinge on the brachial plexus.[7] The wasted hand, with marked weakness and muscular atrophy, is encountered in 2.5% of my patients. This typically occurs in

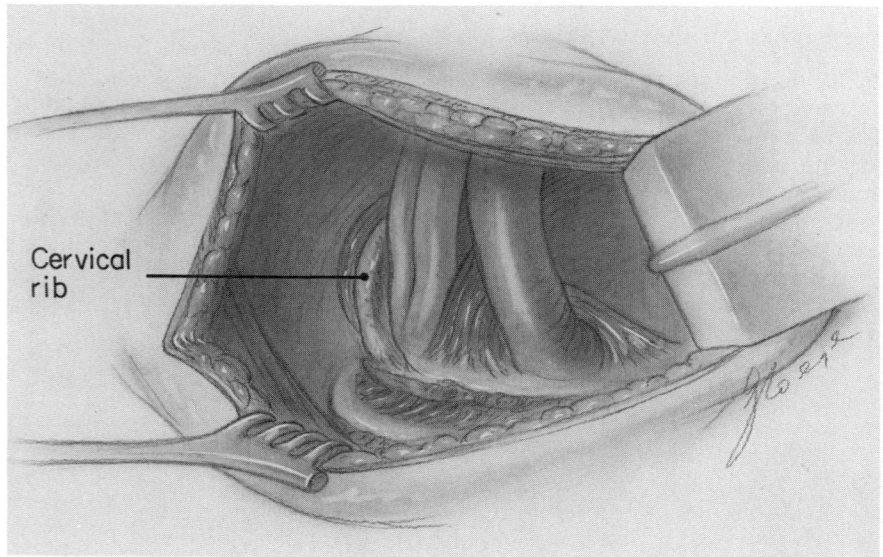

Figure 2 Appearance of a cervical rib articulating with the first thoracic rib as seen from the transaxillary exposure. (From Makhoul RG, Machleder HI. Developmental anomalies at the thoracic outlet: An analysis of 200 consecutive cases. J Vasc Surg 1992; 16:534–545; with permission.)

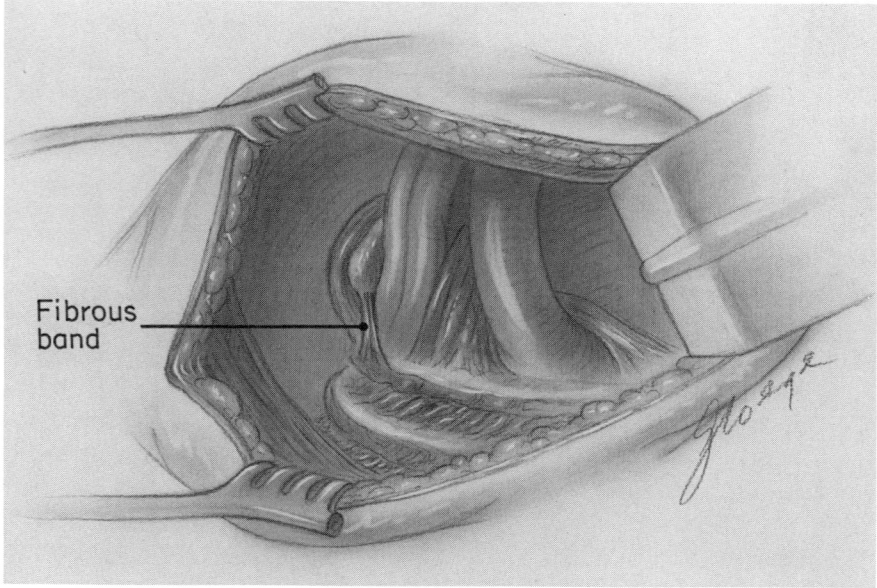

Figure 3 Cervical rib connected to first rib by residual fibrocartilagenous band.

muscles supplied by specific branches of the median and ulnar nerve that are innervated by the C8 through T1 nerve roots.

Scalene Muscle Anomalies

Supernumerary Muscles

Milliez, in his recent studies of scalene muscle in a 2.5 cm embryo, has emphasized the influence of neurovascular structure development on the ultimate configuration of the scalene muscle mass.[8] He recognized a confluent scalene muscle distinguished only by a groove at the site of anterior and middle scalene differentiation. Actual separation into two muscles occurs where the muscle mass is traversed by the roots of the brachial plexus. Rather than the scalenus minimus forming as a separate muscle entity, it represents one form of segmentation of the scalenic mass. The persistence of certain muscle inclusions in the brachial plexus, as well as muscle groups that traverse various elements of the brachial plexus, is related to the original mass of the scalene variously fragmented by the passage of these structures as the limb bud develops. The separation of muscle bundles as they interdigitate between the neurovascular structures accounts for the muscular bridges often seen between the middle and anterior scalene. Roos and Sanders documented these abnormalities of scalene segmentation in anatomic dissections of adult cadavers.[9] Although not pathologic in their own right, these congenital fibers may result in neurogenic symptoms as a consequence of later abnormal growth, peculiarities of occupational or recreational use, or post-traumatic changes.

The scalenus minimus muscle, present in 10% of patients, can be represented by a fully formed muscle or by a residual ligament called the costovertebral or pleurospinal ligament when the muscle has regressed. Roos[4] described these as type 5 or type 6 bands depending on the site of insertion to rib or apical pleura.[4] Lang[10] noted a scalenus minimus or residual ligament in 39% of dissections (Fig. 4).

Abnormalities of Insertion

A number of clinical investigators have described a peculiar crossed insertion of the anterior and middle scalene muscles. This abnormality, which in the extreme is a sling like crossing of the scalene muscles, is often described as a V-shaped deformity that traps the subclavian artery and brachial plexus. It corresponds to the type 4 band described by Roos and is referred to by Makhoul and Machleder[1] as intercostalization, to reflect the embryonic derivation of these muscles (Fig. 5). Roos[11] subdivided these crossing bands into an eighth and ninth abnormality in 1980, the type 8 representing a band from the middle scalene to the costochondral junction and type 9 a fascial band in the concave curve of the first rib.

Despite some common variations of scalene muscle

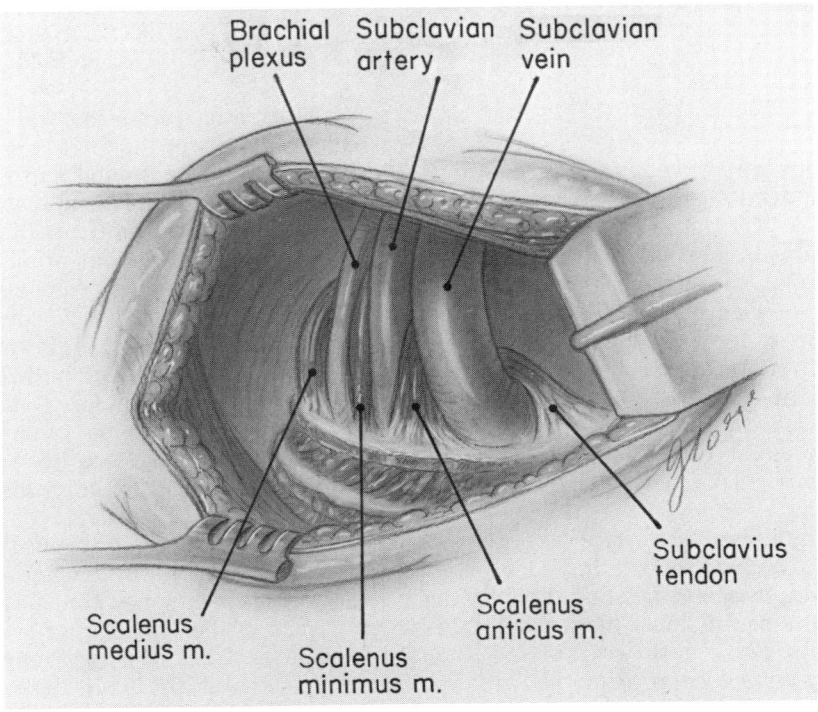

Figure 4 Scalenus minimus muscle.

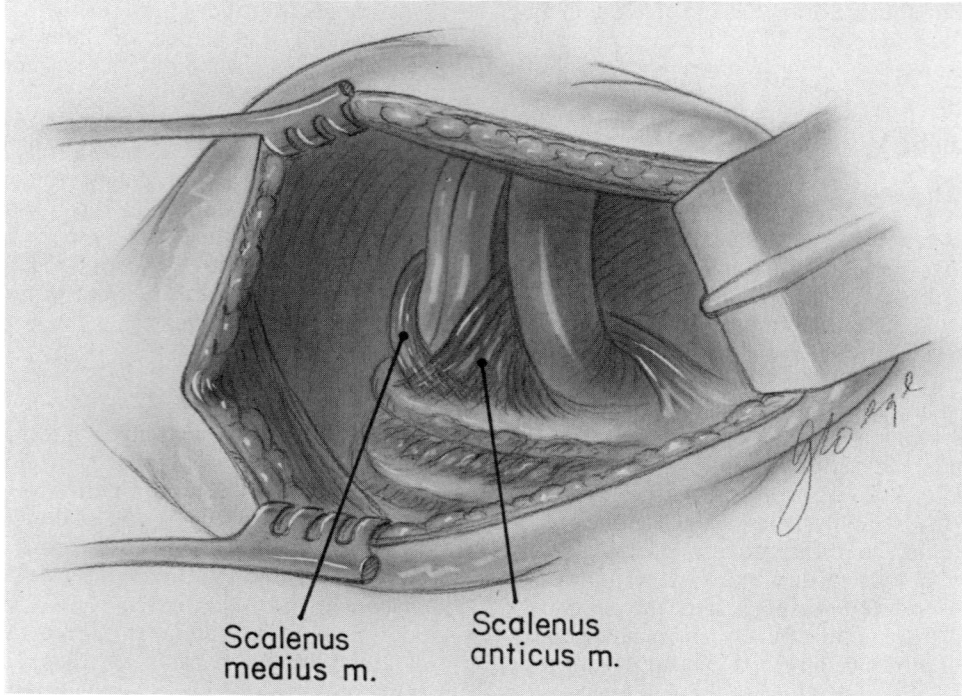

Figure 5 Example of intercostalization, or crossing of the scalenus medius and anticus insertions.

insertion, the unique configurations mentioned above tend to compress the neurovascular structures in the interscalene triangle. They have been identified clinically as accounting for 43% of the variations seen in transaxillary correction of neurovascular compression.

Subclavius Anomalies

Anatomic dissections have documented that during the movements of abduction or retraction of the shoulder, the tendon of the subclavius muscle compresses the subclavian vein against the first rib. In Paget-Schroetter syndrome the striking hypertrophy of the subclavius tendon has been noted. This particular manifestation of compression at the thoracic outlet is related to progressive enlargement of the subclavius muscle system with repetitive compressive trauma to the subclavian vein followed by fibrosis, stricture, and thrombosis. An abnormality in this system was found in 19.5% of our patients, with 15.5% having an exostosis at the subclavius tubercle.

Despite the congenital nature of these deformities, the onset of symptoms in early to mid adult life has been recorded by virtually all physicians treating the clinical disorders. This delay in onset is most likely related to postnatal development. The chest widens and the clavicle continues its growth to approximately age 25, after which the pectoral girdle begins to descend. With loss of strength or tone in the supporting musculature of the thoracic girdle there is further traction on the neurovascular structures at the thoracic outlet.

ULTRASTRUCTURAL STUDIES OF SCALENE MUSCLE

The initial ultrastructural studies of the anterior scalene muscle in the UCLA neuropathology laboratories have been continued and the distinctive fiber type changes seen in post-traumatic compression of the brachial plexus substantiated by further analysis (Fig. 6). The observations, documenting unique fiber type distribution or myosin isoform variation, have been corroborated by other laboratories. There is also an increasing body of evidence that myosin isoforms and muscle fiber phenotype changes occur in response to injury or altered physiologic environments both in the experimental situation and in a number of human disorders.[12] Similar distinctive changes have been described in muscular systems as diverse as the perineum, nasopharynx, and myocardium.

The anterior scalene muscle in patients with post-traumatic thoracic outlet compression symptoms has an extraordinary adaptive transformation and recruitment response in the type 1 fiber system, possibly reflecting chronic increased tone or motor neuron stimulation. It seems particularly likely that in post-traumatic TOS, stretch injury to the muscle initiates a response that if uninterrupted serves to accentuate and perpetuate the

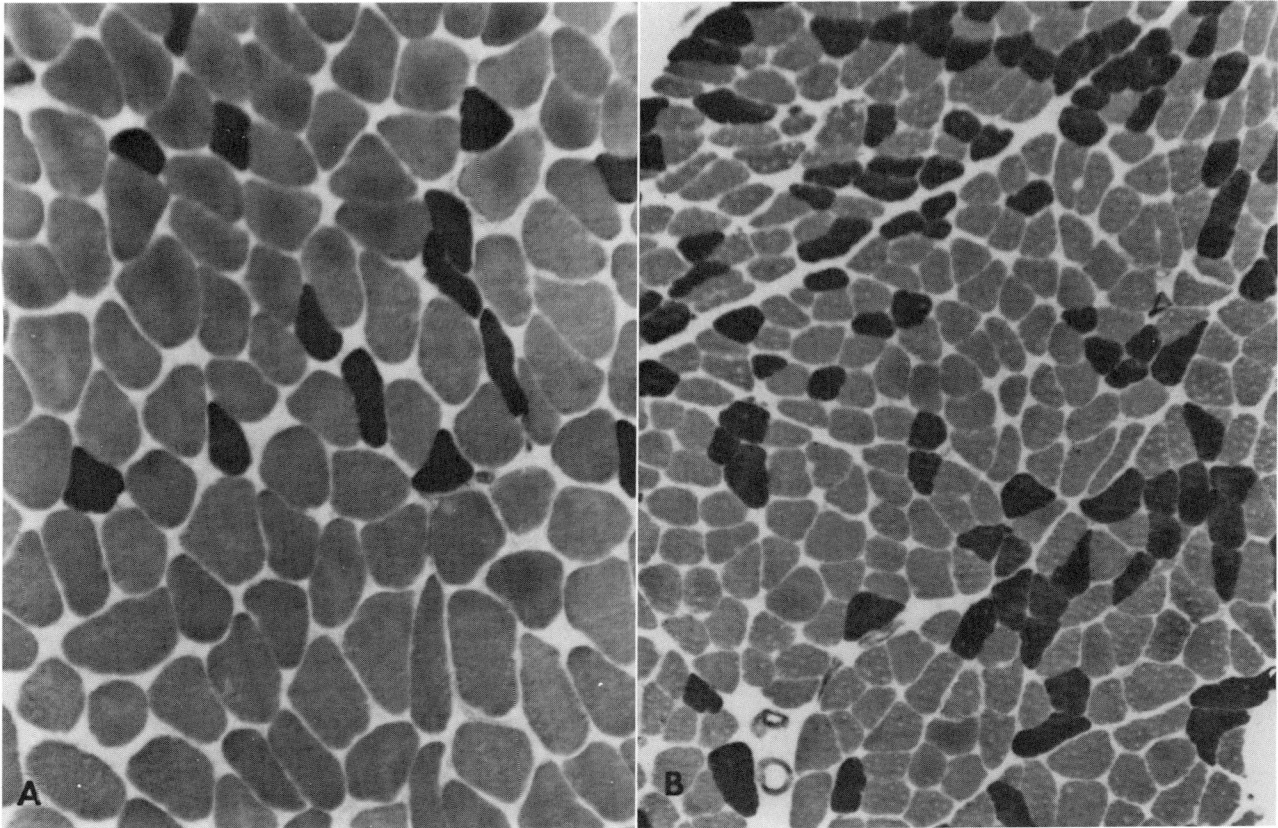

Figure 6 Representative microscopic fields of two anterior scalene muscles, demonstrating the typical mosaic pattern with fiber type staining. *A,* Type 1 fiber *(pale staining)* hypertrophy and predominance, characteristic of patients with post traumatic thoracic outlet compression syndrome. *B,* Muscle after tenotomy with type 1 fiber atrophy and increased proportion of type 2 *(dark staining)* fibers (myosin adenosine triphosphatase stain × 110).

neurovascular compressive phenomenon. In a small percentage of individuals with hyperextension neck injuries there will be gradual development of signs and symptoms of brachial plexus compression in the interscalene triangle. This development will often occur months after resolution of the initial symptoms of musculoligamentous strain. The subtotal replacement of fast acting type 2 fibers with sustained contracting type 1 fibers and the increase in hypertrophy index is thought to be the pathophysiologic mechanism in this delayed onset of neurocompressive symptoms.

REFERENCES

1. Makhoul RG, Machleder HI. Developmental anomalies at the thoracic outlet: An analysis of 200 consecutive cases. J Vasc Surg 1992; 16.534–545.
2. Machleder HI, Moll F, Verity A. The anterior scalene muscle in thoracic outlet compression syndrome: Histochemical and morphometric studies. Arch Surg 1986; 121:1141–1144.
3. Sanders RJ, Jackson CGR, Banchero N, Pearce WH. Scalene muscle abnormalities in traumatic thoracic outlet syndrome. Am J Surg 1990; 159:231–236.
4. Roos DB. Congenital anomalies associated with thoracic outlet syndrome. Am J Surg 1976; 132:771–778.
5. White JC, Poppel MH, Adams R, et al. Congenital malformations of the first thoracic rib: A cause of brachial neuralgia which simulates the cervical rib syndrome. Surg Gyn Obstet 1945; 81:643–659.
6. Kunkel JM, Machleder HI. Treatment of Paget-Schroetter syndrome: A staged multidisciplinary approach. Arch Surg 1989; 124:1153–1158.
7. Gilliatt RW, LeQuesne PM, Longue V, et al. Wasting of the hand associated with a cervical rib or band. J Neurol Neurosurg Psychiatry 1970; 33:615–624.
8. Milliez PY. Contribution a l'etade de l'ontogense des muscles scalenes. Paris: Pantheion-Sorbonne, 1991.
9. Sanders RJ, Roos DB. The surgical anatomy of the scalene triangle. Contemp Surg 1989; 35:11–16.
10. Lang J. Topographische Anatomie des Plexus brachialis and Thoracic-Outlet Syndrom. Berlin: Walter de Gruyter, 1985.
11. Roos DB. Pathophysiology of congenital anomalies in thoracic outlet syndrome. Acta Chir Belg 1980; 79:353–361.
12. Dubowitz V. Responses of diseased muscle to electrical and mechanical intervention. In: Ciba Foundation Symposium 138. Plasticity of the Neuromuscular System. Chichester, U.K.: John Wiley & Sons, 1988:240–250.

DIAGNOSIS OF THORACIC OUTLET SYNDROME

LAZAR J. GREENFIELD, M.D.

Thoracic outlet syndrome (TOS) is a blanket term covering manifestations of both vascular and neurogenic disorders. It is also a term of convenience misapplied to a variety of myofascial and joint disorders. Aside from the advanced neurogenic and vascular manifestations of the syndrome, there are no objective ways of confirming the diagnosis in the majority of patients who present with upper extremity, shoulder, and neck symptoms. This combination of difficulties with the definition and lack of objective tests has led many surgeons to be pessimistic about the role of operation in the management of the disorder. There is more agreement on the potential for improvement when the subclavian vessels are involved, and this is the most appropriate place to begin the diagnostic assessment. Unfortunately, this represents the minority of patients (5%) who present for evaluation.

ARTERIAL TOS

The arterial type of TOS is seen in younger patients with the most significant degrees of mechanical compression, such as by bony abnormalities and cervical ribs or bands. It can also be seen in older patients who have had milder forms of compression for 40 to 50 years, resulting in degenerative changes in the vessel wall. In both groups, the symptoms are ischemic, more typically cramping and muscle fatigue with use of forearm muscles in the younger group. There may also be blanching and sensitivity to cold, which can be confused with reflex sympathetic dystrophy and Raynaud's phenomenon.

The most dramatic presentation of the disorder is acute digit or hand ischemia from an embolic event. The emboli originate from aneurysmal dilation of the post-stenotic subclavian artery. Every patient presenting with such signs and symptoms should have a proximal subclavian artery aneurysm excluded before an extensive workup is undertaken to search for cardiac or other sources.

On examination, the subclavian artery may be prominent and palpable in the supraclavicular fossa, and a bruit may be audible. A discrepancy in systolic blood pressures between the arms greater than 15 mm Hg may be present. The examination of the hand should note the color of the nail beds for any evidence of digital ischemia. Evidence of ischemia may also be present with performance of the elevated arm stress test as popularized by Roos.[1] This test is performed with the arms elevated in the hands-up position, and the patient is asked to open and close the hands slowly over a period of 3 minutes. Reproduction of symptoms with this maneuver helps to confirm the diagnosis, although it is also positive in patients with carpal tunnel syndrome. Simple obliteration of the pulse with the arms abducted is not a reliable sign because most normal persons have this finding. Adson's test, which has achieved more popularity than it deserves, is rarely performed as originally described. The original test was performed by palpating the radial pulse with the hand in the lap, having the patient turn the head to the ipsilateral side, and then tilting it backward while the patient takes a deep breath. Although this test can demonstrate anterior scalene muscle compression of the subclavian artery, it is neither sensitive nor specific enough for the diagnosis of TOS.

Hyperabduction and military maneuvers can also compress the artery, not only at the level of the first rib but also at the pectoralis minor insertion and around the head of the humerus. These tests are similarly positive in many normal patients and should not be used to make the diagnosis of TOS. The appropriate diagnostic study for the patient presenting with signs and symptoms of arterial TOS is a selective arteriogram with the arm in neutral and abducted positions. Noninvasive ultrasound imaging and Doppler studies have proved to be disappointing in these patients. They may be of value, however, in the evaluation of patients with suspected sympathetic over-reactivity.

VENOUS TOS

The first recognition of the potential adverse effects of shoulder movement on the subclavian vein was by von Schroetter, who introduced the term effort thrombosis.[2] Subsequent clinical observations that neither trauma nor thrombosis was required were made by Hughes, who coined the term Paget-von Schroetter syndrome to credit the two individuals who first described the condition.[3] The anatomy of the compression injury is the narrow junction between clavicle and first rib and the pressure of the anterior scalene muscle, which squeezes the vein into the rigid costoclavicular ligament. Young male weightlifters seem to have a particular predisposition to this disorder.

The presenting symptoms of the disorder are pain, swelling, cyanosis, and venous distention in the involved upper extremity. With acute thrombosis, the arm may be tender and dusky with evidence of collateral veins over the shoulder and anterior chest wall. Prior to complete obstruction, patients give a history of being unable to wear rings and of worsening of the symptoms with effort. On examination, the involved extremity is edematous with distended superficial veins that fail to collapse with elevation of the arm. In the absence of thrombotic obstruction, the elevated arm stress test may demonstrate venous congestion in the involved extremity and reproduce the symptoms.

The definitive diagnostic study is a peripheral phlebogram, performed without tourniquet, which either documents the point of compression or confirms the presence of subclavian vein thrombosis by documentation of collateral venous filling. The phlebogram should be performed with the arms abducted because there is physiologic compression of the axillary vein with the arm adducted. Some vein compression can also be seen in about one-third of normal patients at the level of the head of the humerus and in the costoclavicular space. Measurement of venous pressure can be of value in helping to discriminate significant mechanical compression. The finding of acute subclavian vein thrombosis is usually an indication to attempt thrombolytic therapy in order not only to clear the obstruction but also to verify the point of compression in order to facilitate operative correction and prevent rethrombosis.

NEUROGENIC TOS

The typical patient with neurogenic TOS is an asthenic woman with poor posture who presents with shoulder girdle and arm pain radiating down the medial aspect of the arm associated with paresthesias and numbness in the ulnar distribution of the hand and forearm. If there is wasting of the lateral thenar muscles and electromyographic examination documents chronic lower trunk brachial plexopathy, then the patient is considered to have "true" or "classical" neurogenic TOS. It is important to differentiate the C8-T1 radiculopathy from the effects of cervical spondylosis, which is the reason for the electrodiagnostic studies. The characteristic findings of nerve conduction studies include low-amplitude median motor responses, low-amplitude ulnar sensory action potentials, relatively low- or normal-amplitude ulnar motor responses, and normal median sensory responses. Examination of specific muscles of the hand demonstrates weakness of the abductor pollicis brevis and the opponens pollicis, with characteristic guttering along the lateral aspect of the thenar eminence. Fortunately for the patient, very few have progressed to this stage when seen initially because this degree of nerve damage is often irreversible. More than 60% of these patients fail to have return of complete function following thoracic outlet decompression.[4]

Most patients presenting with signs and symptoms of neurogenic TOS do not have evidence of nerve damage by electrodiagnostic testing or by muscle wasting. The description by the patient is usually that of a dull, constant, aching pain that is more diffuse in the shoulder region and spreading down the arm, but not in the C8-T1 dermatomal pattern. It is the paresthesias that are segmental and felt in the inner aspect of the arm and forearm with involvement of the fourth and fifth digits. Occasionally, a burning sensation or even sharp, localized pains may be experienced. Pain is typically worse toward the end of a day of vigorous activity, and many patients are awakened by aching pain at night, particularly if the arm is raised above the pillow. Both pain and paresthesias are aggravated by carrying heavy objects in the hand or by wearing garments or accessories with shoulder straps. Occupations or sports involving abduction and use of the arm above the shoulder are tolerated poorly.

The difference between the distribution of the pain and paresthesia can be explained by known pain pathways in the upper extremity. It is the superficial pain fibers that are involved in the production of paresthesia and hypesthesia in the typical C8-T1 distribution, with more focal involvement of the ulnar side of the forearm and hand. Additional fibers that transmit deep pain sensation from the arm originate from the dorsal root ganglia of the T2-T5 segments and travel in the sympathetic chain, entering the anterior surface of the C8 and T1 roots before they merge to form the lower trunk. Because these deep pain fibers are intermingled with other somatic fibers of the brachial plexus that receive input from the T2-T5 dermatome, the discomfort is recognized over broader areas of chest, shoulder, and arm. Motor changes are also appreciated by the patient prior to the onset of specific weakness and wasting. The hand is described as weak, stiff, and clumsy, with most of the difficulty early in the day. There are usually problems with activities of daily living, such as shampooing hair. It is also helpful to ask the patient about driving because it is usually not possible to use the involved extremity on the steering wheel for any length of time. Some vasomotor symptoms may also be present, such as blanching with exposure to cold and reddish discoloration of the arm and hand when the arm is dependent.

In eliciting the history from the patient, it is important to know whether the symptoms followed specific trauma or a motor vehicle accident. There may be a history of hyperextension injury of the neck with residual myofascial pain that involves the neck, back, and shoulder in addition to the arm symptoms. It is also important to know the quantity and duration of pain medication and whether litigation is in process. These variables add considerable complexity to the management of the patient, and the prior history of trauma is associated with less favorable outcome.[4] The patient's response to previous physical therapy is important because many patients are seen after failure to respond. Often the physical therapy has consisted of range-of-motion and strengthening exercises, which are most likely to aggravate rather than improve the situation. The most appropriate physical therapy for these patients usually involves stretching rather than strengthening exercises and the treatment of trigger points by injection or other modalities. It is not unusual for these patients to have had prior nerve entrapment problems such as carpal tunnel syndrome, and this history should be elicited. Prior assessment in a chronic pain clinic is not unusual, and identification of response to specific treatment should be sought. A detailed work history is important, with demonstration of specific tasks required. Any history of psychological problems should be identified, as well as any evidence of drug dependence. The nonclassical or disputed neurogenic TOS is a diagnosis of exclusion; therefore, diagnostic tests are limited to those that can identify closely related diagnoses. Of particular value are cervical spine x-rays and a chest x-ray look for possible superior sulcus (Pancoast) tumors. In addition to identification of potential nerve root compression, cervical spine x-rays can document prominent transverse processes that are surrogate cervical ribs often found to be associated with fascial bands that produce mechanical compression. Although sensory evoked potentials have been found by some authors to be of value in the identification of patients who will benefit from thoracic outlet decompression,[5,6] it has not been possible to consistently duplicate this experience. Similarly, electromyography is used only to exclude other nerve entrapment syndromes. Although computed tomography and magnetic resonance imaging studies are frequently obtained in these patients, they generally provide less useful information than the x-rays previously mentioned. Routine angiography should not be obtained unless there are specific vascular findings as indicated in the description of arterial and venous TOS.

PHYSICAL EXAMINATION

A careful and complete physical examination is essential not only in the identification of patients with thoracic outlet syndrome but also in monitoring their response to conservative and operative treatment. Particular attention should be paid to the patient's posture, which is often a clue to the problem. Initial attention is focused on range of motion of the head and neck with identification of paracervical muscle spasm. The patient with TOS as opposed to paracervical muscle strain is able to tolerate head turning better than head tilting toward each shoulder. Tilting of the head often reproduces brachial plexus symptoms. Vertex compression can also be used to evaluate for cervical disk. Shoulder shrug and shoulder range-of-motion tests can be used to look for muscle and intrinsic shoulder joint pathology. Thumb compression of the clavicle and all of the supraclavicular structures on both sides usually identifies specific brachial plexus tenderness on the affected side. Ninety-degree abduction of the arm with full eversion often reproduces symptoms, and, as mentioned previously, the elevated arm stress test can be of value. Although Adson's sign is not particularly helpful, Wright's maneuver can confirm the presence of positional vascular compression and may reproduce the symptoms. Direct palpation of the pectoralis minor should also be evaluated because myofascial involvement there can mimic the findings of TOS.[7] Bilateral arm and hand strength should be evaluated and the hands examined for muscle wasting and intrinsic muscle function. Upper extremity reflexes and dermatome response to pin prick complete the evaluation. Some investigators have found other provocative tests, such as Phalens, to be of value. Also, it is thought by some that the initial deficit for nerve compression consists of the loss of the ability to appreciate high-frequency vibration changes, and a vibragram, along with assessment of two-point discrimination, is felt to be of value.

DIAGNOSIS

The diagnosis of classical neurogenic and vascular TOS can be established by the angiographic and neurologic findings described. It is easy to criticize any diagnosis of thoracic outlet syndrome of the disputed neurogenic type because it is a diagnosis of exclusion and

Table 1 Differential Diagnosis of Thoracic Outlet Syndrome

Neurogenic	Vascular	Musculoskeletal
Spinal cord	Arterial	Inflammation
Tumors, cysts	Arteriosclerosis, aneurysm, occlusion	Bursitis
Degenerative disease, syringomyelia,	Embolism	Arthritis
ALS, MS, motor neuron disease	Collagen vascular disease	Myositis
Inflammation	Functional Raynaud's aerocyanosis	Fibrositis
Nerve roots	Erythromelalgia	Tendinitis
Ruptured disk	Venous	Trauma
Degenerative disease	Thrombophlebitis	Rotator cuff
Tumors	Arteriovenous fistula	Visceral
Inflammation	Lymphangitis	Angina pectoris
Brachial plexus	Lymphedema	Esophageal disease
Superior sulcus tumors	Mediastinal venous obstruction	Pulmonary disease
Trauma		Psychogenic
Peripheral nerves		
Entrapment neuropathy of median,		
ulnar, radial nerves		
Trauma		
Tumors		
RSD and causalgia		
Medical neuropathy		

ALS = amyotrophic lateral sclerosis; MS = multiple sclerosis; RSD = reflex sympathetic dystrophy.
From Luoma A, Nelems B. Thoracic outlet syndrome: Thoracic surgery perspective. Neurosurg Clin North Am 1991; 2:187–226; with permission.

based on patient symptoms. However, angina pectoris and other pain syndromes are diagnosed in a similar fashion. It is certainly easier to discount the symptoms and refer the patient, but there is substantial potential value to making the effort on the assumption that the patient truly desires to get better. Based on this assumption, the criteria for diagnosis should include the presence of neck, shoulder, or arm pain, arm paresthesias, and reproduction of these symptoms by provocative arm maneuvers. Evidence of pain on palpation of the brachial plexus also helps to reinforce the diagnosis. The most frequent mimic of the findings is the myofascial pain syndrome, which is not unusual in conjunction with TOS findings. Other considerations in the differential diagnosis are listed in Table 1.[8] All of these patients deserve maximal efforts to relieve the myofascial pain syndrome by conservative measures. Seeing the patients along with an experienced physical therapist and pain psychologist in the clinic has the highest likelihood of success.

REFERENCES

1. Roos DB. Congenital anomalies associated with thoracic outlet syndrome: Anatomy, symptoms, diagnosis and treatment. Am J Surg 1976; 132:771–778.
2. von Schroetter L. Handbuch der allgemeinen pathologie and therapie. Berlin: A Herschwald, 1884. Cited in: Sanders RJ, Hang CE. Thoracic outlet syndrome: A common sequela of neck injuries. Philadelphia: JB Lippincott, 1991.
3. Hughes ESR. Venous obstruction in the upper extremity. B J Surg 1948; 36:155–163.
4. Green RM, McNamara J, Ouriel K. Long term follow-up after thoracic outlet decompression: An analysis of factors determining outcome. J Vasc Surg 1991; 14:739–745.
5. Jerrett SA, Cuzzone LJ, Pasternak BM. Thoracic outlet syndrome: Electrophysiologic reappraisal. Arch Neurol 1984; 41:960–963.
6. Machleder HI, Moll F, Verity A. The anterior scalene muscle in thoracic outlet compression syndrome: Histochemical and morphometric studies. Arch Surg 1986; 121:1141–1144.
7. Hong C-Z, Simons DG. Response to the treatment for pectoralis minor myofascial pain syndrome after whiplash. J Musculoskeletal Pain 1993; 1:89–129.
8. Luoma A, Nelems B. Thoracic outlet syndrome: Thoracic surgery perspective. Neurosurg Clin North Am 1991; 2:187–226.

NONOPERATIVE MANAGEMENT OF THORACIC OUTLET SYNDROME

ROBERT D. DeFRANG, M.D.
LLOYD M. TAYLOR Jr, M.D.
GREGORY L. MONETA, M.D.
JOHN M. PORTER, M.D.

Pathologic compression of upper extremity neurovascular structures has been recognized for more than a century. In 1853, Hilton described upper extremity neurovascular compression related to bony abnormalities, and subsequently Coote reported the first patient relieved of symptoms following first rib removal. Mechanisms of neurovascular compression were hypothesized as early as 1905, when Murphy and later Halsted studied the pathophysiology of subclavian artery aneurysms in patients with cervical ribs. In the following decades multiple compression syndromes located in the thoracic outlet were described as etiologies of upper extremity pain syndromes. Depending on the specific structures affected, the clinical presentation, diagnostic tests, and therapy have varied markedly. Because of this, Gilliatt has preferred the plural term, thoracic outlet syndromes, in that there are defined subgroups of this disorder.[1]

In 1956, however, Peet and associates suggested grouping all these syndromes under a single heading, thoracic outlet syndrome (TOS).[1] Shortly thereafter, Clagett hypothesized that the first rib was the key to both the pathophysiology and surgical treatment of TOS.[2] Reported surgical results of first rib resection combined with the cosmetically acceptable transaxillary approach described by Roos in 1966 led to enthusiastic acceptance of surgical treatment of all forms of TOS by many surgeons.[3]

Thoracic outlet syndrome is assumed to result from compression of either the subclavian artery, the subclavian vein, or the brachial plexus, or a combination of these, at some site between the inferolateral neck and the axilla. Depending upon the hypothesized offending structure, TOS has been known by many names, including first cervical rib syndrome, scalenus anticus syndrome, subcoracoid-pectoralis minor syndrome, hyperabduction syndrome, and costoclavicular syndrome.

To be best understood, TOS should be considered according to the specific structures affected. We find it most convenient to classify TOS as arterial vascular, venous vascular, true neurogenic, or disputed neurogenic. The vascular and true neurogenic subgroups are not controversial. Each is associated with bony abnormalities of the thoracic outlet and is accompanied by objective physical, hemodynamic, and/or electrodiagnostic findings. Treatment is appropriately surgical, and results of these procedures are predictably excellent. Therefore, vascular and true neurogenic TOS are not discussed in this section. Unfortunately, the most frequently diagnosed subgroup, disputed neurogenic TOS

(DN-TOS), is also the only controversial subgroup. It is estimated that more than 95% of TOS patients operated upon in the United States are in this category. It is distinguished from other forms of TOS by lack of the specific objective physical and electrophysiologic findings that are found in the other three subgroups. Instead, its features are unique in the field of peripheral neurology.[4]

Symptoms of DN-TOS are attributed to compression of the brachial plexus at the level of the thoracic outlet. Although surgical therapy has never been proved effective, thousands of operations have been performed to treat this disorder. No consensus has ever been reached regarding any of its basic tenets, and its proponents agree on surprisingly little except that it is common. Given no clear pathophysiology of DN-TOS and the uncertain benefit associated with surgical therapy, we presently favor nonoperative therapy for a diagnosis of DN-TOS.

PRESENTATION

Symptoms attributed to DN-TOS are varied and numerous. Most frequently pain and paresthesias in the distribution of the lower brachial plexus trunk are described. The lower trunk of the brachial plexus carries median nerve motor fibers to thenar muscles, ulnar nerve motor fibers to hypothenar muscles, and ulnar nerve sensory fibers. The vagueness and generality of reported symptoms, many of which defy precise neuroanatomic characterization, are difficult to reconcile.

Typically, symptoms of DN-TOS are associated with monotonous repetitive movements of the shoulder or arms in musicians, assembly line workers, hairdressers, and those operating video display terminals or typewriters. Interestingly, more than 70% of reported cases are in women. Data from the National Center for Health Statistics suggest that in 1985 to 1987, close to 1% of the U.S. population had musculoskeletal impairment of the upper extremity, and nearly 20% were attributed to on-the-job injury.[5,6] Highly repetitive shoulder muscle contractions and work at shoulder level appear to be exposure factors that increase the risk of developing symptoms associated with the diagnosis of DN-TOS.

Pain may be unifocal or multifocal and is often poorly localized in the limb musculature. It is variously described as aching, sharp, dull, burning, squeezing, or stabbing in nature. Weakness and/or numbness in all or parts of the extremity are also reported, in addition to cramping, swelling, and stiffness. Most often paresthesias and aches occur along the medial side of the arm, forearm, and sometimes the hand in primarily a lower trunk distribution but without clear dermatomic reference. In fact, any discomfort of the neck, shoulder, or arm has been considered DN-TOS. Symptoms are usually aggravated by use of the extremity. Motor symptoms are least common and certainly less pronounced than sensory complaints. Many patients have presented with such diffuse complaints as chest and/or shoulder pain, headache, temporomandibular joint discomfort, and/or muscle tension. How presumed pressure on the brachial plexus in the thoracic outlet can produce these symptoms is unclear. A frequent, unsubstantiated assumption is that these subjective symptoms are caused by the patients' occupations.

DIAGNOSIS

In contrast to all other reported peripheral nerve compression syndromes, clinical examination typically reveals no muscle wasting, swelling, or trophic changes. Maneuvers such as Adson's test, EAST (elevated arm stress test) procedure, hyperabduction, and costoclavicular tests are often positive, but these phenomena are also noted in 10% to 74% of normal asymptomatic individuals. For example, a positive EAST, which some authorities consider diagnostic, has been demonstrated in more than 90% of patients with objective confirmation of carpal tunnel syndrome and in 74% of normal asymptomatic controls.[1]

Attempts by proponents to identify diagnostic electrophysiologic abnormalities have not met with success, and there remains no consensus to date. Multiple tests were initially heralded as both highly sensitive and specific. Currently, somatosensory evoked potentials hold center stage, displacing previously favored nerve conduction studies, F waves, F loops, electromyography, thermography, and C-8 root needle stimulation, all of which have been proven to be invalid.[7] Unfortunately, currently described abnormalities in somatosensory evoked potentials are nonspecific and suggest only the presence, but not the cause, of abnormal conduction along large-diameter efferent and afferent nerve fibers.[4] Daube found that the mean conduction velocities, latencies, and amplitude of motor and sensory fibers in the lower cords of the brachial plexus in patients with DN-TOS did not differ significantly from the results of studies performed in normal asymptomatic persons.[8] Similarly, Wilbourn challenged earlier studies describing prolonged conduction across the thoracic outlet in patients with DN-TOS, leading to an admission of fabrication.[4]

TREATMENT

Our approach to patients with presumed TOS or with symptoms suggestive of TOS is as follows: Electrodiagnostic testing is essential. True neurogenic TOS (1 per million population) has characteristic electrical abnormalities that include decreased amplitude of ulnar sensory action potentials and normal nerve conduction velocities. Other nerve entrapment disorders, specifically carpal tunnel syndrome, ulnar neuropathy, brachial plexopathy, and cervical radiculopathy, must be excluded. Additionally, we obtain x-rays to specifically identify thoracic outlet bony abnormalities, including cervical ribs, abnormal first ribs, and hypertrophic clavicle fractures. Venous and arterial diagnostic testing are performed when indicated by history and physical examination. Once a diagnosis of DN-TOS is reached by exclusion, we feel that in the absence of a consensus on treatment, these patients are best managed by rendering no specific treatment. Conversely, many others believe treatment, either operation and/or physical therapy, should be initiated.

Roos, Machleder, and others suggest that all but the least affected patients, those improving with nonoperative treatment, require operative treatment.[3,7] The implication is that untreated patients progress to true neurogenic TOS. This implication appears unfounded, and we are unaware of a single report of such disease progression. Interestingly, most reports describing treatment of DN-TOS indicate excellent results regardless of the type of treatment performed. Good results routinely follow physical therapy and exercise programs in 60% to 90% of patients; similarly, first rib resection also improves nearly 90% of patients.[3,5,9] In most such reports, the operating surgeon, hardly a disinterested observer, has recorded the postoperative assessment. Interestingly, equally good results have been reported by other operations including scalenectomy alone.

Reservations against operation include the risk of major complications, such as brachial plexus injury, as well as persistence of postoperative neck, shoulder, and/or arm pain. Most surgical studies claiming high success rates were reported by the same groups performing the surgical procedures. An alternate view is supplied by Lepantalo and associates, who followed 103 patients an average of 6 years after first rib resection for DN-TOS. One month postoperatively, 77% were improved and remained so for 6 months. However, at 6 years, two independent examiners found a permanent success rate of only 37%.[10]

Physical therapy for DN-TOS consists of exercises and muscle relaxation. Initial treatment emphasizes rest and splinting. Sessions are conducted at least three times per week during the first month and then twice a week for the second month. Additional sessions are occasionally necessary after this. The goal of physical therapy is symptomatic relief, although the exact mechanisms of improvement are not known with certainty. Passive range of motion is maintained and inflammation is reduced with use of nonsteroidal anti-inflammatory agents, ice, massage, and ultrasound. This is followed by a reconditioning phase with therapy to increase strength and posture. At this point, job analysis and work modification, if possible, are begun to facilitate re-entry into the work force. Attention by the patient to both physical and psychological factors in the work place as well as in nonoccupational activities and at home appears important. Carrying heavy loads and prolonged abduction should be avoided. Sports that entail violent shoulder movement are discouraged. If a high suspicion of radiculopathy persists after conservative treatment, a cervical myelogram or magnetic resonance imaging may be indicated.

Relatively little has been published concerning the results of nonoperative treatment of DN-TOS. Nonetheless, available reports document improvement or complete relief of symptoms with physical therapy at 4 years in 66% to 87.5% of patients. Kenney and colleagues prospectively evaluated a supervised physiotherapy program in eight patients with TOS. After only 3 weeks of intervention, symptoms assessed by visual analog scales had significantly improved in all patients (p less than 0.01).[9]

What is strikingly absent in the TOS literature is the natural history of untreated DN-TOS. No treatment may be just as good as either physical therapy or operation. We have noted anecdotally that a number of patients in our referral practice appear worse following operation and/or physical therapy. Our approach has, therefore, been to identify and treat TOS subgroups that include venous vascular, arterial vascular, and true neurogenic TOS in addition to other objectively determined nerve compression syndromes. No specific treatment, either surgical or nonsurgical, is recommended for DN-TOS, a syndrome that as yet defies pathologic characterization.

REFERENCES

1. Wilbourn AJ, Porter JM. Thoracic outlet syndromes. Spine 1988; 2:597–626.
2. Clagett OT. Presidential address: Research and prosearch. J Thorac Cardiovasc Surg 1962; 44:153–186.
3. Roos DB. Transaxillary approach for first rib resection to relieve thoracic outlet syndrome. Ann Surg 1966; 163:354–358.
4. Wilbourn AJ. The thoracic outlet syndrome is overdiagnosed. Arch Neurol 1990; 47:328–330.
5. Lederman RJ. Repetitive motion disorders. Neuroscience Today 1993; 25:1–15.
6. Mandel S. Neurologic syndromes from repetitive trauma at work. Postgrad Med 1987; 82:87–92.
7. Machleder HI, Moll F, Nuiver M, et al. Somatosensory evoked potentials in the assessment of thoracic outlet syndrome. J Vasc Surg 1987; 6:177–184.
8. Daube JR. Nerve conduction studies in the thoracic outlet syndrome. Neurology 1975; 25:347–352.
9. Kenny RA, Traynor GB, Withington D, Keegan DJ. Thoracic outlet syndrome: A useful exercise treatment option. Am J Surg 1993; 165:282–284.
10. Lepantalo M, Lindgren KA, Leino E, et al. Longterm outcome after resection of the first rib for thoracic outlet syndrome. Br J Surg 1989; 76:1255–1256.

TRANSAXILLARY OPERATIVE MANAGEMENT OF THORACIC OUTLET SYNDROME

RICHARD M. GREEN, M.D.

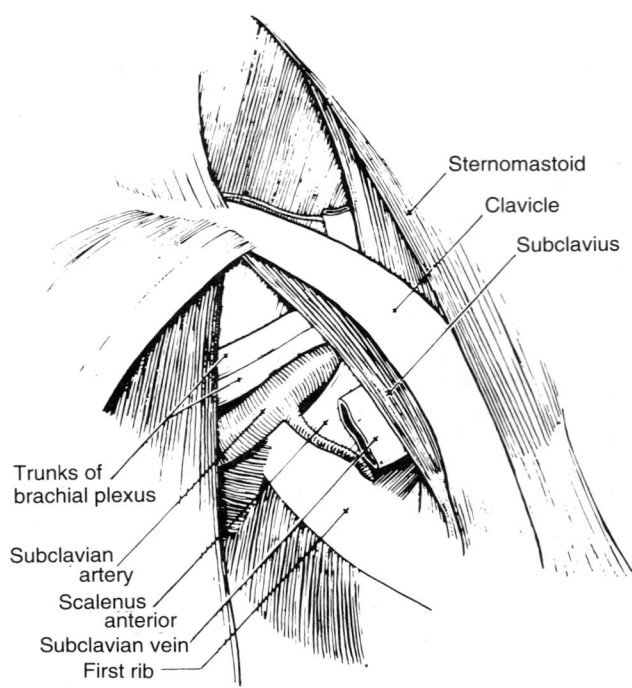

Figure 1 Anatomic relationships of the thoracic outlet. Unfortunately, the operative field does not look anything like this. The space should be thought of in three-dimensional terms. The first rib forms the floor; the clavicle, the roof. The scalene muscles and any anomalous structures serve as walls to subdivide the space. Because everything attaches to the first rib, its removal should decompress the entire region.

The thoracic outlet syndrome (TOS) consists of a variety of conditions caused by compression of the neurovascular structures passing between the clavicle, scalene muscles, and the first rib (Fig. 1). The syndrome may result from a congenital musculoskeletal anomaly such as a cervical rib or from an acquired condition such as a fractured clavicle. Often there is no definable anatomic abnormality. The diagnosis is clear when either the axillary-subclavian artery or vein is involved. Unfortunately, most of the patients are referred because of neurologic symptoms, and the diagnosis is not clear.

The neurologic component of TOS is an entity that has fueled many controversies, not only about the proper treatment but also about its very existence.[1] The controversies exist because the symptoms are subjective and no reproducible diagnostic test is available. When a patient's symptoms warrant operative therapy, transaxillary first rib resection should be performed in most cases. Appropriate diagnostic and therapeutic approaches for the variety of syndromes exist (Table 1). For two basic conditions transaxillary management of TOS is not the approach of choice: (1) fixed vascular pathology that requires direct vessel repair and (2) a broad-based cervical rib. In each instance, supraclavicular incisions with or without claviculectomy provide better exposure. In the former instance, the transaxillary exposure does not allow sufficient control of the vessels. In the latter instance, the broad cervical rib is difficult to remove from the axilla without manipulation of the nerves because of the broad synarthrosis with the first rib.

The subjective nature of the neurologic symptoms and the lack of a specific diagnostic test make patient selection and analysis of results difficult. Although various screening tests have been proposed to identify those patients who would benefit from a first rib resection, none has held up to close scrutiny. The obliteration of the radial pulse with abduction of the shoulder is not diagnostic of TOS. In fact, more than 90% of normal subjects lose at least one radial pulse with this maneuver. Similarly, the elevated arm stress test (EAST) is positive in 92% of patients with carpal tunnel syndrome. Electrodiagnostic testing is not helpful in the diagnosis of TOS but is helpful in excluding other neurologic conditions such as carpal tunnel syndrome or ulnar entrapment. Cervical myelography and/or magnetic resonance imaging is indicated whenever spondylosis is suspected.

Transaxillary first rib resection should be performed in patients with chronic venous TOS when the collateral veins are compressed by shoulder abduction. This diagnosis can be confirmed with phlebograms via the median antecubital vein in the resting and stressed position. These patients develop large collateral veins draining along the chest wall that are compressed by the first rib with shoulder abduction. It is crucial in these patients to remove the entire medial portion of the rib. Some prefer medial claviculectomy in this situation, but this operation may leave an unsightly scar and often results in limitations of shoulder movement. Medial claviculectomy is best reserved for those patients who require exposure of the vein for either thrombectomy or repair.

Transaxillary first rib resection is not often used for arterial involvement. Because these cases are almost always due to a large cervical rib, an anterior approach is preferred. This can be accomplished either by a medial claviculectomy or by combined supraclavicular and infraclavicular incisions. The transaxillary approach should be used only in those rare instances of arterial compression in the absence of a cervical rib and fixed arterial pathology.

Most patients with neurologic TOS requiring operation are best treated by the transaxillary approach. Although some concern exists that a significant number of brachial plexus injuries occur after transaxillary rib resection, plexus damage after transaxillary rib resection

Table 1 Diagnostic and Therapeutic Preferences for the Different Components of TOS

Syndrome	Diagnosis	Preferred Approach	Comments
Venous compression	Phlebogram via median antecubital vein	Transax first rib	Some prefer claviculectomy but more disability and unsightly scar
Venous with thrombosis (chronic)	Phlebogram via median antecubital vein	Transax first rib	Relieves compression of collateral veins; if venous reconstruction is required, the best approach is via a medial claviculectomy
Arterial with cervical rib	C-spine x-rays, arteriogram	Supraclavicular	Cervical ribs associated with arterial pathology are usually very wide and difficult to remove from the axilla
Arterial with aneurysm	C-spine x-rays, arteriogram	Supraclavicular and infraclavicular	Cosmetically better than claviculectomy, which gives same exposure
Arterial without bony or vascular pathology	C-spine x-rays, arteriogram	Transax first rib	Unusual presentation, old anterior scalene syndrome?
Neurologic	Neurology consult, electromyogram, C-spine x-ray, magnetic resonance imaging	Transax first rib	Best decompression with lowest incidence of recurrence
Neurologic with cervical rib	Neurology consult, electromyogram, C-spine x-rays	Transax first rib	These ribs are usually very narrow and can be removed through the axilla along with the first rib

Table 2 Indications for Operation in Neurologic TOS

Condition	Operation	Comments
Atrophy of the ulnar innervated muscles	Transaxillary rib resection with division of fibrous band from C-7	So-called classic TOS; very rare but no one would debate its existence or indication for operation; atrophy persists after operation
Repetitive work-related injury	Poor results, especially in women; operation should be avoided	Makes up part of the "disputed" neurologic TOS; many doubt the existence of this entity
Symptoms reproduced by abduction of the shoulder	Transaxillary rib resection	Patients must be screened carefully but good results can be achieved
Symptoms in the presence of a cervical rib	Large ribs should be removed with a supraclavicular incision; small ribs can be removed from the axilla	Presence of a cervical rib makes the diagnosis of TOS more certain
Symptoms with chronic denervation on electrodiagnostic studies	Poor results with any operation	TOS rarely causes permanent nerve damage

is rare in the large reported series. Scalenectomy has been proposed as an initial procedure because of its relative safety, but good long-term results have not been uniformly achieved. The recurrence rate at the University of Rochester after an initial scalenectomy is five times the recurrence rate after rib resection. Furthermore, early reports of brachial plexus damage during supraclavicular procedures appeared prior to the advent of the transaxillary approach.

Proper patient selection is an important determinant of results after transaxillary rib resection for neurologic symptoms. The decision to operate upon a patient should be made only after a complete neurologic evaluation has excluded any other entity that could cause similar symptoms. The symptoms should be severe enough to prevent employment or required activities. Physical therapy should be tried prior to operation.[2] It should be focused on pain reduction initially and on muscle strengthening once the pain and muscle spasm subside. Patients who have sustained work-related injuries due to repetitive extremity use do not do well after rib resection and should not be offered operation. These injuries appear more in women than in men. Likewise, patients with pain and chronic neural deficits do not do well with operation.

Physical examination should concentrate on any neurologic abnormalities. Atrophy of the ulnar innervated muscles of the hand may occur; it is the one classic sign of fixed compression of the T-1 nerve root. Usually a fibrous band extending from the tip of the seventh cervical rib onto the first rib is found at operation. Abduction of the arm to 60° and greater should reproduce the neurologic symptoms. If not, rib resection is unlikely to provide any meaningful relief. A variety of neurologic situations are listed in Table 2 with recommendations for treatment.

It is very important to discuss the potential outcome of the procedure with the patient. Because many of these patients have ill-defined symptoms, they should not expect complete relief. This is particularly true of the posterior shoulder problems that many patients have, presumably from trapezius muscle spasm. Patients with work-related injuries may not be able to return to the repetitive activities that may have produced the problem in the first place.[3] They should also know that they will probably experience numbness and burning on the inner aspect of the operated arm.

THE OPERATION

The transaxillary first rib resection is performed with the patient in the lateral thoracotomy position.[4] The ipsilateral arm, neck, chest wall, and axilla are prepared. The arm is covered with sterile cotton stockinette and wrapped with a gauze bandage. The second assistant stands on footstools cephalad to the surgeon and elevates the arm and shoulder to provide exposure. The incision is made just below the axillary hair line, which is identified by lifting the shoulder. The incision extends from the pectoralis major to the latissimus dorsi muscle. The incision is carried down to the chest wall. Exposure of the muscles is not necessary. There are usually several small vessels that require ligation and division. The chest wall dissection is done bluntly. The axillary vessels can be readily identified at this point by their characteristic pulsations, which provide a guide to the proper path of dissection. It is better to divide the intercostobrachial nerve than to overstretch it to facilitate exposure. Once divided, the tunnel can be expanded by the dissection of loose areolar tissue from the chest wall. An arterial branch from the axillary artery should be identified penetrating the second intercostal space and divided between hemoclips. This is an essential maneuver prior to exposing the first rib. This branch must not be avulsed. A narrow Deaver retractor can be placed under the pectoralis major muscle to provide exposure. Retractors must never be placed against the nerve roots.

The anatomy of the thoracic outlet can then be defined. The medial scalene muscle can be observed as it courses onto the first and second ribs and wraps itself posteriorly around the T-1 nerve root. The anterior scalene muscle can be identified as it courses from the neck onto the first rib, where it separates the vein and artery. It should be isolated with a gauze dissector and divided with electrocautery once completely freed from the surrounding blood vessels. Another arterial branch may require division between hemoclips during this dissection. Once the anterior scalene muscle has been divided and the vessels are free, one can identify any anomalous structures responsible for the compression syndrome. These structures are usually fibrous bands that attach to the first rib and serve to further compartmentalize the thoracic outlet. The medial scalene muscle should be divided behind the T-1 nerve root. This must be done very carefully because nerve roots may pass through this muscle. After both scalene muscles have been divided, the entire superior surface of the first rib should be free. If not, any anomalous bands should be divided. If a cervical rib is present, it can be identified and removed at this point. A periosteal elevator then can be used to clean the surface and the inferior aspect of the first rib. A finger inserted in the interspace is best for dissecting the pleura off the posterior surface of the rib.

In some patients the tunnel is quite narrow, and the first interspace does not allow insertion of the large rib-cutting instrument. The first rib can be divided in its midportion and the dissection completed back to the vertebral body by grasping the cut end of the rib. This facilitates a complete removal of the rib and makes placement of the rib cutter in this narrow space easy. The anterior segment of the rib is then removed in like fashion. The space is filled with saline and the lung inflated. A chest tube is placed through a midaxillary stab wound and connected to a water-sealed suction system if the pleura has been entered. The tube can be removed in the recovery room after confirmation of complete expansion of the lung by chest x-ray. The wound is closed with absorbable subcuticular sutures and covered with a plastic wound protector. The patient usually requires a day or two of hospitalization. During that time, range-of-motion exercises are begun so that the shoulder can be abducted to 90°. This is the maximal abduction allowed for 1 month following operation.

Patients are seen at 3 weeks following operation. It is most unusual to see a smiling face. They tend to have significant muscle spasm and pain. At this point a month of physical therapy usually provides relief, and the patient can return to preillness activities. Excellent results can be achieved with this approach. Recurrences are uncommon and usually follow some sort of trauma.

REFERENCES

1. Peet RM, Henriksen MD, Anderson TP. Thoracic outlet syndrome: Evaluation of a therapeutic exercise program. Mayo Clin Proc 1956; 31:281–287.
2. Wilbourn AJ. The thoracic outlet syndrome is overdiagnosed. Arch Neurol 1990; 47:328–330.
3. Roos DB. Experience with first rib resection for thoracic outlet syndrome. Ann Surg 1971; 173:429–442.
4. Green RM, McNamara J, Ouriel K, DeWeese JA. Long-term results after thoracic outlet decompression: An analysis of factors determining outcome. J Vasc Surg 1991; 6:739–745.

SUPRACLAVICULAR OPERATIVE APPROACH TO THORACIC OUTLET SYNDROME

LAZAR J. GREENFIELD, M.D.

The controversial nature of the thoracic outlet syndrome extends to the operative approaches used to correct it. Although the original concept of the disorder was focused on the anterior scalene muscle as the etiology, subsequent experience and the work of Clagett[1] shifted the emphasis to the first rib as the fulcrum responsible for the disorder. With the focus on the first rib, the operative approaches evolved to favor a transaxillary approach as the most direct and cosmetically acceptable.[2] Limitations of this approach, however, became evident in follow-up studies that showed a recurrence rate that was attributed to reattachment of the scalene muscle to the residual scar tissue of the resected rib. In response, a combined supraclavicular and transaxillary approach was favored by some authors,[3] but it soon became apparent that the entire procedure could be performed from the supraclavicular approach, adding the advantage of visualization of all of the structures requiring decompression.[4] The remaining limitation to this approach is the clavicle, which can restrict access and decompression of the subclavian vein. To facilitate subclavian vein venolysis, a combined supraclavicular and intraclavicular approach has recently been recommended.[5] Other surgeons with extensive experience continue to recommend claviculectomy.[6]

The lack of agreement on operative approaches is not surprising in view of the lack of agreement on the etiology of the nonvascular manifestations of the syndrome. The surgeon who has made the diagnosis of thoracic outlet syndrome assumes the responsibility for providing optimal decompression of the thoracic outlet structures without risking additional injury. It is this rationale that favors the supraclavicular approach, enabling the surgeon to visualize the cords of the brachial plexus, the subclavian artery, and a portion of the subclavian vein.

OPERATIVE TECHNIQUE

The optimal position of the patient is a semi-Fowler's position with the head turned away from the affected side. Some padding beneath the neck and shoulders facilitates extension of the head and exposure. Some authors have favored placing a pad vertically beneath the spine, but this tends to produce more posterior angulation of the clavicle, reducing the access to the anterior portion of the first rib and the subclavian vein. A curved incision is made one fingerbreadth above the clavicle from the lateral border of the sternocleidomastoid muscle to the anterior border of the trapezius (Fig. 1). After division of the platysma, skin and platysma flaps are elevated to the clavicle inferiorly and for a distance of 4 to 5 cm superiorly. It is better to preserve than divide the external jugular vein to avoid an unsightly bulge in the flap. Dissection is begun at the lateral border of the sternocleidomastoid muscle, which can usually be left intact and retracted. Occasionally it is necessary to divide the clavicular head of the muscle to facilitate exposure, but it should be repaired prior to skin closure. The scalene fat pad is elevated by dissection using cautery, reflecting it laterally from the jugular vein. Spreading a clamp below the fat pad allows visualization of the anterior scalene muscle and the phrenic nerve that runs within its fascial envelope on the surface of the muscle. The omohyoid muscle is divided if it appears in the wound. The fat pad is mobilized from the clavicle anteriorly to the trunks of the brachial plexus posteriorly on a laterally based pedicle, and a self-retaining retractor is used to hold the fat pad out of the incision. Another self-retaining retractor at right angles to the first one holds the skin flaps and facilitates exposure.

The phrenic nerve is unique, running from a lateral to a medial direction across the surface of the anterior scalene muscle, and should be dissected from it with care. Although some authors advocate using a loop around it for retraction, there is less risk of phrenic nerve palsy when it is simply dissected free and gently retracted during division of the anterior scalene muscle. The anterior scalene muscle should be mobilized inferiorly as it proceeds toward its attachment to the first rib. It should be possible to visualize the subclavian artery as it exits lateral to the muscle. The attachment of the muscle should be divided on the first rib, which facilitates exposure and subsequent division of the anterior portion of the rib. A clamp on the transected muscle facilitates its dissection and elevation off the trunks of the plexus and allows visualization of any bridging muscle fibers between the anterior and middle scalene muscles. Additional retraction and palpation superiorly allow identification of the transverse processes of the cervical vertebrae that mark the superior level of division of the muscle. Once the anterior scalene muscle is excised, the artery should be inspected to be sure that it is free of any encircling bands. During the dissection and mobilization of the scalene fat pad, large lymphatic ducts may be identified and transected. These should be ligated to avoid postoperative lymph collections or drainage.

Attention is then directed to the brachial plexus that is gently freed from the middle scalene muscle. Small blood vessels running between the trunks of the brachial plexus can be left intact because they are not usually responsible for pressure symptoms. A small malleable retractor can then be used to hold the brachial plexus anteriorly while the middle scalene muscle is dissected. Dissection along the lateral border of the middle scalene muscle proceeds until the long thoracic nerve is identified. Its course is variable, however, and it can be found either anterior or posterior to the muscle. Once the long

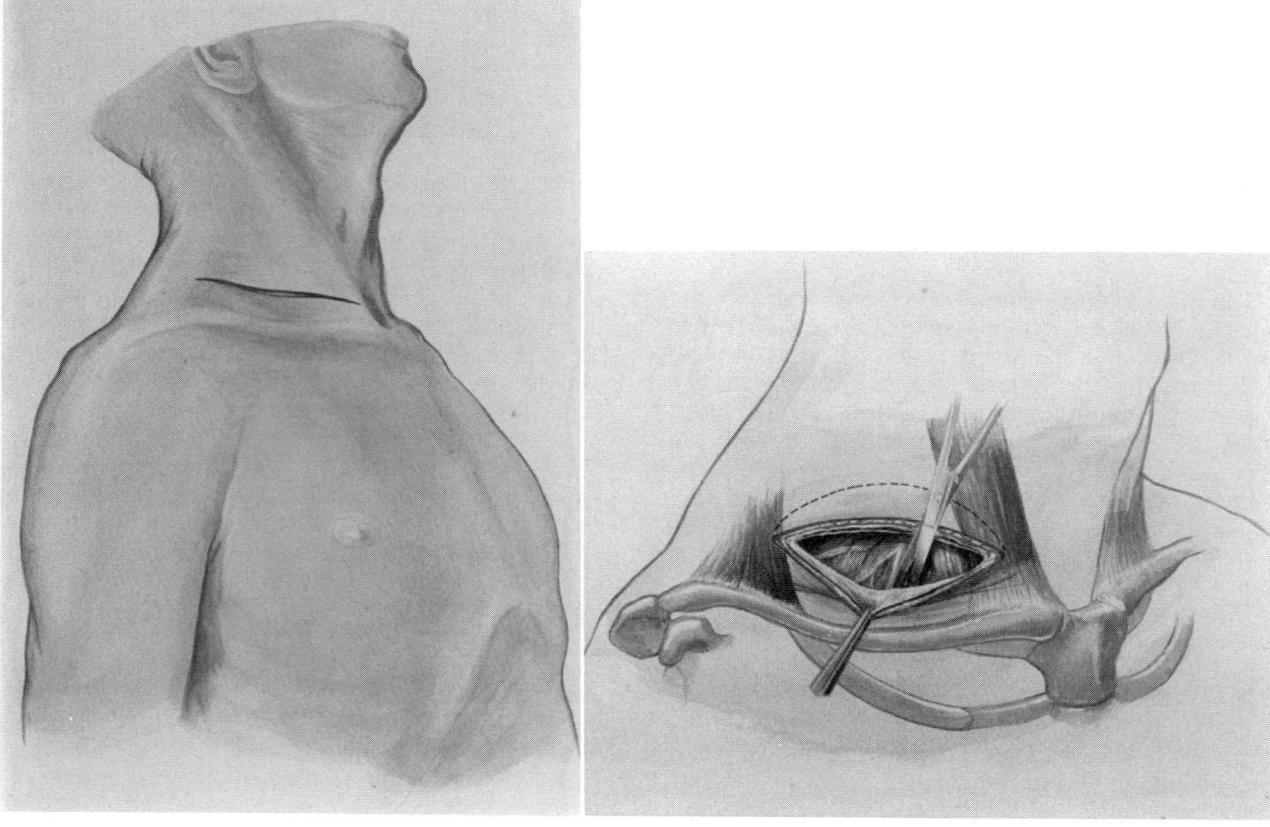

Figure 1 The position of the patient is shown *(A)* with the supraclavicular incision. Subplatysmal flaps are developed *(B)* in both directions.

thoracic nerve is identified, the muscle can be freed and divided inferiorly at its attachment to the first rib. Because the muscle envelops the rib, digital palpation helps to identify the level of muscle division. The divided muscle and long thoracic nerve can then be gently retracted posteriorly to expose the neck of the first rib.

At this point, a blunt periosteal elevator can be used to expose the rib, although elevation of the periosteum is not advisable in that it might allow regrowth of the rib. Before the rib is divided, it is advantageous to bluntly dissect the underlying dome of the lung and some of the lateral intercostal muscle attachments to the rib. This can be done digitally as well as with the blunt elevator. Sibson's fascia, which lies beneath the rib, becomes fused with the pleura, and during this dissection pleural entry may occur. Once the neck of the first rib is mobilized, a small blade on the pneumatic sagittal saw can be used to divide it, positioning the malleable retractors to protect adjacent structures. Once the rib is divided, it can be grasped by a Kocher clamp and elevated to facilitate further dissection of its attachments. Both sharp and blunt dissection can be used to free its lateral and inferior attachments.

Attention is then directed anteriorly to the attachments between the first rib and the subclavian vein. The vein should be handled with care to avoid injury to it or to any small branches. The clavicle is retracted anteriorly to facilitate exposure, and blunt and sharp dissection are used to mobilize the rib. A Raney rongeur can be used to good advantage to divide the rib, beginning laterally and proceeding medially; it allows visualization of all the structures that need to be protected during the division. A duckbill rongeur can then be used to remove additional rib as needed medially to decompress the vein. The first rib can then be elevated and further mobilized, dividing the lateral muscular attachments with scissors. Once the rib is freed, it can be removed either anteriorly or posteriorly by gentle traction.

At this point the wound should be irrigated and inspected for any air leaks. If pleural entry is noted, it can be managed most readily by having the anesthesiologist add 5 cm of positive end-expiratory pressure (PEEP) to keep the lung fully inflated during closure. The divided ends of the ribs are inspected and smoothed with a rongeur. The brachial plexus is inspected for any remaining tethering bands or attachments, which are divided. Following this, the brachial plexus should be loose and untethered. After further inspection for hemostasis, the scalene fat pad is reattached medially to envelop the upper trunks of the plexus and insulate them from the subcutaneous position. The wound is then inspected for any residual bleeding or lymph drainage. If this is difficult to control, closed suction wound drainage can be used, but this is rarely necessary. The head is then turned to a forward position, facilitating wound closure. Following reapproximation of the platysma, the skin is closed with a subcuticular suture, and a bulky elastic adhesive dressing applied. This is usually kept in place for 24 hours. Free movement and use of the arm are allowed postoperatively.

PARACLAVICULAR OPERATIVE APPROACH

In order to facilitate circumferential decompression of the subclavian vein, Thompson and his colleagues have recommended a combined approach.[5] The procedure consists of both supraclavicular and infraclavicular incisions to gain access to the entire first rib and costoclavicular space. This allows access to the proximal subclavian vein where it crosses the costosternal portion of the first rib behind the clavicle. The procedure does not employ any direct approach to the vein in terms of reconstruction, thrombectomy, or bypass. The supraclavicular approach is as previously described, with the addition of a short incision below the clavicle, overlying the insertion of the first rib. After separation of the pectoral muscles, the first rib can be palpated and exposed by blunt and sharp dissection of the overlying muscles. Because the medial attachment of the rib is cartilaginous, it is relatively easy to divide sharply, and the rongeur can be used to complete the resection. Once the rib is freed, it can be removed through the supraclavicular incision. This approach allows for more complete mechanical decompression of the vein and the removal of paravenous scar tissue. It remains to be seen whether it will improve the long-term results in these patients.

COMPLICATIONS

The most common complication of the procedure is pneumothorax, which is usually recognized at the time of operation and can be managed by the use of PEEP to keep the lung inflated during wound closure. In about 20% of patients, some residual pneumothorax is seen on postoperative chest x-rays, but because there is no reason to anticipate a pulmonary air leak, it can usually be observed. Nerve injuries are rare but can be disabling, particularly if either the phrenic or long thoracic nerve is affected. The incidence of phrenic nerve palsy has been reported as 7% and is usually followed by gradual recovery of nerve function.[8] Some type of brachial plexus palsy has been reported in approximately 5% of patients, and there are rare reports of injury to the cervical sympathetic chain or recurrent laryngeal nerve. Vascular and lymphatic injuries have been reported in 2% to 4% of patients, and wound complications are seen in 1% to 2%. Other types of respiratory complications such as atelectasis or pneumonia are seen with a frequency expected following a general anesthetic unless there is a persistent pneumothorax.

RESULTS

In assessing the results of the operation, it is important to recognize the tendency toward deterioration of favorable results with time. There is also no uniform method by which results have been reported or a standard definition of what represents a favorable outcome. Recent results from authors who have had extensive experience is revealing but indicate some of the difficulties with interpretation of the outcomes (Table 1). In general, an early favorable outcome can be expected in about 80% of patients, with subsequent deterioration to 50% to 60% after 3 years. It is also

Table 1 Results of Operation for Thoracic Outlet Syndrome

Author	Procedure	Patients	Outcome (Number of Limbs)	
Lord & Wright[6]	Claviculectomy	28*	Excellent	19 (54%)
			Good	9 (26%)
			Fair	6 (17%)
			Poor	1 (3%)
Green et al[7]	Transaxillary first rib	136	Return to activity	90 (66%)
			Satisfied	107 (66%)
			Not satisfied	29 (21%)
Reilly & Stoney[8]	Supraclavicular	135	Cured	54%
			Improved	32%
			Unchanged	7%
			No data	7%
Hempel et al[4]	Supraclavicular	433	Good	366 (84%)
			Fair	55 (13%)
			Failed	12 (3%)
Sanders & Haug[9]	Supraclavicular	249	Success	75%
			Failure	25%
Greenfield	Supraclavicular	50	Early relief	47 (94%)
			Resume activity	38 (76%)

*The outcome data for this study are based on number of limbs rather than number of patients.

important to note how many patients were operated upon for neurologic as opposed to vascular manifestations of the syndrome; the latter carries a generally more favorable outcome. It is clearly most difficult to define those patients who will benefit from the procedure if their symptoms are not vascular. In our experience since 1990, 187 patients have been evaluated, and 50 have undergone the operative procedure described (27%). The mean age was 35 years and 76% were females. The mean length of follow-up was 24 months, and 64% of patients have had physical therapy postoperatively, which usually correlates with a more favorable course. The type of physical therapy is important, however, because it is an error to provide workload activity. Instead, it is stretching and range-of-motion exercises that seem to produce the best results. Although 47 of the 50 experienced at least some relief of pain and paresthesias (94%), only 76% were able to resume full activity of daily living and/or return to work. These patients require a significantly greater commitment of time and effort to achieve a favorable outcome.

REFERENCES

1. Clagett OT. Presidential address: Research and prosearch. J Thorac Cardiovasc Surg 1962; 44:153–166.
2. Roos DB, Ownes JC. Thoracic outlet syndrome. Arch Surg 1966; 93:71–74.
3. Ovafordt PG, Ehrenfeld WE, Stoney RJ. Supraclavicular radical scalenectomy and transaxillary first rib resection for the thoracic outlet syndrome. A combined approach. Am J Surg 1984; 148:111–116.
4. Hempel GK, Rucher AH Jr, Wheeler CG, et al. Supraclavicular resection of the first rib for thoracic outlet syndrome. Am J Surg 1981; 141:213–215.
5. Thompson RW, Schneider PA, Nelken NA, et al. Circumferential venolysis and paraclavicular thoracic outlet decompression for "effort thrombosis" of the subclavian vein. J Vasc Surg 1992; 16:723–732.
6. Lord JW Jr, Wright IS. Total claviculectomy for neurovascular compression in the thoracic outlet. Surg Gynecol Obstet 1993; 176:609–612.
7. Green RM, McNarmara J, Ouriel K. Long term follow-up after thoracic outlet decompression: An analysis of factors determining outcome. J Vasc Surg 1991; 14:739–746.
8. Reilly LM, Stoney RJ. Supraclavicular operative approach to thoracic outlet syndrome. In: Ernst CB, Stanley JC, eds. Current therapy in vascular surgery, 2nd ed. Philadelphia: BC Decker, 1991:231.
9. Sanders RJ, Haug CE. Thoracic outlet syndrome: A common sequela of neck injuries. Philadelphia: JB Lippincott, 1991:171–191.

SUBCLAVIAN AND AXILLARY ARTERY ANEURYSMS

GLENN C. HUNTER, M.D.
KEVIN A. HALL, M.D.

Aneurysms of the subclavian and axillary arteries are infrequent, accounting for fewer than 1% of all peripheral aneurysms. In a review of the Mayo Clinic experience, Bower and colleagues reported only 38 operations for repair of subclavian artery aneurysms over a 40 year period.[1] Although atherosclerosis is the most common cause of femoropopliteal aneurysms and can be expected to occur with increasing frequency in an aging population, aneurysmal dilation of the subclavian and axillary arteries is seldom seen as a complication of generalized atherosclerosis.

Because of their infrequent occurrence, a clear understanding of the etiology, clinical presentation, and management of subclavian and axillary aneurysms is essential if they are to be recognized early and treated appropriately before limb-threatening ischemia ensues.

ANATOMY

The right subclavian artery arises from the brachiocephalic trunk and the left from the arch of the aorta. Distal to their origins, each subclavian artery arches above the cervical pleura and leaves the root of the neck at the lateral border of the first rib. The subclavian artery continues as the axillary artery to the inferior border of the tendon of the teres major muscle where it becomes the brachial artery (Figs. 1 and 2).

The subendothelial layer of elastic arteries, such as the subclavian and axillary arteries, is composed predominantly of longitudinally arranged collagen and elastic fibers and may comprise up to 20% of the thickness of the arterial wall. In contrast, the subendothelial layer of muscular arteries consists of only a few layers of collagen and elastic fibers bound by an internal elastic lamina. The media of the subclavian and axillary arteries consists chiefly of fenestrated elastic lamellae, collagen, and smooth muscle surrounded by a thin adventitial layer of irregularly arranged connective tissue. The media of muscular arteries consists predominantly of smooth muscle surrounded by an adventitia of comparable thickness. These structural differences between elastic and muscular arteries may explain why the majority of aneurysms involving the proximal vessels of

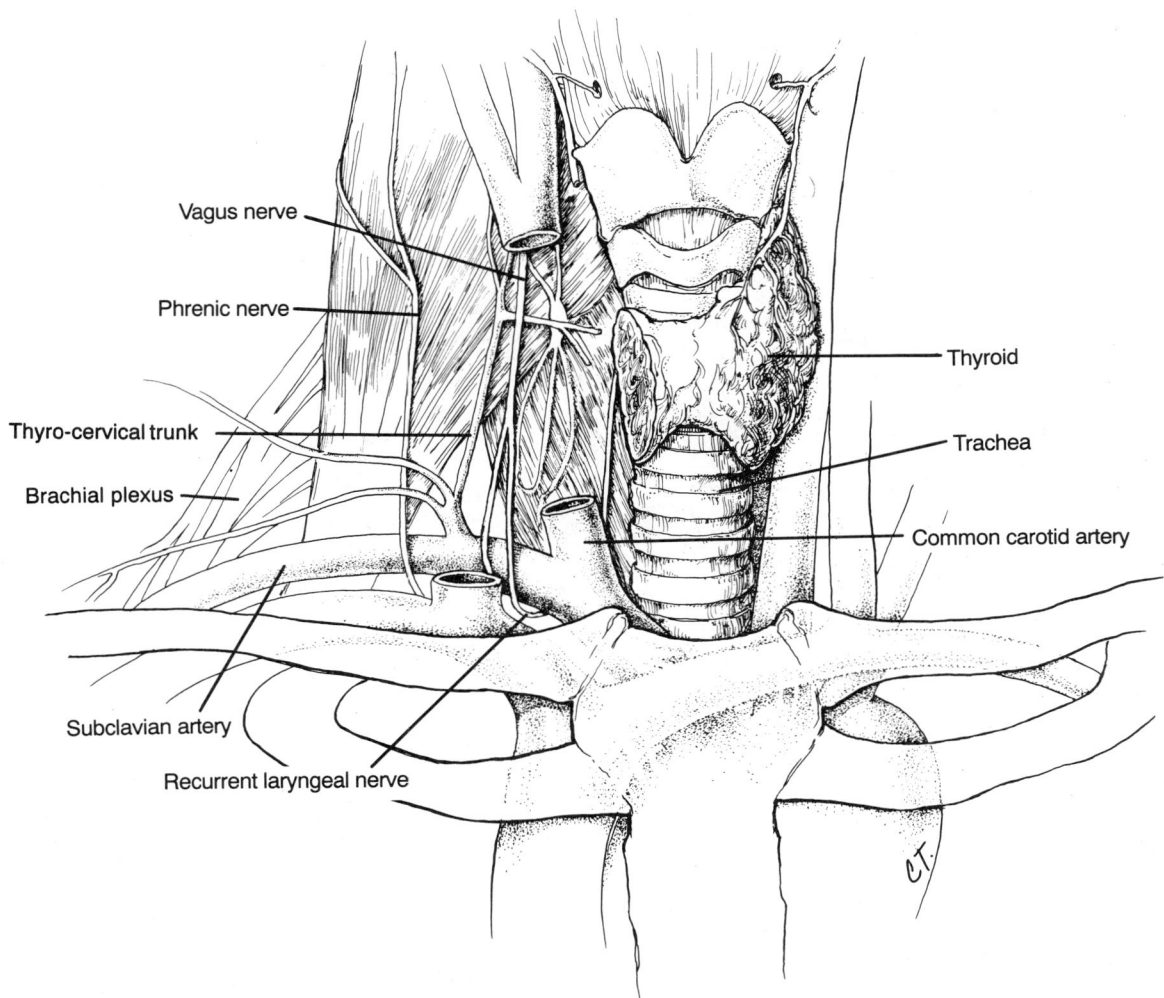

Figure 1 Diagrammatic representation of the anatomic relationships of the right subclavian artery.

the upper extremity are associated with chronic trauma and why aneurysms due to atherosclerosis are infrequent. Furthermore, the absence of a well-defined adventitial layer affords an explanation for the fragility and hence the technical difficulties encountered during repair or bypass grafting of these vessels.

PATHOGENESIS

The causes of these arterial aneurysms are varied (Tables 1 and 2). Hobson and co-workers in an analysis of 195 subclavian and axillary aneurysms reported in the world literature found that aneurysmal disease involved the subclavian artery more often than the axillary artery (88% versus 12%). Chronic trauma as a result of thoracic outlet obstruction or the prolonged use of crutches was the most common etiologic factor implicated in 74% of subclavian and 54% of axillary aneurysms. Atherosclerosis accounted for only 15% of the aneurysms.[2] In contrast, Pairolero and associates observed a slightly higher frequency of axillary aneurysms (54% versus 45%) in a series of subclavian and axillary aneurysms treated over a 20 year period. Fifty-five percent (12 of 22) of the aneurysms were due to atherosclerosis, and 27% (6 of 22) were associated with poststenotic dilation.[3] In the series reported by McCollum and colleagues, 50% (8 of 16) of the subclavian aneurysms were due to atherosclerosis.[4]

In a recent review of the etiology and management of brachiocephalic aneurysms, Bower and co-workers noted a predominance of females and a predilection for the right side in patients with subclavian aneurysms.[1] Aneurysmal dilation of an aberrant right subclavian artery occurred almost exclusively in males. Atherosclerosis (34%) and thoracic outlet obstruction (39%) were implicated with almost equal frequency in the etiology of these aneurysms.

These disparate findings between the studies of the Hobson group and those of the Pairolero, McCollum,

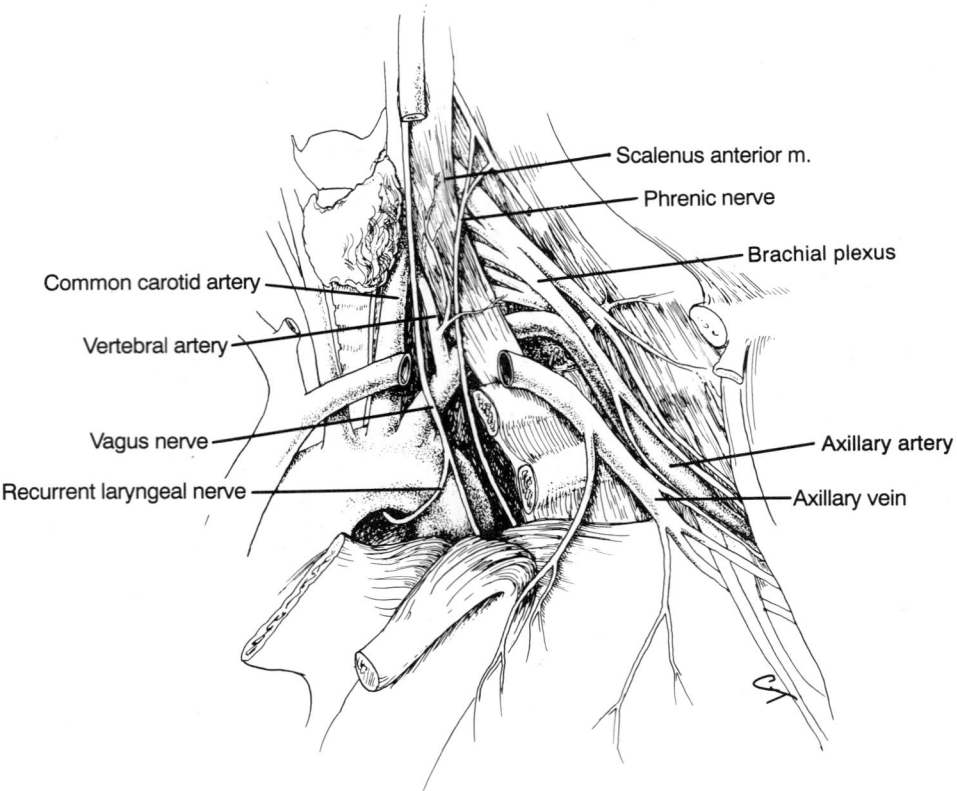

Figure 2 Diagrammatic representation of the anatomic relations of the left subclavian and axillary arteries.

Table 1 Etiology of Subclavian Artery Aneurysms

	Hobson et al (%)[2]	Bower et al (%)[1]
Thoracic outlet obstruction	127 (74)	16 (39)
Atherosclerosis	24 (14)	14 (34)
Trauma	2 (3)	4 (10)
False aneurysm	5 (3)	0 (0)
Anastomotic	0 (0)	2 (5)
Miscellaneous	13 (6)	5 (12)

Table 2 Etiology of Axillary Aneurysms

	Hobson et al (%)[2]	Neumayer et al (%)[6]
Crutch trauma	13 (54)	24 (47)
Atherosclerotic	5 (21)	7 (14)
Thoracic outlet obstruction	1 (5)	6 (12)
Fibromuscular dysplasia	2 (8)	4 (8)
Miscellaneous	3 (13)	4 (8)

and Bower groups presumably reflect the relatively small number of patients in the series reported from individual institutions.[1-4]

Less common causes of subclavian aneurysms include tuberculosis, syphilis, bacterial arteritis (mycotic aneurysms), cystic medial degeneration, and Takayasu's disease. Rarely, axillary artery aneurysms have been described in patients with Kawasaki disease, melorheostosis, tuberous sclerosis, and sarcoidosis. Both subclavian and axillary aneurysms have been reported in patients with Marfan and Ehlers-Danlos syndromes and fibromuscular dysplasia.

Atherosclerotic aneurysms occur most commonly in the proximal portion of the subclavian artery (Fig. 3), whereas arterial dilation associated with thoracic outlet obstruction involves the distal subclavian and proximal axillary arteries.[2]

Poststenotic dilation of the second portion of the subclavian artery usually results from extrinsic compression of the vessel in the interscalene triangle formed by the anterior and middle scalene muscles and the first rib. Approximately 1 cm at its base, this triangle is readily narrowed by a complete cervical rib, healed clavicular fracture, thickened anomalous first rib, or abnormal insertion of the anterior scalene muscle.

The compression and angulation produced by the upward, medial, and anterior displacement of the second part of the subclavian artery by a cervical rib or healed clavicular fracture produce a focal area of stenosis. The hemodynamic disturbances that occur distal to the stenosis result in aneurysmal dilation of the third part of the subclavian proximal axillary arteries. The prolonged

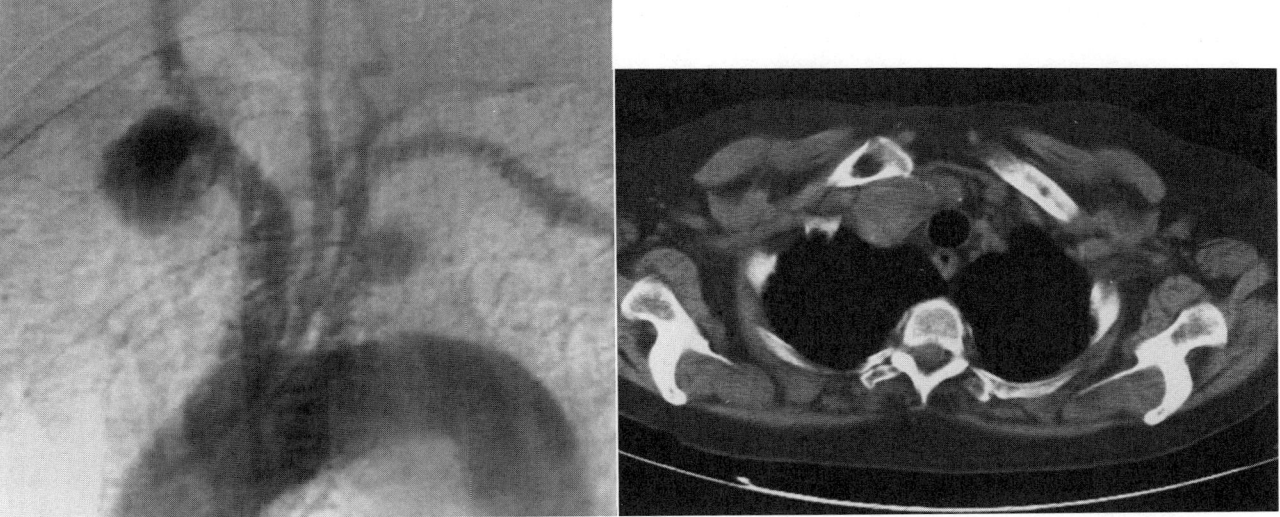

Figure 3 *A,* Arch aortogram showing large right and smaller left subclavian artery aneurysms. *B,* CT scan demonstrating the right subclavian aneurysm.

use of axillary crutches may result in thrombosis or aneurysmal dilation of the axillary artery.

It is often difficult to distinguish true aneurysms from pseudo-aneurysms on the basis of history alone because the initial injury may have been a very minor one, unrecognized at the time by the patient. Furthermore, months or years may have elapsed between the traumatic event and recognition of the aneurysm. Typically, however, patients with pseudo-aneurysms have an antecedent history of trauma, orthopedic procedure, or attempts at cannulation of the artery or the adjacent vein.

ABERRANT SUBCLAVIAN ANEURYSMS AND KOMMERELL'S DIVERTICULUM

Anomalous origin of the right subclavian artery is the most common aortic arch anomaly. In patients with aberrant subclavian arteries, the vertebral arteries arise from either the aortic arch or ipsilateral common carotid artery. The recurrent laryngeal nerve on the affected side takes a direct course to the larynx, and the thoracic duct may similarly be anomalous. The majority of aberrant subclavian arteries are asymptomatic and detected incidentally on radiologic imaging studies. (Fig. 4). Symptoms arise with increasing tortuosity or when aneurysmal dilation of the aberrant subclavian artery and its accompanying aortic diverticulum occurs.[5]

CLINICAL PRESENTATION

The mean age of patients with subclavian or axillary aneurysms is 52 years (range 10 months to 84 years). Commonly they present as an asymptomatic supraclavicular or infraclavicular pulsatile mass. Subclavian and axillary aneurysms may range in size from 1 to 12 cm in diameter (mean 4 cm).[1-3,6] Symptoms arise with progressive enlargement of these aneurysms and manifest as a result of (1) compression of adjacent structures including the cords of the brachial plexus, the recurrent laryngeal nerve, trachea, esophagus, or superior vena cava; (2) thromboembolism from atherosclerotic debris, mural thrombus, or thrombosis with retrograde propagation; and (3) rupture into the soft tissues of the neck, adjacent structures, or pleural cavity.

Symptoms due to compression of the neurovascular bundle include pain and paresthesias usually in the C8-T1 distribution, hoarseness, Horner's syndrome, and swelling of the face and/or arm. Stridor, dysphagia, and chest pain are the usual symptoms elicited in patients with tortuous and aneurysmal aberrant vessels.

Thromboembolism is the major limb-threatening complication of these aneurysms, regardless of etiology. Emboli from axillary or subclavian artery aneurysms, unlike the more frequent cardiac emboli, are usually small and occlude the brachial, radial, ulnar, and palmar digital arteries. Occlusion of the digital vessels may be manifested as temperature change, episodic pallor, paresthesia, absent or diminished pulses, and digital tissue loss. Less frequently, the patients present with arm ischemia or rest pain. Retrograde propagation of thrombus, more common on the right than the left, may result in transient ischemic attacks or stroke.

Rupture of subclavian and axillary aneurysms is uncommon and most frequently occurs with very large atherosclerotic, mycotic, or traumatic pseudo-aneurysms. The rupture may be contained within the tissues of the neck or penetrate adjacent structures such as the subclavian or jugular veins, trachea, esophagus, pleural cavity, or chest wall.

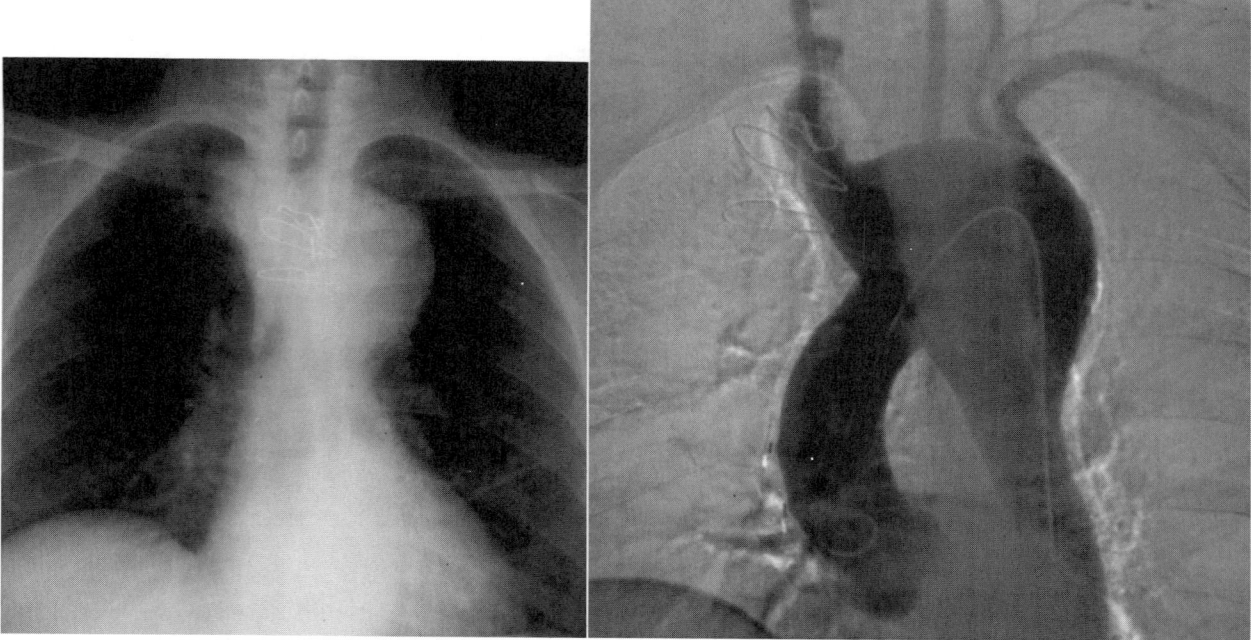

Figure 4 *A*, Chest x-ray demonstrating widening of the mediastinum due to prominence of the aortic arch in a patient with aneurysms of an aberrant right subclavian artery and Kommerell's diverticulum. *B*, Arch aortogram demonstrating the aneurysms.

EVALUATION

A careful history and physical examination excludes other causes of digital ischemia, such as collagen vascular disease, diabetes mellitus, Raynaud's disease, intravenous drug use, or emboli of cardiac origin. The presence of a supraclavicular or mediastinal mass or cervical bruit in association with digital ischemia and absent or diminished pulses should alert the examiner to the presence of an upper extremity aneurysm. Upper extremity pulses, neurologic deficits if present, and extent of tissue loss should be noted in each patient.

Doppler-derived segmental arm blood pressure measurements, insonation of the deep and superficial palmar arches, and digital photoplethysmography usually identify the level of proximal large vessel involvement and the extent of digital occlusion.

Occasionally, bony abnormalities, such as healed clavicular or first rib fractures or cervical ribs associated with these aneurysms are identified on chest radiographs. Arterial lesions of the thoracic outlet and mediastinum in patients of this age group must be distinguished from neoplasms of the lung or mediastinum.

Color-flow duplex scanning is useful in delineating distal subclavian and axillary artery aneurysms, but its utility for proximal subclavian lesions is limited by the clavicle. Contrast-enhanced computed tomography (CT) scanning, magnetic resonance imaging (MRI), and arteriography of the aortic arch and its branches help delineate the size and nature of such lesions. As approximately 35% to 50% of patients with subclavian aneurysms have associated aneurysms, especially in the thoracic and abdominal aorta, careful physical examination and ultrasonographic and radiologic evaluation of the thoracic and abdominal aorta and its branches are essential to exclude associated aortic or peripheral artery aneurysms.[3,4]

PREOPERATIVE EVALUATION

Careful preoperative assessment of cardiac and pulmonary function as well as the extent of pre-existing hand ischemia is essential prior to operation. Cardiac evaluation may include electrocardiography, echocardiography, dipyridamole thallium scintigraphy, and cardiac catheterization as indicated. Pulmonary function studies may be helpful in the occasional patient with severe respiratory disease. Biplanar arch and selective subclavian arteriography using the Seldinger technique with vasodilation and magnified views of the hand delineate the extent of the aneurysms and the severity of digital occlusion. In patients with thoracic outlet obstruction, a second series of radiographs should be taken with the arm in the provocative position.

TREATMENT

Operative intervention for these aneurysms depends on their location and other factors (Table 3). In view of the potential for distal embolization from mural thrombus, asymptomatic aneurysms greater than 2.5 times the

Table 3 Location and Management of Subclavian and Axillary Aneurysms

	Subclavian (Proximal)	Subclavian (Distal)	Axillary (Proximal)	Axillary (Distal)
Histology	Elastic	Elastic	Elastic	Elastic/muscular
Etiology				
Atherosclerotic	X			
Poststenotic/dilation		X	X	
Traumatic/pseudo-aneurysm	X	X	X	X
Kommerell's diverticulum	X			
Treatment	Resection and grafting	Rib—resection and grafting	Resection and grafting	Resection and grafting
Exposure	Right, median sternotomy, left, anterolateral thoracotomy	Supraclavicular and infraclavicular incisions	Supraclavicular and infraclavicular incisions	Supraclavicular and infraclavicular incisions

arterial diameter should be repaired electively.[2-4] Smaller (less than 2.5 times the arterial diameter) asymptomatic aneurysms may be followed with color-flow duplex and/or CT scans. The presence of clinical or noninvasive evidence of decrease or loss of arterial flow in the involved extremity or digit should prompt repair before severe or irreversible ischemia occurs, regardless of aneurysm size.

The elective treatment of large asymptomatic and symptomatic subclavian and axillary artery aneurysms is resection and grafting with either autogenous vein or prosthetic grafts. The operative exposure of subclavian and axillary artery aneurysms depends on their size, location, and underlying pathology. In patients with very large aneurysms of the proximal right subclavian artery, extension of a supraclavicular incision as a median sternotomy is usually necessary. Small aneurysms of the second and third portions of the right subclavian artery can usually be approached initially by transverse supraclavicular and infraclavicular incisions, although the operative field should always be widely prepared to permit extension through the sternum.

Exposure of the intrathoracic portion of the left subclavian artery usually requires a separate third or fourth interspace anterolateral thoracotomy. A second supraclavicular incision is usually necessary to complete the distal anastomosis. Resection of the medial half of the clavicle may improve exposure of distal subclavian and proximal axillary lesions.[1-4,7]

In patients with poststenotic dilation associated with a cervical rib or thoracic outlet syndrome, the offending rib is resected. The anterior supraclavicular approach is the preferred route for resection of cervical ribs because it also allows inspection of the neurovascular bundle. If the poststenotic dilation is minimal and without evidence of embolization, cervical or first rib resection may suffice. However, if the lesion is greater than 2.5 times the arterial diameter or there is evidence of distal embolization, direct repair of the aneurysm is also performed. In some patients with poststenotic dilation, the redundancy of the subclavian artery and the short length of the aneurysm may, on occasion, permit construction of an end-to-end anastomosis. However, an interposition graft is usually necessary.

In patients with symptoms referable to an aneurysm of an aberrant subclavian artery, proximal ligation with anastomosis to the ipsilateral common carotid artery is sometimes feasible. Because of its origin from the posteromedial aspect of the descending aorta, ligation of an aberrant right subclavian artery is best performed using a right anterolateral thoracotomy.[5] Large aneurysms of an aberrant subclavian artery are resected and replaced with prosthetic grafts originating from the aortic arch, the descending aorta, or ipsilateral common carotid artery. Although repair of the aneurysmal dilation associated with Kommerell's diverticulum often can be undertaken directly through a left lateral thoracotomy incision, resection of the aneurysm with placement of an interposition graft (with or without cardiopulmonary bypass) may be required.[5]

Both supraclavicular and infraclavicular incisions with or without division of the clavicle are usually required to provide adequate exposure of the axillary artery.[1,7]

The management of traumatic pseudo-aneurysms depends on their location and presenting symptoms. The operative exposure of traumatic pseudo-aneurysms in hemodynamically stable patients is similar to that employed for elective aneurysm resection. Because associated injuries are common, extension of existing incisions may be necessary to obtain proximal control.

The walls of very large aneurysms are frequently adherent to the cords of the brachial plexus or the axillary vein, and attempts to resect such aneurysms may result in injury to these structures. Proximal and distal ligation with bypass grafting is technically easier and safer. The Matas endoaneurysmorrhaphy should be employed as necessary to reduce the bulk of the mass and relieve compressive symptoms. Balloon catheter occlusion may be helpful if control cannot be readily obtained by direct pressure or by the application of vascular clamps.

Ruptured aneurysms, depending on their location, usually require median sternotomy or left anterolateral thoracotomy to obtain proximal control.

In all patients, the legs should prepared so that a segment of saphenous vein can be obtained. Although saphenous vein is the ideal conduit for bypass grafting from the subclavian and axillary arteries to the brachial artery or its distal branches, the use of saphenous vein more proximally has two major disadvantages. There is often a significant size discrepancy between vein and artery. Furthermore, saphenous vein grafts in this location have a tendency to late aneurysmal dilation, intraluminal thrombus formation, and recurrent digital embolization. We, therefore, favor prosthetic graft material, Dacron, or polytetrafluoroethylene, for repair of proximal subclavian aneurysms. In patients with traumatic pseudo-aneurysms, especially when there has been injury to the trachea or esophagus, ligation alone or with saphenous vein bypass grafting should be undertaken.[2]

In patients with acute upper extremity ischemia due to distal embolization, emergency embolectomy in addition to aneurysm repair is required. Occasionally, thrombotic material cannot be retrieved by use of an embolectomy catheter, and residual occlusion of the palmar arch and digital vessels may produce severe ischemia, resulting in loss of all or part of the hand. In such patients, a catheter-directed infusion of urokinase preoperatively or intraoperatively may minimize digital loss. Rarely, patients with irreversible ischemia may require digital or forearm amputation.

Antithrombotic agents are a useful adjunct following upper extremity bypass in patients with distal grafts and poor runoff, those with known coagulation disorders, or patients undergoing redo bypass grafting. Aspirin or sodium warfarin, in addition to selective use of vasodilator therapy with calcium channel blockers or alpha-adrenergic blockers, may be indicated. In selected patients with digital ischemia and skin loss who have a good response to a stellate ganglion block, cervical sympathectomy may facilitate healing of skin lesions and relief of pain.

RESULTS

The elective repair of distal subclavian and axillary aneurysms can be undertaken with minimal morbidity and mortality; patients with rupture are at far greater risk. Complications associated with repair of these aneurysms include anastomotic bleeding, lymphoceles, Horner's syndrome, phrenic nerve, recurrent laryngeal nerve, brachial plexus palsies, and pneumothorax. We have recently encountered a patient who developed Wallenberg's syndrome, characterized by nystagmus, hearing loss, loss of sensory and motor function of the face, dysmetria, and dysrhythmia following ligation of an atretic vertebral artery during repair of a large subclavian aneurysm.

The long-term survival rates of patients following repair of subclavian and axillary artery aneurysms are usually excellent. The 5 year survival rate is over 90%, and the 10 year survival rate is between 60% and 70%.[1]

REFERENCES

1. Bower TC, Pairolero PC, Hallett JW, et al. Brachiocephalic aneurysm: The case for early recognition and repair. Ann Vasc Surg 1991; 5:125–132.
2. Hobson R, Israel M, Lynch T. Axillosubclavian arterial aneurysms. In: Bergan JJ, Yao JST, eds. Aneurysms: Diagnosis and treatment. New York: Grune & Stratton, 1982:435.
3. Pairolero PC, Walls JT, Payne W, et al. Subclavian axillary artery aneurysms. Surgery 1981; 90:757–763.
4. McCollum CH, DaGama AD, Noon GP, DeBakey ME. Aneurysm of the subclavian artery. J Cardiovasc Surg 1979; 20:159–164.
5. Keiffer E, Bahnini A, Koskas F. Aberrant subclavian artery: Surgical management in thirty-three adult patients. J Vasc Surg 1994; 19:100–111.
6. Neumayer LA, Bull DA, Hunter GC, et al. Atherosclerotic aneurysms of the axillary artery. J Cardiovasc Surg 1992; 33: 172–177.
7. Ernst CB. Exposure of the subclavian arteries. Semin Vasc Surg 1989; 2(4):202–208.

HYPOTHENAR HAMMER SYNDROME

MARK R. NEHLER, M.D.
LLOYD M. TAYLOR Jr, M.D.
JOHN M. PORTER, M.D.

Post-traumatic aneurysm of the ulnar artery in the palm, first described in 1934 by Von Rosen,[1] was termed the hypothenar hammer syndrome by Conn and associates in 1970.[2] Most affected patients are males who typically present with symptoms of digital ischemia resulting from embolization to palmar and digital arteries. Although simple aneurysm excision with or without primary arterial reanastomosis and/or upper extremity sympathectomy have been recommended historically for management of these lesions,[3] recent publications have reported excellent symptomatic improvement and intermediate-term patency rates with aneurysm excision and interposition reversed vein graft replacement.[4,5]

ANATOMY AND PATHOPHYSIOLOGY

The ulnar artery passes through Guyon's canal with the ulnar nerve. At this point the vessel passes adjacent to the hook of the hamate bone and divides into the deep and superficial palmar branches. The deep branch follows the deep branch of the ulnar nerve beneath the hypothenar muscles and terminates as the deep palmar arch. The superficial branch courses over the hypothenar muscles proximal to the protective covering of the palmar aponeurosis and terminates as the superficial palmar arch. The short arterial segment immediately proximal to the superficial palmar arch is prone to damage from acute and chronic blunt trauma to the hypothenar eminence where it lies relatively unprotected between the skin and bone (Fig. 1). Both thrombosis and aneurysm formation of the ulnar artery may occur at this site following repetitive trauma.[6] Much less frequently encountered causes of aneurysms of the hand arteries such as atherosclerosis, tumor, and arteritis are not considered further in this section.

CLINICAL PRESENTATION

The prevalence of traumatic ulnar artery aneurysms is unknown. A study examining the hands of all mechanics from two Australian government vehicle maintenance workshops documented Doppler-determined ulnar artery occlusion in 11 of 79 (14%) workers who gave a history of repetitive use of the hypothenar eminence to strike objects.[7] Interestingly, we have encountered, during a 20 year period, only 10 patients with ulnar artery aneurysms out of more than 1,200 patients referred for evaluation of fixed or vasospastic hand and finger ischemia. This suggests that many of these lesions are asymptomatic.

Most patients diagnosed as having ulnar artery aneurysms are male and between the ages of 20 and 50 years; they are frequently employed in the automotive or construction industries. A history of using pneumatic tools or repetitively striking objects with the dominant hand is characteristic of the syndrome. Associated tobacco use is almost universal. The most frequent presenting symptom is Raynaud's syndrome of the two or three ulnar digits, resulting from moderate digital ischemia incident to common or proper digital artery embolization of aneurysmal debris. Less frequent complaints include ischemic digital rest pain with or without ulceration, pain at the site of the aneurysm, neuropathy from ulnar nerve compression, and asymptomatic palmar mass (Table 1).

DIAGNOSTIC EVALUATION

Initial evaluation in addition to history and physical examination includes the following blood tests: complete blood count, multibiochemical panel, antinuclear antibody, serum protein electrophoresis, and rheumatoid factor to rule out myeloproliferative, autoimmune, or other associated diseases. A variety of noninvasive upper extremity vascular laboratory tests are routinely obtained, including brachial, radial, and ulnar arterial pressure determinations and Doppler waveform recording. In addition, finger photoplethysmography (PPG),

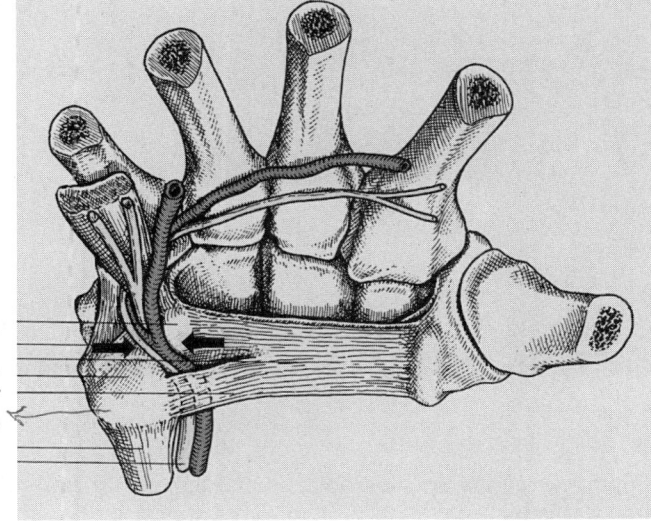

Figure 1 Drawing of the ulnar artery and nerve exiting Guyon's canal demonstrating the anatomic site of artery vulnerability at the hook of the hamate bone (*arrows*). (From An atlas of surgical exposures of the upper extremity. Tubiana R, McCullough CJ, Masquelet AC, eds. Philadelphia: JB Lippincott, 1990; with permission.)

Table 1 Clinical Demographics of Hypothenar Hammer Syndrome at Oregon Health Sciences University

Age (Years)	Sex	Presenting Symptoms	Smoking	Occupation
31	M	Rest pain, fingers 4, 5	No	Steelworker
43	M	Ulcer, finger 3	Yes	Mechanic
46	M	Raynaud's syndrome, finger 4	Yes	Machinist
18	M	Rest pain, fingers 3, 4, 5	Yes	Basketball
44	M	Raynaud's syndrome, finger 2	Yes	Mechanic
25	M	Raynaud's syndrome, fingers 3, 4, 5	Yes	Mechanic
37	M	Raynaud's syndrome, fingers 2, 3	Yes	Mechanic
35	M	Raynaud's syndrome, finger 3	Yes	Construction
37	M	Rest pain, fingers 2, 3, 4	No	Mechanic
26	M	Rest pain, finger 3	Yes	Construction

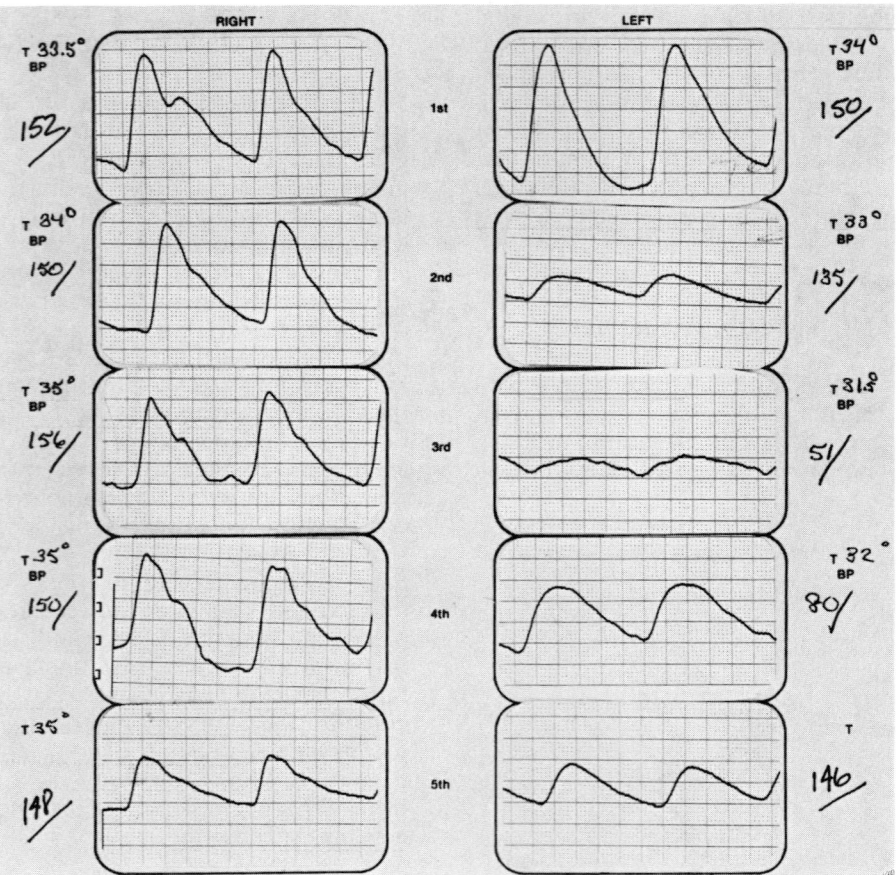

Figure 2 Finger plethysmography and blood pressure recordings from a patient with an ulnar artery aneurysm demonstrating digital artery occlusions in the left ring and middle fingers.

including blood pressure determinations in the index, long, and ring fingers, and digital artery closure testing after cooling are performed.[8] Typically, these patients have normal brachial, radial, and ulnar artery pressures with digital artery obstruction in one or more fingers as shown by obstructive digital PPG waveforms and blood pressure measurements (Fig. 2). Bilateral studies should be performed to detect contralateral lesions. Detailed upper extremity arteriography including magnification hand arteriography is usually reserved for patients who have unilateral digital artery occlusions on noninvasive evaluation (Fig. 3). Bilateral abnormalities suggest a much more diffuse disease process, typically autoimmune arteritis. Hand warming, intra-arterial vasodilators, and magnification views are used routinely in the performance of arteriography.

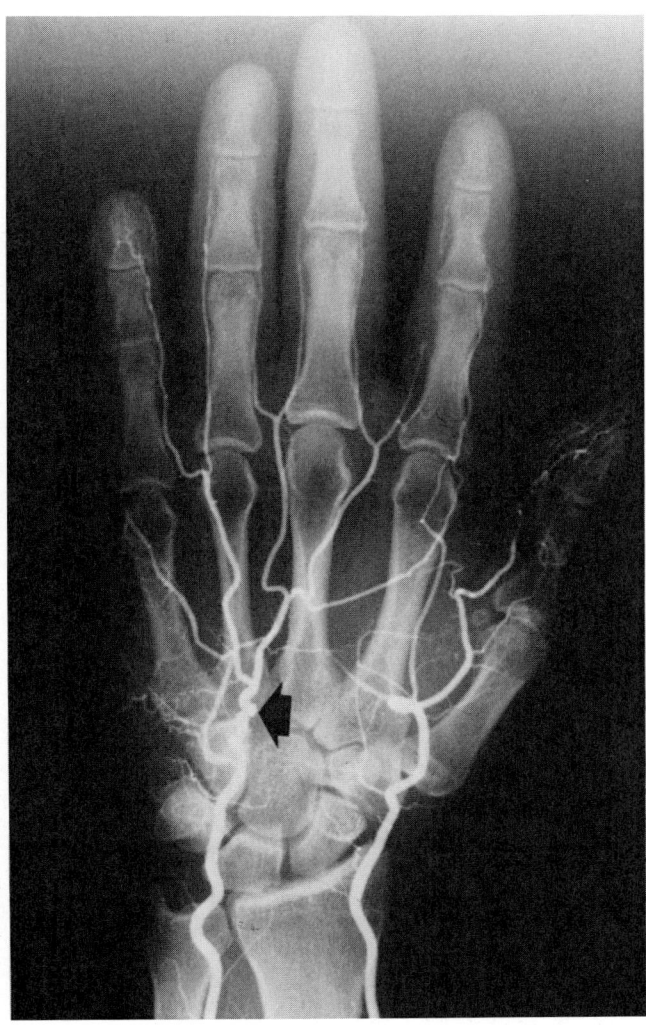

Figure 3 Preoperative arteriogram demonstrating diffuse distal ulnar luminal irregularity indicative of ulnar aneurysm (*arrow*) with multiple digital artery occlusions in fingers 2 through 5. (From Nehler MR, Dalman RL, Harris EJ, et al. Upper extremity arterial bypass distal to the wrist. J Vasc Surg 1992; 16:633–642; with permission.)

TREATMENT

Historically, treatment options for ulnar artery aneurysms have included observation alone, thoracic sympathectomy, and/or aneurysm excision with or without primary arterial anastomosis.[2,5,9] A single case report describes the successful use of intra-arterial thrombolysis followed by resection and primary repair of a patent ulnar aneurysm that had embolized to the digital arteries.[10] Recently we[4] and others[5] have described the results of ulnar aneurysm resection and interposition vein grafting. It has been our practice to consider aneurysm excision and vein grafting the treatment of choice for patients with a patent superficial palmar arch distal to a patent ulnar aneurysm with clinical or radiographic evidence of digital artery embolization or in patients in whom a thrombosed ulnar aneurysm has resulted in significant digital ischemia. A dorsal foot vein is preferentially used as the bypass conduit in order to approximate the size of the arterial segments involved more closely, although aneurysm excision with primary anastomosis has been used successfully by others. The goal is to maintain inflow to the superficial palmar arch while eliminating the source of future embolization. In selected patients, we recommend resection of asymptomatic contralateral ulnar aneurysms discovered incidentally during evaluation of the symptomatic hand because of their embolic potential. An asymptomatic thrombosed ulnar aneurysm probably requires no specific therapy. At Oregon Health Sciences University to date,[4] 10 patients have undergone 11 ulnar aneurysm excisions with interposition vein grafting (Table 1). There were no operative deaths or complications. Symptomatic improvement was noted in 7 of 10 patients, with persistent Raynaud's syndrome documented by Nielsen testing in 3. At mean follow-up of 15 months, 10 of 11 grafts were patent by clinical examination and duplex scanning or repeat arteriography. No routine anticoagulation or antiplatelet therapy was used.

All patients require intensive counseling regarding avoidance of repetitive hand trauma postoperatively as well as smoking cessation. For a significant number of these young men, a change of occupation may be necessary in order to eliminate further arterial injury from learned behavior patterns. The importance of this counseling cannot be overemphasized. These cases are frequently complicated by medical-legal matters, including workers' compensation claims.

REFERENCES

1. Von Rosen S. Ein Fall von Thrombose in der Arteria Ulnaris nach Einwirkung von Stumpfer Gewalt. Acta Chir Scand 1934; 73:500–506.
2. Conn J, Bergan JJ, Belol JL. Hypothenar hammer syndrome: Posttraumatic digital ischemia. Surgery 1970; 68:1122–1128.
3. Koman LA, Urbaniak MD. Ulnar artery insufficiency: A guide to treatment. J Hand Surg [AM] 1981; 6:16–24.
4. Nehler MR, Dalman RL, Harris JE, et al. Upper extremity arterial bypass distal to the wrist. J Vasc Surg 1992; 16:633–642.
5. Mehlhoff TF, Wood MB. Ulnar artery thrombosis and the role of interposition vein grafting: Patency with microvascular technique. J Hand Surg [Am] 1991; 16:274–278.
6. Barker NW, Hines EA Jr. Arterial occlusion in the hands and fingers associated with repeated occupational trauma. Mayo Clin Proc 1944; 19:345–354.
7. Little JM, Ferguson DA. The incidence of hypothenar hammer syndrome. Arch Surg 1972; 105:684–685.
8. Neilsen SI, Lassen NA. Measurement of digital blood pressure after local cooling. J Appl Physiol 1977; 43:907.
9. Gaylis H, Kushlick AR. Ulnar aneurysms of the hand. Surgery 1973; 73:478–480.
10. Lawhorne TW Jr, Sanders RA. Ulnar artery aneurysm complicated by distal embolization: Management with regional thrombolysis and resection. J Vasc Surg 1986; 3:663–665.

AORTIC ANEURYSM

GENETICS OF ABDOMINAL AORTIC ANEURYSMAL DISEASE

ANITA K. GREGORY, M.D.
ANIL P. HINGORANI, M.D.
M. DAVID TILSON, M.D.

Abdominal aortic aneurysm (AAA) is a disorder that affects 1% to 5% of the general population, but the incidence, as studied over a 30 year period, appears to be increasing. Morbidity and mortality remain high and impose increasing burdens on health care resources as the proportion of our elderly population also increases. Several relatively recent observations strongly suggest that many aortic aneurysms are familial and that genetic factors may be important in their pathogenesis. Histologic and biochemical examination of aneurysmal tissue has documented extensive connective tissue matrix remodeling, making the genes controlling synthesis and degradation of these connective tissue proteins potential candidates for the putative aneurysm gene.

Clifton, in 1977, reported three brothers who sustained ruptured AAAs.[1] In 1981, Tilson and Dang postulated a genetic basis for aneurysmal disease and cited the familial predisposition and preponderance of male over female patients as evidence of an inherited disorder.[2] The possibility of an X-linked gene being responsible for familial aneurysms was raised. The pedigrees of 16 families with AAA were published in 1984, but several of these did not support a theory of X-linked inheritance.[3] As this collected series was extended, it became apparent that at least two mechanisms of transmission were present. Twelve of the 50 families studied had apparent inheritance from fathers to sons, making it necessary to postulate an autosomal dominant pattern.[4] A dominant mechanism, however, does not explain the relative sex limitation of the disease. A multigene or multifactorial pattern of inheritance cannot be excluded. As wider pedigrees are obtained and possible phenotypic markers are identified, the true mechanism of inheritance may be elucidated.

Johansen and Koepsell compared the family histories of 250 patients with AAA to a control group of 250 patients with atherosclerotic disease of the abdominal aorta. Control subjects had reported aneurysm disease in 2.4% of first-degree relatives compared to 19.2% of the patients with AAA.[5] This study, because it contained a control group, firmly established that a genetic component exists in AAA disease, as the risk-odds ratio for AAA among first-degree relatives was six times that of the controls. Many studies have since confirmed the familial predisposition in AAA disease. An unpublished prospective study from our research group documented a positive first-order relative in 13 of 50 families studied (26%).

A prospective study of 542 consecutive patients undergoing operation for AAA was carried out by Darling and colleagues.[6] Their results, published in 1989, suggested that 15.1% of patients with AAA had an affected first-degree relative, compared to 1.8% of a control population of similar age and sex. Identification of a female member with an aneurysm in an affected family was strongly correlated with the risk of rupture. The term black widow syndrome was suggested, as female members appear to mark those families at significantly higher risk (63% versus 37%) for developing a potentially fatal ruptured aneurysm. In general, women enjoy a relative protection from AAA disease, with the projected peak in incidence occurring beyond the normal life span. Accordingly, one might speculate that when a woman presents as a proband in a family, it represents a more severe variant of the genetic susceptibility, so that the males in the family may be more adversely affected.

The search to determine the mode of inheritance of AAA disease and to identify a single aneurysm gene continues. Tilson concluded that if only one aneurysm gene exists it is likely to be autosomal, but if there is molecular heterogeneity, other forms may be X-linked.[4] The relatively high incidence of affected first-degree relatives suggests a dominant pattern of inheritance, but a recent statistical evaluation supports recessive inheritance.[7] Segregation analysis was performed on the pedigrees of 91 probands, as was comparison of nongenetic and genetic models using likelihood methods. Statistically significant evidence supported a genetic pattern of inheritance. It was postulated that AAA is controlled by a major autosomal diallelic locus, with the disease-causing allele being recessive, and that susceptibility to AAA can be accounted for by the presence of a major gene without any multifactorial component. Powell and Greenhalgh, however, proposed that the inheritance of AAA is multifactorial with an estimated "heritability factor" of 70%.[8]

Two molecular genetic approaches, which ultimately led to the discovery of the gene responsible for Marfan syndrome, have been used in the search for a genetic cause of AAA disease as well. The "reverse" approach follows the inheritance of different chromosomes among generations of family members using specific polymorphic markers. A particular chromosome must be inherited synchronously with the disease in question in order for it to be the "causative" factor. In a disease that affects individuals late in life, it is difficult to follow multiple generations of affected individuals. It has been estimated that a sib-pair reverse study would require about 1,000 subjects.

The classical approach identifies a candidate protein that is then traced on a molecular level to its gene of origin. Extensive connective tissue matrix remodeling has been documented in the vessel walls of AAA patients. Thus, the genes involved in the synthesis and degradation of connective tissue proteins have been the principal targets of investigation. Genetic loci that have been implicated in the pathogenesis of AAA include those coding for cholesterol-ester transfer protein (CETP), haptoglobin, type III collagen, tissue inhibitor of metalloproteinases (TIMP), alpha-1-antitrypsin, elastin, and fibrillin.

Powell and associates have reported an independent association between two genes on chromosome 16 and AAA.[9] The frequency of the haptoglobin alpha-1 gene was significantly higher in AAA patients than in healthy controls. Variation was also seen at the CETP locus, which could alter lipid metabolism and promote subsequent atherosclerosis. Although neither of these genes encodes connective tissue proteins, the Powell group notes they are both in close proximity to gelatinase A (type IV collagenase), which is known to degrade several connective tissue proteins including elastin. A major family of metallothionein genes also resides between these two loci.

A family with aortic aneurysms but no definitive stigmata of either Ehlers-Danlos syndrome or Marfan syndrome provided the first substantial evidence of an associated, possibly causative, collagen mutation with AAA disease. The report, published in 1990, identified a single-base mutation that converted the codon for glycine at position 619 to a codon for arginine in type III procollagen.[10] This mutation was also found in DNA extracts from pathologic specimens of two family members who had died from ruptured arterial aneurysms. The mutation was shown to decrease the thermal stability of the cleavage product, fragment A, of the type III procollagen molecule. The enthusiasm generated by this report was tempered by a subsequent report in which sequencing of the cDNA from 50 additional patients uncovered only one nucleotide change that altered the structure of type III procollagen.[11] These results suggest that mutations in the triple-helical domain of type III procollagen are an infrequent cause of aortic aneurysms, accounting for only about 2% of the overall population of AAAs.

The gene encoding tissue inhibitor of metalloproteinases (TIMP) has been investigated by our own research group. Western blot analysis and radioimmunoassay detected significantly less immunoreactive TIMP in aortic extracts from AAA patients than from controls.[12] This may promote an environment contributing to the increased proteolysis observed in the AAA matrix. Sequence analysis of the cDNAs from AAA patients suggested an identical point polymorphism in two of the six patients. However, the C to T substitution at the third position of codon 101 did not change the amino acid encoded.[13] These studies did not support the hypothesis that the TIMP deficiency seen in AAA specimens results from a primary genetic defect.

Following Cannon and Read's suggestion that failure of the protease inhibitor system may be a mechanism of AAA development, several studies were published on the altered antiprotease activity in patients with AAA. Cohen and associates examined the elastase, alpha-1-antitrypsin, and total protein in 37 patients who underwent repair of an AAA. They found that patients with ruptured AAA had higher elastase activity and lower alpha-1-antitrypsin activity than patients undergoing elective AAA repair or aortofemoral bypass for occlusive disease.[14] Our group reported an alpha-1-antitrypsin deficiency phenotype in 3 of 13 consecutive AAA patients. When the data were merged with those from Cohen and co-workers, however, the frequency decreased from 23% to 11%. St. Jean and co-workers subsequently screened 65 unrelated AAA patients to determine the association between AAA and three postulated causative loci: alpha-1-antitrypsin (PI), haptoglobin (HP), and type III collagen (COL3A1).[15] No significant association was seen between PI polymorphisms and AAA disease. However, alpha-1-antitrypsin deficiency may be an important genetic susceptibility factor in a small subset of patients, just as the collagen mutation represents only a small subset of the entire population of AAAs.

Loss of elastin is apparently involved in aortic dilation, although a genetic basis for this phenomenon has not been elucidated. Elastin is a very stable protein, with a biologic half-life of approximately 70 years, making it very resistant to degradation by physical or chemical means. Histologic examination of AAA specimens, quantitative analysis of aneurysmal tissue, and the induction of experimental aneurysms using pancreatic elastase support the hypothesis that loss of elastin is associated with aneurysmal dilation.

Fibrillin, a microfibrillar protein discovered by Sakai in 1986, has been found to be an important component of the aorta and other connective tissues. Several mutations that have been discovered in the fibrillin gene affect the functional integrity of the protein in patients with Marfan syndrome. Whether mutations of the fibrillin gene may play a role in the pathogenesis of

AAAs is yet to be determined, but it should be considered an additional candidate for the elusive "aneurysm gene."

Possible candidates for the putative AAA gene have been reviewed.[16] If this gene is found, perhaps a screening test could be developed that would identify patients with a genetic susceptibility early in the course of the disease. Mutations of type III collagen, in relatives of an AAA proband with the GLY-ARG 619 mutation, have already been identified using salivary DNA and polymerase chain reaction technology. Development of a genetic screening test would allow screening of high-risk populations. Not all of these patients may develop aneurysms, as environmental factors may also affect the expression of the gene. However, once the population at risk is identified, serial ultrasound examinations could monitor the development or progression of AAAs, or early intervention, based on the known pathophysiology of the disease, could possibly prevent the disease altogether.

Some evidence suggests that collagen mutations may contribute to the development of arterial aneurysms in Marfan and Ehlers-Danlos type IV syndromes. If a genetic overlap between these syndromes and nonspecific AAA disease is found, screening of relatives of patients with these diseases may also be of benefit.

Based upon the familial studies, relatives of AAA patients should undergo regular ultrasound screening to identify early aneurysmal dilations. First-degree relatives are at high risk for developing an AAA, and early detection may help to decrease the significant morbidity and mortality associated with this entity. This is especially true for the male relatives over the age of 50 of a female AAA proband. It is, therefore, imperative that a detailed family history be obtained whenever a diagnosis of AAA is made. As more is understood about the basic genetics of AAA, perhaps more of an impact can be made in the face of the increasing incidence of this potentially fatal disorder.

REFERENCES

1. Clifton M. Familial abdominal aortic aneurysms. Br J Surg 1977; 64:756–766.
2. Tilson MD, Dang C. Generalized arteriomegaly: A possible predisposition to the formation of abdominal aortic aneurysms. Arch Surg 1981; 16:1030–1032.
3. Tilson MD, Seashore MR. Human genetics of the abdominal aortic aneurysm. Surg Gynecol Obstet 1984; 158:129–132.
4. Tilson MD, Seashore MR. Fifty families with abdominal aortic aneurysms in two or more first-order relatives. Am J Surg 1984; 147:551–553.
5. Johansen K, Koepsell T. Familial tendency for abdominal aortic aneurysms. JAMA 1986; 256:1934–1936.
6. Darling RC III, Brewster DC, Darling RC, et al. Are familial aortic aneurysms different? J Vasc Surg 1989; 10:39–43.
7. Majmunder PP, St Jean PL, Ferrell RE, et al. On the inheritance of abdominal aortic aneurysms. Am J Hum Genet 1991; 48:164–170.
8. Powell JT, Greenhalgh RM. Multifactorial inheritance of abdominal aortic aneurysms. Eur J Vasc Surg 1987; 1:29–31.
9. Powell JT, Bashir A, Dawson S, et al. Genetic variation on chromosome 16 is associated with abdominal aortic aneurysm. Clin Sci 1990; 78:128–138.
10. Kontussari S, Tromp G, Kulvaniemi H, et al. A mutation in the gene for type III procollagen (COL3A1) in a family with aortic aneurysms. J Clin Invest 1990; 86:1465–1473.
11. Tromp G, Wu Y, Prockop DJ, et al. Sequencing of cDNA from 50 unrelated patients reveals that mutations in the triple-helical domain of type III procollagen is an infrequent cause of aortic aneurysm. J Clin Invest 1993; 91:2539–2545.
12. Brophy CM, Marks WH, Reilly JM, Tilson MD. Decreased tissue inhibitor of metalloproteinases (TIMP) in abdominal aortic aneurysm tissue: A preliminary report. J Surg Res 1991; 50:653–657.
13. Tilson MD, Reilly JM, Brophy CM, et al. Expression and sequence of the gene for tissue inhibitor of metalloproteinases in patients with abdominal aortic aneurysm. J Vasc Surg 1993; 18:266–270.
14. Cohen JR, Mandell C, Margolis I, et al. Altered aortic protease and antiprotease activity in patients with ruptured abdominal aortic aneurysms. Surg Gynecol Obstet 1987; 164:355–358.
15. St Jean PL, Ferrell RE, Majmunder PP, et al. Abdominal aortic aneurysm (AAA): Association with alpha-1-antitrypsin, haptoglobin, and type III collagen. J Cardiovasc Surg (Torino) 1991; 32:38.
16. Abdominal aortic aneurysm: Report of a meeting of physicians and scientists, University College London Medical School. Lancet 1993; 341:215–220.

PATHOGENESIS OF AORTIC ANEURYSMS

CHRISTOPHER K. ZARINS, M.D.

During the past 30 years there has been a 25% reduction in deaths from heart attacks and strokes. During this same time, the prevalence of aortic aneurysms has increased 300%. Population-based screening studies suggest that at the present time approximately 10% of men over the age of 70 have aneurysms. This number has stimulated a great deal of interest, not only in the diagnosis and treatment of aortic aneurysms but also in understanding the pathogenesis of aneurysm formation. It has long been recognized that most patients with aortic aneurysms have evidence of significant atherosclerosis; thus, abdominal aortic aneurysms (AAAs) have usually been referred to as atherosclerotic aortic aneurysms. However, a number of investigators have questioned an etiologic relationship between atherosclerosis and aneurysm formation and have suggested alternative hypotheses.

THEORIES OF PATHOGENESIS

A number of theories have been proposed to explain the pathogenesis of infrarenal aortic aneurysms. The most prevalent theory is that aneurysm formation is a manifestation of atherosclerotic aortic wall degeneration.[1] The coexistence of atherosclerosis and aneurysms in patients with shared common risk factors and an increasing incidence of both with increasing age support this notion. However, a number of investigators point out that an etiologic relationship has not been proved and that coexistence of the two disease manifestations is simply coincidental because the patients are elderly. Alternative hypotheses relate to genetic predisposition, proteolytic enzyme activity, abnormalities of connective tissue metabolism, and hemodynamic influences on the artery wall.[2] Interesting new data related to these hypotheses have led some investigators to conclude that there is little evidence to suggest an etiologic relationship between atherosclerosis and aneurysm formation.[2,3] Some argue that the two diseases must be fundamentally different because arteries get larger in aneurysmal disease and become constricted or stenotic in atherosclerosis. These arguments were considered by the Society for Vascular Surgery committee on standards for reporting on arterial aneurysms, which recommended that use of the term "atherosclerotic aneurysm" be abandoned in favor of the term "nonspecific aortic aneurysm."[4] However, increasing knowledge of the atherosclerotic process and its effects on the artery wall and, in particular, recognition of the fact that atherosclerotic arteries tend to enlarge support a pathogenetic relationship between atherosclerosis and aneurysm formation. There is no evidence to support abandoning use of the term "atherosclerotic aneurysm" for the commonly encountered infrarenal AAA. Most likely, the pathogenesis of aortic aneurysms is multifactorial and most of the proposed influences play an important role.

Genetic Predisposition

Familial clustering of aneurysms has been reported by a number of investigators, suggesting a genetic basis for the pathogenesis of aneurysms. Approximately 15% of patients with AAA have a family history of aneurysm formation.[3] Familial aneurysms appear more common in women than in men. Persons with a positive family history for aneurysms are at increased risk and should be screened for aneurysms during the latter decades of life. However, the study of genetic abnormalities in aneurysms using pedigree analysis is complicated by the fact that aneurysms occur only late in life. Thus, most tests of statistical association are based on analysis of first-degree relatives and sibling pairs. Solid information in parents is scarce, and many years will pass before substantial data on children of probands will be available.[5]

The search for a genetic defect in aneurysm formation has centered on abnormalities of matrix proteins, particularly collagenases, elastases, metalloproteinases, and their inhibitors. Patients with familial aneurysms have less type 3 collagen in the aortic media than aneurysm patients with no known affected relative.[6] Polymorphisms have been noted on the gene for pro-αI(III) chain of type 3 collagen, and the haptoglobin α' allele is seen more often in aneurysm patients than in control patients. Powell and Greenhalgh have proposed that haptoglobin binds to elastin in the atherosclerotic aorta to enhance the degradation of elastin of patients with an α-I gene.[6] Rare polymorphisms have also been noted at the cholesterol ester transfer protein locus. Abnormalities on the long arm of chromosome 16 may contribute directly to aneurysm susceptibility. A deficiency of alpha-1-antitrypsin may also promote aneurysm formation, and genetically determined risk has been suggested by the finding of high levels of Lp(a) in the serum of aneurysm patients.[3]

Several specific genetic abnormalities have been identified in "nonatherosclerotic" aneurysm groups such as fibrillin gene abnormalities in patients with Marfan syndrome and procollagen type 3 defects in patients with type 4 Ehlers-Danlos syndrome. It is unclear how relevant these findings in patients with connective tissue disorders are to patients with "atherosclerotic" aneurysms.

Because 85% of patients with aortic aneurysms have no known family history of aneurysmal disease, a single primary genetic etiology is unlikely to be identified for most patients with AAA. Although most patients with atherosclerosis do not develop aneurysms, patients with aneurysms invariably have atherosclerotic involvement. Thus, the relationship must be explained in any unified hypothesis of aneurysm formulation.[5] The late onset of aneurysm disease in affected individuals makes it highly probable that genetic factors create, at best, a predisposition and that the subsequent development of aneurysmal disease depends on environmental factors such as smoking and atherosclerotic plaque formation. Genetic factors play an important role in the development of atherosclerosis, and certain genetic predispositions may determine whether an individual responds to atherogenic stimuli with proliferation and stenosis while others primarily respond with dilation and aneurysmal enlargement.

Proteolytic Enzymes

The major determinant of the structure and functional characteristics of the aorta is the medial layer of the aortic wall. The media consists of groups of similarly oriented smooth muscle cells surrounded by a common basal lamina of type 4 collagen and an interlacing basketwork of type 3 collagen fibrils. Each group of smooth muscle cells is surrounded by similarly oriented elastic fibers. The resulting musculoelastic fascicles appear as layers on transverse histologic sections. Thick bundles of type 1 collagen fibers weave between adjacent layers and provide much of the tensile strength of the media. The elastic fibers, which are relatively extensible, distribute mural tensile stresses throughout the media and provide recoil during the cardiac cycle.[7]

The musculoelastic fascicles provide the primary structural integrity of the aortic media. Thus, for aneurysmal enlargement to occur, the collagen and elastin matrix fibers of the aortic media must first be degraded. Degradation of extracellular matrix and loss of structural integrity of the aortic wall have been the subject of extensive research.[8] Increases in collagenase and elastase activity have been documented in aortic aneurysms, with the greatest increases in rapidly enlarging and ruptured aneurysms. Inflammatory cells may play an important role in the local release of proteolytic enzymes, particularly metalloproteinases. Experimental enzymatic destruction of the medial lammelar architecture of the aorta results in aneurysm formation with dilation and rupture of the aorta.

Whether increased proteolytic enzyme activity in aneurysms is a primary or secondary event is unclear. A primary generalized imbalance of proteolytic activity would probably result in diffuse aneurysmal enlargement with other systemic effects rather than localized enlargement of the infrarenal aorta. Proteolytic enzymes must play a secondary role in conditions that result in arterial enlargement, such as atherosclerosis and arterial enlargement due to increased blood flow and increased wall shear stress. Although clearly proteolytic enzymes play a role in the process of aneurysm formation, their activity is probably stimulated by additional factors that result in localized increases in proteolytic activity and destruction of the aortic wall.

Hemodynamic Influences

Blood flow is the major determinant of artery lumen diameter. Blood flow is sensed on the lumen surface as wall shear stress. Chronic increases in wall shear stress result in arterial enlargement in order to normalize wall shear stress. This process is modulated by the endothelial layer through the release of nitric oxide. Chronic alterations in hemodynamic forces with low shear in the infrarenal aorta have been suggested to predispose the abdominal aorta to increased atherosclerotic plaque deposition.[9] Conversely, abnormal shear stress patterns with localized imbalances in shear stress may result in localized enlargement and tortuosity. The observation that World War II amputees have higher incidence of aortic aneurysms than other veterans has been used to support this hypothesis.[10] Aortic tortuosity and aneurysmal dilation occur in relation to the asymmetric blood flow pattern through the iliac artery. Although hemodynamic forces may play a facultative role in atherosclerosis and aneurysm formation, they are unlikely to be significant primary etiologic factors.

ATHEROSCLEROSIS

The atherosclerotic process includes a complex series of events occurring over a long period involving intimal plaque deposition and compensatory artery wall responses. Plaque deposition usually is focal and involves cellular proliferation and migration, lipid accumulation, inflammation, necrosis, matrix fiber deposition, degradation, and dystrophic calcification. A common misconception is that atherosclerosis is a stenosing or constricting disease of arteries and thus different from aneurysmal enlargement. In fact, atherosclerosis is a dilating disorder of arteries in that the primary response to intimal plaque deposition is artery enlargement. This is felt to be an adaptive mechanism that tends to compensate for intimal plaque encroachment on the lumen.[10]

Plaque Formation

Plaque formation is usually eccentric and is accompanied by artery wall responses and remodeling of the intimal plaque. Lumen contour usually remains round, and the plaque is covered by a fibrous cap that serves to sequester the lipid accumulation and necrotic debris from the lumen. Plaque characteristics change over time, and degeneration of the protective fibrous cap can occur, leading to complications such as ulceration, embolization of plaque contents, and thrombosis. Although intimal plaque enlargement can encroach on the lumen and produce stenosis, it is not inevitable. Plaques form in the arteries of most elderly persons, and most do not cause lumen stenosis because of compensatory arterial dilation or enlargement.

Artery Enlargement

Intimal plaque deposition is accompanied by compensatory arterial dilation or enlargement, which can prevent the development of lumen stenosis. Such enlargement has been documented in human coronary arteries, carotid arteries, aorta, and superficial femoral arteries. Human coronary artery enlargement can maintain a normal or near normal lumen caliber when intimal plaque cross-sectional area does not exceed approximately 40% of the area encompassed by the internal elastic lamina.[10] In the human abdominal aorta, the primary determinant of abdominal aortic size is the amount of intimal plaque. This relationship is not true in the thoracic aorta and may account for the increased propensity of the abdominal aorta to develop aneurysms.[11]

Media Thinning

Thinning of the media with disappearance of the normal artery wall structure underneath a plaque is a common feature of atherosclerotic arteries. Under these circumstances, the structural support of the artery wall may be borne by the fibrocalcific plaque as the media atrophies under the plaque. Similarly, thinning and disappearance of the media are constant features of aortic aneurysm formation. Human atherosclerotic aneurysms characteristically have extensive atrophy of the media with loss of the normal lamella architecture of the media. Elastin layers are markedly reduced, and the aortic wall is replaced by a narrow fibrous band. Atrophic changes are also evident in the overlying atherosclerotic plaques, which are thinned and contain little residual lipid fibrosis.

Plaque Evolution

The atherosclerotic process changes over time with early intimal proliferation, lipid accumulation, fibrous cap formation, and compensatory arterial involvement. The media may become quite thin and atrophic underneath the atherosclerotic plaques. Plaque evolution over time may include fibrosis and calcification, necrosis and ulceration, and the development of lumen stenosis or thrombosis. This heterogeneous change in the plaque and artery wall accounts for the varying clinical and pathologic manifestations of atherosclerosis, including the potential for aneurysmal degeneration.

MECHANISM OF ANEURYSM FORMATION

Consideration of the atherosclerotic process of plaque formation and compensatory arterial response suggests a possible mechanism that may account for localized aneurysm formation in the abdominal aorta.[11] Hemodynamic factors and structural vulnerabilities of the abdominal aorta may increase the propensity of the abdominal aorta to form atherosclerotic plaques. Plaque deposition accompanied by compensatory arterial enlargement acts initially to maintain a normal lumen caliber. Plaque formation and enlargement are accompanied by atrophy of the underlying media, further increasing vulnerability of the abdominal aorta. In later stages of plaque evolution, proteolytic enzymes released from the plaque or cellular inflammatory responses may produce localized destruction of the remaining structural matrix proteins of the aortic wall and result in progressive enlargement. Under certain circumstances, regression or absorption of plaque contents may simultaneously release proteolytic enzymes, which then act on the structural integrity of the aortic wall. Macrophages and inflammatory cells involved with repair processes and resorption or alteration of lipids during regression or evolution of atherosclerotic lesions may be important sources of the proteolytic enzymes that may play an important role in aneurysmal enlargement. Aneurysms appear to be a relatively late phase of plaque evolution, when plaque and media atrophy predominate, rather than at earlier phases of atherosclerosis when cell proliferation and fibrogenesis as well as lipid accumulation and sequestration characterize plaque progression.

EXPERIMENTAL OBSERVATIONS

Experimental observations support all of these proposed theories of aneurysm pathogenesis. Genetic animal models of aneurysm formation exist, and aneurysms can be induced by exogenous cholesterol feeding in nongenetically susceptible primates. Aneurysm formation in diet-induced atherosclerosis is enhanced by regression of the atherosclerotic plaque, supporting the concept that the interaction between the plaque and artery wall in atherosclerosis is an important pathogenic mechanism.[12] Hemodynamic models of arteriovenous fistula formation have documented enlargement in response to increased blood flow and wall shear stress, and animal models utilizing proteolytic enzymes in the aorta result in focal aneurysmal dilation. Enlargement of atherosclerotic arteries can be induced in hypercholesterolemic experimental animals, and such enlargement is associated with destruction of the architecture of the media. This pathologic feature is particularly prominent in those primate species that are susceptible to aneurysm formation. Experimental destruction of aortic medial architecture by mechanical methods alone or by mechanical injury along with hyperlipidemia has also been shown to produce aneurysms. Thus, experimental models have supported all of the hypotheses proposed in the pathogenesis of aneurysms.

REFERENCES

1. Zarins CK, Glagov S. Aneurysms and obstructive plaques: Differing local responses to atherosclerosis. In: Bergan JJ, Yao J, eds. Aneurysms: Diagnosis and treatment. New York: Grune & Stratton, 1982:61.
2. Ernst CB. Abdominal aortic aneurysm. N Engl J Med 1993; 328:1167–1172.
3. Tilson MD. A perspective on research in abdominal aortic aneurysm disease with a unifying hypothesis. In: Bergan JJ, Yao J, eds. Aortic surgery. Philadelphia: WB Saunders, 1989:27.
4. Johnston KW, Rutherford RB, Tilson MD, et al. Suggested standards for reporting on arterial aneurysms. J Vasc Surg 1991; 13:452–458.
5. Kuivaniemi H, Tromp G, Prockop DJ. Genetic causes of aortic aneurysms. J Clin Invest 1991; 88:1441–1444.
6. Powell J, Greenhalgh RM. Cellular, enzymatic, and genetic factors in the pathogenesis of abdominal aortic aneurysms. J Vasc Surg 1989; 9:297–304.
7. Clark JM, Glagov S. Transluminal organization of the arterial wall: The lamellar unit revisited. Arteriosclerosis 1985; 5:19–34.
8. Menashi S, Campa JS, Greenhalgh RM, Powell JT. Collagen in abdominal aortic aneurysm: Typing, content and degradation. J Vasc Surg 1987; 6:578–582.
9. Glagov S. Hemodynamic risk factors: Mechanical stress, mural architecture, medial nutrition and the vulnerability of arteries to atherosclerosis. In: Wissler RW, Geer JC, eds. Pathogenesis of atherosclerosis. Baltimore: Williams & Wilkins, 1972:164.
10. Glagov S, Weisenberg E, Kolettis G, et al. Compensatory enlargement of human atherosclerotic coronary arteries. N Engl J Med 1987; 316:1371–1375.
11. Zarins CK, Glagov S. Atherosclerotic process and aneurysm formation. In: Yao JST, Pearce WH, eds. Aneurysms: New finding and treatments. Norwalk, Conn: Appleton and Lange, 1994; 35.
12. Zarins CK, Xu C, Glagov S. Aneurysmal enlargement of the aorta during regression of experimental atherosclerosis. J Vasc Surg 1992; 15:90–101.

PATHOLOGY OF INFLAMMATORY AORTIC ANEURYSM

MITCHELL H. GOLDMAN, M.D.

Inflammatory aortic aneurysm with perianeurysmal inflammatory response was first described by Walker and associates[1] in 1972. They described a concurrent elevated erythrocyte sedimentation rate (ESR) and believed that an inflammatory abdominal aortic aneurysm (AAA) was unrelated to an atherosclerotic AAA or to other arteridites. Inflammatory AAA seems to occur in 2% to 14% of patients with abdominal aneurysms. The male predominance associated with atherosclerotic aneurysms is retained to a slightly lesser extent in inflammatory aneurysms. The mean age of presentation is the seventh decade, and the range is from 50 to 80 years of age. Inflammatory AAAs (50% to 85% symptomatic) are more likely than atherosclerotic AAAs (17% to 55% symptomatic) to be symptomatic. Abdominal, back, groin, flank, and perineal pain are the most common presenting symptoms.[2] Weight loss may occur in up to 5% of patients. Signs of ureteral obstruction occur in 3% to 4% of patients. Rupture is rare with inflammatory aneurysm, occurring in 4% of patients at most.

Associated with the inflammatory response, the ESR may be elevated to 50 to 100 mm/hr. Peripheral blood may contain an abundance of activated T lymphocytes of the Leu 4 and Leu 5 type expressing interleukin-2 receptors.[3] Because of ureteral involvement, renal function may be impaired. Computed tomographic (CT) scanning often documents a thickened contrast-enhancing rind surrounding the aneurysm and is commonly the method of best differentiating symptomatic AAA from an inflammatory AAA.[4] Similarly, magnetic resonance imaging may aid in the differentiation of leaking aneurysm from symptomatic inflammatory aneurysm without the need of contrast.[5]

PATHOLOGY

The gross appearance of inflammatory AAA is described as porcelaneous, with shiny, pearly-white tissue surrounding the anterior, medial, and lateral walls of the aneurysm. The surrounding viscera and mesentery may be edematous, with the small-bowel mesentery being shortened and thickened. The duodenum, small bowel, ureters, vena cava, renal and iliac veins, and ascending and sigmoid colon are commonly fixed to the inflammatory process surrounding the aorta. The thickened, inflammatory tissue does not usually involve the posterior wall. The back wall may be thin and often is the point of rupture or vertebral erosion, giving rise to the back and flank pain seen with symptomatic aneurysms. Since the duodenum and renal vein are involved in the inflammatory process, mobilization of them for proximal control of the aneurysm is somewhat hazardous. To complicate the dissection, tissue planes are often obliterated. In addition, while rare, inflammatory AAA may extend into the thorax as a thoracoabdominal aneurysm associated with mediastinal fibrosis. Inflammatory aneurysm has also been occasionally associated with coronary arteritis.[6]

Microscopic examination of the inflammatory aneurysm wall reveals a chronic adventitial inflammatory process surrounding advanced atherosclerotic degeneration of the media (Fig. 1). Calcification is often present in the media. The adventitial rind may be as much as 4 to 5 cm thick. Hallmarks of an inflammatory aneurysm are endarteritis and phlebitis of the adventitia and the vessels within perianeurysmal tissue. Associated with the entrapment and vasculitis of adventitial arteries and veins is entrapment of lymph nodes, ganglia, and adipose tissue. There is significant collagen deposition in the adventitia and outer media. The media is thinned, with disruption of normal architecture, including the internal elastic lamina. Loss of myocytes, atherosclerotic plaque, fibrosis, and deposition of collagen in the outer layer of the media are characteristic of inflammatory aneurysm. There is marked subendothelial myointimal hyperplasia and ulcerated surface plaques. Rose and Dent[7] have defined a histologic spectrum of inflammatory responses in atherosclerotic aneurysms from mild to severe based on the amount and type of infiltrate. Their hypothesis is that an inflammatory aneurysm is simply at the severe

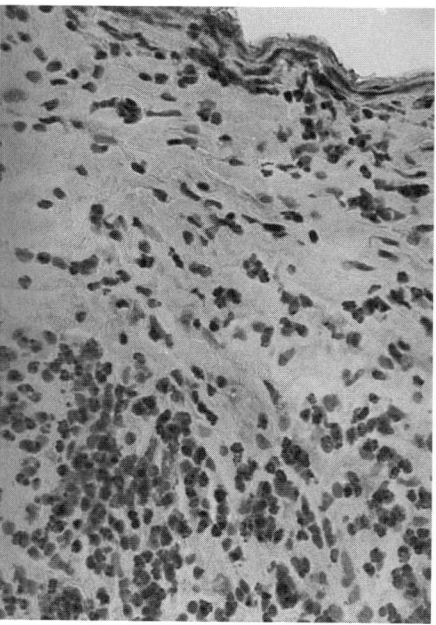

Figure 1 Histologic section of inflammatory aneurysm demonstrating the inflammatory infiltrate in the media and adventitia. (Hematoxylin and eosin staining, original magnification × 125.)

end of the spectrum, showing an unusual accentuation of the inflammatory response observed in relation to an atherosclerotic AAA. In this context inflammatory aneurysms have a marked infiltration of clusters of mononuclear cells, including macrophages and polyclonal plasma cells, activated T lymphocytes, and vacuolated histiocytic cells. The lymphocytes are predominantly CD3 phenotypic cells with many macrophages as well as B lymphocytes staining for kappa chains, lambda chains, IgG, and IgM. Hemosiderin, once thought to be the cause of inflammatory aneurysm and to represent intermittent leak, is not consistently seen. Eosinophilia, a prominent feature of retroperitoneal fibrosis, is rare in the inflammatory aneurysm.

After surgical treatment the ESR and peripheral blood cell phenotypes return to normal, and in over half of the patients followed by serial CT scans, the perianeurysmal rind regresses. However, postoperative regression fails to occur in up to 30% of patients. Regression may be related to the amount of fibrosis of the aneurysm wall, with increased interstitial fibrosis and decreased cellular infiltrate portending a lack of postoperative regression. Also, it seems that the longer the follow-up period, the more the inflammatory response disappears. Because the inflammatory response does often regress, procedures to free up structures such as ureters entrapped in the process have not been generally advocated.

ETIOLOGY

There has been considerable speculation about the cause of inflammatory AAA. Bacteria, viruses, and contained leakage have been implicated as sources of the inflammatory response, but none have supportive pathologic data. Obstructed lymphatics secondary to aortic expansion or wall ischemia due to atheroemboli have also been suggested. However, there is no convincing evidence to support these contentions. Rheumatoid spondylitis, sclerosing lymphogranulomatosis, retroperitoneal fibrosis, and Takayasu's disease have been proposed as mechanisms, but the pathologic features and clinical presentation of an inflammatory aneurysm do not seem to sustain a relationship.

A lingering question has been whether an inflammatory aneurysm is simply a more severe inflammatory reaction to atherosclerosis in AAA or whether it is a unique entity unto itself.[8] The putative development of an inflammatory AAA from an existing AAA has been documented on sequential CT scans and lends credence to the concept that an inflammatory aneurysm may be at one end of a continuum of responses to atherosclerosis.[9] Microscopic evidence that such a gradation of an inflammatory infiltration exists in an AAA supports this hypothesis as well. Findings consistent with an inflammatory aneurysm have been found in aneurysms that were not found clinically or macroscopically to be inflammatory. Among the infiltrating cells are found both activated T lymphocytes and immunoglobulin secreting cells, which suggests that an inflammatory aneurysm is a cellular and serologic response to a component of the atherosclerotic process. One possibility is ceroid, an oxidized low density lipoprotein that has been found closely apposed to increased IgG in histologic sections of inflammatory aneurysm, especially in plaques associated with attenuated media.[10] Circulating antibodies to ceroid and not to native low-density lipoproteins have been found in patients with inflammatory AAAs, chronic periaortitis, and elderly patients with severe atherosclerosis.[11] While ceroid may not be the only initiating factor, evidence suggests that the inflammatory component of an inflammatory aneurysm represents an upregulation of an immune response to some atherosclerotic component of abdominal aneurysm. Perhaps it is triggered by aneurysmal thinning and breaching of the media and the exposure of new antigens to recognition and response by the immune system. An inflammatory AAA, therefore, is the clinical entity of symptomatic atherosclerotic AAA associated with an enhanced pathologic response to components of the aneurysm. This mechanism accounts for the systemic symptoms, immunoglobulin production, infiltration of immunocompetent cells, adventitial fibrosis and vasculitis, and adherence of surrounding tissues and organs characteristic of the unusual but intriguing pathology of an inflammatory aortic aneurysm.

REFERENCES

1. Walker BI, Bloor K, Williams G, Gillie I. Inflammatory aneurysms of the abdominal aorta. Brit J Surg 1972; 59:609–614.
2. Sterpetti AV, Hunter WJ, Feldhaus RJ, et al. Inflammatory aneurysms of the abdominal aorta: Incidence, pathologic, and etiologic considerations. J Vas Surg 1989; 9:643–650.
3. Lieberman J, Scheib JS, Googe PB, et al. Inflammatory abdominal aortic aneurysm and the associated T-cell reaction: A case study. J Vas Surg 1992; 15:569–572.
4. Cullenward MJ, Scanlan KA, Pozniak MA, Acher CA. Inflammatory aortic aneurysm (periaortic fibrosis): Radiologic imaging. Radiol 1986; 159(1):75–82.
5. Rieber A, Allenberg JR. Magnetic-resonance tomography of an inflammatory aneurysm. Thorac Cardiovasc Surg 1991; 39:237–239.
6. Cohle SD, Lie JT. Inflammatory aneurysm of the aorta, aortitis, and coronary arteritis. Arch Pathol Lab Med 1988; 112:1121–1125.
7. Rose AG, Dent DM. Inflammatory variant of abdominal atherosclerotic aneurysm. Arch Pathol Lab Med 1981; 105:409–413.
8. Goldstone J, Malone JM, Moore WS. Inflammatory aneurysms of the abdominal aorta. Surg 1978; 83:425–430.
9. Latifi HR, Heiken JP. CT of inflammatory abdominal aortic aneurysm: Development from an uncomplicated atherosclerotic aneurysm. J Comput Assist Tomogr 1992; 16:484–486.
10. Parums DV, Chadwick DR, Mitchinson MJ. The localization of immunoglobulin in chronic periaortitis. Atherosclerosis 1986; 61:117–123.
11. Parums DV, Brown DL, Mitchinson MJ. Serum antibodies to oxidized low-density lipoprotein and ceroid in chronic periaortitis. Arch Pathol Lab Med 1990; 114:383–387.

PATHOPHYSIOLOGY OF AORTIC DISSECTION

JAMES I. FANN, M.D.
D. CRAIG MILLER, M.D.

Aortic dissection is the most common catastrophe involving the aorta, with approximately 2,000 to 4,500 episodes annually in the United States. Occurring twice as frequently as ruptured abdominal aortic aneurysm, it unfortunately is recognized less frequently antemortem. Aortic dissection is highly lethal if not recognized and treated definitively. Without medical intervention, acute dissection is associated with a mortality of 8% within the first 6 hours, 13% within 12 hours, 21% within 24 hours, and 74% in the first 2 weeks.[1] Primary causes of death in patients with untreated ascending aortic dissection (Stanford type A) include intrapericardial and pleural rupture, aortic regurgitation, or compromised cerebral or coronary blood flow. Those with untreated descending aortic dissection (Stanford type B) die because of pleural rupture or ishemia or infarction of vital organs secondary to compromise of aortic tributaries. Because occlusion of one or more aortic branches may complicate the clinical presentation of acute dissection and thus mimic many other acute medical or surgical illnesses, the physician must maintain a high index of suspicion for this serious condition so that prompt diagnosis and appropriate therapy can be instituted.

CLASSIFICATION

The biologic behavior of dissections pivots on whether the ascending aorta is involved by the dissecting hematoma; the prognosis and therapy are dictated primarily by this feature, and not by location of the primary intimal tear or the extent of distal propagation.[2] Dissections involving the ascending aorta irrespective of the site of primary intimal tear or distal extent are termed type A (Stanford), proximal, ascending, or type I/II (DeBakey); those without ascending aortic involvement are classified as type B (Stanford), distal, descending, or type III (DeBakey). A DeBakey type I dissection involves the ascending aorta and extends to the descending thoracic or abdominal aorta, whereas a type II dissection is limited to the ascending aorta. The dissection is classified as acute if symptoms occurred within 14 days and chronic if greater than 14 days from presentation. Importantly, the acuity and type of dissection determine the appropriate therapeutic approach (i.e., surgical management with median sternotomy and total cardiopulmonary bypass for acute type A dissection versus medical therapy or left thoracotomy with partial cardiopulmonary bypass for acute type B dissection) as well as the overall outcome if the patient is not definitively treated.

PATHOGENESIS

Although aortic dissections can originate at any point along the aorta, two regions (the ascending aorta and the proximal descending aorta just beyond the ligamentum arteriosum) are particularly prone to the development of an intimal tear, probably because of increased hydrostatic, traction, and/or torsional forces.[1,3,4] There are three proposed etiologic mechanisms of aortic dissection. One possibility is an initial intimal tear with secondary extension into the tunica media, lifting the intima from adventitia. An intimal tear by itself, however, does not necessarily lead to aortic dissection. Underlying medial laxity and/or degeneration are essential prerequisites to extension of the dissecting hematoma.[1,4] This concept does not account for all cases, and it has been proposed that the initiating event is hemorrhage into a diseased media, precipitating a secondary tear of the intima. Then again, an intimal tear is not present in some patients. Hirst and colleagues reviewed 505 autopsies and found that 4% of patients had no identifiable intimal tear.[1] One mechanism for what has been termed "aortic dissection without intimal rupture" is rupture of vasa vasora, resulting in a hematoma dissecting between the middle and outer third of the media, which is the layer in which the vasa vasora ramify.[1,4,5] Hemorrhage from the fragile vasa vasora that form during the repair of medial degeneration can be the primary event. Contrast-enhanced computed tomography (CT) scans, magnetic resonance imaging (MRI), and transesophageal echocardiography (TEE) do not document an identifiable intimal tear but do document an intramural hematoma (IMH), which does not communicate with the aortic lumen. Cases of IMH can progress to frank aortic dissection years later, suggesting that this process may represent a precursor to conventional aortic dissection.[6] A rare mechanism of localized aortic dissection is that due to penetrating atherosclerotic ulcer extending into the internal elastic lamina, with resultant hematoma formation within the media.[5] In distinction to the conventional type B aortic dissection, where the intimal defect is typically located immediately distal to the left subclavian artery, dissection due to a penetrating atherosclerotic ulcer originates in the middle or distal descending thoracic aorta. Distinct features as assessed by CT scanning include the presence of an ulcer with a localized hematoma and absence of an intimal flap or extensive propagation of the false lumen.

Because elastic tissue and smooth muscle cells in the tunica media contribute substantially to the tensile strength of the aortic wall, processes that result in degeneration of these components lead to development of aortic dissection. The most common predisposing factor for aortic dissection (particularly type B) is hypertension, affecting 70% to over 80% of patients.[1,3,4] Hypertension accelerates the medial smooth muscle degeneration that normally occurs with aging. Other risk factors for aortic dissection (particularly type A) are heritable connective tissue disorders, such as Marfan syndrome and the Ehlers-Danlos syndrome, which are associated with aortic valvular incompetence, annuloaortic ectasia, mitral valve prolapse, and mitral regurgitation. In some patients with Marfan syndrome, a mutation on chromosome 15 of the fibrillin-1 (FBN-1) gene has been identified.[7] Fibrillin is a critical structural component of connective tissue microfibrils and is important in maintaining the integrity of a variety of organs, including the aortic media. Congenital aortic valvular anomalies (e.g., bicuspid aortic valve) and aortic coarctation are also associated with an increased risk of aortic dissection. Iatrogenic aortic dissection is a rare complication of cardiac surgery and aortic catheterization. After cardiac surgery, aortic dissection may develop in the region of aortic cross-clamp placement, aortotomy, or site of vein graft anastomosis. Blunt chest trauma per se may be a possible cause of aortic dissection, but the extent of dissection in a structurally normal aorta is usually limited. Aortic dissection has been associated with certain genetic and autoimmune disorders, such as Turner's syndrome, Noonan's syndrome, polycystic kidney disease, giant cell aortitis, systemic lupus, and relapsing polychondritis. Overall, aortic dissection affects men more often than women (ratio of 3 to 1). Unfortunately, approximately one-half of dissections in women under the age of 40 occur during the third trimester of pregnancy or during labor.

PATHOPHYSIOLOGY

The most common site of origin of aortic dissection (upwards of 70% of patients) is the ascending aorta, usually just distal to the sinotubular ridge, corresponding to the cephalad extension of the aortic valve commissures.[1,4] The intimal tear typically involves one-half to two-thirds of the aortic circumference, but rarely the entire aorta. Intimal tears are generally transverse, consistent with the circular orientation of the medial smooth muscle fibers. In type A dissection, the tear commonly extends from the right lateral aortic wall coursing along the greater curvature of the ascending, transverse, and descending thoracic aorta. Autopsy series, as opposed to some clinical studies, have confirmed the more frequent involvement of the ascending aorta, reflective of the more lethal nature of type A dissections.

A less common site of origin (about 25% of patients) is in the descending thoracic aorta just distal to the left subclavian artery near the insertion of the ligamentum arteriosum.[1,4] This transitional point between a relatively fixed descending thoracic aorta and the more mobile aortic arch is also prone to traumatic intimal tears. Less common sites of origin of aortic dissection include the aortic arch (10% or more), abdominal aorta (2%), and, rarely, individual aortic branches, such as the carotid and renal arteries. This distribution is just the reverse of atherosclerosis, the incidence of which progressively decreases from the abdominal aorta to the proximal thoracic aorta.

The dissecting hematoma usually propagates distally, but retrograde extension is not uncommon. The dissecting process can render the aortic valve incompetent and/or compromise the inflow to one or many aortic branches. Once blood enters the tunica media, the period required for the pulsatile flow to dissect the entire aorta is usually brief—on the order of a few seconds to minutes.[4] Propagation of the dissection is dependent on multiple factors, including the rate of rise of aortic systolic pressure, diastolic recoil pressure, mean arterial pressure, and the structural integrity and strength of the media. Pathologic studies suggest that stress is sustained in the inner two-thirds of the media, leaving a weakened interface at the external one-third of the media that is prone to further disruption. Re-entry sites connecting the true and false lumina occur in most patients, are multiple in number, and correlate with sheared-off branch ostia. The progression of the dissecting hematoma may be limited by extensive atherosclerosis or anatomic constraints, such as coarctation of the aortic isthmus.[1,4] If aortic coarctation is absent, aortic dissection in younger patients nearly always involves the entire thoracic and abdominal aorta. In older patients the dissection can be somewhat more localized, perhaps because of a greater degree of atherosclerotic disease.

The most frequent cause of death in patients with aortic dissection is aortic rupture, that is often located near the site of primary intimal tear.[1,4] Because the pericardium covers the ascending aorta just up to the origin of the innominate artery, rupture of any portion of the ascending aorta leads to leakage into the pericardial sac. Rupture of the aortic arch is into the mediastinum. Descending aortic dissections commonly rupture into the left pleural space (but can also rupture into the right pleural cavity). Rupture of abdominal aortic dissection involves the retroperitoneum. Retrograde dissection from an ascending aortic tear extending into a coronary artery may lead to acute myocardial ischemia. Dissection involving the aortic valve commissures can result in acute valvular regurgitation (Fig. 1). Other local complications include pulmonary artery compression (Fig. 2) and retrograde perforation into the atria or ventricles leading to aortoatrial or aortoventricular fistulas.

Propagation of the dissection into an artery arising from the aorta may lead to ischemia or necrosis of the organ or tissue normally perfused by that artery (Fig. 3). Although occasionally sheared off, the true lumen of a larger artery tends to be compressed either at its origin or somewhere along its course by the false lumen. Luminal compression may be followed by thrombosis. The orifice of a small artery can be sheared off cleanly so that distal blood flow originates from the false lumen and is unimpeded. Approximately 30% to 50% of patients develop one or more peripheral vascular complications, including stroke, paraplegia, peripheral pulse loss, and impaired renal or visceral perfusion.[8] Depending on the specific pathoanatomic findings, central nervous system involvement may be manifested by syncope, focal neurologic signs, or frank coma. Stroke occurs infrequently, with an incidence of 3% to 7%. Severe peripheral arterial compromise may lead to

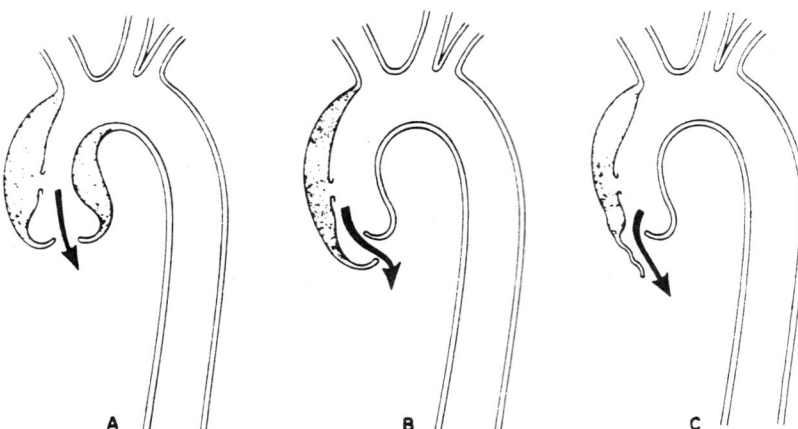

Figure 1 Mechanisms of aortic regurgitation in aortic dissection. *A*, Circumferential tear with widening of aortic root and separation of aortic cusps. *B*, Displacement of one aortic cusp substantially below the level of the others by the pressure of the dissecting hematoma. *C*, Actual disruption of the annular leaflet support leading to a flail cusp. (From Slater EE, DeSanctis RW. The clinical recognition of dissecting aortic aneurysm. Am J Med 1976; 60:625–633; with permission.)

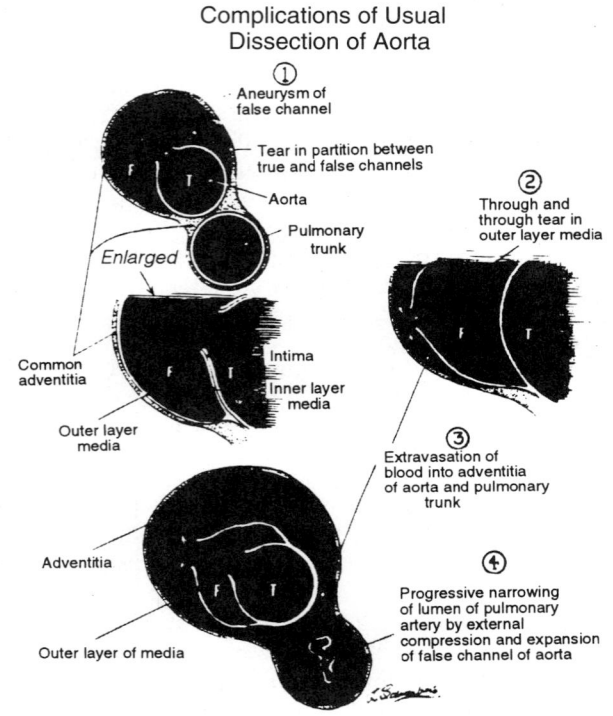

Figure 2 Diagram showing extension of the aortic dissection into the wall of the pulmonary artery, resulting in pulmonary artery luminal narrowing. (From Roberts WC. Aortic dissection: Anatomy, consequences, and causes. Am Heart J 1981; 101:195–214; with permission.)

ischemic peripheral neuropathy involving one limb. The incidence of paraplegia from spinal cord ischemia complicating aortic dissection occurs in 2% to 6% of patients. Loss of a peripheral pulse can occur in one-third to one-half of patients with type A dissection and one-quarter of all patients. These pulse deficits resolve spontaneously in up to one-third of patients, presumably because of re-entry into the true lumen from the false lumen. Because the dissecting hematoma can involve the renal arteries, leading to renal ischemia or infarction, the presence of oliguria, flank pain, and hematuria is of diagnostic and prognostic importance. The incidence of renal artery compromise in patients with aortic dissection is reported to range from 5% to 60%, probably reflecting the method of detection (i.e., angiography versus autopsy) rather than population differences. Acute dissection involving the visceral vessels leading to mesenteric ischemia or infarction is uncommon (occurrence rate of 3% to 5%) but highly lethal.

About 10% of acute dissections "heal" and become chronic dissections.[1,4] Generally, survival after acute dissection and progression to chronic dissection are related directly to the distance of the intimal tear from the aortic valve. The intimal tear in chronic dissection is commonly located beyond the aortic isthmus, and arch vessel and coronary artery involvement are infrequent. Nearly all patients with chronic dissections have an identifiable distal re-entry site, usually in the distal descending thoracic aorta, abdominal aorta, or iliac artery. The false lumen may thrombose, remain patent and endothelialize, or become aneurysmal.

PATHOLOGY

Described approximately 60 years ago by Erdheim, "cystic medial necrosis" has been associated with aortic dissection, arterial rupture, and diffuse aneurysmal degeneration. The significance of this pathologic finding has been questioned, and others have reported no consistent histologic abnormalities of the aortic wall in patients with aortic dissection and without Marfan syndrome.[1,4,9] Hirst and Gore found that, in patients with aortic dissection under the age of 40 years and in

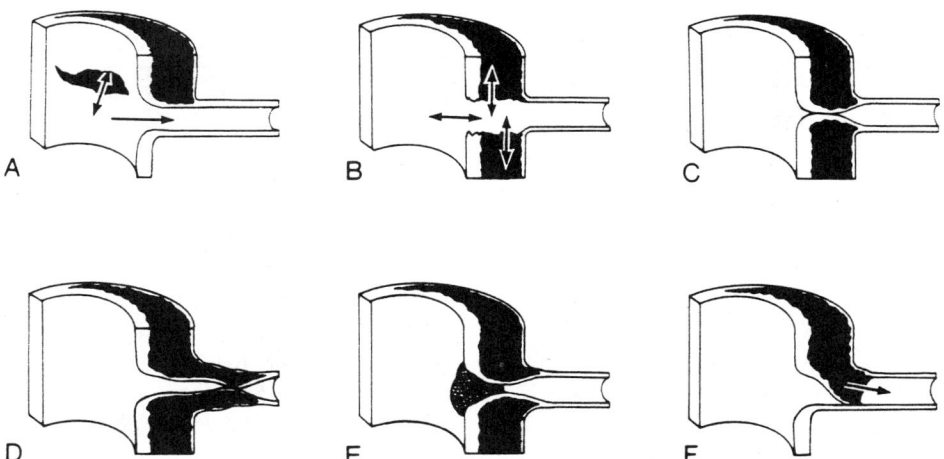

Figure 3 Examples of pathoanatomic complications of aortic dissections. Perfusion of the aortic branch vessel is illustrated in A, B, and F. Perfusion takes place through the true lumen in A and B and through the false lumen in F. Obstruction of the aortic tributary from extrinsic compression is shown in C and D, and compromise of the true lumen and consequent thrombosis is shown in E. In F, re-entry of the dissection at a tributary has created an intimal flap; in chronic dissections, this may become a permanent situation if the flap heals to the opposite wall of the vessel, thus rendering this branch solely dependent upon perfusion from the false lumen. (From Miller DC. Surgical management of aortic dissections: Indications, perioperative management and long-term results. In: Doroghazi RM, Slater EE, eds. Aortic dissection. New York: McGraw-Hill, 1983:198; with permission.)

those with Marfan syndrome, the degenerative changes predominantly involve the medial elastic tissue.[9] Nonetheless, cystic medial necrosis continues to be used by some authors to describe the nonspecific pathologic process characterized by medial smooth muscle cell and elastic lamellar disruption and acid mucopolysaccharide accumulation in mucoid-appearing regions. The term cystic is a misnomer in that these medial lesions do not form true cysts with a distinct lining. Medial "necrosis" is inferred as a result of depletion and degeneration of the medial elements. Elastic fragmentation and smooth muscle cell degeneration are frequently found in the aging aorta and probably represent the morphologic changes associated with repeated aortic wall injury and repair. The term cystic medial necrosis, therefore, should be replaced by more specific terms for the abnormal pathologic features of the aorta relating to elastic tissue lesions or smooth muscle cell degeneration. Generally, the elastic tissue degeneration seen in younger patients with type A dissections is commonly the result of a connective tissue abnormality. In older patients, type B dissections are more common, associated with degeneration and loss of medial smooth muscle cells.

REFERENCES

1. Hirst AE, John VL, Kime SW. Dissecting aneurysm of the aorta: A review of 505 cases. Medicine 1958; 37:217–279.
2. Miller DC. Surgical management of aortic dissections: Indications, perioperative management, and long-term results. In: Doroghazi RM, Slater EE, eds. Aortic dissection. New York: McGraw-Hill, 1983:193.
3. DeSanctis RW, Eagle KA. Aortic dissection. Curr Probl Cardiol 1989; 14:227–278.
4. Roberts WC, Aortic dissection: Anatomy, consequences, and causes. Am Heart J 1981; 101:195–214.
5. Lui RC, Menkis AH, McKenzie FN. Aortic dissection without intimal rupture: Diagnosis and management. Ann Thorac Surg 1992; 53:886–888.
6. Robbins RC, McManus RP, Mitchell RS, et al. Management of patients with intramural hematoma of the thoracic aorta. Circulation 1993; 88:1–10.
7. Tsipouras P, Del Mastro R, Sarfarazi M, et al. Genetic linkage of the Marfan syndrome, ectopia lentis, and congenital contractural arachnodactyly to the fibrillin genes on chromosomes 15 and 5. N Engl J Med 1992; 326:905–909.
8. Fann JI, Sarris GE, Mitchell RS, et al. Treatment of patients with aortic dissection presenting with peripheral vascular complications. Ann Surg 1990; 212:705–713.
9. Hirst AE, Gore I. Is cystic medionecrosis the cause of dissecting aortic aneurysm? Am Heart J 1976; 53:915–916.

ROLE OF ARTERIOGRAPHY IN ASSESSMENT OF ABDOMINAL AORTIC ANEURYSM

MICHAEL J. PETERSEN, M.D.
DAVID C. BREWSTER, M.D.

Table 1 Preoperative Data Required for Safe Repair of Abdominal Aortic Aneurysms

Confirmation of diagnosis
Determination of accurate size
Definition of proximal and distal extent
Renal artery abnormalities
Visceral artery abnormalities
Lower extremity occlusive disease
Associated aneurysmal disease

Use of preoperative arteriography in patients with abdominal aortic aneurysms (AAA) remains unsettled and controversial. Some surgeons emphasize the anatomic information it can provide and recommend its liberal, if not routine, use prior to aneurysm repair.[1-5] Such advocates draw a parallel to the value and importance of an arteriographic road map in facilitating the performance and improving the outcome of vascular reconstruction for occlusive disease and in other revascularization procedures. Advocates of this position contend that the results of operation will be superior if the surgeon has maximal knowledge of arterial anatomy, information that may not be provided by other imaging techniques or determined adequately during operation. Supporters argue that arteriography provides such information with minimal risk and at reasonable cost.

In contrast, other authors either oppose the use of preoperative arteriography or more commonly employ it only in selected circumstances.[6-12] This position emphasizes the risks and expense of arteriography. More important is the contention that important information that will truly modify the operative procedure and that cannot be obtained from other less invasive imaging techniques or determined by an experienced surgeon during the operation itself is rarely gained from preoperative arteriography. The issue then is whether preoperative arteriography prior to repair of an abdominal aortic aneurysm provides sufficiently important information to justify its risk and cost.

INFORMATION NEEDED BY THE SURGEON

To examine these issues, it is important first to define the information required by the surgeon for safe and successful repair of an AAA (Table 1). Clearly, confirmation of the diagnosis and accurate sizing are necessary to determine whether surgical repair is indicated. Once operation is planned, it is important to determine the extent of aneurysmal disease, particularly its cephalad relationship to the renal arteries. It is often the extent of the aneurysm that dictates the appropriate surgical approach and influences determination of operative risk. Therefore, this information must be accurately defined preoperatively. In addition, the surgeon should know about clinically significant renal or visceral artery abnormalities. Accessory renal arteries and high-grade renal or visceral stenoses or aneurysms may warrant concomitant repair, and their unrecognized presence may have profound perioperative consequences. The presence of associated lower extremity occlusive disease may also have important implications to distal aortic reconstructions, and its presence requires complete evaluation prior to aneurysm repair.

With these things in mind, it is possible to group preoperative anatomic data into three major categories: (1) those which may be crucial to the operative procedure, (2) those which are often quite helpful although perhaps not critical, and finally (3) those which are sometimes helpful. Crucial anatomic information includes the proximal extent of the aneurysm, the presence of critical renal artery abnormalities, and severe visceral artery disease. Anatomic information that can be helpful by perhaps increasing efficiency and safety of the planned procedure requires a thorough evaluation of the aneurysm outflow. This includes the presence of outflow occlusive disease involving iliofemoral, profunda femoral, or other infrainguinal arteries. Aneurysmal disease involving the iliac, hypogastric, femoral, or other intraabdominal vessels also falls into this category. Lastly, anatomic information that is sometimes helpful includes unsuspected findings such as occult visceral aneurysms, dissections, arteriovenous fistula, contained leak, and unusual lumbar arteries, which all can influence the surgical approach and operative plan.

ADVANTAGES OF ARTERIOGRAPHY

The value of arteriography is not in the diagnosis of an aortic aneurysm or in determining its exact size. Aortography is generally acknowledged to be relatively inaccurate in this regard because of the well-recognized effects of mural thrombus within the aneurysm resulting in opacification of only the aneurysm lumen. Rather its value and importance are in the anatomic information it provides once the diagnosis is made and operation is recommended. Numerous studies have documented a significant incidence of "positive" findings of arteriograms performed prior to aortic aneurysm repair (Table 2).

The proximal extent of aneurysmal dilation, particularly regarding the renal arteries, is unquestionably of critical importance. The placement of the proximal cross-clamp on a healthy aortic neck is a critical step in successful abdominal aortic aneurysm repair. The incidence of suprarenal aortic involvement in patients with

Table 2 Results of Routine Preoperative Aortography in Patients with AAA

	Brewster[1]	Kwaan[2]	Baur[3]	Nuno[9]	Bell[7]	Couch[8]	Bunt[5]	TOTALS
Number of patients	190	132	100	105	104	110	70	811
Major complications	0%	0%	0%	1%	0%	0%	0%	0.1%
Minor complications	2%	1.5%	1%	5%	3%	5%		3%
Suprarenal extension	5%	8%	9%	0	7%	4%	6%	6%
Celiac/SMA stenosis	10%	26%	27%	13%	5%	19%		16%
Renal stenosis	22%	10%	32%	20%	16%	7%	6%	17%
Accessory renal	17%	5%	37%	3%	10%	1%	7%	12%
Iliac aneurysm	41%	20%	66%	18%	48%		47%	39%
Iliofemoral stenosis	48%	41%	49%	41%	41%		34%	43%
Other aneurysms	Renal 2%			Renal 2%	Femoral 9%		Renal 1% Iliac AVF 1%	

Vascular abnormalities in patients with abdominal aortic aneurysms undergoing routine arteriography during preoperative evaluation. SMA, Superior mesenteric artery. AVF, Arterial venous fistula.

AAAs ranges from 0 to 9% (average 6%) and was 5% among our own patients. Often with AAA there is also lengthening tortuosity and significant atherosclerosis of the proximal infrarenal aorta. When this occurs, the neck of the aneurysm may actually lie in a posterior to anterior plane and be of sufficient length for infrarenal repair and yet appear as a juxtarenal or suprarenal aneurysm on computed tomography (CT) or ultrasound. If the aneurysm extends to or above the renal arteries, a medial visceral rotation or a thoracoabdominal retroperitoneal approach may be required to allow safe and secure clamping. Biplane aortography, especially the lateral view, will not only allow accurate measurement of the aneurysm neck length but also clarify the geometry and quality of the aorta in this area.

The presence of aneurysmal disease of the iliac, hypogastric, or femoral vessels may also influence the surgical plan. In our series, 41% of AAA patients had iliac aneurysmal degeneration, and an additional 15% had associated hypogastric, femoral, or popliteal aneurysms.[1] Overall, iliac aneurysm involvement was noted on average in 39% of patients studied by arteriography (Table 2). Although some associated aneurysms may be detected preoperatively by physical examination, iliac or hypogastric aneurysmal disease may not be found until operation. In our prospective study comparing CT and arteriography, common iliac aneurysm or lack thereof was correctly identified by CT in only 42 (84%) of 50 patients and hypogastric aneurysms were correctly diagnosed in only one of three (33%) patients. Todd and co-workers,[11] using CT, failed to detect preoperatively 3 of 22 (16%) iliac aneurysms associated with abdominal aortic aneurysms. Although these were detected at the time of operation and repaired without incident, it is possible that a right iliac or hypogastric aneurysm may be overlooked or difficult to correct if a retroperitoneal approach is used.

Associated renal artery abnormalities are another important finding of arteriography. In AAA patients the incidence of such findings averaged 17% (Table 2). In our study, 22% of patients had significant renal occlusive disease and of these 24% underwent concomitant renal revascularization.[1] Certainly routine repair of all stenotic renal arteries is unnecessary and ill advised, but high-grade lesions associated with significant hypertension or diminished renal function need careful consideration for concomitant correction at the time of AAA repair. Routine operative dissection and exposure for standard aneurysm repair afford little ability to evaluate renal or mesenteric arteries for occlusive disease intraoperatively, much less repair them. The surgeon should not overestimate his or her ability accurately to assess and evaluate the severity or clinical importance of intra-abdominal occlusive disease intraoperatively. Whether preoperative clinical criteria will identify all patients with renal artery abnormalities who require preoperative arteriography is still open to question. In one series by Valentine and associates[13] 10% of AAA patients were noted to have severe renal artery stenosis (at least 75%), and all patients in this group had identifiable clinical criteria (renal insufficiency or severe hypertension). Patients are occasionally found with severe preocclusive (more than 90%) renal artery stenoses and minimal hypertension or renal dysfunction. Because of the usual natural history of progression of such lesions to occlusion, with subsequent loss of functioning renal mass, it is our preference to carry out simultaneous repair of such lesions even in the absence of classic indications.

Accessory renal arteries are found with varying frequency in patients with AAA (1% to 37%). In our series significant multiple or accessory renal arteries were noted in 17% of patients (Table 2). These vessels may arise from the aneurysm, and if not anticipated, they may be injured or ligated during aneurysm dissection and repair, with subsequent segmental renal infarction. This may cause postoperative impairment of function or hypertension. It has been our policy to preserve and reimplant accessory renal arteries arising from the aneurysm if they are over 2 mm in diameter.

Visceral artery occlusive disease is a fairly frequent, usually asymptomatic associated arteriographic finding in patients with aortic aneurysms. Although we noted a 10% incidence of significant superior mesenteric artery (SMA) or celiac stenoses, others have observed a higher incidence, 13% to 27%.[1] An average of 16% of AAAs were found to have significant narrowing of the SMA or celiac (Table 2). Although associated visceral artery disease usually does not warrant concomitant repair in the asymptomatic patient undergoing aneurysm repair, such knowledge gained from preoperative aortography may be of importance for some patients to minimize the risk of postoperative bowel and particularly colonic ischemia, with its known high morbidity and mortality. In such circumstances the surgeon is alerted to the possible need to reimplant a patent inferior mesenteric artery and preserve pelvic blood flow. In some instances visceral artery reconstruction by bypass or endarterectomy may be appropriately combined with aneurysm repair. This may be the case if the patient has symptoms of possible chronic intestinal ischemia or will likely lose important sources of collateral blood flow to the bowel, as when the hypogastric circulation cannot be maintained because of the pattern of aneurysmal disease.

Iliofemoral outflow occlusive disease is the most common associated vascular abnormality in patients with AAA. In our series we noted significant iliac or femoral artery stenosis in 48% of patients (Table 2). Such findings may influence the distal anastomotic sites and surgical approach. Although many of these patients will have clinical symptoms or findings on pulse examination or noninvasive studies to suggest such associated occlusive disease, an occasional patient will have outflow disease that is not yet clinically apparent. However, this may still cause technical difficulties with distal graft anastomoses if unrecognized, particularly if the operative approach does not easily lend access to the more distal arterial segment, as for example with right iliac disease and a left retroperitoneal incision. Furthermore, if distal anastomoses are constructed proximal to developing occlusive disease, the patient may later become symptomatic, or worse, develop an iliac limb occlusion in late follow-up, both of which might have been prevented with a more distal femoral anastomosis.

A moderate number of miscellaneous lesions are regularly discovered on arteriography (Table 2). These lesions include renal and visceral artery aneurysms, unusual lumbar arteries, and arterial venous fistula. In none of these patients was antecedent clinical history available to suggest the diagnosis. Operative discovery of these lesions may not occur, or correction may require a significant alteration of the operative plan and prove difficult or dangerous. It is far better to know of their presence preoperatively.

DISADVANTAGES OF ARTERIOGRAPHY

Development of other imaging modalities and emphasis on cost containment have intensified the debate over the use of preoperative arteriography prior to aneurysm repair. The major arguments against routine contrast arteriography revolve around its cost, invasiveness, and potential for procedure-related complications. Although the exact cost of aortography depends upon the extent of the study and varies from hospital to hospital, use of preoperative arteriography at our hospital adds approximately $2000 to $2500 to the hospital bill if all technical and professional charges are included. This is unquestionably more than CT scans ($800 to $1000) and magnetic resonance angiography (MRA) studies ($1200 to $1500). However, charges for both of these modalities approximately double if more extensive imaging of the aorta from above the renal arteries to below the proximal iliac level is performed, as is routine in many centers. Alternatively, if two-level CT or MRA studies are not done, it is likely that important surgical information will be overlooked.

An additional criticism of the use of preoperative arteriography is that it adds the expense of an additional hospital day. However, increasing use of outpatient studies is largely eliminating this consideration.

Moreover, operating room charges are high, averaging approximately $1200 per hour, or $20 per minute, at our hospital. The time-saving and, therefore, cost-reducing value of an expeditious operation based upon full preoperative anatomic information gained from arteriography can be considerable. Furthermore, the value of avoiding postoperative complications such as renal failure, colon ischemia, and graft thrombosis because of indispensable knowledge gained from preoperative arteriography is difficult to quantify but must be recognized.

As with any invasive procedure, arteriography has an inherent risk of procedure-related complications. However, when it is performed by experienced personnel with appropriate equipment, its hazards are quite low. Our own experience parallels that of the literature, showing low overall incidences, approximately 0.5% for major complications and 1% to 3% for minor complications. The risk of mortality is practically nonexistent. The possibility of contrast-induced renal failure is often cited as a significant danger of preoperative arteriography. With today's contrast agents and widespread appreciation of the importance of periprocedural hydration, clinically significant renal failure is infrequent in patients with normal renal function. In higher-risk patients such as diabetics with varying degrees of pre-existing renal insufficiency, the incidence of this problem rises to approximately 10%. However, such contrast-related renal dysfunction is almost always transient and self-limited. The increased use of outpatient arteriography and digital subtraction techniques has further reduced the risk of renal toxicity by spacing the diagnostic and surgical procedures further apart and limiting contrast loads.

RECOMMENDATIONS

From a thoughtful appraisal of all data and arguments for and against the use of preoperative arteriography prior to aortic aneurysm repair, it is evident that it is not possible or appropriate to establish a blanket

Table 3 Indications for Preoperative Arteriography in AAA Patients

Suspected suprarenal extension
Suspected renovascular disease
Suspected visceral artery disease
Iliofemoral occlusive disease
Associated aneurysmal disease
Renal anomalies

policy. A decision to employ arteriography must be individualized, based upon a thorough history and physical examination, other forms of conventional preoperative evaluation, and sound clinical judgment. In addition, some surgeons will feel more confident and better prepared with the information provided by arteriography, a reasonable and legitimate reason for its use in our opinion.

There is no question that aneurysm repair can be successfully accomplished in many patients without an arteriogram. However, in some instances it does provide critically important anatomic information. Even opponents of frequent or routine preoperative arteriography acknowledge its value and importance in certain patients. The key to selective use of arteriography is identification of such patients. Certain clinical findings or indications can single out patients for whom arteriography is advisable. Unfortunately, however, no entirely reliable, infallible clinical criteria for this purpose exist, and the policy of selective arteriography in relatively few patients will undoubtedly omit the study in some who would likely have benefited from its performance. Therefore, our approach is liberal use of preoperative arteriography in most but not all aneurysm patients (Table 3).

REFERENCES

1. Brewster DC, Retana A, Waltman AC, et al. Angiography in the management of aneurysms of the abdominal aorta. N Engl J Med 1975; 292:822–825.
2. Kwaan JH, Connolly JE, Vander Molen R, et al. The value of arteriography before aneurysmectomy. Am J Surg 1977; 134:109–114.
3. Baur GM, Porter JM, Eidemitter LR, et al. The role of arteriography in abdominal aortic aneurysm. Am J Surg 1978; 136:184–189.
4. Porter JM. The role of preoperative arteriography in patients with abdominal aortic aneurysms. In: Najarian JS, Delaney JP, eds. Advances in vascular surgery. Chicago: Year Book Medical Publishers, 1983:275.
5. Bunt TJ, Cropper L. Routine angiography for abdominal aortic aneurysm: The case for informed operative selection. J Cardiovasc Surg 1986; 27:725–727.
6. Gaspar MR. Role of arteriography in the evaluation of aortic aneurysms: The case against. In: Bergan JJ, Yao JST, eds. Aneurysms: Diagnosis and treatment. New York: Grune & Stratton, 1982:243.
7. Bell DD, Gaspar MR. Routine aortography before abdominal aortic aneurysmectomy: A prospective study. Am J Surg 1982; 144:191–193.
8. Couch NP, O'Mahoney J, McIrvine A, et al. The place of abdominal aortography in abdominal aortic aneurysm resection. Arch Surg 1983; 118:1029–1034.
9. Nuno IN, Collins GM, Bardin JA, et al. Should arteriography be used routinely in the elective management of abdominal aortic aneurysm? Am J Surg 1982; 144:53–57.
10. Campbell JJ, Bell DD, Gaspar MR. Selective use of arteriography in the assessment of aortic aneurysm repair. Ann Vasc Surg 1990; 4:419–423.
11. Todd GJ, Nowygrod R, Benvenisty A, et al. The accuracy of CT scanning in the diagnosis of abdominal and thoracoabdominal aortic aneurysms. J Vasc Surg 1991; 13:302–310.
12. Friedman SG, Kerner BA, Krishnasastry KV, et al. Abdominal aortic aneurysmectomy without preoperative angiography: A prospective study. NY J Med 1990; 90:176–178.
13. Valentine RJ, Myers, SI, Miller GL, et al. Detection of unsuspected renal artery stenoses in patients with abdominal aortic aneurysms: Refined indications for preoperative aortography. Ann Vasc Surg 1993; 7:220–224.

MAGNETIC RESONANCE IMAGING, ULTRASONOGRAPHY, AND COMPUTED TOMOGRAPHY IN ASSESSMENT OF ABDOMINAL AORTIC ANEURYSM

DAVID ROSENTHAL, M.D.

Noninvasive vascular imaging is an essential part of the evaluation of patients with an abdominal aortic aneurysm (AAA). A clinical diagnosis of AAA may be made by physical examination, and lateral lumbar x-ray films can confirm the diagnosis, but these methods are inadequate to plan a safe operation. Aortography has been advocated to establish a diagnosis of AAA; however, aortography often defines only the inner lumen of the aneurysm and may grossly underestimate the overall aneurysm size. Aortography should not, therefore, be the primary diagnostic procedure but rather an adjunctive study to delineate the presence of occlusive lesions in the visceral, renal, and iliofemoral vessels.

Ultrasonography, computed tomography (CT), and magnetic resonance imaging (MRI) can provide invaluable information that allows the surgeon to anticipate technical difficulties, know the safe locations for vascular clamp placement, and often avoid venous or organ injuries due to unsuspected anatomic anomalies.

ULTRASONOGRAPHY

Ultrasonography is readily available and is the least expensive of the noninvasive imaging studies. These two features have made ultrasonography the preferred examination for establishing the diagnosis of AAA, for surveillance of small aneurysms, and for use in aneurysm screening programs.[1] An image is obtained by reflecting an ultrasound beam off different tissues; the detected echoes produce images on a video screen. The echo characteristics of the tissues in relation to the transducer position provides a two-dimensional image (B-mode scanning). The transducer may be moved in any plane to provide a two-dimensional echo image.

With the advent of gray-scale real-time sonography the diagnostic accuracy of the ultrasonography was expected to improve significantly. However, despite early optimistic reports,[2] experience gathered from multicenter studies documented that sizing inaccuracies were common.[3] These inaccuracies included both overestimation of aneurysm size because of oblique scanning and underestimation of size when mural thrombus was not appreciated. B-mode ultrasonography has sufficient accuracy to size the abdominal aorta for the purpose of diagnosing an aneurysm, but it fails to provide reliable information concerning the relation of the aneurysm to the renal, visceral, and iliac vessels because sound is attenuated by intervening bowel gas. With a full bladder providing a sonographic window, it may occasionally be possible to visualize the external iliac arteries, but documenting continuity with the aortic bifurcation is often impossible. In obese patients or patients with extensive bowel gas, the examination may be impossible.[4]

Recent improvements in deep abdominal Doppler scanning with the addition of real-time color flow mapping may overcome the limitations of duplex and B-mode systems. Color flow mapping systems display in real time velocities throughout the entire lumen of vessels studied. This capability is useful in aneurysm imaging because it facilitates identification of visceral and renal vessels, intraluminal thrombus, venous anomalies, and sites of blood flow abnormality produced by arterial occlusive disease.[5] However, the more detailed information provided by CT and MRI has relegated ultrasound primarily to a screening and surveillance technique.

COMPUTED TOMOGRAPHY

Improved CT technology has broadened its use for scanning, diagnosis, and preoperative evaluation of AAA to the point where it is recognized as the gold standard in the investigation of aneurysm disease. CT imaging is performed with highly sensitive x-ray detectors placed in a 360° array around the patient and aligned with an x-ray tube. The intensity of the x-ray beam from each radial is altered by tissue absorption, and the detectors convert this information into electric signals that are digitized and computer processed to produce a two-dimensional cross-sectional image. This image is displayed on a video system, and transverse scans are obtained at 1 to 3 cm intervals. Scanning time and skin surface radiation have been reduced, and contrast enhancement and improved-resolution scanners have continued to improve the accuracy and anatomic definition in aneurysm assessment. CT is highly predictive of aneurysm size, has no false-negative results, and can generally localize the proximal extent of the aneurysm.[6] Infrequently, the renal arteries cannot be confidently defined in juxtarenal aneurysms if the upper end of the aneurysm overlies the renal artery origin because of tortuosity of the aorta at this level. In these patients and in patients who are suspected of having accessary renal arteries, MRI or aortography performed in the lateral position will most accurately identify the renal vessels (Fig. 1).[7]

If no contraindication to a contrast agent exists, a contrast enhancement CT scan is preferred. Patients are infused intravenously with a bolus of contrast medium (50 to 100 ml of nonionic diatrizoate), which allows

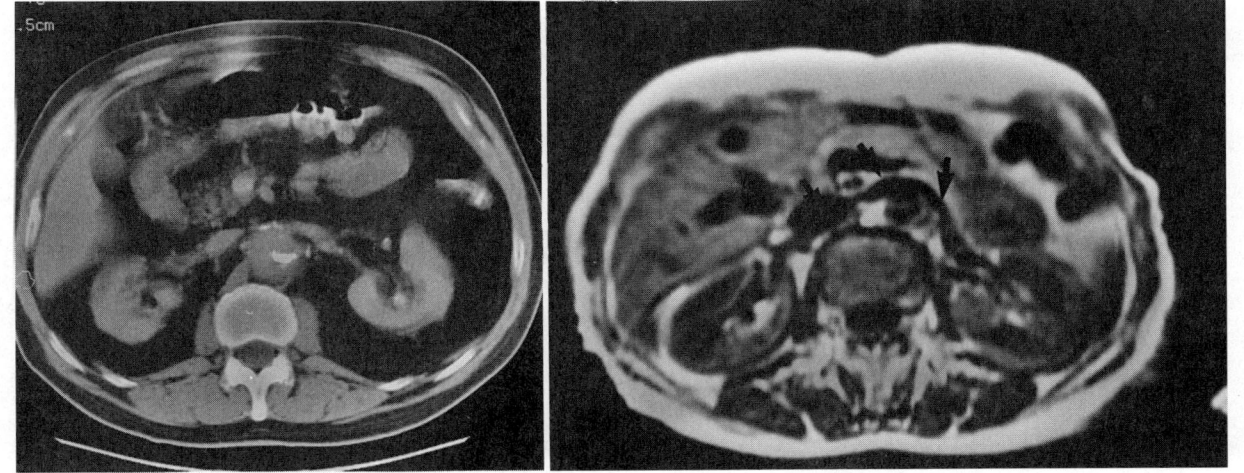

Figure 1 *A,* CT scan of a juxtarenal AAA that could not delineate renal artery involvement. *B,* MRI juxtarenal AAA in the same patient; renal arteries (*arrows*) are separate from aneurysm.

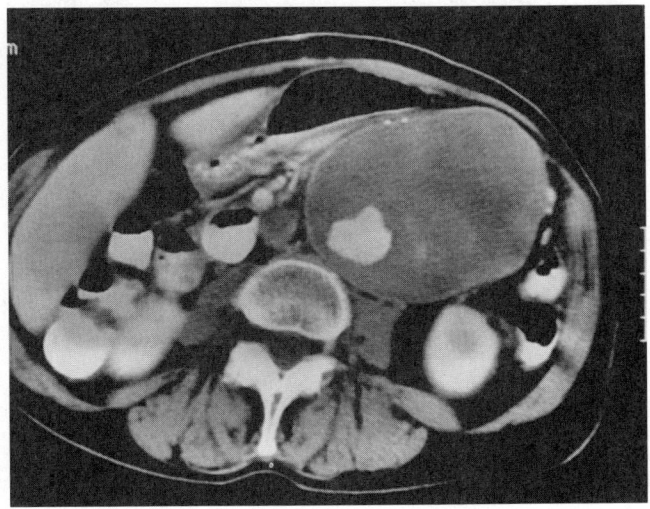

Figure 2 Contrast-enhanced CT scan of AAA. Note minimal thrombus between the medial wall and lumen, which suggests the possibility of early rupture.

definition of thrombus within the aneurysm and can provide information on renal status by identifying anomalies in renal parenchyma (i.e., renal cysts, horseshoe kidney), in contrast excretion (i.e., renal artery occlusion), or outflow obstruction (i.e., hydronephrosis, nephrolithiasis).[6]

The contrast-enhanced aortic lumen is typically located posteriorly in the aneurysm sac with thrombus laminated anteriorly (Fig. 2). CT scans are superior to ultrasonography in defining aneurysm wall integrity, relationship of the aneurysm to the inferior vena cava (Fig. 3*A*) and other major venous anomalies (Fig. 3*B*), detection of an inflammatory aneurysm (Fig. 4), and contained rupture (Fig. 5). CT imaging, even without contrast, documents the presence of blood in the retroperitoneal space. A leaking or ruptured aneurysm appears as a high-density CT substance most commonly posterior to the aneurysm, which disrupts the integrity of the aneurysm wall and normal configuration of the surrounding retroperitoneum (Fig. 6).

CT scans are safe and easy to interpret, and they produce an accurate measurement of the aneurysm diameter while defining the lumen and laminated thrombus if contrast enhancement is used. Obesity and bowel gas are not problems, and CT can readily evaluate the visceral, renal, and iliac vessels. Barium in the gastrointestinal tract or surgical clips adjacent to the aneurysm can produce artifact. CT scans require only moderate technical skill and can be performed with sufficient speed when evaluating symptomatic but hemodynamically stable patients with suspected rupture. Although radiation exposure and cost remain drawbacks, the detailed delineation of the abdominal aorta, retroperitoneum, and intraperitoneal organs make CT the preferred noninvasive method of preoperative evaluation.[6]

MAGNETIC RESONANCE IMAGING

MRI is a new noninvasive technique that provides both anatomic images in multiple planes and information about tissue characteristics.[8] Images are obtained by placing the patient in a static magnetic field. Magnetized protons (hydrogen nuclei) within the patient are bombarded by radiofrequency pulses that create an oscillating magnetic field. The hydrogen nuclei absorb this energy and migrate from a state of excitation to relaxation, and a complex computer-processed algorithm translates this activity into anatomic density. The

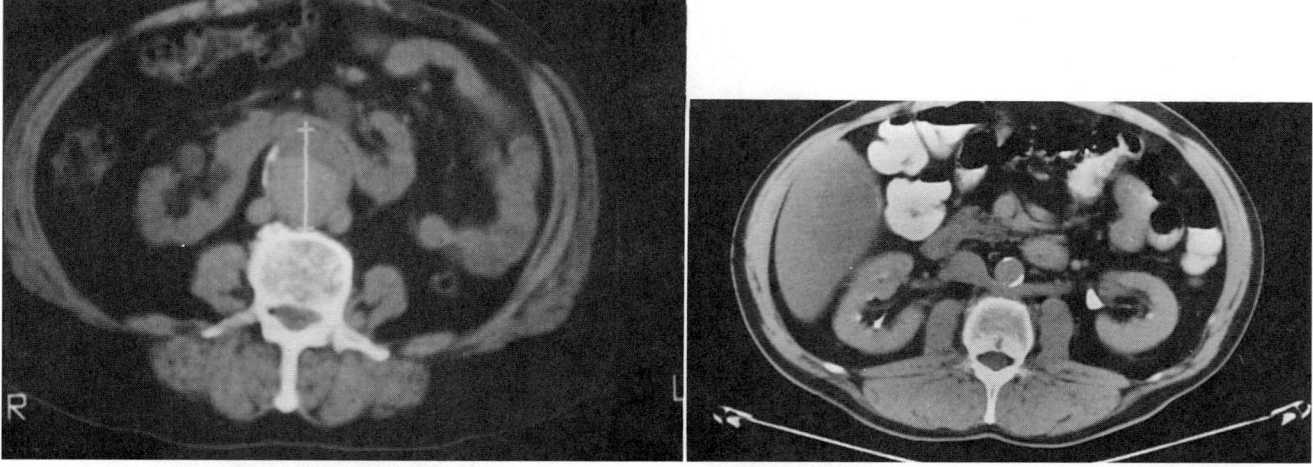

Figure 3 *A*, CT scan of AAA with double inferior vena cavas and horseshoe kidney. *B*, CT scan of retroaortic left renal vein at the neck of an AAA.

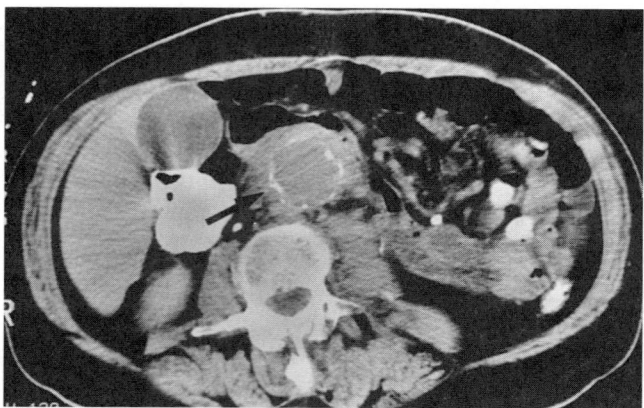

Figure 4 CT scan of an inflammatory aneurysm. A thick mantle of tissue lies around the aneurysm lumen (*arrow*).

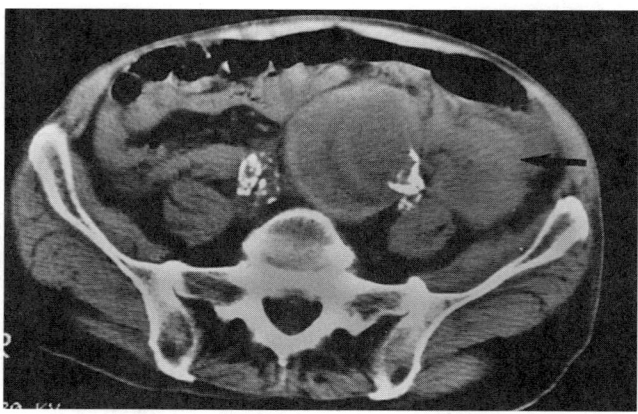

Figure 6 CT scan of ruptured AAA with retroperitoneal hematoma (*arrow*). Note the loss of aortic wall integrity.

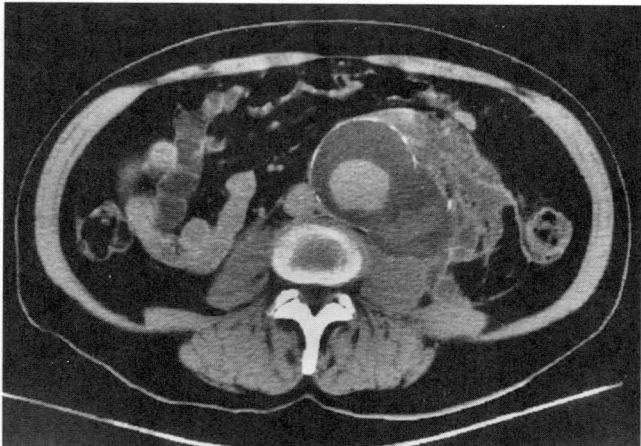

Figure 5 Contrast-enhanced CT image of chronic contained-rupture aneurysm. Patient complained of severe back pain of 4 weeks' duration.

multiplaner reconstruction of arterial anatomy by MRI yields information that cannot be obtained by ultrasound or CT imaging, both of which provide images in axial (transverse) planes. The three-dimensional imaging by MRI (axial, sagittal, and coronal planes) allows the most precise preoperative assessment of the patient with an aortic aneurysm (Fig. 7).[9]

Anatomic information includes lumen dimensions, rate of blood flow, quality of the aortic wall, cephalad and caudal extension of the aneurysm, involvement of arterial branches, and an accurate distinction between dissection and thoracoabdominal aneurysm. MRI does not use ionizing radiation, does not depend on operator skill or habitus of the patient, and can penetrate bone without significant attenuation. Its resolution is somewhat inferior to that of CT imaging, but the contrast resolution of soft tissue is superior. Intravenous injection of contrast media is unnecessary with MRI because flowing blood provides a natural contrast between static

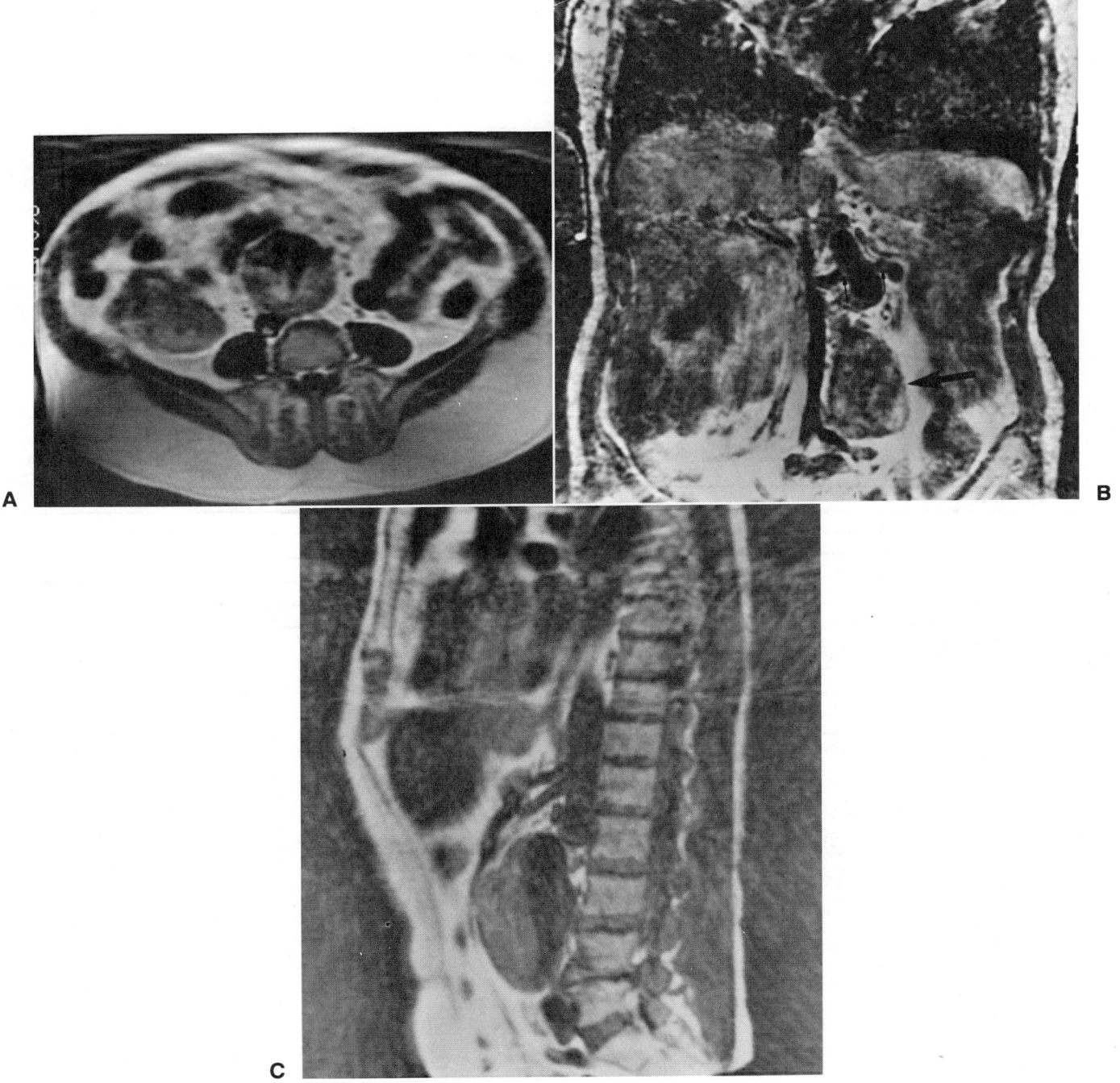

Figure 7 MRI images of AAA. *A,* axial, *B,* coronal (*small arrows* identify renal arteries, large arrow the aneurysm and adjacent inferior vena cava), and *C,* sagittal views. (Note identification of celiac and superior mesenteric arteries above AAA.)

blood and fixed structures. Some disadvantages of MRI for aneurysm imaging include slow scanning time resulting in image degradation with cardiovascular motion, inability to recognize calcification, and claustrophobia. Accessory renal and/or occlusive disease in mesenteric and main renal arteries may not be well visualized, but with more sophisticated scanning techniques these problems may be resolved in the near future. However, MRI scans are expensive; scanners may be inaccessible; critically ill patients cannot cooperate well or be properly monitored; and vascular surgical clips and pacemakers are contraindications to scanning.

SURGICAL TREATMENT OF NONRUPTURED INFRARENAL AND JUXTARENAL AORTIC ANEURYSMS

CALVIN B. ERNST, M.D.

It can be argued with some merit that the modern era of aneurysm treatment began on March 29, 1951, when Charles Dubost performed the first successful aortic reconstruction for an abdominal aortic aneurysm (AAA). Prior to this landmark accomplishment, aortic aneurysms had been treated by ligation, wrapping, and intraluminal foreign body thrombosis. Within approximately a year American vascular surgical pioneers such as DeBakey, Julian, and Szilagyi had duplicated Dubost's feat and established graft repair as the definitive treatment of infrarenal AAA.

Operative mortality rates have continued to decline over the 4 decades since aortic reconstruction was introduced.[1] Few will dispute that all significant aortic aneurysms should be repaired unless compelling contraindications exist. With contemporary surgical and anesthetic technology, even aneurysms encroaching upon the renal arteries can be safely repaired. This chapter reviews contemporary management of infrarenal and juxtarenal aortic aneurysms.

DEFINITIONS

An aortic aneurysm is a focal dilation of the aorta at least 50% greater than the expected normal diameter.[2] A pararenal aneurysm involves the renal artery origins but originates below the superior mesenteric artery. A juxtarenal aortic aneurysm is a pararenal aneurysm that encroaches upon the origins of the renal arteries with no infrarenal aortic segment suitable for clamping and anastomosis (Fig. 1).[2] Juxtarenal aneurysms pose challenges with regard to exposure, site of proximal aortic clamping, and prevention of renal dysfunction.

MAGNITUDE OF THE PROBLEM

In 1988 AAAs were responsible for almost 15,000 deaths in the United States among individuals 55 years of age and older. Aneurysms accounted for 9,874 deaths in men and 5,108 deaths in women in this age group.[1]

All reports cite major differences in mortality rates between elective and emergency aneurysm repairs, but such data do not reflect the true lethality of ruptured aortic aneurysms. Including prehospital deaths, the overall mortality for ruptured aortic aneurysms may exceed 90%. Clearly, AAA is a highly lethal lesion, and it presents a formidable clinical challenge in view of the increasing age of the population.

Aside from the cost of lives, ruptured aneurysms impose an onerous financial burden on hospitals. Diagnostic group cost reimbursement data suggest that emergency aortic reconstruction may result in a financial loss of almost $25,000 per patient.

PATHOGENESIS AND NATURAL HISTORY

A unified concept of aortic aneurysm pathogenesis has not yet emerged. Characterizing aortic aneurysms as arteriosclerotic may be an oversimplified view of pathogenesis, and it has been suggested that AAAs be designated nonspecific.[2] The true natural history of untreated AAA is debatable, since all natural history studies are from referral-based clinical practices, which

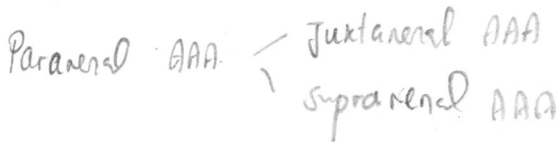

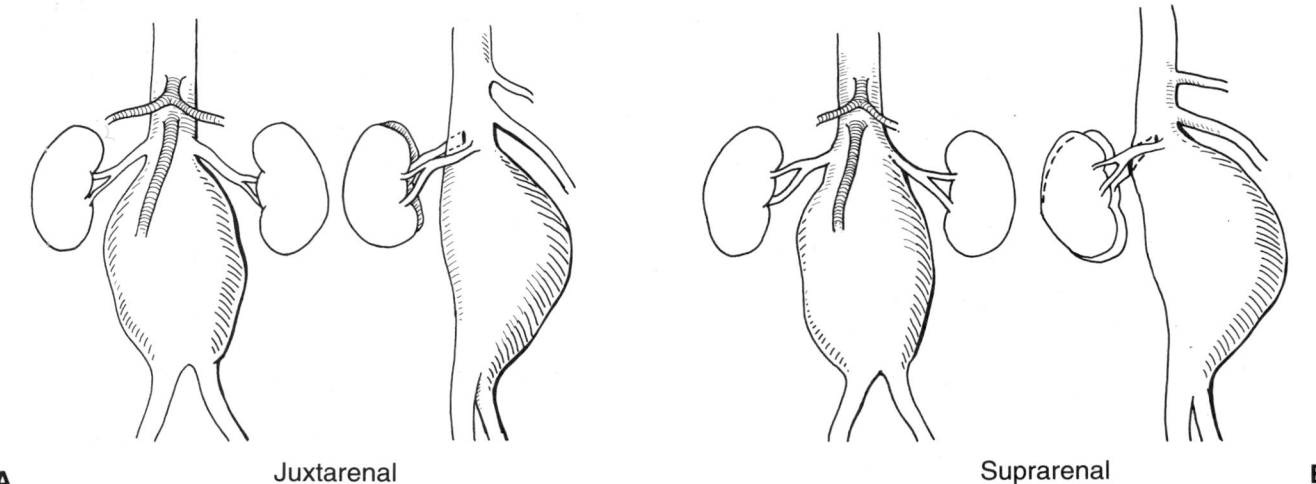

Figure 1 Classification of pararenal AAA. *A,* Juxtarenal AAA extends up to the origins of the renal arteries. *B,* Suprarenal AAA involves the origin of at least one renal artery but not the superior mesenteric artery. (From Nypaver TJ, Shepard AD, Reddy DJ, et al. Repair of pararenal abdominal aortic aneurysms: An analysis of operative management. Arch Surg, 1993; 128:803–813, with permission.)

are confounded by treatment selection bias. There are no published randomized clinical trials comparing surgical with nonsurgical management, although three are under way. Until such natural history data are available, the decision for or against aortic reconstruction must be based on the patient's life expectancy, aneurysm size, and the relation of rate of expansion to risk of rupture.

Expansion rate data from population-based studies suggest an annual increase of about 0.2 cm in aneurysm diameter, and referral-based studies record annual expansion rates averaging 0.4 cm. The 5 year risk of rupture of aneurysms 5 cm or greater ranges from 25% to 41%. Data for 4 to 5 cm aneurysms are sparse, but lesions in this size range have been reported to have a 5 year rupture rate of 3% to 12%. In one analysis, 74% of patients with aneurysms greater than 4 cm and under 69 years of age at entry into the study eventually underwent operation. This suggests that good-risk patients with reasonable life expectancies and small aneurysms will eventually come to aortic reconstruction.[3] The risk of rupture of an aneurysm less than 4 cm is about 2%.

The patient's age as it relates to elective aortic reconstruction is an independent risk factor for perioperative death. In Crawford's comprehensive study,[4] age-related operative mortality rates were as follows: less than 60 years, 3.3%; 60 to 69 years, 4.6%; 70 to 79 years, 5.4%; and 80 to 89 years, 12%. If the patient's life expectancy is reasonable, age is not a contraindication to operation. Actuarial data suggest that life expectancies for men aged 75, 80, and 85 years are 11.7, 9, and 6.8 years, respectively. For women aged 75, 80, and 85 years, life expectancies are 14, 10.6, and 7.8 years, respectively.

Provided comorbid conditions do not preclude operation, most vascular surgeons recommend aortic reconstruction for all symptomatic or ruptured aneurysms and for all asymptomatic aneurysms greater than 5 cm in diameter. If the patient has mild chronic obstructive pulmonary disease and hypertension, aneurysm repair becomes even more compelling.[5] Operation for aneurysms measuring 4 to 5 cm remains controversial. Data from a Markov decision model analysis suggest that early operation is preferred to observation for aneurysms 4 to 5 cm in diameter.[5] My personal approach, confirmed by an ad hoc committee of the Society for Vascular Surgery and North American Chapter of the International Society for Cardiovascular Surgery,[6] is to repair aneurysms greater than 4 cm in young, healthy patients with the knowledge that the majority will eventually come to operation.

PREOPERATIVE EVALUATION AND PREPARATION

Comorbid conditions, particularly coronary artery disease, must be identified and treated preoperatively to achieve optimal results. In a comprehensive analysis of the effects of coronary artery disease on surgical management of aortic aneurysms, Hertzer documented that myocardial infarction caused 37% of early postoperative deaths.[7] Furthermore, 39% of late deaths resulted from coronary artery disease. That these data have been confirmed by others suggest that studies to identify correctable symptomatic coronary artery disease are justified. Such studies include ECG, exercise myocardial imaging, pharmacologic stress myocardial imaging, multigaited ejection fraction scintigraphy (MUGA), continuous Holter monitoring, and two-dimensional transesophageal echocardiography. If significant coronary artery disease is identified, serious consideration should be given to myocardial revascularization prior to aneurysm repair.

Other complicated problems such as pulmonary or renal disease must also be addressed and corrected when possible. Marginal renal function manifest by serum creatinine elevations of greater than 3 mg/dl and pulmonary insufficiency reflected by a vital capacity and FEV_1 of less than 50% predicted may preclude elective aortic reconstruction.

Correctable renal artery occlusive disease may contribute to impaired renal function. Marginal renal function may be seriously compromised in patients with juxtarenal aneurysms. Consequently, it is important that biplanar arteriography be obtained in all patients with suspected ischemic nephropathy or with juxtarenal aneurysms when adjunctive renal revascularization or suprarenal or supraceliac aortic clamping is anticipated during aneurysm repair. Lateral aortography is particularly helpful in determining the proximal extent of the juxtarenal aneurysm and to document absence or presence of pararenal aortic atherosclerosis. Such preoperative data are critical in planning the operative approach and details of aneurysm repair. For example, a disease-free suprarenal aorta may be safely clamped, but extensive suprarenal aortic atherosclerosis mandates supraceliac aortic clamping (Fig. 2). Preoperative aortography for management of routine infrarenal aortic aneurysms is controversial. Some surgeons obtain aortography routinely, some almost never, and some selectively. If there are no compelling contraindications such as severe contrast medium allergy or severe renal dysfunction, biplanar aortography should be obtained under the following circumstances: suspected juxtarenal or suprarenal aneurysms, suspected renovascular hypertension or ischemic nephropathy, suspected splanchnic artery occlusive disease, and associated iliofemoral arterial occlusive disease.

Most patients deposit 2 to 3 units of their own blood in the blood bank preoperatively for use during aortic reconstruction. In addition, operative blood salvage and reinfusion are used in all patients undergoing aneurysm repair. Such adjuncts materially decrease need for banked blood during aortic reconstruction and thereby limit transmission of blood-borne infections due to non-A and non-B hepatitis viruses and human immunodeficiency virus.

The night before operation the colon is mechanically cleansed by giving the patient oral polyethylene glycol (Colyte). Supplemental intravenous fluid is given to assure adequate hydration. Preoperative measurement and plotting of left ventricular function curves are not performed unless serious myocardial compromise is evidenced by left ventricular ejection fractions of less than 25%. The surgeon who is managing juxtarenal aneurysms with need for suprarenal or supraceliac aortic clamping must direct special attention to adequate hydration and optimal cardiac performance. The morning of operation, patients receive 1 g of a second-generation cephalosporin with the anesthetic premedication.

OPERATIVE MANAGEMENT

Without equivocation, graft replacement of the aorta is the standard of care for infrarenal and juxtarenal aortic aneurysms. Feasibility of transfemoral endovascular graft implantation for infrarenal aortic aneurysms

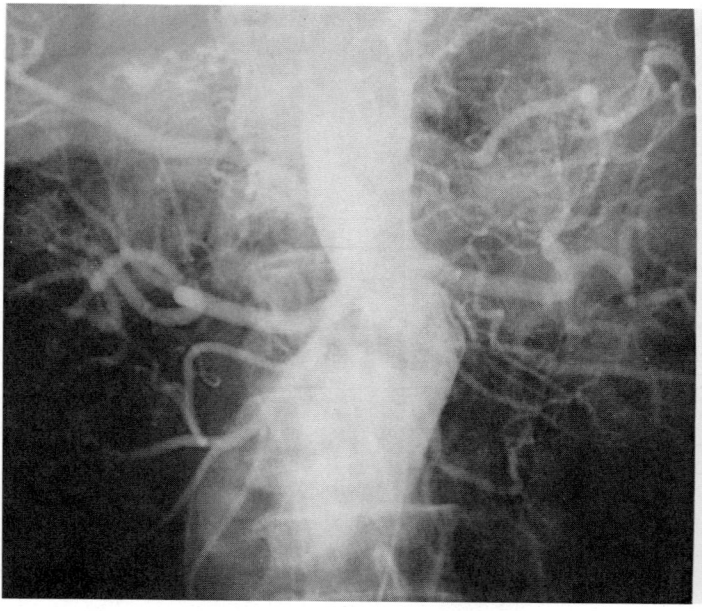
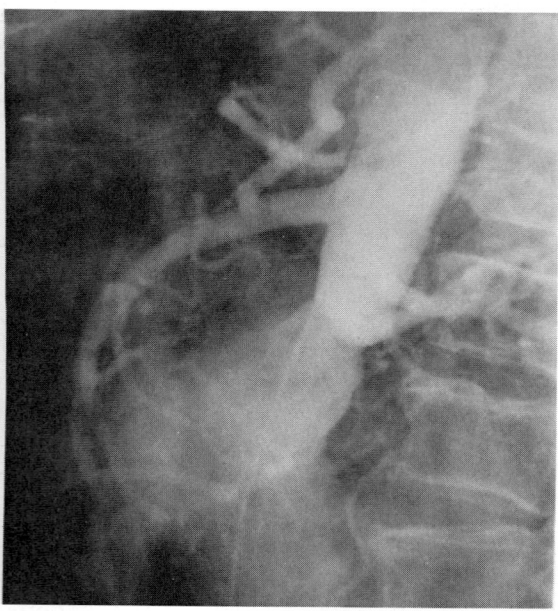

Figure 2 *A,* Anteroposterior projection of an aortogram documenting a large juxtarenal abdominal aortic aneurysm. *B,* Lateral aortogram documenting a disease-free suprarenal aorta and adequate segment of aorta between renal artery and superior mesenteric artery (SMA) for suprarenal clamping without encroachment of clamp on SMA osteum.

has recently been documented.[8] However, before widespread adoption is appropriate, such innovative techniques must await adequate clinical trials and proof of both short-term and long-term success.

Monitoring and Anesthetic Support

Modern anesthetic and surgical techniques have enhanced safety and success of aortic reconstruction for infrarenal as well as juxtarenal aneurysms. A radial artery cannula simplifies continuous recording of blood pressure and arterial blood sampling. A flow-directed pulmonary artery balloon-tipped (Swan-Ganz) catheter facilitates optimal blood volume management, determination of cardiac output and left ventricular end-diastolic pressure, and pulmonary artery pressure measurements, particularly during aortic clamping and declamping.

Epidural anesthesia supplemented with general endotracheal anesthesia has been proven beneficial both operatively and postoperatively, particularly in pain management. If, when repairing a juxtarenal aneurysm, supraceliac aortic clamping more than 30 to 45 minutes is anticipated, cerebrospinal fluid drainage is performed prior to aortic clamping. However, it is unusual that aortic occlusion times exceed 30 to 45 minutes during repair of a juxtarenal aneurysm. Cerebrospinal fluid drainage is not performed when suprarenal clamping is required.

Vasodilating agents, primarily nitroglycerin and nitroprusside, are used both as coronary artery vasodilators and to decrease left ventricular work. Modulation of left ventricular preload and afterload is important during aortic clamping and declamping. Nitroglycerin lessens both preload and afterload, and nitroprusside is more effective for afterload reduction. The decrease in preload after declamping is managed by infusion of crystalloid and colloid solutions.

Operative Technical Considerations

The various operative approaches, methods of aortic exposure, and sites of proximal aortic clamping are based on extent of aneurysmal disease and presence of associated aortic and/or renal disease. For uncomplicated infrarenal aneurysm repairs, unless there are mitigating circumstances such as a hostile abdomen, extreme obesity, a horseshoe kidney, or abdominal stomata, the transperitoneal approach is preferred with the patient supine. In some patients left flank retroperitoneal exposure is superior to transperitoneal exposure. The retroperitoneal approach has been used in approximately 25% of infrarenal aneurysm repairs and in about two-thirds of patients with pararenal aneurysms.[9,10] Although the transperitoneal approach may provide adequate exposure for some juxtarenal aneurysms, and although suprarenal or supraceliac aortic clamping can be obtained, it may prove difficult. Consequently, a left flank retroperitoneal approach is preferred for juxtarenal aneurysms despite its limitations. Access to the right renal artery beyond its origin is limited, and exposure of the distal right iliac vessels may be compromised. The left retroperitoneal approach does allow easy exposure of the right distal iliac artery through a short right lower quadrant extraperitoneal incision.

For management of juxtarenal aneurysms, the patient is placed in about a 60° right lateral decubitus position and the operating table is flexed. An oblique flank incision beginning at the lateral border of the rectus muscle is extended into the tenth intercostal space with radial division of about 10 to 12 cm of the diaphragm. The diaphragmatic incision is not usually extended to the aortic hiatus, but such a short diaphragmatic incision prevents tearing of the costal attachment of the diaphragm during opening of the rib spreader. After ligation and division of the lumbar branch of the left renal vein, a dissection plane behind the left kidney is developed to reflect the kidney, left renal vein, and ureter anteromedially. After ligation and division of the lymphoareolar tissue over the aorta and partial division of the left crus of the diaphragm, the aorta is exposed from the celiac level to the aortic bifurcation. This occasionally requires reflection of the spleen and tail of the pancreas medially. If the distance between the superior mesenteric artery and renal arteries is at least 2 cm and this segment of aorta is free of extensive atherosclerosis as documented by preoperative biplane aortography, the suprarenal aorta is dissected for clamp application. If the suprarenal aorta is not suitable for clamping, the supraceliac segment is selected (Fig. 3). Circumferential aortic dissection at the proximal clamp site is limited. Only enough aorta is dissected to admit the blades of the aortic clamp. About 15 minutes prior to proximal clamp application, 12.5 to 25 g of mannitol is given intravenously to ensure a brisk diuresis. Immediately before aortic clamping, heparin sodium is judi-

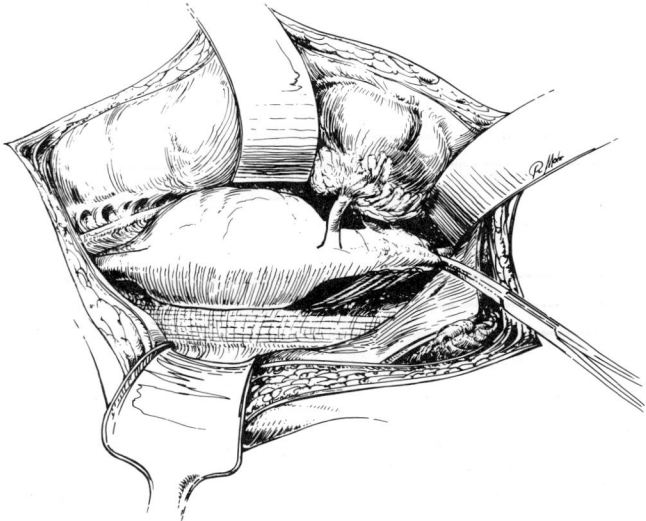

Figure 3 Exposure of the suprarenal and supraceliac aorta provided by the left flank retroperitoneal approach. The vascular clamp is illustrated across supraceliac aorta.

Table 1 Results of Operation for Nonruptured Infrarenal Abdominal Aortic Aneurysm

Author	Year	Source	Study Interval	N	Deaths	% Mortality
Crawford	1981	Baylor University	1955–1980	860	41	4.8
McCabe	1981	Massachusetts General Hospital	1972–1977	364	9	2.5
Diehl	1983	Cleveland Clinic	1974–1978	350	18	5.1
Hertzer	1984	Cleveland Vascular	1978–1981	840	55	6.5
Donaldson	1985	Hartford Hospital	1972–1983	476	24	5.0
Reigel	1987	Mayo Clinic	1980–1985	499	14	2.8
Green	1989	University Rochester	1983–1987	379	8	2.1
Johnston	1989	Canadian Vascular	1986	666	32	4.8
Leather	1989	Albany Medical College	NS	299	11	3.7
Sicard	1989	Washington University	1983–1988	213	3	1.4
Golden	1990	Brigham and Women's	1973–1989	500	8	1.6
Abu Rahma	1991	Charleston, West Virginia	1983–1987	332	12	3.6
Ernst	1993	Henry Ford Hospital	1980–1989	710	25	3.5
TOTAL				6488	260	4.0

NS = Not stated.
From Ernst CB. Abdominal aortic aneurysm. N Engl J Med 1993; 328:1167–1173; with permission.

ciously given and monitored by activated clotting times. However, no more than 50 units/kg is recommended because of the coagulopathy that may be associated with visceral ischemia. For this reason, heparin sodium is not given when supraceliac clamping is required but only when suprarenal or infrarenal clamping is used.

After the aneurysm is incised and the mural thrombus is evacuated, the orifice of the inferior mesenteric artery is identified. If vigorously backbleeding, it is oversewn from within the aneurysm sac. Bleeding lumbar arteries are similarly managed. The proximal anastomosis is fashioned with the inclusion technique for both juxtarenal and infrarenal aneurysms. For juxtarenal aneurysms the proximal anastomosis is constructed immediately infrarenal, adjacent to and frequently involving the inferior margins of the renal artery ostea. When the aorta is clamped above the renal arteries, backbleeding is usually minimal, and what there is can be suctioned with the autotransfusor, providing a clear operative field. More troublesome backbleeding can be controlled by threading a 30 cc Foley balloon catheter through one of the limbs of the graft into the proximal aorta and temporarily inflating it. After the aortic anastomosis is complete, the obturator catheter is removed (if one was required). When the aorta has been flushed to remove any accumulated clot or debris, the graft is clamped below the anastomosis and the suprarenal clamp is removed.

Isolated aortic aneurysms are repaired by tube grafting with either knitted Dacron or expanded polytetrafluoroethylene (ePTFE) prosthesis. PTFE suture is preferred when using an ePTFE graft to minimize graft suture hole bleeding. Small common iliac aneurysms 2 to 3 cm in diameter in high-risk patients in whom limited pelvic dissection is desired do not require repair. Aortic aneurysms with large common iliac components require aortoiliac grafting, usually end to end, to the distal common iliac vessels. If disease extends into the common iliac bifurcation, the distal anastomoses are made to the external iliac arteries after the iliac bifurcations are stapled, preserving retrograde hypogastric perfusion. Occasionally, distal anastomoses must be to the common femoral vessels.

After the anastomoses are secure and hemostasis is complete, the aneurysm sac is debrided and sutured around the prosthesis separating it from the bowel. Although the retroperitoneal approach precludes most of the bowel from coming into contact with the graft, the graft must be enveloped with debrided aneurysm wall to isolate the fourth portion of the duodenum from the graft. The heparin sodium effect is usually not reversed unless troublesome oozing persists. If the left chest has been entered, the diaphragm and chest are closed over a 20 Fr catheter in the left pleural space. After the lung is inflated and the residual pleural space air is evacuated, the catheter is removed and the remainder of the wound is closed in layers.

POSTOPERATIVE CARE

Postoperative care for juxtarenal aneurysm repair is similar to that for uncomplicated infrarenal repair except that the more extensive dissection and potential for greater blood loss accompanying juxtarenal repair complicates fluid management within the first 24 to 48 hours. After juxtarenal repair the patient is maintained on a ventilator overnight and extubated the following morning. Following transperitoneal infrarenal aneurysm repair, patients are occasionally extubated the day of operation but frequently not until the following morning. Epidural catheter analgesic injection facilitates pain management and ease of postoperative recovery.

Table 2 Results of Pararenal Abdominal Aortic Aneurysm Repairs

Author/Year	Number of Patients	Aneurysm Type	Morbidity (%)	Mortality (%)	Postoperative Renal Insufficiency (%)	Dialysis (%)
Crawford (1985)	101	JR	NS	8 (7.9)	16 (16)	8 (7.9)
Qvarfordt (1985)	77	JR/SR	22 (28)	1 (1.2)	18 (23)	2 (2.5)
Poulias (1992)	38	JR	11 (29)	2 (5.3)	9 (24)	4 (10.5)
Allen (1993)	65	JR/SR 19 TA	23 (35)	1 (1.5)	8 (12)	2 (3.1)
Nypaver (1993)	53	JR/SR	19 (36)	2 (3.8)	12 (23)	3 (5.6)
Total	334	—	75 (32)	14 (4.2)	62 (19)	19 (5.7)

JR = juxtarenal, SR = suprarenal, TA = total abdominal (Crawford type IV thoracoabdominal)
Not stated
From Shepard AD, Nypaver TJ, Ernst CB. Pararenal abdominal aortic aneurysm repair. In: Yoo JST, Pearce WH, eds. Aneurysms: New findings and treatments. Norwalk, Conn: Appleton & Lange, 1994; with permission.

Renal dysfunction is distinctly uncommon following juxtarenal aneurysm repair, particularly when aortic occlusion time is under 30 to 40 minutes. Nonetheless, adequate hydration must be maintained to ensure a brisk postoperative diuresis.

Prophylactic antibiotics are continued for 24 to 48 hours postoperatively.

RESULTS

Over the past 4 decades elective infrarenal aortic reconstruction has become a very safe operation. Improved preoperative preparation and postoperative care and improvements in surgical and anesthetic techniques have reduced operative mortality for elective aneurysm repair from approximately 20% to 4%.[1] Review of contemporary results from representative North American reports dating from 1980 reveals excellent results (Table 1). Perioperative mortality for 6,488 nonruptured aneurysm repairs ranged from 1.4% to 6.5% and averaged 4% (median 3.6%).

Perioperative mortality and morbidity for pararenal aneurysm repairs, which include juxtarenal aneurysms, tend to be slightly higher than for infrarenal aneurysm repairs (Table 2). In our experience among 53 patients with pararenal aneurysms, 42 of which were juxtarenal, mortality and morbidity rates were 3.8% and 36%, respectively. Perioperative mortality and morbidity rates for 65 randomly selected patients undergoing elective infrarenal aneurysm repairs during the same time period were 1.5% and 25%, respectively.[10]

Although contemporary indications and results for aneurysm repair help define who should undergo operation, it is important to consider each patient individually because some patients with aneurysms less than 5 cm in diameter will merit operation and others with aneurysms greater than 5 cm may not.

REFERENCES

1. Ernst CB. Abdominal aortic aneurysm. N Engl J Med 1993; 328:1167–1173.
2. Johnston KW, Rutherford RB, Tilson MD, et al. Suggested standards for reporting on arterial aneurysms. J Vasc Surg 1991; 13:452–458.
3. Brown PM, Pattenden R, Gutelius JR. The selective management of small abdominal aortic aneurysms: The Kingston study. J Vasc Surg 1992; 15:21–27.
4. Crawford ES, Saleh SA, Babb JW III, et al. Infrarenal abdominal aneurysm: Factors influencing survival after operation performed over a 25-year period. Ann Surg 1981; 193:699–709.
5. Katz DA, Littenberg B, Cronenwett JL. Management of small abdominal aortic aneurysms. Early surgery versus watchful waiting. JAMA 1992; 268:2678–2686.
6. Hollier LH, Taylor LM, Ochsner J. Recommended indications for operative treatment of abdominal aortic aneurysms. J Vasc Surg 1992; 15:1046–1056.
7. Hertzer NR: Fatal myocardial infarction following abdominal aortic aneurysm resection: Three hundred forty-three patients followed 6-11 years postoperatively. Ann Surg 1980; 192:667–673.
8. Parodi JC, Palmaz JC, Barone HD. Transfemoral intraluminal graft implantation for abdominal aortic aneurysms. Ann Vasc Surg 1991; 5:491–499.
9. Shepard AD, Tollefson DFJ, Reddy DJ, et al. Left flank retroperitoneal exposure: A technical aid to complex aortic reconstruction. J Vasc Surg 1991; 14:283–291.
10. Nypaver TJ, Shepard AD, Reddy DJ, et al. Repair of pararenal abdominal aortic aneurysms: An analysis of operative management. Arch Surg 1993; 128:803–813.

SURGICAL TREATMENT OF RUPTURED INFRARENAL AORTIC ANEURYSM

MOHAMMED M. MOURSI, M.D.
JAMES C. STANLEY, M.D.

Abdominal aortic aneurysm (AAA) rupture is often a catastrophic and lethal event. It has been among the 15 most frequent causes of death in the United States during the past decade and is likely to become more common in our aging population.[1] Bleeding with rupture usually occurs into the retroperitoneum or the peritoneal cavity proper, with bleeding into the gastrointestinal (GI) tract or inferior vena cava (IVC) being very rare. The only effective means of preventing AAA rupture is elective surgical treatment prior to rupture. Elective aneurysmectomy has been associated with a constant decline in operative mortality to nearly 5% during the past decade.[1-3]

Unfortunately, a similar decline in mortality following emergent aneurysmectomy for AAA rupture has not occurred, with mortality rates persisting in the 50% range.[1-3] This does not reflect the actual overall risk of death from ruptured AAA. In a 10 year study of 260 patients with the diagnosis of ruptured AAA, only 101 reached the hospital alive (38%), and of these only 52 survived, for an overall mortality rate of more than 80%.[4] Even in a community with an exceptional prehospital delivery system and expedient early hospital care (12 minutes from the emergency room to the operating room), the overall mortality for AAA rupture approached 70%.[5] Clearly, the considerable mortality of this disease is appropriately attributed to the prehospital setting.

FACTORS AFFECTING SURVIVAL

Numerous studies have focused on factors affecting surgical survival after AAA rupture. In general terms, normotensive patients with a small, contained periaortic hematoma have an operative mortality of approximately 20%. The mortality is closer to 40% in those presenting with hypotension, who respond well to resuscitation with restoration of blood pressure and normalization of urine output but have a more extensive periaortic hematoma. The mortality is 60% among those with hypotension who respond incompletely to resuscitation or who are unstable during operation. The mortality increases to 80% if urine output ceases during the operation.[6]

Certain factors contributing to operative and overall mortality can be classified as either uncontrollable or controllable variables.[7] The former are patient-related and include age, gender, and medical comorbidities, as well as aneurysm size, location, and rupture site. The latter are physician-related variables that are potentially alterable and include duration and efficacy of prehospital resuscitation and transport, time taken to diagnose AAA rupture, time in transit to the operating room, time in the operating room before control of bleeding, hemodynamic status during the preoperative and postoperative course, technical intraoperative complications, and volume of blood and fluids needed.

Wakefield and his colleagues at the University of Michigan[8] observed seven preoperative factors to be reasonable predictors of ruptured AAA mortality: (1) heart disease, (2) hypertension, (3) flank ecchymosis, (4) pulsatile abdominal mass, (5) preoperative hypotension, (6) renal dysfunction evidenced by a blood urea nitrogen level greater than 30 mg/dl or a serum creatinine level greater than 3 mg/dl, and (7) a hematocrit less than 33%. Seven intraoperative factors were also found to be predictive of mortality: (1) duration of operation greater than 400 minutes, (2) hypotension lasting longer than 110 minutes, (3) estimated blood loss greater than 11,000 ml, (4) blood transfusion in excess of 17 units, (5) fluid administration in excess of 7,000 ml, (6) blood pressure less than 100 mm Hg at the conclusion of the operation, and (7) intraoperative cardiac arrest.

DIAGNOSIS AND PRESENTATION

The triad of a palpable abdominal mass, excruciating, knifelike abdominal pain or back pain, and hypotension is often thought to be pathognomonic of ruptured AAA. Wakefield and colleagues, in a review of 116 patients with ruptured AAA, documented the presence of a palpable pulsatile abdominal mass in 83%, abdominal and back pain in 72%, and hypotension in 45%.[8] Thus, fewer than 50% of patients with AAA rupture present with this complete triad.

Patients presenting with a ruptured AAA are often misdiagnosed, and fewer than half of the patients experiencing rupture have a known, pre-existing, intact AAA. The issue of misdiagnosis is critical. In the Cleveland Vascular Registry experience, the mortality was 35% when the initial diagnosis was correct or suspected, but when the diagnosis was incorrect the mortality rate was 75%.[9]

Nearly 10% of patients with a ruptured AAA present with urologic-like signs and symptoms, including flank pain with radiation to the hip, genitalia, or thigh, similar to ureteral colic. Acute unilateral painful neuropathy involving the femoral and/or obturator nerves secondary to extrinsic compression may also occur. Flank and paraumbilical ecchymoses (Cullen's sign) may be seen in patients having more chronic ruptures. An AAA rarely ruptures into the intestinal tract. When this occurs, it is usually into the duodenum or the colon, resulting in major upper or lower GI bleeding. Rupture into the IVC with development of an aortocaval fistula is manifested by systemic venous overload, congestive heart failure, and lower extremity edema.

Other clinical entities such as a perforated viscus or mesenteric ischemia, as well as other causes of intraabdominal hemorrhage, may present with signs and symptoms highly suggestive of AAA rupture. These patients should undergo emergent operation not only to establish a diagnosis but also as lifesaving treatment. One does not need to encounter a ruptured AAA at every exploration in patients suspected of rupture to justify such an aggressive approach.

A diagnostic dilemma may exist in patients who present with abdominal or back pain without hypotension or a pulsatile abdominal mass and who have a stable hematocrit. This clinical setting affords the clinician a chance to perform well-thought-out and useful diagnostic studies, but it is critical that these patients be followed very closely. Any deterioration in their hemodynamic status requires immediate cessation of diagnostic testing and emergent operative intervention.

Computed tomography (CT) with intravenous contrast medium is an important diagnostic tool for evaluation of suspected AAA rupture in stable patients with equivocal clinical findings.[10] Relevant findings of AAA rupture on CT include unilateral hematomas and mass lesions in the region of the psoas muscle, ventral or ventrolateral displacement of the kidney, abnormal soft tissue collections along the posterior border of the aneurysm, effacement of the normal fat plane between the aneurysm and juxtaposed intestine, indistinct margins of the aortic wall, and presence of retroperitoneal fluid collections with or without extravasation of contrast material. The CT has 70% sensitivity, 100% specificity, and greater than 90% accuracy in establishing a diagnosis of AAA rupture. In the stable patient with suspicion of a ruptured AAA, the initial abdominal CT should be performed with a limited number of cuts to simply identify any obvious evidence of a leaking or ruptured AAA. Once a diagnosis of an AAA rupture is excluded, a more complete study can be undertaken.

Cross-table lateral abdominal roentgenograms are often used to identify the anterior rim of calcification in abdominal aneurysms of asymptomatic patients but are not very useful in evaluating suspected ruptured AAA. Similarly, abdominal ultrasound may be useful in establishing a diagnosis of an AAA but is of marginal value in differentiating a ruptured aneurysm with minimal extravasation of blood from an intact aneurysm. Arteriography has no role in the evaluation of rupture of an AAA.

If an intact AAA exists without objective signs of rupture but the patient's symptoms suggesting expansion persist for 24 hours, operation should be undertaken. A very high incidence of AAA rupture occurs in symptomatic patients, and longer delays in surgical therapy are unjustified.

THERAPY

The critical issue in treating a ruptured AAA is the application of an aortic clamp to control blood loss, followed by graft replacement of the diseased aorta. Just as diagnostic maneuvers should not delay the prompt transfer of the patient to the operating room, no prolonged effort should be made to resuscitate and stabilize a patient with a ruptured AAA in the emergency room. Such efforts are often futile because replacement of blood being lost into the retroperitoneal or peritoneal cavity is frequently not feasible.

Once a diagnosis of AAA rupture is made, standard care for patients in hemorrhagic shock, including placement of large-bore peripheral intravenous lines and judicious crystalloid fluid resuscitation, should be carried out en route to the operating room. Blood for cross-match purposes should be drawn. An electrocardiogram can be obtained in the operating room.

The patient with a presumed AAA rupture should be prepped and draped from the neck to toes while awake prior to anesthetic induction. The surgeon should be prepared to make an incision once anesthesia is induced because of the frequent hypotension associated with anesthetic-induced reductions in vascular tone. A midline incision from xiphoid to pubis is preferred and provides excellent operative exposure. However, if renal artery involvement is suspected, a transverse supraumbilical incision may be more appropriate.

Once blood is available, it should replace crystalloid solutions for resuscitative purposes. The use of an autotransfusion device is advocated and should be available for use upon entering the abdominal cavity. Coagulopathies are a major problem associated with the operative treatment of AAA rupture and must be avoided by careful control of unnecessary blood loss and avoidance of hypothermia. The latter can be accomplished by heating the operating room, placing warming blankets on all exposed body areas, using a heated ventilator circuit, and heating all intravenous fluids. Many patients with a ruptured AAA develop both consumption and dilution coagulopathies during the course of operative therapy. Anticipation of such problems and the early procurement of needed blood products, including fresh frozen plasma and platelets, may be lifesaving.

Cross-clamping or occluding the aorta can be undertaken by several methods. In extreme circumstances, it can be accomplished through a left thoracotomy with clamping of the descending thoracic aorta. This is most successful when undertaken in the operating room such that rapid infrarenal clamping can follow, before irreparable ischemic injury to the liver and kidneys occurs. Remote aortic control can also be gained by using a balloon catheter threaded centrally through a peripheral artery. However, this approach may be unsuccessful and consume precious time in patients who might better be managed operatively. Intraluminal control can also be gained by direct placement of a large aortic balloon catheter or a Foley catheter into the proximal aorta through the aneurysm itself.

Aortic control in the operating room is usually gained at the supraceliac level just beneath the diaphragm, first by a direct compression with the surgeon's fingers and then with either a clamp or a specialized **T** device specifically designed for aortic occlusion. Attention is then directed to the infrarenal neck of the aneurysm, and a second clamp is placed at this lower level to allow removal of the supraceliac clamp or occlusion device. Occasionally, the infrarenal aorta may be clamped initially, thus avoiding occlusion of the aorta above the renal arteries. Care must be taken during aortic dissection to avoid potential injury to small arterial branches, as well as the IVC or left renal vein. These vessels are particularly subject to injury when they are obscured by periaortic hematoma. The left renal vein can be ligated near the IVC and transected, if need be, for added exposure without major additional morbidity. Distal control of the iliac arteries can be obtained by using conventional vascular clamps or with intraluminal balloons if it appears that potentially hazardous dissections are otherwise required.

Intravenous heparin sodium should be administered prior to aortic clamping, if possible, or soon thereafter. Antibiotics should be given early and, if there is a large amount of ongoing blood loss, repeatedly. A first-generation cephalosporin is preferred by the authors.

A ruptured suprarenal AAA poses a more serious problem. Management must be individualized and an operative decision made regarding the suprarenal component. If these aneurysms are in fact juxtarenal or pararenal, proximal aortic control may be obtained at the supraceliac level and the graft placed in a conventional manner, incorporating the renal ostia in the suture line or using an inclusion patch for reimplantation of these vessels, if needed. In certain instances, if the infrarenal neck is not larger than 4 cm in diameter, a large-diameter graft can be placed at this level. Although this might represent a compromise in standard technique, it may represent the only reasonable therapeutic option in an otherwise unstable patient who would not tolerate an extensive proximal aortic reconstruction. The alternative, when faced with a suprarenal aneurysm extending above the diaphragm, is to expose the proximal aorta through an extension of the incision into the thorax, with subsequent medial visceral rotation and conventional placement of an interposition aortic graft with patch inclusion of the intestinal and renal arteries.

In the rare case of an aortoduodenal fistula due to AAA rupture, the duodenal fistula should be taken down, the intestinal wall repaired in two layers, and, after copious irrigation of the operative area, the aortic reconstruction should take place in a standard manner. The interposition of healthy tissue between the graft and duodenal repair should minimize the incidence of postoperative graft infection. In cases of extensive retroperitoneal infection, aneurysmectomy with oversewing of the infrarenal aorta would be more appropriate, followed by performance of a nonanatomic bypass, such as an axillofemoral reconstruction.

Woven Dacron grafts, collagen- or albumen-impregnated knitted Dacron grafts, or expanded polytetrafluoroethylene grafts may be used for these reconstructions. Porous knitted grafts require preclotting, a time-consuming step. A straight tube aortoarotic graft is sufficient for repair of most ruptured aneurysms. However, it is necessary to place a bifurcated aortoiliac or aortofemoral graft in 10% to 15% of patients with AAA rupture. Small to moderate iliac aneurysms are usually not treated in the setting of a ruptured AAA.

The postoperative complications attending operation for a ruptured AAA are the same as for elective AAA repair and are directly related to the same factors that contribute to overall mortality. Complications following operation for AAA rupture, when compared to those attending elective aneurysm repair, occur more frequently and are usually more severe. The three most common organ systems involved are the heart, kidneys, and lungs. Myocardial infarction and acute renal failure account for most early deaths following operation for AAA rupture. Nevertheless, timely and carefully executed operative therapy has proven successful in the treatment of ruptured infrarenal aortic aneurysms and represents one of the more important lifesaving efforts undertaken by vascular surgeons.

REFERENCES

1. Ernst CB. Abdominal aortic aneurysm. N Engl J Med 1993; 328:1167–1172.
2. Katz DJ, Stanley JC, Zelenock GB. Operative mortality rates for intact and ruptured abdominal aortic aneurysms in Michigan: An eleven-year statewide experience. J Vasc Surg 1994; 19:804–817.
3. Mannick JA, Whittemore AD. Management of ruptured or symptomatic abdominal aortic aneurysms. Surg Clin North Am 1988; 68:377–384.
4. Ingoldby CJH, Wujanto R, Mitchell JE. Impact of vascular surgery on community mortality from ruptured aortic aneurysms. Br J Surg 1986; 73:551–553.
5. Johansen K, Kohler TR, Nicholls SC, et al. Ruptured abdominal aortic aneurysm: The Harborview experience. J Vasc Surg 1991; 13:240–247.
6. Rutherford RB, McCroskey BL. Ruptured abdominal aortic aneurysms. Surg Clin North Am 1989; 69:859–868.
7. Donaldson MC, Rosenberg JM, Bucknam CA. Factors affecting survival after ruptured abdominal aortic aneurysm. J Vasc Surg 1985; 2:564–570.
8. Wakefield, TW, Whitehouse WM, Wu S, et al. Abdominal aortic aneurysm rupture: Statistical analysis of factors affecting outcome of surgical treatment. Surgery 1982; 91:586–596.
9. Hoffman M, Avellone JC, Plecha FR, et al. Operation for ruptured abdominal aortic aneurysms: A community-wide experience. Surgery 1982; 91:597–602.
10. Weinbaum FI, Dubner S, Turner JW, et al. The accuracy of computed tomography in the diagnosis of retroperitoneal blood in the presence of abdominal aortic aneurysm. J Vasc Surg 1987; 6:11–16.

MANAGEMENT OF SMALL ABDOMINAL AORTIC ANEURYSMS

JOHN W. HALLETT Jr, M.D.

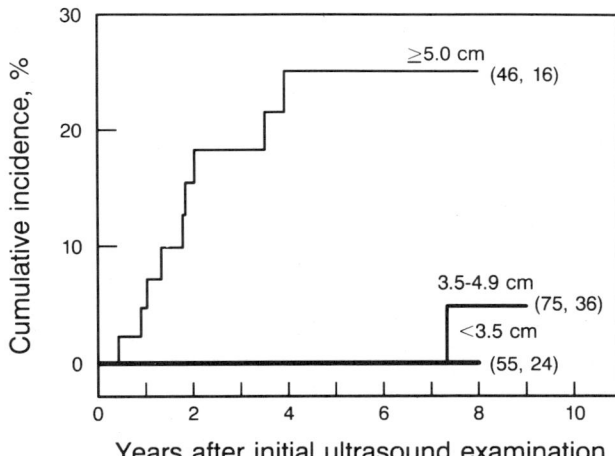

Figure 1 Cumulative incidence of rupture of abdominal aortic aneurysm according to aneurysm diameter at initial ultrasound. (From Nevitt MP, Ballard DJ, Hallett JW Jr. Prognosis of abdominal aortic aneurysms: A population-based study. N Engl J Med 1989; 321:1011; with permission.)

Management of small (less than 5 cm in diameter) abdominal aortic aneurysms (AAAs) has become more problematic in recent years. Aneurysms of all sizes are being recognized incidentally by ultrasound and computed tomography used to evaluate other abdominal complaints. Reports of safer surgical therapy have also influenced the propensity to repair more aneurysms, especially smaller ones. However, escalating health care costs in the elderly may eventually force a more selective approach to all types of cardiovascular and interventional therapy. Small aneurysms are likely to remain in the midst of these controversies.

BACKGROUND OF CURRENT CONTROVERSY

What is a small AAA? The definition has shifted slightly over time. Studies between 1960 and the late 1970s referred to small aneurysms as those with a diameter less than 6 cm. This number was based on the perception that aneurysms less than 6 cm seldom rupture. This perception remains reasonable, but the current definition centers around 5 cm. This threshold is based on several modern autopsy and population-based studies.

The interest in small AAAs intensified with Darling and colleagues' provocative autopsy study from the Massachusetts General Hospital in 1977.[1] They reported that 34 of 265 (12.8%) nonresected AAAs less than 5 cm at autopsy had ruptured. This rupture rate increased to 23% for AAAs of 4 to 5 cm. The limitations of autopsy studies, however, prevent direct application to clinical practice.[2] These limitations include measurement of aneurysm size in a nonpressurized and deformed state after rupture. Autopsy studies are also limited by the bias of examining only patients who died and had an autopsy, an increasingly rare clinicopathologic practice in American hospitals today. Consequently, autopsy studies have given way to population-based studies in living patients followed in clinical practice.

Studies based on serial ultrasound have repeatedly confirmed that rupture risk begins to accelerate above 5 cm in diameter and exceeds a truly dangerous threshold at 7 cm.[3,4] Although a smaller AAA may occasionally rupture, this is an unusual clinical event (Fig. 1). In an attempt to predict which small AAAs may acutely expand or rupture, Cronenwett and colleagues have analyzed numerous clinical and aneurysm characteristics and emphasized that the eventual need for operation is increased for patients with three predominant features: larger initial size, longer follow-up, and widened pulse pressure.[3] Patients with chronic lung disease and alpha-1-antitrypsin (antiprotease activity to balance destructive elastases) deficiency may also be more likely to experience aneurysm expansion.

In addition, six recent population-based analyses confirm that AAA rupture is higher for those aneurysms greater than 5 cm in diameter.[4] Reliable numbers for clinical management include rupture risks at 5 years of 5% for less than 5 cm, 25% for 5 to 7 cm, and at least 50% for greater than 7 cm. It must be emphasized that nearly all small AAAs that eventually rupture have expanded to over 5 cm. All of these studies have found that slightly over one-third of patients being followed with small AAAs come to elective repair by 5 years. Another one-third die of other causes, and the remaining one-third remain relatively stable.

THE EPIDEMIOLOGIC DILEMMA

During the past three decades, the age- and sex-adjusted incidence of AAAs has tripled.[4] Incidence changes have varied considerably for different sizes of AAAs. For example, the incidence of small aneurysms (5 cm) has increased ten fold. In contrast, the incidence of medium-sized (5 to 7 cm) and large (greater than 7 cm) has risen only by a factor of two to three. Small AAAs now account for about 50% of all clinically recognized aneurysms. This is an important epidemiologic finding because many physicians are uncertain about the appropriate management of a newly discovered small aneurysm.

Several other demographic facts must also be considered in developing strategies for small AAAs.[4] First, approximately 3% to 5% of those over 65 years of age harbor an AAA. This calculates to at least a million AAAs in the United States. Second, currently, less than 100,000 aneurysm repairs per year are being performed in this age group. To add the remaining 400,000 to 500,000 small AAAs to the future operative agenda may not be a fiscally acceptable strategy.

Population-based data on statewide operative mortality for AAAs also document higher elective mortalities than the results of referral centers.[5,6] Most AAAs are still being repaired in community hospitals by surgeons doing fewer than 25 AAA repairs per year with an elective mortality of 5% to 10%, not the lower rates of 2% to 3% in selected referral centers.[5]

MANAGEMENT OPTIONS

Essentially two choices exist: (1) early operation when a small AAA is found[6,7] or (2) close observation and repair for expansion, symptoms, or associated aortic occlusive disease.[2,8,9] Although inability to return for follow-up and patient anxiety about the aneurysm are mentioned as other surgical indications, our recent community analysis found these latter factors in fewer than 10% of patients with small AAAs.[9]

The immediate operation approach is based on three primary assumptions: (1) inevitable AAA expansion and worsening operative risk with age, (2) improved late survival if the repair is performed earlier in life, and (3) a low operative mortality in experienced surgical hands.[10] Although all aneurysms tend to expand with time, the rate does not fit a biologically normal distribution.[2] In fact, about 80% of AAAs enlarge at a relatively slow median rate of 2 to 3 mm yearly, sometimes remaining stable for several years.[2] The remainder enlarge faster, at a rate of 4 mm or more yearly. It is rare for an aneurysm to enlarge more than 10 mm in 1 year. About one-third of small AAAs expand to greater than 5 cm over 5 years' follow-up.[3,8-10]

Worsening of health with time makes common sense, but we currently have very little longitudinal health data for patients with small AAAs. About one-third die of other cardiovascular events in 5 years.[3,8] Our population-based data suggest that patients undergoing repair of small AAAs are younger than patients with large AAAs and have less clinically evident coronary heart disease (small versus large, 28% versus 48%).[9] The assumption, however, that late survival of patients undergoing repair of small AAAs is equal to or better than the general age-matched population or patients having large AAA repairs has not been proved. In fact, late survival of both small and large AAA repair patients remains significantly worse than the age-matched general population without aneurysms (5-year survival: general population, 83%; large AAA repairs, 60%; small AAA repairs, 62%).[9]

The influence of elective operative mortality is emphasized by a recent Markov decision tree analysis of early operation versus watchful waiting.[7] This analysis concludes that the key determinants of the decision to perform early operation are (1) risk of rupture (low, 0.4%/year; higher, 3.3%/year), (2) elective operative mortality (4% to 5% at 30 days), (3) age at presentation (younger than 70 years is better), and (4) size threshold for repair. This analysis favors early operation if the rupture risk is moderately high (3.3%/year) in younger (less than 70 years) patients in low-risk surgical hands (less than 5% mortality) for a threshold size of 4.7 cm. Few surgeons would argue with this recommendation in the idealized setting. But, if the annual rupture risk is lower (0.5% per year) as several studies suggest, early operation will provide benefit (more quality-adjusted life years, QALYs) only when operative mortality is less than 1%, an unrealistic expectation in most community and tertiary hospitals.

The second option, which is the one most commonly followed by most physicians is close observation and selective operation of small aneurysms.[3,4] This approach is especially appropriate for elderly patients (greater than 70 years) with other serious medical comorbidity. Anticipating that about one-third of small AAAs will eventually reach 5 to 6 cm in 5 years, primary care physicians should focus their efforts on measuring the severity of the medical comorbidity and improving the functional status of the patient. For example, patients with progressive or unstable angina pectoris should be considered for cardiac evaluation and coronary revascularization before elective AAA repair. Likewise, steps to reduce smoking and alcohol use should be undertaken. Simply starting sedentary, deconditioned patients on a regular exercise program (e.g., walking 30 minutes, 3 to 5 days weekly) can also improve operative outcome.

If the observational approach is selected for patients with small AAAs, good-risk patients should be encouraged to undergo elective repair when their AAA approaches or enters the 5 to 6 cm range. High-risk patients should generally undergo elective AAA repair only when the AAA reaches the more dangerous size of 6 to 7 cm or becomes symptomatic. Bernstein and Chan documented that such a selective strategy in high-risk patients with small (less than 6 cm) AAAs resulted in a very low rupture risk (1%/year) and reassuring elective mortality of 4.9%.[10] In this series 40% eventually underwent elective repair. This selective approach resulted in only four deaths (4%), two from rupture and two from elective operation in 99 patients.

QUALITY OF LIFE ISSUES

Despite the controversy of small AAA management, no randomized clinical trials have been completed. Consequently, reliable quality of life data are essentially nonexistent. A recent analysis suggested that QALYs may be improved, but only moderately (+0.63 QALYs), when operative risks are low (less than 5%) and when risk of rupture or acute expansion is moderately high (3.3%/year).[8] For higher operative mortality (10%) and lower rupture risk (0.5%/year), early operation may actually be a loser (−0.3 QALYs).

CLINICAL TRIALS

The small AAA controversy has attracted enough recent international attention to generate three clinical trials that randomize small (4 to 5.5 cm) AAAs to immediate operation or serial observation with selective repair.[4] These trials (Canadian, British, and American Veterans Administration) are underway but will not yield definitive results and recommendations for several more years. Until randomized clinical trials on the management of small abdominal aortic aneurysms are completed, most small AAAs should be monitored for expansion and operated electively when they approach or enter the range of 5 to 6 cm in good-risk patients.

REFERENCES

1. Darling RC, Messina CR, Brewster DC, Ottinger LW. Autopsy study of unoperated abdominal aortic aneurysms. The case for early resection. Circulation 1977; 56:161–164.
2. Nevitt MP, Ballard DJ, Hallett JW Jr. Prognosis of abdominal aortic aneurysm: A population-based study. N Engl J Med 1989; 321:1009–1014.
3. Cronenwett JL, Sargent SK, Wall MH, et al. Variables that affect the expansion rate and outcome of small abdominal aortic aneurysms. J Vasc Surg 1990; 11:260–269.
4. Hallett JW Jr. Abdominal aortic aneurysm: Natural history and treatment. Heart Disease Stroke 1992; 1:303–308.
5. Katz DJ, Stanley JC, Zelenock GB. Operative mortality for intact and ruptured abdominal aortic aneurysms in Michigan: An 11-year statewide experience. J Vasc Surg 1994; 19:804–817.
6. Hollier LH, Taylor LM, Ochsner J. Recommended indications for operative treatment of abdominal aortic aneurysms. Report of a subcommittee of the Joint Council of the Society for Vascular Surgery and the North American Chapter of the International Society for Cardiovascular Surgery. J Vasc Surg 1992; 15:1046–1056.
7. Katz DA, Littenberg B, Cronenwett JL. Management of small abdominal aortic aneurysms. Early surgery vs watchful waiting. JAMA 1992; 268:2678–2686.
8. Brown, PM, Pattenden R, Gutelius JR. The selective management of small abdominal aortic aneurysms: The Kingston study. J Vasc Surg 1992; 15:21–27.
9. Hallett, JW, Naessens JM, Ballard DJ. Early and late outcome of surgical repair for small abdominal aortic aneurysms: A population-based analysis. J Vasc Surg 1993; 18:684–691.
10. Bernstein EF, Chan EL. Abdominal aortic aneurysm in high-risk patients. Outcome of selective management based on size and expansion rate. Ann Surg 1984; 200:255–263.

SURGICAL TREATMENT OF INFLAMMATORY ABDOMINAL AORTIC ANEURYSMS

SAMUEL R. MONEY, M.D.
LARRY H. HOLLIER, M.D., F.A.C.S., F.A.C.C.

In 1935, James described a patient who was dying of uremia secondary to bilateral ureteral obstruction due to an inflammatory reaction that centered around an abdominal aortic aneurysm.[1] This is apparently the first case report of an inflammatory aortic aneurysm. Initially, surgical treatment was directed toward relief of the ureteral obstruction. The aneurysm was not replaced, but nephrostomy tubes were placed bilaterally and ureterolysis performed. In 1955, Shumacker and Garrett reported successful treatment of a patient by ureterolysis and graft replacement of the abdominal aortic aneurysm.[2] This patient initially had presented with pulmonary edema secondary to uremia. In addition, he also had a 10 cm abdominal aortic aneurysm. It is described that large amounts of bowel were found adherent to the dense perianeurysmal inflammatory mass. The operation performed involved replacing the aneurysm with a bifurcated graft in that not only was the aorta involved but, in addition, the common iliac arteries were involved. The patient did well postoperatively.

The term inflammatory aneurysm was coined in 1972 by Walker and colleagues, who described 19 patients with such aneurysms, which represented 10% of their patients with abdominal aortic aneurysms.[3] In Pennell and co-workers' review of 2,816 consecutive abdominal aortic aneurysms, 127 (4.5%) were inflammatory aneurysms.[4] The incidence of inflammatory aneurysms has been reported from 2% to 20% of infrarenal aortic aneurysms; however, it is generally thought to be approximately 5% of abdominal aortic aneurysms.[4-7] In an effort to stress the gross pathologic description, inflammatory aneurysms also have been called porcelain aneurysms because of the white, glistening appearance of the anterior aortic wall. The hallmark of this condition is the significant amount of inflammation surrounding the aortic aneurysm.

CLINICAL PRESENTATION

Patients with inflammatory abdominal aortic aneurysms differ from patients with routine abdominal aortic aneurysms in several ways. There is a significant male predominance in inflammatory aneurysms. Females generally account for less than 5% of patients with inflammatory aneurysms, whereas they ordinarily account for approximately one-third of patients with routine abdominal aneurysms.[4] Most patients with inflammatory aneurysms present with symptoms of either back or flank pain. Inflammatory aneurysms tend to be more easily palpable at the time of diagnosis because of their large size. In addition, many of these patients have tenderness on palpation of the aneurysm. Sterpetti and co-workers found a significant difference in age between patients with inflammatory and those with noninflammatory aortic abdominal aneurysms.[8] Patients with inflammatory aneurysms tend to be younger (mean age 62.2 years), whereas those with noninflammatory aneurysms are older (68.2 years). Erythrocyte sedimentation rates (ESR) are elevated in approximately 75% of patients with inflammatory aneurysms. If one could define the classic patient with an inflammatory abdominal aortic aneurysm, the patient would be male, in his early 60s, with a large abdominal aneurysm, pain on palpation, weight loss, and an elevated ESR. Aside from the elevated ESR, this presentation can mimic an acute rupture of an abdominal aortic aneurysm, or even an acute dissection.

DIAGNOSIS

Ultrasound can be used preoperatively to diagnose an inflammatory aneurysm.[9] The ultrasound documents an echogenic and thickened wall with a hypoechoic anterior and anterolateral rim around the aorta. Ordinarily, however, the diagnosis of inflammatory aortic aneurysms is made preoperatively by computed tomography (CT). The CT scan documents thickening and contrast enhancement of the aorta in the periadventitial region[10] (Fig. 1). Frequently, calcifications are present in the media, and they are easily discernible from the adventitial inflammatory response. The adventitial thickening lies outside of the calcific rim of the media. The periaortic inflammatory reaction can extend up to 5 cm in thickness and frequently shows a uniform enhancement. The reaction is ordinarily absent in the posterior portion of the aorta. To inexperienced observers, it may be difficult to differentiate an inflammatory aneurysm from aneurysm rupture. However, it must be kept in mind that the attenuation value of retroperitoneal blood on CT imaging is higher than that of the inflammatory rim of the aneurysm. Frequently, hydronephrosis is also noted on the CT scan. The ureters may be displaced medially due to the inflammatory aneurysm. This is in sharp contrast to the typical lateral deviation of the ureters due to large aneurysm. Aortograms or plain abdominal flat plate x-rays offer little information about the extent of the inflammatory reaction or the true size of the aneurysm.

Corticosteroids may help reduce the reaction in patients with inflammatory aneurysms. Some authors have recommended steroid treatment prior to or in lieu of operation.[11] Certain patients with inflammatory aneurysms present with excessive risks for surgical replacement of the aneurysm. Corticosteroids may abolish the abdominal pain caused by the inflammatory reaction and may even reduce some of the inflammatory reaction in the retroperitoneum, thereby relieving some of the ureteral obstruction. The one major limitation of corticosteroid treatment is that it does not treat the

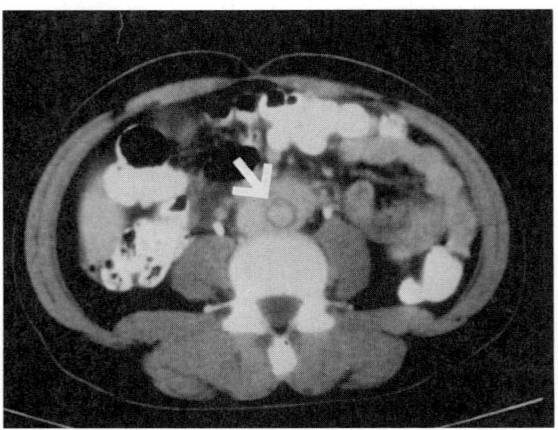

Figure 1 Computed tomography scan of a patient with an inflammatory aortic aneurysm. Note the large, contrast-enhanced inflammatory mass (*arrow*) around the aortic lumen.

diseased aneurysmal aorta. Unfortunately, patients are committed to chronic corticosteroid dependence with an aortic aneurysm in place. Discontinuation of corticosteroid therapy usually leads to recurrence of symptoms. It may be preferable to place only selected, very high-risk patients on corticosteroid treatment rather than operate. Consensus today is that replacement of the aneurysm with a synthetic graft is the treatment of choice; it not only reduces the retroperitoneal fibrosis but also treats the dilated diseased aortic segment.

OPERATIVE MANAGEMENT

The most striking feature of inflammatory aneurysms is the focus of the inflammatory process. The anterior and lateral borders of the abdominal aneurysm may be covered by a dull pink or glistening white connective tissue. The duodenum is almost always adherent to the aneurysm wall. In addition, the colon, the mesentery of the small bowel, and the jejunum are frequently adherent and involved in this large inflammatory process. Despite patients in whom the inflammatory process extends cephalad and may involve the suprarenal aorta, most of the time the inflammatory process is confined to the infrarenal aorta.[7] Most of the inflammatory process involves the anterior and/or lateral walls of the aorta. The posterior wall is frequently spared. Therefore, rupture of this aneurysm can occur, and if it occurs, it generally ruptures posterolaterally into either the flank or along the area around the vertebral column. Surgical treatment for inflammatory aneurysms consists of a graft insertion performed from within the aneurysm sac. This is done to simplify the operative dissection and to avoid injury to the structures that are involved in the inflammatory process. The periaortic inflammatory reaction is highly vascular, and multiple vessels transverse it. The tenacity with which the organs and loops of bowel are fixed to the aneurysmal mass makes mobilization of these structures quite difficult and dangerous. Therefore, mobilization of these structures should not be attempted because it will cause significant bleeding and may cause injury and denudation to the bowel wall.

Many authors suggest the use of the extraperitoneal approach to facilitate aneurysm repair. Surgeons should use the method with which they are most familiar. If a surgeon uses the extraperitoneal approach only for inflammatory aneurysms, we feel that the anterior midline approach may be more successful.

Proximal control of the aorta usually can be obtained below the level of the renal arteries. If it cannot be obtained there, then supraceliac control may be required. Another alternative for proximal control of the aorta is the use of an intra-aortic occlusion balloon. Distal control of the aneurysm can usually be obtained in the common iliac arteries. If the common iliac arteries are involved in the inflammatory process and obtaining control is difficult, then the external iliac arteries are usually uninvolved. Hypogastric control can be obtained with balloon catheters after the aneurysm sac is opened. Once proximal and distal control are obtained, the patient is fully anticoagulated and the aneurysm is opened in an area that does not risk injury to the adherent structures. Care is taken not to open the aneurysm close to the adherent duodenum or small bowel. Because of the vascularity of the inflammatory mass surrounding the aneurysm, we use electrocautery to open the aneurysm. Once the aneurysm is opened, the mural thrombus is removed and the lumbar arteries are ligated from within. An appropriate-sized graft is then sutured in place to an uninvolved proximal segment of aorta with standard continuous monofilament suture. We frequently use a larger-than-standard needle for this repair. Frequently, to support the posterior wall of the repair, we use felt pledgets. After the proximal anastomosis is complete and checked, the proximal clamp can be removed and placed on the graft distal to this anastomosis. If a suprarenal or supraceliac aortic cross-clamp was used, it can be moved down expeditiously following the proximal anastomosis. The distal anastomosis is usually performed in a standard fashion. When the surgeon is confident that hemostasis has been obtained, the native aortic sac is closed over the graft. Frequently this cannot be done because of the thickness and rigidity of the inflammatory mass. We suggest covering the graft with retroperitoneal tissue if possible. If not, the use of a polytetrafluoroethylene (ePTFE) membrane should be considered.

If the preoperative diagnosis of an inflammatory aneurysm has been made, it is prudent to place ureteral stents. They allow identification of the ureters during the operative procedure, and therefore may minimize injury to the ureters. In addition, they might also improve renal function by reducing obstruction of the ureters. Operative treatment of the ureteral obstruction is dependent upon the degree of obstruction and renal function. If the patient has severe hydronephrosis, it may be prudent to place ureteral stents or even percutaneous nephrostomy tubes several days before operation to allow time for renal function to improve prior to operation. For severe obstruction, ureterolysis is recommended. It must be kept in mind, however, that many authors have reported a decrease in the fibrosis involving ureters following replacement of the aortic aneurysm with a graft. Most patients who have minimal compression of their ureters due to fibrosis have resolution of ureteral obstruction following the repair of the aneurysm.

In the original report by Walker and associates, 6 of the 19 patients operated upon with inflammatory aneurysms did not survive the procedure.[3] Now only a 3% to 4% operative mortality is reported.[4,6,7] By avoiding extensive dissection and following the methods described, we believe that acceptably low morbidity and mortality can be achieved.

REFERENCES

1. James TGI. Uremia due to aneurysm of the abdominal aorta. Br J Urol 1935; 7:157.
2. Shumacker HB Jr, Garrett R. Obstructive uropathy from abdominal aortic aneurysm. Surg Gynecol Obstet 1955; 100:758–761.
3. Walker DI, Bloor K, Williams G, et al. Inflammatory aneurysms of the abdominal aorta. B J Surg 1972; 59:609–614.
4. Pennell RC, Hollier LH, Lie JT, et al. Inflammatory abdominal aortic aneurysms: A thirty-year review. J Vasc Surg 1985; 2:859–869.
5. Feiner HD, Raghavendra BN, Phelps R, et al. Inflammatory abdominal aortic aneurysm: Report of six cases. Hum Pathol 1984; 15:454–459.
6. Goldstone J, Malone JM, Moore WS. Inflammatory aneurysms of the abdominal aorta. Surgery 1978; 83:425–430.
7. Crawford JL, Stowe CL, Safi HJ, et al. Inflammatory aneurysms of the aorta. J Vasc Surg 1985; 2:113–124.
8. Sterpetti AV, Hunter WJ, Feldhaus RJ, et al. Inflammatory aneurysms of the abdominal aorta: Incidence, pathologic and etiology considerations. J Vasc Surg 1989; 9:643–650.
9. Cullenward MJ, Scanlan KA, Pozniak MA, et al. Inflammatory aortic aneurysm (periaortic fibrosis): Radiologic imaging. Radiology 1986; 159:75–82.
10. Ramirez AA, Riles TS, Imparato AM, et al. CAT scans of inflammatory aneurysms: A new technique for preoperative diagnosis. Surgery 1982; 91:390–393.
11. Baskerville PA, Browse NL: Peri-aortic fibrosis: Progression and regression. J Cardiovasc Surg (Torino) 1987; 28:30–31.

SURGICAL TREATMENT OF INFECTED ABDOMINAL AORTIC ANEURYSMS

MARTIN I. ELLENBY, M.D.
CALVIN B. ERNST, M.D.

Infected aneurysms, a rare subset of abdominal aortic aneurysms, were present in only 0.65% of the 2,009 abdominal aortic aneurysms operated upon at the Henry Ford Hospital from 1960 through 1989. However, the incidence increased from 0.13% in the first decade to 1.61% in the third decade of this study period.[1] Intravenous drug abuse and a growing population of immunocompromised individuals may account in part for the rising incidence.

Infected abdominal aortic aneurysms are universally fatal without operative excision. Although the outcome following operation has improved, the associated morbidity and mortality remain formidable.[1-4] There are new trends in the etiology and bacteriology of infected abdominal aortic aneurysms,[2-4] and alternative surgical approaches, such as in situ aortic grafting, are being advocated.[5]

CLASSIFICATION

In 1885, William Osler described a patient with infectious endocarditis who was found to have aneurysms of the aortic arch, which he attributed to "mycotic endarteritis." Subsequently, the term mycotic aneurysm was applied to all varieties of infected aneurysm, regardless of the cause or circumstances. In order to alleviate confusion related to this ambiguity, a more precise nomenclature has been proposed to classify infected aneurysms: (1) mycotic aneurysms, as originally described by Osler, developing when a septic embolus of cardiac origin infects an artery; (2) microbial arteritis, in which hematogenous bacteria infect nonaneurysmal, but typically atherosclerotic arteries, leading to aneurysmal degeneration; (3) infection of a pre-existing aneurysm; and (4) a false aneurysm resulting from arterial trauma with concomitant microbial inoculation.

Microbial arteritis is now the predominant cause of infected abdominal aortic aneurysms, responsible for approximately 80% of infected abdominal aortic aneurysms.[3,4] Post-traumatic infected aneurysms secondary to illicit drug injections, the most common type of infected aneurysm at all anatomic locations, infrequently involve the abdominal aorta.[2,3]

The exact incidence of infection in pre-existing aneurysms is unclear. Ernst and colleagues obtained intraoperative cultures from the aneurysm contents of 80 consecutive patients undergoing abdominal aortic aneurysmectomy. Although cultures were positive in 15%, subsequent graft infection developed in only 2.5%. Of note, bacterial cultures were positive in 38% of ruptured aneurysms.[6] These data, which have been confirmed by other investigators, suggest that some aneurysms are colonized with bacteria that apparently pose a minimal threat of subsequent graft infection as compared to overtly infected aneurysms.

BACTERIOLOGY

In the preantibiotic era, when classic mycotic aneurysms predominated, the responsible pathogens were typically nonhemolytic streptococci, pneumococci, or staphylococci. In contemporary studies, *Salmonella* is the most common organism, identified in almost 40% of patients with infected abdominal aortic aneurysms.[2-4] Other commonly isolated organisms are *Streptococcus, Staphylococcus, Bacteroides, Arizona hinshawii, Escherichia coli,* and *Pseudomonas aeruginosa*.[1-5,7] Infections with gram-negative organisms are more likely to be associated with aneurysm rupture.[2-4] Recent reports suggest that gram-positive organisms are increasing in frequency in all types of infected aneurysms, but to a lesser extent in abdominal aneurysms than in aneurysms of the extremities.[2-4]

Infections with atypical organisms are appearing with greater regularity, possibly as a result of the growing population of immunocompromised individuals. Abdominal aortic aneurysms infected with *Salmonella, Haemophilus influenzae,* and *Mycobacterium tuberculosis* have been reported in individuals with the acquired immunodeficiency syndrome (AIDS).[8] Of particular concern is the observation that 25% of patients over 50 years old with a pre-existing aneurysm and an episode of *Salmonella* enteritis, a common malady associated with AIDS, developed a *Salmonella* infection of their aneurysm.[9]

CLINICAL PRESENTATION AND DIAGNOSIS

Early recognition and prompt surgical treatment are essential for the successful management of infected abdominal aortic aneurysms. However, early diagnosis is difficult because the clinical manifestations of an infected abdominal aortic aneurysm are usually insidious. The typical patient is elderly with generalized atherosclerosis. The most common symptoms are fever, abdominal pain, or back pain. A pulsatile abdominal mass or embolization to peripheral arteries may be evident.[1-4,7] A history of a recent febrile or enteric illness, endocarditis, arterial catheterization, abdominal trauma, or accelerated aneurysm expansion may be clues to the presence of an infected abdominal aortic aneurysm.[4,7]

Laboratory data lack sensitivity and specificity. Leukocytosis greater than $10,000/mm^3$ is found in 50% of patients with infected abdominal aortic aneurysms.

Blood cultures are positive in approximately 36% to 50% of patients.[4,7] Negative blood cultures do not exclude the diagnosis of an infected aneurysm, however.

Computed tomography (CT) is the best study for diagnosis of an infected abdominal aortic aneurysm. The CT findings that suggest an aortic infection include the presence of an enhancing and eccentric periaortic mass, an aneurysm at an atypical location, periaortic fluid or gas, retroperitoneal soft tissue edema, prominent periaortic lymphadenopathy, and evidence of aneurysmal rupture.[2,7]

Aortography helps confirm the diagnosis of aortic aneurysm infection. Aneurysms that are saccular, eccentric, multilobular, or situated at an atypical location should signal concern for infection (Fig. 1). Furthermore, infection should be suspected when a discrete aneurysm or multiple aneurysms are noted in an aorta that is otherwise smooth or minimally diseased. Aortography is also valuable to plan the details of operation.

Ultrasonography is not recommended when an infected abdominal aortic aneurysm is suspected because of inadequate sensitivity and specificity. The utility of magnetic resonance imaging and nuclear imaging studies, such as the indium-111 labeled leukocyte scan, remain to be determined.

During operation, certain findings are suggestive of an infected abdominal aortic aneurysm. It is usually thin walled and saccular and may involve an unusual site in an otherwise relatively normal aorta. The likelihood of infection is increased in the presence of periaortic inflammatory changes, prominent lymphadenopathy, infection involving nearby or contiguous tissues, aortoenteric fistula, aortovenous fistula, or rupture.

MANAGEMENT

When the diagnosis of an infected abdominal aortic aneurysm is entertained, broad-spectrum antibiotics should be administered, followed by urgent operation. Operation should not be deferred in order to "sterilize" the aneurysm, an approach that may prove disastrous.

Principles of operative management are (1) control of hemorrhage, (2) removal of infected tissues, and (3) restoration of visceral and lower extremity perfusion. The abdominal aorta may be exposed through either a transperitoneal or a retroperitoneal approach, depending on the location and extent of the aneurysm and involvement of visceral arteries. A midline transperitoneal approach is preferred for most infected ruptured aneurysms. The aorta is controlled proximally at a level that appears noninfected using standard techniques. Thoracotomy to gain proximal aortic control should be avoided unless absolutely necessary because of the risk of contaminating the thorax.

It is imperative to obtain proper specimens of the aneurysm wall, the aneurysm contents, and the aorta at the margin of resection for Gram staining and cultures of aerobic and anaerobic bacteria, fungus, and mycobacteria. Microscopic evaluation of the aneurysm is positive in

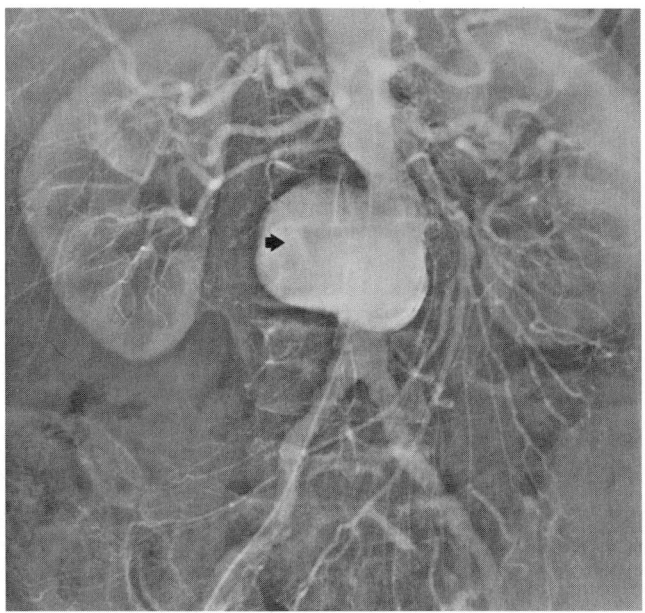

Figure 1 Transfemoral aortogram demonstrates an eccentric saccular infected infrarenal aortic aneurysm (From Reddy DJ, Ernst CB. Infected aneurysms. In: Rutherford RB, ed. Vascular surgery, 3rd ed. Philadelphia: WB Saunders, 1989: 987; with permission.)

approximately 50% to 82% of infected aneurysms. These studies are more likely to be positive in the case of a ruptured aneurysm.[2,3,6,7] A negative intraoperative Gram stain does not exclude the diagnosis. Culture results will direct long-term antibiotic therapy.

Major postoperative morbidity is related to persistent infection, subsequent graft infection, or dehiscence of the proximal aortic closure. Therefore, all infected tissues must be excised, including infected visceral vessels or a densely adherent vena cava.

The method of arterial reconstruction is influenced by intraoperative Gram stains. Recent data suggest that in situ grafting may be safe in the absence of frank suppuration.[4,5] Although in situ grafting may be a viable option when minimal localized inflammation and negative Gram stains are found, we favor in situ reconstruction only when the suprarenal aorta is involved. In all other patients, aneurysm excision and extra-anatomic bypass such as an axillofemoral graft are recommended. The optimal prosthetic material for in situ grafting has not been determined. Expanded polytetrafluoroethylene grafts and Dacron grafts impregnated with antibiotics may have better resistance to infection, but this has not been clinically substantiated.

When preoperative CT scans document suppuration limited to the infrarenal aorta and no evidence of rupture, extra-anatomic bypass precedes aneurysm repair in the stable patient. All skin incisions are closed prior to aneurysm resection. Bacteremic seeding of a newly constructed bypass during debridement of the aorta has not proved to be a problem.

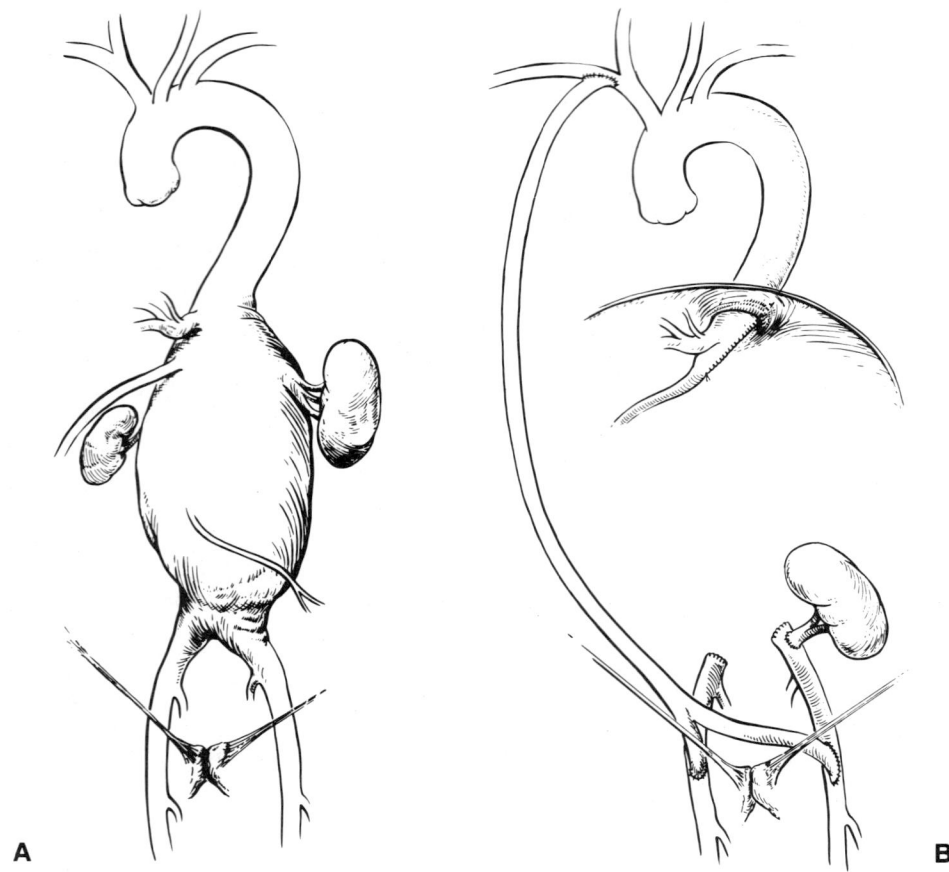

Figure 2 *A,* Diagram demonstrating extensive infected suprarenal aortic aneurysm. *B,* Reconstruction with tapered aortoplasty beginning above the level of the celiac trunk, autotransplantation of the left kidney into the pelvis, and extra-anatomic axillobifemoral bypass. (Adapted from Reddy DJ, Lee RE, Oh HK. Suprarenal mycotic aortic aneurysm: Surgical management and follow-up. J Vasc Surg 1986; 3:919; with permission.)

When rupture cannot be excluded, the aneurysm is resected first, followed by extra-anatomic reconstruction. After aneurysm excision, aortic stump closure, aortic bed debriding and irrigating, and abdominal closure, the patient is reprepped and redraped. The extra-anatomic bypass is constructed with personnel using fresh instruments, gowns, and gloves. It is prudent to place initial axillofemoral bypasses on the right side, to permit a left flank retroperitoneal approach for future aortic reconstruction. In addition to axillofemoral bypass, a bypass from the descending thoracic aorta to the iliac or femoral vessels through uninvolved tissue planes has also proven useful.[10]

Involvement of the pararenal or suprarenal aorta presents special challenges. When infection is limited to the posterior wall of the suprarenal aorta, it may be possible to maintain perfusion of the viscera by constructing a tapered conduit from the anterior wall of the aorta (Fig. 2). If the celiac, superior mesenteric, or renal arteries require debridement, grafts to these arteries must be constructed, originating from the proximal uninvolved aorta or from an aortic prosthesis placed in situ. Autogenous tissue is preferred for visceral bypass grafts. Kidney autotransplantation to the pelvis with the blood supply derived from the iliac vessels may be required (Fig. 2).

To minimize the risk of catastrophic aortic stump dehiscence, the proximal aorta must be securely closed with a double row of monofilament sutures through healthy-appearing tissue. Aortic suture lines, be they stump closures or anastomoses, should be covered with a pedicle of omentum transposed through the transverse mesocolon. Retroperitoneal closure is often impossible because of the lack of adequate tissue following debridement. The aortic bed should be thoroughly irrigated. Retroperitoneal drains are recommended in the presence of frank suppuration. Concomitant cholecystectomy has been advised if *Salmonella* is known to be the pathogen.[7]

LONG-TERM MANAGEMENT

Initially, broad-spectrum antibiotic therapy against gram-negative, gram-positive, and anaerobic organisms is recommended. If a pathogen is identified, organism-specific antibiotics should be administered. The duration of the antibiotic therapy is dictated by the virulence of the organism, the extent of the infection, and the method of arterial reconstruction. In most patients, 6 weeks of intravenous therapy is recommended. When the infection is localized and the responsible organism is not identified or proves to be a less virulent gram-positive organism, a 4 week course of parenteral antibiotics may be adequate. After in situ aortic graft reconstruction, 6 weeks of parenteral antibiotics followed by lifelong oral antibiotics are advised.

Blood cultures are obtained upon cessation of parenteral antibiotics. Intravenous antibiotics are reinstituted if these cultures are positive or for any other manifestation of residual infection.

During follow-up, patients must be scrutinized for evidence of persistent infection with frequent physical examinations and CT scans. A baseline CT scan should be obtained approximately 2 weeks postoperatively, followed by scans at regular intervals thereafter.

If the axillofemoral bypass fails postoperatively, in situ aortic reconstruction is acceptable if there was no evidence of persistent infection during the preceding 6 months. Alternatively, bypasses from the ascending aorta may be placed ventrally to avoid previously infected tissue planes. The descending thoracic aorta or supraceliac aorta may be accessible through a left thoracoabdominal or retroperitoneal flank approach.[10]

RESULTS

At the Henry Ford Hospital from 1960 to 1989, 4 of 13 patients (31%) with infected abdominal aortic aneurysms died within 30 days of operation.[1] Other investigators have reported mortality rates of 14% to 75%, depending on the type of infected aneurysm.[1-5]

The safety of in situ aortic reconstruction remains controversial. Ewart and associates reported a 23% rate of reoperation following in situ grafting, which increased to 63% for infection with gram-negative organisms.[7] In contrast, based on a literature review of 109 cases of infected abdominal aortic aneurysms, Fichelle and co-workers reported perioperative mortality rates of 26% and 28% following in situ and extra-anatomic bypass, respectively. However, the incidence of septic aortic complications was greater for in situ reconstruction (22%) than for extra-anatomic bypass (14%).[5]

REFERENCES

1. Reddy DJ, Shepard AD, Evans JR, et al. Management of infected aortoiliac aneurysms. Arch Surg 1991; 126:873–879.
2. Reddy DJ, Ernst CB. Infected aneurysms. In: Rutherford RB, ed. Vascular surgery, 3rd ed. Philadelphia: WB Saunders, 1989:983.
3. Brown SL, Busuttil RW, Baker JD, et al. Bacteriologic and surgical determinants of survival in patients with mycotic aneurysms. J Vasc Surg 1984; 1:541–547.
4. Oz MC, Brener BJ, Buda JA, et al. A ten-year experience with bacterial aortitis. J Vasc Surg 1989; 10:439–449.
5. Fichelle JM, Tabet G, Cormier P, et al. Infected infrarenal aortic aneurysms: When is in situ reconstruction safe? J Vasc Surg 1993; 17:635–645.
6. Ernst CB, Campbell HC, Daugherty ME, et al. Incidence and significance of intraoperative bacterial cultures during abdominal aortic aneurysmectomy. Ann Surg 1977; 185:626–633.
7. Ewart JM, Burke ML, Bunt TJ. Spontaneous abdominal aortic infections: Essentials of diagnosis and management. Am Surg 1983; 49:37–50.
8. Gouny P, Valverde A, Vincent D, et al. Human immunodeficiency virus and infected aneurysm of the abdominal aorta: Report of three cases. Ann Vasc Surg 1992; 6:239–243.
9. Cohen PS, O'Brien TF, Schenbaum SC, Medeiros AA. The risk of endothelial infection in adults with salmonella bacteremia. Ann Intern Med 1978; 89:931–932.
10. Criado E, Johnson G, Burnham SJ, et al. Descending thoracic aorta-to-iliofemoral artery bypass as an alternative to aortoiliac reconstruction. J Vasc Surg 1992; 15:550–557.

MANAGEMENT OF CONCURRENT INTRA-ABDOMINAL DISEASE AND ABDOMINAL AORTIC ANEURYSM

S. TIMOTHY STRING, M.D.

The decision to perform primary, concomitant, or delayed operative procedures for concurrent intra-abdominal disease with aortic aneurysm repair requires well-informed clinical judgment. The performance of other procedures during aortic aneurysmectomy remains controversial. The two central debated issues are the propensity for graft infection following aneurysmectomy and the determination that a concomitant procedure is beneficial. Primary or delayed procedures are influenced by the acuteness or potential for acuteness of the associated pathology, the size and type of aneurysm, the possibility for subsequent graft infection, and the type of associated intra-abdominal disease.

ANEURYSM

Potential aneurysm rupture following the correction of intra-abdominal pathology is a consideration for a surgeon contemplating primary, concomitant, or delayed procedures. No large study delineates the parameters or frequency of aneurysm rupture when the associated abdominal pathology becomes the primary procedure and the aneurysm remains intact. Swanson suggested that increased collagenase activity occurs following major intra-abdominal surgical procedures.[1] Aneurysmal rupture was observed 6 to 21 days following cholecystectomy, small bowel resection, and vagotomy and pyloroplasty. Circumstantial evidence exists that aneurysm size influences the propensity for rupture in the postoperative period. An aneurysm 5 cm or greater in diameter, as well as saccular or "bleb" aneurysms, influences the decision to perform an aneurysmectomy in the face of associated nonemergent intra-abdominal pathology.

Ruptured aneurysms are almost always a contraindication to a second procedure. A contained ruptured aneurysm in a patient who has been hemodynamically stable through the preoperative and intraoperative periods might be the only instance when a second procedure would be considered.

If the nonaneurysmal pathology is emergent or semiemergent and needs to be primarily corrected, the patient requires close observation during the immediate postoperative period. The aneurysmectomy should be performed at the earliest medically expeditious time.

HERNIAS

Ventral, umbilical, incisional, and inguinal hernias are occasionally associated with the population undergoing abdominal aortic aneurysmectomy. As long as there are no intraoperative mitigating factors, repair of such hernias is appropriate at the conclusion of the aneurysmectomy, sparing the patient the attendant morbidity of a second procedure. These are repaired intra-abdominally or as part of the abdominal closure.

APPENDICITIS

Ochsner, Cooley, and DeBakey reported results of concomitant procedures for intra-abdominal disease along with aortic procedures.[2] They performed incidental appendectomy with aneurysmectomy without additional morbidity and mortality.

The probability of developing appendicitis with an otherwise normal appendix diminishes with age (1 in 100 patients at age 65). The presence of a fecalith or an appendiceal tumor may justify appendectomy as a concomitant procedure.

SMALL BOWEL DISEASE

Concomitant small bowel resection for such nonacute pathology as a carcinoid tumor or Meckel's diverticulum was performed without a significant increase of morbidity or mortality. No significant study exists regarding other types of nonacute, subacute, or acute small bowel pathology, although additional morbidity has not been noted with the repair of primary aortoduodenal fistula.

GASTRIC DISEASE

Peptic ulcer disease has been identified in 5% to 10% of the population prone to abdominal aortic aneurysms, but no direct association of the two diseases has been identified. When bleeding, perforation, or obstruction occurs with an associated symptomatic abdominal aortic aneurysm, a gastric procedure may be considered necessary.

Gastrostomy rather than nasogastric tube suction is suggested to decrease postoperative morbidity. In Morris and co-workers' study, patients with gastrostomy did not develop postoperative graft infections, whereas patients with nasogastric suction did.[3] If concomitant gastrostomy is deemed beneficial, the morbidity of the procedure appears minimal.

No large studies provide a basis for a decision to proceed with a concomitant procedure for peptic ulcer disease. It would be unusual not to have identified peptic ulcer disease preoperatively. The more usual situation would be identification of an associated aortic aneurysm during a gastric procedure. The occurrence of perforation would preclude an aneurysmectomy, as would unstable bleeding or obstruction.

Postaneurysmectomy peptic ulcer complications of bleeding, obstruction, perforation, or an unhealed lesser curvature ulcer increase morbidity and mortality. Therefore, if resection of a symptomatic aortic aneurysm is imperative in a patient with active symptomatic peptic ulcer disease, selective vagotomy and pyloroplasty with a decompressive gastrostomy are the procedures of choice. This therapeutic approach carries a low associated morbidity and mortality. A closed procedure such as a highly selective vagotomy might further lessen the chance for graft contamination but has a higher incidence of lesser curvature ischemia and perforation.

When a malignant nonobstructing gastric tumor is encountered with a 5 cm or larger aneurysm, the aneurysm is resected then and the tumor resected at a later time. However, if local invasion or evidence of metastasis (biopsy confirmed) is present, then strong consideration is given to performing no procedure and closing the abdomen. Resection of a benign gastric tumor without associated bleeding, perforation, or obstruction could be considered following aneurysmectomy because small bowel resection for benign tumors has no increased morbidity.

COLONIC DISEASE

Malignant or benign colonic disease associated with an aortic aneurysm is a management challenge with no consensus of surgical opinion.[4] The incidence of colonic cancer with aneurysmal disease is greater than other colonic pathology and is as high as 4%. Szilagyi and colleagues offered general principles of treatment for associated colon cancer:[5] (1) aneurysm resection in presence of symptoms or rupture; (2) resection of a malignant colonic lesion associated with complication of hemorrhage, perforation, or obstruction; (3) in the absence of these factors, treatment is based on the size of the aneurysm (large aneurysms are resected and the colon lesion resected at a later date, but with small aneurysms the colon cancer is treated first, followed by aneurysm repair); (4) presence of metastatic disease under effective control justifies aneurysm resection if it is symptomatic, ruptured, or large.

Acute diverticulitis has been reported following aneurysmectomy but can usually be managed conservatively. However, when acute diverticular disease requires surgical correction and is associated with aneurysmal disease, mortality may be high because of postoperative aneurysm rupture.

Because concomitant aneurysmectomy is not recommended during operation for acute diverticular disease, aneurysmectomy is performed within 1 week. Beyond the first week, the incidence of aneurysm rupture increases. These same principles apply to other inflammatory bowel conditions.

BILIARY TRACT DISEASE

Concomitant cholecystectomy with aortic reconstruction has been advocated by several authors.[2,6-10] Others have questioned the performance of the two procedures during the same operation. The concerns of critics focus on immediate or delayed postoperative infection of the prosthetic graft, the development of cholecystitis requiring a subsequent cholecystectomy, the possibility of increased morbidity and mortality of a concomitant procedure in an older population, and prolongation of operative time.

A collection of the reported studies[8] plus my own 51 unreported patients total 314 patients. Only one instance of a graft infection occurred following concomitant cholecystectomy, an incidence of 0.32%. The infection occurred when the aortic graft was not reperitonealized prior to cholecystectomy. Even though the incidence of positive bile cultures is high, no delayed morbidity has been encountered during long-term follow-up. The concerns of graft infection and increased mortality and morbidity attributable to the concomitant cholecystectomy appear to be unsubstantiated.[2,6,7,9,10] However, increased morbidity and mortality were noted in some studies of concomitant cholecystectomy and aortic reconstruction as compared to those of only aortic reconstruction.[8,11]

It is well documented that patients with cholelithiasis undergoing aortic reconstruction may require future cholecystectomy.[6,7,12] Immediate postoperative cholecystectomy for acute calculus cholecystitis may result in up to 47% mortality.[6,9,12,13]

Elective aneurysmectomy is not recommended in the presence of acute cholecystitis. Aneurysmectomy should be performed once the patient has recovered from the cholecystectomy.

OTHER

Needle biopsy of the liver, ovary, or kidney has been performed concomitantly without incident. Removal of ovarian or tubal disease at the completion of an aneurysmectomy has occurred without additional morbidity. Also, nephrectomy for the small, nonfunctioning, hypertensive kidney has been performed without adverse efects, as has splenectomy.

OPERATIVE TECHNIQUE

Aneurysmectomy should be the primary procedure when concomitant procedures are contemplated. However, if a small bowel enterotomy is made, the sequence is reversed. The area is packed off with surgical pads, and the instruments for repair of the small bowel enterotomy are segregated from other instruments. These instruments are removed at the completion of the bowel closure. Gowns and gloves are changed, and the affected area is copiously irrigated before the aneurysmectomy is begun. If a colon enterotomy with spillage occurs, the aortic procedure is abandoned, and the colon is repaired. However, if there is no colonic spillage and the patient has undergone a preoperative mechanical or antibiotic bowel prep, the colotomy could be primarily closed, the area copiously irrigated, and the aneurysmectomy performed, if the surgeon's judgment so dictates.

When a surgeon performs a concomitant procedure, retroperitonealization of the entire graft is imperative prior to the performance of the second procedure. The area of associated pathology is isolated with surgical packs. During cholecystectomy, care is exercised not to perforate the gallbladder, although this has occurred with no untoward side effects. The ligated cystic duct is transected with electrocautery. Once the secondary procedure is performed, the area is copiously irrigated with normal saline. Antibiotic solution lavage is an option. Drains are not used.

REFERENCES

1. Swanson RJ, Littooy FN, Hunt TK, et al. Laparotomy as a precipitating factor in the rupture of intra-abdominal aneurysms. Arch Surg 1980; 115:299–304.
2. Ochsner JL, Cooley DA, DeBakey ME. Associated intra-abdominal lesions encountered during resection of aortic aneurysm. Dis Colon Rectum 1960; 3:485–490.
3. Morris T, Bouhoutsos J, Martin P. The value of gastrostomy in the surgery of aortic aneurysms. Br J Surg 1974; 61:662–664.
4. Lobbato VJ, Rothenberg RE, LaRaja RD, et al. Coexistence of abdominal aortic aneurysm and carcinoma of the colon: A dilemma. J Vasc Surg 1985; 2:724–742.
5. Szilagyi DE, Elliott JP, Berguer R. Coincidental malignancy and abdominal aortic aneurysm. Arch Surg 1967; 95:402–412.

6. String ST. Cholelithiasis and aortic reconstruction. J Vasc Surg 1984; 1:664–667.
7. Ouriel K, Ricott JJ, Adams JT, Deweese JA. Management of cholelithiasis in patients with abdominal aortic aneurysm. Ann Surg 1982; 198:717–719.
8. Thomas JH. Abdominal aortic aneurysmorrhaphy combined with biliary or gastrointestinal surgery. Surg Clin North Am 1989; 69:807–815.
9. Ameli FM, Provan JL, Johnston KW. Safety of cholecystectomy with abdominal aortic surgery. Can J Surg 1987; 30:170–173.
10. Tompkins WC Jr, Chavez CM, Conn JH, Hardy JD. Combining intra-abdominal arterial grafting with gastrointestinal or biliary tract procedures. Am J Surg 1973; 126:598–600.
11. Bickerstaff LK, Hollier LH, Van Peenen HJ, et al. Abdominal aortic aneurysm repair combined with a second surgical procedure: Morbidity and mortality. Surgery 1984; 95:487–491.
12. Ottinger LW. Acute cholecystitis as a postoperative complication. Ann Surg 1976; 184:162–165.
13. Franko E, Cohen JR. General surgical problems requiring operation in postoperative vascular surgery patients. Am J Surg 1991; 162:247–250.

RETROPERITONEAL APPROACH FOR ELECTIVE ABDOMINAL AORTIC ANEURYSMECTOMY

ROBERT P. LEATHER, M.D.
R. CLEMENT DARLING III, M.D.
BENJAMIN B. CHANG, M.D.
DHIRAJ M. SHAH, M.D.

The retroperitoneal approach for repair of abdominal aortic aneurysm (AAA) has been advocated by many.[1,2] Surgeons regard the retroperitoneal approach to be indicated under certain circumstances, such as high-risk patients. We have used this approach exclusively for AAA repair in an effort to minimize operative trauma, blood loss, intensive care unit requirements, and hospital stay.[3] The posterolateral exposure from the left side affords the most flexible and widest exposure of the aorta. The retroperitoneal approach can be used with several variations: from the left side, varying the level of incisions along the lower intercostal spaces, and from the right side, depending on indications. Although there is controversy, many feel that the retroperitoneal approach has some physiologic benefits and also under certain circumstances it is indicated to provide superior exposure and versatility.[3-7] In this chapter we present our current techniques of left and right retroperitoneal approach for elective AAA repair.

RATIONALE

The advantages of the retroperitoneal approach in our experience are both technical and physiologic. It allows minimum dissection, minimum blood loss, a stable operative field, and excellent exposure of the aneurysm neck and aortic branches. Physiologic advantages include less pain, less requirement for ventilator support, less fluid shift, shorter and smoother postoperative course, and early return of bowel function. When exclusion bypass technique is used with the retroperitoneal approach, a decrease in blood loss has been observed.[8] Approximately a third of our patients did not require blood transfusions, another third of the operations were done using the patient's own blood, and the remaining patients required an average of 1.5 units of banked blood transfusions. Although we consider the retroperitoneal approach appropriate for all patients with AAA, there are certain circumstances in which this approach is excellent, including redo operations, inflammatory aneurysms, aneurysms associated with horseshoe kidney, patients with pulmonary insufficiency, obese patients, and patients who have had multiple intra-abdominal operations.

LEFT RETROPERITONEAL APPROACH

After the induction of anesthesia, the patient is positioned by use of a suction bean bag with the left side up (Fig. 1). The chest is elevated 30° to 60°, and the pelvis is minimally rotated to provide access to the right groin and right retroperitoneal area. The left arm is supported by a folded blanket or with a cross-arm sling. The left thigh is elevated and the knee flexed with a folded blanket or a second bean bag. Such flexion is important to relax the iliopsoas muscles. Finally, the table is flexed 20° to 30° in a reverse V position to open the space between the ribs and the iliac crest.

The incision can be made from the tenth intercostal space to the twelfth, depending on whether suprarenal aortic cross-clamping is needed. By dividing the left crus of the diaphragm, one can cross-clamp the aorta above the celiac axis without entering the chest. The incision is carried from the posterior to midaxillary line to the rectus muscle sheath, which is not divided. All the flat muscles of the abdomen are divided; then the retroperitoneum is entered (Fig. 2). The left kidney and viscera are retracted forward and medially. The aorta is approached posterolaterally behind the kidney (Fig. 3). If needed, intercostal muscles are divided along the top of the rib, to avoid the intercostal nerve and vessels. It is wise to block or divide the intercostal nerve to avoid intercostal neuralgia. There are a few collateral venous connections between the peritoneum and the retroperitoneum that should be carefully divided. The aneurysm neck, position of the left renal artery, and iliac arteries are identified, as well as the ureter, which is retracted forward. A self-retaining retractor is used for maintaining the intended exposure throughout the remainder of the operation. Prior to aneurysm manipulation, usually the outflow vessels are controlled. The left iliac artery is

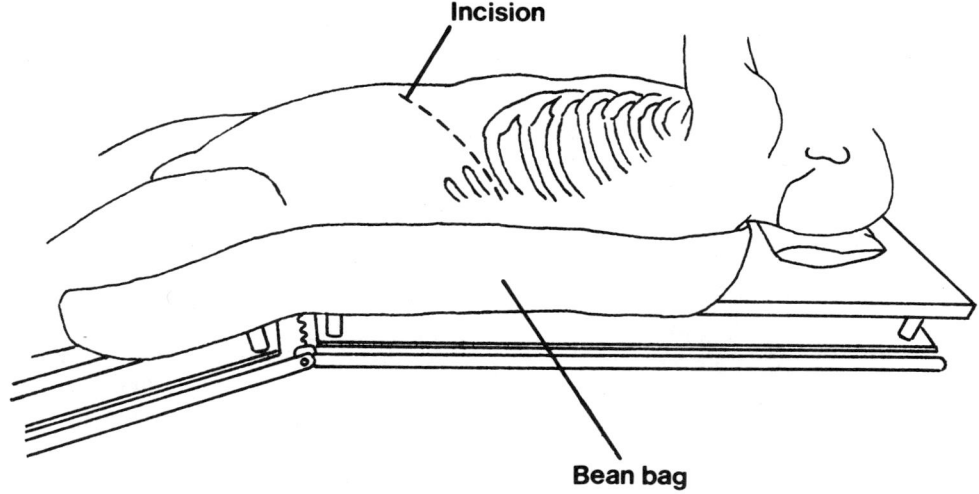

Figure 1 Placement of the patient in right lateral decubitus position.

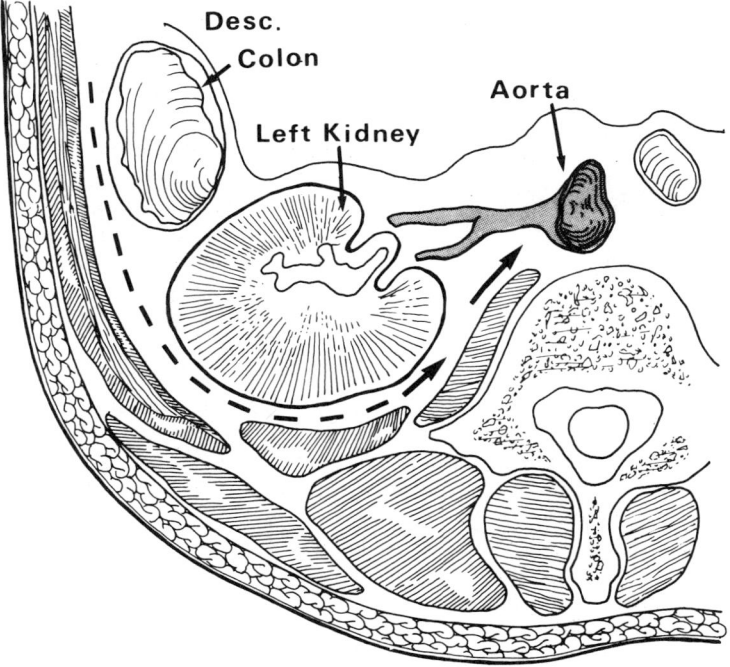

Figure 2 Intended path in the retroperitoneal dissection to the aorta (dotted line).

dissected through the same incision. The proximal 1 to 2 cm of the right iliac artery can be exposed from the left side if it is not aneurysmal. Otherwise, the right iliac artery is exposed by a separate incision above the inguinal ligament from the right side, using the right retroperitoneal approach. The patient usually receives heparin sodium, 30 units/kg of body weight.

Two landmark structures identify the aneurysm neck area, the lumbar branch of the left renal vein and the left renal artery (Fig. 4). The lumbar branch is identified and is ligated in continuity and divided. The left renal artery is at the level of the arcuate end of the left crus of the diaphragm. Dissection of the renal artery is not necessary unless a renal artery bypass is contemplated. Lymphoareolar tissues are divided, and the aneurysm neck is dissected anteriorly and posteriorly about three-quarters of the circumference. Lumbar arteries in the area are ligated and divided as necessary. The aorta is cross-clamped. If the aneurysm is repaired by open conventional endoaneurysmorrhaphy, bleeding is controlled by suture ligating the lumbar and inferior mesenteric arteries, and the graft is anastomosed in the usual manner from inside the aneurysm sac.

We have used aortic exclusion and bypass technique to minimize the dissection and blood loss. This procedure is conceptually similar to an aortobifemoral bypass performed for occlusive disease (Fig. 5). Aneurysm ex-

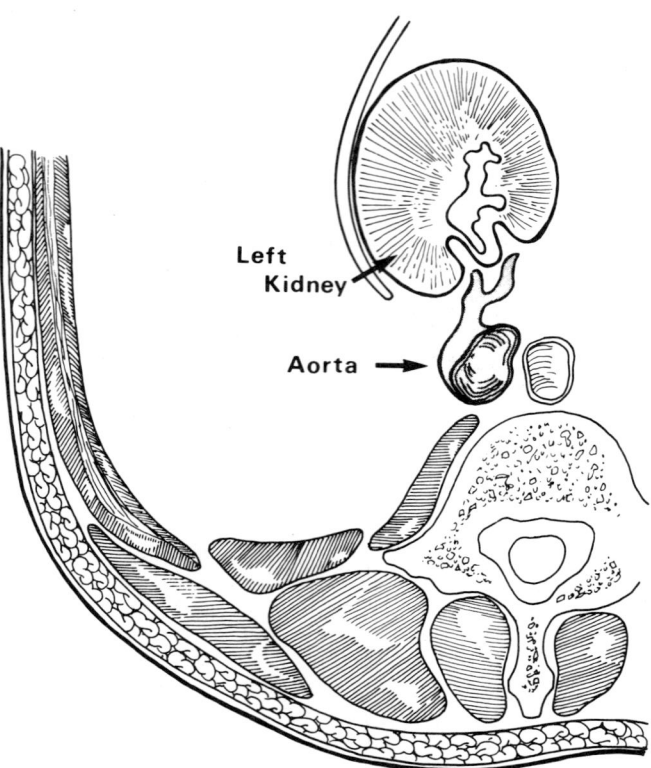

Figure 3 Aorta is approached posterolaterally.

clusion requires two clamps placed across the neck of the aneurysm, leaving about 1 to 2 cm between the clamps for anastomosis of the graft. If the aortic aneurysm extends up to the renal artery and there is not sufficient neck, the distal clamp can be applied on the aneurysm sac itself because it is going to be oversewn and excluded. The aorta is transected between the two clamps, usually flush with the distal clamp. The transection requires care at the right corner of the aorta so that injury to vena cava does not occur. Once two-thirds to three-quarters of the aorta is divided, the rest of the aorta is divided from inside. As soon as the limiting adventitial wall of the aorta is visible, small snips with scissors are taken. The distal aorta is oversewn with two layers of continuous 3-0 polypropylene suture under and over the clamp, and then the clamp is removed and the suture is tied. The oversewn aneurysm sac is now flaccid and is retracted distally.

The proximal anastomosis is usually performed in an end-to-end fashion using a parachute technique with 3-0 polypropylene continuous suture. After completion of the proximal anastomosis, the anastomosis is tested, taking a repair suture if needed. When a tube graft is used, another clamp is applied at the distal end of the aneurysm and the aorta is divided between the iliac bifurcation and the aneurysm. The aneurysm sac is oversewn. The aneurysm sac is retracted cephalad to visualize the distal transected aorta for distal anastomosis in an end-to-end fashion. Care is taken not to injure the vena cava during both dividing the aorta and the anastomosis.

When a bifurcated graft is used, the left common iliac artery or external iliac artery anastomosis is done through the same left incision. The iliac artery is divided or ligated in continuity so the aneurysm is excluded from retrograde perfusion. The distal anastomosis is performed in an end-to-end or end-to-side fashion, using 5-0 or 6-0 polypropylene suture in a continuous manner using the parachute technique. The right limb of the graft is tunneled retroperitoneally, in front of the iliac artery and behind the ureter. If this space is not usable, it could be passed along the space of Retzius or even anteriorly. Tunneling is done under direct vision from the left side to the right. The right iliac artery, usually the external iliac artery, is either ligated or divided, the proximal end is oversewn, and the distal anastomosis is done with 5-0 or 6-0 polypropylene continuous suture in an end-to-end or end-to-side fashion.

RIGHT RETROPERITONEAL APPROACH

When it is necessary to repair the right renal artery or the left side is not accessible because of prior incision, left colostomy, or other reasons, the right retroperitoneal approach may be used. This approach is analogous to the anterolateral approach; the aorta is exposed either anterior to the right kidney or below the right kidney, depending on the level of the neck of the aneurysm. The only difference between the left- and the right-sided approaches is the vena cava. Usually the aorta is exposed in front of the vena cava. The right gonadal vein is usually divided, and the aorta is approached below the renal artery. The limitation of this approach is that one might not be able to reach the aorta cephalad to the renal arteries because of the liver. If more proximal exposure is necessary, then one may have to identify, mobilize, retract, or divide the left renal vein. Aneurysm repair can be done either by endoaneurysmorrhaphy technique or by exclusion. If a bifurcation graft is needed, the left iliac vessels are exposed counterincision.

CLINICAL EXPERIENCE

During the past 14 years we have used the retroperitoneal approach in 774 patients for elective aneurysm repair. Although we initially started using the retroperitoneal approach selectively, as our experience increased it was used exclusively. The retroperitoneal approach has been used with the aneurysm exclusion technique in more recent years.

RESULTS

Operative mortality was 2.3%. It did not vary according to technique or change year to year. Most deaths were due to myocardial infarctions. The second most common cause of death was multiple organ failure. The major morbidity was also associated with myocardial disease. The excluded aneurysm sacs usually thrombosed within 3 to 6 months. During a 10 year follow-up, there was no deterioration of the graft, formation of false

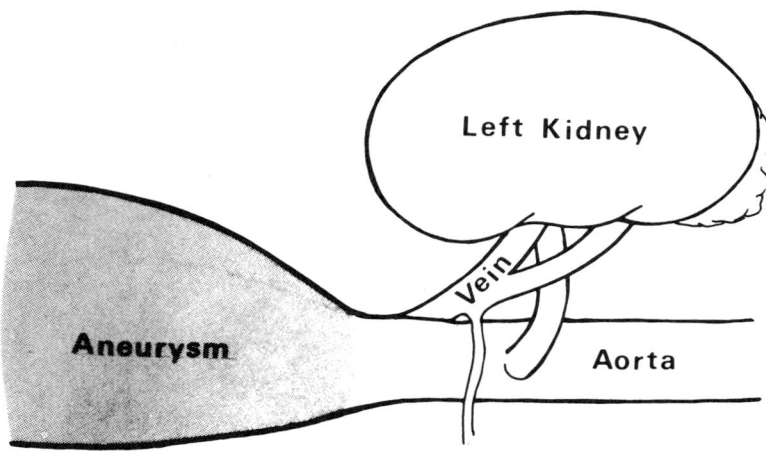

Figure 4 Lumbar branch of left renal vein and left renal artery as landmarks.

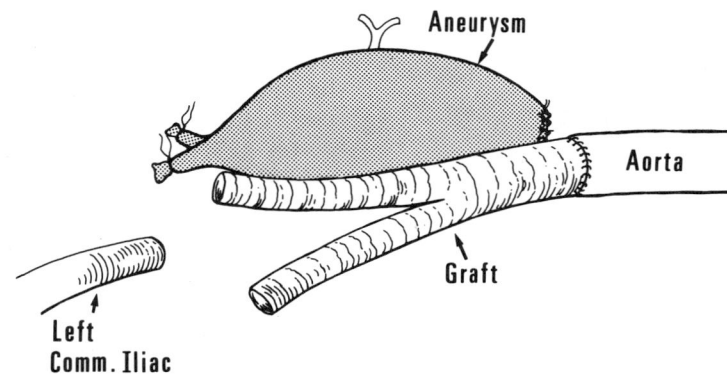

Figure 5 Diagram for aneurysm exclusion.

aneurysm, or infection of the aneurysm sac. In one patient, the aneurysm sac continued to expand because of a patient lumbar artery. The patient refused operation, and this aneurysm sac ruptured. Following operation, the patient survived. In two other patients the aneurysm sac was not completely excluded by dividing the iliac artery, and the aneurysm showed continued flow and wall motion by ultrasound. These patients were reoperated upon, and the iliac arteries were divided to exclude the aneurysm sac, which then thrombosed.

One interesting aspect of this operation is inability to evaluate the inferior mesenteric artery. The left colon is inspected clinically at the end of the procedure by making a small opening in the peritoneal cavity. We did not reimplant the inferior mesenteric artery except in one patient who had both the superior mesenteric and celiac arteries occluded. There was no instance of transmural colonic ischemia in these elective aneurysm repairs.

The only complication associated with the incision was incisional bulge or hernia, but not significantly more frequent than hernia formation or wound disruption with the transperitoneal approach. Intercostal neuralgia has been a nuisance rather than a problem that was usually resolved by intercostal nerve block, and in a minority of patients by neurectomy.

REFERENCES

1. Rob C. Extraperitoneal approach to the abdominal aorta. Surgery 1963; 53:87–89.
2. Williams GM, Ricotta JJ, Zinner M, Burdick JF. The extended retroperitoneal approach for the management of extensive atherosclerosis of the aorta and renal vessels. Surgery 1980; 88:846–855.
3. Leather RP, Shah DM, Kaufman JL, et al. Comparative analysis for retroperitoneal and transperitoneal aortic replacement for aneurysm. Surg Gynecol Obstet 1989; 168:387–393.
4. Cambria RP, Brewster DC, Abbott WM, et al. Transperitoneal versus retroperitoneal approach for aortic reconstruction: A randomized prospective study. J Vasc Surg 1990; 11:314–325.
5. Sicard GA, Freeman MB, Van der Woude JC, Anderson CB. Comparison between transabdominal and retroperitoneal approach for reconstruction of the infrarenal aorta. J Vasc Surg 1987; 5:19–27.
6. Hudson JC, Wurm WH, O'Donnell TF, et al. Hemodynamics and prostacyclin release in the early phases of aortic surgery. Comparison of transabdominal and retroperitoneal approaches. J Vasc Surg 1988; 7:190–198.
7. Nypaver TJ, Shepard AD, Reddy DJ, et al. Repair of pararenal abdominal aortic aneurysms: An analysis of operative management. Arch Surg 1993; 128:803–813.
8. Shah DM, Chang BB, Paty PSK, et al. Treatment of abdominal aortic aneurysm by exclusion and bypass: An analysis of outcome. J Vasc Surg 1991; 13:15–20.

AORTIC ANEURYSM REPAIR WITH COEXISTENT VISCERAL AND RENAL ARTERY DISEASE

DAVID F. J. TOLLEFSON, M.D.
CHARLES A. ANDERSEN, M.D.

Criteria for elective abdominal aortic aneurysm (AAA) repair are now well defined. Likewise, criteria for elective repair of symptomatic renal or visceral arterial lesions are well established. Adjunctive repair of renal or visceral vessels with aortic reconstruction, although accepted, is uncommon. Indications for renal and visceral arterial repair with AAA repair are less clear, particularly when asymptomatic renal or visceral arterial disease is found incidentally during preoperative arteriography.

INDICATIONS FOR RENAL REVASCULARIZATION

Although the operative mortality for repair of AAA ranges from 1% to 5%, the operative mortality for aortic reconstruction in conjunction with renal revascularization ranges higher, from 3% to 25%. Hence, prior to contemplating adjunctive renal revascularization with aortic reconstruction, certain criteria are required to justify the increased risk (Table 1). Certain anatomic situations coincident with an AAA make renal and visceral revascularization mandatory. Proximal aneurysmal extension to involve renal or visceral arterial ostia or the presence of a horseshoe kidney requires repair of those involved vessels.

Accepted indications exist for isolated renal revascularization, and these apply for adjunctive renal revascularization during aortic aneurysm repair. Isolated or bilateral renal artery stenosis causing renovascular hypertension requires repair. Determination of unilateral renal artery stenosis causing hypertension has relied on lateralization of split-function renal studies, renal vein renin ratios, or renal-systemic renin indices.[1] We utilize the latter two studies to assess the significance of a unilateral stenosis. Renal vein renin ratios, comparing effluent from each kidney, are suggestive of renovascular disease if greater than 1.4. However, these ratios can be less sensitive if renin secretion from the contralateral kidney is also elevated. Although renal vein renin values can vary considerably, comparison of renal vein renin activity from an individual kidney to systemic activity usually is 0.24, with combined activity from both kidneys related to systemic activity usually 0.48. When the renal-systemic renin index from the ischemic kidney is greater than 0.48 and the contralateral kidney renal-systemic renin index approaches zero, beneficial response to renal revascularization to the ischemic kidney can be expected. Recently, we have employed an angiotensin converting enzyme inhibitor, captopril, to stimulate renin production and enhance the differential between renal vein renins.[2] This does not require any special preparation or the withholding of antihypertensive medication. Duplex scan analysis of the renal arteries is utilized to help determine stenotic involvement of the renal arteries. Renal artery stenosis greater than 60% is present if a renal artery-aorta peak systolic velocity ratio is greater than 3.5.

Although renal vein renin assays are helpful in prediction of success in bypass to unilateral stenoses, their value is limited in patients with bilateral renal artery stenoses. Bilateral renal artery stenoses that lateralize by renal vein renin analysis to one side undergo adjunctive renal revascularization only to the side with elevated renin. When renal vein renin analysis does not lateralize in patients with bilateral renal artery stenoses, arteriographic analysis is critical. Arteriography is used to assess the hemodynamic significance of bilateral renal artery stenoses and as support of the contribution of unilateral renal artery stenosis toward renovascular hypertension. Arteriographic evidence of collateral blood flow circumventing a high-grade renal artery stenosis documents its hemodynamic significance. Bilateral adjunctive renal revascularization is advocated in patients with clinical evidence of renovascular disease, nonlateralizing renal vein renins, and bilateral high-grade renal artery stenoses.

Revascularization of kidneys with bilateral renal artery stenoses in conjunction with chronic renal insufficiency can produce a salutary effect. Dean and associates have suggested that these effects are primarily evident only in severely azotemic (serum creatinine of 3 mg/dl or greater) individuals with bilateral correctable disease.[3] We have taken a more liberal approach and perform adjunctive renal revascularization in patients with bilateral preocclusive stenoses and modest creatinine elevation whose kidney size is greater than 7 cm in length and who have evidence of some function by isotopic renography.

Uncertainty exists in the proper management of

Table 1 Indications for Renal or Visceral Revascularization in Conjunction with Aortic Aneurysm Reconstruction

Renal revascularization
  Aneurysmal involvement of renal artery ostia
  Renovascular hypertension
  Renal failure with bilateral preocclusive stenoses or solitary kidney with preocclusive stenosis
  Bilateral asymptomatic preocclusive stenoses (>80%)
  Renal artery aneurysm >2 cm
Visceral revascularization
  Chronic mesenteric ischemia with both superior mesenteric and celiac artery high-grade stenosis or occlusion
  Preoperative preocclusive stenoses or occlusions of both the superior mesenteric and celiac arteries with evidence of meandering mesenteric artery flow from the inferior to superior mesenteric artery
  Intraoperative colonic and/or small bowel ischemia

asymptomatic renal artery disease discovered during preoperative assessment by either duplex imaging or aortography. Renal artery stenoses have been found in almost one-fourth of patients with AAA, and over half were asymptomatic. Rates of progression of renal artery stenoses have ranged as high as 53% with the incidence of occlusion ranging from 9% to 16%.[4,5] Tollefson and Ernst and Schreiber and colleagues have suggested that lesions that are preocclusive in nature (greater than 80% stenosis) are at a high risk to proceed to occlusion.[4,5] In view of this, we repair asymptomatic bilateral renal artery preocclusive stenoses (greater than 80%) or preocclusive stenosis in a solitary kidney in conjunction with aortic aneurysm repair in patients who are otherwise good risks medically.

There is a small subgroup of patients with documented renovascular hypertension from a small kidney who have nonreconstructible vessels and negligible or no residual excretory function. In these patients we advocate aortic aneurysm repair with adjunctive nephrectomy of the nonfunctional kidney. As reported initially by Sonkodi and co-workers, nephrectomy not only can improve blood pressure control but also may improve total renal function.[6]

Some renal artery aneurysms require repair in conjunction with aortic aneurysmorrhaphy. Renal artery aneurysms greater than 2 cm, especially those contributing to renovascular hypertension, those that are embolizing, or those that are expanding on serial duplex scans or arteriographic studies, warrant adjunctive reconstruction during aortic aneurysm repair.

INDICATIONS FOR VISCERAL REVASCULARIZATION

Indications for visceral artery repair in conjunction with aortic aneurysm repair are mainly twofold (Table 1). The first are those accepted indications for visceral revascularization for chronic mesenteric ischemia. The second is visceral revascularization to prevent or treat postoperative intestinal ischemia.

Visceral revascularization for chronic mesenteric ischemia is recommended for individuals who have the typical constellation of progressive weight loss, postprandial abdominal pain, no other intra-abdominal pathology, and high-grade stenoses or occlusions of both the superior mesenteric artery (SMA) and celiac artery. Although the need for adjunctive mesenteric revascularization with aortic reconstruction was described by Connolly and Kwaan over ten years ago, the need for it is relatively uncommon.[7] Mesenteric duplex imaging is utilized to help assess these patients preoperatively. Duplex scan criteria for mesenteric arterial stenoses greater than 70% is a fasting peak systolic velocity in the celiac artery and SMA of greater than 200 cm/second and 275 cm/second, respectively. Adjunctive mesenteric revascularization is generally performed in individuals with symptomatic chronic visceral ischemia or in asymptomatic individuals who have preocclusive or occlusive disease of the SMA and celiac artery, documented by lateral aortography, and evidence of significant collateral blood flow with meandering mesenteric artery flow from the inferior mesenteric artery (IMA) to the SMA.[8]

Some individuals have no evidence clinically of chronic mesenteric ischemia, but upon completion of aortic reconstruction, have evidence of colonic ischemia. The incidence averages 2% but has been reported to be higher, averaging 9.3%, if postoperative colonoscopy is utilized.[9] Intraoperative assessment that can foreshadow the possibility of postoperative colon ischemia is a widely patent IMA that has minimal or no backbleeding upon opening the aneurysm. Readily available intraoperative maneuvers that can be performed to assist in the determination of inadequate blood flow to the colon include the loss of Doppler signals in the colon with IMA occlusion and IMA stump blood pressure measurements less than 40 mm Hg. Loss of arterial pulsation with unmeasurable transcolonic oxygen saturations using a pulse oximeter probe also suggest inadequate colonic blood flow.[8] Restoration of blood flow to at least one hypogastric artery is generally adequate to prevent colonic ischemia. However, if the blood flow to both hypogastric arteries is in jeopardy or collateral flow is inadequate, reimplantation of a patent IMA is usually sufficient treatment. If the IMA is not patent, and the blood flow from the SMA and celiac artery is compromised, alternative methods of visceral reconstruction are required. Our preference is to expose the SMA in the root of the small bowel mesentery and perform a bypass from the aortic graft to the SMA.

PREOPERATIVE ASSESSMENT

A decision for AAA repair with or without concomitant renal or visceral reconstruction must be made in the context of the patient's overall medical condition. The single most important determinant of successful outcome in aortic reconstruction is cardiac status. Thirty-one percent of patients undergoing aortic reconstruction for aneurysmal disease have been found to have significant, reconstructible coronary artery disease.[10] Thus, all patients considered for AAA repair undergo complete cardiac evaluation including history, physical examination, and usually some type of physiologic stress test, either a graded exercise stress test or thallium stress test. For those individuals unable to exercise, dipyridamole thallium-201 myocardial imaging or, more recently, adenosine thallium-201 is utilized. Adenosine, a potent direct coronary vasodilator, is now preferred over dipyridamole because of its rapid onset of action and very short half-life of less than 2 seconds. Cardiac catheterization is performed in individuals identified at risk, with coronary angioplasty or coronary artery bypass grafting performed prior to aortic reconstruction, should critical coronary artery disease be identified.

Individuals with significant nonreconstructible coronary artery disease, or other severe comorbid diseases require balanced judgment regarding what intervention,

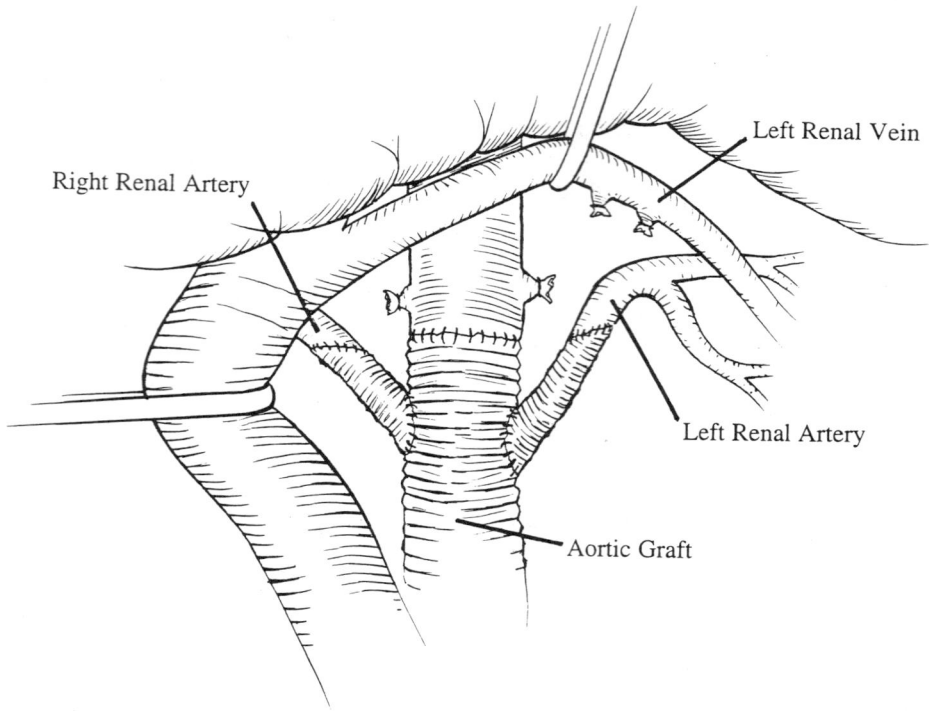

Figure 1 Bilateral aortorenal bypass. Note renal anastomoses are spatulated and end-to-end.

if any, should be entertained. Renal and visceral artery duplex imaging is performed if there is evidence of renovascular hypertension, renal failure, or chronic mesenteric ischemia. Patients routinely donate three units of their own blood prior to operation to decrease the requirement for banked blood.

OPERATIVE MANAGEMENT

All patients receive a preoperative bowel preparation with polyethylene glycol to reduce the fecal load and oral simethicone to minimize intestinal distention. Antibiotics, usually cefazolin, are given on induction of anesthesia and maintained postoperatively until all lines and catheters are removed. Intraoperative management involves close monitoring with a radial artery catheter, urinary catheter, and a Swan-Ganz pulmonary artery catheter. Transesophageal two-dimensional echocardiography is used in patients with severely compromised cardiac function. Patients undergoing aortic aneurysm repair and concomitant renal or visceral arterial reconstruction uniformly receive heparin sodium and mannitol prior to aortic cross-clamping. Protamine sulfate is given subsequently for heparin effect reversal. Operative autotransfusion is used routinely. Spinal catheter drainage is not utilized. Transient renal arterial infusion is occasionally performed, using a chilled balanced salt solution containing heparin sodium and mannitol, if a long renal cross-clamp time is expected.

The approach to the aorta is generally transabdominal for aneurysms that are infrarenal or juxtarenal. Suprarenal and supraceliac aneurysms are exposed by a

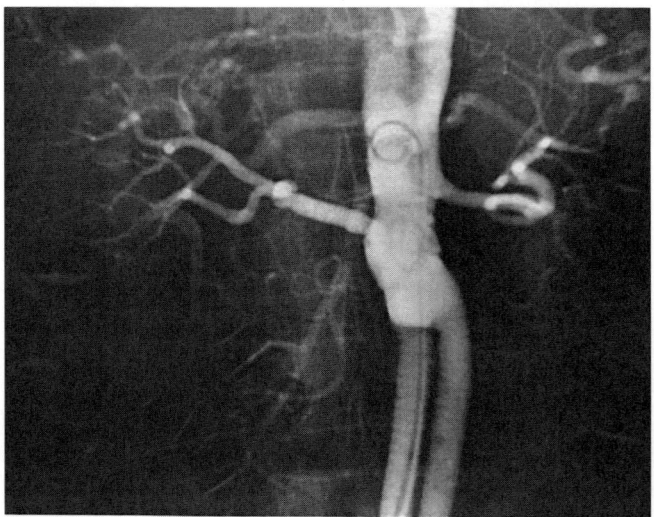

Figure 2 Postoperative arteriography demonstrating right aortorenal artery bypass with saphenous vein.

left flank retroperitoneal approach with an inclusion technique of revascularization for the renal and visceral vessels.

A collagen-impregnated Dacron graft requiring no preclotting is used for the aortic graft with the proximal anastomosis performed in an end-to-end fashion and the distal anastomoses performed end-to-end for aortic straight grafts and generally end-to-side for bifurcated grafts. Methods for renal revascularization must be tailored to the situation encountered, and many methods

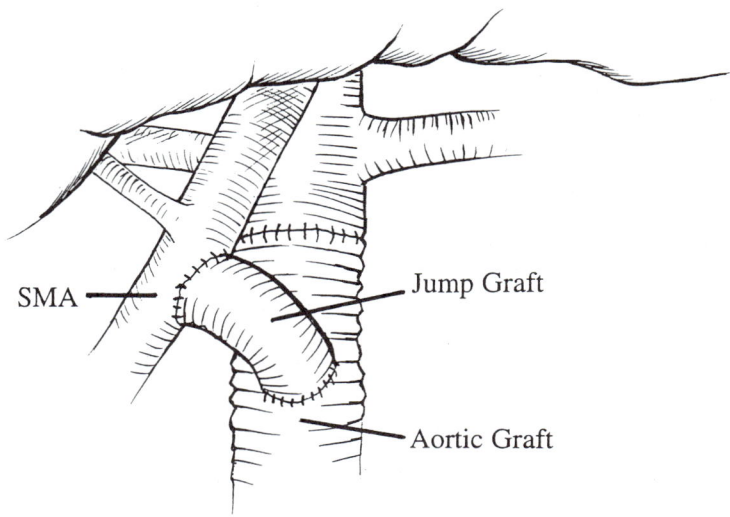

Figure 3 Aortic graft to superior mesenteric artery *(SMA)* bypass. Note short graft length with preferential use of prosthetic material as the conduit.

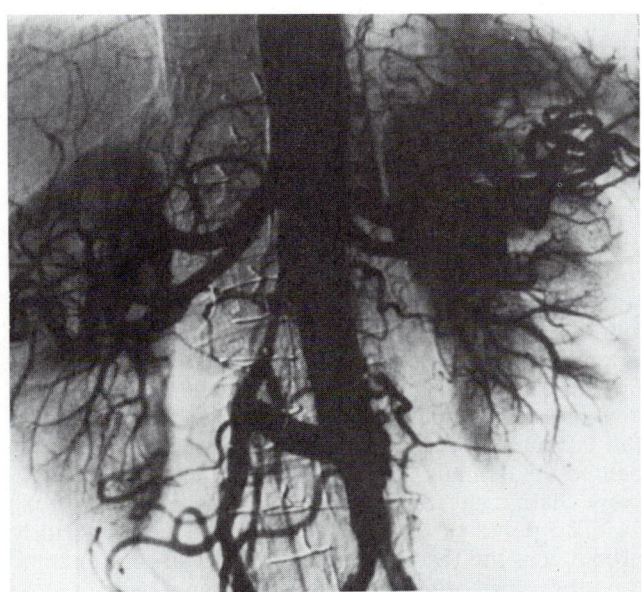

Figure 4 Postoperative arteriography demonstrating patent aortosuperior mesenteric artery bypass.

should be in the surgeon's armamentarium, including endarterectomy and bypass. If direct reimplantation is not possible, our preference is to use reversed saphenous vein as the conduit with polytetrafluoroethylene (PTFE) utilized if inadequate vein is present. The proximal end of the renal bypass is end-to-side to the aortic graft, and the distal anastomosis to the renal artery is spatulated and end-to-end. The right renal bypass should ideally lie behind the vena cava, although this is not always advantageous (Figs. 1 and 2).

Visceral vessel reconstruction, if performed for intraoperative colonic ischemia, may require only IMA reimplantation into the side of the aortic graft. However, if the patient has had preoperative evidence of chronic mesenteric ischemia, an aortic graft to SMA bypass using PTFE or Dacron is preferred. It is our bias to use a prosthetic graft for the aortic graft to SMA bypass, keeping the graft short and having it lie straight to minimize the risk of kinking of the graft when the intestines are restored to the abdominal cavity (Figs. 3 and 4). It is essential to perform the distal anastomosis to the SMA first, in an end-to-side fashion, to facilitate a meticulous distal anastomosis with the graft then placed end-to-side into the side of the aortic graft. If the IMA is patent, it too should be reimplanted.

REFERENCES

1. Stanley JC, Fry WJ. Surgical treatment of renovascular hypertension. Arch Surg 1977; 112:1291–1297.
2. Lyons DL, Streck WF, Kem DC, et al. Captopril stimulation of differential renins in renovascular hypertension. Hypertension 1983; 5:615–622.
3. Dean RH, Englund R, Dupont WD, et al. Retrieval of renal function by revascularization. Study of preoperative outcome predictors. Ann Surg 1985; 202:367–375.
4. Tollefson DFJ, Ernst CB. Natural history of atherosclerotic renal artery stenosis with aortic disease. J Vasc Surg 1991; 14:327–331.
5. Schreiber MJ, Pohl MA, Novick AC. The natural history of atherosclerotic and fibrous renal artery disease. Urol Clin North Am 1984; 11:383–392.
6. Sonkodi S, Abraham G, Mohalsi G. Effects of nephrectomy on hypertension, renin activity and total renal function in patients with chronic renal artery occlusion. J Hum Hypertens 1990; 4:277–279.
7. Connolly JE, Kwaan JHM. Prophylactic revascularization of the gut. Ann Surg 1979; 190:514–521.
8. Tollefson DFJ, Ernst CB. Gastrointestinal and visceral ischemic complications of aortic reconstruction. In: Bernhard VM, Towne JB, eds. Complications in vascular surgery. St Louis: Quality Medical Publishing, 1991:135.
9. Tollefson DFJ, Ernst CB. Colon ischemia following aortic reconstruction. Ann Vasc Surg 1991; 5:485–489.
10. Young JR, Hertzer NR, Beven EG, et al. Coronary artery disease in patients with aortic aneurysm: A classification of 302 coronary angiograms and results of surgical management. Ann Vasc Surg 1986; 1:36–42.

RENAL ECTOPIA AND RENAL FUSION IN PATIENTS REQUIRING ABDOMINAL AORTIC OPERATIONS

MAX R. GASPAR, M.D.
HARRIS J. WATERS, M.D.
ALLEN W. AVERBOOK, M.D.

Table 1 Classification of Renal Ectopia

I. Anomalies of position
  A. Simple ectopia
    1. Pelvic kidney
    2. Iliac kidney
    3. Abdominal kidney
    4. Thoracic kidney
II. Anomalies of form and fusion
  A. Horseshoe kidney
  B. Crossed renal ectopia without fusion
    1. Solitary crossed renal ectopia
    2. Bilaterally crossed renal ectopia
  C. Crossed renal ectopia with fusion
    1. Unilateral fused kidney with inferior ectopia
    2. Unilateral fused kidney with superior ectopia
    3. Sigmoid or S-shaped kidney
    4. Lump kidney
    5. L-shaped kidney
    6. Disk kidney

Adapted from Perlmutter AD, Retik AB, Bauer SB. Anomalies of the upper urinary tract. In: Walsh PC, Gittes RF, Perlmutter AD, Stamey TA, eds. Urology, 5th ed. Philadelphia: WB Saunders, 1986: 1665.

Congenital variations in renal anatomy challenge the ingenuity of surgeons operating on the abdominal aorta. Renal ectopia and renal fusion create problems with exposure and surgical dissection, and pose dangers with regard to aberrant blood supply, abnormal venous return, and abnormally located ureters. An ectopic kidney can be found anywhere from the thorax to the pelvis, and can be contralateral to the side of entry of its ureter into the bladder. Once the ectopic kidney crosses the midline, there is potential for fusion with the opposite kidney.

CLASSIFICATION AND ANATOMY

A classification has been adapted by the authors (Table 1) for ease of application in vascular surgery.[1]

Simple Renal Ectopia

The pelvic kidney is opposite the sacrum and below the level of the aortic bifurcation. The lumbar kidney rests opposite the sacral promontory in the iliac fossa and anterior to the iliac vessels. The abdominal kidney is located above the iliac crest and adjacent to the second lumbar vertebra. A thoracic kidney partially or completely protrudes above the diaphragm into the posterior mediastinum at the foramen of Bochdalek and is very rare.

In simple renal ectopia, the kidney can be supplied by one or more main renal arteries from the distal aorta or aortic bifurcation, with one or more aberrant arteries from the common or external iliac arteries or even from the inferior mesenteric artery. The kidney can be supplied entirely by multiple arteries, none of which arise from the aorta. The ureter is usually short and tortuous but enters the bladder on the ipsilateral side.

Horseshoe Kidney

The horseshoe kidney is a form of fusion consisting of two distinct renal masses that lie vertically on either side of the aorta and are connected by a parenchymatous or fibrous isthmus at the midline of the body. The lower poles are fused in 95% of patients, and the upper poles in 5%. The isthmus can be high on the aorta or very low in the pelvis and can pass between the inferior vena cava and the aorta or even behind both vessels.[2]

Variations in the vasculature of the horseshoe kidney are numerous. The more common varieties of arterial anomalies can be summarized as follows: (1) a single artery to each half of the kidney, (2) a single artery to each half plus an additional artery to the isthmus, (3) two renal arteries to each half and two arteries to the isthmus, (4) multiple renal arteries, numbering from four to ten, to all portions of the renal parenchyma. Vessels supplying the horseshoe kidney may arise anywhere along the aorta, occasionally from the common or external iliac arteries, and even from the sacral or mesenteric vessels. The isthmus has the most aberrant arterial origins, including the aorta either above or below the isthmus or from multiple small arteries entering behind the isthmus. In general, as the arterial pattern is more chaotic, the venous pattern is also more abnormal.

The pelvis of each kidney segment lies anteriorly, probably as the result of incomplete renal rotation, and the ureter may originate high on the renal pelvis and lie laterally. The ureter courses downward anterior to the isthmus and may deviate laterally if the midline fusion is thick. Accessory ureters are not uncommon.

Crossed Renal Ectopia Without Fusion

Crossed renal ectopia is a renal anomaly in which an ectopic kidney is located on the opposite side from its ureteral insertion into the bladder. The two subdivisions are solitary and bilaterally crossed renal ectopia (Fig. 1).

Crossed Renal Ectopia With Fusion

Crossed renal ectopia with fusion may take several forms (Fig. 2). The fused kidney can be a single elongated mass or variously configured. If the crossed ureter comes from the lower portion of the fused mass,

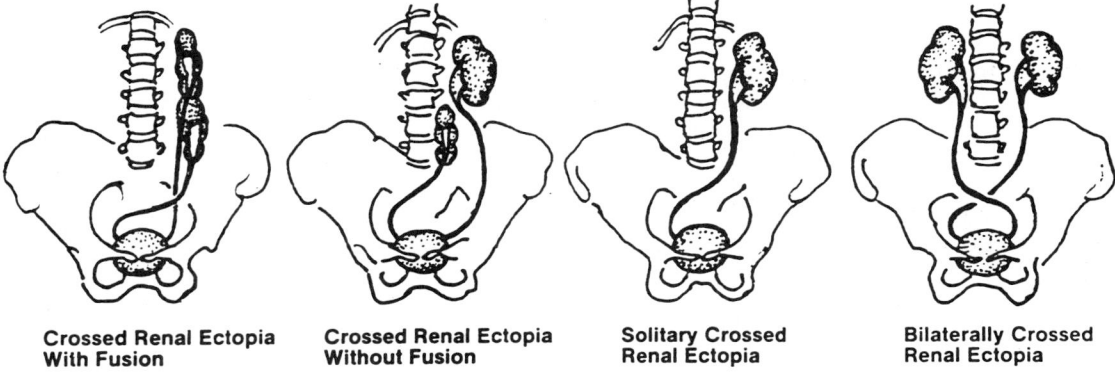

Figure 1 Four types of crossed renal ectopia. (From McDonald JH, McClelland DS. Am J Surg 1957; 93:995–1001; with permission.)

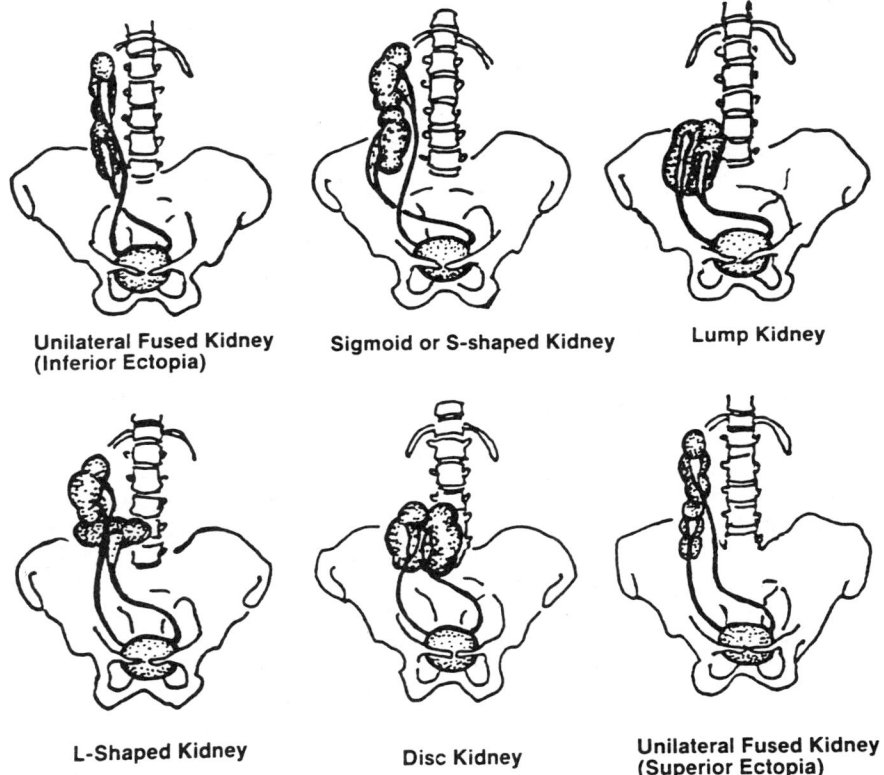

Figure 2 Six forms of crossed renal ectopia with fusion. (From McDonald JH, McClelland DS. Am J Surg 1957; 93:995–1001; with permission.)

it is classified as unilateral fused kidney with inferior ectopia. If it comes from the upper portion of the fused masses (the rarest configuration), it is classified as unilateral fused kidney with superior ectopia. The fused kidney may be S-shaped or L-shaped. The kidneys may be fused side by side, in which case they are called a lump kidney, or they may be fused at the superior and inferior poles, in which case they are called a disk or doughnut kidney.

Crossed renal ectopia is notorious for variability in vascular supply to the kidneys.[3] Of the arteries, 75% arise from the upper abdominal aorta, and the remainder from the lower portion of the aorta or from the common iliac arteries. Only in rare instances do the arteries arise from other sources, such as mesenteric or sacral vessels. The total number of arteries may vary from one to six, but most have two to four. In solitary crossed renal ectopia, the blood supply usually is from a single renal artery that originates from the common iliac artery on the same side as the kidney. In a crossed renal ectopia with fusion, the superior kidney usually receives one or two arteries from the abdominal aorta, and the inferior ectopic kidney receives one or more arteries from the lower aorta or common iliac artery. Attempts to classify arterial supply serve little purpose because it is so variable. The more variable the arterial supply, the more the venous anatomy tends to be altered.

PREOPERATIVE EVALUATION

When aortic reconstruction for aneurysm or occlusive disease is contemplated, the surgeon occasionally palpates an abnormal abdominal mass that might represent an ectopic kidney. Any preoperative noninvasive imaging techniques such as ultrasound, computed tomography (CT), or magnetic resonance imaging is capable of documenting such abnormal masses or, equally important, may note the absence of a normally located kidney. When ultrasound is performed to estimate aneurysm size, radiologists and surgeons should check for kidneys in the usual location. Most patients scheduled for abdominal aortic reconstruction have one or more imaging studies. Particularly helpful is CT with contrast. Thoughtful radiologists and surgeons are aware of the possibility of abnormalities in the urinary system and pay particular attention to this aspect of the scan. Intravenous pyelography, although performed less frequently, is very sensitive in uncovering abnormal renal anatomy but is poor for delineating renal blood supply.

Aortography before aneurysm resection is not always necessary, but it is imperative to delineate the blood supply when urinary anomalies are suspected. Multiple views, including occasional selective arterial catheterization, may be needed for an adequate outline of the renal arteries. The late renal excretory phase should be obtained to opacify the renal collecting system, including the course of the ureters. Venous phase imaging is also helpful. Identifying aberrant renal arteries is the single most important issue to be confronted in determining surgical management.

The detection of ectopic kidneys may cause the surgeon to re-evaluate the indications for aortic reconstruction because the risk of operation is increased for such patients. However, aortic reconstruction can be done in the presence of abnormal renal anatomy with little increase in mortality, providing the operation is carefully planned and superbly executed.

OPERATIVE MANAGEMENT

The location of the ectopic renal tissue, the presence or absence of fusion, and the number, origin, and course of aberrant arteries dictate the best surgical approach. The surgeon should have a primary operative plan but must also have enough experience to be flexible and capable of altering the plan. This is often the place for surgical innovation.

Basically, there are three approaches for exposure: transperitoneal, retroperitoneal, and transperitoneal with medial rotation of viscera.

The traditional transperitoneal approach via a midline incision is probably the least useful, although it is adequate in instances of nonfused ectopia or fusion with no or few aberrant vessels. It has been used extensively for horseshoe kidney, but the difficulty in this situation is the lack of exposure of the segment of aorta posterior to the isthmus. If the renal mass is easily mobile after it is dissected off the anterior aortic wall, it can be mobilized superiorly and inferiorly as needed for exposure. An aortic graft may be passed behind the kidney once the proximal anastomosis is complete. The fewer aberrant vessels and the more proximal they are on the aorta, the more mobile the ectopic kidney is, as well as the isthmus of a fused or horseshoe kidney. Renal mobility becomes limited and exposure difficult as the number of aberrant arteries arising from the distal aorta or the iliac vessels increase.

If the isthmus of a horseshoe kidney is thin and fibrous, it may be divided and oversewn. However, in a thick isthmus the renal pelvis may extend across the midline. Some surgeons have transected and oversewn the isthmus in such situations, but it is not recommended because of the risk of urine leak.

The left-sided retroperitoneal approach is particularly useful for horseshoe kidney.[4,5] It facilitates preservation of the blood supply to the renal mass by utilizing Crawford's inclusion technique when there are multiple arteries supplying the parenchyma.[6] Such an approach also allows endarterectomy or bypass of an occluded or severely stenotic aorta. Difficulty arises when there is extensive arterial or occlusive disease of the right common or external iliac arteries. This can be overcome by an auxiliary incision in the right lower quadrant of the abdomen for extraperitoneal exposure of the right iliac vessels. If necessary, grafts can be tunneled to the femoral arteries from the retroperitoneal approach.

The most versatile approach for crossed renal ectopia with fusion, and the one we favor, is a midline transperitoneal incision with medial rotation of viscera from either the left or the right side. This was a common method of operating upon abdominal aortic aneurysms in the 1950s, when aneurysms were resected rather than treated with inlay grafts. Superb exposure of the infrarenal aorta and all of its branches, including any aberrant renal arteries, can be obtained by rotating the entire ascending colon and transverse colon to the left after incising the posterior parietal peritoneum lateral to the ascending colon. Similarly, superb exposure of the entire abdominal aorta and iliac arteries can be obtained by rotation of the viscera from left to right after incision of the posterior parietal peritoneum lateral to the descending colon. If the fused ectopic renal mass is located on the right side of the aorta, its arterial supply can be exposed by rotation of the viscera from left to right without disturbing the renal tissue. Conversely, if

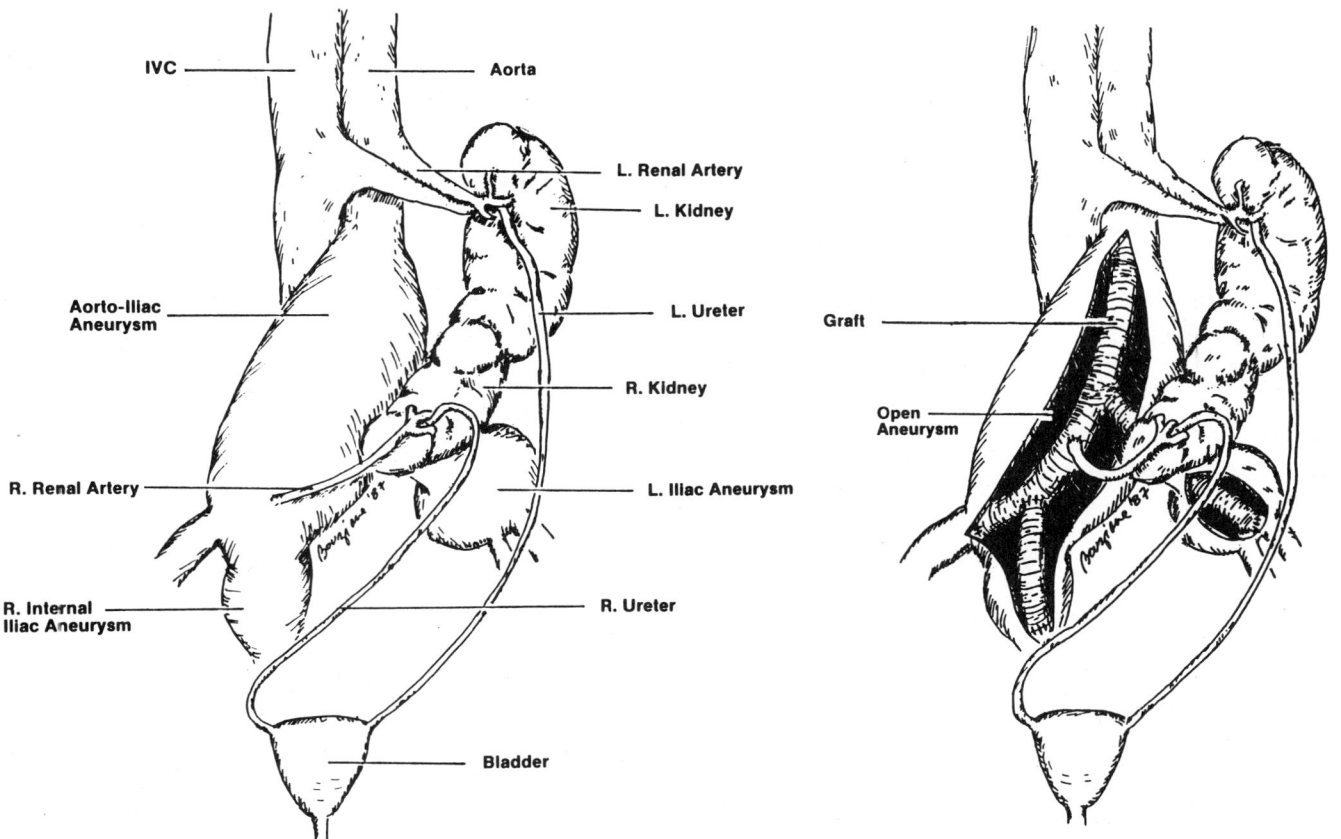

Figure 3 *A,* Artist's rendition of abdominal aortic aneurysm with right common iliac and hypogastric aneurysms and left common iliac aneurysm in patient with crossed renal inferior ectopia with fusion. *B,* Entire pathology exposed by transperitoneal midline incision and rotation of ascending and transverse colon from right to left. Aneurysms replaced with Dacron graft with reimplantation of anomalous right renal artery without disturbing aberrant renal tissue. (From Waters, HJ, Gaspar MR. J Vasc Surg 1989; 9:172–176; with permission.)

the ectopic fused renal mass is on the left, its arterial supply can be exposed by rotation from right to left. If there are multiple aneurysms, as in a case we reported,[7] the transperitoneal medial visceral rotation approach is ideal. It allows full exposure of the aberrant vascular anatomy and the renal anomalies (Fig. 3).

Reimplantation of aberrant vessels by means of a Carrel patch is preferred. This is especially appropriate for multiple vessels whose orifices can be included in one patch, as well as for a small-caliber vessel whose orifice might otherwise be narrowed by direct anastomosis. Endarterectomy of associated renal arterial occlusive disease can also be performed at the time of implantation, if necessary. If the aberrant vessel to be reimplanted is too short, an interposition graft of synthetic or autogenous material can be used.

Various renal preservation techniques can be used. Cold perfusate used for long-term preservation is not necessary or practical for short-term renal protection, but cold perfusion by instilling 4°C Ringer's lactate solution directly into the renal vessels for up to 120 minutes will protect from ischemia. Ureteral catheterization for ease of identifying ureters is optional.

REFERENCES

1. Perlmutter AD, Retik AB, Bauer SB. Anomalies of the upper urinary tract. In: Walsh PC, Gittes RF, Perlmutter AD, Stamey TA, eds. Urology, 5th ed. Philadelphia: WB Saunders, 1986:1665.
2. Bietz DS, Merendino KA. Abdominal aneurysm and horseshoe kidney: A review. Ann Surg 1975; 181:333–341.
3. Rubenstein ZJ, Hertx M, Shamin N, Deutsch V. Crossed renal ectopia: Angiographic findings in six cases. Am J Roentgenol 1976; 126:1035–1038.
4. Crawford ES, Coselli JS, Safi HJ, et al. The impact of renal fusion and ectopia on aortic surgery. J Vasc Surg 1988; 8:375–383.
5. O'Hara PJ, Hakaim AG, Hertzer NR, et al. Surgical management of aortic aneurysm and coexistent horseshoe kidney: Review of a 31-year experience. J Vasc Surg 1993; 17:940–947.
6. Crawford SE, Crawford JL. Diseases of the aorta. Baltimore: Williams & Wilkins, 1984.
7. Waters HJ, Gaspar MR. Abdominal aortic and multiple iliac aneurysms with crossed-fused ectopia of the kidney: A case report and review. J Vasc Surg 1989; 9:172–176.

AORTIC RECONSTRUCTION IN RENAL TRANSPLANT PATIENTS

GARY W. GIBBONS, M.D.
CHRISTOPHER J. KWOLEK, M.D.

Table 1 Methods of Renal Graft Perfusion During Aortoiliac Reconstruction in Renal Transplant Patients

Permanent axillofemoral graft
Ascending aorta to femoral bypass
Transluminal angioplasty
Intraluminal stent for aneurysm
Temporary axillo or brachial shunt to ipsilateral femoral or iliac artery
Temporary upper abdominal aorta to ipsilateral iliac or femoral artery shunt
Proximal aortic graft to ipsilateral iliac or femoral artery with temporary Pruitt-Inhara shunt
Pump oxygenator by way of ipsilateral femoral artery and vein
Hypothermic perfusion of ipsilateral iliac artery
Removal, mechanical perfusion, and reimplantation of transplanted kidney
Aortoiliac reconstruction without renal transplant protection

The initial and long-term cost-effective success and survival of patients undergoing renal transplantation has extended its indications to include more complicated patients with end-stage renal disease, including diabetic and elderly patients. Many of these patients have accelerated atherosclerosis secondary to chronic renal failure and prolonged dialysis, arterial hypertension, and other vascular disease risk factors. Despite renal transplantation, atherosclerotic vascular disease may progress and later result in limb- or life-threatening complications. It has been shown that despite the concern about potential prosthetic graft infection in patients receiving post-transplant immunosuppression, subsequent vascular reconstruction in these patients can be accomplished with acceptable risks.[1,2]

Regarding aortic reconstruction in renal transplant patients, a major concern addresses optimal renal graft perfusion during vascular reconstruction. It has been shown that a normal kidney cannot tolerate more than 30 minutes of normothermic ischemia without tubular damage. The assumption that temporary warm ischemia of the renal transplant is poorly tolerated has been questioned. As early as 1956, Morris and co-workers had shown experimentally that kidneys perfused at a low arterial pressure of only 25 mm Hg remain viable.[3] Crawford and Vaccaro's experience with significant periods of proximal aortic occlusion for surgical treatment of thoracoabdominal aneurysms, without protective measures for the kidneys, documented an incidence of renal insufficiency of only 10%, and this insufficiency was usually transient.[4] Prolonged aortic occlusion times had an adverse effect on renal function after resection of thoracoabdominal aneurysms.

Lacombe has pointed out that the transplanted kidney is not completely ischemic and is still partially perfused during aortic cross-clamping by the retrograde flow from the lumbar, inferior mesenteric, and iliac arteries.[5] He maintains that this flow ensures sufficient perfusion of the kidney with pressures greater than 35 mm Hg. His results as well as those of Harris and May lead them to conclude that aortoiliac repair without protection of the kidney transplant did not entail excessive risk.[6,7] This opinion, however, appears to be in the minority. These authors also concluded that the transplanted kidney must not have functional impairment, that careful technique is mandatory, and that vascular occlusion time must be kept at a minimum. One would also have to question this technique when the collateral circulation to the transplanted kidney would be sparse, as in the patient with concomitant iliac occlusive disease.

All would agree that protection of renal function is of the utmost importance during an aortic reconstruction in renal transplant recipients. Various methods for maintaining renal perfusion have been described (Table 1). In 1977 Sterioff and Parks reported on the use of a polyvinyl tubing shunt between the upper abdominal aorta and the ipsilateral common iliac artery to maintain perfusion of a renal transplant during abdominal aortic aneurysmectomy.[8] Hughes and associates, using a temporary Gott shunt from suprarenal to ipsilateral common femoral artery, noted the advantage that dissection near the renal graft is minimal or avoided.[9] Cox and Sabiston recommended the use heparin sodium–bonded shunts in the preservation of renal artery blood flow during correction of complicated abdominal aortic aneurysms.[10] O'Mara and associates described a Gott shunt from the suprarenal abdominal aorta to the ipsilateral superficial femoral artery that allowed retrograde perfusion to the transplanted kidney while allowing repair of coexisting common iliac artery aneurysms.[11] All of the methods utilizing a suprarenal aortic shunt carry the risk of atheromatous embolization, and careful flushing is required. Extensive atherosclerosis may also preclude placement of a aortic shunt.

Campbell and colleagues in 1981 reported using a pump-oxygenator for perfusion of the transplanted kidney by way of the ipsilateral femoral artery and vein during aortic aneurysm repair.[12] Some hospitals may not be equipped with extracorporeal circulatory support, and the added expense may be unnecessary. In centers where this option is available, it may be preferable for the hypotensive patient with a leaking aortic aneurysm, especially in that it can be done with local anesthesia prior to commencement of aortic reconstruction.

Laborde and colleagues used a Pruitt-Inahara shunt to perfuse the transplanted kidney during aortic aneurysm repair.[13] Although this technique is simple, there is some renal ischemia time because the proximal anastomosis must be completed before the shunt can function.

Nghiem and Lee in 1982 described in situ hypothermic preservation of the renal graft by perfusion of the ipsilateral iliac artery with 4°C Ringer's lactate solution.[14] The technique of removing and mechanically perfusing a transplanted kidney during aortic reconstruction with subsequent renal reimplantation, while an option, carries the risk of injury to the transplanted kidney and is not recommended.

The ascending aorta also presents a possible origination site for aortofemoral grafting. Under appropriate circumstances in a patient with severe aortoiliac occlusive disease, this option could be used without interrupting the flow to the renal graft. End of graft to side of abdominal aorta is another possibility under certain circumstances. Transluminal angioplasty may be considered an option for isolated, short-segment occlusive disease. Intraluminal stents for aneurysmal disease require further investigation in transplant patients.

In 1982 we described a temporary axillofemoral bypass graft to maintain transplant perfusion during aortoiliac reconstruction.[15] This method of temporary heparin-bonded tube shunting from the axillary or brachial artery to the femoral artery carries a low risk of atheromatous emboli to the renal graft and allows minimal dissection around the transplant. The disadvantages include possible trauma to the axillary or brachial artery and the additional time necessary for exposure and isolation of these arteries. Permanent axillofemoral bypass may be the only suitable method if prosthetic material should not be placed, such as in patients with a septic retroperitoneum.

Many therapeutic alternatives exist for the management of renal transplant patients requiring aortoiliac reconstruction for aneurysmal or occlusive disease. Each alternative has specific advantages and disadvantages. Except in certain instances, aortoiliac reconstruction without renal protection appears to carry an excessive risk to the transplanted kidney. The alternative chosen should allow (1) physiologic perfusion of the kidney transplant, (2) minimal or no ischemic time for the kidney, (3) minimal or no dissection near the renal transplant, and (4) and a technique that is available and cost-effective. Most important is a carefully planned preoperative strategy considering the specific risk-benefit ratio of each technique to allow individual successful aortoiliac reconstruction for occlusive or aneurysmal disease in the renal transplant patient.

REFERENCES

1. Benvenisty AI, Todd GJ, Argenziano M, et al. Management of peripheral vascular problems in recipients of cardiac allografts. J Vasc Surg 1992; 16:895–902.
2. Sterioff S Jr, Zachary JB, William GM. Dacron vascular grafts in the renal transplant patients. Am J Surg 1974; 127:525.
3. Morris GC Jr, Heider CF, Moyer JH. The protective effect of subfiltration arterial pressure on the kidney. Surg Forum 1956; 6:623–624.
4. Crawford ES, Vaccaro PS. Thoracoabdominal aortic aneurysm. In: Bergan JJ, Yao JST, eds. Aneurysms: Diagnosis and treatment, New York:Grune & Stratton, 1982:151.
5. Lacombe M. Abdominal aortic aneurysmectomy in renal transplant patients. Ann Surg 1986; 203:62–68.
6. Lacombe M. Aortoiliac surgery in renal transplant patients. J Vasc Surg 1991; 13:712–718.
7. Harris JP, May J. Successful aortic surgery after renal transplantation without protection of the transplanted kidney. J Vasc Surg 1987; 5;457–461.
8. Sterioff S, Parks L. Temporary vascular by-pass for perfusion of a renal transplant during abdominal aneurysmectomy. Surgery 1977; 82:558–560.
9. Hughes JD, Milfeld DJ, Shield CF III. Renal transplant perfusion during aortoiliac aneurysmectomy. J Vasc Surg 1985; 2:600–602.
10. Cox JL, Sabiston DC. The use of heparin bonded shunts for perfusion of the renal artery during resection of complex abdominal aortic aneurysms. Surg Gynecol Obstet 1978; 147:859–864.
11. O'Mara CS, Flinn WR, Bergan JJ, Yao JST. Use of a temporary shunt for renal transplant protection during aortic aneurysm repair. Surgery 1983; 94:512–517.
12. Campbell DA, Lorber MI, Arneson WA, et al. Renal transplant protection during abdominal aortic aneurysmectomy with pump oxygenator. Surgery 1981; 90:559–562.
13. Laborde AL, Hoballah JJ, Sharp WJ, et al. A simple technique of renal transplant preservation during aortic reconstruction. Ann Vasc Surg 1992; 6:550–552.
14. Nghiem DD, Lee HM. Insitu hypothermic preservation of a renal allograft during resection of abdominal aortic aneurysm. Am Surg 1982; 48:237–238.
15. Gibbons GW, Madras PN, Wheelock FC, et al. Aortoiliac reconstruction following renal transplantation. Surgery 1982; 91:435–437.

VENOUS ANOMALIES ENCOUNTERED DURING AORTIC RECONSTRUCTION

JOSEPH M. GIORDANO, M.D.

Aortic reconstruction has become a safe and effective procedure because of impressive advances in surgical technique, anesthesia, cardiac assessment, and postoperative management. Despite a low complication rate, improvements in morbidity and mortality are a constant goal. Although unusual today, massive bleeding during aortic dissection is always a risk and can cause death. This bleeding can occur if the surgeon is unaware of venous anomalies that can complicate the aortic dissection.

DEVELOPMENT OF THE INFERIOR VENA CAVA

The inferior vena cava (IVC) forms during the first trimester from three parallel pairs of veins that appear during different periods of gestation (Fig. 1).[1,2] After forming extensive anastomotic channels, the veins undergo partial regression, and the remaining segments form the iliac veins and the IVC. Located on the posterior aspect of the fetus, the posterior cardinal veins appear first. However, most of the cardinal veins disappear, with the most proximal and distal sections forming the azygous system and the iliac bifurcation. The subcardinal veins form anterior and medial to the regressing posterior cardinal veins. The left subcardinal vein completely disappears, but the right subcardinal vein forms the suprarenal IVC. Posterior to the abdominal aorta, the supracardinal veins form last. The left supracardinal vein regresses, but the right remains to form the infrarenal IVC. At the level of the renal veins extensive anastomotic channels form between the subcardinal and supracardinal systems. These coalesce to form a large vein anterior and posterior to the aorta that drains the left kidney. Eventually the vein posterior to the aorta disappears and the anterior vein becomes the left renal vein.

This complex process understandably can produce venous anomalies, four of which are clinically relevant.[3-5] First, duplication of the IVC, with a reported incidence of 0.2% to 3%, consists of large veins on both sides of the infrarenal aorta that usually join anterior or posterior to the aorta at the level of the renal arteries. The anomaly occurs from failure of the left supracardinal vein to regress. Second, transposition, or left-sided IVC, with an incidence of 0.2% to 0.5%, consists of a large vein to the left of the aorta and an absent right-sided IVC. The left-sided IVC crosses to the right at the level of the renal arteries to form the suprarenal IVC. Because of the transposition the left adrenal and gonadal veins empty into the IVC, and the right adrenal and gonadal veins empty into the right renal vein, the mirror image of the normal anatomy. Third, circumaortic left renal vein, with an incidence of 1.5% to 8.7%, consists of a vein anterior and posterior to the aorta. This anomaly occurs from failure of the vein posterior to the aorta to regress, forming a venous collar around the aorta just before the renal vein enters the IVC. Fourth, a retroaortic left renal vein, with an incidence of 1.2% to 2.4%, occurs from regression of the vein anterior to the aorta and persistence of the posterior vein so that the left renal vein crosses posterior to the aorta to join the IVC. Both duplications and the left-sided IVC are frequently associated with anomalies of the renal vein. Therefore, a left-sided IVC can be accompanied by a circumaortic or a retroaortic left renal vein.

DIAGNOSIS

Prior to the routine use of computed tomography (CT) imaging, most venous anomalies were diagnosed at operation during the dissection of the aorta. Sonography can sometimes detect duplication or left-sided IVC, but this is not common.[6] Since forewarned is forearmed, CT scans are performed on all patients scheduled for resection of abdominal aortic aneurysm but not routinely for patients who undergo other infrarenal aortic procedures. This helps diagnose venous anomalies and other unusual complicating problems such as inflammatory aneurysms, horseshoe kidney, extension of the aneurysm above the renal arteries, and iliac artery aneurysms. The surgeon should systematically consider each venous anomaly as part of the review of the CT scan.[7,8] Is the IVC in its normal location just to the right of the abdominal aorta? Is there an identical structure to the left of the abdominal aorta, indicating a duplication of the IVC (Fig. 2)? If the IVC is not present in its usual location, a tubular structure to the left of the aorta suggests a left-sided IVC. Contrary to some reports, it is almost always possible to identify on CT scan the left renal vein in its normal location anterior to the aorta. If this is not present, a structure posterior to the aorta represents retroaortic left renal vein. On CT scan the retroaortic left renal vein does not appear as well defined as the left renal vein in its normal anterior location. A circumaortic renal vein may be missed if the surgeon sees the anterior component only and does not consider the presence of the posterior component of the collar.

If the diagnosis of a venous anomaly is made on CT scan, a phlebogram of the IVC should be performed. This should be done through the left femoral vein, since this will most likely opacify a left-sided venous structure such as a duplication or left-sided IVC. The phlebogram will document the anomalies but also unusual communications between venous structures to alert the surgeon about these hazards during the aortic dissection. Also,

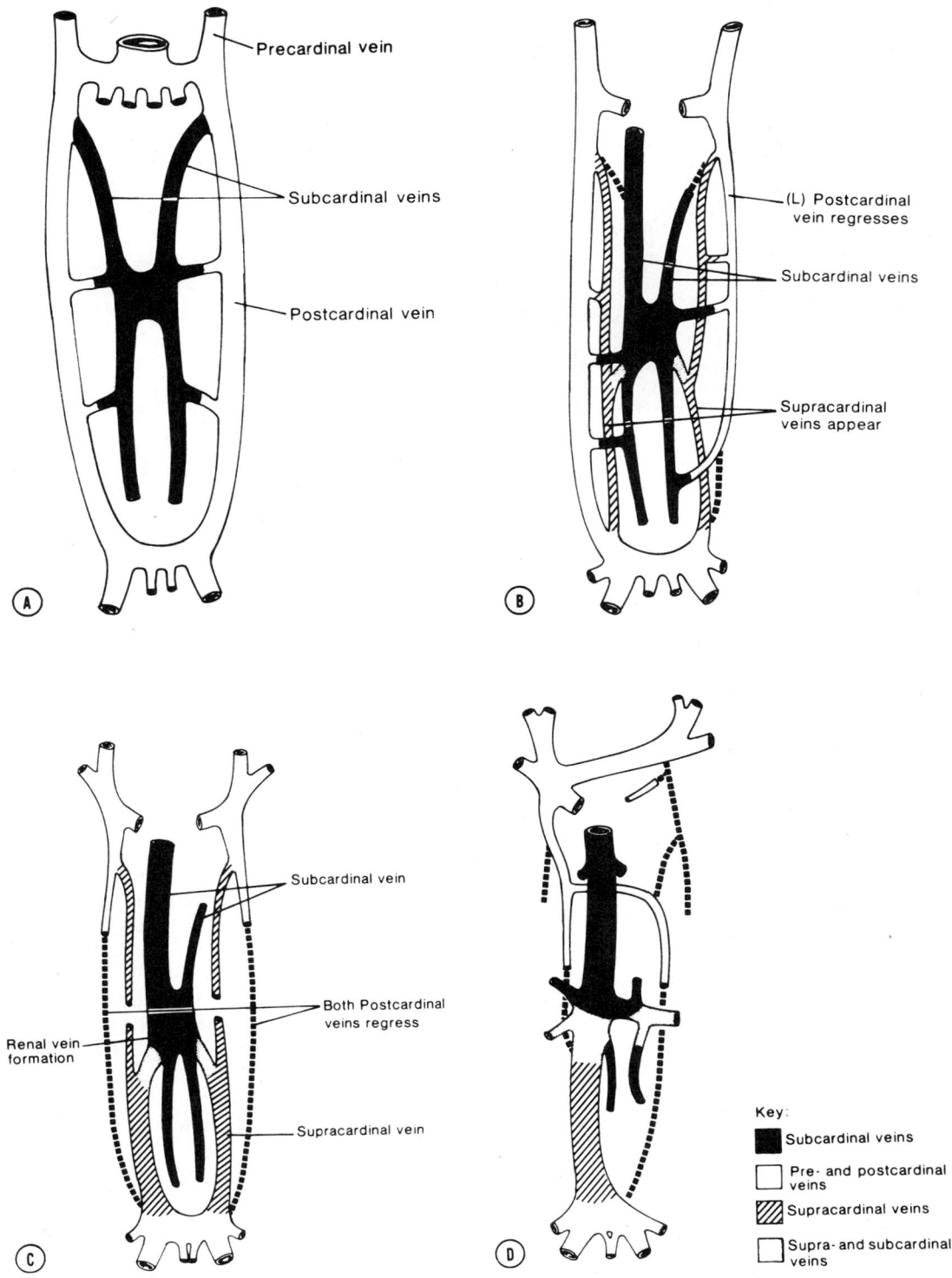

Figure 1 *A,* Gestation at 6 weeks; posterior cardinal veins dominant. *B,* Gestation at 7 weeks; subcardinal veins dominant, postcardinal veins begin to regress. *C,* Gestation at 8 weeks; supracardinal veins dominant; subcardinal system forms prerenal IVC. *D,* Adult inferior vena cava. (From Giordano GM, Trout HH. Anomalies of the inferior vena cava. J Vasc Surg 1986; 3:927; with permission.)

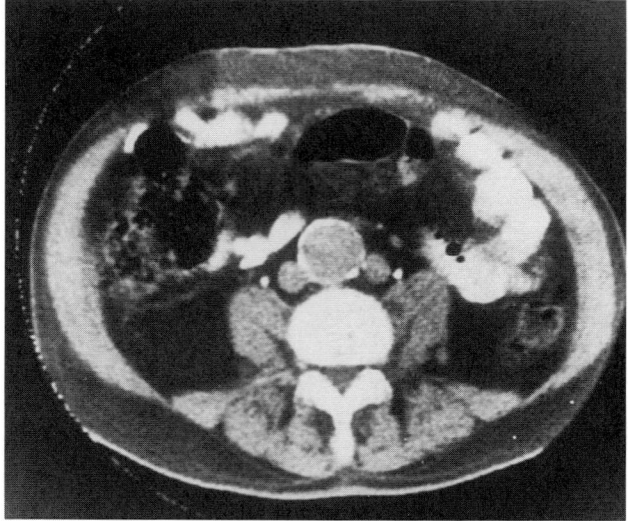

Figure 2 CT scan with tubular structure on both sides of the aorta, indicating a duplication of the IVC.

the anatomy of the left renal vein, more likely to be aberrant with IVC anomalies, will be seen.

For patients undergoing aortic reconstructive procedures who do not have a preoperative CT scan, the first encounter with venous anomalies may be at the time of the aortic dissection. Initially, neither duplication nor left-sided IVC may be obvious. As the normal IVC is not seen during dissection, an IVC on the left side may not be appreciated initially. However, as the dissection proceeds proximally, a left IVC will be encountered as it crosses the midline at the aorta just below the renal arteries. Hopefully, this is identified without injury to the vein. If this is not seen, the patient probably has a retroaortic left renal vein. If the left renal vein is seen, a circumaortic collar is still possible.

TREATMENT OPTIONS

A left-sided IVC and duplication present technical problems in the dissection of the proximal infrarenal abdominal aorta during aneurysm resection. A left-sided IVC usually crosses to the right side anterior to the aorta at the level of the renal arteries (Fig. 3). Occasionally the crossing occurs behind the aorta. This complicates exposure of the proximal abdominal aorta. Ligation and division may cause significant lower leg edema and should be avoided. Transection of the IVC with repair of the aneurysm followed with reanastomosis of the transected left-sided IVC is an option. This approach presents technical problems because the crossing IVC is broad and under tension from external pressure of the expanded aneurysmal wall. However, after repair the tension is less, allowing an easier reanastomosis. Careful dissection and mobilization of the left-sided IVC allows tight but adequate exposure of the proximal aorta, eliminating the need for transection.

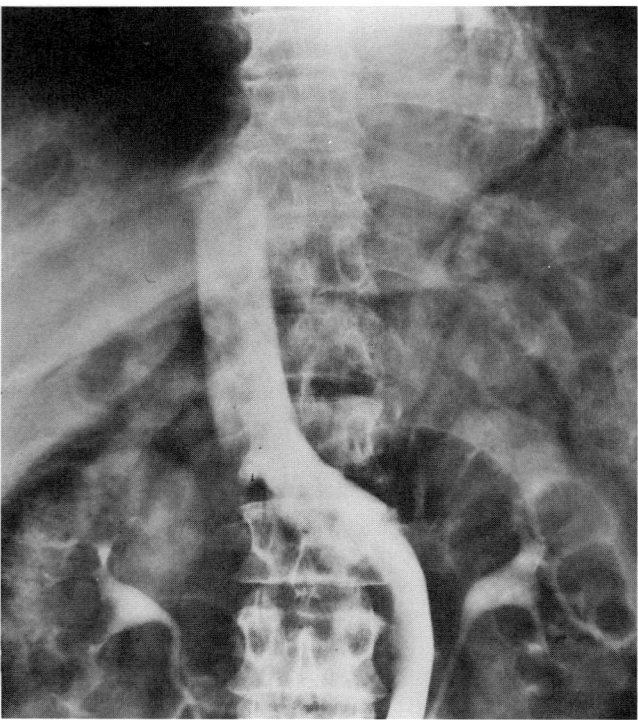

Figure 3 A phlebogram showing a left-sided IVC crossing to the right side at the level of the renal arteries. Note the width of the IVC as it crosses over.

This mobilization may include division of the right renal vein. Since the left-sided IVC is a mirror image of the normal anatomy, the adrenal and gonadal veins enter directly into the right renal vein instead of the IVC. Thus, division of the right renal vein adjacent to the IVC with preservation of the adrenal and gonadal outflow can be performed, just as the left renal vein can be divided in patients with normal anatomy.

A double IVC unites anterior to the aorta, again complicating proximal aortic exposure. If the diagnosis was made preoperatively on CT scan and then confirmed with a phlebogram, communications between both IVCs and iliac veins will appear. These communications almost always occur, and they allow division of the left IVC, with the left leg draining into the right IVC through the communicating veins. This will facilitate exposure and allow for a safe dissection of the proximal aorta.

Retroaortic and circumaortic renal veins are potential sources of bleeding complications if injuries occur during aortic dissection. The preoperative diagnosis of these common anomalies is helpful in avoiding injury to these structures. The left renal vein is routinely identified during aortic dissection. If renal vein anomalies are unsuspected, injuries can still be avoided by keeping dissection of the aorta confined to the anterior surface and sides of the aorta. However, even without circumferential dissection of the aorta, injury to a retroaortic and circumaortic renal vein may still occur with the placement of a proximal aortic clamp. Control of this bleeding is difficult requiring transection of infrarenal aorta for posterior exposure as one technical solution. If the left renal vein is not in its anterior location, there should be suspicion of a posterior left renal vein. The presence of an anterior left renal vein does not preclude a circumaortic renal collar with its posterior vein component.

Venous anomalies can complicate other common procedures performed by the vascular surgeon. A left sympathectomy can be hazardous if a left-sided IVC is present. The placement of a filter device in the IVC may not prevent pulmonary emboli if a left-sided IVC as part of IVC duplication is present draining the left leg. Sampling of the renal vein for renin assay to diagnose renovascular hypertension may be inaccurate if renal vein anomalies are present.

Most surgeons do not accumulate an enormous experience with venous anomalies that can complicate aortic dissection. Consequently, simple aortic aneurysm resection may become a difficult, life-threatening procedure if inadvertent injury to anomalous veins occurs. Since CT scans for aneurysms are commonly performed preoperatively, checking for easily identifiable venous anomalies and following the approaches listed should preclude serious bleeding complications.

REFERENCES

1. Giordano JM, Trout HH. Anomalies of the inferior vena cava. J Vasc Surg 1986; 3:924–928.
2. Giordano JM. Embryologic development of the vascular system. In: Giordano JM, Trout HH, DePalma eds. Basic science of vascular surgery. Mount Kisco, NY: Futura, 1988:3.
3. Chaung VP, Mena CE, Hoskins PA. Congenital anomalies of the left renal vein: Angiographic consideration. Br J Radio 1974; 47: 214–218.
4. Brener BJ, Darling C, Frederick PL, Longton RR. Major venous anomalies complicating abdominal aortic surgery. Arch Surg 1974; 108:160–165.
5. Mayo J, Gray R, SJ Louis E, Grossman H, et al. Anomalies of the inferior vena cava. Am J Roentgenol 1983; 140:339–345.
6. Richardson ML, Kinnard RE, Levesque PH. Inferior vena cava duplication: Demonstration by sonography. J Clin Ultrasound 1983; 11:225–228.
7. Royal SA, Collen P. CT evaluation of the anomalies of the inferior vena cava and left renal vein. Am J Roentgenol 1979; 132:759–763.
8. Siegfried MS, Rochester D, Bernstein JR, Miller JW. Diagnosis of inferior vena cava anomalies by computerized tomography. Comput Radiol 1983; 7:119–123.

MANAGEMENT OF THORACOABDOMINAL AORTIC ANEURYSM

G. MELVILLE WILLIAMS, M.D.

Adapting the techniques pioneered by Crawford[1,2] for managing thoracoabdominal aortic aneurysms (TAAA) has led to progress in the management of patients with this condition. However, mortality remains high (10%), and paraplegia occurs in 5% to 32% of patients with the most extensive disease. Multisystem organ failure and intraoperative bleeding, largely from the failure of tissues to retain suture, remain the leading the causes of death. Paraplegia, although not the most common cause of morbidity, is certainly the one most feared by patient and surgeon, and its etiology remains unclear.

A review of mechanisms and means of prevention of paraplegia should lead the surgeon to a rational course of action in managing patients with extensive TAAAs. The aim is to reduce mortality and eliminate paraplegia and other significant complications, such as renal failure and multisystem organ failure. The author proposes the following specific recommendations for operative indications, preoperative evaluation, operative management, and adjunctive therapy in the management of these patients.

OPERATIVE INDICATIONS

Operative indications should be more conservative for TAAA than those we apply in the treatment of infrarenal abdominal aortic aneurysms. Although rupture is a major threat to patients with large descending thoracic aortic aneurysms, the descending thoracic aorta is normally 3 cm in diameter in elderly patients. We have taken expansion to twice the normal diameter (6 cm) as the marker for elective repair. Operative repairs are best done electively, with the full complement of skilled anesthesiologists and after arteriographic evaluation. Patients with symptoms most commonly complain of high epigastric and back pain situated between the scapulae. When this pain is unremitting, representing expansion of periaortic tissue, urgent operation is justified, particularly if the computed tomographic scan documents any evidence of a hematoma. However, many large aneurysms initiate an inflammatory reaction creating adhesions to the lung with partial atelectasis. These changes should not be confused with hematoma.

MEDICAL MANAGEMENT

The therapy for most patients with acute DeBakey type IIIB dissecting aneurysms is medical, as is the case of patients with small fusiform aneurysms. The principal aim is normalizing blood pressure under carefully monitored conditions.[3] Operation should be limited to patients whose symptoms persist, whose aneurysms enlarge, and who develop evidence of bleeding. Although the medical approach risks death from acute rupture of dissections, operation is even more hazardous, as freshly dissected aorta holds sutures poorly. Limited repairs of the torn proximal thoracic aorta have proven to be temporary, and a sizable proportion of patients return later with expanding aneurysms of the lower thoracic and abdominal aorta. However, tailoring operations in the dissected but nondilated abdominal aorta to correct perfusion defects of the viscera, kidneys, and lower extremities may be undertaken in the acute situation in older patients. The dissected tissue in the nondilated abdominal aorta frequently retains sutures well with the exception of young patients with metabolic aortic diseases.

PREOPERATIVE EVALUATION

Virtually all patients presenting with TAAAs require extensive cardiac evaluation. The young patient with an aortic dissection may have concomitant aortic valve disease. The older patient, particularly those with hypertension, merit echocardiography and some form of stress testing as a minimum. All patients who are candidates for repairs of the aortic arch should undergo cardiac catheterization and have their coronary arteries repaired if diseased. This position is different from our approach to patients with infrarenal abdominal aortic aneurysms, concerning which we base testing on the patients' symptomatology and electrocardiography.

Arteriographic localization of the great radicular artery (GRA) or artery of Adamkiewicz supplying blood flow to the spinal cord is not as difficult or time-consuming as one might think. Patients with fusiform aneurysms have mural thrombus occluding many of the intercostal arteries. The patent arteries are identified by an aortic flush injection and then are catheterized selectively. A small GRA, originating from intercostal collateral vessels, is likely to be insignificant; a major artery arising from the main intercostal itself (Fig. 1) may be crucial and its attachment to the aortic graft vital to prevent paraplegia. In the case of DeBakey IIIB dissecting aneurysms, the "tailoring technique"[4] restores blood flow through all of the inferior intercostal vessels as well as all lumbar vessels (Fig. 2 and 3), obviating the need to identify the specific intercostals requiring reattachment. For this reason, selective catheterization is not done in patients with dissections.

It is also important to assess the patency of the visceral, renal, and lower extremity vessels. This point is dramatized by the following example.

Mrs. G. presented with unremitting upper abdominal pain thought to represent aneurysmal expansion of a large TAAA. She had limited studies because of the need for an

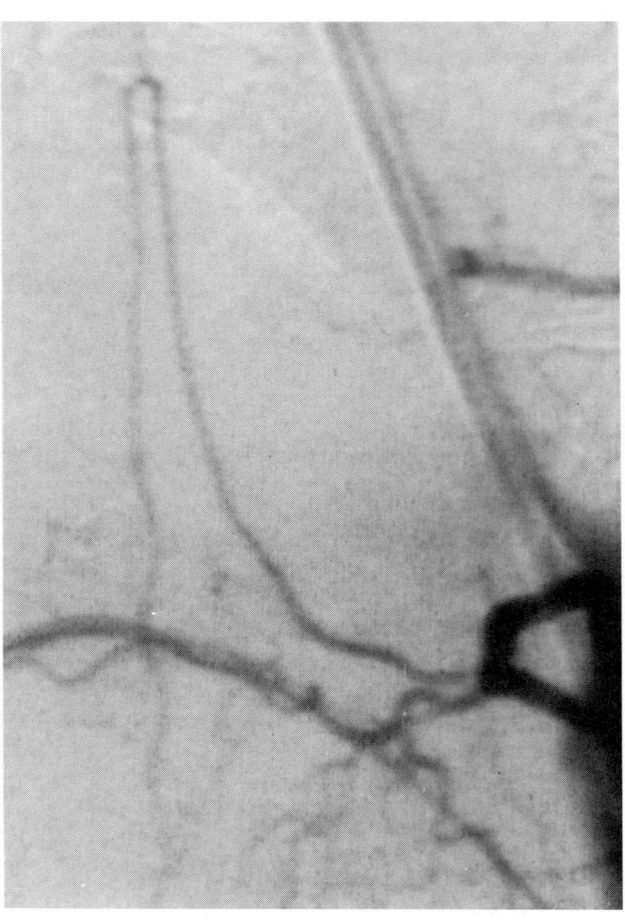

Figure 1 A large artery of Adamkiewicz. Note that this vessel making the characteristic hairpin turn originates directly from the intercostal vessel. There is also cephalad as well as caudad blood flow, indicating a low perfusion pressure in the anterior spinal artery superiorly. Evoked potentials were lost after a 10 minute aortic cross-clamp in this patient.

expeditious operation. At operation, the orifice of the superior mesenteric artery (SMA) was patent, and the celiac axis was occluded. The SMA was implanted into the prosthesis, along with the right renal artery. At the conclusion of the operation, there was blood flow assessed by Doppler within the small bowel mesentery. However, pulsations at the base of the mesentery were weak. After an initial postoperative good recovery, the patient deteriorated and at celiotomy widespread intestinal ischemia was evident. Aorto-SMA reconstruction of the stenotic SMA did not salvage the gut, and the patient succumbed. In retrospect, her abdominal pain was probably caused by mesenteric ischemia and not aneurysm expansion.

OPERATIVE MANAGEMENT

Monitoring. A catheter is placed in the lumbar subarachnoid space to drain cerebrospinal fluid (CSF) at pressures greater than 10 cm of water. Electrodes are placed adjacent to the posterior tibial nerve at the ankle

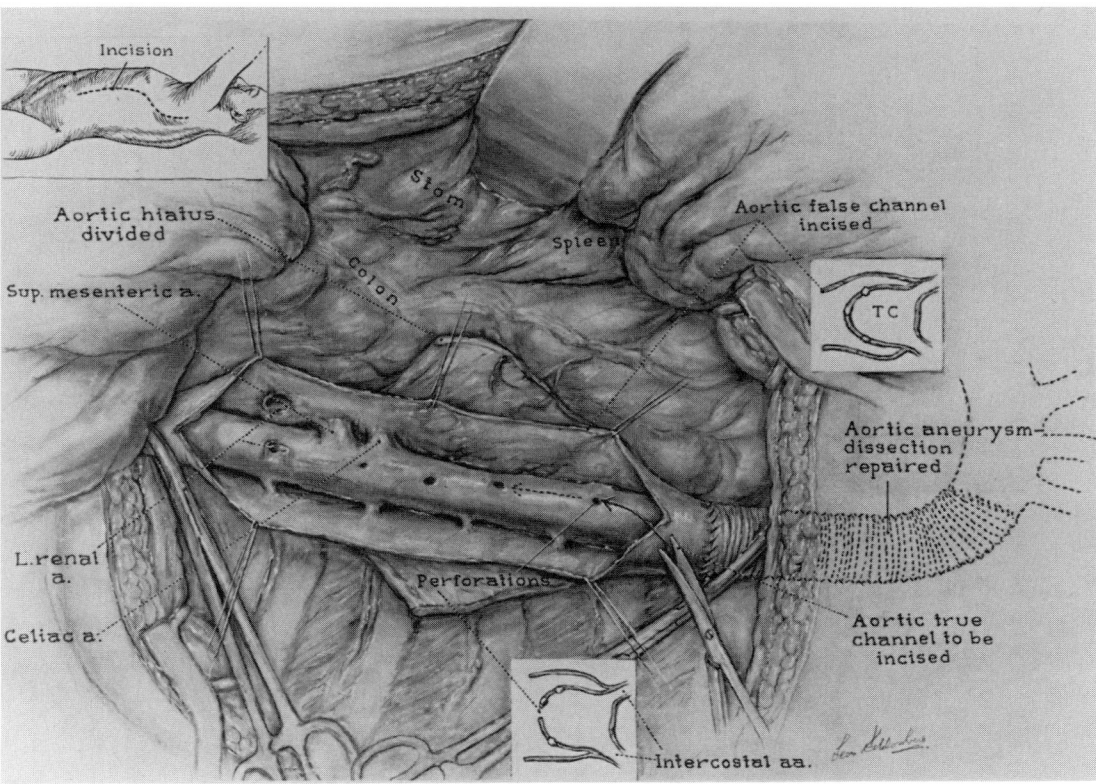

Figure 2 Tailoring extensive dissecting aneurysms. A long aortotomy has been made through the false lumen to expose the true lumen within. Most often, several small openings represent communications between the true and false lumens. Probing these allows the surgeon to discriminate between such communications and the orifices of visceral or renal vessels, allowing safe entry into the true lumen.

and on the scalp for monitoring of sensory evoked potentials. Motor evoked potentials are achieved with electrodes placed in the neck.[5] A Swan-Ganz catheter is inserted and the patient is intubated to provide single-lung ventilation. Large intravenous catheters are placed, and a rapid infuser connected. The radial artery and the aorta or iliac artery distal to the inferior aortic clamp are catheterized to record arterial pressures proximal and distal to the site of aortic occlusion. Rectal and nasopharyngeal temperatures are monitored.

Exposure. The patient is placed on the right side, and the skin of the entire left chest, left flank, abdomen, and both groins prepped. For the repair of Crawford type I aneurysms,[1] a standard incision is made for a posteriolateral thoracotomy. Proximal exposure is gained by excision of the fifth rib and "notching" of the fourth. Distal exposure is achieved through a second thoracotomy in the ninth interspace, but through the same skin incision. The diaphragm need not be taken down, but is incised at the crus to provide exposure at least to the celiac axis. For Crawford type II aneurysms, the identical skin incision is extended across the costal margin inferiorly and lateral to the rectus abdominus muscle. The costal margin is divided at the ninth interspace and the diaphragm divided peripherally, developing the entire extraperitoneal space posterior to the left kidney. Control of the common iliac arteries is achieved by extending the incision further inferiorly or by making a second small left lower quadrant incision.

Patients presenting with Crawford type III aneurysms are managed with an incision in the eighth or ninth intercostal space, extending across the costal margin and onto the abdomen lateral to the rectus abdominus muscle. Again, the diaphragm is incised peripherally providing exposure of the aorta from mid-descending thoracic aorta to its bifurcation. The left common femoral artery or left external iliac artery is cannulated by making a separate incision. A catheter for monitoring distal arterial pressure is placed in the most convenient area, usually the infrarenal aorta. The left atrium is exposed by opening the pericardium posterior to the phrenic nerve and cannulating it with a large venous cannula secured with a pursestring suture. The left femoral artery and aorta, when indicated, are cannulated with the 22 Fr arterial cannulae and connected to a centrifugal pump and heat exchanger.

Operative Procedure. During this extensive preparation of the patient by the anesthesia team, the patient's body temperature is allowed to drift downward. Atriofemoral bypass is initiated after giving heparin sodium, 100 units/kg, and the heat exchanger is used to lower and sustain the core temperature at 30° to 33°C. This risk of

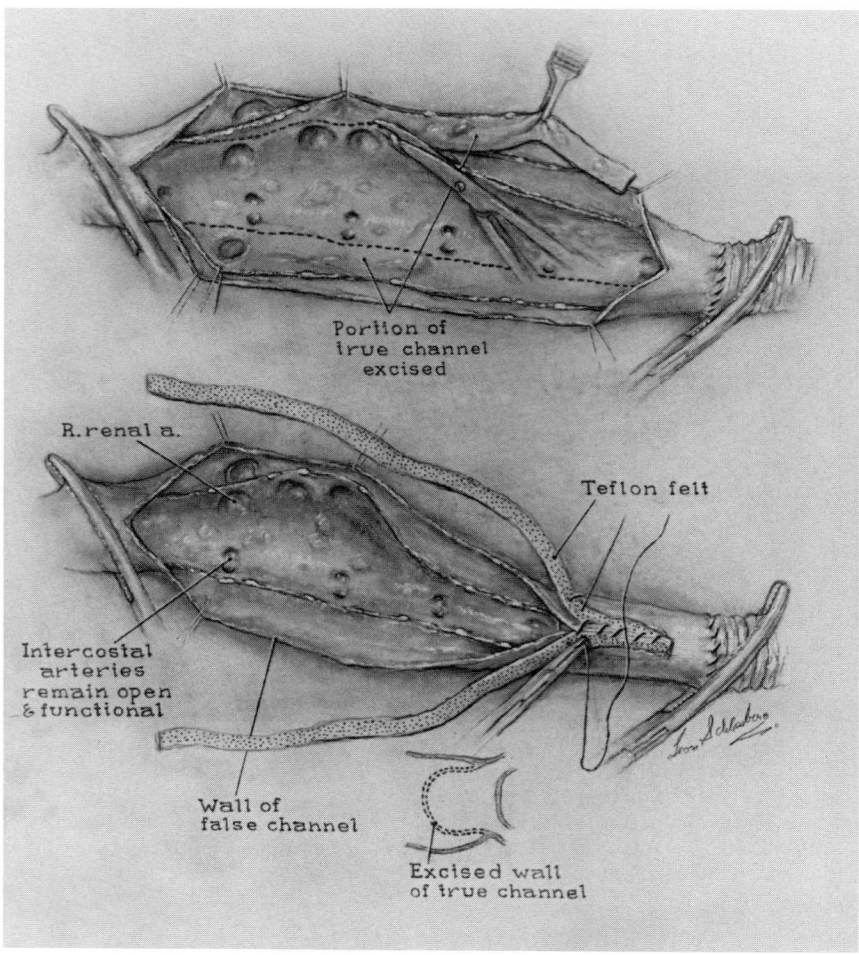

Figure 3 Excision of the nonattached intima of the true lumen to construct a single lumen. The single lumen is closed with Teflon felt to buttress the suture line.

cardiac dysrhythmia is justified in managing Crawford type I and II aneurysms. However, patients with lesser problems are maintained at 33°C. During the period of cooling, begun after achieving proximal and distal control, additional dissection of the aorta is carried out, achieving control at several points for the staged repair. Frequently, the final dissection of the aortic arch for the placement of the proximal clamp is best carried out with the bypass in place. At blood flows of 2 to 3 L/minute, ventricular ejection is reduced enough to "soften" the arch. Circulation is maintained to all body parts during the performance of the proximal anastomosis, which can be conducted in a careful manner, buttressing the aortic tissue with Teflon felt as needed (Fig. 4).

Stage 2 involves the attachment of intercostal arteries. This is done in all patients with one exception. Patients with limited patent vessels, all of which were studied arteriographically and found not to supply a GRA, are treated by intercostal ligation. In every other instance, large intercostal vessels when surrounded by relatively normal aorta are attached to the prosthesis. The inclusion technique is used (Fig. 5). The surgeon must be prepared to control backbleeding from nonessential intercostals rapidly, for in some patients this bleeding is torrential. Allis clamps are used to occlude the orifices until they can be oversewn.

Stage 3 is begun by changing the distal clamp from its position just above the diaphragm to an infrarenal position and clamping the graft distal to the intercostal anastomosis. This allows perfusion of the intercostal vessels and is safe in the heparinized patient. The remaining distal thoracic and abdominal aorta is opened longitudinally, and the visceral and renal vessels are attached as described by Crawford[2] (Fig. 6). Midway through stage three, rewarming is begun but is not very effective as only the pelvis and extremities are being perfused. However, enough blood flow is generated to prevent overdistention of the left ventricle, and nitrates are seldom needed.

Stage 4 is accomplished with an anastomosis to the terminal aorta iliac or to femoral vessels, as required (Fig. 7). The atrial-femoral bypass may be stopped, provided the patient is adequately heparinized. Prior to the restoration of blood flow to the lower extremities,

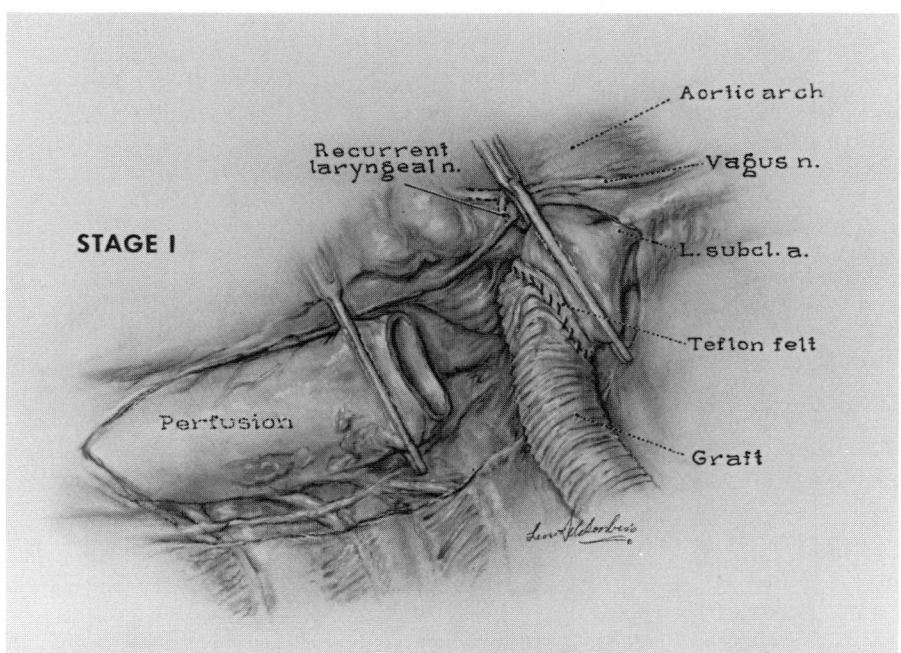

Figure 4 Stage 1 in the repair of type II aneurysms. The proximal descending thoracic aorta has been transected, and the proximal anastomosis completed, employing atrial-femoral bypass to maintain normal mean perfusion blood pressures distal to the aortic clamp. A careful, accurate, and hemostatic anastomosis can be constructed without haste. Tympanic membrane and bladder temperatures are reduced and held at 30°C.

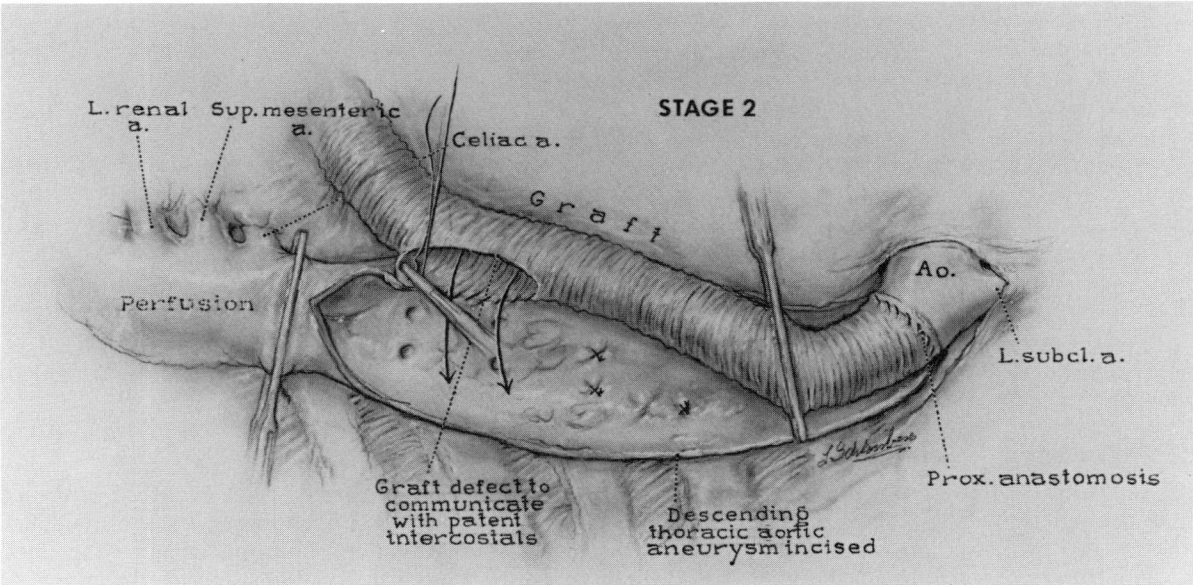

Figure 5 Stage 2 in the repair of type II aneurysms. Stage 2 is the attachment of two pairs of intercostal arteries at T-8 and T-9 to the prostheses. At this level of intercostal attachment, a clamp may be applied to the aorta above the celiac axis to allow perfusion of the viscera and kidneys during the performance of this anastomosis. When the intercostal vessels at T-11 and T-12 are dominant, providing visceral and renal perfusion during intercostal attachment may not be possible.

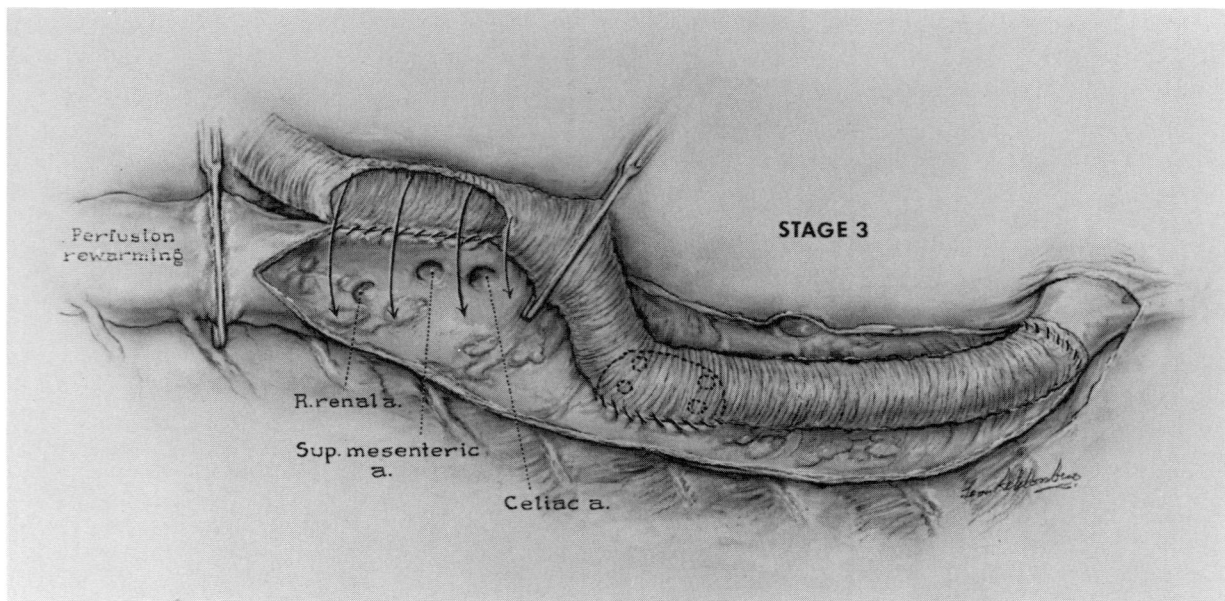

Figure 6 Stage 3 in the repair of type II aneurysms. Stage 3 consists of visceral and renal attachment, allowing intercostal perfusion and rewarming of the lower extremities and pelvis.

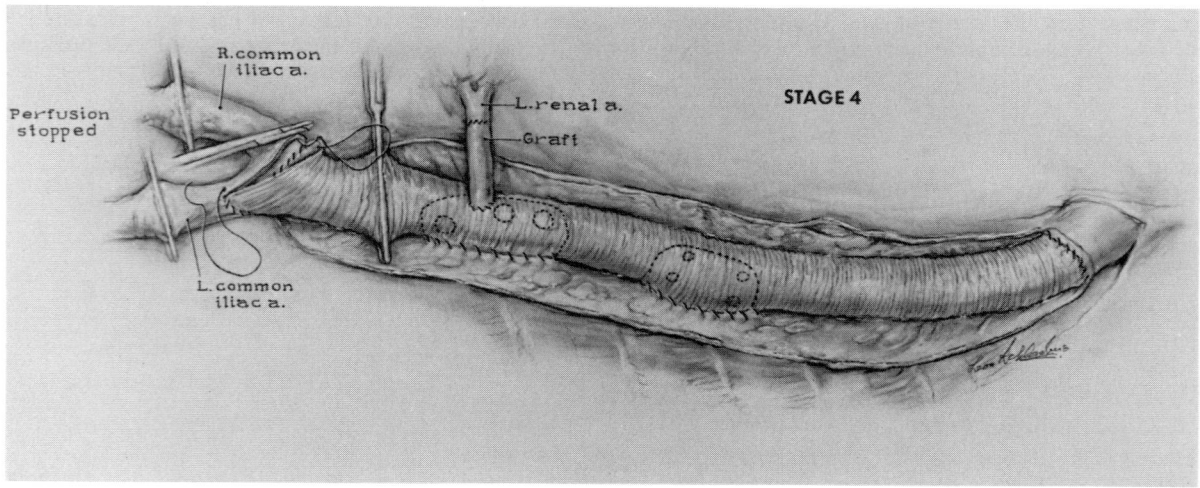

Figure 7 Stage 4 in the repair of type II aneurysms. Stage 4 completes the procedure by restoring circulation to the legs and commonly the left kidney. When the common iliac arteries require reconstruction, bypass is discontinued temporarily, and the bypass circuit must be "flushed" when it is reinstituted for rewarming.

appropriate flushing is carried out not only through the vessels but through the bypass tubing as well. Lost blood is rescued by the cell saver and returned to the rapid infuser. With the repair completed, the heat exchanger is utilized to increase body temperature to 37.5°. Once this is accomplished, the cannulae are removed and the heparin effect reversed. The double thoracotomy is closed in standard fashion.

The tailoring procedure utilized for the repair of expanding DeBakey type IIIB dissecting aneurysms is accomplished through the same exposure. In the majority of patients, expansion has occurred in the proximal two-thirds of the descending thoracic aorta. This area is not appropriate for tailoring because the aneurysmal tissue frequently contains mural thrombus and the intima has degenerated. Thus, this portion of the aorta should be replaced with a Dacron graft that terminates in an area where the aorta is a more normal size (4 cm or less in diameter). Whenever possible, an end-to-end anastomosis is constructed between the dissected distal, thoracic aorta and the graft at the junction of the middle and lower thirds of the descending thoracic aorta; it allows preservation of all intercostal vessels distal to T7. The anastomosis is constructed between the outer wall of the dissection and the Dacron graft, buttressing the anastomosis with Teflon felt. During the construction of this anastomosis, the inferior intercostal arteries are perfused through the bypass circuit.

The distal clamp is then moved to occlude the aorta several inches inferior to the renal artery, and the aorta incised longitudinally. The dissected membrane is excised, and the portion of the intima still attached to the wall of the aorta is left undisturbed (Fig. 2). When intercostal backbleeding is torrential, the lower thoracic aorta is reconstructed rapidly, reducing the lumen to 2.5 cm. The proximal clamp is placed across the reconstructed aorta at the diaphragm, and the descending thoracic aorta is perfused by the heart. Tailoring is concluded most frequently by construction of an end-to-end anastomosis to a Dacron graft. Body temperature is returned to 37.5°, employing atrial-femoral bypass and the heat exchanger. During this time, hemostasis is secured, the peritoneum is opened, and the abdominal contents are examined by inspection and the hand-held Doppler.

The principal postoperative complication is bleeding, and there have been two sources meriting special attention prior to closure. The first is from an intercostal or lumbar artery. The sutures at the orifices of these vessels are often placed hurriedly, and many encompass plaque. With reperfusion, delayed exsanguinating backbleeding may ensue. Thus, prior to wrapping the graft with the aneurysm sac, the oversewn orifices should be inspected carefully. Second, we have had three delayed hemorrhages from ruptures of "contained" splenic hematomas. Therefore, the peritoneum must be opened at the conclusion of the operation, and its contents thoroughly examined.

We still rely heavily on opiates for analgesia but believe anesthetic management will slowly change as advocated by Acher and his colleagues, employing thiopental and naloxone.[6] Blood replacement should consist of providing equal amounts of fresh frozen plasma to cell-saved blood. Platelets are infused after the cannulae are removed. Prior to departure from the operating room, a standard single-lumen endotracheal tube should replace the double-lumen tube to provide selective lung ventilation.

Postoperative Care. On the basis of three case reports documenting return of spinal cord function in patients with delayed-onset paraplegia by removal of CSF, we maintain CSF drainage for 2 to 3 days by using a device that drains fluid whenever the CSF pressure exceeds 10 cm H_2O. Additionally, whenever patients are unstable hemodynamically, we sustain drainage for 5 days.

REFERENCES

1. Crawford ES, Crawford JL, Safi HJ, et al. Thoracoabdominal aortic aneurysms: Preoperative and intraoperative factors determining immediate and long-term results of operations in 605 patients. J Vasc Surg 1986; 3:389–404.
2. Crawford ES, Snyder DM, Cho GC, Rhoem JO. Progress in treatment of thoraco-abdominal aneurysms involving celiac, superior mesenteric and renal arteries. Ann Surg 1978; 188:404.
3. Wheat MW, Palmer RF, Bartley TD, et al. Treatment of dissecting aneurysms of the aorta without surgery. J Thorac Cardiovasc Surg 1965; 50:364–373.
4. Williams GM. Treatment of chronic expanding dissecting aneurysms of the descending thoracic and upper abdominal aorta by extended aortotomy, removal of the dissected intima, and closure. J Vasc Surg 1993; 18:441–449.
5. Laschinger JC, Owen JH, Rosenbloom M, et al. Direct non-invasive monitoring of spinal cord function during thoracic aortic occlusion: Use of motor evoked potentials. J Vasc Surg 1988; 7:161–171.
6. Acher CW, Wynn MM, Hoch JR, et al. Combined use of cerebral spinal fluid drainage and naloxone reduces the risk of paraplegia in thoracoabdominal aneurysm repair. J Vasc Surg 1994; 19:236-249.

SURGICAL TREATMENT OF ABDOMINAL AORTIC ANEURYSM — INFERIOR VENA CAVA FISTULA

JOHN E. CONNOLLY, M.D.

Abdominal aortic aneurysms usually rupture into the retroperitoneal space; rupture directly into the free peritoneal cavity is the next most common course. A few will perforate into the gastrointestinal tract, most commonly the duodenum, and on rare occasions the fistula occurs with the inferior vena cava (IVC). Hypovolemic shock is the consequence of all of these complications except for perforation into the IVC, which produces an arteriovenous fistula resulting in high-output congestive heart failure, peripheral edema, and renal insufficiency. Diversion of flow from high to low resistance raises the venous pressure and both cardiac output and plasma volume. The magnitude of heart failure depends on the size of the fistula, its duration, and the cardiac reserve of the patient. Venous hypertension in the legs may be accentuated because of compression of proximal veins by the aneurysm. Arteriovenous fistula between the aorta and the IVC was initially described by Syme[1] in 1831 and was first successfully treated surgically by Cooley[2] in 1954. Prompt recognition and early surgical repair of the fistula and aneurysm are the key elements to successful treatment of this relatively rare lesion.

The clinical picture typically is one of low back or abdominal pain followed by progressive cardiac, renal, and hepatic decompensation.[3] Physical examination documents a pulsating abdominal mass, often with a continuous bruit, a wide pulse pressure with systolic accentuation, and varying degrees of swelling of the lower extremities and even the lower trunk. The venous hypertension may also cause hematuria and rectal bleeding. Some patients present with anorexia, nausea, and vomiting. Treatment by digitalis and diuretics of the high-output heart failure commonly seen with this lesion is universally unsuccessful, and the subsequent course without operation is uniformly fatal.

Preoperative diagnosis is usually made by aortography but has also been reported to be confirmed by peripheral venous digital angiography, computed tomography, color Doppler ultrasonography, and magnetic resonance imaging. While confirmation of the diagnosis is desirable in stable patients, it should not delay operation. A simple and expeditious method of making the diagnosis of an aortocaval fistula is by insertion of a Swan-Ganz catheter through a groin vein.[4] Either elevated blood pressure recording or high blood oxygen content should confirm arteriovenous fistula. A correct diagnosis gives forewarning against fluid overloading, prevention of which is perhaps the most important preoperative maneuver to improve survival.

TREATMENT

Once the diagnosis has been made or suspected, early operation should be performed. Autotransfusion is important, as it is in all cases of abdominal aortic aneurysmectomy. The operation is carried out as with standard abdominal aortic aneurysmectomy, except that if preoperative or operative confirmation of an aortocaval fistula is made, the proximal and distal IVC should be controlled at the time of opening of the aneurysm. This maneuver helps prevent embolization of intra-aneurysmal clot into the vena cava, with possible fatal pulmonary emboli, before the fistula is closed. In some patients intra-aortic clot may be occluding the fistula, and great care is necessary to avoid dislodging clot into the vena cava. Since the diagnosis of an aortocaval fistula may not have been made before operation, such a diagnosis should always be considered before opening a large aneurysm.[5] Palpation may reveal a thrill or pulsating veins and alert the surgeon to the correct diagnosis. If so, gradual clamping of the aorta is advised, since a sudden increase in cardiac afterload combined with a sudden fall in venous return has been reported to cause cardiac arrest. Standard repair of the fistula is carried out by continuous suture of the venous edge of the fistula from within the opened aneurysm followed by standard aortic reconstruction. If the fistula edges cannot be readily sutured, the IVC may be ligated proximally and distally.

REFERENCES

1. Syme J. Case of spontaneous varicose aneurysm. Edinburgh Medical Surgical Journal 1831; 36:104.
2. Cooley DA. Discussion of David M, Dye WS, Grove JW, et al. Resection of ruptured aneurysms of the abdominal aorta. Ann Surg 1955; 142:623.
3. Gilling-Smith GL, Mansfield AO. Spontaneous abdominal arteriovenous fistulae: Report of eight cases and review of the literature. Brit J Surg 1991; 78:421–426.
4. Kwaan JHM, McCart PM, Jones SA, Connolly JE: Aortocaval fistula detection using a Swan-Ganz catheter. Surg Gynec Obstet 1977; 144:919–921.
5. Calligaro KD, Savarese RP, DeLaurentis DA. Unusual aspects of aortovenous fistulas associated with ruptured abdominal aortic aneurysms. J Vasc Surg 1990; 12:586–590.

MANAGEMENT OF PRIMARY AORTOENTERIC FISTULA

SCOTT S. BERMAN, M.D.
VICTOR M. BERNHARD, M.D.

Fistulas between aneurysms of the abdominal aorta and the gastrointestinal tract were first identified as a source of hemorrhage by Sir Astley Cooper in 1829.[1] Despite this early recognition, fewer than 200 cases have been reported, establishing the relatively infrequent presentation of this clinical entity.[2-6] In most patients the underlying pathology is erosion of an atherosclerotic aneurysm into the adherent third or fourth portion of the duodenum. Other pathophysiologic processes, including infections (tuberculosis, syphilis), vasculitis, carcinoma, diverticulitis, appendicitis, and cholecystitis, have been described as causative factors in approximately 20%.[2-6] The most frequent of these latter factors is primary aortocolic fistula due to diverticulitis.[3] From a review of autopsy series, the reported incidence of primary aortoenteric fistulas (AEF) is between 0.04% and 0.07%.[6] Secondary aortoenteric fistulas are more common, occurring as a complication of prosthetic aortic replacement in 0.1% to 2% of patients.[7] In contrast to primary AEF's, secondary aortoenteric fistulas are a major consideration in the differential diagnosis of a patient with a previous aortic graft who has gastrointestinal bleeding. Despite this difference in incidence, primary and secondary aortoenteric fistulas represent similar challenges for the vascular surgeon, whose management must address the problems of diagnosis, removal of a focus of vascular infection, and revascularization of the limbs and pelvis.

DIAGNOSIS

Paramount to the successful management of primary AEF are a high index of suspicion and expedient investigation to establish the diagnosis. Presenting symptoms of primary AEF may include abdominal or flank pain, fever, and anemia. Unfortunately, the diagnostic triad of abdominal pain, gastrointestinal hemorrhage, and a pulsatile abdominal mass is seen infrequently.[2-6] Taheri and co-workers[6] cited an incidence of 0 to 40% for this symptom complex in their review of the literature. Abdominal, back, or flank pain, symptoms common to abdominal aortic aneurysms, were present in fewer than 50% of patients. The most common presenting symptom of primary AEF is gastrointestinal hemorrhage. This may appear as melena in up to 55% or hematemesis in up to 64% of patients.[5,6] A phenomenon described in both primary and secondary AEFs is the herald bleed. An initial nonexsanguinating hemorrhage that ceases spontaneously, it is predictably followed by further hemorrhagic episodes until one culminates in fatal exsanguination. Hypovolemic shock as the initial presentation is rare in the absence of an antecedent bleeding event and accounted for less than 5% of 189 patients reviewed by Sweeney and Gadacz.[5] Thus, sudden aortic rupture into the gastrointestinal tract with continued massive bleeding as the initial pathologic process is an unusual scenario for primary AEF.[5]

In the collected series reviewed, the majority of patients presenting with primary AEF are men (80%).[2-6] The average age of both men and women at presentation is 62 years. These findings which are consistent with the demographics of abdominal aortic aneurysm in patients without AEF, explain the incidence of comorbid atherosclerotic, inflammatory, and gastrointestinal conditions that may share in the etiology of primary AEF. Moreover, patients with abdominal aortic aneurysms may have an incidence of peptic ulcer disease as high as 25%, which may contribute to the frequent misdiagnosis of the presenting signs and symptoms.[5] A palpable abdominal mass is reported to occur in up to 70% of patients.[2-6]

The successful preoperative diagnosis of a primary AEF is elusive. Unless a high index of suspicion is present, the diagnosis is usually arrived at fortuitously during evaluation of gastrointestinal bleeding. This often occurs at the time of operative exploration for persistent or severe gastrointestinal hemorrhage. Plain abdominal x-ray film may reveal calcifications in the wall of the aortic aneurysm in roughly 50% of patients, which suggests primary AEF in a patient with gastrointestinal bleeding.[5] Esophagogastroduodenoscopy may be completely normal in up to 30% of patients and has been incriminated in delaying the diagnosis by documenting gastritis and duodenitis. Considering the significant incidence of peptic ulcer disease in patients with aortic aneurysms, these findings not uncommonly terminate further evaluation of the patient with primary AEF and have contributed to delays of up to 1 week between presentation and operation.[5] However, bleeding seen in the third portion of the duodenum strongly suggests AEF. Endoscopy should be considered negative for primary AEF only if an actively bleeding peptic or neoplastic lesion is found in the stomach or proximal duodenum. Otherwise the diagnosis of primary AEF must remain a consideration, especially in patients with evidence of an aortic aneurysm by physical examination or imaging techniques, including ultrasound, computed tomography (CT), or magnetic resonance imaging (MRI). Passage of the endoscope through the entire length of duodenum may document ulceration, erosion, thrombus, or active bleeding at the site of the AEF. This establishes the diagnosis if the fistula is in this segment of bowel. The surgical team should be prepared for an immediate celiotomy before commencing endoscopy, since manipulation of a quiescent fistula may promote recurrent massive hemorrhage.

Upper and lower gastrointestinal contrast studies are usually not helpful in making the diagnosis. The only findings suggestive of primary AEF on upper gastrointestinal barium studies are a persistent filling defect and/or an ulcer in the third or fourth portion of the duodenum.[5,6] Barium enema may reveal inflammatory strictures of the sigmoid colon consistent with diverticulitis.[3] In a patient with lower gastrointestinal bleeding, it is unlikely that this finding will suggest that an AEF is the cause of hemorrhage in the presence of acute diverticulitis.

Arteriography has also been disappointing in its ability to detect primary AEF. Presumptive evidence is documentation of the fistula on lateral aortography or intravascularly injected contrast within the lumen of the bowel. Since these are infrequent findings and arteriography has the potential for dislodging the clot within the fistula, which may reactivate bleeding, enthusiasm for its application in the evaluation of primary AEF has waned.

The modern imaging techniques of CT scanning and MRI may provide more accurate diagnostic information to identify primary AEF preoperatively by documenting an aneurysm, particularly if it appears to merge with or be intimately adherent to a loop of bowel. However, only a few cases have been reported, as CT and MRI have been available for too short a time to be assessed for their roles in the diagnostic evaluation of primary AEF.

SURGICAL MANAGEMENT

Primary AEF is uniformly fatal without surgical intervention.[2-6] The issues that must be addressed at the time of operation are closure of the defect in the gastrointestinal tract, removal of the underlying vascular and/or gastrointestinal pathology, and revascularization with either in situ replacement using a prosthetic aortic graft or bypass using the axillobifemoral route. Appropriate adjunctive antibiotic therapy completes the management algorithm for primary AEF.

The first attempt at surgical repair for a primary AEF was made in 1956, but success was not achieved until a year later. These early efforts used aneurysmorrhaphy to manage the aneurysm.[2] The first successful prosthetic replacement of the aorta for primary AEF took place in 1961. In their review of this topic in 1991, Taheri and associates[6] noted that only 29% of reported patients were treated surgically, so operative experience with this clinical entity is limited.

Closure of the gastrointestinal defect can be accomplished by adhering to basic principles of intestinal surgical procedures. This includes debridement of diseased bowel, with primary closure in two layers. If necessary, resection and primary anastomosis can be performed. Breakdown of intestinal suture lines has not been a significant problem in patients who have been operated upon for primary AEF.[2-6]

A more important decision in the treatment of primary AEF is whether to place a prosthetic aortic graft in situ or to perform extra-anatomic bypass. The need for revascularizing the pelvis and lower extremities is preeminent in primary AEF, just as it often is for secondary AEF involving grafts placed for aneurysmal disease. By contrast, if significant collateralization is present, revascularization may not be required in the treatment of secondary AEF involving grafts placed for occlusive disease. Consideration for performing in situ replacement with a prosthetic graft is based upon anecdotal experience and collected reviews of primary AEF as well as recently reported series of secondary AEF managed in this manner.[2,6,8] This approach is predicated on the absence of gross infection and necrosis at the time of exploration and on specific antibiotic therapy directed against cultured organisms. Development of a recurrent AEF after in situ grafting for primary AEF may be prevented by interposition of the omentum between the proximal suture line and the duodenum. Survival rates up to 76% have been achieved using this technique.[5,6] In a thorough review of in situ replacement for primary AEF reported by Daugherty and associates,[9] including three patients that they managed, no graft-related complications occurred in 13 of 14 patients (93%) treated in this manner. In their review of the literature, the survival rate of the 28 patients subjected to surgical intervention was 61%. However, the overall survival of the 52 patients with the confirmed diagnosis of primary AEF was only 32%.

The choice of prosthetic material may influence the rate of recurrent infection, as polytetrafluoroethylene (PTFE) has shown the potential to be more resistant to infection than the more commonly used Dacron grafts in both animal and human reports.[10] The use of PTFE aortic prostheses in infected fields may prove to be a factor in improving outcome as more experience is gained with these grafts.

Experience using extra-anatomic bypass to revascularize primary AEF is widespread in the literature.[2-6] The rationale for this approach rests on the presumed high risk of infection and recurrence with in situ grafting. Absolute indications for extra-anatomic bypass include primary AEF that results from inflammatory and infectious processes originating in the lower gastrointestinal tract, which may account for up to for 20% of cases. Mortality and morbidity appearing in historical reviews of both secondary and primary AEF using extra-anatomic bypass range from 28% to 65% and 10% to 31%, respectively.

The duration of perioperative and postoperative antibiotic therapy may affect persistent or recurrent infectious complications. Extrapolating the data available for the management of vascular graft infections suggest that it is reasonable to continue culture specific antibiotics for 6 months (parenteral for 6 weeks followed by oral) if intraoperative cultures of the residual aortic wall are positive.[11] This approach seems appropriate particularly if in situ grafting is chosen as the route of revascularization.

REFERENCES

1. Cooper A. Lectures on the Principles and Practices of Surgery, 5th ed. London: Renshaw, 1837.
2. Evans D, Webster J. Spontaneous aortoduodenal fistula. Br J Surg 1972; 59:369–372.
3. Wilson SE, Owens ML. Aortocolic fistula: A lethal cause of lower gastrointestinal bleeding. Dis Col Rect 1976; 19:614–617.
4. Reiner MA, Brau SA, Schanzer H. Primary aortoduodenal fistula: Case presentation and review of literature. Am J Gastroenterol 1978; 70:292–297.
5. Sweeney MS, Gadacz TR. Primary aortoduodenal fistula: Manifestation, diagnosis, and treatment. Surgery 1984; 96:492–497.
6. Taheri SA, Kulaylat MN, Grippi J. Surgical treatment of primary aortoduodenal fistula. Ann Vasc Surg 1991; 5:265–270.
7. Piotrowski JJ, Bernhard VM. Management of vascular graft infections. In Bernhard VM, Towne JB, eds. Complications in Vascular Surgery. St. Louis: Quality Medical Publishing, 1991:235.
8. Walker WA, Cooley DA, Duncan JM. The management of aortoduodenal fistula by in situ replacement of the infected abdominal aortic graft. Ann Surg 1987; 205:727–732.
9. Daugherty M, Shearer GR, Ernst CB. Primary artoduodenal fistula: Extra-anatomic vascular reconstruction not required for successful management. Surgery 1979; 86:399–401.
10. Stone KS, Walshaw R, Sugiyama GT. Polytetrafluoroethylene versus autogenous vein grafts for vascular reconstruction in contaminated wounds. Am J Surg 1984; 147:692–695.
11. Malone JM, Lalka SG, McIntyre KE. The necessity for long-term antibiotic therapy with positive arterial wall cultures. J Vasc Surg 1988; 8:262–267.

TREATMENT OF ABDOMINAL AORTIC ANEURYSM BY ENDOVASCULAR GRAFTING

TIM CHUTER, M.D.
JAMES A. DeWEESE, M.D.

DEVELOPMENT

The goal of endovascular treatment of aortic aneurysms is no different from that of conventional treatment, namely, the insertion of a durable graft to convey blood through the aneurysm and protect its walls from risk of rupture.

The main advantage of the endovascular approach is the avoidance of an abdominal operation. The graft is introduced through the femoral artery and passed cephalad into the aorta under fluoroscopic guidance. When the graft reaches its desired position, attachment devices are used to fix it to the nondilated vessels proximal and distal to the aneurysm. This division of function applies to all the systems in clinical use, although several experimental systems combine the barrier functions of a graft with the structural functions of a stent in a single component. The design of the delivery system depends mainly on the characteristics of the stent, which may be self-expanding, balloon-expandable, or both.

The concept of a remotely inserted endovascular graft to treat aneurysms was suggested and developed almost a decade ago by Maas and associates,[1] Balko and colleagues,[2] Wright and co-workers,[3] and Lazarus and associates.[4] The first clinical application of this approach was performed by Parodi in Argentina.[5] The Parodi system employs a balloon-expandable Palmaz stent attached to a thin-walled, weft-knit polyester graft. The early results in a variety of high-risk patients have been excellent. However, in other hands a similar technique failed to achieve graft placement in half the patients. The Lazarus device is the only system approved by the FDA for clinical studies in the United States. Rigid selection criteria have slowed the accrual of patients to this study, and at the time of writing little information about the results was generally available.

Morphology

None of these endovascular systems works well if the morphology of the distal vasculature lies outside certain relatively narrow limits. The remoteness of the manipulations involved in endovascular graft placement makes the technique less invasive than conventional surgical methods, but it also impairs the ability to accommodate variant anatomy intraoperatively. During endovascular graft insertion there is little opportunity to change the size of the graft or the location of distal implantation. Moreover, the implantation of a stent requires a larger margin of normal artery than construction of a sutured anastomosis, and the often tortuous iliac arteries have to be traversed by the rigid delivery system. Therefore, endovascular techniques depend on the morphology of the aneurysm and its branches. Variations in arterial anatomy must be known and accommodated in advance. Important factors include the length of the segment between the aneurysm and the renal arteries, the length of the segment between the aneurysm and the iliac arteries, the tortuosity of the iliac arteries, and the presence of iliac aneurysms.

We studied these variables by reviewing three-dimensional reconstructions of computed tomography (CT) data in 22 patients.[6] Profiles of the axial skeleton, the aneurysm, the aorta, the renal arteries, the mesenteric arteries, and the iliac arteries were outlined manually on conventional CT slices and processed to form a three-dimensional virtual object, which was represented as shaded surface displays on hard copy. We were most interested in the length of nondilated aorta available for stent implantation between the renal arteries and the proximal end of the aneurysm and between the aortic bifurcation and the distal end to the aneurysm. For the purposes of this study the aneurysm was said to begin where the walls of the aorta started to diverge and to end where they became parallel again. Having defined the proximal neck as a segment with parallel walls, we were not surprised to find that the diameter of this segment changed very little from the level of the renal arteries (24.9 ± 1.4 mm) to the proximal end of the aneurysm (27.1 ± 1.5 mm). The mean length of the proximal neck was 26.7 ± 4.1 mm. The proximal neck was longer than 20 mm in 14 patients and longer than 10 mm in 18. There was an inverse relationship between the length of the proximal neck and the size of the aneurysm. Only 38% of patients with an aneurysm wider than 60 mm had a proximal neck longer than 20 mm.

It is hard to use this information to predict the proportion of patients who will be excluded from endovascular repair because of the length of the proximal neck, because the actual exclusion criteria depend on the type of fixation mechanism used and the accuracy of implantation. Indeed, several modifications of prosthesis design may permit implantation in a shorter segment of aorta. One approach is to augment the effect of friction between the artery and the stent by using short barbs. This may permit stents to be implanted even where the aortic walls are not parallel but may not be entirely reliable when the aorta is heavily calcified, as it often is in the presence of an aneurysm. Another approach is to use a shorter stent, although shortening the stent also reduces the length of the zone of apposition between the graft and the aorta. Alternatively, the uncovered part of a longer stent or a second stent may be implanted in a suprarenal segment of aorta. A stent in this location will probably not occlude the renal or superior mesenteric arteries (SMA) immedi-

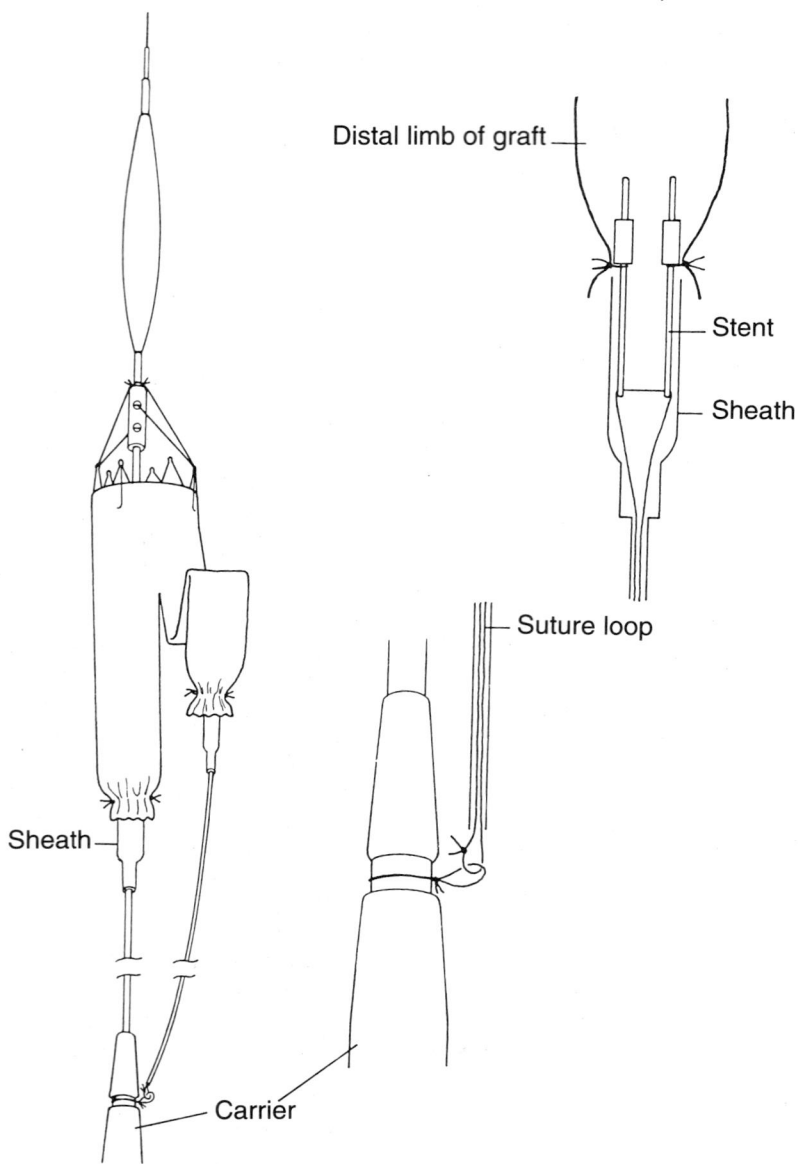

Figure 1 The bifurcated graft, showing the small sheaths and catheters used to control the stents at the distal ends of the graft limbs.

ately, but it may not be advisable when long-term implantation is anticipated.

In our group of 22 patients the distal cuff was usually relatively short (mean 4.2 ± 1.6 mm). In only one patient was the cuff longer than 20 mm, and in only four was it greater than 10 mm. The same caveats apply to interpretation of cuff length as a determinant of the feasibility of distal stent implantation, but this is a major obstacle to distal stent implantation.

Only four patients would have been excluded from consideration for bifurcated graft placement because of iliac aneurysms. In these patients the distal ends of a bifurcated graft could not have been implanted proximal to the iliac bifurcation.

Any delivery system for aneurysm repair must negotiate the often tortuous iliac arteries. Our study of aneurysm morphology documented deviation of the right common iliac artery of more than 45° in seven patients and the deviation of the left iliac common artery of more than 45° in nine. We have not found this degree of tortuosity to be a problem with our delivery system, but iliac tortuosity may limit the usefulness of larger, less flexible systems, particularly those that do not employ a guide wire.

Although the cutoff points for patient selection depend as much on the technical capabilities of the different systems as on the anatomy of the aorta, it is instructive to consider the effects of various selection

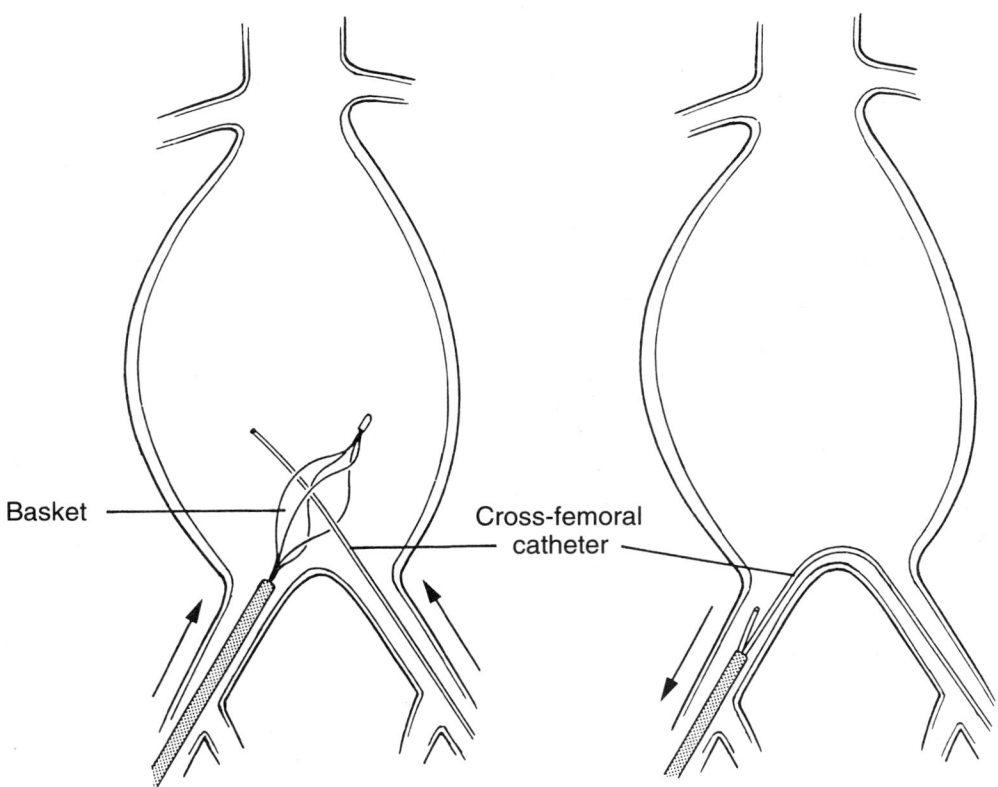

Figure 2 Placement of the cross-femoral catheter using the stone retrieval basket.

criteria in the 22 patients in the morphologic study. We found that 42% of the patients in this study would have been excluded by one of the following: a neck shorter than 10 mm, iliac angulation of more than 60°, or extensive iliac aneurysms. Requiring a 10 mm distal cuff for distal stent implantation would have excluded an additional 49%, leaving only 9% as candidates for straight graft repair. In contrast, 58% would have been suitable for repair with a bifurcated graft, because this type of graft does not depend on the anatomy of the distal cuff. Therefore, we decided to use bifurcated grafts in most cases of endovascular aneurysm repair and have since focused our efforts on the development of a bifurcated system.

Animal Studies

We use a polyester fabric graft that is fixed to the walls of the aorta by barbed Gianturco stents. Our early animal studies with a straight version of this system suggested that the prosthesis could be implanted in the aorta of a dog accurately and securely.[7] We have since performed long-term implantations in animal models of aortic aneurysm with similar results. Canine experiments with a bifurcated version of our system suggested that distal stents were needed to ensure complete opening of the graft limb orifices.[8] Our current system (Fig. 1) uses three stents, one at each orifice, all sutured to the graft prior to delivery. Small sheaths ensure that the distal stents remain collapsed until both distal limbs of the graft are in position. The steps in bifurcated graft insertion are as follows:

1. Placement of a cross-femoral catheter with a stone retrieval basket (Fig. 2)
2. Insertion of a guide wire through one lumen of a double-lumen sheath while the cross-femoral catheter occupies the other, preventing twisting in the iliac artery
3. Insertion of an angiographic catheter over the guide wire
4. Arteriography for identification of the renal arteries and the upper end of the aneurysm
5. Guide wire exchange of the angiographic catheter for the delivery system
6. Extrusion of the graft by removal of the outer sheath of the delivery system
7. Connection of the cross-femoral and distal limb catheters (Fig. 3)
8. Placement of the contralateral distal limb by traction on the cross-femoral catheter (Fig. 4)
9. Release of the contralateral distal limb stent by transecting the associated catheter and suture

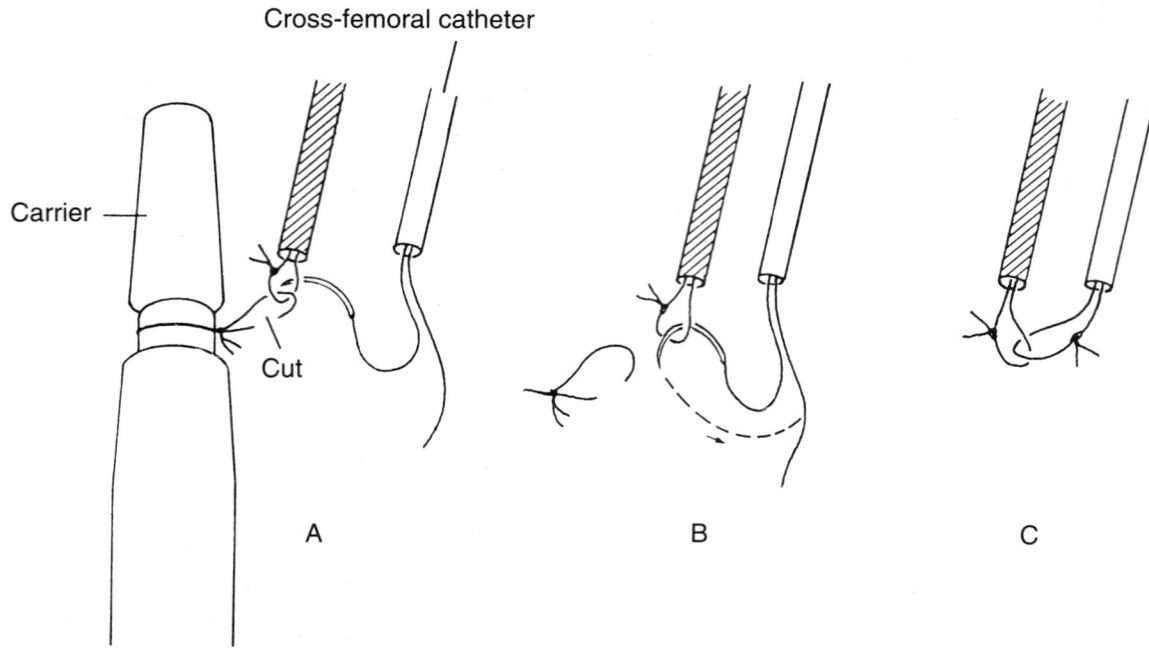

Figure 3 Steps in suturing a connection between the cross-femoral catheter and the other small catheter.

10. Release of the prosthesis from the delivery system by removal of the inner catheter
11. Removal of the delivery system
12. Completion arteriography

CLINICAL TRIALS

We have just begun a multicenter clinical trial in Europe and Australia. All the centers are following a standard protocol that defines the selection criteria, operative procedure, and follow-up.

Patient Selection

Patient selection always centers on an analysis of risk versus benefit. In the case of endovascular aneurysm repair, the patients who have the greatest potential for benefit are those whose medical condition precludes conventional repair. However, these patients also have the highest risk, since unsatisfactory endovascular repair will require operative correction, for which they are unfit. Patients who would otherwise be candidates for conventional repair risk little by undergoing endovascular repair, assuming that any complications are diagnosed and treated promptly. For this reason we include only patients who have sufficient risk of rupture to justify conventional repair and sufficient cardiopulmonary reserve to tolerate an abdominal operation should it be necessary.

We do not consider that sophisticated three-dimensional CT reconstruction is entirely necessary to evaluate patients for endovascular repair. These exclusion criteria for clinical studies are based entirely on the findings of conventional CT scanning and arteriography:

1. Proximal neck shorter than 20 mm
2. Iliac artery aneurysm
3. Iliac artery stenosis with a diameter of less than 6 mm
4. Arteriographic signs that the inferior mesenteric artery (IMA) is indispensable, including opacification of a large IMA, filling of the SMA via collaterals, and stenosis of the celiac or SMA on oblique views

The grafts are custom made for the diameter of the neck and the length of the aneurysm. These measurements are also based on the findings of conventional CT scanning and arteriography.

Study Design

The goals of the first phase of clinical trials are to assess the technical limitations of the system and to refine criteria for patient selection or stratification to be used in subsequent studies. It must be shown that preoperative testing can be used to select patients for whom the technique is safe and effective. This phase of the study will include 20 patients.

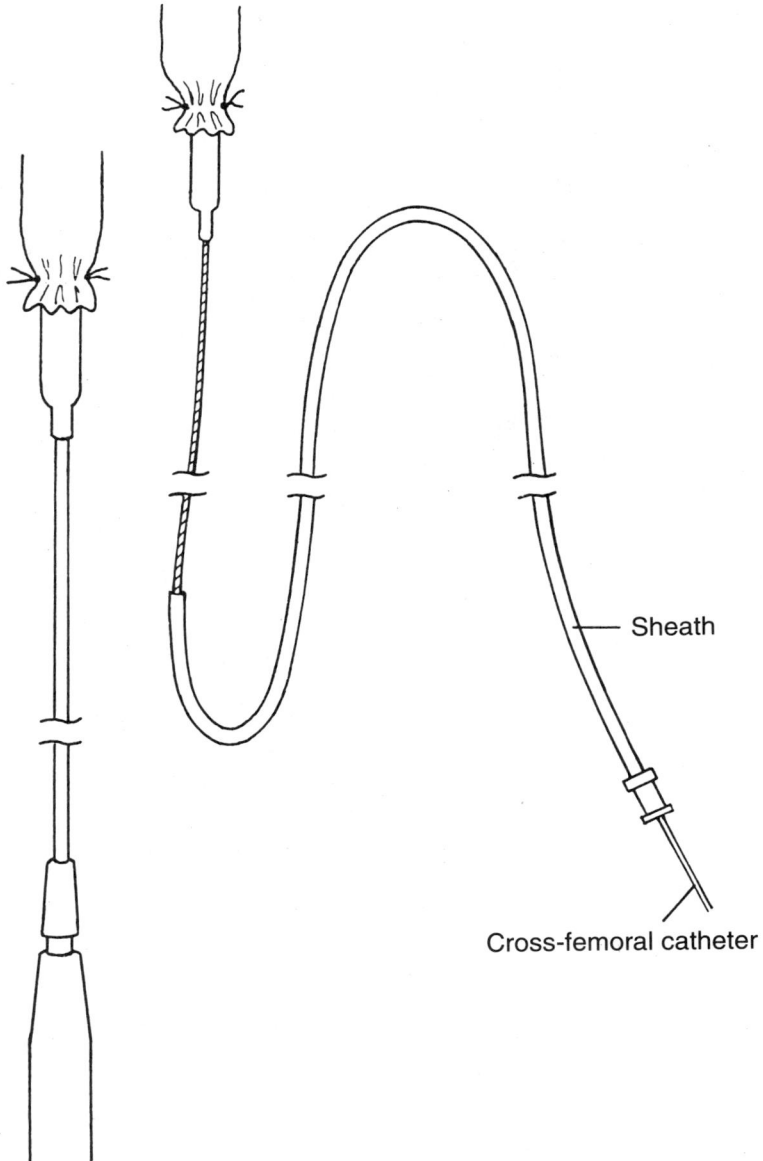

Figure 4 The bifurcated graft and associated catheters at the start of distal limb translocation.

The goal of subsequent phases is to determine the role of endovascular technique by comparing its results with those of conventional repair. To be clinically useful in the broadest range of patients endovascular repair must provide complete protection from risk of rupture and entail lower complication rates than conventional repair. The number of patients must be adequate to reflect the relative rarity of many of the complications of conventional repair. We plan to enroll 200 patients in the second phase, which will make it unlikely that any complication occurring at a rate of 3% or more will fail to be detected (confidence limits 0.6% to 5.4%). All 200 patients in phase 2 will have endovascular repair, and the results will be used to design a larger third phase, in which patients will be randomized to conventional and endovascular therapies, with stratification according to fitness for operation and arterial anatomy.

Procedure

At the time of writing only a week has elapsed since the first two patients were treated in Aachen, Germany.

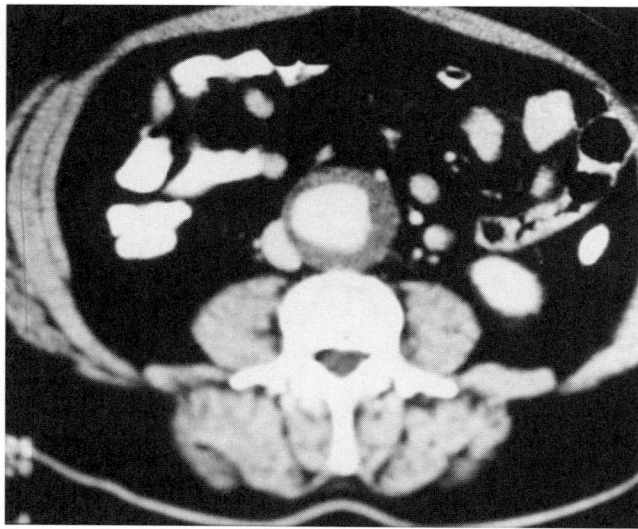

Figure 5 CT scan showing thrombus within the aneurysm.

In both patients the iliac arteries contained angulations greater than 90°. The proximal neck was 30 mm long in the first patient and 28 mm long in the second. Neither patient had a cuff between the distal end of the aneurysm and the iliac arteries according to the findings of CT scanning.

Graft placement followed the series of maneuvers described in the section on animal experimentation. The only difference was the use of a wire to guide the sheath of the stone retrieval basket through the tortuous iliac arteries.

The second patient had large quantities of mural thrombus lining the aneurysm (Fig. 5) and iliac arteries that were almost parallel to one another (Fig. 6). The orientation of the iliac arteries directed the cross-femoral catheter away from the stone retrieval basket, necessitating several minutes of manipulation with the basket and catheter in the aneurysm. We were not, therefore, surprised to see fragments of thrombus floating in the blood flushed from the aorta and also caught in the tip of the basket.

Both proximal stents were placed within 2 mm of the desired position at the distal margin of the renal arterial ostia. On arteriograms and plain abdominal radiographs obtained in the first postoperative week, neither stent was seen to have migrated from the initial position. After distal graft limb deployment both patients had brisk flow at the femoral level, and after closure of femoral arteriotomies both patients had normal pedal pulses. Completion arteriograms documented bilateral flow into the iliac arteries without signs of perigraft leakage. In addition, intravenous digital subtraction arteriograms were performed in the radiology suite on the first postoperative day. These provided more detailed views, which confirmed the findings of completion arteriography and showed no kinking of the grafts despite the sharply angulated iliac arteries (Fig. 7).

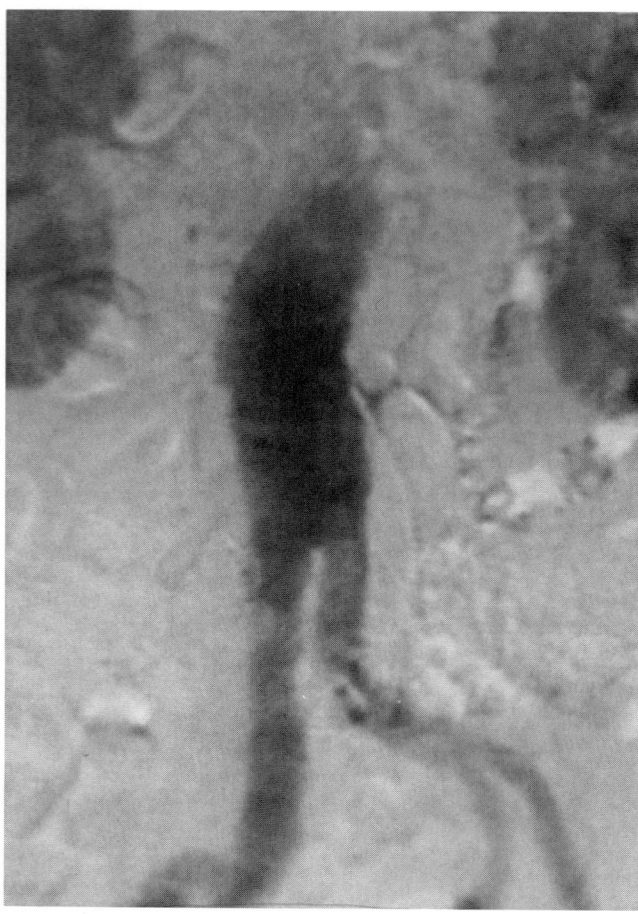

Figure 6 Angiogram showing the configuration of the iliac arteries.

Both patients were eating normally and walking the day after operation. Neither had any signs of embolism or of colon ischemia.

The precision of proximal stent placement and successful graft insertion in the presence of very tortuous iliac arteries suggests that a long proximal neck and straight iliac arteries may not be as important as we supposed. However, we still expect to exclude approximately 30% of patients from endovascular repair because of a proximal neck shorter than 10 mm or iliac artery aneurysms.

Follow-up

These patients will be followed primarily by duplex scanning to assess changes in the graft, the aneurysm, and the flow through lumbar and mesenteric arteries. Close follow-up is important because the long-term fate of endovascular grafts is unknown. Endovascular grafting employs different means of attachment from conventional repair, results in different hemodynamic patterns, leaves the thrombus in place, and leaves the aneurysm intact. The only experience with aneurysm exclusion suggests aneurysm thrombosis in all but a small

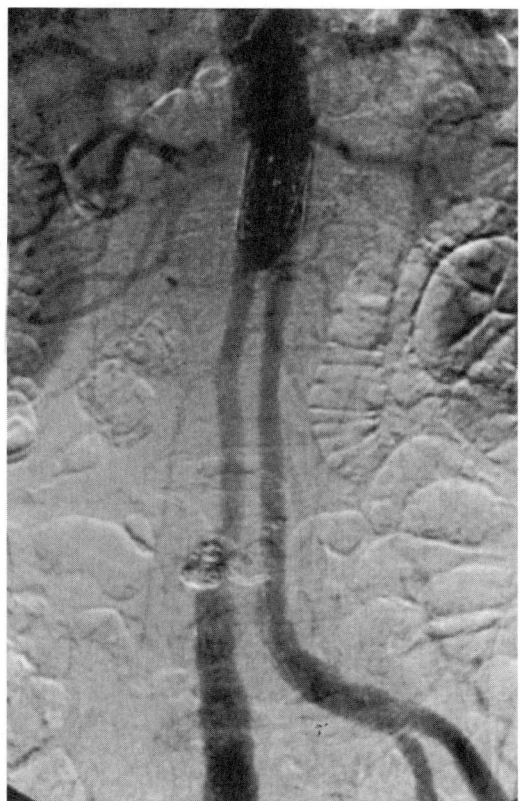

Figure 7 Postoperative angiogram.

minority of patients, no instances of infection in the residual thrombus, and no instances of rupture.[9]

There remain many unanswered questions concerning the long-term fate of patients with aneurysms repaired using endovascular grafts. Even if endovascular techniques prove to be highly effective, some patients will require the standard operation because endovascular repair is limited by anatomic constraints. On the other hand, the potential for lower morbidity of the endovascular approach may broaden the range of candidates to include those with small aneurysms and poor general health.

REFERENCES

1. Maas D, Zollikofer CL, Largiarder F, et al. Radiological follow-up of transluminally inserted vascular endoprosthesis: An experimental study using expanding spirals. Radiology 1984; 152:659–663.
2. Balko AB, Shah DM. Process for restoring patency to body vessels. US Patent No. 4512338, 1985.
3. Wright KC, Wallace S, Charnsangavej C, et al. Percutaneous endovascular graft: Experimental evaluation. Radiology 1987; 163:357–360.
4. Lazarus HM. Intraluminal graft device: System and method. US Patent No. 4787899, 1988.
5. Parodi JC. Palmaz JC, Barone HD. Transfemoral intraluminal graft implantation for abdominal aortic aneurysms. Ann Vasc Surg 1991; 5:491–499.
6. Chuter TAM, Green RM, Ouriel K, DeWeese JA. Infrarenal aortic aneurysm morphology: Implications for transfemoral repair. J Vasc Surg 1993; 17:1120–1121.
7. Chuter TAM, Green RM, Ouriel K, et al. Transfemoral aortic aneurysm repair: Straight and bifurcated grafts in dogs. J Vasc Surg 1993; 17:233.
8. Chuter TAM, Green RM, Ouriel K, et al. Transfemoral endovascular aortic graft placement. J Vasc Surg 1992; 16:300–301.
9. Shah DM, Chang BB, Paty PS, et al. Treatment of abdominal aortic aneurysm by exclusion and bypass: an analysis of outcome. J Vasc Surg 1991; 13:15–22.

ACUTE LIMB ISCHEMIA FOLLOWING AORTIC RECONSTRUCTION

RICHARD E. CARBALLO, M.D.
JONATHAN B. TOWNE, M.D.

The morbidity and mortality of aortic reconstruction for aneurysmal and occlusive disease of the aorta has been reduced by improvements in patient selection, perioperative care, and surgical technique. Peripheral thromboembolism has been recognized as a complication of aortic reconstruction since the beginning of modern vascular surgery. In 1959, Body and Pastel reported a 25% incidence of arterial thromboembolic complications.[1] Since that time there has been a significant reduction of thromboembolic complications, with most series reporting an incidence of 2% to 8%. A recent multicenter prospective study from the Canadian Aneurysm Study Group recorded a 3.3% incidence of distal thromboembolism and a 3.5% incidence of intraoperative ischemia secondary to graft thrombosis.[2] Acute limb ischemia complicating aortic reconstruction prolongs recovery, often necessitates additional operative procedures, and increases morbidity and mortality.[3] In our study there was a 10.3% incidence of acute limb ischemia, which was detected at the conclusion of the operation in 19% of patients and within 48 hours in the remaining 81%. The mortality for patients with ischemia complications was 22%, compared with 3% in patients without limb ischemia.[3] This complication is usually secondary to technical error in the construction of the anastomosis, embolization secondary to mobilization and clamping of a diseased aortoiliac segment, or inadequate runoff to support the intended revascularization. Careful preoperative planning, meticulous surgical technique, and prompt recognition can all lead to minimizing the risk of postoperative limb ischemia and thus minimize the morbidity and mortality of aortic reconstruction.

CAUSES AND PREVENTION OF THROMBOEMBOLIC COMPLICATIONS

Distal Embolization

Distal embolization is the most common cause of acute limb ischemia after aortic reconstruction, accounting for 44% of ischemic complications (Table 1).[3] Macroembolization and microembolization can both occur within the lower extremity. Macroembolization, or large vessel occlusion, presents with an ischemic limb. The foot is cold, pale, pulseless, and mottled. In contrast, in microembolization, or trash foot, the foot is ischemic secondary to microembolic showers to digital vessels; however, pedal pulses are usually palpable. Imparato[4] also stresses embolization as a primary cause of ischemic complications and describes appropriate surgical techniques that are critical in reducing the incidence to a minimum, 0.57% in his analysis.

Distal thromboembolization during aortic reconstruction can occur during dissection of the aneurysm, at the time of aortic clamping, and at the time of restoration of flow. Prevention of this complication begins during the preoperative period. Preoperative examination must include a thorough evaluation of the peripheral pulses and Doppler-derived ankle brachial indices. An accurate baseline examination is crucial to assess the patient's postoperative peripheral circulation. A preoperative arteriogram should be obtained in patients with an abdominal aortic aneurysm who have evidence of lower extremity arterial occlusive disease.

The technical conduct of aortic reconstruction is of utmost importance in preventing thromboembolic complications. Imparato[4] stresses obtaining distal vascular control first and avoiding dissection of the common iliac arteries, which are frequently the site of aneurysmal degeneration. Distal control is obtained at the level of the external iliac arteries and the hypogastric arteries.

Table 1 Causes and Incidence of Acute Limb Ischemia

Cause	*Incidence*
Embolus	44%
Coagulopathy	26
Intimal flaps	18
Inadequate heparin sodium	8

The external iliac artery is clamped first, then the hypogastric artery. The hypogastric artery is at times aneurysmal, and this clamping sequence minimizes the chance of embolization down an open external iliac artery upon clamping of the hypogastric artery. After bilateral distal control is obtained, dissection proceeds at the neck of the aneurysm, and a nonaneurysmal segment of the aorta is chosen for proximal clamping. After the aneurysm is open and the backbleeding lumbar arteries controlled with suture ligatures, the proximal anastomosis is performed and tested for hemostasis. A well-constructed hemostatic proximal anastomosis eliminates the need for reclamping and placing additional sutures, all of which increase the chance of embolization. The iliac anastomosis is performed to the distal common iliac artery 2 to 3 mm proximal to the bifurcation. This area is rarely aneurysmal but may be heavily calcified. This calcification can create a problem in suturing; however, searching the arterial wall for a soft area that allows passage of the needle is usually successful. This anastomosis must be done under direct vision for all suture placement to avoid the creation of an intimal flap. Before the anastomosis is complete, the proximal clamp should be released to allow any debris from the aortic clamp site or from the proximal graft anastomosis to be flushed out of the contralateral limb of the aortic prosthesis. After flushing, the graft is forcefully irrigated with heparinized saline. It is important to clear all blood from the graft after preclotting or flushing of the proximal aorta. If blood is allowed to remain in contact with the prosthesis, it can form thrombi which can embolize after restoration of flow. After the graft has been forcefully irrigated, distal vascular control should be released to allow backbleeding. If there is no distal backbleeding when the hypogastric and external iliac clamps are released, Fogarty catheters should be passed cautiously to retrieve any thrombus or atherosclerotic debris. When the anastomosis is complete, flow should be restored to the hypogastric artery first and subsequently to the external iliac artery.

After completion of both anastomoses, the iliac and femoral pulses should be assessed prior to closing the abdomen. Upon completion of the procedure and with normal femoral pulses, it is essential to assess the remainder of the distal circulation. Early detection of distal embolic complications is important for good results. What would have been a simple problem to rectify in the operating room, if detected early, can propagate into more extensive distal ischemia in the early postoperative period. The distal circulation can be assessed by observation of cutaneous changes, by evaluating distal pulses, and by obtaining Doppler-derived ankle brachial indices in the operating room. These data are compared with preoperative values.

THROMBOTIC COMPLICATIONS

Thrombotic complications may be secondary to inadequate heparinization, a hypercoagulable state, technical errors in construction of the anastomosis, or inadequate runoff to support the intended aortic reconstruction. Associated aortoiliac and femoro-popliteal arterial occlusive disease predisposes to acute ischemia secondary to thrombotic problems. In our study acute ischemia occurred in 9.5% of the patients undergoing abdominal aortic aneurysm repair, 8% of patients undergoing aortobifemoral bypass, and 17% of patients with combined abdominal aortic aneurysm and occlusive disease.[3] These data suggest that concomitant aortic occlusive disease in patients with abdominal aortic aneurysms increases their risk of lower extremity ischemic complications.

Heparinization and Hypercoagulable States

The use of systemic heparinization during aortic reconstruction is well accepted. This is especially critical when aortic clamp time is prolonged.[3,4] However, the absolute need for heparin sodium in the absence of prolonged aortic clamp time is debated. Some studies documented no significant difference in thrombotic complications after aortic reconstruction in patients receiving systemic heparinization compared with those receiving regional heparinization.[2] It is our practice to give 5,000 units of heparin sodium systemically prior to aortic clamping. If the clamp time is prolonged beyond an hour, we give an additional 1,000 units. Serial activating clotting times should be obtained to ensure that anticoagulation is adequate. Paradoxic thrombotic complications with heparin sodium therapy are uncommon but can be responsible for intraoperative graft occlusion. In our study 26% of all ischemic complications were secondary to inadequate heparinization or a hypercoagulable state.

Heparin Sodium–Induced Thrombocytopenia

Heparin sodium–induced thrombocytopenia is common, with 30% of patients exhibiting thrombocytopenia after the institution of heparin therapy. However, thrombotic complications are observed in only 5%.[5] Two types of heparin sodium–induced thrombocytopenia exist. Type I is a non–immune mediated thrombocytopenia thought to be secondary to the direct effect of heparin sodium on platelets, causing aggregation. This form occurs early and runs a benign course, with improvement in the platelet count after the discontinuation of heparin therapy. Type 2 is an immune-mediated form of heparin sodium–induced platelet aggregation. It occurs 5 to 14 days after the administration of heparin sodium and is reported to have a 23% to 60% thrombotic or hemmorhagic complication rate and a 12% to 18% mortality rate.[6] Any patient who has thrombotic complications while receiving heparin sodium should have heparin sodium–induced aggregation of platelets considered as a possible cause. Unexplained thrombosis of an aortic graft in the immediate postoperative period should alert the surgeon to the possibility of heparin sodium–induced thrombosis. At the time of thrombectomy, the finding of white clot composed of the aggregated platelets devoid of any significant red cells is characteristic.[7] Treatment consists of discontinuing all heparin sodium and the use of alternative means of anticoagulation. The defibrinogenating drug ancrod has been proposed as the agent of choice if continued anticoagulation is necessary.[8]

Antithrombin III Deficiency

Antithrombin III (AT III) deficiencies may be another reason for seemingly unexplained thrombotic episodes. AT III, is an alpha-2 globulin produced by the liver, is a potent inactivator of thrombin and factors XII, XI, X, and VII. It also functions as a heparin cofactor necessary for heparin sodium's anticoagulant activity. A common presentation of AT III deficiency is a patient with a thrombotic event who fails to be adequately anticoagulated with heparin sodium. AT III deficency results primarily in venous thrombosis, but it has been reported as a cause of arterial thrombosis, including graft thrombosis after aortic reconstruction.[9] The diagnosis can be confirmed by measurement of plasma AT III levels. It should be kept in mind that AT III deficency can be associated with several conditions, including diffuse intravascular coagulation, liver disease, and the administration of heparin sodium. Treatment of AT III deficency requires sodium warfarin, since warfarin has been reported to increase the level of AT III.[5] Acute treatment in a patient with thrombosis requires the replacement of AT III using fresh frozen plasma and heparin sodium anticoagulation until adequate oral anticoagulation is achieved.

TREATMENT

Treatment of an ischemic limb complicating aortic reconstruction depends on the cause of the ischemia. All efforts should be made to assess the graft-iliac anastomoses and ensure adequate inflow before the abdomen is closed. If the femoral pulse is absent postoperatively, abdominal exploration is required. After heparinization and application of vascular clamps, the anastomosis is examined for technical defects through a linear incision in the limb of the prosthesis just proximal to the anastomosis. If no technical error is found, a Fogarty catheter is carefully passed proximally and distally to remove any thromboembolic debris. It is important to clamp the contralateral prosthetic limb to avoid embolization of debris. If satisfactory flow to the groin level cannot be restored, the graft should be extended to the femoral vessels. Thrombosis of the graft is likely to be secondary to latent iliac disease if no technical flaw is appreciated at the iliac anastomosis. If there is not prompt return of foot color with pedal pulses, an operative femoral arteriogram should be obtained. Orificial stenosis at the level of the profunda femoris artery is an indication to incorporate a profundaplasty into the distal anastomosis. A difficult situation arises when the superficial femoral artery is occluded and there is diffuse disease of the profunda femoris artery. Under these circumstances, profundaplasty alone will not provide sufficient outflow to maintain patency of the aortofemoral limb, and a distal bypass to achieve adequate outflow is indicated.

Thromboembolism can also occur to the femoropopliteal or tibial vessels. If there is acute limb ischemia with a normal femoral pulse, femoral exploration is indicated. Femoral thromboembolectomy should be performed and followed by an operative arteriogram. There may be clot in the distal popliteal artery or tibial vessels that cannot be cleared from the common femoral artery. If this is the case, dissection of the infrageniculate popliteal artery, the tibioperoneal trunk, and the anterior tibial artery will allow an arteriotomy in the distal popliteal artery and direction of a Fogarty catheter selectively down the tibial vessels.

When embolization occurs to the distal tibial or pedal arteries or when propagation of thrombus leads to thrombosis of the vessels, severe distal ischemia and possibly tissue loss that is not amenable to catheter thromboembolectomy may develop. The systemic use of thrombolytic therapy in the immediate postoperative period is contraindicated. One option reported by Camerota[10] is the use of high-dose isolated limb perfusion with urokinase. The extremity is elevated and an esmarch bandage applied to drain the venous system. A tourniquet is applied, and selective infusion of the distal circulation is performed, with the effluent drained at the level of the popliteal vein. There is no systemic thrombolytic effect. This approach is effective only if the majority of the occluding material is thrombotic clot. When atheromatous debris occludes the distal circulation, intraoperative thrombolytics are ineffective.

In instances of repeated thrombosis where no technical error is found, patients should be evaluated for a coagulation disorder. A platelet count should be obtained to assess the possibility of heparin sodium–induced platelet aggregation. If thrombocytopenia is present, a specimen should be sent for heparin sodium–induced platelet antibodies, and the heparin sodium should be discontinued. If the platelet count is normal, fresh frozen plasma should be administered and the heparin sodium continued while evaluating the patient for an AT III deficency. Protein C and S levels should also be determined. All patients with unexplained thrombosis of either the arterial or venous systems should undergo complete evaluation of the coagulation system.

REFERENCES

1. Body DP, Pastel H. Results of treatment of aneurysms of the abdominal aorta. Postgrad Med 1959; 25:238–243.
2. Johnston KW. Multicenter prospective study of nonruptured abdominal aortic aneurysms, part 2: Variables predicting morbidity and mortality. J Vasc Surg 1989; 9:437–446.
3. Strom JA, Bernhard VM, Towne JB. Acute limb ischemia following aortic reconstruction: A preventable cause of increased mortality. Arch Surg 1984; 119:470–473.
4. Imparato AM. Abdominal aortic surgery: Prevention of lower limb ischemia. Surgery 1983; 93:112–116.
5. Silver D. Heparin-induced thrombocytopenia. Semin Vasc Surg 1988; 1:228.
6. Jacobs DL, Towne JB. Hemostasis and coagulation. In: White R, Hollier L, eds. Vascular surgery: Basic science and clinical correlation (in press).
7. Towne JB, Bernhard VM, Hussey C, Garancis JC. White clot syndrome: Peripheral vascular complications of heparin therapy. Arch Surg 1979; 114:372–377.
8. Cole CW, Fournier LM, Bormanis J. Heparin-associated thrombocytopenia and thrombosis: Optimal therapy with ancrod. Can J Surg 1990; 33:207.
9. Towne JB, Bernhard VM, Hussy C, Garancis JC. Antithrombin III deficiency: A cause of unexplained thrombosis in vascular surgery. Surgery 1981; 89:735–742.
10. Camerota, AJ. Intra-arterial thrombolytic therapy. In: Camerota AJ, ed. Thrombolytic therapy. New York: Grune & Stratton, 1988:125.

INTESTINAL ISCHEMIA AS A COMPLICATION OF ABDOMINAL AORTIC RECONSTRUCTION

MASSIMO M. NAPOLITANO, M.D.
ALEXANDER D. SHEPARD, M.D.

The first case of intestinal ischemia following aortic reconstruction was described only 2 years after the first successful resection of an abdominal aortic aneurysm (AAA).[1] Since then intestinal ischemia has become a well recognized but infrequent complication of abdominal aortic reconstruction. Because of the significant morbidity and mortality associated with transmural intestinal ischemia, prevention remains the key. To avoid this complication vascular surgeons must thoroughly understand the anatomy of the visceral circulation and its pathophysiology.

INTESTINAL CIRCULATION ANATOMY

The distribution of the three major visceral arteries corresponds to the embryologic development of the gut. The celiac trunk and its branches supply the foregut organs (stomach, duodenum, liver, and spleen); the superior mesenteric artery (SMA) supplies the midgut (jejunum, ileum, and right and transverse colon); and the inferior mesenteric artery (IMA) supplies the hindgut (distal transverse, descending, and rectosigmoid). The SMA has two collateral connections with the IMA. The better known but hemodynamically less important is through the marginal artery of Drummond, which originates from the left branch of the middle colic artery and courses along the margin of the transverse mesocolon to join the ascending branch of the left colic artery at the splenic flexure. A second and more important collateral channel originates from the proximal portion of the left branch of the middle colic artery and terminates in the proximal third of the left colic artery. This vessel is present in two-thirds of individuals; it has many eponyms but is best known as the meandering mesenteric artery (MMA). In the presence of a chronically occluded IMA the MMA may enlarge significantly and be clearly visible angiographically. When present, the MMA is a vital collateral channel to the hindgut, and its injury or ligation leads almost invariably to colonic ischemia. With SMA occlusion this vessel may also be critical for perfusion of the small bowel, and failure to reimplant a patent IMA during aortic reconstruction in this situation can lead to midgut ischemia. Important collateral connections are also present at the level of the rectum between branches of the IMA (superior hemorrhoidal arteries) and branches of the hypogastric arteries (middle and inferior hemorrhoidal arteries).

PATHOPHYSIOLOGY

Visceral ischemia after aortic reconstruction results from mesenteric hypoperfusion or less commonly embolism of atheromatous debris. Hypoperfusion is usually due to interruption of blood flow through a hemodynamically important feeding vessel. Ligation of a patent, poorly collateralized IMA is the most common cause of rectosigmoid ischemia following aortic reconstruction.[2] Even with preexisting IMA occlusion, however, ischemic colitis can occur if the hypogastric circulation is excluded or important collaterals like the MMA are damaged. Midgut ischemia results from failure to reimplant a patent IMA in the presence of significant SMA disease and a large MMA or from iatrogenic SMA injury. Hypoperfusion can also be nonocclusive, a problem usually associated with periods of prolonged hypotension or other low flow states. The visceral circulation is particularly sensitive to low flow, which can result in persistent mesenteric vasoconstriction and redistribution of blood flow to other vital organs. This nonocclusive process is a rare cause of intestinal ischemia following aortic reconstruction. Atheroembolism to the small bowel may result from manipulation of a diseased suprarenal aorta. Similar atheroembolism through the IMA can also occur with infrarenal aortic manipulation but is a less frequent cause of ischemic colitis. Patchy transmural necrosis is the usual result.

Three degrees of ischemic bowel injury can be recognized. Mucosal ischemia is characterized by patchy sloughing of the mucosa with submucosal edema; the bowel wall remains intact and distensible. When the muscularis is involved, endoscopic findings include thinned-out mucosa with visible submucosal vessels and islands of ulcerated mucosa. The most severe injury, transmural necrosis, is recogized by gray mucosa coupled with a stiff, nondistensible bowel wall. Mucosal ischemia alone usually resolves without sequelae. Involvement of the muscularis also heals but frequently leaves a residual stricture. Transmural necrosis invariably progresses to gangrene and perforation if left untreated.[2]

INCIDENCE AND ASSOCIATED RISK FACTORS

Left colon and sigmoid ischemias are the most common visceral ischemic syndromes following aortic reconstruction. The incidence of ischemic colitis in the literature ranges from 0.2% to 10%, with a rate of clinically significant ischemia between 1% and 2% in most recent series. This figure may be an underestimate of the overall incidence because of exclusion of minor and asymptomatic ischemia. In a prospective study using routine postoperative colonoscopy, Ernst and colleagues[3] found an incidence of 6%. Small-bowel ischemia after aortic reconstruction occurs less frequently, with reported rates varying from 0.15% to 0.6%. Review of our experience at Henry Ford Hospital over the past 20 years with 1,473 abdominal aortic reconstruction procedures revealed 16 (1.08%) patients with transmural infarction of the left colon and 2 (0.13%) patients with combined small-bowel and colon ischemia.

Ischemic colitis somewhat less frequently follows operation for aortoiliac occlusive disease than for aneurysmal disease, probably because of the greater number of collaterals in patients with occlusive disease. The highest incidence of colon ischemia follows ruptured AAA repair, in which probable contributing factors include perioperative hypotension, IMA ligation, and a large mesenteric hematoma that can compress collateral blood vessels. Other risk factors for colon ischemia include prior colon resection and total redo aortic grafting, both of which raise the potential for interruption of normal collateral circulation.[4] Small-bowel ischemia resulting from SMA injury or embolism usually follows complex aortic reconstructions requiring suprarenal aortic clamping. Both of our instances of small-bowel ischemia were in patients requiring suprarenal aortic clamping in whom manipulation of a diseased pararenal aorta led to atheroembolism of the SMA and IMA.

OPERATIVE RECOGNITION AND PREVENTION OF INTESTINAL ISCHEMIA

Prevention of intestinal ischemic complications requires good operative planning and attention to technical details. All patients undergoing elective aortic reconstruction in our institution undergo preoperative aortography to document patency of the SMA and IMA and the presence of an MMA. In addition, aortography provides information about the status of the hypogastric circulation and the pararenal aorta. Knowledge of any significant atheromatous disease in the pararenal aorta as well the relationship of the SMA to the renal arteries is particularly important for complex aortic reconstruction in which suprarenal aortic clamping may be required.

Preservation of hypogastric blood flow is important to the prevention of ischemic colitis, particularly in patients with known IMA occlusion. In patients with occlusive disease undergoing aortofemoral grafting, retrograde blood flow from the femoral arteries is usually sufficient to maintain blood flow to the hypogastric arteries. In the occasional patient with bilateral external iliac artery occlusions, a proximal end-to-side aortic anastomosis should be considered. This configuration preserves prograde blood flow to patent hypogastric arteries and the IMA. During AAA repair, blood flow to at least one hypogastric artery should be preserved; hence, end-to-end anastomoses to both external iliac arteries should be avoided.

If the IMA is found to be patent during AAA repair, it is necessary to decide whether revascularization is necessary. Since most patients tolerate IMA ligation safely, routine reimplantation is unnecessary. An accurate test for detecting colon ischemia intraoperatively will allow selective IMA reconstruction when appropriate. Visual inspection of the colon is notoriously unreliable, so a variety of detection methods have been devised. These include measurement of IMA stump blood pressure, detection of Doppler flow signals along the mesenteric and antimesenteric borders of the colon, photoplethysmography of the colon, and measurement of intraluminal colonic pH (Table 1). Regardless of the method used, if colon ischemia is detected, every effort should be made to restore IMA flow. IMA reconstruction should also be considered if there is significant occlusive disease of the SMA, particularly in the presence of a large MMA, or aneurysmal disease of the hypogastric arteries necessitating bilateral aneurysm exclusion. A history of colon resection has not been an absolute indication in our experience, but it suggests the need for objective documentation of adequate colonic blood flow.

Certain technical details are important to the prevention of intestinal ischemia. During initial exposure care should be taken to avoid injury to the visceral arteries and collateral channels, particularly when using unyielding mechanical retraction devices, which may damage vessels by prolonged compression. The SMA is especially vulnerable to injury when it originates close to the renal arteries and suprarenal aortic clamping is attempted. Careful assessment of the aorta at the site of proposed cross-clamp is also necessary to minimize the risks of atheroembolism. Temporary clamping of a patent IMA prior to manipulation and clamping of a significantly diseased infrarenal aorta can prevent hindgut atheroembolism. When atheromatous disease extends to involve the pararenal aorta, we have found clamping the usually disease-free supraceliac aorta to be a safer alternative.[5]

Table 1 Intraoperative Detection of Colonic Ischemia

Method	Critical Value
IMA stump pressure*	Less than 40 mm Hg (mean)
Doppler flow in colonic mesentery†	Absence of flow signal
Photoplethysmography‡	Loss of pulsatile flow
Tonometric measurement of colonic mucosal pH§	pH not more than 6.86

*Ernst CB, Hagihara PF, Daugherty ME, et al. Inferior mesenteric artery stump pressure: A reliable index for safe IMA ligation during abdominal aortic aneurysmectomy. Ann Surg 1978;187:641–646.
†Hobson RW, Wright DB, Rich NM. Assessment of colonic ischemia during aortic surgery by doppler ultrasound. J Surg Res 1976; 20:231–235.
‡Ouriel K, Fiore WM, Geary JE. Detection of occult colonic ischemia during aortic procedures: Use of an intraoperative photoplethysmographic technique. J Vasc Surg; 1988; 7:5–9.
§Fiddian-Green RG, Amelin PM, Herrmann JB. Prediction of the development of sigmoid ischemia on the day of aortic operations. Arch Surg 1986; 121:654–660.

On opening the anterior wall of an AAA, the IMA orifice should be preserved so that a Carrel patch can be constructed in case IMA reimplantation becomes necessary. When IMA backbleeding is pulsatile, its origin can be safely oversewn from within the aneurysm. If there is any doubt of the adequacy of backbleeding, an IMA backpressure can be measured from within the opened aneurysm. This measurement is obtained only after distal blood flow has been restored to take advantage of any contribution the hypogastric circulation may have to IMA blood flow. Backbleeding from the IMA can be controlled with a 3 Fr balloon occlusion catheter passed from within the opened aneurysm or by application of a small occluding clamp applied to the proximal artery. Backpressure is measured with a small ball-tipped cannula connected to pressure tubing and passed through the ostium of the IMA for 3 to 4 mm. A mean pressure less than 40 mm Hg is an indication for IMA revascularization.

The easiest way to restore flow to the IMA is by reimplanting a small excised button of aortic wall containing the origin of this vessel into the side of the prosthesis. With this technique it is frequently necessary to perform a limited endarterectomy of the aortic wall and IMA orifice to remove friable calcific plaque. Rarely is a vein graft necessary.

DIAGNOSIS AND TREATMENT OF POSTOPERATIVE INTESTINAL ISCHEMIA

Despite careful efforts to recognize and prevent intestinal ischemia during aortic reconstruction, such complications occur. Prompt diagnosis is mandatory to minimize morbidity and mortality. Significant small bowel ischemia usually becomes apparent in the immediate postoperative period through refractory acidosis, increased fluid requirements, and hemodynamic instability. Both of our patients with significant small-bowel ischemia had persistent postoperative hypotension and oliguria unresponsive to intravenous fluids associated with a low peripheral vascular resistance. Significant physical findings are usually absent in the immediate postoperative period. A high index of suspicion and prompt celiotomy are necessary to prevent progression to midgut infarction. Mesenteric atheroembolism is usually fatal unless limited to short segments of bowel. Injury and/or thrombosis of the SMA should be treated by thrombectomy and repair followed by resection of nonviable bowel.

Ischemic colitis and lesser degrees of small-bowel ischemia are usually not manifest until the second or third postoperative day, occasionally even later. The diagnosis is suggested most frequently by diarrhea. Bloody stool is an ominous sign, almost invariably signifying transmural necrosis. However, diarrhea can be guaiac-negative, as in four of our patients with endoscopically documented colon ischemia. Physical findings include abdominal distention and tenderness with signs of peritoneal irritation when ischemia has progressed to transmural infarction. In the postoperative period, however, these signs may be difficult to appreciate. Increased postoperative fluid requirements or failure to mobilize normal third space fluid losses on the third or fourth postoperative day was present in 9 of our 16 patients with transmural colonic involvement. Persistent leukocytosis and mild acidosis were also common (Table 2).

Flexible sigmoidoscopy is a simple, safe, and reliable test for identifying colonic ischemia, and it should be used liberally early in the evaluation of postoperative diarrhea and/or unexplained early sepsis following aortic reconstruction. This examination, which can be performed at the bedside to determine the extent and severity of the ischemic insult, is valuable in planning therapy.

Once the diagnosis of ischemic colitis is established, treatment depends on the degree of ischemia. Mucosal ischemia usually resolves without sequelae and is treated conservatively with bowel rest, broad-spectrum intravenous antibiotics, and total parenteral nutrition. These measures are continued until bowel activity returns to normal, abdominal findings or signs of sepsis resolve, and repeat sigmoidoscopy documents resolution of the injury. More extensive ischemia with involvement of the muscularis can be treated similarly. Long-term follow-up is necessary because stricture formation is common. In patients with transmural infarction, celiotomy with colon resection, end colostomy, and Hartmann's procedure are mandatory. Broad-spectrum antibiotics are given preoperatively. The entire left colon should be removed along with the distal transverse colon back to the middle colic artery. The rectal closure is best performed below the peritoneal reflection, where the blood supply is via the hemorrhoidal arteries, to reduce the risk of delayed necrosis. To minimize contamination of the recently placed aortic prosthesis, the colonic mesentery is divided immediately adjacent to the bowel wall, taking care to avoid opening any previous retroperitoneal incisions.

Table 2 Findings Associated with Transmural Ischemic Colitis (N = 16)

Finding	Patients	(%)
Diarrhea	11	(69)
Grossly bloody	7	(44)
Guaiac negative	1	(6)
Increased fluid requirements*	9	(56)
Abdominal findings†	8	(50)
Peritoneal irritation	5	(31)
Leukocytosis (WBC greater than 15,000)	7	(44)
Fever (temperature 38.5° C or above)	7	(44)
Persistent metabolic acidosis (pH less than 7.32)	5	(31)

*Requirement for at least 2.5 times the calculated daily maintenance dose of intravenous fluids on the first and second postoperative days in the absence of any obvious ongoing fluid losses *or* failure to mobilize third space fluid losses on the third and fourth postoperative days.
†Distention and/or tenderness with or without peritoneal signs.

Mortality for transmural intestinal ischemia is significant, ranging from 50% to 80%. In our experience the mortality was 56%, with sepsis and multiorgan failure being the most common cause of death. Complications included renal failure in five patients; respiratory failure, rectal abscess, myocardial infarction, and liver failure in two patients each; and congestive heart failure and stroke in one patient each. There were no episodes of delayed graft infection in our series.

Intestinal ischemia following aortic reconstruction remains an infrequent but potentially catastrophic complication. However, our recent experience and that of others[6] suggest that the incidence of this problem can be minimized by good preoperative planning, careful surgical technique, and adherence to accepted surgical principles for preserving visceral blood flow.

REFERENCES

1. Moore SW. Resection of the abdominal aorta with defect replaced by homologous graft. Surg Gynecol Obstet 1954; 99:745–747.
2. Ernst CB. Prevention of intestinal ischemia following abdominal aortic reconstruction. Surgery 1983; 93:102–106.
3. Ernst CB, Hagihara PF, Daugherty ME et al. Ischemic colitis following abdominal aortic reconstruction: A prospective study. Surg 1976; 80:417.
4. Brewster DC, Franklin DP, Cambria RP et al. Intestinal ischemia complicating abdominal aortic surgery. Surgery 109: 1991; 447–454.
5. Nypaver TJ, Shepard AD, Reddy DJ et al. Supraceliac aortic cross-clamping: Determinants of outcome in elective abdominal aortic reconstruction. J Vasc Surg 1993; 17:868–876.
6. Zelenock GB, Strodel WE, Knol JA, et al. A prospective study of clinically and endoscopically documented colonic ischemia in 100 patients undergoing aortic reconstructive surgery with aggressive colonic and direct pelvic revascularization, compared with historic controls. Surgery 1989; 106:771–780.

NEUROLOGIC COMPLICATIONS OF ABDOMINAL AORTIC RECONSTRUCTION

ELLIOT L. CHAIKOF, M.D., PH.D.
ATEF A. SALAM, M.D.

Spinal cord ischemia is a devastating complication of abdominal aortic reconstruction. The first such case was reported in 1956 by McCune,[1] but it was not until the comprehensive review by Szilagyi and associates[2] in 1978 that estimates of the frequency of this complication, the neurologic presentation, and postulated pathophysiologic mechanisms were clearly stated. The most common cause of spinal cord damage was considered to be a direct interruption of the blood supply of the spinal cord due to an anomalously placed great radicular artery. Although attempts at prevention were suggested, for the most part the avoidance of this complication was considered impossible. Szilagyi's most recent review of the world literature[3] confirms the estimated incidences observed in both the original and a later report[4]: 1 in 400 after abdominal aortic aneurysmectomy and 1 in 5,000 after reconstruction for aortoiliac occlusive disease. Notwithstanding the infrequent occurrence of this complication, the presumption that all such cases are unpreventable may be incorrect. Indeed, studies in the past decade suggest that a failure to appreciate the significance of collateral sources of spinal cord blood flow may be responsible for at least some cases of postoperative paraplegia.

ANATOMY

Despite the inherent variability of the spinal cord's blood supply and the lack of a single extraspinal source, numerous anatomic studies have characterized several consistent features, including proximal, intermediate, and terminal arterial divisions (Fig. 1). The rostral portion of the cord is supplied by branches arising from the vertebral arteries and the costocervical and thyrocervical trunks. The thoracic and lumbar regions receive their blood supply from intercostal and lumbar vessels, and the caudal portion of the cord receives branches from the lumbar, iliolumbar, and lateral sacral arteries of the hypogastric circulation. These primary aortic branches can be considered the proximal division of the cord arterial circulation.

Radicular arteries and their associated anterior or posterior radicular branches are derived from the primary aortic branches and constitute an intermediate pathway. Although there may be as many as 31 pairs of radicular arteries, most end within the nerve roots, the dura, or the pia mater. Below the upper cervical segments six to eight anterior radicular arteries supply most of the anterior cord blood supply, giving rise to ascending and descending branches that constitute the anterior spinal artery. The middle cervical segments are supplied by two or three anterior radicular arteries that arise from the vertebral arteries. The lower cervical and upper two or three thoracic segments are supplied by an anterior radicular artery from the costocervical trunk. A small radicular branch enters the vertebral column between T5 and T7 and supplies the midthoracic segments. The largest and most constant anterior radicular artery, the arteria radicularis magna (ARM), also known as the great radicular artery or the artery of Adamkiewicz, originates from a lower intercostal or an upper lumbar artery. In 75% of patients it accompanies the ninth, tenth, eleventh, or twelfth thoracic nerve root and in two-thirds lies to the left of the midline.[4] The ARM supplies primarily caudad blood flow in the anterior spinal artery. Some 18 to 22 smaller posterior radicular arteries give rise to interrupted and irregular anastomosing vessels, known as the paired posterior spinal arteries.

The anterior and paired posterior spinal arteries and their associated intraspinal branches are considered the terminal division of the cord blood supply. Although this terminology suggests continuous vessels running along the anterior or posterior surfaces of the cord, functionally there is little longitudinal flow. However, these vessels are continuous at the tip of the conus medullaris, where an anastomotic loop is formed between the anterior and posterior spinal arteries. The regions of poorest collateralization in the anterior spinal artery are between T4 and T9 and between T12 and L5. The terminal nature of higher-order arterial branching characterizes the intraspinal arterial network (Fig. 2). Anterior sulcal arteries originate from the anterior spinal artery and pass posteriorly through the anterior median fissure, where they branch at right angles to supply either the left or right side of the cord. An exception to this has been noted in the lumbar and sacral regions, where in an occasional patient the anterior sulcal arteries will bifurcate and supply both sides. Similarly, the paired posterior spinal arteries give rise to penetrating posterior sulcal arteries. Anastomotic connections by way of the vasa corona are present but do not provide significant collateral flow between the anterior and posterior circulations, and so these penetrating vessels act as end arteries. Thus, sulcal branches that arise from the anterior spinal artery supply all the cord gray matter except for the posterior horns and most of the anterior and lateral white matter columns. A superficial rim of white matter and the posterior horns are supplied by penetrating rami from the posterior sulcal arterial plexus.

CLINICAL CORRELATION

The practicing vascular surgeon must consider several important factors. First, although collateral

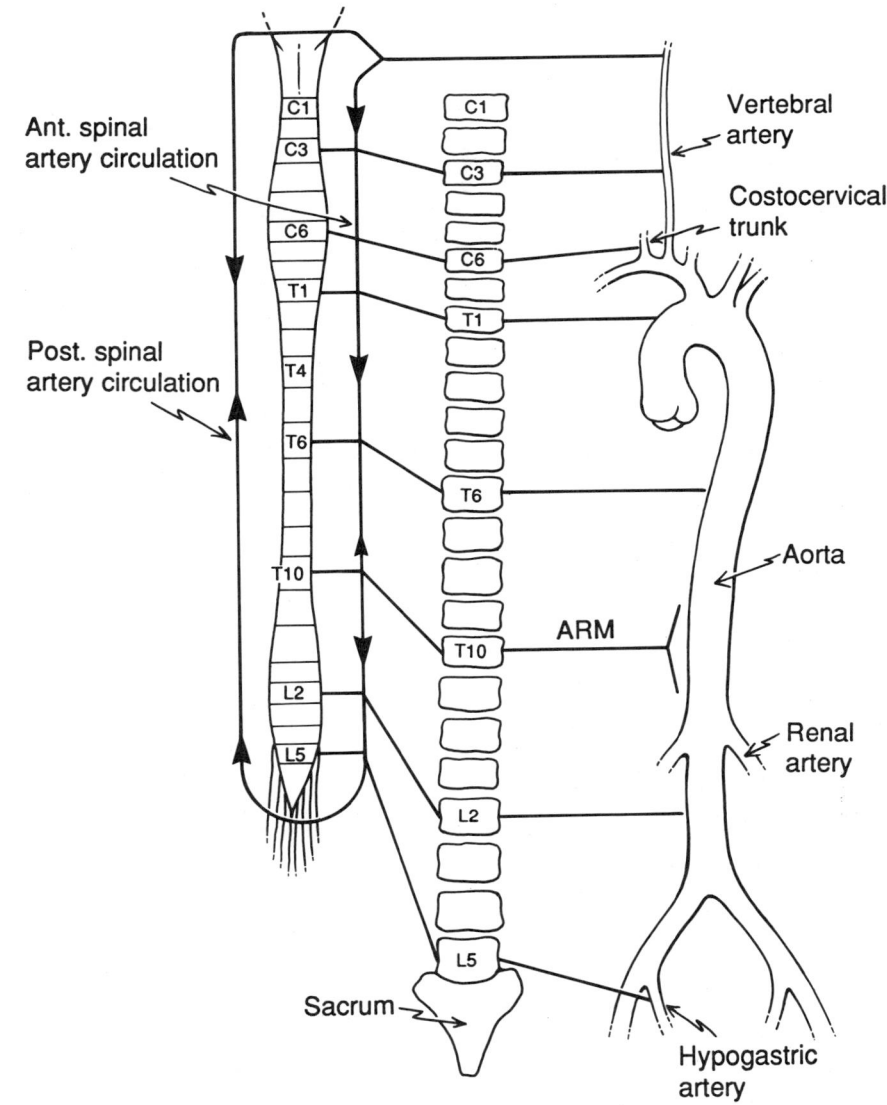

Figure 1 Components of spinal cord blood supply. (Adapted from Picone AL, Green RM, Ricotta JR, et al. Spinal cord ischemia following operations on the abdominal aorta. J Vasc Surg 1986; 3:94–103; with permission.)

blood flow is limited within and immediately surrounding the cord, functionally significant anastomotic channels exist between aortic extraspinal arteries. As a consequence, the closer an arterial obstruction is to its origin from the aorta, the greater is the possibility of adequate collateral circulation. Thus, the lack of spinal ischemia despite the absence of observed backbleeding from multiple intercostal or lumbar vessels during many instances of aortic reconstruction emphasizes the significance of extraspinal collateral flow. Second, the surgeon must be aware of the potential importance of the ARM and particularly its relationship to the origin of the renal arteries, which defines the site of aortic cross-clamping in most patients. Because the ARM typically originates between T9 and T12, occlusion of this pathway would be expected to produce ischemia in an anterior spinal artery territory of poor collateral blood flow. Characteristically, the watershed area in the midthoracic region between T4 and T9 is most susceptible. A low origin of the ARM has been documented at the L1 level in 10% and at the L2 and L3 levels in 12% of patients.[5] Thus, in perhaps 10% of aortic reconstructions the ARM may be occluded during infrarenal aortic clamping. The rarity of postoperative spinal ischemia cannot be attributed to the infrequency of a low ARM. Rather, the presence of either a low thoracic radicular artery or alternate sources of collateral blood flow, principally via the hypogastrics, most likely preserves spinal perfusion.[6–9]

In this regard the importance of mesenteric collaterals in maintaining pelvic circulation bears emphasis (Fig. 3). In the event of chronic bilateral interruption of

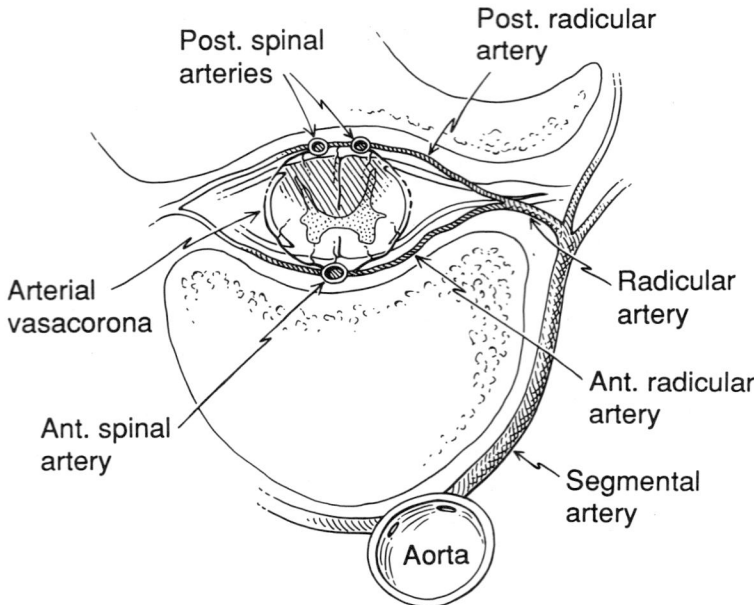

Figure 2 Terminal branching of the intraspinal arterial network.

the hypogastric and inferior mesenteric (IMA) arteries, a meandering mesenteric artery may provide important collateral blood flow to the internal iliac vessels. In addition, although the marginal artery of Drummond is not generally considered an important collateral pathway to hypogastric arteries, it may occasionally serve in this capacity after acute interruption of prograde flow. Therefore, patients who have lost mesenteric collateral either through direct ligation or previous colectomy may be at increased risk for spinal cord ischemia in the event of bilateral hypogastric artery ligation. Failure to maintain a critical hypogastric collateral pathway typically produces ischemia in the watershed region of the anterior spinal artery at the thoracolumbar level between T12 and L5.

Occlusion of the anterior spinal artery usually leads to infarction of the anterior two-thirds of the cord. On the other hand, prolonged hypotension more often results in fusiform infarction of the central portion of the spinal cord at the watershed region of the posterior and anterior circulations. Both lesions, however, can produce an identical clinical picture, the anterior spinal artery syndrome. This syndrome is characterized by flaccid weakness, sphincter dysfunction, and decreased or absent pain and temperature sensation. Vibratory sense and proprioception remain intact. Initial spinal shock is followed by hypertonia, hyperreflexia, and extensor plantar responses. Occlusion of the posterior spinal artery is rare, perhaps as a consequence of better collateralization within the arterial plexus.

Posterior column infarction results in diminished sensation to position and vibration, although the patient may complain of pain or dysthesia. If there is associated edema or extension of the lesion, the infarct may extend into the posterior horns and corticospinal tracts, leading to paresis or paralysis, sphincter dysfunction, and eventual loss of sensation and reflexes. In general, clinical recovery is greater among patients with either ischemic injury of the lumbosacral plexus or injuries associated with incomplete paralysis or sensory loss.

CAUSES

Infarction of the spinal cord may result from direct interruption of the cord blood supply, a critical collateral, or systemic hypoperfusion. Atheromatous embolic infarction has been implicated in several reports. Additionally, spontaneous thrombosis of an atherosclerotic radicular artery has been suggested as a cause of cord infarction. Theoretically, this may occur under conditions of stagnant flow, but that is considered a rare event. The role of aortic cross-clamping and the significance of the hypogastric circulation have been noted. However, it bears reemphasis that while an occasional low ARM may be occluded by infrarenal or suprarenal clamping, loss of prograde flow in the internal iliac arteries may be the most common cause of paraplegia following aortic reconstruction. Typically, this occurs with complex aortic reconstruction in association with either hypogastric occlusive or aneurysmal disease.

The significance of maintaining adequate blood pressure is documented by the higher rates of paraplegia associated with repairs of ruptured aneurysms as a consequence of hypotension, prolonged clamp times, or both. As in direct radicular artery occlusion, severe sustained decreases in perfusion pressure may result in infarction in any one of three possible watershed regions, the midthoracic level, the central cord, and the lumbosacral region. In a series of postmortem examinations,

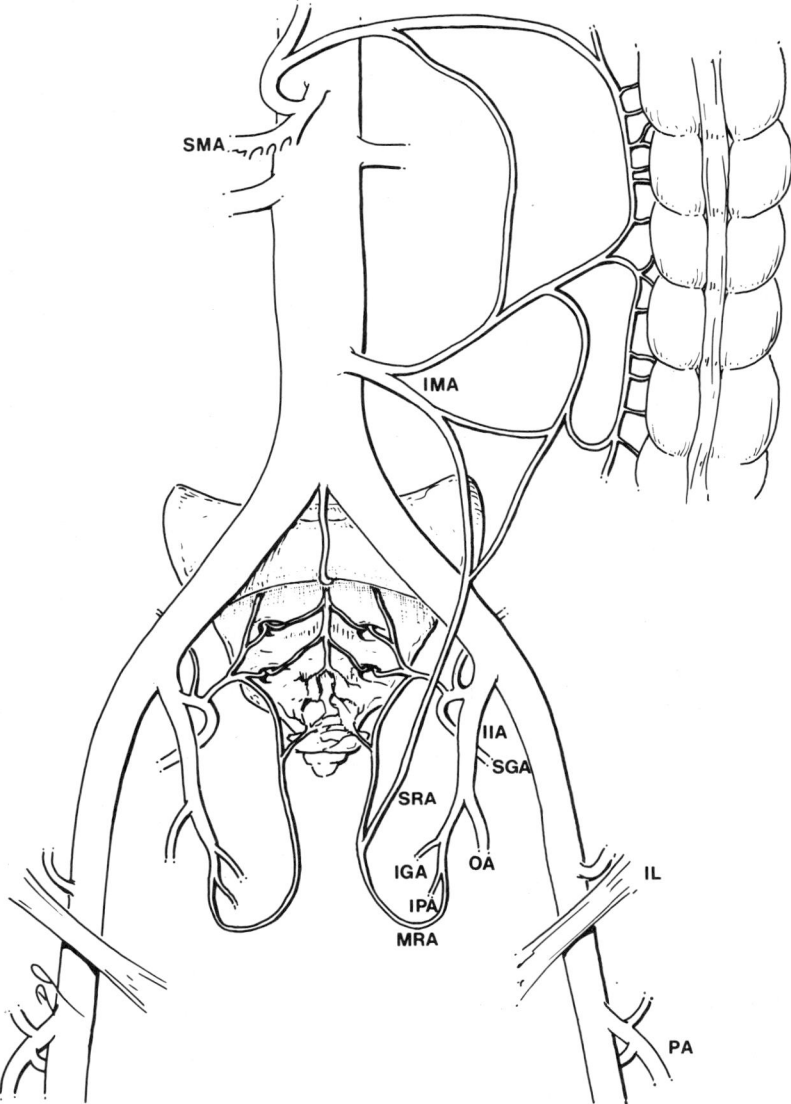

Figure 3 Mesenteric collateral circulation and vessels perfusing the caudal portion of the spinal canal. SMA-Superior mesenteric artery; IIA-internal iliac artery; SGA-superior gluteal artery; SRA-superior rectal artery; IGA-inferior gluteal artery; OA-obturator artery; IL-inguinal ligament; IPA-internal pudendal artery; MRA-middle rectal artery; PA-profunda artery. (From Salam AA, Sholkamy SM, Chaikof EL. Spinal cord ischemia after abdominal aortic procedures: Is previous colectomy a risk factor? J Vasc Surg 1993; 17:1108-1110; with permission.)

Azzarelli and Roessman[10] documented that the lumbosacral region was most susceptible to infarction after sustained hypoperfusion.

DIFFERENTIAL DIAGNOSIS AND EVALUATION

Paraplegia following aortic reconstruction generally results from spinal ischemia. Nonetheless, if the patient's condition is stable, magnetic resonance imaging of the spine should be obtained to exclude a compressive lesion of the cord. Hematomyelia should be considered if a preoperative epidural or spinal anesthetic was administered, particularly if a bloody tap was noted. Additionally, failure to perform a complete preoperative evaluation may cause misdiagnosis of the occasional patient who presents with neurogenic claudication in association with aortic disease.

PREVENTION

Until recently spinal ischemia after abdominal aortic reconstruction was considered entirely unpreventable. General recommendations included delicate handling of tissues; systemic heparinization; and the avoidance of intraoperative hypotension and prolonged or suprarenal aortic clamping. Selective preoperative arteriography of the lumbar and intercostal arteries to localize the cord blood supply has been used in patients with thoracic or thoracoabdominal aneurysms. However, it remains impractical and certainly not cost effective for most routine abdominal aortic operations. Likewise, hypothermia, low-molecular-weight dextran, thiopental anesthesia, and cerebrospinal fluid drainage have all been reported as possibly beneficial. Nonetheless, without an adequate means of determining risk preoperatively, the institution of any given maneuver, including lumbar artery reimplantation, is haphazard at best.

The significance of the pelvic circulation in relation to cord ischemia has been emphasized in a number of reports. It may well be the most important factor in avoiding neurologic complications after abdominal aortic reconstruction. Pelvic blood flow can be maintained in the majority of patients by either IMA reimplantation or the construction of a limb anastomosis to allow at least unilateral hypogastric perfusion. Options include performing end-to-end anastomosis to a cuff of the common iliac artery, end-to-side anastomosis distal to an intact iliac artery bifurcation, graft interposition, and direct hypogastric reimplantation. Thus, with adequate preoperative planning and intraoperative care, the risk of paraplegia following abdominal aortic reconstruction can be minimized.

REFERENCES

1. McCune WS. Discussion. In: Adams HD, Geetruyden HH. Neurologic complications of aortic surgery. Ann Surg 1956; 144:574–610.
2. Szilagyi DE, Hageman JH, Smith RF, Elliott JP. Spinal cord damage in surgery of the abdominal aorta. Surgery 1978; 83:38–56.
3. Szilagyi DE. A second look at the etiology of spinal cord damage in surgery of the abdominal aorta. J Vasc Surg 1993; 17:1111–1113.
4. Lazorthes G, Gouaze A, Zadeh JO, et al. Arterial vascularization of the spinal cord. J Neurosurg 1971; 35:253–262.
5. Priscol K. Die Blutversorgung des Rückenmarkes und ihre klinische Relevanz. Berlin-Heidelberg-New York: Springer-Verlag, 1972:27.
6. Lazorthes G, et al. La vascularisation du renflement lombaire. Étude des variations et des suppléances. Rev Neurol Paris 1966; 122:109–122.
7. Picone AL, Green RM, Ricotta JR, et al. Spinal cord ischemia following operations on the abdominal aorta. J Vasc Surg 1986; 3:94–103.
8. Gloviczki P, Cross SA, Stanson AW, et al. Ischemia injury to the spinal cord or lumbosacral plexus after aortoiliac reconstruction. Am J Surg 1991; 162:131–136.
9. Salam AA, Sholkamy SM, Chaikof EL. Spinal cord ischemia after abdominal aortic procedures: Is previous colectomy a risk factor? J Vasc Surg 1993; 17:1108–1110.
10. Azzarelli B, Roessman V. Diffuse "anoxic myelopathy." Neurology 1977; 27:1049–1052.

PREVENTION OF SPINAL CORD ISCHEMIA DURING THORACOABDOMINAL AORTIC RECONSTRUCTION

ROBERT Y. RHEE, M.D.
PETER GLOVICZKI, M.D.

Alexis Carrel stated at the turn of the century that "the main danger of the aortic operation does not come from the heart or from the aorta itself, but from the central nervous system." Unfortunately, even with modern techniques, paraplegia remains a devastating complication following thoracoabdominal aortic aneurysm (TAAA) repair. The etiology of this complication is multifactorial. Paraplegia can result from anatomic, physiologic, and technical factors. The most important event is alteration in perfusion and oxygenation of the thoracolumbar spinal cord during and following aortic cross-clamping. This could occur by way of changes in regional spinal cord blood flow caused by either temporary (aortic cross-clamping) or permanent (thrombosis, embolization, and trauma) occlusion of the arteries supplying the spinal cord. Reperfusion injury after a period of ischemia to the spinal cord can further exacerbate the damage. Failure to restore the major blood supply to the cord is another critical factor in determining outcome. Essentially, any change in local cerebrospinal fluid dynamics, in the spinal cord's autoregulatory mechanism controlling spinal vascular resistance, and in the microvascular environment of the spinal cord–blood barrier can affect the extent of spinal cord injury.

The incidence of spinal cord ischemia following thoracoabdominal aortic reconstruction ranges from 0.4% to 40%. Unfortunately, the problem remains unpreventable even in the largest series. In a recent report by Svensson et al. on 1,509 patients operated upon by E. Stanley Crawford for TAAA, the paraplegia-paraparesis rate was 16% (234/1,509).[1] Risk factors for paraplegia included urgency of the operation, presence of rupture or dissection, duration of aortic cross-clamping, extent of the aneurysm, age of the patient, and perioperative hypotension.

In the Mayo Clinic experience of 181 patients who underwent TAAA repair between 1980 and 1992, the incidence of paraparesis and paraplegia was 8% (15/181).[2] The highest rate of paraplegia occurred in patients with extensive type II aneurysms (29%) and the lowest rate affected those with distal type IV aneurysms (2%) (Table 1).

Despite exhaustive experimental and clinical research directed at preventing spinal cord ischemia and subsequent paraplegia, no single or unified approach appears to be effective. Currently used techniques either enhance perfusion to the cord during aortic cross-clamping or protect the cord via pharmacologic or thermoregulatory means. Attempts are also made to identify critical blood supply to the cord preoperatively to facilitate revascularization during TAAA repair.

METHODS OF SPINAL CORD PROTECTION

Aortic Cross-Clamp Time

Expeditious operation with swift reimplantation of the visceral branches and critical intercostal arteries is crucial for good clinical results. The maximum safe aortic cross-clamp time for prevention of spinal cord ischemia during TAAA repair is not known. Clinical experience with dissecting thoracic aneurysms has shown that if aortic cross-clamp times exceeds 30 to 40 minutes, the incidence of spinal cord ischemia increases sharply[2] (Fig. 1). The median time in our thoracoabdominal aneurysm series to complete the aortic reconstruction with revascularization of the lower extremities was 60 minutes (range, 15 to 264 minutes). It is imperative that a vascular surgeon be highly experienced and skilled in aortic reconstruction techniques in order to minimize aortic cross-clamp times.

Control of Proximal Hypertension and Spinal Fluid Pressure

High aortic cross-clamping results in proximal hypertension. This increases cerebrospinal fluid (CSF) pressure and decreases spinal cord perfusion. The perfusion pressure of the spinal cord is defined as the difference between arterial perfusion pressure and CSF pressure. Thus, any intervention that lowers CSF pres-

Table 1 Spinal Cord Complications Following Repair of Thoracoabdominal Aortic Aneurysms in 181 Patients at the Mayo Clinic (1980-1992)

	Paraplegia and/or Paraparesis*	
	No.	%
Type I		
Nondissecting (n = 34)	2	6
Dissecting (n = 2)	0	0
Total (n = 36)	2	6
Type II		
Nondissecting (n = 12)	2	17
Dissecting (n = 5)	3	60
Total (n = 17)	5	29
Type III		
Nondissecting (n = 55)	5	9
Dissecting (n = 9)	2	22
Total (n = 64)	7	11
Type IV		
Nondissecting (n = 64)	1	2
Dissecting (n = 0)	0	0
Total (n = 64)	1	2
Type I-IV		
Nondissecting (n = 165)	10	6
Dissecting (n = 16)	5	31
Total (n = 181)	15	8

*Unable to assess in 26 patients because of death within 24 hours.

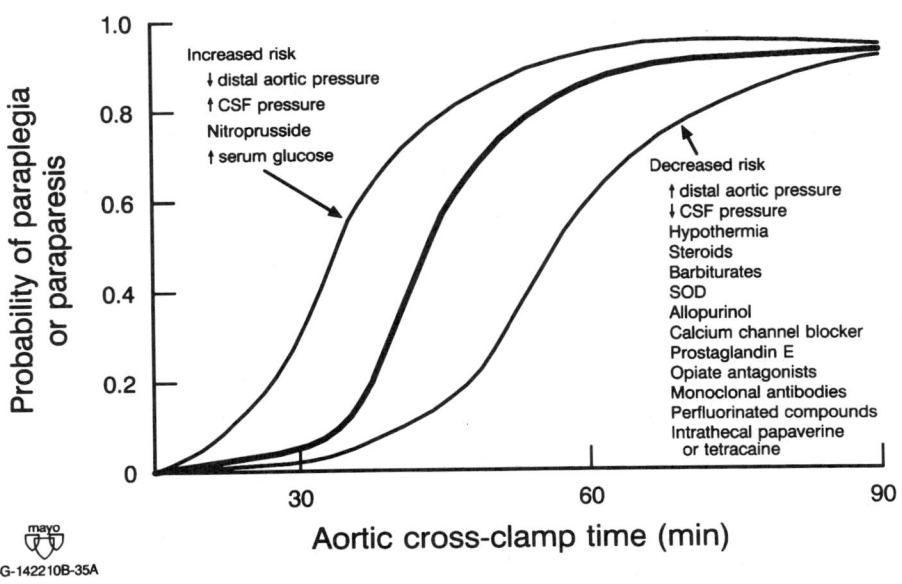

Figure 1 The probability of ischemic spinal cord injury during occlusion of the thoracic aorta. (Adapted from Svensson LG, Loop FD. Prevention of spinal cord ischemia in aortic surgery. In: Bergan JJ, Yao JST, eds. Arterial surgery: New diagnostic and operative techniques, Orlando: Grune & Stratton, 1988:273; with permission.)

sure should augment spinal cord perfusion pressure. There is significant experimental evidence that CSF drainage improves spinal cord blood flow, decreases reperfusion injury, and improves neurologic outcome after thoracic aortic cross-clamping.[3] Using a canine model, we have shown that spinal cord blood flow increased significantly in dogs that underwent CSF drainage during aortic cross-clamping (Fig. 2).

Spinal fluid drainage in patients was introduced by Hollier, and it continues to be one of the techniques used in the multimodality approach with excellent clinical results.[4] In 68 patients who underwent CSF drainage during TAAA repair at the Mayo Clinic, the CSF pressure was carefully monitored with spinal catheters and approximately 50 to 100 cc (mean 67.2 cc) of CSF was removed. An intrathecal catheter is introduced in the L2–L3 space and advanced proximally 5 to 10 cm until a stable reading is obtained. The spinal fluid is withdrawn just before aortic cross-clamping as well as during and after the procedure to maintain the CSF pressure at less than 10 mm Hg. The spinal catheter is usually maintained for 48 to 72 hours postoperatively for further drainage, if the pressure should rise above 10 mm Hg. It should be noted, however, that the clinical trial of Crawford and the Mayo experience have failed to demonstrate statistically significant improvement in neurologic outcome for patients in the CSF drainage group.[5,6] Then again, CSF drainage is a relatively safe and effective method of decreasing the microenvironmental pressure of the spinal canal.

Hypothermia

Hypothermia reduces the metabolic rate and oxygen requirements of ischemic neural tissue. Reduction of core temperatures in humans to 12° to 20°C can extend safe ischemia time of brain tissue to 60 minutes in patients undergoing thoracic aortic operations. However, in the spinal cord, there does not appear to be a clear, linear relationship between temperature and duration of ischemia tolerated in the spinal cord. In addition, profound reduction of body core temperature without cardiopulmonary bypass (CPB) would increase the risk of arrhythmia and bleeding. Because total CPB with deep hypothermia and cardiac arrest requires full heparinization and is not without risk, it appears that suitable clinical techniques of regional or local hypothermia have to be developed to take advantage of the protective effect of spinal cord cooling. At our institution, only mild (32° to 34°C) systemic hypothermia is used throughout the operation because of the risks described. The core body temperature reduction is monitored closely via a pulmonary artery catheter thermistor, and warming fluids or inspired gases during cross-clamping are avoided.

Reimplantation of Intercostal Arteries

Although the mechanism of spinal cord injury is complex, the alteration of blood flow to the cord itself is ultimately responsible for ischemic changes. The major source of blood supply to the cord is the anterior spinal artery, which receives its branches from the intercostal arteries in the thoracolumbar region (Fig. 3). The largest artery supplying blood flow to the lumbar region of the spinal cord in humans is the great radicular artery or the artery of Adamkiewicz. It usually originates from the T9 to T12 level in 75% of patients, from T5 to T8 in 15%, and from L1 to L2 in 10%. This vessel provides the majority of spinal cord blood flow below the midthoracic level. Therefore, preservation of this important artery is vital to the prevention of perfusion-related spinal cord ischemia. However, clinical studies with preoperative spinal cord angiography failed to identify this artery in a

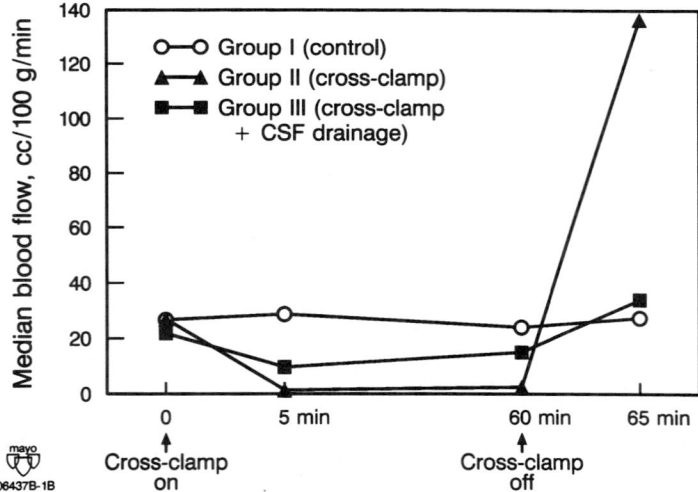

Figure 2 Temporal changes of gray matter blood flow in lumbar segment of spinal cord. (From Bower TC, Murray MJ, Gloviczki P, et al. Effects of thoracic aortic occlusion and cerebrospinal fluid drainage on regional spinal cord blood flow in dogs: Correlation with neurologic outcome. J Vasc Surg 1989; 9:135–144; with permission.)

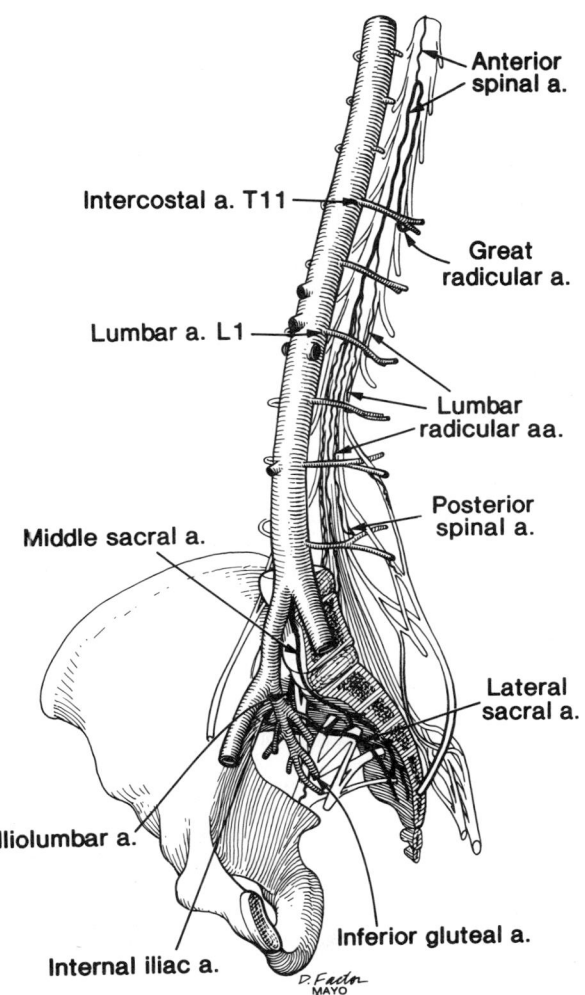

Figure 3 Blood supply to the spinal cord. (From Gloviczki P, Cross SA, Stanson AW, et al. Ischemic injury to the spinal cord or lumbosacral plexus after aortoiliac reconstruction. Am J Surg 1991; 162:131–146; with permission.)

significant subset of patients, either because of technical problems or because the main intercostal artery was chronically occluded or stenosed.[7] Moreover, the collateral blood supply to the cord in this group of patients was unpredictable.

Although preoperative identification of the spinal arterial anatomy would be ideal, angiography is often incomplete. Hence, operative reimplantation of intercostal arteries during TAAA repair is based on the fact that most great radicular arteries arise at the T8-L1 levels. Crawford, in a prospective randomized study, found that intercostal artery reimplantation did not improve postoperative paraplegia rates.[5] Then again, analysis of a subset of patients showed that the paraplegia rate was significantly higher if the intercostal arteries arising from a segment of the cord at the T11 to L1 levels were found patent and were not reimplanted. We continue to reimplant all patent intercostal arteries at T8–L1 level.

Mechanical Shunt or Bypass

Several types of shunts and bypass techniques are available for increasing distal aortic perfusion. The aortoaortic (Gott) shunt, femorofemoral bypass, and left atrial or pulmonary vein to femoral artery bypass with centrifugal pumps are the techniques used during TAAA reconstruction. Experimental evidence supports shunting in special situations.[8] If critical intercostal arteries originate from the aorta distal to the excluded segment, partial shunts or bypasses may be beneficial, if cross-clamp time exceeds about 30 minutes. Total CPB is advocated by some if these vessels originate from the excluded, cross-clamped segment. The potential problems associated with total circulatory arrest and systemic hypothermia limit their routine use. Frequently the distal perfusion produced by the shunt or bypass may be too far distal to increase flow to the critical segment of the spinal cord. In the Mayo experience, the only patients who clearly benefited from such mechanical support devices were those with dissection of the descending thoracic aorta.[2] Our indications for external circulatory support include aortic dissections, anticipated prolonged clamp time (greater than 60 minutes), very extensive segmental aneurysms that allow isolated clamping to specific regions of the aorta, and patients with limited cardiac reserve or valvular disease (e.g., aortic insufficiency) to decrease afterload during aortic clamping. Currently, we use the atriofemoral bypass very selectively in TAAA reconstruction.

INTRAOPERATIVE METHODS OF EVALUATING SPINAL CORD ISCHEMIA

Measurement of Somatosensory Potentials

Measurement of somatosensory evoked potentials (SSEP) monitors cortical responses to stimulation of peripheral nerves. Somatosensory evoked potentials rely on transmission of impulses through posterior column pathways. Changes in latency and amplitude of signals that are monitored from the cerebral cortex indicate decreased function of the spinal cord tissue due to ischemia. Because peripheral nerve ischemia during aortic cross-clamping may alter the results, this technique should be employed in conjunction with distal aortic perfusion whenever possible. Another problem with SSEP is that impulses that do not travel along the motor pathways are not documented by the sensors. In a prospective randomized study by Crawford on 198 patients with TAAA, measurement of SSEP failed to show any significant benefit. Using SSEP to predict spinal cord injury, the false positive rate was 67% and the false negative rate was 13%.[9]

Measurement of Motor Evoked Potentials

Motor evoked potentials (MEP), which directly reflect the activity of motor tracts of the spinal cord, are more accurate indicators of the cord's perfusion status.

The electrical impulses are generated at the level of the cerebral cortex and propagated to the lower motor neurons of the spinal gray matter. The MEP are less affected by peripheral nerve ischemia because the conduction pathways are more direct and do not rely on peripheral nerve function. However, the use of intraoperative muscle relaxants may affect the tracings. Despite its theoretical advantages, in our laboratory MEP failed to produce accurate and reliable records of spinal cord ischemia. Using our canine model for spinal cord ischemia, the overall accuracy was 59% in predicting neurologic outcome, with a sensitivity of only 67%.[10] We continue to evaluate the efficacy of different techniques of SSEP and MEP in experiments and in patients to determine their exact role in the detection of spinal cord ischemia.

SUMMARY OF EXPERIMENTAL METHODS OF PROTECTION

Many etiologic factors have been implicated in the development of spinal cord ischemia during high aortic cross-clamping. Because ischemic damage is affected by insufficient aerobic metabolism and by the by-products of consequent anaerobic metabolism, experimental studies should address the issue of the spinal cord's complex microenvironment and tissue hypoxia. Drugs, either introduced intravenously or intrathecally, should be examined in an attempt to modify the local effects of toxic metabolites such as oxygen-derived free radicals and lactic acid on the spinal cord. It is well documented that the predictive curve of spinal cord ischemia can be shifted to the right in experiments by various agents such as steroids, barbiturates, superoxide dismutase, and calcium channel blocking agents (Fig. 1).

Intrathecal papaverine has also been shown to decrease ischemic and reperfusion injury. The mechanism of action of papaverine is related to its ability to selectively dilate the anterior spinal artery, resulting in increased blood flow to the spinal cord. Slow infusion of a 1% solution via an intrathecal route after drainage of 20 to 30 cc of native CSF is sustained throughout the aortic cross-clamping period. Because CSF is allowed to drain freely throughout the procedure, one cannot clearly differentiate the effects of CSF drainage from the effects of papaverine. At present we do not employ intrathecal papaverine in patients.

Ongoing laboratory and clinical research on the prevention of spinal cord ischemia is essential to improving patient outcome. The thrust of future research should concentrate on three main areas. First, the problem of intercostal anatomy and its unpredictability must be solved via more precise imaging techniques. This would allow the vascular surgeon to minimize the overall aortic cross-clamp time by selectively reimplanting only those critical intercostal arteries that supply the spinal cord. Second, a reliable and clinically usable technique of monitoring spinal cord perfusion must be developed. Somatosensory evoked potentials, as employed today, have limited accuracy and are fraught with inconsistencies. We are currently experimenting with improved techniques to monitor SSEP and MEP in experiments and have used the laser flow Doppler successfully as a new method of directly measuring spinal cord perfusion. The third area of investigation should focus on finding methods to prolong the ischemia tolerance and decrease reperfusion injury to the spinal cord. We believe that certain drugs such as nimodipine (a neuroselective calcium channel blocking agent) and regional spinal cord cooling may decrease further damage to the ischemic cord by altering its metabolic microenvironment.

REFERENCES

1. Svensson LG, Crawford ES, Hess KR, et al. Experience with 1509 patients undergoing thoracoabdominal aortic operations. J Vasc Surg 1993; 17:357–370.
2. Gloviczki P, Bower TC. Visceral and spinal cord protection during thoracoabdominal aortic reconstructions. Semin Vasc Surg 1992; 5:163–173.
3. Bower TC, Murray MJ, Gloviczki P, et al. Effects of thoracic aortic occlusion and cerebrospinal fluid drainage on regional spinal cord blood flow in dogs: Correlation with neurologic outcome. J Vasc Surg 1988; 9:135–144.
4. Hollier LH, Money SR, Naslund TC, et al. The risk of spinal cord dysfunction in patients undergoing thoracoabdominal aortic replacement. Am J Surg 1992; 164:210–214.
5. Murray MJ, Bower TC, Oliver WC, et al. Effects of cerebrospinal fluid drainage in patients undergoing thoracic and thoracoabdominal aortic surgery. J Cardiothorac Vasc Anesth 1993; 7:266–272.
6. Crawford ES, Svensson LG, Hess KR, et al. A prospective randomized study of cerebrospinal fluid drainage to prevent paraplegia after high-risk surgery on the thoracoabdominal aorta. J Vasc Surg 1990; 13:36–46.
7. Kieffer E, Richard T, Chiras J, et al. Preoperative spinal cord arteriography in aneurysmal disease of the descending thoracic and thoracoabdominal aorta: Preliminary results in 45 patients. Ann Vasc Surg 1989; 3:34–46.
8. Elmore JR, Gloviczki P, Harper CM, et al. Spinal cord injury in experimental thoracic aortic occlusion: Investigation of combined methods of protection. J Vasc Surg 1992; 15:789–799.
9. Crawford ES, Mizrahi EM, Hess KR, et al. The impact of distal aortic perfusion and somatosensory evoked potential monitoring on prevention of paraplegia after aortic aneurysm operation. J Thorac Cardiovasc Surg 1988; 95:357–367.
10. Elmore JR, Gloviczki P, Harper CM, et al. Failure of motor evoked potentials to predict neurologic outcome in experimental thoracic aortic occlusion. J Vasc Surg 1991; 14:131–139.

AUTOTRANSFUSION IN AORTIC RECONSTRUCTION

DANIEL J. REDDY, M.D.

Over the last decade, surgeons, sharing their patients' concerns with the potential added operative risk associated with transfusion-related diseases, have revived interest in autotransfusion. Reports from busy vascular surgery services have confirmed the safety, cost-effectiveness, and benefits of intraoperative blood salvage with autotransfusion.[1-3] Whereas surgeons have underscored the utility of intraoperative blood salvage, others have emphasized the need for a comprehensive blood transfusion program to minimize patient exposure to homologous blood while adding autologous blood to the blood bank's resource pool.[4-6] In vascular surgery, autotransfusion is most effective in support of aortic aneurysm operations.[1]

The three key elements of a comprehensive blood transfusion program in aortic operations are (1) autologous preoperative blood deposit for elective operations, (2) routine use of intraoperative blood salvage in elective and emergency operation, and (3) adherence to patient-specific indications for transfusions.

Other potential future supporting measures not part of our current protocol include deliberate intraoperative hemodilutional anemia following induction of general anesthesia and perioperative treatment of patients who predeposit blood with parenteral recombinant human erythropoietin. Some authors advocate platelet-rich plasma sequestration collection to fashion autologous fibrin glue for topical intraoperative hemostasis. This latter practice is finding its greatest application in cardiac surgery but is not widely used in aortic reconstructions. Strict adherence to optimal operative hemostatic technique is indispensable in aortic operations, particularly from the standpoint of minimizing homologous transfusions.[7]

Although the risk of acquired immunodeficiency syndrome (AIDS) seems overstated in the minds of some patients, much of the impetus for autologous blood transfusions has come from the high likelihood of contracting and dying of AIDS following receipt of a single unit of contaminated homologous blood. The actual risk of a particular unit being contaminated with the AIDS virus, however, is estimated to be as low as 1 in 1 million.[6] Then again, the risk of post-transfusion hepatitis C presents a more likely risk, estimated at approximately 1 in 100 as recently as 1988.[6] Fortunately, the incidence of post-transfusion hepatitis C has decreased markedly with recent improvements in the blood banks' ability to screen blood donors. The contemporary risk of post-transfusion hepatitis is estimated to be about 3 per 10,000 units transfused.[8]

Although avoiding transmitted infectious complications from homologous transfusion has received the most attention, additional advantages favor autologous over homologous transfusions are: avoiding transfusion mismatch and compatibility reactions, recipient isoimmunization, and immune suppression. Moreover, homologous blood collected and stored weeks prior to transfusion has less effective oxygen-carrying capacity.[9]

In addition to the advantages enumerated, the formal endorsements of the American Medical Association Council on Scientific Affairs and the National Institutes of Health (NIH) encourage the prudent vascular surgeon to consider incorporating autologous blood transfusion in the management plan for appropriate patients undergoing aortic reconstruction. As a measure of the general public's heightened awareness of autotransfusion, during its 1992 legislative session, the State of Michigan House of Representatives, reacting to patients' demands, entertained a bill (HB5144) requiring physicians who perform operative procedures to inform all patients for whom blood transfusion may be anticipated, of the option of preoperatively storing their own blood for transfusion. This governmental intrusion in medical practice illustrates the level of general interest and emotion surrounding this topic.

AUTOLOGOUS PREOPERATIVE DEPOSIT

This procedure is typically undertaken by blood bank personnel following established protocols in response to the surgeon's request. It is applicable when there is both a likely need for perioperative blood transfusions and sufficient time to allow repeated outpatient phlebotomies. A hemodynamically unstable patient requiring an urgent or emergency operation, such as a symptomatic abdominal aortic aneurysm, is an unsuitable candidate for autologous predeposit. Moreover, patients with limited cardiac reserve owing to coronary or valvular heart disease should undergo phlebotomy only after consideration of the possible adverse cardiac effects of anemia and the compensatory blood volume shifts associated with phlebotomies. Patients being considered for aortic operations may already be scheduled for cardiac stress testing. The results of this evaluation could guide the decision to predeposit blood, as well as its timing and the optimal number of units.

The blood bank standards requiring volunteers to wait at least 2 months between donor phlebotomies is relaxed for autologous predeposit patients. In good-risk patients, we allow only 4 to 7 days between phlebotomies, timing the final donation for approximately 3 days prior to the planned procedure. Oral iron supplements are administered throughout the predeposit period. The hemogram is monitored to keep the patient's preoperative hemoglobin at least 10 g/dl and hematocrit no less than 30 vol %.

The age guidelines for autologous predeposit are less stringent than those for volunteer donors for homologous blood transfusion. This fact maintains autologous predeposit a practicality in the aged vascular surgery population.

It is important to avoid an implied or stated guarantee that autologous predeposit protects against the need for any homologous blood or blood products. Rather, autologous predeposit is an effective method to lower the likelihood that homologous blood may be needed.

When predeposited blood exceeds the blood volume needed for transfusion during the perioperative period, we do not infuse the remaining predeposited blood simply because it is available. An unindicated blood transfusion, albeit autologous, carries some unnecessary risks and costs. There is the risk of bacterial contamination in any stored blood. Although remote, a potentially disastrous labeling error causing a mismatched transfusion can occur. These problems can be avoided altogether if unindicated transfusions, even autologous, are not given. At our institution, unused autologous blood is either frozen for future use or discarded. We do not release unused units to the general resource pool for use as donated homologous units.

Most patients scheduled for elective abdominal aortic and thoracoabdominal aortic aneurysm repairs predeposit 2 to 4 units of autologous blood. In contrast, patients scheduled for carotid or femoral popliteal bypass are not expected to need blood transfusion and, accordingly, are not candidates for predeposit and are referred to the blood bank only when they insist.

INTRAOPERATIVE AUTOTRANSFUSION IN ELECTIVE AND EMERGENCY AORTIC PROCEDURES

Of the various types of devices available for retrieving shed blood for retransfusion during aortic operations, we employ only those that process salvaged blood for retransfusion as washed packed red blood cells.[1] The responsibility to set up and operate the equipment is assigned to a skilled operator who is on call 24 hours daily. The machine operator is dedicated to processing salvaged blood and does not have additional anesthetic or circulating nurse duties that may distract attention from blood salvage.

The protocol calls for shed blood to be suctioned into a standard cardiology reservoir via a double lumen suction catheter. Integral to the suction line is a parallel heparin sodium solution line that mixes heparin-saline with suctioned blood as it leaves the operative field. Every effort is made by the surgeon to suction pooled blood rather than aspirate at the blood-air interface, as this latter technique is associated with increased erythrocyte hemolysis. Moreover, negative pressure at the suction line should be maintained under 100 torr to minimize hemolysis. The aspirated and anticoagulated blood is macrofiltered through a 120 micron filter and then pumped into a centrifuge bowl, which is then spun at approximately 45,000 rpm. The supernatant is discarded and the packed red cells mass resuspended in 1 L of 0.9N sodium chloride to be "washed" by repeat centrifugation. The discarded solutions contain the saline wash, plasma proteins, free hemoglobin, cellular debris, platelets, leukocytes, activated clotting factors, anticoagulants, and any extravascular debris suctioned from the operative field. The resulting product is a 220 ml unit of fresh autologous packed red blood cells with a hematocrit of 0.50 vol %. This unit is given to the anesthesia team for retransfusion as needed.

Alternative whole blood salvage methods that are less expensive and do not require a dedicated operator are available. Concerned by the potential for coagulopathy caused by transfusion of unwashed anticoagulated whole blood, however, we have avoided these alternative devices. Although there have been reports favoring these devices with small-volume transfusion, we do not believe that the risk-benefit ratio justifies their use, as the infusion of activated procoagulants may paradoxically increase bleeding by causing diffuse intravascular coagulation, particularly with larger transfusion volumes.

We have employed these conservative protocols in hundreds of abdominal aortic aneurysm repairs and scores of thoracoabdominal aortic aneurysm repairs and have not detected complications or death related to the use of intraoperative autologous transfusion. In particular, we detected no instances of air embolism, diffuse intravascular coagulopathy, or bleeding attributed to intraoperative autotransfusion.

The volume of blood salvage in elective and nonelective abdominal aortic aneurysm repairs was 0.87 ± 0.53 L and 1.45 ± 1.50 L, respectively.[1] For elective and nonelective thoracoabdominal aortic aneurysm repairs, the volume of blood salvage was 2.47 ± 1.36 L and 2.15 ± 1.61 L, respectively. Of patients undergoing elective abdominal aortic aneurysm repairs, 40% received no homologous red cells during operation.[1] Moreover, at the time of this study, we had not yet initiated autologous blood predeposit and now estimate that more than 65% of patients can undergo elective abdominal aortic aneurysm repairs without needing homologous transfusions.[10] In our institution, the costs of providing intraoperative autotransfusion, as described, can be met by the savings enjoyed by limiting blood bank costs when 2.3 units are salvaged.

When the surgeon doubts that operative blood loss will be sufficient to net blood salvage volumes that are cost-effective but is concerned about the unpredictability of blood loss in any given operation, an intermediate protocol can be followed. In this circumstance, the cardiology reservoir, heparin sodium solution, and double lumen suction line are set up in the usual manner. The relatively expensive disposable harness that interfaces with the cell-washing machine is kept on standby but left unopened. By holding the sterile harness in reserve until it is evident that the blood volume in the cardiology reservoir exceeds a unit or more, the costs of the disposable harness and the skilled operator are not incurred unless needed. At the same time, however, the potential to use intraoperative blood salvage has been maintained, as the blood suction for the field has not been discarded but rather is heparinized in the standard cardiology reservoir to be processed only if needed.

INDICATIONS FOR TRANSFUSION

Adherence to specific indications for transfusion may be an underutilized component of many blood transfusion programs. In our study we noted in retrospect that our transfusion practice had been to maintain both operative and postoperative blood hemoglobin and hematocrit values at preoperative levels.[1] If the hemoglobin or hematocrit can safely be allowed to drift to lower levels without triggering a transfusion that may not be strictly needed, fewer homologous blood products will be utilized. The percentage of patients avoiding perioperative homologous blood and blood product transfusions can be increased, if transfusions are ordered only for positive indications rather than to maintain a hemoglobin of 10 g/L or some other arbitrary level. Responding to the challenge issued by the NIH report, we now attempt to allow postoperative hemoglobin levels to drift down to approximately 8 g/L. This lower transfusion trigger is tolerable to most patients but requires that the patient have sufficient cardiac reserve to maintain hemodynamic stability. This practice mandates more physiologic and careful monitoring as one would put a patient at unnecessary cardiac risk not to replenish needed oxygen-carrying capacity by transfusion when indicated. Standard monitoring parameters in current use in surgical intensive care units will suffice to guide this decision.

Close cooperation and communication between anesthetic and surgical teams are essential if unnecessary transfusions are to be avoided while necessary transfusions are to be given. This is particularly true when preoperative autologous blood predeposits have made a patient relatively anemic prior to operation. A comprehensive management plan incorporating autologous blood predeposit and intraoperative blood salvage for autotransfusion coupled with adherence to specific indications for transfusion has the potential of minimizing homologous blood exposure while ensuring that adequate oxygen-carrying capacity is maintained.

REFERENCES

1. Reddy DJ, Ryan CJ, Shepard AD, et al. Intraoperative autotransfusion in vascular surgery. Arch Surg 1990; 125:1012–1016.
2. Hallet JW, Popovsky M, Ilstrup D. Minimizing blood transfusions during abdominal aortic surgery: Recent advances in rapid autotransfusion. J Vasc Surg 1987; 5:601–606.
3. O'Hara PJ, Hertzer NR, Santilli PH, et al. Intraoperative autotransfusion during abdominal aortic reconstruction. Am J Surg 1983; 145:217–220.
4. AMA Council on Scientific Affairs. Autologous blood transfusions. JAMA 1986; 256:2378–2380.
5. Maffei LM, Thurer RL, eds. Autologous blood transfusion: Current issues. Arlington, Va: American Association of Blood Banks, 1988.
6. Consensus Conference. Perioperative red blood cell transfusions. JAMA 1988; 260:2700–2703.
7. Cutler BS. Avoidance of homologous transfusion in aortic operations: The role of autotransfusions, hemodilution, and surgical technique. Surgery 1984; 95:717–722.
8. The declining risk of post-transfusion hepatitis C virus infection. N Engl J Med 1992; 327:369–373.
9. Williamson KR, Taswell HF. Intraoperative blood salvage: A review. Transfusion 1991; 31:662–675.
10. O'Hara PJ, Hertzer NR, Krajewski LP, et al. Reduction in the homologous blood requirement for abdominal aortic aneurysm repair by the use of preadmission autologous blood donation. Surgery 1994; 115:69–76.

ANEURYSMAL DETERIORATION OF ARTERIAL PROSTHESES

DANIEL B. NUNN, M.D.

In general, two categories of vascular prostheses are used to replace or bypass diseased or injured segments of large and medium-sized vessels. One is the various textile grafts that are constructed of polyethylene terephthalate, PET (Dacron), and the other is nontextile grafts made of expanded polytetrafluoroethylene, or PTFE (Teflon).

Despite the generally successful use of both types of prostheses, graft-related complications continue to occur sporadically. The most common are suture line disruption, excessive dilatation, thrombosis, bleeding, and infection. In PET grafts, particularly knitted fabrics, dilatation is by far the most prevalent complication and may result in intrinsic graft failure manifested by aneurysmal formation. Although aneurysms developed in some of the early PTFE grafts manufactured between 1975 and 1976,[1,2] subsequent changes in the manufacturing process that increased the strength of the grafts appear to have eliminated the problem. Today PTFE grafts exhibit little tendency to dilate, and there are no reports of true aneurysmal deterioration.

PET GRAFT STRUCTURES AND PHYSICAL PROPERTIES

As textile structures, PET grafts may be classified as either woven or knitted, with subclassification into smooth or velour surfaces and triaxial constructions.

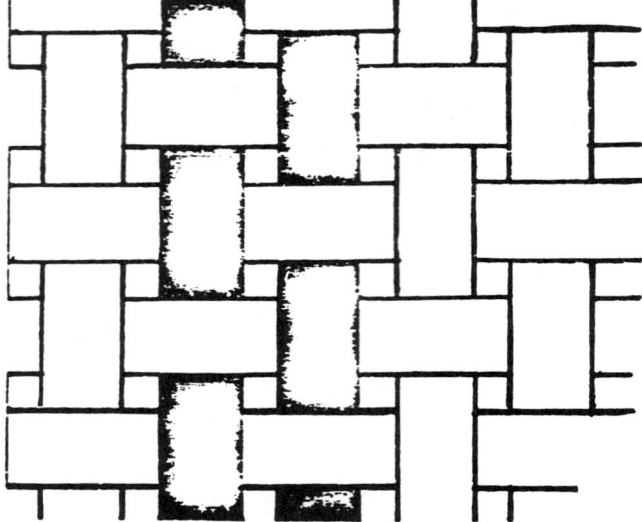

Figure 1 Structure of plain woven fabric.

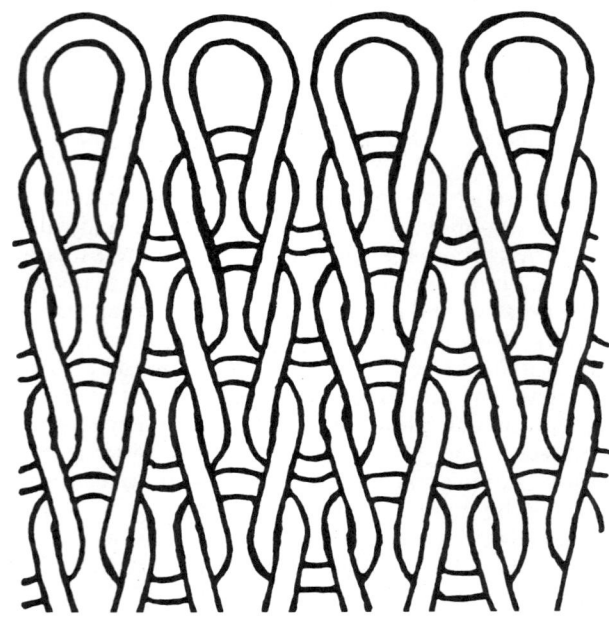

Figure 3 Weft knit.

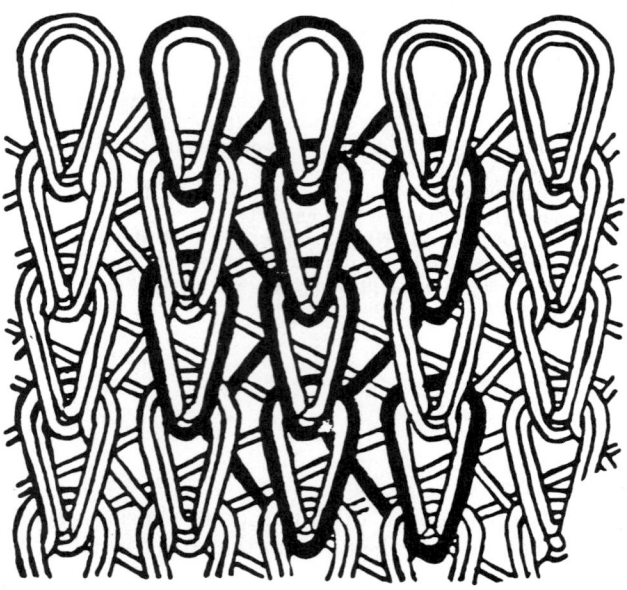

Figure 2 Warp knit.

Since the basic material is the same, the differences in physical properties are primarily a function of the fabric construction.

Woven fabrics by virtue of their structure, are for the most part dimensionally stable. They exhibit little tendency to dilate and have low porosity and high bursting strength (Fig. 1). However, they are less compliant and comfortable than knitted fabrics, more difficult to handle and suture, and they tend to fray at the edges.

Because of their looped structure, knitted fabrics have little resistance to extension, and the loops can readily straighten, with resultant deformation in the line of highest stress. Knitted grafts are categorized according to the direction of the loops. If the yarns lie predominately lengthwise, the fabric is a warp knit (Fig. 2), and if they lie mostly transverse, it is a weft knit (Fig. 3). Warp knits are more dimensionally stable and unlike weft knits do not unravel, curl up, or fray at the edges. Lightweight fabrics manufactured with thin yarns and filaments and grafts with increased porosity and long loops are likely to stretch most.

Velour is a woven or knitted fabric with a soft filamentous surface on one or both sides as a consequence of additional pile yarns or a napped finish. Manufacturers use that term to describe a graft made of finer texturized yarns with bundles separated by mechanically deforming the yarn and heat setting to provide smaller interstices and more surface area. The velours are easy to handle, preclot effectively, conform readily to the suture line, and have excellent bonding to surrounding tissues. All velour grafts are lightweight fabrics and so subject to dilation.

In triaxial construction the extra yarn is woven or knitted into the basic fabric. In triaxial knits the extra yarn provides greater dimensional stability and significantly reduces porosity, obviating the need for compaction, a process used to shrink a knitted fabric either by chemical agents or heat to reduce porosity to an acceptable level.

POSTOPERATIVE DILATION OF PET GRAFTS

All PET grafts dilate after implantation. The primary initial dilation of crimped prostheses is due to flattening of the crimps when the graft is pressurized. Contributing factors include type of crimp, method of setting the crimp, and number of crimps per unit of graft length. Subsequently the grafts undergo a further increase in diameter and decrease in length as the textile structure shifts.

Although structural properties are largely responsible for dilatation, the extent is also influenced by the amount of longitudinal tension applied to the graft during implantation. The higher the tension, the greater the restriction of dilatation. Since dilatation is a function of the level of applied stress, it may become a problem in hypertensive patients in a relatively short time.

Dilatation may be exacerbated by mechanical fatiguing and biodegradation of the yarns, manufacturing flaws, damage to material during graft processing (compaction, crimping, cleaning), inappropriate surgical handling of the graft (e.g., use of unpadded vascular clamps to occlude the graft, use of cutting needles for anastomoses, and needle and catheter punctures to obtain arteriograms), and improper resterilization and/or storage of grafts.

Associated complications with dilatation include bleeding through graft interstices, fiber breakdown with resultant holes and tears, deposition of mural thrombus with possible graft occlusion and/or distal embolization, and anastomotic aneurysms.

Clinical studies have documented that PET knitted grafts often dilate more than 10% to 20%, previously considered the normal or expected range of postoperative dilatation.[3-8] The tendency to dilate continues, and since it has several causes, the extent of dilatation may vary widely among patients with different types of grafts as well as those with the same graft type and implantation times.

In a study of patients with knitted PET aortic bifurcation grafts evaluated by computed tomography (CT) scanning, all grafts were found to have dilated. However, the three parts of each graft did not always dilate uniformly or undergo the same percent change in diameter. Five basic patterns of dilatation were identified: uniform dilatation of all graft parts, disproportionate dilatation of the aortic portion, one limb, the aortic portion and one limb, and both limbs.

DILATATION AND GRAFT FAILURE

The structural integrity of an implanted synthetic arterial prosthesis for the life of the patient depends upon the inherent strength of the graft material and fabric construction. Accordingly, intrinsic failure may be defined as the inability of a graft to maintain its integrity in the environment of host tissues. However, the various types of grafts have significantly different physical properties that may account for alterations in postimplantation behavior. The lack of in vitro tests and animal studies that can reliably predict dilatation, long-term strength, or durability of synthetic grafts after implantation further complicates the problem.[9] Moreover, there are insufficient clinical data regarding the usual dilative characteristics for specific grafts.

Dilatation is an inherent feature to a greater or lesser degree in all PET arterial prostheses. Consequently, impending graft failure is difficult to identify in the presence of uncomplicated generalized dilatation. A specific degree of generalized dilatation for the various PET grafts that constitutes a significant hazard and warrants replacement cannot be defined at this time.

The diagnosis of intrinsic PET graft failure manifested by aneurysmal deterioration should be based on the proven existence of either a localized aneurysm within the body of a graft or generalized dilatation complicated by bleeding through graft interstices or a tear, anastomotic aneurysms, or graft thrombosis. Although nonuniform generalized dilatation of different parts of the same aortic bifurcation graft probably should be viewed as possible failure, the cause and significance of this unusual pattern are still unclear.

Aneurysmal deterioration of PET arterial prostheses with or without rupture has been reported among these graft types: Wesolowski Weavenit (Meadox Medicals, Inc., Oakland, N.J.), Ultralightweight (Bard Cardiosurgery Division, Billerica, Mass.), DeBakey Standard Weight (Bard), Microknit (Golaski Laboratories, Philadelphia, Pa.), Sauvage External Velour (Bard), Cooley Double Velour (Meadox), Microvel (Meadox), Vasculour-D Internal Velour (Bard), Cooley I Knit (Meadox), low-porosity woven Dacron, and unspecified Dacron grafts. Graft failure occurred at 6 to 144 months post implantation with an average time of 59 months, or 4.9 years.[7] With the exception of the Golaski grafts (Milliknit and Microknit), all weft-knit grafts (Wesolowski Weavenit, Sauvage External Velour, Ultralightweight, DeBakey Standard Weight, Vasculour-D Internal Velour) have been replaced with warp-knit grafts.

MANAGEMENT

PET arterial grafts may continue to dilate after implantation, and inherent serious complications may

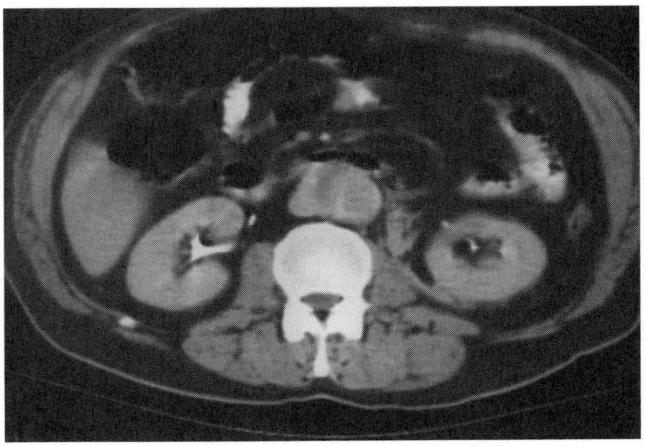

Figure 4 Saccular aneurysmal formation in aortic portion of PET knitted aortic bifurcation graft.

occur 5 or more years post implantation. Therefore, patients should be followed for life with periodic physical examinations and CT evaluation of the entire graft.

Clearly, operation is indicated for aneurysmal deterioration, i.e., a localized aneurysm within the body of a graft (Fig. 4) or generalized dilatation complicated by bleeding through interstices or a tear, anastomotic aneurysms, or graft thrombosis. Patients with uncomplicated generalized dilatation should be followed closely to detect rapid and/or significant changes in graft size or other problems that require operative intervention. Since the prognostic significance of nonuniform generalized dilatation of different parts of aortic bifurcation grafts is unknown, decisions regarding management must be based on individual considerations.

Whenever evidence of aneurysmal deterioration is detected, the entire graft should be carefully assessed with CT scanning and arteriography. The final decision regarding the amount of graft to be replaced depends upon clinical and radiologic findings as well as the patient's general medical condition.

REFERENCES

1. Campbell CD, Brooks DH, Webster MW, et al. Aneurysm formation in expanded polytetrafluoroethylene prostheses. Surgery 1976; 79:491–493.
2. Mohr LL, Smith LL. Polytetrafluoroethylene graft aneurysms: A report of five aneurysms. Arch Surg 1980; 115:1467–1470.
3. Nunn DB, Freeman MH, Hudgins PC. Postoperative alterations in size of Dacron aortic grafts. Ann Surg 1979; 189:741–745.
4. Nunn DB, Carter MD, Donohue MD, Hudgins PC. Postoperative dilation of knitted Dacron aortic bifurcation graft. J Vasc Surg 1990; 12:291–297.
5. Kim GE, Imparato AM, Nathan I, Riles TS. Dilation of synthetic grafts and junctional aneurysms. Arch Surg 1979; 114:1296–1303.
6. Clagett GP, Salander JM, Eddleman WL, et al. Dilation of knitted Dacron aortic prostheses and anastomotic false aneurysms: Etiologic consideration. Surgery 1983; 93:9–16.
7. Nunn DB. Dilatation tardive des prostheses en Dacron. In: Kieffer E, ed. Le Remplacement arterial: principes et applications. Paris: A.E.R.C.V. 1992.
8. Mikati A, Marache P, Watel A, et al. End-to-side aortoprosthetic anastomoses: Long-term computed tomography assessment. Ann Vasc Surg 1990; 4:584–591.
9. American national standard for vascular graft prostheses. Developed by the association for the advancement of medical instrumentation. Approved 7 July 1986 by the American National Standards Institute, Inc.

AORTIC ANEURYSM, ARTERIOMEGALY, AND ANEURYSMOSIS

CHARLES L. MESH, M.D.
LINDA M. GRAHAM, M.D.

Abdominal aortic aneurysms and multiple concomitant peripheral aneurysms (aneurysmosis) develop in the setting of normal, occluded, and enlarged adjacent native vessels. When diffusely enlarged arteries (arteriomegaly) are discovered in patients with abdominal aortic aneurysms, the incidence of concomitant multiple peripheral aneurysms increases dramatically, and the distinction between aneurysmal and native vessel may become blurred.

DEFINITIONS

Normal Arteries

The ad hoc subcommittee on reporting standards for arterial aneurysms of the Society for Vascular Surgery and the North American Chapter of the International Society for Cardiovascular Surgery (SVS-ISCVS) has published ranges of diameters for normal human arteries based on computed tomography (CT), B-mode ultrasound, and arteriographic studies.[1] The diameter of the normal human infrarenal aorta ranges from 1.2 to 2.05 cm and is remarkably constant whether measured by angiography, B-mode ultrasound, or direct examination at autopsy. Recent studies document that normal arteries are consistently larger in men than in women and that arterial size increases with age.[2]

Arteriomegaly

Diffusely enlarged arteries were first described by Leriche[3] as "dolicho et méga artère" (elongated and enlarged arteries). Other terms to describe enlarged arteries include ectasia, arteria magna, and arteria magna et dolicho. In 1971 Thomas[4] coined the descriptive term arteriomegaly, implying the generalized enlargement of the entire arterial system. The ad hoc subcommittee on reporting standards for arterial aneurysms of the SVS-ISCVS has suggested that arteriomegaly be used to describe diffuse arterial enlargement involving several arterial segments (nonfocal) with an increase in diameter above 50% by comparison with the expected normal diameter (Fig. 1). Mild dilation, less than 50% of the

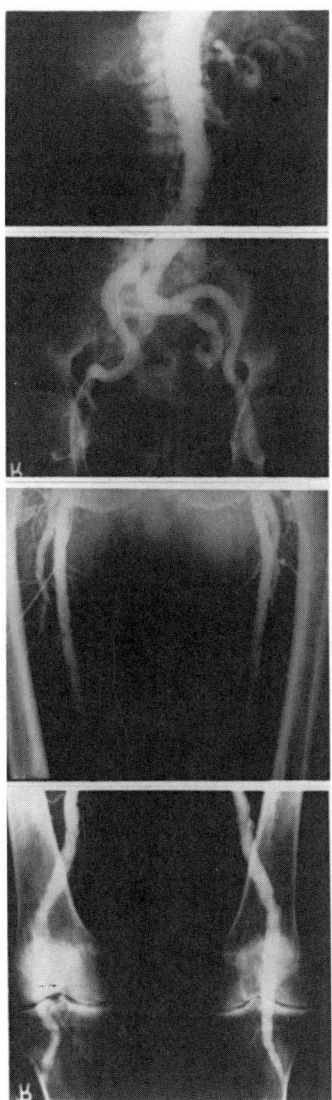

Figure 1 Composite arteriogram demonstrating the tortuous and elongated abdominal aorta, iliac, femoral, and popliteal arteries of arteriomegaly.

normal expected arterial diameter, has been classified as ectasia.[1]

Aneurysm

The ad hoc subcommittee on reporting standards for arterial aneurysms of the SVS-ISCVS suggests that aneurysm be defined as a permanent localized (focal) dilation of an artery having at least a 50% increase in diameter compared with the expected normal diameter of the artery in question.[1] In the setting of arteriomegaly an aneurysm should be considered a localized increase in arterial diameter of 50% compared with the diameter of the proximal adjacent vessel.

Aneurysmosis

The term aneurysmosis, attributed to Trippel, implies multiple contiguous aneurysms at different levels of the vascular tree.[5] In contrast to its classic definition, aneurysmosis is commonly used to describe multiple combined aneurysms separated by normal, occluded, or arteriomegalic arteries. Aneurysmosis in the context of arteriomegaly can be classified into three categories.[6] Type 1 accounts for 11% of patients and consists of aortic, iliac, and common femoral artery aneurysms with distal arteriomegaly. Type 2 classifies 7.7% of patients and is defined as aortic and iliac arteriomegaly with aneurysms of the common femoral, superficial femoral, and popliteal arteries (Fig. 2). The large majority of patients (81.3%) have aortoiliac, femoral, and popliteal aneurysms with arteriomegaly of intervening arteries and are classified as type 3.

EPIDEMIOLOGY AND PATHOLOGY

The true incidence of arteriomegaly is unknown, since this diagnosis has conventionally been made using arteriography. In patients undergoing arteriography for the evaluation of lower extremity pathology, arteriomegaly is a relatively rare finding, noted in 5% to 6% of studies.[6,7] The arteriographic incidence of aneurysmosis is similar, occurring in 4% of examinations.[8] While the combination of aneurysmosis and arteriomegaly occurs in only 1.6% of all arteriograms, 30% of patients with arteriomegaly will have concomitant aneurysmosis.[6]

The cause of aneurysmosis is assumed to be the same as that of isolated aneurysm. The histopathologic examination of the component aneurysms found in aneurysmosis differs little from that of isolated aneurysms. In both situations there is fragmentation and loss of elastic laminae. Alpha$_1$-antitrypsin, a major inhibitor of elastase, has been noted to be lower in patients with aneurysmosis than in those with isolated aortic aneurysm.[9] It has therefore been theorized that isolated aortic aneurysm and aneurysmosis are different points in the progression of a systemic disease that is characterized by prolonged and/or unchecked elastin digestion.

CLINICAL PATTERNS

Aneurysmosis, arteriomegaly, and aneurysmosis in the presence of arteriomegaly all occur predominantly in men during the sixth and seventh decades of life and are associated with tobacco use and hypertension. In contrast to isolated aneurysms, women do not develop aneurysmosis,[8] and there is no familial predisposition to either aneurysmosis or arteriomegaly. The incidence of underlying cardiac disease is approximately 40% for patients with isolated aneurysm and for those with aneurysmosis,[8] but it is higher (60%) in the group with both aneurysmosis and arteriomegaly.[6]

The natural history of patients with aneurysmosis reflects that of the component aortic and peripheral

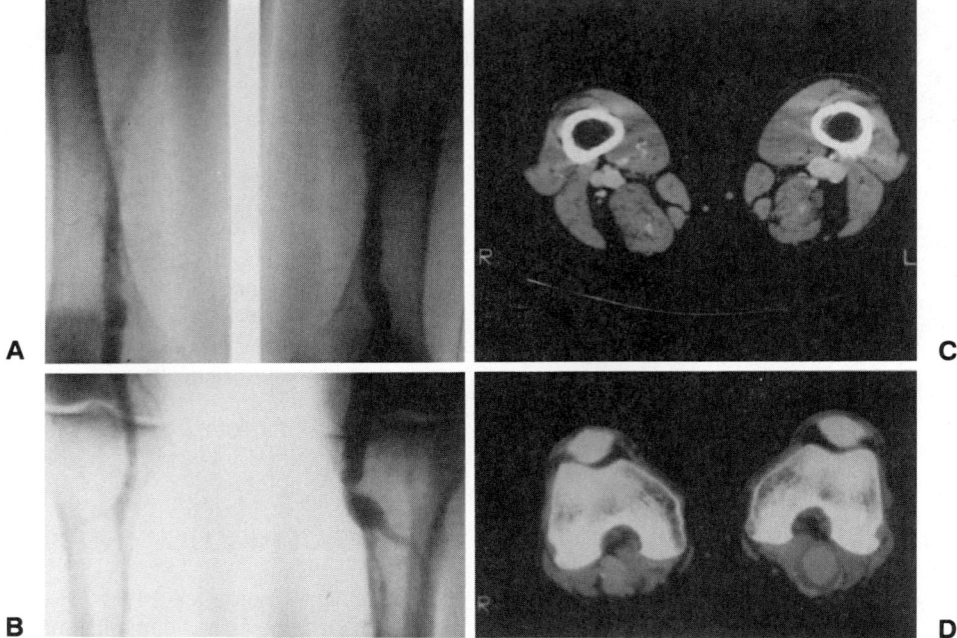

Figure 2 *A, B,* Composite preoperative arteriogram. *C, D,* Representative computed tomographs. Top views show arteriomegaly and bottom views show aneurysms characteristic of type III arteriomegaly and aneurysmosis.

aneurysms. Femoral and popliteal aneurysms may thrombose and/or embolize. More importantly, life-threatening aortic aneurysms are present in up to 95% of patients and are almost always asymptomatic.[8] Patients may present with aortic rupture or with symptoms ranging from acute lower extremity ischemia to rest pain, tissue loss, claudication, and even Raynaud's phenomena. Both femoral and popliteal aneurysms can cause local pain as they enlarge. They rupture only rarely, most often at the femoral position. Delayed surgical therapy for peripheral aneurysmal disease is uniformly disappointing. This observation is most compelling in the setting of aneurysmosis and arteriomegaly. Some 35% of patients with this condition will present with symptoms of acute ischemia, with as many as 44% ultimately requiring major amputation.[6]

DIAGNOSTIC APPROACH

The diagnostic approach to aneurysmosis, with or without concomitant arteriomegaly, should be directed at the detection, localization, and accurate sizing of all aneurysms. Many patients with aneurysmosis have no complaints. Their disease is most often discovered as an incidental finding on either routine physical examination or radiologic study.

Most femoral and popliteal artery aneurysms are detectable on physical examination. In contrast, accurate diagnosis of aortoiliac aneurysms necessitates either B-mode ultrasound or CT. These modalities are also applicable for detection and measurement of femoral and popliteal artery aneurysms.

Arteriomegaly may often be mistaken for aneurysmal degeneration on both physical examination and ultrasonic imaging. Therefore, to distinguish these entities, study of the entire arterial system from the infrarenal aorta to the tibial arteries is required. CT, magnetic resonance imaging (MRI), and arteriography have all been used for this purpose. Arteriography may depict the strikingly slow flow of contrast medium classical of arteriomegaly.[3] However, this sluggish flow and the effective capacitance of arteriomegalic arteries make arteriographic visualization difficult and necessitate nephrotoxic doses of contrast medium. The contrast medium load can be reduced with digital subtraction techniques, but the presence of muralluminal thrombus may lead arteriography to underestimate aneurysm size. Thus, arteriography can detect the diffuse nature of both aneurysmosis and arteriomegaly, but it cannot reliably distinguish between these conditions.

Late-generation CT can provide sequential high-definition transverse images along a single corporal axis, which makes it the ideal modality with which to diagnose multiple aneurysms, define their diffuse nature, and distinguish arteriomegaly from aneurysmosis. MRI should provide all the information of CT as well as data regarding arterial flow rates. However, MRI is more expensive than CT and is neither as widely available nor as well studied.

Aneurysmosis should be suspected in three typical clinical scenarios: in the asymptomatic patient with a pulsatile lower extremity mass; in the patient with an aortic aneurysm and arteriomegalic iliac arteries discovered either on radiologic examination or at emergency operation for aortic rupture; and in the patient with acute lower extremity ischemia requiring emergent vascular reconstruction. The first case should be treated as a typical peripheral aneurysm with careful physical examination and B-mode ultrasound inspection of all possible sites of aneurysmal development, including the aorta, iliac, femoral and popliteal arteries. Further investigation with arteriography should be based on the type of aneurysms detected and the necessary reconstructions. In the second setting, the arteriomegalic iliac vessels should suggest the risk of aneurysmosis. Extension of arteriography to determine lower extremity runoff is helpful to define the extent of arteriomegaly and/or aneurysmosis. However, as in the first case, arteriomegaly demands physical examination and B-mode ultrasound imaging of all potential sites of aneurysmal degeneration. In the third setting, time is of the essence, and therefore, most studies should be performed in the operating room. On-table arteriography—an absolute component of any vascular reconstruction for acute ischemia—and direct operative examination of vessels will usually define either multiple aneurysms or infrainguinal arteriomegaly. If these studies prove equivocal, the use of angioscopy or intraoperative duplex scanning may be diagnostic. If either arteriomegaly or aneurysmosis is noted, postoperative physical examination and B-mode ultrasound investigation of all potential aneurysmal sites, especially of the contralateral extremity and the abdominal aorta are necessary.

THERAPY

Arteriomegaly by itself requires no treatment. Since patients with this condition are thought to develop aneurysms eventually, they should be evaluated annually for such progression with B-mode ultrasound. In contrast, aneurysmosis demands prompt surgical therapy. Treatment is dictated by the acuity of symptoms, the location of the aneurysms, and the presence of diffuse aneurysmal dilation. The principles of therapy for aneurysmosis are those of routine aneurysm repair: exclusion of the aneurysm from arterial circulation and arterial reconstruction with anastomoses to undiseased vessels. The surgical therapy of the aortic aneurysm and the individual peripheral aneurysms found in patients with multiple noncontiguous arterial aneurysms lends itself to staged arterial reconstruction.

The patient with classical aneurysmosis has diffuse arterial dilation extending from the infrarenal aorta to the below-knee popliteal artery and requires both aortic and infrainguinal reconstruction. It is distinctly unusual for a patient to have a symptomatic aortic aneurysm and simultaneous limb-threatening lower extremity ischemia. Therefore, the aortic and infrainguinal repairs can almost always be staged. The life-threatening aortic aneurysm should be treated first and the necessary infrainguinal reconstruction performed later. In the setting of acute lower extremity ischemia complicating either a femoral or popliteal aneurysm, this sequence is reversed.

The aortic reconstruction is performed with standard techniques. Since the external iliac system is frequently spared focal aneurysmal dilatation, the distal anastomoses can usually be performed in the pelvis. These anastomoses are sewn end to end to the common iliac bifurcation at the origin of the internal and external iliac arteries or end to side to the external iliac artery after the distal common iliac artery has been oversewn. Every effort is made to maintain pelvic and distal colonic perfusion by preserving at least one internal iliac artery or the inferior mesenteric artery. In cases of bilateral internal iliac aneurysms and inferior mesenteric artery occlusion, this can be accomplished by a short bypass from one of the iliac limbs of the aortic graft to uninvolved internal iliac artery. In cases with extensive internal iliac degeneration and a patent inferior mesenteric artery, it is often easiest to preserve the inferior mesenteric artery as a Carrel patch for reimplantation into the aortic graft.

If the external iliac arterial system is aneurysmal, the distal anastomosis is performed in the groin during repair of any coexisting femoral artery aneurysms. In the case of a common femoral artery aneurysm, the graft limb can usually be anastomosed end to end to the bifurcation at the origin of the superficial and profunda femoral arteries. Aneurysmal extension into the superficial or profunda femoral arteries is usually limited. This situation lends itself to end-to-end anastomosis of the graft to the superficial femoral artery with deep femoral artery preservation by either direct implantation or short bypass. Pelvic revascularization is by direct implantation of the internal iliac artery into the graft limb, by short bypass from the graft limb to the internal iliac artery, or by Carrel patch implantation of the inferior mesenteric artery into the aortic graft.

Infrainguinal reconstruction in a patient with aneurysmosis almost always involves repair of a popliteal artery aneurysm. Femoral artery aneurysms are repaired during either aortic or infrainguinal reconstruction. During infrainguinal reconstruction femoral aneurysm repair is accomplished with a short prosthetic graft from the distal external iliac artery to the profunda femoral artery, sewn end to end at each anastomosis. Invariably popliteal aneurysm repair requires bypass from the femoral artery prosthesis to the below-knee popliteal artery or to a tibial vessel, and so the conduit of choice is autogenous saphenous vein. In the case of diffuse aneurysmosis or particularly large aneurysms, the in situ technique avoids tunneling along the aneurysm with its attendant risks of distal embolization and laceration of venous structures adherent to the aneurysm. Proximal and distal anastomoses are performed with standard techniques. The popliteal artery aneurysm should always be excluded from the circulation by proximal and distal ligation. In the setting of acute ischemia, urokinase may be instilled into the infrapopliteal vasculature to enhance recovery of runoff.

REFERENCES

1. Johnston KW, Rutherford RB, Tilson MD, et al. Suggested standards for reporting on arterial aneurysms. J Vasc Surg 1991; 13:444–450.

2. Ouriel K, Green RM, Donayre C, et al. An evaluation of new methods of expressing aortic aneurysm size: relationship to rupture. J Vasc Surg 1992; 15:12–20.
3. Leriche R. Dilatation pathologique des alteres en dehors des artères aneurysmes vie tissulaire des artères. Presse Med, 1942; 50:641–642.
4. Lea M. Arteriomegaly. Br J Surg 1971; 58:690–694.
5. Beal JM. Aneurysmosis. Ill Med J 1968; 133:157–160.
6. Hollier LH, Stanson AW, Gloviczki P, et al. Arteriomegaly: Classification and morbid implications of diffuse aneurysmal disease. Surgery 1983; 93:700–708.
7. Callum KG, Lea M, Browse NL. A definition of arteriomegaly and the size of arteries supplying the lower limbs. Br J Surg 1983; 70:524–529.
8. Dent TL, Lindenauer SM, Ernst CB, Fry WJ. Multiple arteriosclerotic arterial aneurysms. Arch Surg 1972; 105:338–344.
9. Cohen JR, Mandell C, Chang JB, Wise L. Elastin metabolism of the infrarenal aorta. J Vasc Surg 1988; 7:210–214.

ISOLATED ILIAC ANEURYSM

WILLIAM C. KRUPSKI, M.D.

The first operation for an iliac artery aneurysm was performed by Sir Astley Paston Cooper in 1817.[1] The patient was a 37-year-old man who presented with a traumatic aneurysm of the external iliac artery that was eroding through the skin. Cooper ligated the aorta above the aneurysm. Although the patient survived the operation, he died 40 hours later. In 1827, Valentine Mott performed the first successful operation for a common iliac artery aneurysm in a 33-year-old farmer "of temperate and regular habits." Mott ligated the proximal iliac artery rather than the aorta, and 18 days later he found that the aneurysm was nonpulsatile when he removed the ligature percutaneously.

Halsted, in his formidable work on the results of ligating the common iliac arteries in 1912, collected 15 reported cases in the literature in which ligation had been performed for aneurysm. In 1913 MacLaren successfully ligated an internal iliac aneurysm secondary to trauma in a young woman after a difficult instrumental delivery. More than a century after Astley Cooper's innovative operation, Rudolph Matas performed the first successful proximal ligation of an aortoiliac aneurysm in 1923. Matas's endoaneurysmorrhaphy presaged the current prevailing method of "internal" or intrasaccular reconstruction.

ETIOLOGY

Isolated iliac artery aneurysms are most commonly degenerative or nonspecific in etiology, and they typically occur in elderly individuals. Atherosclerosis may be simply coexistent rather than causative. Reports of infected aneurysms of the iliac vessels have appeared from time to time, and the pathologic changes in such aneurysms of the iliac arteries do not differ from mycotic aneurysms in other major vessels. Iliac artery aneurysms even less commonly occur as congenital abnormalities or due to the following disorders: Marfan syndrome, Kawasaki disease, Ehlers-Danlos syndrome, Takayasu syndrome, cystic medial necrosis, and spontaneous dissection.

INCIDENCE

The incidence of solitary iliac aneurysms is difficult to ascertain. In autopsy studies as well as clinical reports, there is a great deal of variability. In a recent study specifically designed to estimate the frequency of occurrence of solitary iliac arterial aneurysms, Brunkwall and colleagues found seven cases in 26,251 hospital autopsies over a 15-year period, for an incidence of 0.03%.[2] Another report examined surgically treated isolated iliac aneurysms and described 16 cases in a 12-year period.[3] These two studies provide conflicting information, but regardless of the precise incidence, it is clear that solitary iliac aneurysms are rare.

Most iliac artery aneurysms accompany abdominal aortic aneurysms (AAA), coexisting with from 10% to 20% of AAAs.[4] In general, iliac aneurysms emanate from the distal extent of aortic aneurysms. In the Brunkwall autopsy series, there were 202 iliac aneurysms among 1,287 aortic aneurysms, for a prevalence of 16%.[2] Richardson and Greenfield, who reported the largest number of patients with iliac aneurysms (55) from one institution, indicated that iliac aneurysm comprised 2.2% of all intra-abdominal aneurysms.[5] Such discrepancies in reported frequencies may be explained in part by differences in definitions of iliac aneurysms, inclusion of aortoiliac aneurysms in the number of iliac aneurysms, and derivation of cases from autopsy versus clinical practice.

ILIAC ANEURYSMS AFTER REPAIR OF ABDOMINAL AORTIC ANEURYSMS

An important clinical question involves the late development of iliac artery aneurysms after repair of AAA. Concern over potential long-term degeneration of iliac arteries has led some to recommend bifurcated graft replacement of most AAAs. In 1985, the Mayo clinic group reported their experience with long-term follow-up of 1,087 patients who underwent AAA repair.[6] After 6 to 12 years, only six iliac aneurysms developed, equally distributed between patients who had a tube graft and those who had a bifurcated graft. Late occurrence of thoracic aneurysms was most common, affecting 24 patients. A 1991 report from the same institution retrospectively reviewed a 35-year experience with AAA repair. In 78 patients, half of whom had a tube graft and half of whom had a bifurcated graft, only 1 (who had a bifurcated graft originally) developed an iliac aneurysm 14 years after the initial procedure. Provan and colleagues in Canada performed serial abdominal ultrasound studies 3 to 5 years postoperatively in 23 patients who had tube graft replacement of AAAs. Iliac arteries, even nine vessels that were enlarged to 1.5 to 3 cm at the time of AAA repair, remained stable in size. Thus, based on what little information is available, late development of iliac aneurysms after tube graft repair of AAAs does not appear to be a major clinical problem.

ANATOMY OF SOLITARY ILIAC ANEURYSMS

Approximately 70% of iliac aneurysms are located in the common iliac artery (Table 1). Rarely do common iliac aneurysms extend into the external iliac, although they often involve the internal iliac. The reason for this predilection is unknown. Solitary aneurysms occur in the internal iliac artery in about 20% of patients, and the remainder are in the external iliac. Richardson and Greenfield emphasized the multiplicity of iliac aneurysms.[5] In their report, 67% of patients were noted to have two or more vessels involved, which underscores the need to evaluate the entire iliac system thoroughly when a patient presents with one aneurysm. When iliac aneurysms appear singularly, they are most likely to involve the hypogastric artery, whose concealed location within the pelvis contributes to delayed recognition.

CLINICAL PRESENTATION

Solitary iliac artery aneurysms most commonly occur in elderly men. The average patient presents in his mid-70s, slightly older than the average patient with an AAA. The male-female ratio is about 6:1 or 7:1, an even greater preponderance of men than for AAAs, in which the ratio averages 2:1 to 4:1, with women "catching up" to men in very old age.

The clinical manifestations of iliac aneurysms depend upon the etiology, size, location, and confounding factors (e.g., connective tissue disorders, hypertension, or intravenous drug abuse). About half of patients in surgical reports presented with symptoms related to their aneurysms, and symptoms are almost always present in clinical reports of hypogastric artery aneurysms.[7] Compression or erosion of surrounding structures and rupture are the most frequent methods of presentation. About one-third of patients complain of lower abdominal pain, often associated with genitourinary symptoms. Sepsis from ureteral obstruction and subsequent pyelonephritis is a common presentation, and erosion or rupture into the ureter or bladder can

Table 1 Location of Solitary Iliac Aneurysms*

First Authors	Year	Location	Total Number†	Common	Internal	External
Frank	1961	University of Rochester	2	0	2	0
Markowitz	1961	Columbia	30	—	—	—
Silver	1967	Duke	11	8	3	0
Lowry	1978	Michigan	8	8	0	0
Victor	1979	Washington University, St. Louis	4	0	4	0
Nelson	1980	Medical University of South Carolina	3	0	3	0
Verta	1982	University of Illinois	2	0	2	0
Kasulke	1982	University of Missouri	2	0	2	0
Brin	1982	University of California at Los Angeles	6	0	6	0
McCready	1983	Mayo Clinic	71 (50)	63	7	1
Perdue	1983	Emory	6	0	6	0
Plate	1985	Mayo Clinic	6	—	—	—
Netto	1986	Sao Paulo, Brazil	2	0	2	0
Hagen	1986	Berlin, Germany	4	3	1	0
Richardson	1988	Medical College of Virginia	72 (55)	48	22	2
Bolin	1988	Linköping, Sweden	22 (16)	16	0	6
Krupski	1989	UCSF and Scripps Clinic	3	0	3	0
Arenson	1989	Toronto, Canada	6	—	—	—
Weber	1989	Zurich, Switzerland	23	15	5	3
Brunkwall	1989	Malmo, Sweden	14	9	4	1
Staniszewski	1990	Vienna, Austria	9	—	—	—
Schroeder	1991	University of Virginia	55 (30)	—	—	—
Nachbur	1991	Berne, Switzerland	53	—	—	—
Sacks	1992	Surrey, United Kingdom	18 (11)	12	5	1
Total			432	182 (67%)	77 (28%)	14 (5%)

*Series reporting two or more patients.
†Number in parentheses is number of patients if it is not the same as number of aneurysms.

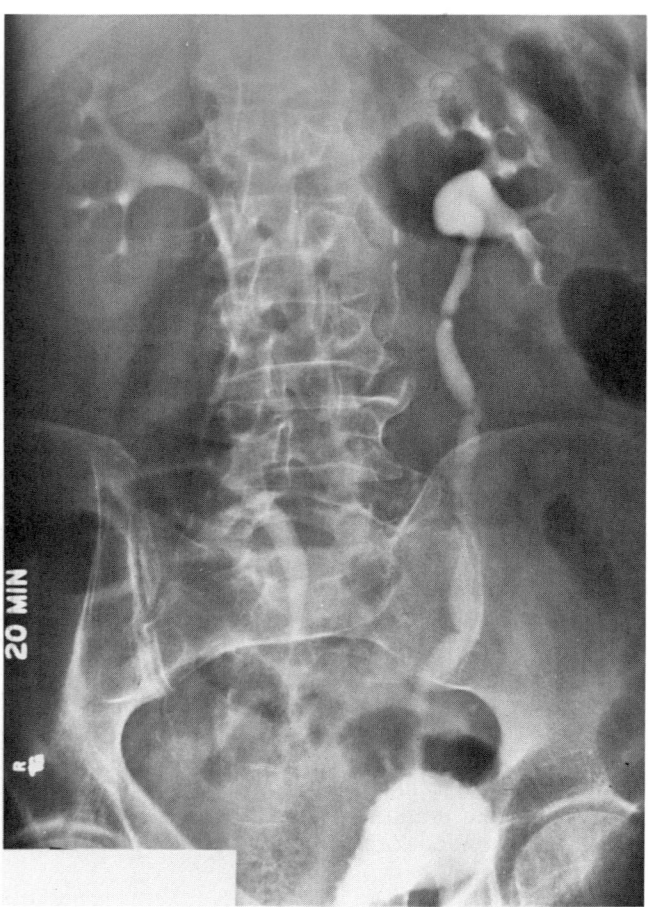

Figure 1 Intravenous pyelogram shows displacement of the right ureter and bladder by a large internal iliac artery aneurysm. The left ureter and collecting system are partially obstructed by a left internal iliac artery aneurysm. This aneurysm eventually eroded and ruptured into the genitourinary system.

cause microscopic or massive hematuria (Fig. 1).[7] One-fifth of patients have gastrointestinal complaints, and an equal number develop neurogenic symptoms owing to compression of femoral, obturator, or sciatic nerves. Nerve compression from iliac aneurysms can cause weakness and paresthesia of the lower extremity, simulating lumbar disk herniation (Fig. 2).[7] About 15% of patients describe both gastrointestinal and genitourinary symptoms. Lower extremity edema from venous compression occurs in 5%. Massive leg swelling and congestive heart failure may arise from spontaneous rupture of an iliac artery aneurysm into the adjacent vein that produces a large arteriovenous fistula. When contained or free rupture occurs, symptoms of severe abdominal or back pain, often radiating into the scrotum or perineum, and associated hypovolemic shock mimic a ruptured AAA.

Physical examination can establish the diagnosis of iliac artery aneurysms if the physician recognizes the patient's symptoms and has a high index of suspicion. More than two-thirds of iliac aneurysms that present clinically can be palpated on abdominal or rectal examination as pulsatile masses.[5,7] Gynecologic examination may be of additional help in women with iliac artery aneurysms, although this is relatively unusual. Other findings associated with aneurysms, such as bruits, thrills, and hypotension, are not specific for those involving the iliac arteries. Perianal ecchymosis, signifying dissection of blood through the retroperitoneal space, and anal sphincter paralysis have been reported after rupture of iliac aneurysms.[4]

DIAGNOSTIC STUDIES

In addition to the clinical features, iliac aneurysms may be confirmed by ultrasonography (US), computed tomography (CT) scans, magnetic resonance imaging (MRI), and arteriography. When the aneurysm is identified by these studies, there is probably very little difference in utility between them. Ultrasonography is substantially less expensive than the other modalities but has the disadvantages of (1) operator dependence, (2) ambiguity because of the depth of the arteries in the pelvis in conjunction with overlying intestinal gas, and (3) inaccuracy with respect to perianeurysmal fluid that

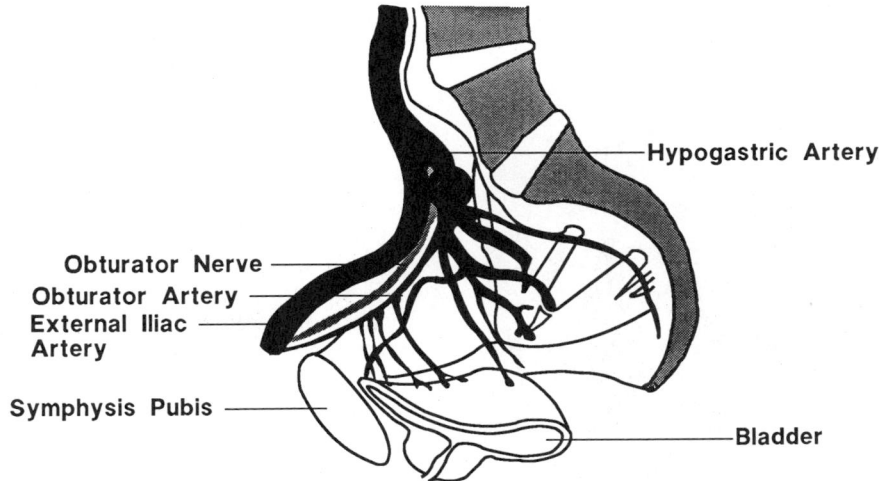

Figure 2 Diagram of lateral view of the relationship of the hypogastric artery and the obturator nerve. (From Krupski WC, Bass A, Rosenberg GD, et al. The elusive hypogastric artery aneurysm: Novel presentations. J Vasc Surg 1989; 10:557–562.)

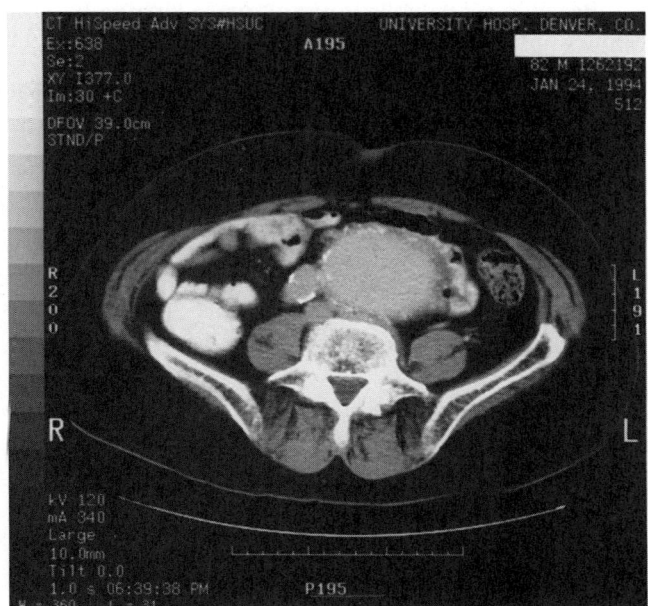

Figure 3 Computed tomography scan shows 10 cm common iliac artery aneurysm.

suggests leakage. For example, a study comparing US, CT, and intravenous digital subtraction arteriography for study of AAAs recorded that US did not detect iliac aneurysms in 19 of 25 patients. Transanal ultrasound theoretically might be of use for diagnosing internal iliac aneurysms. There does not appear to be much dissimilarity between the ability of CT scans and MRI for providing architectural information about iliac aneurysms (Fig. 3). Arteriography may overlook iliac artery aneurysms because of the well-known propensity for thrombus to fill the aneurysmal sac. However, in contrast to the controversy over routinely obtaining arteriograms to evaluate AAAs, there is general agreement that arteriography is essential for planning elective repair of iliac aneurysms in order to assess the pelvic circulation (Fig. 4).

NATURAL HISTORY

The indications for surgical repair and a rational approach to management of iliac aneurysms should be dictated by the natural history or untreated course of the aneurysm. This determination must also include the ease of exposure and vascular control, the consequences of interrupting flow through the arterial segment, technical features of the repair, and the general status of the patient. Unfortunately, there is no large prospective study describing the natural history of solitary iliac aneurysms. The limited number of patients reported, all either anecdotal or retrospective analyses, makes the recommendation for treatment largely empirical.

It seems reasonable to assume that iliac aneurysms are similar to AAAs, with rupture possible at smaller diameters than for AAAs. In fact, rupture has been reported in aneurysms as small as 2 cm.[5] However, most authors define iliac aneurysms as larger than 2.5 cm in diameter, and it is very unusual for one to rupture under 3 cm. Like AAAs, iliac aneurysms tend to enlarge unpredictably, with an estimated average expansion rate of 4 mm/year.[8] In the Mayo Clinic experience, 19 patients with iliac aneurysms ranging from 2 to 9 cm (mean 3.4 cm) were followed for 3 months to 11 years.[8] Ten patients did not have enlargement of the aneurysm. There was only one death from ruptured iliac aneurysm in this group (from a 4.5 cm aneurysm that had expanded to 6 cm in 4.5 years). In the Medical College of Virginia report, aneurysm expansion was documented in 36% of patients.[5]

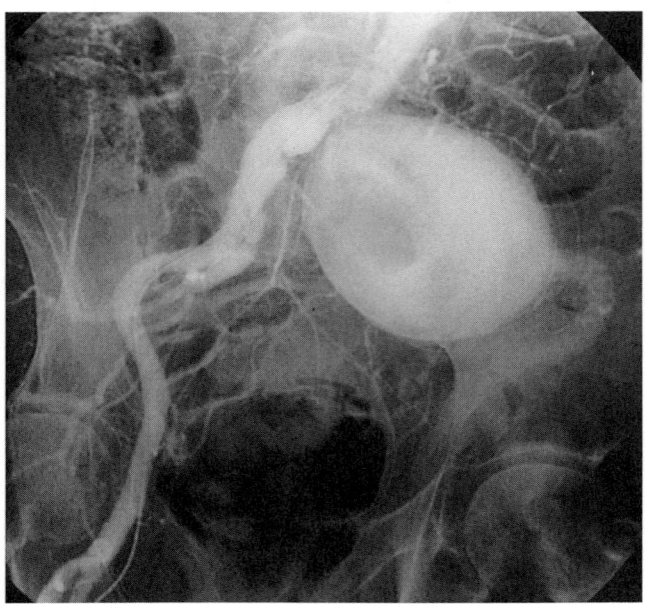

Figure 4 Arteriogram of aneurysm shown in Figure 3. Note redundant, uninvolved external iliac aneurysm arising from the distal extent of the aneurysm.

In striking contrast to the benign course of the serially observed patients in the Mayo Clinic report, most studies cite a high incidence of ruptured iliac aneurysms. Approximately one-third of patients with iliac aneurysms present with rupture (Table 2). In the 55 patients (with 72 aneurysms) reported by Richardson and Greenfield, there was a 33% rupture rate, including 1 of 11 (9%) aneurysms managed nonoperatively.[5] In this report, the mean diameter of ruptured aneurysms was 5.6 cm, but the smallest aneurysm to rupture was 3.5 cm. Although aneurysms in the common iliac artery occur more frequently than in the internal iliac, the frequency of rupture is equivalent.

Size seems to be an important risk factor for rupture of iliac aneurysms. Lowry and Kraft reported that 75% of their patients presented with ruptured aneurysms; the mean arterial diameter in this series was 7.5 cm.[4] In what amounts to a natural history pilot study, Schuler and Flanigan found that 9 of 13 patients (69%) died of ruptured aneurysms within just slightly more than 4 months of making the diagnosis.[9] The average size of aneurysms in this report was 8.5 cm, but the authors did not specifically correlate size with rupture.

Based on available information, all patients with isolated iliac artery aneurysms larger than 3 cm in

Table 2 Rupture and Survival Rates for Solitary Iliac Aneurysms*

First Authors	Year	Number of Patients	Number of Aneurysms	Ruptures	Deaths Related to Aneurysms
Frank	1961	2	2	2	1
Markowitz	1961	30	30	5	5†
Silver	1967	11	11	0‡	—
Lowry	1978	8	8	8	4
Victor	1979	4	4	2	4
Nelson	1980	3	3	1	1
Verta	1982	2	2	2	2
Kasulke	1982	2	2	0	0
Brin	1982	5	6	3	2
McCready	1983	50	71	7	5
Perdue	1983	6	6	2	1
Plate	1985	6	6	2	3
Netto	1986	2	2	0	0
Hagen	1986	4	4	2	1
Richardson	1988	55	72	18§	11
Bolin	1988	16	22	9	5
Krupski	1989	2	3	2	0
Arenson	1989	5	6	0	NS
Weber	1989	23	23	19	5
Brunkwall	1989	13	14	6	4
Staniszewski	1990	9	9	2	NS
Schroeder	1991	30	55	0	4
Nachbur	1991	53	53	15	3
Sacks	1992	11	18	3	1
Total		352	432	110 (31% ruptures per patient)	62 (18%)

*Series reporting two or more patients.
†Five of 12 operated patients (42%) died.
‡No ruptures in three hypogastric aneurysms.
§Emergency operations for "suspected" rupture.

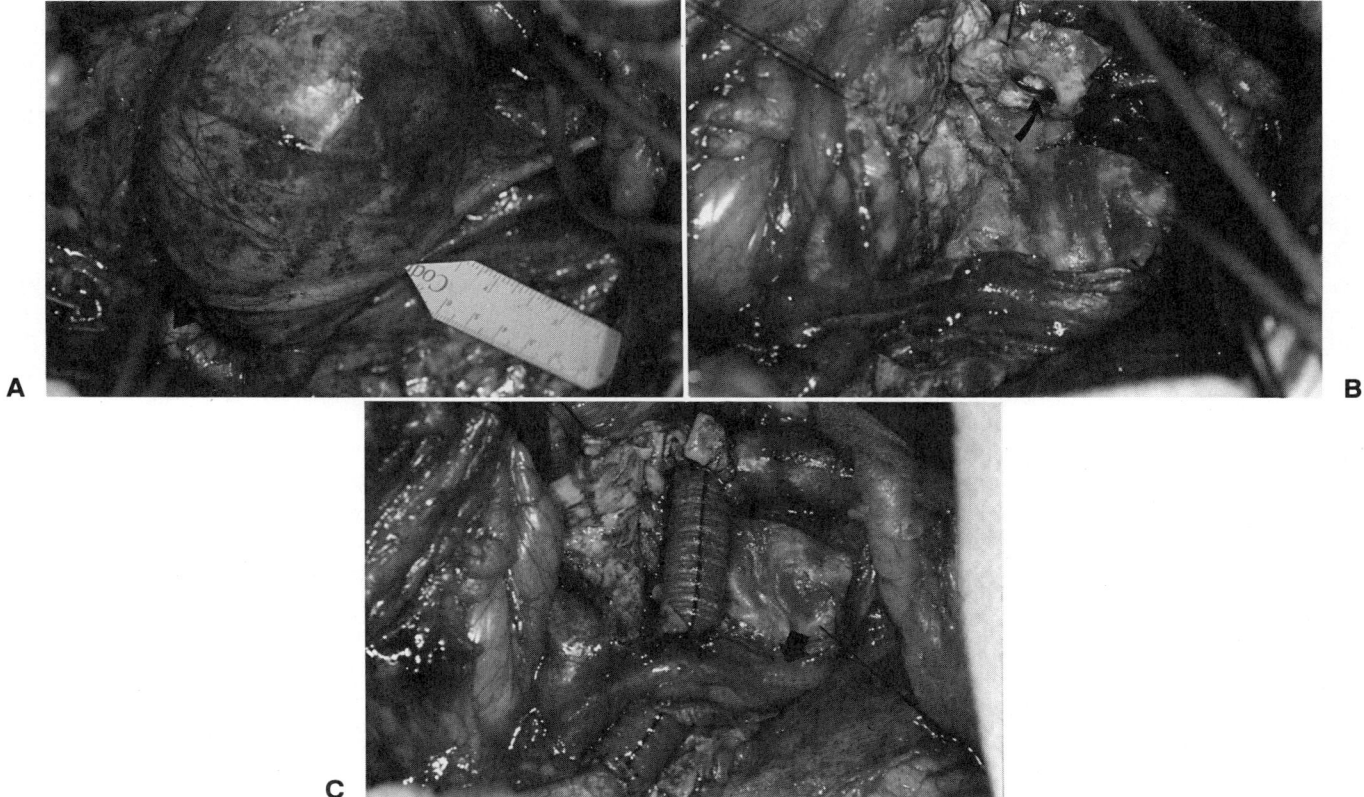

Figure 5 *A,* Large common iliac artery aneurysm with ureter stretched over the anterior surface (indicated by ruler). Note redundant external iliac artery arising from the aneurysm encircled by a loop in the left lower corner of the photograph (*black arrow*). *B,* After proximal and distal arterial control is obtained, the aneurysm sac is opened longitudinally with placement of stay sutures. The orifice of the common iliac artery is indicated by the curved arrow. *C,* An interposition graft is in place between the common and external iliac arteries. The ureter can be seen coursing over the graft (*black arrow*). Before closure of the retroperitoneum, the aneurysm sac is reapproximated over the graft.

diameter who otherwise are in good health should undergo elective repair. In patients who are poor surgical risks or who have aneurysms smaller than 3 cm, observation should be performed in much the same manner that AAAs are monitored. In contrast to sonography for AAAs, computed tomography is the technique of choice for detecting iliac aneurysmal enlargement.

OPERATIVE TECHNIQUES

Surgical treatment should be tailored to the clinical presentation. Ruptured and symptomatic aneurysms demand emergent or urgent repair. When aneurysms are treated electively, in addition to operative repair, thrombosis using embolization with available gelatin sponges (Gelfoam), steel coils, or cyanobucrylate by means of interventional radiologic techniques may be considered for high-risk patients. Operative strategy depends on which arteries are involved and the presence or absence of multiple aneurysms, particularly bilateral ones.

Solitary common iliac artery aneurysms are best treated by retroperitoneal exposure and replacement by interposition prosthetic grafts (Fig. 5). If the contralateral internal iliac artery is undiseased, the ipsilateral internal iliac can be safely ligated. If the ipsilateral hypogastric artery is also aneurysmal, it is usually safest to open the sac and ligate the branches of the artery from within the aneurysm rather than risk injury to the many dilated veins surrounding the external surface of the aneurysm. After graft interposition is completed, the graft should be covered by the aneurysm sac, as is usually done for repair of AAAs.

Solitary internal iliac aneurysms should be removed from in-line blood flow and either resected, if they are very small, or, more commonly, excluded from circulation with oversewing of branches from within the aneurysm. Often the external iliac artery is redundant and a primary end-to-end common-to-external iliac artery anastomosis can be accomplished. Alternatively, interposition of a prosthetic graft can be performed.

Bilateral common iliac artery aneurysms are generally most expeditiously treated by exclusion using a bifurcated prosthetic interposition graft originating from the abdominal aorta (even though the aorta is undiseased). A transperitoneal approach is best in this situation. At least one distal anastomosis should incorporate the lumen of the hypogastric artery. Alternatively, a "jump" graft can be taken to one of the internal iliac arteries. If both internal iliac arteries are excluded from circulation, as may be the case with bilateral hypogastric artery aneurysms, one should ensure that the inferior mesenteric artery is patent. Reimplantation of the inferior mesenteric artery into a prosthetic graft may be required when an aortic replacement is performed in such instances. Impotence should be anticipated when both internal iliac arteries are removed from in-line blood flow.

Aneurysms of the external iliac artery are rarely encountered. Retroperitoneal in-line replacement is optimal, although proximal and distal ligation and femorofemoral bypass is an option.

OUTCOME

Death is predictable if operative treatment of ruptured iliac aneurysms is delayed. Reported operative mortality of ruptured iliac artery aneurysms ranges from 0 to 100%, but in general perioperative death occurs in one-quarter to one-third of patents in larger series. The reason for the better outcome after ruptured iliac artery aneurysms than for ruptured AAAs is unclear. In contrast to the improved prognosis for survival after repair of ruptured iliac artery aneurysms, the elective operative mortality is slightly worse for iliac aneurysms than for AAAs, averaging about 10%. The range of reported elective mortality is wide, from 0 to 50%. Late survival rates are infrequently reported. In a study of 53 repaired isolated iliac artery aneurysms, the 5-year survival was 66% overall, 70% for nonruptured aneurysms, and 55% for ruptured aneurysms.[10]

REFERENCES

1. Haeger K. The illustrated history of surgery. New York: Bell, 1988.
2. Brunkwall J, Hauksson H, Bengtsson H, et al. Solitary aneurysms of the iliac arterial system: An estimate of their frequency of occurrence. J Vasc Surg 1989; 10:381–384.
3. Bolin T, Lund K, Skau T. Isolated aneurysms of the iliac artery: What are the chances of rupture? Eur J Vasc Surg 1988; 2:213–215.
4. Lowry WF, Kraft RO. Isolated aneurysms of the iliac artery. Arch Surg 1978; 113:1289–1293.
5. Richardson JW, Greenfield LJ. Natural history and management of iliac aneurysms. J Vasc Surg 1988; 8:165–171.
6. Plate G, Hollier LA, O'Brien P, et al. Recurrent aneurysms and late complications following repair of abdominal aortic aneurysms. Arch Surg 1985; 120:590–594.
7. Krupski WC, Bass A, Rosenberg GD, et al. The elusive isolated hypogastric artery aneurysm: Novel presentations. J Vasc Surg 1989; 10:557–562.
8. McCready RA, Pairolero PC, Gilmore JC, et al. Isolated iliac artery aneurysms. Surgery 1983; 93:688–693.
9. Schuler JJ, Flanigan DP. Iliac artery aneurysms. In: Bergan J, Yao JST, eds. Aneurysms: Diagnosis and treatment. New York: Grune & Stratton, 1982:469.
10. Nachbur BH, Inderbitzi RGC, Bar W. Isolated iliac aneurysms. Eur J Vasc Surg 1991; 5:375–381.

VASCULAR COMPLICATIONS OF EHLERS-DANLOS SYNDROME AND MARFAN SYNDROME

THOMAS A. WHITEHILL, M.D.

Many conditions known to affect the strength and stability of collagen or elastin result in arterial wall abnormalities. They all have in common the presence of compositional defects of the media because the collagen and elastin fibers essential for normal arterial strength, integrity, and resilience reside there. The pathologic changes of cystic medial necrosis, with the resultant clinical problems of aortic dissection, spontaneous arterial rupture, and disseminated aneurysm formation, result from a variety of metabolic conditions and syndromes, the most common of which are Ehlers-Danlos syndrome and Marfan syndrome. Spontaneous arterial dissection, aneurysmal degeneration, and hemorrhage due to vessel wall structural defects make these patients challenging to manage, as they are prone to catastrophic vascular complications.

EHLERS-DANLOS SYNDROME

The Ehlers-Danlos syndrome is a heterogeneous condition characterized by hyperelastic skin, hypermobile joints, fragile tissues, easy bruising, and abnormal scarring. Eleven different variants of Ehlers-Danlos syndrome have now been described. Each has its own clinical characteristics, documented genetically determined abnormality of collagen biosynthesis and structure, variable genetic molecular defect, and pattern of inheritance.[1] The clinical manifestations of the syndrome vary between different pedigrees. The true incidence of Ehlers-Danlos syndrome is unknown; however, the syndrome is accepted as being one of the most frequently inherited connective tissue disorders.

Clinical Manifestations

Three types of Ehlers-Danlos syndrome (I, III, and IV) frequently have arterial complications, especially type IV (arterial-ecchymotic type, Sack-Barabas syndrome). These patients produce little or no type III collagen, which is of major structural importance in vessels, viscera, and skin. The skin and soft tissues are easily disrupted, tend to fragment and tear with manipulation, and hold sutures and heal poorly. Postoperative wound dehiscence is common. The fragility of the tissues in these patients underlies the life-threatening complications to which they are prone, including catastrophic bleeding from rupture of large and medium-sized arteries and rupture of the colon. The arteries of patients with type IV Ehlers-Danlos syndrome may rupture spontaneously or become aneurysmal with subsequent rupture or dissection. As expected, affected patients frequently describe relatives who have died of these complications.

It is now recognized that type IV Ehlers-Danlos syndrome is actually a group of clinically similar, but genetically distinct disorders. Each involves a defect in the metabolism of type III collagen, resulting in decreased or absent type III collagen in the skin and other affected tissues. Because any number of different biochemical mechanisms could produce the same end result, it is not surprising that several distinct alterations in type III collagen metabolism have been implicated in Ehlers-Danlos syndrome. Some are related to abnormalities of collagen secretion, whereas others are caused by decreased or absent collagen synthesis. A total of 36 patients with type IV Ehlers-Danlos syndrome have been reported in the literature; this comprises 4% of the total number of known cases.

Vascular Complications

Patients with type IV Ehlers-Danlos syndrome present a formidable surgical challenge because of their varied clinical presentations and the difficulty of vascular repair. Arterial rupture in patients with Ehlers-Danlos syndrome occurs most commonly in the region of the hip joint and shoulder girdle and often follows minor trauma, but it may occur spontaneously. Any artery may be affected, and rupture of the aorta or a visceral vessel carries a particularly high mortality. If the artery is in a confined space, a false aneurysm may form, and spontaneous arteriovenous fistula is also described. Isolated venous complications have not been reported, although several authors refer to severe venous hemorrhage encountered during arterial reconstruction in these patients.

Vascular complications often present as life-threatening emergencies, and there may not be time for diagnostic studies. If the patient's condition permits, vascular imaging is helpful in planning treatment, but the emphasis must be on noninvasive techniques. Arteriography used in type IV patients is associated with a high complication rate. Uncontrollable arterial laceration or dissection can occur at puncture sites or at remote sites. Of patients undergoing arteriography, 67% have had procedure-related complications, and 17% have died. There are numerous reports in the literature of bleeding, limb loss, and death resulting from arterial puncture.[2] Intravenous digital subtraction angiography is believed to be safer, although perforation of the superior vena cava has been reported. Therefore, conventional arteriographic techniques should be avoided in these patients, and noninvasive imaging with computed tomography (CT) scan, duplex scan, or intravenous digital subtraction angiography (IVDSA) should be used to localize and characterize bleeding sites.[3] If arteriography is unavoidable, small-diameter catheters and atraumatic technique are mandatory.

All authors who have operated upon Ehlers-Danlos type IV patients describe the extreme friability of the vessels encountered. Sutures pull through, ligatures cut through, and conventional arterial clamps tear. Major arterial branches may be sheared from their origins with minimal manipulation. Overall resultant surgical mortality is high. As such, management of spontaneous bleeding episodes should be nonoperative, consisting of compression, bed rest, careful monitoring, and transfusion. Hematomas should be allowed to resolve, and varicose veins should be treated with compression hosiery. Arteries that rupture in confined spaces can sometimes be treated conservatively, and this option is preferable when feasible.[4]

In other circumstances, operation is essential. In such cases, extreme delicacy is required, the use of vascular clamps should be avoided if possible, and simple measures to control bleeding are preferable to complex reconstructions. Standard arterial repair with suture or bypass grafts is difficult if not impossible. Gentle dissection, proximal vessel control with external tourniquets or internal balloon catheters, and carefully applied heavy sutures or umbilical tapes buttressed with a second layer of fine vascular sutures are emphasized. There should be no tension on suture lines.[3]

The prognosis in type IV Ehlers-Danlos patients is poor, with 44% dying before surgical intervention and another 19% dying during the perioperative period for an overall mortality rate of 63%. All reported aortic hemorrhages have been fatal. The occasional intra-abdominal bleeding episodes from sources other than the aorta have been controlled in 50% of patients.[1]

All patients with known Ehlers-Danlos syndrome must be readily identifiable so that appropriate precautions can be taken, should the patient present with a potential arterial catastrophe. This approach will decrease improper application of hazardous diagnostic studies. All patients with this condition should be advised to make their diagnosis known to every physician they consult and to wear a warning bracelet.[4]

MARFAN SYNDROME

Marfan syndrome is a well-recognized, heritable autosomal dominant disorder of connective tissue that is serious largely because of cardiovascular complications. The incidence of Marfan syndrome is estimated at 1 in 10,000. At least 25% occur in the absence of a family history, and there has been no tendency to inordinately affect members of any race or either gender. The syndrome shows full penetrance, but there is considerable clinical variability both between and within affected families.

Until recently, the precise nature of the biochemical defect of Marfan syndrome was unknown. The clinical features of the disease suggested an abnormality in collagen, or perhaps elastin, yet detailed analyses of the structural collagen genes and less intensive evaluation of the elastin genes in patients with the disorder failed to yield any clues. The microfibrillar system, which often is associated with elastin, is widely distributed in the extracellular space. Microfibrils are prominent in the ocular ciliary zonule containing the suspensory ligament of the lens; they have also been detected in the aortic media and in the periosteum of bone.

Hollister and colleagues investigated fibrillin levels in patients with Marfan syndrome, initially detecting diminished levels of fibrillin in skin biopsies and cultured fibroblasts using an immunoassay technique.[5] Subsequent genetic linkage studies have identified a causal relationship between missense mutations in the gene on chromosome 15 encoding fibrillin (FBN1), a glycoprotein component of extracellular microfibrils, and the Marfan phenotype.[6] It is probable that a variety of mutations of this gene will be detected among patients with Marfan syndrome. Perhaps a class of fibrillins exists with several subtypes, similar to that of collagen, and the abnormal type determines the phenotypic expression, much the same way as the different collagen abnormalities determine the types of Ehlers-Danlos syndromes. Pereira and associates have recently documented that not all family members who satisfy the classic diagnostic criteria for Marfan syndrome are at equal risk for life-threatening cardiovascular manifestations.[7] As such, patients with major clinical manifestations of Marfan syndrome may be more accurately assessed for their presymptomatic cardiovascular risk by using familial gene linkage analysis.[7]

Clinical Manifestations

In its classic form, the syndrome is easily recognized and consists of abnormalities of the eye (subluxation of the lens), of the skeleton (arachnodactyly, extreme limb length, pectus excavatum or carinatum, joint laxity), and of the cardiovascular system (ascending aortic aneurysmal dilation, aortic valvular incompetence, mitral valve prolapse, mitral valvular incompetence). Initially, dilation of the aortic root occurs and may be particularly pronounced in the region of the sinuses of Valsalva. This dilation often involves the aortic valvular area, resulting in aortic insufficiency. The aneurysmal dilation is progressive and eventually results in aortic dissection or rupture (Fig. 1). Mild coarctation of the aortic isthmus may also occur. Generally, it is of little significance, but proximal aortic dissection is common in the presence of coarctation, in part due to hypertension in those patients with significant coarctation.

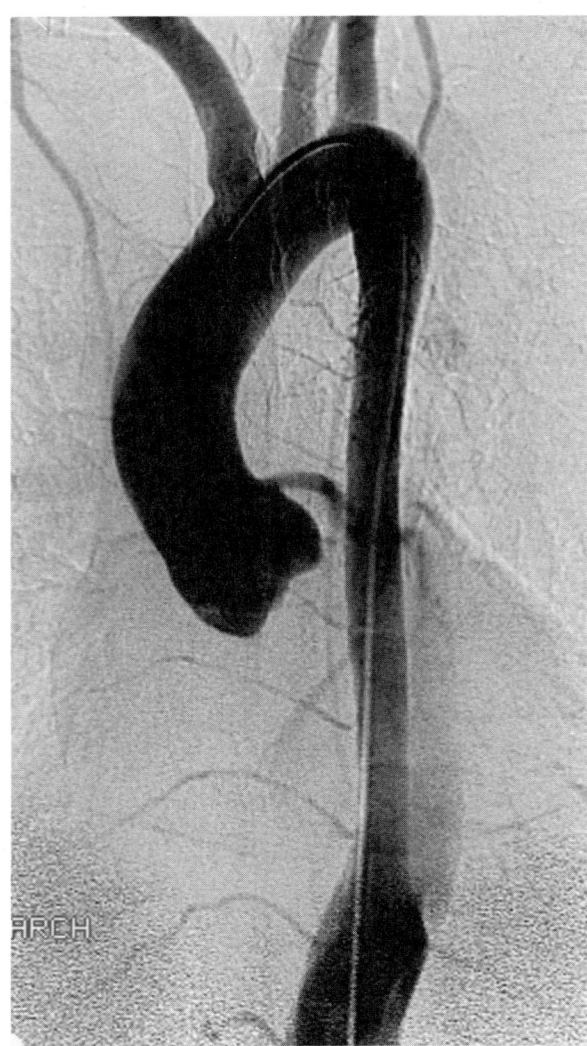

Figure 1 Arch aortogram documenting dilated ascending aorta with dissection involving the descending thoracic aorta to the level of the diaphragm. The false lumen is faintly visible; its entry point is just proximal to the innominate artery orifice.

Histopathologic evaluation of aortic segments of Marfan syndrome patients has revealed degenerative cystic medial necrosis with disruption of collagen fibers and fibrosis of the media. Decreased tensile strength has also been documented in the aortic segments obtained after death from Marfan syndrome patients dying from cardiovascular complications. A recent study measured aortic distensibility and aortic stiffness indices of the ascending aorta and the midabdominal aorta in Marfan syndrome patients and age-matched controls. The values were determined by indirectly measuring changes in echocardiographic diameter and arterial pulse pressure. Compared to normal subjects, the Marfan syndrome patients had decreased aortic distensibility and increased aortic stiffness indices in both aortic segments, irrespective of the aortic diameter.[8]

Vascular Complications

The cardiovascular abnormalities of surgical importance in Marfan syndrome have been well studied. Clinically and in terms of prognosis, dilation of the aortic root is the key manifestation of the syndrome because it predisposes the patient to the risk of aortic dissection with fatal rupture, or severe aortic valvular incompetence and resultant heart failure. Some patients develop mitral valvular prolapse, which is often the cause of significant mitral valvular insufficiency. Aneurysmal dilation and dissection of numerous other vessels including the pulmonary, coronary, carotid, and splenic arteries have also been reported, albeit at a much lower frequency. If untreated, the life expectancy of a patient with Marfan syndrome is about 40 years, with 95% of deaths related to cardiovascular causes.

Because of the predictably progressive nature of aortic dilation, all patients with Marfan syndrome should be followed from childhood with annual echocardiograms to detect the onset and continuation of aortic root dilation; CT scanning can also be utilized to follow the progression of the aortic disease. Hypertension, if present, should be aggressively controlled; this reduces the aortic pressure impulse (dP/dt) of left ventricular ejection and the heart rate. It has been documented that long-term beta-adrenergic blockade therapy (propranolol, atenolol), initiated before the onset of aortic valvular incompetence, retards the onset of valvular failure, slows the rate of aortic aneurysmal dilation, and reduces the overall rate of aortic complications associated with Marfan syndrome.[9]

Elective repair of the aortic valve and ascending aorta should be accomplished prophylactically before severe aortic insufficiency compromises left ventricular function or the ascending aorta exceeds 55 to 60 mm in diameter, at which point the risk of dissection and rupture increases. Composite aortic valve-graft replacement of the ascending aorta and valve has become the procedure of choice for patients with Marfan syndrome. Occasionally, mitral valve replacement is required. With this combination of expectant management, aggressive antihypertensive control, and modern surgical techniques, the life expectancy of these patients can be improved considerably, as emphasized by recent reports with low operative mortality, even in severely symptomatic patients.[10,11]

REFERENCES

1. Cikrit DF, Miles JH, Silver D. Spontaneous arterial perforation: The Ehlers-Danlos specter. J Vasc Surg 1987; 5:248–255.
2. Beighton P, Horan FT. Surgical aspect of the Ehlers-Danlos syndrome. A survey of 100 cases. Br J Surg 1969; 56:255–259.
3. Hunter GC, Malone JM, Moore WS. Vascular manifestations in patients with Ehlers-Danlos syndrome. Arch Surg 1982; 117:495–498.
4. Brearley S, Fowler J, Hamer JD. Two vascular complications of the Ehlers-Danlos syndrome. Eur J Vasc Surg 1993; 7:210–213.
5. Hollister DW, Godfrey MP, Sakali LY, et al. Immunohistologic abnormalities of the microfibrillar-fiber system in the Marfan syndrome. N Engl J Med 1990; 323:152–159.
6. Dietz HC, Cutting GR, Pyeritz RE, et al. Marfan syndrome caused by a recurrent de novo missence mutation in the fibrillin gene. Nature 1991; 352:337–339.
7. Pereira L, Levran O, Ramirez F, et al. A molecular approach to the stratification of cardiovascular risk in families with Marfan's syndrome. N Engl J Med 1994; 331:148–153.
8. Hirata K, Triposkiadis F, Sparks E, et al. The Marfan syndrome: Abnormal aortic elastic properties. J Am Coll Cardiol 1991; 18:57–63.
9. Shores J, Berger KR, Murphy EA, et al. Progression of aortic dilatation and the benefit of long-term β adrenergic blockade in Marfan's syndrome. N Engl J Med 1994; 330:1335–1341.
10. Gott VL, Pyeritz RE, Cameron DE, et al. Composite graft repair of Marfan aneurysm of the ascending aorta: Results in 100 patients. Ann Thorac Surg 1991; 52:38–45.
11. Taniguchi K, Nakano S, Matsuda H, et al. Long-term survival and complications after composite graft replacement for ascending aortic aneurysm associated with aortic regurgitation. Circulation 1991; 84(suppl 3):31–39.

MEDICAL MANAGEMENT OF ACUTE AORTIC DISSECTION

MARVIN M. KIRSH, M.D.
CONSTANCE NEWMAN, R.N.

Aortic dissection is a common aortic pathologic lesion. It occurs in approximately 5 to 10 patients per million of population per year. The incidence is higher in male patients 50 to 70 years of age and is rare in patients under 40 years except in those with familial predisposition, such as Marfan syndrome, other connective tissue disorders, congenital heart lesions such as bicuspid aortic valve or coarctation of the aorta, and in young pregnant women. Acute aortic dissection if untreated is almost invariably lethal, with 21% of individuals dying within 24 hours, 60% within 2 weeks, and 90% in 3 months.[1]

PATHOGENESIS

The process of aortic dissection begins at a site of an intimal tear, after which the dissection propagates. Over 95% of the tears occur either in the ascending aorta just distal to the aortic valve (type A) or in the distal descending thoracic aorta immediately beyond the left subclavian artery (type B). The principle cause of death is not the intimal tear but is related to the propagation of the dissection.[2]

Two main interrelated hemodynamic forces are responsible for both the initial intimal tear and subsequent propagation. First are forces originating from the heart responsible for pulsatile flow (dp/dt). This impulse force is a function of the acceleration of the cardiac output, which in turn is a function of the rate of ventricular fiber shortening. The second are forces related to the mean systemic blood pressure that act for the most part in diastole.[3]

MEDICAL MANAGEMENT

The goal of pharmacologic treatment is to lessen the forces that initiated the dissection, preventing propagation. This is accomplished with pharmacologic agents that affect the rate of ventricular fiber shortening, hence reduce the impulse. These negative inotropic agents when used with potent antihypertensive agents reduce the major forces tending to increase the dissection.[3]

As soon as the diagnosis of acute aortic dissection is suspected, intravenous drug therapy should be started. It should continue while diagnostic procedures are being performed even in patients who are to undergo immediate surgical repair.

It is generally agreed that optimal management in patients with acute type A dissection is immediate surgical intervention, because fatal rupture or cardiac tamponade can occur at any time. In addition, the results with surgical therapy are superior to those with medical therapy.[3]

The method of management, surgical versus medical, for acute type B dissection is controversial. However, intense pharmacologic therapy is considered by most centers to be the treatment of choice for patients with acute type B dissection.[4] The rationale behind medical management in patients with type B dissection is based on these observations: (1) Drugs that affect the rate of ventricular fiber shortening reduce the impulse (dp/dt) and in conjunction with control of the blood pressure reduce the major forces tending to increase the dissection and its disastrous sequelae; (2) Medical therapy prevents early death in the majority of patients; (3) The operative mortality has been relatively high, since these patients tend to be elderly and have associated complicating illnesses such as generalized arteriosclerosis, pulmonary, and renal disease; (4) The long-term outcome has been similar in surgically and medically treated patients.

Acute Medical Management

Intensive continuous monitoring of the patient is mandatory, and it includes the following: arterial cannula for arterial blood pressure measurements, pulmonary arterial and wedge pressure measurements with a Swan-Ganz catheter, a Foley urinary catheter, and a pulse oximeter to monitor the patient's oxygenation. Baseline chest roentgenograms and electrocardiograms should be obtained.

For initial treatment a prompt onset of action necessitates intravenous administration of fast-acting agents. It is important to reduce the cardiac output and blood pressure to the lowest possible level consistent with maintaining adequate cerebral, coronary, and renal perfusion. In hypertensive patients nitroprusside sodium is effective and should be infused initially at 1 to 2 µg/kg/min, with dosage varying to maintain the systolic blood pressure between 100 and 120 mg Hg. At times the blood pressure should be reduced to 80 or 90 mm Hg if necessary to control the patient's pain. Since nitroprusside sodium alone can cause an increase in dp/dt it is essential that adequate simultaneous adrenergic beta blockade be used as well. If nitroprusside is ineffective or poorly tolerated, the ganglionic blocking agent trimethaphan camsylate (Arfonad) can be used. The initial infusion rate is 1 mg/min with the dosage titrated to achieve the desired systolic blood pressure of 100 to 120 mm Hg.

To reduce dp/dt acutely, propanolol or a comparable intravenous beta-blocker such as esmolol should be administered until there is evidence of a satisfactory beta-adrenergic blockade indicated by a pulse rate less than 70 beats/min. Propranolol should be given in incremental dosages of 1 to 5 mg every 5 minutes until the desired pulse rate is achieved. Additional dosages of 5 mg of propranolol should be given intravenously every 4 to 6 hours to maintain adequate beta-adrenergic blockade. Esmolol administered as a bolus (100 µg/kg/min) followed by a continuous infusion of 25 to 50 µg/kg/min is effective in controlling the heart rate. It has the added advantages of not requiring frequent bolus injections and having a short half-life, which is advantageous if over–beta blockade occurs. Many other intravenous beta-blockers can be used (Table 1).

An alternative agent to reduce both blood pressure and dp/dt is reserpine 1 to 2 mg intramuscularly every 4 to 6 hours. When reserpine is used, concomitant cimetidine 300 mg orally or intravenously is required to reduce the likelihood of gastric ulceration.

Calcium channel antagonists such as diltiazem and nifedipine can be used if the other measures fail, since these agents lower the blood pressure and decrease dp/dt as well. The recommended intravenous dosages are 0.1 mg/kg/hr of diltiazem and 10 µg/kg/hr of nifedipine.

In patients who are normotensive on admission to the hospital, intravenous beta-adrenegic blockade is all that is necessary acutely (Table 2).

One of the frequent associated problems of elderly patients with type B dissection is chronic obstructive pulmonary disease. The administration of beta-adrenergic blockers; nitroprusside, which causes intrapulmonary shunting; sedation; and bed rest frequently lead to respiratory complications. Therefore, these patients should receive bronchodilators and incentive spirometry to prevent atectelasis and pneumonia. At times it may be necessary to add intravenous theophylline or another bronchodilator to the regimen.

Daily chest roentgenograms should be obtained to

Table 1 Intravenous Therapy for Acute Aortic Dissection

Drug	Dosage
Nitroprusside sodium	1 to 2 mcg/kg/min
Trimethaphan camsylate	1 mg/min
Reserpine	1–2 mg-1. mg 4-6h
Methyldopa (Aldomet)	250–500 mg q6h
Esmolol	150 mcg/kg bolus
	100 µg/kg/min continuous
Labetalol	5 to 20 mg bolus over 2 min
	2 to 5 mg/min continuous
Metoprolol	5 mg q 2 min × 3

Table 2 Oral Therapy for Acute Aortic Dissection

Drug	Dosage
Atenolol	50–100 mg q.d.
Metoprolol	50 mg b.i.d.
Labetalol	100 mg b.i.d.
Propranolol	10–40 mg q.i.d.
Nifedipine	10 mg t.i.d.
Diltiazem	30–60 mg t.i.d.
Verapamil	80 mg t.i.d.
Lisinopril	20–40 mg q.d.
Captopril	12.5–25 mg t.i.d.
Clonidine	0.1–0.2 mg b.i.d.
Methyldopa (Aldomet)	250–500 mg q.i.d.

detect changes in mediastinal or aortic contour as well as any pleural fluid.

Long-Term Medical Management

Long-term pharmacologic therapy is indicated for all patients with type A dissection who survive surgical repair and for those with type B dissection who stabilize after initial therapy.

When patients with type B dissections are pain free and the blood pressure and pulse rate have been controlled, the intravenous medications can be gradually withdrawn and oral antihypertensive and negative inotropic medications added to the regimen. The preferred negative inotropic agents are the beta-adrenergic blockers (atenolol, metoprolol, labetalol, propranolol). Calcium channel blockers (verapamil, nifedipine, diltiazem) can be used if the beta-blockers are poorly tolerated. Calcium channel blockers should be used with one or more of the potent antihypertensive medications such as clonidine, methyldopa (Aldomet), lisinopril, and captopril. If lisinopril or captopril is used, renal function must be carefully monitored. Hydralazine should be avoided, since it is incorporated into the mucopolysaccharide in the aortic media and may weaken the aortic wall.

Once the patient is ambulatory, the degree of blood pressure and pulse rate control can be evaluated. In elderly patients, especially those with pre-existing cerebrovascular or renal disease, a blood pressure higher than 120 mm Hg may have to be accepted to avoid the sequalae of drug-induced hypotension.

Meticulous follow-up is mandatory. During the first few weeks these patients require frequent office evaluation. Attention should be focused on blood pressure and pulse rate control and cardiac, cerebral, and renal function to be certain that the hypotensive drug therapy is well tolerated. Serial chest roentgenograms and ultrasound studies should be obtained every 3 to 6 months. It must be emphasized to the patients that they must comply with their regime. If they do not, surgical resection should be contemplated.

NONFATAL COMPLICATIONS OF MEDICAL THERAPY

Changes in mental status manifested by somnolence or agitation are the most common early complications of medical therapy. These result from too-rapid lowering of blood pressure, especially in elderly patients with pre-existing hypertension, and from the use of potent sympatholytic agents. These complications have no influence on survival. Other complications include orthostatic hypotension, hypotensive induced azotemia, and peptic ulceration when reserpine is used without antacids or H_2 blocking agents.

RESULTS

Although long-term medical therapy for acute type B dissections has been available since 1965, there are no randomized prospective studies comparing medical with surgical therapy. In addition, few studies address the long-term survival of patients with acute type B dissections treated with medical therapy. Wheat[4] in 1983 culled from the literature 66 patients from six medical centers treated with intensive drug therapy with an 83% (n = 55) survival rate (Table 3). At these same institutions 44 patients were treated with immediate operation with only 55% (n = 24) surviving. Of the medically treated patients 22 were followed for at least 3 years and showed a survival rate of 91%.

Doroghazi and associates[5] reported on 35 patients treated with medical therapy from 1963 to 1978 at the Massachusetts General Hospital with 80% (n = 28) surviving initially. This was considerably superior to the surgical mortality, almost 50%. Of those discharged alive, 27 were followed for a mean period of 48.4 months. Of these patients 64% were alive at the time of follow-up. There were no deaths related to drug therapy or failure of drug therapy. Most of the deaths resulted from complications of the dissection present at the time of initiation of drug therapy.

This study as well as that of Wheat documented that the good initial results obtained by the use of intensive drug therapy are maintained over the long term follow-up period. Interestingly, Doroghazi and his colleagues noted that the life expectancy of any patient with

Table 3 Results of Medical Therapy for Acute Type B Dissection 30-day Mortality

	Year Reported	Number	Survival
Daily	1970	5	4
Attar	1971	8	4
Dalen	1974	6	6
Strong	1974	19	15
Balooki	1979	14	13
Doroghazi	1983	35	28
Wheat	1983	14	13
Glower	1990	56	46
Total		157	129 (83%)

an aortic dissection was inferior to that of age-matched control population. Therefore, over the long term patients with type B dissections were just as likely to die of an unrelated cause as of a sequela of the dissection. This is true because of their advanced age and the many medical problems prevalent in patients with type B dissections.

Further support for these conclusions has been reported by Glower and co-workers,[6] who evaluated a relatively large retrospective cooperative study from Duke and Stanford comparing the medical and surgical therapy in patients with acute type B dissections. Of the 89 patients with acute dissections, 56 were treated medically. The medically treated patients tended to have more associated illnesses than the surgical cohort. For the 56 patients managed with intense pharmacologic therapy, the 30-day hospital mortality rate was 18%, much lower than the 33% surgical mortality. By multivariate analysis the independent predictors of mortality were complications of the dissection at presentation, pleural rupture, age, and cardiac disease. There were 12 early deaths in the medically treated group. The causes of death were unrelated to the dissection in 8 patients, with only 4 patients dying of rupture. An additional 3 patients required graft replacement for aortic expansion or rupture 9 days and 2 and 16 months later. For patients presenting without compelling indications for emergency operation (n = 49) the 30-day mortality was only 10% for the medically treated patients but 19% for the surgically treated. Among patients without cardiac or renal disease, the 30-day medical and surgical mortality was 16% and 9%, respectively. (p = N.S.) In contrast to these results are those in patients with coexisting medical problems. The 30-day mortality in the medically treated group was only 7%, and it was 40% in the surgically treated patients.

Long-term survival rates for patients with acute type B dissections, whether treated medically or surgically, are similar. The probability of survival for those with uncomplicated type B aortic dissections managed medically at 1, 5, and 10 years was 94%, 87%, and 32%, and the survival probability for the surgically treated patients was 90%, 80%, and 50%, respectively.

These studies support the use of intensive pharmacologic therapy as the definitive treatment of uncomplicated acute type B dissection, especially in patients with cardiac and other medical illnesses. Surgical therapy should be reserved for patients with complications of the dissection.

These patients should be closely monitored, with careful regulation of their medication and periodic surveillance of the thoracic aorta with computed tomographic or magnetic resonance imaging or transesophageal echocardiography. This is necessary because of the increased evidence of cardiovascular disease and residual aortic pathology in these patients.[6]

REFERENCES

1. Fuster V and Ip J. Medical aspects of acute aortic dissection. Semin Thorac Cardiovasc Surg 1991; 3:219–224.
2. Roberts C, Roberts W. Aortic dissection with the entrance tear in the descending thoracic aorta. Ann Surg 1991; 213:356–368.
3. Crawford ES. The diagnosis and management of aortic dissection. JAMA 1990; 264:2537–2541.
4. Wheat M. Evolution of intensive drug therapy in aortic dissection. In: Doroghaza R, Slater, E, eds. Aortic Dissection. McGraw-Hill, 1983:165.
5. Doroghazi R, Slater E, De Sanctis R, et al. Long term survival of patients with treated aortic dissections. J. Am Coll Cardiol 1983; 3:1026–1034.
6. Glower D, Fann J, Speier R, et al. Comparison of medical and surgical therapy for uncomplicated descending aortic dissection. Circulation 1990; 82 (suppl 4):39–46.

SURGICAL TREATMENT OF ACUTE AND CHRONIC THORACIC AORTIC DISSECTIONS

JOSEPH S. COSELLI, M.D.

That aortic dissection is a serious disorder requiring emergent medical and surgical management is beyond dispute. It is the most common catastrophic process affecting the thoracic aorta. Early reports documented high mortality, particularly when the disorder is associated with untreated proximal aortic dissection.[1,2] Some 35% of such patients expired within the first 24 hours and 50% in 48 hours. The condition carried a mortality of 70% in 1 week, and only 20% survived 2 weeks. Of those surviving 2 weeks, half died within 3 months and an additional 10% within a year. Distal aortic dissection, with a somewhat less dismal prognosis, nevertheless has only a 60% survival rate at 1 month. The fortunate patients who progress to chronic aortic dissection have a yearly mortality rate of approximately 20%.

PATHOLOGY

Aortic dissection is the result of an intimal tear producing a longitudinal cleavage propagating through the aortic media, most commonly between the inner third and the outer half, producing a false channel. Most intimal tears are single and transverse. Secondary or re-entry tears, usually distal, are frequently multiple. The false channel occupies half to two-thirds of the circumference of the aorta and compresses or narrows the true lumen. On occasion the entire circumference is involved. Propagation of the false channel is primarily distal, with a variable amount of proximal progression. Dissection originating beyond the left subclavian artery generally extends proximally only 1 to 3 cm but may occasionaly reach the aortic valve.

Besides aortic rupture into the pericardium resulting in cardiac tamponade, death from proximal aortic dissection is related to complications at the aortic root. Proximal involvement of the ascending aorta produces aortic valvular insufficiency as a result of a dehiscence of one or more commissures of the aortic valve. Progression of the dissection may compromise coronary artery blood flow and any branch vessel, producing cerebral, renal, visceral, spinal cord, or lower extremity ischemia. Distal rupture is less common, and although it may occur at any site, it is most frequent at the proximal descending thoracic aorta into the left chest.

CLASSIFICATION

Patients with aortic dissections within 14 days of initial occurrence are considered to have acute aortic dissections, and those beyond 2 weeks are arbitrarily classified as chronic.

The extent of aortic involvement is critical in determining prognosis and establishing the course of management. In the DeBakey classification, patients with type 1 dissection have involvement of the ascending, arch, and thoracoabdominal aortas and those with type 2 have the false channel limited to the ascending aorta (Fig. 1). Patients with type 3 dissection are divided into 3a (those that terminate above the diaphragm) and 3b (those that extend into the abdominal aorta). The Stanford classification considers all patients with ascending aortic involvement as type A and all patients without ascending aortic involvement as type B. Both classifications appropriately disregard the site of intimal tear and focus on the amount of aortic involvement, which is more closely related ultimately to prognosis.

DIAGNOSIS

Severe chest pain, the most common presenting symptom, occurs in 90% of patients and is frequently

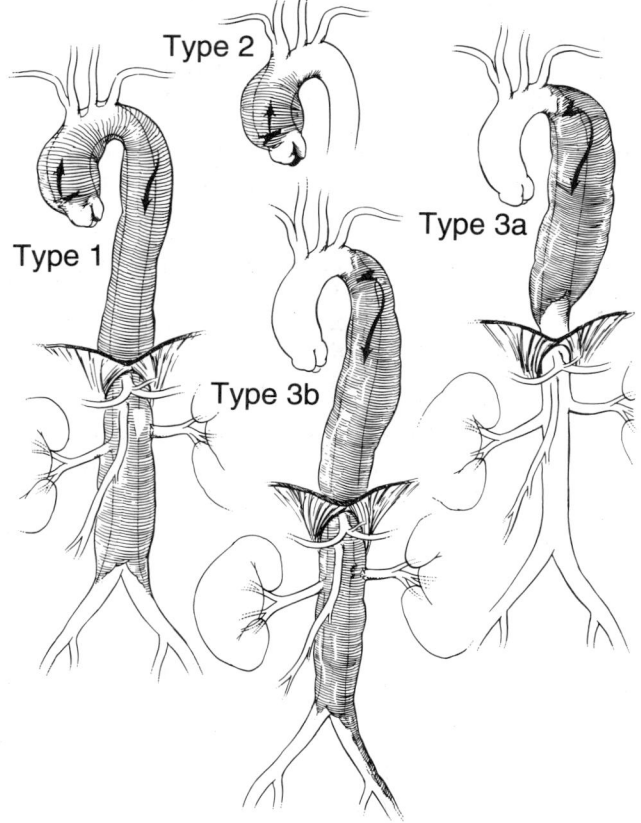

Figure 1 The DeBakey classification of aortic dissection.

difficult to differentiate from acute myocardial infarction. A plain roentgenogram of the chest may document a dilated aorta, widened mediastinum with cardiomegaly, pulmonary edema, or pleural effusion. A normal chest x-ray film is extremely unusual. Electrocardiographic (ECG) abnormalities are variable but generally are not diagnostic of acute myocardial infarction. Patients with chest pain, an abnormal chest x-ray film with or without aortic valvular insufficiency, a normal electroencephalogram (EEG), and evidence of branch vessel occlusion have a high index of suspicion for acute aortic dissection and must be rapidly evaluated.

The combination of transthoracic (TTE) and transesophageal (TEE) echocardiography constitutes an exquisitely sensitive method for diagnosing aortic dissection.[3,4] Major limitations include the inability to image the entire thoracic aorta, lack of coronary artery visualization, and operator dependency. Combined echocardiography (TTE and TEE) is noninvasive, requires no contrast media administration, frequently identifies the site of intimal tear, evaluates global and regional systolic myocardial function, quantifies valvular insufficiency, and can identify a pericardial effusion. In many instances echocardiography can provide all the information needed to make a diagnosis and carry out operative management.

Aortography has long been considered the study of choice for the evaluation of patients with suspected aortic dissection. Although it has the disadvantage of requiring the administration of intravenous nephrotoxic contrast media, it allows evaluation of the entire aorta and its branches. False-negative aortography, however, is not uncommon in the presence of a thrombosed false lumen.

Computed tomography (CT) scanning is widely available, relatively fast, sensitive, and operator independent. Although the entire aorta may be imaged, the site of intimal tear may not be readily identified. Magnetic resonance imaging (MRI), similar to aortography and CT scanning in that it evaluates the entire aorta, is more expensive, time-consuming, and less widely available. Gated MRI scanning, unlike CT, can be used to semi-quantify aortic regurgitation and evaluate left ventricular function. In patients with acute dissections who are hemodynamically unstable, intubated and monitored, MRI scanning is relatively inaccessible. In patients with proximal aortic dissections requiring aortic valvular repair, TEE is used intraoperatively to assess valvular competency and for distal repairs to monitor cardiac function.

TREATMENT

Surgical Management

In all patients with acute proximal aortic dissection (Stanford type A, DeBakey type 1 and type 2) operative repair is undertaken as an emergency. Operative intervention is carried out through a median sternotomy (Fig. 2A). Cardiopulmonary bypass (CPB) is established with femoral arterial cannulation for pump return. In the absence of occlusive disease, either femoral artery is satisfactory. Only rarely does aortic dissection extend to the distal common femoral artery, compromising perfusion into the true lumen from either side. Bicaval cannulation for cardiac isolation and myocardial protection is preferred, although single atrial cannulation is quite satisfactory.

Systemic cooling for profound hypothermic circulatory arrest is used in all patients. EEG monitoring is used and cardiac arrest is induced only after the development of electrocerebral silence. When EEG is unavailable, cooling should be carried out for at least 20 minutes and until a core temperature of 18° to 20°C (64.4° to 68°F) is reached.

Circulatory arrest obviates the need for placement of an aortic clamp while the distal aortic anastomosis is carried out (Fig. 2B,C). This allows for an open distal anastomosis providing visual examination of the internal aspects of the transverse aortic arch. During circulatory arrest intimal tears along the greater curvature of the transverse aortic arch may be repaired and those along the lesser curvature resected. The placement of a distal aortic clamp limits aortic resection and may fracture the delicate tissue that separates the true from the false lumen, producing a new re-entry point beyond the distal anastomosis.

The distal anastomosis is fashioned using running 4-0 or 5-0 polypropylene suture. The suture line is used to obliterate the false lumen and direct all flow into the true lumen. A collagen-impregnated woven double velour Dacron graft is used. Alternatively, a woven Dacron tube graft may have its interstices sealed by saturating the material with 25% albumen and autoclaving it for 3 minutes at 121°C (250°F). Generally 26 to 30 mm diameter grafts are necessary. In very rare instances, when the aortic wall is particularly friable, the aortic tissue may be buttressed with Teflon felt strips using 5-0 or 6-0 polypropylene suture.

After completion of the distal aortic anastomosis, the aorta and graft are filled via the femoral arterial cannula to remove all air. If upon restoration of pump perfusion there is any concern that the inflow is not entirely isolated to the true lumen, transference of the arterial cannula to the distal portion of the aortic graft for antegrade flow is carried out. Regardless, CPB is resumed along with rewarming, with a clamp placed on the distal portion of the aortic graft.

Proximally the aorta is transected immediately distal to the coronary artery origins. Cardioplegic solution may be administered directly into the coronary artery origins for myocardial protection or alternatively by retrograde coronary sinus approach. The redundant aortic wall is usually excised, saving the posterior portion and protecting the anterior portion of the right pulmonary artery. At this point the aortic valve and root are carefully evaluated. When the aortic valve is involved by proximal progression of the dissection, the result is separation of one or more commissures from the aortic

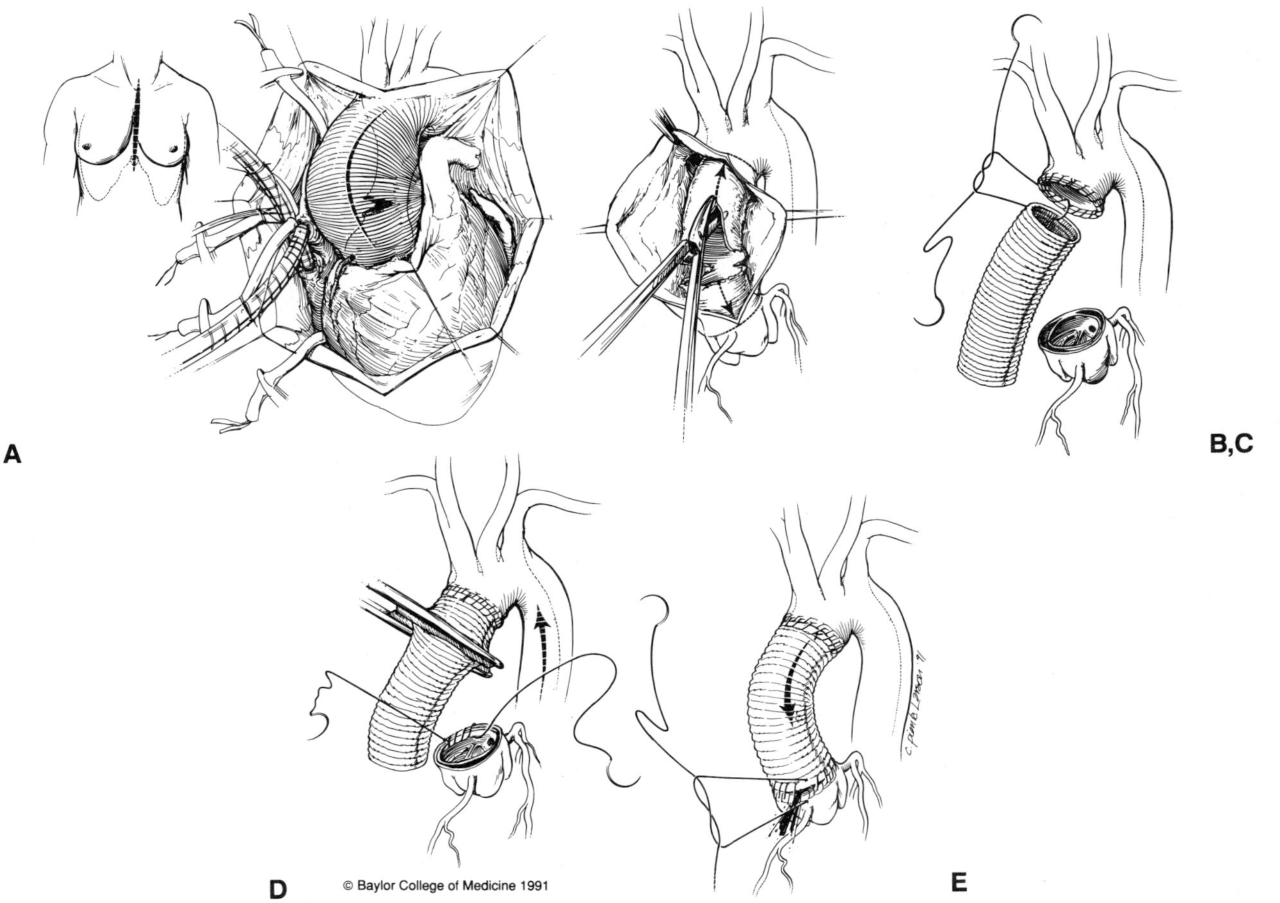

Figure 2 Technique for surgical repair of acute DeBakey type 1 aortic dissection.

wall. The commissure between the noncoronary and right coronary cusp is most frequently involved. Prolapse of this commissure and the aortic valve leaflets during diastole produces a central aortic valvular insufficiency. If the aortic root anatomy was normal before dissection, a competent aortic valve may be restored in most patients, even if all three commissures are involved.[5]

Aortic valve resuspension is carried out to restore the anatomic position of the commissure using transmurally placed Teflon pledgeted reinforced mattress sutures at the apex of each. In patients with Marfan syndrome and non-Marfan annuloaortic ectasia composite valve graft replacement of the aortic root is performed. Patients with calcific aortic valvular stenosis and a normal caliber aortic sinus segment are treated by separate aortic valvular replacement. Proximal graft anastomosis is carried out with a running 4-0 or 5-0 polypropylene suture, again obliterating the false lumen in the proximal suture line (Fig. 2D,E). As much aortic tissue in the noncoronary sinus is removed as is feasible. Only rarely, with markedly friable aortic tissues, has it been necessary to sandwich the proximal aortic wall between Teflon felt strips before anastomosis. Since the originating intimal tear in most patients with proximal aortic dissection arises within 1 to 2 cm of the aortic valve, this technique eliminates the site of tear, which is considered the point of greatest weakness and most susceptible to rupture.

Distal aortic involvement by the dissection is present in most patients. Despite the re-establishment of blood flow into the true lumen, up to 75% of patients maintain some patency of the distal false lumen. Consequently, patients with proximal dissection (DeBakey type 1 and Stanford A) are in effect converted to acute distal aortic dissection (DeBakey 3, Stanford B), requiring ongoing intensive medical management of blood pressure with intravenous antihypertensive medication in the immediate postoperative period. They are converted to oral alternatives as soon as feasible.

All patients with distal aortic dissection (DeBakey type 3, Stanford B) are treated initially with intensive medical management.[6] If uncomplicated, such patients are carried into the chronic phase and periodically evaluated. Indications for operative intervention include failure to control hypertension, particularly with continued pain, expansion of the aneurysm, signs or symptoms of rupture, waxing and waning neurologic deficits, or evidence of compromise of major arterial branches to the arm, viscera, kidneys, or lower extremities.[7] A left pleural effusion develops in 12 to 72 hours and is ubiquitous, frequently blood tinged, and not to be confused with rupture.

Operative treatment when required is carried out via left posterolateral thoracotomy either through the fifth intercostal space or with resection of the sixth rib. The objective of surgical treatment is to remove the site of intimal tear and aneurysmal dilatation and to reroute blood flow to the true lumen. Cardiofemoral bypass from the left atrium to the left common femoral artery with a biomedicus pump protects the visceral and renal circulation during aortic cross clamping. Bypass of this type provides preload reduction, simplifies anesthetic management, and may reduce the risk of spinal cord ischemia in some patients.

It is frequently necessary to cross-clamp the aorta between the left common carotid and left subclavian arteries for access to enough aorta proximal to the aortic tear. The phrenic and recurrent laryngeal nerves should be protected. After isolation of the proximal aorta between clamps the aneurysm is opened generally into the false lumen, and the wall between the true and the false lumen is excised (Fig. 3A,B). The aortic wall is generally thin, and consequently, to avoid the esophagus, it may be necessary to transect the aorta completely before constructing the posterior portion of the anastomosis. A woven Dacron graft is inserted, fashioning both proximal and distal anastomoses with continuous 4-0 or 3-0 polypropylene suture. The proximal anastomosis is performed proximal to the aortic tear, and the distal anatomosis is used to obliterate the false lumen (Fig. 3C,D). All dilated aorta is removed at the initial operation. Thoracoabdominal aortic replacement may be necessary, particularly if acute dissection is superimposed upon a chronic medial degenerative aneurysm. Consequently, reattachment of multiple intercostal arteries as well as the visceral and renal arteries may be required, depending upon distal extent of aneurysmal involvement (Fig. 4).

Patients with chronic aortic dissection are followed closely and for the rest of their lives for the development of complications. The most frequent complication is aneurysm of the false lumen. Other manifestations include compression of the recurrent laryngeal nerve, producing hoarseness; compression of the trachea or bronchus with stridor, dyspnea, or pneumonia; and compression of the superior vena cava resulting in superior vena caval syndrome. In patients with chronic type 1 and type 2 dissections, significant aortic valvular insufficiency has been encountered in 52% of patients.[8]

The surgical principles are similar for acute and chronic dissection. However, due to the rigidity of the aortic wall and the dependency of major arterial branches on perfusion from the false lumen, the distal anastomosis is constructed so as to allow for flow into both the true and the false lumen distally. In good-risk patients, resection and replacement for all segments with an overall combined diameter of 6 cm is recommended. Of the patients with thoracic aortic aneurysms secondary to dissection with rupture, 88% have been less than 10

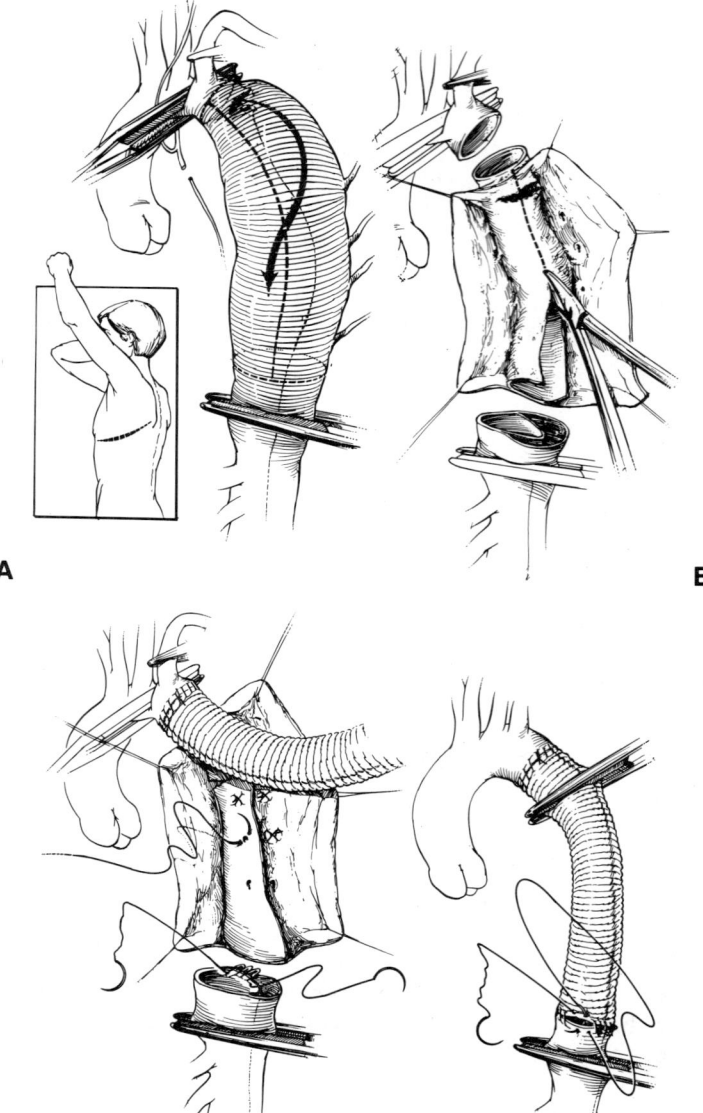

Figure 3 Technique for surgical treatment of acute DeBakey type 3 aortic dissection.

cm and 23% have been less than 6 cm in diameter.[9,10] An aggressive approach to extensive aortic replacement is recommended for the initial operation, resecting all dilated segments of the dissected aorta and substantially reducing the likelihood of reoperation.[11]

RESULTS

Aggressive surgical intervention for acute dissection with modern operative technique has substantially improved early and late survival. Current 30-day survival

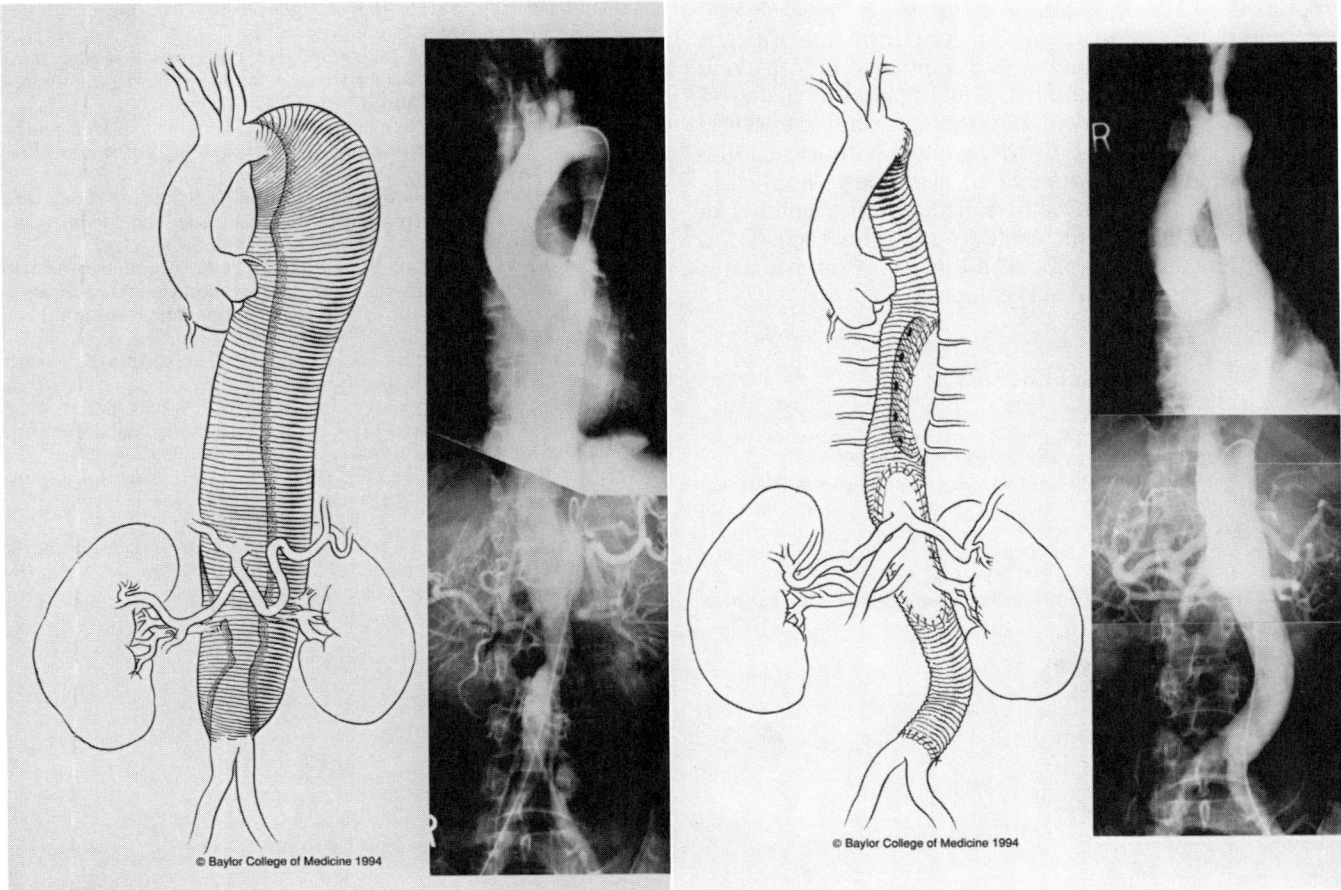

Figure 4 Aortogram and drawing of patient with chronic dissection of the thoracoabdominal aorta. *A,* Preoperative. *B,* Postoperative.

rates for patients undergoing operation on the ascending and/or transverse aortic arch for acute and chronic dissection approaches 95% and 92%, respectively.[8] Factors predictive of a 30-day mortality include increasing age, severe aneurysm symptoms, diabetes, previous proximal aortic operation, need for cardiac support, postoperative tracheostomy, postoperative heart dysfunction, and stroke. Survival probability for patients undergoing an initial operation for type 1 dissection has been reported to be 81%, 73%, 66%, and 57%, respectively at 1, 3, 5, and 7 years.[10]

When the entire transverse aortic arch was included in the initial resection, the 30-day survival was 84% as compared with 97% when only the ascending aorta is involved.[11] Consequently, repair of the entire aortic arch is not systematically included unless the intimal tear arises in the transverse arch, dissection extending from the ascending or descending thoracic aorta has resulted in rupture of the arch segment, the false channel in the aortic arch segment is severely dilated, or dissection is superimposed on a coexisting fusiform aneurysm of the transverse arch.

Except in patients with Marfan syndrome or significant annuloaortic ectasia, aortic valve reconstruction by resuspension of the valve commissures was undertaken whenever possible. The long-term durability of this approach has been well substantiated by the Stanford group.[5]

Current 30-day survival rates for patients undergoing surgical resection and replacement of the descending thoracic aorta for acute and chronic dissection are 94% and 96%, respectively.[8,9] Predictors of early mortality include symptoms directly related to the aneurysm, acuity, postoperative cardiac problems, and reoperation for bleeding. The survival rate for surgical treatment of acute and chronic dissection involving the thoracoabdominal aorta approaches 95%. Comparable results for medical or early surgical treatment of patients with distal aortic dissection is to be anticipated and will support a complication-specific approach to the treatment of such patients. Uncomplicated dissection is treated medically, and complicated dissection is treated surgically. Overall survival at 1, 5, and 10 years is 73%, 58%, and 25%, respectively.

Patients with aortic dissections must never be considered to be completely cured, and consequently must be followed for life. The incidence of late reoperation, which was related to dissection, has been reported by Haverich and associates[12] to be 13% at 5 years and 23% at 10 years. For long-term surveillance, serial CT or MRI scanning at 3 months, 6 months, and then yearly is recommended. Any segment of the aorta dilating to 6 cm, regardless of symptoms, should undergo elective replacement. Aortic segments with lesser dilatation with the development of symptoms should undergo aggressive treatment. Further improvements in early survival rates will result from earlier recognition and treatment; improvement in long-term survival rates will result from careful surveillance.

REFERENCES

1. Hirst AE Jr, Johns VJ Jr, Kime SW Jr. Dissecting aneurysms of the aorta: A review of 505 cases. Medicine 1958; 37:217–219.
2. Lindsay J, Hurst JW. Clinical features and prognosis in dissecting aneurysms of the aorta: A reappraisal. Circulation 1967; 35:880–888.
3. Khandheria BK. Editorial comment: Aortic dissection, the last frontier. Circulation 1993; 87:1765–1768.
4. Erbel R. Role of transesophageal echocardiography in dissection of the aorta and evaluation of degenerative aortic disease. Cardiol Clin 1993; 11:461–473.
5. Fann JI, Glower DD, Miller DC, et al. Preservation of aortic valve in type 1 aortic dissection complicated by aortic regurgitation. J Thorac Cardiovasc Surg 1991; 102:62–75.
6. Glower D, Fann JI, Speier RH, et al. Comparison of medical and surgical therapy for uncomplicated descending aortic dissection. Circulation 1990; 82(5, suppl 4):39–46.
7. Elefteriades JA, Hartleroad J, Gusberg RJ, et al. Long-term experience with descending aortic dissection: The complication-specific approach. Ann Thorac Surg 1992; 53:11–21.
8. Crawford ES, Svensson LG, Coselli JS, et al. Surgical treatment of aneurysm and/or dissection of the ascending aorta, transverse aortic arch, and ascending aorta and transverse aortic arch. J Thorac Cardiovasc Surg 1989; 98:659–674.
9. Svensson LG, Crawford ES, Hess KR, et al. Dissection of the aorta and dissecting aortic aneurysms: Improving early and long-term surgical results. Circulation 1990; 82(5, suppl 4):24–38.
10. Crawford ES, Svensson LG, Coselli JS, et al. Aortic dissection and dissecting aortic aneurysms. Ann Surg 1988; 208:254–273.
11. Crawford ES, Kirklin JW, Naftel DC, et al. Surgery for acute dissection of ascending aorta: Should the arch be included? J Thorac Cardiovasc Surg 1992; 104:46–59.
12. Haverich A, Miller G, Scott WD, et al. Acute and chronic aortic dissections: Determinants of long-term outcome for operative survivors. Circulation 1985; 72 (suppl 2):22–33.

LOWER EXTREMITY ANEURYSM

ARTERIOSCLEROTIC FEMORAL ARTERY ANEURYSM

BRUCE S. CUTLER, M.D.

Aneurysms of the femoral arteries are comparatively rare but important because of their limb-threatening potential due to acute thrombosis or rupture and their frequent association with aneurysms in other locations. The combined results of the four largest studies of femoral aneurysms documents that the likelihood of a second aneurysm involving the aortoiliac segment is 67%, the popliteal artery 37%, and the contralateral femoral artery 52%.[1-4] Conversely, 3.2% of patients with aortic aneurysms will also have a femoral aneurysm. Although femoral aneurysms are histologically similar to atherosclerotic aneurysms in other locations, the reason for their association with other aneurysms is not known. It may be part of a generalized arterial degenerative process, since the frequency of multiple aneurysms increases with age. In addition, there is speculation about a possible enzymatic defect in collagen or elastin synthesis, causing widespread arterial wall weakness and aneurysm formation. The average age at the time of diagnosis of a femoral aneurysm is 67 years. As with other peripheral aneurysms, there is a strong male preponderance, with men affected 45 times as frequently as women.[5]

DIAGNOSIS

In the early publications most patients with femoral aneurysms were symptomatic at the time of diagnosis. More recently most patients are asymptomatic, and their aneurysms are discovered because of their known association with aortic or popliteal aneurysms. The diagnosis is usually easily made on physical examination by detection of a superficial pulsatile swelling of the common femoral artery distal to the inguinal ligament. Duplex imaging, ultrasound, and computed tomographic scanning are not usually required except in the obese patient or to determine the dimensions or extent of the aneurysm. Ultrasound should be employed routinely to look for associated popliteal and aortic aneurysms. Arteriography is not necessary to make the diagnosis of femoral aneurysm but is useful prior to operative treatment to define the extent of the aneurysm and to evaluate the distal runoff when the aneurysm is thrombosed or there has been distal embolization.

Femoral aneurysms may become symptomatic by acute or chronic thrombosis, compression of adjacent structures including the femoral nerve or vein, distal embolization, or rupture. Acute thrombosis usually results in the sudden onset of ischemia, manifest by coolness, hypesthesia, and eventually pain in the extremity, and is observed in about 8% of patients. It may be mistaken for a femoral embolus, but the presence of a firm, sometimes tender, pulseless mass involving the femoral artery should distinguish the two diagnoses. Chronic thrombosis occurs in 8% of patients and often mimics atherosclerotic occlusion of the superficial femoral artery, producing calf claudication or ischemic rest pain. Again, a pulseless mass in the inguinal region together with absent distal pulses should differentiate it from the much more common superficial femoral artery occlusion.

Large aneurysms may produce pain or paresthesias on the medial aspect of the thigh as a result of femoral nerve compression. Impingement on the femoral vein has been reported to produce limb edema. Even small aneurysms may produce a nonspecific dull aching sensation centered over the inguinal area.

Femoral aneurysms may also produce limb ischemia from distal embolization, although the precise incidence is difficult to determine because of their frequent association with popliteal aneurysms, an even more common source of atheroembolization. From a practical point of view any patient with blotchy cyanosis or cutaneous infarction of the toes should be closely examined for an embolic source due to an aneurysm at the aortic, femoral, or popliteal levels.

Rupture is the rarest complication, occurring in less than 5% of patients. It usually produces a painful expanding pulsatile mass and eventually develops a large inguinal and thigh ecchymosis.

CLASSIFICATION

Common femoral aneurysms may be divided into two types, that occur with equal frequency, based on the involvement of the origin of the profunda femoris artery.[2] Type 1 aneurysms are confined to the common femoral artery, and in type 2 aneurysms the profunda femoris originates from the aneurysm. The anatomic difference is important because surgical reconstruction of the second type is technically more challenging. Isolated aneurysms of the profunda femoris or superficial femoral artery account for only 5% of femoral aneurysms. Profunda femoris aneurysms usually extend distally and involve the medial and lateral femoral circumflex branches. Superficial femoral aneurysms may occur anywhere in the artery and are often seen in conjunction with diffuse arterial dilatation (aneurysmosis) and popliteal aneurysms.

NATURAL HISTORY

Most of the data about femoral aneurysms come from surgical studies, which are biased in favor of operative treatment of acute limb-threatening complications, exceeding 70% in some reports.[2,3] For this reason and because of the comparative rarity of femoral aneurysms, the natural history of these lesions is not well known. However, it seems likely that the risk of either acute thrombosis or rupture is substantially less than implied by the surgical reviews. In the only large series of patients with asymptomatic aneurysms followed without operation, 3 of 58 patients developed limb-threatening complications during the follow-up period, which averaged 28 months.[4] Further, the average size of the aneurysms that became symptomatic did not differ from those that remained without symptoms, reflecting the fact that femoral aneurysms are more likely to thrombose than rupture. Since the risk of thrombosis in general is unrelated to aneurysm diameter, no size criteria have been established to estimate the risk of complications developing in an asymptomatic patient. While the natural history of asymptomatic femoral aneurysms may be less ominous than that of aortic or popliteal aneurysms, femoral aneurysms are nonetheless unpredictable. Since elective surgical repair is usually well tolerated, it seems reasonable to recommend elective operation for asymptomatic aneurysms greater than twice the size of the external iliac artery, in good risk patients.

SURGICAL TREATMENT

Except in the rare case of life- or limb-threatening rupture of a femoral aneurysm, an arteriogram should be obtained prior to operation. The surgical strategy depends on the patency of the superficial femoral artery. If this vessel is patent, the treatment of type 1 femoral aneurysms usually requires only a short interposition graft for the aneurysmal segment of the common femoral artery (Fig. 1). Small aneurysms may be safely excised, but for larger aneurysms it is safer to place the graft within the aneurysm sac using the Creech technique commonly employed for aortic aneurysms, avoiding possible injury to the femoral vein or nerve.[5] The superficial epigastric and the superficial circumflex iliac arteries should be preserved, as they are important

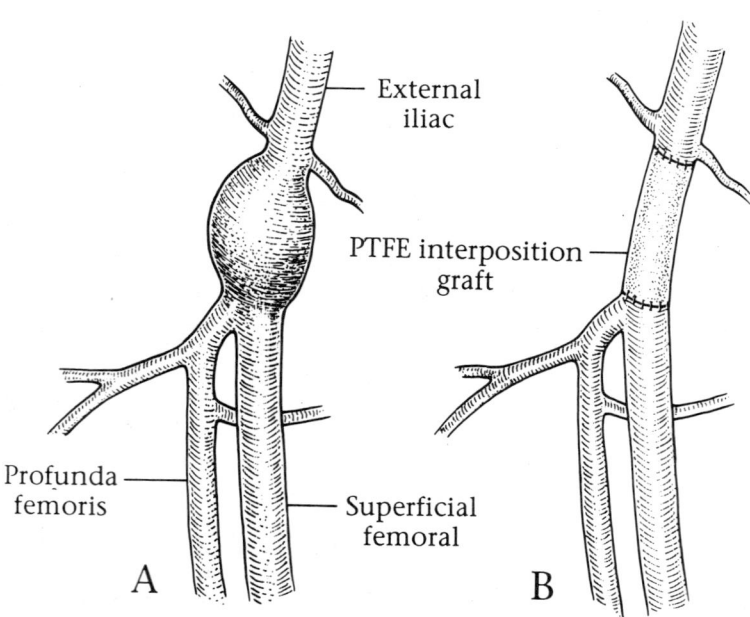

Figure 1 *A*, Type 1 common femoral artery aneurysm, in which the aneurysm does not involve the origin of the profunda femoris artery. *B*, Resection of type 1 aneurysm with PTFE interposition graft.

collateral vessels. Grafts of Dacron or polytetrafluoroethylene (PTFE) are preferable to saphenous vein because of a better size match with the usually large caliber femoral artery. The long-term patency of prosthetic grafts appears to be equivalent to that of the saphenous vein in this location.[6] If the superficial femoral artery is occluded, the interposition graft may be used as the origin for a femoropopliteal or femorotibial bypass graft.

In type 2 aneurysms the profunda femoris artery originates from the aneurysm. If the superficial femoral artery is patent, an interposition graft should be placed between the proximal common and superficial femoral arteries and the origin of the profunda implanted into the side of the graft. Occasionally a separate graft may be necessary if the origin of the profunda femoris is dilated (Fig. 2). If the superficial femoral artery is occluded, the graft should be interposed between the common and the deep femoral arteries. If the limb remains ischemic, the interposition graft may be used as the origin for a saphenous vein femorodistal bypass graft.

Because of their deep location, isolated aneurysms of the profunda and superficial femoral arteries are usually not detected until they become symptomatic, usually because of rupture. This emergency frequently requires ligation of the branches of the profunda femoris artery for control of hemorrhage, which precludes an anatomic vascular reconstruction. Femoropopliteal grafting is usually not necessary unless the superficial femoral artery is occluded. Aneurysms of the superficial femoral artery can usually be treated with a prosthetic interposition graft.

Because of the frequent association of aortic and femoral aneurysms, the treatment of combined lesions at one operation is a consideration. Attempts to treat aortic and femoral aneurysms with an aortofemoral graft, in which the ventral wall of the femoral aneurysm is excised and the femoral limb of the graft is implanted end-to-side to the femoral artery have resulted in a high incidence of false aneurysm formation.[4] It is preferable to treat combined aortic and femoral aneurysms as separate lesions but at the same operation. The aortic aneurysm can usually be managed with an aortoaortic or aortobiliac graft and the femoral aneurysm treated separately with one of the techniques noted. If aortoiliac occlusive disease requires an aortofemoral graft, a graft should be placed for the femoral aneurysm first and the distal limb of the aortofemoral graft implanted into the side of the femoral graft (Fig. 3A).

Femoral and popliteal aneurysms may also be treated concurrently. The femoral aneurysm should be resected first, with placement of a prosthetic femoral interposition graft. This graft can then be used as the source of inflow for a saphenous vein femoropopliteal bypass (Fig. 3B). Anastomosis of the saphenous vein to the aneurysmal femoral artery, even after aneurysmorraphy, carries the risk of recurrent aneurysm formation and is not recommended. Blood flow to the popliteal aneurysm should be interrupted by ligation proximally and distally. If the aneurysm is large and may compress either the bypass graft or surrounding structures, its contents should be evacuated and side branches suture-ligated from within the sac.

The results of elective operation are excellent for all types of solitary asymptomatic femoral aneurysms, which usually employ short, large-caliber grafts. In contrast, the amputation rate for emergency procedures is significant, 22% for rupture and 10% for acute thrombosis. Morbidity and mortality are increased for combined procedures, with added risks usually attributable to operation on the concomitant aortic or popliteal aneu-

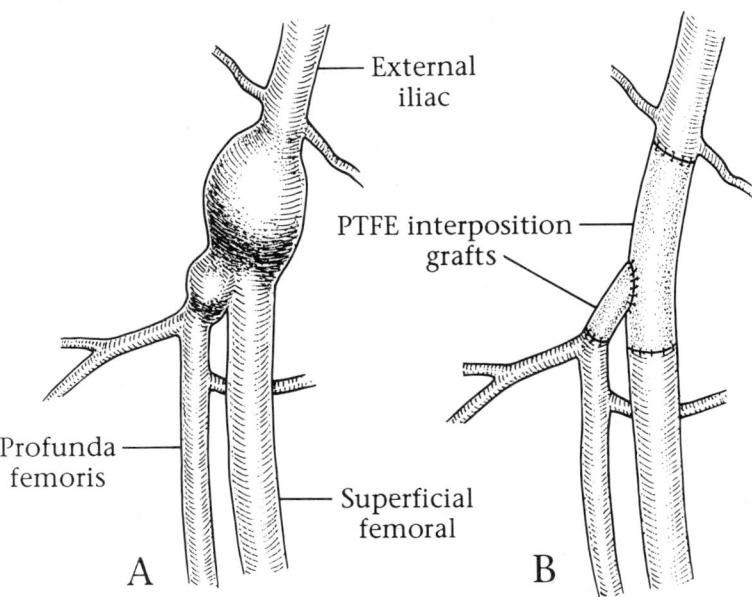

Figure 2 *A*, Type 2 common femoral artery aneurysm, in which the aneurysm involves the origin of the profunda femoris artery. *B*, Resection of type 2 aneurysm, with implantation of profunda femoris artery using a second PTFE interposition graft.

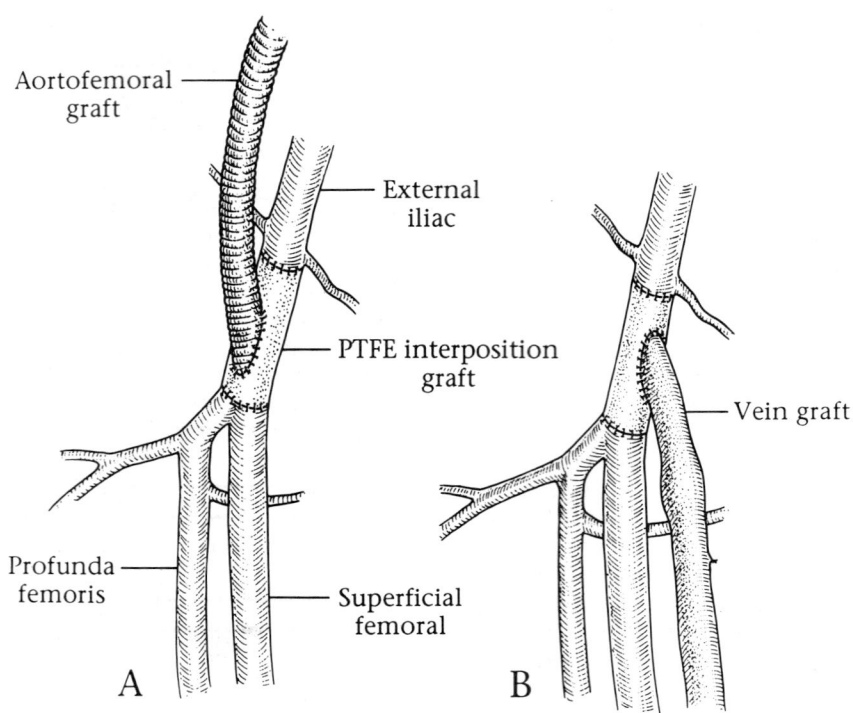

Figure 3 *A,* Treatment of combined aortic and femoral aneurysms, with the femoral limb of the aortic graft implanted into the side of a separate femoral graft to avoid late pseudoaneurysm formation. *B,* Femorodistal bypass grafts should take their origin from a femoral interposition graft to avoid late pseudoaneurysms.

rysm. Since most patients with femoral aneurysms are elderly and have significant associated coronary artery disease, a staged approach to multiple aneurysms may be the safest choice for the high-risk patient. Lastly, it is important to remember that a patient with a femoral aneurysm has a high likelihood of developing additional aneurysms in other locations and should be carefully followed for life.

REFERENCES

1. Pappas G, Janes JM, Bernatz PE, Shirger A. Femoral aneurysms: Review of surgical management. JAMA 1964; 190:489–493.
2. Cutler BS, Darling RC. Surgical management of arteriosclerotic femoral aneurysms. Surgery 1973; 74:764–773.
3. Baird RJ, Gurry JF, Kellam J, Plume SK. Arteriosclerotic femoral artery aneurysms. Can Med Assoc J 1977; 117:1306–1307.
4. Graham LM, Zelenock GB, Whitehouse, WM Jr, et al. Clinical significance of arteriosclerotic femoral artery aneurysms. Arch Surg 1980; 115:502–507.
5. Brown OW, Hollier LH. Atherosclerotic aneurysms of the femoral artery. In: Bergan JJ, Yao JST, eds. Aneurysms: Diagnosis and treatment. New York: Grune & Sratton, 1982; 505.
6. Graham LM, Rubin JR. Arteriosclerotic femoral artery aneurysm. In: Ernst CB, Stanley JC, eds. Current therapy in vascular surgery, ed 2. Philadelphia: BC Decker, 1991; 347.

INFECTED FEMORAL ARTERY FALSE ANEURYSM ASSOCIATED WITH DRUG ABUSE

FRANK T. PADBERG Jr., M.D.

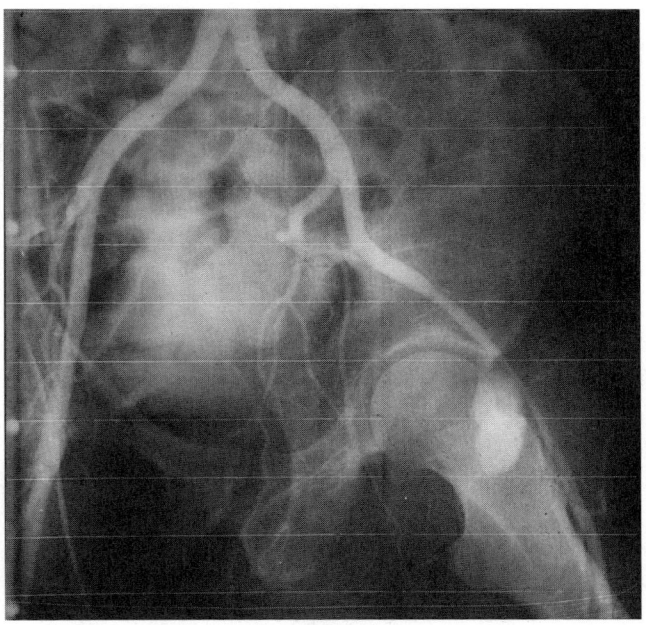

Figure 1 The infected pseudoaneurysm originates from the common femoral artery. Delineation of femoral arterial anatomy is enhanced with the hip flexed and rotated laterally.

Infected femoral artery pseudoaneurysm from needle trauma by intravenous drug abusers may lead to life-threatening hemorrhage, loss of limb, and death. Ligation of the common (CFA), superficial (SFA), or profunda femoris (PFA) artery offers definitive local treatment usually uncomplicated by significant ischemia.[1-3] However, when the preoperative status of limb viability is unclear, it may be determined intraoperatively. When an ankle Doppler signal cannot be detected after ligation, reconstruction may be considered to prevent ischemic gangrene. While the results of arterial reconstruction have improved dramatically, the potential for morbidity is not clearly balanced by the risk of limb loss and other secondary complications in this population.[1,2]

PRESENTATION AND DIAGNOSIS

Femoral venous injection is usually employed by experienced drug users who have exhausted other access sites. The mean age of these patients has been reported to be 34 to 37 years and the mean duration of drug use was 16 years.[1,3,4] Regular physician contact generally has been avoided by these patients and care is often not sought until the infectious process is far advanced. Many patients recognize an error in injection technique wherein the artery is entered rather than the vein and can often remember the time of the inciting event. Such a misadventure is called a "miss," "red blood," a "hot line," or "hitting the pink." Despite knowing this the average delay between onset of symptoms and vascular surgical consultation was 17 days in our patients. The analgesic effect of continued opiate use contributes to prehospital delays in management. Self-administration of antibiotics by drug abusers is common and may temporarily mask or control the infectious symptoms. It is not unusual for the patient to persist with injection into the site.

A tender groin mass, almost invariably present, is pulsatile in only 50% of patients. When sought, a bruit is evident in over 90%. An open punctate skin lesion draining serosanguinous fluid is characteristic. The contralateral groin may also exhibit the inactive lesion as a depressed circular scar. Other stigmata of chronic drug use may be present; however, an occasional patient presents with evidence of groin injection only. Evidence of distal embolization may be present in 5% to 10% of patients.[1,4,5] Since these aneurysms are not readily distinguished from abscesses, ill-advised incision and drainage are a trap for the unwary.[1,2,4] Rupture occurs in 5% to 15%.[1,3,4] The infected aneurysm is often not recognized in the early stages of the process, and extensive damage may be present at the first contact with vascular surgical personnel.

Systemic infection and bacteremia are common but not always present. *Staphylococcus aureus* is recovered most frequently. *Pseudomonas aeruginosa* is common, and unusual microbiologic organisms are also cultured.[1-4,6] Other communicable infectious diseases are endemic in this patient population, and caution should be exercised in their medical and surgical care.

Adjacent structures are commonly involved by the pseudoaneurysm that has progressed for several weeks. Femoral nerve compression resulted in substantial morbidity with little subsequent recovery in our patient population. This alone accounted for major disability following treatment of the infected aneurysm. Likewise, with chronic injection, localized thrombosis of the femoral vein is common. Inability to extend the hip fully indicates extension of the infection deep into the thigh, and such patients present with their hip flexed and externally rotated.

Arteriography distinguishes abscess from pseudoaneurysm and localizes the arterial defect anatomically (Figs. 1 and 2). It is obtained in all patients with a suspicious groin mass and a history of injection in the area unless precluded by life-threatening hemorrhage. The anatomic location of the aneurysm determines which and how many arteries must be ligated and may be useful in predicting the probability of limb ischemia.[3]

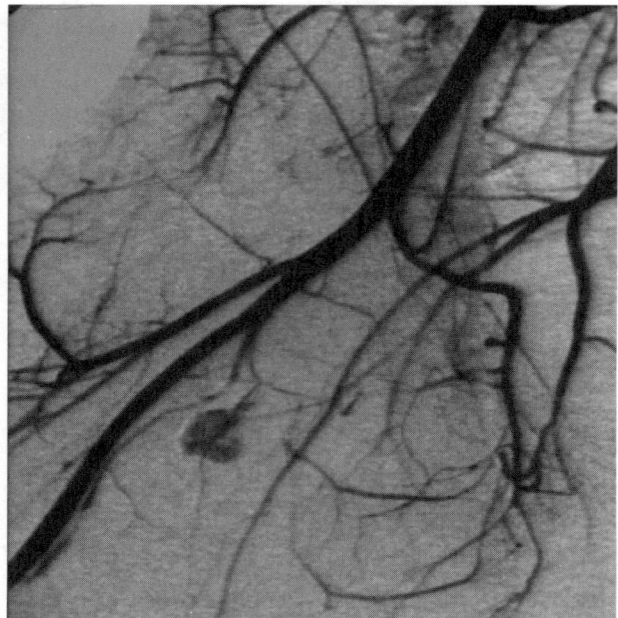
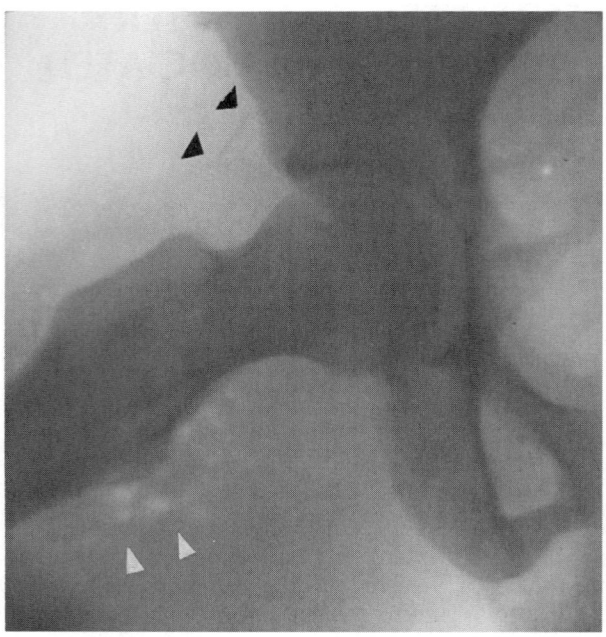

Figure 2 *A,* An infected aneurysm originating from a branch of the profunda femoris artery. The proximal and distal ends of the branch were ligated. While the limb is not at risk from ligation of the PFA or its branch, subsequent arterial rupture may occur. *B,* A scout film detected a broken needle fragment (*black triangles*) embedded in the soft tissue anterior to the aneurysm which was recovered at the time of operation. Air in the soft tissue indicates gas-forming organisms (*white arrows*). Peptostreptococcus micros and *Staphylococcus aureus* were cultured from a foul-smelling hematoma.

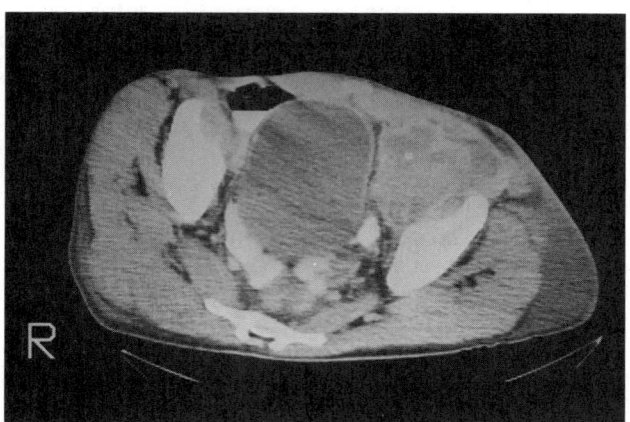

Figure 3 This computed tomographic image is taken in a horizontal plane superior to the symphysis pubis, inguinal ligament, and acetabulum. This is the same patient illustrated in Figure 1. Extension of the abscess cavity deep into the pelvis is marked by the white square.

Occasionally an aneurysm will originate from a branch of the PFA (Fig. 2). This arteriographic information may substantially alter operative management. Since occult thromboembolism may be an important determinant of the final outcome of the limb, visualization of the distal arterial tree is important.[1] If bypass is considered, delineation of distal arterial anatomy facilitates preoperative planning.

Computed tomography (CT) may be used to assess the extent of the pseudoaneurgsm or abscess. It is especially helpful when extension proximal to the inguinal ligament is suspected (Fig. 3). However, the anatomic origin of the aneurysm is not accurately defined by CT imaging. Duplex and color flow ultrasound have become increasingly useful in management. Although increasing success has been reported with ultrasound-guided compression for pseudoaneurysms following catheterization procedures, this is unlikely to assist in management of the infected femoral artery pseudoaneurysm. The site is generally quite tender, and these patients have a low tolerance for discomfort. Furthermore, the arterial wall may have disintegrated at the site of injury. Inaccurate and imprecise images further reduce the utility of ultrasound in this condition.[3] In addition, the examination may be complicated by active drainage and concern for probe contamination.

LIGATION

Arterial ligation and debridement alone are appropriate for most patients with infected femoral artery pseudoaneurysms. Ligation offers definitive local treatment, removes the threat of hemorrhage, and controls the septic process. Uncorrected hypotension or hypovolemia at the time of ligation increases the probability of ischemic complications. The involved arterial segment is excised to anatomically normal artery, which is oversewn or ligated. Debridement is performed to remove all nonviable tissue, which may include skin, nerve, muscle, ligament, and adjacent vein. Bacterial cultures are obtained from the purulent drainage and arterial wall. A distal arterial signal at the ankle is confirmed with a sterile 9.5 mHz Doppler transducer.

Emergent reoperation for secondary ligation may be required. In my experience this has occurred twice after ligation of a PFA branch. In this situation SFA or bifurcation ligation was required to control subsequent bleeding.[1,2,4,5] Presumably the dissection for control of the main arteries predisposes to subsequent rupture.[1] Thus, even though the initial procedure may not require ligation of the main arterial supply, there is significant risk of this occurring subsequently.

A postligation arterial Doppler signal at the ankle correlated with limb viability. The mean Doppler-derived ankle to brachial index (ABI) following ligation was 0.63. In another study an ABI of 0.41 was reported for triple ligation (CFA, SFA, and PFA) and 0.58 after single ligation.[2] Patients with ligation as the primary treatment fared better than those undergoing reconstruction.[1,2]

Recommended management for infected pseudoaneurysms of the femoral artery has included ligation alone,[2,5,7] ligation with selective revascularization,[1,3] and routine revascularization.[6] Various reports have documented that isolated arterial segment ligation is well tolerated and revascularization is not usually required.[1-4] However, a subgroup of patients undergoing ligation of all three femoral arteries had a worse prognosis.[3] When revascularization is selected, prosthetic grafts are often required and frequently result in secondary septic complications and death.[1,3,4,5]

RECONSTRUCTION

When limb viability cannot be assured and arterial reconstruction is deemed necessary, it must be initiated immediately, since there is a relatively short tolerance for profound ischemia. Extra-anatomic bypass has been used through clean operative fields, but this usually requires prosthetic grafts.[1,4,5,8-10] If an adequate vein can be found, the patient may benefit from a short autogenous graft placed in the bed of the resected aneurysm.[3] Prosthetic grafts in the bed of the aneurysm have performed poorly.[1] The obturator foramen bypass is useful, but when the aneurysm is extensive, especially if it extends into the retroperitoneum, ipsilateral iliac based grafts may be contraindicated. It is inadvisable to use the contralateral iliac or femoral artery, since secondary infection would then threaten bilateral limb loss. Thus, an axillofemoral or axillopopliteal graft becomes attractive. These may be tunneled along the flank and the distal anastomosis constructed using an entirely lateral approach.[1,9,10]

Intermittent claudication presents little problem in postoperative management, and if present, it may reasonably be addressed during follow-up.[1,2,4] For individuals with chronic substance abuse, the risk of prosthetic reconstruction for claudication clearly outweighs the benefits.[3,5] Thus, it is difficult to justify routine revascularization.[6]

Revascularization may be accompanied by numerous complications. Additional operative procedures for hemorrhage, acute thrombosis, and graft infection are often required.[1,3-5,7] Thrombosis of the reconstruction may not mandate graft replacement, since collateral circulation continues to develop following ligation. However, the patent subcutaneous prosthesis provides a worrisome opportunity for the recidivist patient to use it for drug injection.[6] Infection of the prosthetic conduit is common, requires excision, and may be complicated by bleeding, sepsis, and distal septic embolization. Such secondary infections may require ligation of donor arteries and may result in limb loss despite patent grafts. Most recent articles report no operative deaths in the treatment of infected femoral pseudoaneurysms associated with drug abuse.[1,3,6,7]

Since these aneurysms infrequently require arterial reconstruction, it is important to define clinical criteria to identify limbs threatened by ischemia. After ligation and debridement, limb viability is determined intraoperatively by identification of an audible arterial Doppler signal at the ankle. When this finding was present, acute ischemia did not develop and limbs survived without tissue loss. However, audible recognition of the Doppler signal is a qualitative assessment that may not be infallible.

REFERENCES

1. Padberg FT, Hobson RW II, Lee BC, et al. Femoral artery pseudoaneurysm: Ligation vs. revascularization. J Vasc Surg 1991; 15:642–648.
2. Cheng SWK, Fok M, Wong J. Infected femoral pseudoaneurysm in intravenous drug abusers. Br J Surg 1992; 79:510–512.
3. Reddy DJ, Smith RF, Elliott JP, et al. Infected femoral artery false aneurysms in drug addicts: Evolution of selective vascular reconstruction. J Vasc Surg 1986; 3:718–724.
4. Johnson JR, Ledgerwood AM, Lucas CE. Mycotic aneurysm, new concepts in therapy. Arch Surg 1983; 118:577–582.
5. Feldman AJ, Berguer R. Management of an infected aneurysm of the groin secondary to drug abuse. Surg Gynecol Obstet 1983; 157:519–522.
6. Patel KR, Semel L, Clauss RH. Routine revascularization with resection of infected femoral pseudoaneurysms from substance abuse. J Vasc Surg 1988; 8:321–328.
7. Yellin AE. Ruptured mycotic aneurysm. Arch Surg 1977; 112:981–986.
8. Fromm SH, Lucas CE. Obturator bypass for mycotic aneurysm in the drug addict. Arch Surg 1970; 100:82–83.
9. Padberg FT. Lateral approach to the popliteal artery. Ann Vasc Surg 1988; 4:397–401.
10. Gupta SK, Veith FJ, Ascer E, et al. Fell SC. Five year experience with axillopopliteal bypasses for limb salvage. J Cardiovasc Surg 1985; 26:321–324.

OBTURATOR FORAMEN BYPASS GRAFTS IN GROIN SEPSIS

S. MARTIN LINDENAUER, M.D.

Infection involving the femoral artery in the groin may occur in a variety of circumstances, including contamination by an intravenous drug abuser; percutaneous cannulation of the femoral vessels for diagnostic or therapeutic cardiac or vascular procedures; an ulcerating neoplasm involving the inguinal lymph nodes; wound healing complications following radical groin lymph node resection for neoplasm; and infection involving the femoral end of a femoropopliteal, axillofemoral, femorofemoral, or aortofemoral prosthetic bypass. The most common circumstance is related to infection of a prosthetic bypass in the groin that occurs most often in the femoral anastomosis of an aortofemoral bypass. However, infection related to arterial cannulation and intravenous drug abuse is increasing in frequency.

The most important principle in the management of an infected arterial prosthesis is removal of the prosthetic bypass and replacement with an alternate bypass through an uninfected area, avoiding cross-contamination.[1,2] These alternate bypass routes usually are in nonanatomic locations and include such procedures as iliosuperficial femoral or iliopopliteal bypass placed lateral to the groin vessels, axillopopliteal bypass, or bypass to the distal profunda femoris and bypass through the obturator foramen. The obturator foramen bypass is perhaps the most anatomic of these alternatives because it follows the course of the obturator artery.

PREOPERATIVE STUDIES AND PREPARATION

In selected instances of a groin abscess associated with extensive cellulitis, incision and drainage of the abscess may cautiously be undertaken. Such an abscess must be distinguished from a pulsating hematoma or pseudoaneurysm. This can usually be accomplished by means of a color flow duplex scan. Operative exploration should be pursued cautiously and if the nature of the pulsating fluctuant groin mass is not fully resolved, the procedure should be accomplished in the operating room. If time permits, other imaging procedures, such as arteriography and computed tomography (CT), can be useful to define more clearly the nature of the groin mass. As incision and drainage are performed, if a nonbleeding artery or anastomosis is uncovered, it should not be disturbed.

In a patient who has a groin wound with an exposed artery or anastomosis, the required diagnostic procedures and operation should be accomplished expeditiously because bleeding is the inevitable outcome. If there is bleeding from the groin wound, control of the groin vessels must be accomplished as an emergency. This may require ligation of a patent iliac artery or the femoral end of a patent aortofemoral bypass. Cautious anticoagulation with heparin sodium should be considered to preserve the patency of outflow vessels, which may be necessary for a subsequent alternate bypass.

After incision and drainage of a groin abscess, operative cultures usually direct specific antibiotic therapy. Although *Staphylococcus aureus* and *S. epidermidis* are the most common organisms, comprising approximately 50% of such cultures, gram-negative organisms and infection with multiple species are common; therefore, broad-spectrum, multidrug antibiotic therapy is required. Once groin hemorrhage or groin cellulitis is controlled, critically important diagnostic studies can be undertaken. These include arteriography to ascertain the appropriate sites for a subsequent alternate bypass and thin-slice CT scanning of the involved area to document gas bubbles or perigraft lucencies that may help to define the extent of the infection. If preliminary operative control of bleeding is required, the exposed vessels should be covered using adjacent soft tissue, if possible, or by rotation of the sartorius muscle to avoid desiccation of the vessels and further hemorrhage. After control of bleeding from an infected groin wound, definitive operative intervention should occur, if possible within 2 or 3 days. In the absence of bleeding and with extensive cellulitis, 7 to 10 days may be required to control the local infection; remember that it cannot be totally eradicated until the involved prosthetic material is removed. Associated cardiopulmonary problems or other comorbidities must be treated but must not delay definitive treatment.

TECHNIQUE OF OBTURATION BYPASS

The patient is placed supine upon the operating table with the affected extremity slightly abducted and externally rotated to provide ready access to the medial thigh. The groin wound is carefully isolated with impervious adherent drapes and covered with a sterile towel secured to the skin with staples. The skin preparation includes the area normally prepared for an aortofemoral and femoropopliteal bypass. The exposed skin, groin towel, and genital drapes are covered with impervious, adherent, antiseptic-impregnated drapes.

A lower quadrant transverse curvilinear incision extending into the flank muscles similar to that used for renal transplantation provides excellent retroperitoneal exposure of the pelvis and pelvic vessels. Complete muscle relaxation, a mild degree of Trendelenburg position, and the use of a self-retaining retractor greatly enhance exposure of the vessels.

The preliminary information provided by a CT scan suggesting that infection does not extend to the common iliac artery or the proximal end of the femoral limb of an aortofemoral bypass must be confirmed. Although extension of a groin infection to involve the native iliac vessels is uncommon, attention to their integrity and the status of the surrounding periarterial tissue should document an absence of periarterial inflammation, which can be confirmed by arterial biopsy from the site of the proposed proximal end of the new bypass graft. Extension of a groin infection involving an arterial prosthesis is more common and can usually be documented by lack of graft incorporation and the presence of perigraft mucoidlike material. Particular attention should be paid to the portion of the aortofemoral limb adjacent to the graft bifurcation. A smear of the perigraft tissue should be obtained for immediate examination to detect the presence of bacteria, and a small portion of the prosthesis and perigraft tissue is submitted for culture examination. *Staphylococcus epidermidis* is frequently difficult to culture, and the likelihood of recovery of this organism can be enhanced by sonication of graft and tissue specimens. If the proximal prosthesis is clinically infected, the contemplated obturator foramen bypass procedure should be aborted because discovery of unsuspected infection involving the body of the prosthesis excludes definitive unilateral management. However, if the proximal end and body of the prosthesis are well incorporated, one may proceed. Even if the proximal culture grows organisms, in the absence of clinical signs of infection, one is not obliged to remove the entire prosthesis. Such patients have received long-term (6 to 12 months) antibiotic therapy with good results. Such a decision may be controversial but clinical assessment of the prosthesis is more reliable than smear and culture results.

The ureter should be clearly identified and displaced anteriorly out of harm's way. Attention is then directed to the distal pelvis, where the superior ramis of the pubis is identified and traced laterally to the obturator foramen containing the obturator artery, vein, and nerve. Alternatively, the junction of the internal and external iliac arteries can be identified laterally at the pelvic brim. Slightly inferior are the junction of the internal and external iliac veins. There is almost always a large lymph node in the bifurcation of the internal and external iliac veins. This lymph node should be handled carefully because it contains multiple fragile venous connections to the iliac venous system. Beneath this node, coursing anteriorly and applied to the lateral pelvic wall, is the obturator nerve that is 2 to 4 mm in diameter. Its stark, white appearance stands out clearly against the lateral pelvic wall. One may easily follow the obturator nerve in a caudad direction and observe its exit from the pelvis through the obturator foramen.

Arising from the internal iliac artery and vein are the obturator artery and vein, which are inferior to the nerve, proceed in a similar direction adjacent to the lateral pelvic wall, and exit the pelvis with the obturator nerve through the obturator canal. Not infrequently these vessels may be joined by branches arising from the external iliac vessels or from the inferior epigastric vessels directly. There may be pubic branches that descend inferiorly over the superior pubic ramis and overlie the obturator aponeurosis and the obturator internus muscle. Familiarity with these variations is essential to avoid undue bleeding and injury to the obturator nerve.

The fascial edge of the obturator fossa can be easily felt. The roof of the fossa is formed by the inferior lateral portion of the superior ramus of the pubis. In this area, the neurovascular structures are crossed by the vas deferens, which crosses the pubic ramis and runs posteriorly. The internal obturator muscle lines the anterolateral portion of the pelvis, forming the obturator fossa, extending from the ischial tuberosity posteriorly, where it is more muscular, to insert anteriorly into the bony superior ramus of the pubis. The anterior fascia in this area is dense and tough, must be sharply incised, and cannot be penetrated bluntly. An incision, therefore, is made through this aponeurotic fascia medial and inferior to the obturator vessels and nerve but superior to the more inferiorly located muscular portion of the obturator internus muscle. With a blunt instrument, the incised fascia can be easily penetrated and the opening enlarged.

The site of the distal anastomosis is ascertained by examination of the preoperative arteriogram. Most often the distal anastomosis is to the proximal popliteal or distal superficial femoral artery. However, if necessary, the anastomosis can be made to the popliteal below the knee. A posteromedial incision is made in the lower thigh to expose the above-the-knee portion of the popliteal artery. A blunt instrument, such as curved ring forceps or uterine packing forceps, is passed from above and below to begin the tunnel beneath the pectineus, adductor brevis, adductor longus, and adductor magnus. A curved graft tunneler is then passed from below up through the obturator foramen. The development of this dissection plane is facilitated by bimanual blunt dissection through the enlarged obturator foramen, staying anterior to the hamstring muscles. A proximal medial thigh incision is to be avoided because it would place the new graft perilously close to the base of the contaminated femoral triangle.[3,4]

The popliteal artery is identified and controlled, and the tunnel developed to the region of the adductor hiatus. If the anastomosis is to be made to the distal superficial femoral artery, the tunnel is placed slightly more superficially to expose the superficial femoral artery just before it enters the adductor hiatus. Externally supported 8 mm diameter polytetrafluoroethylene is a suitable material for the bypass. Ordinarily the tunnel is sufficiently posterior to the femoral infection site so that there is no question regarding the sterility of the tissues adjacent to the new graft site. However, if there is uncertainty about extension of the inflammatory process to the anticipated location of the bypass graft, an autogenous saphenous vein is a better choice of graft material. The new bypass is passed through the tunneling device, and care is taken to ensure that it is not twisted. The stripe present on most prosthetic materials is helpful in this regard. A similar stripe can be placed on a saphenous vein with a sterile marking pen. Flushing the graft with heparinized saline, with the opposite end

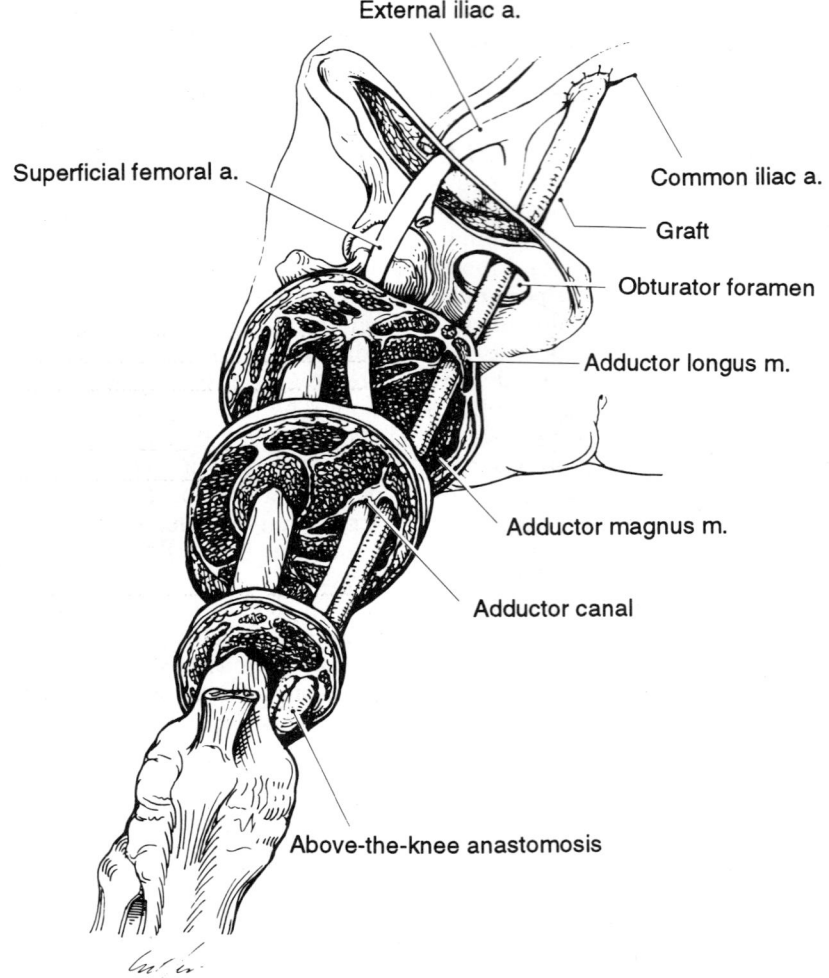

Figure 1 Path of obturator bypass graft. Note distance between obturator bypass and femoral artery in groin.

free to rotate, helps to straighten any inadvertent twists. The graft can originate from the contralateral iliac vessels by establishing a dissection plane in the space of Retzius anteriorly between the symphysis and the bladder. This route is circuitous and should be avoided if at all possible.

After this dissection and after systemic heparinization, a 1 to 2 cm segment of the proximal prosthesis is excised and the ends of the divided prosthesis are oversewn. The oversewn distal end is then displaced caudad for a short distance in the perigraft canal, and adjacent soft tissue is used to obliterate the perigraft tunnel. The graft should arise from the proximal common iliac or the most proximal portion of the limb of the aortofemoral bypass (Fig. 1). This forms a straight path for the new prosthesis to the distal superficial femoral or popliteal artery. If the proximal anastomosis is to a prosthesis, the anastomosis should be end to end so that the distal infected limb of the graft can be removed. However, if the proximal anastomosis is to a native artery, an end-to-side anastomosis to the common iliac artery is preferred because it allows continued perfusion of the hypogastric artery.

After completion of the proximal anastomosis, the clamp is briefly released to assure adequate inflow through the prosthesis. The distal anastomosis is constructed in an end-to-side fashion to allow both antegrade and retrograde perfusion of the femoropopliteal system. Retrograde perfusion is particularly important in this circumstance to maintain continuity of the profunda femoris artery, which is subsequently ligated at its origin in the groin. Occasionally, perfusion of the profunda collateral network results in bleeding from the groin wound that may necessitate proximal popliteal ligation. Similarly, ligation of the common iliac artery distal to the proximal anastomosis should be avoided to allow perfusion of hypogastric collaterals. This can usually be accomplished with subsequent ligation of the common femoral artery unless intraoperative bleeding from the groin wound necessitates proximal iliac ligation. Under *no* circumstance should the infected groin wound be approached directly at this time because this would result in cross-contamination of the new bypass.

When adequate perfusion through the new bypass is assured, the wounds are closed in layers and the skin approximated with a subcuticular suture. Heparinization is maintained during this period when there is parallel flow through existing channels to avoid inadvertent thrombosis of the new bypass. The incisions are isolated with impervious adherent plastic drapes, and only then is the groin wound uncovered. Appropriate debridement is undertaken, and the femoral vessels exposed and controlled. The distal portion of the infected aortofemoral limb is retrieved and removed in its entirety. Because of the precarious status of the femoral vessels, it might be tempting to leave a "cuff" of graft material to close; however, all of the prosthesis must be removed to prevent recurrent hemorrhage and to ensure healing of the groin wound.

Secure ligation of the femoral vessels may sometimes prove to be difficult. The infected femoral artery must be debrided to facilitate secure arterial closure. Usually all three femoral arteries require individual ligation with monofilament suture. The wound is packed open. Residual exposed vessels must be covered with adjacent soft tissue to prevent recurrent bleeding. The sartorius muscle may be mobilized to facilitate vessel coverage.

Results of obturator bypass are generally satisfactory, with overall patency of collected small series in the range of 60% to 80% when the distal anastomosis is above the knee and the outflow is satisfactory.[5,6]

REFERENCES

1. Shaw RS, Baue AE. Management of sepsis complicating arterial reconstructive surgery. Surgery 1963; 53:75–86.
2. Fry WJ, Lindenauer SM. Infection complicating the use of plastic arterial implants. Arch Surg 1967; 94:600–609.
3. Wood RFM. Arterial grafting through the obturator foramen in secondary hemorrhage from the femoral vessels. Angiology 1982; 33:385–392.
4. Lai DTM, Huber D, Hogg J. Obturator foramen bypass in the management of infected prosthetic vascular grafts. Aust N Z J Surg 1993; 63:811–814.
5. VonDet RJ, Brands LC. The obturator foramen bypass: An alternative procedure in iliofemoral artery revascularization. Surgery 1981; 89:543–547.
6. Nevelsteen A, Mees U, Deleersnijder J, Suy R. Obturator bypass: A sixteen year experience with 55 cases. Ann Vasc Surg 1987; 1:558–563.

POPLITEAL ARTERY ANEURYSM

ROBERT W. HOBSON II, M.D.

Popliteal artery aneurysms are the most common peripheral arterial aneurysms managed by vascular surgeons. Since aneurysmal disease of the arterial system has common cause, the relationships between the incidence of popliteal arterial aneurysms and aneurysms of the abdominal aorta and iliofemoral system are fascinating. For example, a patient with a unilateral popliteal artery aneurysm has approximately a 50% chance of a contralateral aneurysm and a 30% or more chance of having an abdominal aortic aneurysm. Patients with abdominal aortic aneurysms should be carefully evaluated for peripheral artery aneurysms, as a high incidence of popliteal artery aneurysm can be anticipated. Of the patients with bilateral popliteal artery aneurysms, over half have aortic, iliac, or femoral artery aneurysms. More than 90% of these aneurysms occur in men.[1-3] In one series of 233 popliteal artery aneurysms, 231 were considered to be atherosclerotic.[3] As reported in most clinical series, the average patient is identified during the sixth or seventh decade of life.

DIAGNOSIS

Physical examination is accurate for the diagnosis of popliteal artery aneurysm in asymptomatic patients as well as those with abdominal aortic aneurysm or other peripheral artery aneurysms. However, most routinely employ duplex scanning of the popliteal fossa to confirm the diagnosis.[4] A popliteal artery is considered aneurysmal if its diameter exceeds 2 cm or is 1.5 times the diameter of the proximal nonaneurysmal arterial segment.[1] In that case arteriography is performed to evaluate the proximal and distal vasculature prior to reconstruction. Some authors have suggested that magnetic resonance imaging (MRI) will replace arteriography in the future and it may reduce the need for duplex scanning[5]; however, most will continue to rely on duplex scanning and contrast arteriography.

CLINICAL PRESENTATION AND SURGICAL MANAGEMENT

The clinical presentation of popliteal artery aneurysm is variable. Perhaps as many as half of the patients are asymptomatic. Results of surgical management among this patient population have been excellent, and routine repair of the asymptomatic aneurysm has been recommended.[1-3] Clinical follow-up also has been remarkably good. In this group of patients, routine practice has been to employ an operative plan as outlined in Figure 1.[6] The extremity is explored medially (Fig. 1A) with performance of proximal and distal ligation and bypass grafting, generally employing reversed autogenous saphenous vein. In some patients distal tibial bypass has been required for limb salvage when the popliteal aneurysm is accompanied by distal tibial occlusive disease, particularly in diabetics. When the aneurysm is larger and ligation might result in a symptomatic mass effect in the popliteal fossa, the technique of endoaneurysmorrhaphy followed by reconstruction of the popliteal artery is preferred. Using this technique, the redundant portion of the aneurysm is generally excised, avoiding trauma to the adjacent popliteal vein (Fig. 1D), if the dissection (Fig. 1B,C) between the artery and vein is difficult. In elderly patients division of the medial musculature and tendons has not been associated with postoperative disability.

In a recent study, however, Michaels and Galland[7] employed Markov decision tree analysis and suggested advantages for elective repair dependent on the selected rate of follow-up complications and estimated months of complication-free survival after repair. Although analyses of this type are difficult to interpret because of widely variable rates of complications in surgical series, a final answer on operative efficacy will require a randomized, prospective clinical trial evaluating the natural history of untreated asymptomatic popliteal artery aneurysm versus that of elective operative management.

The complications of popliteal arterial thrombosis, distal embolization, or rupture resulting in lower limb ischemia occur in 50% to 70% of reported series and are associated with amputation rates as high as 20%.[8] Evans and Vermilion[2] documented complications in 70% of patients from their series of popliteal artery aneurysms. In 15 extremities with embolization, 3 amputations ultimately were required. Aneurysmal rupture was unusual in this series, occurring in only 7% of patients; however, two of the four patients required amputation.

In managing the acutely ischemic limb, immediate heparinization and selective arteriography are indicated. Recent data suggest that the use of thrombolytic therapy in these patients prior to definitive surgical management is effective in reducing amputation rates and overall morbidity.[9,10] Carpenter and colleagues[9] recently reported on the management of 54 popliteal artery aneurysms among 33 patients treated between 1979 and 1992. Seven patients with aneurysm thrombosis as well as limb ischemia due to thrombosis of the distal vasculature received preoperative thrombolytic therapy (urokinase, n-5; streptokinase, n-2). Six of seven patients developed vessel recanalization with subsequent revascularization and limb salvage in all. No amputations were required in this group. The recommendation for initial thrombolytic therapy in patients with popliteal artery aneurysm and limb-threatening ischemia secondary to thrombosis or distal emboli rather than emergency operative intervention is appropriate. Pharmacologic control of the postoperative ischemia-reperfusion syndrome may also have a future role in the management of these patients.

Finally, endovascular placement of synthetic prostheses, usually polytetrafluoroethylene, has been presented and discussed in individual case reports. The role of these catheter-based interventions remains speculative, and larger case studies will be required to evaluate their efficacy and long-term value when compared with the usually recommended operative management.

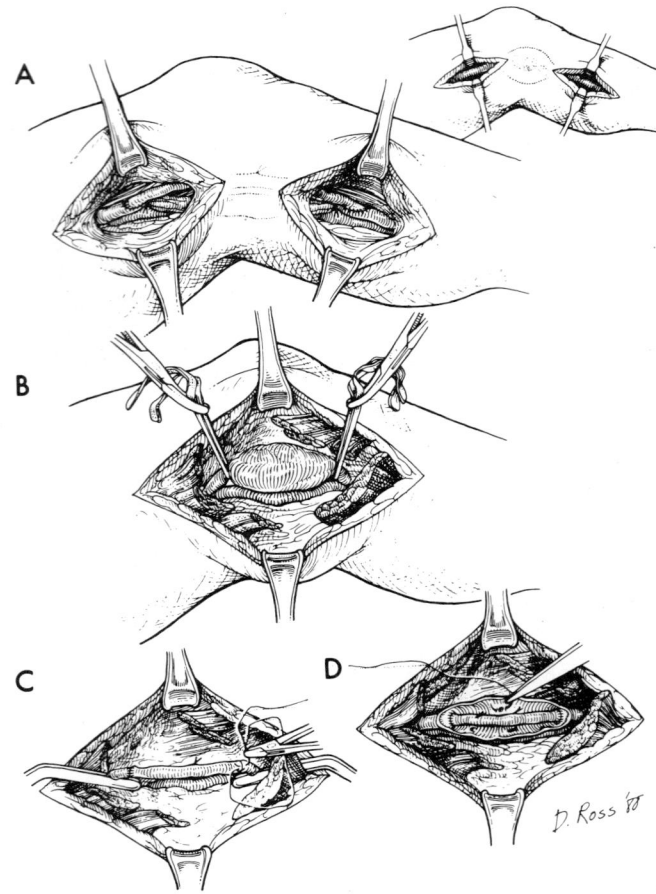

Figure 1 Surgical exploration of the extremity is performed from the medial aspect of the leg with the patient supine. *A*, Proximal and distal arterial ligation with bypass grafting using reversed autogenous saphenous vein is recommended. *B,C,D*, After transection of the medial head of the gastrocnemius muscle as well as the tendons of the gracilis, semitendinous, and semimembranous muscle, the aneurysm can be resected or the technique of endoaneurysmorrhaphy can be employed. (From Hobson RW II, Jamil Z, Lynch TG: Peripheral arterial aneurysms. In Bergan JJ, Yao JST, eds. Operative techniques in vascular surgery. New York: Grune & Stratton, 1980:177; with permission.)

REFERENCES

1. Szilagyi DE, Schwartz, RL, Reddy, DJ. Popliteal arterial aneurysms. Arch Surg 1981; 116:724–728.
2. Evans WE, Vermilion BD. Popliteal aneurysms. In: Bergan JJ, Yao JST, Eds. Aneurysms: Diagnosis and treatment. New York: Grune & Stratton, 1982:487.
3. Wychulis AR, Spittell JA Jr, Wallace RB. Popliteal aneurysm. Surg 1970; 68:942–952.
4. Collins GJ, Rich NM, Hobson RW. Ultrasound diagnosis of popliteal arterial aneurysms. Am Surg 1976; 42:853.
5. Abbott WM. Popliteal artery aneurysm. In: Ernst CB, Stanley JC, eds. Current therapy in vascular surgery, ed 2. Philadelphia: BC Decker, 1991:357.
6. Hobson RW, Jamil Z, Lynch TG. Peripheral arterial aneurysms. In: Bergan JJ, Yao JST, Eds. Operative techniques in vascular surgery. New York: Grune & Stratton, 1980:175.
7. Michaels JA, Galland RB. Management of asymptomatic popliteal aneurysms: The use of a Markov decision tree to determine the criteria for a conservative approach. Eur J Vasc Surg 1993; 7:136–143.
8. Reilly MK, Abbott WM, Darling RC. Aggressive surgical management of popliteal artery aneurysms. Am J Surg 1983; 145:498–502.
9. Carpenter JP, Barker CF, Roberts B, et al. Popliteal artery aneurysms: Current management and outcome. J Vasc Surg 1994; 19:65–73.
10. Giddings AEB. Influence of thrombolytic therapy in the management of popliteal aneurysms. In: Aneurysms: New findings and treatments. Norwalk, Conn.: Appleton & Lange, 1974:493.

AORTOILIAC OCCLUSIVE DISEASE

ANATOMIC DISTRIBUTION AND NATURAL HISTORY OF AORTOILIAC AND INFRAINGUINAL ATHEROSCLEROSIS

MARK F. FILLINGER, M.D.
JACK L. CRONENWETT, M.D.

ANATOMIC DISTRIBUTION

Atherosclerosis is a diffuse process, but it is accentuated in certain locations, giving rise to recognizable disease patterns in the lower extremities. Throughout the circulation, bifurcations are focal points for accelerated atherosclerosis, presumably because of hemodynamic disturbances and shear stress changes that occur at these sites. The proclivity for stenoses in the proximal common iliac and profunda femoral arteries are good examples of this phenomenon. Beyond this general observation concerning arterial bifurcations, other specific disease patterns have been repeatedly observed in the lower extremities. Early atherosclerotic changes are most frequently found in the superficial femoral artery (SFA) at the adductor canal, a finding that has led to speculation that chronic, repetitive, local arterial trauma may accelerate these changes (Fig. 1). Alternatively, it has been suggested that the adductor canal restricts expansion of the SFA that occurs elsewhere in the artery as intimal plaques develop. Whatever the mechanism, SFA atherosclerosis at the adductor canal is one of the earliest and most frequent locations of occlusive disease in the leg.

Certain atherosclerotic risk factors may result in different anatomic disease distributions. The best-characterized example is diabetes mellitus, which predisposes to occlusive disease in the tibial and peroneal arteries, more diffuse profunda femoral disease, and less aortoiliac involvement than in nondiabetic, atherosclerotic patients.[1] In fact, distal, segmental occlusive disease of the profunda femoral artery (as opposed to localized, orificial disease) is so characteristic of patients with diabetes mellitus that it may occasionally lead to the discovery of previously undetected hyperglycemia (Fig. 2). Furthermore, focal tibial-peroneal artery disease, with a preserved SFA-popliteal segment, is very characteristic of diabetic patients, whereas nondiabetic patients with atherosclerosis seldom develop severe tibial-peroneal disease without concomitant SFA-popliteal involvement. The explanation has not been elucidated, but this difference has been observed repeatedly. Finally, the lower incidence of aortoiliac atherosclerosis (and aortic aneurysmal disease) in diabetic patients has been widely observed, but not explained. Of importance for the treatment of diabetic ulcers has been the refutation of the previously accepted theory that diabetic patients had "small vessel disease" of the foot that prevented successful revascularization. Careful histologic studies, as well as multiple successful distal revascularizations, have dispelled this myth and resulted in markedly improved limb salvage despite the presence of aggressive tibial-peroneal disease in diabetic patients.[2]

Although other atherosclerotic risk factors, such as smoking and hyperlipidemia, have not been associated with such specific disease patterns as diabetes mellitus, it is clear that the presence of multiple risk factors over a prolonged period leads to more diffuse atherosclerotic involvement of multiple arterial segments of the lower extremities. Thus, young patients who develop symptoms of arterial occlusive disease are much more likely to have isolated aortoiliac or focal SFA involvement, and elderly patients with the same risk factors usually present with diffuse disease involving the aortoiliac, SFA, popliteal, and tibial arteries.

Several disease patterns occur in the aortoiliac (A-I) segment. Young patients who present with A-I disease not only have focal disease but also often have an underlying small-diameter A-I segment (Fig. 3). These smaller arteries provide less margin for the development of atherosclerosis, leading to earlier symptoms at a time when the occlusive disease is focal. The "small aorta syndrome" has been described most frequently in women, although men can also present with symptoms associated with localized atherosclerosis in a small A-I segment at a young age.

In a study of women with symptomatic aortoiliac

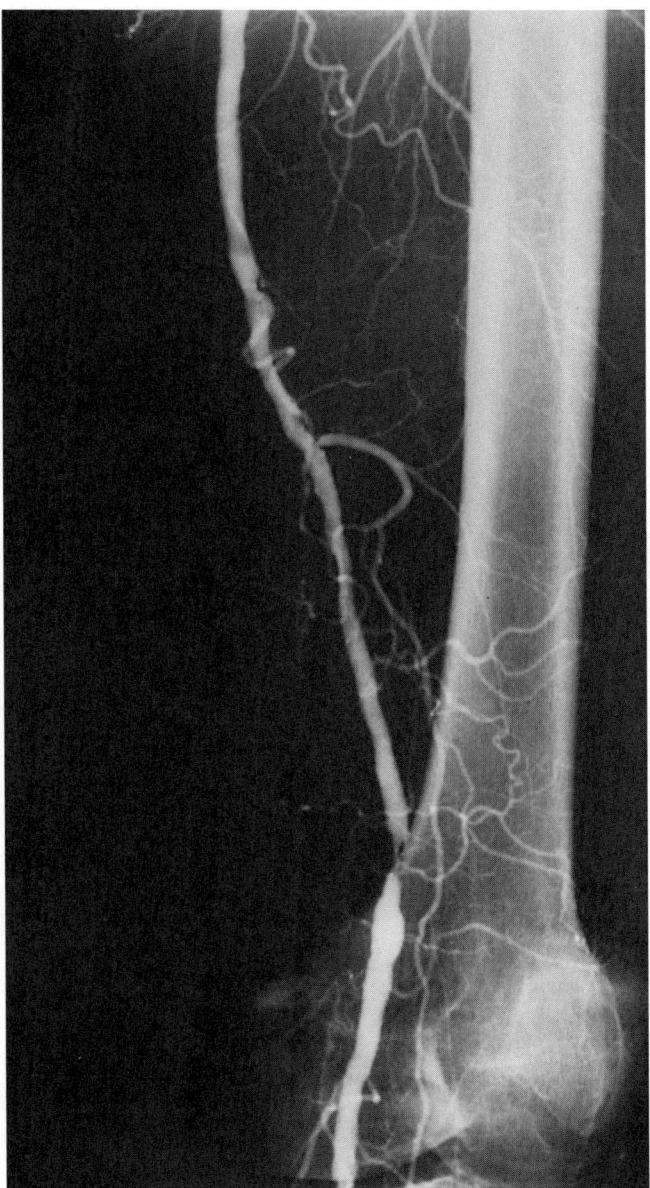

Figure 1 Superficial femoral artery lesion in the region of the adductor canal.

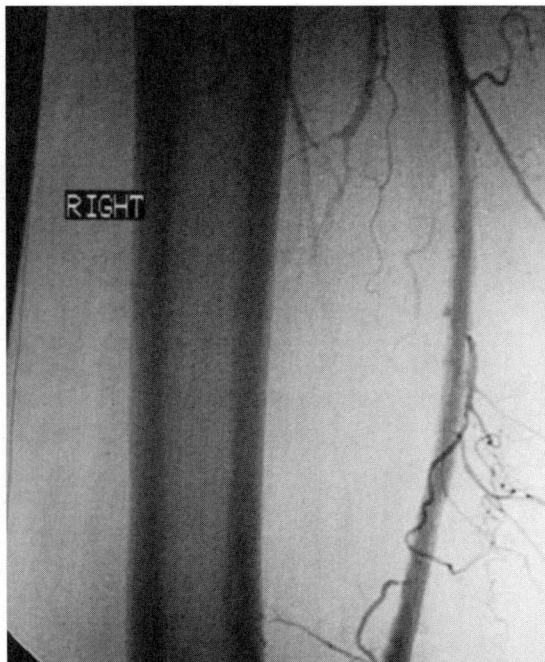

Figure 2 Distal profunda disease in a diabetic despite a lack of disease in vessels from the external iliac to the distal SFA. Note the faint calcification of the occluded profunda segment.

disease, we found that a distinct subset of women with small arteries did not exist, but that women with small arteries presented with symptoms at a young age, had localized aortoiliac disease, had few systemic atherosclerotic complications, and were small in overall body size, especially height.[3] A second example of aortic disease that seems to have a gender predilection is the "coral reef" syndrome, which consists of highly calcified, exuberant shaggy plaque in the suprarenal aorta (Fig. 4). This condition has been found almost exclusively in women, although not in smaller aortas. The mechanism for female gender predilection is not known, but this disease pattern is distinct.

Different anatomic disease patterns are important because of the implications concerning the type of intervention to be performed. In the case of focal aortic and proximal iliac disease in young patients, endarterectomy is often the procedure of choice. This is especially true for suprarenal, coral reef atherosclerosis. As the aortoiliac disease becomes diffuse with disease that involves the external iliac arteries, however, endarterectomy becomes less attractive and much more technically demanding than aortofemoral bypass. For patients with a small aortoiliac segment (aorta immediately below the renal arteries less than 13 mm and the aorta just above the bifurcation less than 10 mm diameter),[3] we prefer bypass with commensurately sized grafts as opposed to endarterectomy because of the lower tolerance for recurrent disease at the endarterectomy site in these small vessels. Focal common iliac disease is effectively treated with balloon angioplasty, also emphasizing the importance of specific patterns of disease location. Although arteriography has always been required to define disease location, the increasing accuracy of duplex ultrasound imaging, even in the pelvis and abdomen, will add much to our understanding of the evolution of specific disease patterns.

Because arterial disease patterns have been previously defined by arteriography, it is important to note the tendency for atherosclerotic disease to accumulate asymmetrically in an artery, usually along the outer, concave surface. Thus, significant lesions can be missed unless oblique or lateral arteriographic views are obtained, or some type of hemodynamic assessment, such

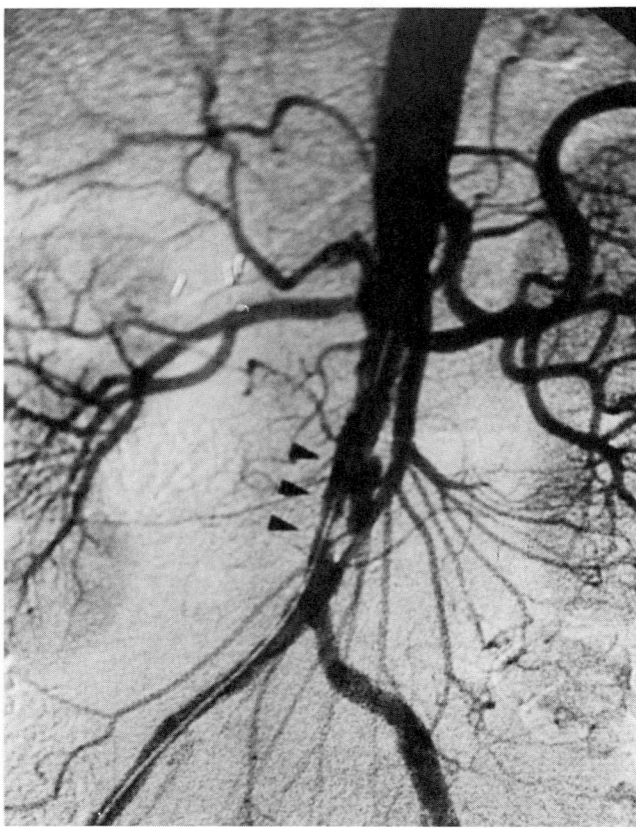

Figure 3 Localized aortoiliac disease in a young patient with an abnormally small aortoiliac segment.

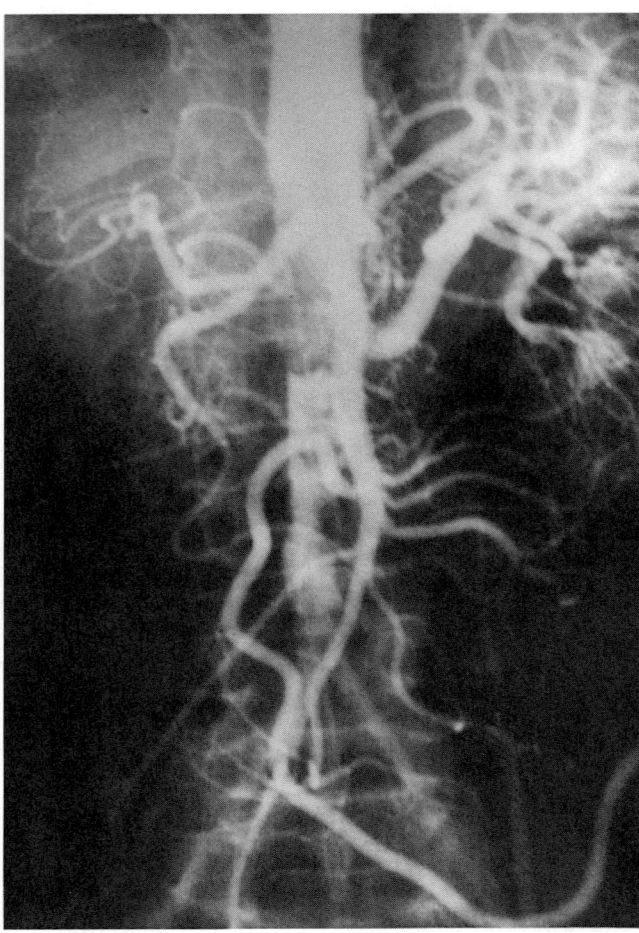

Figure 4 Large suprarenal coral reef plaque in an elderly patient with diffuse aortoiliac disease.

as pressure measurement, is also performed. The best example of this is in the iliac arteries, where disease tends to accumulate on the posterior surface and is often undetected by anteroposterior arteriograms.

Internal iliac and inferior mesenteric arteries (IMA) are frequently involved in patients with "aortoiliac" disease and must be considered in surgical planning. Pelvic perfusion may be compromised by aortofemoral reconstruction if a proximal end-to-end anastomosis is constructed and severe external iliac disease prevents retrograde pelvic perfusion. In such patients, internal iliac or IMA revascularization is advisable to avoid potential pelvic or sigmoid colon ischemia. Alternatively, in the presence of severe external iliac disease but minimal distal aortic and common iliac disease, pelvic perfusion may be preserved with a proximal end-to-side aortic anastomosis. In a follow-up study of such patients, we have shown that the distal aorta usually occludes after a period of weeks to months, but such gradual occlusion may allow collateral development, in that we have not seen pelvic ischemia.[4] Occasionally, isolated internal iliac disease may lead to impotence or local buttock claudication without diffuse aortoiliac disease, although this disease pattern is unusual.

Infrainguinal disease patterns also have important clinical implications. In previous years surgeons were hesitant to use the popliteal artery as an inflow source for tibial bypass grafts, because of an expected high frequency of SFA disease progression in such patients. However, diabetic patients often have a relatively undiseased SFA, especially if they are nonsmokers, and it is now known that bypass grafts originating below a relatively normal SFA are no more prone to failure than bypasses originating at the common femoral artery.[5] Similarly, it was long feared that bypass grafts to the very distal vessels in diabetic patients would be prone to failure because "small vessel disease" would cause poor runoff. However, bypass grafting is now commonly performed for this pattern of disease with excellent results since the concept of "small vessel disease" has been refuted.[2] In diabetic patients with infragenicular disease, the anterior tibial and posterior tibial arteries are usually affected first.[1] Thus, these patients commonly present with only the peroneal or pedal arteries for a bypass. These vessels are adequate for the outflow of a distal bypass, however, with similar graft patency and limb salvage rates for bypass to the tibial, peroneal, or pedal vessels.[5]

NATURAL HISTORY BY ANATOMIC DISTRIBUTION

Most of our knowledge of the natural history of atherosclerosis is based on patients' symptoms rather than anatomy because arteriography has usually been performed only when therapeutic intervention is being considered. This biases our historical observations toward patients with more severe, diffuse disease patterns. Accepting this shortcoming, the majority of patients who present with significant symptoms from A-I occlusive disease also have substantial infrainguinal atherosclerosis. Patients with such "tandem" or multilevel disease are more likely to develop subsequent disease progression than those with isolated aortic or iliac lesions, and are more likely to eventually require operative intervention.[6,7] Diabetic patients with minimal SFA disease are unlikely to experience rapid progression of proximal disease in the near term, making the SFA a good inflow source for distal bypass.[2] Likewise, the distal calf and foot vessels of diabetic patients are no more prone to rapid disease progression than other vessels in the lower extremity, making them useful vessels for bypass.

The utilization of duplex ultrasound imaging has afforded an opportunity to obtain information concerning the natural history of specific anatomic lesions. This is important because of the availability of angioplasty and other endovascular techniques, which, unlike surgical intervention, are more effective for treating arterial stenoses than occluded arteries. In fact, proponents of these techniques have suggested that minimally symptomatic but severe stenoses should undergo balloon angioplasty before occlusion occurs, which might thwart successful treatment. To determine whether this proposal is appropriate, a knowledge of the natural history of specific atherosclerotic lesions is necessary. To address this question, Walsh and colleagues followed the anatomic disease progression of 45 superficial femoral arteries in 38 patients who had undergone arteriography for pathology in the abdomen or the contralateral leg.[8] In all patients, symptoms in the ipsilateral "study" leg were minimal. Patients were subsequently re-evaluated by repeat arteriography (if symptoms progressed) or duplex ultrasound imaging. After a mean follow-up of over 3 years, 72% of SFA stenoses did not progress, 28% did progress, and 17% occluded. For lesions that progressed, the average rate of stenosis progression was 12% diameter reduction per year, with a maximum predicted progression rate of 30% diameter reduction per year. When all lesions were considered (including those that were stable), the average rate of progression and the maximum predicted progression rate were 5% and 15% diameter reduction per year, respectively. Importantly, this study documented that anatomic disease progression was highly correlated with symptom progression. Other than symptom progression, only smoking history and contralateral SFA occlusion were predictive of accelerated stenosis progression in this series. Although this was a small study, we concluded that intervention for most asymptomatic SFA stenoses is not warranted because few would progress to occlusion, especially without new warning symptoms that could prompt endovascular intervention. Based on the maximum predicted stenosis progression rate, it is clear that stenoses of less than 70% diameter reduction can be safely followed by duplex scanning on an annual basis.

In an effort to better predict the natural history of individual SFA stenoses, we recently assessed the effect of SFA stenosis morphology on the rate of stenosis progression. For this study, we selected patients who initially underwent arteriography for occlusive disease in another location that documented asymptomatic SFA lesions, but who later required repeat arteriography for treatment of a symptomatic SFA stenosis or occlusion. We followed 98 distinct lesions in 19 patients for a mean of 32 months. Each lesion was characterized by location, length, percent stenosis, and initial morphologic appearance on arteriogram. Surprisingly, most lesions (78%) that progressed arose from areas of minimal disease (less than 20% stenosis), rather than from areas of pre-existing severe stenoses. Nearly all lesions (90%) progressing to occlusion were found in the adductor canal, and these lesions progressed at a more rapid rate than lesions in other areas (19% versus 10% diameter reduction/year). The length of these SFA stenoses, the details of morphology, and even the severity of the initial stenosis were not useful predictors of disease progression. Only lesion location in the adductor canal predicted both progression and subsequent occlusion. These data suggest that SFA occlusion is likely the result of rapid expansion of the diseased area, probably by plaque rupture or hemorrhage. These results also suggest that balloon angioplasty of asymptomatic SFA stenoses outside the adductor canal is unnecessary. Furthermore, even within the adductor canal, most occlusions arose from initially mildly stenotic lesions, while the more severe stenoses remained stable.

NATURAL HISTORY BY SYMPTOMS

Much more is known about the natural history of lower extremity atherosclerosis as it relates to patients' symptoms, although the estimates in different reports vary because of differences in presenting symptoms, atherosclerotic risk factors, anatomic disease location, and referral sampling bias of specific populations. Because patients with rest pain or tissue loss at the time of presentation are likely to undergo urgent surgical intervention, most natural history studies involve patients with intermittent claudication. We studied 91 patients with intermittent claudication who had been stable for at least 6 months.[6] In this group, the majority of patients had symptom progression within 2.5 years mean follow-up, with a surgical intervention rate of 9%/year. Of potential risk factors for symptom progression, only tobacco use, exercise, and ankle brachial indices (ABI) were helpful in predicting clinical outcome. Patients who had smoked at least 40 pack-years were 3.3 times more likely to have surgical intervention.

Patients who exercised to the limits of claudication once or twice daily were significantly less likely to have symptom progression. A decrease in ABI of 0.15 during follow-up was associated with a symptom progression rate twice that of patients with stable ABIs. Furthermore, patients with a significant decrease (greater than 0.15) in ABI were also 2.5 times more likely to require operations. These results have been reproduced in several other studies. In a review of 48 articles relating to the natural history of claudication, we found that smoking and reduced ABI at follow-up were consistently associated with a worse outcome in claudicants, whereas exercise was associated with improved outcome.[7] Regular exercise was associated with an average improvement in walking distance of 67%. Operative intervention in these compiled studies (representing over 1,600 patients) was 6%/year, with an amputation rate of 1%/year. Mortality in claudicants averages 6%/year, with the majority of deaths due to vascular causes such as myocardial infarction or stroke.

Risk factors clearly have prognostic significance in terms of the natural history of this patient population. Smoking cessation reduces the likelihood of symptom progression by 25%, the probability of amputation to nearly zero, the chance of tissue loss or operation by 75%, and mortality by over 50%.[7] Diabetics have a sevenfold higher amputation rate, a 100% greater chance of progression to tissue loss or operation, and a 100% higher mortality rate than the nondiabetic claudicant. Lower extremity atherosclerosis is an important marker for systemic disease that leads to death by myocardial infarction or stroke. One recent study documented that even a mildly abnormal ABI (0.9 or less) is a predictor for increased mortality (relative risk 4.1) and cardiovascular disease mortality (relative risk 3.7).[9] Thus, risk factor intervention has important implications for overall health as well as for lower extremity disease.

In contrast to intermittent claudication, much less is known about the natural history of patients presenting with ischemic rest pain or tissue loss. Although it is generally accepted that virtually all patients with "limb threat" eventually progress to limb loss, this is not borne out by the limited studies available. Prospective, randomized studies to evaluate the effect of prostaglandins on patients with ischemic rest pain or gangrenous ulcers have documented ulcer healing and/or improvement of rest pain in up to 50% of the placebo group. These short-term studies of patients with minimal tissue loss indicates that not all such patients truly have irreversible limb threat. Noninvasive testing in these patients can be helpful in determining the prognosis and the urgency of therapy. For instance, patients without pedal Doppler signals have high rates of limb loss and mortality, with or without revascularization. As with claudicants, patients presenting with ischemic rest pain or tissue loss are likely to have severe systemic atherosclerosis, and the previous statements regarding cardiovascular mortality and risk factor intervention apply. As one might expect, mortality rates for patients presenting with rest pain or tissue loss are worse than for claudicants, with 5 year survival rates approximating only 40%. Because patients presenting with severe lower extremity symptoms generally have more severe systemic disease, risk factor modification for asymptomatic patients with abnormal ABIs deserves attention. A great deal can be learned about the natural history, prognosis, indications for therapy, comorbidities, and mortality rates in these patients by performing a simple history and physical examination with attention to the peripheral arteries.

REFERENCES

1. Haimovici H. Patterns of arteriosclerotic lesions of the lower extremity. Arch Surg 1967; 95:918–933.
2. Logerfo FW, Coffman JD. Vascular and microvascular disease of the foot in diabetes. N Engl J Med 1984; 311:1615–1618.
3. Cronenwett JL, Davis JT Jr, Gooch JB, Garrett HE. Aortoiliac occlusive disease in women. Surgery 1980; 88:775–784.
4. O'Connor SE, Walsh DB, Zwolak RM, et al. Pelvic blood flow following aortobifemoral bypass with proximal end-to-side anastomosis. Ann Vasc Surg 1992; 6:493–498.
5. Schneider JR, Walsh DB, McDaniel MD, et al. Pedal bypass versus tibial bypass with autogenous vein: A comparison of outcome and hemodynamic results. J Vasc Surg 1993; 17:1029–1040.
6. Cronenwett JL, Warner KG, Zelenock GB, et al. Intermittent claudication: Current results of nonoperative management. Arch Surg 1984; 119:430–436.
7. McDaniel MD, Cronenwett JL. Basic data related to the natural history of intermittent claudication. Ann Vasc Surg 1991; 3:273–277.
8. Walsh DB, Gilbertson JJ, Zwolak RM, et al. The natural history of superficial femoral artery stenoses. J Vasc Surg 1991; 14:299–304.
9. Newman AB, Sutton-Tyrrell K, Vogt MT, Kuller LH. Morbidity and mortality in hypertensive adults with a low ankle/arm blood pressure index. JAMA 1993; 270:487–489.

SMOKING AND VASCULAR DISEASE

DAN J. HIGMAN, F.R.C.S
JANET T. POWELL, M.D., Ph.D.
ROGER M. GREENHALGH, M.D., M.Chir., F.R.C.S.

Cigarette smoking has been recognized as a risk factor for the development of atherosclerosis since the 1950s. The vascular surgeon considers smoking the single most important etiologic factor in patients with peripheral arterial disease or occlusive or aneurysmal aortic disease. This is perhaps in contrast to the experience of cardiologists and cardiac surgeons, who also recognize hyperlipidemia and a strong family history as common factors predisposing to coronary atherosclerosis. It is the central role of smoking, particularly in noncardiac vascular disease, that provides the need for an increased understanding of the effects of smoking on the vasculature.

BIOLOGY OF SMOKING INJURY

Precise mechanisms by which smoking induces the development of atherosclerosis are poorly understood, but injury to the vascular endothelium by the circulating products of smoking is probably the initial event. The effect of smoking to potentiate arterial thrombosis compounds the endothelial damage. One critical function of the endothelium is the control of vascular tone through the production of endothelium-derived relaxing factor (EDRF), which is known to be nitric oxide. The EDRF, in addition to being the major modulator of vasomotor tone, decreases platelet aggregation and adhesion and may have an important role in the maintenance of the endothelium as a permeability barrier. Studies on young, healthy volunteers have suggested that the endothelium-dependent relaxation of the superficial femoral artery is decreased in heavy smokers.[1] Our own research has documented that a similar reduction in endothelium-dependent relaxation occurs in the saphenous vein endothelium of smokers and that this is attributable to a diminished production of EDRF. The decrease in the production of EDRF is reversible, but several months of smoking cessation appear to be necessary before full endothelial function is restored. Similarly, the increases in plasma fibrinogen concentration and plasma viscosity associated with smoking are reversed after several months of smoking cessation. Platelet function also is adversely influenced by smoking, but there is no evidence concerning the reversal of this effect. Morphologic differences in the vascular endothelium between smokers and nonsmokers have been identified by transmission electron microscopy. The endothelial basal lamina of saphenous vein is grossly thickened and contains accumulations of fibronectin in smokers. Thickened basal lamina also have been reported from studies of the umbilical vasculature from babies born to smoking mothers. In addition to being a pathologic marker of smoking injury to the vascular endothelium, this thickening may interfere with the nutrient transport and normal signaling between the endothelium and the underlying vessel wall.

DETECTION OF SMOKING AMONG VASCULAR DISEASE PATIENTS

Nearly all patients with peripheral arterial disease have a long history of smoking. Many of these patients continue to smoke, even after medical advice to stop smoking. These patients may prefer to deceive the clinician about their current smoking habit rather than confess to not wanting to stop smoking or not being able to stop smoking. Nicotine is a powerful addictive drug. However, if accurate data about the complex relationship between smoking and vascular disease are to be obtained, objective measures of smoking habits among patients are required. Patients' accounts of their own smoking habits may be unreliable. For instance, in a study of patients undergoing femoropopliteal bypass, approximately 25% of patients had their claims to have stopped smoking refuted by the evidence from the measurement of smoking markers.[2] Objective markers of smoking include expired carbon monoxide, carboxyhemoglobin, and plasma and urinary cotinine. Cotinine is the principal metabolite of nicotine and has a half-life of about 18 hours. Therefore, cotinine provides a specific and convenient marker of smoking. Sometimes it is necessary to use a marker with a longer half-life. In these circumstances, plasma thiocyanate becomes the marker of choice because it has a half-life of over 6 days.

BENEFIT OF IDENTIFYING SMOKERS

Identification of patients with peripheral vascular disease who are still smoking can improve patient care and increase understanding of the natural history of arterial disease. In the clinical setting, the knowledge among patients that current smoking can be detected may provide an incentive for some to stop smoking. For those who continue, their identification allows for more effective targeting of antismoking counseling and assistance. Accurate information concerning current smoking habits allows the clinician to decide whether a deterioration in symptoms represents a real failure of maximal conservative measures such as cessation of smoking and increasing the amount of walking or whether continued covert smoking may be contributing to the deterioration. In Britain there has been considerable debate as to whether patients with intermittent claudication, which is inconvenient but not limb-threatening, should be eligible for arterial reconstruction or other palliative procedures if they continue to smoke. With this debate being public knowledge, there is an increased risk that current smokers will not admit to continuing tobacco usage. In this context it is more important than ever for the clinician to identify smokers accurately.

SMOKING AND DEVELOPMENT OF PERIPHERAL ARTERIAL DISEASE

Increasing awareness of the damaging effects of smoking upon health has caused the tobacco industry to modify its cigarettes and other products. Today cigarettes contain less tar and nicotine than in the past. However, there is no evidence that this modification of tobacco products has resulted in a reduced prevalence or severity of peripheral arterial disease. On the contrary, the incidence of another smoking-related disorder, abdominal aortic aneurysm, is increasing alarmingly. Interestingly, the smoking of hand-rolled, rather than manufactured, cigarettes has been associated particularly with death from ruptured aortic aneurysm.

Does the mode of smoking or the type of tobacco influence the development of peripheral arterial disease? From a case control study, just completed, of smokers with and without peripheral arterial disease, it is evident that two aspects of smoking are particularly associated with the development of peripheral arterial disease: an increased number of pack-years of smoking and the increasing depth of inhalation. The tar yield of cigarettes and age of onset of smoking appeared not to be contributory to the development of peripheral arterial disease.

SMOKING AND PROGRESSION OF ARTERIAL DISEASE

The relationship between the continuation of smoking and the progression of arterial disease is controversial. Some studies have documented marked benefits for smoking cessation, whereas others have failed to document any effect of secondary prevention. One condition where the necessity of stopping smoking is uncontroversial is in Buerger disease.

Commonly, peripheral arterial disease is just one manifestation of generalized atherosclerosis. Not surprisingly, patients with peripheral arterial disease have an increased cardiovascular morbidity and mortality. Peripheral arterial disease itself is not usually life-threatening. Several studies have indicated that smoking has most influence on the prognosis of intermittent claudication by increasing both cardiovascular and all-cause mortality. The British Regional Heart Study documented that the rate of heart attacks, stroke, and cardiovascular mortality increased significantly with increasing severity of calf pain, which itself was very strongly associated with current smoking.[3]

Stopping smoking and keeping active may reduce cardiovascular events in patients with established peripheral atherosclerosis. The advice to "stop smoking and keep walking" should be heeded.[4]

RECURRENCE OF DISEASE AFTER VASCULAR RECONSTRUCTION

The repertoire of vascular surgery includes carotid endarterectomy, aortic aneurysm repair, and distal revascularization procedures. In each instance the diseased artery is subjected to endarterectomy to leave exposed arterial media on the luminal surface or bypassed by autogenous vein or prosthetic material. The prosthetic aortic graft is of large diameter, and late complications of graft occlusion are rare. In contrast, there is a significant failure rate of the narrower femoropopliteal prosthetic graft. The failure rate increases further when the distal anastomosis extends to below the knee. The results of the United Kingdom Femoropopliteal Bypass Trial, where objective markers of smoking were used, documented the clear advantage of stopping smoking after a prosthetic distal bypass. Graft patency (polytetrafluororthylene or human umbilical vein) 2 years after bypass was 78% in nonsmokers and 57% in smokers.[5] For most surgeons, saphenous vein is the conduit of choice for femoropopliteal bypass. Approximately half the saphenous vein endothelium is lost or damaged in preparation for grafting. After transplantation into the arterial circulation, the vein "arterializes" or adapts to the new pressures and shear stresses. The saphenous vein bypass graft is vulnerable to occlusion from stenosis, intimal hyperplasia, or thrombosis during this period of adaptation. This vulnerability to occlusion appears to be greater in continuing smokers. Again, results from the U.K. Femoropopliteal Bypass Trial documented the superior patency of saphenous vein grafts after 1 year in nonsmokers (84%) as compared to smokers (63%) (Fig. 1).[2]

Some restenosis following carotid endarterectomy is common, but it is usually benign and asymptomatic. Severe restenosis is uncommon, and symptomatic restenosis is very uncommon. Nevertheless, the wide availability of duplex scanning has resulted in careful documentation of restenosis after carotid endarterectomy. Again, when objective markers of smoking have been used, the effect of smoking to potentiate restenosis has been documented. One year following endarterectomy, restenoses of greater than 50% developed twice as often in smokers as in nonsmokers.[6] The proliferation of smooth muscle cells, which causes restenosis after endarterectomy, also is the cause of restenosis after balloon angioplasty. The risk of restenosis following distal balloon angioplasty or atherectomy also may be higher in smokers, but the appropriate studies have not yet been performed.

Although in many patients the need for vascular reconstruction and the consequent period of hospitalization provide the necessary shock for stopping smoking, this may not be soon enough. Where vein is used as a bypass, the endothelium takes several months to repair the damage caused by smoking. Perhaps more impor-

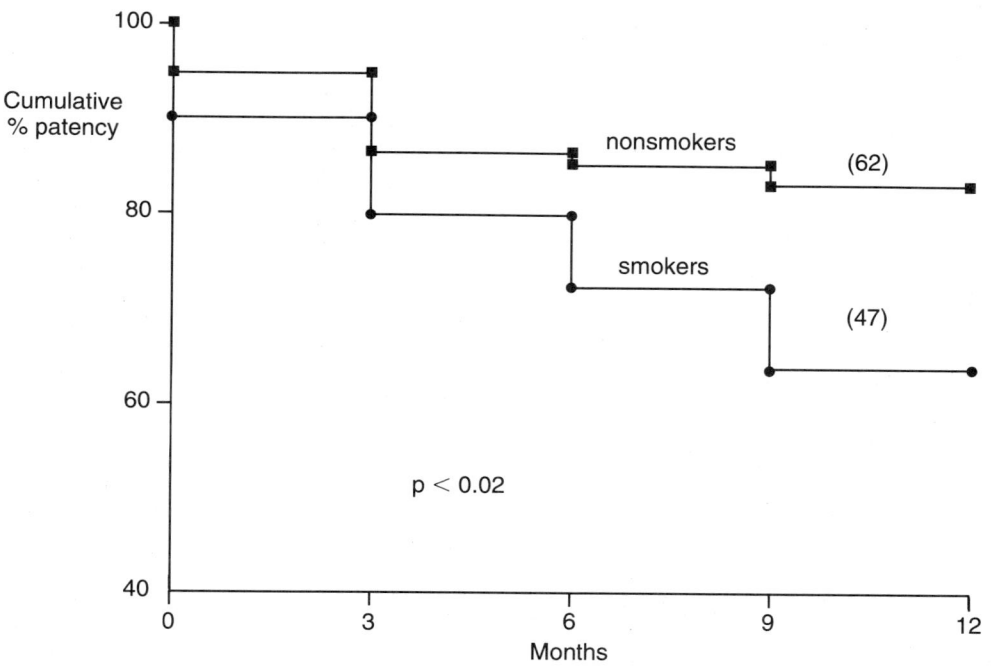

Figure 1 The patency of femoropopliteal vein bypass grafts. Smokers have serum thiocyanate concentration greater than 70 micromoles per liter, and nonsmokers have serum thiocyanate concentration less than 70 microcoles per liter. The number of patients with patent grafts is given in parentheses.

tant, smokers are at increased risk of postoperative pulmonary complications following anesthesia.[7,8] The benefits of smoking cessation, in the patient facing vascular reconstruction, are clear and overwhelming.

REFERENCES

1. Celermajer DS, Sorensen KE, Gooch VM, et al. Non-invasive detection of endothelial dysfunction in children and adults at risk of atherosclerosis. Lancet 1992; 340:1111–1115.
2. Wiseman S, Kenchington G, Dain R, et al. Influence of smoking and plasma factors on patency of femoropopliteal vein grafts. Br Med J 1989; 299:643–646.
3. Shaper AG, Wannamethee SG, Walker MK. Calf pain on walking, risk factors and cardiovascular outcome in middle aged British men. In: FGR Fowkes, ed. Epidemiology of peripheral vascular disease. New York: Springer-Verlag, 1991:127.
4. Housley E. Treating claudication in five words. Br Med J 1988; 296:1483.
5. Wiseman S, Powell JT, Greenhalgh RM, et al. The influence of smoking and plasma factors on prosthetic graft patency. Eur J Vasc Surg 1990; 4:57–61.
6. Cuming R, Worrell P, Woolcock NE, et al. The influence of smoking and lipids on restenosis after carotid endarterectomy. Eur J Vasc Surg 1993; 7:572–576.
7. Svensson LG, Hess KR, Coselli JS, et al. A prospective study of respiratory failure after high risk surgery on the thoracoabdominal aorta. J Vasc Surg 1991; 14:271–282.
8. Forrest JB, Rehdr K, Cohalan MK, Goldsmith CH. Multicenter study of general anaesthesia, III. Predictors of severe perioperative adverse outcomes. Anesthesiology 1992; 76:3–15.

TREATMENT OF HYPERLIPIDEMIA

DOROTHY M. KAHKONEN, M.D.

Over the past 10 years several primary prevention trials have documented that a decrease in cholesterol levels is associated with decreased cardiovascular morbidity and mortality.[1-3] The decreases in cholesterol ranged from 8.5% to 19%, with decreases in cardiovascular events from 10.6% to 34%. During the past 5 years, several secondary arteriographic trials have documented a lack of progression and/or regression of atherosclerosis with aggressive treatment of hypercholesterolemia.[4-6] The decreases in cholesterol ranged from 22.6% to 33.8% with more significant decreases in the LDL cholesterol and, in some instances, increases in HDL cholesterol. Evidence for regression of atherosclerotic lesions ranged from 16% to 18% in treated patients compared to 2% to 6% in patients on placebos.

At the present time it is evident that lowering cholesterol makes a difference in the risk of developing cardiovascular complications, and the only continuing controversy seems to be who should be treated. The question of whether to treat hypertriglyceridemia is not as easily answered. There is little controversy regarding the need for treatment of triglyceride levels greater than 1,000 mg/dl to prevent pancreatitis. There is some evidence in support of treating milder elevations of triglycerides from the Helsinki Heart Study.[3] The most significant improvement in this study was noted in patients with a combined elevation of cholesterol and triglycerides. Of note also is the 11% increase in HDL cholesterol in this study. The reciprocal changes in triglycerides and HDL cholesterol have been documented repeatedly.

Evaluation of patients with hyperlipidemia to determine whether any underlying conditions are producing a secondary form of hyperlipidemia is important. The most common of these conditions are diabetes mellitus, hypothyroidism, and renal disease. If any such conditions are identified, they need to be addressed, recognizing that the hyperlipidemia may also need to be treated. Complete resolution of some underlying or contributing conditions such as diabetes and renal diseases can be difficult; therefore, the secondary component of hyperlipidemia cannot be eliminated completely. The other problem is that a primary hyperlipidemia can exist and is exacerbated by one of these causes of secondary hyperlipidemia. In these situations, the hyperlipidemia will persist in spite of therapy and require specific therapy.

LIPOPROTEINS

The major lipoproteins are very-low-density lipoprotein (VLDL), which is the primary carrier for triglycerides; low-density lipoprotein (LDL), which is the primary carrier for cholesterol; intermediate-density lipoprotein (IDL), which carries almost equal amounts of cholesterol and triglycerides; and high-density lipoprotein (HDL), which is involved in reverse cholesterol transport and has an inverse correlation with coronary artery disease. Excess levels of LDL and IDL are associated with premature atherosclerosis. The relationship of VLDL to atherosclerosis remains uncertain. The contribution of VLDL to atherosclerosis may occur through its effects on HDL (decrease) or its effects on the LDL to produce small, dense particles that are atherogenic. Elevations of VLDL, whether directly or indirectly, may contribute to atherosclerosis in diabetics and seem to deserve a more aggressive approach in that population.

The small, dense LDL-cholesterol particles are a subclass of LDL cholesterol that contain a greater proportion of protein (Apo B-100) than the more lipid-rich normal particles. These small particles are associated with elevations of triglycerides, LDL, and IDL cholesterol, decreased levels of HDL cholesterol, and a threefold increase in the risk of coronary artery disease. These small particles are more susceptible to oxidation than the normal particles, which may be the link to the development of atherosclerosis. It is of interest that these small, dense LDL particles are increased in individuals with non–insulin-dependent diabetes mellitus, the population at increased risk for atherosclerosis.

CLINICAL EVALUATION OF LIPID DISORDERS

Measurements of serum total cholesterol, triglycerides, and HDL cholesterol with calculation of the LDL cholesterol provide the basis for institution of treatment in virtually all patients. Screening cholesterol measurements in population studies can be nonfasting; however, if levels are elevated, fasting studies will be required so that accurate triglyceride and HDL cholesterol measurements are obtained and the LDL cholesterol can be calculated. The technology for direct LDL cholesterol measurement is developing rapidly, and a reliable test suitable for clinical use should soon be widely available.

If patients are being evaluated because of the presence of vascular disease or have a family history of premature vascular disease (younger than 55 years in men and 65 years in women), fasting studies are recommended initially. They provide the HDL cholesterol, and being certain it is not low in these individuals is important. The measurements of cholesterol can vary within a laboratory coefficient of variation of 3% to 5% in the best of laboratories and an additional 4% to 12% biologic variation. If triglyceride levels are also in-

Table 1 Classification Based on Total and LDL Cholesterol Levels

Cholesterol Level	LDL Cholesterol Level	Classification
< 200 mg/dl	< 130 mg/dl	Desirable levels
200–239 mg/dl	130–159 mg/dl	Borderline-high levels
≥ 240 mg/dl	≥ 160 mg/dl	High levels

Table 2 Coronary Heart Disease Risk Factors

Positive
  Age
    Men ≥ 45 years
    Women ≥ 55 years or premature menopause without estrogen replacement
  Family history of premature CHD
  Smoking
  Hypertension
  HDL cholesterol < 35 mg/dl
  Diabetes mellitus
Negative
  HDL cholesterol ≥ 60 mg/dl

Table 3 Treatment Based on LDL Cholesterol Levels

Patient Category	Initiation Level	LDL Goal
Dietary Therapy		
Without CHD and < 2 risk factors	≥ 160 mg/dl	< 160 mg/dl
Without CHD and ≥ 2 risk factors	≥ 130 mg/dl	< 130 mg/dl
With CHD or other atherosclerosis	> 100 mg/dl	≤ 100 mg/dl
Drug Therapy		
Without CHD or other atherosclerosis and < 2 risk factors	≥ 190 mg/dl	< 160 mg/dl
Without CHD or other atherosclerosis and ≥ 2 risk factors	≥ 160 mg/dl	< 130 mg/dl
With CHD or other atherosclerosis	≥ 130 mg/dl	≤ 100 mg/dl

CHD = Coronary heart disease.

creased, the measurements can be even more variable. Triglycerides can change remarkably within 24 to 48 hours of dietary changes, the use of alcohol, or the addition or subtraction of medications. Both total and HDL cholesterol levels can be affected by hypertriglyceridemia. For these reasons, repeat studies are recommended to confirm the presence of high-risk status prior to initiation of treatment.

Isolated elevation of cholesterol levels is present in familial hypercholesterolemia, which occurs as a heterozygous abnormality in 1 in 500 people. At present, four classes of genetic mutations that produce defective LDL cholesterol have been identified. However, these account for only approximately 20% of the hypercholesterolemia identified. The remaining 80% are considered polygenic hypercholesterolemia secondary to a combination of genetic and environmental factors or familial combined hyperlipidemia, which is due to elevated apo B and can present with increased VLDL levels, increased LDL levels, or a combination of both. In familial combined hyperlipidemia the family history is less significant than in familial hypercholesterolemia, and different phenotypes can occur within a single family. This form of hypercholesterolemia is rarely associated with xanthomas. The prevalence of familial combined hyperlipidemia is estimated at five times that of familial hypercholesterolemia and affects approximately 1% of the population.

The National Cholesterol Education Program (NCEP) Adult Treatment Panel II published updated recommendations for cholesterol management in June 1993.[7] The classification of total and LDL cholesterol levels remains the same (Table 1). The major changes are in the emphasis on coronary heart disease (CHD) risk status as a guide to therapy and more attention to HDL cholesterol as a CHD risk factor. The CHD risk is deemed increased in men over the age of 45 and in women who are over the age of 55 or postmenopausal (Table 2). The presence of CHD, cerebrovascular disease, or occlusive peripheral vascular disease identifies patients who are at highest risk, and lower target levels for LDL cholesterol are recommended (Table 3). The results of the secondary arteriographic trials have provided the impetus for more aggressive treatment of patients with documented vascular disease. The latest NCEP guidelines also emphasize, along with diet, physical activity and weight loss as components of the initial therapeutic approach to management of high blood cholesterol levels.

DIETARY THERAPY

The major dietary concerns regarding cholesterol levels are the intake of cholesterol and saturated fat and the presence of obesity. Dietary intake of cholesterol affects synthesis and ultimately numbers of LDL receptors. Dietary sources of saturated fat affect the affinity or binding ability of the LDL receptors. Obesity leads to overproduction of lipoproteins. The usual American diet in the 1990s contains 300 to 400 mg of cholesterol, 35% to 40% of total calories as fat, and 14% to 20% of total calories as saturated fat. The American Heart Association has recommended a step I diet with 30% of total calories as fat, 10% of total calories as saturated fat, and less than 300 mg of cholesterol. A more restricted diet, step II, includes less than 20% of total calories as fat, less than 7% of total calories as saturated fat, and less than 200 mg of cholesterol. Finally, the most restricted diet limits total fat to 15% to 20% of calories, saturated fat to 5% of calories, and cholesterol to 100 mg/day. Total caloric recommendations should be designed to promote the achievement or maintenance of ideal body weight.

Additional issues to consider with regard to diet include replacement of saturated fat with monounsaturated or polyunsaturated fatty acids; the use of increased fiber, antioxidants, and garlic; and the addition of omega-3 supplements. Studies comparing polyunsaturated fatty acids with monounsaturated fatty acids have documented variable results. Both lower cholesterol, with a more beneficial effect on triglycerides with polyunsaturated fatty acids and a more beneficial effect on HDL cholesterol levels with monounsaturated fatty acids. The interest in soluble fiber has been long-standing and may account for an additional 5% to 10% reduction in cholesterol levels. The use of antioxidants (beta-carotene, vitamins C and E) has been encouraged by some because of the evidence indicating that oxidation of LDL cholesterol facilitates development of atherosclerosis. It is recommended that increased amounts of fruit and vegetables be included in the diet and a vitamin E supplement of 400 I.U./day can be added. The prospective scientific data supporting the use of antioxidant supplements are lacking. The data available are from small, poorly controlled studies using vitamin E or retrospective data from the U.S. Physician's and Nurse's Health Studies, where dietary intake of these items was assessed and intake inversely correlated with coronary disease was found. The evidence for a small (5% to 10%) reduction in cholesterol by garlic seems real. The omega-3 supplements decrease VLDL synthesis, and whether there are any antiatherogenic effects not related to lipids remains unanswered.

Overall predictions for cholesterol reductions with dietary therapy range from 15% to 30%, depending on the amount of cholesterol and saturated fat ingested prior to modification of the diet. Individuals with associated triglyceride elevations respond better to diet than those with isolated elevations of cholesterol. If the abnormalities are mild to moderate and patients are well motivated and disciplined, dietary therapy may be all that is required.

PHARMACOLOGIC THERAPY

If treatment goals are not achieved in asymptomatic individuals after 6 to 18 months of diet and lifestyle changes, drug therapy should be considered. The LDL cholesterol levels, along with the CHD risk status, determine who should be treated. The LDL cholesterol level is also used to monitor drug therapy, with adjustments in dose or changes in drugs dependent upon the response and ability to achieve the target level (Table 3). The lowest-risk individuals are men younger than 35 years of age and premenopausal women who have no CHD risk factors. Drug therapy can be delayed in these individuals or initiated at LDL cholesterol levels greater than 220 mg/dl. The highest-risk individuals are those with CHD or other atherosclerotic disease, for whom the initiation of drug therapy is recommended at LDL cholesterol levels greater than 130 mg/dl and the target LDL cholesterol level less than 100 mg/dl. In my practice these individuals are frequently started on dietary therapy and drug therapy concomitantly.

There are two other groups to consider for drug therapy. The first is a moderately high-risk group without CHD or other atherosclerosis but with two or more risk factors. Drug therapy is recommended for persistent LDL cholesterol levels above 160 mg/dl. The second group is considered low risk without CHD or other atherosclerosis and one or no risk factors. Drug therapy is recommended in this group for LDL cholesterol levels greater than 190 mg/dl.

The HMG-CoA reductase inhibitors or statins (lovastatin, pravatatin, and simvastatin) provide the greatest efficacy with the fewest side effects in lowering cholesterol. Twenty percent to 40% reductions in LDL cholesterol can be achieved with these drugs.

They can be used safely if one remembers the potential for hepatic toxicity and myositis. Their single disadvantage is cost. A recent report is the first to document slower progression and increased frequency of regression of coronary artery lesions in patients treated with a statin (lovastatin) and diet.[8] These drugs are used whenever possible as the initial drug in patients with CHD or other atherosclerosis. They are likely to be the first choice also in patients with severe hypercholesterolemia. The frequency and severity of myositis with these drugs increase when they are used in combination with gemfibrozil, cyclosporine, and, less frequently, nicotinic acid.

Nicotinic acid is also a potent cholesterol-lowering drug with reported decreases from 20% to 30%. It also lowers triglycerides 20% to 50% and has a beneficial effect on HDL cholesterol, increasing it 15% to 25%. It is inexpensive, but the side effects and toxicity limit its use (Table 4).

Bile acid sequestrants or resins produce more modest decreases in cholesterol (15% to 20%), are very safe, and are intermediate to expensive in cost. However, they produce significant side effects. The most appropriate use of these drugs seems to be in smaller doses in mild hypercholesterolemia or in combination with either a statin or nicotinic acid.

Probucol is considered a minor cholesterol-lowering drug. It decreases total and LDL cholesterol levels 10% to 15%. Experimental studies have documented an ability to block oxidation of LDL, which may be of value in the prevention of atherosclerosis. The side effects are few, with only occasional mild gastrointestinal symptoms and reports of effects on cardiac conduction in animals.

Fibric acid derivatives are most effective in lowering triglycerides (30% to 50%) and increasing HDL cholesterol (10% to 20%), with only modest changes in total and LDL cholesterol (10% to 20%). Gemfibrozil and clofibrate are available in the United States. Fenofibrate is used widely in Europe and is also available in Canada. These drugs are well tolerated and should be considered first-line drugs for the treatment of hypertriglyceridemia. Gemfibrozil is generally used first because it is more potent than clofibrate and less lithogenic. These drugs are considered minor cholesterol-lowering drugs and are used to lower cholesterol only when there is an associated elevation of triglycerides. Combination of fibric acid derivatives and statins is not recommended

Table 4 Doses and Side Effects of Lipid-Lowering Drugs

	Initial Dose	Maximum Dose	Side Effects and Toxicity
Statins			
Lovastatin	20 mg q.d.	80 mg q.d.	Hepatic toxicity, myositis
Pravastatin	10 mg q.d.	40 mg q.d.	Hepatic toxicity, myositis
Simvastatin	10 mg q.d.	40 mg q.d.	Hepatic toxicity, myositis
Nicotinic acid	250–500 mg/day	3–4 g/day	Hepatic toxicity, skin and GI symptoms
Resins			
Cholestyramine	4–8 g/day	20–24 g/day	GI symptoms and hypertriglyceridemia
Colestipol	5–10 g/day	25–30 g/day	GI symptoms and hypertriglyceridemia
Probucol	500–1,000 mg/day	1,000 mg/day	GI symptoms, possible conduction effects
Fibric acids			
Gemfibrozil	600–1,200 mg/day	1,200 mg/day	GI symptoms, hepatic toxicity, potentiates myositis, cholelithiasis
Clofibrate	500–1,000 mg/day	2,000 mg/day	Effects same as gemfibrozil

GI = Gastrointestinal.

because of the increased risk of myositis and rhabdomyolysis.

Estrogen replacement therapy can be used in postmenopausal women to achieve a more favorable lipid profile. The effects generally are to decrease the LDL cholesterol and increase the HDL cholesterol. Women with hypertriglyceridemia can exhibit an adverse effect with estrogen therapy, resulting in even higher triglycerides, increased total and LDL cholesterol, and decreased HDL cholesterol. Once estrogen replacement has been instituted, triglyceride levels should be monitored along with the cholesterol during the early weeks of treatment.

Aggressive management of hyperlipidemia in the primary prevention trials has been shown to decrease cardiovascular morbidity and mortality with no improvement in all-cause mortality at the time the studies were completed. This seems to be a time-related phenomenon, and review after an extended time period in three studies (Coronary Drug Project, Multiple Risk Factor Intervention Trial, and the Program on the Surgical Control of Hyperlipidemia) has now documented a decrease in both overall mortality and cardiovascular mortality. Effective therapeutic options are now available and should be utilized.

REFERENCES

1. Lipid Research Clinics Program. The lipid research clinics coronary primary prevention trial results 1. Reduction in the incidence of coronary heart disease. JAMA 1984; 251:351–364.
2. Multiple Risk Factor Intervention Trial Research Group. Multiple risk factor intervention trial: Risk factor changes and mortality results. JAMA 1988; 248:1465–1477.
3. Manninen V, Elo MO, Frick MH, et al. Lipid alterations and decline in the incidence of coronary heart disease in the Helsinki Heart Study. JAMA 1988; 260:641–651.
4. Blankenhorn DH, Nessim SA, Johnson RL, et al. Beneficial effects of combined colestipol-niacin therapy on coronary atherosclerosis and coronary venous bypass grafts. JAMA 1987; 247:3233–3240.
5. Brown G, Albers JJ, Fisher LF, et al. Regression of coronary artery disease as a result of intensive lipid-lowering therapy in men with high levels of apolipoprotein B. N Engl J Med 1990; 323:1289–1298.
6. Kane JP, Mallory MJ, Ports TA, et al. Regression of coronary atherosclerosis during treatment of familial hypercholesterolemia with combined drug regimens. JAMA 1990; 264:3007–3012.
7. Expert Panel on Detection Evaluation and Treatment of High Blood Cholesterol in Adults. Summary of the second report of the NCEP expert panel (Adult Treatment Panel II). JAMA 1993; 269:3015–3023.
8. Blankenhorn DH, Azen SP, Kramsch DM, et al. Coronary angiographic changes with lovastatin therapy. Ann Intern Med 1993; 119:969–976.

HYPERTENSION AS A RISK FACTOR IN ATHEROSCLEROTIC CARDIOVASCULAR DISEASE

ALAN B. WEDER, M.D.

Hypertension is one of the major remediable risks for atherosclerotic cardiovascular disease. Atherosclerotic complications of this risk factor, primarily coronary heart disease, represent the most common fatal and nonfatal outcomes of long-standing hypertension. The National Health and Nutrition Examination Survey III (NHANES III), conducted between 1988 and 1991, documented that some 50 million Americans have elevated blood pressures, defined as a sustained systolic blood pressure (SBP) of 140 mm Hg or greater and/or a diastolic blood pressure (DBP) of 90 mm Hg or greater and/or current treatment with antihypertensive medications.[1] Of these, some 65% have been told by a physician of their condition, and 49% are taking medications. These figures represent improvements in the rates for detection and treatment of hypertensive individuals over previous surveys performed in the 1970s, but distressingly, from NHANES III findings, it is estimated that only 21% of hypertensive individuals are actually controlled at acceptable blood pressure levels.[1] Thus, untreated and poorly controlled hypertension continues to contribute importantly to cardiovascular morbidity and mortality.

ATHEROSCLEROTIC CARDIOVASCULAR RISK FACTORS IN HYPERTENSION

Epidemiologic studies, most importantly the Framingham Heart Study, documented that the cardiovascular risk associated with increasing blood pressure is continuous and graded in both sexes and at all ages and is related to both the systolic and diastolic components of blood pressure. These same studies established that the cardiovascular risk associated with hypertension is additive to that of multiple other risk factors; thus, the prediction of coronary and cerebrovascular risk in hypertensive patients requires evaluation of historical, demographic, biochemical, and structural cardiovascular characteristics.

Although in the determination of risk, blood pressure level is treated as an independent, additive contributing variable, it has long been recognized that hypertension is rarely found in isolation. Recent findings in the Tecumseh Blood Pressure Study of young adults suggest that in borderline hypertensive patients (and even in patients with "office" or "white coat" hypertension, whose blood pressure is actually normal in natural settings and elevated only during clinic visits), hypertension is frequently accompanied by a spectrum of other risk factors.[2] Based on data from the Tecumseh Blood Pressure Study, it appears that there are multiple interrelationships of blood pressure and other cardiovascular risk factors (Fig. 1).

Why hypertension is so commonly associated with other risk factors for cardiovascular disease remains unknown, but the possibility that this clustering reflects some common underlying mechanism has led to much current interest in identifying links between the metabolic and hemodynamic features of hypertension. Recently, attention has focused on the intimate relationship of hypertension and insulin resistance. Insulin resistance is a state in which insulin-stimulated glucose uptake by tissues is impaired, resulting in a need for higher blood insulin concentrations in order to maintain glucose homeostasis. There is wide agreement that insulin resistance and hypertension commonly coexist, and two theories have been proposed to explain the link. The first suggests that insulin resistance is the prime mover and that elevated plasma levels of insulin resulting from insulin resistance act on cardiovascular effector systems such as vascular smooth muscle cells, renal tubules, and sympathetic neurons to promote hypertension and also to lead to hyperlipidemia. Julius and co-workers have proposed an alternative hemodynamic explanation in which the vasoconstriction of skeletal muscle vascular beds in hypertensive patients impedes delivery of insulin and glucose and causes insulin resistance.[2] In this construct, insulin resistance is a consequence rather than a cause of hypertension. Both theories have support. Although neither is proven, the controversy created by the competing hypotheses has provided impetus to investigators attempting to explain the clustering of risk factors so frequently observed in hypertensives.

Our present understanding of the elements contributing to cardiovascular risk in individual hypertensive patients remains incomplete, and the list of risk factors continues to grow. As noted, hyperinsulinemia frequently accompanies hypertension, and levels of plasma insulin as well as plasma glucose have been identified as risk factors for heart disease in several studies. Other common concomitants of hypertension, including elevated serum uric acid and creatinine levels and the presence of microalbuminuria, are also associated with increased cardiovascular risk. Increased activity of the renin-angiotensin system, which has long been thought to be a possible causal agent in hypertension, has been linked to adverse cardiac outcomes. In an analysis of hypertensive men initially classified by renin profiling, it was noted that after 8 years those with high plasma renin activity were 5.3 times more likely to have suffered heart attacks than those with low renin levels.[3] The atherogenic potential of elements of the hemostatic system has continued to receive attention. Fibrinogen level has been shown to be directly related to blood pressure, and elevated fibrinogen seems to confer an increased risk for coronary heart disease that is roughly equivalent to the other major traditional risk factors. Lipoprotein (a), which shares structural homology with plasminogen, is

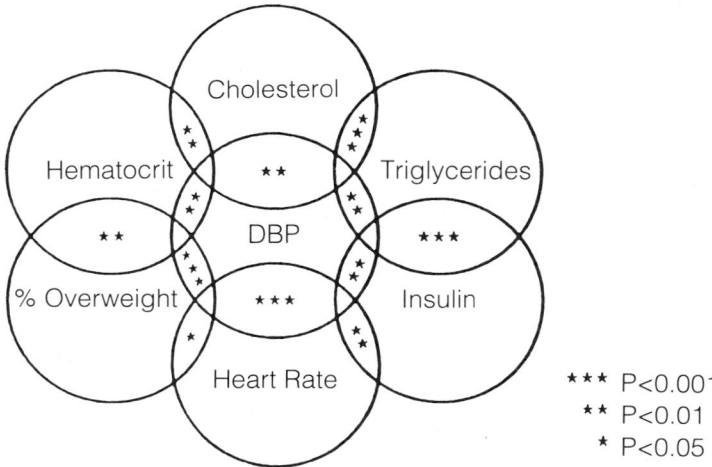

Figure 1 The constellation of coronary heart disease (CHD) risk factors associated with diastolic blood pressure (DBP) level.

also emerging as a significant modifier of cardiovascular risk. The list of new risk factors is growing and, with it, our ability to predict risk. Some of the exciting future areas will derive from our increasingly detailed understanding of the genetics of hypertension.

GENETICS OF HYPERTENSION

Observations of the clustering of hypertension in twins, relatives, and families has led to considerable interest in the genetic basis of hypertension. All approaches have yielded rather consistent evidence that hypertension is a heritable disease in which about 20% to 40% of blood pressure variability can be explained by polygenic factors, and genetic syndromes contributing to cardiovascular risk are beginning to be identified. Recently described is the syndrome of familial dyslipidemic hypertension, defined as a familial occurrence of early onset (before age 60) hypertension in two or more siblings coupled with the presence of one or more blood lipid abnormalities (high total cholesterol, LDL cholesterol or triglycerides or low HDL cholesterol).[4] Persons with familial dyslipidemic hypertension have substantially increased risk of coronary heart disease, and they and their relatives should be screened early for lipid abnormalities and hypertension with consideration toward aggressive follow-up and treatment.

Recently, specific genes contributing to hypertension and cardiovascular risk have been identified, and considerable future effort will be required before there is understanding of the genetic architecture of hypertension. Already, however, new insights into the role of individual gene products in mediating cardiovascular risk are emerging. One particularly intriguing observation concerns a polymorphism in the structure of the angiotensin-converting enzyme (ACE) gene. Two alleles defined by the insertion or deletion of a piece of DNA within the ACE gene have been identified, and genetic epidemiologic studies have documented that in subjects otherwise at low coronary risk as defined by traditional risk factors, homozygosity for the deletion polymorphism increases heart attack risk 3.2-fold compared to heterozygotes or individuals homozygous for the insertion genotype.[5] Whether such observations will be confirmed is unknown, and the application of this kind of genetic analysis to risk stratification is still in its infancy. Still, the ability to define risk genotypically, perhaps before phenotypic traits develop and begin to cause harm, would be a great boon to preventive strategies.

IMPORTANCE OF CARDIOVASCULAR ADAPTATIONS IN HYPERTENSION

Regardless of the cause of hypertension, almost as soon as blood pressure rises, the cardiovascular system begins to undergo adaptive changes, most importantly, vascular and cardiac hypertrophy. In most blood vessels such hypertrophy concentrically thickens vessel walls, causing encroachment on the vascular lumen and resulting in an increased wall-lumen ratio. The geometry of this vascular adaptation serves to amplify vasoconstrictor influences, thereby facilitating the maintenance of hypertension through increased vascular resistance.

The heart also undergoes adaptive changes in hypertension. As with blood vessels, concentric hypertrophy is common, although other geometries are also observed, such as eccentric hypertrophy and concentric remodeling. Studies in Framingham, Massachusetts, documented that the presence of left ventricular hypertrophy (LVH) increases atherosclerotic heart disease risk, but the method used to detect LVH in those studies, electrocardiography, was quite insensitive. The application of echocardiography to studies of the hypertensive heart led to marked improvement in the ability to detect LVH, and recent data suggest that echocardiographically defined LVH is a potent risk factor for cardiovascular disease.[6] Whether routine echocardiographic evaluation of all hypertensives is warranted is debatable, but the demonstrable risk associated with echocardiographically detected LVH, the tendency for LVH to regress during effective antihypertensive therapy, and results from early intervention trials suggesting that there may be differences in the ability of the various classes of antihypertensive drugs to promote regression all suggest that echocardiography will become increasingly important in the evaluation and treatment of hypertension.

TREATING HYPERTENSION TO REDUCE CARDIOVASCULAR RISK

Pharmacologic antihypertensive therapy is a remarkable triumph of empiricism because with no certain understanding of the underlying cause of hypertension, treating its only obvious manifestation by lowering blood pressure has provided protection against adverse outcomes. It is as if treating fever cured pneumococcal pneumonia. However, therapeutic success has not been unqualified. Whereas early intervention trials examining the impact of pharmacologic antihypertensive therapy documented a definite reduction in stroke, the evidence for reduction in heart attack risk was not as compelling. This observation led to the concept that stroke is a "pressure-related" complication, whereas coronary artery disease is multifactorial and less amenable to antihypertensive treatment. A recent meta-analysis of the large treatment trials confirms this to be the case. MacMahon and colleagues confirmed, in a review of populational surveys, that the risk of stroke and heart attack is directly and continuously related to the level of blood pressure, with no threshold below which lower blood pressure is not associated with lower risk.[7] They used survey data to estimate the effect to be expected from antihypertensive treatment in intervention trials. In the 14 trials reviewed in their meta-analysis, which included some 37,000 individuals randomized chiefly to either diuretics or beta-blockers and followed for an average of about 5 years, DBP fell on average some 5 to 6 mm Hg.[8] Using risk estimates from the epidemiologic observational studies, this magnitude of blood pressure lowering would be expected to confer a 35% to 40% reduction in stroke risk. In fact, the trial outcomes showed a reduction of 42% in stroke incidence. Thus, stroke risk related to hypertension apparently can be fully reversed by effective antihypertensive therapy with diuretics or beta-blockers. The story with coronary disease is different. Lowering blood pressure did reduce the heart attack rate but did not fully reverse the risk. Observational data suggested that a 5 to 6 mm Hg reduction in blood pressure should be associated with an approximately 20% to 25% reduction in coronary risk, but the trial data documented only a 14% reduction in actual heart attacks.[8] Thus, the suspicion that not all coronary risk associated with hypertension is mediated by the level of blood pressure seems correct.

Such analyses have led some to suggest that the specific therapeutic agents employed in the large randomized trials, diuretics and beta-blockers, have side effects, such as their modest but rather consistently reported dyslipidemic effects and their negative impact on insulin sensitivity, that could counterbalance part of the expected benefit of blood pressure lowering. Such thinking has led to increasing use of the newer classes of agents, the angiotensin-converting enzyme inhibitors, calcium channel blockers, and alpha-blockers, as primary therapy because of their beneficial effects on lipids and glucose-insulin metabolism. Often overlooked is that none of these new agents has been examined rigorously for effects on heart attack or stroke rates in large randomized controlled trials similar to those in which the efficacy of diuretics and beta-blockers has been established. Nevertheless, it is argued that it is logical to expect that the apparently salutary effects of the newer antihypertensives on surrogate end points will translate into improved survival and fewer morbid events. Although such speculations are rational and attractive, they are fueled in large part by hope and pharmaceutical industry money, and the results of several ongoing trials evaluating the impact of these new agents on cardiovascular outcomes will be welcome. In the meantime, the Joint National Committee on the Detection, Evaluation, and Treatment of Hypertension has recommended the use of diuretics and beta-blockers as first-line therapy in milder degrees of hypertension in the patients with no contraindications to those agents.[1]

TREATING HYPERTENSION IN THE ELDERLY

Another controversial therapeutic issue has been that of treating hypertension in the elderly. With aging, SBP rises continuously; DBP peaks in the sixth decade and remains unchanged or declines slightly thereafter. Systolic accentuation leads to progressive widening of the pulse pressure in patients with diastolic hypertension (disproportionate systolic hypertension) and to the development of elevated SBP in many individuals with normal DBP, termed isolated systolic hypertension. It was held for many years that isolated elevated SBP in the elderly was merely a surrogate for progressive aortic stiffening from atherosclerosis and that specific therapy was unwarranted except in extreme cases. Some even contended that elevated blood pressure represented a useful adaptation to serve the needs of diseased coronary and cerebral vascular beds and worried that lowering blood pressure could precipitate heart attacks and strokes. This concern was fueled by the demonstration of a "J-curve" for mortality in treated hypertensives. In one study, patients with the lowest DBP during treatment had somewhat higher cardiac mortality than those with "optimally controlled" levels (DBP between 85 and 90 mm Hg). Above those levels, such as in poorly controlled hypertensives, mortality rose as expected. Thus, it was suggested that it could be harmful to patients, particularly those with extant coronary disease, to lower DBP somewhat below conventional goals, which is often a necessary consequence of lowering SBP in patients with isolated or disproportionate systolic hypertension.

Several of the early major trials of hypertension treatment included elderly individuals, but none was large enough to prove definitively either a benefit of treatment or an absence of harm in potentially susceptible subgroups. Recently, however, three large trials of the treatment of hypertension in the elderly have been completed, and the results are clear and consistent. Treatment of elderly individuals with either combined systolic-diastolic or isolated systolic hypertension prevents strokes and heart attacks[1] (Table 1). Regarding the debate on whether there is an optimal target level of blood pressure to strive for, none of these trials is conclusive. The common clinical scenario in which treatment for isolated hypertension results in a decline in DBP well below 90 mm Hg is one for which we still have no definite resolution. Current recommendations are to target treatment for DBP to 90 mm Hg in combined systolic-diastolic hypertension and SBP to 140 to 160 mm Hg in isolated or disproportionate systolic hypertension, accepting whatever DBP results.

A NEW EMPHASIS: PRIMARY PREVENTION OF HYPERTENSION

Essential hypertension and atherosclerosis are diseases of acculturation. The high prevalence of hypertension and atherosclerosis in the modern world is a direct result of the population-wide impact of the changes humans have experienced as we moved from a nomadic hunter-gatherer lifestyle to stable, initially agriculture-based and subsequently urbanized and industrialized societies. In reality, diseases such as hypertension and atherosclerosis are part of the price we pay for an environment of dietary excess, prolonged longevity, and diminished physical activity. Although studies of primitive populations and migrations establish that the biology of humans does not dictate that any of us must have hypertension or atherosclerosis, our biology apparently does result in a high incidence of hypertension, hypercholesterolemia, and other atherosclerotic risk factors if we choose to live as we currently do.

It is important to recognize how the environment contributes to the epidemic of hypertension and atherosclerosis in our society. In many environmentally induced diseases, such as those produced by toxins or infectious agents, where the exposure of individuals to the disease-producing agent is the direct cause of disease, individual factors such as susceptibility and

Table 1 Effects of Therapy in Older Hypertensive Patients

	EWPHE	MRC	SHEP
Number of patients	840	4,396	4,736
Age range, years	>60	65–74	≥60
Mean blood pressure at entry (mm Hg)	182/101	185/91	170/77
Relative risk of event (treated vs control)			
Stroke	0.64	0.75*	0.67*
CAD	0.80	0.81	0.73*
CHF	0.78	—	0.45*
All CVD	0.71*	0.83*	0.68*

EWPHE = European Working Party on High Blood Pressure in the Elderly; MRC = Medical Research Council; SHEP = Systolic Hypertension in the Elderly Program; CAD = coronary artery disease; CHF = congestive heart failure; CVD = cardiovascular disease.
*Statistically significant.
Adapted from Joint National Committee on Detection, Evaluation, and Treatment of High Blood Pressure. The fifth report of the Joint National Committee on Detection, Evaluation, and Treatment of High Blood Pressure (JNCV). Arch Intern Med 1993; 153:154–183; with permission.

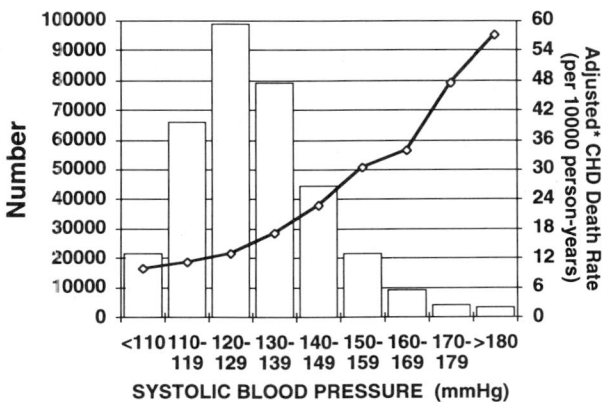
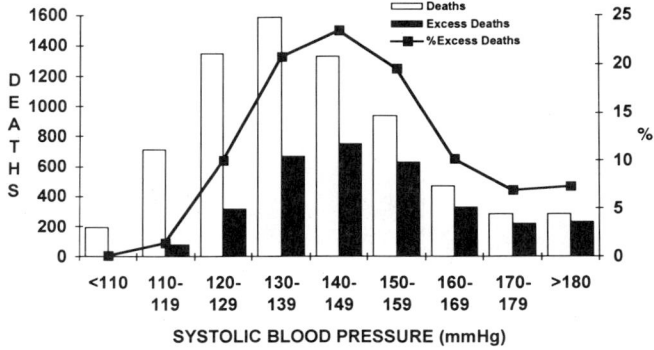

Figure 2 A, Relationship of systolic blood pressure (SBP) to coronary heart disease (CHD) risk in male screenees of the Multiple Risk Factor Intervention Trial (MRFIT). Number of individuals in each systolic blood pressure interval is indicated by height of bar. Adjusted CHD risk indicated by line. B, Relationship of CHD deaths to level of SBP in MRFIT screenees expressed as absolute deaths (*open bars*), excess deaths attributed to SBP with SBP < 110 mm Hg taken as baseline (*closed bars*) and % excess deaths (*line*). (Adapted from Stamler J, Stamler R, Neaton JD. Blood pressure, systolic and diastolic, and cardiovascular risks. Arch Intern Med 1993; 153:598–615; with permission.)

duration of exposure are critical determinants of whether one contracts disease. However, for hypertension and probably for many other diseases of civilization, agents implicated in promoting disease, such as calorie and salt excess, are essentially universally and continuously active. It has been shown that the prevalence of a disease like hypertension, which is defined by an arbitrary limit drawn within the continuous distribution of blood pressure, is directly and closely dependent on the populational mean value.[9] Thus, the high prevalence of hypertension in societies such as the United States reflects a shift of the entire population to high blood pressure levels, probably as the result of environmental factors.

The importance of populational thinking in assessing risk is documented by assessing the risk of cardiovascular death in relation to levels of SBP for 361,662 men screened for participation in the Multiple Risk Factor Intervention Trial (Fig. 2A).[10] Risk is continuous and graded. At each level of increasing SBP, even within the normotensive range, an individual's cardiovascular risk increases. As clinicians, our usual medical approach to hypertension is to focus most of our efforts on identifying and treating those individuals at greatest risk, those with the highest blood pressure. However, from a population perspective, risk is a function not only of the relative risk of any individual, but also of the number of people at risk. Accordingly, small individual risks can contribute significantly to the total cardiovascular burden borne by the population. For instance, there is a small increase in relative risk associated with high normal blood pressures (130 to 139 mm Hg systolic), but because there are many individuals at risk, the total number of deaths attributable to blood pressure in this range, called the population attributable risk, is substantial (Fig. 2B). At very high levels of SBP, relative risk for individuals is high, but because few individuals have such extremely elevated blood pressures, population attributable risk is modest.

Based on such populational thinking, it has been said that for diseases such as hypertension, there are sick populations as well as sick individuals. The therapeutic charge derived from such thinking is that there may be

Table 2 Lifestyle Modifications for Hypertension Control and/or Overall Cardiovascular Risk

Lose weight if overweight
Limit alcohol intake to ≤1 oz/day of ethanol (24 oz beer, 8 oz wine, or 2 oz 100-proof whiskey)
Exercise (aerobic) regularly
Reduce sodium intake to <100 mmol/day (<2.3 g sodium or approximately <6 g sodium chloride)
Maintain adequate dietary potassium, calcium, and magnesium intake
Stop smoking and reduce dietary saturated fat and cholesterol intake for overall cardiovascular health; reducing fat intake also helps reduce caloric intake, important for control of weight and type II diabetes

From Joint National Committee on Detection, Evaluation, and Treatment of High Blood Pressure. The fifth report of the Joint National Committee on Detection, Evaluation, and Treatment of High Blood Pressure (JNCV). Arch Intern Med 1993; 153:154–183; with permission.

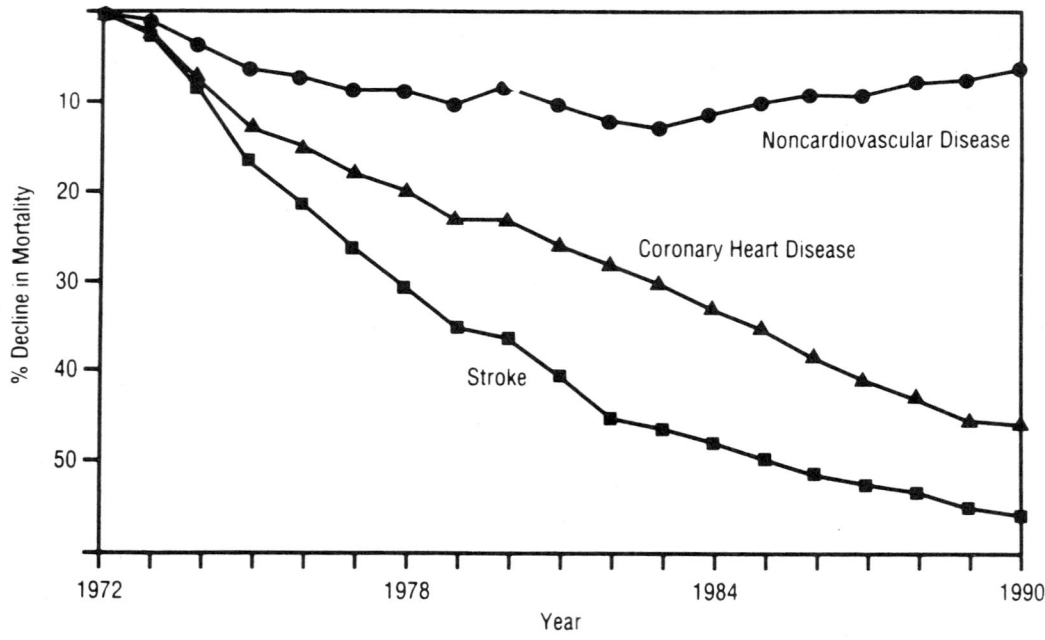

Figure 3 Trends in age-adjusted mortality in the United States for cardiovascular and noncardiovascular diseases. (From Joint National Committee on Detection, Evaluation, and Treatment of High Blood Pressure. The fifth report of the Joint National Committee on Detection, Evaluation, and Treatment of High Blood Pressure (JNC V). Arch Intern Med 1993; 153:154–183; with permission.)

considerable benefits to be derived from treating the population as well as the individual. Thus, it has been calculated that a populational intervention that shifted the entire blood pressure distribution to values 7 to 8 mm Hg lower would yield the same benefit as treating all individuals with DBP of 105 mm Hg or above with a 100% effective drug.[11] Increasingly, therefore, attention is being paid to lifestyle interventions as a way of preventing cardiovascular disease, and recommendations for the primary prevention of hypertension have been proposed[1,10] (Table 2). An important element of these recommendations is that they are proposed for population-wide application and necessitate efforts not only in traditional medical settings such as the office and hospital but also in lobbying the food industry, educating the public at large via mass media, and altering medical education efforts to stress prevention as well as treatment. Clearly, such activities should not replace but rather should complement our efforts to identify and treat high-risk individuals. Without such lifestyle changes, we will be fighting a never-ending battle against hypertension, but can we actually achieve healthful behaviors in the population at large? Some are skeptical, but the rather dramatic decline in coronary heart disease mortality in this country over the past several decades (Fig. 3), which cannot be attributed only to improved detection and treatment of conditions contributing to atherosclerotic risk, suggests that populational behavioral change is possible and that further efforts in the public health arena could have lasting benefits.

REFERENCES

1. Joint National Committee on Detection, Evaluation, and Treatment of High Blood Pressure: The fifth report of the Joint National Committee on Detection, Evaluation, and Treatment of High Blood Pressure (JNC V). Arch Intern Med 1993; 153:154–183.
2. Julius S, Jamerson K, Mejia A, et al. The association of borderline hypertension with target organ changes and higher coronary risk. JAMA 1990; 264:354–358.
3. Alderman MH, Madhavan S, Ooi WL, et al. Association of the renin-sodium profile with the risk of myocardial infarction in patients with hypertension. N Engl J Med 1991; 324:1098–1104.
4. Williams RR, Hunt SC, Hopkins PN, et al. Familial dyslipidemic hypertension. Evidence from 58 Utah families for a syndrome present in approximately 12% of patients with essential hypertension. JAMA 1988; 259:3579–3586.
5. Camblen F, Poirier O, Lecerf L, et al. Deletion polymorphism in the gene for angiotensin-converting enzyme is a potent risk factor for myocardial infarction. Nature 1992; 359:641–644.
6. Levy D, Garrison RJ, Savage DD, et al. Prognostic implications of echocardiographically determined left ventricular mass in the Framingham Heart Study. N Engl J Med 1990; 322:1561–1566.
7. MacMahon S, Peto R, Cutler J, et al. Blood pressure, stroke, and coronary heart disease. Part 1, prolonged differences in blood pressure: Prospective observational studies corrected for the regression dilution bias. Lancet 1990; 335:765–774.
8. MacMahon S, Peto R, Cutler J, et al. Blood pressure, stroke and coronary heart disease. Part 2, short-term reductions in blood pressure: Overview of randomised drug trials in their epidemiological context. Lancet 1990; 335:827–838.
9. Rose G, Day S. The population mean predicts the number of deviant individuals. BMJ 1990; 301:1031–1034.
10. Stamler J, Stamler R, Neaton JD. Blood pressure, systolic and diastolic, and cardiovascular risks. Arch Intern Med 1993; 153:598–615.
11. Rose G. Strategy of prevention: Lessons from cardiovascular disease. BMJ 1981; 282:1847–1851.

ASSESSMENT AND IMPORTANCE OF CORONARY ARTERY DISEASE IN PATIENTS WITH AORTOILIAC OCCLUSIVE DISEASE AND ABDOMINAL AORTIC ANEURYSMS

RICHARD P. CAMBRIA, M.D.

Associated coronary artery disease (CAD) is the principal cause of both perioperative morbidity and long-term limitation on life expectancy in patients who require treatment of aortoiliac occlusive (AIOD) and aneurysmal (AAA) disease. Although cardiac-related morbidity and mortality have improved substantially in current practice, such complications still account for the bulk of operative mortality after aortic reconstruction. Cherry summarized numerous clinical studies representing 3,000 AAA repairs over the past 20 years and noted an overall 4.8% operative mortality. More than half the deaths were due to cardiac complications.[1] In the Canadian multicenter study of more than 600 elective AAA operations, overall mortality was also 4.8%, and two-thirds of these operative deaths were cardiac related.[2] Similarly, studies that examine long-term prognosis after successful AAA repair emphasize that, even with the threat of aneurysm rupture removed, long-term survival after AAA repair does not equal that of an age-matched cohort unless patients with evidence of coronary disease are excluded. Furthermore, those with obvious clinical evidence of CAD at the time of initial presentation have a measurably worse prognosis than those without CAD. In follow-up studies of our patients who have undergone aortic reconstruction, those who have also undergone coronary artery bypass grafting (CABG) have a prognosis that equals that for an age-matched "normal" population.

The modern era of coronary risk assessment in

vascular surgery patients can be traced to the study by Hertzer and colleagues from the Cleveland Clinic.[3] They reported basic data with respect to angiographically documented CAD in patients presenting for peripheral vascular interventions. In their study of 1,000 coronary arteriograms, 31% of 263 patients with AAA with a mean age of 67 years were found to have severe correctable CAD. In addition, another 29% of these AAA patients had advanced but compensated CAD, and 5% harbored severe inoperable CAD.[3] Because this study was performed prospectively on all patients presenting for treatment of AAA, it provided basic information documenting that nearly two-thirds of patients with AAA have significant coexistent CAD. This sobering figure coincides with data from our unit on more than 300 patients, which indicate that approximately 40% will have reversible thallium defects and an additional 40% have fixed defects indicating prior infarction.

With these background data, efforts began in earnest both to develop less invasive methods of identifying CAD and to define which patients should be tested prior to vascular operations. Although few would dispute the importance of CAD in the vascular surgical patient, there remains no consensus on the appropriate role of cardiac risk stratification prior to aortic reconstruction. This is reflected in the wide spectrum of practice in this regard, from those who advocate preoperative cardiac testing in virtually all candidates for aortic reconstruction to those who cite the safety of modern vascular operations and argue against any preoperative testing. However, the concept of cardiac risk assessment (CRA) should no longer be viewed in the narrow context of perioperative safety but include the issue of patient longevity after operation. Indeed, a number of recent reports corroborate our own data, which suggest that preoperative CRA can also afford valuable prognostic information relative to cardiac morbidity and mortality in the months and years following vascular surgical intervention. Our data on more than 300 aortic operations performed during the interval 1984 to 1990 document that late myocardial infarction occurred in 11% of patients. Furthermore, a perioperative myocardial infarction at the original aortic operation was a powerful predictor of late cardiac events. Thus, the concept of CRA has matured over the past decade from an assessment to improve operative safety to an evaluation that places a potential aortic replacement in an appropriate context of overall cardiovascular prognosis.

PRINCIPLES OF CARDIAC RISK ASSESSMENT

Most surgeons and cardiologists would agree that aortic reconstruction has greater potential for physiologic stress when compared to infrainguinal and/or carotid reconstruction. The perspective of the vascular surgeon is necessary to provide insight as to the extent, urgency, and indication for the intervention. Despite the fact that our own data suggest that the "hard" end points of cardiac death and nonfatal myocardial infarction occur more frequently after infrainguinal reconstruction than after aortic reconstruction, these data cannot be used to argue for an equally aggressive posture with respect to cardiac testing between these two patient groups. In fact, this apparent dichotomy is illustrative of an important and often overlooked component, that is, the patients' clinical presentation, in the decision to obtain CRA. The fundamental question for the clinician is whether further knowledge of the patient's coronary anatomy will affect management (Fig. 1). It is obvious to the vascular surgeon, but may not be to the cardiologist, that the diabetic patient with tissue necrosis in the foot requires urgent attention to forestall limb loss irrespective of the results of CRA. Alternatively, the patient presenting with a 5 cm AAA may be a potential candidate for either coronary angiography and CABG or indefinite delay of aneurysm repair. Simply stated, the more elective the vascular procedure, the lower should be the threshold for obtaining CRA.

Although an extensive discussion of the numerous clinical scoring systems and noninvasive modalities available to detect CAD is beyond the purview of this chapter, it is noteworthy that clinical factors have assumed increasing importance in our practice with respect to obtaining CRA. Clinical scoring systems such as that devised by Goldman and later modified by Detsky are useful but are associated with inferior sensitivity for identifying patients felt to be at low risk who develop major cardiac complications. Presumably, this group of patients coincides with the 18% of AAA patients Hertzer and associates identified with severe, correctable, unsuspected CAD.[3]

Noninvasive tests for the detection and quantification of CAD have been greatly refined over the past decade. A variety of tests are available, all of which involve a provocative stress mechanism with subsequent identification of potentially ischemic myocardium by either electrocardiographic criteria, dynamic radioisotopic imaging, or ventricular wall motion analysis. These noninvasive studies have been particularly useful in aortic surgical patients whose capacity to achieve an adequate, standard treadmill test is often limited by claudication and/or advanced age. Impressive data have documented that a variety of these tests including dipyridamole-thallium scintigraphy (D-THAL), Holter ECG monitoring, and dobutamine echocardiography are highly sensitive for the detection of CAD. In our unit, a decade of favorable experience with D-THAL imaging has evolved to the point where it is a highly quantitative assessment of CAD with important implications for perioperative risk and long-term prognosis. Most would agree that a determination of resting ejection fraction (EF) is inadequate in this regard, although a substantially reduced EF (as a major marker of CAD) both has important implications for long-term prognosis and influences the decision to proceed with CRA (Fig. 1).

It is important to emphasize that with CRA the surgeon is hoping to detect the potential for periopera-

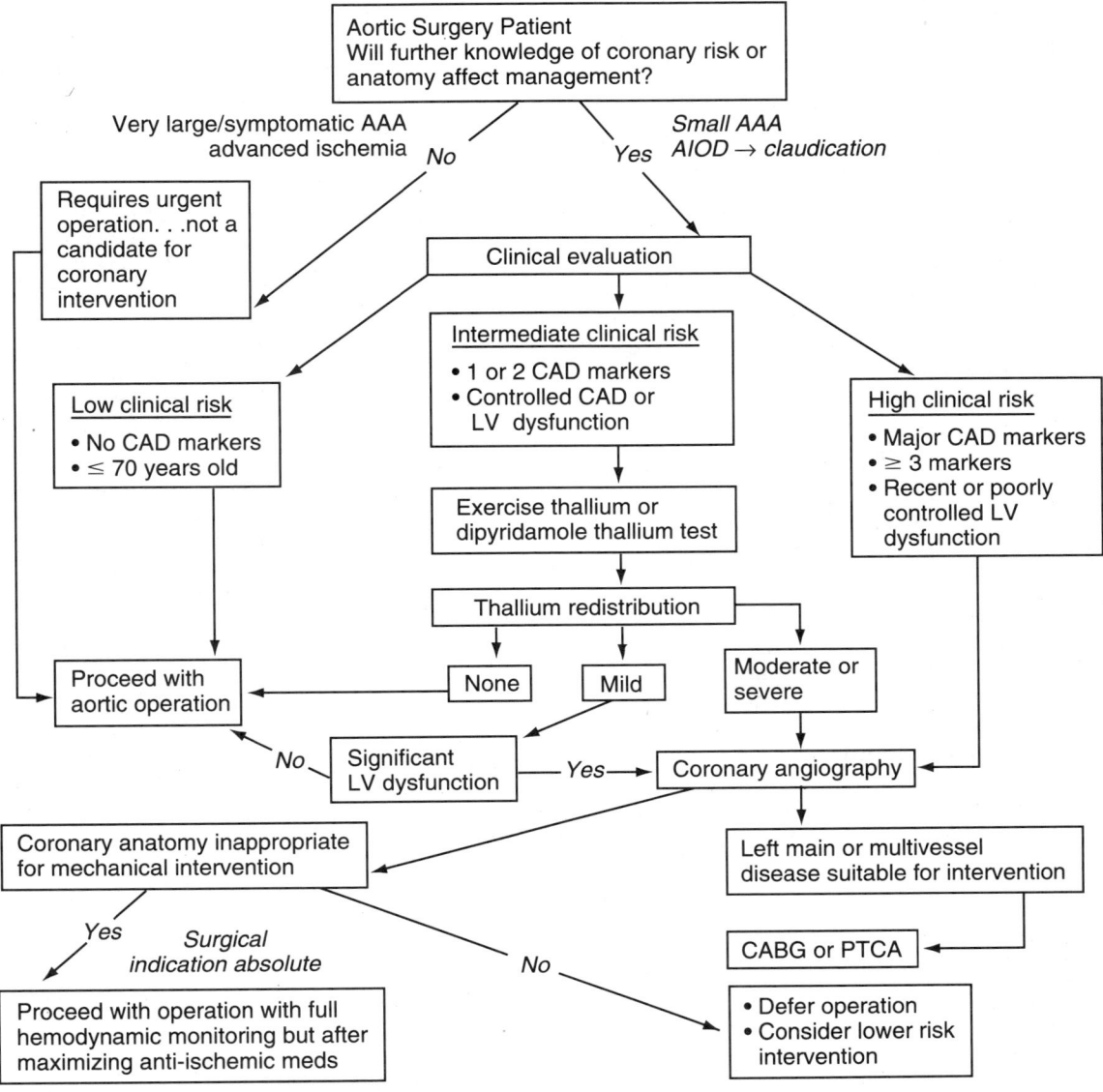

Figure 1 Algorithm for selective cardiac risk stratification prior to aortic reconstruction. Major coronary artery disease (CAD) markers: recent myocardial infarction (MI) complicated by angina, congestive heart failure, or positive stress test; unstable or new-onset angina; recent anterior MI; three or more CAD markers in selected patients. AAA = Aneurysmal disease; AIOD = aortoiliac occlusive disease; LV = left ventricular; CABG = coronary artery bypass grafting; PTCA = percutaneous coronary angioplasty.

tive ischemic events as predicted by some quantitative assessment of the amount of myocardium at risk. An extension of this concept relates to the nature and severity of the projected perioperative events and emphasizes both the quantitative aspects of CRA and our preference for D-THAL in this regard. The latter test, when properly performed, is not interpreted as positive or negative but rather gives information with respect to (1) the number and distribution of coronary artery territories at risk, (2) evidence of fixed ventricular scarring indicative of prior infarction, and (3) dynamic information about dipyridamole-induced left ventricular dysfunction, which may correlate with global ischemia and/or triple-vessel CAD. The quantitative information available from D-THAL, reflecting the amount of jeopardized myocardium, is perhaps the most important factor in both predicting major postoperative cardiac complications and selecting patients for preoperative coronary arteriography. In our unit, patients with pressing indications for peripheral vascular intervention who are discovered to have single coronary territory redistribution on D-THAL routinely undergo the indicated vascular operation without further cardiac evaluation, whereas patients with evidence of more diffuse CAD on D-THAL may be considered for coronary arteriography.

Presuming that a patient considered for aortic

reconstruction has undergone CRA, how might the surgeon react to the acquired information? Indefinite delay of the surgical therapy may be appropriate for patients with claudication alone or modest-sized aneurysms. Selection of a less invasive form of therapy is often available for patients with AIOD and may soon be a reality for patients with AAA in the form of endoluminal graft placement. If formal aortic reconstruction is the only option, further evaluation with coronary arteriography may be desirable in accordance with an algorithm (Fig. 1). In fact, D-THAL imaging that suggests need for coronary arteriography generally predicts diffuse CAD seldom amenable to balloon angioplasty. Thus, surgeon and physician should consider the desirability of recommending CABG prior to recommending coronary angiography. Many patients in need of aortic reconstruction are inappropriate candidates for antecedent CABG.

Information available from CRA may affect anesthetic management, the desirability for invasive monitoring in the perioperative period, and the decision to institute anti-ischemic medical therapy prior to operation. In fact, a common scenario is that of the patient who needs aortic reconstruction and is discovered to have reversible defects on D-THAL imaging. Institution of anti-ischemic therapy in such patients, including, at least, beta-blockers, often ameliorates the ischemic potential as evidenced by improvement in the D-THAL perfusion abnormalities. Thus, we believe an important component of preoperative CRA is the level of awareness required for perioperative medical therapy of the associated CAD.

SELECTION OF PATIENTS FOR PREOPERATIVE TESTING

Given an elective vascular operation where knowledge of the patient's coronary anatomy might affect management, several strategies are possible for preoperative cardiac evaluation. The extreme position of routine coronary arteriography and CABG or percutaneous coronary angioplasty (PTCA) for appropriate lesions is neither cost-effective nor in the best interests of patient safety. At the opposite end of the spectrum are those who contend that contemporary aortic reconstruction is conducted with as low a risk as can be reasonably expected in a population with diffuse vascular disease.[4] Intermediate positions consist of either routine or selective noninvasive testing with subsequent coronary arteriography based on noninvasive testing.

Following the initial report of Boucher and colleagues documenting that redistribution on D-THAL was predictive of cardiac ischemic events after vascular operations, other investigations confirmed these findings.[5] Common to all of these reports are the limitations of D-THAL in predicting perioperative cardiac ischemic events. These tests lack specificity. Although the negative predictive value is excellent (patients without redistribution on D-THAL seldom have perioperative ischemic events), the positive predictive value for perioperative ischemic events is poor, which is not surprising because many patients with significant CAD safely undergo indicated vascular repairs.

In an effort to improve the specificity of CRA with D-THAL, Eagle and co-workers reported that certain clinical markers of CAD could identify patients at risk for postoperative ischemic events and be used to select patients for preoperative CRA.[6] In a recent prospective study, these investigators studied 254 patients prior to vascular reconstruction with D-THAL and delineation of a variety of clinical CAD markers. Using multivariate analysis, five clinical markers of CAD were identified as predictive of postoperative cardiac events: (1) age greater than 70 years, (2) Q-waves on ECG, (3) history of ventricular arrhythmias, (4) diabetes mellitus, and (5) angina pectoris. Absence of all five of these clinical markers was associated with freedom from postoperative cardiac complications. At the other extreme was the 50% cardiac event rate among 20 patients with three or more of the critical clinical markers.[6] This high complication rate occurred irrespective of thallium redistribution during preoperative testing. However, the predictive value of redistribution was again documented in that 13 of 15 patients with end points of cardiac death or myocardial infarction had redistribution on preoperative D-THAL. Combining readily apparent clinical markers with D-THAL variables increased the overall specificity to 81%, whereas use of clinical or D-THAL variables alone produced specificities in the 66% to 69% range.

Based on the five clinical markers alone, low-risk (absence of markers) and high-risk groups (greater than three markers) could be identified. For patients at intermediate levels of risk (one or two clinical markers) D-THAL proved most useful for the prediction of perioperative ischemic events. Of the 116 patients in the intermediate clinical risk category, 62 had no redistribution and their event risk (3.2%) was similar to the low risk found in patients with no clinical markers. However, the other 54 patients had redistribution on D-THAL and a cardiac event rate of nearly 30%. Based on these data, we adopted a selective approach to preoperative CRA, depending on the presence or absence of critical clinical markers of CAD. Such an approach appears cost-effective in that formal CRA could be eliminated in patients deemed to be at low risk for cardiac complications on the basis of clinical markers alone. Furthermore, D-THAL scintigraphy could also be eliminated in patients at high risk based on the presence of three or more of the clinical CAD markers. In addition to patients with three or more markers, others with an unstable or threatening coronary status are best served by eliminating the preliminary step of noninvasive cardiac testing. If such patients are potential candidates for therapy of their CAD prior to vascular reconstruction, or if further knowledge of CAD anatomy would affect management, proceeding directly to coronary arteriography would be our preference (Fig. 1).

Table 1 Clinical Markers of Coronary Artery Disease in Aortic Surgery Patients

Number of Markers*	AAA Number of Patients (%): Mean Age		AIOD Number of Patients (%): Mean Age		Totals Number of Patients (%)	
0	46	(30) 65.4	18	(35) 57.1	64	(32)
1	63	(42) 72	19	(37) 63	82	(40.5)
2	30	(20) 73.7	14	(27) 65.8	44	(22)
3	10	(7) 69.5	—		10	(5)
4 or 5	2	(1) 71	—		2	(1)
Totals	151	70 yrs	51	62 yrs	202	

*Age 70 yrs or older, diabetes, history of angina, Q-wave on ECG, history of ventricular ectopy.

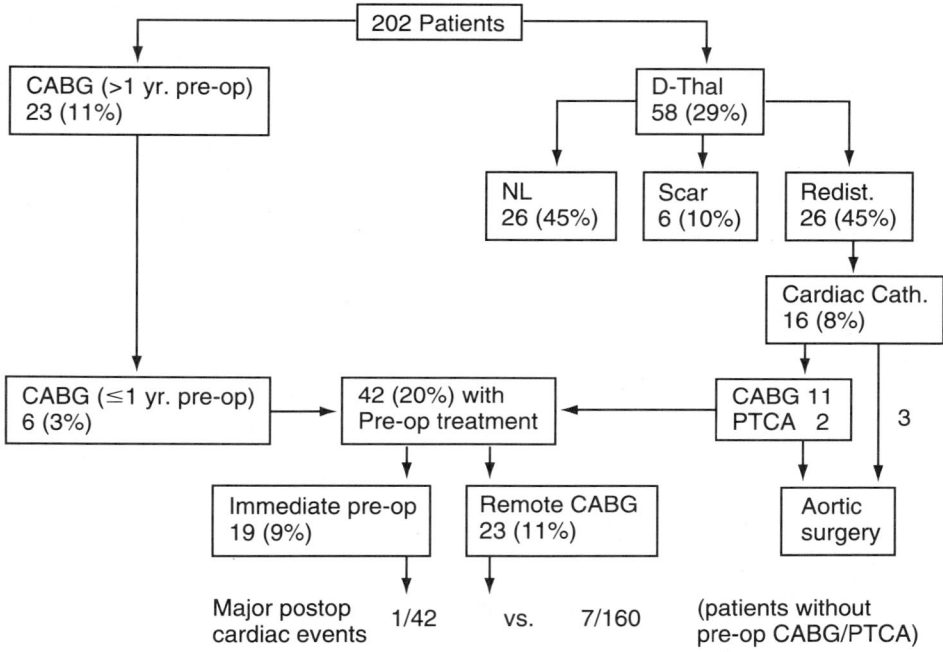

Figure 2 Evaluation and treatment of coronary artery disease in 202 abdominal aortic reconstructions. Aneurysmal disease, 151; aortoiliac occlusive disease, 51. CABG = coronary artery bypass grafting; PTCA = percutaneous coronary angioplasty; NL = normal. RP, Brewster DC, Abbott WM, et al. (From Cambria The impact of selective use of dipyridamole-thallium scans and surgical factors on the current morbidity of aortic surgery. J Vasc Surg 1992; 15:43; with permission.)

CURRENT PRACTICE OF RISK ASSESSMENT IN AORTIC SURGICAL PATIENTS

When viewed from the perspective of early postoperative outcome, aortic reconstruction is a safe undertaking, with most contemporary series recording operative mortality rates of less than 4%. In our unit, 567 elective aortic aneurysm operations were carried out between 1989 and 1993. Overall cardiac death rate was 1.4%, with an additional 1.9% of patients sustaining major but nonfatal cardiac complications.

In applying a selective approach to CRA in more than 200 consecutive aortic surgery patients, it appeared that their cardiac risk profiles, based on the five clinical markers of CAD, were perhaps less ominous than most would assume. More than 70% of our patients had none or only one clinical marker of CAD (Table 1). Thus only 28% of these patients would undergo D-THAL preoperatively, and approximately 20% would come to operation with antecedent treatment of their CAD. The timing and type of CAD treatment was such that roughly half of the interventions for CAD were conducted in the year prior to the aortic reconstruction, with the balance representing CABG carried out more than 1 year prior to the vascular operation (Fig. 2). Cardiac catheterization was felt necessary immediately prior to operation in 8% of our patients, and most (13 of 16) of these had PTCA or CABG prior to their aortic reconstruction. No major morbidity was associated with invasive CAD therapy in these patients, and such therapy appeared to be protective of perioperative ischemic events in that seven of eight major cardiac complications occurred in patients without treatment of CAD. Overall cardiac-related morbidity after aortic reconstruction was very low with but one cardiac-related death and a 3% rate of nonfatal perioperative myocardial infarction.[7] Thus, selective application of CRA can be accomplished safely and with cost advantages when compared to a policy of routine preoperative CRA. In studies detailing routine preoperative CRA, more coronary arteriography has been performed to achieve the same results. McEnroe and associates performed routine D-THAL and subsequent coronary arteriography in 29% of 100 AAA patients.[8] Their use of preoperative CABG (8%) and the perioperative cardiac death and/or myocardial infarction (4%) are similar to our own. Other contemporary studies, including those using selective testing, continue to report what we believe to be excessive use of preoperative coronary arteriography. Suggs and colleagues performed preoperative coronary arteriography in 33% of 263 AAA patients with preoperative CABG required in 8%.[9] In current practice, the quantitative information available from D-THAL should serve to restrict coronary arteriography to patients with truly threatening diffuse CAD, that is, those individuals who would have indications for CABG on its own merits.

REFERENCES

1. Cherry KJ. Management of patients with abdominal aortic aneurysms and coronary artery disease: Current trends. Perspect Vasc Surg 1988; 1:21–33.
2. Johnson WK. Multicenter prospective study of nonruptured abdominal aortic aneurysm. Part II: Variables predicting morbidity and mortality. J Vasc Surg 1989; 9:437.
3. Hertzer N, Beven E, Young J, et al. Coronary artery disease in peripheral vascular patients: A classification of 1000 coronary angiograms and results of surgical management. Ann Surg 1984; 199:223.
4. Taylor LM, Yeager RA, Moneta GL, McConnell DB. The incidence of perioperative myocardial infarction in general vascular surgery. J Vasc Surg 1992; 15:52.
5. Boucher CA, Brewster DC, Darling RC, et al. Determination of cardiac risk by dipyridamole-thallium imaging before peripheral vascular surgery. N Engl J Med 1985; 312:389.
6. Eagle KA, Coley CM, Newell JB, et al. Combining clinical and thallium data optimizes preoperative assessment of cardiac risk before major vascular surgery. Ann Intern Med 1989; 110:859.
7. Cambria RP, Brewster DC, Abbott WM, et al. The impact of selective use of dipyridamole-thallium scans and surgical factors on the current morbidity of aortic surgery. J Vasc Surg 1992; 15:43.
8. McEnroe CS, O'Donnell TF Jr, Yeager A, et al. Comparison of ejection fraction and Goldman risk factor analysis to dipyridamole-thallium 201 studies in the evaluation of cardiac morbidity after aortic aneurysm surgery. 1990; J Vasc Surg 11:497.
9. Suggs WD, Smith RB, Weintraub WS, et al. Selective screening for coronary artery disease in patients undergoing elective repair of AAA. J Vasc Surg 1993; 18:349–357.

PHYSIOLOGIC STUDIES TO DOCUMENT SEVERITY OF AORTOILIAC OCCLUSIVE DISEASE

JOSEPH P. ARCHIE Jr, M.D.

The severity of aortoiliac occlusive disease is determined clinically by the signs and symptoms it produces, anatomically by the degree, length, location, and number of stenoses, and physiologically by the limitations it produces on blood flow at rest and with exercise. There is little agreement on what constitutes an anatomic or a physiologic hemodynamically significant aortoiliac stenosis. The estimated range is between 30% and 75% diameter stenosis. Stenoses greater than 75% are usually easily detected. Stenoses less than 30% produce symptoms only with strenuous exercise.

Physiologic studies are valuable for qualitating and quantitating the severity of an aortoiliac stenosis, making clinical decisions regarding interventions, evaluating the effect of interventions, and providing short- and long-term follow-up. Such studies indirectly or directly measure blood pressures, blood flow velocities, and the pulsatile pressure or flow waveforms. The principle noninvasive technologies utilized are Doppler ultrasound and air plethysmography. Invasive methods focus on direct measurement of systolic or mean blood pressures proximal and distal to stenotic aortoiliac segments. Although much information on invasive aortoiliac blood pressure measurements has accumulated, reports of clinical outcomes of interventional procedures guided by these measurements are sparse and constitute a fertile area for investigation.

Physiologic studies help to answer a number of clinical questions such as, Are the patient's signs and symptoms due to atherosclerotic occlusive disease? Are they due to aortoiliac disease, infrainguinal occlusive disease, or a combination of both? In patients with combined disease, which arterial segment is the major determinant of the signs or symptoms? In patients with combined disease, is the aortoiliac stenosis severe enough to jeopardize an infrainguinal reconstruction?

NONINVASIVE PHYSIOLOGIC STUDIES

Separation of hemodynamically significant isolated aortoiliac occlusive disease from isolated infrainguinal

Table 1 Simplified Overview of Noninvasive Segmental Limb Doppler-Derived Blood Pressures and Waveforms and Air Plethysmography for Determining Isolated Aortoiliac, Isolated Infrainguinal, and Combined Suprainguinal and Infrainguinal Stenoses

Study	Isolated Aortoiliac	Isolated Infrainguinal	Combined
Segmental systolic pressures	Equal	Equal, or thigh > calf, ankle	Equal, or thigh > calf, ankle
Femoral, popliteal, tibial Doppler waveforms	Monophasic or damped monophasic	Monophasic or damped monophasic	Monophasic or damped monophasic
Segmental air plethysmography amplitude	Equal, or thigh < calf, ankle	Thigh > calf, ankle	Equal, or thigh > calf, ankle
Common femoral artery end-diastolic Doppler velocity	>0	0	>0

occlusive disease is usually straightforward with good-quality conventional noninvasive vascular testing. However, the degree of aortoiliac disease is difficult to determine when both supra and infrainguinal stenoses are present. The simplest and most frequently employed noninvasive physiologic tests are segmental Doppler-derived thigh, calf, and ankle systolic blood pressure measurements. The use of high thigh blood pressures to separate aortoiliac from infrainguinal arterial stenoses has been a much debated issue, with little convincing supporting evidence. The addition of segmental thigh, calf, and ankle air plethysmography (pulse volume recordings) and femoral, popliteal, and tibial artery Doppler velocity waveforms is helpful in delineating the level and severity of disease, particularly in distinguishing aortoiliac from infrainguinal stenoses. Common femoral artery Doppler velocity waveform analysis adds significantly to lower extremity noninvasive arterial testing. Failure of the end-diastolic velocity to return to 0 as well as the amount of elevation from the zero velocity baseline relative to the peak systolic velocity are qualitative indications of the presence and degree of aortoiliac stenosis.

Noninvasive Doppler ultrasound and air plethysmography studies are useful in eliminating the presence of hemodynamically significant infrainguinal stenosis. For example, a patient with intermittent claudication and similar segmental thigh, calf, and ankle blood pressures, similar monophasic femoral, popliteal, and tibial artery velocity waveforms, an end-diastolic common femoral artery velocity greater than 0, and a higher-amplitude calf than thigh air plethysmography signal has a very high probability of isolated aortoiliac stenosis (Table 1). This conclusion is reached not because the location or degree of aortoiliac stenosis is identified, but rather by the elimination of significant infrainguinal occlusive disease. Severe common femoral artery stenosis or combined superficial and profunda femoral artery stenoses can produce Doppler and plethysmographic results identical to those of aortoiliac stenosis. Although standard noninvasive studies give a reasonable estimate of the presence and severity of aortoiliac disease, they are not truly quantitative, even when the disease is isolated to this segment. In patients with combined aortoiliac and infrainguinal stenoses, the ability to quantitate the significance of aortoiliac stenosis by noninvasive methods becomes much less accurate.

More sophisticated common femoral artery Doppler waveform analyses utilizing the frequency or velocity spectrum are reported to aid in determining the presence and significance of aortoiliac stenosis. These include inspection of the frequency or velocity spectrum, calculation of the pulsatility index (ratio of peak systolic velocity to mean velocity), and measuring the time rate of increase of early systolic velocity. Duplex scanning of the femoral arteries aids in the diagnosis and quantitation of an aortoiliac stenosis because unusual conditions that mimic aortoiliac stenosis, such as severe isolated common femoral artery stenosis or combined superficial and profunda femoral artery stenoses, can be identified. Exercise testing is sometimes necessary in symptomatic patients with mild stenosis and normal or near normal resting noninvasive studies. However, exercise testing is not particularly helpful in localizing the level of disease.

Unlike the infrainguinal and extracranial carotid arteries, duplex scanning of the aortoiliac segments is not currently an effective method of determining the degree of iliac disease. Measurements of peak systolic blood flow velocities in or just distal to an iliac stenosis have been used to estimate the pressure gradient across the stenosis by using a simplified Bernoulli equation (pressure gradient equals 4 times the square of maximum systolic velocity). However, analysis of the rationale for this technique reveals a major flaw in the application of this equation. It is an estimate of the peak kinetic energy produced by the stenosis. The assumption is that all of the kinetic energy is dissipated, thereby producing the pressure gradient. Although some of the kinetic energy may be dissipated, it is clear that much is converted to potential energy or blood pressure. When this formula was applied to the much more easily studied carotid stenosis, it proved to be invalid.

INVASIVE STUDIES

In 1956, Haimovici and Escher[1] reported measurements of aorta to common femoral artery pressure gradients in 16 limbs at rest. They pointed out that both systolic and mean aortic to femoral blood pressure

Table 2 Recommended Numeric Criteria for Five Pressure Variables and Their Associated Degree of Iliac Artery Diameter Stenosis

Pressure Variable	Numerical Criteria	References	Percent Iliac Stenosis* (Mean ± SD)
Resting systolic aortic to femoral pressure gradient	15 mm Hg	1, 3, 8	31 ± 27
	59 mm Hg	1	88 ± 21
Resting mean aortic to femoral pressure gradient	1 mm Hg	1	23 ± 26
	17 mm Hg	1	81 ± 15
Hyperemic mean aortic to femoral pressure gradient	10 mm Hg	5, 7	45 ± 25
Resting systolic ratio of femoral to aortic pressure	0.9	6	27 ± 25
	0.74	1	54 ± 26
	0.7	9	57 ± 27
Percent change from rest to hyperemia in systolic ratio of femoral to aortic pressure	10%	4	38 ± 25
	15%	4, 6	45 ± 37

*Obtained from same data base.
From Archie JP. Analysis and comparison of pressure gradients and ratios for predicting iliac stenosis. Ann Vasc Surg 1994; 8:271-279.

gradients are excellent physiologic variables for estimating the degree of aortoiliac stenosis. Since then, a number of techniques to measure these blood pressures have been reported, including percutaneous femoral artery needle puncture, proximal and pull-back femoral catheter pressure measurements at the time of angiography, and direct operative measurements. The pressure gradient across one or more stenotic arterial segments is determined by the equation: Pressure gradient equals resistance times flow, where the resistance is determined primarily by the degree of stenosis. A number of methods have been employed to increase blood flow during blood pressure measurements and hence increase the pressure gradient across an aortoiliac stenosis. These include papaverine hydrochloride injection into the common femoral artery, pedal ergometry, and reactive hyperemia following temporary limb ischemia by thigh blood pressure cuff inflation. All of these techniques produce limb hyperemia due to vasodilation. Vasodilation of the distal arterial tree lowers vascular resistance and increases blood flow. The amount of blood flow increase is determined by the degree of aortoiliac stenosis and the amount of distal vasodilation. The latter is highly variable; accordingly, these techniques cannot be relied upon to produce a uniform increase in blood flow across the stenosis. It is interesting that superficial femoral artery occlusion only slightly decreases the effect of papaverine hydrochloride on common femoral artery blood flow.[2]

Early investigators used systolic or mean central-to-femoral artery blood pressure gradients to estimate the hemodynamic significance of aortoiliac stenosis. More recently, the ratios of femoral to systemic blood pressure and the percent change in these ratios from rest to hyperemia have been reported. Five different pressure gradient or pressure ratio variables have been reported, each with one or more recommended numeric criteria for determining the hemodynamic significance of aortoiliac stenosis[1,3-9] (Table 2). With one exception, the validity of the various recommended pressure variables and their numerical criteria have not been confirmed by evaluation of the results of interventional procedures based on decisions using these criteria.[5] Even though directly measured femoral artery pressures are considered the gold standard for determining the hemodynamic significance of aortoiliac stenosis, the widespread use of these techniques is questionable. This may be due in part to the confusion and controversy over what constitutes a hemodynamically significant aortoiliac pressure gradient or ratio, which pressure variable to use, and what numeric criteria to use. This is further complicated by the difficulty of accurately measuring the degree of stenosis from arteriograms.

Analysis of Pressure Variables

To investigate which aortofemoral pressure variables are optimal and what numeric criteria to apply to estimate various degrees of stenosis, femoral artery and radial artery blood pressures were measured in 144 limbs and six pressure variables calculated over the range of aortoiliac stenoses.[10] The results suggest first that resting systolic and mean blood pressure gradients are as good as hyperemic blood pressure gradients, except perhaps for estimating low grades of stenosis; second, that resting systolic and mean blood pressure gradients are equal to or better than pressure ratios, and superior to the change in pressure ratios produced by hyperemia; and, third, that the recommended numeric criteria for most pressure variables correspond to a low degree of aortoiliac stenosis. High-grade (75%) diameter stenosis is predicted with 95% confidence by a resting pressure gradient of at least 52 mm Hg systolic and at least 16 mm Hg mean. Hyperemia is not necessary for predicting aortoiliac stenoses of 50% or greater. Moderate (50%) stenosis is predicted with 95% confidence by resting systolic pressure gradients of at least 34 mm Hg and resting mean pressure gradients of at least 7 mm Hg (Figs. 1 and 2). Characteristic curves may be generated for resting systolic blood pressure gradients and resting mean blood pressure gradients for 30%, 50%, and 75% iliac stenoses (Figs. 3 and 4).[10] These data illustrate the

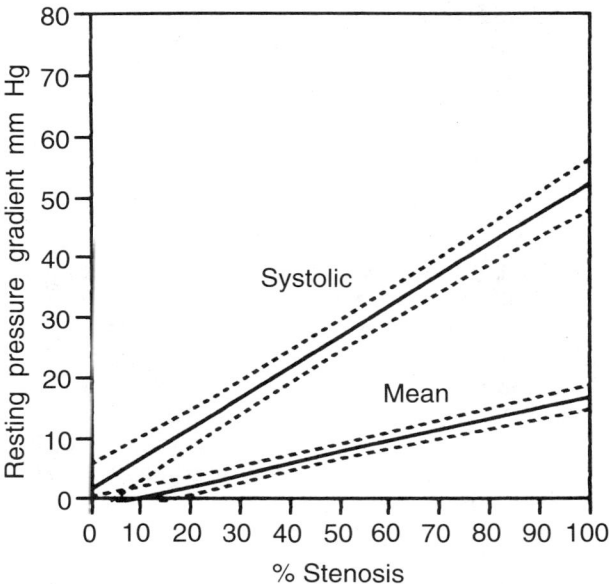

Figure 1 The linear regression line between resting systolic and mean blood pressure gradients versus percent iliac stenosis for 144 measurements.[10] The 95% confidence intervals for the means are shown as dashed lines.

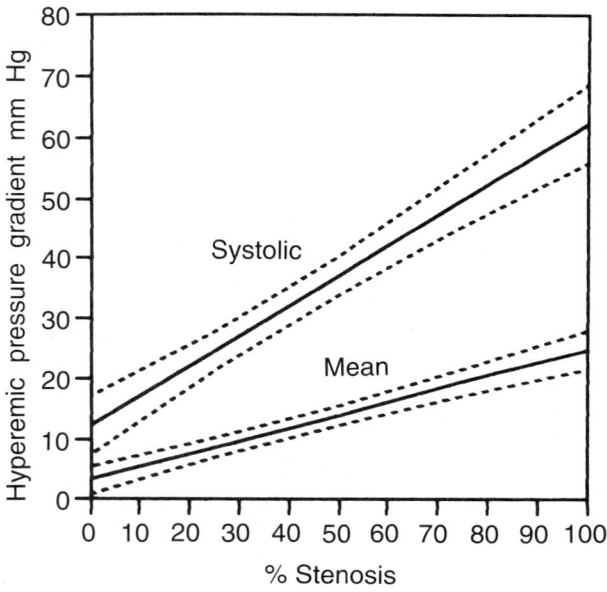

Figure 2 The linear regression line between papaverine hydrochloride–induced hyperemic systolic and mean blood pressure gradients versus percent iliac stenosis for 119 measurements.[10] The 95% confidence intervals for the mean are shown as dashed lines.

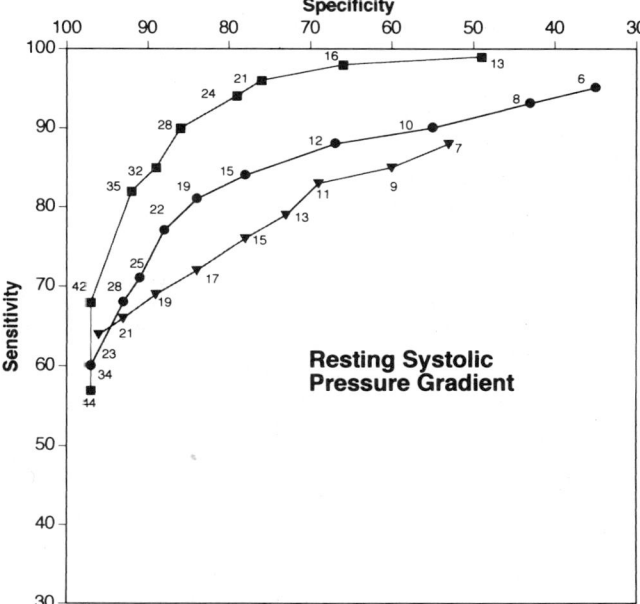

Figure 3 Receiver operating characteristic curves for resting systolic blood pressure gradients for three degrees of iliac stenosis: triangle is 30% stenosis, circle is 50% stenosis, and square is 75% stenosis. The numbers adjacent to each data point are the values of the pressure gradient.

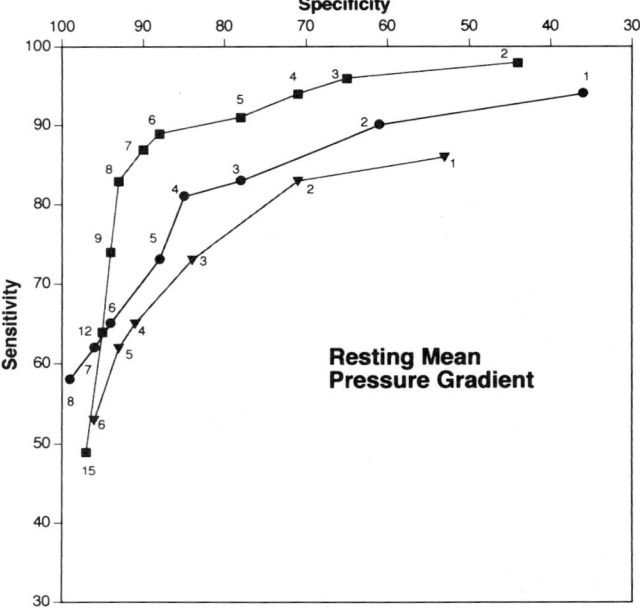

Figure 4 Receiver operating characteristic curve for resting mean blood pressure gradients for three degrees of stenoses: triangle is 30% stenosis, circle is 50% stenosis, and square is 75% stenosis. The numbers adjacent to each data point are the values of the pressure gradient.

probabilities of various measured blood pressure gradients correctly predicting a specific level of stenosis. Other variables such as pressure ratios and percent changes in ratios with hyperemia do not improve on these results and in most cases are inferior.[10]

Technique of Blood Pressure Measurements

The method of measuring central arterial blood pressure varies. Clearly, the optimal location is in the aorta proximal to the stenosis. This can be done at the time of arteriography. Most investigators use direct brachial or radial artery blood pressure measurements. Doppler-derived brachial artery systolic pressure has been used.[6] However, when this technique is compared to direct arterial blood pressure measurements, there is a fair amount of variability; accordingly, this is probably not the optimal method.[10] Needles or cannulas of 20 or 21 gauge are used for direct measurements; 22-gauge needles or cannulas produce some damping and, accordingly, systolic values may not be accurate. Needles larger than 20 gauge are not necessary for accurate systolic pressure measurements. If two separate cannulas or needles are used, the rigid connecting tubing should be of identical length and type. A single transducer for measuring both central and common femoral artery pressures is advisable because of the induced error of separate transducers. If two transducers are used, both should be calibrated, the zero reference levels must be identical, and the connecting tubing should be switched on the transducers to be sure that identical pressures are measured on each. Use of a single transducer switching back and forth between the aortic, radial, or brachial arteries and the femoral artery eliminates most errors induced by transducer calibration and all errors due to zero reference. There is a slight amplification of systolic pressure as the arterial pulse travels distally. The brachial artery systolic blood pressure is slightly higher than the systolic aortic blood pressure and is lower than the radial artery systolic blood pressure. One point in favor of mean over systolic blood pressures is that pressure wave amplification does not affect mean pressure. If systolic blood pressures are used, the transducer's impedance should be matched to the tubing catheter-needle system to prevent overdamping or underdamping. Impedance mismatch does not influence mean blood pressures. In addition, the tubing and cannulas or needles should be flushed clear of blood because backbleeding into the tubing can produce systolic blood pressure damping. It is advisable to average three to five pressure readings while the blood pressure is stable.

Injection of 30 mg of papaverine hydrochloride directly into the common femoral artery is sufficient to produce hyperemia. Depending on the outflow resistance, it takes 10 to 30 seconds for maximum vasodilation and minimum femoral artery blood pressure changes to occur. Papaverine hydrochloride may lower the systemic arterial blood pressure, and accordingly both systemic and femoral artery blood pressures must be measured during peak limb blood flow. Electromagnetic or transit-time Doppler blood flowmeter measurements of common femoral artery flow are helpful when using papaverine hydrochloride.[2]

REFERENCES

1. Haimovici H, Escher DHW. Aortoiliac stenosis. Diagnostic significance of vascular hemodynamics. Arch Surg 1956; 72:107–117.
2. Archie JP. Some determinants of papaverine-induced femoral artery pressure gradients. J Surg Res 1990; 48:211–216.
3. Weismann RE, Upson JP. Intraarterial pressure studies in patients with arterial insufficiency of lower extremities. Ann Surg 1963; 157:501–506.
4. Brener BJ, Raines JK, Darling RC, Austen WG. Measurement of systolic femoral artery pressure during reactive hyperemia. Circulation 1974; 49, 50, (suppl 2):259–267.
5. Archie JP, Feldtman R. Intraoperative assessment of the hemodynamic significance of iliac and profunda femoris artery stenosis. Surgery 1981; 90:876–880.
6. Flanigan DP, Ryan TJ, Williams LR, et al. Aortofemoral or femoropopliteal revascularization? A prospective evaluation of the papaverine test. J Vasc Surg 1984; 1:215–223.
7. Breslau PH, Jorning PJG, Greep JM. Assessment of aortoiliac disease using hemodynamic measurements. Arch Surg 1985; 120:1050–1052.
8. Baker JD. Preoperative assessment of the extent and severity of aortoiliac occlusive disease. Surgical Rounds 1989; 5:27–32.
9. VanAsten WNJC, Beijneveld WJ, Pieters BR, et al. Assessment of aortoiliac obstructive disease by Doppler spectrum analysis of blood flow velocities in the common femoral artery at rest and during reactive hyperemia. Surgery 1991; 109:633–639.
10. Archie JP. Analysis and comparison of pressure gradients and ratios for predicting iliac stenosis. Ann Vasc Surg 1994; 8:271–279.

AORTOFEMORAL BYPASS FOR ATHEROSCLEROTIC AORTOILIAC OCCLUSIVE DISEASE

WILLIAM M. ABBOTT, M.D.
CHRISTOPHER J. KWOLEK, M.D.

The modern surgical treatment of aortoiliac occlusive disease (AIOD) dates back to the reports of thromboendarterectomy by dos Santos in 1947 and Wylie in 1951. During the same period, excision and graft replacement for aortic disease was described by Julian and colleagues, Dubost and colleagues, and Oudot in 1951 and DeBakey in 1952. Shortly thereafter, DeBakey described the use of aortoiliac and aortofemoral bypass grafting in the treatment of AIOD. The results of treatment have continued to improve with time, but the patterns of distribution of disease, the incidence of disease in women, and the preferred methods of treatment have changed.[1] Currently, the aortobifemoral bypass graft is considered the gold standard for the treatment of AIOD, and all other treatment options must be compared to it with respect to both long-term patency and complication rates.

PRESENTATION

Leriche was the first to describe the clinical presentation of patients with end-stage AIOD or aortic occlusion. These patients often present with the triad of intermittent claudication, impotence, and absence of femoral pulses commonly referred to as Leriche syndrome. Today, the typical patient presenting with aortoiliac occlusive disease is a male smoker in his early 60s presenting with complaints of impotence, distal calf claudication or rest pain, and signs of distal ischemia on physical examination. In addition, he is likely to have a significant history of coronary artery disease, hypertension, or other comorbid disease related to systemic atherosclerosis. Further evaluation reveals that he has diffuse atherosclerotic involvement of the vessels both above and below the inguinal ligament, what we have previously referred to as type III disease (Fig. 1).[2] In comparison, the classic female patient is a smoker who is a decade younger than her male counterpart. She typically presents with symptoms of buttock, hip, or thigh intermittent claudication and is less likely to have a history of significant comorbid disease. Further evaluation in this patient often reveals that her disease is limited to the distal aorta and iliac arteries. We refer to this segmental pattern of atherosclerosis in the aorta and common iliac arteries as type I disease (Fig. 1). As the incidence of AIOD in women continues to increase, however, the pattern of disease seems to be shifting toward that seen in men. Patients with type II disease have involvement of the aorta, internal iliac, and external iliac vessels (Fig. 1). They tend to present with mixed symptoms combining those found in type I and III patients.

Several reports from the Massachusetts General Hospital suggest that the percentage of patients presenting for operation with segmental disease limited to the aortoiliac region has decreased over time. Duncan reported in a 1971 review that one-third of patients presented with a type I distribution and that one-half had type III disease.[2] Our most recent review included 582 patients seen between 1963 and 1977. Patients presenting with type I lesions had decreased to 13%; those with diffuse type III lesions had increased to 66%. Most large series of aortobifemoral bypass grafting report that between one-half and two-thirds of patients present with type III disease and that two-thirds of the patients are operated upon for disabling intermittent claudication.[3]

A careful physical examination also provides important information when evaluating patients with atherosclerotic disease of the aorta. Absent or weakened femoral artery pulses can be noted in at least one-third of patients with AIOD, and bruits over the aortoiliofemoral regions of the lower abdomen can sometimes be appreciated. Signs of severe peripheral ischemia or tissue loss can also be seen. Other presentations such as the blue toe syndrome, characterized by the presence of ischemic blue toes in the presence of intact peripheral pulses, are believed to represent atheromatous emboli from more proximally located ulcerated aortic lesions and constitute an indication for surgical repair.

Once the diagnosis of AIOD has been made, further evaluation with noninvasive techniques and arteriography is usually indicated. We have traditionally obtained segmental limb Doppler pressure measurements and pulse volume recordings to physiologically quantify the severity of the disease. These measurements also provide a baseline for comparison in the postoperative monitoring of our patients. Contrast arteriography provides a useful roadmap and allows the surgeon to plan more effectively the optimal operative procedure, particularly for patients who may have associated renal, mesenteric, or peripheral vascular arterial lesions. We have also found that the presence of a significant drop in femoral arterial pressure across a radiographically documented lesion is one of the best predictors of a successful outcome in patients with multilevel occlusive disease. A good result is obtained in more than 90% of patients undergoing proximal bypass when the difference in resting systolic blood pressure between the distal aorta and the common femoral artery is at least 10 mm Hg or a 15% drop occurs in response to reactive hyperemia.

One of the newer vascular imaging techniques being developed is magnetic resonance angiography (MRA). We have found this technique useful in selected patients for the evaluation of peripheral vascular disease.[4] As the sensitivity and speed of these machines continue to

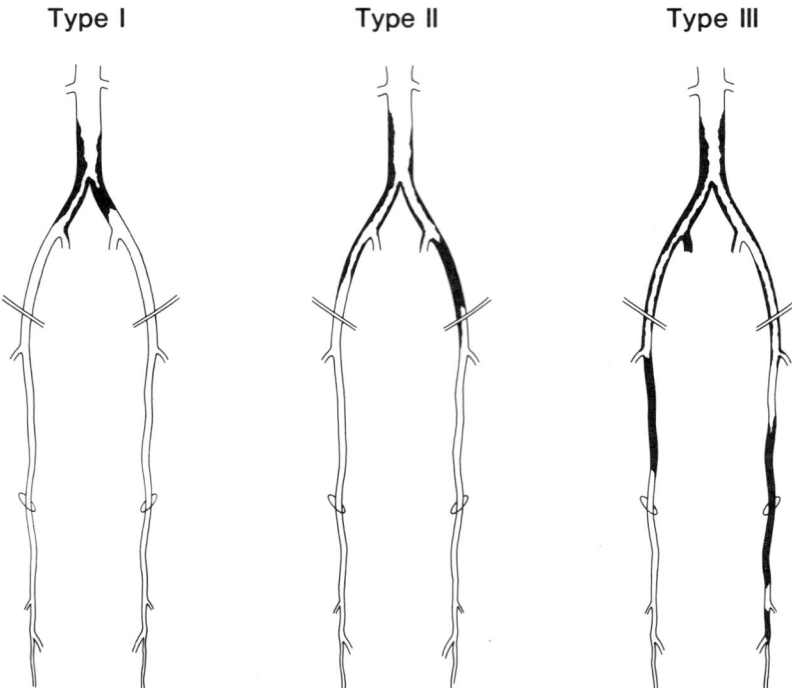

Figure 1 Types of aortoiliac occlusive disease. Type I disease is confined to the distal abdominal aorta and common iliac arteries. The type II pattern demonstrates more widespread intra-abdominal disease. Type III disease involves a diffuse pattern of disease with extension below the inguinal ligament. (From Brewster DC. Direct reconstruction for aortoiliac occlusive disease. In: Rutherford RB ed. Vascular surgery, 3rd ed. Philadelphia: WB Saunders, 1989: 667; with permission.)

improve, MRA will play an increasingly important role in the evaluation of patients with both aneurysmal and occlusive disease of the aortoiliac system, particularly those patients with a history of contrast-induced allergy or renal insufficiency.

HISTORIC TREATMENT

Early reports concerning the treatment of atherosclerotic disease of the aortoiliofemoral system emphasized the use of aortoiliac and even aortoiliofemoral endarterectomy. Later reports for the treatment of AIOD all document a marked preference for the use of aortobifemoral bypass grafting. In part, this is due to the poor long-term results of endarterectomy of the external iliac system. The incidence of recurrent disease requiring reoperation in these patients approaches 32% at 10 years. In addition, the percentage of patients with limited type I disease, who are suitable candidates for aortoiliac endarterectomy, has decreased over time. Currently, fewer than 10% of the patients are candidates for aortoiliac endarterectomy. These patients should have disease that terminates just beyond the aortic bifurcation, extending no more than 1 to 2 cm into the common iliac arteries. In addition, patients with aortic occlusion extending to the level of the renal arteries, those with evidence of aneurysmal changes in the aorta or iliac vessels, and patients with significant disease of the external iliac vessels should not be considered for this procedure.

CURRENT TREATMENT

Most current surgical reports describe aortofemoral bypass as the preferred method of treatment for atherosclerotic AIOD. Reasons for this preference over endarterectomy include improved late patency rates, lower initial failure rates, lower overall mortality rates, decreased operative time, less blood loss, and a less technically demanding procedure than endarterectomy.

In early surgical reports, aortoiliac bypass was advocated as a preferred method of treatment for AIOD. This was primarily due to concerns about the long-term potential for graft infection and pseudoaneurysm formation when bringing the limbs of the graft across the inguinal ligament into the groin. Fortunately, these concerns have not been significant in any of the modern analyses of aortobifemoral bypass grafting. Thus, the technically easier aortobifemoral graft has become the preferred method for treating AIOD.

The results of aortofemoral bypass grafting have continued to improve for several reasons. Perioperative anesthesia management and hemodynamic monitoring techniques have limited the risk of cardiac-related morbidity and mortality in this high-risk group of patients.

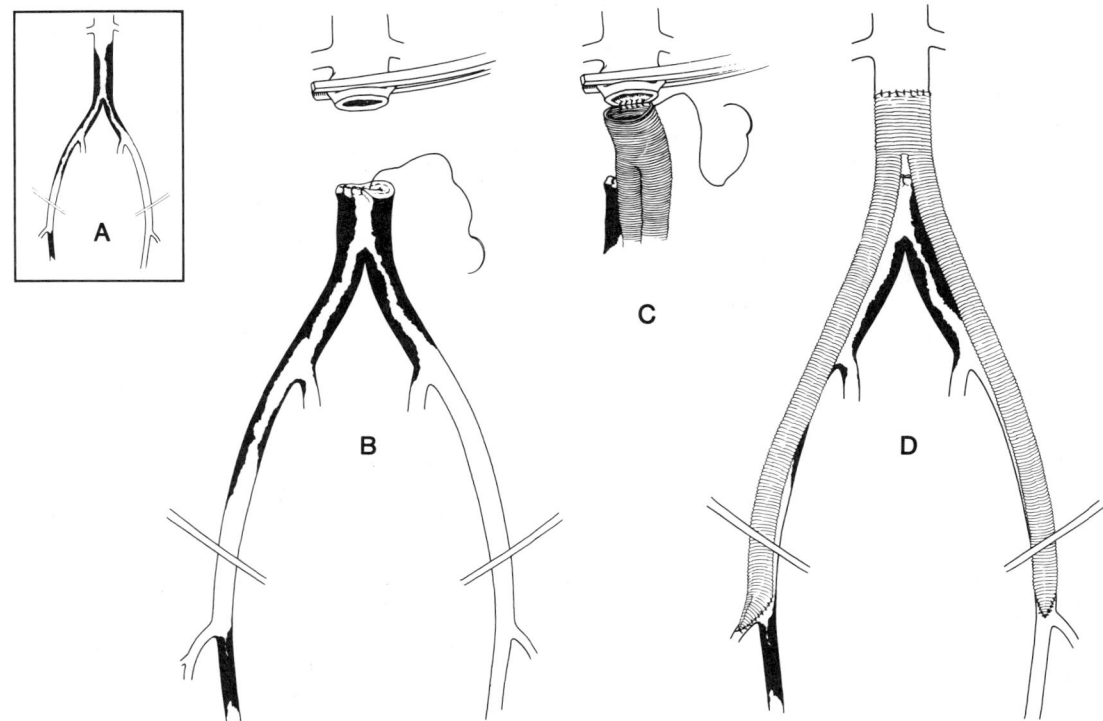

Figure 2 Technique of aortobifemoral bypass grafting. *A,* Preoperative aortogram. *B,* Segment of diseased aorta is resected and distal aortic stump oversewn. *C,* End-to-end proximal anastomosis. *D,* Completed reconstruction. (From Brewster DC. Direct reconstruction for aortoiliac occlusive disease. In: Rutherford RB, ed. Vascular surgery, 3rd ed. Philadelphia: WB Saunders, 1989: 667; with permission.)

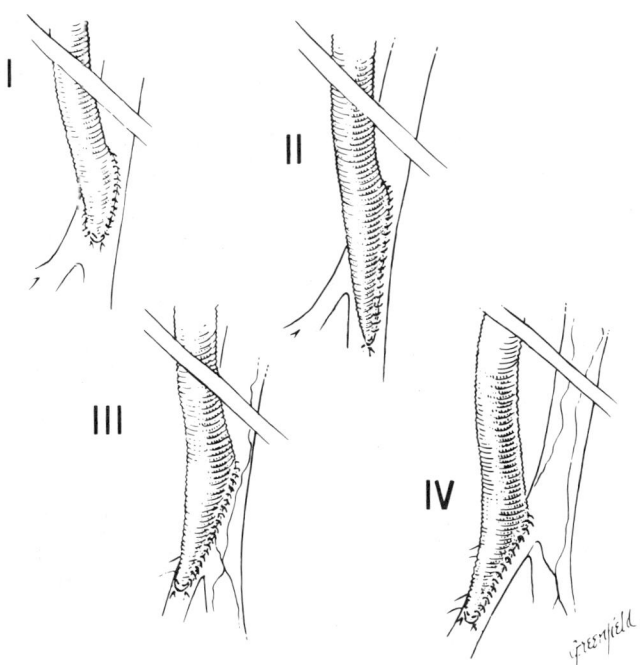

Figure 3 The four types of distal anastomosis for aortofemoral grafts. (From Darling RC, Brewster DC, Hallett JW Jr, et al. Aortoiliac reconstruction. Surg Clin North Am 1978; 59:565–579; with permission.)

Attention to several operative technical details have improved the outcome of bypass even in patients with multilevel occlusive disease. Current operative technique involves exposure of the abdominal aorta through a midline incision, with exposure of the aorta to the level of the left renal vein (Fig. 2). The femoral vessels are exposed through separate longitudinal groin incisions. The patient is systemically heparinized prior to the placement of the vascular clamps. The proximal anastomosis is performed high on the infrarenal aorta, where there tends to be less disease, in an end-to-end fashion. In order to facilitate this anastomosis, part of the proximal aorta is routinely resected to allow the graft to lie in the correct anatomic position, and proximal endarterectomy is performed if necessary. In patients who are found to have aortic occlusion, the proximal aorta is controlled just below the renal arteries. Vascular bulldog clamps can be placed on both renal arteries when the thrombus extends proximally to the level of the renal vessels to prevent embolization of any clot. Thrombectomy is then performed to the level of the renal arteries and completed with a blunt clamp, allowing the organized cap of thrombus that terminates the occlusion to be extruded. The use of interrupted mattress sutures to perform the proximal anastomosis is particularly useful in patients with small aortas in order to avoid compromising the lumen. We believe that the end-to-end anastomosis provides superior hemodynamic

Table 1 Aortobifemoral Bypass Graft Results

Authors	Years	Number of Grafts	Indications	Cumulative Patency (5 Years)	Cumulative Patency (10 Years)
Brewster & Darling[1]	1963–1977	241	65% Claudication 35% Limb salvage	88%	75%
Szilagyi et al.[5]	1954–1983	1186	70% Claudication 30% Limb salvage	77%	76%
Crawford et al.[6]	1955–1981	396	76% Claudication 24% Limb salvage	83%	71%
Malone et al.[7]	1959–1974	180	60% Claudication 40% Limb salvage	85%	66%
Martinez et al.[8]	1967–1977	376	72% Claudication 28% Limb salvage	88%	78%

flow characteristics, minimizes kinking of the graft because of its correct anatomic positioning, eliminates the possibility of competitive flow from patent common iliac vessels, and provides for better soft tissue coverage of the graft, and therefore, less risk of fistula formation or erosion into adjacent structures. Ultimately, end-to-end anastomoses should provide better long-term graft patency, although this has not been proven by any prospective randomized trials. Indications for use of a proximal end-to-side anastomosis include patients with extensive disease of the external iliac arteries where retrograde hypogastric perfusion is questionable, women with small aortas where even a 12 mm prosthesis cannot be used, and occasionally patients undergoing redo aortic procedures who have extensive scarring that prevents the safe circumferential control of the proximal aorta.

We routinely perform the distal anastomosis to the femoral vessels to maximize limb blood flow. This is particularly important in patients undergoing bypass with severe infrainguinal disease or superficial femoral artery (SFA) occlusion. The deep femoral artery provides the major source of outflow for the aortic graft in many of these patients. Thus, if there is any question of narrowing at the origin of the deep femoral artery, the distal toe of the graft is sutured onto the profunda as a patch angioplasty to widen the orifice (Fig. 3). In patients with minimal disease of the femoral vessels, a type I anastomosis can be performed to the common femoral artery. In patients with SFA disease or occlusion, a type III or type IV anastomosis can be performed. We have found that a type IV anastomosis to the isolated deep femoral artery can sustain the inflow from an aortic graft limb if the vessel accepts a 4 mm probe with good backbleeding and allows the passage of a noninflated catheter for a distance of approximately 20 cm. The type II anastomosis is the least commonly performed but is useful for preserving the origin of the SFA.

Finally, the improvement of prosthetic grafts, including increased flexibility, improved tissue incorporation, and a decreased tendency for pseudo-aneurysm formation, has also contributed to the excellent long-term results obtained with aortobifemoral grafting. We currently tend to use knitted Dacron grafts because of their conformability. This is particularly important when performing a type III or IV distal anastomosis in the groin. However, none of the currently available prosthetics has provided better long-term patency rates than any of the others. The more important factors are meticulous attention to operative technique and selection of the proper size of femoral limbs to match the outflow vessels.

Current results document that 5 year cumulative patency rates approach 88%, with 10 year rates approaching 75% and perioperative mortality rates well under 5% (Table 1).[1,5-8] Early complication rates approach 5% to 10%, including a 3% to 5% incidence of nonfatal myocardial infarction. Other complications such as bleeding, graft thrombosis, distal embolization, bowel ischemia, spinal chord ischemia, wound infection, and pulmonary injury occur much less frequently. Late complications include a 10% to 20% incidence of graft limb occlusion with most related to problems with outflow. Thrombectomy of occluded graft limbs has been effective and, when combined with distal bypass and repeat thrombectomies, can provide an extended limb patency rate of 74% at 5 years with a 30 day mortality rate of only 2%.[9] The incidence of aortoenteric fistula, graft infection, and anastomotic pseudo-aneurysm formation has fortunately been low in our series and should not be higher than 1% to 2%. The most serious long-term complication is death related to the high incidence of coronary artery disease. Five-year survival rates are in the 70% to 80% range, whereas 10 year survival drops to 40% to 50%.

A certain number of patients with type III disease and SFA occlusion require an outflow procedure in order to obtain satisfactory results. In our recent review of 181 such patients undergoing aortobifemoral bypass grafting, 4% of the patients required synchronous distal grafting, and another 13% required a distal bypass at an average of 2.5 months after the first operation. An additional 4% of patients who initially had a good result required a distal bypass at an average of 3 years after the first operation due to progression of distal disease, for a total additional graft rate of 21%.

REFERENCES

1. Brewster DC, Darling RC. Optimal methods of aortoiliac reconstruction. Surgery 1978; 84:739–748.
2. Duncan WC, Linton RR, Darling RC. Aortoiliofemoral atherosclerotic occlusive disease: Comparative results of endarterectomy and Dacron bypass grafts. Surgery 1971; 70:974–984.
3. Brewster DC. Clinical and anatomic considerations for surgery in aortoiliac disease and results of surgical treatment. Circulation 1991; 83(suppl 1):42–52.
4. Cambria RP, Yucel EK, Brewster DC, et al. The potential for lower extremity revascularization without contrast arteriography: Experience with magnetic resonance angiography. J Vasc Surg 1993; 17:1050–1057.
5. Szilagyi DE, Elliot JP, Smith RF, et al. A thirty year survey of the reconstructive surgical treatment of aortoiliac occlusive disease. J Vasc Surg 1986; 3:421–436.
6. Crawford ES, Bomberger RA, Glaeser DH, et al. Aortoiliac occlusive disease: Factors influencing survival and function following reconstructive operation over a twenty-five year period. Surgery 1981; 90:1055–1067.
7. Malone JM, Moore WS, Goldstone J. The natural history of bilateral aortofemoral bypass grafts for ischemia of the lower extremities. Arch Surg 1975; 110:1300–1306.
8. Martinez BD, Hertzer NR, Beven EG. Influence of distal arterial occlusive disease on prognosis following aortobifemoral bypass. Surgery 1980; 88:795–805.
9. Brewster DC, Meir GH, Darling RC, et al. Reoperation for aortofemoral graft limb occlusion: Optimal methods and long-term results. J Vasc Surg 1987; 5:363–374.

COARCTATION AND HYPOPLASIA OF THE SUBISTHMIC THORACIC AND ABDOMINAL AORTA

CHARLES J. SHANLEY, M.D.
JAMES C. STANLEY, M.D.

Focal developmental narrowings of the distal thoracic and midabdominal aorta are rare anomalies accounting for less than 2% of all aortic coarctations (Fig. 1). Most physicians have limited experience with the management of these unusual lesions. A more common entity, aortoiliac hypoplasia, is responsible for the "small aorta syndrome." Such a diffusely narrowed infrarenal aorta and iliac arterial system may evolve initially as a developmental lesion (Fig. 2). It occurs in a distinct subgroup of patients, mostly younger women, with atherosclerosis often affecting the narrowed segment. In fact, slightly more than 20% of women with arteriosclerotic aortoiliac occlusive disease manifest this entity.[1] Regardless of the particular nomenclature utilized, most evidence suggests that these diseases represent a spectrum of developmental abnormalities. Variations in their presentation relate more to different anatomic locations and secondary pathologic events than underlying etiologic differences.

ETIOLOGY

The most widely accepted hypothesis as to the cause of these narrowings relates to abnormal fetal aortic development, including faulty fusion of the two primitive dorsal aortae near day 25 of intrauterine life.[2] Indirect evidence in support of this is derived from the fact that multiple renal arteries occur in 70% of patients with

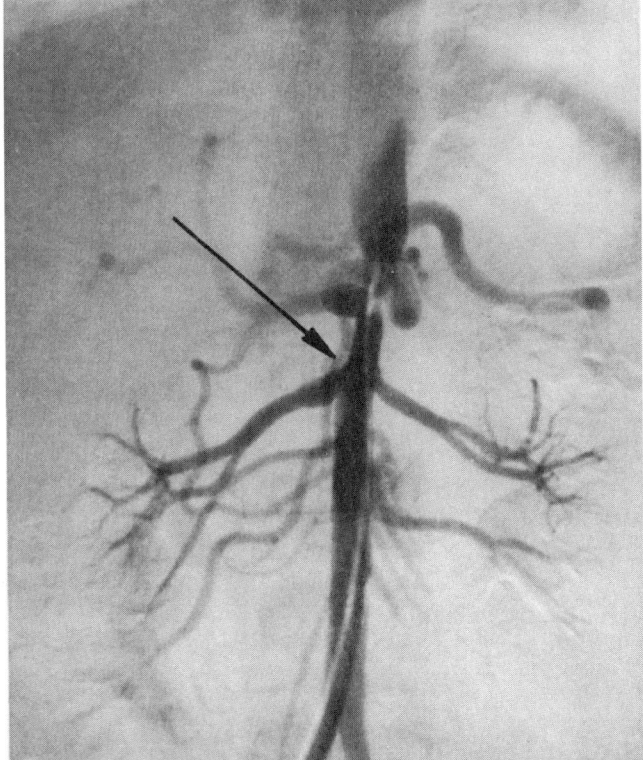

Figure 1 Midabdominal aortic coarctation with concomitant ostial stenoses of the celiac, superior mesenteric, and right renal arteries. Poststenotic dilation with aneurysmal changes were most evident in the renal artery (*arrow*). (From Stanley JC, Graham LM, Whitehouse WM Jr, et al. Developmental occlusive disease of the abdominal aorta, splanchnic and renal arteries. Am J Surg 1981; 142:190–196; with permission.)

narrowings of the midabdominal aorta.[3,4] This is two to three times the expected frequency of multiple renal arteries in the general population. These renal arteries often exhibit ostial narrowings (Figs. 3 and 4). The basis for this presentation is rather complex.

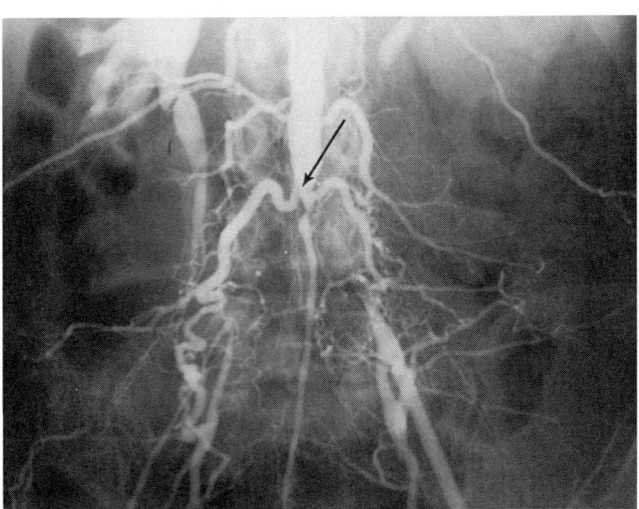

Figure 2 Aortoiliac hypoplasia with secondary arteriosclerotic terminal aortic occlusion in an adult female. Note the common orifice of the distal lumbar artery (*arrow*).

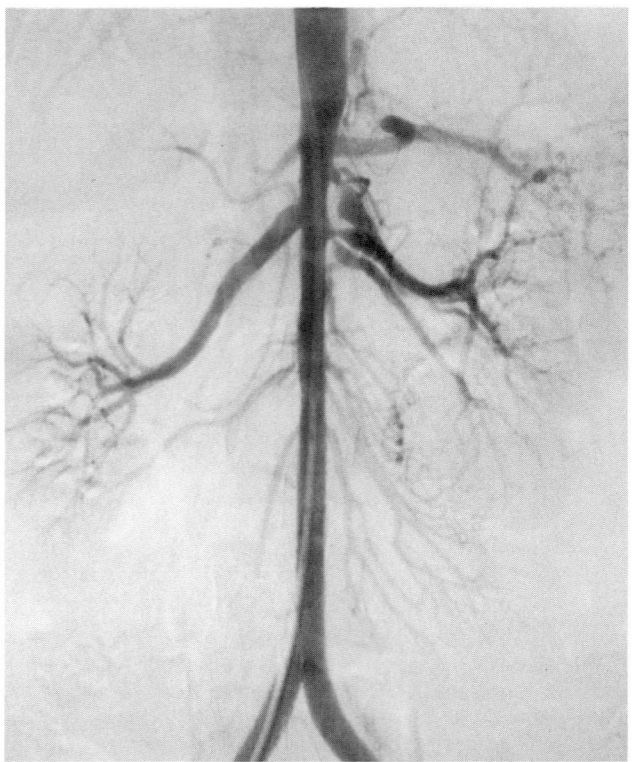

Figure 3 Diffuse aortic hypoplasia extending from the level of the celiac artery to the infrarenal aorta. Severe renal arterial occlusive disease is most apparent, affecting the ostia of two left renal arteries. (From Graham LM, Zelenock GB, Erlandson EE, et al. Abdominal aortic coarctation and segmental hypoplasia. Surgery 1979; 86:519–529; with permission.)

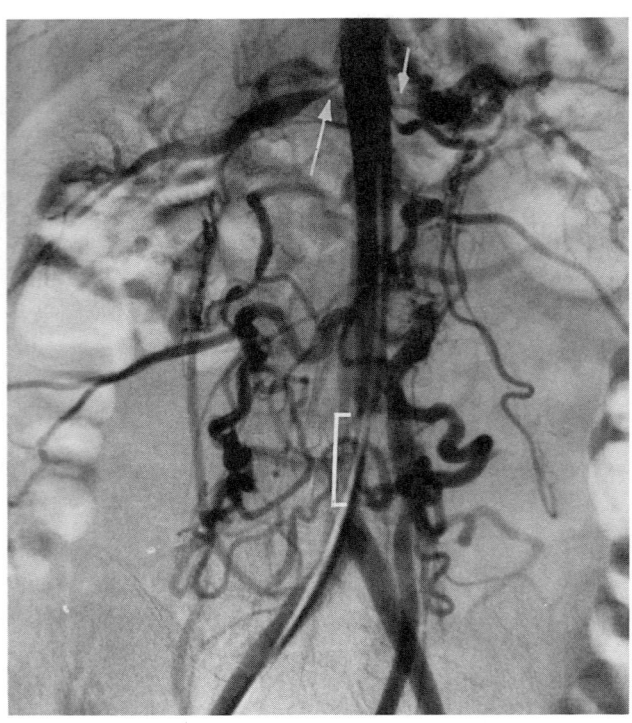

Figure 4 Bilateral renal artery stenoses (*arrows*) and an infrarenal abdominal aortic coarctation (*bracket*). (From Stanley JC, Wakefield TW. Arterial fibrodysplasia. In: Rutherford RB, ed. Vascular surgery. ed 3. Philadelphia: WB Saunders, 1989: 245; with permission.)

During normal development, fusion of the paired dorsal aortae occurs simultaneously, with regression of all but one dominant metanephric vessel to each kidney. This results in a single main renal artery on each side in 65% to 75% of fetuses. Development of this single renal artery occurs because of its obligate hemodynamic advantage over adjacent metanephric vessels. By creating local blood flow disturbances with an aortic fusion abnormality, this obligate hemodynamic advantage is lost and multiple metanephric channels persist. When the aortic coarctation is distant from the upper abdominal aorta, multiple renal arteries are less likely to develop (Fig. 4). Support for an overfusion of the two fetal aortas comes from the finding of a single bifurcating distal lumbar artery in up to 55% of patients with diffuse infrarenal aortoiliac hypoplasia (Fig. 2), compared to less than 5% in normal individuals.[5,6]

Theoretically, any event that alters the normal transition or organization of fetal mesenchymal cells into vascular smooth muscle may result in abnormalities of aortic, splanchnic artery, or renal artery development. This may explain the existence of aortic coarctation or hypoplasia following viral infections such as gestational rubella, or as a late consequence of certain inflammatory diseases such as Takayasu aortitis. Abnormalities in the growth and development of vascular smooth muscle have also been implicated in the frequent association of aortic hypoplasia with neurofibromatosis.[7] Finally, the occurrence of aortic hypoplasia and multiple aortic branch stenoses following infantile hypercalcemia lends further support to their developmental etiology.[8] Coincident with the aortic narrowings in these patients are accompanying visceral artery narrowings. These vessels are truly diminutive. It is more than happenstance that, of patients with midabdominal aortic narrowings, renal arterial stenoses were seen in 81% and splanchnic arterial occlusive disease in 22%.[3,4]

CLINICAL MANIFESTATIONS

Developmental narrowings of the distal thoracic and midabdominal aorta generally become evident during the first or second decade of life, with a mean age at initial diagnosis of 22 years.[3,4] There does not appear to be a gender predilection. The classic triad in these young patients consists of severe hypertension, diminished or absent femoral pulses, and an abdominal bruit. Lower extremity intermittent claudication occurs in approximately 25% of these patients.[3]

The natural history of patients with developmental narrowings of the distal thoracic or midabdominal aorta appears directly related to the severity of their hypertensive vascular disease. The prognosis for untreated patients is dismal, with most patients dying in early adulthood from cardiac failure or cerebrovascular accidents. In one review, 55% of untreated patients died at a mean age of 34 years.[3] Thus, all patients with coarctation or segmental hypoplasia of the distal thoracic or midabdominal aorta must be considered at risk for serious complications of their disease.

The most common location for developmental narrowings of the abdominal aorta is interrenal, occurring in 52% of patients. Isolated narrowings affect the suprarenal aorta in 11% of patients, the infrarenal aorta in 25% of patients, and diffuse involvement of the entire abdominal aorta in an additional 12% of patients.[3,4] Aortography with both anterior-posterior and lateral projections is essential to define the precise extent of aortic narrowing and associated aortic branch disease.

In contrast to focal developmental lesions at or above the renal arteries, infrarenal narrowings usually become symptomatic in the third or fourth decade of life as a result of secondary atherosclerotic occlusive disease. There is a universally recognized predilection for women to exhibit hypoplastic aortoiliac lesions. Although the genetic basis for this phenomenon is unknown, anecdotal evidence suggests a higher incidence among women with red hair. The primary site of involvement is generally the distal aorta just above its bifurcation. Presenting symptoms are usually those of progressive lower extremity intermittent claudication. Among patients with atherosclerotic occlusive disease, those with infrarenal aortoiliac hypoplasia present with symptoms approximately 10 years earlier than those having normal-sized arteries.[5,6,9] This probably relates to earlier encroachment by arteriosclerotic plaque on the patient's already narrowed aortic lumen. The life expectancy of patients with developmental narrowings of the infrarenal aorta parallels the extent of their systemic arteriosclerotic disease.

MANAGEMENT

There is no role for long-term medical management of patients with severe hypertension secondary to developmental narrowings of the distal thoracic and midabdominal aorta. Conventional drug interventions for control of hypertension have been largely unsuccessful, and angiotensin converting enzyme inhibitors have potentially deleterious effects on renal function in these patients. Because the developmental narrowings represent true hypoplastic vessels, percutaneous transluminal renal artery dilatation has met with limited success and poses a significant risk for extensive vessel fracture with overly zealous attempts at angioplasty. In other instances, because of the increased content of elastic tissue in the vessel wall, balloon dilation may initially appear successful with stretching of the vessel, only to be followed by immediate return of the stenosis with balloon deflation. Thus, percutaneous angioplasty has not been favored for treatment of this disease.

The surgical approach to these complex developmental anomalies must be individualized, based on the aortic pathology and extent of renal and splanchnic arterial disease. An important goal is to restore normal renal perfusion in order to relieve hypertension. A single-staged reconstruction is currently favored to avoid the technical difficulties that may accompany secondary staged operations. Thoracoabdominal bypass or patch aortoplasty with concomitant renal revascularizations have been preferred in treating these patients.

Extensive anatomic exposure of the distal thoracic and midabdominal aorta is essential to achieve a technically satisfactory result. Exposure of the suprarenal aorta is facilitated by a thoracoabdominal incision through the left sixth or seventh intercostal space. This incision is generally extended from the left posterior axillary line across the costal margin, either to the right of the umbilicus or along the midline to the suprapubic region. A circumferential incision of the left hemidiaphragm near its periphery facilitates exposure of the distal thoracic aorta. An extraperitoneal medial rotation of the abdominal viscera following incision of the lateral parietes provides exposure of the abdominal aorta and its branches. For lesions confined to the pararenal region, a transverse supraumbilical abdominal incision extended laterally to the posterior axillary lines, combined with medial rotation of the viscera, is preferred to a midline incision and transmesenteric approach.

Prior to aortic clamping, systemic anticoagulation is achieved with intravenous heparin sodium (150 units/kg). A brisk diuresis is established with administration of intravenous mannitol. In the past, thoracoabdominal bypasses employing expanded polytetrafluoroethylene (ePTFE) or knitted Dacron prostheses, in conjunction

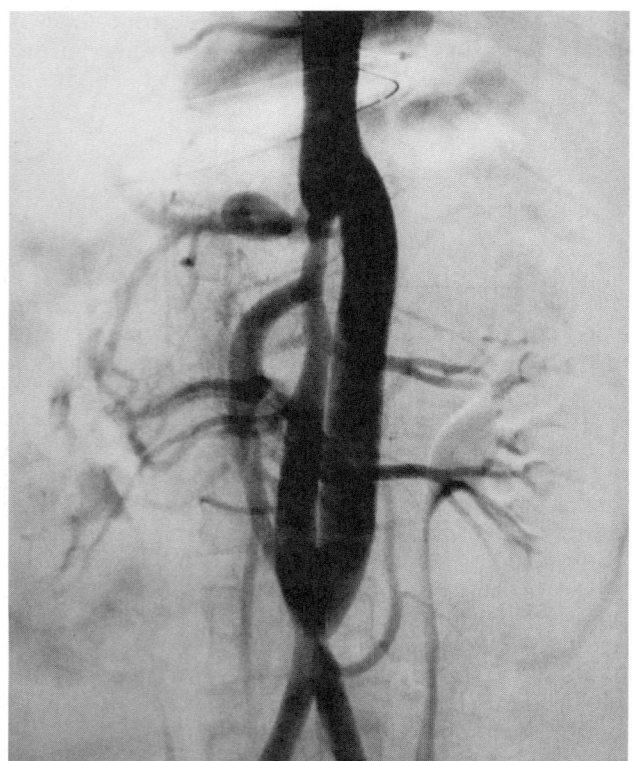

Figure 5 Thoracoabdominal bypass (Dacron velour graft) and aortorenal bypass to right renal artery in a 14-year-old patient who had a suprarenal abdominal aortic coarctation and ostial stenosis of the right renal artery. (From Graham LM, Zelenock GB, Erlandson EE, et al. Abdominal aortic coarctations and segmental hypoplasia. Surgery 1979; 86:519–529; with permission.)

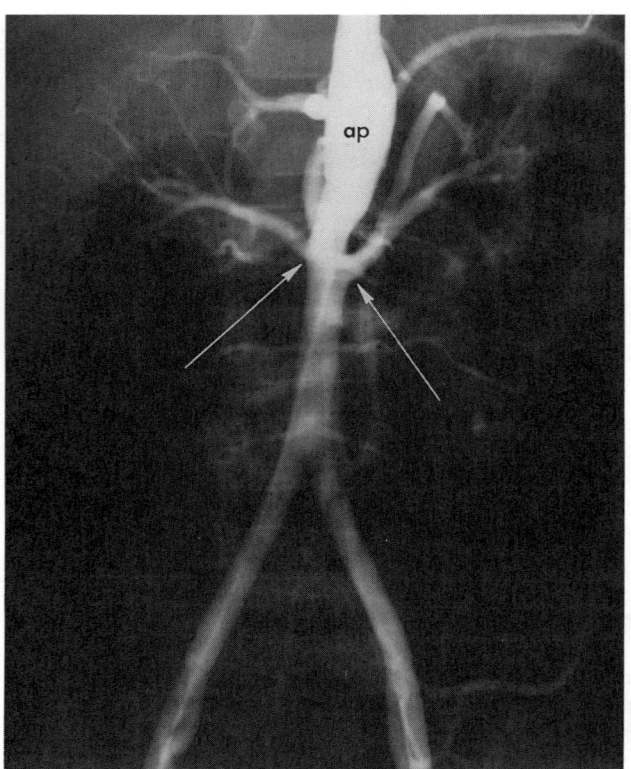

Figure 6 Aortoplasty (*ap*) of midabdominal aortic coarctation (ePTFE patch) with bilateral reimplantation of renal arteries (*arrows*) in a 5-year-old patient who had a suprarenal abdominal aortic coarctation and bilateral renal artery ostial stenotic disease. (From Stanley JC, Brothers TE. Midabdominal aortic coarctations and hypoplasia associated with renal artery stenosis. In: Ernst CB, Stanley JC, eds. Current therapy in vascular surgery. ed 2. Philadelphia: BC Decker, 1991: 856; with permission.)

with renal or visceral revascularization, were the most common procedures undertaken (Fig. 5). The proximal aortic anastomosis is constructed first, in an end-to-side fashion using continuous 3-0 or 4-0 polypropylene suture above the level of the coarctation. The bypass graft is tunneled through the posterior hemidiaphragm behind the left kidney to the level of the infrarenal aorta. The distal anastomosis is subsequently constructed in a similar fashion. Lesions of the splanchnic and renal vessels are invariably ostial in location. Autogenous saphenous vein, internal iliac artery, and small-diameter ePTFE are the bypass conduits that have been used for visceral arterial reconstructions. These grafts may originate from the thoracoabdominal graft or the native aorta, with origination from the latter preferred.

The optimal technique for treating younger children with these aortic anomalies is a primary aortoplasty employing a Dacron or ePTFE patch, combined with direct implantation of the normal splanchnic or renal arteries, beyond their diseased segments, into the native aorta (Fig. 6). In these patients the aorta, as well as its visceral branches, are controlled, and the patch is sewn into place with 3-0 or 4-0 polypropylene before undertaking the visceral artery reimplantations. The patch should be generous enough to allow for normal growth but not so large as to be aneurysmal with mural thrombus formation and possible subsequent embolization. Advantages of this technique include avoidance of competitive parallel arterial flow within the native aorta and thoracoabdominal bypass graft, the absence of free visceral interposition grafts, and a reduction in the number of required anastomoses.

In patients with infrarenal aortoiliac hypoplasia, medical management should center around reduction of risk factors for atherosclerosis, especially the cessation of cigarette smoking. The primary goal of operative therapy in this subgroup of patients is improvement of lower extremity perfusion and alleviation of disabling intermittent claudication. Percutaneous transluminal angioplasty is generally not recommended due to the diffuse nature of the aortic hypoplasia and the high risk of recurrence. The use of intralumenal stents may obviate certain failures attributed to percutaneous balloon angioplasty, but experience with this technology in this particular subgroup of patients is currently too limited to support its routine use.

Aortofemoral bypass is generally considered the operative treatment of choice in these patients. A standard transperitoneal approach to the infrarenal aorta is used. Small-caliber bifurcated ePTFE grafts are favored for these reconstructions. An end-to-end proximal graft-to-aorta anastomosis is preferred, although in patients with very small aortas an end-to-side anastomosis should be used. The graft-to-femoral artery anastomoses are constructed in a conventional end-to-side fashion. When an aortofemoral bypass is not feasible, other techniques have been employed, including axillofemoral or thoracofemoral bypasses and aortoiliac endarterectomy. Endarterectomy and patch angioplasty are not favored in treating most infrarenal aortoiliac lesions because of their predisposition to restenosis. Exceptions exist with exceedingly focal lesions at the terminal aorta, where a limited aortic endarterectomy would be appropriate.

RESULTS

Surgical treatment of midabdominal aortic coarctation and hypoplasia provides excellent results. At the University of Michigan Medical Center, thoracoabdominal bypass or patch aortoplasty combined with visceral arterial reconstructions has yielded good to excellent results in 93% of younger patients with these developmental lesions. There have been no operative deaths in this experience. Aortofemoral bypass and occasional endarterectomy with patch closure for infrarenal aortoiliac hypoplasia in the older patient exhibiting secondary atherosclerosis carry a 90% patency at 5 years, despite the tiny caliber of the outflow vessels.

REFERENCES

1. Cronenwett JL, Garrett HE. Arteriographic measurement of the abdominal aorta, iliac, and femoral arteries in women with atherosclerotic occlusive disease. Radiology 1983; 148:389–392.
2. Arnot RS, Louw JH. The anatomy of the posterior wall of the abdominal aorta: Its significance with regard to hypoplasia of the distal aorta. S Afr Med J 1973; 47:899–902.
3. Graham LM, Zelenock GB, Erlandson EE, et al. Abdominal aortic coarctation and segmental hypoplasia. Surgery 1979; 86:519–529.
4. Stanley JC, Graham LM, Whitehouse WM Jr, et al. Developmental occlusive disease of the abdominal aorta and the splanchnic and renal arteries. Am J Surg 1981; 142:190–196.
5. Caes F, Cham B, Van den Brande P, Welch W. Small artery syndrome in women. Surg Gynecol Obstet 1985; 161:165–170.
6. Palmaz JC, Carson SN, Hunter G, Weinshelbaum A. Male hypoplastic infrarenal aorta and premature atherosclerosis. Surgery 1983; 94:91–94.
7. Greene JF, Fitzwater JE, Burgess J. Arterial lesions associated with neurofibromatosis. Am J Clin Pathol 1974; 62:481–487.
8. Wiltse HE, Goldbloom RB, Antia AU, et al. Infantile hypercalcemia syndrome in twins. N Engl J Med 1966; 275:1157–1160.
9. DeLaurentis DA, Friedmann SO, Wolferth CC Jr. Atherosclerosis and the hypoplastic aortoiliac system. Surgery 1978; 83:27–37.

ENDARTERECTOMY FOR ATHEROSCLEROTIC AORTOILIAC OCCLUSIVE DISEASE

ALLAN R. DOWNS, M.D.

Thromboendarterectomy of the femoral artery was the first effective method of direct arterial reconstruction introduced by Dos Santos in 1947.[1] Early reports by Wylie[2] and Rob and Downs[3] documented the efficacy of aortoiliac thromboendarterectomy. Over the past two decades, prosthetic grafts have replaced endarterectomy as the preferred procedure for aortoiliac reconstruction, and endarterectomy is now infrequently used.[4]

In our experience with aortoiliac reconstruction for occlusive disease from 1958 to 1968, 40% of patients with aortoiliac occlusive disease were treated with endarterectomy and about two-thirds of these were unilateral iliac or iliofemoral endarterectomies performed by the open or semiclosed technique. Between 1968 and 1979 our group performed 335 reconstructions for aortoiliac disease, including only 50 (14%) endarterectomies. The remainder were treated with prosthetic bypass grafts. The 5 year patencies of aortofemoral grafts and aortoiliac endarterectomies were almost identical at 86%. From 1982 to 1987, 471 patients were operated upon for aortoiliac occlusive disease, with endarterectomies performed in only 4.8% of patients.[5] This has decreased to 2% in the past 5 years. Except for our early experience, extensive aortoileofemoral endarterectomies, as reported by Inahara, has not been performed.[6]

Aortoiliac endarterectomy is now reserved for occlusive disease localized to the distal infrarenal aorta and common iliac arteries in patients younger than 50. A rare indication would be limb-threatening ischemia due to aortoiliac occlusion in a septic patient in whom a prosthetic graft would be undesirable. We had such an experience recently when aortoiliac endarterectomy obviated need for prosthetic reconstruction in the presence of infection. The advantages of endarterectomy remain those related to autogenous tissue, primarily an absence of late complications including infection, false aneurysm development, and prosthetic aortointestinal fistulas.

CLINICAL PRESENTATION

Generally only patients under 50 years of age have atherosclerotic occlusive disease localized to the aortoiliac segment. This is particularly so in young women with midabdominal aortic lesions that are amenable to endarterectomy. These patients usually present with claudication in the calves, thighs, and buttocks, but occasionally the symptoms are limited to the thighs and buttocks. Rarely this is described as weakness or paralysis of the legs on exercise rather than claudication. Impotence is usually present in males with bilateral iliac arterial involvement. Occasionally the patient presents with toe ischemia due to embolization, even in the absence of claudication. When there is aortoiliac stenosis, femoral pulses may be present along with abdominal, iliac, and femoral bruits. Segmental thigh, calf, and ankle Doppler-derived pressures may be helpful in determining the severity and level of occlusive disease. Treadmill testing may be necessary to document hemodynamically significant blood pressure decreases at the ankles. Arteriography is performed by either the translumbar or transfemoral route to determine the site and extent of disease. Biplane arteriography may be necessary to document discrete eccentric stenotic lesions.

PROCEDURE

General anesthesia with epidural analgesia for postoperative pain management is generally used. The patient is draped in a supine position with exposure from xiphoid to thighs to allow access to the groins if bypass should be necessary. The abdomen is explored through a long midline incision, and the external iliac arteries are assessed. If there is significant external iliac arterial disease, the procedure is abandoned and an aortofemoral bypass grafting is performed. In the absence of external iliac disease, the aorta and common iliac arteries are exposed from below the left renal vein to the common iliac bifurcations. In the male the sympathetic plexus across the left common iliac artery is preserved in an attempt to avoid postoperative impotence and retrograde ejaculation. The aorta is mobilized proximal to the inferior mesenteric artery until the wall feels relatively normal. The common, internal, and external iliac arteries are mobilized distally, and the lumbar and medial sacral arteries are identified for control with clips. The patient is given 5,000 units of heparin sodium systemically, and the aorta and iliac arteries are clamped.

The aorta and right common iliac artery are opened with one longitudinal incision that should extend to the distal limits of the plaque. A posterior tongue of plaque often extends into the external iliac orifice. The internal iliac artery is endarterectomized blindly by a blunt dissector. The left common iliac artery is opened with a separate longitudinal incision distal to the sympathetic plexus. The endarterectomy from the aorta to the bifurcation of the right common iliac artery is completed. The proximal left common iliac artery is endarterectomized from the aortic bifurcation to the separate incision distally. Endarterectomy beyond the first 1 cm of the external iliac artery is not recommended. The external iliac arteries should accept a 4 mm dilator following the endarterectomy. If the origin of the external iliac artery is narrow or if tacking stitches are necessary to secure a posterior plaque, a short saphenous vein patch should be used for the distal 2 to 3 cm of closure. The remainder of the common iliac artery and aorta are closed with running 5-0 or 6-0 polypropylene suture.

Blood flow is re-established into the right leg, and the separate left common iliac arteriotomy is similarly closed starting distally. Again, if the external iliac artery is small, it may require a vein patch. After re-establishing blood flow into the left leg, protamine sulfate is given to reverse the heparin effect. When hemostasis has been attained, blood flow should be assessed with a Doppler intraoperatively, and the femoral arteries should be palpable.

RESULTS

Results following aortoiliac endarterectomy in our early experience were comparable to aortofemoral grafting, with a 5 year patency rate of 80% to 90%. Inahara and Vitale have continued to report excellent results with extensive iliofemoral endarterectomy.[7,8] During the past 15 years the operation has been restricted to only 2% to 5% of our patients with very localized disease so that the results cannot be compared with patients treated with aortofemoral grafts, 65% of whom have associated superficial femoral disease. However, late failures following aortoiliac endarterectomy can be treated with bypass grafting with little additional morbidity, and the patients will not have risked the complications of prosthetic grafting such as graft infection, anastomotic false aneurysm, and prosthetic intestinal fistulas. Aneurysm development following abdominal aortic endarterectomy has rarely been reported, but an abdominal aortic aneurysm has been successfully repaired in a patient who underwent an aortoiliac endarterectomy 25 years earlier.

REFERENCES

1. Dos Santos JC. Sur la desobstion des thromoses arterielles anciennes. Mem Acad Chir 1947; 73:409–411.
2. Wylie EJ. Thromboendarterectomy for arteriosclerotic thrombosis of major arteries. Surgery 1952; 32:275–292.
3. Rob CG, Downs AR. Chronic occlusive disease of the aorta and iliac arteries (treatment and results). J Cardiovasc Surg 1960; 1:57–64.
4. Brewster DC. Direct reconstruction for aorto-iliac occlusive disease. In: Rutherford RB, ed. Vascular surgery, 3rd ed. Philadelphia: WB Saunders, 1989:667.
5. Johnston KW, Rae M, Hogg-Johnston SA, et al. Five-year results of a prospective study of percutaneous transluminal angioplasty. Ann Surg 1987; 106:403–413.
6. Inahara T. Eversion endarterectomy for aortoiliofemoral occlusive disease: A 16-year experience. Am J Surg 1979; 138:196–204.
7. Vitale GF, Inahara T, Extraperitoneal endarterectomy for iliofemoral occlusive disease. J Vasc Surg 1990; 12:409–415.
8. Inahara T. Endarterectomy for atherosclerotic aortoiliac and aortofemoral occlusive disease. In: Ernst CB, Stanley JC, eds. Current therapy in vascular surgery, 2nd ed. Philadelphia: BC Decker, 1991:398.

PERCUTANEOUS ARTERIAL DILATION FOR ATHEROSCLEROTIC AORTOILIAC OCCLUSIVE DISEASE

KYUNG J. CHO, M.D.
THOMAS PFAMMATTER, M.D.

Percutaneous transluminal angioplasty (PTA) has become an important method of treating atherosclerotic aortoiliac occlusive disease (AIOD). Since the initial reports by Dotter and Judkins in 1964 and Grüntzig and Kumpe in 1979, much experience has accumulated utilizing this method.[1,2] More recently, the introduction of intravascular stents has expanded the application of PTA from focal stenoses to more complex aortoiliac occlusive lesions.[3-5] Balloon angioplasty and stent placement may be used in a complementary fashion in a given patient, but stents are more often used when PTA has failed or seems unlikely to be successful.

ARTERIOGRAPHY

Arteriography should always be performed prior to PTA to provide a vascular roadmap and to define the sites and degrees of occlusive disease, distal runoff vessels, and collateral circulation. Because PTA and stent placement can be performed at the same session of arteriography, we obtain the patient's informed consent for both procedures. Both groins are prepared when arteriography and/or PTA is to be performed. The right femoral approach is preferable to the left femoral approach, which is used for patients in whom the right femoral artery cannot be used or in whom arterial dilation is to be performed in the left iliac artery. The distal left axillary or proximal brachial artery may also be used for arteriography and PTA for patients in whom neither femoral artery can be used. Because the femoral arteries are usually patent in the presence of aortoiliac occlusion, the nonpalpable femoral artery can be punctured by using the bony landmark or Doppler ultrasound.

The Seldinger percutaneous technique is used for arteriography and percutaneous arterial dilation for atherosclerotic AIOD. The technique involves percutaneous puncture of the common femoral artery with either an 18 or 19 gauge Seldinger-type needle, insertion of a 0.035 inch guide wire through the needle, dilation of the puncture site, and introduction of a 5 Fr catheter (usually pigtail type) into the abdominal aorta. After the catheter is positioned at the level of the renal arteries, biplane aortography is obtained with an injection of 76% contrast medium (15 to 18 ml/second for 2 seconds for cut-film arteriography and 15 ml for 1 second for digital subtraction arteriography). The catheter is then retracted to the distal abdominal aorta for evaluation of the iliac and femoral arteries and their outflow vessels. Either biplane or oblique projections are used for evaluation of the iliac and femoral arteries. For evaluation of one extremity, the catheter is positioned in the external iliac artery for unilateral injection of contrast medium to improve visualization of the outflow vessels. Intra-arterial pressure measurement is used to assess the functional significance of the obstruction before and after an intra-arterial injection of a vasodilator such as tolazoline. Cut-film and intra-arterial digital subtraction arteriography (IA DSA) are used in complementary fashion. Recent advances in equipment have increased the use of IA DSA for evaluation of peripheral arterial occlusive lesions. It is particularly useful in evaluating the results of arterial dilation. When the examination is completed, the catheter is removed, and manual pressure is applied to the puncture site for 10 to 15 minutes. After adequate hemostasis is achieved, the patient is kept in bed for 8 hours. During this period the patient's vital signs and peripheral pulses are monitored, and the puncture site is visually inspected for bleeding.

Atherosclerotic disease can produce a wide spectrum of arteriographic abnormalities that usually reflect the gross morphologic changes. The nonocclusive form of the disease produces irregular wall and filling defects of the contrast opacified arteries, often associated with vessel elongation and tortuosity. The occlusive atheromatous plaques produce focal or long occlusion of the arteries. Aortic occlusions occur initially at or just above the aortic bifurcation and propagate proximally to the level of the renal arteries and distally to the common iliac arteries. The collateral pathways associated with AIOD vary with the site and length of the obstruction and the patency of collateral vessels.

PERCUTANEOUS ARTERIAL DILATION

It is essential for interventional radiologists and vascular surgeons to review the clinical situations and arteriograms of each patient before percutaneous arterial dilation. Selection of the proper catheterization method and equipment for percutaneous arterial dilation is important in obtaining successful results. It should depend on the location and type of the occlusive lesions, the availability of arterial access, and the angiographer's experience. Balloon catheters are usually used for dilation of focal, circumferential stenoses of the infrarenal abdominal aorta and the iliac arteries. Intravascular stents have been developed to supplement PTA and prevent restenosis. The two major types of intravascular stents that are currently used in the infrarenal abdominal aorta and iliac arteries are the Palmaz balloon-expandable stent and self-expanding Wallstents. The Palmaz stent is rigid and requires a 10 Fr sheath for placement. It is approved by the FDA for use in the

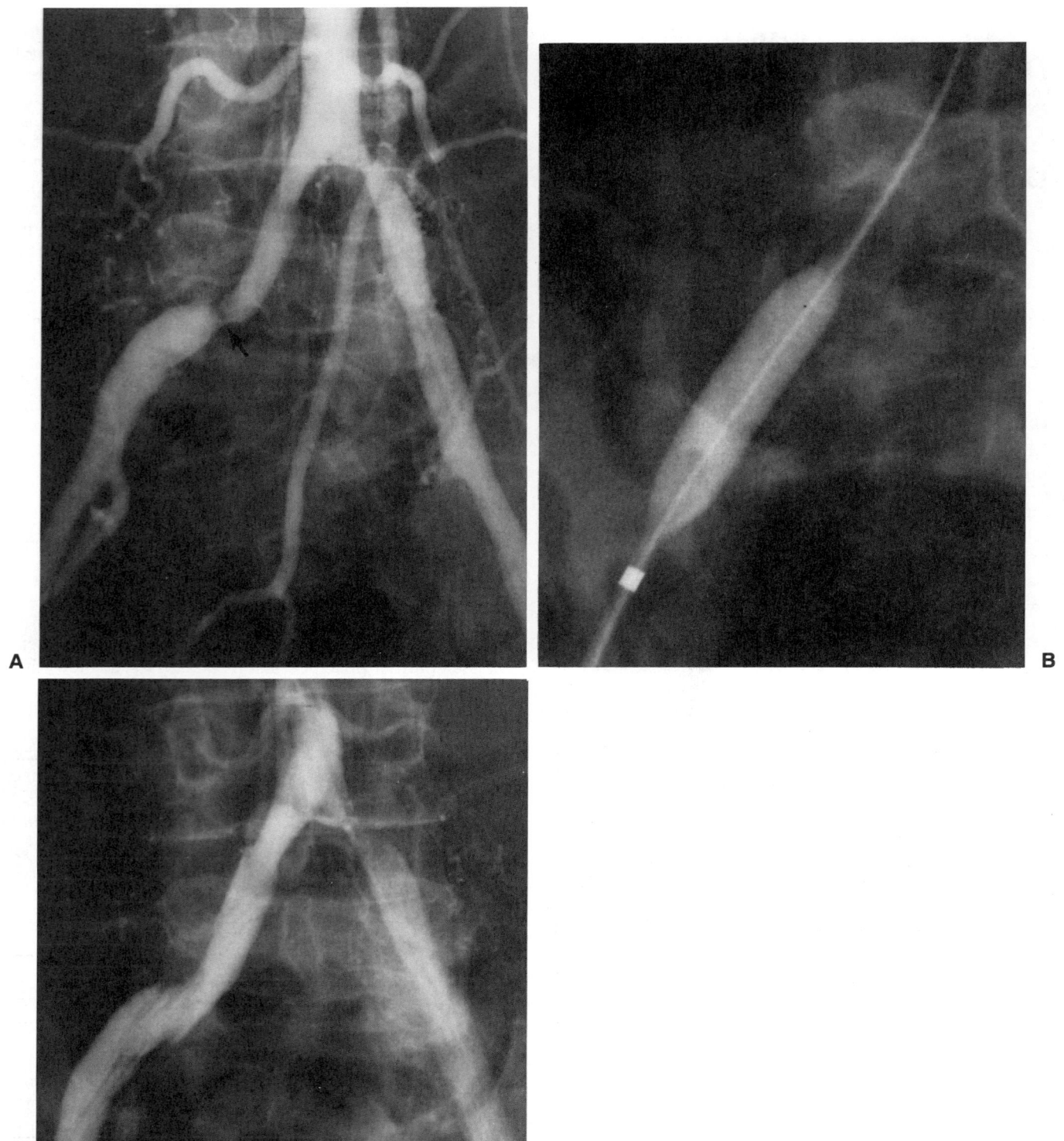

Figure 1 Iliac artery percutaneous transluminal angioplasty (PTA). *A*, Iliac arteriogram in a patient with right lower extremity claudication demonstrating high-grade stenosis of the common iliac artery *(arrow)*. *B*, The balloon catheter has been inflated at the site of the common iliac artery lesion. *C*, Post-PTA angiogram demonstrating a good angiographic result.

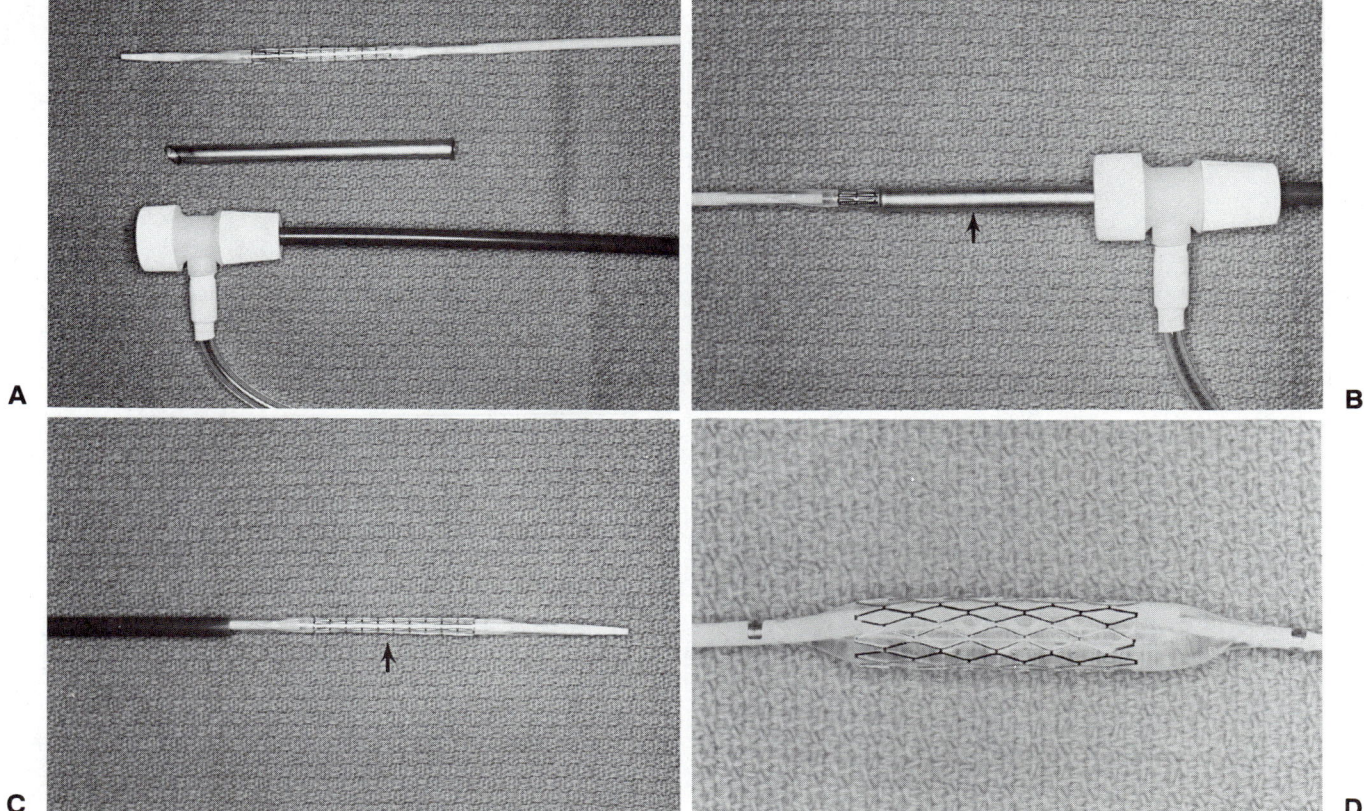

Figure 2 Palmaz balloon-expandable stent and required equipment for stent implantation. *A,* A Palmaz stent is mounted on a balloon catheter *(top)* using a crimping tube and crimping tool (not shown). Introducer tube *(middle),* 30 cm long introducer sheath *(bottom). B,* Insertion of stent-balloon assembly through introducer tube *(arrow),* which has been inserted through the hemostatic valve of the sheath, *C,* Stent-balloon assembly *(arrow)* has exited from the introducer. *D,* The balloon catheter is inflated to expand the stent. Length of unexpanded stent is 30 mm. Length of stent after expansion to 8 m is 28.9 mm.

treatment of common and external iliac arterial lesions in the United States and other countries. The Wallstent is flexible and requires an 8 Fr sheath for deployment. Clinical experience with atherectomy devices and lasers in the iliac artery is quite limited.

Abdominal Aortic PTA

Circumferential, focal, distal abdominal aortic atherosclerotic stenoses can be treated by PTA. The aortic PTA technique is the same as that used for iliac PTA. If the aortic stenosis to be dilated involves the aortic bifurcation, two balloon catheters are introduced from each femoral artery and inflated simultaneously to prevent displacement of the plaques and downstream embolization.[6] The diameter of the balloon catheter should be the same as that of the aorta to be dilated and is estimated by measuring the aorta proximal or distal to the lesion. During the procedure the patient is administered 3,000 to 5,000 units of heparin sodium. Anticoagulant therapy is not usually required afterward. Antiplatelet agents, such as aspirin and dipyridamole, may be useful in maintaining long-term patency following angioplasty. In several reports over a 12 year period, the rate of technical success of aortic PTA has been 93% to 100%, and the long-term patency was 75% to 100%.[6-9] The benefit of stent placement following successful aortic PTA remains unknown. However, stenting is generally indicated for the treatment of complex, abdominal aortic stenoses.

Focal abdominal aortic atherosclerotic occlusions can be treated with PTA and stenting. The technique involves the intra-aortic infusion of a lytic agent, balloon dilation, and stent placement. Experience is still too limited to assess the safety and long-term patency of such treatment. At present PTA is used only for the patient with focal aortic occlusion at high risk for surgical therapy.

Iliac Artery PTA

Since the late 1970s, reports have documented the efficacy and long-term patency of iliac PTA. Current indications for iliac PTA are (1) focal, concentric stenoses of the common and/or external iliac arteries (Fig. 1); (2) to increase inflow in patients in whom either

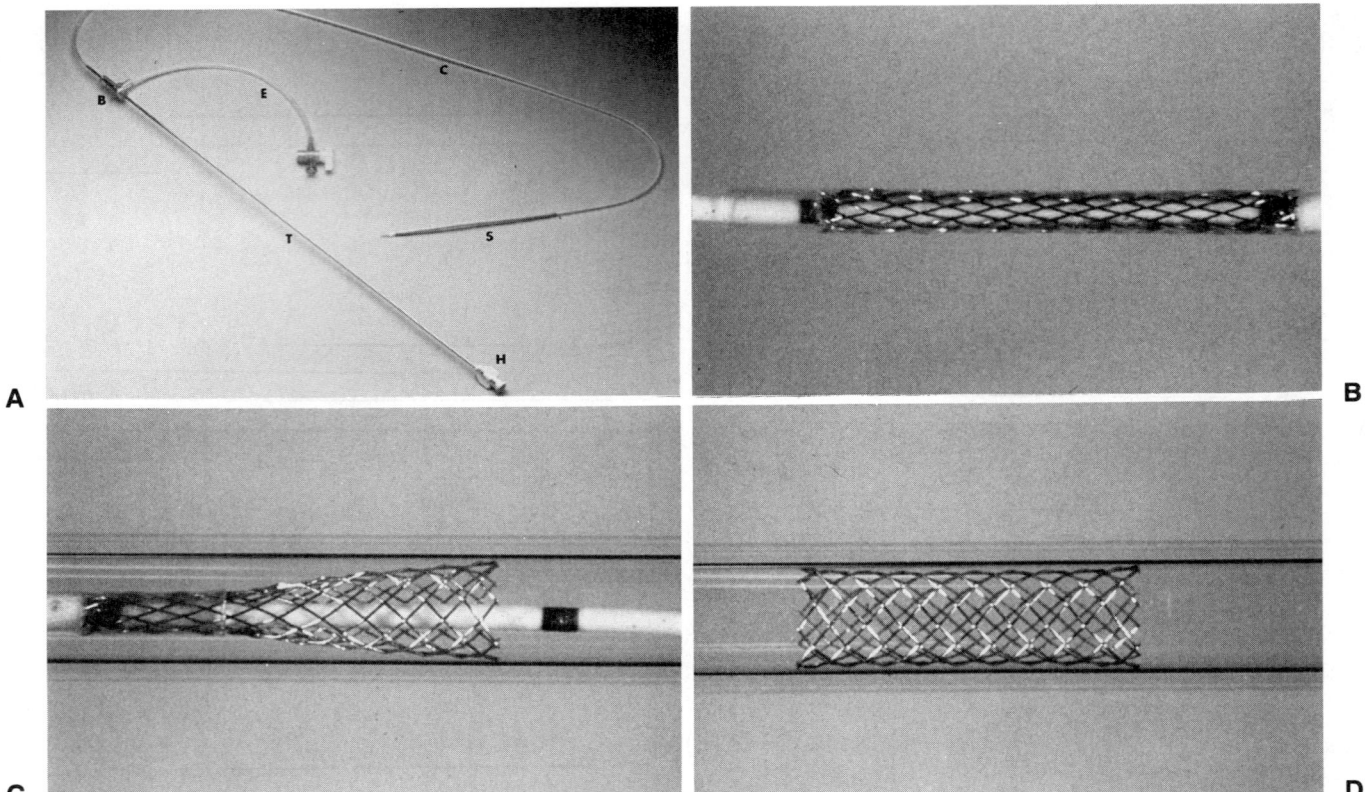

Figure 3 The Schneider Wallstent with the Unistep delivery device and mechanism of deployment. *A,* The delivery system (110 cm in length) consists of coaxial catheters *(C)*, stent *(S)*, valve body *(B)*, stainless steel tube *(T)*, and extension tube *(E)*. Sterile saline is injected into the extension tube to facilitate deployment of the stent. The stent is released by retracting the valve body of the outer tube along the stainless steel tube toward the hub *(H)*. *B,* The stent mounted between the inner and outer tubes is introduced through a 8 Fr sheath over a 180 cm, 0.035 inch guide wire. *C,* The stent has been partially released. A partially deployed stent can only be pulled back for precise stent placement or removed from the patient. Note that the stent is shortened upon release. *D,* Stent release has been completed and the delivery system was removed.

PTA or surgical bypass is considered for infrainguinal arterial occlusive disease; and (3) to increase inflow for limb salvage in the patient with severe infrainguinal arterial disease. There are no absolute contraindications to iliac PTA. Diffuse iliac artery stenoses and heavily calcified lesions should not be treated by PTA.

The patient to undergo iliac PTA should be evaluated by arteriography following a noninvasive Doppler study. Because precise positioning of the balloon catheter is important, a cut-film arteriogram or digital roadmapping capability should be available in the procedure room. The ipsilateral femoral approach is preferred for iliac PTA and stenting. If the artery to be dilated involves the external iliac artery, the femoral artery should be punctured below the inguinal ligament to avoid dilating the puncture hole of the artery. If the femoral artery is not palpable, Doppler ultrasound guidance, digital roadmapping technique, or other landmarks such as the femoral head or femoral arterial calcification are used to facilitate the arterial puncture.

The technique of PTA is similar to that used in percutaneous arteriography. After the femoral artery has been punctured, a 0.035 inch guide wire is advanced to the level of the lesion, and over the guide wire a catheter is advanced. Then a flexible-tip torque guide wire such as Glide wire is used to traverse the lesion. After the guide wire has crossed the lesion, the catheter is advanced into the abdominal aorta, and contrast medium is injected for an arteriogram and digital roadmapping. The catheter is then exchanged for a balloon catheter of the appropriate balloon size over the guide wire. After precise placement of the balloon catheter at the site of the lesion under fluoroscopy, the balloon is inflated until balloon waist resulting from the stenosis is effaced. The balloon may be inflated two to three times for 30 to 40 seconds at each inflation. If the stenosis to be dilated is longer than the length of the balloon, dilation should proceed from proximal to distal portion of the lesion. Extreme care must be taken when crossing the previously dilated stenosis to prevent arterial damage. This is especially important when stenting is to be performed for the treatment of PTA-induced dissection. Therefore, the guide wire must be left in place through the angioplasty site until the

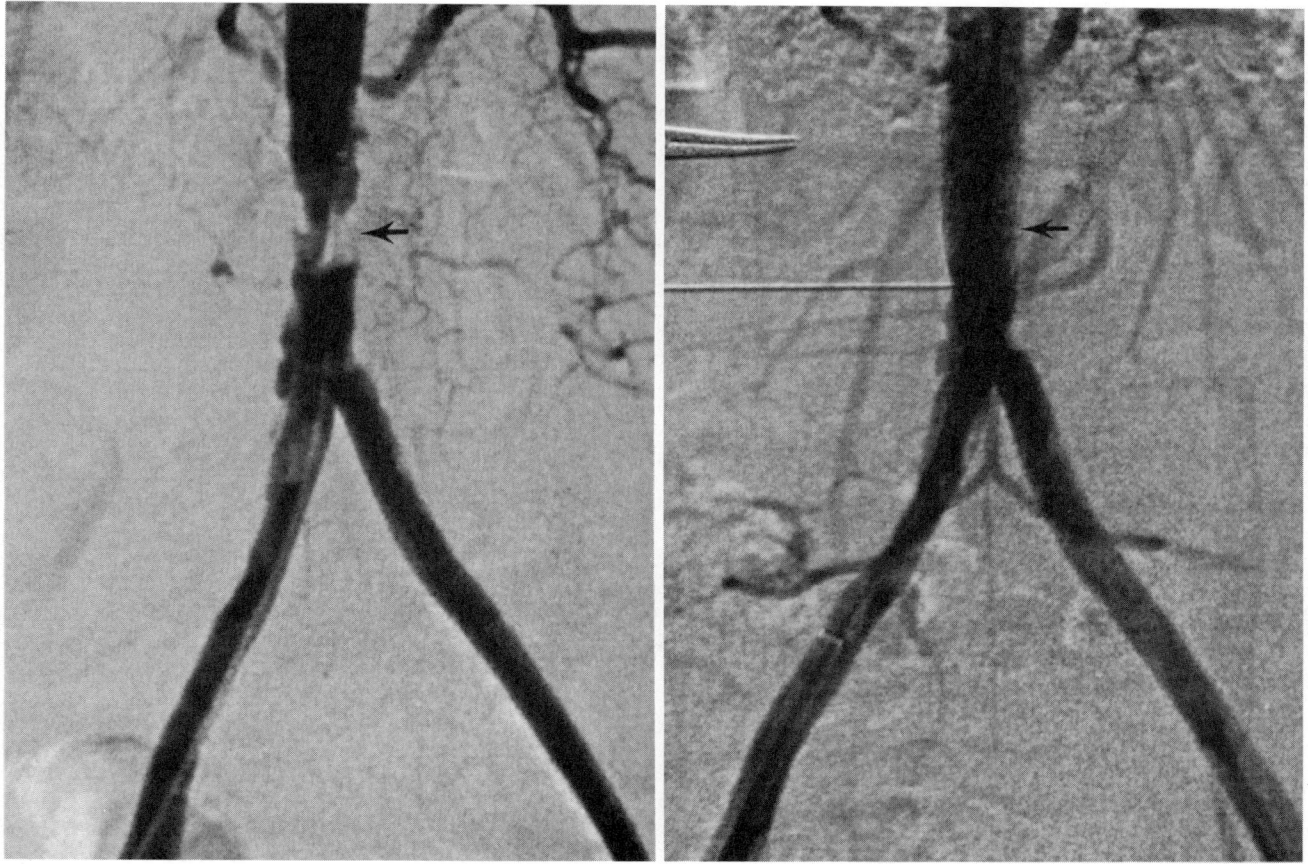

Figure 4 Infrarenal abdominal aortic stent placement. *A,* Digital subtraction abdominal aortogram in a 60-year-old female with right buttock and thigh claudication demonstrating irregular high-grade atherosclerotic stenosis of the distal abdominal aorta *(arrow)*. *B,* After a Palmaz stent mounted on a 8 mm balloon catheter was released, it was further expanded to 12 mm using a Blue Max balloon catheter. Repeat digital subtraction aortogram demonstrates a good result *(arrow)*. After stent placement, pressure gradient was zero. (Courtesy Michael Sarosi, M.D., St Joseph Hospital, Ann Arbor, Michigan.)

procedure is completed. If stenosis persists following the initial dilation, the balloon size should be increased by 1 or 2 mm to increase the diameter of the lesion. If the stenosis has not been completely eliminated following the second dilation, stent placement is indicated.

In a review of reported series over a 10 year period, the technical success rate of iliac PTA has been 50% to 96% (mean, 92%), and the long-term patency rates were 65% to 93% (mean, 81%) for 2 years and 50% to 87% (mean, 72%) for 5 years.[10] The patencies reported in the literature compare well with those of aortobifemoral grafting. The risks of the procedure include groin hematoma, distal embolization, arterial occlusion, arterial dissection, arteriovenous fistula, and iliac artery rupture. Patients may experience pain during the inflation of the balloon catheter. If they do after deflation of the balloon, contrast medium is injected immediately after deflation of the balloon to exclude arterial rupture. When extravasation is identified, the balloon catheter is inflated at the site of the rupture to prevent exsanguination. Surgical repair is necessary for iliac arterial rupture caused by PTA.

Balloon angioplasty has been used for the treatment of iliac artery occlusions. The technique involves traversal of the occlusion and dilation of the artery. When traversal of the occlusion fails, thrombolytic therapy may be used prior to PTA. Recanalization of the occlusion by thrombolysis not only facilitates traversal of the occlusion but also reduces the potential risk of vessel perforation during crossing of the lesion. The results of PTA in 56 occluded iliac arteries documented a 71% initial success rate, a 76% primary patency rate, and 81% secondary patency rate for 72 months. The overall patency including failures was 63%.[11]

Infrarenal Aortic Stent Placement

Balloon angioplasty and stenting using the Palmaz stent and the Wallstent have been used to treat infrarenal abdominal aortic stenoses and occlusions

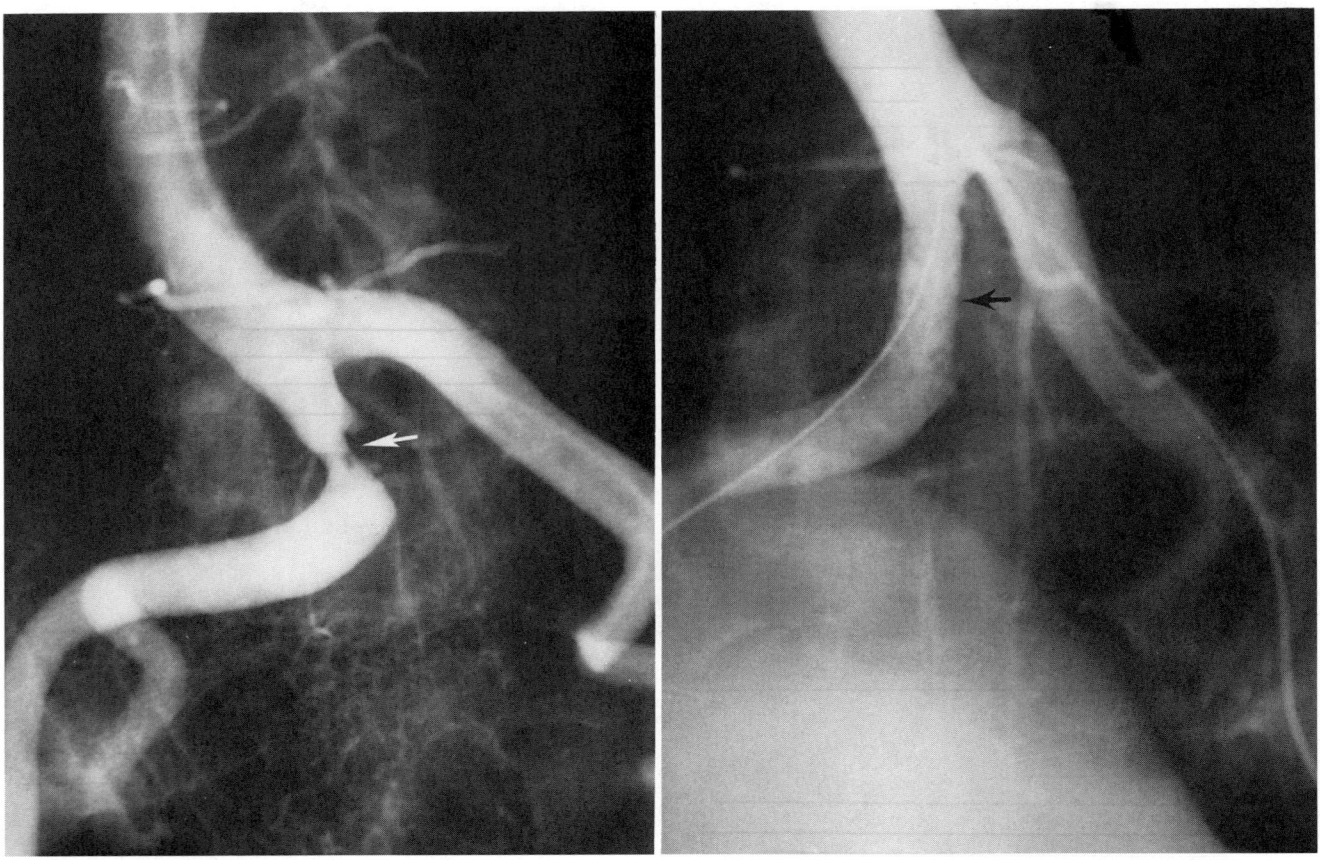

Figure 5 Iliac artery stent placement. *A*, Iliac arteriogram in a 75-year-old female with right lower extremity claudication demonstrating an irregular atherosclerotic stenosis of the right common iliac artery. *B*, After predilation with an 8 mm balloon catheter, a Palmaz stent was implanted and expanded to 10 mm in diameter. Repeat arteriogram demonstrates a good result *(arrow)*. The use of a superstiff guide wire in this patient facilitated stent placement through such a tortuous iliac artery.

(Figs. 2 and 3). Stenting is indicated in patients with complex atherosclerotic aortic stenosis (Fig. 4) and occlusion(s) and following unsuccessful balloon angioplasty. The currently available Palmaz stent is designed to expand to 8 to 12 mm in diameter. If necessary, the stent can be further expanded by a larger balloon catheter after deployment. The stent shortens upon expansion. A 30 mm long unexpanded stent shortens to 28.9 mm upon expansion to 8 mm in diameter and to 26.2 mm upon expansion to 12 mm in diameter. Shortening of the stent should be taken into consideration to ensure correct stent placement and stent overlapping when multiple stents are to be implanted. The Wallstent is currently available in 8 to 12 mm diameter with a range of 20 to 90 mm in length.

Long and colleagues reported successful stent placement in seven patients with aortic stenosis (five patients) and occlusion (two patients) using the Wallstent and Palmaz stents.[12] The patency rate for a mean of 15.1 months (range 12 to 24 months) was 100%. Because overlapping stents may compromise the origin of the aortic branches, stents should be used only for the infrarenal abdominal aorta. Overlapping of the inferior mesenteric artery origin must be avoided in patients with stenoses of the internal iliac and superior mesenteric arteries.

Iliac Artery Stent Placement

The results of multicenter studies documented the safety and efficacy of the intravascular stents for the treatment of atherosclerotic aortoiliac occlusive disease. The current indications for iliac stent placement include (1) atherosclerotic stenosis with ulcerated plaques (Fig. 5), (2) iliac artery occlusion (Fig. 6), (3) post-PTA arterial dissection, (4) failure of balloon angioplasty (residual stenosis of greater than 30% and/or a pressure gradient of greater than 5 mm Hg), and (5) recurrent stenosis following PTA. Contraindications to stent placement include densely calcified lesions, stenoses associated with aneurysmal dilation of the iliac artery, poor distal outflow, and extravasation of contrast media at the site of balloon dilation.

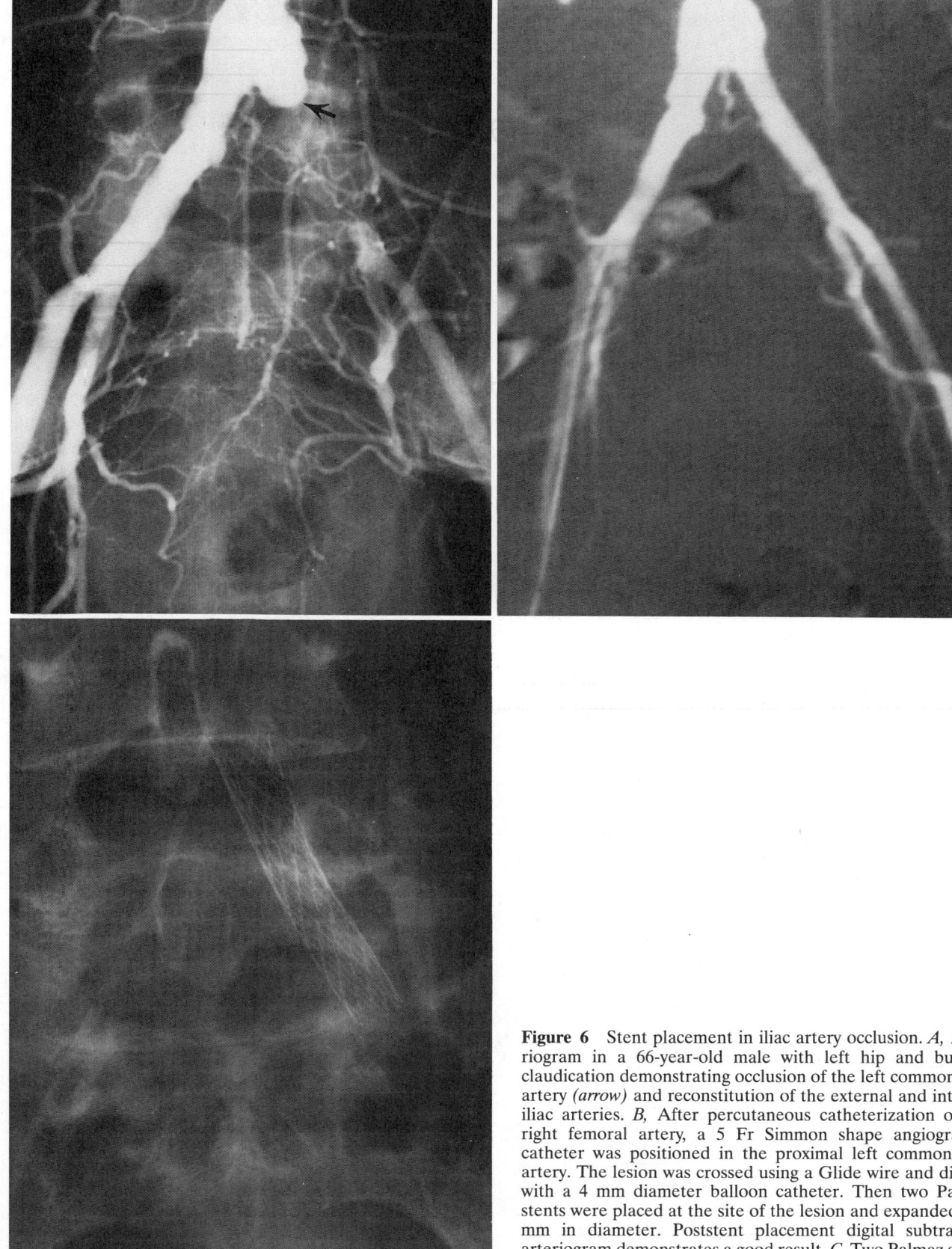

Figure 6 Stent placement in iliac artery occlusion. *A,* Arteriogram in a 66-year-old male with left hip and buttock claudication demonstrating occlusion of the left common iliac artery *(arrow)* and reconstitution of the external and internal iliac arteries. *B,* After percutaneous catheterization of the right femoral artery, a 5 Fr Simmon shape angiographic catheter was positioned in the proximal left common iliac artery. The lesion was crossed using a Glide wire and dilated with a 4 mm diameter balloon catheter. Then two Palmaz stents were placed at the site of the lesion and expanded to 8 mm in diameter. Poststent placement digital subtraction arteriogram demonstrates a good result. *C,* Two Palmaz stents implanted in the iliac artery demonstrating approximately 5 mm overlap.

The technique of Palmaz stent placement is the same, regardless of whether stenting is performed as the initial treatment or following an unsuccessful balloon angioplasty. Because the Palmaz stent is rigid, the ipsilateral femoral approach should be used for stent implantation. Prestent dilation of the lesion is usually necessary to facilitate traversing the lesion. After the lesion has been crossed using a guide wire, a heavy-duty guide wire such as Amplatz superstiff guide wire is passed into the abdominal aorta through the diagnostic angiographic catheter. Then the puncture site is dilated to a 10 Fr diameter. A 30 cm, 10 Fr sheath with dilator is advanced across the site of the lesion and the dilator is removed. The stent-balloon assembly is then advanced through the sheath and positioned at the intended placement site. The stent is exposed by retracting the sheath along the balloon catheter toward its hub. During this procedure, the catheter must be held in place to prevent stripping of the stent. Contrast medium may be injected through the side arm of the sheath to ensure that the stent has been exposed beyond the sheath tip. If repositioning of the stent is necessary, the sheath is advanced beyond the stent to prevent stent dislodgement. After precise placement of the stent, the balloon catheter is inflated to expand the stent. After deflation of the balloon, the catheter is removed over the guide wire. When multiple stents are to be implanted, the proximal stent is implanted first, with the more distal stent deployed second. If a second stent needs to be placed proximal to the first stent, the sheath with a dilator is advanced through the lumen of the proximal stent and the dilator is removed. The same procedure is repeated as that used for initial placement. Each stent should overlap the previous one by 2 to 3 mm. A 5 Fr straight catheter is advanced through the sheath for a poststent placement angiogram and pressure measurement. If the pressure gradient is greater than 5 mm Hg, the stent is further expanded with a 9 or 10 mm diameter balloon catheter.

Aortic bifurcation stenoses, where the plaques in the iliac arteries extend into the aorta, require stenting of both common iliac arteries. The lesions are dilated simultaneously using two balloon catheters introduced from each femoral artery before stent implantation. Stents are implanted sequentially one side at a time while the balloon remains inflated in the contralateral common iliac artery.

Occluded iliac arteries should be recanalized prior to stent implantation. Recanalization may be achieved by balloon angioplasty after traversing the lesion with a guide wire or after thrombolytic therapy with urokinase at a rate of 4,000 units/minute for 1 to 3 hours. After the occluded artery has been recanalized, the ipsilateral femoral artery is punctured for stent placement using the technique described. Stent placement at the origin of the internal iliac may result in occlusion of the artery. If there is no significant pressure gradient after stent placement, the sheath is removed and hemostasis is achieved by direct pressure to the puncture site. The patient is expected to be in bed for 8 hours, to limit mobility for the following 24 hours, and to be discharged from the hospital the third day. Regimen for stent placement includes aspirin before and 3 months after stent placement, 5,000 units of heparin sodium during the procedure, and antibiotics if indicated.

The Palmaz stent has undergone a multicenter study to evaluate its safety and efficacy.[3] For a 4 year period, a total of 486 patients underwent 587 procedures. Stents were placed unilaterally in 83% and bilaterally in 17%. Their follow-up ranged from 1 to 48 months (mean 13.3 ± 11 months). The angiographic patency rate was 92% with clinical benefits in 68.6% of treated patients at 43 months. The complication rate was 9.9%; 8% related to the procedure and 1.9% related to the stent. Complications requiring surgical and percutaneous intervention occurred in 1.6%. There was no mortality associated with stent placement.

A clinical trial with the Wallstent in iliac arteries included 125 patients (63 iliac occlusions and 62 complex iliac stenoses).[4] Once the lesions were traversed, stents were placed in all patients. Traversal was unsuccessful in 26% of the 85 patients with iliac occlusions. There was a technical success rate of 98%. Cumulative patency was 100% for 6 months and 89.4% for 24 months. Complications related to stent placement occurred in 4% of patients but only two (1.6%) required surgical or percutaneous intervention. Complications occurring in patients with iliac artery occlusion included two with contralateral embolism and one each with ipsilateral embolism, aortic dissection, and septicemia.

The Strecker stent has been used clinically since 1987. It is a tubular network knitted from tantalum wire and dilated by a balloon for deployment. It is mounted on a 5 Fr or 6 Fr Ultrathin balloon catheter and expands to 4 to 12 mm upon balloon inflation. The flexibility of the stent allows placement in curved vessels. Liermann and associates reported results from a clinical study with the Strecker stent in the iliac and femoropopliteal arteries.[5] Of 100 patients, 52 had stents placed in the iliac arteries with a 98% patency rate for a mean of 20 months after stent implantation (range 8 to 48 months). Their indications for stent placement included acute dissection with occlusion, reocclusion immediately or less than 6 months after successful PTA, and restenosis after PTA less than 6 months of second restenosis.

REFERENCES

1. Dotter CT, Judkins MP. Transluminal treatment of arteriosclerotic obstruction. Description of a technique and a preliminary report of its application. Circulation 1964; 30:654–670.
2. Grüntzig A, Kumpe DA. Technique of percutaneous transluminal angioplasty with the Grüntzig balloon catheter. Am J Roentgenol 1979; 132:547–552.
3. Palmaz JC, Laborde JC, Rivera FJ, et al. Stenting of the iliac arteries with the Palmaz stent: Experience from a multicenter trial. Cardiovasc Intervent Radiol 1992; 15:291–297.
4. Vorwerk D, Günther RW. Stent placement in iliac arterial lesions: Three years of clinical experience with the Wallstent. Cardiovasc Intervent Radiol 1992; 15:285–290.

5. Liermann D, Strecker EP, Peters J. The Strecker stent: Indications and results in iliac and femoropopliteal arteries. Cardiovasc Intervent Radiol 1992; 15:298–305.
6. Tegtmeyer CJ, Kellum CD, Kron IL, et al. Percutaneous transluminal angioplasty in the region of the aortic bifurcation. Radiology 1985; 157:661–665.
7. Morag B, Garniek A, Bass A, et al. Percutaneous transluminal aortic angioplasty: Early and late results. Cardiovasc Intervent Radiol 1993; 16:37–42.
8. Tadavarthy AK, Sullivan WA Jr, Nicoloff E, et al. Aorta balloon angioplasty: 9-year follow-up. Radiology 1989; 170:1039–1041.
9. Yakes WF, Kumpe DA, Brown SB, et al. Percutaneous transluminal aortic angioplasty: Technique and results. Radiology 1989; 172:965–970.
10. Becker GJ, Katzen BT, Dake MD. Noncoronary angioplasty. Radiology 1989; 170:921–940.
11. Gupta AK, Ravimandalam K, Rao VRK, et al. Total occlusion of iliac arteries: Results of balloon angioplasty. Cardiovasc Intervent Radiol 1993; 16:165–177.
12. Long AL, Gaux JC, Raynaud AC, et al. Infrarenal aortic stents: Initial clinical experience and angiographic follow-up. Cardiovasc Intervent Radiol 1993; 16:203–208.

MANAGEMENT OF JUXTARENAL AORTIC OCCLUSIVE DISEASE BY TRANSABDOMINAL EXPOSURE OF THE PARARENAL AND SUPRARENAL AORTA USING MEDIAL VISCERAL ROTATION

LINDA M. REILLY, M.D.

The difficulty in obtaining adequate exposure of the pararenal aorta is well known. In the past this technical challenge has led to the development of indirect operative approaches for the management of arterial disease affecting this segment of the aorta and its branches, approaches designed specifically to avoid direct exposure of this region.[1] However, these indirect methods limit the options for reconstruction, and cumulative experience raised questions about their durability.[2,3]

Shirkey and colleagues first described the technique of transabdominal medial visceral rotation (MVR) in a plane anterior to the left kidney to provide exposure of an injury to the proximal superior mesenteric artery (SMA).[4] Two years later Buscaglia, Blaisdell, and Lim reported their experience in treating patients with penetrating abdominal vascular injuries involving the aorta, its major visceral branches, and the vena cava.[5] They advocated the use of left-to-right medial rotation of the viscera to approach the aorta and its branches and the use of right-to-left medial rotation of the viscera to approach the inferior vena cava (IVC). They also described modifications to augment the exposure, with rotation of the left kidney anteriorly and medially to access the posterolateral aorta and the extension of the incision into the thorax to expose the distal thoracic aorta. Subsequently, this exposure became popular for the treatment of traumatic injuries to this proximal aortic segment, varying only in whether the plane was developed anterior or posterior to the kidney. During this time the only published description of this approach in the elective setting came from Crawford, who used it to expose complex aneurysms involving the proximal abdominal aorta.[6]

Our search for the optimal method of exposure for this segment of the aorta began with the thoracoretroperitoneal technique which was actually a combination of DeBakey's thoracoabdominal approach and the retroperitoneal approach first used in the repair of abdominal aortic aneurysms.[7] This method provides unrestricted access to the full length of the aorta, but at the cost of a two-body cavity incision. An analysis of our own patients undergoing visceral reconstruction for chronic mesenteric ischemia documented a substantially greater morbidity, especially pulmonary, in the thoracoretroperitoneal group, than in the transabdominal group.[8] This prompted us to determine if we could obtain adequate aortic exposure without the thoracic portion of the incision. Recently we have begun to expose this midabdominal aorta by performing transabdominal MVR rather than attempting to obtain adequate exposure with the standard infracolic approach. Our initial use of this approach was prompted by the difficulty of obtaining adequate exposure of juxtarenal and pararenal aortic aneurysms through the infracolic approach. Currently, aortic aneurysmal disease remains a more common indication for this approach in our patients, but the extensive exposure it provides has led us to apply it to pararenal and paravisceral occlusive disease affecting the aorta, its visceral branches, or both.[9]

CLINICAL EXPERIENCE

Between July 1987 and November 1992, 65 patients underwent MVR exposure of the midabdominal aorta to allow treatment of occlusive disease of the aorta and/or its visceral branches (Table 1). A quarter of the patients had symptomatic coronary artery disease. Twelve patients had preoperative evidence of impaired renal

Table 1 Patient Profile

	Number	Percent
Risk Factors		
Diabetes	7	10.8
Hypertension	44	67.7
Hypercholesterolemia on treatment	2	3.1
Smoking	45	69.2
Associated Illnesses		
Cardiac	17	26.2
Pulmonary disease requiring treatment	3	4.6
Elevated liver enzymes	4	6.2
Elevated creatinine	12	18.5
Prior Surgery		
Aortic/aortic branch	24	36.9
Nonvascular intra-abdominal	16	24.6

Table 2 Operative Details

	Number	Percent
Technique		
Bypass	24	36.9
Endarterectomy	18	27.7
Bypass + endarterectomy	23	21.3
Infected graft removal	2	3.1
Dilation	1	1.5
Bypass + excision/1° reanastomosis	1	1.5
Reimplantation + excision/1° reanastomosis	1	1.5
Transposition + reimplantation	1	1.5
Bypass + angioplasty + transposition	1	1.5
Bypass + endarterectomy + transposition	1	1.5
Arteries Repaired		
Renal only	18	27.7
Visceral only	13	20.0
Aorta + renal	10	15.4
Aorta only	9	13.8
Renal + visceral	7	10.8
Aorta + renal + visceral	7	10.8
Aorta + visceral	1	1.5
Aortic Cross-clamp Level		
Supraceliac	33	20.8
Supra superior mesenteric artery	8	12.3
Suprarenal	8	12.3
Infrarenal	4	6.2
Partial occlusion	4	6.2
None*	8	12.3

*Aortic branch clamped only.

function, as indicated by an elevated serum creatinine. About half the patients had previously undergone either aortic or aortic branch reconstruction or other major nonvascular, intraabdominal operations.

Of the procedures, 55 were elective, 7 were urgent, and 3 were emergent. Twenty-seven patients required some aortic reconstruction, either alone or more commonly in combination with renal or visceral repair or both (Table 2). Thirty-eight patients required no aortic procedure and underwent reconstruction of the renal arteries, visceral arteries, or both. The aortic procedures were performed to treat intermittent claudication, rest pain, graft infection, a combination of intermittent claudication with infrarenal aneurysm, and incidentally to allow renal or visceral repair (Table 3). Most of the 42 patients who underwent renal revascularization were hypertensive, had impaired renal function, or both. However, seven asymptomatic stenoses were treated. Of the 28 patients who underwent visceral reconstruction, the most common indication was chronic symptoms, but five patients were asymptomatic.

The most common techniques used for aortic or aortic branch reconstruction were, first, bypass, followed by endarterectomy, and then bypass plus endarterectomy (Table 2). Other techniques, including reimplantation, transposition, excision with primary reanastomosis, angioplasty, and dilation, were usually used in combination with either bypass or endarterectomy.

Table 3 Indication for Operation

Indication	Number
For Aortic Procedures	27
Rest pain	4
Claudication	17
Graft infection	4
Incidental	2
For Renal Artery Procedures	42
Hypertension	16
Elevated creatinine	1
Hypertension + elevated creatinine	11
Asymptomatic	7
Renal artery aneurysms	5
Involved by infected aortic graft	1
Incidental	1
For Visceral Artery Procedures	28
Acute symptoms	4
Chronic symptoms	17
Chronic + acute symptoms	1
Asymptomatic	5
Involved by aortic graft infection	1

OPERATIVE TECHNIQUE

Left Medial Visceral Rotation

We currently prefer a standard, full-length, midline transabdominal incision, although initially a modified left subcostal incision was used. The small bowel is enclosed in an intestinal bag and displaced to the right. Mobilization of the descending and sigmoid colon is begun in the standard manner by incising the lateral peritoneal reflection. This peritoneal incision is carried cephalad through the phrenocolic and lienorenal ligaments. Using gentle, blunt and occasional sharp dissection, a plane is developed between the pancreas and

Gerota's fascia. The descending colon, pancreas, spleen, and stomach are then rotated anteriorly and medially, leaving the gonadal vein, ureter, left kidney, and adrenal gland in situ. Maintaining the correct plane during this mobilization avoids bleeding, pancreatic injury, and adrenal or renal injury. Left adrenal injury occurs if one does not stay in the same plane anterior to the kidney from the level of the left renal vein all the way up to the aortic hiatus in the crus of the diaphragm. The spleen and pancreas are protected with moistened pads, and a self-retaining retractor system is positioned to hold all of the anteriorly mobilized viscera to the right. The peritoneum is reflected from the left crus of the diaphragm, and the triangular ligament and left lobe of the liver is freed. The esophagophrenic ligament is left intact to protect the anterior and posterior trunks of the vagus nerve. The aorta is now clearly in view, crossed by the left renal vein, the autonomic ganglia tissue, and the left crus of the diaphragm.

Exposure of the upper abdominal aorta requires circumferential dissection of the left renal vein to its junction with the IVC so that it can be widely displaced as needed. Caudal retraction of the left renal vein facilitates the exposure of the origin of the renal arteries. The left renal artery can easily be freed from its origin to the renal hilum. Right lateral retraction of the IVC allows exposure of the proximal 2 to 3 cm of the right renal artery. The SMA and celiac axis are exposed by incising the dense autonomic ganglia on the left lateral surface of the aorta, as well as the crus of the diaphragm. As this neural and muscular tissue is mobilized to the right in the plane of Leriche, the supraceliac aorta becomes visible. Resection of the median arcuate ligament and separation of the muscle fibers of the diaphragm expose the distal thoracic aorta within the lower mediastinum. The MVR approach allows only restricted exposure of the right side of the aorta; therefore, care must always be taken that the crus and median arcuate ligament tissue are completely divided and retracted in order to allow sufficient mobilization of the right side of the aorta to safely place a clamp. Failure to mobilize the paramesenteric aorta adequately increases the risk that the aorta will be injured during placement of the occluding clamp. Mobilization of the lower abdominal aorta proceeds by incising the loose areolar tissue along its left lateral surface. Reflection of this tissue to the right reveals the origin of the inferior mesenteric artery, with the course of the vessel now vertical as a result of the colon displacement. The aortic bifurcation and the iliac arteries are easily accessible for mobilization, if necessary.

Modified Left Medial Visceral Rotation

The technique of left MVR may be modified according to the required level of aortic exposure and the planned revascularization technique. If a large upper abdominal aortic aneurysm must be replaced, the mobilization plane is developed posterior to the left kidney. When the proximal extent of aortic exposure is below the SMA, the visceral rotation may be confined to the colon, leaving the pancreas, spleen and stomach in situ—a partial or limited left MVR. In this case the incision in the lateral peritoneal reflection is extended only up to the splenic flexure, dividing the phrenocolic ligament but leaving the lienorenal ligament intact. Instead, the lienocolic ligament is then incised, allowing the splenic flexure and descending colon segments to be rotated anteriorly and medially. The pararenal and infrarenal aorta can then be exposed as previously described.

Right Medial Visceral Rotation

An incision is made in the lateral peritoneal reflection along the ascending colon and is carried cephalad to the hepatocolic ligament, which is then transected. This enables the hepatic flexure and ascending colon segments to be rotated anteriorly and medially. The second portion of the duodenum is then in view and can be mobilized along with the head of the pancreas, using a traditional Kocher maneuver. This exposes the IVC and the pararenal aorta. Circumferential dissection of the IVC, as well as the right and left renal veins, allows for safe retraction of these vessels as necessary. Retraction of the IVC to the left and of the right renal vein caudally exposes the origin of the right renal artery, which can be mobilized from the aorta to the hilum of the kidney. However, this approach does limit exposure of the left renal artery to the proximal 2 to 3 cm. The distal aorta can then be exposed as previously described.

Although it is unusual to need simultaneous extensive bilateral exposure, it is nonetheless feasible to perform left and right MVR at the same operation. This was required in five patients, three of whom had left complete and right partial MVR; the remaining two patients had left partial and right partial MVR.

The extensive exposure of the aorta provided by MVR is reflected in the varied levels of the aortic cross-clamp in this series of operations. In almost half the patients, it was the supraceliac aorta, and in two patients the distal thoracic aorta was the clamp site. Overall, about 75% of these procedures required aortic clamping at some level above the renal arteries. The resulting interval of visceral ischemia averaged 37.1 ± 18.3 minutes and of renal ischemia averaged 38.2 ± 23.9 minutes. The mean operative time for these complex repairs was 8.2 ± 2.8 hours. The mean operative weight gain was 8.3 ± 4.5 kg.

RESULTS

Mortality

Two patients died intraoperatively (3.1%), and 10 patients died postoperatively (15.4%). Mortality was greatest among the 10 patients undergoing urgent or emergent operations (40%) and substantially less (14.5%) for elective procedures in 55 patients. Elective primary procedures involving only aortic or renal or visceral reconstruction were associated with a perioperative mortality of 4.2%, whereas reoperative procedures had a mortality of 10.5% and elective combined aortic and aortic branch repairs had a mortality of 27.3%.

The leading cause of death was visceral infarction with sepsis, occurring in five patients. The second most common cause of death was hemorrhage. In three patients, massive hemorrhage due to coagulopathy occurred intraoperatively during elective procedures involving combined aortic, renal, and visceral reconstruction or renal and visceral revascularization. Two patients died intraoperatively, and one died a few days following operation because of the resultant multisystem organ failure. The fourth patient bled from a spontaneous hepatic rupture 1 day after antegrade aortovisceral bypass to both the SMA and celiac artery. The etiology of the liver bleeding was never established. All four of these patients required supraceliac aortic cross-clamping, and the resulting period of visceral ischemia was 37.5 minutes, which was not different from the group as a whole.

Morbidity

The most frequent intraoperative complication was splenic injury, which necessitated splenectomy in all but one instance (Table 4). Seven patients developed excessive bleeding intraoperatively and, as previously described, in four it was fatal. Five of these patients had undergone some visceral reconstruction, with an average ischemia time of 38 minutes. Only four of these patients received heparin sodium.

Although most patients were extubated within 24 hours of operation, the most common postoperative complications were pulmonary (Table 5). No patient died as a direct consequence of a pulmonary complication. Sixteen patients were treated for pneumonia, and two patients required drainage of pleural effusions that were not associated with a concurrent pulmonary or intra-abdominal process.

Cardiac complications occurred in 12 patients, and most of them were arrhythmias of little significance. Three patients had postoperative myocardial infarctions. One led to fatal nonocclusive visceral infarction, and one was fatal in spite of coronary artery grafting.

Nine patients developed a rising creatinine postoperatively, but six of these were patients who later died. Similarly, all patients who required dialysis postoperatively were among those who died. Of the surviving 53 patients, 51 (96.2%) were discharged with creatinine levels equal to or less than their admission creatinine levels.

Clinically evident pancreatitis occurred in three patients, requiring operative debridement in one patient and percutaneous drainage to control a pancreaticocutaneous fistula in another. Also, peripancreatic inflam-

Table 4 Intraoperative Complications

Complication	Number
Splenic Injury	9
Splenectomy	8
Splenorraphy	1
Hemorrhage	7
Technical	4
Celiac–superior mesenteric artery intimal flap	1
Celiac axis injury	3
Thrombosis	3
Aorta	1
Renal	1
Aortofemoral bypass graft limb	1
Embolization	2
Small bowel	1
Femoral	2
Miscellaneous	2
Graft required revision	2

Table 5 Postoperative Complications

Complication	Number
Cardiac	12
Arrhythmia requiring treatment	9
Myocardial infarction	3
Pulmonary	16
Pneumonia	9
Respiratory failure requiring reintubation	4
Pleural effusion	2
Pulmonary edema	1
Renal	7
New onset dialysis	4
Among survivors	0
Among nonsurvivors	4
Elevated creatinine at discharge (survivors only)	2
Neurologic	2
Cerebrovascular accident	1
Lower extremity paralysis	1
Gastrointestinal	8
Bowel ischemia/infarction	5
Pancreatitis	3
Infection (Nonpulmonary)	11
Urinary tract	3
Gastrointestinal	2
Intravascular catheter	2
Intra-abdominal/retroperitoneal	1
Wound	2
Unknown source	1
Limb Ischemia	5
Requiring fasciotomy	3
Wound	2
Dehiscence	1
Hematoma requiring drainage	1

mation was found at autopsy in a fourth patient. Among these four patients, three had combined aortorenal reconstruction, and only one had aortorenovisceral reconstruction. Of note, although serum amylase levels were not routinely measured postoperatively, in the 27 patients whose data were available, 15 were elevated.

DISCUSSION

The advantages associated with the use of MVR are unlimited exposure and the lack of any constraint on the choice of arterial reconstruction technique. This exposure provides the surgeon with the most operative options to manage complex arterial lesions of the upper abdominal aorta and its branches, regardless of extent. This approach is particularly appealing when the patient has previously undergone aortic reconstruction or other major intra-abdominal procedures. It is not the technique of choice for transient proximal aortic control to allow infrarenal aortic reconstruction. As a consequence, it is rarely needed when the only planned reconstruction is for aortic occlusive disease.

In analyzing the outcome of such operations, an attempt was made to identify deaths and complications that are related to the MVR exposure versus those that are related to the arterial reconstructions that were performed. The complications that may be related to the dissection would include injuries to structures in the field and possibly the development of a coagulopathy. Among the recorded injuries, those that seem clearly related to the MVR technique are the splenic injuries. Splenic injuries almost always occurred during the early phase of mobilization of the spleen itself or during mobilization of the splenic flexure of the colon.

The etiology of the coagulopathy has never been defined; therefore, it is difficult to determine exactly what the contribution of the method of exposure is, as opposed to the contribution of the procedure itself. Proposed mechanisms include prolonged hepatic-visceral ischemia, hypothermia, and hemodilution, none of which is specific to any one method of exposure. To minimize the risk of developing a coagulopathy, we prefer to maintain some visceral perfusion by placing the aortic clamp at the lowest level that allows safe performance of the indicated repair. Thus, we do not routinely place a supraceliac clamp, even though it is often technically easier, if a lower level clamp is adequate. We also try to maintain core temperature throughout the operation and have minimized or eliminated the use of heparin sodium.

Complications that might be related to retraction of the viscera include pancreatitis and visceral ischemia-infarction. During mobilization of the viscera, progressively more medial retraction is placed on the pancreas until finally, when the viscera are fully mobilized to the midline, retractors are placed on the pancreas at about the level of the neck. During this mobilization, increasing traction is exerted on the visceral vessels until the proximal vessels have been exposed over an adequate length to allow reconstruction. This retraction and traction have the potential for injury to the pancreas as well as the visceral vessels or may create a low flow state in the viscera by compressing or occluding the SMA and, to a lesser extent, the celiac axis. Although most patients who developed pancreatitis had a supravisceral aortic cross-clamp, there was no correlation between aortic clamp level and pancreatitis. Therefore, we believe retraction injury was the mechanism responsible for at least some of the cases of pancreatitis that occurred.

Both these complications, pancreatitis and visceral infarction, emphasize the necessity for appropriate handling of the viscera during mobilization and retraction. Mobilization should be complete in order to allow the viscera to be uniformly retracted without being scissored against remaining fixed points. Furthermore, retractors should be well padded and, if mechanical retraction is used, the retractors should be released intermittently. Finally, the appearance of the retracted viscera should be assessed at regular intervals to be sure that adequate perfusion is maintained during all phases of the exposure.

REFERENCES

1. Morris GC Jr, Crawford ES, Cooley DA, DeBakey ME. Revascularization of the celiac and superior mesenteric arteries. Arch Surg 1962; 84:113–125.
2. Stoney RJ, Ehrenfeld WK, Wylie EJ. Revascularization methods in chronic visceral ischemia caused by atherosclerosis. Ann Surg 1977; 186:468–476.
3. Rapp JH, Reilly LM, Qvarfordt PG, et al. Durability of endarterectomy and antegrade grafts in the treatment of chronic visceral ischemia. J Vasc Surg 1986; 3:799–806.
4. Shirkey AL, Quast DC, Jordan GL Jr. Superior mesenteric artery division and intestinal function. J Trauma 1967; 7:7–24.
5. Buscaglia LC, Blaisdell FW, Lim RC Jr. Penetrating abdominal vascular injuries. Arch Surg 1969; 99:764–769.
6. Crawford ES. Thoraco-abdominal and abdominal aortic aneurysms involving renal, superior mesenteric, and celiac arteries. Ann Surg 1974; 179:763–772.
7. Stoney RJ, Wylie EJ. Surgical management of arterial lesions of the thoracoabdominal aorta. Am J Surg 1973; 126:157–164.
8. Cunningham CG, Reilly LM, Rapp JH, et al. Chronic visceral ischemia: Three decades of progress. Ann Surg 1991; 214:276–288.
9. Reilly LM, Ramos TK, Murray SP, et al. Optimal exposure of the proximal abdominal aorta: A critical appraisal of transabdominal medial visceral rotation. J Vasc Surg 1994; 19:375–390.

ACUTE AORTIC OCCLUSION

ALEXANDER D. SHEPARD, M.D.
CHRISTOS D. DOSSA, M.D.

Acute aortic occlusion (AAO) is an infrequent but often catastrophic vascular emergency. Severe lower extremity ischemia combined with an acute sustained increase in cardiac afterload, usually in a compromised heart, places the mortality of this entity in a range similar to that of ruptured abdominal aortic aneurysm (AAA). Successful treatment requires prompt diagnosis and agressive early operation.

CAUSES

Acute occlusion of the abdominal aorta is caused by either a large embolus lodging in the infrarenal aorta, usually at the aortic bifurcation, or by thrombosis of the distal aorta. Embolic occlusion appears to be the most common cause, occurring in 65% of patients in a recent review of 46 patients with AAO.[1] However, thrombotic occlusion is increasing in frequency; nearly two-thirds of the patients presenting with AAO over the last decade of the former study had it. In the majority of patients the occlusion is limited to the infrarenal aorta.

Most emboli originate from the heart, and the most common associated cardiac abnormalities are atrial fibrillation, congestive heart failure, mitral valve disease, and myocardial infarction. Women are much more likely than men to be affected by embolic AAO. This finding may result from the smaller caliber of the female infrarenal aorta, which can trap emboli that would travel further distally in larger male arteries. Aortoiliac occlusive disease accounts for most (75% in our series) cases of thrombotic AAO. Other causes include hypercoaguability, AAA, aortic dissection, and trauma. Not uncommonly, the acute thrombosis in patients with aortoiliac disease is precipitated by a state of transient hypoperfusion such as accompanies dehydration or severe congestive heart failure.

DIAGNOSIS

Prompt diagnosis of AAO is crucial to a good outcome. Patients have classic symptoms and signs of acute arterial occlusion involving both lower extremities. All patients in our study complained of acute onset of lower extremity pain and/or paresthesias, and over 80% had lower extremity weakness or paralysis. Femoral and distal pulses are absent bilaterally. Mottling of the feet and lower legs is common, and not infrequently cyanosis extends to the umbilicus. Despite these findings, the diagnosis of AAO can be challenging for the nonsurgeon clinician. Since most patients present with acute pain, numbness, weakness, and sometimes paralysis of the lower extremities, physicians may focus on possible neurologic causes while overlooking the clinical signs of acute ischemia. In our experience 11% of patients were first referred for neurologic or neurosurgical evaluation before a vascular surgeon was consulted. A similar pattern of confusion has been reported by others.

Distinguishing between embolic and thrombotic occlusion is sometimes difficult. Besides the female predilection, patients with embolic occlusions have a higher incidence of heart disease (100% versus 25% in our experience) than those with thrombotic occlusions and commonly give a history of prior arterial embolism. Patients with thrombotic occlusions did not have a significantly higher incidence of claudication, although they were more frequently cigarette smokers. Typically, patients with embolic AAO present earlier for medical evaluation than do patients with thrombotic occlusion. In our 46 patients the median duration of ischemia, defined as the interval from onset of symptoms to time of revascularization, was 7 hours for the embolic group and 17 hours for the thrombotic group. The most likely reason for this difference was a greater degree of pre-existing collateral circulation in the thrombotic group. However, clinical differentiation between embolic and thrombotic AAO is not always possible and is not necessary prior to operation.

Preoperative aortography has not proved useful with most cases of AAO, and usually it only delays definitive therapy.[2,3] Possible exceptions are patients with acute renal failure and/or abdominal pain, which suggest concomitant renal and/or visceral involvement. The only two such patients in our study both presented with abdominal pain and had visceral emboli documented by aortography. Only their aortic emboli were treated, however, because of hemodynamic instability secondary to recent myocardial infarctions.

TREATMENT

Once the diagnosis of AAO has been made clinically, the patient should be prepared for operation. Treatment usually begins with 10,000 units of heparin sodium intravenously to prevent local propagation of clot and to maintain patency of collateral channels. Central venous access is usually best accomplished prior to heparinization; later conversion to a pulmonary artery catheter can be performed without complications. If a significant delay is anticipated prior to operation continuous heparin sodium infusion should be instituted to maintain the partial thromboplastin time at 2 to 2½ times normal. A pulmonary artery catheter, radial artery cannula, urinary bladder catheter, and at least one large-bore peripheral venous line should be inserted. Attention is focused on the patient's cardiac status and appropriate steps taken to control associated heart failure, arrhythmias, and myocardial ischemia. In patients with severe lower extremity ischemia, maintenance of urine output of at least 100 ml/hr using volume loading or diuretics is important to minimize renal dysfunction from possible myoglobin. Administration of intravenous sodium bicarbonate, to alkalinize the urine, and mannitol should also be considered in this circumstance. However, prolonged preoperative resuscitation efforts are inappropriate.

Occasional high-risk patients with minimal ischemia can be treated nonoperatively with continued anticoagulation. Intra-arterial thrombolysis is another possible therapy, though its role in AAO has not yet been clearly defined. Factors militating against its routine use are the severity of lower extremity ischemia and the extent of clot. In patients with irreversible limb ischemia manifested by rigidity of major muscle groups, primary amputation should be performed.

Operative Therapy

Wide prepping and draping are necessary to allow for the possibilities of aortic reconstruction, axillobifemoral grafting, distal limb exploration and fasciotomy. Regardless of the type of AAO, all patients should undergo an initial attempt at retrograde balloon catheter embolectomy or thrombectomy via bilateral femoral arteriotomies (Fig. 1). In high-risk patients this procedure can be performed with local anesthesia. Blood loss can be substantial, and the use of an autotransfusion device is recommended. It is important to achieve brisk, pulsatile blood flow; otherwise the possibility of early reocclusion is high. Poor blood flow signifies either retained thrombus or proximal occlusive disease and requires further intervention.

For most patients with embolic AAO catheter embolectomy is usually successful in restoring blood flow. Catheters should also be passed down the superficial and deep femoral arteries, although in our experience the incidence of concomitant distal thromboemboli is low. If catheter thromboembolectomy is unsuccessful, direct aortic thromboembolectomy with aortic reconstruction or extra-anatomic bypass can be performed, depending on the patient's condition. For embolic occlusion necessary aortic exposure can usually be obtained through a limited retroperitoneal approach. If there is any doubt as to the cause of AAO, midline exposure is safest. Extracted embolic material should be examined microscopically and cultured for bacteria to verify its composition and source.

When thrombosis is the cause of AAO, arterial reconstruction is almost always required. Only one patient in our thrombotic group was treated successfully by catheter thrombectomy alone, and this patient had an underlying hypercoaguable state. If the patient is hemodynamically stable and an acceptable operative risk, aortic reconstruction is favored over axillobifemoral bypass. When aortofemoral grafting is performed, care must be taken when clamping the infrarenal aorta because of the frequent propagation of thrombus to a level immediately below the renal arteries. In this situation we have used temporary supraceliac aortic clamping as a quick and safe method of proximal control.

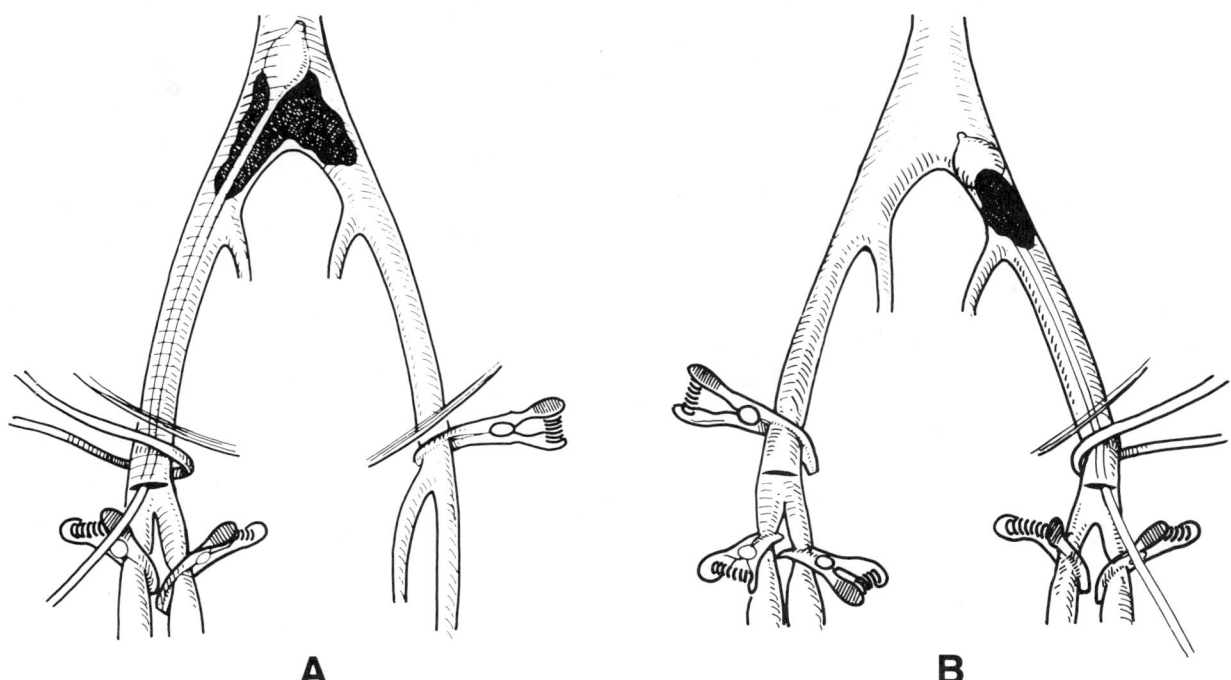

Figure 1 Method of retrograde aortic balloon catheter thrombectomy or embolectomy through bilateral femoral arteriotomies. *A,* A large (6 Fr) Fogarty catheter is passed up one iliac artery into the aorta and withdrawn. *B,* The same procedure is performed on the opposite side to remove residual thrombus. (From Shepard AD, Ernst CB. Arterial embolectomy and arteriovenous fistula repair. In: Nora PF, ed. Operative surgery. Philadelphia: WB Saunders, 1990:975; with permission.)

Following transection and thrombectomy of the aorta below the renal arteries, the clamp can be moved to an infrarenal location, minimizing the risk of dislodging thrombotic debris into the renal arteries.

Regardless of method of revascularization used to treat AAO, restoration of blood flow to the lower extremities should be carefully controlled. Reperfusion of a severely ischemic limb can result in dangerous metabolic derangements that can produce myocardial depression, arrhythmias, and cardiac arrest. Careful communication between the surgeon and anesthetist is important to avoid such problems. Additional administration of sodium bicarbonate and mannitol may be helpful.

Following restoration of blood flow, the lower extremities are assessed for perfusion and development of compartment compression syndrome. If there is any doubt regarding the adequacy of distal circulation, operative arteriograms are helpful in identifying retained distal emboli. However, in many of these high-risk patients, return of good Doppler flow signals to the extremity should be considered a success, and further efforts at distal revascularization should be limited. Any extremity with doughy or firm distal musculature should undergo fasciotomy.

Postoperative Care

Postoperatively, attention is directed to the status of the lower extremities, possible sequelae of a reperfusion syndrome, treatment of underlying medical conditions, and in the case of embolic occlusion, prevention of recurrent emboli. Urine is examined for myoglobin in cases of moderately severe to severe ischemia and appropriate treatment instituted as necessary. Patients with embolic occlusions should be anticoagulated with heparin sodium as soon as safely possible postoperatively and should have lifelong sodium warfarin therapy because of the high incidence of both early and late recurrent arterial emboli.[4] Three patients in our study had recurrent embolism (two mesenteric, one cerebral) in the early postoperative period, and two died of it. Embologenic conditions should also be sought and corrected when possible. In nearly 40% of our embolic occlusion survivors it was possible to treat a cardiac source of emboli by mitral valve reconstruction.

OUTCOME

Morbidity and mortality for AAO remain high despite advances in anesthetic and postoperative care. Overall mortality in our study was 35% and morbidity was 74%, which is similar to other recent reports in the literature.[2,3,5,6] Cardiac complications are the most common cause of death and morbidity, as expected given the high incidence of underlying cardiac disease in these patients and the acute sustained increase in cardiac afterload associated with occlusion of the infrarenal aorta. Myoglobinuria, renal failure, respiratory insufficiency, and other complications related to the reperfusion syndrome are also common. Limb morbidity is suprisingly low in published reports, with limb salvage rates exceeding 95%.[1-3,5,6] Excluding the one patient in our study who underwent primary amputations, only four legs were lost in three patients; six patients required fasciotomies, of whom three had persistent ischemic neuropathy. Both survival and functional outcome were more closely related to severity of ischemia on presentation than to absolute duration, contradicting some previous reports in the literature that emphasized a 6- to 8-hour "golden period" of ischemia before irreversible damage occurs.

Despite the high incidence of associated cardiac disease, survivors of AAO have a reasonable long-term prognosis. In our study 5 year survival approached 75%, with a slight trend toward better survival in the thrombotic group. Distressingly, 37% (7 of 19) of embolic AAO survivors had an episode of late recurrent arterial embolism, and 3 of these were recurrent AAO. These emboli occurred despite continued sodium warfarin administration, though no patient had a therapeutic prothrombin time at the time of representation. This finding underscores the importance of careful monitoring of anticoagulation status in this high-risk group.

REFERENCES

1. Dossa CD, Shepard AD, Reddy DJ, et al. Acute aortic occlusion: A 40 year experience. Arch Surg 1994; 129:603–608.
2. Littooy FN, Baker WH. Acute aortic occlusion: A multifaceted catastrophe. J Vasc Surg 1986; 4:211–216.
3. Busuttil RW, Keehn G, Miliken J, et al. Aortic saddle embolus: A 20 year experience. Ann Surg 1983; 197:698–706.
4. Elliott JP, Hageman JH, Szilagyi DE, et al. Arterial embolization: Problem of source, multiplicity, recurrence, and delayed treatment. Surgery 1980; 88:833–845.
5. Babu SC, Shah PM, Sharma P, et al. Adequacy of central hemodynamics versus restoration of circulation in the survival of patients with acute aortic thrombosis. Am J Surg 1987; 154:206–210.
6. Tapper SS, Jenkins JM, Edwards WH, et al. Juxtarenal aortic occlusion. Ann Surg 1992; 215:443–450.

DESCENDING THORACIC AORTA TO FEMORAL BYPASS

WALTER J. McCARTHY, M.D.

The descending thoracic aorta to femoral artery bypass can be defined as a bypass from the aorta just proximal to the diaphragmatic hiatus with either a bifurcated or tube graft reaching the iliac or femoral arterial system. This operation was first performed in 1956 by Sauvage, who used an aortic homograft for a patient who had standard aortoiliac graft failure.[1] In 1961 Blaisdell used the thoracofemoral bypass for reconstruction after removing an infected infrarenal aortic prosthesis.[2] Increasing acceptance of this operation by the surgical community is reflected by reports of 166 similar cases in the literature by 1992.[3]

INDICATIONS

This operation is simple in concept but should be restricted to very special settings in which conventional arterial grafting configurations are inadequate. As a general rule, if simpler or more commonly used operations can achieve the same end, they should be used preferentially to the thoracofemoral bypass. Thus, although the thoracic aorta provides excellent inflow for treatment of an infrarenal aortic occlusion, the routine intraabdominal approach remains preferred. Although the thoracofemoral operation has been described for situations of acute aortic infection, one might more reasonably use axillary femoral bypass instead. The reason is that, in the septic patient, if the extra-anatomic repair were to become infected, the axillary based graft is easier to manage than one anastomosed to the descending thoracic aorta. Therefore, in the relatively common setting of infected infrarenal aortic bypass removal, axillary femoral bypass is still recommended.

Three specific indications have coalesced from the Northwestern University experience.[3] The first is the rare situation of a hostile abdomen, usually after either extensive previous operations or radiation in the periaortic region. Circumstances including inflammatory bowel disease or abdominal wall deficiencies may enter into this decision. In such patients, aortic inflow from the left chest may be less traumatic than an abdominal exploration. The second general indication is for repeated failure of abdominal aortic grafting. As a general rule, failure after a single aortofemoral bypass is appropriately managed with another intra-abdominal aortic graft. After two failures, one may reasonably consider moving to the thoracic aorta for inflow. Finally, the thoracofemoral bypass has been useful for patients with multiple failed extra-anatomic bypasses. They include individuals with axillopopliteal and axillofemoral grafts having had multiple graft thrombectomy operations. Many of these patients were first seen at the time of infected aortic graft removal, and reconstruction was performed in the usual way with axillary-based inflow grafts. Following removal of their infected grafts, many such patients enjoy a potentially long life and are gravely affected by their repeated axillary graft thromboses. A reconstruction providing an uninhibited inflow source such as the descending thoracic aorta and the intracavitary tunnel of the thoracofemoral bypass seems reasonable in this setting.

SURGICAL TECHNIQUE

The patient is positioned to maintain adequate surgical access to both femoral arteries.[4] The pelvis is left reasonably flat with a rotation of the thorax to about 30° (Fig. 1). A thoracotomy incision is made in the sixth or

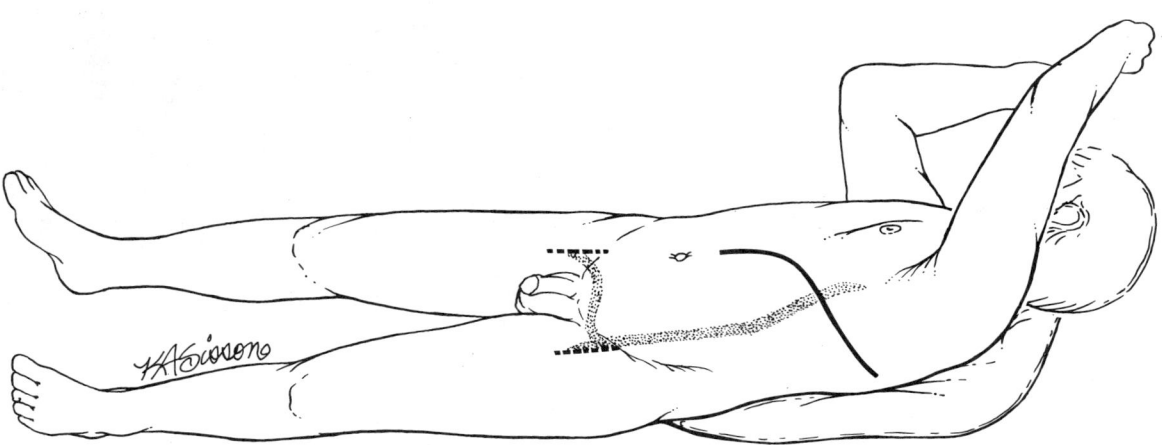

Figure 1 Rotation of the left chest to 30° allows level positioning of the femoral regions. (From McCarthy WJ, Rubin JR, Flinn WR, et al. Descending thoracic aorta-to-femoral artery bypass. Arch Surg 1986; 121:681–688; with permission.)

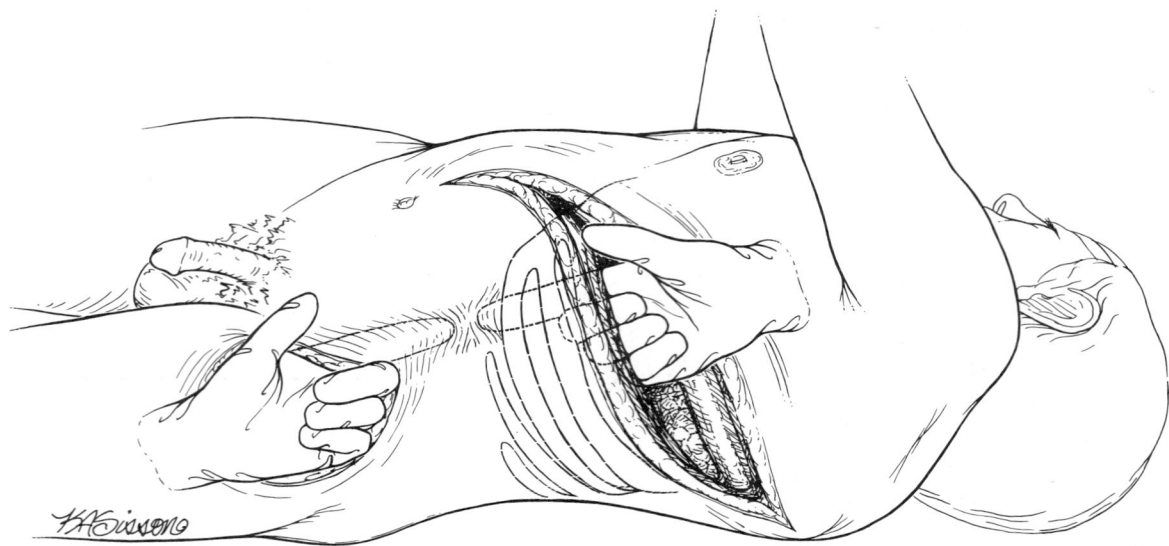

Figure 2 Blunt index finger dissection allows atraumatic tunneling along the anterior or midaxillary line. (From McCarthy WJ, Rubin JR, Flinn WR, et al. Descending thoracic aorta-to-femoral artery bypass. Arch Surg 1986; 121:681–688; with permission.)

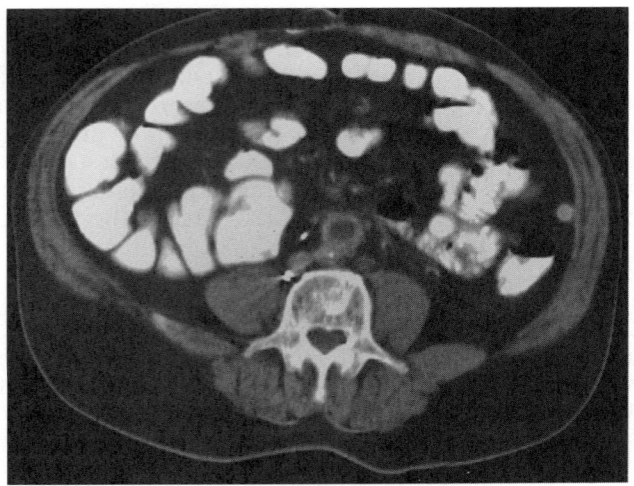

Figure 3 The 10 mm graft is visible retroperitoneally along the midaxillary line anterior to the kidney and spleen.

seventh intercostal space and brought across the costal cartilage for several centimeters onto the abdominal wall. After the chest is opened, the diaphragm is incised for several centimeters in a radial fashion. Later, the bypass graft will pass through this short incision. Left lung retraction with either conventional retractors or selective deflation with a double-lumen endotracheal tube is followed by incision of the inferior pulmonary ligament to expose the aorta. The aorta is circumferentially dissected just above the diaphragm to allow placement of a bypass graft several centimeters above the diaphragmatic hiatus. A nasal gastric tube allows identification of the esophagus by palpation during this dissection, and an elastic sialastic sling is left around the aorta for control.

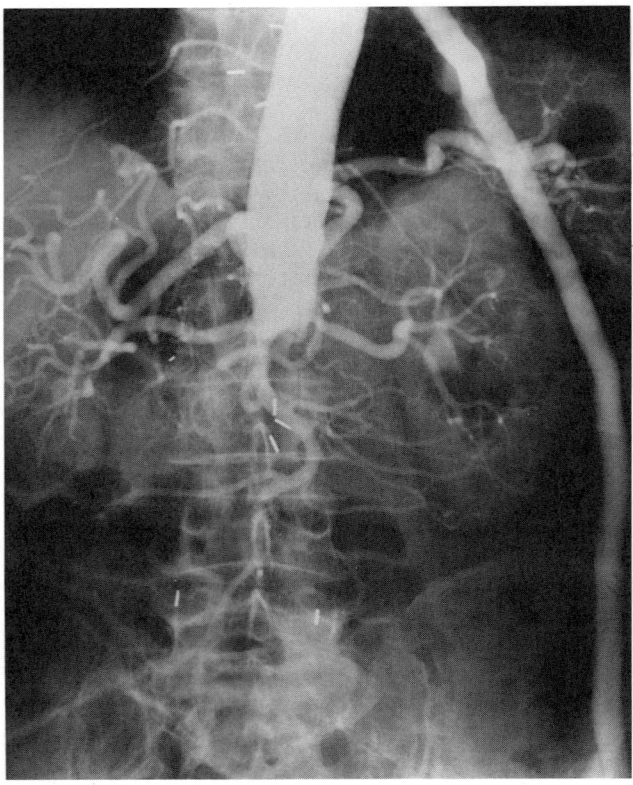

Figure 4 The bypass graft is visible coursing over the diaphragm and along the lateral abdominal wall retroperitoneally. This patient had undergone removal of an infected aortic graft 2 years previously.

Table 1 Patency Features from Representative Reports

Authors	Year	No. of Patients	Mean Follow-up (Months)	Patency (%)	Time (Months)
Feldhaus et al.[5]	1985	18	Not given	85	60
Schultz et al.[6]	1986	15	37	80	60
Bowes et al.[7]	1990	26	53	86	42
Criado et al.[8]	1992	16	24	83.3	24
Branchereau et al.[9]	1992	27	26.3	72.6	24
McCarthy et al.[3]	1993	21	44	86	48

Tunnels are formed from the retroperitoneum just beneath the costal cartilage incision to the left groin. This process is aided by transecting the left inguinal ligament and achieved with blunt bimanual index finger dissection. Remarkably, finger dissection usually provides enough length for this tunnel (Fig. 2). The tunnel is beneath the lateral abdominal musculature but extraperitoneally along the anterior or midaxillary line (Fig. 3). After heparinization, the proximal aortic anastomosis is performed after partial occlusion of the aorta. Selection of just the right J-shaped clamp may require some experimentation. Patients are well served with a 10 mm graft, but 8 or 12 mm grafts may be used, depending upon patient size. Suture with 3-0 or 4-0 polypropylene or polytetrafluoroethylene is appropriate. Chest tube drainage for 1 or 2 days is instituted after standard closure of the thoracotomy.

Tunneling techniques differ among surgeons. The aforementioned method is the simplest available and allows tunneling anterior to the left kidney and spleen (Fig. 4). Perfusion of the right lower extremity is provided by standard femorofemoral grafting based from the thoracofemoral graft. Alternative tunneling techniques involve using a more posterior tunnel often with a bifurcated aortic graft. The posterior tunnel method often requires a left flank counterincision and considerable blind tunneling to reach the right femoral region. Either approach should yield a good result.

RESULTS

The 5 year patency characteristics for several series range from 72% patency at 2 years to 85% patency at 5 years (Table 1).[3,5-9] Not all of these studies were published with standard lifetable techniques, but it seems that the expected patency is consistently in the lower 80th percentile at 5 years. This is slightly lower than what is reported for standard aortofemoral bypass grafting but is achieved in patients who are almost always undergoing reoperation rather than primary repair. A review of 166 patients reported in the literature documents a perioperative mortality rate of 6.6%. Many of these patients died of septic complications. Patient survival data are unavailable from most reports but was 65% at 60 months for 21 patients in the Northwestern study.[3] Six of the eight patients who died in the follow-up period had myocardial infarction as cause of death at a mean of 39 months after their operation.

Review of the functional outcome for 21 patients in the Northwestern study documented that additional arterial operations were necessary for limb salvage.[3] In this group 15 subsequent infrainguinal surgical procedures were required. These included five femoral popliteal, three femoral tibial, and two operations involving the deep femoral artery. There were two femorofemoral bypass operations, and three patients underwent leg amputation but never because of failed arterial inflow. Patients require careful surveillance of their legs and also particular attention to cardiac risk factors for long-term success after this operation.

REFERENCES

1. Stevenson JK, Sauvage LR, Harkins HN. A bypass homograft from thoracic aorta to femoral arteries for occlusive vascular disease: Case report. Ann Surg 1961; 27:632–637.
2. Blaisdell FW, DeMattei GA, Gauder PJ. Extraperitoneal thoracic aorta to femoral bypass graft as replacement for an infected aortic bifurcation prosthesis: Case reports. Am J Surg 1961; 102:583–585.
3. McCarthy WJ, Mesh CL, McMillan WD, et al. Descending thoracic aorta to femoral bypass: Ten years' experience with a durable procedure. J Vasc Surg 1993; 17:336–348.
4. McCarthy WJ, Rubin JR, Flinn WR, et al. Descending thoracic aorta-to-femoral artery bypass. Arch Surg 1986; 121:681–688.
5. Feldhaus RJ, Sterpetti AV, Schultz RD, Peetz DJ Jr. Thoracic aorta-femoral artery bypass: Indications, technique, and late results. Ann Thorac Surg 1985; 40:588–592.
6. Schultz RD, Sterpetti AV, Feldhaus RJ. Thoracic aorta as source of inflow in reoperation for occluded aortoiliac reconstruction. Surgery 1986; 100:635–644.
7. Bowes DE, Youkey JR, Pharr WP, et al. Long term follow-up of descending thoracic aorto-iliac/femoral bypass. J Cardiovasc Surg (Torino) 1990; 31:430–437.
8. Criado E, Johnson G Jr, Burnham SJ, et al. Descending thoracic aorta-to-iliofemoral artery bypass as an alternative to aortoiliac reconstruction. J Vasc Surg 1992; 15:550–557.
9. Branchereau A, Magnan P-E, Moracchini P, et al. Use of descending thoracic aorta for lower limb revascularisation. Eur J Vasc Surg 1992; 6:255–262.

AXILLOFEMORAL BYPASS

LESTER R. SAUVAGE, M.D.
SHERIF EL-MASSRY, M.D.

In 1959, a patient with a ruptured abdominal aortic aneurysm was successfully treated by exclusion of the aneurysm and placement of a composite graft (a straight nylon prosthesis sutured to an aortic bifurcation homograft), which was joined to the proximal end of the left subclavian artery above and to the distal ends of the external iliac arteries below. This case demonstrated for the first time that an upper extremity artery could successfully supply blood to both lower extremities. Three years later a surgeon in South Africa and another in the United States independently and almost simultaneously performed the first unilateral axillofemoral bypasses for severe unilateral iliac occlusive disease in poor-risk patients. In 1966 it was documented that a single axillofemoral bypass could supply blood to both lower extremities by the addition of a graft limb to the opposite femoral artery.[1] In the ensuing years, axillobifemoral bypass has become an important method of augmenting the circulation to the lower limbs of poor-risk patients with severe ischemia due to aortoiliac occlusive disease.

INDICATIONS AND PATIENT SELECTION

With the proper indications axillofemoral bypass is a good operation. These indications are the patient's general condition and the hemodynamic relationship between the axillary and femoral arteries. The frail patient with severe diffuse aortoiliac occlusive disease who has disabling claudication, rest pain, impending tissue loss, or a small extent of actual tissue breakdown is a proper candidate for this procedure, provided there is a continuous pressure gradient between the axillary and femoral arteries at rest. However, if the axillary inflow is impaired as evidenced by a weak radial pulse, a decreased brachial artery pressure in relation to the opposite side, and the presence of a supraclavicular murmur, the affected axillary artery may not be capable of supplying an adequate quantity of blood to even one lower extremity. On the other hand, if there is a good radial pulse, a brachial pressure at least equal to that of the other side, and no murmur above the clavicle, the inflow is adequate not only for the arm but also for both lower extremities in patients whose walking needs are only modest.

Without a continuous pressure gradient at rest, the axillofemoral procedure should not be done, because this graft cannot compete successfully with a significant iliac inflow for long periods. To remain patent the axillofemoral graft needs substantial flow throughout systole and diastole, both at rest and with exercise. If there is diastolic flow only during exercise, early closure is likely.

The elderly patient who needs an axillofemoral graft rarely requires it to sustain strenuous exercise. The physical activity of these patients is usually restricted by age, arthritis, and general weakness in addition to the impaired blood supply to their lower extremities. They need only a moderately improved blood supply to sustain their legs in a pain-free and reasonably functional state for the remainder of their lives.

The axillofemoral operation is also indicated for selected healthy patients with severe symptoms who meet the hemodynamic criteria and in whom the aortofemoral procedure would be substantially riskier, because either exposing the aorta or anastomosing the graft to it would be unduly hazardous due to extensive adhesions, severe calcification, or marked atheromatous degeneration. In addition, axillofemoral bypass is an essential procedure for many of the patients in whom an infected aortofemoral graft must be removed and may also be advisable for patients with an infected abdominal aortic aneurysm. Axillopopliteal bypass is indicated in some patients with infected aortofemoral grafts when the infection extends distally to involve the groin. This procedure is less popular than axillofemoral grafting, and the results are less favorable.

GRAFT SELECTION

At least seven generic graft types are available, and there are many more specific types. Grafts that do not require preclotting are favored by most surgeons. This is an important attribute of polytetrafluoroethylene (PTFE), woven Dacron, and coated knitted Dacron prostheses. Supported grafts are recommended for axillofemoral bypass to avoid compression during sleep, should the patient turn on the side of the graft. While there are no prospective trials comparing either nonsupported with supported PTFE prostheses or crimped, nonsupported with noncrimped, supported knitted Dacron prostheses for axillofemoral bypass, most surgeons use supported prostheses. The theoretic advantages of these grafts are that they are resistant to compression and kinking and in the case of Dacron prostheses provide a noncrimped surface to the blood. Most surgeons use PTFE prostheses for axillofemoral bypass, even though several retrospective studies and the preliminary results of the only prospective trial have not shown it to have higher patency rates than Dacron.

An externally-supported knitted Dacron graft that is converted by preclotting into a highly sophisticated bioprosthesis is preferred by the authors. The wall of this composite graft is approximately 600 μm thick and consists of a Dacron yarn framework with a fibrin-thrombus matrix dispersed throughout its structure that fills all interstices, coats all filaments, and forms the surfaces presenting to the blood internally and to the perigraft tissues externally. It is believed that these biologic components, which make the graft wall impervious to bleeding, provide the chemotactic properties and growth factors necessary to promote healing by the arterial wall to which it will be attached, by the perigraft tissues that will surround it, and by the blood that will flow over its surface. We prefer an 8 mm diameter prosthesis. In our experience a 6 mm diameter graft is too small for most patients because of reduced flow capacity and greater pressure head loss.

AXILLOUNIFEMORAL VERSUS AXILLOBIFEMORAL BYPASS

The choice between axillounifemoral and axillobifemoral configuration is determined by the hemodynamic conditions on the two sides. If there is severe obstruction on both sides, an axillobifemoral procedure is indicated. However, if the obstruction is severe on only one side but the contralateral iliac inflow is not adequate to support a femorofemoral bypass, an axillounifemoral procedure is indicated.

The volume of blood flow in an axillobifemoral graft is greater than in the axillounifemoral graft because of the flow in the femorofemoral bypass. In our experience the mean operative blood flow in the main limb of 29 axillobifemoral grafts was 694 ± 430 ml/min, and the flow in the crossover component was 335 ± 306 ml/min. The flow in 50 axillounifemoral grafts was 525 ± 381 ml/min.[2]

Several older studies reported higher patency rates for axillobifemoral grafts than for axillounifemoral grafts. However, the only prospective study of axillofemoral grafts, and some recent retrospective studies, have shown similar patency rates for both configurations.[2-4] It is not clear whether this trend is related to the exclusive use of externally supported grafts.

PREOPERATIVE EVALUATION

An aortogram with runoff, often with oblique views, is required to establish a definitive diagnosis of the extent of aortoiliac occlusive disease and to provide an arterial road map to assist in planning the surgical strategy. A preoperative subclavian-axillary arteriogram is not needed unless there is clinical suspicion of stenosis. Calligaro and colleagues[5] reported a 25% incidence of a 50% or more inflow stenosis when preoperative arteriograms were routinely done without reference to the clinical findings. They also reported a 16% incidence of such inflow stenosis in failed axillofemoral grafts. If both axillary arteries are good, the artery ipsilateral to the most severely impaired lower limb should be used.

IMPLANTATION TECHNIQUE

Though the axillofemoral procedure is not difficult, the technique employed is important. If the operation is done poorly, the results are likely to be poor. These are the broad technical objectives we believe to be important for successful implantation of axillofemoral grafts (Figs. 1 and 2).

Axillounifemoral Bypass

Incisions

The femoral incision may be made either along the common femoral artery or just below and parallel to the inguinal ligament. The axillary incision runs parallel to the lower border of the middle portion of the clavicle.

Exposure

We expose the common femoral artery from the inguinal ligament down to and including the upper portion of the profunda femoris and superficial femoral arteries and bare the axillary artery by splitting the fibers of the pectoralis major and dissecting inward. We free the artery superior to the axillary vein as far medially as possible without injury to the brachial plexus.

Tunnel

Development of the tunnel in the anterior axillary line proceeds upward from the femoral incision and downward from the axillary incision. The upper portion lies in the areolar tissue between the pectoralis major and minor muscles, and the middle and lower portions lie in the areolar tissue beneath the fatty layer of the subcutaneous tissues of the torso and groin. Transection of the pectoralis minor has been recommended, but we have not found this necessary. The only difficult part of constructing the tunnel is breaking through the fascial envelopments of the inferolateral border of the pectoralis major. Generally this necessitates two short incisions following the skin lines below the pectoral level.

During this procedure it is vital to avoid hematoma formation so that the subcutaneous tissues can come in direct contact with the outer graft wall. This proximity of the tissues promotes healing and greatly decreases the possibility of perigraft infection or seroma formation.

Femoral Anastomosis

If the common femoral artery is a good length, we make the lower anastomosis to an opening in its distal portion. However, if the common femoral is short, and especially if the patient has an obese, overhanging abdomen, we make the anastomosis to an opening that extends from the lower portion of this artery out into the profunda femoris artery. Local pathology may necessitate performing the anastomosis entirely to the profunda. It is important to place the anastomosis distally enough that the lower portion of the graft will not be angulated when the patient flexes the hip in sitting, bending over, or lifting the leg.

At least 5 to 6 cm of the crimped, nonsupported

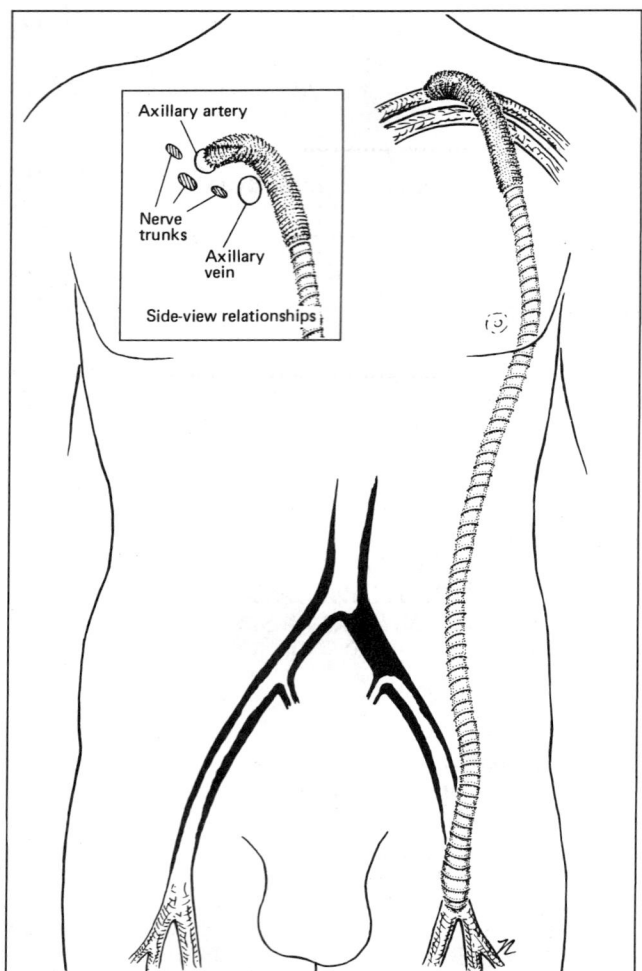

Figure 1 Unilateral lower extremity revascularization by axillofemoral bypass using preclotted 8-mm-diameter externally supported warp-knit Dacron graft. The graft is placed in the tunnel and then the lower anastomosis is performed. The graft is cut to preserve as much of the supported, noncrimped portion as possible, leaving at least 5 to 6 cm of the crimped, nonsupported portion at the upper end. The proper length is determined and the graft is cut to assure that it has at least 5 cm of slack, as compared with the tightly extended state. The upper anastomosis is then performed to an opening in the anterior wall of the axillary artery as far medially as possible. Inset shows side view of upper end of graft demonstrating proper tension. The graft must not be tight.

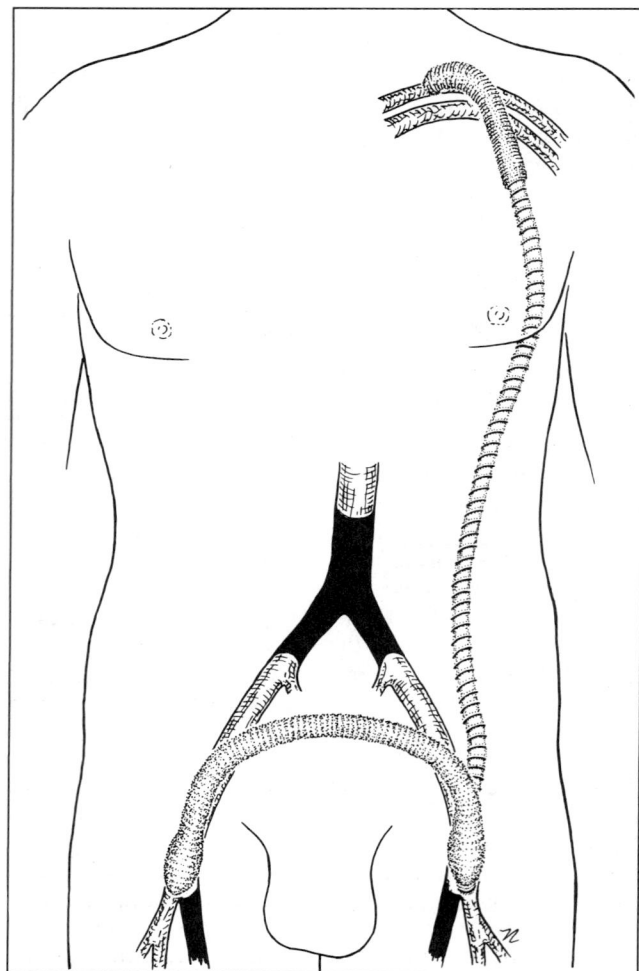

Figure 2 Bilateral lower extremity revascularization by a unilateral axillofemoral bypass combined with a cross-over femorofemoral bypass. Both grafts are placed in their respective tunnels, after which the lower anastomoses may be performed simultaneously. The inflow anastomoses of both grafts may be performed at the same time, with the femorofemoral graft anastomosed to an opening in the hood of the femoral anastomosis of the axillofemoral graft.

upper portion of an EXS Dacron graft and as much of the supported, noncrimped (45 cm long) middle portion as possible are retained. To retain this length of crimped graft at the upper end, we transect the graft for the lower anastomosis at the proper level. If the torso is long, we retain all of the supported middle portion and begin the anastomosis at its distal end, including the last support coil with the heel stitch. Then we complete the anastomosis to the noncrimped, nonsupported lower portion. How much of the crimped upper portion of the graft we retain depends on the length of the torso. If the torso is short, we transect the graft in the supported portion at a level that will leave the desired length of the crimped section at the upper end.

We have not found that performing the femoral anastomosis to the supported portion of the prosthesis causes problems. We have observed 2 closures in 25 supported anastomoses and 10 closures in 54 nonsupported anastomoses (p = .12).[2] Blaisdell[6] in fact has recommended that the femoral anastomosis be made to the supported portion of the graft.

Graft Tension

Surface measurements have shown that maximum flexion of the thoracolumbar spine to the opposite side, combined with abduction of the arm, increases the distance between the groin and the axilla in the midaxillary line by 15%. Axillofemoral grafts lie more in the anterior axillary line and are probably subjected to a little less elongation, perhaps 10% with spine flexion and arm abduction. For this additional length of about 5 cm to be available, the graft must be loosely placed at implantation.

The graft must be long enough to emerge from the upper anastomosis nearly at right angles to the axillary artery and pass superior to and then downward in front of the vein without compressing it even to a slight degree (see Fig. 1).

The residual crimp in the upper portion of the graft should be at least 50% of its original nonstressed height. There should be laxity in the graft throughout its length. We have placed grafts that were too tight but never one that was too loose.

Axillary Anastomosis

Never place the graft behind the axillary vein because if a repair of the upper end becomes necessary later, the adhesions that will have formed between the graft and the vital structures in this area may make a secondary operation impossible.

The more lateral the graft is to the axillary artery, the greater this anastomosis elevates with raising of the arm and the more the graft must elongate. Therefore, if the graft is short with the arm at the side, the tension on the suture line with abduction increases markedly and may disrupt the anastomosis. For this reason the axillary anastomosis should always be performed as far medially as possible.

This anastomosis is made to an opening in the anterior wall of the axillary artery. If the graft is too tight, divide it and interpose an appropriate segment to provide the desired additional length. It is well to recall that a graft that is too short at implantation will become more so over time from contraction of the fibrous tissue that invades its wall.

Axillobifemoral Bypass

All of the technical factors that are important for an axillounifemoral graft are important for an axillobifemoral graft. The only additional features involve the cross-over femorofemoral graft. We believe this arrangement is hemodynamically better than converting the lower portion of the axillofemoral graft into a bifurcation prosthesis by running a side limb to the opposite femoral artery. This configuration diverts about 50% of the flow to the opposite femoral system and decreases the flow in the distal axillofemoral segment to an equivalent degree. We have observed distal graft thrombosis under these circumstances.

An 8 mm diameter graft is used for both the axillofemoral and femorofemoral bypasses. However, we do not use a supported graft for the cross-over because it is not necessary in this location, where the graft is relatively short and subject to neither compression nor kinking. Instead we use a crimped knitted graft and preclot it in the same manner as the axillofemoral graft.

The axillofemoral and crossover grafts are placed in their respective tunnels in the areolar tissue beneath the fatty layer of the anterolateral region of the trunk, of the lower anterior abdominal wall, and of both groins. The anastomosis of the femorofemoral graft, like that of the axillofemoral graft, is sufficiently distal that there will be no kinking of the graft when the patient's hip is flexed.

If there are two surgical teams, the femoral dissections for both grafts can be started simultaneously. The proper length of this graft is determined after the femoral anastomosis of the axillofemoral graft is complete. Then we perform the inflow anastomoses of both grafts at the same time. The femorofemoral graft is anastomosed to an opening in the hood of the axillofemoral graft during the axillary anastomosis of this graft.

OPERATIVE MORTALITY AND LONG-TERM SURVIVAL

Operative mortality is directly related to the indications for the axillofemoral procedure and the degree of urgency of the operation. Patients with infected aortofemoral grafts, aortoenteric fistulas, or infected aneurysms have been reported to have perioperative mortalities as high as 24%.[7] Furthermore, emergency operations for acute ischemia have even higher mortalities, with reports of 26% to 67%.[8,9] However, elective axillofemoral bypasses have been reported to have mortalities ranging from 2.8% to 12% (Table 1). The 5 year survival of these patients has been reported to be only 38% to 50%, reflecting their impaired physical status.[2,10]

UPPER EXTREMITY COMPLICATIONS

Disruption of the axillary anastomosis has been reported. Embolization to the arm has been reported with thrombosed tight grafts that pull the axillary artery downward. Steal occurs only when there is proximal stenosis in the subclavian artery. Thrombosis of the axillary artery has been reported as a late complication of thrombosed grafts. However, these complications are uncommon.

PATENCY RATES

The 30-day mortality for 77 patients (79 grafts) since 1978 is 5%. The primary patencies at both 5 and 10 years for axillofemoral grafts with and without a cross-over component were 78% and 73%, respectively (Figs. 3 to 5). There was no statistical difference between procedures done for limb salvage and for disabling claudication. Table 1 summarizes the patency findings reported in the recent literature. The 5 year primary patency rates

Table 1 Clinical Results for Axillofemoral Grafts

	Number of Grafts	Graft Type	Critical Ischemia	5-Year Primary Graft Patency (%)			Perioperative Mortality (%)	5-Year Actuarial Survival of Patients (%)	Infection (%)
				All	AxUnifem	AxBifem			
El-Massry, et al.[d]	79	Dacron	62	78	79	76	5	50	4
Porter, et al., 1993[e]	106	PTFE	[a]	76	none	76	3.7	[c]	[c]
Schneider, et al., 1992[f]	34	PTFE	94	63[b]	67[b]	62[b]	9	35[b]	3
De, et al., 1991[g]	131	Dacron	80	[c]	43	73	5.3	[c]	[c]
Johnson, et al., 1991[h]	103	PTFE	75	[c]	14	55	[c]	[c]	[c]
Dujardin, et al., 1991[i]	85	Dacron/PTFE	87	74[b]	[c]	[c]	12	77[b]	[c]
Schroe, et al., 1990[j]	83	Dacron/PTFE	90	49[b]	[c]	[c]	12	38	[c]
Naylor, et al., 1990[k]	38	PTFE	100	68	50	80	11	44	[c]
Rutherford, et al., 1987[l]	42	PTFE	89	47	19	62	12	[c]	[c]
Kallman, et al., 1987[m]	90	Dacron	67	68[b]	58[b]	77[b]	9	50[b]	[c]

[a]No percentage is given, but the majority of the cases were done for limb salvage.
[b]These rates are at 3 years.
[c]Not given.
[d]El-Massry S, Saad E, Sauvage LR, et al. Axillofemoral bypass with externally supported, knitted Dacron grafts: A follow-up through 12 years. J Vasc Surg 1993; 17:107–115.
[e]Porter JM, Harris JE, Taylor LM, Moneta GL, Yeager RA. Extra-anatomic bypass: a new look (supporting view). Adv Surg 1993; 26:133–149.
[f]Schneider JR, McDaniel MD, Walsh DB, et al. Axillofemoral bypass: Outcome and hemodynamic results in high-risk patients. J Vasc Surg 1992; 15:952–963.
[g]De P, Hepp W. Present role of extraanatomic bypass graft procedures for aortoiliac occlusive disease. International Angiology 1991; 10:224–228.
[h]Johnson WC, Squires JW. Axillofemoral (PTFE) and infrainguinal revascularization (PTFE and umbilical vein): Vascular Registry of the New England Society of Vascular Surgery. J Cardiovasc Surg 1991; 32:344–349.
[i]Dujardin P, Lavigne JP, Defraigne JO, et al. Axillounifemoral and axillobifemoral bypasses. Retrospective study of 85 cases. Acta Chirurg Belg 1991; 91:155–160.
[j]Schroe H, Nevelsteen A, Suy R. Extra-anatomical grafting for aorto-occlusive disease: The outcome in 133 procedures. Acta Chirurg Belg 1990; 240–243.
[k]Naylor AR, Ah-See AK, Engeset J. Axillofemoral bypass as a limb salvage procedure in high-risk patients with aortoiliac disease. Brit J Surg 1990; 77:659–661.
[l]Rutherford RB, Patt A, Pearce WH. Extra-anatomic bypass: A closer view. J Vasc Surg 1987; 6:437–446.
[m]Kalman PG, Hosang M, Cina C, et al. Current indications for axillounifemoral and axillobifemoral bypass grafts. J Vasc Surg 1987; 5:828–832.

in the series combining both axillounifemoral and axillobifemoral procedures series have varied from 47% to 78%. These findings are lower than the 5 year patencies of 85% to 90% reported for aortofemoral grafts. Axillopopliteal grafts have a less favorable primary patency, with a 3 year result of 43%, than axillofemoral grafts.

PATENCY OF THE SUPERFICIAL FEMORAL ARTERY

It has been suggested that ipsilateral occlusion of the superficial femoral artery compromises the distal runoff and adversely affects the patency rates of axillofemoral grafts. However, our recent observations show similar patencies for grafts whether the superficial femoral artery is open or closed.[2] Moreover, the mean operative flow for our 46 axillofemoral grafts proximal to patent superficial femoral arteries or femorodistal bypasses (603 ± 399 ml/min) was not significantly different from that for the 33 grafts proximal to occluded superficial femoral arteries (543 ± 420 ml/min). These observations underline the importance of the profunda femoris artery when the superficial femoral artery is occluded.

PERIGRAFT SEROMA

A perigraft seroma forms around a small percentage of axillofemoral grafts. The fluid is usually clear with no demonstrable organisms and is contained in a nonsecretory fibrous pseudomembrane. The graft literally floats in this fluid. There is no tissue ingrowth into the outer wall of the graft. The fluid has been studied in a few cases by biochemical and electrophoretic means and found to resemble serum, suggesting that it arises from the plasma and seeps through the graft wall. In these cases there were neither acute nor chronic inflammatory cells. The fluid usually recurs after aspiration but seldom progresses to frank infection. Sometimes, when the fluid is turbid, low-grade infection with *Staphylococcus epidermidis* has been documented by broth cultures of either ultrasonated or minced graft specimens. A conservative, watchful policy for these collections is recommended in older, poor-risk patients, and graft replacement may be advised in good-risk patients.

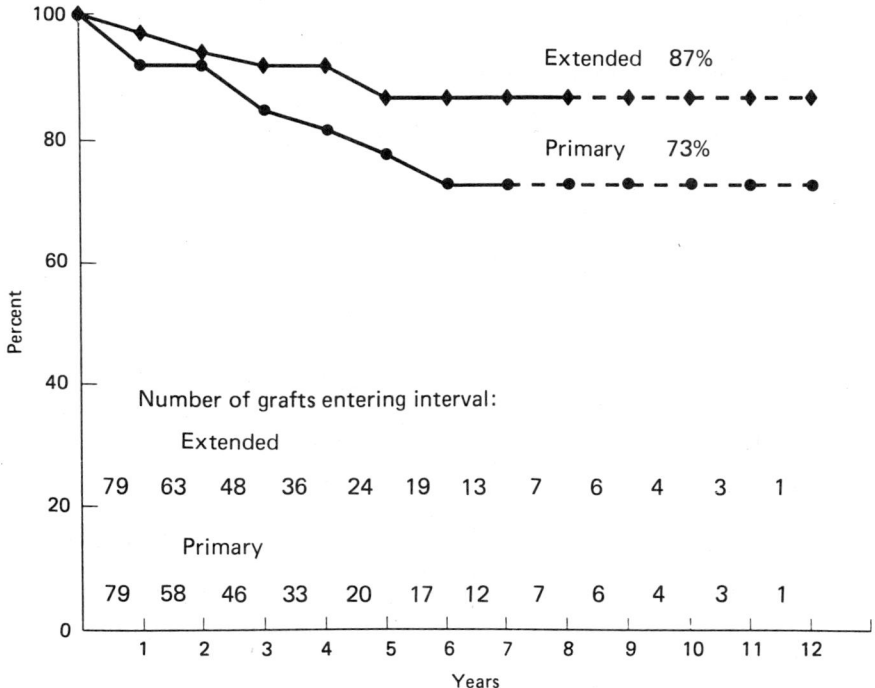

Figure 3 Primary and extended patency rates for 79 axillofemoral grafts. Broken line indicates SE of at least 10%. (From El-Massry S, Saad E, Sauvage LR. Axillofemoral bypass with externally supported, knitted Dacron grafts: A follow-up through 12 years. J Vasc Surg 1992; 17:110; with permission.)

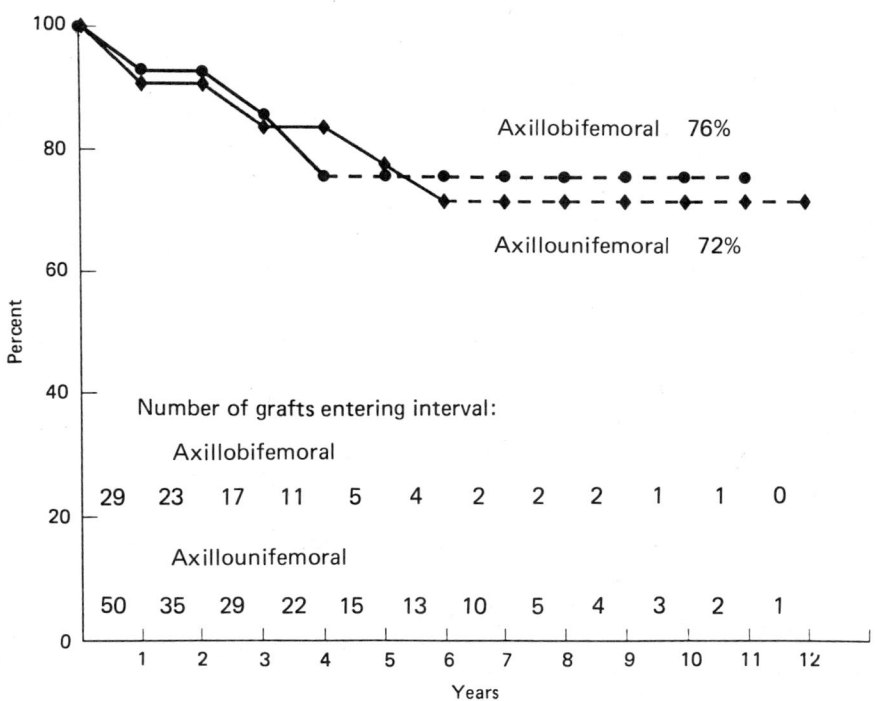

Figure 4 Primary patency rates for 50 axillounifemoral and 29 axillobifemoral grafts. Broken line indicates SE of at least 10%. (From El-Massry S, Saad E, Sauvage LR. Axillofemoral bypass with externally supported, knitted Dacron grafts: A follow-up through 12 years. J Vasc Surg 1992; 17:109; with permission.)

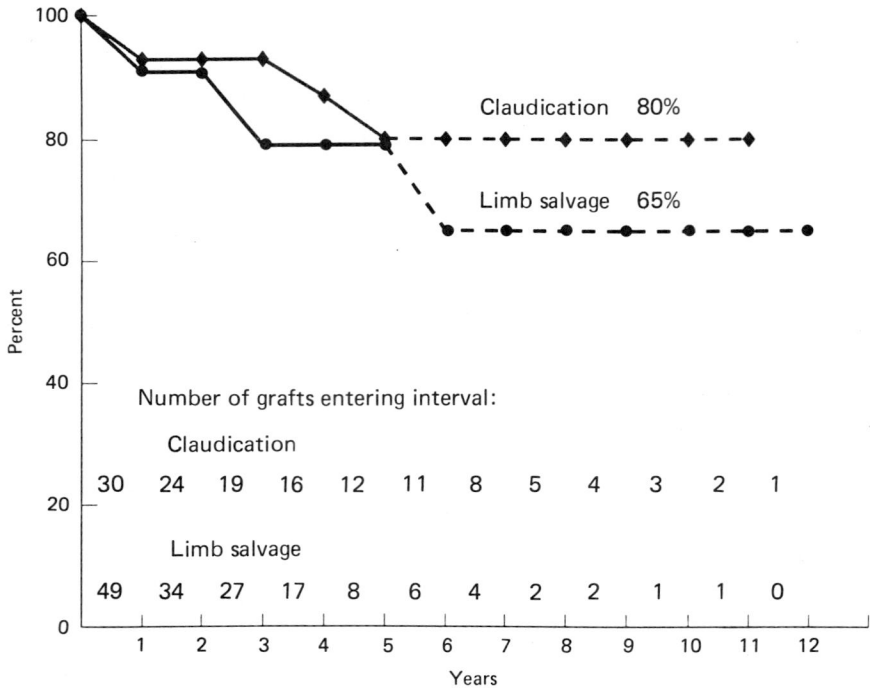

Figure 5 Primary patency rates for 49 grafts used for limb salvage and 30 grafts used for disabling claudication. Broken line indicates SE of at least 10%. (From El-Massry S, Saad E, Sauvage LR. Axillofemoral bypass with externally supported, knitted Dacron grafts: A follow-up through 12 years. J Vasc Surg 1992; 17:110; with permission.)

GRAFT INFECTION

Graft infection is an uncommon but grave complication of vascular reconstruction. Axillofemoral grafts are at a higher risk for infection than aortofemoral or femoropopliteal grafts. This may be attributed to the relatively large operative field, which provides greater opportunity for graft-skin contact, to the frequent use of these grafts in patients with sepsis, and to the need for multiple thrombectomies to keep the grafts functioning. The age and overall poor general condition of the typical candidate for such an operation also suggest a compromised immune response and a decreased capacity to combat infection. The incidence of graft infection is related to the indications for the axillofemoral operation. Infection rates as high as 13% to 27% have been reported in several recent series of infected aortofemoral grafts managed by axillofemoral bypass and graft excision. On the other hand, grafts implanted for indications other than abdominal sepsis have lower infection rates, 3% to 9% (see Table 1).

REFERENCES

1. Sauvage LR, Wood SJ. Unilateral axillary bilateral femoral bifurcation graft: A procedure for the poor risk patient with aortoiliac disease. Surgery 1966; 60:573–577.
2. El-Massry S, Saad E, Sauvage LR, et al. Axillofemoral bypass with externally supported, knitted Dacron grafts: A follow-up through 12 years. J Vasc Surg 1993; 17:107–115.
3. Ascer E, Veith FJ, Gupta SK, et al. Six year experience with expanded polytetrafluoroethylene arterial grafts for limb salvage. J Cardiovasc Surg 1985; 26:468–472.
4. Schneider JR, McDaniel MD, Walsh DB, et al. Axillofemoral bypass: Outcome and hemodynamic results in high-risk patients. J Vasc Surg 1992; 15:952–963.
5. Calligaro KD, Ascer E, Veith FJ, et al. Unsuspected inflow disease in candidates for axillofemoral bypass operations: A prospective study. J Vasc Surg 1990; 11:832–837.
6. Blaisdell FW. Extra-anatomic bypass procedures. World J Surg 1988; 12:798–804.
7. Bacourt F, Koskas F. Axillobifemoral bypass and aortic exclusion for vascular septic lesions: A multicenter retrospective study of 98 cases: French University Association for Research in Surgery. Ann Vasc Surg 1992; 6:119–126.
8. Agee JM, Kron IL, Flanagan T, Tribble CG. The risk of axillofemoral bypass grafting for acute vascular occlusion. J Vasc Surg 1991; 14:190–194.
9. Savrin RA, Record GT, McDowell DE. Axillofemoral bypass: Expectations and results. Arch Surg 1986; 121:1016–1020.
10. Schroe H, Nevelsteen A, Suy R. Extra-anatomical grafting for aorto-occlusive disease: The outcome in 133 procedures. Acta Chirurg Belg 1990; 90:240–243.

UNILATERAL RETROPERITONEAL ILIOFEMORAL BYPASS

DHIRAJ M. SHAH, M.D.
R. CLEMENT DARLING III, M.D.
BENJAMIN B. CHANG, M.D.
ROBERT P. LEATHER, M.D.

Treatment of significant occlusive disease of the suprainguinal arteries presents the vascular surgeon with several reconstructive options. The individual occlusive pattern, the patient's medical status and life expectancy, and the surgeon's experience and training must be weighed carefully to select the most appropriate reconstructive procedure. In good-risk patients with occlusive disease involving the infrarenal aorta, either aortobifemoral bypass or aortoiliac endarterectomy may be employed with expectations of 90% 5 year patency rates and operative mortality rates of 2% to 3%.[1]

In patients without hemodynamically significant aortic disease, isolated ilioarterial occlusive disease may be treated with any of several types of bypass or endarterectomy procedures. Truly unilateral iliac occlusive disease is often treated with femorofemoral crossover bypass, especially in high-risk patients. However, these grafts carry a relatively poor patency rate (55% to 68% over 5 years) in most series.[2,3] Axillofemoral bypass grafts perform even more poorly (19% to 57% 5 year patency). These extra-anatomic bypasses are probably best reserved for patients with truly limited life expectancy.

As an alternative to either of these two reconstructive procedures, some patients with iliac occlusive disease may be treated with unilateral iliofemoral bypass. Indications for this procedure include isolated unilateral iliac occlusive disease with disabling claudication or critical ischemia plus mild or relatively asymptomatic occlusive disease of the contralateral iliac artery and unilateral symptoms when an extensive aortic reconstructive procedure is contraindicated.

EVALUATION OF INFLOW

Proper patient selection is imperative for unilateral iliac reconstruction. The most important aspect of unilateral iliac reconstruction is ensuring adequacy of inflow. Preoperative pulse volume recordings and segmental blood pressure measurements are generally not useful for determining inflow adequacy. Arteriography may be useful in documenting patency of the aorta and the common iliac artery in the affected limb, but dense posterior plaque makes definitive surgical decisions based on the study of single plane arteriograms hazardous. Measurement of blood pressures within the iliac artery, ideally after the administration of 60 to 120 mg of papaverine, may be done at the time of arteriography to estimate the adequacy of inflow.

SURGICAL TECHNIQUE

Exposure of the iliac and femoral arteries is performed two ways. If the occlusive process is restricted to the external iliac and femoral arteries, a vertical groin incision may be carried cephalad through the inguinal ligament and lower abdominal wall. More often the iliac artery is exposed through an anterior extraperitoneal incision in the appropriate lower quadrant. This incision usually starts between the anterior superior iliac spine and the twelfth rib and carries medially to the edge of the rectus abdominus muscle 2 to 3 inches above the pubic ramus. Maintaining extraperitoneal exposure makes retraction of the bowel simple and coverage of the reconstruction automatic.[4]

After the arteries are exposed, arterial blood pressures may be measured by direct puncture and augmented with papaverine if there is any doubt about the adequacy of inflow.

Bypass is usually preferred for extensive disease, small arteries, and reoperative procedures. In particular, disease extending into the profunda femoris and/or the superficial femoral arteries makes bypass a technically easier option. If the aortic bifurcation is undiseased, the common iliac artery may be clamped. If not, the terminal aorta and contralateral iliac may have to be controlled. Either an end-to-end or end-to-side proximal anastomosis may be performed, although the latter is usually technically easier in partially diseased arteries. Endarterectomy of the inflow artery may facilitate the anastomosis as well as improve the hemodynamic results. Either 8 or 6 mm prosthetic grafts are used for bypass. The graft is tunneled anatomically into the groin after completion of the proximal anastomosis. Usually an end-to-side anastomosis is performed to the distal common femoral artery extending across any orifice stenosis of the profunda femoris artery.

RESULTS

We retrospectively evaluated our results with iliofemoral reconstruction compared with aortofemoral bypasses for occlusive disease.[5] Patients with significant aortofemoral or hemodynamically significant bilateral iliac disease underwent aortofemoral bypasses. Patients with hemodynamically unobstructed iliac arteries had an iliac-based procedure. When preoperative blood pressure measurements were inconclusive because of significant distal disease, pressure measurements were repeated after the bypass. All operations were performed through the extraperitoneal route. We performed 248 bypasses using aortobifemoral grafts. In the same period we did 454 arterial reconstructions using the iliac arteries as donor vessels. Risk factors, demographics, and indications for operation were similar in both groups. The 30 day mortality for the aortobifemoral bypass group was 3.6% compared with 1.6% for the iliac based inflow group (P < .05). Postoperatively, all patients undergoing aortic reconstruction were admitted to the intensive care unit and were intubated with monitoring. However, fewer than 15% of patients undergoing iliac-based procedures required admission to the intensive care unit, and even fewer had general anesthesia for their operations. The 30 day primary patency rate for aortobifemoral grafts was 95%. The 30 day primary patency rate for the iliac-based group was 97%. Cumulative patency rates at 1 and 5 years were 91% and 77% respectively for patients undergoing aortobifemoral bypass. Cumulative patency rates for iliac-based reconstructions were 92% and 79%, respectively (Table 1). We had a slightly better patency rate for iliofemoral endarterectomies, with a 94% cumulative patency rate at 1 year and 89% at 5 years. This was probably because favorable morphology caused a selection bias in patients chosen for endarterectomy. Also, if we did not consider the endarterectomy technically satisfactory, it was converted to an iliofemoral bypass. The 5 year patency rate for iliofemoral bypass of 82% was comparable to the 77% 4 year patency rate reported by others.[6,7,8] Other authors concluded that if patients have suitable arterial anatomy, iliofemoral bypass is a viable alternative to aortofemoral reconstruction.[6-8] The common femoral and profunda femoris arteries were used as outflows with equal frequency in our study. The superficial femoral artery was patent in 45% of patients in the iliofemoral group and 38% of patients undergoing aortofemoral bypass. We restored profunda femoris outflow by extending the distal anastomosis across the profunda femoris orifice. It is essential not to hesitate to add a distal bypass procedure if the outflow system is inadequate.

In comparison with femorofemoral bypass, iliofemoral bypass has numerous technical advantages. Iliofemoral bypass can be performed easily through a suprainguinal renal transplant incision. The graft lies deeper and is protected by muscle and fascia. The iliofemoral bypass graft is shorter than the femorofemoral bypass graft and it avoids bilateral femoral incisions, which may decrease the risk of infection. The femorofemoral bypass is a hemodynamically disadvantaged procedure because of retrograde flow when using the inverted "U" configuration. Although many have reported good patency rates with femorofemoral bypass, we have found our iliofemoral bypass results superior to those of our femorofemoral bypasses.

Table 1 Patency of Iliofemoral Reconstructions: Life Table Analysis

Follow-up (Months)	At Risk	Occluded	Initial Patency (%)	Cumulative Patency (%)
<1	454	14	97	97
1–6	440	12	97	94
7–12	426	10	98	92
13–18	340	10	97	89
19–24	285	12	96	85
25–30	259	6	98	83
31–36	241	1	99	82
37–42	169	3	98	80
43–48	143	1	99	79
49–52	108	0	100	79
53–60	52	0	100	79

REFERENCES

1. Brewster DC, Darling RC. Optimal methods of aortoiliac reconstruction. Surgery 1978; 84:739–748.
2. Mannick JA, Maini BS. Femorofemoral grafting: Indications and late results. Am J Surg 1978; 136:190–192.
3. Perler BA, Burdick JF, Williams MG. Femorofemoral or iliofemoral bypass for unilateral inflow reconstruction. Am J Surg 1991; 161:426–430.
4. Vitale GF, Inahara T. Extraperitoneal endarterectomy for iliofemoral occlusive disease. J Vasc Surg 1990; 12:408–415.
5. Darling RC III, Leather RP, Chang BB, et al. Is the iliac artery a suitable inflow conduit for iliofemoral occlusive disease: An analysis of 514 aortoiliac reconstructions. J Vasc Surg 1993; 17:15–19.
6. Piotrowski J, Pearch WH, Jones DN, et al. Aortobifemoral bypass: Operation of choice for unilateral iliac occlusion? J Vasc Surg 1988; 8:211–218.
7. Kalman PG, Hosana M, Johnson RW, et al. Unilateral iliac disease: The role of iliofemoral bypass. J Vasc Surg 1987; 6:139–143.
8. Couch NP, Clowes AW, Whittemore AD, et al. The iliac-origin arterial graft: A useful alterative for iliac occlusive disease. Surgery 1985; 97:83–87.

FEMOROFEMORAL BYPASS FOR AORTOILIAC OCCLUSIVE DISEASE

SUSHIL GUPTA, M.D.
RAUL LANDA, M.D.
FRANK VEITH, M.D.

Femorofemoral bypass is widely accepted for the treatment of patients with unilateral iliac artery lesions. Although Freeman and Leeds [1] in 1952 were the first authors to report the use of femorofemoral bypass, this operation was popularized by Vetto,[2] who reported on this procedure in 10 high risk patients with unilateral iliac artery obstruction.

Initially, femorofemoral bypass was used for treatment of symptomatic unilateral iliac disease in high-risk patients. Later, prompted by its technical simplicity and early good results, it was advocated for good-risk patients to avoid more extensive aortic reconstructions.[3,4] Despite widespread use, femorofemoral bypass has become controversial because several authors have documented better patency rates with direct aortofemoral or iliofemoral reconstructions and have criticized use of femorofemoral bypass in low-risk patients.[5,6]

Patients for any procedure should be selected by weighing the operative risk and the life expectancy of the patient against durability and effectiveness of the procedure under consideration. Other factors that affect graft patency and limb salvage should also be taken into consideration. The obvious indications for femorofemoral bypass are rather narrow: patients with normal aorta, normal iliac artery on one side, and occluded or stenotic iliac artery on the symptomatic side. In practice, this operation is employed in a variety of circumstances to facilitate complex primary or secondary vascular reconstructions, and its utility should be viewed with these broadened applications in mind. For example, the femorofemoral bypass has become the procedure of choice for treatment of unilateral thrombosis of aortobifemoral grafts when thrombectomy of the occluded limb fails. It has also been used to provide inflow to femoropopliteal or femorodistal bypasses when there is ipsilateral iliac artery disease as well as to provide outflow for failing or failed axillary, femoral, or aortic procedures.

In the past 15 years we have been involved in a total of 233 reconstructions in which femorofemoral bypass was performed as an isolated procedure or part of other complex vascular reconstructions.

PATIENT SELECTION

The usual candidate for a primary femorofemoral bypass is a patient with relatively normal abdominal aorta and iliac arteries on one side and advanced arteriosclerotic disease of the iliac arteries on the symptomatic side. The ischemic symptoms may range from disabling claudication to rest pain, ischemic ulcerations, and tissue necrosis. On physical examination the femoral pulse is found to be diminished or absent on the diseased side and normal on the contralateral side. Noninvasive evaluation of the arterial system should include pulse volume recordings and Doppler pressure measurements at rest and after exercise. Although these tests may not help in selecting the type of reconstruction, they are valuable in confirming the extent of disease on the symptomatic side and in postoperative follow up. On the donor side, minor iliac disease or disease distal to the common femoral artery does not preclude femorofemoral grafting but should be documented to assess postoperative changes.

EVALUATION OF DONOR ILIAC ARTERY

One of the most important criteria for ensuring a successful femorofemoral bypass is the hemodynamic adequacy of the donor iliac artery. Normal femoral pulse and Doppler waveforms on the donor side and normal appearance on arteriography may not be adequate for assessing hemodynamically significant iliac disease at rest. Several methods such as reactive hyperemia, pedal exercise, and injection of papaverine while measuring interarterial pressures in the femoral artery, have been proposed to increase the accuracy of this evaluation. The last method is the standard practice in most institutions. We use the Seldinger technique for femoral puncture and employ the usual technique to visualize the arterial tree from the renal arteries down to the tibial and pedal arteries. If aortoiliac disease is suspected, multiple views are obtained and a catheter is placed in the pararenal aorta. Systolic blood pressures are measured while withdrawing the catheter through potential stenosis down to the femoral artery. In addition, blood pressure measurements are repeated after injection of 60 mg of papaverine into the ipsilateral iliac artery. These blood pressures are compared with simultaneous measurements of brachial systolic pressures, and if there is a gradient of more than 15 mm Hg or a difference greater than 10% between the femoral artery and the brachial artery pressure, the adequacy of the donor iliac artery is in doubt.

ROLE OF PERCUTANEOUS TRANSLUMINAL ANGIOPLASTY IN PREPARING THE DONOR ILIAC ARTERY

Although minor disease, less than 30% to 35% as evident arteriographically, in the donor iliac artery may not disqualify a patient for femorofemoral bypass, a hemodynamically significant stenosis will adversely affect patency. In this instance, some surgeons elect to perform aortofemoral bypass, particularly in a good-risk patient; others choose to dilate the stenosis in the donor iliac artery to ensure good inflow for a planned femorofemoral bypass. The decision to use percutaneous transluminal angioplasty (PTA) depends on the location as well as the extent (single versus multiple, occlusion versus stenosis) of the disease. If there is a single stenotic lesion in the common iliac artery, the chances of success are good, and excellent long-term results can be expected of PTA.[7] These results can be further improved by use of intraluminal stents.[8] In high-risk patients this approach merits attention before selection of a more invasive aortic surgical procedure or an axillary procedure with relatively poorer results.

EVALUATION OF COMBINED DISEASE

In patients with simultaneous suprainguinal disease and infrainguinal disease on the symptomatic side, it is often difficult to assess whether proximal reconstruction to the groin level will provide symptomatic relief. If the patient has necrosis, a proximal reconstruction to the groin level usually will not suffice. A combined reconstruction consisting of femorofemoral bypass and femoropopliteal or femorodistal bypass on the symptomatic side should be planned. This combined reconstruction is well tolerated, but occasionally, in patients with prohibitive risk, it may be staged. In patients with minor symptoms such as claudication with rest pain, proximal femorofemoral reconstruction may be attempted first, with distal bypasses performed later if the symptoms do not resolve.

In some patients undergoing distal bypass, the extent of inflow disease is not apparent until the bypass is complete and a gradient is noticed.[9] In these patients, if the contralateral iliac artery is suitable, a femorofemoral bypass may be added to guarantee the success of the distal reconstruction.

EVALUATION OF RISK

Femorofemoral bypasses have traditionally been reserved for high-risk patients. However, indications can be liberalized to include good-risk patients with anatomically favorable unilateral iliac disease. Patients who are considered high risk because of severe cardiac or pulmonary disease should have appropriate preoperative evaluation. If the procedure is limited to a femorofemoral bypass, we do not employ Swan-Ganz catheters for intraoperative monitoring except for extremely sick cardiac patients. However, if additional inflow or outflow procedures are planned, we use Swan-Ganz catheters routinely.

TECHNIQUE

Spinal or epidural anesthesia is preferred, although some patients prefer general anesthesia. If the patient's risk is high, local anesthesia can be used. In some patients the adequacy of the donor iliac artery may be in doubt. In these patients general anesthesia is used, since the aorta or ipsilateral axillary artery may have to be used for inflow.

A radial artery catheter is placed to take arterial pressure measurements. A Foley catheter is inserted and intravenous antibiotics are given prophylactically. Regardless of the type of anesthesia used, the skin over one subclavian and axillary region as well as abdomen and both groins and thighs is prepared. If distal procedures are planned, the entire lower extremity to the ankles should be prepared and draped.

We make bilateral longitudinal groin incisions, preferably slightly lateral to the femoral arteries, to lessen lymphatic dissection. The common femoral arter-

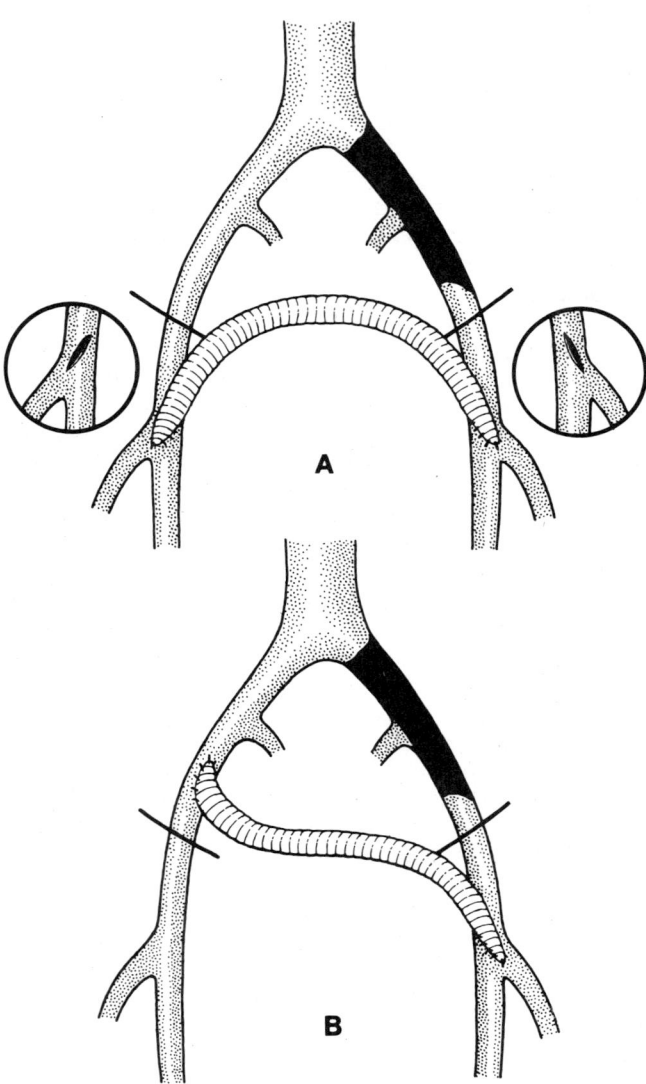

Figure 1 *A*, Usual C configuration of femorofemoral bypass. Inset shows slight angle of the incision in the CFA to prevent kinking of the graft. *B*, S configuration as a result of placing the donor anastomosis high in the CFA or external iliac artery.

ies (CFA) are dissected to the level of the inguinal ligaments, then both the superficial and deep femoral arteries. If lesions in the deep femoral artery are identified by arteriography, more dissection of this artery is necessary for an additional procedure such as a profundoplasty or endarterectomy. A subcutaneous tunnel in the suprapubic area is made to allow the graft to follow a gentle arch. The tunnel is created by digital dissection from each side of the groin and should be wide enough to avoid extrinsic compression on the graft.

Although saphenous vein can be used, we prefer prosthetic grafts. Knitted or woven Dacron grafts can be used, but we prefer polytetrafluoroethylene (PTFE) grafts with rings to avoid compression or kinking. The size of the graft, which depends on the size of the native arteries, varies from 6 to 10 mm in diameter. The most common sizes of grafts are 6 and 8 mm.

After the patient receives systemic heparin sodium, we clamp the recipient femoral arteries and make an arteriotomy in the common femoral artery opposite the origin of the deep femoral artery at a slight angle (Fig. 1A, inset). This prevents the slight kinking of the graft that may occur with conventional axial arteriotomies. If the origin of the deep femoral artery is stenotic, we carry the arteriotomy from the common femoral artery into the anterior wall of the deep femoral artery. A common femoral artery endarterectomy may also be necessary. We bevel the PTFE graft end and do an end-to-side anastomosis with monofilament polypropylene nonabsorbable sutures.

After the recipient-side anastomosis is finished, we remove the clamps. The graft passes through the subcutaneous tunnel into the opposite groin incision, ensuring no twisting or kinking. Then we apply a clamp to the graft close to the anastomosis and do an anastomosis in the donor common femoral artery close to the inguinal ligament. The arteriotomy is extended accordingly if additional procedures are necessary (profundoplasty, common femoral endarterectomy). Generally, the finished reconstruction assumes a C shape with the heads of the two anastomoses pointed at the feet (Fig. 1A). Occasionally the donor artery anastomosis is higher in the external iliac artery, and then the graft assumes a S shape (Fig. 1B). After removal of clamps and restoration of circulation, we generally confirm the adequacy of donor iliac artery, particularly if the donor side was treated with angioplasty or arteriographic evaluation of the donor iliac artery documented diseased areas. For this purpose we place a needle in the proximal anastomosis and compare blood pressures with that in the radial artery with and without clamping the graft.[9] If the difference in blood pressures is at least 15%, we

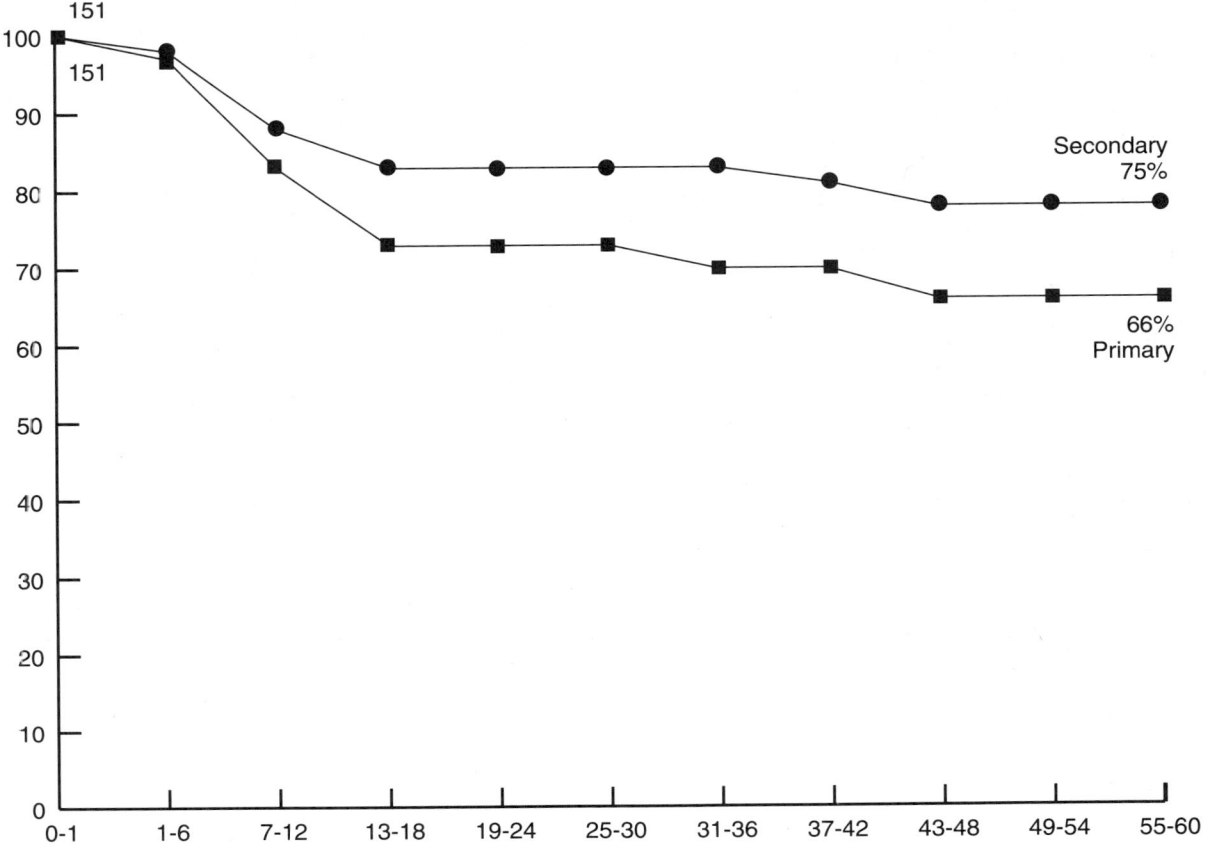

Figure 2 Primary and secondary patency rates for 151 isolated femorofemoral bypasses at 5 years.

assume proximal inflow disease is likely and the patency of the graft may be compromised. If this is the case, we recommend an additional procedure to improve the inflow, such as axillofemoral, ileofemoral, or aortofemoral bypass in a good-risk patient. PTA in the postoperative period may be used for the poor-risk patients.

Postoperative evaluation of bypass patency is important. This evaluation is done with pulse volume recordings and ankle brachial index (ABI) pressures. A temporary decrease of ABI in the donor side may be apparent but usually improves with time. Our policy is to survey these grafts routinely every 3 months for the first 2 years and thereafter every 6 months. A duplex examination of the graft is also done every 6 months. Recognition of a failing graft and prompt correction of the problem will improve patency rates.

RESULTS

Some 233 femorofemoral bypasses were constructed at Montefiore Medical Center between 1977 and 1991. Of these, 151 grafts were isolated femorofemoral grafts for unilateral iliac disease. Of the patients, 62% had rest pain or claudication as the major symptom, and 38% had tissue necrosis or a nonhealing ulcer. Indications for the other 82 grafts were as follows: 45 bypasses were performed to improve the inflow for femoropopliteal or femorodistal reconstructions, and 16 were performed to augment the outflow of failing axillary or aortofemoral reconstructions. Another 21 femorofemoral grafts were performed for miscellaneous indications such as occluded limbs of aortofemoral bypasses, during repair of femoral artery injury, or for acute thrombosis or embolic disease superimposed on pre-existing iliac disease.

The 5 year cumulative life table primary patency rate for 151 isolated femorofemoral bypass grafts was 66% and secondary patency rate was 75% (Fig. 2). The primary patency for all 82 grafts performed to provide inflow or outflow was 58%. The primary patency of 45 grafts used to provide inflow to distal bypasses was 53%.

Femorofemoral reconstruction offers a safe and effective alternative to aortic reconstruction in managing unilateral iliac disease. Success of these reconstructions depends on hemodynamic adequacy of the donor iliac artery. In our experience such adequacy cannot always be assessed in the preoperative period, since 18% of our patients undergoing femorofemoral reconstruction had significant residual gradients measured intraoperatively following completion of the bypass. Therefore, it is essential that inflow gradients be measured during operation to correct gradients if found and to improve the overall patency of these reconstructions.

Although the long-term patency of this procedure may not be as good as the traditional aortic procedure, femorofemoral bypass offers many advantages such as lower mortality and morbidity, technical simplicity, and preservation of potency. Furthermore, it does not interfere with subsequent aortoiliac reconstructions. Femorofemoral bypass may also facilitate other complex reconstructions such as femorodistal bypasses to provide inflow and may be used to improve outflow of proximal procedures. Theoretic disadvantages such as pelvic steal or steal from the donor limb have not proven to be major problems.

REFERENCES

1. Freeman NE, Leeds FH. Operations on large arteries: Application of recent advances. Calif Med 1952; 77:229–233.
2. Vetto RM. The treatment of unilateral iliac artery obstruction with a transabdominal, subcutaneous femorofemoral graft. Surgery 1962; 52:342.
3. Davis RC, O'Hara ET, Mannick JA, et al. Broadened indications for femorofemoral grafts. Surgery 1972; 72:990.
4. Parsonnet V, Alper JA, Brief DK. Femorofemoral and axillofemoral grafts: Compromise or preference. Surgery 1970; 67:26–33.
5. Piotrowski JJ, Pearce WH, Jones DN, et al. Aortobifemoral bypass: The operation of choice for unilateral iliac occlusion? J Vasc Surg 1988; 8:211–218.
6. Ricco JB. Unilateral iliac artery occlusive disease: A randomized multicenter trial examining direct revascularization versus crossover bypass. Ann Vasc Surg 1992; 6:209–219.
7. Brewster DC, Waltman AC, Darling RC, et al. Long term results of combined iliac balloon angioplasty and distal surgical revascularization. Ann Surg 1989; 210:324–331.
8. Palmaz JC, Laborde JC, Rivera FJ. Stenting of the iliac arteries with the Palmaz stent: Experience from a multicenter trial. Cardiovascular and Interventional Radiology 1992; 15:291–297.
9. Gupta SK, Veith JF, Kram HB, et al. Significance and management of inflow gradients unexpectedly generated after femorofemoral, femoropopliteal, and femoroinfrapopliteal bypass grafting. J Vasc Surg 1990; 12:278–283.

VASCULOGENIC IMPOTENCE

JAMES S. T. YAO, M.D., PH.D.

Table 1 Major Disease Categories in Impotence

Neurogenic
Endocrinologic
Psychogenic
Vasculogenic
Drug-induced
Diabetic

In the first report on obliteration of the terminal aorta, Rene Leriche described inability to maintain an erection as one of the five characteristic symptoms.[1] In that report, he suggested insufficient blood flow to fill the corpora cavernosa as the cause of sexual impotence. Since then, several surgeons have called attention to the importance of sexual function and its relationship to aortic reconstruction.[2] Objective assessment of pelvic hemodynamics as well as the effect of aortic reconstruction on sexual function was not achieved until the introduction of penile pressure measurement using the Doppler ultrasound technique. The Doppler technique provides a simple method to study impotence of vascular origin. Although a decrease of blood flow may contribute to sexual impotence, inability to maintain or to obtain an erection is a complex clinical problem. Vascular surgeons must not be tempted to expect that restoration of blood flow by aortic bypass will automatically restore sexual potency. The role of the vascular surgeon in dealing with impotence in patients with arterial occlusive disease is (1) to preserve or to enhance pelvic perfusion and (2) to minimize disturbance of ejaculatory function from surgical dissection. For evaluation of a patient with sexual impotence, vascular surgeons must possess a complete knowledge of the pathophysiology of erectile and ejaculatory function.

ARTERIAL SUPPLY

The blood supply of the penis derives from the paired internal iliac arteries through the internal pudendal artery, which subdivides into major branches: an artery to the bulb of the corpus spongiosum, an artery to the corpus cavernosum, and the dorsal penile artery, which passes to the glans and the urethral artery. The dorsal penile artery, which supplies the penile skin and the glans, also gives perforating branches to the mid and distal part of the corpus cavernosum. Anatomic variation of penile blood supply is common. Normal variation includes the origin of both cavernosal arteries from one side, hypoplasia or absence of one dorsal penile artery, and variation in internal pudendal arteries. Venous drainage is largely from the deep dorsal vein and also through the cavernosal and crural veins.

NEURAL REGULATION

The erectile function is under both sympathetic and parasympathetic control. The latter involves a reflex arc in which stimuli (mainly tactile) from the genital area pass through synapses in the spinal cord, in the region S2 to S4, and return to the penis via the parasympathetic nerves. Sensory afferent fibers from the penile skin and the glans, as well as the efferent motor fibers to the bulbocavernous and ischiocavernous muscles, are part of the pudendal nerve, which arises from the second, third, and fourth sacral nerves. The pudendal nerve leaves the pelvis through the great sacrosciatic foramen, follows the internal pudendal vessels through the lesser sacrosciatic foramen and Alcock's canal, and divides into the perineal nerve and the dorsal nerve of the penis.

INCIDENCE AND CAUSES OF IMPOTENCE

In the process of evaluation of vasculogenic impotence, the vascular surgeon must be familiar with the incidence and, in particular, the causes of impotence. It is estimated that 10 million American men are impotent.[3] Impotence is an age-dependent disorder, with an incidence of 1.9% at 40 years of age and 25% at 65 years of age.[3] In diabetes, the prevalence of impotence is estimated at 35% to 50%.[4] The essential causes of impotence are multiple (Table 1). Quite often, erectile failure may be due to more than one mechanism, and a combination of neurogenic, arteriogenic, venous leakage, and psychogenic mechanisms is not uncommon. The combination of two etiologic factors may account for more cases than previously believed.[5]

INVESTIGATION OF SEXUAL DYSFUNCTION

In the last decade, significant improvement has occurred in screening and diagnostic techniques in the evaluation of patients with impotence. History taking remains the most important step to guide the evaluation. A detailed sexual history conducted in a private and confidential manner must be sought in patients with arterial occlusive disease, especially those with aortoiliac occlusive disease or aneurysm. Complete documentation of sexual function is essential before surgical correction because the surgical procedure itself may induce sexual dysfunction. Current investigational techniques for impotence are as follows.

Doppler and Duplex Ultrasonography

Penile blood pressure measurement is the most commonly used noninvasive screening test for penile arterial insufficiency. It is performed with an inflatable cuff around the base of the penis with a transcutaneous ultrasound probe as the sensor. The technique is simple and can be performed in the office or by the bedside. In general, a penile-brachial blood pressure index (PBI) less than 0.6 is indicative of arterial insufficiency. In normal potent men with a median age of 54 years (range 35 to 70 years), the mean value of PBI was 0.86 ± 0.08 (range: 0.7 to 1.02).[5] The PBI decreases with age. The 95% confidence levels of a PBI determination are $\pm$ 0.05, and the predictive value of a positive test (PBI less than 0.6) is 91% in patients with atherosclerotic occlusive disease, whereas the predictive value of a negative test is 72%. This suggests that a determination of the PBI may establish the diagnosis of penile arterial insufficiency as the cause of impotence, but it is unable to exclude the diagnosis. Other limitations of penile blood pressure measurement include (1) inability to measure the blood pressure in the cavernosal artery consistently and (2), because testing is done in a flaccid state as opposed to the dynamic state, the ability of the cavernosal artery to dilate during erection may not be assessed accurately. Nevertheless, the technique is simple enough to remain as an initial screening test in patients with impotence.

Recently, duplex ultrasonography has been added to provide more diagnostic information. Both the diameter of the penile artery and velocity can be recorded and may be used in conjunction with intracavernosal administration of vasoactive agents to determine changes in the diameter of the cavernosal artery and the velocity of blood flow. Cavernosal arteries with atherosclerosis have minimal changes in diameter and low blood flow velocity in the dynamic state.

Provocative Testing

Instead of a resting study, a provocative test such as the pelvic steal test or pharmacologically induced hyperemic test may help to further evaluate erectile dysfunction in a dynamic state. Pelvic steal has been cited as one of the causes for vasculogenic impotence. The test consists in measuring penile blood pressure before and after exercise involving femoral and gluteal muscles. The mean change in PBI in normal potent subjects after exercise is -0.06 ± 0.04, yielding a normal limit for a decrease of 0.14. This test helps to elucidate further the cause of vasculogenic impotence. Recently, a provocative test has been introduced in which erectile response is observed after intracavernosal injection of vasoactive agents. Papaverine is the best evaluated drug for this purpose. A normal rigid erection should develop within 5 to 10 minutes and last approximately 1 hour. A normal response in an impotent patient implies normal vasculature, and neurogenic or psychological factors should be pursued. If only partial, short-lived, or no erection results, then altered pelvic hemodynamics may be suspected. The test, however, is not foolproof, and failure to produce an erection in this setting may be due to excessive adrenergic constrictor tone as a result of anxiety. Thus a negative response from a single injection may not be conclusive.[3]

Other Investigations

Erectile failure is often a result of more than one defect, and in patients who present with impotence as the chief complaint, the following tests must be evaluated prior to arterial reconstructive surgery.

Nocturnal Penile Tumescence Measurement. Nocturnal penile tumescence measurement (NPT) is probably one of the most widespread investigations in impotence. The test is often conducted in a sleep laboratory, where the penile circumferential changes are recorded by strain gauge plethysmography during 1 to 3 nights' sleep. The duration and degree of tumescence are helpful to differentiate between psychogenic and organic impotence. Others have, however, questioned the validity of this investigation.

Dynamic Infusion Cavernosography. Dynamic infusion cavernosography is a radiologic examination of the cavernous body and its venous drainage. The test is done by slow infusion of contrast medium through a cannula into the cavernous body during fluoroscopic observation and simultaneous recording of the intracavernous pressure. The intracavernosal pressure is determined by the rate of infusion required to maintain a blood pressure level equal to or greater than penile systolic blood pressure recorded by the Doppler technique. Venous drainage through the deep dorsal vein can be observed to determine venous leakage. In impotence, this examination serves primarily to define the routes of venous leakage.

Bulbocavernous Reflex Latency. Bulbocavernous reflex latency is performed by bipolar electromyographic electrodes. A stimulating electrode is placed around the glans of the penis, and a coaxial needle is placed in the bulbocavernous muscle to register the conduction of the dorsal pudendal nerve. Latencies greater than 40 msec are considered abnormal and indicative of penile neuropathy.

Arteriography. Most routine arteriography of the aorta and its runoff vessels will provide information on the patency of the internal iliac artery. Detailed information on the internal pudendal artery, especially penile blood supply, must be done with a selective magnification penile pharmacoarteriogram.[6] Patients who are candidates for reconstructive surgery solely for impotence must undergo this selective study. This technique gives detailed information of intrapenile arterial anatomy.

VASCULOGENIC IMPOTENCE

In the majority of patients with vasculogenic impotence, the cause is atherosclerotic occlusive disease of the aortoiliac system (Table 2). Erectile failure usually develops insidiously over months or years. It often starts with failure of maintaining erection. Interestingly, erectile failure bears no chronologic relationship to the onset of symptoms of intermittent claudication. One-third of the patients suffered from impotence for more than 6 months before the onset of claudicating symptoms. In a Danish study, Metz found that 9 of 47 patients with

Table 2 Causes of Vasculogenic Impotence

Arteriosclerosis
Congenital arterial dysplasia of internal iliac artery
  Hypoplasia
  Agenesis
Pelvic arteriovenous fistula
  Acquired
  Congenital
Pelvic fracture with injury to pudendal artery
Ligation of internal iliac arteries prior to cystectomy
Ligation of internal iliac arteries in conjunction with renal transplantation

arteriogenic impotence had no symptoms of intermittent claudication.[5]

The incidence of preoperative erectile impotence in patients with aortoiliac disease has varied from 46% in retrospective medical record surveys[2] to as high as 80% in prospective studies.[7,8] Patients with aortic aneurysms have a higher incidence of impotence than those with occlusive disease, probably because of the age factor, as patients with aneurysms are much older.

Aortoiliac Reconstruction and Sexual Function

Sexual dysfunction may be affected by aortoiliac revascularization, and the incidence has been reported to range from 21% to 88%.[5,7,8] In prospective studies the incidence is much lower, ranging from 5% to 18%.[8,9] The two mechanisms thought to be responsible for sexual dysfunction following reconstructive surgery are ischemia secondary to diversion of pelvic blood flow and/or autonomic nerve injury from dissection. Further support for this may be found in the fact that approximately 25% of impotent patients who undergo aortoiliac reconstruction regain sexual function postoperatively.[7-9] In our study using penile blood pressure measurement before and after operation,[7] we documented that diversion of pelvic blood flow could result in impotence and that increased pelvic blood flow as a result of aortoiliac revascularization could lead to improved sexual function.[7-9]

Disturbance of the ejaculation mechanism from inadvertent division or operative trauma of the hypogastric neural plexus can cause retrograde ejaculation. The incidence of retrograde ejaculation is variable but has been reported as high as 63% by May and his colleagues in patients following aneurysm repair versus 49% in those with occlusive disease.[2] Others, however, have reported an incidence of 30% to 33%.[8]

Assessment and evaluation of a patient with aortoiliac occlusive disease or aneurysm must include a detailed inquiry of sexual function and special attention paid to patency of the internal iliac artery and pelvic collaterals. In the planning of a procedure to restore blood flow to the extremity, consideration must be given to (1) preservation of or ways to increase pelvic blood flow and (2) avoidance of ejaculatory dysfunction. To prevent ejaculatory dysfunction, the use of a femorofemoral graft may be preferred in patients with unilateral iliac artery occlusion. Not only is ejaculatory function preserved, but femorofemoral bypass has been reported to improve erectile function in these patients. Percutaneous balloon dilatation of a stenotic lesion of the iliac artery may be the procedure of choice, especially in terms of preserving ejaculatory function. In considering femorofemoral bypass, balloon dilatation of a stenotic donor iliac artery can also be done in selected patients.

If aortic reconstruction is needed, such as for bilateral iliac occlusions or aneurysms, several surgical maneuvers need to be exercised: (1) end-to-end versus end-to-side aortic anastomosis of an aortofemoral bypass graft, (2) internal iliac artery revascularization, (3) prevention of atheromatous debris embolizing into the internal iliac artery, and (4) nerve-sparing technique. End-to-side aortic anastomosis retains blood flow through the native distal aorta into the internal iliac arteries and is preferred in patients with external iliac artery stenosis, which may prevent retrograde perfusion to the pelvic region. When aortic anastomosis is fashioned in end-to-end manner, as required in aneurysms, distal reconstruction is needed to preserve pelvic perfusion if there is coexistent external iliac disease. Several authors have reported that improvement of sexual function can be achieved by adjunctive endarterectomy of the internal iliac artery. In the atheromatous aorta, vascular clamps must be applied to the common iliac arteries before manipulating the aorta. On blood flow restoration, both the internal and external iliac arteries must be flushed openly and profusely rather than closely into the internal iliac artery. The latter maneuver causes impotence due to atheromatous embolization. The nerve-sparing technique advocated by DePalma and colleagues is designed to preserve ejaculatory function.[8] The capacity for ejaculation depends specifically on the sympathetic nerves, particularly those lying in front of the aortic bifurcation. It is generally acknowledged that the L2 and L3 nerves in the presacral and hypogastric plexus are most important; if these are divided, retrograde ejaculation occurs. The nerve-sparing technique calls for aortotomy to be made at the right lateral side of the aorta, avoiding the nerve plexus surrounding the inferior mesenteric artery. In the dissection of the aortic bifurcation and the left common iliac artery, care must be taken to avoid damage to the hypogastric plexus. The hypogastric sympathetic plexus innervates the so-called internal sphincter of the bladder, and division results in retrograde ejaculation. The entire nerve plexus can be dissected free and elevated as a flap rather than divided.

The effect of aortic reconstruction on erectile function can be predicted by matching arteriograms to the intended surgical procedure. In general, changes of erectile capability are followed by corresponding changes in penile blood pressure measurement.[5]

Pelvic Steal Syndrome

The pelvic steal syndrome or the external iliac steal syndrome is a special type of arteriogenic erectile impotence. The syndrome is characterized by symptoms related to acute changes in the pelvic hemodynamics following activation of the gluteal and femoral muscles. The classic arterial lesion leading to this syndrome is unilateral common iliac artery occlusion. The symptoms are either pain in the buttock during sexual intercourse or an improved maintenance of the erection in certain coital positions.[5] The pelvic steal phenomenon can be confirmed by the pelvic steal test and by arteriography documenting large collaterals between the pelvic area and the lower extremity and reverse blood flow in the internal iliac artery in serial arteriographic exposures. Restoration of blood flow by femorofemoral or aortofemoral bypass is effective in eliminating the symptoms. In addition to common iliac artery occlusion, we have identified "femoral steal syndrome." Common arteriographic findings in this syndrome are (1) an obstructed external iliac artery with (2) an ipsilaterally patent internal iliac artery whose branches supply blood to a distally ischemic limb and (3) an occluded contralateral internal iliac artery. Flow through the unobstructed hypogastric artery and its collaterals is then mainly directed at supplying blood to the distal ischemic limb. The result of such altered pelvic hemodynamics is impotence. Revascularization of the ischemic extremity reverses the steal and restores sexual capability and pelvic perfusion.

Vascular Procedures Specially Designed for Impotence

Procedures designed solely for correction of erectile failure often involve the use of microvascular techniques. Two types of arterial microvascular bypasses are now used: (1) bypass into the dorsal penile artery and (2) arterialization of the deep dorsal veins. In bypass to the dorsal artery, either the inferior epigastric artery or a vein graft from the aorta is used as the source of inflow. All these patients require selective penile arteriography prior to the procedure. In addition to bypass, venous interruption to stop venous leakage has also been used in treatment of erectile failure. Variable results of these procedures have been reported by several investigators.[10] The long-term result of dorsal artery bypass, however, remains unknown.

REFERENCES

1. Leriche R. De la resection du carrefour aortico-iliaque avec double sympathectomie lombaire pour thrombose arteritique de l'aorte: Le syndrome de l'obliteration termino-aortique par arterite. Presse Med 1940; 48:601–604.
2. May AG, Deweese JA, Rob CG. Changes in sexual function following operation on the abdominal aorta. Surgery 1969; 65:41–47.
3. Krane RJ, Goldstein I, De Tejada IS. Impotence. N Engl J Med 1989; 321:1648–1659.
4. McCulloch DK, Campbell IW, Wu FC, et al. The prevalence of diabetic impotence. Diabetologia 1980; 18:279–283.
5. Metz P. Arteriogenic erectile impotence. Copenhagen: Laegeforeningens Forlag, 1986.
6. Bookstein JJ. Penile angiography: The last angiographic frontier. Am J Roentgenol 1988; 150:47–54.
7. Queral LA, Whitehouse WM, Flinn WR, et al. Pelvic hemodynamics after aortoiliac reconstruction. Surgery 1979; 86:799–809.
8. DePalma RG, Levine SB, Feldman S. Preservation of erectile function after aortoiliac reconstruction. Arch Surg 1978; 113:958–962.
9. Flanigan DP, Schuler JJ, Keifer T, et al. Elimination of iatrogenic impotence and improvement of sexual function after aortoiliac revascularization. Arch Surg 1982; 117:544–560.
10. Michal V, Kramar R, Hejhal L. Revascularization procedures of the cavernous bodies. In: Zorgniotti AW, Rossi G, eds. Vasculogenic impotence. Springfield, Ill: Charles C. Thomas, 1980:239.

DIAGNOSIS OF AORTIC GRAFT INFECTION

THOMAS W. WAKEFIELD, M.D.

Prosthetic arterial vascular graft infections affect between 1% and 6% of patients, with an average incidence of approximately 1% for aortoiliac grafts and 1.5% to 2% for aortofemoral bypass grafts. Mortality from infected grafts in the aortoiliac or aortofemoral position has been reported to be above 50%.

Factors contributing to graft infection include skin contact of the graft during insertion, contaminated lymphatics, breaks in sterile technique during graft insertion, extension from wound sepsis or wound contamination, arterial wall infection, and transient bacteremias before a complete pseudointima has developed on the prosthetic surface. Bacteria have been found in the contents of aortic aneurysms. More than 40% of arterial walls cultured during routine vascular surgical procedures have been found to harbor organisms, the most common being *Staphylococcus epidermidis*. An increase in graft infection occurs in patients with positive arterial wall cultures undergoing secondary operations.

There has been a recent shift in the bacteriology of arterial graft sepsis. In the 1970s *Staphylococcus aureus* was the leading pathogen. Today *S. epidermidis* is the most likely cause of infection. For the identification of this organism, grafts should be sonicated to loosen the bacteria from the slime that is produced by *S. epidermidis* for maximal recovery.

Tests for the diagnosis of prosthetic arterial graft

infections include radionuclide tests such as indium-111-labeled white blood cell scans, new indium and technetium tests, ultrasound, computed tomography (CT), magnetic resonance imaging (MRI), and arteriography. However, the definitive diagnosis of prosthetic vascular graft infection may still require operative inspection of the graft to establish the presence or absence of infection. Failure of graft incorporation, accumulation of perigraft fluid or debris, and Gram stain evidence of bacteria or leukocytes all suggest infection.

RADIONUCLIDE TECHNIQUES

Radionuclide techniques primarily require gallium-67 and indium-111. The problems with gallium compared with indium include enhanced uptake of gallium by the gastrointestinal tract and kidney, with activity obscuring the location of the aortic graft, and poorer gamma emission of gallium. Nevertheless, cases of graft infection were diagnosed by gallium as early as 1980 and in a recent study of 16 patients with 25 grafts (16 in the aortic position), gallium imaging after the injection of 5 mCi of Gallium-67 citrate had a sensitivity of 78% and a specificity of 94%.[1] In fact, the overall specificity of gallium was greater than that of CT scanning in this study (94% versus 72%). The advantages of gallium over indium when tagged to white blood cells include less cost, no special tagging to blood elements necessary, wider use, and localization to a focus of infection more quickly than indium-labeled white blood cells.

Indium-111 oxine has been used extensively in the evaluation of intra-abdominal abscesses with good accuracy. In 1981 the first reports appeared of aortic graft infection detected by indium-111 oxine leukocyte scanning in both laboratory animals and patients. We also documented in dogs that this technique, used in the evaluation of graft infections of 3 months' duration, provided a sensitivity of 67% and a specificity of 100%. A number of clinical series suggest that this technique is useful. These include the largest clinical experience, of 70 patients with 57% abdominal grafts and 27% thoracic grafts. In this study the overall sensitivity was 100% (14 of 14) with a specificity of 85% and an overall accuracy of 88%.[2] If three equivocal scans are considered false positives, these figures become 100%, 80% and 84%, respectively (Fig. 1). Other authors have recorded similar results. Lawrence and co-workers[3] reported on 31 scans in 21 patients (more than half involving an aortic graft) with a sensitivity of 100% and specificity of 87%.[3] Reilly and associates[4] reported 23 patients with suspected graft sepsis and found a sensitivity of 82%, specificity of 83% and accuracy of 83%.

The discrepancy in specificities between the canine and clinical studies most likely relates to the differences in endothelial graft coverage between dog and man. Complete endothelial coverage occurs on the surface of short infrarenal canine aortic grafts. Endothelial coverage does not develop on human aortic grafts, but a

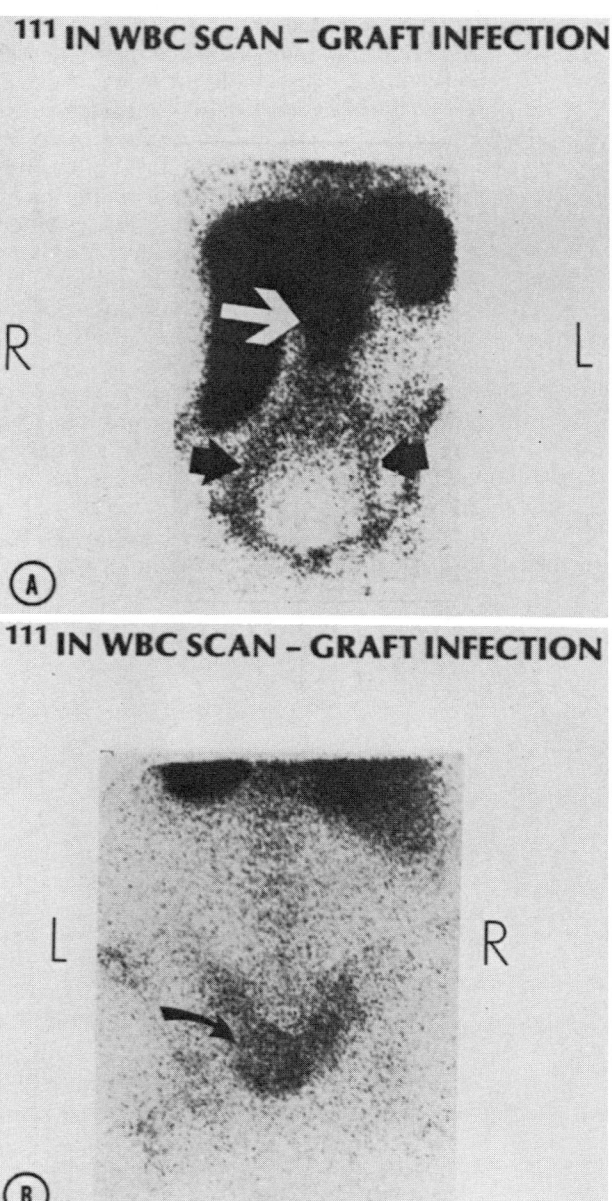

Figure 1 Indium-111 white blood cell scans. *A*, True positive (AP projection). White arrow indicates involvement of central limb of graft; involvement of both femoral graft limbs was also present (*black arrows*). *B*, True negative (PA projection). Arrow indicates positive indium uptake in left tubo-ovarian abscess but no uptake in aortic graft. (From Brunner MC, Mitchell RS, Baldwin JR, et al. Prosthetic graft infection: Limitations of indium white blood cell scanning. J Vasc Surg 1986; 3:45; with permission.)

surface consisting of a platelet-fibrin coagulum remains thrombogenic, attracting platelets over the life of the graft and patient. Most labeling techniques are performed with differential centrifugation, resulting in the labeling not only of white blood cells but also of platelets and red blood cells, elements that are normally attracted to the surface of noninfected grafts. False-positive results have been reported in up to 50% of patients early after graft implantation, most likely for this reason.

In an attempt to improve labeling and reduce the false-positive rate, Forstrom and colleagues[5] have reported a technique of gravity sedimentation followed by Ficoll-hypaque double-density centrifugation producing purified autologous granulocytes. These pure granulocytes were then labeled with indium-111 tropolone. Sensitivity was reported as 70% (7 of 10) and specificity improved to 91% (10 of 11), with the only false-positive result in a patient with an inflammatory abdominal aortic aneurysm. Such techniques hold promise for improving the specificity of indium scanning.

Newer radionuclide techniques that have yet to be evaluated more than once in large clinical studies include indium-111-labeled human IgG (sensitivity 91%, specificity 100%, Fig. 2),[6] technetium-99m-hexametazime white blood cell scanning (sensitivity 100%, specificity 94%),[7] and technetium-99m-hexamethyl-propyleneamine oxine (Tc-99m-HMPAQ) leukocyte scanning (Fig. 3).[8] Possible advantages of indium-111-labeled IgG imaging over indium-111-labeled white blood cell scanning include less indium accumulation in the spleen, allowing the use of approximately six times as much indium, a longer shelf life, ease of preparation, improved safety as no blood is used, less variability, no inadvertent platelet labeling, and minimal accumulation in the bowel.[6] Advantages of technetium techniques include greater availability of technetium than indium, lower cost, and shorter interval between radioisotope injection and scan acquisition. The short 6 hour half-life of technetium compared with 2.8 days for indium allows administration of isotope with higher activity. Additionally, technetium has higher affinity than indium for granulocytes and produces less radiation-induced cellular damage than indium. Furthermore, technetium-99m-hexametazime labeled white blood cell scanning has the capability to detect low-grade graft infection more readily than indium techniques.[7] The exact role of these

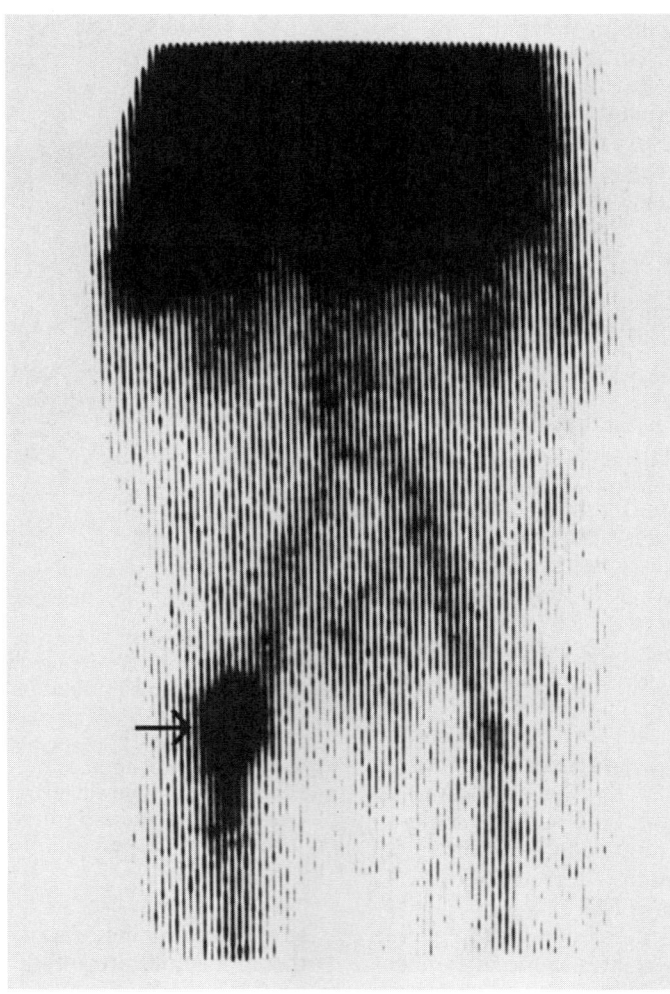

Figure 2 Indium-111-IgG scan shows positive accumulation of tracer (*arrow*) at the proximal anastomosis of a prosthetic femoropopliteal graft. The patient was found to have an infected anastomotic aneurysm caused by Pseudomonas. (From LaMuraglia GM, Fischman AJ, Strauss HW. Utility of the indium-111-labeled human immunoglobulin G scan for the detection of focal vascular graft infection. J Vasc Surg 1989; 10:25; with permission.)

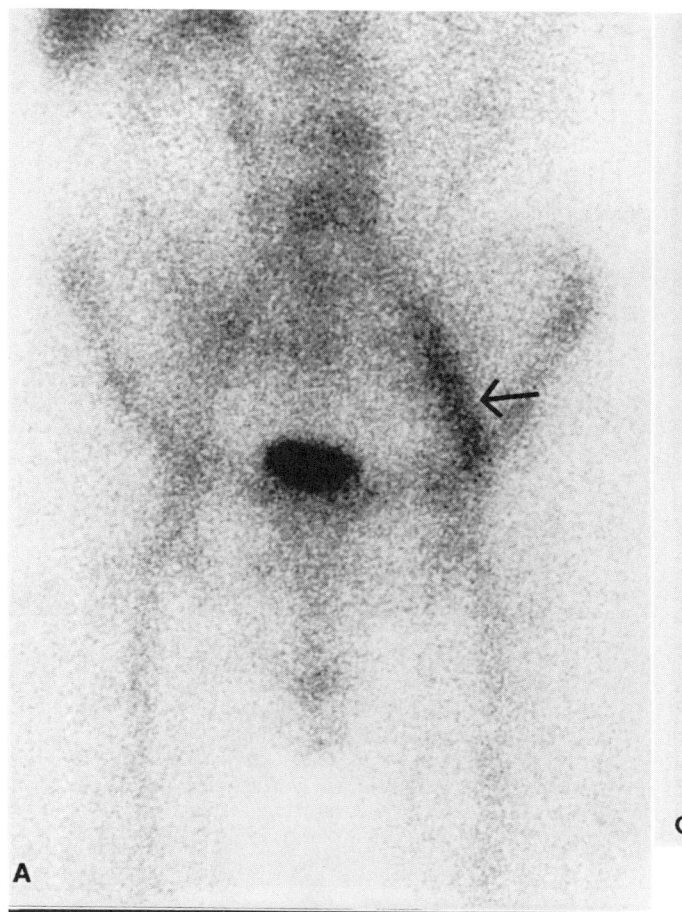
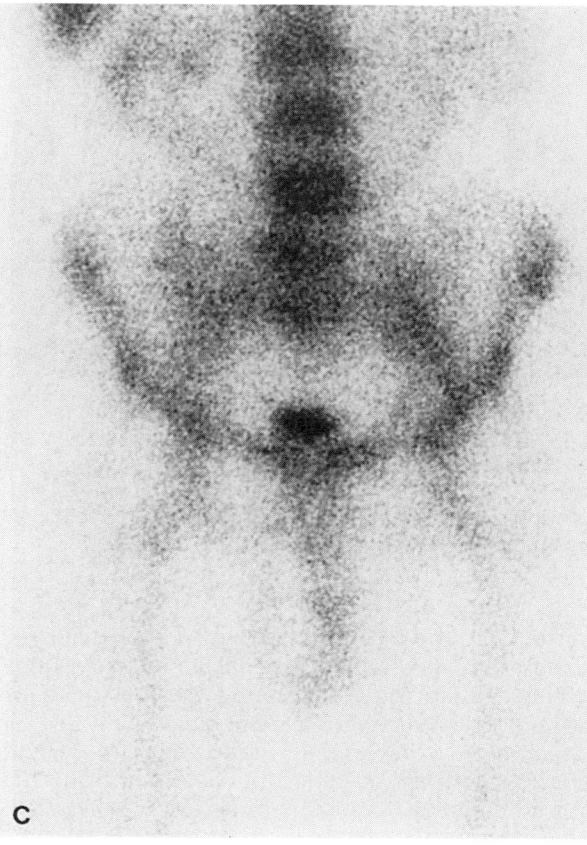
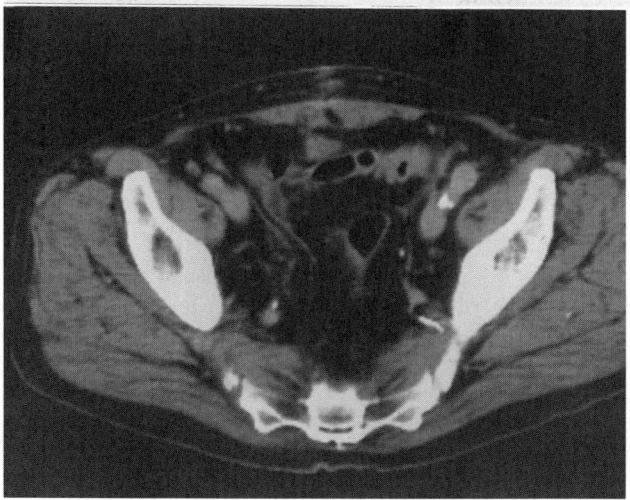

Figure 3 Patient with aortobifemoral graft had clinical infection with a draining groin wound and sepsis. *A,* A strong accumulation of Tc-99m-HMPAQ labeled white blood cells was observed (*arrow*). *B,* CT scan was normal. *C,* After antibiotic treatment, the accumulation was markedly diminished, and no clinical signs of infection were noted 6 months postoperatively. (From Romo OJ, Vorne M, Lantto E. Postoperative graft incorporation after aortic reconstruction: Comparison between computerized tomography and Tc-99m-HMPAQ labelled leukocyte imaging. Eur J Vasc Surg 1993; 7:125; with permission.)

alternative radionuclide techniques requires further clinical evaluation.

CT, MRI, AND ARTERIOGRAPHIC TECHNIQUES

Ultrasound provides limited information about prosthetic vascular graft infection. Perigraft fluid suggests infection, and ultrasound-guided aspiration may be performed. However, CT scanning is preferred over ultrasound for this purpose. Changes on CT scanning suggestive of infection include perigraft fluid, ectopic gas, soft-tissue swelling, focal bowel wall thickening, increased soft tissue between the graft and wrap, and false aneurysm formation (Fig. 4). Bowel wall thickening of more than 5 mm suggests graft-enteric fistula. In a study of 55 patients referred for CT scanning to detect possible prosthetic vascular graft infection or aortoen-

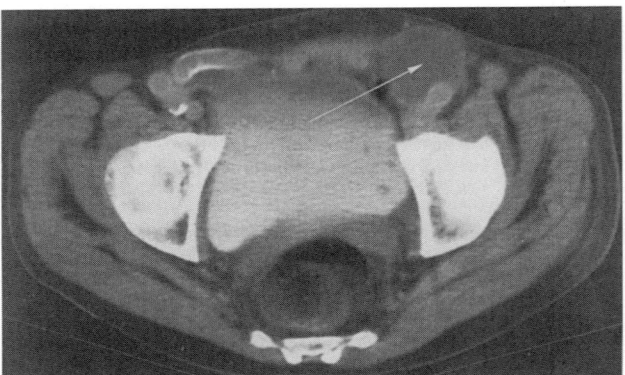

Figure 4 CT scan of perigraft fluid associated with an infected limb of a prosthetic aortofemoral bypass graft (*arrow*). (From Stanley JC, Messina LM, Wakefield TW. Complications of Vascular Surgery and Trauma. In: Greenfield LJ, ed. Complications in Surgery and Trauma, ed 2. Philadelphia: JB Lippincott; 1990:361; with permission.)

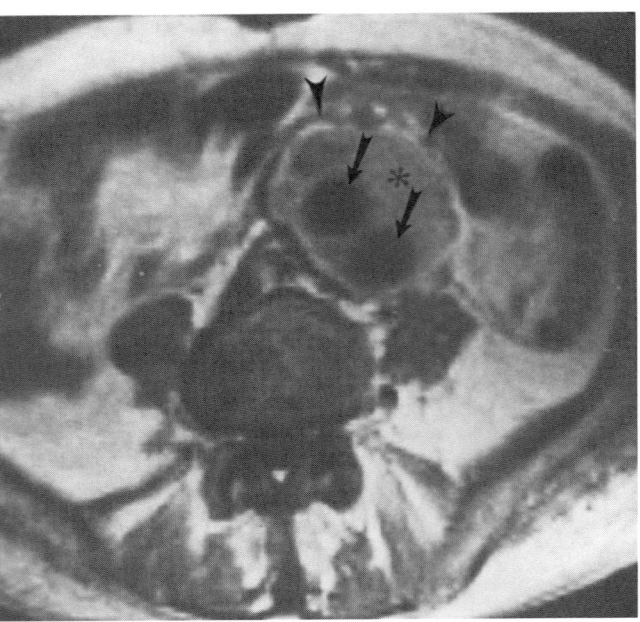

Figure 5 Protein density MRI of retroperitoneal portion of aortobifemoral graft surrounded by noninfected large pseudoaneurysm. Note fibrous capsule (*arrowheads*) and low-intensity signal of clotted blood(*). Graft is marked by arrows. (SE, TE, = 30 milliseconds; TR = 1,000 milliseconds). (From Olofsson PA, Auffermann W, Higgins CB et al. Diagnosis of prosthetic aortic graft infection by magnetic resonance imaging. J Vasc Surg 1988; 8:104; with permission.)

teric fistula, CT was 94% sensitive and 85% specific for detecting either of these two complications.[9] In the study comparing gallium and CT scanning, the sensitivity for CT scanning was 100% with a specificity of 72%.[1] Mark and associates[10] compared CT scanning with indium imaging in eight patients clinically suspected of having aortic graft infection because of groin infection, sepsis or both. CT scanning correctly identified all five patients with aortic graft infection by documenting perigraft fluid, gas in the graft bed, or both. Extension of infection into the retroperitoneum was diagnosed correctly in three patients with groin infection, whereas the indium white blood cell study showed extension into the retroperitoneum in only one. Likewise, the use of antibiotics normalized one abnormal indium scan. CT scanning provided safer and more precise drainage of perigraft fluid collections. Overall, CT scanning appears to be equal to or greater in sensitivity than radionuclide techniques for the diagnosis of prosthetic aortic graft infection.

Perhaps the most exciting new technique for making the diagnosis of aortic prosthetic graft infection is MRI (Fig. 5). In a study of 18 patients with a history and clinical findings suggestive of prosthetic aortic graft infection, 16 had infection verified at operative exploration, 14 with infection in the retroperitoneal portion of the graft and two in the groins.[11] Perigraft infection was correctly diagnosed on the basis of MRI findings in 14 of 16 patients. One was a false-negative scan, and one was questionable. In two negative explorations, MRI correctly excluded graft infection. MRI also defined the extent of infection in 14 of 16 patients. The diagnostic ability of MRI was based on its capability to differentiate fluid from surrounding tissue and to provide information about inflammatory reactions involving surrounding tissues in all phases of graft incorporation. Additionally, MRI holds promise for differentiating perigraft fluid and inflammatory changes in surrounding structures from subacute or chronic hematoma, although MRI cannot determine the difference between infected and sterile fluid. On the other hand, abscesses and necrotic material give a relatively high signal intensity on T2 weighted images, quite different from chronic hematomas. In this study MRI was much more sensitive than CT scanning. However, MRI failed to reveal aortoenteric fistulas in five patients.

The inability of MRI to differentiate between infected and sterile fluid limits its usefulness in the early postoperative period. In a natural history study of MRI in patients undergoing aortic reconstruction, 90% of patients studied 1 week postoperatively had perigraft fluid collections, in 22% at 12 weeks it was the same, and it was not until 24 weeks that this fluid disappeared in all patients.[12] A similar shortcoming has been observed for CT scanning.

Arteriography and sinography complete the various imaging tests available for making the diagnosis of prosthetic aortic graft infection. Although some have recommended that sinograms be performed in all instances of open wound or draining sinuses,[13] this technique carries the risk of spreading infection to noninfected areas of the graft. Arteriography usually provides little additional diagnostic help unless it documents the presence of a pseudoaneurysm and should be considered a preoperative study for helping to determine the type of vascular reconstruction necessary.

Among patients with gastrointestinal bleeding who have an aortic graft, endoscopy to include the third and fourth portions of the duodenum is mandatory and in up to 50% of patients documents a nonvascular source of the bleeding. Ultimately, the only definitive means to exclude the presence of an aortoenteric fistula is operative exploration.

REFERENCES

1. Johnson KK, Russ PD, Bair JH, et al. Diagnosis of synthetic vascular graft infection: Comparison of CT and gallium scans. Am J Roentgenol 1990; 154:405–409.
2. Brunner MC, Mitchell RS, Baldwin JC, et al. Prosthetic graft infection: Limitations of indium white blood cell scanning. J Vasc Surg 1986; 3:42–48.
3. Lawrence PF, Dries DJ, Alazarki N, et al. Indium 111-labeled leukocyte scanning for detection of prosthetic vascular graft infection. J Vasc Surg 1985; 2:165–173.
4. Reilly DT, Grigg MJ, Cunningham DA, et al. Vascular graft infection: The role of indium scanning. Eur J Vasc Surg 1989; 3:393–397.
5. Forstrom LA, Dewanjee MK, Chowdhury S, et al. Indium-111-labeled purified granulocytes in the diagnosis of synthetic vascular graft infection. Clin Nucl Med 1988; 13:859–862.
6. LaMuraglia GM, Fischman AJ, Strauss HW, et al. Utility of the indium 111-labeled human immunoglobulin G scan for the detection of focal vascular graft infection. J Vasc Surg 1989; 10:20–28.
7. Fiorani P, Speziale F, Rizzo L, et al. Detection of aortic graft infection with leukocytes labeled with technetium 99m hexametazime. J Vasc Surg 1993; 17:87–96.
8. Ramo OJ, Vorne M, Lantto E, et al. Postoperative graft incorporation after aortic reconstruction—Comparison between computerized tomography and Tc-99m-HMPAQ labelled leukocyte imaging. Eur J Vasc Surg 1993; 7:122–128.
9. Low RN, Wall SD, Jeffrey RB Jr, et al. Aortoenteric fistula and perigraft infection: Evaluation with CT. Radiology 1990; 175:157–162.
10. Mark AS, McCarthy SM, Moss AA, et al. Detection of abdominal aortic graft infection: Comparison of CT and indium-labeled white blood cell scans. Am J Roentgenol 1985; 144:315–318.
11. Olofsson PA, Auffermann W, Higgins CB, et al. Diagnosis of prosthetic aortic graft infection by magnetic resonance imaging. J Vasc Surg 1988; 8:99–105.
12. Spartera C, Morettini G, Petrassi C, et al. Role of magnetic resonance imaging in the evaluation of aortic graft healing, perigraft fluid collection, and graft infection. Eur J Vasc Surg 1990; 4:69–73.
13. O'Brien T, Collin J. Prosthetic vascular graft infection. Br J Surg 1992;79:1262–1267.

TREATMENT OF AORTIC GRAFT INFECTION

DENNIS F. BANDYK, M.D.

Infection involving an aortic prosthesis constitutes one of the most challenging diagnostic and therapeutic challenges in arterial reconstruction. Delays in treatment invariably increase morbidity, particularly if sepsis or hemorrhage occurs prior to intervention. Despite aggressive surgical and antibiotic therapy, more than one-third of patients will die or require a major amputation, especially if a virulent infection develops within 4 months of graft implantation.[1-3] The spectrum of aortic graft infection dictates that therapy be individualized based upon clinical presentation and the microbiology of the infectious process. The preferred treatment for most patients is graft excision with lower limb revascularization by ex situ bypass or autogenous reconstruction. Carefully selected patients with localized low-grade infections, i.e. late-appearing infection caused by *Staphylococcus epidermidis,* may be safely treated by in situ graft replacement. Similarly, if primary healing of a groin wound fails and a distal aortofemoral graft limb is exposed, local debridement and muscle flap coverage may provide satisfactory graft coverage and secondary wound healing.[4,5] Prolonged survival can be expected in the majority of patients successfully treated for aortic graft infection, but surveillance of retained graft segments for recurrent infection is required. Successful management relies on a prompt diagnosis, thorough assessment of the extent of graft involvement, identification of the infecting pathogen(s), and a treatment plan that eradicates the infectious process and yet maintains, if feasible, adequate distal tissue perfusion.

CLASSIFICATION AND PATHOGENESIS

Aortic graft infections can be grouped according to differences in clinical presentation, extent of graft involvement, and infecting pathogen (Table 1).[6] Such a classification, although arbitrary, is useful clinically, since the appropriate treatment option depends on the anatomy and microbiology of the infectious process. Early graft infections, defined as those treated within 4 months of implantation, typically are perigraft in nature and present no major problem in diagnosis, since most follow unsuccessful treatment of a wound infection or another procedure-related problem such as gastrointestinal tract perforation, ischemia, or ureter injury. Failure to adequately treat a noninfectious wound complication such as hematoma, perigraft lymphocele, or necrosis of incisional skin margins invariably leads to extension of a superficial infection to deeper tissue surrounding the graft. When grafts are confined to the abdomen, the

Table 1 Classification of Aortic Graft Infections

Time of Onset	Clinical Signs	Pathogen(s)	Graft Involvement
Early, < 4 mo.	Wound infection Sepsis Anastomotic bleeding	S. aureus Streptococcus E. coli Klebsiella sp. Pseudomonas sp.	Diffuse infection
Late, > 4 mo.	UGI hemorrhage Perigraft infection Anastomotic aneurysm Groin sinus tract Hydronephrosis	S. epidermidis E. coli* Klebsiella sp.* Candida sp.	Localized or diffuse infection

*Following gastrointestinal tract involvement by erosion.

diagnosis of "early" infection is more difficult. Unexplained sepsis, prolonged postoperative ileus, or abdominal distention and tenderness may be the only clinical signs.

Patients with early graft infections demonstrate systemic and local signs including fever, leukocytosis, bacteremia, perigraft purulence, a pulsatile groin mass, or a graft-artery anastomotic dehiscence. Predisposing factors include emergent operation for ruptured aortic aneurysm, concomitant remote infection, impaired immunocompetence, and postoperative development of colon ischemia. If the prosthetic graft material is visible following drainage of a wound or abdominal abscess, diffuse involvement of the prosthesis should be assumed, since graft incorporation and tissue ingrowth occur only after several months of implantation. *Staphylococcus aureus* is the prevalent organism causing early graft infections, although gram-negative organisms (*Escherichia coli,* Klebsiella, Enterobacter, Pseudomonas, Bacteroides species) will be isolated when the pathogenesis of infection involved direct contamination due to adjacent bowel ischemia or injury.

Most aortic graft infections are recognized late, more than a year after implantation.[7] Common clinical manifestations include an inflammatory process (e.g., sinus tract, perigraft air or exudate with cavity) involving the groin incision of an aortofemoral graft, anastomotic false aneurysm, hydronephrosis, or graft-enteric fistula or erosion (GEF-GEE). Approximately one-half of patients with GEF-GEE will present with a herald hemorrhage, manifest as hematemesis or melena, and hypotension. One-third of patients with proven graft-enteric communications will exhibit no evidence of bleeding, and the remaining patients present with chronic gastrointestinal tract bleeding extending over weeks to months. Failure to diagnose an aortic graft infection can be associated with secondary complications such as exsanguination from anastomotic rupture or fistula, organ failure, and fatal outcomes. It is usually the responsibility of the consulting surgeon to prove aortic graft infection is not present in patients with gastrointestinal tract hemorrhage or sepsis.

The prevalent organisms responsible for late aortic graft infections are coagulase-negative staphylococci (CNS), including *S. epidermidis, S. hominis,* and *S. warneri.* However, with involvement of the gastrointestinal tract, gram-negative organisms, particularly *E. coli* and Klebsiella, are typically recovered from excised graft material. The pathobiology of graft infection caused by CNS is a complex process involving biomaterial surface colonization, adherence-mediated growth, and chronic activation of host defenses. Pathogenetic strains of CNS have been termed slime or mucin producing because of the large amounts of capsular glycoproteins produced.[8] This growth characteristic is strain specific, mediates adherence to biomaterial, and protects the organisms against antibodies, antibiotics, and phagocytes. Unlike *S. aureus* and gram-negative bacteria, infecting CNS strains do not produce toxins or products capable of tissue autolysis, and when host immunity is normal, bacterial invasion of perigraft tissue is difficult to document by routine microbiologic or histologic analysis. Since the infectious process is perigraft and confined primarily to the graft surfaces, it has been termed a bacterial biofilm infection. Clinical signs of this process include formation of a perigraft cavity with subsequent anastomotic false aneurysm formation or fistula development to the skin or bowel.

MICROBIOLOGIC DIAGNOSTIC METHODS

Recovery of microorganisms from culture of the vascular prosthesis is necessary to guide antibiotic therapy. The method of processing material for culture is especially important for recovery of *S. epidermidis,* the prevalent pathogen of late-appearing aortic graft infections. Routine microbiologic techniques frequently will not isolate a microorganism from perigraft tissue of these graft infections because of the sequestration of bacteria within a surface biofilm on the prosthesis and the absence of perigraft tissue invasion by the bacteria. The sampling error of a swab culture taken from perigraft tissue or graft surfaces, transported in thioglycollate media to the laboratory and imprinted on agar plates is low if the bacteria concentration is high and perigraft tissue invasion has occurred. If Gram stain of perigraft tissue or exudate documents many polymorphonuclear leukocytes but no bacteria, an agar plate culture will frequently not isolate a microorganism, and culture of the prosthetic material in broth media is necessary to confirm biomaterial colonization. Mechanical disruption of prosthetic surface biofilms can further increase the recovery of microorganism from vascular prostheses with graft healing complications and minimal or no anatomic signs of graft infection.[9] Microbiologic recovery techniques that employ broth medium with or without surface biofilm disruption are necessary to identify graft colonization in patients with late-appearing aortic graft infections. In vitro testing confirmed that a biofilm bacterial concentration of less than 100 colony forming units/cc of graft material can be identified reliably with these methods.

Graft Biofilm Culture

A 1 to 2 cm^2 specimen of graft is placed in glucose-supplemented (0.25% dextrose) tryptic soy broth (TSB). The culture tube containing the broth medium and graft specimen is incubated at 35°C (95°F). This method will in 90% of cases recover the infecting microorganism when anatomic signs of infection such as inflammation, perigraft exudate, Gram stain showing many white blood cells with or without bacteria are present. Two methods of mechanical surface biofilm disruption can be used: ultrasonic oscillation and tissue grinding. Graft specimens are placed in a culture tube containing TSB. During the sonication or tissue grinding process, the bacteria biofilm, if present, is detached from the prosthetic surfaces, and any sequestered microcolonies are disrupted and dispersed into the surrounding media. Although broth and agar media have a similar biochemical composition, the nutrient and growth environment afforded by broth medium exerts less stress for continued growth of an inoculum containing a small number of microorganisms.

PREPARING THE PATIENT FOR OPERATION

Patients with sepsis or hypovolemic shock due to anastomotic bleeding can tolerate only a brief period of resuscitation prior to intervention. Administration of intravenous fluids, blood products, and clotting factors; perioperative cardiopulmonary monitoring; broad-spectrum antibiotics; and planning the surgical approach form the essential elements of urgent preoperative treatment of critically ill patients.

Although most patients with aortic graft infections allow time for adequate preoperative preparation, many are debilitated by infection, malnutrition, dehydration, and prior surgical procedures in addition to having chronic pulmonary, cardiac, and renal problems. Patients should be prepared physiologically and psychologically for the most extensive operation that may be required.

Arterial circulation to the upper and lower extremities should be assessed by Doppler-derived pressure measurements and arteriography for determination of appropriate revascularization alternatives to maintain limb perfusion after graft excision. Review of previous operative reports is important for planning treatment, since insight into graft anatomy and the technical details of the prior reconstruction can assist in safe graft excision or replacement. Systemic antibiotics should be selected according to isolated or suspected pathogens. Other sites of infection, such as urinary tract, lung, and soft tissue, should be appropriately evaluated and treated.

TREATMENT OPTIONS

Effective treatments of an infected aortic graft include several options depending on clinical presentation and extent of graft involvement (Table 2). Established surgical tenets include graft excision; wide debridement of infected tissue, including the artery adjacent to the infected graft; antibiotic irrigation and placement of closed suction drains; reconstruction of vital arteries through uninfected tissue planes; and prolonged antibiotic administration. The surgeon should consider all surgical options and select the safest treatment for the patient. If graft excision can be accomplished without limb loss, it is always preferred. Most aortoiliac grafts have been implanted for aneurysmal disease, and graft removal will result in critical limb ischemia. By comparison, aortofemoral grafts are more commonly implanted for occlusive disease, and collateral circulation may be adequate to avoid amputation if native vessel patency can be maintained. It is preferable to revascularize the limb before removing the infected graft, but in the presence of anastomotic bleeding and hypovolemic shock, control of hemorrhage takes precedence.

Excision of the entire infected graft accompanied by ex situ bypass (femorofemoral, axillofemoral, obturator) is the most commonly required treatment. Total graft excision is essential in patients who are septic or have anastomotic bleeding or complete graft involvement with a virulent organism. Attempts at graft preservation with antibiotic therapy and wound drainage have been reported, but persistence of infection is common and patients remain at risk for exsanguination during the observation period.

Dissatisfaction with the complexity, morbidity (20% to 30% amputation rate), and mortality (up to 40%) of total graft excision with simultaneous revascularization has prompted use of alternative methods such as in situ revascularization with autologous conduits (endarterectomized iliac or femoral arteries, superficial femoral vein), allograft, or a new vascular prosthesis.[4,10] In situ prosthetic graft replacement appears to be a safe option for the treatment of low-grade late-appearing infections with the anatomic and microbiologic features of a bacterial biofilm infection. Central to all treatment strategies is the successful eradication of the infectious process surrounding and involving the biomaterial.

Graft excision with extra-anatomic bypass, either

Table 2 Treatment Options for Aortic Graft Infection Based on Appearance Time and Extent of Graft Involvement

Early, <4 mo.		
	Graft limb only	Excise, ex situ bypass unilateral Ax-SFA–deep femoral obturator bypass
		Excise alone (adequate collaterals, thrombosed graft)
	Diffuse graft involvement	Excise, ex situ bypass bilateral Ax-femoral bypass axillobifemoral bypass
	Exposed femoral segment	Nonexcisional therapy with muscle flap coverage
Late, >4 mo.		
	GEE-GEF	Excise, ex situ bypass
		Excise, autogenous reconstruction (endarterectomy, superficial femoral veins)
	Biofilm infection	Excise, in situ reconstruction

simultaneous or staged, is recommended for early infections with diffuse aortic graft involvement or late infections presenting with GEF-GEE.[1-3, 11,12] Graft excision alone or aortoiliac endarterectomy of the previous arterial segments is feasible in fewer than 10% of patients. Autologous reconstruction of the aortic bifurcation using endarterectomized superficial femoral artery or superficial femoral vein have been reported, as has allograft replacement, but these options should be avoided in patients with virulent infections.

If the diagnosis can be established preoperatively, the preferred treatment is preliminary right-sided axillobifemoral bypass followed by graft excision at the same operation if the patient is hemodynamically stable. If this bypass should fail, the left axillary artery and supraceliac or descending thoracic aorta are available for secondary revascularization of the lower limbs. A 8 mm diameter ringed polytetrafluoroethylene (PTFE) graft is recommended for the axillofemoral graft or the rarely necessary axillopopliteal bypass graft. The femorofemoral conduit can be either a PTFE graft or autologous greater saphenous vein, depending on the presence and severity of infection in the groin(s) and the ability to route the cross-over graft through clean tissue planes and avoid contaminated tissue. In patients with appropriate anatomy, the common iliac arteries can be anastomosed end to end to provide cross pelvic flow.

Several reports have documented a trend toward decreased morbidity and mortality with staged treatment. Preliminary lower limb revascularization can be performed without increasing the risk of death, ex situ bypass infection, or bleeding complications when total graft excision is delayed 1 or 2 days. The physiologic stress on the patient may be reduced with this approach, which has been applied primarily for treatment of aortofemoral graft infections. After ex situ bypass, the groins are explored, debrided, and reconstructed. The aortic graft limbs are ligated and retracted into the retroperitoneum. O'Hara and associates[1] reported a decrease in limb loss with staged (7%) versus simultaneous procedures (41%) but no difference in mortality.

In the case of aortofemoral graft infection with groin involvement, extra-anatomic graft outflow cannot be established at the common femoral artery. Lateral placement of axillofemoral limb medial and deep to the anterior iliac spine is used in routing the graft to the superficial or profunda femoris artery in the thigh. The site of the femoral anastomoses and type of groin reconstruction depends on whether the superficial femoral artery is patent or occluded (Fig. 1). In general, anastomosis to the superficial or profunda femoris artery is possible and maintenance of retrograde pelvic blood flow via a reconstructed common femoral artery using autologous tissue is highly desirable.

Graft Removal and Aortic Stump Closure

Obtaining safe proximal control of the aorta and secure aortic stump closure are critical features of graft excision and must be executed with unhurried diligence. Hemorrhage and aortic stump blowout remain the most common causes of death. Achieving proximal control at the supraceliac aorta before exposure of the proximal anastomosis is recommended. Total aortic encirclement is not necessary for secure clamp placement. Likewise, control of distal vessels can be achieved by ventral and lateral dissection, with backup use of balloon catheter occlusion to prevent backbleeding from distal vessels via axillofemoral graft inflow. In general, the appearance of the aorta on CT imaging can be used as guide for areas of safe dissection and clamp placement. A nonaneurysmal aortic segment not involved with inflammation or scar tissue or harboring mural thrombus can be safely exposed, clamped, and occluded. Scalpel dissection should be used to mobilize the duodenum from the graft and encircle the adjacent aorta for closure or repair. Aggressive aortic debridement to histologically normal wall, aortic closure in multiple layers, omental coverage, and 3 months or more of antibiotic therapy provide excellent protection against aortic stump blowout due to persistent infection. A specimen of the normal-appearing, debrided aorta should be submitted for culture, since a positive result mandates prolonged antibiotic administration and careful patient follow-up. Aortic stump closure technique should use two rows of interlocking 3-0 polypropylene sutures. A pedicle of omentum should be passed through the transverse mesocolon and positioned around the aortic stump and into the bed of the excised aorta and graft. If necessary, the aorta can be excised to above the renal arteries, with renal revascularization via saphenous vein bypasses originating from the hepatic or splenic arteries. Closed suction drains should be placed in the infected graft bed and brought out the flank opposite from the axillofemoral graft limb.

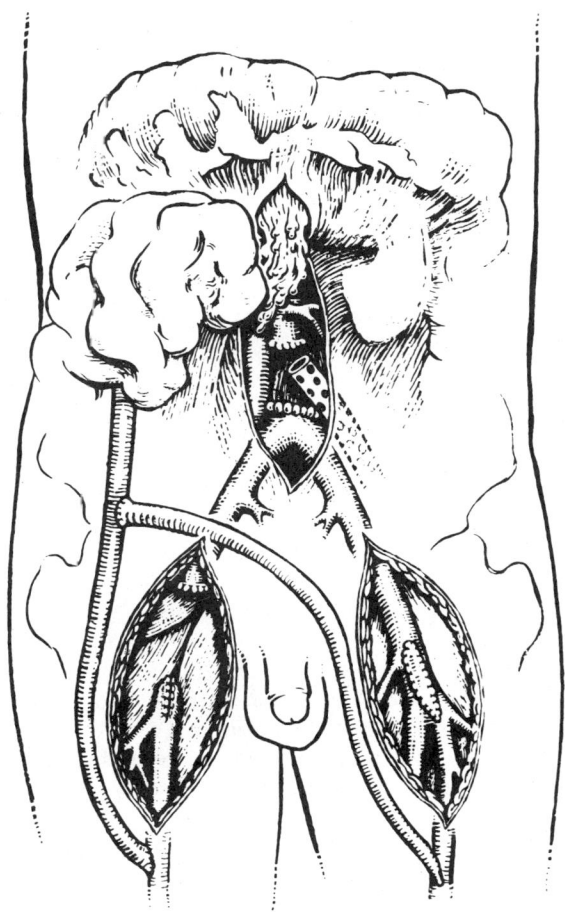

Figure 1 Excision of an infected aortofemoral graft with right-sided axillofemoral bypass to right superficial femoral artery (SFA) and cross-over graft to left profunda femoris artery (PFA). Left femoral artery reconstructed with vein-patch angioplasty. Right femoral artery ligated with end-to-end anastomosis of SFA to PFA. Aortic stump closed and covered with omentum brought through the transverse mesocolon. Closed suction drain placed in bed of infected graft.

The distal aorta and iliac arteries should also be closed with monofilament suture. Preoperative placement of ureteral stents can be helpful, but they are not necessary unless hydronephrosis is present. The site and method of iliac artery ligation should be selected to maintain adequate perfusion to the colon, pelvic organs, and buttock musculature. With infrarenal aortic ligation, pelvic circulation can be maintained via retrograde blood flow from the axillobifemoral bypass through the external and internal iliac arteries. Flow to iliac artery usually provides adequate pelvic blood flow because of the extensive collateral flow via the visceral and profunda femoris arteries.

Results of Treatment

Operative mortality and amputation rates of less than 20% and prolonged survival in two-thirds of patients have been reported to follow graft excision and ex situ bypass (Table 3). By contrast, local treatment, primary repair of a GEF, excision, and aortic ligation have all resulted in a mortality in excess of 50%. Mortality associated with total graft excision is the result of myocardial infarction, persistent infection, and aortic stump blowout. Reilly and her associates[2] reported that 43% of early deaths and 71% of late deaths were due to aortic stump blowout. Patients with graft-enteric fistula are at greatest risk for this complication. Newer methods of treatment such as in situ or in-line graft replacement and arterial allografts have resulted in comparable operative mortality but a reduction in limb loss.[10,13,14] Infection of the replacement graft has occurred in fewer than 10% of patients. In situ revascularization has been limited to treatment of patients with late-appearing graft infections demonstrating no frank purulence in the retroperitoneum. Aggressive aortic debridement and prolonged antibiotic administration, in some instances lifelong, are important features of successful in situ graft replacement procedures.

Treatment of Low-Grade Graft Infections

In situ replacement, preservation, and segmental excision of the graft can be considered in patients whose grafts are exposed or have a bacterial biofilm infection.[4] When biofilm infection caused by CNS is suspected, excision of the involved portion of the graft, typically an aortofemoral limb, with in situ autologous or prosthetic reconstruction is safe and effective. We have successfuly treated 20 patients with aortofemoral graft infections that manifested as a groin abscess, sinus tract, or false aneurysms using in situ revascularization with a PTFE prosthesis. Resolution of the infectious process was achieved in all patients. During follow-up, 5 patients died of causes unrelated to graft infection, and in 2 the retained aortic graft exhibited persistent infection requiring additional in situ replacement. A clear understanding of the pathogenesis and microbiology of bacterial biofilm infections is crucial in selecting patients suitable for this less aggressive therapy. Gram stain of the perigraft exudate should document only leukocytes, no bacteria. The technique of in situ replacement must be executed to treat the known pathobiology of biofilm graft infection (Table 4).

Graft segments circumferentially involved with mucinous biofilm infection should be excised with adjacent anastomotic sites. The extent of graft involvement mirrors findings on CT imaging, with uninvolved graft segments having no perigraft fluid and adherence to the surrounding graft capsule. The transected proximal graft segment and graft bed should be irrigated with pulsed irrigation system and antibiotic solution. A preference for grafts constructed of PTFE as opposed to Dacron as in situ replacement is based on experimental data documenting reduced bacterial adherence to PTFE surfaces and a decreased reinfection rate

Table 3 Outcome Following Treatment of Aortic Graft Infection

Reference	No. of Patients	Mortality (%)	Early Amputation (%)	Stump Blowout (%)	Survival >1 yr (%)	Infection of EAB* (%)
Excision/EAB						
Bandyk, 1984[7]	18	11	11	0	66	17
O'Hara, 1986[1]	84	18	27	22	58	25
Reilly, 1987[2]	92	14	25	13	73	20
Schmitt, 1990[3]	20	15	5	6	75	6
Yeager, 1990[12]	38	14	21	4	76	22
Quinones-Baldrich, 1991[15]	45	24	11	0	63	20
Ricotta, 1991[11]	32	25	13	10	70	–
Taylor, 1992[16]	18	4	4	0	–	–
In Situ Replace						
Walker, 1987[13]	23	26	0	–	83	–
Kieffer, 1993†[14]	43	12	0	–	82	–
Clagett, 1993[10]	17	10	10	0	88	–

*EAB = Ex situ arterial bypass graft.
†Arterial allograft.

Table 4 Components of In Situ Graft Replacement for Biofilm Infection

Preoperative and perioperative administration of vancomycin
Gram stain of perigraft fluid to exclude bacteria
Wide debridement of inflamed perigraft tissue
Excision of involved graft segment and adjacent anastomotic sites
Cleansing and debridement of tissues with a wound irrigation system
Use of PTFE prosthesis for graft replacement
Muscle flap coverage of replacement graft if feasible

in an animal model.[8] Where appropriate, profundaplasty or endarterectomy of vessels should be used to enhance the graft outflow tract. During treatment of infected aortofemoral graft limbs the sartorius muscle is mobilized at its origin and rotated laterally to medially, being careful not to injure its segmental blood supply. Surgical wounds are closed in layers with closed suction drainage positioned laterally at the site of sartorius muscle transposition. Muscle-flap coverage has also been successfully used to cover exposed aortofemoral grafts in the groin following debridement of a superficial wound infection or skin and subcutaneous tissue necrosis.[5]

SURVEILLANCE OF THE PATIENT

Patients treated by total graft excision or in situ replacement of an aortic graft infection should be followed at regular intervals (initially every 3, then every 6 months) to detect life- and limb-threatening complications, including false aneurysm, graft-enteric erosion, and anastomotic stenosis. Patients should not be considered cured until a postoperative imaging study confirms normal perigraft healing. If deterioration in anastomotic integrity or hydronephrosis is detected, graft infection should be suspected and the patient considered for graft replacement or excision based on the bacteriology of the perigraft process. The role of labeled leukocyte scanning to aid in decision making is not known. In our series of patients treated with in situ replacement, persistent infection of retained graft segments was documented in approximately 10% of patients with long-term follow-up.

REFERENCES

1. O'Hara PJ, Hertzer NR, Beven EG, et al. Surgical management of infected aortic grafts: Review of a 25-year experience. J Vasc Surgery 1986; 3:725–731.
2. Reilly LM, Stoney RJ, Goldstone J, et al. Improved management of aortic graft infections: The influence of operation sequence and staging. J Vasc Surg 1987; 5:421–431.
3. Schmitt DD, Seabrook GR, Bandyk DF, et al. Graft excision and extra-anatomic revascularization: The treatment of choice for the septic aortic prosthesis. J Cardiovasc Surg 1990; 31:327–331.
4. Bandyk DF, Bergamini TM, Kinney EV, et al. In situ replacement of vascular prostheses infected by bacterial biofilms. J Vasc Surg 1991; 13:575–585.
5. Calligaro KD, Veith FJ, Gupta SK, et al. A modified method for management of prosthetic graft infections involving an anastomosis to the common femoral artery. J Vasc Surg 1990; 11:485–490.
6. Bandyk DF. Aortic graft infection. Semin Vasc Surg 1990; 3:122–132.
7. Bandyk DF, Berni GA, Thiele BL, et al. Aortofemoral graft infection due to Staphylococcus epidermidis. Arch Surg 1984; 119:102–108.
8. Bergamini TM, Bandyk DF, Govostis D, et al. Infection of vascular prosthesis caused by bacterial biofilms. J Vasc Surg 1988; 7:21–30.
9. Bergamini TM, Bandyk DF, Govostis D, et al. Identification of Staphylococcus epidermidis vascular graft infection: A comparison of culture techniques. J Vasc Surg 1989; 9:665–670.
10. Clagett GP, Bowers BL, Lopez-Viego MA, et al. Creation of a neoaortoiliac system from lower extremity deep and superficial veins. Ann Surg 1993; 218:239–249.
11. Ricotta JJ, Faggioli GL, Stella A, et al. Total excision and extra-anatomic bypass for aortic graft infection. Am J Surg 1991; 162:145–149.

12. Yeager RA, Moneta GL, Taylor LM, et al. Improving survival and limb salvage in patients with aortic graft infection. Am J Surg 1990;159:465–469.
13. Walker WE, Cooley DA, Duncan JM, et al. The management of aortoduodenal fistula by in situ replacement of the infected abdominal aortic graft. Ann Surg 1987; 205:727–732.
14. Kieffer E, Bahnini A, Koskas F, et al. In situ allograft replacement of infected infrarenal aortic prosthetic grafts: Results in 43 patients. J Vasc Surg 1993; 17:349–356.
15. Quinones-Baldrich WJ, Hernandez JJ, Moore WS. Long-term results following surgical management of aortic graft infection. Arch Surg 1991; 126:507–511.
16. Taylor SM, Mills JL, Fujitani RM, Robison JG. The influence of groin sepsis on extra-anatomic bypass patency in patients with prosthetic graft infection. Ann Vasc Surg 1992; 6:80–84.

AORTIC GRAFT–ENTERIC FISTULA

JOHN W. SMITH, M.D.

The diagnosis and treatment of aortic graft–enteric fistula is one of the most challenging problems the surgeon faces. Such problems are fortunately rare, affecting 0.3% to 1.5% of aortic grafts, but they are fatal if untreated. Mortality in treated patients is high, with morbidity common in the survivors.

Two types of fistulas occur. The first and more common is direct communication between bowel lumen and a graft suture line. Disruption of the suture line leads to hemorrhage.

The second is paraprosthetic fistula, in which the bowel lumen is in contact with the body of the graft and not with a suture line. These patients have a small amount of bleeding from the mucosal ulceration. With time the enteric enzymes and bacteria spread along the graft. The patient will then exhibit features of graft infection such as fever and malaise. When the suture line is reached and disrupted by the infection, the fistula involves the arterial lumen. Since both forms of fistula are managed in a similar manner and vary mostly by the degree of urgency, they will be considered as a single entity.

DIAGNOSIS

The patient with an aortic graft–enteric fistula usually has gastrointestinal bleeding and also may have features of a graft infection. The usual situation is small amounts of bleeding at first, followed at a variable interval by massive hemorrhage.

The time since the original operation may be as short as a few weeks or months or as much as 20 years. The index of suspicion must be very high. Any patient with gastrointestinal bleeding in the presence of an aortic graft must be assumed to have a graft-enteric fistula until proved otherwise.

The difficulty in diagnosis is illustrated by the experience of Goldstone and Cunningham.[1] In their study of 53 aortic graft–enteric fistulas, the diagnosis was established preoperatively in less than one-third, and there was no gastrointestinal bleeding in one-third.

An aggressive search for the cause of bleeding in these patients is necessary unless the hemodynamic status of the patient forbids it. The unstable patient should proceed directly to operative exploration.

If time permits, upper gastrointestinal endoscopy should be the first study performed. It is essential to see the esophagus, stomach, and all parts of the duodenum. If all is normal except for a bleeding area in the third or fourth part of the duodenum, the diagnosis is established. There is no characteristic appearance for the duodenal lesion. It may be only a small red area. Rarely, graft material can be seen in an ulcerated mucosal lesion. Unfortunately, the identification of another cause of upper gastrointestinal bleeding does not rule out aortoenteric fistula, and it may delay the diagnosis and treatment.

Abdominal computed tomography (CT) may be useful, particularly if endoscopy does not document a lesion. CT permits visualization of the graft and adjacent areas. A collection of fluid, perigraft air, and perhaps alteration of tissue planes in the retroperitoneum may suggest graft infection. Ultrasound is generally less useful for visualizing details around a retroperitoneal graft but can document false aneurysm at a suture line. Magnetic resonance imaging (MRI) may be helpful in the future but is now less useful than CT. Aortography usually will not document a fistula but can demonstrate false aneurysms and is very helpful for planning arterial reconstruction. The subclavian and axillary arteries can be studied as well to evaluate possible inflow arteries for revascularization.

The decision to operate is straightforward in the unstable patient and in the one in whom the diagnosis has been established preoperatively. The decision is made on clinical suspicion in the other patients. Exploration of the aortic graft in these patients is seldom negative, and the consequences of failing to operate are catastrophic.

TREATMENT

The goals of treatment are as follows: (1) Stop the bleeding. (2) Close the opening in the intestine. (3)

Remove the infected graft and any septic surrounding tissues. (4) Restore arterial circulation.

The variability of presentation and stability of these patients requires modification of the treatment as appropriate in the circumstance. The standard treatment is well described by Ernst.[2] This begins with gaining control of the aorta proximal to the proximal suture line, most often at the aortic hiatus. The old graft is dissected out, the enteric opening repaired, and the graft removed. The aortic stump is debrided back to healthy tissue and closed with two rows of monofilament suture. If the aorta is infected to the level of renal arteries, reconstruction or reimplantation at a higher level may be required. Any infected surrounding tissue is debrided, and the bed is drained, keeping the drain away from contact with the aortic stump and the duodenal closure. After closure of the abdomen, the patient is reprepared and new drapes, gowns, gloves, and instruments are used to perform the extra-anatomic reconstruction of the lower extremities. Since most of these patients had their first operation for aneurysm, the initial graft is placed in the aortoiliac position, and axillofemoral and femorofemoral bypass is the appropriate reconstruction.

These operations are accompanied by fluid shifts and hemodynamic instability. Monitoring will require at minimum arterial and pulmonary artery catheters. A midline incision from xiphoid to pubis permits the extensive exposure needed. Some technical details are important. Control of the aorta at the level of the diaphragm is done by division of overlying muscle fibers of the right crus. Dissection on both sides of the aorta can be limited to just enough room to place a vascular clamp. Dissection behind the aorta is not necessary. Closure of the duodenum often requires wide dissection to permit a tension-free suture line. The consequence of failure to remove all infected aortic wall is later disruption of the aortic stump closure with exsanguinating hemorrhage.

If the graft placement was for occlusive disease, particularly if the indication was claudication, it may be possible to remove the infected graft without immediate reconstruction. Autogenous reconstruction with endarterectomy and vein grafts may be possible as well.

The "standard treatment" is a prolonged operation in a sick patient and necessarily imposes a period of ischemia on the lower extremities. There is evidence that performing the extracavitary bypass first with staged removal of the aortic graft after several days leads to better results, with reduction of mortality from 26% to 13% in the series at the University of California at San Francisco. Obviously, this cannot be done in the hemodynamically unstable patient, but most are stable. A theoretic concern with this method is that the parallel arterial circuit will not stay open during the few days before the primary graft is removed.

There have been reports of placement of a new graft in the retroperitoneum after removal of the infected graft. Walker and associates[3] reported 23 patients with 75% long-term survival using knitted Dacron replacements. Miller[4] reported 15 aortic graft segments replaced with polytetrafluoroethylene (PTFE) grafts in an adjacent clean or debrided area. The whole graft was removed in only five of these. There were two deaths in this series.

Another approach is direct repair of the fistula. Eastcott[5] reported 16 cases of aortic graft–enteric fistula in 1982. Five patients died without operations, and 10 had direct repair. Two of these had early signs of infection and were treated by graft excision and axillofemoral bypass. Two others had false aneurysms at the repair site and were also treated with excision and remote bypass. The decision in favor of direct repair was based on the appearance of the graft. Eastcott noted that most of these grafts did not appear to be infected, and these were the ones that underwent direct repair. Those that appeared to be infected were excised.

Stoney[6] has suggested the following modification of the treatment plan for the actively bleeding patient. Rapid exploration and control of the aorta allow stabilization of the patient and identification of the fistula. The aortic graft anastomosis and the enteric opening are directly repaired. The patient is closed and permitted to stabilize and begin recovery. After a few days the extra-anatomic bypass is performed as a second stage. The third stage is removal of the graft with appropriate debridement and closure. This plan changes a long, complicated, high-risk procedure into a series of smaller, less stressful operations. Stoney has not reported any data on patients treated in this manner.

PREVENTION

Since aortic graft–enteric fistula is such a catastrophic complication, efforts to prevent it are mandatory. Meticulous dissection with prevention of injury to the duodenum followed by care in retraction should avoid ischemic injury. In cases of inflammatory aneurysm, the thickened, fibrotic area should be left adherent to the duodenum with dissection proximal and distal to the inflammatory area. All contents of the aortic aneurysm should be cultured, especially those from ruptured aneurysms, so that pre-existing infection or contamination can be treated.

Living soft tissue must be interposed between the graft and the duodenum. In aneurysm operations, the aneurysm wall can be tailored to cover the graft. In operations for occlusive disease, the adjacent soft tissues or a pedicle of omentum can serve as the buffer.

There are no controlled studies, nor are there likely to be, comparing graft material and the incidence of aortoenteric fistula. However, some reports concerning bowel-graft reaction and healing of anastomoses suggest that graft material may make a difference. The W. L. Gore Company[7] is aware of only two aortic graft–enteric fistulas following the implantation of approximately 70,000 PTFE grafts in the aortic position. Cavallaro and associates[8] studied the reaction between bowel wall and graft material in dogs and found that Dacron became intensely adherent with inflammatory change and progression toward penetration of the bowel. The PTFE remained nonadherent to the bowel under the same circumstance. Quinones-Baldrich and his colleagues[9] found that anastomotic tensile strength was higher for PTFE grafts in their dog experiments than for various formulations of Dacron grafts. They thought this helped explain why so few false aneurysms are seen after implantation of PTFE grafts. Hollier[10] has reported using PTFE membrane to prevent adherence of lung and bowel after thoracoabdominal aneurysm replacement.

REFERENCES

1. Goldstone J, Cunningham CC. Diagnosis, treatment and prevention of aortoenteric fistulas. Acta Chir Scand Suppl 1990; 555:165–172.
2. Ernst CB. Aortoenteric fistulas. In: Haimovici H, ed. Vascular emergencies. New York: Appleton-Century-Crofts, 1982:365.
3. Walker, WE, Cooley DE, Duncan JM, et al. The management of aortoduodenal fistula by in situ replacement of the infected abdominal aortic graft. Ann Surg 1987; 205:727–732.
4. Miller JH. Partial replacement of an infected arterial graft by a new prosthetic polytetrafluoroethylene segment: A new therapeutic option. J Vasc Surg 1993; 17:546–558.
5. Eastcott HHG. Aortoenteric fistula: Possibilities for direct repair. In: Greenhalgh RM, ed. Extra-anatomic and secondary arterial reconstruction. London: Pitman, 1982:58.
6. Stoney RJ. Discussion of Peck JJ, Eidemiller LR, aortoenteric fistulas. Arch Surg 1992; 127:1191–1194.
7. WL Gore Co., Flagstaff, Ariz.: Personal communication, May 24, 1993.
8. Cavallaro A, Sciacca V, Cisternino S, et al. Experimental study of the interaction between aortic grafts and the intestine: Dacron versus PTFE. Vasc Surg 1987; 4:243–247.
9. Quinones-Baldrich WJ, Ziomek S, Henderson T, Moore WS. Primary anastomotic bonding in polytetrafluoroethylene grafts? J Vasc Surg 1987; 5:311–318.
10. Hollier LH. Management of thoracoabdominal aortic aneurysm. In: Ernst CB, Stanley J, eds. Current therapy in vascular surgery, ed 2. Philadelphia: B.C. Decker, 1991, 292–297.

MANAGEMENT OF GROIN LYMPHOCELE AND LYMPH FISTULA

MARK C. RUMMEL, M.D.
MORRIS D. KERSTEIN, M.D.

Lymphocele and lymphorrhea are rare but acknowledged complications of peripheral vascular operations. Lymphoceles, lymph-filled cavities that do not have a distinct epithelial lining, arise in 1.8% to 4% of patients.[1,2] Lymphorrhea is the drainage of lymph fluid from disrupted lymphatic channels. Their appearance is associated with prolonged drainage, wound infection, graft contamination, graft infection, loss of graft, and sometimes loss of limb.

PATHOPHYSIOLOGY

Lymphoceles are associated with different events including retroperitoneal lymphadenectomy, renal transplants, and peripheral surgical procedures such as saphenous vein ligation, femoral vein interruption, lymph node biopsy, thighplasty, and femoral vessel reconstruction. The lymphatics are often cut during these procedures. Usually, open lymph vessels seal within 24 to 48 hours and begin to regenerate within 8 days. Regeneration does not occur if the disrupted segment exceeds 3 to 5 cm. The adherence of surrounding tissue and collagen fibers to the open lymphatics can result in the nonhealing of the lymph vessels and persistent lymphorrhea.[2] Additionally, lymphatic fluid has poor clotting characteristics. Inadequate tissue approximation allows a potential dead space that can develop into a lymphocele. Other factors that have been implicated in formation of a lymphocele are radiation therapy, anticoagulants, infection, diuretics, and hematoma.[3]

PRESENTATION

The diagnosis of a lymphocele should be entertained when a persistent, pulseless, cystic mass arises in the groin after surgical exploration. These masses are painless and are not inflamed unless infected. Lymphoceles may present at any time after exploration; however, they appear most often in the immediate postoperative period. A differential diagnosis of groin masses should include femoral artery false aneurysm, urinoma, seroma, hematoma, or abscess, in addition to lymphocele. Lymphatic complications appear to be associated with re-exploration in the groin. In Kwaan and colleagues' study of 12 patients, 5 had undergone previous groin dissections.[1] Other factors that may play a role in the development of lymphatic complications include poor wound healing, inadequate subcutaneous tissue approximation, and excessive postoperative limb motion.[1]

Aspiration of these masses produces a clear, thin, straw yellow fluid. Purulent aspiration indicates a secondary infection, with *Staphylococcus Aureus* the most common etiology.[4] Analysis of the fluid shows a total protein in the range of 0.5 to 2 g/dl. This may be used to distinguish a lymphocele, which has a low protein content, from a seroma.[3] Microscopic examination demonstrates a majority of lymphocytes, with only a few red blood cells, polymorphonuclear leukocytes, and in some cases fat globules.[5]

Lymphoceles may be imaged by both ultrasound and computed tomography (CT) scans. Ultrasound is felt to be an excellent method to document lymphoceles. Examination documents an anechoic or hypoechoic mass with occasional internal septa and debris. An increase in the debris and internal echoes is associated with an increased likelihood of infection.[5] A lymphocele can also be diagnosed by CT imaging. Examination documents a mass with low density and characteristically negative CT values.[5] The CT numbers increase into higher ranges when a hematoma or an abscess is present.

THERAPY

Nonoperative treatment of lymphocele consists of bed rest, gradient support stockings, analgesics, and antibiotics, if appropriate. Conservative therapy of lymphoceles and groin fistulas has consisted of simple packing with dressing changes, aspiration and pressure dressings, catheter drainage, or radiation therapy. An additional form of therapy used with some success is the introduction of sclerosing agents into abdominal lymphatic collections.

Kwaan and associates treated a group of seven patients who had undergone a variety of vascular surgical procedures that had involved a groin dissection.[1] Treatment in this group consisted of pressure dressings, local application of providone-iodine, systemic antibiotics, diet control, and immobilization. The lymph fistulas persisted for a period of 4 to 6 weeks in six of the seven patients. Positive wound cultures developed in three of the seven patients. The one patient who had a persistent lymph leak developed a graft infection and subsequently underwent removal of the prosthetic graft and below-knee amputation.

Other experience with nonoperative treatment of lymphoceles has been as dismal. Roberts and co-workers reported their experience with lymphorrhea complicating femoral revascularization.[2] In their series seven patients developed eight lymphoceles with otherwise uncomplicated hospital courses. One of the patients had immediate surgical correction of the lymphocele. Three of the patients underwent percutaneous aspiration and compression dressings. One of these patients developed a wound dehiscence and infection. Three additional patients were observed as outpatients. All three lymphoceles enlarged, and two drained spontaneously. All seven patients required surgical intervention to manage their lymphoceles and lymph fistulas. It was noted that a increased number of lymphatic complications were seen in patients who had oblique groin incisions (6 of 132 oblique incisions versus 2 of 182 vertical incisions), although this was not statistically significant.

Other groups have attempted to use catheter drainage of abdominal lymphoceles. In one study this was successful in 11 of 14 patients; however, catheter placement averaged 18 days and extended to 5 weeks in one patient.[5] Tetracycline sclerosis of abdominal lymphocele cavities also has been successfully used.[6] Others have reported success with irradiating a draining groin fistula.[7]

OPERATIVE THERAPY

Operative intervention in lymphoceles and lymphorrhea has produced more gratifying results than nonoperative therapy. Lymphoceles should be explored under general anesthesia. The lymphocele cavity is lined by a gray fibrinous material that is residual from the lymph fluid. The draining lymph channel can usually be identified without difficulty. If necessary, massage of the thigh can help reveal the leaking lymph vessel. Another adjunct that may be used is the injection of aqueous dyes to help identify the area of leakage.

Evans blue dye (5% aqueous solution) and isosulphan blue dye have both been used to delineate leaking lymph channels.[8] The dye is injected into the web spaces of the foot on the ipsilateral side approximately 30 minutes preoperatively. The dye is absorbed and transported by the lymphatics. On exploration, the dye can be seen leaking from the damaged lymphatic channels, which can then be ligated. Isosulphan blue dye may be preferable for this use because it does not stain the surrounding tissues. The lymphocele cavity is then excised, and the wound is meticulously closed in layers.

Infected lymphoceles with exposed graft material pose a special problem. Soots and colleagues used sartorius muscle myoplasties to treat benign and infected lymphoceles.[9] In a group of seven patients with either positive cultures or abscess formation around the graft, they were able to preserve six of the seven grafts. One graft, which was involved in a suppurative wound, was lost 19 months after the sartorius myoplasty.

The results of operative exploration of lymphoceles have been gratifying. Kwaan and associates reported that in patients who underwent immediate lymphatic ligation that their hospital course shortened and they had a lower incidence of wound infection than the nonoperative group.[1] Roberts and co-workers reported similar results.[2] All of the patients who had an attempt at nonoperative management subsequently required operative intervention to heal their lymphoceles.

REFERENCES

1. Kwaan JHM, Bernstein JM, Connolly JE. Management of lymph fistula in the groin after arterial reconstruction. Arch Surg 1979; 114:1416–1418.
2. Roberts JR, Walters GK, Zenilman ME, Jones CE. Groin lymphorrhea complicating revascularization involving the femoral vessels. Am J Surg 1993; 165:341–344.
3. Leitner DW, Sherwood RC. Inguinal lymphocele as a complication of thighplasty. Plast Reconstr Surg 1983; 72:878–881.
4. Fergusson JH, Maclure JG. Lymphocele following lymphadenectomy. Am J Obstet Gynecol 1961; 82:783.
5. VanSonnenberg E, Wittich GR, Casola G, et al. Lymphoceles:

Imaging characteristics and percutaneous management. Radiology 1986; 161:593–596.
6. McDowell GC 2nd, Babaian RJ, Johnson DE. Management of symptomatic lymphocele via percutaneous drainage and sclerotherapy with tetracycline. Urology 1991; 37:237–239.
7. Croft RJ. Lymphatic fistula: A complication of arterial surgery. BMJ 1978; 2:205 (letter).
8. Weaver FA, Yellin AE. Management of postoperative lymphatic leaks by use of isosulphan blue. J Vasc Surg 1991; 14:566–567.
9. Soots G, Mikati A, Warembourg H Jr, Noblet D. Treatment of lymphorrhea with exposed or infected vascular prosthetic grafts in the groin using sartorius myoplasty. J Cardiovasc Surg 1988; 29:42–45.

ANASTOMOTIC ANEURYSM

CALVIN B. ERNST, M.D.

Arterial reconstructive procedures have become commonplace over the past 40 years. With the remarkable advances in surgical and anesthetic techniques, operative mortality and morbidity have progressively declined. Despite the evolutionary improvements toward achieving perfection, late complications continue to threaten the durability of arterial reconstructive procedures. Some complications such as graft infection or aortoenteric fistulas threaten both life and limb. Others, such as anastomotic aneurysms, jeopardize limb viability.

Development of an anastomotic aneurysm is very rare following autogenous tissue reconstruction. For practical purposes, anastomotic aneurysms occur only after prosthetic reconstructive procedures, mainly following aortofemoral bypass for aneurysmal or occlusive disease. A femoral or popliteal anastomotic aneurysm rarely follows femoral popliteal prosthetic bypass. Because they are obscure and difficult to detect clinically, reports of aortic and iliac anastomotic aneurysms are uncommon.[1,2] Consequently, data on the natural history and management of aortic and iliac anastomotic aneurysms are virtually nonexistent. Therefore, here the focus is primarily on femoral anastomotic aneurysms (FAAs).

INCIDENCE

From a 30 year experience ending in 1987 at the Henry Ford Hospital, 6,090 aortoiliofemoral anastomoses were performed. Of these, 15 aortic and 21 iliac anastomotic aneurysms were recognized, an incidence of 0.4% and 0.8%, respectively. Seven of the aortic and 14 of the iliac anastomotic aneurysms were repaired. Over the same period, 145 FAAs were repaired.[3] However, this low incidence, particularly of aortic and iliac anastomotic aneurysms, which is confirmed by the paucity of published reports, probably represents an underestimation of the frequency of anastomotic aneurysms because routine postoperative screening and detection have not been employed. One study that routinely employed postoperative ultrasound surveillance documented incidences of 4.8% aortic, 3.6% iliac, and 13.6% FAAs.[4]

PATHOGENESIS

Causes of anastomotic aneurysms are multifactorial and include failure of suture material, prosthetic graft dilation, anastomotic stress from compliance mismatch between prosthesis and artery, arterial wall degeneration, hypertension, graft-artery size mismatch, end-to-side anastomoses, excessive graft tension, hip motion, redo operations, direct trauma, postreconstruction anticoagulation, inguinal ligament tethering of the graft, wound healing complications, and graft infection. With discontinuing the use of biodegradable silk suture for anastomoses, the incidence of FAAs was anticipated to decline dramatically, but such has not been the case. Host vessel degeneration has been the most commonly cited cause in contemporary reports. It should be noted, however, that although many causes have been suggested for development of FAAs and several may continue to be operational following aortofemoral bypass, more than 90% of all femoral anastomoses do not develop aneurysms.

A FAA may develop in the immediate postoperative period as a result of technical inadequacy, in the early postoperative period as a result of healing complications such as infection, lymphoceles, or hematomas, or in the late follow-up period as a result of the above cited causes.

Of particular note was the observation that an occult bacterial infection may influence development of FAAs.[5] Such infections usually involve *Staphylococcus* species and require special culturing techniques to isolate the organisms. No doubt such occult infections have gone undetected among some FAA repairs. Even when documented, however, these infections appear to have little or no influence on reinfection of the replacement grafts or recurrence of FAAs.[5] Clinically obvious infections with grossly purulent material and lack of graft incorporation associated with a FAA, however, must be treated with graft excision and extra-anatomic reconstruction.

DIAGNOSIS AND INDICATIONS FOR OPERATION

In that most anastomotic aneurysms involve the femoral vessels, diagnosis is usually obvious. Most FAAs become clinically apparent about 4 to 6 years after operation. Acute limb ischemia may result from graft occlusion (2% to 30%) or distal embolization (4% to 14%) of aneurysmal thrombotic debris. Although many FAAs are asymptomatic when first discovered, the potential for progressive occlusion of outflow vessels from microemboli and macroemboli should signal need for correction. Femoral anastomotic aneurysms rarely rupture. Because aortic and iliac anastomotic aneurysms are obscure, many such lesions are symptomatic, with a rupture rate of approximately 33% when first recognized.

If the FAA is at least 50% larger than the diameter of the host artery, it is usually easily diagnosed by palpation unless the patient is very obese. Duplex imaging is virtually 100% diagnostic. For the more obscure intra-abdominal anastomotic aneurysms, conflicting results have been reported with ultrasound; consequently, contrast computed tomography (CT) imaging is preferred.

Principles of management of anastomotic aneurysms have evolved over four decades of experience with such lesions.[3] Site of involvement influences management. If the aneurysm is obvious, cautious observation may be appropriate, particularly if the lesion is small and the patient appears to be high risk for operation. If, however, the aneurysm is obscure, cautious observation is contraindicated and early operation is indicated, provided the patient is an acceptable risk. It is important to recognize that some FAAs are not progressive and are not serious risks. Those FAAs less than 2 cm in diameter may be treated expectantly and with regular follow-up examinations. If progressive enlargement is documented and the patient is a candidate for operation, then repair is indicated. If the aneurysm is greater than 2 to 2.5 cm in diameter, it should be repaired. All symptomatic FAAs require repair, provided the patients are acceptable operative risks. Clearly, tender, expanding, embolizing, or thrombosed aneurysms require operation.

PREOPERATIVE EVALUATION AND PREPARATION

Beyond noninvasive imaging studies to document the presence of a FAA, arteriography is required to plan the approach and details of operative repair for all patients. If sepsis is suspected, precise, CT-guided fine-needle aspiration, under absolutely aseptic precautions, may prove helpful in planning the operation. However, not finding clinical evidence of sepsis does not conclusively exclude infection because slime-producing staphylococcal organisms may defy preoperative detection. Nevertheless, in the absence of clinical evidence of infection, the surgeon may proceed with relative assurance that the nature of the occult infective process does not preclude successful in situ arterial reconstruction.[5]

Surgical treatment of an aortic or iliac anastomotic aneurysm is more complicated than that of a FAA. Preoperative evaluation proceeds as when undertaking treatment of nonruptured infrarenal and juxtarenal aortic aneurysms. The retroperitoneal approach is preferred for such intra-abdominal anastomotic aneurysms.

Prophylactic antibiotics are administered preoperatively by giving 1 g of a second-generation cephalosporin with the anesthetic premedication.

OPERATIVE TECHNIQUE

When operating upon a FAA, the type of repair is dictated by arteriographic findings with the caveat that preoperative plans may require modification by operative findings. Because of perivascular scar tissue, technical vicissitudes coincident to FAA repairs present challenges beyond those encountered during routine arterial reconstructive procedures. Consequently, the operation must be simplified and confined to the groin whenever possible. Although some surgeons recommend the addition of an outflow procedure,[6] in our experience, extended revascularization procedures, such as simultaneous femoral-popliteal bypasses, have not been required during FAA repairs.

With the patient supine, both lower extremities and the lower abdomen are draped into a sterile operative field. A sterile transparent plastic bag is used to cover the ipsilateral foot to monitor peripheral perfusion.

Although technical details may vary among surgeons, certain standardized principles have been regularly and successfully employed. They include early proximal control of the prosthetic graft, minimal dissection of the anastomotic aneurysm, only partial excision of the aneurysm, intraluminal balloon obturator occlusion of the deep and superficial femoral arteries from within the opened aneurysm, systemic heparinization, anastomosis to as healthy arterial tissue as possible to avoid suturing to scar or aneurysmal tissue, and expanded polytetrafluoroethylene (ePTFE) graft replacement because ePTFE appears resistant to slime-producing bacterial infections.[5] Because the superficial femoral artery is frequently occluded, the only available outflow vessel is the deep femoral artery. As a result of scar tissue, dissection and mobilization of the deep femoral artery are not only tedious but also potentially hazardous to surrounding structures such as the femoral nerve; consequently, limited dissection is suggested.

The aneurysm is exposed through a vertical groin incision. Scalpel dissection facilitates exposure of the aneurysm and the old prosthesis. When necessary, the inguinal ligament may be incised to obtain adequate proximal exposure. Occasionally, when a suitable length of the old prosthesis cannot be exposed through the groin, a short transverse experitoneal suprainguinal incision is required. Once proximal control is obtained, distal control of the outflow vessels may be attempted,

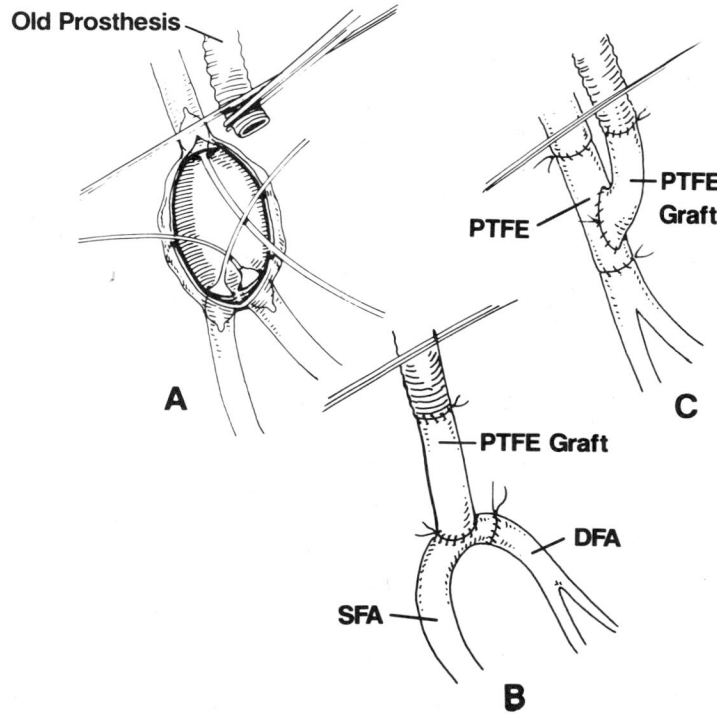

Figure 1 *A*, Method of obtaining proximal and distal control through the ostia of the common femoral, superficial femoral (SFA), and deep femoral arteries (DFA) with balloon obturator catheters. The old prosthesis has been detached and is occluded with a vascular clamp. *B*, The superficial and deep femoral arteries have been anastomosed end to end, thereby constructing a new common femoral bifurcation. The ePTFE graft is anastomosed to the end of the old graft proximally and to the side of the superficial femoral artery distally. *C*, Method of reconstructing the femoral vessels when the host common femoral and external iliac arteries are patent. The ePTFE graft has been interposed between the proximal common femoral artery and the distal common femoral artery. A second ePTFE graft is interposed between the old graft and the interposed ePTFE graft.

but if scar tissue precludes safe dissection, distal control with intraluminal balloon catheters is recommended (Fig. 1). Dissection of a patent proximal common femoral artery may also prove difficult, and intraluminal balloon catheter occlusion is required for this vessel as well.

After giving 50 to 100 units/kg of heparin sodium intravenously, the proximal prosthetic limb is clamped, the aneurysm is opened, and balloon catheters are inserted and inflated. The previous anastomosis is dismantled, and the old prosthesis is trimmed appropriately. One usually finds that the prosthesis is detached from most or all of the host vessel. Intraluminal thrombus is evacuated and a segment of the old prosthesis and thrombus are sent to the laboratory for bacterial culture. When available, sonication of the specimen increases yield of bacterial cultures by freeing the organisms from the encapsulating glycocalyx associated with slime-producing staphylococcal infections.[5]

The distal anastomosis is performed first. The site of the distal anastomosis depends upon the extent of involvement of the common, superficial, and deep femoral arteries. If the distal common femoral artery is not suitable and the superficial femoral artery is patent, an end-to-end anastomosis between the proximal deep femoral and proximal superficial femoral arteries is performed, thereby functionally constructing a new common femoral bifurcation. Following this, an ePTFE graft is anastomosed to the side of the superficial femoral artery and the end of the old prosthesis, restoring blood flow to both the deep and superficial femoral territories (Fig. 1). If the superficial femoral artery is occluded, which is the usual finding, an end-to-end anastomosis is performed to the ostium of the deep femoral artery. When necessary, distal control is obtained by a balloon catheter threaded through a segment of 8 mm ePTFE graft and into the deep femoral artery (Fig. 2). The distal end-to-end anastomosis to the rim of the ostium of the deep femoral artery is constructed with polypropylene or PTFE suture (Fig. 2). The balloon catheter is then deflated and removed, and the ePTFE graft is occluded with an atraumatic clamp. The ePTFE graft is trimmed appropriately, and an end-to-end anastomosis is constructed to the old graft (Fig. 2).

In order to maintain retrograde flow into the external and internal iliac arteries, when the host proximal common femoral artery is patent, a segment of ePTFE graft is interposed between the two ends of the common femoral artery or the proximal common femoral and deep femoral arteries. A second 8 mm ePTFE graft is then anastomosed end to side to the interposed ePTFE graft and finally end to end to the old graft (Fig. 1).

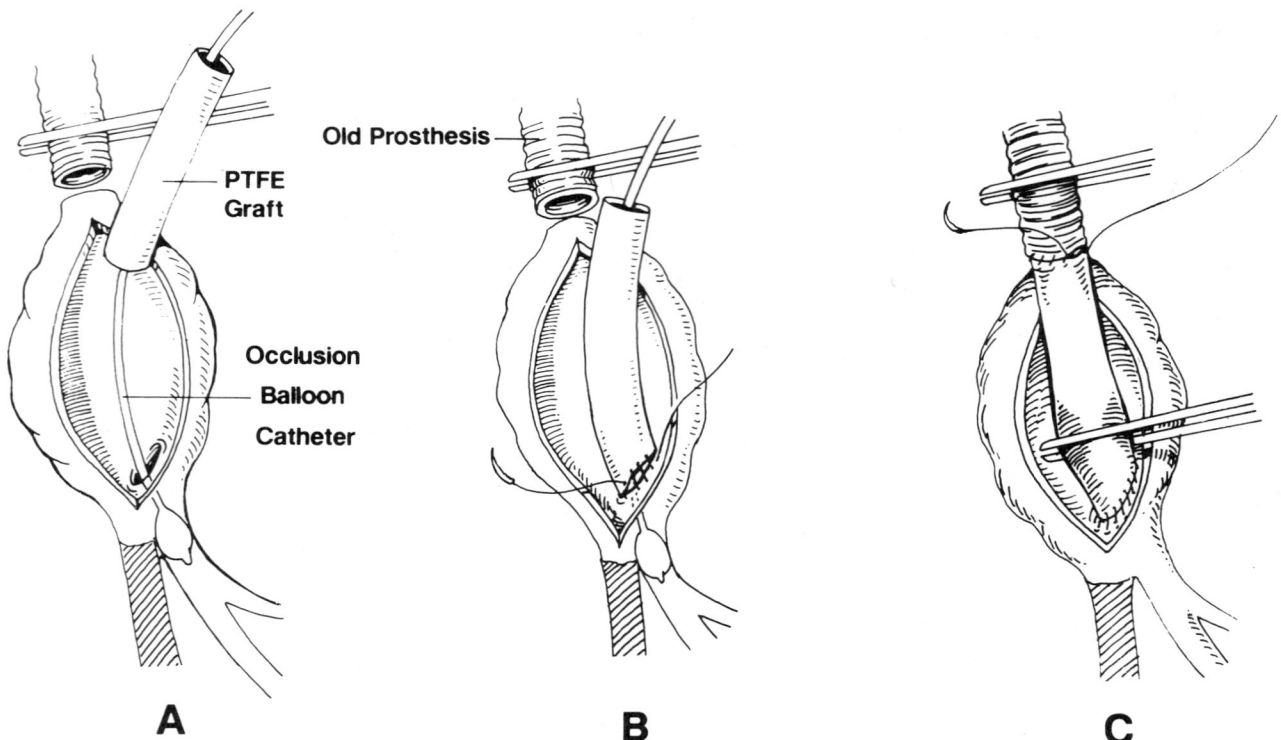

Figure 2 *A,* Segment of ePTFE graft is threaded over occlusion balloon catheter, which is placed into the ostium of the deep femoral artery. The superficial femoral artery is thrombosed. *B,* The distal anastomosis between the ePTFE graft and the rim of the ostium of the deep femoral artery is completed with the occlusion balloon catheter in place. *C,* The distal anastomosis has been completed, the occlusion balloon catheter has been removed, and the ePTFE graft is clamped while the proximal anastomosis is completed.

After completion of the various anastomoses and restoration of blood flow, the foot is examined and, confirming adequate perfusion, the wound is meticulously closed in two to three layers. Judicious excision of scar tissue is performed, leaving sufficient healthy tissue to cover the ePTFE prosthesis. It is particularly important to suture ligate oozing lymphatics to prevent groin lymph complications. When adequate healthy tissue is not available to cover the prosthesis, the sartorius muscle may be detached from its origin and transposed over the repaired vessels. Drains are not used.

Aortic anastomotic aneurysms are repaired using a retroperitoneal approach. Retroperitoneal exposure facilitates supraceliac aortic clamping, which may be required during such repairs. The same principles are followed when repairing aortic and iliac anastomotic aneurysms as for FAAs, namely, minimal dissection, balloon obturator control of involved vessels when necessary, and interposition ePTFE grafting between the old prosthesis and as healthy a host artery as possible.

RESULTS

Results vary depending upon the site of the anastomotic aneurysm and the indications for and urgency of operation. Of the 21 patients with aortic and iliac anastomotic aneurysms operated upon at the Henry Ford Hospital, four patients died, an operative mortality rate of 19%. Three of the 14 iliac aneurysms had ruptured, forcing operation, but none of the seven aortic aneurysms had. Eight aortic and seven iliac anastomotic aneurysms were observed because prohibitive risk factors precluded operation. Three (20%) of these patients died of rupture during follow-up. This confirms that aortoiliac aneurysms are potentially lethal lesions requiring repair when possible. However, such repairs are predictably complicated, which contributes to the high mortality and morbidity.

No convincing data are available regarding screening of patients who may harbor aortic and iliac anastomotic aneurysms; therefore, practical recommendations regarding screening are not available. Although data are lacking regarding routine screening for intraabdominal anastomotic aneurysms in every patient following aortoiliac or aortofemoral reconstruction, aortoiliac CT or duplex imaging is justified among patients with FAAs because they may be prone to aneurysms for reasons yet to be defined. The policy we follow is, if the patient is a reasonable operative risk and if it appears that the anastomotic aneurysm can be safely repaired, operation is recommended for those greater than 50% the normal vessel diameter, those proved to be enlarging, or those that are symptomatic.

Less extensive aortic and iliac aneurysms are cautiously observed.

Results following elective operation for FAAs are, in general, excellent. Combined mortality and amputation rates are less than 5%, despite the inclusion of many patients who are high risks.[3,6] Among patients presenting with complications of FAAs, mortality and morbidity rates are approximately double that for prophylactic repair. A small number of FAAs recur.[3] Significant variables related to recurrence include female gender, local wound healing complications following the initial FAA repair, and a short time interval between the original operation and the first appearance of an FAA. Recurrent FAAs should be managed like other FAAs, and comparable results can be expected.

REFERENCES

1. Treiman GS, Weaver FA, Cossman DV, et al. Anastomotic false aneurysms of the abdominal aorta and the iliac arteries. J Vasc Surg 1988; 8:268–273.
2. Edwards JM, Teefey SA, Zierler RE, et al. Intra-abdominal paraanastomotic aneurysms after aortic bypass grafting. J Vasc Surg 1992; 15:344–353.
3. Ernst CB, Elliott JP Jr, Ryan CJ, et al. Recurrent femoral anastomotic aneurysms: A 30-year experience. Ann Surg 1988; 208:401–409.
4. Vanden Akker PJ, Brand R, Van Schilfgaarde R, et al. False aneurysms after prosthetic reconstructions for aortoiliac obstructive disease. Ann Surg 1989; 210:658–666.
5. Seabrook GR, Schmitt DD, Bandyk DF, et al. Anastomotic femoral pseudoaneurysm: An investigation of occult infection as an etiologic factor. J Vasc Surg 1990; 11:629–634.
6. Schellack J, Salam A, Abouzeid MA, et al. Femoral anastomotic aneurysms: A continuing challenge. J Vasc Surg 1987; 6:308–317.

AORTIC GRAFT LIMB OCCLUSION

DAVID C. BREWSTER, M.D.

Despite the well-established effectiveness and durability of aortic reconstruction for aortoiliac occlusive disease, problems may recur both early and late following operation. In virtually all studies, the most common complication is thrombosis of one limb of an aortofemoral bifurcation graft.[1] Although the exact frequency of graft limb occlusion varies from one report to another, it is recognized to affect approximately 10% to 20% of patients, depending upon the duration of follow-up. Specifically, graft limb thrombosis occurs in approximately 10% of patients within the first 5 years after primary operation and may be anticipated in 15% to 30% of patients if follow-up is in excess of 10 years.[2,3] In our review of this problem, the average interval from original graft insertion to occlusion was 33.8 months.[3]

Management of this problem is often difficult, frequently requiring an urgent reoperation in the densely scarred groin of an elderly, high-risk patient with complex patterns of extensive multilevel occlusive disease. Careful clinical judgment is necessary, and the technical demands of operation require an experienced vascular surgeon. Nonetheless, successful results can usually be achieved if treatment is based upon the likely cause of graft failure as well as a clear understanding of the arterial anatomy and clinical circumstances of each patient.

CAUSES OF GRAFT OCCLUSION

Early (less than 30 days after operation) thrombosis of an aortic graft limb affects 1% to 3% of patients and is generally attributable to technical or judgmental errors. Problems such as twisting or kinking of the graft limb, incorrect tunneling of the graft, or anastomotic obstruction due to a poorly performed anastomosis or mechanical flaps secondary to disrupted plaque or intima at the anastomotic site may be responsible. The surgeon may not have adequately flushed fresh clot developing within the graft limb prior to completion of the distal anastomosis. Inadequate heparinization or an unrecognized hypercoagulable state may contribute to such difficulties. Finally, the surgeon may have underestimated the severity of outflow disease and failed to establish good blood flow into the profunda femoris artery in a patient with multilevel disease. Typically in these circumstances, the distal anastomosis has been made to the common femoral artery in a patient with chronic superficial femoral artery (SFA) occlusion who also has a diseased profunda origin. Early graft limb thrombosis is not surprising in this situation and underscores the well-recognized importance of a profundaplasty as part of the original procedure to ensure long-term patency.

Similar graft outflow problems are the cause of the majority of late graft limb occlusions as well. In the first several years following graft implantation, this is often

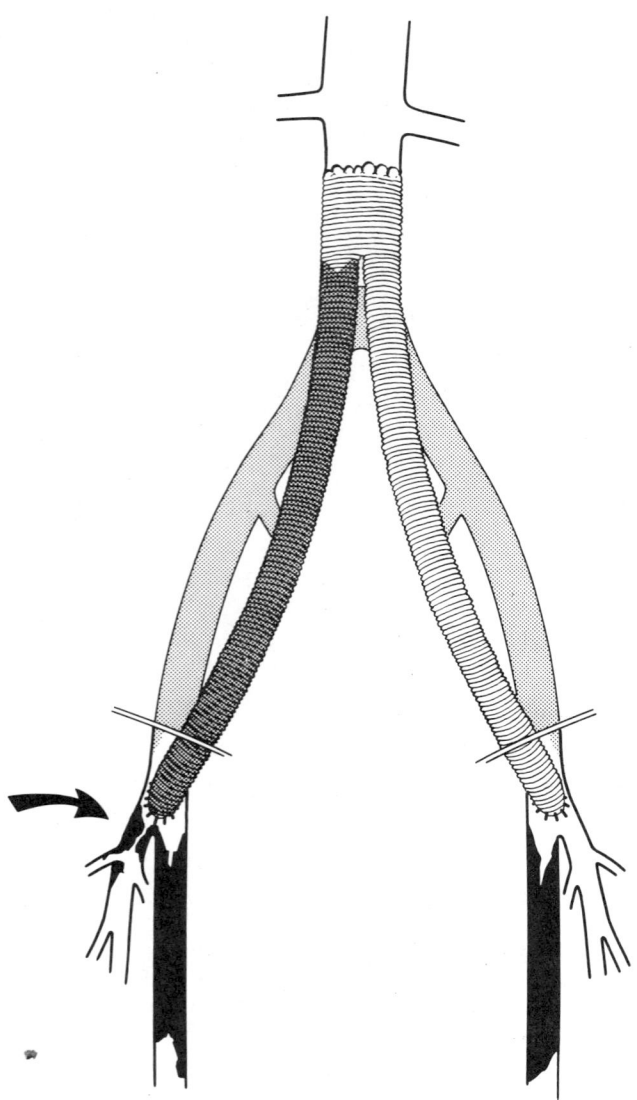

Figure 1 Unilateral thrombosis of one limb of aortofemoral graft is usually due to progressive stenosis of proximal profunda femoris (*arrow*) just below femoral anastomosis in patient with pre-existent superficial femoral artery occlusion.

due to development of fibrous neointimal hyperplasia at or just beyond the distal anastomotic site. Progressive atherosclerotic disease compromising the outflow vessels is usually responsible for graft failures occurring at later intervals beyond 2 to 3 years. Because the majority of patients undergoing aortofemoral grafts have coexistent SFA occlusion, causative occlusion lesions are most often found in the proximal profunda femoris (Fig. 1). Worsening profunda stenosis results in diminution of blood flow through the graft limb, progressive deposition of concentric layers of thickened fibrin or "pseudointima," and eventually graft thrombosis.

Less commonly, outflow obstruction may be due to thrombosis of an anastomotic aneurysm or to an arterial embolus in a patient with cardiac problems. Rarely, systemic causes such as a low output state from a variety of conditions or various problems associated with hypercoagulability may be responsible. Iatrogenic injuries to host vessels or the graft itself during cardiac catheterization or other interventional radiographic procedures are occurring more frequently with the increased application of such studies.

Impaired inflow is a distinctly unusual etiology of failure of one limb of a bifurcation graft. Such proximal causes of graft occlusion usually lead to failure of the entire reconstruction (Fig. 2). Residual or progressive atherosclerotic disease at the proximal graft anastomosis is less frequent in current practice with general recognition of the necessity to place the aortic anastomosis of a graft as close to the renal artery origins as possible in order to minimize the changes of such subsequent difficulties. Aortic anastomotic aneurysms may also compromise the proximal graft anastomosis but occur relatively infrequently.

DIAGNOSIS

Recognition of aortic graft occlusion is usually straightforward. It is readily apparent to the patient, who notes an abrupt onset of ischemic symptoms, and to the surgeon, who detects loss of a previously palpable femoral pulse. In some instances of gradual graft occlusion, sufficient collateral circulation may have developed to maintain a weak femoral pulse that may be felt in a thin patient. If an end-to-side proximal anastomosis had been utilized, some blood flow may be maintained through stenotic but patent host iliofemoral vessels. Diagnosis may be facilitated by Doppler pressure indices and pulse volume recordings, particularly if previous studies done when a functioning graft was present are available for comparison. Suspected graft occlusion is confirmed by arteriography.

MANAGEMENT

In most instances of aortic graft occlusion, the resultant limb ischemia necessitates further efforts at revascularization. The majority of patients with acute graft failure have ischemic symptoms worse than those at the time of initial operation. In our review of graft limb failures, 81% had limb-threatening symptoms, and nearly half required urgent operation within 48 hours of admission.[3] In some patients with more gradual failure, sufficient collateral circulation may have developed so that reoperation may not be mandatory. Because all methods of reoperation for aortic graft failure are technically demanding, associated with greater risk of complications or mortality, and less likely to have good long-term results, the surgeon may elect a nonoperative approach in certain poor-risk or inactive patients if recurrent limb-threatening ischemia is not present.

Acute perioperative graft limb thrombosis is best managed by expeditiously returning the patient to the

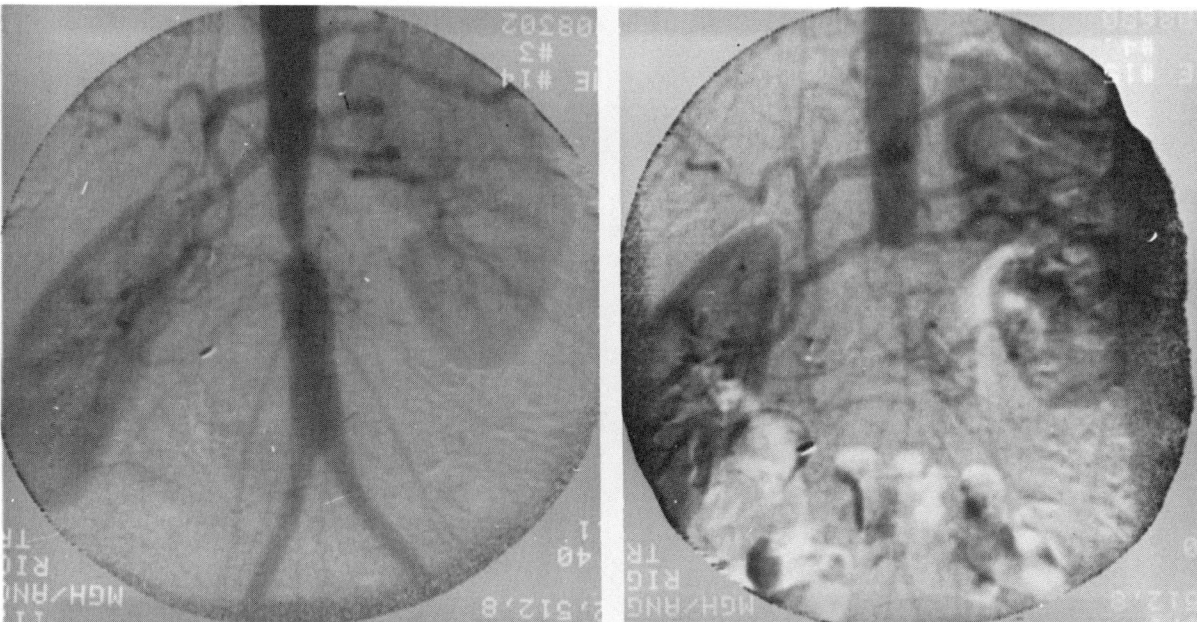

Figure 2 Left is progressive aortic atherosclerosis compromising proximal anastomosis of aortobifemoral graft. Right is the same patient 2 months later, with occlusion of entire graft and retrograde aortic thrombosis to juxtarenal level. (From Brewster DC. Surgery of late aortic graft occlusion. In: Bergan JJ, Yao JST, eds. Aortic surgery. Philadelphia: WB Saunders, 1989; with permission.)

operating room for immediate reoperation. Preoperative arteriography is generally unnecessary and rarely helpful. The involved groin incision is reopened, and the femoral anastomosis inspected through an incision in the distal graft hood. Any technical error or local pathology is corrected and graft limb thrombectomy is carried out with a No. 4 or 5 Fogarty balloon embolectomy catheter. This will successfully remove fresh thrombus and restore inflow in almost all instances. Following closure of the incision in the graft hood, some means of intraoperative assurance of a satisfactory result should be obtained by use of completion arteriography, angioscopy, or intraoperative hemodynamic monitoring. If no clear technical faults or mechanical reasons for acute graft failure are found and poor outflow is judged to be the primary cause of acute thrombosis, distal bypass grafting to the popliteal or tibial levels should be considered if the deep femoral artery is small or if uncorrectable disease in the more distal deep femoral artery exists.

Treatment of late graft limb occlusions, defined as those occurring at varying intervals after discharge following aortic reconstruction, is usually complex and challenging. Determination of the probable cause of graft occlusion and evaluation of the status of inflow and runoff vessels requires preoperative arteriography in almost all instances. Although this may be omitted in a small number of patients who present with signs of profound limb ischemia, particularly if they have not come to medical attention for some time after the onset of graft occlusion, complete preoperative arteriography is extremely important in the management of late occlusions.

Several key elements of anatomic information are sought by preoperative arteriography and serve to guide subsequent reoperative decisions. The abdominal aorta and proximal anastomosis are visualized, preferably in two planes, to assure adequate inflow and the integrity of the proximal anastomosis. Abnormalities of the aorta or proximal anastomosis require direct aortic reoperation or selection of an appropriate extra-anatomic method of inflow revascularization. If any uncertainty exists about the possibility of a proximal anastomotic aneurysm, a computed tomography scan can also be obtained. If unilateral graft limb failure is documented, the presence of clot in the graft body, condition of the contralateral graft limb, and status of reconstituted distal vessels are all evaluated (Fig. 3). This helps to determine whether graft limb thrombectomy may be attempted, documents the feasibility of femorofemoral grafting, and suggests the possible need for concomitant distal bypass grafting as part of the reoperative plan.

It should be stressed, however, that failure to visualize contrast medium in the groin or distal arterial bed of the involved extremity does not necessarily preclude attempts at reoperation or imply the absence of any patent runoff vessels. Therefore, it is advisable to explore the groin vessels of patients with acute graft occlusion even if runoff vessels are not adequately seen on preoperative arteriography. These can be assessed by exploration and operative arteriography.

A variety of reoperative methods have been suggested to restore and maintain patency of the occluded graft limb. In general, reoperation requires a combination of techniques to restore inflow as well as re-establish

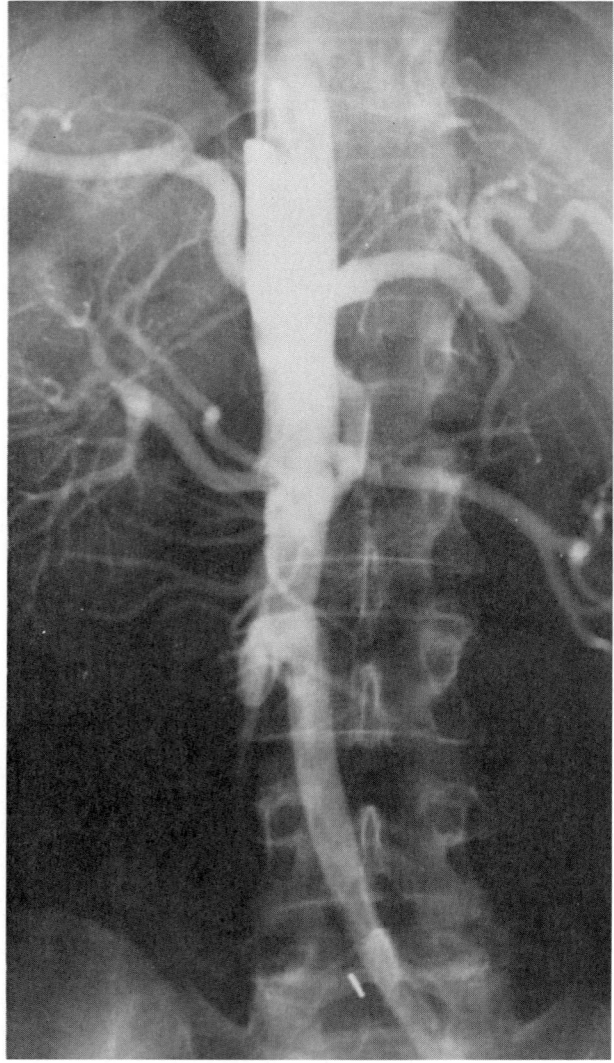

Figure 3 Typical arteriographic appearance of unilateral occlusion of aortofemoral graft limb. Thrombus is limited to the involved right limb, terminating below the origin of the limb. The proximal aorta, body of the graft, and contralateral graft limb appear normal.

Table 1 Options for Reoperation for Occluded Aortic Graft Limb

Inflow	Outflow
Graft limb thrombectomy	Profundaplasty
Femorofemoral graft	Graft extension to more distal profunda
Replace graft limb	
Redo entire aortic graft	Addition of femorodistal bypass
Thrombolytic therapy	

mented the absence of proximal aortic disease, an adequate aortic anastomosis, and a patent, normal-appearing contralateral graft limb, it is usually possible to re-establish inflow by graft limb thrombectomy. Favorable experience with retrograde thrombectomy of the occluded graft limb via a groin incision has been reported with approximately 90% success by many authors, and it is therefore worthwhile to utilize this as an initial step in almost all patients.[3-5] The obvious appeal of such an approach is that reoperation may be accomplished through a single groin incision, thereby reducing the potential morbidity and mortality of more complex methods of revascularization. In addition, as most failures are caused by recurrent or progressive occlusive lesions in the groin, such an approach focuses attention upon reconstruction of the outflow tract, a crucial component of any successful reoperative procedure.

Unquestionably, thrombectomy is more likely to be successful for graft occlusions of short duration. Nonetheless, there is no agreement on a time period beyond which thrombectomy is certain to fail or ill advised. Thrombectomy has succeeded in a high percentage of chronic occlusions of up to 7 months when appropriate techniques were utilized.[3,4]

Either regional or general anesthesia may be employed. The patient should be widely prepped and draped so that the sterile field includes the entire abdomen, both groins, and involved lower extremity, in the event that thrombectomy is not possible and other means of re-establishing inflow to the leg are necessary or concomitant distal bypass grafting is required. The old femoral incision is opened as required for adequate exposure, particularly the proximal several centimeters of the profunda femoris artery. The occluded graft limb is divided immediately proximal to the femoral anastomosis. The distal stump of the graft is then opened longitudinally to expose the orifices of the runoff vessels and determine the probable cause of outflow obstruction. Thrombectomy of the occluded limb is then carried out with a No. 4 or 5 embolectomy catheter introduced about 15 cm, and thrombus removed. The catheter is then reintroduced and advanced about 5 cm further, again withdrawing thrombus. Such serial passages and extractions are done in an attempt to minimize the chances of "pushing" thrombus over the aortic bifurcation into the uninvolved limb. By removal of most of the thrombus, the surgeon hopes that systemic pressure will blow out the proximal cap of thrombus. The apex of the

reliable outflow (Table 1). Some aspects of surgical strategy remain controversial, particularly regarding the best method of restoring inflow to the ischemic limb and how often a concomitant distal bypass must be performed to augment outflow. It should be emphasized that there is no single standard operation for aortic graft occlusion. The surgical approach must be carefully individualized.

Restoration of Inflow

Graft Limb Thrombectomy

If graft failure involves one limb of an aortobifemoral graft and preoperative arteriography has docu-

thrombotic material can usually be reliably identified by examination of the removed thrombus. Extraction of this final bit of organized thrombus is usually followed by a vigorous, pulsatile arterial blood flow and is generally a reliable indication of satisfactory clearance of the graft limb.

An additional maneuver that may help prevent cross-embolization to the contralateral graft limb is compression over the graft pulse in the opposite groin. The intention is to reduce blood flow in the uninvolved limb and encourage flushing of all thrombotic debris out the thrombectomized graft limb. Thromboembolic compromise of the uninvolved graft limb did not occur in our series of 106 graft limb thrombectomies.[3]

If the graft limb occlusion is longstanding, simple balloon catheter embolectomy may not adequately remove all the densely organized and adherent laminated thrombus. In such instances, additional maneuvers are required to remove the tenacious thrombotic plug. This obstructing material is frequently located at the origin of the graft limb. As originally described by Ernst and Daugherty,[6] a Cannon loop endarterectomy stripper can dislodge tenaciously adherent fibrinous material (Fig. 4). Recently, development of a Fogarty graft thrombectomy catheter has simplified and extended this concept (Fig. 5).[7] This device utilizes a wire helix instead of a Latex balloon at its retrieval tip. The spiral-wire tip has an adjustable diameter of approximately 4 to 16 mm, controlled by a sliding knob on its handle, and functions similarly to a variable-diameter ring stripper. The surgeon passes the device with its wire helix in a low-profile position through the graft limb and then, by continuously adjusting the pitch of the spiral-wire tip, withdraws the device with appropriate traction on the graft wall. The wires of the helical tip scrape adherent neointima and thrombus from the graft wall and greatly facilitate restoration of adequate inflow through more chronically occluded graft limbs.

Upon completion of the thrombectomy, it is important to confirm adequate clearing of occluding fibrinothrombotic debris from the graft. The surgeon may estimate the force of arterial inflow after thrombectomy or measure arterial pressure in the distal graft limb at completion of the procedure. However, more direct

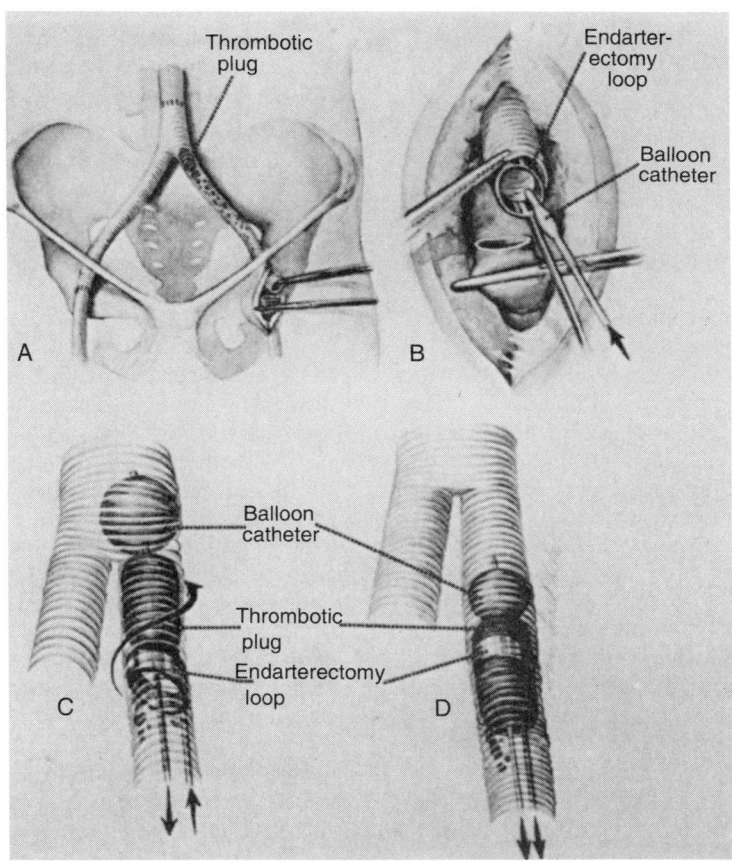

Figure 4 Method of extracting adherent thrombus. *A,* Tenacious thrombotic plug occluding graft limb. *B,* Embolectomy catheter passed through loop endarterectomy stripper into transected graft limb. *C,* Exerting downward countertraction of the inflated balloon catheter, the surgeon advances the stripper with a gentle twisting motion. *D,* Catheter, loop, and thrombotic debris removed together. (From Ernst CB, Daugherty ME. Removal of a thrombotic plug from an occluded limb of an aortofemoral graft. Arch Surg 1978; 113:301–302; with permission.)

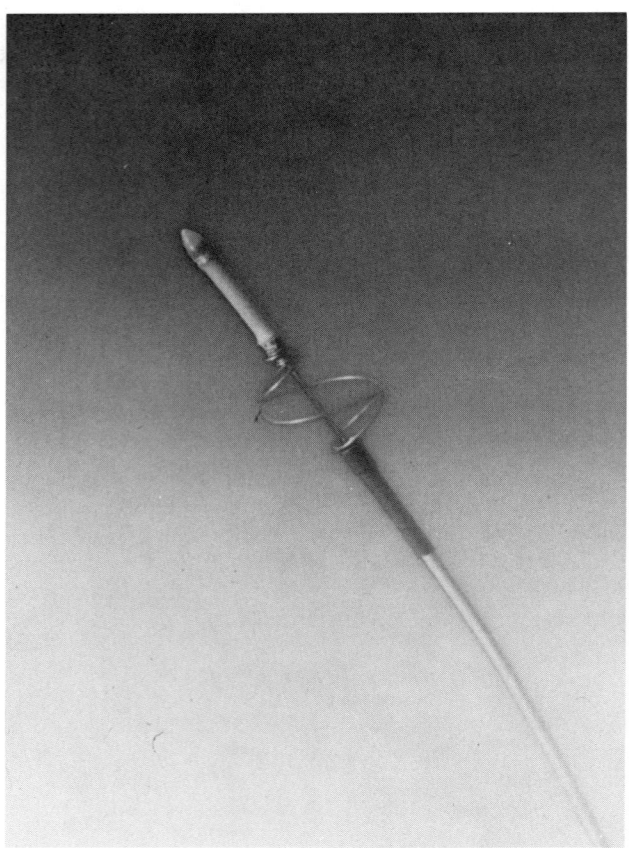

Figure 5 Helical wire retrieval tip of Fogarty graft thrombectomy catheter, with variable diameters adjustable by changing the pitch of the spiral configuration.

methods are generally recommended. Retrograde flush arteriography via a large-bore catheter inserted in the distal end of the thrombectomized graft limb can provide excellent visualization of the involved limb and its origin from the body of the graft, a frequent location of persistent organized thrombotic material. In recent years, angioscopic examination of the graft limb following thrombectomy has also been successful.[8]

Alternative Inflow Procedures

If graft thrombectomy is not successful in restoring adequate inflow, alternative methods must be employed. The most common alternative for unilateral graft limb occlusion is a femorofemoral bypass based upon the normal contralateral graft limb. Such an alternative is usually safer for the patient and technically easier for the surgeon than direct replacement of the occluded graft limb. Other types of extra-anatomic reconstruction, such as an axillofemoral bypass, are rarely performed for unilateral graft limb failures.

Direct in-line replacement of the occluded graft limb or a redo procedure to insert an entirely new aortic bifurcation graft has been advocated by some and may be performed by either ipsilateral retroperitoneal or standard transabdominal approach. However, the technical challenges and risks of such reoperative procedures should not be underestimated, with the potential for injuries to major adjacent veins, ureter, or duodenum secondary to scarring in the periaortic operative field. In general, direct redo aortic procedures are best reserved for those cases of aortic graft failure clearly caused by proximal aortic disease, anastomotic complications, or significant dilation or degeneration of the original prosthesis.

Limited experience with thrombolytic therapy has suggested that an acutely thrombosed aortic graft may sometimes be reopened with this method. However, if ischemia is severe, time constraints may not permit use of lytic therapy. It is also clear that lytic therapy may result in significant complications. Most important, surgical revision of the graft outflow tract is required in most patients. For all of these reasons, there seems to be little support for frequent use of lytic therapy in the management of failed aortic graft limbs.[3] Its one advantage is that clearing of clot from the occluded limb does allow more precise arteriographic definition of the exact anatomic cause of graft thrombosis and thereby can facilitate decisions regarding reoperation. As such, a brief initial attempt at lytic therapy may be justfied for patients seen early after graft limb thrombosis who do not have advanced ischemia, particularly high-risk patients.

Revision of Graft Outflow

Because approximately 80% of late graft limb occlusions are caused by progressive outflow obstructions, appropriate revision of the outflow tract is usually the most important aspect of a successful and durable reoperative procedure. Because the SFA is occluded in most patients requiring reoperation of graft limb failure (85% in our series), establishment of unobstructed blood flow into the deep femoral artery is usually the primary focus of outflow revision.

A variety of techniques may be employed to restore runoff, depending upon the local anatomy (Fig. 6). Most often, profundaplasty with or without local endarterectomy is sufficient.[3,4] Our preference is to add a short segment of a new graft to the original graft limb with end-to-end anastomosis distally to the profunda beyond significant occlusive disease (Fig. 6A). If the proximal profunda is extensively diseased or scarred, an extension to more distal portions of the profunda, with end-to-side anastomosis, may be employed (Fig. 6B). In such instances, the surgeon may prefer to expose the second or third portion of the profunda through more normal tissues and develop an intermuscular plane lateral to the sartorius muscle, which is retracted medially.

If profunda endarterectomy is elected and the surgeon wishes to preserve retrograde iliac blood flow, patch closure of the arteriotomy may be performed with reimplantation of the aortic graft limb just above the patch or into the patch itself (Fig. 6C1). In our experience, arteriotomy closure is best accomplished by

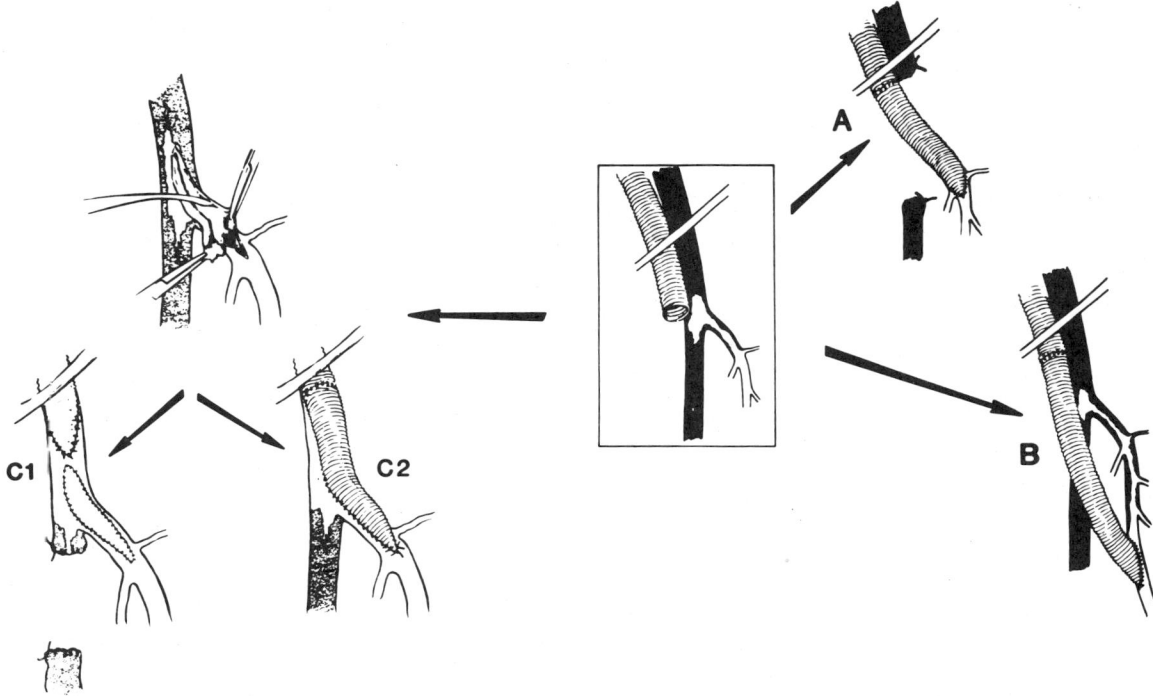

Figure 6 Options for outflow tract reconstruction. *A,* Addition of short extension of new prosthetic material with end-to-end anastomosis to profunda below diseased proximal segment. *B,* Longer bypass to more distal profunda. *C,* If the surgeon wishes to maintain femoral and retrograde iliac artery flow, formal endarterectomy may be performed, with separate patch closure employing autogenous or prosthetic material (*C1*), or use of long beveled tongue of new graft segment (*C2*).

addition of a new segment of graft material with distal anastomosis of a long beveled tongue of the graft tip over the profunda arteriotomy (Fig. 6*C2*).

If profundaplasty proves impossible or the profunda is too small or diseased to serve as an effective outflow vessel, it may be necessary to carry out a synchronous distal bypass to the popliteal or tibial level. Preoperative or intraoperative arteriographic findings may help in this judgment, but such decisions are usually made on the basis of several intraoperative criteria of the adequacy of the deep femoral artery.[3] If the profunda accepts a 4 mm probe and measures 20 to 25 cm in length, as determined by gentle passage of a noninflated embolectomy catheter or similar measuring device, the surgeon may usually be confident of a well-developed deep femoral outflow tract capable of sustaining aortic graft blood flow. If such criteria are not met, synchronous distal grafting seems advisable. Complementary distal grafts were used in our series in 32% of all procedures (26% of initial reoperations and 53% of repetitive reoperations for recurrent failures).[3] Other investigators, however, feel that supplementary distal bypass is seldom necessary.[4,9] Although disagreement persists on this issue and the practice is often taught to wait 24 to 48 hours to see if profunda revascularization alone will suffice, it seems easier and more appropriate to proceed with distal graft insertion at the time of initial reoperation if the various factors outlined here suggest a high likelihood that such grafts will be needed for a successful outcome. Harris also has emphasized the advisability of adding a distal graft in more than 50% of procedures for aortic graft limb occlusion.[10]

RESULTS

Early and late results of 157 reoperative procedures for aortic graft limb occlusion in our study are representative of those reported by other authors.[3-5,9] Despite the frequent associated cardiovascular disease and other comorbid conditions, operative mortality was only 1.9%. Graft limb patency was ultimately maintained in 78% of patients and limb salvage achieved in 67%. Recurrent graft occlusion may occur, however, and 26% of the patients required repetitive reoperation (two to five reoperations) to maintain the limb. Nonetheless, an aggressive policy toward reoperation and perseverance by the surgeon appear justified by satisfactory long-term results and acceptable morbidity and mortality rates.

REFERENCES

1. Brewster DC. Complications of aortic and lower extremity procedures. In: Strandness DE, Van Breda A, eds. Vascular

diseases: Surgical and interventional therapy. New York: Churchill Livingstone, 1994:1151.
2. Brewster DC, Cooke JC. Longevity of aortofemoral bypass grafts. In: Yao JST, Pierce WH, eds. Long-term results in vascular surgery. East Norwalk, Conn: Appleton & Lange, 1993:149.
3. Brewster DC, Meier GH III, Darling RC, et al. Reoperation for aortofemoral graft limb occlusion: Optimal methods and long-term results. J Vasc Surg 1987; 5:363–374.
4. Bernhard WM, Wray LI, Towne JB. The reoperation of choice for aortofemoral graft occlusion. Surgery 1977; 82:867–874.
5. Hyde GL, McCready RA, Schwartz RW, et al. Durability of thrombectomy of occluded aortofemoral graft limbs. Surgery 1983; 94:748–751.
6. Ernst CB, Daugherty ME. Removal of a thrombotic plug from an occluded limb of an aortofemoral graft. Arch Surg 1978; 113:301–302.
7. Fogarty TJ, Hermann GD. New techniques for clot extraction and managing acute thromboembolic limb ischemia. In: Veith FJ, ed. Current critical problems in vascular surgery. Vol 3. St Louis: Quality Medical Publishing, 1991:197.
8. LaMuraglia GM, Brewster DC, Moncure AC, et al. Angioscopic evaluation of aortic graft limb thrombectomy: Is it helpful? J Vasc Surg 1993; 17:1069–1076.
9. Legrand DR, Vermilion BD, Hayes JP, Evans WE. Management of the occluded aortofemoral graft limb. Surgery 1983; 93:818–821.
10. Harris PL. Aorto-iliac-femoral re-operative surgery. Supplementary surgery at secondary operations. Acta Chir Scand 1987; 538:51–55.

MANAGEMENT OF CHYLOPERITONEUM AND CHYLOTHORAX AFTER AORTIC RECONSTRUCTION

MARK A. MATTOS, M.D.
DAVID S. SUMNER, M.D.

Chyloperitoneum and chylothorax are rare but potentially life-threatening complications of reconstruction of the abdominal or thoracic aorta. Chyloperitoneum occurs when the cisterna chyli or adjacent lymphatics are injured during aortic dissection, allowing lymph to leak into the peritoneal cavity. Injuries to the thoracic duct or lymphaticovenous collaterals are responsible for chylothorax. The identifying characteristic of these conditions is the "milky" fluid that collects within the abdomen or pleural space.

Because most of the literature concerning chyloperitoneum and chylothorax consists of single case reports, the true frequency of these conditions is unknown. The reported incidence of chylous ascites following abdominal aortic reconstruction ranges from 0.03% to 0.1%.[1] At present, only 29 cases of chyloperitoneum following aortic reconstruction have been recorded in the English literature.[1,2] Postoperative chylothorax probably occurs even less frequently. The estimated incidence ranges from 0.2% to 0.56% of all intrathoracic operations, including both cardiovascular and noncardiovascular.[3,4]

ANATOMY AND PHYSIOLOGY

Because of their proximity to the great vessels, major components of the lymphatic system are vulnerable to injury during aortic dissection. The cisterna chyli lies on the anterior surface of the L1 or L2 vertebra, posterior and somewhat medial to the aorta at the level of the renal arteries. It serves as the major lymphatic outflow tract below the diaphragm, receiving chyle from the right and left lumbar lymphatic trunks, which drain the lower extremities, mesenteric lymphatic trunk, and multiple lymphatic channels from the liver. Beginning at the cisterna chyli, the thoracic duct ascends extrapleurally through the aortic hiatus. From there, it continues upward in the right posterior mediastinum, along the anterior surfaces of the T12 and T8 vertebrae between the azygous vein and the aorta. At the level of the T6 to T4 vertebrae, the duct crosses the midline to the left posterior mediastinum; passes behind the esophagus, aortic arch, and more superiorly, the left subclavian artery; and ultimately drains into the left subclavian vein. This "classic anatomy," however, is present in only 40% to 60% of individuals. The cisterna chyli, for example, may be replaced by a rich plexus of retroperitoneal lymphatics that coalesce to form the thoracic duct. Furthermore, the thoracic duct may empty as a single channel on the right side or ascend as a duplicated trunk.

The composition, volume, and rate of chyle production also vary, depending on dietary content, bowel activity, and the level of physical activity. Chyle is characterized by a high concentration of long-chain triglycerides and the presence of chylomicrons, which give the fluid its milky white appearance. Chylomicrons are absorbed through the intestinal lymphatics, collected in the cisterna chyli, transported through the thoracic duct, and emptied into the venous system. Normal chylous flow ranges from 1,500 to 2,000 ml/day. Although lymphatic flow in the thoracic duct of resting, fasting subjects has been reported to be less than 1 ml/minute, rates as high as 225 ml/minute have been recorded in the postprandial period. Ingestion of carbohydrates and proteins has little effect on lymph flow; starvation decreases flow to a barely perceptible rate. However, ingesting fat, particularly long-chain fatty acids, or water produces remarkable increases in thoracic duct flow.

PATHOGENESIS

Although transection, laceration, or tears of the intestinal lymphatics, cisterna chyli, or thoracic duct provide an obvious explanation for the lymphatic leak, the mechanism responsible for chyloperitoneum and chylothorax remains elusive. Because chyle leaks are often observed during operation on patients who never develop these conditions, additional factors must be involved. The rich network of collateral lymphatics above and below the diaphragm makes it improbable that a simple increase in chyle production could alone lead to chyloperitoneum or chylothorax. Similarly, obstruction of lymphatic outflow by trauma to the thoracic duct, enlarged lymph nodes, lymphatic endothelial hyperplasia, or major venous obstruction is unlikely to be totally responsible. Rather, it would appear that a combination of lymphatic injury, increased chyle production, and some degree of ductal obstruction, partial or complete, is necessary.

Chyloperitoneum occurs more frequently following aortic aneurysm replacement than after reconstruction for aortoiliac occlusive disease. Of the 29 reported cases in which chylous ascites developed after aortic operations, 22 were for aneurysmal disease, 16 elective and six ruptured aneurysms. In contrast, only five cases of chylous ascites have been reported following reconstruction for occlusive disease. Two others followed removal of infected aortic grafts.[1] Thus, it appears that chyle-containing abdominal lymphatics are particularly vulnerable to injury during hurried or difficult aortic resections, particularly when extensive juxtarenal dissections are required for large or ruptured aneurysms or for secondary aortic reconstructions.

Chylothorax occurs in both the presence and absence of thoracic duct trauma.[5] Mobilization of the aortic arch, the left subclavian artery, and the great vessels in the mediastinum exposes the duct to injury. Thoracic aortic rupture and the complexity of thoracic aortic resection place both the duct and the adjacent lymphaticovenous network at increased risk. Although operations for congenital heart disease are frequently implicated, chylothorax is seldom a complication of coronary bypass grafting. Chylothorax can develop on either the left or right side and may even be bilateral, depending on the level of injury to the thoracic duct or the lymphaticovenous collaterals. Injuries below T4 to T6 produce a right-sided chylothorax, whereas injuries above this level produce a left-sided chylothorax. Simultaneous injuries above and below the T4 to T6 level may cause bilateral chylous effusions.

CLINICAL PRESENTATION AND DIAGNOSIS

Abdominal distention is the hallmark of chyloperitoneum. Twenty-eight (97%) of the 29 cases reported following aortic operations presented with ascites and abdominal distention.[1,2] Abdominal pain as an isolated symptom is infrequent. Other symptoms and signs include early satiety, nausea, vomiting, anorexia, weight loss or gain, malnourishment, weakness, edema, and dyspnea. Distention seldom becomes evident immediately after operation, owing to the low volume of lymph flow during the postoperative period. Instead, patients usually present 2 to 4 weeks after aortic reconstruction with dyspnea and progressively worsening abdominal distention and discomfort. Return to a normal dietary intake is probably necessary to increase chyle flow sufficiently to produce ascites. The mean time to the onset of abdominal distention following operation is approximately 19 days (range 7 to 120 days). Only three (10%) of 29 patients first developed distention later than 28 days after operation.

Although ultrasound or computed tomography confirms the presence of intraperitoneal fluid, the definitive diagnostic test is abdominal paracentesis. Paracentesis yields a milky-colored fluid that is odorless and sterile, resists putrefaction, and separates into a creamy layer on standing. This fluid is alkaline, with a specific gravity exceeding 1.012, a total protein content greater than 3 g/dl, a total solid content in excess of 4%, and a fat content higher than any other body fluid, ranging between 0.4 and 4 g/dl. Triglyceride levels are elevated, but the exact value depends on the patient's recent dietary intake. Sudan III staining reveals fat globules. A predominance of lymphocytes is evident on the differential white blood cell count. Other diagnostic modalities include lymphography, which is used infrequently, and lymphoscintigraphy, which may have a role in the identification of a lymph leak in patients with persistent chylous ascites.

Chylous pleural effusion is the distinguishing characteristic of postoperative chylothorax. Chylothorax typically develops during the first 2 weeks following a major thoracic operation. Presenting symptoms relate to compression of the lung and include diminished pulmonary function and subsequent respiratory embarrassment, if pleurocentesis is not performed. Occasionally, chest x-rays document widening of the superior mediastinum prior to the development of pleural effusion, an indication that chyle is trapped within the mediastinal pleural envelope. When the pleura is intact, "chylomas" of the posterior mediastinum may persist for several days until the accumulated fluid ruptures into the pleural space.[4] If the mediastinal pleura is damaged or defective at the time of aortic reconstruction, pleural effusion or chylothorax develops immediately following lymphatic injury.

Milky fluid retrieved on thoracentesis establishes the diagnosis. Like chylous ascites, chylous pleural effusions are sterile, odorless, alkaline, usually high in triglycerides, and low in cholesterol and reveal a cholesterol-triglyceride ratio greater than 1 with a specific gravity exceeding 1.012. Sudan III stain shows fat globules and a large number of lymphocytes, with cell counts ranging from 400 to 6,000/ml.[3] Lipoprotein electrophoresis identifies the presence of chylomicrons. Chyle is nonirritating and bacteriostatic and thus does not produce inflammation or infection of the pleura. Not all chylous effusions are milky in appearance. Approximately 12% of patients have serous or serosanguinous effusions, an observation consistent with restriction of enteric feeding during the immediate postoperative period.[4] With the resumption of oral intake and an increase in dietary fat content, the effusion becomes turbid or milky.

TREATMENT

Initial therapy for chyloperitoneum and chylothorax should be directed toward reducing intra-abdominal pressure to improve respiration and relieve discomfort and toward decompressing the pleural space to avoid respiratory compromise. Long-term treatment goals should focus on preventing the continued leakage of chyle, returning chyle to the body, maintaining electrolyte balance, providing adequate nutritional support to prevent a catabolic state, and establishing normal immunologic function.

Chyloperitoneum

Several methods have been used to treat chyloperitoneum following aortic reconstruction. Most patients (96%) have required a combination of two or more modalities, including single or multiple therapeutic paracenteses, diuretics, low-fat–high-protein diets, medium-chain triglyceride (MCT) diets, total parenteral nutrition (TPN), intravenous reinfusion of chyle, peritoneovenous shunting, and re-exploration with surgical repair of the lymphatic leak. Management begins with the initial paracentesis, which is both diagnostic and therapeutic (Fig. 1). Multiple therapeutic paracenteses should be avoided because serious complications may occur, such as cutaneous lymph fistulas, peritonitis, anasarca, and infection of the aortic graft. Moreover, repeated aspiration of chylous fluid may result in severe electrolyte and metabolic imbalance, cachexia (hypoalbuminemia, hypoproteinemia, weight loss), anemia, lymphocytopenia, and immunologic abnormalities, ultimately resulting in a state of inanition and immunosuppression that places the patient at risk for septic complications and possibly death. Chylous ascites has never resolved with paracentesis alone, although there is one reported success with intravenous reinfusion of chyle.[1] To foster spontaneous healing of injured lymphatics, a low-fat–high-protein diet is recommended. Low dietary fat regimens reduce the flow of chyle by decreasing production of long-chain triglycerides (LCT), which are transported through the intestinal lymphatics to the cisterna chyli and thoracic duct. A medium-chain triglyceride (MCT) diet has been advocated by many authors. MCTs are broken down in the intestinal wall and, unlike LCTs, are transported directly to the liver via the portal vein rather than having to pass through the intestinal lymphatics. A low-fat diet with MCT supplementation achieves the lowest possible flow of chyle during enteral intake.

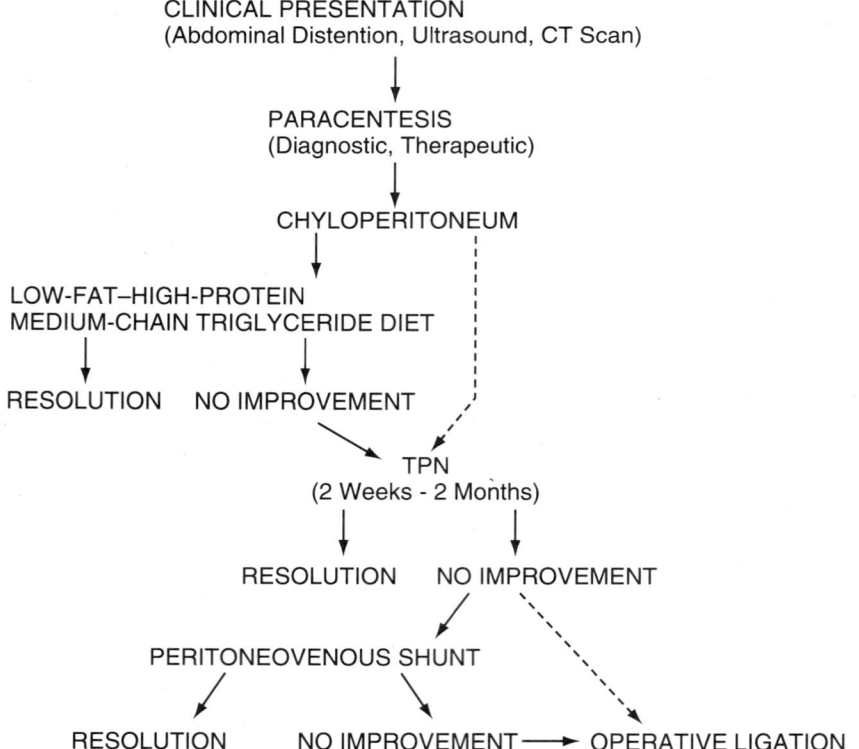

Figure 1 Algorithm for treatment of chyloperitoneum following abdominal aortic reconstruction.

If chylous ascites does not resolve with enteric feeding, the next step is to institute TPN, which places the bowel at rest and further reduces intestinal lymph flow (Fig. 1).[1,6] This allows uninterrupted healing of intestinal lymphatics, simultaneously corrects electrolyte and immunologic abnormalities, and maintains adequate fluid and nutritional support. Unfortunately, resolution of chylous ascites has been achieved in only 56% of patients when TPN was used alone or in combination with paracentesis and/or dietary manipulation (Table 1). Moreover, long-term use of TPN increases the risk of catheter-related sepsis and associated aortic graft infection.

Surgical therapy is indicated for patients who fail to respond to paracentesis, dietary management, and TPN (Fig. 1). Operative intervention, however, should be delayed in the nutritionally stable patient for at least 2 weeks to 2 months to allow for spontaneous closure of lymphatic leaks, the development of collaterals, and possible resolution of chylous ascites. If no improvement is noted during this period, peritoneovenous shunting or direct surgical repair is recommended.

Intravenous transfusion of chylous ascites is mentioned only to be condemned because it carries a prohibitive risk of complications, including infection, peritonitis, intravascular coagulopathy, and death. A more attractive alternative to autotransfusion is the use of a peritoneovenous shunt.[7,8] This minimally invasive procedure was successful in resolving chylous ascites in four (80%) of five patients who failed previous nonsurgical treatment (Table 1). Not all authors recommend the use of peritoneovenous shunting, citing possible, albeit infrequent, complications such as disseminated intravascular coagulopathy, sepsis, and subsequent death. Because most patients with chylous ascites are not optimal candidates for a major surgical procedure, peritoneovenous shunting remains the next logical step or at least an attractive alternative to suture repair of the lymphatic leak (Fig. 2).

Operative ligation of the lymphatic leak should be restricted to low-risk patients or to those in whom all other therapeutic options have failed (Fig. 1). An advantage of ligation is that it may avoid protracted hospitalization.[7] Identification of the lymph fistula can be improved by feeding the patient a preoperative meal of cream, lipophilic dyes, or nontoxic coal tar dyes. Lymph fistulas were successfully closed and ascites resolved in all five reported patients who underwent ligation (Table 1).

Although other causes of chylous ascites are associated with a grim prognosis (43% to 88% mortality),[8] chyloperitoneum following aortic reconstruction generally has a favorable outcome. There have been five reported deaths (mortality rate, 17%), three of which were directly attributable to chyloperitoneum. One patient died from inanition and two from septic complications.[1] Chylous ascites resolved in 18 (64%) of 28 patients with nonoperative treatment alone, and subsequent surgical therapy was successful in 9 of 10 patients in whom nonoperative therapy failed, for an overall success rate of 90% (Table 1). The time to complete resolution of chyloperitoneum has been quite variable and is usually prolonged, ranging from 2 weeks to 5 months (mean, 2 months).

Chylothorax

Owing to its infrequent occurrence and variable presentation, there is no consensus regarding the ideal method for treating postoperative chylothorax. Once the diagnosis has been made by thoracentesis or by the appearance of turbid or milky pleural drainage from an existing chest tube, therapy should begin with a low-fat–high-protein diet, supplemented with an MCT diet (Fig. 3). If this regimen is unsuccessful in resolving the effusion, continuous tube drainage should be used to maintain expansion of the lung. Continued loss of large amounts of chylous fluid does, however, lead to signifi-

Table 1 Results of Treating Chyloperitoneum Following Aortic Reconstruction (29 Patients)

Modality	Successful			Unsuccessful	
	N	Alive	Died	Alive	Died
Paracentesis alone	1	1	0	0	0
Diet alone	11	7	1 PE	2 (2 Lig)*	1 Inanition
TPN alone	5	1	1 Sepsis	3 (1 Lig, 2 PVS)*	0
TPN plus diet	11	6	1 MI	3 (1 Lig, 2 PVS)*	1 (1 PVS)* Sepsis
TOTAL nonoperative	28	15	3	8	2
Peritoneovenous shunt†	5	4	0	0	1 Sepsis
Ligation‡	5	0	0	0	0
TOTAL operative	10	4	0	0	1

*Subsequent therapy after failure of nonoperative management.
†All had previously unsuccessful nonoperative management.
‡Four had previously unsuccessful nonoperative management.
PE = Pulmonary embolism; MI = myocardial infarction; Lig = fistula ligation; PVS = peritoneovenous shunt; TPN = total parenteral nutrition.
Data from Pabst TS, McIntyre KE, Schilling JD, et al. Management of chyloperitoneum after abdominal aortic surgery. Am J Surg 1993; 166:194–199; and Varekamp AP, Spruit M, Bosman CHR: Chylous ascites after aortic replacement. Eur J Surg 1992; 158:623–625.

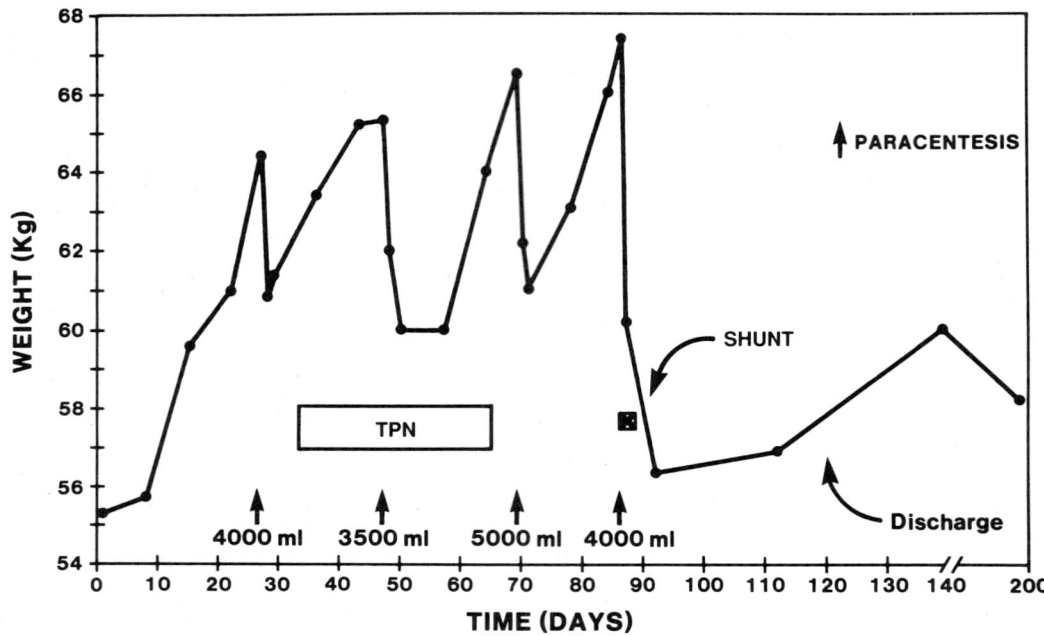

Figure 2 Effect of paracenteses and peritoneovenous shunt on the weight of a patient with chylous ascites following resection of a 10 cm abdominal aortic aneurysm. Ascites was refractory to repeated paracenteses and TPN but responded to shunt placement. (From Fleisher HL, Oren JW, Sumner DS. Chylous ascites after abdominal aortic aneurysmectomy: Successful management with a peritoneovenous shunt. J Vasc Surg 1987; 6:403–407.)

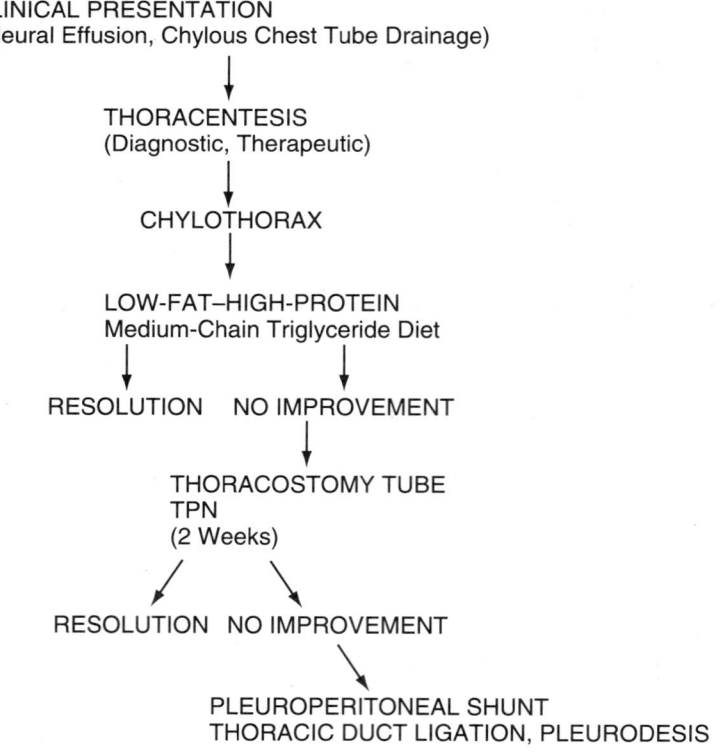

Figure 3 Algorithm for treatment of chylothorax following thoracic aortic reconstruction.

cant electrolyte, nutritional, and immunologic derangements similar to those encountered in the treatment of chyloperitoneum. Total parenteral nutrition with complete bowel rest may be used to circumvent these serious and potentially fatal complications. Several authors recommend instituting TPN and tube thoracostomy drainage at the onset of chylothorax without a trial of enteral feeding in an effort to decrease the time to closure of the lymph leak and to shorten hospitalization. Nonoperative therapy should be tried for at least 1 or 2 weeks before undertaking surgical treatment (Fig. 3).

Indications for surgical repair of chylothorax include chylous drainage greater than 1,500 ml/day in adults and greater that 100 ml/year of age in children for more than 5 days, continuous chylous flow for 14 days or more, and the development of unremitting metabolic complications or immunologic deterioration.[3,4] Although fibrin glue, talc, or tetracycline pleurodesis and pleurectomy have been used to treat chylothorax, most authors prefer pleuroperitoneal shunting[9] or thoracic duct ligation.[3,4] Pleuroperitoneal shunting, a minimally invasive procedure that is fairly well tolerated in most postoperative patients, indirectly returns chyle to the circulation and prevents the loss of important nutritional and immunologic factors. It may be particularly advantageous in children. When nonoperative therapy fails or when pleuroperitoneal shunting is tried and does not control the chylous effusion, the thoracic duct should be ligated. Ligation is performed just caudal to the lymphatic leak if the site of injury is easily identified or at the aortic hiatus if the leak cannot be visualized. A right thoracotomy is recommended if ligation of the duct at the hiatus is necessary. The thoracic duct is easily accessible at this level, where it typically exists as a single structure. Occasionally, re-exploration on the side of the original thoracotomy may be required when it is necessary to repair multiple injuries to the duct or to the lymphaticovenous collaterals.

REFERENCES

1. Pabst TS, McIntyre KE, Schilling JD, et al. Management of chyloperitoneum after abdominal aortic surgery. Am J Surg 1993; 166:194–199.
2. Varekamp AP, Spruit M, Bosman CHR. Chylous ascites after aortic replacement. Eur J Surg 1992; 158:623–625.
3. Marts BC, Naunheim KS, Fiore AC, Pennington G. Conservative versus surgical management of chylothorax. Am J Surg 1992; 164:532–535.
4. Valentine VG, Raffin TA. The management of chylothorax. Chest 1992; 102:586–591.
5. Ferguson MK, Little AG, Skinner DB. Current concepts in the management of postoperative chylothorax. Ann Thorac Surg 1985; 40:542–545.
6. Meinke AH III, Estes NC, Ernst CB. Chylous ascites following abdominal aortic aneurysmectomy. Management with total parenteral hyperalimentation. Ann Surg 1979; 190:631–633.
7. Williams RA, Vetto J, Quiñones-Baldrich W, et al. Chylous ascites following abdominal aortic surgery. Ann Vasc Surg 1991; 5:247–252.
8. Fleisher HL, Oren JW, Sumner DS. Chylous ascites after abdominal aortic aneurysmectomy: Successful management with a peritoneovenous shunt. J Vasc Surg 1987; 6:403–407.
9. Murphy MC, Newman BM, Rodgers BM. Pleuroperitoneal shunts in the management of persistent chylothorax. Ann Thorac Surg 1989; 48:195–200.

LOWER EXTREMITY OCCLUSIVE DISEASE

DOPPLER PRESSURE ASSESSMENT OF INFRAINGUINAL OCCLUSIVE DISEASE

J. DENNIS BAKER, M.D.

The qualitative evaluation of an arterial pulse provides a limited determination of the status of the cardiovascular system. Of the three parameters related to arterial circulation—pressure, volume flow, and peripheral resistance—pressure is by far the easiest to quantitate. Since the turn of the century, cardiac function has been estimated by the indirect measure of blood pressure, using the sphygmomanometer developed by Rova-Ricci. In 1950 Winsor introduced the indirect measure of extremity blood pressure at different levels as a tool in the assessment of peripheral arterial occlusive disease. Although Winsor used an air plethysmograph, the detection of the systolic end point was simplified with the introduction of the Doppler velocity detector in the 1960s. The ease of determination of segmental extremity blood pressures by this technique has resulted in this test being the most commonly performed noninvasive test.

PHYSIOLOGY

The indirect measurement of systolic blood pressure with a sphygmomanometer is based upon the principle that the occluding pressure within the pneumatic cuff is equal to the pressure causing the artery to collapse. For this assumption to be met, the width of the cuff should be 20% greater than the diameter of the limb segment studied. The systolic end point is determined as the pressure at which blood flow is first detected beyond the cuff during deflation. The measurement is an overall estimate of perfusion pressure under the cuff and cannot determine blood pressure in specific vessels or distinguish collateral vessel contributions. As a main conduit artery develops a progressive stenosis, there is an increasing contribution to distal blood pressure by collateral branches, so that even with an occlusion the gradient may be only 30 to 50 mm Hg. With stenoses in tandem, the majority of the gradient results from the tightest stenosis. The other lesions produce some additional gradient, but the effect is not a linear one and cannot be estimated mathematically.

There are two important sources of error in the use of the sphygmomanometer. If the cuff width is less than 120% of the limb diameter, the pressure required to collapse the underlying arterial segment is greater than the intra-arterial pressure. This becomes a problem most commonly with thigh measurements. The second type of error is found in arteries with pathologic stiffening, most common in diabetics, although it can occur with other conditions. Under such circumstances, the force required to collapse the artery is a combination of the intra-arterial pressure and the wall stiffness, so that the sphygmomanometer measurement is artifactually high. In extreme cases, it is not possible to arrest the flow even with the cuff inflated to 300 mm Hg.

Peripheral blood pressures are measured primarily to identify an occlusive lesion by the pressure gradient it produces. Normally, there is no significant blood pressure gradient in the main conduit arteries of an extremity. In a steady flow model the pressure drop (ΔP) across a stenosis is defined by Poiseuille's law,

$$\Delta P = \frac{Q \times 8LN}{\pi R}$$

where Q = volume flow, L = length of stenosis, N = viscosity, and R = the internal radius of the stenosis. For resting extremity blood flow rates, there is no significant pressure gradient until the diameter of the vessel is reduced more than 50%. However, at the higher blood flows that occur during exercise, a greater gradient results from the same degree of stenosis. This change in gradient is the basis for exercise testing.

ANKLE PRESSURE MEASUREMENT

Technique

The patient is examined in the supine position after resting for 15 minutes. In most situations it is important to obtain true resting measurements in order to reduce the variability resulting from changes in peripheral resistance after walking. A Doppler velocity detector with a frequency of 8 to 10 MHz is optimal. A 12 cm wide (standard arm size) blood pressure cuff is placed just above the malleoli. The Doppler probe is adjusted to obtain an optimal signal from the dorsalis pedis or the posterior tibial arteries at the level of the ankle joint. The cuff is inflated until flow stops and is then slowly deflated until flow returns. The cuff pressure at this point defines the systolic value. Diastolic blood pressure is not detected with this technique. The measurement is repeated several times to ensure a constant value. In some cases of severe ischemia, there may not be blood flow detected in the dorsalis pedis or the posterior tibial vessels, so that the anterior branch of the peroneal artery must be used. The highest blood pressure obtained at the ankle level is recorded. Bilateral brachial artery blood pressures are then measured and the higher of the two systolic values recorded.

Interpretation

The ankle blood pressure provides an overall assessment of the extent of occlusive disease in an extremity. An isolated value for an ankle blood pressure is not helpful but must be considered in the context of the patient's central blood pressure, as indicated by the higher brachial value. The usual procedure is to normalize the ankle pressure by dividing it by the brachial pressure to obtain the ankle brachial index (ABI). In a healthy person the ankle blood pressure is actually higher than that in the arm, so that normally the ABI is in a range of 1.1 to 1.2. An ABI less than 0.95 is abnormal, and in general terms, the lower the value, the more severe the occlusive disease. It is important to realize that there is overlap in ABI values of patients with intermittent claudication and those with more severe disease (Fig. 1). In general, ABI values less than 0.5 are found in patients with multilevel disease.

Often ABI values are used for determination of progression of disease or for postoperative follow-up. In some people the ankle index remains quite constant; in others there is day-to-day variation. This range of blood pressure responses in the lower extremities may be related to differences in sympathetic activity due to temperature or stress, levels of recent exercise, or reaction to smoking. Unless one has previous data to document a constant level of ABI, a change in the ratio of 0.15 is required to be considered significant.[1]

There are potential errors in measuring the ABI. The most common problem is the artifactually elevated index found in patients with pathologically stiff vessels. This condition precludes the use of ankle blood pressures in 5% to 15% of these patients. In some patients the error is obvious for the vessels may be so stiff that blood flow persists in spite of the cuff being inflated to 300 mm Hg. In others the problem is more subtle, and patients with significant occlusive disease may have ABIs in the normal range. A simple step to identify this source of error is to palpate the ankle pulses. An artery with a normal ABI should have a full, easily palpable pulse. Failure to palpate a pulse in a vessel with a normal index indicates an artifact, and the blood pressure measurements should not be used to assess the severity of occlusive disease. In these patients assessment is usually possible by measuring blood pressure in the toe or forefoot because the foot vessels are not as commonly affected by severe stiffening. Forefoot blood pressure is measured with a cuff around the forefoot and Doppler detection of blood flow in one of the distal branches. Toe blood pressure is measured with a 1 inch cuff around the first toe. Although the blood pressure end point can be determined with a Doppler device, this is often difficult, so a plethysmographic technique is commonly used.

SEGMENTAL PRESSURES

Technique

Blood pressures are measured at different levels of the leg to provide an estimate of level of occlusive disease. For the lower leg, 12 cm wide cuffs are placed just below the knee and above the malleoli. Thigh determinations are done either with a single thigh cuff (18 cm or greater) or with 12 cm cuffs, one placed just above the knee and the second as high on the thigh as possible. The single cuff technique is used to obtain an accurate thigh blood pressure determination. By contrast, the two-cuff technique must account for the artifact produced by a narrow cuff but is intended to distinguish between occlusive lesions above and below the superficial femoral artery. The high cuff is taken as reflecting the blood pressure at the common femoral artery; the low thigh cuff is used to assess the superficial

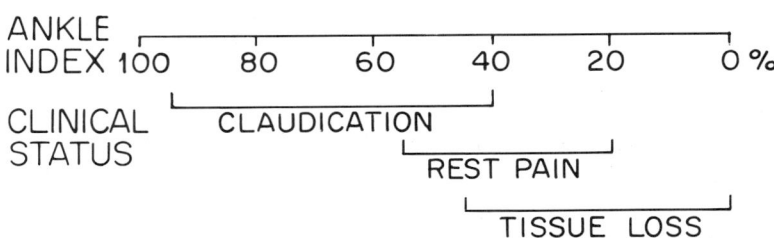

Figure 1 Range of ABI values for patients in different clinical categories.

femoral and upper popliteal levels. Most laboratories use the ankle artery with the best Doppler signal as the distal sensing site for segmental blood pressure measurements. Franzeck and associates compared thigh blood pressure measurements obtained using the popliteal artery and an ankle artery as sensing sites. They found that the blood pressures were significantly lower in 23% of patients using the ankle level for Doppler detection.[2] In spite of this report, few laboratories use the popliteal artery as the sensing site for thigh blood pressures.

Interpretation

A wide thigh cuff has the advantage of avoiding an artifact. Normally the thigh blood pressure should equal the brachial pressure. Flanigan and colleagues[3] and Francfort and co-workers[4] have defined the normal thigh-brachial ratio as being above 0.9. Some investigators have arbitrarily defined the high thigh artifacts as 30 mm Hg so that a normal high thigh blood pressure is 30 mm Hg or more above the brachial pressure.[5,6] The other approach is to use a high thigh-brachial ratio, with normal usually considered above 1.[3,4] Gradients of 20 mm Hg or more reflect occlusive disease between cuff levels. When tandem lesions exist, the effect of the severity of the distal lesion may be underestimated if a tight proximal stenosis or occlusion is combined with poor collateral. The limited blood flow reaching the second lesion does not cause as large a pressure gradient as would result in the absence of the proximal one.

Segmental leg blood pressures measured at four levels fail to distinguish the level of occlusive disease in about one-fourth of patients. Studies addressing this question report accuracies between 70% and 78% in correct identification of level.[4,5,7] The variable level of superficial femoral artery lesions and the presence or absence of deep femoral artery disease account for the limitations of the pressure measurements. Whereas an abnormal thigh blood pressure does not always distinguish between disease above and below the inguinal ligament, it is important to note that a normal thigh pressure essentially rules out aortoiliac disease.[3,7]

EXERCISE TESTING

Routine screening studies are performed at rest to assess baseline status; however, in some patients these tests may miss early, symptomatic occlusive disease. In such cases there may not be a significant pressure drop at rest. The Poiseuille equation predicts that the gradient across a stenosis is proportional to the flow. With exercise the femoral artery blood flow normally rises threefold to fivefold, and the hemodynamic effect of a moderate stenosis increases accordingly. If there is a flow-limiting stenosis, the pressure taken immediately after exercise is reduced, with gradual return to resting baseline (Fig. 2).

Exercise testing is usually performed by having the patient walk on a treadmill. A common protocol has the patient walk for 5 minutes at 2 mph on a 12% incline.[8] This represents a relatively low level of exercise compared to a cardiac stress test. Patients with severe, multilevel disease are so limited by claudication that they cannot walk for 5 minutes, in which case they walk until symptoms force them to stop. Some patients are forced to stop by angina or shortness of breath. It is important to note these limiting factors, for they suggest that the patient's main limitation is the result of an etiology other than the arterial insufficiency. Baseline ABIs are measured before walking. Repeat pressures are measured as soon as possible after the end of exercise and at 1 minute intervals for 5 minutes. Although patients with severe disease may not return to baseline within 5 minutes, collecting data beyond this point does not add significantly to the test. Also, it is

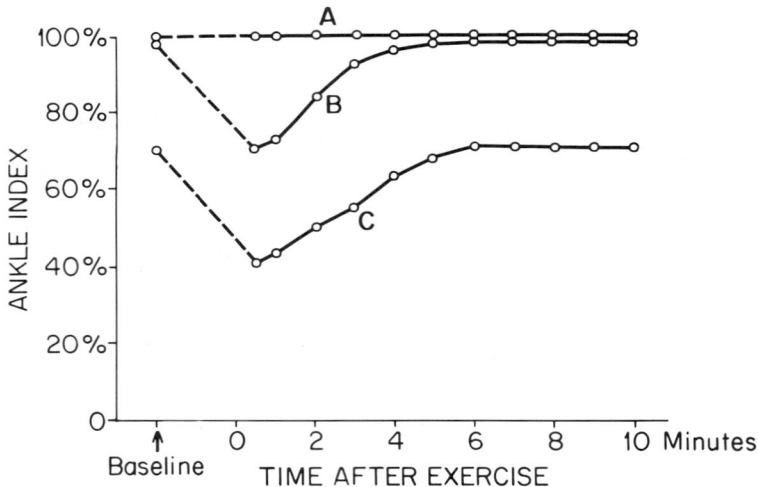

Figure 2 Change in ABI following 5 minutes of treadmill exercise. *A*, Normal subject; *B*, early disease with limited claudication and normal resting ABI; *C*, more severe occlusive disease.

unlikely that a treadmill test is indicated in patients with this severity of disease.

A normal person has no drop in the ankle index. The severity of arterial insufficiency is reflected by both the magnitude of the blood pressure drop and the duration of the recovery phase. Patient B with a normal resting ABI has a gradient brought out by the walking, and the recovery phase is typical of mild claudication (Fig. 2). Patient C, with advanced occlusive disease has an abnormal resting value, which has both a greater drop and a slower recovery. For patients who cannot walk because of cardiac or other limitations, an alternative stress test can be carried out by using the reactive hyperemia that follows a period of pneumatic cuff occlusion at the thigh.[8]

In clinical practice, exercise testing is only indicated in a small proportion of patients. It is most helpful in patients with symptoms of intermittent claudication and normal or borderline resting ABI values. A normal exercise test rules out vascular insufficiency as the cause of the complaints.

ADJUNCTIVE TESTS

In practice, extremity blood pressures are rarely used as the only technique. Experience has shown that adding a second study improves the accuracy of lower extremity evaluation. A common adjunct is the pulse volume recorder (PVR), a calibrated air plethysmograph. The device records the change in the blood volume during the cardiac cycle of the portion of the extremity under a pneumatic cuff. In most laboratories the contour of the tracing is assessed qualitatively and assigned to one of several categories. Rutherford and associates[9] and Kempczinski[10] have reported improved diagnostic accuracy when extremity blood pressures are combined with PVR recordings. Another approach is to obtain Doppler velocity recordings at the femoral, popliteal, and ankle levels. These recordings are either evaluated qualitatively or by a quantitative analysis such as pulsatility index or LaPlace damping index. Both of these adjunctive techniques are valuable because they are not affected by arterial wall stiffening.

CLINICAL APPLICATIONS

The primary use of extremity blood pressure measurements is for screening both in initial assessment and follow-up. It is important to remember that these tests provide an overall evaluation rather than giving specific information about discrete arteries. In past years great efforts were made to improve the accuracy of the correct identification of level of occlusive disease; however, duplex scanning now provides the ideal tool for comprehensive evaluation. The duplex scan can accurately detect the anatomic location of disease but can also distinguish stenosis from occlusion. Then again, the simplicity of instrumentation and examination makes Doppler blood pressure measurement an inexpensive yet objective evaluation. A large proportion of patients can be examined with this method, and the more expensive alternatives reserved for specific situations identified by the screening.

REFERENCES

1. Baker JD, Dix D. Variability of Doppler ankle pressures with arterial occlusive disease: An evaluation of ankle index and brachial-ankle pressure gradient. Surgery 1976; 79:134–137.
2. Franzeck UK, Bernstein EF, Fronek A. The effect of sensing site on the limb segmental blood pressure determination. Arch Surg 1981; 116:912–916.
3. Flanigan DP, Gray B, Schuler JJ, et al. Utility of wide and narrow blood pressure cuffs in the hemodynamic assessment of aortoiliac occlusive disease. Surgery 1982; 92:16–20.
4. Francfort JW, Bigelow PS, Davis JT, Berkowitz HD: Noninvasive techniques in the assessment of lower-extremity arterial occlusive disease. Arch Surg 1984; 119:1145–1148.
5. Heintz SE, Bone GE, Slaymaker EE, et al. Value of arterial pressure measurements in the proximal and distal part of the thigh in arterial disease. Surg Gynecol Obstet 1978; 146:337–343.
6. Lynch TG, Hobson RW, Wright CB, et al. Interpretation of Doppler segmental pressures in peripheral vascular occlusive disease. Arch Surg 1984; 119:465–467.
7. Beijneveld WJ, van Asten WNJC, Rutten WEAM, et al. How accurate are high thigh narrow cuff pressure measurements in the assessment of aorto-iliac obstructive disease? Eur J Vasc Surg 1989; 3:523–527.
8. Baker JD. Stress testing. In: Kempczinski RF, Yao JST, eds. Practical noninvasive diagnosis. Chicago: Year Book, 1987:127.
9. Rutherford RB, Lowenstein DH, Klein MF. Combining segmental systolic pressures and plethysmography to diagnose arterial occlusive disease of the legs. Am J Surg 1979; 138:211–218.
10. Kempczinski RF. Segmental volume plethysmography in the diagnosis of lower extremity arterial occlusive disease. J Cardiovasc Surg (Torino) 1982; 23:125–129.

DUPLEX IMAGING OF INFRAINGUINAL OCCLUSIVE DISEASE

GREGORY L. MONETA, M.D.

The preferred noninvasive test for evaluation of patients with suspected chronic lower extremity ischemia depends upon individual circumstances. Doppler-derived ankle-brachial systolic blood pressure indices (ABI) provide an accurate and reproducible measure of overall blood supply to the foot in patients without extensive mural calcification. Simple ABIs are clinically most useful for confirming the presence but not the location of occlusive disease.

Treatment decisions are frequently influenced both by the degree and location of occlusive lesions. Four-cuff segmental blood pressures can be used to grossly localize hemodynamically significant lower extremity arterial stenoses. Accuracy of four-cuff blood pressures is, however, significantly reduced by multilevel disease and is suboptimal for detection of iliac occlusive disease. In addition, four-cuff pressures cannot distinguish between long- and short-segment occlusions or between those vessels that remain patent but highly stenotic, distinctions that are important in screening patients for possible endovascular procedures. Many of these limitations can be overcome by using color duplex scanning.

EQUIPMENT AND TECHNIQUE

Lower extremity arterial color flow duplex imaging is performed with a variety of ultrasound transducers. For iliac vessels 3 mHz transducers are optimal, whereas a 5 mHz transducer suffices for most infrainguinal vessel examinations. Distal tibial arteries occasionally are best examined with a 7.5 or 10 mHz transducer. Angle correction is necessary. Not all lower extremity arteries can be readily insonated at the ideal Doppler angle of 60°. Angles between 30° and 70° can, however, always be

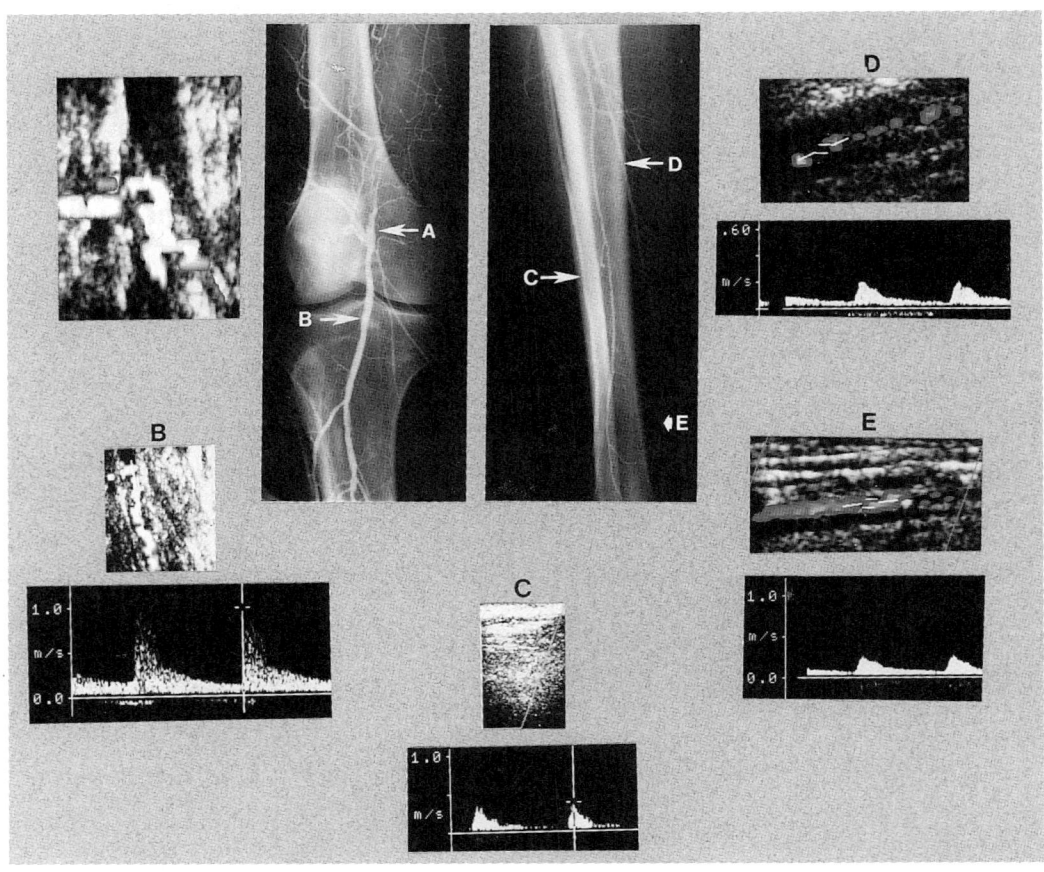

Figure 1 Arteriogram and duplex mapping from a patient with a distal superficial femoral artery (SFA) occlusion. Duplex mapping correctly identified the SFA occlusion, site of reconstitution of the popliteal artery, and intact anterior and posterior tibial artery runoff. (From Moneta GL, Yeager RA, Antonovic R, et al. Accuracy of lower extremity arterial duplex mapping. J Vasc Surg 1992; 15:275–284; with permission.)

obtained. The results obtained within this range of Doppler angles in lower extremity arterial duplex mapping provide information sufficiently accurate for clinical purposes, provided only velocity waveforms obtained at similar angles are compared.

Color flow greatly aids duplex examination of lower extremity arteries, particularly the iliac and tibial arteries. It facilitates vessel location, helps in identification of points of turbulence associated with stenoses, and can determine the length of arterial occlusions while identifying sites of reconstitution of occluded vessels (Fig. 1). Accurate quantification of stenosis, however, requires spectral analysis. Color column measurements are less accurate than spectral analysis in quantifying stenoses. It is important to remember that color is a display of average, not peak, velocity shifts and that it changes with changes in the angle of insonation. Clinical application of duplex mapping to the lower extremity arteries, therefore, begins with color flow to identify the arteries and ensure a reliable Doppler angle. Depending on the color settings, it may help to localize areas suspicious for stenoses, but only elevated peak systolic velocities can be used reliably as an indication of a significant stenosis. Points within a vessel that do not fill on color flow and do not have an associated Doppler signal indicate occlusion.

A complete lower extremity arterial duplex examination extends from the aorta to the ankle and is best performed in the morning after an overnight fast, which reduces the amount of intra-abdominal gas present at the time of examination and facilitates evaluation of the iliac arteries. All arteries, with the exception of the popliteal, are examined moving proximal to distal with the patient supine. The femoral bifurcation is more easily visualized with the leg slightly externally rotated. The popliteal artery is best insonated in the prone position to avoid confusion with large geniculate collateral vessels. Tibial arteries, when occluded proximally, are examined by identifying the vessel at the ankle and moving cephalad. With persistence, adherence to this protocol, and well-trained, experienced vascular technologists, adequate visualization of the lower extremity vessels to the level of the ankle is almost always possible[1] (Table 1). Complete examination of both legs requires 1 to 2 hours, and difficult examinations take even more time. However, complete examinations are unusual except as a research protocol. Most examinations are shortened by focusing on only clinically suspicious areas.

VELOCITY WAVEFORMS AND CRITERIA DEFINING STENOSES

Lower extremity arterial velocity waveforms are triphasic in the absence of significant upstream stenosis. Systolic forward flow is followed by a short reverse flow component, and then diastolic forward flow declines to or near zero at the end of diastole. Peak systolic velocities in normal lower extremity arteries gradually decrease from the aortic bifurcation to the knee[2] (Table 2). Velocities in continuously patent tibial arteries in the absence of proximal occlusive disease are about 50 cm/second and remain relatively constant from proximal to distal with no differences between the peroneal, anterior, and posterior tibial arteries.[3]

Jäger and colleagues first proposed duplex criteria for grading isolated stenoses in the iliac, femoral, and popliteal arteries[4] (Table 3). These criteria depend heavily on analysis of spectral broadening for detection of stenoses of less than 50% diameter reduction. Because apparent spectral broadening is difficult to quantify in clinical studies and can be increased by increasing sample volume size and/or the gain control of the duplex scanner, clinicians have not found spectral broadening to be useful in quantifying mild lower extremity arterial stenoses. However, the criteria for 50% to 99% stenosis have proven quite accurate in prospective blinded clinical studies (Table 4). In addition, color flow duplex scanning is very reliable in distinguishing stenosis from occlusion in iliac and

Table 1 Visualization by Color Flow Duplex Scanning of Arterial Segments in 286 Lower Extremities Also Studied with Arteriography

Artery	Number of Segments Satisfactorily Visualized by Angiography	Percent of Angiographic Visualized Segments Also Visualized by Color Flow Duplex
Common iliac	269	95
External iliac	265	98
Common femoral	261	100
Deep femoral (origin)	246	99
Superficial femoral*	616	100
Popliteal†	380	99
Anterior tibial*	539	94
Posterior tibial*	525	96
Peroneal*	506	83

*Represents total of separate analysis of proximal, middle, and distal segments of the vessel.
†Represents total of separate analysis of above- and below-knee segments of the vessel.

Table 2 Peak Systolic Velocities in Normal Lower Extremity Arteries

Artery	Peak Systolic Velocity (cm/second)
Common iliac	111 ± 17
External iliac	112 ± 49
Common femoral	90 ± 41
Superficial femoral (proximal)	89 ± 23
Superficial femoral (distal)	74 ± 21
Popliteal	59 ± 12

From Sacks D. Peripheral arterial duplex ultrasonography. Semin Roentgenol 1992; 27:28–38; with permission.

femoropopliteal arterial segments, with accuracies of 98% to 100%.[1,5]

To date we have not attempted to quanitate tibial artery stenoses but rather have sought to predict patency of a tibial artery from the popliteal trifurcation to the ankle. Sensitivities and specificities for duplex scanning in predicting interruption of anterior and posterior tibial artery patency are 90% to 93%. Those for the peroneal artery are 82% and 74% respectively.[1]

Table 3 Original Spectral Criteria for Duplex Identified Stenoses in Lower Extremity Arteries

Percent Stenosis	Criteria
0	Normal waveforms and velocities
1–19	Normal waveforms and velocities; spectral broadening primarily on the downslope of the systolic portion of the velocity curve
20–49	Normal triphasic waveform with marked spectral broadening; there is at least a 30% increase in peak systolic velocity
50–99	Loss of end systolic reverse flow; 100% or more increase in peak systolic velocity
Occluded	No detectable Doppler signal in an adequately visualized vessel

From Jäger KA, Phillips DJ, Martin RL, et al. Noninvasive mapping of lower limb arterial lesions. Ultrasound Med Biol 1985; 11:515–521.

CLINICAL APPLICATIONS

Color Flow Duplex Scanning Versus Segmental Doppler Blood Pressures

An obvious use of lower extremity arterial color duplex scanning is as an alternative to lower extremity segmental Doppler blood pressures. We have compared the ability of arterial duplex mapping and segmental blood pressures to detect a 50% to 100% stenosis in above-knee arteries from 151 lower extremities.[8] We found the ability of duplex to detect a 50% to 100% lesion in the iliac, common femoral, superficial femoral, and popliteal arteries to be superior to segmental pressures at every level (Table 5). In addition, there was complete agreement between duplex mapping and arteriography in 82% of the limbs studied. Complete agreement between arteriography and segmental blood pressures was found in only 34% of limbs ($p < 0.0001$). Further advantages of duplex over segmental pressures include the ability to distinguish a stenosis from occlusion and to measure the lengths of occluded segments.

It is, however, not practical to replace segmental blood pressures with duplex scanning. In most clinical settings, segmental pressures have provided a reasonable estimate of arterial disease distribution. Research protocols designed to assess progression of lower extremity arterial disease should, however, employ duplex scan-

Table 4 Sensitivities, Specificities, Positive (PPV), and Negative Predictive (NPV) Values for Duplex Scanning in Detecting ≥50% Stenoses in Lower Extremity Arteries Proximal to the Tibial Vessels*

Author	Number Patients	Iliac	Common Femoral	Deep Femoral	Superficial Femoral	Popliteal
Kohler, et al[5]		89/90	67/98	67/81	84/93	75/97
		75/96	80/96	53/88	90/88	86/93
Moneta, et al[1]	150	89/99	76/99	83/97	87/98	67/99
		94/97	93/96	83/97	97/89	93/94
Cossman, et al[6]	61	81/98	70/97	71/95	87/85	84/97
		94/92	78/96	56/97	86/72	93/93
Legemate, et al[7]†	40	92/98	NA	NA	88/98	
		90/98	NA	NA	94/97	

*Sensitivity/specificity.
†NA = Data not available; superficial femoral and popliteal arteries combined for data analysis.

Table 5 Comparison of Segmental Doppler Pressures (SDP) and Duplex Mapping (DM) in Detection of 50% to 100% Stenoses in Arterial Segments from 151 Lower Extremities

Arterial Segment	Correct Findings (n)		Incorrect Findings (n)		p Value
	SDP	DM	SDP	DM	
Iliac/common femoral ($n = 151$)	114	140	37	11	<0.0001
Superficial femoral ($n = 151$)	113	146	38	5	<0.0001
Popliteal ($n = 151$)	82	137	69	14	<0.0001

Adapted from Moneta GL, Yeager RA, Lee RW, Porter JM. Noninvasive localization of arterial occlusive disease: A comparison of segmental Doppler pressures and arterial duplex scanning. J Vasc Surg 1993; 17:578–582.

ning as a means of following individual arteries or arterial segments.

As a clinical tool, lower extremity arterial duplex scanning is used in our vascular laboratory primarily to answer precise questions about specific arterial segments that are suspected to have changed from a previous noninvasive or arteriographic examination. Others with a particular interest in the application of endovascular techniques to the treatment of arterial occlusive disease have suggested arterial duplex scanning may be used to screen patients for an endovascular procedure.

Color Flow Duplex Scanning in Preparation for Endovascular Therapy

Advocates of endovascular treatment point out that some moderately claudicating patients who do not respond to conservative measures and who do not want the discomfort and more prolonged recovery of an operative procedure may be candidates for endovascular therapy. This is obviously contrary to traditional vascular surgical practice, in which therapy is based on severity of symptoms and not the availability of a procedure to correct an anatomic defect. Nevertheless, a number of centers have begun to evaluate duplex mapping as a screening procedure prior to arteriography, with the goal of determining if it can identify patients for endovascular therapy.

Jäger and colleagues first reported a series of patients selected for transluminal angioplasty based on symptoms, physical examination, and lower extremity arterial duplex mapping.[9] Later, Cossman and associates also documented the accuracy of duplex mapping in the identification of lesions anatomically suited for a endovascular intervention.[6]

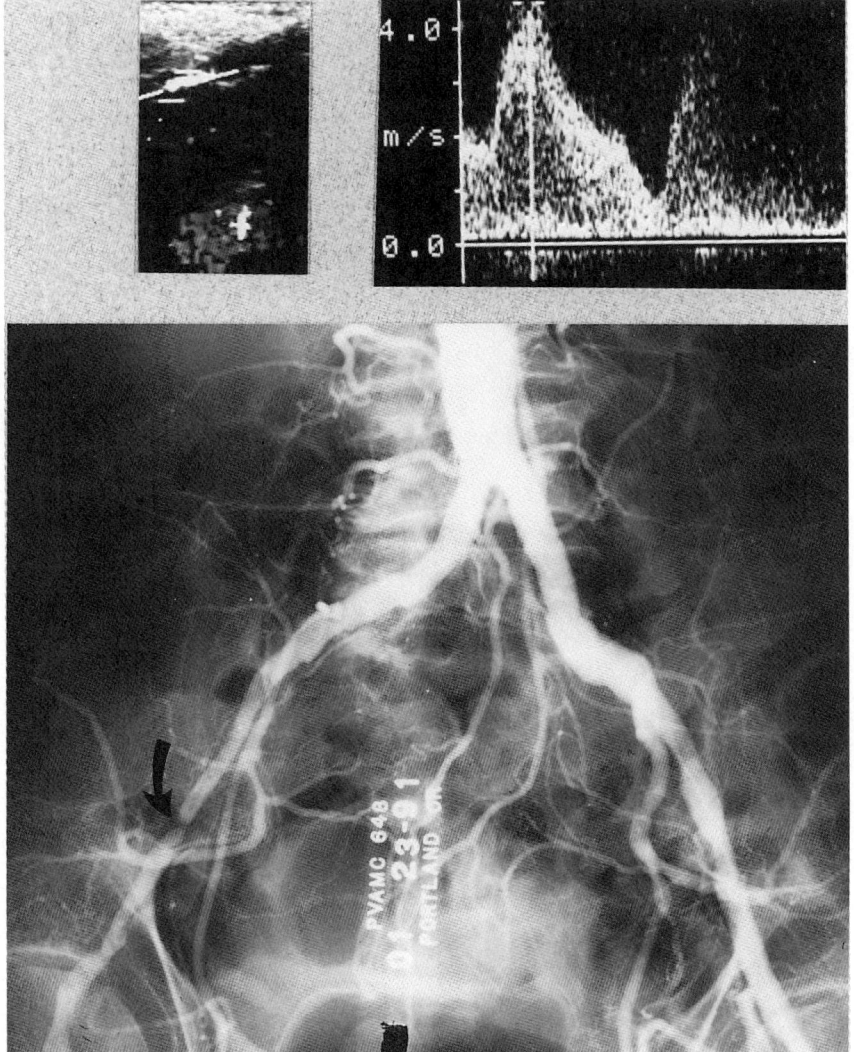

Figure 2 Duplex mapping documenting a high-grade focal external iliac stenosis felt suitable for transluminal angioplasty in a patient with short-distance right leg claudication.

Edwards and co-workers reported 110 patients with lower extremity arteriography preceded by arterial duplex mapping.[10] Fifty patients were scheduled for a percutaneous intervention based on the duplex mapping study. In 47 of the 50 patients (94%), an anticipated endovascular procedure was performed.[10] Van der Heijden and colleagues also reported 31 patients with 51 arterial lesions determined by arterial duplex mapping to be suitable for transluminal angioplasty.[11] In 48 of 51 lesions, duplex mapping accurately predicted the location and character of the lesion as subsequently determined by arteriography. These authors also noted that duplex mapping was useful in determining puncture sites and catheter routes for percutaneous angioplasty[11] (Fig. 2).

Intra-arterial Pressure Gradients

The ability of duplex imaging to predict blood pressure gradients across an arterial stenosis is not established. However, the Bernoulli equation is used to calculate pressure gradients across heart valves. With certain assumptions the equation is simplified to

$$P = 4(Vmax)^2,$$

where P is the pressure gradient in mm Hg across a stenosis and $Vmax$ is the maximum intrastenosis systolic flow velocity.

Clinical studies comparing iliac artery blood pressure gradients determined by duplex scanning and the simplified Bernoulli equation to arteriographic pull-back catheter gradients are inconclusive. In one study of 18 patients, correlation was poor ($R = 0.54$);[12] in another study of 11 patients, it was very good ($R = 0.9$).[13] A larger prospective study of 60 patients produced intermediate results ($R = 0.62$).[11]

Arterial Duplex Mapping Instead of Arteriography Prior to Operation

We have performed a small number of elective lower extremity arterial reconstructions based only on physical examination and duplex mapping. No obvious complications have been noted. These procedures were performed in the setting of very strong relative contraindications to arteriography. We continue to believe that arteriography is required for optimal preoperative planning. Although duplex mapping can accurately screen for hemodynamically significant lesions above the knee and predict patency of tibial arteries, its ability to identify the best distal anastomotic site, particularly in a tibial vessel, has not been established. However, Kohler and colleagues have suggested that individual vascular surgeons will, in many cases, make similar preoperative plans regardless of whether the patients' arterial anatomy was determined by arteriography or duplex mapping.[14] Determination of the particular circumstances in which surgical reconstruction may be based on duplex mapping alone will require careful prospective study.

REFERENCES

1. Moneta GL, Yeager RA, Antonovic R, et al. Accuracy of lower extremity arterial duplex mapping. J Vasc Surg 1992; 15:275–284.
2. Sacks D. Peripheral arterial duplex ultrasonography. Semin Roentgenology 1992; 27:28–38.
3. Caster JD, Cummings CA, Moneta GL, et al. Accuracy of tibial artery duplex mapping (TADM). J Vasc Tech 1992; 16:63–68.
4. Jäger KA, Phillips DJ, Martin RL, et al. Noninvasive mapping of lower limb arterial lesions. Ultrasound Med Biol 1985; 11:515–521.
5. Kohler TR, Nance DR, Cramer MM, et al. Duplex scanning for diagnosis of aortoiliac and femoropopliteal disease: A prospective study. Circulation 1987; 76:1074–1080.
6. Cossman DV, Ellison JE, Wagner WH, et al. Comparison of contrast arteriography to arterial mapping with color flow duplex imaging in the lower extremities. J Vasc Surg 1989; 10:522–529.
7. Legemate DA, Teeuwen C, Hoeneveld H, et al. The potential of duplex scanning to replace aortoiliac and femoropopliteal angiography. Eur J Vasc Surg 1989; 3:49–54.
8. Moneta GL, Yeager RA, Lee RW, Porter JM. Noninvasive localization of arterial occlusive disease: A comparison of segmental Doppler pressures and arterial duplex mapping. J Vasc Surg 1993; 17:578–582.
9. Jäger KA, Johl H, Seifert H, et al. Perkutane transluminale angioplastic (PTA) ohne vorausgehude diagosische arteriographic. VASA 1986; 15 (suppl):24 (abstract).
10. Edwards JM, Coldwell DM, Goldman ML, et al. The role of duplex scanning in the selection of patients for transluminal angioplasty. J Vasc Surg 1991; 13:69–74.
11. Van der Heijden FHWN, Legemate DA, vanLeeuwen MS, et al. Value of duplex scanning in the selection of patients for transluminal angioplasty. Eur J Vasc Surg 1993; 7:71–76.
12. Kohler TR, Nicholls SC, Zierler RE, et al. Assessment of pressure gradient by Doppler ultrasound: Experimental and clinical observations. J Vasc Surg 1987; 6:460–469.
13. Langsfeld M, Nepute J, Hershey FB, et al. The use of deep duplex scanning to predict hemodynamically significant aortoiliac stenoses. J Vasc Surg 1988; 7:395–399.
14. Kohler TR, Andros G, Porter JM, et al. Can duplex scanning replace arteriography for lower extremity arterial disease? Ann Vasc Surg 1990; 4:270–278.

CONVENTIONAL ARTERIOGRAPHIC DIAGNOSIS OF INFRAINGUINAL OCCLUSIVE DISEASE

P.C. SHETTY, M.D.
DAVID J. KASTAN, M.D.

Conventional arteriography remains the gold standard for imaging blood vessels in patients with peripheral vascular occlusive disease. Recording of the images during arteriography currently includes film-screen combination and digital, as well as digital subtraction. In most instances, infrainguinal occlusive disease is a local manifestation of a more generalized disease process. For this reason, it is important to evaluate the entire vascular tree with supplemental imaging as indicated.

PREARTERIOGRAPHIC EVALUATION

Arteriography for evaluation of infrainguinal occlusive disease is performed on an outpatient basis unless there are reasons for the patient to be admitted to the hospital. Knowledge of the patient's medical history with particular regard for associated cardiac and cerebral vascular disease, renal insufficiency, coagulation abnormalities, and allergy history is crucial to minimize the risks of arteriography.[1] It is important for optimal care that good communication be established with the referring vascular surgeon, who should provide results of any noninvasive studies,[2] the likely arteriographic findings, and possible treatment options so that one may design an appropriate arteriographic procedure. Peripheral vascular occlusive disease is a dynamic process, and a stenosis may progress to occlusion quickly. Recent data suggest that arteriography may accelerate the occlusive disease process.[3] For this reason, it is important to perform a dedicated, limited clinical examination of the patient with special attention to the lower extremity pulses just before and after arteriography.[1] We routinely obtain serum creatinine, blood urea nitrogen, prothrombin time, partial thromboplastin time, hemoglobin, and platelet counts prior to arteriography. In addition, bleeding time may be obtained if the patient is receiving antiplatelet medication such as aspirin, particularly if a transaxillary or translumbar approach is required for catheter insertion.

PREMEDICATION

Sedative and analgesic drugs, in conjunction with verbal reassurance, are used to reduce patient anxiety and pain during peripheral arteriography, although universal agreement on the ideal premedication and pain control protocol does not exist. Hence, selection of appropriate medication should be based on the patient's physical condition, response to previous medication, and procedural requirements. We recommend that all patients receive 0.4 mg of atropine sulfate as part of premedication, 30 minutes before the procedure. For sedative and amnestic effects, we recommend midazolam, allowing at least 5 minutes between doses. Midazolam is rapidly metabolized by the liver and has a plasma half-life of 30 to 60 minutes, which is significantly less than diazepam and lorazepam. Fentanyl is used as an analgesic because it has a shorter half-life and less myocardial depressant action than morphine and meperidine. Fentanyl is also given intravenously in incremental doses. Response to intravenous fentanyl begins within 2 minutes and lasts for 45 to 60 minutes.[4]

Vital signs, electrocardiogram, and peripheral oxygen saturation are monitored continuously. The importance of appropriate patient monitoring during the procedure and in the immediate postprocedural period cannot be overemphasized. Indeed, it is a must for the prompt diagnosis of untoward effects of arteriography, such as contrast reaction or other adverse cardiac or pulmonary events.

TECHNICAL CONSIDERATIONS

Arterial Puncture and Catheterization

Retrograde catheter insertion by percutaneous puncture of the common femoral artery (CFA) is considered the safest method of performing peripheral arteriography. Because antegrade femoral artery puncture is often more time-consuming and technically difficult, we reserve this approach for interventional procedures such as fibrinolytic therapy or angioplasty. We discourage the redirecting of a retrograde transfemoral catheter to an antegrade direction because of the increased incidence of local complications such as hematoma and vessel dissection. With bilaterally normal CFA pulses, puncture and retrograde catheterization of the right CFA are performed for a bilateral lower extremity arteriography simply because most angiographic suites are better suited to this arrangement. The left CFA approach is used if there is a decreased right femoral pulse.

When both femoral artery pulses are significantly decreased, we utilize a high left brachial approach. Better hemostasis can be obtained after puncture of the proximal segment of the brachial artery rather than the axillary artery. Not infrequently, a significant amount of manipulation is required to catheterize the descending aorta via puncture of the right brachial artery. For this reason, the right brachial approach is used only in the presence of significant disease in the left brachial, axillary, or subclavian arteries.

An uncomplicated aortobifemoral graft can be punctured and catheterized 6 months after placement for performing arteriography, although our surgeons prefer transaxillary access where possible. A complication of the latter is more easily handled than graft injury. Similarly, an uncomplicated axillofemoral graft can be punctured using a 18 gauge sheathed needle. We do not recommend catheter manipulation within axillofemoral grafts because of a high incidence of graft complications.

When transfemoral and transbrachial catheterization are not possible, translumbar aortography (TLA) may be used. We recommend utilizing a sheathed needle for translumbar aortography, primarily for reasons of safety, but also for improving the quality of the study. Injection through the sheath can be performed proximal or distal to the puncture site by directing the sheath cephalad or caudad. This technique also minimizes damage to the aortic wall at the puncture site and minimizes the risk of injection of contrast outside the aortic lumen, which may occur as a result of inadvertent patient motion.

Except for TLA, we use 18 gauge, short-beveled, single-wall arterial puncture needles for arterial access. A floppy guide wire with 3 mm J-tip for Seldinger vessel access is used to minimize the chance of vessel dissection. Our incidence of dissection with single-wall needles is no different than that reported for double-wall needles. A 5 Fr pigtail catheter is generally used for aortic flood injections. A 4 Fr or 5 Fr straight multihole catheter is used for injections in the external iliac artery to evaluate the ipsilateral lower extremity, and a 5 Fr end-hole catheter is used for injections in the femoral or popliteal arteries via contralateral or antegrade femoral artery puncture.

Contrast Material and Injection Parameters

Currently, it is reasonable to use low-osmolar contrast material (LOCM) for aortography with runoff. It reduces discomfort and minimizes the adverse effects of contrast on the kidneys and the heart. For a patient with known serious reaction to iodinated contrast material, carbon dioxide may be an alternative contrast agent. In all new patients being evaluated for infrainguinal occlusive disease, we prefer to study the renal

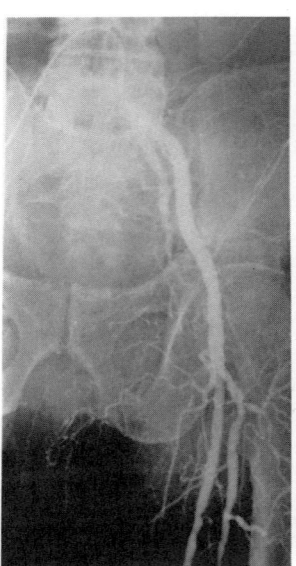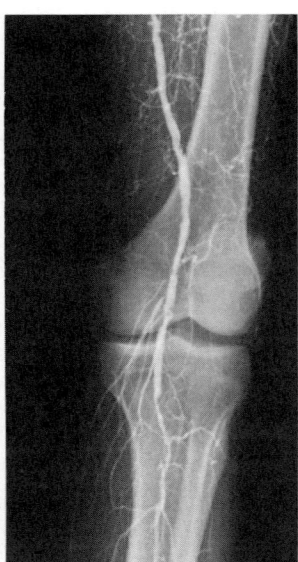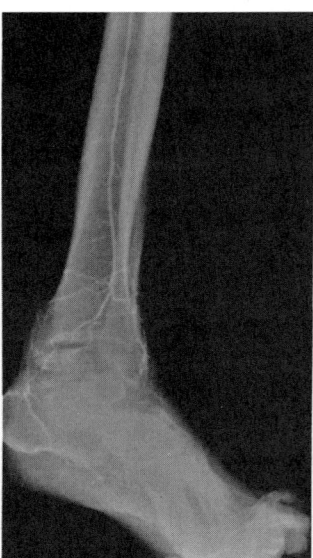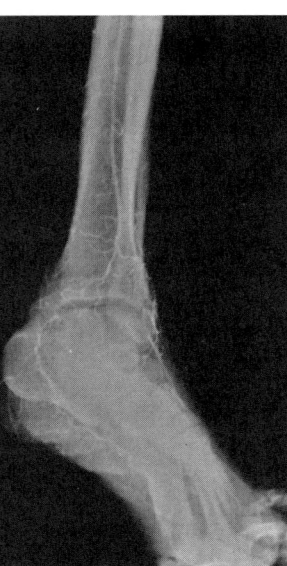

Figure 1 Diabetic patient with multiple stenoses of the superficial femoral artery and occlusions involving the infrapopliteal vessels. In spite of multiple stenoses and occlusions, injection of 45 cc of contrast at the rate of 4 cc per second into the left common iliac artery opacifies vessels of the foot without the aid of digital subtraction angiography.

Table 1 Injection Parameters (Low-Osmolar Contrast Material with 300 mg Iodine/ml)

Catheter Position	Volume	Rate	Imaging
Abdominal aorta at the level of renal arteries	30–40 ml	15–20 ml/sec	Abdominal aorta using DSA or cut film
Just above the aortic bifurcation	25–30 ml	12–15 ml/sec	Iliac arteries and bifurcation of common femoral arteries using DSA (anterior-posterior and/or obliques)
Just above the aortic bifurcation	100–120 ml	8–12 ml/sec	Both lower extremities using long film-screen
External iliac lower artery	35–50 ml	4–6 ml/sec	Ipsilateral extremity

DSA = Digital subtraction angiography.

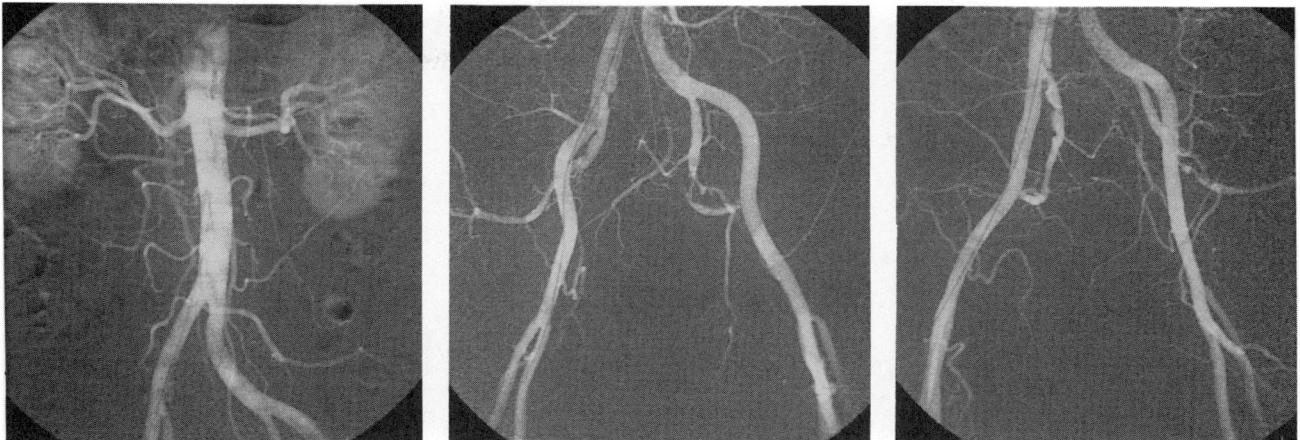

Figure 2 *Left,* DSA of the abdominal aorta demonstrating the renal arteries and the aortic bifurcation. *Center,* DSA of the pelvis in right anterior oblique projection ideally demonstrating the left common iliac bifurcation and right common femoral artery bifurcation. *Right,* DSA of the pelvis in left anterior oblique projection ideally demonstrating the right common iliac artery bifurcation and left common femoral artery bifurcation. DSA, Digital subtraction angiography.

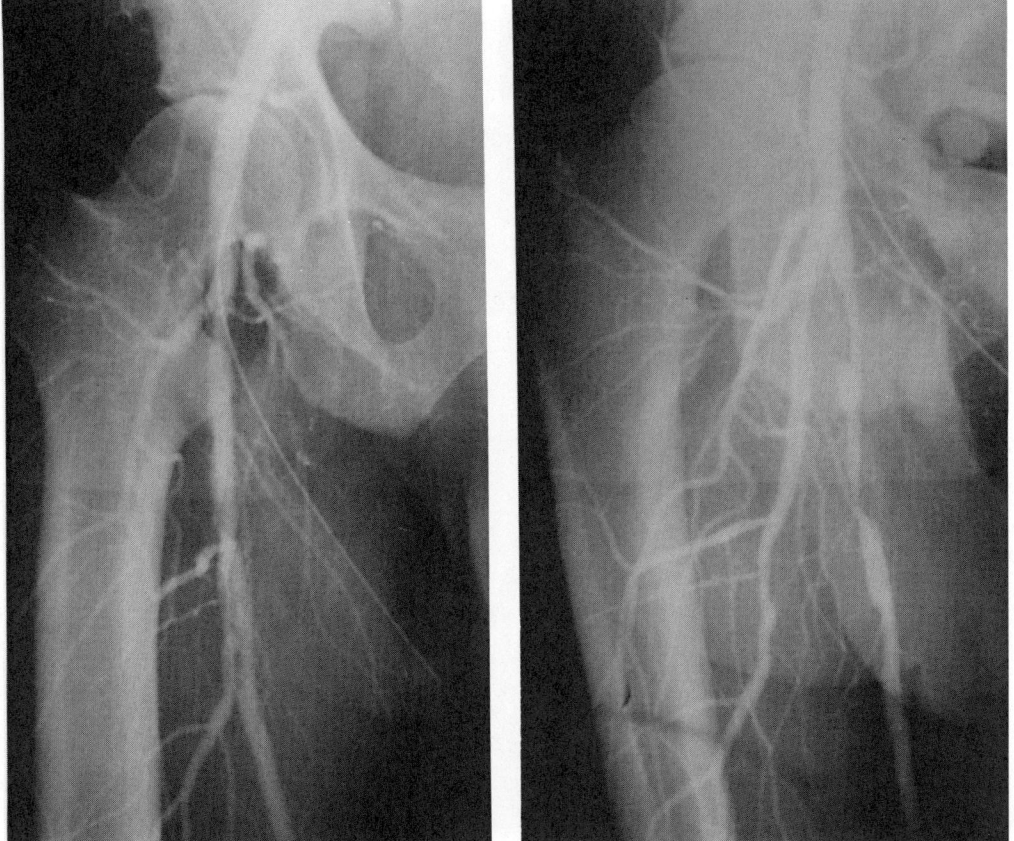

Figure 3 *Left,* Right femoral arteriogram in anterior-posterior projection demonstrating minimal plaque in the proximal superficial femoral artery. *Right,* Same patient in right anterior oblique projection demonstrating significant stenosis of superficial femoral artery by "opening up" the common femoral artery bifurcation.

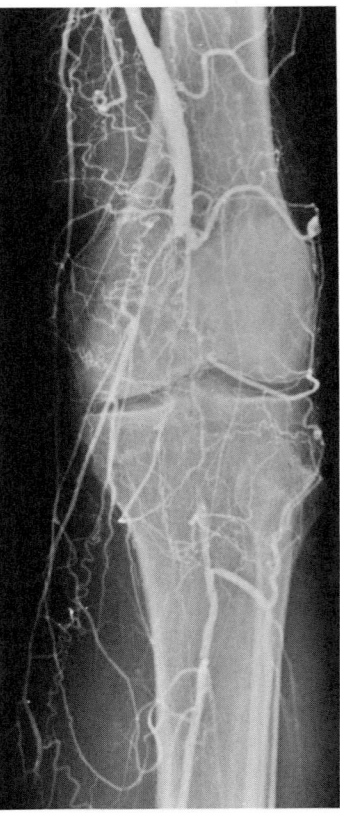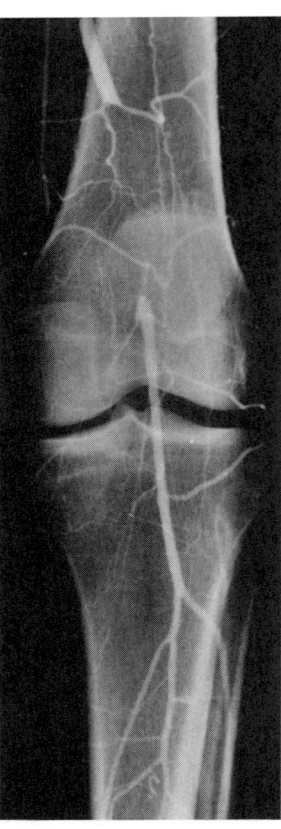

Figure 4 *Left,* Atherosclerotic occlusion of the popliteal artery with well-formed collaterals. *Right,* Embolic occlusion of the distal superficial femoral artery with poorly formed collaterals.

arteries, infrarenal aorta, and iliac arteries with bilateral runoff to the feet for the following reasons. First, it is not uncommon to have clinically undiagnosed atherosclerotic disease in the aorta and iliac arteries, especially ulcerated plaques. Second, information about the inflow is crucial in planning a distal bypass. For example, preoperative or intraoperative angioplasty of a moderate stenosis of the iliac artery is often performed before femoral-popliteal grafting.

A large amount of contrast material is used, slowly injected at a remote site proximal to a stenosis or to an occlusion to provide better opacification of the distal vessels via collaterals, as opposed to distal selective catheterization and injection close to the site of the stenosis or occlusion, beyond the origins of the collateral vessels. Injection in this manner usually demonstrates vessels of the foot, even in the presence of multiple stenoses and/or occlusions (Fig. 1). An exception to this rule is patients with arteriomegaly, who often require the use of distal selective injections to opacify the peripheral vasculature because of markedly slowed blood flow.

Vasodilatory Agents

Vasodilators in peripheral arterial occlusive disease are used to improve the opacification of the distal arteries, to help distinguish between spasm and stenosis, and in the treatment of nonocclusive vasospastic changes. The two most commonly used vasodilators in our practice are tolazoline and nitroglycerin. To relieve spasm and/or for opacification of the distal vessels, an intra-arterial injection of 25 mg of tolazoline is performed over 10 to 15 seconds close to the site of spasm and/or stenosis. Injection of tolazoline farther away from the site of abnormality produces vasodilation in the proximal vessels and their branches, thus increasing the amount of contrast flowing to the proximal vessels and decreasing contrast flow to the distal vessels.[5] An intra-arterial bolus of 50 to 100 µg of nitroglycerin produces vasodilation by acting on the smaller arteries and veins. Sublingual (0.4 mg) nitroglycerin is useful in preventing catheter and guide wire–induced spasm.

Imaging Sequence

First, imaging of the renal arteries and the abdominal aorta in the anterior-posterior projection, supplemented with a lateral view of the aorta as needed, is performed (Table 1). Second, imaging of the aortic bifurcation, iliac arteries, and common femoral arteries, including bifurcations, with bilateral oblique projections is done. Third, imaging of the arteries of both lower extremities is performed to include arterial opacification of the feet (feet externally rotated). We prefer digital

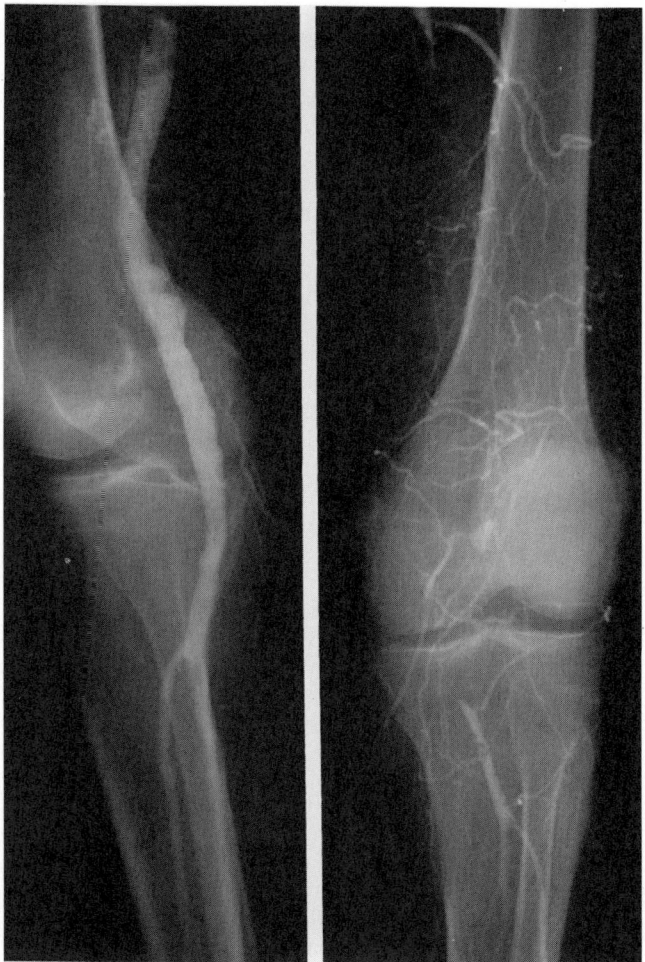

Figure 5 *Left,* Patient with bilateral popliteal artery aneurysms. Right popliteal aneurysm demonstrated by arteriography. *Right,* Thrombosed left popliteal artery aneurysm with emboli in the distal popliteal artery. Bilateral popliteal artery aneurysms were confirmed by ultrasound.

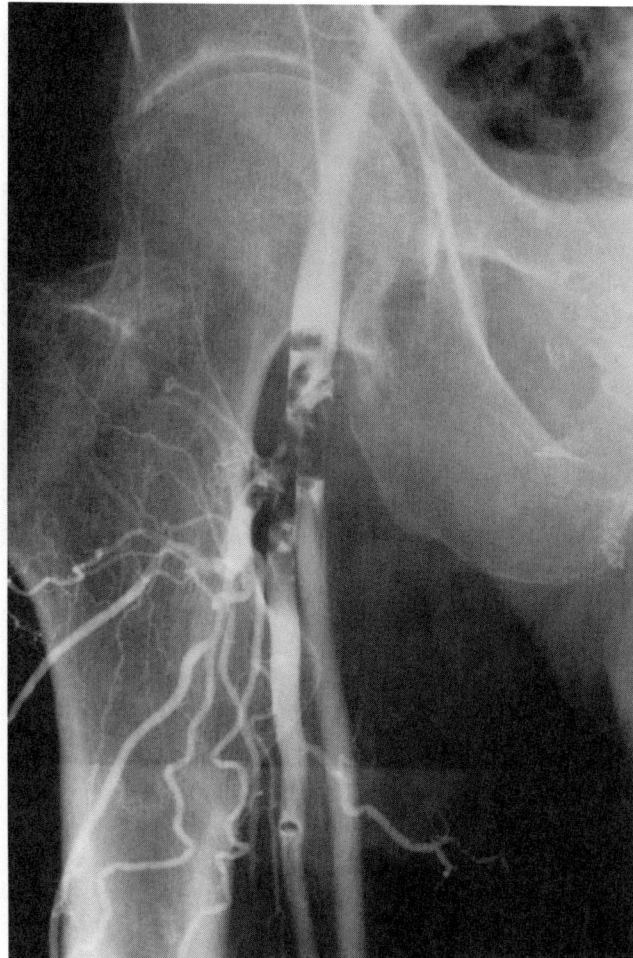

Figure 6 Patient with sudden onset of right lower extremity pain and loss of distal pulses. Femoral arteriogram demonstrates multiple, partially occluding emboli involving the right common femoral artery bifurcation.

subtraction angiography (DSA) for imaging of the aorta and the oblique views of the pelvis in conjunction with long film cassette changer with 8 foot x-ray tube–film changer distance for imaging the lower extremity arteries (Fig. 2). Oblique views at bifurcations and sites of overlapping vessels are critical to detect stenoses[6] (Fig. 3). In addition, we prefer a large volume of contrast injected at a slow rate in the external iliac artery for imaging the distal vessels of the leg and foot rather than using DSA for segmental imaging of the lower extremity vessels and feet. Although DSA has higher contrast resolution, details of the small vessels including patency and quality of the vessel wall are better evaluated with conventional film-screen imaging. Very few patients have the capacity to satisfactorily hold their feet motionless, which is required for high-quality DSA imaging of these small vessels.

During follow-up arteriography or in a patient presenting with either renal insufficiency or local acute severe symptoms, arteriography may be restricted to a particular region. In the case of compromised renal function, normal blood pressure measurements in the external iliac arteries, even after injection of vasodilators to mimic exercise, may allow avoidance of the aortogram and pelvic arteriogram portions of the study in the evaluation of infrainguinal occlusive disease.

ARTERIOGRAPHIC DIAGNOSIS

Atherosclerosis remains the most common cause of infrainguinal occlusive disease. Atherosclerosis produces segmental or diffuse plaque formation resulting in varying degrees of stenosis, some of which may progress to occlusion. Varying degrees of calcification in the arterial wall are also associated with atherosclerosis. It is more pronounced in patients with chronic renal failure. Occlusion due to slow progression of a stenosis produces

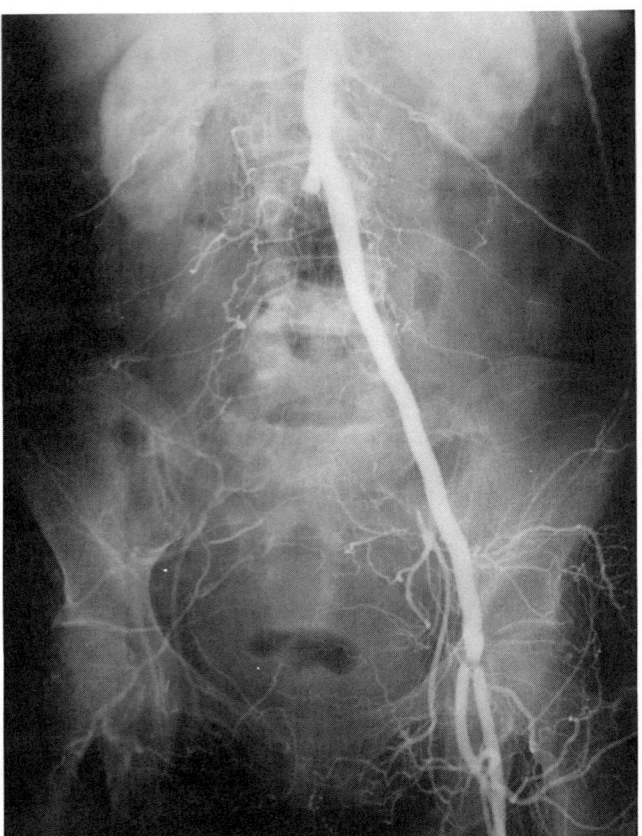

Figure 7 Occluded right limb of the aortobifemoral graft with significant stenosis of the origin of deep and superficial femoral arteries secondary to neointimal hyperplasia at the distal anastomosis in the left groin.

well-developed collaterals in most patients. Embolic occlusion rarely has well-formed collaterals (Fig. 4).

Atherosclerosis can also result in aneurysmal disease such as arteriomegaly and popliteal artery aneurysm (Fig. 5). Arteriomegaly is a generalized enlargement, often with adjacent aneurysms of the arterial tree. Popliteal artery aneurysms may be difficult to visualize on arteriography if the lumen is partially or totally thrombosed.

Occlusive disease due to emboli produces one or more filling defects or an abrupt cutoff of the vessel with a convex margin, often in an otherwise normal-appearing artery with poorly developed collaterals (Figs. 4 and 6). Most emboli originate in the heart but can arise from other sources such as aneurysms or ulcerated plaques of the aorta, iliac, femoral, and popliteal arteries. Emboli often lodge at vessel bifurcations.

In patients who have undergone bypass grafting for occlusive disease, late graft failure is most commonly due to progression of atherosclerotic disease proximal or distal to the graft. Graft problems such as anastomotic neointimal fibrous hyperplasia (Fig. 7) may also occur.

Vasculitides such as thromboangiitis obliterans (Buerger's disease), scleroderma, polyarteritis nodosa, and lupus erythematosus can also produce occlusive disease of the lower extremity vessels. The angiographic findings in the vasculitides, including long, smooth stenoses or occlusions, often with tortuous, well-developed collaterals, are very similar regardless of etiology, and clinical correlation and histology are necessary for making the definitive diagnosis.

Popliteal vascular entrapment syndrome is an uncommon cause of occlusive disease. It typically occurs in young individuals and is manifested arteriographically

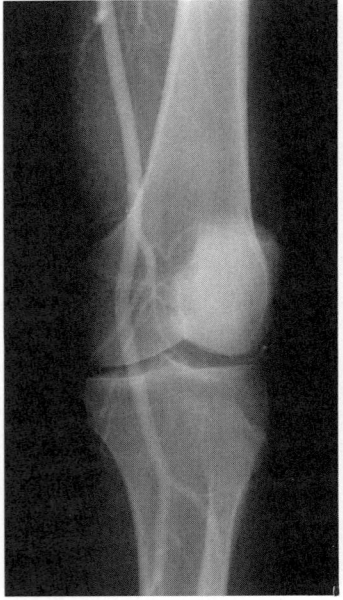 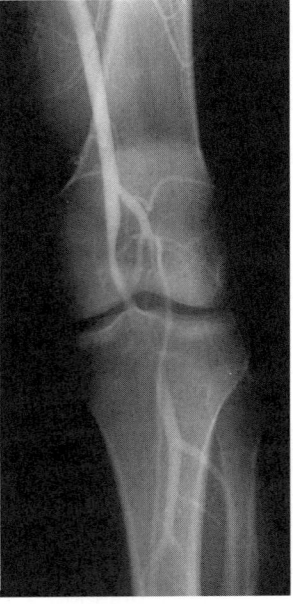

Figure 8 *Left*, Medial deviation of the left popliteal artery by the gastrocnemius muscle in a patient with popliteal artery entrapment syndrome. *Right*, Extrinsic compression by the medial head of the gastrocnemius muscle results in significant reduction of flow during flexion of the foot against resistance in the same patient.

most often as medial deviation of the popliteal artery, usually displaced by the medial head of the gastrocnemius muscle (Fig. 8).

Adventitial cystic disease of the popliteal artery is another uncommon cause of popliteal artery stenosis or occlusion. Arteriography may document an eccentric or central stenosis or occlusion of the popliteal artery with lack of atherosclerotic changes elsewhere in the arteries.

REFERENCES

1. Nelson JP. The vascular history and physical examination. Clin Podiatr Med Surg 1992; 9:1–17.
2. Barnes RW. Noninvasive diagnostic assessment of peripheral vascular disease. Circulation 1991; 83 (2 suppl):I20–27.
3. Fellmeth BD, Bookstein JJ, Lusie AL, Dillard JP. Rapid progression of peripheral vascular disease after diagnostic angiography. Radiology 1990; 175:71–74.
4. Hurlbert BJ, Landers DF. Sedation and analgesia for interventional radiologic procedures in adults, Semin Interventional Radiol 1987; 4:151–160.
5. Jacobs JB, Hanafee WN. The use of Priscoline in peripheral arteriography. Radiology 1967; 88:957–960.
6. Freiman DB, Oleaga JA, Ring EJ. Angiography of the femoral bifurcation. Prediction of the correct oblique projection. Radiology 1979; 131:254.

MAGNETIC RESONANCE ARTERIOGRAPHY FOR ASSESSMENT OF INFRAINGUINAL OCCLUSIVE DISEASE

JEFFREY P. CARPENTER, M.D.
RICHARD A. BAUM, M.D.

Magnetic resonance angiography (MRA) is a noninvasive vascular imaging technique that directly images flowing blood without the need for intravascular contrast agents. It can detect blood flow in arteries as slow as 2 cm/second and can display reconstructed images as conventional arteriograms, with excellent demonstration of the infrainguinal arteries, including the small vessels of the foot. It is particularly useful for visualization of the distal vessels of the leg and foot in patients with severe proximal occlusive disease.

Since its inception in the 1950s, arteriography has been the mainstay of preoperative vascular evaluation. Arteriography, however, is not without hazards and limitations. Nearly 10% of patients undergoing arteriography sustain a minor complication such as a hematoma, and a very small percentage have a major complication such as contrast-induced renal failure, heart failure, or even death.[1] Studies comparing preoperative arteriographic findings with findings at operation or on operative arteriograms have noted that in up to 70% of patients, the preoperative study fails to opacify all of the patent distal vessels. Even with the use of adjunctive maneuvers such as selective distal arterial injections, reactive hyperemia, delayed filming, and intra-arterial vasodilators, conventional arteriography fails to visualize 10% to 21% of calf arteries[2-4] and 40% to 86% of calf and foot arteries that are seen on operative arteriograms. Intra-arterial digital subtraction angiography is generally thought to improve detection of distal vessels, but the evidence for this is scant and a recent prospective study comparing intra-arterial digital subtraction angiography to conventional arteriography in 50 patients detected no difference with respect to the number of distal arteries visualized or the accuracy of grading stenotic lesions.[5] This limitation is inherent to contrast-based imaging techniques, as the demonstration of patency of a distal vessel in a patient with severe proximal occlusive disease necessitates that a bolus of proximally injected contrast medium traverse multiple segmental occlusions before it can opacify the patent downstream vessels. In the process, there are multiple dilutions and reconstitutions of contrast medium as it crosses arteriolar and capillary beds via circuitous collaterals to the distal circulation. In patients with limb-threatening ischemia and severe occlusive disease, opacification of small distal vessels presents a great challenge to contrast-based imaging techniques. Recently, MRA has been compared to conventional arteriography and found to be more sensitive than arteriography for the detection of patent distal vessels.[6]

FUNDAMENTAL PRINCIPLES OF MRA

In the two-dimensional time-of-flight technique for MRA, the patient is placed in a strong magnetic field in which all of the patient's protons became aligned with the applied field. The patient's tissue (protons) is then irradiated with a radio frequency pulse. The irradiated tissue emits a radio frequency echo, which is detected as the signal from which the magnetic resonance image is constructed. If the tissue is rapidly and repeatedly irradiated, giving it little time to relax, the tissue becomes saturated, and the echo signal becomes progressively weaker (Fig. 1). If, however, the tissue includes a vessel through which blood is flowing, "relaxed" blood will continuously enter this vessel. The relaxed blood,

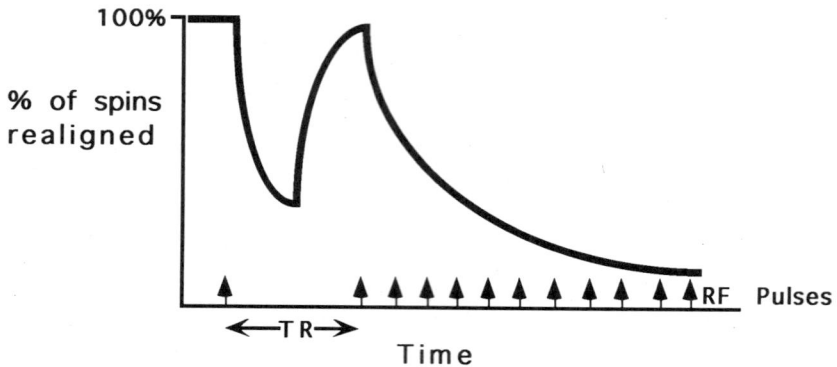

Figure 1 Saturation of spins. In the presence of a strong externally applied magnetic field, the proton spins are aligned in accordance with the direction of the applied magnetic field. When electromagnetic radiation in the radiofrequency (RF) range is used to bombard the protons, they absorb energy sufficient to disturb their alignment with the applied magnetic field. With time, the protons realign with the magnetic field. The interval between the RF pulses is known as the repetition time (TR). If the protons are rapidly and repeatedly irradiated with RF pulses (short TR), there is not sufficient time to realign with the magnetic field and the spins are in disarray. This is known as *saturation*. Saturated spins yield weak signals on MRA images.

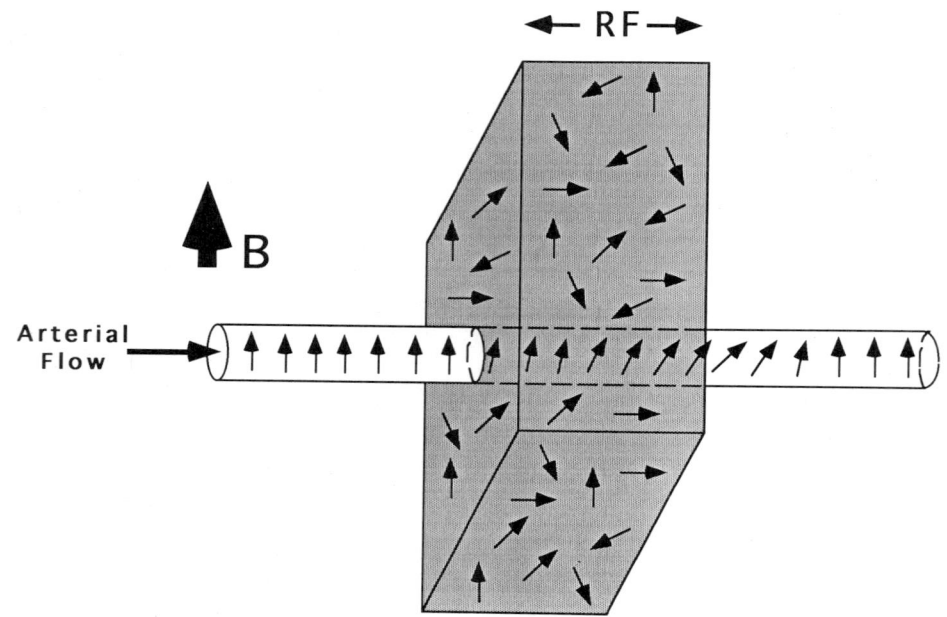

Figure 2 Time-of-flight effects. Soft tissue within the MR scanner, which has been repeatedly irradiated with radiofrequency (RF) pulses, has become saturated and yields a weak echo signal, causing it to appear dark on MR images. However, fresh blood containing protons that are fully aligned with the externally applied magnetic field, having not been exposed to the RF pulses within the imaging plane of the scanner, produces a large echo signal in response to an RF pulse. This fully magnetized blood produces a bright signal in contrast to the saturated surrounding soft tissue, selectively imaging flowing blood. This is known as *flow-related* enhancement.

which has not yet been irradiated, emits a strong signal (Fig. 2).

By saturating the tissue on one side of the slice to be examined, arteries or veins can be imaged selectively (Fig. 3). If the tissue below the slice of interest is saturated, only arterial blood, descending into the slice from unsaturated superior regions, yields a strong signal when the slice of interest is irradiated. Venous blood, ascending into the slice from the saturated inferior region, emits only a weak signal. Conversely, venous flow can be selectively imaged and arterial signals suppressed by superior saturation. This technique is known as magnetic resonance venography.

Data collected by any of these strategies are acquired as axial slices through the body (Fig. 4). A computer reconstruction of stacked axial images forms a projection magnetic resonance angiogram, which appears similar to a conventional contrast arteriogram. However, the information available from a reconstruction of stacked cross-sectional images is considerably

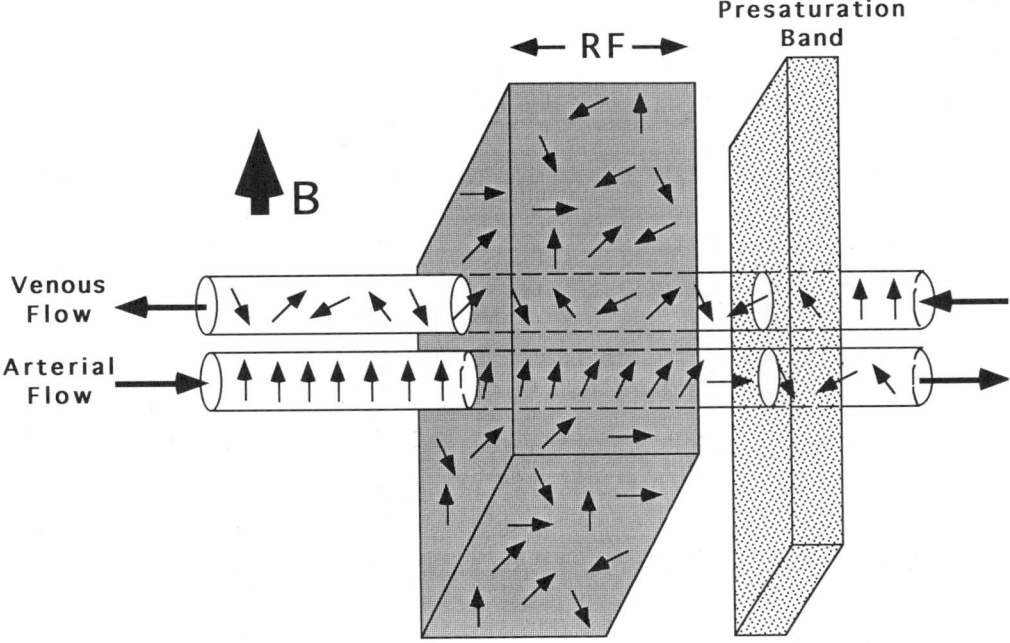

Figure 3 Presaturation. Selective imaging of arteries or veins is accomplished by the use of presaturation with radio frequency (RF) either inferior or superior to the imaging plane. To image arteries selectively, inferior saturation is chosen to suppress the magnetization of venous blood flowing from inferior to superior to reach the imaging plane. The venous blood, which is fully magnetized prior to reaching the presaturation band, becomes saturated in the presaturation band prior to entering the imaging plane. Thus, it yields little or no signal in the imaging plane itself. By contrast, arterial blood flowing from superior to inferior is fully magnetized upon entering the imaging plane and still yields a strong echo signal in respond to RF pulses in the imaging plane.

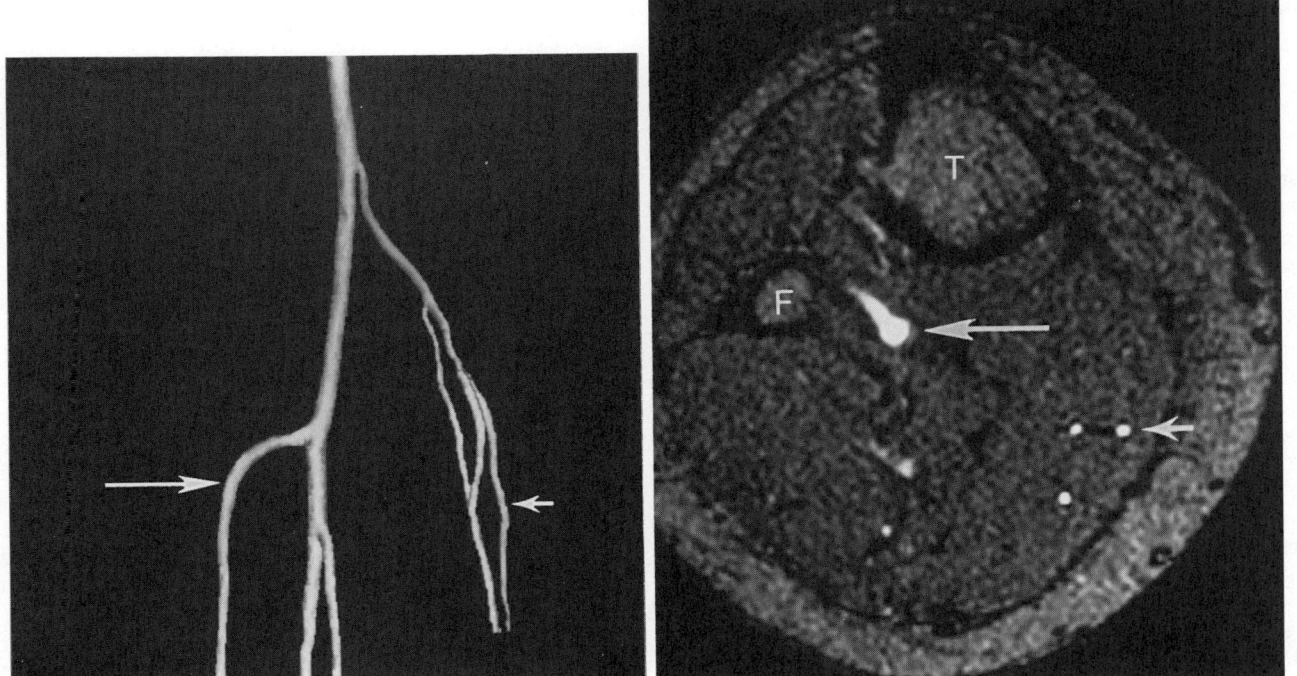

Figure 4 Normal magnetic resonance angiogram of the popliteal and runoff vessels. *A*, A normal popliteal artery and runoff vessels as well as collateral branches *(short arrow)* are demonstrated. The long arrow indicates the level through which the cross-sectional image *(B)* is taken. *B*, Computer-reconstructed projection arteriograms are comprised of stacked axial images. The origin of the anterior tibial artery from the popliteal artery *(long arrow)* and the collaterals seen in cross-section *(short arrow)* are appreciated on the axial image. The tibia (T) and fibula (F) are seen.

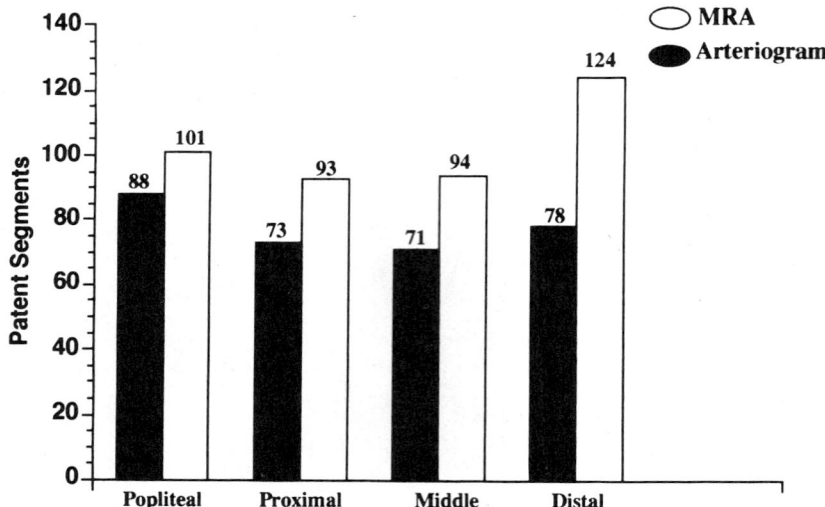

Figure 5 Comparison of patent vessel segments imaged by MRA and contrast arteriography by location. Increased sensitivity of MRA is noted at every location but is greatest in distal segments (49% greater sensitivity). (From Carpenter JP, Owen RS, Baum RA, et al. Magnetic resonance angiography of peripheral runoff vessels. J Vasc Surg 1992; 16:807–815; with permission.)

greater than that from conventional biplanar arteriography. Because the precise three-dimensional anatomy of a patent vessel segment can be determined, the exact location in space of a patent vessel segment is possible. Review of individual axial images indicates the level at which a target vessel resumes its patency, facilitating the placement of incisions. Cross-sectional images also allow the appreciation of irregular and eccentric atherosclerotic plaques.

CLINICAL EXPERIENCE WITH MRA

In a study of 55 limbs of 51 patients with severe symptomatic peripheral vascular disease, patients were examined by MRA from the mid-thigh through the foot by both imaging modalities.[7] Verification of vessel patency was provided by direct surgical inspection and/or operative or postbypass arteriography in 40 of the 55 limbs. The MRA was performed with two-dimensional time-of-flight technique using a standard 1.5 Tesla superconducting system with a transmit-receive extremity coil and commercially available pulse sequences. Inferior saturation pulses to suppress signals from venous blood flow were employed. Three hundred to 400 axial images were acquired from the mid-thigh through the foot and were reconstructed into projection arteriograms using maximum-intensity pixel technique. Conventional arteriograms were performed according to standard techniques, with filming continued for 40 seconds after the end of contrast medium injection. Opacification of distal arteries was enhanced by the use of vasodilators, delayed filming, reactive hyperemia, and intra-arterial digital subtraction arteriography.

For purposes of comparison, the arteries of the lower extremity were divided into three equal segments defined as proximal, middle, and distal artery. The MRA and conventional arteriograms were graded for patency at each location.

In 29 of 55 limbs (52%), there was exact agreement between the MRA and arteriographic studies. In the remaining 26 limbs (48%), MRA identified all of the vessels visualized by arteriography but also noted 106 (24%) additional patent vessel segments not seen by conventional arteriography. This increased detection of patent runoff vessels was not uniformly distributed through the leg but was most pronounced in the distal arterial segments (Fig. 5).[7] Additional patent runoff vessels were detected by MRA at every location in the leg. Whereas 13% more popliteal segments were identified by MRA, 49% more distal vessel segments were identified. These findings were confirmed by operative or postbypass arteriography or direct surgical inspection.

The explanation of the greater sensitivity of MRA than contrast arteriography is based on the mechanism of image formation in each of the two techniques. Instead of relying on contrast medium to fill the vessel lumen, MRA directly images flowing blood, allowing detection of patent vessels that are distal to severe proximal occlusive disease with extremely slow blood flow.

In this study, the results of MRA and arteriography, combined with the clinical characteristics for each patient, were used to formulate two separate interventional plans based on each imaging technique. These plans were identical in 40 (78%) of 51 patients. However, in 9 patients (18%) no runoff vessels suitable for use in a limb salvage procedure were identified by arteriography. In each of these patients MRA identified a patent vessel suitable for use in bypass grafting (Fig. 6). All of these patients had successful limb-salvage procedures guided by the MRA results. Had the arteriograms been the only available preoperative studies, these patients would have undergone blind exploration of vessels with

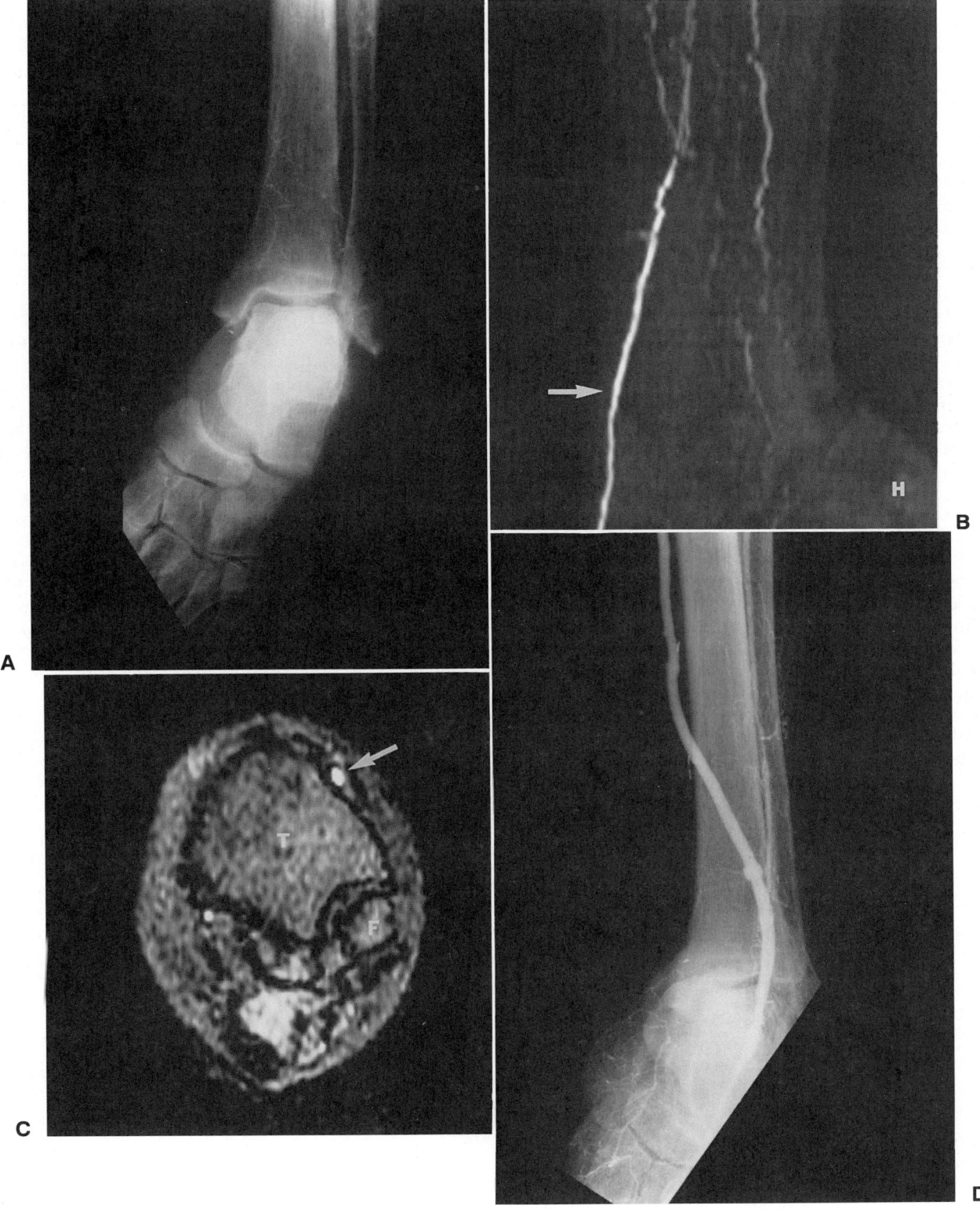

Figure 6 Results of imaging by arteriography and MRA in a 73-year-old man with a nonhealing ulcer of the left foot. *A,* Arteriogram shows only small collateral vessels in the distal foot and no vessels suitable for use in a distal bypass procedure. *B,* The MRA is shown in a lateral projection (H, heel). A patent anterior tibial artery is seen *(arrow). C,* The axial MRA section from the level of the distal leg shows the anterior tibial artery *(arrow).* The tibia (T) and fibula (F) can be seen. The anterior tibial artery was explored and found to be patent. A successful limb salvage procedure was performed based on these findings. *D,* The completion arteriogram. (From Carpenter JP, Owen RS, Baum RA, et al. Magnetic resonance angiography of peripheral runoff vessels. J Vasc Surg 1992; 16:807–815; with permission.)

operative arteriography. Either a bypass or an amputation would have resulted, depending upon the findings at operation. Thus, the identification of additional patent vessels detected by MRA was clinically important, altering the preoperative surgical plan in 18% of patients. Although these "angiographically occult" runoff vessels, unopacified by contrast material but detected by MRA, might have been found at operation, the need for multiple incisions in an ischemic limb with the resultant morbidity of poor wound healing would have been a disadvantage. Operation guided by MRA findings allowed an expedient bypass procedure with a minimum of dissection.

Other advantages of MRA were noted during this study as well. In two patients (4%) MRA findings directed bypasses to runoff vessels different from those suggested to be most suitable on the arteriogram. In one patient a reconstituted anterior tibial artery was mistakenly identified as a peroneal artery by arteriography. The cross-sectional MR image identified this artery correctly, and this was confirmed by operation and bypass to this artery. In the second patient a significant stenosis was not appreciated by arteriography because the arterial segment containing the stenosis was obscured by its position overlying cortical bone. This lesion was correctly identified by MRA, and a bypass was performed to an alternative patent runoff vessel. The postbypass arteriogram confirmed the presence of this stenosis. The definitive identification of patent runoff vessels and their locations in the leg, as well as the absence of signal from cortical bone, offer advantages over conventional arteriograms. In addition, the hazards of arterial puncture and contrast media are avoided in MRA studies, which are noninvasive.

Further studies with MRA have evaluated its ability to reliably image the proximal inflow vessels.[8] In a comparative study of arteriography and MRA of the aorta, iliac, and femoral arteries, MRA was shown to accurately identify patent and occluded arterial segments, as well as reliably identify significant stenoses. Reliable imaging of the proximal vasculature, however, requires more sophisticated pulse sequences than are commercially available.

In addition to the ability of MRA to detect patency of inflow and runoff vessels, it has recently been shown to accurately assess peripheral arterial stenoses.[9] In a comparative study of arteriography and MRA, 48 arterial stenoses (19 patients) were identified, from the distal aorta through the crural vessels. A high degree of interobserver agreement was noted in the readings of arteriograms and MRA studies. Measurement of degree of stenosis as evaluated by MRA and arteriography was analyzed by linear regression (Fig. 7) and Spearman-ranked correlation, both of which showed a high degree of correlation between the two diagnostic modalities ($r = 0.83$, $p < 0.001$; $r_s = 0.84$, $p < 0.001$). Decreases in cross-sectional area, which can be measured directly from MRA images, may provide better functional information than simple measurements of diameter stenosis.

Thus, MRA allows noninvasive evaluation of the inflow vessels and provides imaging of the runoff vessels, which is more sensitive than conventional arteriography. It also accurately evaluates stenotic lesions of the peripheral vasculature. In addition, MR technology is capable of measuring blood flow velocity quantitatively. This quantitative information may be combined with qualitative vascular imaging to provide a complete noninvasive vascular assessment of the lower extremity.

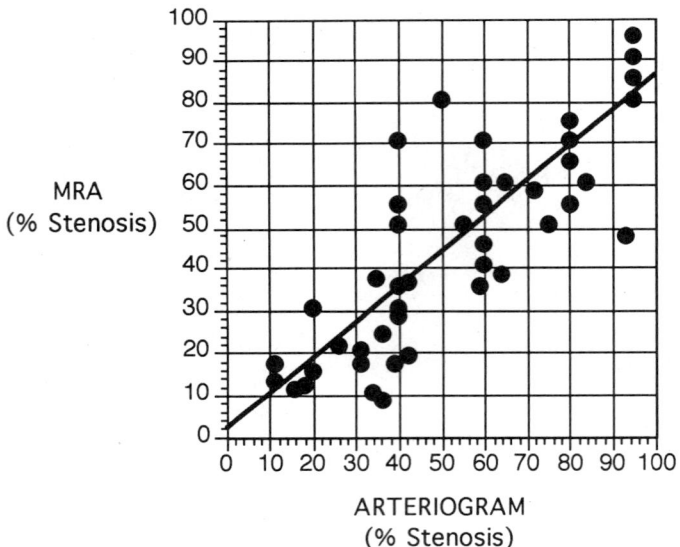

Figure 7 Correlation of MRA and contrast arteriographic measurement of stenosis. Pearson correlation coefficient *(r)* equals 0.83 *(p < 0.001)*. (From Hertz SM, Baum RA, Owen RS, et al. Peripheral arterial stenosis: Comparison of magnetic resonance and contrast arteriography. Am J Surg 1993; 166:112–116; with permission.)

CURRENT RECOMMENDATIONS FOR MRA

As magnetic resonance hardware and software continue to develop, MRA's role in noninvasive vascular assessment of the lower extremity will increase. In its present state of development, however, MRA of the lower extremities is viewed as an adjunct to arteriography rather than a replacement for it. Its greatest utility is its application in instances where suitable distal arterial segments are either absent or inadequately visualized on arteriograms. It can serve as an alternative to exploration of vessels with prebypass operative arteriography. Because MRA can be performed on an outpatient basis, it can eliminate the need for inpatient evaluation of patients for whom there is a question of distal arterial patency. Because the need for contrast medium is obviated, it is apparent that MRA is valuable for patients with renal insufficiency who are at high risk for contrast-induced renal failure.

Magnetic resonance arteriography can be implemented on a wide variety of currently available magnetic resonance scanners by using commercially available software and extremity coils. At present, the time required to perform an MRA study from the knee through the foot is 30 minutes. This time continues to decrease as hardware and software improve. The cost for the examination is equivalent to that of arteriography, unless nonionic contrast agents are used or the cost of an overnight stay for conventional arteriography is included in the analysis, in which case arteriography is more expensive than MRA. There may be an eventual cost saving with MRA if it completely replaces arteriography. Used as an adjunct to arteriography, however, MRA represents an incremental cost. There is no known morbidity attached to MRA, although an occasional patient is too claustrophobic for the examination to be completed. The only contraindications are those that apply to magnetic resonance imaging in general (e.g., the presence of a pacemaker, cerebral aneurysm clips, or metal in the eye). It is hoped that the increased sensitivity of this noninvasive technique and its ability to delineate vascular pathology may improve the overall limb salvage rate and decrease morbidity in patients with occlusive peripheral vascular disease.

REFERENCES

1. Waugh JR, Sacharias N. Arteriographic complications in the DSA era. Radiology 1992; 182:243–246.
2. Patel PR, Semel L, Clauss RH. Extended reconstruction rate for limb salvage with intraoperative prereconstruction angiography. J Vasc Surg 1988; 7:531–537.
3. Ricco J-B, Pearce WH, Yao JST, et al. The use of operative prebypass arteriography and Doppler ultrasound recordings to select patients for extended femor-distal bypass. Ann Surg 1983; 198:646–653.
4. Scarpato R, Gembarowicz R, Farber S, et al. Intraoperative preconstruction arteriography. Arch Surg 1981; 116:1053–1055.
5. Smith TP, Cragg AH, Berbaum KS, Nakagawa N. Comparison of the efficacy of digital subtraction and film-screen angiography of the lower limb: Prospective study in 50 patients. Am J Roentgenol 1992; 158:431–436.
6. Owen RS, Carpenter JP, Baum RA, et al. Magnetic resonance imaging of angiographically occult runoff vessels in peripheral arterial occlusive disease. N Engl J Med 1992; 326:1577–1581.
7. Carpenter JP, Owen RS, Baum RA, et al. Magnetic resonance angiography of peripheral runoff vessels. J Vasc Surg 1992; 16:807–815.
8. Carpenter JP, Owen RS, Holland GA, et al. Magnetic resonance angiography of the aorta, iliac and femoral arteries. Surgery 1994; 116:17–23.
9. Hertz SM, Baum RA, Owen RS, et al. Peripheral arterial stenosis: Comparison of magnetic resonance and contrast arteriography. Am J Surg 1993; 166:112–116.

SUPERFICIAL FEMORAL ARTERY ENDARTERECTOMY FOR ATHEROSCLEROTIC LOWER EXTREMITY OCCLUSIVE DISEASE

FRITZ R. BECH, M.D.
DANIEL B. WALSH, M.D.

Superficial femoral artery endarterectomy and femoral popliteal bypass with reversed saphenous vein were proposed over 40 years ago as solutions for chronic lower extremity ischemia due to atherosclerotic occlusion of the superficial femoral artery (SFA). Debate concerning the comparative efficacy of the two procedures continued for two decades. Only in the 1970s was vein bypass firmly established as the procedure of choice because of superior results that may have been partly related to the easier standardization of the bypass technique. By contrast, SFA endarterectomy evolved as two distinct techniques, open and semiclosed, which confused the interpretation of published results and contributed to its reputation as a difficult procedure to perform. Additional confusion resulted from the wide variety of disease patterns treated by SFA endarterectomy, ranging from 2 cm stenoses to axial occlusions of the entire SFA. A fair reassessment of the effectiveness of SFA endarterectomy depends on clear definition of the operative techniques and detailed analysis of both remote and recent reports.

OPEN ENDARTERECTOMY

The open technique of endarterectomy, often referred to as the Edwards procedure, employs a single longitudinal arteriotomy that traverses the entire diseased segment, an endarterectomy under direct vision, and closure of the artery with a long saphenous vein patch. The method is comparable to standard carotid endarterectomy. Although initially applied even to long (longer than 25 cm) lesions, this technique came to be regarded as too time-consuming for any but very localized lesions. Closure of a long arteriotomy with a vein patch was especially tedious, required the sacrifice of substantial lengths of vein, and sometimes resulted in aneurysmal dilation of the patch, creating the potential for thromboembolic complications. Open endarterectomy is, therefore, not performed for long segment occlusions.

Short segment disease of the SFA, in contrast, is often ideally suited to open endarterectomy. Inahara and Scott, in describing their experience with 100 patients (85% for claudication), emphasized proper patient selection by arteriography (15 cm maximum length), a deep endarterectomy plane (removal of all but the adventitia), beveling and tacking points of transition between endarterectomized and untreated segments, and in most patients application of a vein patch extending 1 to 2 cm beyond both end points.[1] As would be expected from the usual distribution of SFA disease, 75% of their procedures were confined to the distal one-third of the artery. The mean length of endarterectomy was 9.7 cm, and multiple arteriotomies were required for longer lesions. Routine adjunctive measures to prevent early thrombosis included the use of both low-molecular-weight dextran and dipyridamole and peripheral vasodilation using an epidural catheter for anesthetic agent injections.

All reconstructed arteries were patent at discharge in the Inahara and Scott series, allaying theoretic concerns raised by the combination of the high resistance of SFA runoff with the thrombogenic arterial surface created by a deep dissection plane. There were no suture line dehiscences. Cumulative patency by the life table method was 70% at 5 years and 50% at 10 years. Thirty endarterectomies failed. Of them, 14 patients required no treatment and 16 underwent femoral-popliteal bypass. One bypass failed, in a patient who initially presented with rest pain, resulting in the single major amputation in the study.

SEMICLOSED ENDARTERECTOMY

Cannon and Barker first described the semiclosed technique in 1955, in a report that introduced the fine wire loop stripper on which this technique depends.[2] Because of the usual structural characteristics of SFA atherosclerotic plaque, they found that once a cleavage plane was established between the lesion and the underlying media or adventitia at any point along the SFA, the plane could be safely developed and advanced within segments of unopened artery by insinuating a wire loop. The entire length of the SFA, therefore, could be disobliterated without opening the entire artery. Short proximal and distal arteriotomies would usually suffice.

Vein patch closure of two short arteriotomies reduced operative time and vein usage compared with the open technique. Cannon and Barker reported success, defined as improvement of symptoms and return of the popliteal and one pedal pulse, in 20 of 23 patients with intermittent claudication and more limited success in patients with established gangrene, who apparently had severely compromised outflow.

Walker and colleagues reported one of the larger American experiences with semiclosed SFA endarterectomy.[3] Just under 50% of these 123 endarterectomies were performed for claudication, the remainder for more severe ischemic symptoms. Diabetics comprised 33% of the patient population. The study spanned 12 years. In the early period, endarterectomy was performed preferentially; later, endarterectomy was used only when adequate saphenous vein was not available. All patients had long segment SFA occlusions, a patent popliteal artery, and at least one runoff vessel patent from its origin to pedal arch. If arteriography documented disease extension to the insertion of the gastrocnemius, the distal incision was carried across the knee; otherwise, a standard above-knee popliteal medial exposure was used. The adductor magnus tendon was routinely divided to facilitate passage of the stripper. A deep endarterectomy plane between media and adventitia was preferred. In contrast to Cannon and Barker's approach, this was begun in the proximal SFA and progressed distally. A third arteriotomy was made at the level of the adductor hiatus if the plaque was particularly adherent. The end point was routinely managed with tacking sutures. All arteriotomies were closed with a vein patch, and a completion arteriogram was always performed.

Patency of the endarterectomized segment was 76% at 1 year and 46% at 5 years for the entire group.[3] Subgroup analysis suggested trends toward an effect on 5 year patency for operative indication (claudication 59.6% versus 30.6% advanced ischemia) and the presence of diabetes (32.3% versus 52% nondiabetics). Other authors noted that the poor results in diabetic patients may be caused by the medial calcification, common in diabetics, which makes development of a consistent endarterectomy plane difficult.

The results of this series of unselected patients with long segment SFA disease are representative of most reports of semiclosed endarterectomy. The 50% to 60% 5 year patency rate, when performed for claudication, although not up to the expected outcome after vein bypass, compares favorably to that of prosthetic bypass.

COMPARISON OF ENDARTERECTOMY TO SAPHENOUS VEIN BYPASS

In the era in which the supremacy of vein bypass had not yet been established, a number of published reports compared SFA endarterectomy to vein bypass. That these techniques were thought to be worth comparing by 10 or more authors is an indication that endarterectomy had demonstrated efficacy considerable enough to be taken seriously. The studies, all of which were nonrandomized, suffered from selection bias. In most, SFA endarterectomy was performed only when bypass was abandoned because of inadequate vein. These comparisons had conflicting outcomes, also reflecting considerable variation in operative indications, divergent surgical technique and experience, and varying perioperative management. Nevertheless, because these studies are often cited as evidence for the inferiority of SFA endarterectomy, the best among them are worth reviewing.

Gutelius and associates, in an early study, compared his experience with 20 open SFA endarterectomies, most for short stenoses, with 60 reversed vein bypasses over the same period.[4] Criteria for choice of operation were not noted. Indications for operation in both groups were claudication in 50% and rest pain or gangrene in 50%. After 16 months, patency in the vein bypass group was 80% and in the endarterectomy group 55%. The poor short-term outcomes for both procedures likely reflected the omission of perioperative anticoagulation and completion arteriography, common during that period. Operative indications made no difference in patency among vein grafts, but claudication predicted greater success for endarterectomy. The vast majority of occlusions after endarterectomy occurred early in the postoperative period. Endarterectomy failed in all three diabetics in whom it was performed, but diabetes had no clear effect on vein bypass patency. Poor runoff appeared to be more detrimental to patency of endarterectomies than to bypass. The authors, who concluded that vein bypass was the superior operation, speculated that endarterectomy failures were due to a sudden ledge between the endarterectomized segment and "normal" but thickened artery, an observation that may have indicated that the endarterectomies performed were of insufficient length.

DeWeese and co-workers compared 55 SFA endarterectomies with 111 vein bypasses.[5] Extent of disease documented by arteriography determined which procedure was performed, with endarterectomy performed for short or moderate-length occlusions and bypass performed for extensive SFA occlusions. Semiclosed endarterectomy was accomplished through three arteriotomies, the most distal of which was transverse. Early patency of endarterectomy surpassed that of bypass: 85% versus 72%. Late follow-up, defined as greater than 2 years, was available in 97% of patients. Of endarterectomized segments patent at discharge, 77% remained patent at late follow-up, compared with 85% of vein bypasses. Despite a lack of statistical analysis, the authors concluded that vein bypass is the best method of reconstructing the femoral-popliteal segment. It is also noteworthy that during the same period 18 synthetic femoral-popliteal bypasses were performed, only 5 of which were open after 1 year.

Darling and Linton's 1972 review of femoral-popliteal revascularizations probably contributed most to the decline of SFA endarterectomy.[6] They preferentially performed reversed vein bypass, which was chosen for 345 reconstructions. In 87 patients, in whom the saphenous vein was insufficient or unavailable, endarterectomy was used. Approximately one-half of these employed the open technique, and half were semiclosed. Indications for operation were identical in the two groups (60% claudication, 40% rest pain or tissue loss) as was the status of the popliteal outflow tract on preoperative arteriography.

Thirty-day patency was identical (94% bypass versus 97% endarterectomy), but by the life table method, patency was inferior for endarterectomy at every late time point (79% bypass versus 45% endarterectomy at 3 years; 72% bypass versus 36% endarterectomy at 5 years). Number of patent outflow vessels did not substantially affect patency in either group. Endarterectomy performed for claudication fared better than if performed for limb salvage (42% versus 29% 5 year patency). No claudicant in either treatment group underwent amputation. The report also includes a parallel series of 49 prosthetic femoral-popliteal bypasses from the same institution with a 20% 5 year patency rate.

The poor 5 year patency rate of endarterectomy in this group represents the low for all published reports on the operation. However, the authors confessed a bias against the procedure at the outset, performed it only when the vein was inadequate for bypass, and performed bypass eight times more often as either open or semiclosed endarterectomy. Although the groups were well matched with respect to operative indications, it is possible that a lack of experience and enthusiasm for endarterectomy may have affected the technical results.

EFFECTS OF VARIABLES

A number of clinical parameters have been examined to determine whether successful SFA endarterectomy can be predicted prospectively. Diabetes has been shown to adversely affect outcome, probably because of the tendency of SFA plaque in diabetics to include calcified, adherent media. Diabetic patients also have a greater likelihood of having SFA disease accompanied by compromised runoff. Multiple stenoses are less likely than occlusion to be successfully treated with endarterectomy because of the difficulty in maintaining a continuous endarterectomy plane. Although lesion length and lesion location have been studied, neither consistently correlates with outcome.

As is true for bypass grafts, most studies suggest greater success when SFA endarterectomy is performed for intermittent claudication than for more advanced ischemia. A related question is whether popliteal artery runoff affects patency. Morton and co-workers reported 84 SFA or popliteal endarterectomies with an analysis of the effect of concurrent occlusive disease on long-term patency.[7] A 75% 3 year patency was achieved in patients with at least two normal runoff vessels. Poor runoff, defined as narrowing or occlusion of all vessels, resulted in a surprisingly good 47% patency rate. In contrast, Inahara and Scott found no correlation between number of runoff vessels and long-term patency in their series of 100 relatively short open endarterectomies.

RECENT SERIES

In the United States, SFA endarterectomy has been relegated to the rank of second- or third-line procedure by most surgeons, and contemporary data are accordingly sparse. However, in some European centers SFA endarterectomy continues to be performed as a procedure of choice.[8] In the recent report by van der Heijden and associates of 10 years of experience, endarterectomy was chosen as the primary procedure if the arteriogram documented reconstitution of the popliteal artery and did not identify extensive calcification of the SFA, which, in the authors' experience, frequently precluded technical success.

In 231 of 259 patients (89%), endarterectomy was technically possible. Failures, defined as either an inability to establish a cleavage plane or perforation of the vessel, were treated with immediate vein bypass. Of the procedures 80% were performed for claudication and 20% for more severe ischemia. A variety of arteriographic disease patterns were present: 64% of SFAs were occluded, and in 35% the occlusion was longer than 30 cm. The percentage of patients who were diabetic was not reported.

Five-year patency after successful endarterectomy was 71% as measured by life table analysis. Of 82 vein bypasses performed for either immediate or late endarterectomy failure, 61% were patent at 5 years. Tertiary patency, defined as patency of either endarterectomy or secondary bypass, was 79% at 5 years. Of 13 major amputations, only three were performed in patients whose initial indication was claudication.

Perioperative rates of mortality (1%) and morbidity (10%) in this as in all other series of SFA endarterectomy were similar to perioperative mortality and morbidity rates in series of bypass grafts.

ENDARTERECTOMY IN PERSPECTIVE

Superficial femoral artery endarterectomy, which has been performed and carefully studied for more than four decades, continues to have a role in current vascular surgical practice. Infrainguinal revascularization to the above-knee popliteal artery can be safely and reliably achieved with acceptable long-term results. For short stenoses, open endarterectomy is effective, and semiclosed endarterectomy can achieve long-term patency rates of up to 70% for long segment disease. By comparison, percutaneous atherectomy, enthusiastically promoted as a potential solution for SFA occlusion in recent years, has to date failed to achieve even a 30% 1 year patency rate.[9]

The SFA endarterectomy has a number of advantages over bypass with prosthetic material. Theoretically, greater resistance to infection makes endarterectomy potentially useful as a replacement for an infected femoral-popliteal bypass or in the presence of soft tissue infection in the limb. Many authors have noted the phenomenon of pseudo-occlusion, in which the popliteal outflow occludes, but the endarterectomized SFA remains patent because of the continued patency of branches.[10] Endarterectomy has also been said to preserve SFA-based collateral vessels, which may account for the benign fate of limbs after occlusion of the endarterectomized segment, with few or no amputations resulting in any reported experiences.

No study has prospectively compared SFA endarterectomy with polytetrafluoroethylene (PTFE) bypass above the knee, but a number of older reports document significantly inferior patency for the prosthetic procedure.[11] Even the best reported patency rates for PTFE do not exceed those of endarterectomy.

POINTS OF EMPHASIS IN SURGICAL TECHNIQUE

Open endarterectomy should be reserved for short (less than 10 cm) stenoses and occlusions. We have had occasional success with this technique, even in the popliteal artery and tibial-peroneal trunk. Successful semiclosed endarterectomy performed for long segment disease depends on initially establishing a natural plane, distal-to-proximal passage of the endarterectomy loop, additional arteriotomies to re-examine the dissection plane when resistance is met, and careful tacking of the distal end point. The endarterectomy should be examined for residual plaque and technical adequacy with arteriography or angioscopy. Judicious perioperative anticoagulation with heparin sodium or dextran is a logical adjunct.

INDICATIONS FOR SFA ENDARTERECTOMY

SFA endarterectomy should be considered in the following circumstances: (1) When lower extremity ischemia is predominantly due to short stenosis or occlusion of the SFA, and open endarterectomy and patch can be effective; (2) to maintain circulation when an infected femoral-popliteal graft must be removed, or when vein is not available to revascularize a limb that is still substantially infected; (3) when vein is inadequate for femoral-popliteal bypass in a nondiabetic; and (4) in a young patient with femoral-popliteal disease who appears to have a high likelihood of requiring a long vein bypass in the future. The utility of staged reconstruction is as yet unproven, but endarterectomy would appear to be a logical "vein-sparing" procedure if this philosophy were adopted.

REFERENCES

1. Inahara T, Scott CM. Endarterectomy for segmental occlusive disease of the superficial femoral artery. Arch Surg 1981; 116:1547–1553.
2. Cannon JA, Barker WF. Successful management of obstructive femoral arteriosclerosis by endarterectomy. Surgery 1955; 38:48–60.
3. Walker PM, Imparato AM, Riles TS, et al. Long-term results in superficial femoral artery endarterectomy. Surgery 1981; 89:23–30.
4. Gutelius JR, Kreindler S, Luke JC. Comparative evaluation of autogenous vein bypass graft and endarterectomy in superficial femoral artery reconstruction. Surgery 1965; 57:28–35.
5. DeWeese JA, Barner HB, Mahoney EB, Rob CG. Autogenous venous bypass grafts and thromboendarterectomies for atherosclerotic lesions of the femoropopliteal arteries. Ann Surg 1966; 163:205–214.
6. Darling RC, Linton RR. Durability of femoropopliteal reconstructions. Endarterectomy versus vein bypass grafts. Am J Surg 1972; 123:472–479.
7. Morton DL, Ehrenfeld WK, Wylie EJ. Significance of outflow obstruction after femoropopliteal endarterectomy. Arch Surg 1967; 94:592–599.
8. van der Heijden FHWM, Eikelboom BC, van Reedt Dortland RWH, et al. Long-term results of semiclosed endarterectomy of the superficial femoral artery and the outcome of failed reconstructions. J Vasc Surg 1993; 18:271–279.
9. Ahn SS, Eton D, Mehigan JT. Preliminary clinical results of rotary atherectomy. In: Yao JST, Pearce WH, eds. Technologies in vascular surgery. Philadelphia: WB Saunders, 1992; 388.
10. Ouriel K, Smith CR, DeWeese JA. Endarterectomy for localized lesions of the superficial femoral artery at the adductor canal. J Vasc Surg 1986; 3:531–534.
11. Kouchoukos NT, Levy JF, Balfour JF, Butcher HR Jr. Operative therapy for femoral-popliteal arterial occlusive disease. A comparison of methods. Cardiovasc Surg 1967; 35/36:174–182.

PROFUNDAPLASTY

DONALD L. JACOBS, M.D.
JONATHAN B. TOWNE, M.D.

The importance of the profunda femoris artery (PFA) as a collateral network allowing perfusion of the lower leg in iliac or femoral-popliteal occlusive disease has been known for more than 30 years. That the PFA as an important outflow vessel for inflow reconstruction has been well established. In the presence of superficial femoral artery occlusion, a profundaplasty performed to treat defined PFA stenosis at the time of an inflow procedure such as aortofemoral, femoral-femoral, or axillofemoral bypass relieves lower extremity ischemia and increases blood flow velocity in the inflow reconstruction, enhancing patency.

Profundaplasty alone as a primary means of treating femoral-popliteal occlusive disease has been debated in the literature.[1-5] The role of profundaplasty in the therapy of lower extremity occlusive disease has changed with the evolution of increasingly successful techniques of distal arterial bypass using autogenous saphenous vein. Profundaplasty as an isolated procedure for lower extremity revascularization is infrequently used. However, profundaplasty is useful as an alternative in patients who have failed previous distal bypass or do not have adequate vein for distal reconstruction. Profundaplasty with autogenous material may provide adequate blood flow to achieve limb salvage in patients requiring removal of a distal bypass for groin sepsis. Also, the use of the distal PFA as a site for inflow reconstruction in patients requiring removal of an infected aortofemoral bypass in the groin permits placement of an inflow prosthesis remote from the infected field. Although use of profundaplasty has changed over the years, PFA reconstruction continues to be an important option for the vascular surgeon when dealing with complex arterial disease of the lower extremity.

ANATOMY

The PFA is the primary blood supply for the thigh and accounts for an average blood flow of 240 ml/minute in the resting state. The PFA arises from the common femoral artery 2 to 4 cm below the inguinal ligament. The usual course of the PFA is deep and lateral to the superficial femoral artery, yet in 10% of patients it courses medial to the superficial femoral artery. The branches of the PFA are variable. In 58% of patients the medial and lateral circumflex vessels arise from the common trunk. However, the common femoral artery is the origin for the medial femoral circumflex in 18% of patients and is the origin for the lateral femoral circumflex in 15%. When the lateral femoral circumflex artery arises from the common femoral artery, the PFA usually takes a more medial course in relation to the superficial femoral artery. The lateral femoral circumflex divides into the superior, transverse, and inferior branches. The medial femoral circumflex passes posteromedial toward the obturator foramen. The main trunk of the PFA gives off perforator branches to the thigh muscles, which run deep and medial to the femur. Typically there are four perforator branches. The fourth branch is designated as the terminal branch of the PFA.

The PFA becomes an important collateral pathway in external iliac, common femoral, or superficial femoral artery occlusions by serving as the major link in a collateral chain that can run from the internal iliac to the popliteal artery. With external iliac or common femoral artery occlusion, the medial and lateral circumflex femoral arteries provide the connection between the PFA and the inferior gluteal and obturator branches of the internal iliac artery (Fig. 1). The geniculate branches

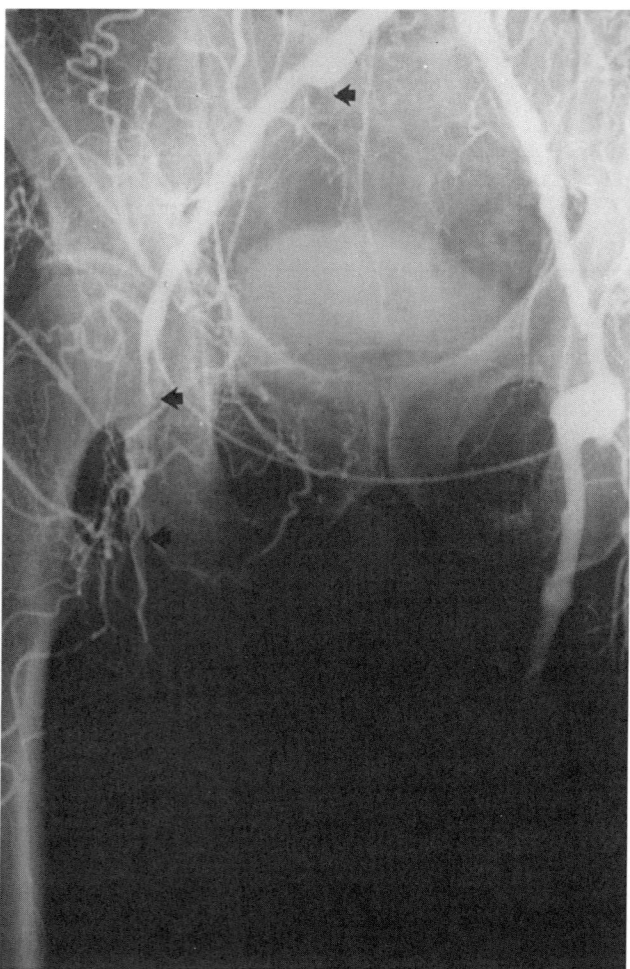

Figure 1 Arteriogram demonstrating an internal iliac occlusion (*upper arrow*), tapering of the common femoral artery to an occlusion of the proximal PFA (*middle arrow*), and reconstitution of the PFA (*lower arrow*) with large collateral vessels from the lateral descending branch.

of the popliteal artery provide the pathway to connect the PFA and its distal branches with the popliteal and tibial vessels in long segment superficial femoral artery occlusions (Fig. 2).

Arterial occlusive disease involves the PFA to a lesser degree than the superficial femoral artery in the majority of patients. Beales and colleagues reported that 59% of 209 limbs undergoing arteriography for ischemic disease had some occlusive disease in the profunda.[6] This study also noted 39% of the limbs had disease of the orifice; however, only 9.3% of the limbs had a greater than 50% stenosis of the proximal PFA. Others have reported a lower frequency of PFA disease ranging from 18% to 30%.[7,8] The distribution of disease in the PFA has been consistently reported to involve the orifice or proximal PFA in 68% to 76% of the affected limbs, with distal disease being much less common.[9]

Adequate arteriographic visualization of the PFA, particularly the orifice, requires lateral or oblique views

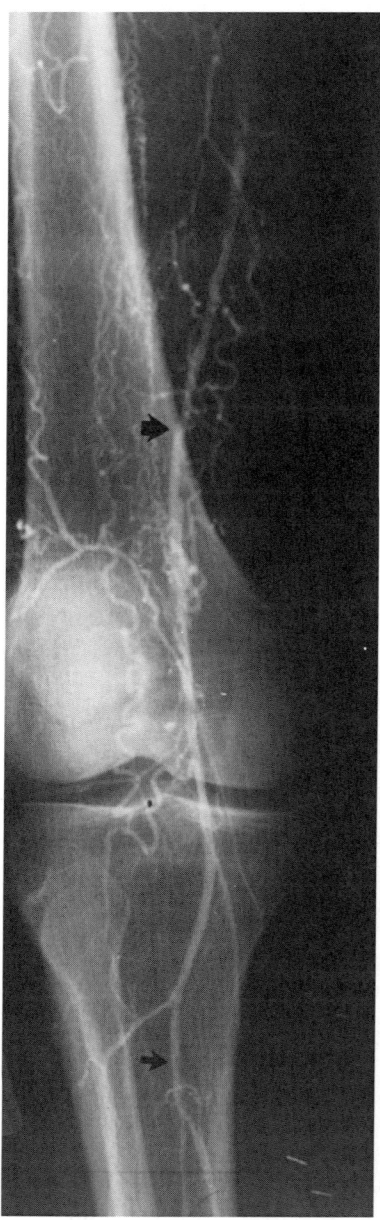

Figure 2 A continuation of the arteriogram in Figure 1 showing reconstitution of the superficial femoral via the lateral descending branch and the distal PFA perforator branches (*upper arrow*). There is continuous flow to the tibioperoneal trunk (*lower arrow*) and only single vessel runoff to the foot via the posterior tibial artery (not shown). This patient had 50 foot claudication and a preoperative ABI of 0.24. His saphenous vein had been previously used for coronary bypass. After a common femoral and PFA endarterectomy with patch closure using endarterectomized superficial femoral artery, his ABI increased to 0.64 and his symptoms resolved.

to rotate the origin of the PFA away from the overlying common femoral and superficial femoral arteries, which can obscure the takeoff of the PFA on anterior-posterior views. The Beales group reported that 85% of the significant PFA orifice stenoses were seen only on the lateral or oblique views.⁶ It is also important to visualize the collaterals that may exist between the distal PFA branches and the popliteal and tibial vessels because the character of these vessels has prognostic significance in predicting the success of profundaplasty.

INDICATIONS

The most common indication for profundaplasty is as an adjunct to an inflow procedure such as an aortofemoral, femoral-femoral, or axillofemoral bypass. This is of primary importance when there is occlusion of the superficial femoral artery and the PFA is the only outflow for the inflow reconstruction. It is imperative that the PFA is assessed and that any identified stenosis in the PFA be corrected at the time of the inflow procedure to ensure the long-term patency of the reconstruction. This is most often achieved by extending the toe of the inflow graft onto the PFA origin as a patch angioplasty. If an extended profundaplasty is required, it is recommended that autogenous material be utilized as the patch material and the prosthetic material of the inflow graft not be used to patch the distal PFA.

A much less frequent clinical situation is consideration of profundaplasty as an isolated procedure to treat lower limb ischemia. To determine whether patients are likely to benefit from an isolated profundaplasty requires knowledge of the extent and distribution of their occlusive disease. As with all lower limb revascularizations, adequate inflow must be present. Also, for a profundaplasty to have significant effect on lower leg perfusion, there must be superficial femoral artery occlusion and a hemodynamically significant (greater than 50%) stenosis in the proximal PFA that can be corrected.⁵ Furthermore, there must be adequate collaterals between the PFA branches and the popliteal or tibial arteries to allow for sufficient blood flow to the foot. Although successful outcome is more frequent in patients with a patent popliteal artery, successful profundaplasty can be performed in the presence of popliteal occlusion if the geniculate collaterals to the tibial vessels are adequate.

Arteriographic evaluation of the collateral network is critical. Ideally, if large, disease-free collaterals are visualized, their adequacy is certain. An alternative method to evaluate the adequacy of collaterals is by Doppler examination of the segmental thigh, calf, and ankle blood pressures. This allows for the calculation of the profunda-popliteal collateral index (PPCI), which is an index of the resistance in the collaterals across the knee joint,¹⁰ calculated as

$$PPCI = \frac{\text{Above-knee pressure} - \text{Below-knee pressure}}{\text{Above-knee pressure}}$$

We have shown that the resistance across the knee joint calculated as the PPCI is the most important determinant of success of profundaplasty. A PPCI of greater than 0.5 implies a high resistance in the collateral bed and is predictive of profundaplasty failure. In a group of 54 patients having an isolated profundaplasty for limb-threatening ischemia, the mean PPCI of the failures was 0.46, compared to 0.19 in those that achieved limb salvage ($p < 0.01$).² McCoy and co-workers reported the use of a similar index, which was calculated by subtracting the ankle pressure from the low thigh pressure and dividing by the low thigh pressure to obtain the thigh ankle gradient index (TAGI).⁴ The TAGI reflects not only the resistance in the geniculate collaterals but also the resistance in the tibial vessels. In the McCoy group's study, patients with a successful profundaplasty had a mean TAGI of 0.39, compared to 0.79 in patients in whom profundaplasty was not successful.⁴

The clinical presentations of lower limb ischemia are prognostic for the success of profundaplasty. Patients with claudication, rest pain, or tissue loss may be candidates for an isolated profundaplasty, provided the appropriate anatomic and physiologic criteria as noted previously are present. However, the success rate is higher in claudication patients than in those with limb-threatening ischemia. In a series of 68 isolated profundaplasties performed from 1970 to 1980, 12 were in patients with claudication, and follow-up revealed an 87% patency at 5 years.³ In the 54 isolated profundaplasties performed for rest pain or tissue loss, the 5 year patency was only 21%.² When the patients with limb-threatening ischemia were stratified by clinical presentation, ischemic ulcers healed in 53%, ischemic necrosis resolved in 35%, and rest pain remained resolved during follow-up in only 32%. In other studies of isolated profundaplasty for limb-threatening ischemia, success rates of approximately 50% have been reported on long-term follow-up. Kalman and associates reported that the outcome for patients with rest pain was not consistently different than the outcome for those with tissue loss.¹ Others have described poor results for profundaplasty in limbs with tissue loss and do not recommend an isolated profundaplasty in such patients. The limb with significant pedal gangrene is frequently not adequately revascularized by an isolated profundaplasty. In these patients, the principal reason to consider a profundaplasty is to provide adequate blood flow for successful healing of a below-knee amputation. Indeed, all patients who are to have a below-knee amputation should have some assessment of the PFA if there is any question of adequacy to heal the amputation. It is possible to lower the anticipated level of amputation from above the knee to below the knee in a patient who has a profundaplasty to correct significant PFA stenosis.

Treatment of a new or previously unrecognized PFA stenosis in a patient who has failed previous vein bypass or whose veins are inadequate or have been used for coronary revascularization may provide limb salvage if the appropriate criteria are present.

OPERATIVE TECHNIQUES

Through a vertical groin incision, the PFA is isolated after obtaining control of the common femoral and superficial femoral arteries. Because of the extent of dissection required for a long profundaplasty and the

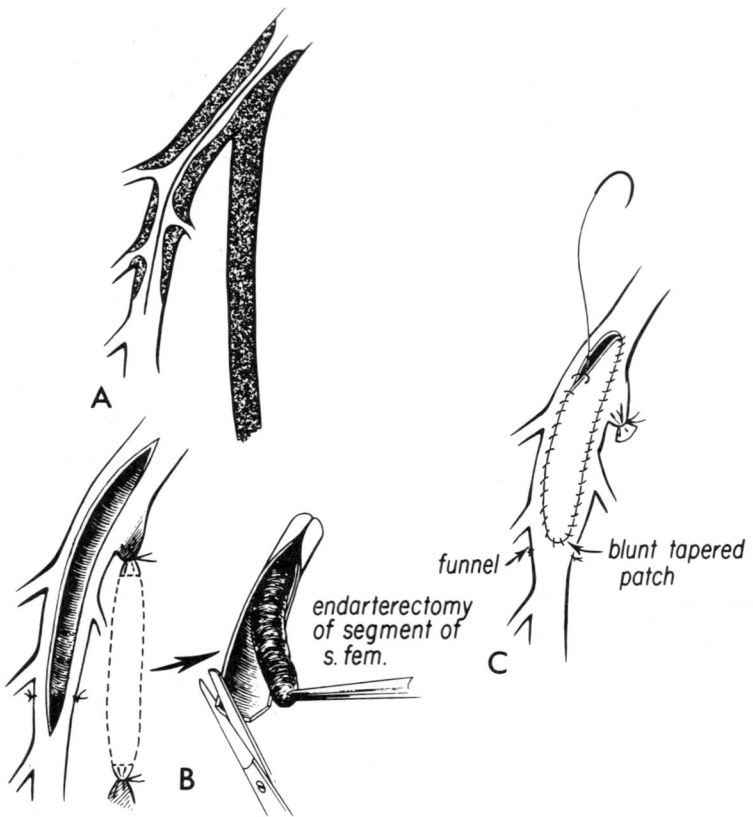

Figure 3 *A*, Arteriotomy extending from the common femoral onto the PFA to the end point of disease. *B*, Tacking sutures at the break point of the distal intima and harvesting of the superficial femoral for use as a patch. *C*, Completion of the patch closure with even tapering of the repair for ideal hemodynamics.

risk of lymphatic leak, all superficial lymphatic tissue must be carefully ligated. The dissection of the common femoral artery should be performed with care to preserve the medial and lateral femoral circumflex arteries that occasionally arise from the common femoral artery. The PFA is usually found branching deep and lateral to the superficial femoral artery. The large femoral circumflex vein crosses the PFA 1 to 2 cm from its origin and must be ligated in continuity and divided to expose the anterior surface of the proximal PFA. Dissection should continue until normal-appearing artery is encountered. The atherosclerotic disease typically ends at a bifurcation. Once the branches distal to the end point of the occlusive disease are controlled, the patient is given heparin sodium and the common femoral, superficial femoral, and PFA branches are clamped. The arteriotomy should start on the common femoral and is extended down the PFA, taking care to avoid the crotch of the common femoral bifurcation and any major PFA branches (Fig. 3). The arteriotomy extends to the bifurcation where the gross disease ends. Endarterectomy of the involved common femoral and PFA is performed as needed. Any plaque that involves the branches (particularly the medial and lateral circumflex branches) is removed completely, as it rarely extends past the branch orifice. Care is taken to achieve a clear break point, and any distal intimal dissection is tacked with 7-0 suture, if required.

Patch closure of the arteriotomy is achieved with the toe of the inflow prosthetic graft material if the profundaplasty is an adjunct to an inflow procedure and the arteriotomy on the PFA is short (2 to 4 cm) (Fig. 4). If the profundaplasty is extended or performed as an isolated procedure, the material of choice for the patch repair is autogenous tissue. The use of endarterectomized occluded superficial femoral artery is recommended (Fig. 3). This is easy to prepare, performs as well as saphenous vein, and saves the vein for subsequent distal arterial bypass or coronary revascularization. The use of autogenous repair in extended profundaplasty is thought to result in less neointimal reaction and have better patency than expanded polytetrafluoroethylene or Dacron repairs. The size of the patch should achieve a smooth taper in the size of the PFA to allow for optimal hemodynamic flow characteristics of the repair.

RESULTS

More than 70% of profundaplasties are performed in conjunction with an inflow procedure such as an aortofemoral, axillofemoral, or femoral-femoral bypass.

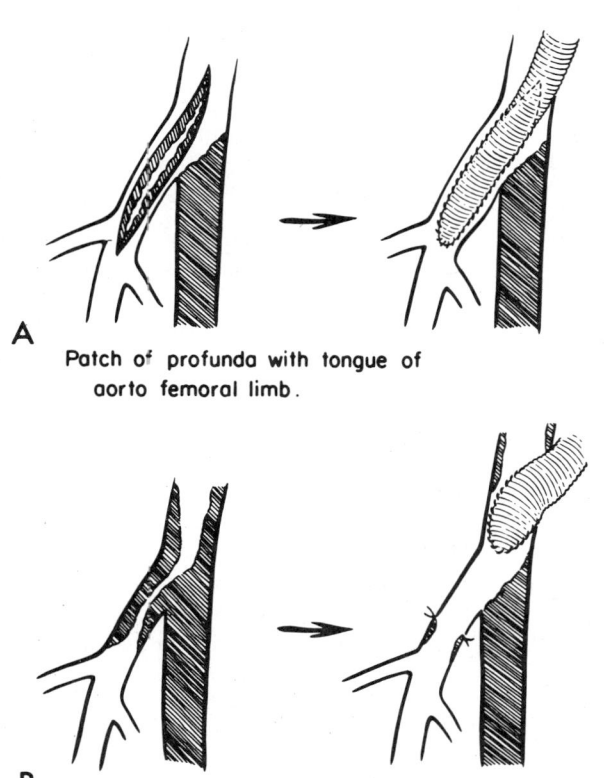

Figure 4 *A*, Short patch on the PFA using the toe of an inflow graft. *B*, Inflow graft and a short endarterectomy into the PFA with tacking sutures but no patch.

In our study reported in 1981, 169 of the 237 profundaplasties were part of an inflow procedure, and the resulting clinical success rate, defined as a patent repair and relief of presenting symptoms, was 55% and limb salvage rate was 80% at 5 years.[3] In our more recent series of 68 profundaplasties performed from 1987 to 1992, 49 (72%) were as adjuncts to inflow procedures. The clinical success rate in these was 54%, and the limb salvage rate was 96% at 4 years. The improved limb salvage rate is attributed to improved techniques in distal bypass used to salvage profundaplasty failures.

When an isolated profundaplasty is performed to treat limb ischemia, the clinical success and limb salvage rates are lower than for inflow and profundaplasty. In our study reported in 1981, the 68 isolated profundaplasties had a 27% clinical success rate and a 36% limb salvage rate at 5 years. When the patients were categorized by their clinical presentation, patients with claudication had a 73% patency at 5 years compared to patients with limb-threatening ischemia, who had 21% patency at 5 years. In our more recent study, six isolated profundaplasties were performed with only one requiring a distal bypass and the other five remaining clinically successful during a mean follow-up of 21 months. Kalman and co-workers report a 49% 3 year clinical success rate and a 76% limb salvage rate after isolated profundaplasty with no significant difference in the outcome of patients with claudication versus patients with limb-threatening ischemia.[1] The degree of ischemia relates to the severity and distribution of occlusive disease. Patients with diffuse disease in the PFA collaterals and the popliteal-tibial vessels have severe ischemia on presentation and, therefore, have poorer results after profundaplasty.

REFERENCES

1. Kalman PG, Johnston KW, Walker PM. The current role of isolated profundaplasty. J Cardiovasc Surg 1990; 31:107–111.
2. Rollins DL, Towne JB, Bernhard VM. Isolated profundaplasty for limb salvage. J Vasc Surg 1985; 2:585–590.
3. Towne JB, Bernhard VM, Rollins DL. Profundaplasty in perspective: Limitations in the long-term management of limb ischemia. Surgery 1981; 90:1037–1046.
4. McCoy DM, Sawchuk AP, Schuler, et al. The role of isolated profundaplasty for the treatment of rest pain. Arch Surg 1989; 124:441–444.
5. Mitchell RA, Bone GE, Bridges R, et al. Patient selection for isolated profundaplasty: Arteriographic correlates of operative results. Am J Surg 1979; 138:912–919.
6. Beales JSM, Adcock FA, Frawley JS, et al. The radiological assessment of disease of the profunda femoris artery. Br J Radiol 1971; 44:854–859.
7. Haimovici H, Shapiro JH, Jacobson HG. Serial femoral arteriography in occlusive disease: Clinical-roentgenologic considerations with a new classification of occlusive patterns. Am J Roentgenol 1960; 83:1042–1048.
8. Margulis AR, Nice CM Jr, Murphy TO. Arteriographic manifestations of peripheral occlusive disease: With the report of two new signs. Am J Roentgenol 1957; 78:273–282.
9. Martin P, Frawley JE, Barabas AP, et al. On the surgery of atherosclerosis of the profunda femoris artery. Surgery 1972; 71:182–189.
10. Boren CH, Towne JB, Bernhard VM, et al. Profundapopliteal collateral index: A guide to successful profundaplasty. Arch Surg 1980; 115:1366–1372.

LUMBAR SYMPATHECTOMY FOR LOWER EXTREMITY CUTANEOUS ISCHEMIC ULCERS

TIMOTHY J. RANVAL, M.D.
ROBERT W. BARNES, M.D.

In 1924, Julio Diez in Buenos Aires performed the first lumbar sympathectomy for rest pain secondary to thromboangiitis obliterans. Trimble reported the use of lumbar sympathectomy for arteriosclerosis obliterans in 1932. These reports culminated a colorful historical interest in sympathetic denervation that included Jaboulay, Leriche, Hunter, Royle, Adson, and Brown, among others. It ushered in a period when lumbar sympathectomy rapidly gained popularity until direct arterial reconstruction began in the 1950s. Early indications for sympathectomy included intermittent claudication, ischemic rest pain, ischemic ulceration, and gangrene, as well as vasospastic disorders. Its indiscriminant use led to mixed results and eventual disillusionment with the procedure.

Lower extremity cutaneous ulcers that occur with atherosclerotic occlusive disease tend to present initially after a minor wound that fails to heal. Left untreated, these superficial wounds can progress to deep ulceration, invasive infection, and, if unchecked, eventual loss of the extremity.

The mainstays of treatment for cutaneous foot ulcers due to vascular disease are revascularization, debridement, and local wound care. Correction of associated medical conditions, cessation of smoking, and initial treatment of infection with debridement, drainage, and antibiotics are simultaneously undertaken. Early in the treatment of such patients, noninvasive and arteriographic evaluation should be undertaken in search of arterial lesions amenable to standard arteriographic and surgical reconstructions.

A small group of patients with unreconstructible arterial disease and marginal foot blood flow with rest pain, pregangrenous changes, and/or superficial ulcers may benefit from lumbar sympathectomy. The small increase in blood flow associated with the procedure may tip the balance in favor of healing the ulcer.

If we are to rationally select patients for this operation, the role of the sympathetic innervation on the vascular system must be understood so that sympathetic ablation can be applied in a logical fashion.

ANATOMY AND PHYSIOLOGY

Preganglionic sympathetic fibers arise from cell bodies in the lateral gray substance of the thoracolumbar spinal cord. These fibers emerge via the anterior (ventral) roots of the thoracic and lumbar nerves and reach the sympathetic chain via the white rami communicantes. After synapsing with cells in the sympathetic ganglia, the postganglionic fibers course through the gray rami communicantes to join the somatic nerves to be distributed to the peripheral blood vessels and sweat glands.

The sympathetic trunks are paired and consist of a series of ganglia connected to intervening fibers. The chain extends from the first cervical vertebra to the tip of the sacrum. The sympathetic ganglia are not strictly segmental, and preganglionic fibers may synapse above or below the root from which they emerge. In the lumbar region there may be five or more ganglia, but four are typical. The sympathetic ganglia are dependent on their synaptic relations to the preganglionic fibers. Sympathectomy denervates the postganglionic fibers by cutting off the connection to the central nervous system.

The lower limb receives all preganglionic fibers through the upper lumbar nerves by way of the lumbar sympathetic trunk. The lumbar portions of the paired sympathetic trunks lie on the anterior-lateral portion of the vertebral bodies. The trunks enter the abdomen from behind the medial arcuate ligament. The L1 ganglia typically lie behind the crura of the diaphragm. The left and right trunks lie posterior-lateral to the aorta and vena cava, respectively. The lumbar arteries and veins may lie in front of or behind the trunks.

Despite the relatively long history of sympathectomy and a large volume of observational and experimental evidence, the effects of sympathectomy on the ischemic leg are controversial. There is little doubt that sympathectomy increases blood flow in a normal limb. However, the effect of sympathectomy on the chronically ischemic limb is less well defined.

Sympathetic tone is one of several factors that control peripheral vasomotor tone, particularly in small arteries and arterioles. The redistribution of postsympathectomy blood flow is of critical importance. Blood flow to muscle is not increased.[1] Hence, the use of sympathectomy for intermittent claudication is not reasonable.

Controversy exists over the nutritive value (capillary flow) of the increased blood flow to skin. It is known that sympathetic nerves function in vasoconstrictive control of the arteriole end of arteriovenous shunts in the skin. The characteristic warm pink flush in the distal skin of the sympathectomized limb is mostly due to an increase in flow through the shunts. The nutritive value of this increased blood flow has been questioned. Moore and Hall, using xenon-133 clearance in ischemic limbs, documented an increase in nutritive blood flow in sympathectomized limbs.[2] Other researchers have failed to document a significant increase in nutritional blood flow.[3] The effect on collateral blood flow seems to be an increase in flow in individuals with inappropriate vasoconstrictions; however, the increase is small and transient.[4]

Two other effects of sympathectomy are the control of sweating and sympathetic pain transmission. The ablative effect on sweating by sympathectomy has led to the use of the operation in the treatment of hyperhidrosis. Likewise, the loss of extremity perspiration, as seen in the diabetic limb, implies "autosympathectomy" and hence has implications in patient selection.

It is known that sympathectomy may relieve ischemic rest pain. The exact physiology of this is unknown. It does not seem to be due to an increase in blood flow.[5] Based on animal data it is thought that sympathectomy decreases pain perception by decreasing tissue norepinephrine as well as reducing spinal augmentation of painful stimuli.[6]

INDICATIONS AND PATIENT SELECTION

In view of the limited augmentation of nutritive blood flow following lumbar sympathectomy, the procedure's indiscriminant use is to be discouraged. Proper patient selection based on arteriographic, clinical, and physiologic criteria is necessary to select candidates likely to respond favorably to the procedure.

The first selection criterion must include nonreconstructible vascular disease. If arterial reconstruction or arteriographic intervention is possible, these interventions should be performed. Once it has been determined that nonreconstructible vascular occlusive disease is present, objective evidence should be gathered to document a potential positive response to sympathectomy.

Clinically, the patient cannot have extensive tissue loss or deep infection. Sympathectomy has not been found to be of use in these situations where amputation is inevitable in all but a few patients. Appropriate clinical settings for sympathectomy are rest pain with pregangrenous changes or superficial ulceration involving only the skin of the forefoot.

The second consideration prior to performing a sympathectomy is the adequacy of collateral reserve. We use a capillary refilling time of 20 seconds or less and an ankle-brachial index of greater than 0.3.

The third assessment to be made regards residual vasomotor tone. The most useful test in our hands are digit or foot plethysmography. Tests of skin temperature, resistance, or sweating and the effect of diagnostic therapeutic nerve blocks are cumbersome, and we generally do not use them when ischemic ulcers are present.

We have found that photoplethysmography is the simplest and most sensitive method to obtain digit pulse waveforms, digit blood pressures, and the effects of sympathetic vasomotor tone and reactive hyperemia on the digit pulse waveforms. The normal digit pulse waveform has a sharp upstroke, a narrow peak, and a dicrotic wave on the downslope, which is concave toward the baseline. The digit pulse waveform distal to the arterial obstruction has a damped waveform, a more gradual upslope, a rounded peak, and loss of the dicrotic wave on the downslope, which may be convex relative to the baseline. Sympathetic vasomotor tone may be assessed by having a patient take a deep breath. The resultant increased sympathetic activity results in vasoconstriction and diminution of the digit pulse waveform. Patients with loss of sympathetic function such as diabetics with advanced neuropathy may show no change in digit pulse amplitude in response to a deep breath. Similarly, patients with advanced arterial occlusive disease may have no vasodilatory reserve and may not vasoconstrict in response to a deep breath. Finally, the presence of vasodilatory reserve may be assessed by recording the response of the digit pulse amplitude during reactive hyperemia following 3 minutes of ischemia induced by the digit cuff. Normally the digit pulse amplitude should increase markedly during the ensuing reactive hyperemia. Patients with advanced peripheral arterial occlusive disease may have lost this vasodilatory reserve. The most severe digit ischemia may result in no digit pulsation either at rest or during reactive hyperemia. Patients with such findings are rarely improved by lumbar sympathectomy.

Buerger's Disease (thromboangiitis obliterans) in general does not respond to sympathectomy.

The blue toe syndrome may benefit from sympathectomy, more in terms of pain relief than in terms of healing of the lesions, which generally heal without surgical intervention.

Vasospastic disorders respond to sympathectomy, but this treatment has largely been replaced by various pharmacologic vasodilators, although in selected patients sympathectomy can be of benefit.

Last, the use of sympathectomy at the time of aortoiliac reconstruction or as an adjunct to distal bypass has been proposed. In 1977 we published a prospective, randomized study of 50 patients undergoing aortoiliac reconstruction with or without concomitant lumbar sympathectomy.[7] No differences were found in graft patency, limb survival, or ankle-brachial indices. There were significant reductions in foot vascular resistances in patients with multilevel disease as measured by plethysmography.[7] Currently we add a sympathectomy to aortoiliac reconstruction in patients with multilevel disease and pregangrenous changes or minor superficial tissue loss.

SURGICAL TECHNIQUE

Lumbar sympathectomy is most commonly performed as a surgical procedure or as a percutaneous chemical sympathectomy.[5] The operation can be carried out before, during, or after vascular reconstruction. It can be performed as an isolated procedure or at the time of aortoiliac reconstruction. A surgical lumbar sympathectomy can be performed as a retroperitoneal or as a transperitoneal procedure.

The patient is positioned supine, with the knees elevated on a pillow to relax the psoas muscles. A transverse skin incision extends from the lateral border of the rectus muscle to the midaxillary line midway between the costal margin and the iliac crest. Through a muscle-splitting incision in the external and internal oblique muscles, the transversus abdominis muscle is exposed. The transversus abdominis muscle and fascia are incised laterally to expose the properitoneal fat. Incision of the transversalis fascia anteriorly must be performed carefully to avoid entry into the peritoneal cavity. The peritoneum is mobilized medially, clearing it from the properitoneal fat pad at the lateral border of the incision. One must be careful not to carry the blunt dissection behind the quadratus lumborum muscle. Care should be taken not to injure the genitofemoral nerve, which lies on the psoas muscle. Likewise, the ureter must not be injured as it is mobilized anteriorly and medially with the peritoneum.

The lumbar sympathetic chain can be palpated as a firm cord on the anterolateral bodies of the lumbar vertebrae, between the psoas muscle and the inferior vena cava on the right or psoas muscle and the aorta on the left. Lumbar veins or arteries, which may course either in front of or behind the lumbar sympathetic chain, may be ligated. The gray-white lumbar sympathetic chain is initially exposed lying on the vertebral column.

The sympathetic chain can be dissected from the surrounding tissues using the dissector end of a Smithwick instrument. The Smithwick hook is then used to elevate the sympathetic chain. A hemoclip is applied to the proximal end of the sympathetic chain between the first and second lumbar ganglia. The sympathetic chain is then transected between the first and second lumbar ganglia while avoiding the first lumbar ganglion to minimize the risk of sexual dysfunction. We routinely remove the second throught the fourth lumbar ganglia. The presence of ganglion cells should be confirmed by microscopic examination of the resected specimen.

COMPLICATIONS

The most common complication of lumbar sympathectomy is neuralgia of the thigh, which occurs in approximately one-third of patients (Table 1). Usually it is temporary and resolves spontaneously. Initial treatment with oral analgesics usually suffices. Patients with severe neuralgia can be treated with a single epidural injection of fentanyl and methylprednisolone.[8] Ejaculatory dysfunction can usually be avoided by preserving the first lumbar ganglion. Paradoxic gangrene is rare and probably the result of atheroembolism and not the result of a hemodynamic steal syndrome, as originally thought. Paraplegia is a rare complication of the procedure, possibly due to the ligation of a critical lumbar artery while exposing the sympathetic chain.

RESULTS

Results of lumbar sympathectomy are predicated on preoperative selection criteria and the definition of success. Criteria for success are relief of pain, healing of skin ulceration, and limb salvage for at least 6 months. Persson and associates performed lumbar sympathectomy on 22 patients with ulceration who were deemed anatomically unreconstructible or whose general medical conditions precluded major vascular reconstruction. In 15 of 16 patients without deep infections, ulcerations healed. The lowest ankle-brachial index (ABI) was 0.27 in this group. One patient with an ABI of 0 was "improved" but expired 2 months postoperatively. None of the 16 patients required amputation in the follow-up period, which was up to 58 months.

Yao and Bergan reported on sympathectomy in 84 unreconstructible patients with severe tissue ischemia, rest pain, or pregangrenous changes in the feet or toes.[10] Forty-nine patients had a favorable response to sympathectomy, 37 of whom had a preoperative ABI greater than 0.25. Twenty-seven patients required amputation, 26 of whom had an ABI of less than 0.2. All patients with ABIs greater than 0.35 responded well to sympathectomy. The authors did not specifically mention the number of patients with ulcers. Less optimistic results for sympathectomy were observed by Collins and coworkers, who reported an amputation rate of 56% (10 of 18), no change in 17% (3 of 18), and good results in only 28% (5 of 18). Skin changes included both ulceration and gangrene.[11]

RECOMMENDATIONS

We currently limit lumbar sympathectomy to a select group of patients with intolerable ischemia of the foot, with or without superficial ulceration or minimal gangrene limited to the toes and forefoot. If revascularization is not feasible, we evaluate the patient for digit vasoreactivity by using the plethysmographic tests that have been described. If there is no evidence of residual sympathetic vasomotor tone, then sympathectomy is not offered. If residual vasomotor tone is present and the ABI is greater than 0.3, sympathectomy is considered. For patients with reconstructible vessels, if the arterial occlusive disease involves only one anatomic level, we proceed with arterial reconstruction. However, patients

Table 1 Complications of Lumbar Sympathectomy

Neurogenic
   Neuralgia (33%)
   Ejaculatory dysfunction
   Nerve injury
   Paraplegia
Vascular
   Paradoxical gangrene
   Postural hypotension
   Aortojejunal fistula
   Vascular injury
Gastrointestinal
   Ileus
   Fecal fistula
Genitourinary
   Ureteral injury

with intolerable pedal ischemia usually have multilevel disease. If the patient is a candidate for aortofemoral reconstruction, we usually recommend a sympathectomy as a concomitant procedure.

REFERENCES

1. Hoffman DC, Jepson RP. Muscle blood flow and sympathectomy. Surg Gynecol Obstet 1968; 127:12–16.
2. Moore WS, Hall AD. Effects of lumbar sympathectomy on skin capillary blood flow in arterial occlusive disease. J Surg Res 1966; 6:423–434.
3. Welch GH, Leiberman DP. Cutaneous blood flow in the foot following lumbar sympathectomy. Scand J Clin Lab Invest 1985; 45:621–626.
4. Ludbrook J. Collateral artery resistance in the human lower limb. J Surg Res 1966; 6:423–434.
5. Cross FW, Cotton LT. Chemical lumbar sympathectomy for ischemic rest pain, a randomized, prospective controlled clinical trial. Am J Surg 1985; 150:341–345.
6. Loh L, Nathan PW. Painful peripheral states and sympathetic blocks. J Neurol, Neurosurg, Psychiatry 1978; 41:664–671.
7. Barnes RW, Baker WH, Shanik G. Value of concomitant sympathectomy in aortoiliac reconstruction. Arch Surg 1977; 112:1325–1330.
8. Buche M, Randour P, Mayne A, et al. Neuralgia following lumbar sympathectomy. Ann Vasc Surg 1988; 2:279–281.
9. Persson AV, Anderson LA, Padberg FT Jr. Selection of patients for lumbar sympathectomy. Surg Clin North Am 1985; 65:393–403.
10. Yao JST, Bergan JJ. Predictability of vascular reactivity relative to sympathetic ablation. Arch Surg 1973; 107:676–680.
11. Collins GJ Jr, Rich NM, Clagett GP, et al. Clinical results of lumbar sympathectomy. Am Surgeon 1981; 47:31–35.

REVERSED AUTOGENOUS VEIN GRAFT FOR ARTHEROSCLEROTIC LOWER EXTREMITY OCCLUSIVE DISEASE

PHILIPPE A. MASSER, M.D.
LLOYD M. TAYLOR Jr., M.D.
GREGORY L. MONETA, M.D.
JOHN M. PORTER, M.D.

Reversed autogenous vein graft (RVG) for lower extremity bypass, popularized by Jean Kunlin over 4 decades ago, has an enviable record of versatility and durability and continues to be our graft of preference for leg bypass. In our practice we have a firm policy of using autogenous conduits for limb bypass whenever possible. In our recent experience with more than 1,200 leg bypasses, we have accomplished an all-autogenous bypass in 94% of patients, despite many multiple redo bypasses. An in situ bypass would have been possible in only 50% of our patients because of multiple redos and saphenous vein inadequacy. Because of both frequent saphenous vein unavailability and a remarkable absence of convincing evidence of in situ superiority, we continue to use and advocate the RVG for lower extremity bypass.

INDICATIONS FOR LOWER EXTREMITY BYPASS

Smoking cessation and daily 1 mile walking are uniformly recommended as initial therapy for patients presenting with intermittent claudication. Patients are routinely advised to walk in shopping malls or city parks where they can sit as often as necessary. They are specifically told to rest when leg pain occurs and that they are not to try to "walk through" claudication discomfort. Pentoxifylline provides clinically significant improvement in about 40% of claudicants and is used occasionally. Cilostazol and carnitine are two investigational drugs in phase III trials that may be of future value in the treatment of claudication. Both have appeared beneficial in preliminary trials. Bypass for claudication is never considered until after a generous trial of nonoperative treatment.

Patients presenting with severe ischemia manifested by rest pain or tissue loss are considered for early arterial reconstruction. At Oregon Health Sciences University (OHSU), 80% of lower extremity bypasses are performed for limb salvage and 18% for claudication. Using modern arteriographic techniques, we are presently able to demonstrate a reasonable recipient artery for bypass in more than 99% of patients.[1] Primary amputation for advanced limb ischemia is recommended only in neurologically impaired, bedridden individuals. The dismal results following amputation are so overwhelming that vigorous attempts at limb salvage are indicated in almost everyone with a threatened limb. Alternatives to operation, such as transluminal balloon angioplasty or catheter endarterectomy, have so far failed to demonstrate sufficient effectiveness and durability to be considered for routine use in the treatment of infrainguinal arterial occlusive disease.

PREOPERATIVE PREPARATION

The optimal preoperative cardiac evaluation of vascular surgical patients remains controversial. All patients with peripheral arterial occlusions sufficiently severe to require operation are presumed to have significant coronary artery disease. Full hemodynamic monitoring and prophylactic nitroglycerin are used routinely. Extensive preoperative diagnostic cardiac examination is limited to patients with coronary symptoms sufficiently severe to warrant further study based on their own merits, without consideration of impending peripheral vascular reconstruction. We do not advocate extensive prophylactic evaluation or treatment of associated cardiac disease. Perioperative cardiac morbidity and mortality data from centers employing aggressive policies of extensive preoperative cardiac evaluation, including prophylactic coronary artery bypass grafting or percutaneous transluminal coronary angioplasty, do not show a lower perioperative myocardial infarction rate or death rate than our own.[2]

All patients undergoing operation for lower extremity occulusive disease are appropriate candidates for screening for associated carotid artery disease and abdominal aortic aneurysm, as vascular patients have a 5% to 10% prevalence of aortic aneurysms and greater than 80% carotid stenoses. All preoperative vascular patients are screened for hypercoagulable states, including anticardiolipin antibody, lupus anticoagulant, protein C, protein S, antithrombin III, and lipoprotein Lp(a). A 15% to 20% prevalence of one or more of these abnormalities has been found in recent years, many of which mandate long-term warfarin anticoagulation. We have not specifically addressed the cost-effectiveness of this program of coagulation screening and are not presently recommending its widespread adoption.

Adequate arteriographic visualization of inflow vessels and distal vessels is essential for optimal surgical planning. With selective use of pharmacologic intraarterial vasodilators, digital subtraction techniques, and reactive hyperemia, adequate distal arteries for grafting are opacified on preoperative arteriography in 99% of patients.[3] A limb is regarded as having no adequate distal vessel only if small, unnamed arteries are seen in the leg and foot. In recent years we have recommended primary amputation because of the absence of distal graftable vessels in less than 1% of patients. The widely published practice of routinely performing operative arteriography to define distal graftable arteries strikes us as inappropriate and indicating the need for improved preoperative arteriography.

Autogenous vein, used either in the reversed or in situ configuration, has proven to be the best arterial conduit and in contemporary reports has routinely produced 5 year patency rates of 75% to 85% in the femoropopliteal position.[3-5] Prosthetic grafts have much lower patency rates than vein grafts.[6,7] Although some have proposed that prosthetic grafts be used preferentially for above-knee bypass and vein reserved for below-knee and redo bypass, we find no justification for this recommendation.[8] All patients undergoing preferential above-knee polytetrafluoroethylene (PTFE) bypass grafting presumably have adequate saphenous vein available and are undergoing their first ipsilateral limb bypass. When only patients undergoing their first leg bypass with an adequate saphenous vein to the above-knee popliteal artery are considered, we have experienced a 5 year patency of 96%, clearly twice as good as preferential above-knee PTFE results. We continue to believe one should do the best operation first.

We prefer RVG for all extremity bypasses. We find no reason to employ the in situ technique, as it has failed to perform in a superior manner in randomized studies,[9-11] and is clearly less versatile than the RVG. Its use results in considerably more endothelial damage,[12] and in our opinion is more difficult to perform well. Experience has shown that in situ grafts require more frequent early secondary procedures to maintain patency. On a practical level, the performance of an in situ graft obviously requires an adequate ipsilateral greater saphenous vein (GSV) that was absent in more than 50% of our patients.[3]

The preoperative clinical examination is generally adequate to evaluate the condition of saphenous veins as potential conduits. Prior thrombosis or inability of the vein to dilate to at least 3.5 mm intraoperatively excludes a vein from consideration. If preoperative evaluation shows that neither GSV is available, duplex vein mapping of alternative veins, such as the lesser saphenous veins, basilic, and cephalic veins, is used.

OPERATIVE TECHNIQUE

Two surgical teams are routinely employed for lower extremity bypass procedures. Loupes and headlights are helpful. A separate back table is used for vein-graft preparation. The cell-saver autotransfusion device is routinely used for reoperative procedures, but not for primary operations.

The vein is fully exposed and side branches carefully ligated while preserving axial flow. Branches are usually ligated with 5-0 silk. Once removed, the vein is gently dilated with chilled autologous heparinized blood with added papaverine (0.2 mg/ml). The vein should dilate to greater than 3.5 mm in diameter. Sclerosed areas are excised if necessary, and a venovenostomy performed with running 6-0 or 7-0 PTFE suture. Leaks are repaired with 8-0 suture. Vein preparation usually requires 10 to 15 minutes, and the vein is implanted at once with the proximal and distal anastomotic sites having been readied by others during vein preparation.

The medial approach to the popliteal, posterior tibial, and peroneal arteries is routinely used, and the anterolateral approach to the anterior tibial artery. The bypass is kept as short as possible, frequently using the distal superficial femoral or profunda femoris arteries for graft inflow. This allows use of a shorter length of vein and reduces the need for venovenostomies. We used a site other than the common femoral artery for graft origin in 58% of patients. With the graft distended to avoid twisting, the RVG is routed in the anatomic position using a specially constructed Oregon tunneler. For distal anastomosis to the anterior tibial artery, an incision in the interosseous membrane is required, together with a medial counterincision in the below-knee popliteal fossa. Reoperative routing to the anterior tibial artery frequently is performed through a lateral subcutaneous route.

For the proximal anastomosis, PTFE suture is used, incorporating a venous side branch whenever possible to minimize heel narrowing (Fig. 1). Profunda femoris endarterectomy is performed if a high-grade stenosis is

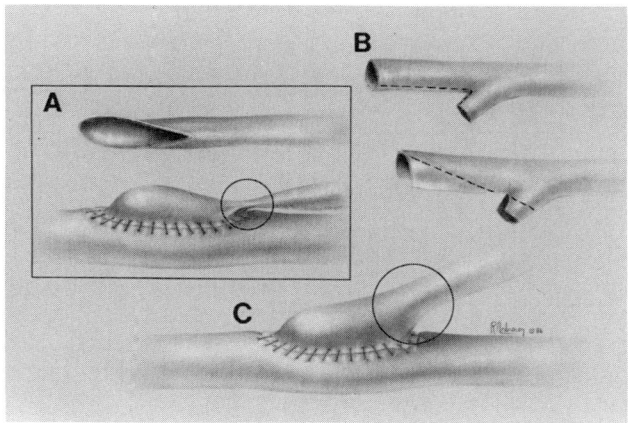

Figure 1 *A,* End-to-side anastomosis with constriction at heel. *B,* Incorporation of vein side branch into proximal anastomosis prevents constriction (*C*). (From Taylor LM Jr, Edwards JM, Phenney ES, Porter JM. Reversed vein bypass to infrapopliteal arteries. Ann Surg 1987; 205:90–97; with permission.)

present. For the distal anastomosis, 6-0 to 8-0 PTFE suture is used. PTFE suture is routinely used in preference to polypropylene for our autogenous vein bypasses. For operative bypass assessment, we insonate the anastomoses with CW Doppler to detect areas of increased frequency as well as confirm unobstructed arterial flow signals at the ankle. The electromagnetic flowmeter is used before and after graft injection of 30 mg of papaverine. We expect minimal mean flow of more than 50 ml/minute and doubling of flow after papaverine administration. Completion arteriography is performed only if the Doppler or the flowmeter suggests a problem (Fig. 2).

After reversal of the heparin effect with protamine sulfate, the incisions are closed in layers with absorbable suture, completing the skin closure with a running subcuticular absorbable suture. The subcuticular technique has almost eliminated the wound healing problems occasionally experienced with prior closure techniques, including staples and adhesive strips. Closed suction drains are routinely used for reoperative sites or with extensive dissections.

POSTOPERATIVE MANAGEMENT

Patients are begun preoperatively on aspirin, 325 mg/day, and this is continued postoperatively. For patients with low flow grafts (less than 75ml/minute), infrainguinal prosthetic bypass, or extensive proximal endarterectomy, 6% Dextran 70 is administered for several days postoperatively, giving 500 ml each 24 hours. Patients with redo bypasses and those with defined hypercoagulable states are routinely maintained on long-term warfarin anticoagulation. Early ambulation is encouraged. All patients are placed in below-knee 20 to 30 mm Hg gradient elastic stockings for 6 weeks to 3 months

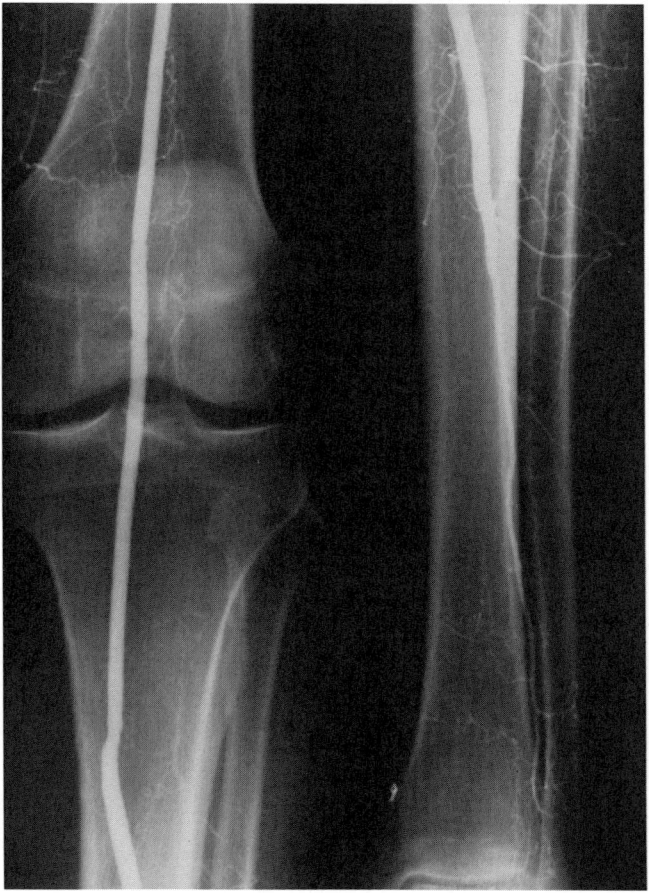

Figure 2 Completion arteriogram of common femoral to peroneal artery reversed vein graft bypass. (From Taylor LM Jr, Edwards JM, Phenney ES, Porter JM. Reversed vein bypass to infrapopliteal arteries. Ann Surg 1987; 205:90–97; with permission.)

postoperatively to assist in management of the invariable postoperative edema that follows leg bypass. Duplex vein graft surveillance is performed every 3 months during the first year and every 6 months thereafter.

RESULTS

It is important to remember that comparison of patencies between reported series is affected by demographic characteristics. A study reporting a large number of redo bypasses, as in most RVG series, almost always has lower patency rates than a study consisting exclusively of first-time bypasses, such as almost all in situ reports. We achieved 5 year primary patency rates at OHSU using exclusively RVG: above-knee femoropopliteal, 77%; below-knee femoropopliteal, 80%; infrapopliteal, 69% (Fig. 3). Leg veins performed better than arm veins. Whereas saphenous vein bypasses had 80% 5 year patency rates, non-GSV grafts had only 68% 5 year primary patency rates (Fig. 4). However, with

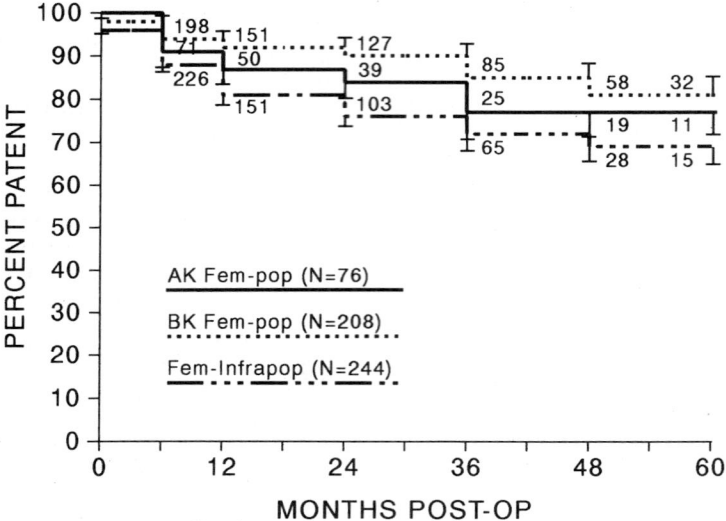

Figure 3 Life table primary patency for grafts grouped according to site of distal anastomosis. Bars indicate standard error. AK, above knee; BK, below knee.

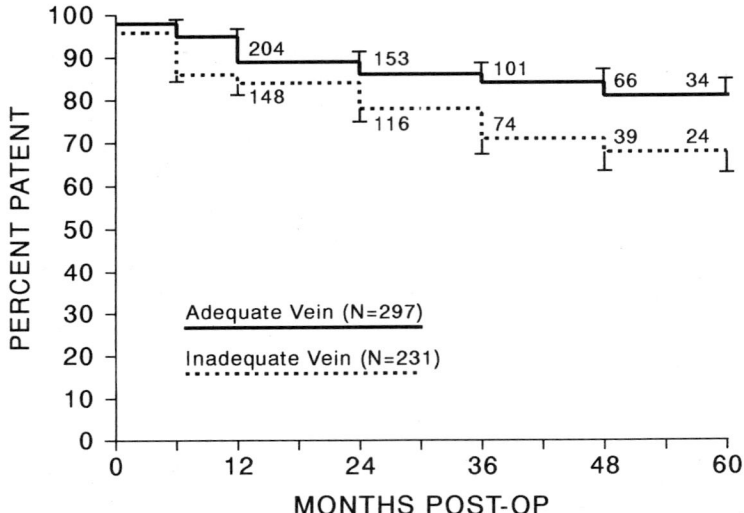

Figure 4 Life table primary patency for grafts performed with adequate intact ipsilateral greater saphenous vein compared to primary patency for grafts when this conduit was not available. Bars indicate standard error.

Table 1 Reversed Versus In Situ Vein Bypass

Series	n	Primary Patency			Secondary Patency		
		1 year	3 years	5 years	1 year	3 years	5 years
Taylor, et al[3]	285	89%	84%	80%	90%	86%	84%
Leather, et al[4]	1,000	—	—	59%	—	—	76%
Bandyk, et al[5]	192	68–74%*	45–58%*	—	86–98%*	80–89%*	—

*Range of patency depending upon site of distal anastomosis.
From Taylor LM, Edwards JM, Porter JM. Present status of reverse vein bypass grafting: Five-year results of a modern series. J Vasc Surg 1990; 11:193–206; with permission.

secondary procedures, there was no significant difference in ultimate 5 year patency between GSV and non-GSV grafts. There were no patency differences between grafts originating from the common femoral artery or those originating from a more distal site. When our patencies are stratified and calculated for patients undergoing their first bypass with a good GSV, a situation comparable to in situ series, there is no difference between our 5 year patency rates and those from comparable in situ series (Table 1). Patients in our series undergoing their first bypass with a good-quality saphenous vein to the above-knee popliteal artery had 5 year primary patency rates of 96%. This emphasizes both the importance of demographic stratification when comparing patencies of different reports and underscores the excellent performance of RVG.

The reversed autogenous vein continues to be the most versatile, available, and durable conduit for lower extremity bypass. We suspect that a well-performed in situ bypass is as good as RVG, but certainly not superior, and not applicable to as many patients. Many points are important in the performance of a leg bypass, including careful patient selection, excellent-quality preoperative arteriography, and meticulous attention to operative technical details. In recent years the importance of routine postoperative duplex graft surveillance has been established, at least for autogenous grafts. In fact, one should not perform leg bypass at all if unable to provide detailed postoperative graft flow surveillance.

REFERENCES

1. Kozak BE, Bedell JE, Rosch J. Small vessel leg angiography for distal vessel bypass grafts. J Vasc Surg 1988; 8:711–715.
2. Taylor LM, Yeager RA, Moneta GL, et al. The incidence of perioperative myocardial infarction in general vascular surgery. J Vasc Surg 1991; 15:52–61.
3. Taylor LM, Edwards JM, Porter JM. Present status of reverse vein bypass grafting: Five-year results of a modern series. J Vasc Surg 1990; 11:193–206.
4. Leather RP, Shah DM, Chang BB, et al. Resurrection of the in situ saphenous vein bypass: 1000 cases later. Ann Surg 1988; 208: 435–442.
5. Bandyk DF, Kaebnick HW, Stewart GW, et al. Durability of the in situ sapenous vein arterial bypass: A comparison of primary and secondary patency. J Vasc Surg 1987; 5:256–268.
6. Quiñones-Baldrich WJ, Busuttil RW, Baker JD, et al. Is the preferential use of polytetrafluoroethylene grafts for femoropopliteal bypass justified? J Vasc Surg 1988; 8:219–288.
7. Veith FJ, Gupta SK, Ascer E, et al. Six-year prospective multicenter randomized comparison of autologous saphenous vein and expanded polytetrafluoroethylene grafts in infrainguinal arterial reconstructions. J Vasc Surg 1986; 3:104–114.
8. Park TC, Taylor LM, Porter JM. Choice of graft material for femoropopliteal bypass: The case against preferential use of PTFE. In: Veith FJ, ed. Current critical problems in vascular surgery, 4th ed. St Louis: Quality Medical Publishing, 1992:29.
9. Harris PL. Prospective randomized comparison of in situ and reversed infrainguinal vein grafts: Status report of a three-center study. In: Veith FJ, ed. Current critical problems in vascular surgery, 4th ed. St. Louis: Quality Medical Publishing, 1992:40.
10. Harris PL, How TV, Jones DR. Prospectively randomized clinical trial to compare in situ and reversed saphenous vein grafts for femoro-popliteal bypass. Br J Surg 1987; 74:252–255.
11. Veterans Administration Cooperative Study Group 141. Comparitive evaluation of prosthetic, reversed and in situ vein bypass grafts in distal popliteal and tibial-peroneal revascularization. Arch Surg 1988; 123:434–438.
12. Sayers RD, Watt PAC, Muller S, Thurston H. Endothelial cell injury secondary to surgical preparation of reversed and in situ saphenous vein bypass grafts. Eur J Vasc Surg 1992; 6:354–361.

IN SITU SAPHENOUS VEIN GRAFT FOR LOWER EXTREMITY OCCLUSIVE DISEASE

JOHN A. MANNICK, M.D.
A. D. WHITTEMORE, M.D.
M. C. DONALDSON, M.D.

The autologous greater saphenous vein has remained the most successful and viable conduit for revascularization below the inguinal ligament, from the time of the first femoral popliteal bypass graft reported in the late 1940s.[1] Originally, all saphenous vein grafts were placed in reversed fashion to properly align the valves. However, the vein was left in situ beginning in the late 1950s by Hall and a few others who employed various approaches to valve lysis.[2] Because of the apparent tediousness and complexity of the in situ method, wider adaptation of this technique did not occur until the introduction of the modified Mills valvulotome by Leather and co-workers in the late 1970s.[3] Since then, a number of centers have developed extensive experience with the in situ method of saphenous vein bypass. However, over the past decade, significant advances have also been made in surgical instrumentation and technique for small vessel anastomosis that have enhanced the success of all methods of vein bypass. The optimal approach to infrainguinal autologous revascularization remains controversial.

In 1983, a policy of preferential use of the in situ greater saphenous vein for all infrainguinal arterial reconstructions was adopted on our service. This policy was instituted because of the success rates reported by Leather and associates[3] for infrapopliteal bypass grafts using the in situ method and because of the appeal of this technique for bypass to the infragenicular arteries. Simple transposition of the distal end of the vein to a small adjacent artery is logical, direct, and apparently minimally traumatic. The in situ technique also has the advantage of allowing the large proximal end of the greater saphenous vein to be attached to the common femoral artery, which is itself frequently thick walled and involved with atherosclerosis. The small distal end of the vein can be used for anastomosis with a tibial artery, which again permits much greater compatibility in size between the graft and the host vessel.

This has made possible successful use of distal saphenous veins with an external diameter of approximately 2.5 mm. Many surgeons, including ourselves, would find it difficult to perform successful anastomoses of veins of that caliber to the common femoral or proximal superficial arteries if the reversed technique of saphenous vein grafting were elected. Because of this feature of the in situ technique, vein utilization in extremities in which a saphenous vein is present has increased from approximately 70% to approximately 90% in our practice.

Whether the segment of the greater saphenous vein left in situ is protected from damage and subsequent myointimal hyperplasia by being left in its natural bed is arguable. However, our experience suggests that stenoses from myointimal hyperplasia in the in situ vein grafts almost invariably occur in the proximal or distal portions of the vein that have been mobilized to permit anastomosis with the host arteries and not in the portion of the vein left in situ.

Potential disadvantages of the in situ technique include failure to lyse all valves, possible intimal damage from the valvulotome, and arteriovenous fistulas from unligated branches of the in situ vein. However, we believe these disadvantages are outweighed by the aforementioned advantages of the in situ technique, particularly when the vein graft needs to originate in the groin and extend to the infrapopliteal vessels. Certainly under these circumstances, it seems simpler and less time-consuming to simply mobilize the proximal and distal ends of the vein graft, lyse the valves, and control all major branches of the intervening vein with hemaclips rather than laboriously dissecting out the entire length of required vein.

TECHNIQUE

Routine preoperative arteriography is employed in all patients using digital techniques, when indicated, to delineate the distal tibial arteries at the ankle level and the foot. Preoperative phlebography or vein mapping with duplex ultrasound is not routinely used. The greater saphenous vein is exposed through a single incision over a sufficient length to reach the chosen recipient artery. The distal recipient artery is isolated through the vein-harvesting incision in the case of the distal popliteal, posterior tibial, and proximal peroneal arteries. The anterior tibial and distal peroneal arteries are exposed through counterincisions over the anterior compartment. Fibulectomy is sometimes used for exposure of the distal peroneal artery. For an anterior tibial anastomosis, the vein graft is ordinarily passed subcutaneously over the fibula. Dorsalis pedis exposure is obtained through a vertical incision just medial to the artery with care to avoid creating too narrow a skin bridge between this incision and the vein-harvesting incision at the ankle. After exposure, the vein is protected with gauze pads soaked in balanced electrolyte solution containing heparin sodium and papaverine.

After systemic heparinization, the saphenofemoral junction is detached, followed by lateral suture closure of the common femoral vein. The most proximal saphenous valve or valves are excised under direct vision, and a suitable anastomosis of the proximal end of the vein graft with the common femoral, proximal superficial, or deep femoral arteries is performed.

After removal of occluding clamps, the Leather-modified Mills valvulotome is introduced sequentially through side branches to incise the valve leaflets. Success of this venture is confirmed by vigorous arterial flow through the distal end of the graft at the conclusion of the procedure. The distal end of the vein graft is ordinarily gently dilated with papaverine-containing solution in order to prevent damage from the valvulotome as it is inserted into the small end of the vein. In some patients, angioscopy has been used to guide a long-handled valvulotome introduced through the distal end of the vein and passed through the full length of the graft. However, we have not been able to show superior results with this technique.

After successful valvulotomy, the distal end of the vein is controlled with a hemaclip to allow dilation of the entire graft under arterial pressure. All major visible tributaries of the vein are then clipped. Finally, the distal anastomosis is performed using loupe magnification and 6-0 polypropylene suture for popliteal or 7-0 for tibial anastomoses. Microsurgical clamps are usually used for tibial arterial control. In some patients, to avoid vein kinking, the infrageniculate popliteal anastomoses are performed after passing the vein through the popliteal fossa in an anatomic position.

Upon completion, sterile continuous wave Doppler ultrasonography is used to assure adequate flow signals and to check for residual arteriovenous fistulas. Following this, completion arteriography is performed in all patients. Any abnormalities, including anastomotic defects, uncut valves, unexpected areas of vein graft stenosis, and arteriovenous fistulas are corrected.

All patients receive perioperative prophylactic intravenous antibiotics, and most patients with infrapopliteal bypasses receive low-molecular-weight Dextran, 500 ml/day for the first 48 hours after operation. Daily aspirin is recommended for all patients. Patients are ordinarily discharged between the fifth and the eighth postoperative days.

Because detection of vein graft stenosis prior to vein graft thrombosis is critically important in long-term vein graft function, patients are evaluated in the office and the vascular laboratory 1 month after discharge and at 3 month intervals for the first year, after which they are seen yearly. Vascular laboratory examinations are performed on each occasion. In the early part of our experience with in situ grafts, such examinations consisted of segmental limb pressures and pulse volume recordings. Recently, follow-up includes a measurement of ankle-brachial indices and a color duplex ultrasound evaluation of the graft. Areas of critical stenosis that cause an increased peak systolic velocity more than double the adjacent segment or an area of the graft with a peak systolic flow velocity below 40 cm/second are sought. Such findings have prompted arteriography and vein graft repair if a stenotic lesion is confirmed.

Using follow-up duplex ultrasound, we have found that approximately 15% of in situ vein grafts within the first year have a lesion requiring operative intervention. We have been impressed by the report of Bandyk and co-workers, who succeeded in enhancing 4 year in situ vein graft primary patency of 62% to a secondary patency of 85% by reoperating on 28% of their patients.[4] Several reports make it clear that revision of a vein graft stenosis before occlusion yields long-term patency similar to that vein grafts not requiring revision.

RESULTS

A review of 440 consecutive in situ saphenous vein grafts performed on 371 patients between March 1983 and June 1990 documented that in 299 instances critical limb ischemia was the indication for operation, with rest pain in 148, ischemic ulceration in 87, and gangrene in 64.[5] Disabling claudication was the indication in the remaining 32% of operations. In approximately 10% of patients, a previous infrainguinal revascularization procedure had been performed in the same limb. Seventy-eight patients had the arterial inflow to the ipsilateral groin corrected prior to the vein graft. The proximal anastomosis was at the groin level in all instances, and the popliteal artery was the site of distal anastomosis in 240 (55%) procedures. The infrapopliteal artery was the site of distal anastomosis in 200 (45%) of procedures, including 18 grafts at the ankle level or below (Table 1).

Table 1 Location of Distal Anastomosis in 440 In Situ Saphenous Vein Grafts

Location	Number (%)
Popliteal above-knee	79 (18)
Popliteal below-knee	161 (37)
Tibioperoneal trunk	12 (3)
Anterior tibial	46 (10)
Posterior tibial*	79 (18)
Peroneal	54 (12)
Dorsalis pedis	9 (2)

*Includes 9 at inframalleolar level.

Thirty-day operative mortality was 2% caused principally by myocardial infarction. Operative complications occurred in 104 patients (24%) (Table 2). Systemic complications included myocardial infarction in 6.3% of operations, congestive heart failure in 2.5%, and arrhythmia in 4.5%. Wound complications occurred in 8% of patients, including infection, seroma, hematoma, and skin slough. Only two grafts were lost because of sepsis, in both instances secondary to wound sepsis. Graft thromboses occurred in 27 instances (6%) within 30 postoperative days. Eighteen of these early failures were in infrapopliteal grafts. The most common causes of early failure appeared to be hypercoagulability, chiefly heparin sodium–associated platelet activation and lupus anticoagulant, and poor distal runoff.

Mean postoperative follow-up was 20.4 months, and 352 grafts (80%) were followed to known end points. Graft surveillance identified 18 grafts with stenotic lesions that were revised while still patent, usually by venous patch angioplasty or distal bypass extension.

Life table analysis documented 5 year in situ graft primary patency of 72%, which was improved to a 5 year secondary patency of 83%, chiefly by revision of stenotic but still patent grafts (Table 3). We have found that long-term patency of thrombosed vein grafts treated either by thrombectomy or thrombolysis is discouragingly small; in general, we now replace thrombosed vein grafts. The secondary graft patency rates for patients operated upon for chronic claudication and critical ischemia were not significantly different, nor were the secondary patency rates of popliteal and infrapopliteal grafts in this series.

The overall limb salvage rate was 88%. Limb salvage in patients operated upon for critical ischemia was 85% at the 5 year interval. The 5 year cumulative patent survival was 66%. Patients operated upon for claudication had a 5 year survival of 73% compared with a survival rate of 63% for patients presenting with critical ischemia.

Table 2 Thirty-Day Operative Morbidity Rate after 440 In Situ Saphenous Vein Grafts

Complications	Rate (%)
Systemic	
Myocardial infarction	16 (3.6)
Congestive heart failure	11 (2.5)
Arrhythmia	20 (4.5)
Renal failure*	8 (1.8)
Pulmonary failure	8 (1.8)
Stroke	2 (0.4)
Transient ischemic attack	2 (0.4)
Deep vein thrombosis	2 (0.4)
Local	
Wound infection/seroma/hematoma	37 (8.4)
Graft occlusion	27 (6.1)
Reoperation for bleeding	5 (1.1)
Unplanned major amputation	3 (0.7)
Compartment syndrome	1 (0.2)

*Creatinine increase more than 1 mg/100 ml.

Table 3 Five-Year Cumulative Patency for In Situ Saphenous Vein Bypass, 1983 to 1990*

Subgroup	n	Primary (%)	Secondary (%)
All grafts	440	72	83
Femoropopliteal	240	78†	86
Above knee	79	72	88
Below knee	161	82	85
Infrapopliteal	200	63†	78
Claudication	141	81†	87
Critical ischemia	299	66†	81
Diabetes	168	76	81
No diabetes	272	70	80

*Standard error <7%.
†$p < 0.05$.

COMMENT

Although a number of solutions to the problem of venous valve lysis and arteriovenous fistula control in in situ vein grafts have been reported, the techniques described here have worked well in our hands. Exposure of the saphenous vein through a continuous incision allows safe and controlled valve lysis using the modified Mills valvulotome with minimal apparent vein injury. In addition, this open method greatly facilitates the ligation of venous branches. Although all fistulas may not need ligation and most of the lateral branches connect only to the subcutaneous capillary network, some of these branches, if left open, can cause stasis thrombosis resulting in painful postoperative superficial phlebitis. Consequently, we recommend ligation of all visible venous tributaries.

There is growing recognition of the importance of postoperative graft surveillance in the detection of early and midterm myointimal hyperplasia within the vein graft or within the anastomotic regions. The subcutaneous location of in situ saphenous vein grafts facilitates monitoring with duplex ultrasound to sample graft velocities and interrogate areas of stenosis. As the duplex method has come into routine use, we have found that our rate of revision of patent grafts has increased, and we believe that, in concert with the experience of Bandyk and co-workers,[4] this will ultimately yield improvement in long-term graft patency.

Large series of in situ saphenous vein grafts have been published recently by Leather and Bandyk and their colleagues with results comparable to our own.[4,6] Contemporary reports of reversed greater saphenous vein have also documented excellent results, testimony to the general impact of advances in anastomotic technique and vein graft handling.[7] Taylor and co-workers in a randomized prospective trial reported in situ and reversed greater saphenous vein bypasses are equally effective at 3 years in the femoral popliteal position.[7] Our own experience with the two techniques of vein grafting over the past 10 years suggests that both the reversed and in situ saphenous veins have comparable long-term performance in the femoral popliteal position. We have found that, for long bypasses to the tibial vessels, the in situ vein graft has proved noticeably superior with regard to long-term patency and simplicity of operative management.

REFERENCES

1. Kunlin JL. Le traitement de L'arterite obliterante par le greffe veineuse. Arch Mal Coeur 1949; 42:371–374.
2. Hall KV. The great saphenous vein used "in situ" as an arterial shunt after extirpation of vein valves. Surgery 1962; 51:492–495.
3. Leather RP, Powers SR, Karmody AM. A reappraisal of the in situ saphenous vein arterial bypass: Its use in limb salvage. Surgery 1979; 86:453–460.
4. Bandyk DF, Schmitt DD, Seabrook GR, et al. Monitoring functional patency of in situ saphenous vein bypasses: The impact of a surveillance protocol and elective revision. J Vasc Surg 1989; 9:286–296.
5. Donaldson MC, Mannick JA, Whittemore AD. Femoro-distal bypass with in situ greater saphenous vein: Long-term results using the Mills valvulatome. Ann Surg 1991; 213:457–465.
6. Leather RP, Shah DJ, Chang BB, et al. Resurrection of the in situ saphenous vein bypass: 1,000 cases later. Ann Surg 1988; 208:435–442.
7. Taylor LM, Edwards JM, Porter JM. Present status of reversed vein bypass grafting: Five-year results of a modern series. J Vasc Surg 1990; 11:193–206.

SEQUENTIAL BYPASS PROCEDURES FOR ATHEROSCLEROTIC LOWER EXTREMITY DISEASE

PAUL FRIEDMANN, M.D.
DOMINIC A. DeLAURENTIS, M.D.

Revascularization of the lower extremities with autogenous saphenous vein is the mainstay of reconstruction for distal ischemia. The principles of bypass grafting have been well established, and the technical limits of operation have been extended as our understanding of the disease process has increased. The patient population now often presents with multilevel arterial disease and with increasingly severe distal disease. Although bypassing all atherosclerotic disease is not necessary, most surgeons tend to perform more distal bypasses in order to minimize outflow resistance and to provide direct perfusion to severely ischemic tissues. The techniques of in situ bypass have lent themselves to these long distal procedures, whose success is predicated upon meticulous surgical technique and attention to detail. Proponents of the use of the reversed saphenous vein or nonreversed translocated saphenous vein also claim good results. The surgeon must maintain a flexible approach to the operative management of limb-threatening ischemia.

Unfortunately, the saphenous vein is not always available for use in its entirety. It may be diseased, absent, or inadequate for use because of anatomic or structural defects. In the absence of a satisfactory saphenous vein, other autogenous conduits and prosthetic devices have been tried. Brachiocephalic veins and lesser saphenous veins are available, but often are not long enough. Splicing vein segments with direct veno-venous anastomosis may produce adequate lengths of a venous conduit. Graft materials such as Dacron, polytetrafluoroethylene (PTFE), and umbilical vein have been used with varying degrees of success in above-knee bypass procedures but have produced inferior results in infrageniculate procedures.

Reasons for failure of prosthetic grafts below the knee may relate to their length and thrombogenicity, to high outflow resistance, or perhaps to the kinking of the prosthetic material as it crosses the knee joint. To provide adequate length and utilize whatever segment of vein is satisfactory, composite grafts have been constructed with a direct end-to-end anastomosis between prosthesis and vein. Unfortunately, clinical results with the use of these composite grafts have been disappointing.

TECHNICAL FACTORS

We first developed the concept of sequential grafting to avoid some of the problems inherent in the use of composite grafts or inadequate saphenous veins. In this procedure, a prosthetic graft is anastomosed to the femoral artery in the groin and to the popliteal artery above the knee. A vein graft is then placed between the prosthetic and the infrageniculate outflow vessel. (Fig. 1) By providing a point of fixation to the popliteal artery, we could provide stability to the vein-graft anastomosis and construct it in such a fashion as to avoid or minimize late problems related to subintimal fibrosis or to pseudointimal hyperplasia. The prosthetic could provide a conduit with little resistance to blood flow, would be relatively short, and would not be subject to the stress related to kinking of the graft across the knee joint. The saphenous vein would provide an endothelium-lined

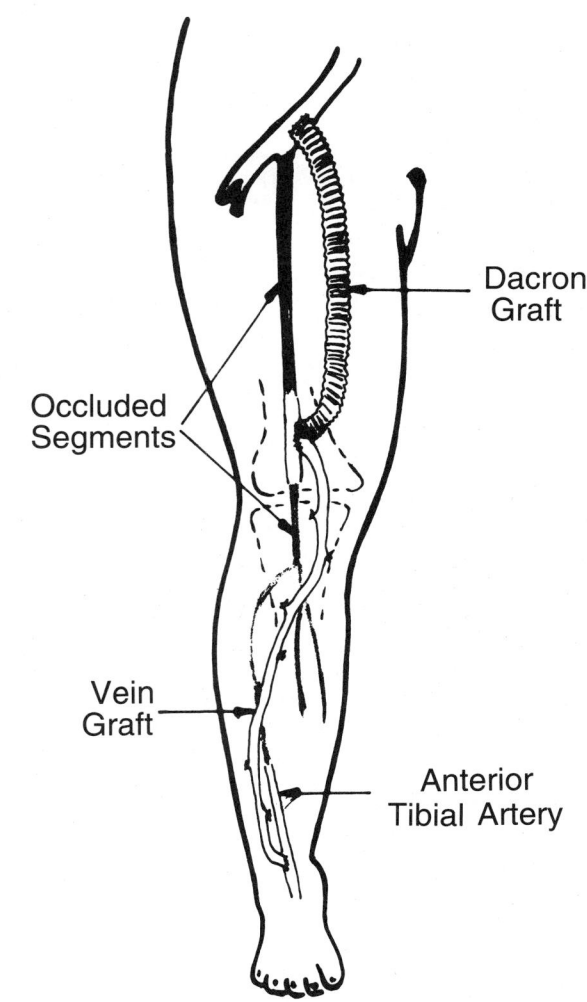

Figure 1 Sequential grafting with both prosthetic graft and vein graft. (From Friedmann PF. The sequential femoropopliteal bypass graft. Am J Surg 1976; 131:453; with permission.)

conduit across the knee joint and would minimize the problems related to size or compliance mismatch with the distal or tibial vessels. Inadequate sections of saphenous vein would not be used. If the saphenous veins are absent or not usable, segments of brachiocephalic or lesser saphenous can be used. In patients with occluded distal superficial femoral arteries, a localized endarterectomy is performed. This not only provides a short segment of arterial conduit but also provides access to major collateral branches, which could help to decrease peripheral resistance and thereby help to enhance graft patency. The distal vein is anastomosed to the most suitable outflow artery in a standard fashion.

Several techniques to construct the anastomosis between prosthetic and vein have been described. In our early experience we used a functional side-to-side anastomosis, with both prosthetic and vein sewn directly in end-to-side fashion to the above-knee popliteal artery (Fig. 2). An alternative approach is to complete the distal end-to-side anastomosis between the popliteal artery and the prosthesis and then to use the distal prosthesis as the point of origin for the saphenous vein graft. This is also an acceptable technique, but care should be taken to use the most distal segment of the prosthesis as the takeoff point of the vein graft. Some authors have placed the prosthetic graft across the knee joint, but this tends to negate one of the principles previously described, and the results tend to be worse. In our initial experience, we used knitted Dacron grafts as the prosthetic conduit. More recently we have used PTFE grafts. The results do not appear to be influenced by the use of either one of these graft materials. We have not used collagen, umbilical vein, or other types of prosthetic materials.

CLINICAL RESULTS

When composite sequential bypasses are performed with the techniques we have described, clinical results indicate that they are effective and durable and can be satisfactory alternatives for vascular reconstruction when the saphenous vein is inadequate. The literature is confusing in this regard because not all sequential grafts are constructed properly and not all composite grafts are constructed in a sequential fashion. It is therefore difficult to compare results in the various reports of composite or sequential grafts.

We reported our 10-year experience in 55 procedures performed in 52 patients in 1981.[1] Thirty-three procedures were femoral-popliteal bypasses. In this group, the 30-day crude patency rate was 76%. The interval patency rates at 60 and 72 months were 100% and 86%, respectively, and cumulative patency rates were 48% and 41% at those same intervals. In the 22 femoral-tibial bypass procedures, the 30-day crude patency rate was 86%, the interval patency rates at 60 and 72 months were 100%, and the cumulative patency rates were 42% at those same intervals. We noted similar results in an update of our experience with this technique in 1987.[2]

In 1984, Verta reported his results in 54 composite sequential bypasses followed for up to 4 years.[3] Life table analysis indicated an 81% patency rate at 2 years and a 72% patency rate at 4 years. He noted that the composite sequential grafts took an average of 51 minutes longer to perform but concluded that the excellent patency rates made sequential bypasses a reasonable option for limb salvage.

Flinn and associates compared composite sequential graft techniques with sequential bypasses using reversed saphenous vein alone or PTFE graft alone.[4] All patients had a significant improvement in lower limb arterial perfusion regardless of the techniques or graft materials used. The 1- and 2-year patency rates for the composite sequential grafts were 80% and were not statistically different from the results with autogenous saphenous vein alone. The patency rates for bypasses performed with PTFE alone were 52% and 47% at 1 and 2 years, respectively, and were statistically significantly worse than those for the composite sequential grafts.

McCarthy and associates described 67 composite sequential bypasses performed over a 7-year period.[5]

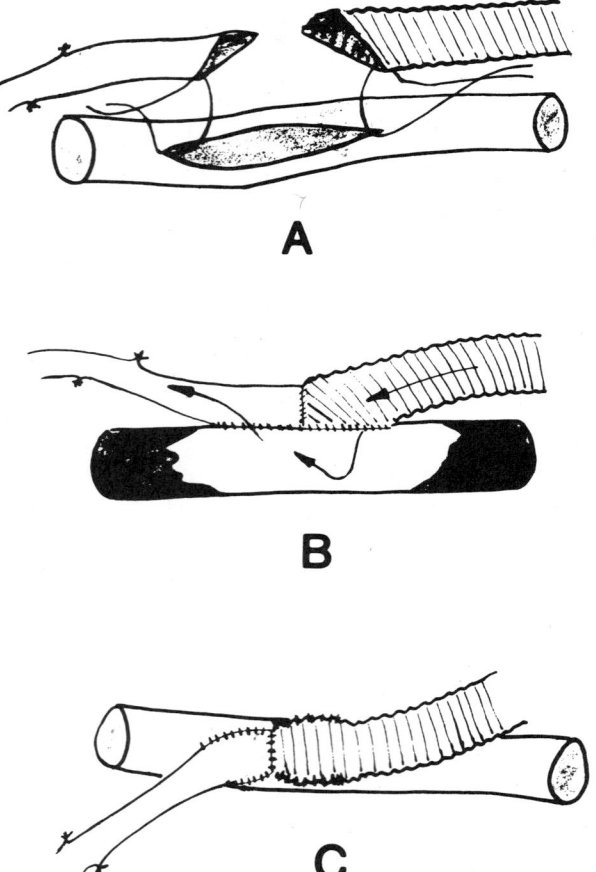

Figure 2 Construction of anastomosis between prosthetic graft and vein. (From Friedmann PF. The sequential femoropopliteal bypass graft. Am J Surg 1976; 131:453; with permission.)

These procedures were used for primary, secondary, and complex tertiary reconstructions. Above-knee prosthetics were placed in 44 instances, and below-knee prosthetics were placed in 23. The cumulative life table primary patency rates were 72% at 1 year, 64% at 2 years, and 48% at 3 years. In patients with the popliteal anastomosis above the knee, the 2-year patency rate was 72%, compared to 46% for those with below-knee anastomoses. This difference suggested a trend but did not reach statistical significance. The authors concluded that composite sequential grafts provide predictable patency rates when reconstruction with all-autogenous tissue is not possible, and are superior to all-prosthetic tibial bypass grafts.

Sequential techniques can also be applied to reconstructive procedures that use only autogenous tissues. The rationale for these procedures is based on the concepts that it is desirable to perfuse more than one distal vascular bed and that the performance of multiple distal anastomoses reduces peripheral resistance and increases blood flow through the graft. Perler and co-workers reported 35 patients undergoing 39 sequential bypass procedures.[6] Thirty-one of these procedures were performed with all autogenous tissues. Life table analysis indicated a primary patency rate of 70% at 1 year, 61% at 3 years, and 52% at 7 years. Cumulative limb salvage rates were 91% at 1 year, 85% at 5 years, and 61% at 7 years. The authors concluded that the multiple sequential distal bypass graft is durable and highly efficacious in achieving limb salvage. Lamberth and colleagues also found improved results when they used the sequential autogenous vein graft technique in femoropopliteal-tibial reconstructions instead of a femoral-tibial bypass technique. They attributed their good results to increased flow in the sequential grafts.[7]

FLOW FACTORS

The question of whether there is increased flow through sequential grafts has been addressed experimentally by Jarrett and colleagues, who found in an animal model that graft flows were augmented in all instances by the addition of a sequential anastomosis.[8] However, findings to the contrary were presented by Hadcock and associates, who hypothesized that the intermediate anastomosis acted to create competitive collateral flow and thereby decreased flow in the distal graft.[9] In their experimental study, proximal graft flows increased, but flows in the distal grafts decreased significantly. The role of this "steal" phenomenon and its significance in our clinical experience remain unsettled at the present time. Perler and associates felt that if arterial inflow was adequate and if the distal recipient beds were sufficiently isolated, the "steal" phenomenon was not clinically significant.[6] There is, however, no consensus that it is necessary to bypass into two or more separate tibial vessels, and most surgeons remain content to bypass into a single distal vessel, if the runoff from that vessel is adequate.

COMMENT

Our overall experience with sequential grafting techniques is now in excess of 20 years. This period has seen the development of techniques involving and extending the use of the saphenous vein as a bypass conduit. In situ techniques, nonreversed translocated techniques, and the standard reversed saphenous vein bypass have all provided excellent results because of improved vein handling techniques, use of fine suture material, and optical magnification. The saphenous vein remains the graft of choice if it is available and if it is adequate. If the ipsilateral saphenous vein is not available or is segmentally inadequate, we continue to use a composite sequential graft. Clinical results with this approach have continued to show satisfactory graft patency and limb survival rates. If the patient requires a below-knee bypass and sufficient autogenous tissue is not available, the composite sequential graft provides very satisfactory and durable results and remains our procedure of choice.

REFERENCES

1. Rosenfeld JC, Savarese RP, Friedmann P, DeLaurentis DA. Sequential femoropopliteal and femoro-tibial bypasses, a ten-year follow up study. Arch Surg 1981; 116:1538–1543.
2. Raviola CA, Savarese RP, DeLaurentis DA. Composite sequential graft. In: Bergan JJ, Yao JST, eds. Arterial surgery: New diagnostic and operative techniques. New York: Grune & Stratton, 1988: 541.
3. Verta MJ. Composite sequential bypass to the ankle and beyond for limb salvage. J Vasc Surg 1984; 12:381–386.
4. Flinn WR, Ricco JB, Yao JST, et al. Composite sequential grafts in severe ischemia, a comparative study. J Vasc Surg 1984; 1:449–454.
5. McCarthy WJ, Pearce WH, Flinn WR, et al. Long-term evaluation of composite sequential bypass for limb threatening ischemia. J Vasc Surg 1992; 15:761–770.
6. Perler BA, Burdick JF, Williams GM. The multiple sequential distal bypass graft: Seven year follow-up. J Vasc Surg 1987; 6:296–300.
7. Lamberth WC, Karkow WS. Sequential femoro-popliteal-tibial bypass grafting: Operative technique and results. Ann Thorac Surg 1986; 42(suppl 6): 31–35.
8. Jarrett F, Perea A, Begelman K, Burch J. Hemodynamics of sequential bypass grafts in peripheral arterial occlusions. Surg Gynecol Obstet 1980; 150:377–378.
9. Hadcock MM, Ubatuba J, Littooy FN, Baker WH. Hemodynamics of sequential grafts. Am J Surg 1983; 146:170–173.

ARM VEINS FOR LOWER EXTREMITY REVASCULARIZATION

NORMAN R. HERTZER, M.D.
MARK E. SESTO, M.D.

Availability of autogenous graft material often is imperative to the long-term success of distal lower extremity revascularization. Countless reports have documented conclusively that the early results and late patency rates of either reversed or in situ bypass using the greater saphenous vein (GSV) are superior to those attained by any synthetic graft for below-knee (BK) popliteal or tibioperoneal arterial reconstruction. Lacking a clear alternative, thoughtful surgeons generally have adopted four general options in the absence of an appropriate GSV in the ipsilateral leg:

First, employ nonoperative management unless advanced ischemia or unconditionally disabling claudication is present. Despite the foresight implicit in this policy, the referral experience at most major medical centers suggests that synthetic grafts still are frequently employed in many patients presenting elsewhere with claudication of only moderate severity, often of recent onset.

Second, procure the contralateral GSV for transposition as a reversed graft in the threatened limb. Although this approach is appropriate in some patients, it may compromise subsequent revascularization of the donor extremity in others who already have marginal arterial circulation on that side as well.

Third, utilize additional measures, including adjunctive arteriovenous fistulas or postoperative oral anticoagulation, when synthetic femoropopliteal or femorotibial grafts are unavoidable. Although such precautions have been reported to enhance the durability of synthetic grafts, none is sufficient to attain results that are comparable to the GSV.

Fourth, construct unconventional autogenous grafts using the lesser saphenous or arm veins. Possibly the most important consideration regarding arm veins is whether their performance warrants the additional time and effort that are necessary to harvest and prepare them for infrainguinal bypass grafting. The purpose of this chapter is to place their results in perspective to those that have been reported for GSV and synthetic materials, especially polytetrafluoroethylene (PTFE).

CLINICAL APPLICATIONS

The first description of arm veins as conduits for lower extremity revascularization was published in 1969.[1] On the basis of preliminary dissections in 20 male and 5 female cadaver specimens, Kakkar initially predicted that his measurements of the length (mean, 54 cm), diameter (mean, 7.6 mm), and minimum bursting pressure (430 mm Hg) of the cephalic vein indicated that it "is always long enough, wide enough, and strong enough to be used as an arterial substitute in the leg." Kakkar also constructed femoropopliteal bypass grafts employing the cephalic veins in a pilot study of seven patients, all of whose grafts remained patent during follow-up intervals ranging from 4 to 12 months. With understandable but perhaps premature enthusiasm, he stated: "It is too early to draw definite conclusions, but if the long term results prove satisfactory in a large number of patients, the cephalic vein will provide an alternative and perhaps better autologous graft than the great saphenous vein."

Only a few additional reports of cephalic vein grafts appeared throughout the decade following Kakkar's original work, and all were characterized by small series of patients, short follow-up periods, and generally modest results.[2] Nevertheless, during the past 10 to 15 years a number of factors may have contributed to a perceived renewal of interest in arm veins for infrainguinal revascularization. First, limb salvage using tibioperoneal and even pedal artery bypass has become much more commonplace than was the case in the 1970s. Furthermore, clinical experience with several generations of synthetic materials during this time confirmed that autogenous grafts remain preferable for infrageniculate arterial reconstruction. Finally, a substantial minority of candidates for BK popliteal or tibioperoneal bypass already have undergone coronary bypass procedures or previous femoropopliteal operations in the same extremity for which the ipsilateral GSV has been employed. Probably as the result of these considerations, some studies that now are available contain sufficient information to clarify the relative success of arm vein grafts at least with respect to intermediate-term patency rates.

We reviewed data from four representative reports,[2-5] together with cumulative 3 year primary patency rates for comparable saphenous vein and PTFE grafts collected from a comprehensive review of the literature,[6] a prospectively randomized multicenter trial,[7] and the Cleveland Vascular Registry[8] (Table 1). The cephalic vein was used either exclusively or predominantly in all four reports of arm vein grafts, although the basilic vein occasionally was employed in three of them.[2-4] Thirty-seven of the 43 grafts constructed by Harward and co-workers[4] and 11 of the 35 reported by Sesto and associates[5] included composite segments of the GSV or the lesser saphenous system. Insofar as can be determined, however, the remaining studies describe "full-length" infrageniculate bypass performed entirely with arm veins. Cumulative patency rates were calculated independently according to the level of the distal anastomosis by Schulman and Badhey[2] and by Andros and co-workers.[3] Both the Harward[4] and Sesto[5] groups limited their analyses to collective results regarding patency, but the peroneal or tibial arteries represented the outflow vessels for 59 (76%) of the 78 operations in these two reports.

Table 1 Representative Primary Patency Rates for Infrageniculate Arterial Reconstruction Performed with Arm Veins, the Greater Saphenous Vein, and PTFE

Graft Material	Distal Anastomosis	Number	Cumulative Patency Rates		
			1 Year	2 Years	3 Years
Arm veins					
Schulman and Badhey[2]	BK popliteal	41	62%	47%	31%
	Tibioperoneal	16	43%	31%	31%
Andros, et al[3]	BK popliteal	33	±88%	±75%	±68%
	Tibioperoneal	43	±73%	±62%	±58%
Harward, et al[4]	All infrageniculate	43	67%	58%	49%
Sesto, et al[5]	All infrageniculate	35	49%	49%	40%
Saphenous vein					
Dalman and Taylor[6]	BK popliteal	Collected series	84%	79%	78%
	Tibioperoneal		77%	70%	66%
Veith, et al[7]	BK popliteal	62	±85%	±85%	±85%
	Tibioperoneal	106	±65%	±60%	±56%
Rafferty, et al[8]	BK popliteal	120	84%	84%	69%
	Tibioperoneal	98	63%	58%	43%
PTFE					
Veith, et al[7]	BK popliteal	80	±85%	±85%	54%
	Tibioperoneal	98	±45%	±35%	±30%
Rafferty, et al[8]	BK popliteal	107	50%	32%	32%
	Tibioperoneal	76	31%	±25%	19%

BK, Below-knee; PTFE, Polytetrafluoroethylene; ±, figures estimated from graphic illustrations.

Table 2 Representative Secondary Patency Rates for Infrageniculate Arterial Reconstruction Performed with Arm Veins, the Greater Saphenous Vein, and PTFE

Graft Material	Distal Anastomosis	Number	Cumulative Patency Rates		
			1 Year	2 Years	3 Years
Arm veins					
Andros, et al[3]	BK popliteal	33	±90%	±90%	±78%
	Tibioperoneal	43	±81%	±70%	±64%
Harward, et al[4]	All infrageniculate	43	74%	64%	64%
Sesto, et al[5]	All infrageniculate	35	68%	58%	44%
Saphenous vein					
Dalman and Taylor[6]	BK popliteal	Collected series	96%	89%	86%
	Tibioperoneal		84%	80%	78%
Rafferty, et al[8]	BK popliteal	120	NA	NA	69%
	Tibioperoneal	98	NA	NA	43%
PTFE					
Dalman and Taylor[6]	BK popliteal	Collected series	68%	61%	44%
	Tibioperoneal		46%	32%	NA
Rafferty, et al[8]	BK popliteal	101	NA	NA	32%
	Tibioperoneal	69	NA	NA	19%

BK, Below-knee; NA, Data not available; PTFE, Polytetrafluoroethylene; ±, figures estimated from graphic illustrations.

With the possible exception of the remarkable results attained by Andros and co-workers,[3] the data generally suggest that 3 year primary patency rates for arm vein grafts surpass those for PTFE (especially with respect to tibioperoneal bypass), even though they fail to meet the expectations traditionally reserved for saphenous vein grafts (Table 1). The average intermediate-term primary patency rates for infrageniculate cephalic and/or basilic vein grafts are approximately 50%, and secondary patency rates may be enhanced on the order of another 10% when elective reoperations prove to be necessary (Table 2). Andros and co-workers[3] attribute much of their singular success to a vigorous surveillance program during the first postoperative year, consisting of a clinical assessment every 4 to 6 weeks, segmental limb plethysmography every 8 to 12 weeks, and Doppler ultrasound (duplex) scanning to detect potentially correctable lesions whenever graft stenosis is suspected on the basis of the physical examination or a reduction in the ankle-brachial pressure index. Using a similar follow-up protocol every 3 months during the first postoperative year, Harward and co-workers[4] were able to improve their secondary patency rate by a relative factor of 30% (from 49% to 64%).

Whereas hyperplastic stenosis is the cardinal late complication after conventional saphenous vein bypass, ectasia or even pathologic dilation also can occur in cephalic and other arm vein grafts.[2,3,5] Schulman and Badhey[2] discovered ectasia or "elongation" in all six of their patients who subsequently underwent follow-up arteriography, and Sesto and co-workers[5] speculated that dilation may be a harbinger of spontaneous thrombosis or distal embolization. Andros and co-workers obtained a total of 73 follow-up arteriograms for 56 grafts in their study and described atypical features in 32%, including enlargement in 11, aneurysms in 6, and elongation in 1.[3] These observations seem to imply that the tensile strength of some cephalic vein grafts eventually deteriorates. But in the absence of obvious aneurysms, their therapeutic implications are not entirely clear when the clinical results of such grafts otherwise appear to be quite satisfactory. Nevertheless, the unpredictable consequences of arm vein ectasia probably warrant periodic surveillance by duplex scanning and, at least in selected patients, may support the liberal use of long-term oral anticoagulation that is seemingly favored by Harward and colleagues.[4]

TECHNICAL CONSIDERATIONS

Schulman and Badhey found that arm veins were inadequate for bypass purposes in 29% of the patients for whom they initially were considered as an alternative source for autogenous grafts.[2] Although enough cephalic vein ordinarily is available for limited revisions of previous saphenous vein grafts, the availability of a sufficient number of segments to perform "full-length" infrageniculate reconstruction is often uncertain. Salles-Cunha and colleagues investigated the utility of duplex scanning for preoperative assessment in a group of 10 patients.[9] They determined that the mean in situ diameter of the cephalic vein was 2 mm larger than its ultrasound measurement, and they concluded that arm veins exceeding 1.5 to 2 mm in size on a duplex scan deserved surgical exploration. Sesto and colleagues subsequently documented that even small cephalic veins could be matured for BK popliteal or tibioperoneal bypass by the construction of a temporary arteriovenous fistula in the upper extremity 7 to 10 days earlier (Fig. 1).[5] They adopted this approach for 23 (68%) of the 35 grafts in their series.

As a practical matter, cephalic vein bypass procedures are greatly expedited by the availability of two surgical teams so that dissection and incisional closure may proceed simultaneously in the upper and lower extremities. General anesthesia always is convenient for this purpose, but local anesthesia usually is sufficient for exposure of the cephalic vein(s) in cooperative patients for whom epidural anesthesia otherwise would be preferable for infrainguinal revascularization. Virtually every technical step throughout the operation must be guided by the recognition that the handling characteristics of arm veins are distinctly inferior to those of the GSV. They are flimsy, easily torn beyond salvage by lateral repair, and subject to twisting either at the heel of each anastomosis or within the deep subsartorial tunnel through which they conventionally are routed. The following observations address some common pitfalls and precautions for preventing complications.

Side Branches

Branches of the cephalic vein often are very small but must be securely ligated with 6-0 or even 7-0 sutures—not hemostatic clips—in order to prevent sudden intraoperative or postoperative bleeding under arterial pressure. Moreover, a constrictive band is easily produced by gathering too much adventitia unless the suture ligature is placed 1 to 2 mm beyond the origin of each branch.

Vein Preparation

Unsecured branches and adventitial bands should be identified by gentle distention of the harvested vein with heparinized blood. Because full-length femoropopliteal or femorotibioperoneal bypass is rarely feasible without using the cephalic veins from at least both upper arms, a spatulated end-to-end venovenostomy almost always is necessary to provide a conduit of adequate length. This anastomosis is complicated because arm veins possess so little surface tension that their walls always tend to coapt, a feature that sometimes makes it difficult to obtain watertight approximation without graft stenosis. The anastomosis may be facilitated by performing it with the veins mounted on a mandril such as a straight urethral sound of appropriate diameter, with stay sutures at the "toe" and both lateral midpoints of the projected suture line.

Arterial Anastomoses

The outflow anastomosis should be constructed first because it is much simpler to reposition the inflow anastomosis to the profunda femoris artery or to a patent, proximal segment of the superficial femoral artery in the event the length of the reversed vein graft is insufficient to reach the common femoral level. Optical magnification is nearly indispensable, and triangulated stay sutures are helpful to display the full circumference of each anastomotic hood.

Once the distal anastomosis has been completed except for a small aperture that is closed after entrapped air is vented at the conclusion of the procedure, the graft again is gently distended with heparinized blood and carefully oriented on the surface of the leg to eliminate twisting when it is drawn proximally through its deep tunnel toward the groin. Even slight axial rotation easily can cause a corkscrew deformity adjacent to the outflow anastomosis when blood flow is restored in an arm vein. For this reason, it often is prudent to mark the longitudinal axis of the graft with a biocompatible marking pen so that misalignment does not occur in the

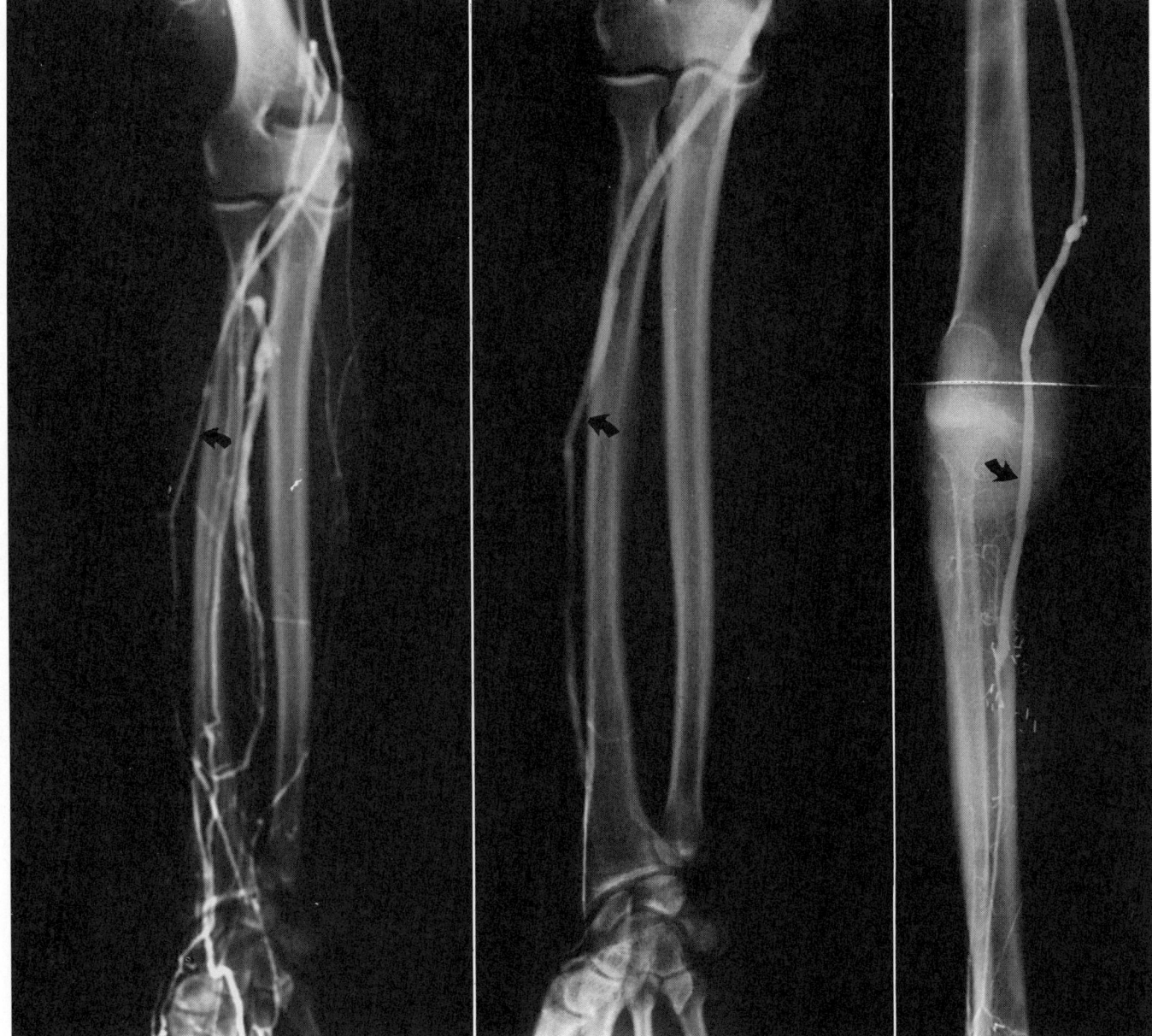

Figure 1 *A,* Preoperative phlebogram revealing a diminutive cephalic vein *(arrow)* in the forearm. *B,* Another contrast study showing enlargement of the same vein *(arrow)* 2 weeks after an arteriovenous fistula had been constructed at the wrist. *C,* The harvested vein *(arrow)* after revascularization of the peroneal artery. The proximal segment of this composite cephalic vein graft was obtained from the contralateral upper extremity. (From Sesto ME, Sullivan TM, Hertzer NR, et al. Cephalic vein grafts for lower extremity revascularization. J Vasc Surg 1992; 15:543–549; with permission.)

anatomic tunnel. In this particular respect, completion arteriography also appears to be indicated.

There is evidence to suggest that some of the structural liabilities of arm vein grafts influence their early outcome. Marcaccio and colleagues recently performed fiberoptic angioscopy to detect intraluminal defects in 109 such grafts, 70 (64%) of which were used for reoperative lower extremity revascularization.[10] Arm veins alone were employed for 78 (72%) of these procedures; the remainder included composite segments of other graft materials. Intraluminal disease or thrombus was discovered in 71 arm veins (63%), intimal webs being the most prevalent lesions. On the basis of the information obtained by angioscopy, 66% of the diseased veins were revised either endoscopically or by resection and reanastomosis. The cumulative patency rate for all grafts in this study was 90% at 30 days and 70% at 1 year. Most importantly, 30 day and 1 year patency rates were

96% and 75%, respectively, for normal and revised grafts (total of 89) in comparison to 70% and 30% for diseased arm veins that were not revised (total of 20). Provided these results eventually extend beyond the first postoperative year and are confirmed by others, adjunctive angioscopy may contribute to the success of arm vein grafts that was predicted by Kakkar[1] nearly two decades earlier.

REFERENCES

1. Kakkar VV. The cephalic vein as a peripheral vascular graft. Surg Gynecol Obstet 1969; 128:551–556.
2. Schulman ML, Badhey MR. Late results and angiographic evaluation of arms veins as long bypass grafts. Surgery 1982; 92:1032–1040.
3. Andros G, Harris RW, Salles-Cunha SX, et al. Arm veins for arterial revascularization of the leg: Arteriographic and clinical observations. J Vasc Surg 1986; 4:416–427.
4. Harward TRS, Coe D, Flynn TC, et al. The use of arm vein conduits during infrageniculate arterial bypass. J Vasc Surg 1992; 16:420–427.
5. Sesto ME, Sullivan TM, Hertzer NR, et al. Cephalic vein grafts for lower extremity revascularization. J Vasc Surg 1992; 15:543–549.
6. Dalman RL, Taylor LM Jr. Basic data related to infrainguinal revascularization procedures. Ann Vasc Surg 1990; 4:309–312.
7. Veith FJ, Gupta SK, Ascer E, et al. Six-year prospective multicenter randomized comparison of autologous saphenous vein and expanded polytetrafluoroethylene grafts in infrainguinal arterial reconstructions. J Vasc Surg 1986; 3:104–114.
8. Rafferty TD, Avellone JC, Farrell CJ, et al. A metropolitan experience with infrainguinal revascularization: Operative risk and late results in northeastern Ohio. J Vasc Surg 1987; 6:365–371.
9. Salles-Cunha SX, Andros G, Harris RW, et al. Preoperative noninvasive assessment of arm veins to be used as bypass grafts in the lower extremities. J Vasc Surg 1986; 3:813–816.
10. Marcaccio EJ, Miller A, Tannenbaum GA, et al. Angioscopically directed interventions improve arm vein bypass grafts. J Vasc Surg 1993; 17:994–1004.

EXPANDED POLYTETRAFLUOROETHYLENE GRAFT FOR ATHEROSCLEROTIC LOWER EXTREMITY OCCLUSIVE DISEASE

WILLIAM D. SUGGS, M.D.
FRANK J. VEITH, M.D.

Expanded polytetrafluoroethylene (ePTFE) was initially developed for industrial purposes as a chemically inert tubing and was modified for use as a vascular prosthesis. In 1972, ePTFE was used to replace the inferior vena cava in experimental animals. In 1976, Campbell and colleagues reported the first clinical application of ePTFE as a bypass graft for the treatment of a lower extremity arterial occlusion.[1] They used ePTFE grafts as femoropopliteal or femorotibial bypasses for critical ischemia in 15 patients in whom the autogenous saphenous vein was not available, and they achieved limb salvage in 13. Since its initial application as a vascular graft, the use of ePTFE has expanded to include many purposes in vascular surgery. These applications include dialysis grafts, extra-anatomic bypasses, grafts for repair of abdominal aortic aneurysms, bypasses of aortoiliac occlusive disease, and infrainguinal bypasses.

PTFE, also known as Teflon, is a nontextile polymer of carbon and fluorine that is inert, highly electronegative, and hydrophobic. Its production includes heating and mechanical stretching that result in a microporous material. The structure of ePTFE is characterized by a series of solid nodes interconnected by small fibrils. The fibril length can be varied in the manufacturing process to determine pore size. Currently available ePTFE grafts have a pore size averaging 30 microns. After its initial use as a bypass graft, aneurysmal formation occurred and an external wrap was added to the ePTFE graft to increase its burst strength and prevent aneurysm formation. Other modifications have also been introduced, including a thin-walled ePTFE graft, a ringed graft to provide external support, a tapered graft, and most recently a longitudinally stretchable graft.

FEMOROPOPLITEAL AND FEMOROTIBIAL BYPASS

For the past two decades autologous vein has been the conduit of choice for most infrainguinal arterial bypass procedures. These lower extremity bypasses are indicated for limb-threatening ischemia or disabling claudication. Such bypasses are generally not justified for mild to moderate claudication.

The exact role of ePTFE in infrainguinal arterial reconstruction remains controversial. In patients who require a bypass to the above-knee popliteal artery, some surgeons preferentially employ ePTFE grafts to preserve the saphenous vein for later use.[2] By contrast, others have adhered to a policy of employing only autologous vein for infrainguinal bypasses.[3] For the last decade our attitude in choosing an infrainguinal graft has tended to be intermediate between these two positions. We have used autologous vein for most of our infrainguinal arterial reconstructions, if the patient had a good ipsilateral greater saphenous vein. However, we perform a primary femoropopliteal bypass with ePTFE when the ipsilateral saphenous vein is diseased or previously harvested. In addition, elderly or debilitated patients with limited life expectancies may benefit from a less complex operation and are therefore candidates for a bypass with ePTFE.

Bypasses for limb salvage to the infrapopliteal vessels should be performed with autologous vein whenever possible. This includes utilization of the contralateral greater saphenous vein if the limb is not ischemic and lesser saphenous vein or arm vein, if they are of good quality. If the amount of vein is limited, a composite sequential bypass with ePTFE and vein should be considered for bypasses to the tibial vessels. All effort should be made to construct the distal ePTFE anastomosis to the patent above-knee popliteal artery. This technique allows the vein to cross the knee joint and should improve the patency of the composite graft.[4] If no autologous vein is available, bypasses to infrapopliteal vessels should be performed with ePTFE and adjuvant anticoagulation therapy should be instituted. Construction of these bypasses is preferential to performing a primary major amputation for limb-threatening ischemia.[5]

A 6 mm diameter ePTFE graft is usually used for infrainguinal arterial bypasses done with prosthetic material. If the distal anastomosis is below the knee or to an infrapopliteal vessel, then a ringed 6 mm ePTFE graft is used. Rarely, in a bypass to a small tibial artery, a 5 mm graft is used. The graft is tunneled under the sartorius muscle and follows the anatomic path of the superficial femoral artery to the above-knee or below-knee popliteal artery. For bypasses to the anterior tibial artery, the graft is tunneled subcutaneously lateral to the knee. Bypasses to the peroneal and posterior tibial arteries are tunneled subfascially along the medial aspect of the leg.

Patency of infrainguinal ePTFE bypass grafts is related to the location of the distal anastomosis. In 1986, a large randomized prospective trial comparing autologous saphenous vein to ePTFE grafts in all infrainguinal bypass operations was completed.[5] Equivalent patency rates at 2 years were noted between autologous vein grafts and ePTFE grafts to the popliteal artery at the same level. Thereafter, patency rates diverged and the differences became significant after 4 years with a patency rate of 68 ± 8% for autologous veins versus 47 ± 9% for ePTFE. Four-year patency rate differences were not statistically significant for above-knee grafts, but they were significant for below-knee grafts (Fig. 1). In a large retrospective review reported by the group from the University of California, Los Angeles (UCLA), primary femoropopliteal bypasses done preferentially with ePTFE had 5 year patency rates of 61.5%.[2] These authors base their recommendations to use ePTFE grafts preferentially on their superior patency results with autologous veins for secondary femoropopliteal bypasses and their poor results with ePTFE grafts in this setting.

Because most surgeons employ saphenous vein as the primary conduit for femoropopliteal bypasses and these bypasses sometimes fail, the role of ePTFE for secondary femoropopliteal bypasses should be examined. Some groups concluded that ePTFE is a poor option when employed as a secondary bypass when suitable vein is not available. The vein remaining after a failed bypass may be insufficient in length or may be damaged or thrombosed as a result of previous incisions or scarring. In addition, use of the vein from the contralateral limb may be undesirable in situations when ischemia exists in that limb. An ePTFE bypass may therefore be required, and it is important to know how effective these secondary femoropopliteal ePTFE bypasses can be. Our group reported on 73 patients in whom secondary femoropopliteal bypasses were performed for limb salvage.[6] The primary 4 year patency rate was only 38%, but with aggressive follow-up and reintervention the secondary patency rate increased to

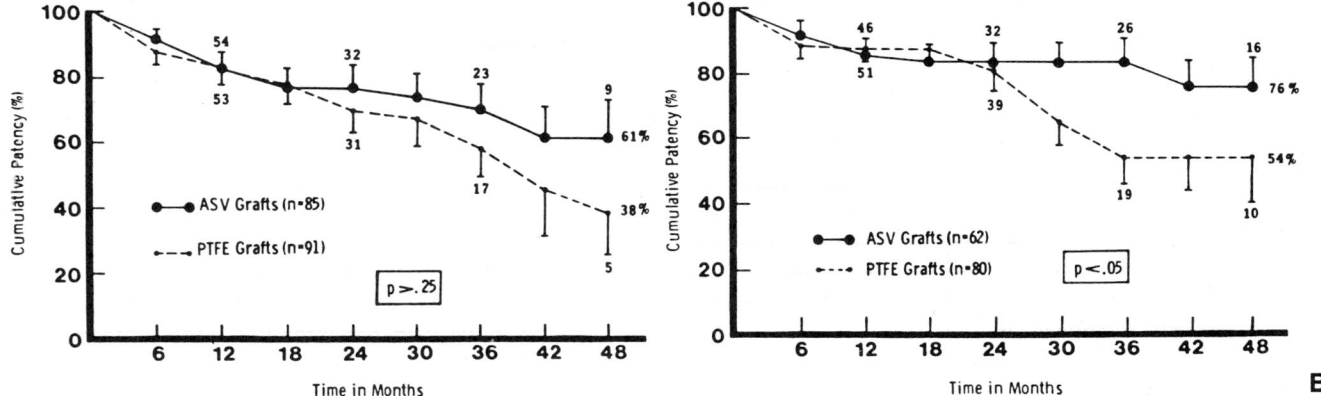

Figure 1 Cumulative life table primary patency rates for all randomized autologous saphenous vein *(ASV)* and polytetrafluoroethylene *(PTFE)* bypasses performed to the popliteal artery *(A),* above-knee, *(B),* below-knee. Number with each point indicates number of patent grafts observed for that length of time. Standard error of each point is shown. (From Veith FJ, Gupta SK, Ascer E, et al. Six-year prospective multicenter randomized comparison of autologous saphenous vein and expanded polytetrafluoroethylene grafts in infrainguinal arterial reconstructions. J Vasc Surg 1986; 3:104–114; with permission.)

55%, with an acceptable limb salvage rate of 74%. Therefore, secondary bypasses with ePTFE may provide reasonable results in this setting when autologous vein is not available. Moreover, these data prompt us to disagree with the UCLA group's recommendation to use ePTFE as a primary graft because it performs so poorly as a secondary bypass.

Bypasses to the tibial vessels with ePTFE have results inferior to bypasses done with autologous vein. In a prospective randomized trial, the 4 year patency rate for autologous saphenous vein was 49% versus 12% for ePTFE grafts.[5] Patency of distal ePTFE grafts is possibly improved with the use of anticoagulant drugs such as warfarin. With this drug, Flinn and colleagues reported a 4 year patency rate of 37% for infrapopliteal ePTFE bypasses.[7] Examination of our own experience since 1986 with 90 patients who underwent femoral-to-infrapopliteal artery bypasses with ePTFE and long-term postoperative anticoagulation revealed a life table 3 year primary patency rate of 57%. The 3 year limb salvage rate after these ePTFE crural bypasses was 76%. Thus ePTFE bypass to infrapopliteal arteries in this setting is a better option than a major amputation.

The construction of a vein cuff (Miller cuff) or a vein patch (Taylor patch) at the distal anastomosis has been suggested to increase the patency of ePTFE tibial artery bypasses. Taylor and co-workers reported a 5 year patency rate of 54% in 83 tibial grafts with an anastomotic vein patch.[8] Harris and co-workers recently reported a 2 year patency rate of 52% in 42 grafts employing a Miller vein cuff at the distal anastomosis.[9] The results of these retrospective studies indicate the need for randomized prospective trials to evaluate the benefit of adjunctive procedures such as vein cuffs and patches. Currently, one such trial is underway in Britain and Ireland, and a prospective trial is proposed in the United States. The results of these trials should provide valuable information concerning the optimal technique for distal prosthetic grafting.

FAILING ePTFE GRAFTS

Like vein grafts, ePTFE grafts may present in the failing state with the responsible lesion in inflow arteries, outflow arteries, at the proximal or distal anastomoses, or occasionally even within the graft. These failing grafts can be identified by changes in ankle-brachial index, pulse volume recordings, pulse examinations, or alterations in the blood flow velocities on duplex scanning. Detection of lesions associated with failing ePTFE grafts mandates early intervention, which greatly improves patency and limb salvage rates.[10] Invariably, the corrective procedure required to repair a failing graft is simpler than the secondary operation would be, if the graft went on to thrombose. Thus, we believe a routine surveillance program that includes duplex scanning should be employed for monitoring ePTFE grafts. In a review of our own experience with failing ePTFE grafts in 85 patients, 87% of the 144 lesions identified were the result of progression of atherosclerotic disease, either proximal or distal to the graft.[10] Only eight anastomotic lesions were identified. Surgical intervention such as patch angioplasty, short graft extensions, or lesion excision was required for 69% of lesions. Treatment of failing grafts was achieved with percutaneous balloon angioplasty as the initial treatment in 28% of the lesions (Fig. 2). Balloon angioplasty was effective in the management of 44% of the inflow lesions, but it was not as beneficial for the treatment of outflow lesions, as evidenced by the fact that 83% required surgical treatment with an extension to distal arteries because the lesions were diffuse, long, or inaccessible to balloon angioplasty. Thus, balloon angioplasty was applicable to focal arterial lesions, particularly those within the iliac arteries, whereas operative interventions were better for the more extensive lesions found in the outflow tract. The 5 year secondary patency rate for treated ePTFE grafts was 71%.[10] These results suggest that anastomotic intimal hyperplasia and progressive atherosclerotic disease are both important causes of graft failure.

COMPLICATIONS

The major complications of ePTFE grafts include early and late thrombosis, graft infection, and aneurysm formation.

Graft thrombosis is the most common complication. Early graft failure (within 30 days of operation) is usually due to a technical flaw or poor choice of inflow or outflow sites. However, early graft thrombosis is not always related to easily defined anatomic problems and may be related to the inherent thrombogenicity of the ePTFE graft or to a transient fall in cardiac output. Aggressive treatment of these early occlusions is justified. After an early graft thrombosis, the patient should be returned promptly to the operating room for graft thrombectomy and operative arteriogram to examine the distal anastomosis for technical problems or distal stenotic or occlusive lesions that were not appreciated on the original arteriogram. These reoperations with correction of any technical problems or residual lesions can result in good long-term patency and limb salvage.[11]

Graft failure may be secondary to either progression of atherosclerotic disease or anastomotic intimal hyperplasia. If late failure is accompanied by a threatened limb, then reintervention should be undertaken. Prior to operation, a new arteriogram should be performed to examine for progression of inflow or outflow disease. If this reveals the cause of graft failure, the appropriate angioplasty or graft extension can be coupled with graft thrombectomy to preserve graft function. Acceptable incremental 3 year patency rates have been reported for this strategy of graft salvage for failed femoral to above-knee popliteal ePTFE grafts.[11] However, other strategies may be employed, including performance of a new vein or ePTFE secondary bypass using virginal, patent arterial segments. Alternatively, catheter-directed thrombolytic therapy may be used to lyse the

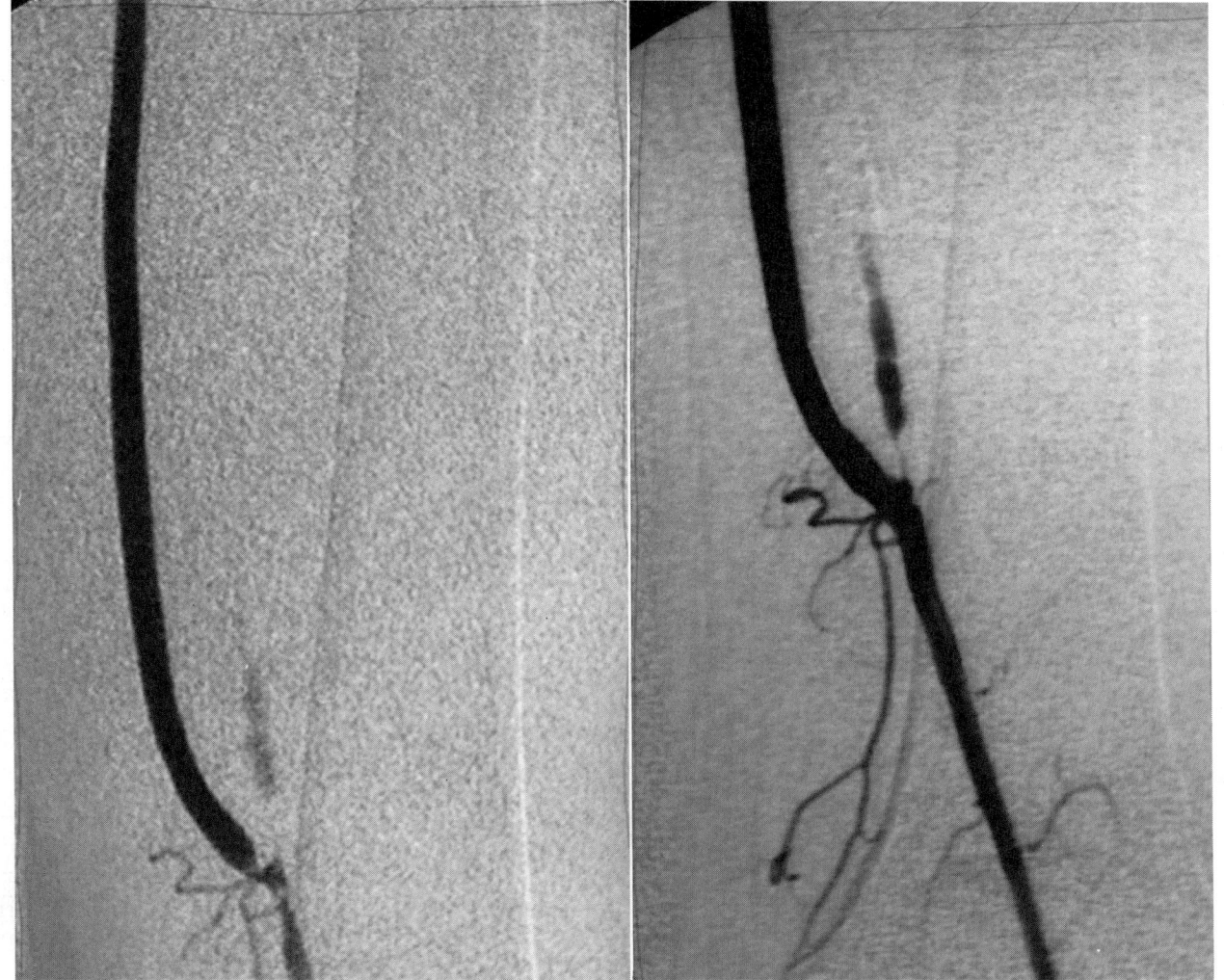

Figure 2 Arteriogram of a patient with a failing ePTFE femoropopliteal graft 7 months after the initial operation. The arteriogram was performed because of loss of distal pulses. *A*, The PTFE graft was patent despite a severe stenosis of the distal anastomosis. *B*, This lesion was successfully treated with percutaneous balloon angioplasty as shown. The graft is patent 2 years after the intervention.

clot and reveal the cause of failure, which can then be corrected by the appropriate endovascular or operative procedure. In addition, if the distal circulation appears occluded on arteriography after graft failure, treatment with thrombolytic agents may restore distal runoff vessels, thereby improving the results of any subsequent intervention.

Thrombectomy of failed ePTFE bypasses to the below-knee popliteal artery and infrapopliteal arteries has not yielded results comparable to new secondary procedures. Therefore, secondary procedures should be performed in preference to graft thrombectomy whenever possible. These secondary procedures should be performed by utilizing previously undissected segments of artery for the origin and insertion of the graft and autologous vein if it is available. One can expect a better than 40% 2 year patency rate with this strategy.[11]

REFERENCES

1. Campbell CD, Brooks DH, Webster MW, et al. The use of expanded microporous polytetrafluoroethylene for limb salvage: A preliminary report. Surgery 1976; 79:485–491.
2. Quinones-Baldrich WJ, Prego AA, Ucelay-Gomez R, et al. Long-term results of infrainguinal revascularization with polytetrafluoroethylene: A ten-year experience. J Vasc Surg 1992; 16:209–217.
3. Kent KC, Whittemore AD, Mannick JA. Short term and mid-term results of an all-autogenous tissue policy for infrainguinal reconstruction. J Vasc Surg 1989; 9:107–114.
4. McCarthy WJ, Pearce WH, Flinn WR, et al. Long-term evaluation of composite sequential bypass for limb-threatening ischemia. J Vasc Surg 1992; 15:761–770.
5. Veith FJ, Gupta SK, Ascer E, et al. Six-year prospective multicenter randomized comparison of autologous saphenous vein and expanded polytetrafluoroethylene grafts in infrainguinal arterial reconstructions. J Vasc Surg 1986; 3:104–114.

6. Yang PM, Wengerter K, Veith FJ, et al. Value and limitations of secondary femoropopliteal bypasses with polytetrafluoroethylene. J Vasc Surg 1991; 14:292–298.
7. Flinn WR, Rohrer M, Yao JST, et al. Improved long-term patency of infragenicular polytetrafluoroethylene grafts. J Vasc Surg 1988; 7:685–690.
8. Taylor RS, Loh A, McFarland RJ, et al. Improved technique for polytetrafluoroethylene bypass grafting: Long-term results using anastomotic vein patches. Br J Surg 1992; 79:348–354.
9. Harris PL, Bakran A, Enabi L, et al. ePTFE grafts for femorocrural bypass: Improved results with combined adjuvant venous cuff and arteriovenous fistula. Eur J Vasc Surg 1993; 7:528–533.
10. Sanchez LA, Suggs WD, Veith FJ, et al. Is surveillance to detect failing PTFE bypasses worthwhile? Twelve-year experience with 91 grafts. J Vasc Surg 1993; 18:981–990.
11. Ascer E, Collier P, Gupta SK, et al. Reoperation for polytetrafluoroethylene bypass failure: The importance of distal outflow site and operative technique in determining outcome. J Vasc Surg 1987; 5:298–310.

UMBILICAL VEIN GRAFTS FOR ATHEROSCLEROTIC LOWER EXTREMITY OCCLUSIVE DISEASE

HERBERT DARDIK, M.D.

Current indications for using particular graft materials in lower extremity revascularization procedures have become reasonably standardized, but variations exist in the patterns of use of alternative materials to the autologous saphenous vein. The primacy of the greater saphenous vein is acknowledged, but the choice and order of use of other autologous veins or the use of prosthetic materials are currently based on individual experience and preference. Some investigators have documented their commitment to autologous vein by use of lesser saphenous and upper extremity veins if ipsilateral or contralateral greater saphenous vein is unavailable or unsuitable. In practice, most surgeons proceed directly to prosthetic materials, which avoids additional incisions and potential for wound complications and is technically easier. Additionally, there can be a significant shortening of the operating time.

Polytetrafluoroethylene (PTFE) has enjoyed popularity, but critical studies have made it clear that this material is inferior to autologous vein with regard to durability and complication-free patency rates. To date few randomized prospective studies in the literature compare PTFE with autologous saphenous vein or the efficacy of PTFE with other alternative prosthetic materials, particularly the human umbilical vein graft.[1-5] Thus, the primacy of PTFE as the alternative material of choice invites challenge.

The glutaraldehyde stabilized human umbilical vein graft (UV) is now nearing completion of its second decade of human use. Numerous misconceptions exist about its clinical utility. Therefore, it is necessary to emphasize that UV is useful and functional, even though indications for use have changed over the years. On a personal note, having continuously used this material prior to and since its commercial introduction in 1979, I still find it valuable in many instances where bypasses are required to the popliteal and crural arteries.

The indications for UV use are subject to individual interpretation. In patients requiring limb salvage whose autologous vein is unavailable or unsuitable, UV should be considered as an alternative graft material. It may be appropriate in other situations such as the need to minimize the duration of an operation or borderline status of vein with regard to quality or even age of the patient. Depending on referral patterns, up to 20% of lower extremity reconstructions require alternative material to greater saphenous vein. In this circumstance, one should consider autologous vein from another site or a prosthetic material. In an additional 5% to 10% of patients, considering a prosthetic in the femoral above-knee popliteal position may also be appropriate, based on some current data suggesting advantage for preserving autologous saphenous vein for later use.[6] The patient's life expectancy, operative risk factors, and quality of runoff are important to use in deciding autologous vein or prosthetic material in the above-knee position.

Twenty years have elapsed since the initial concept and development of the human UV graft. Experience with more than 1,000 UV grafts forms the basis of this report as the indications for this prosthesis have been refined and its performance defined. In 1988, a 10 year (1975–1985) experience with UV was published, describing the results of 907 bypasses constructed in 715 patients (799 limbs).[7] The primary and secondary cumulative graft patency rates, as well as half-life patencies for popliteal, tibial, and peroneal reconstructions, the latter being 6.5, 2.3, and 1.7 years respectively, were acceptable (Fig. 1). There were no significant differences between primary and secondary graft patency rates for any of the major reconstruction groups, a secondary patency rate of 57% achieved for femoropopliteal bypass at 5 years and 33% for femorocrural bypasses. We concluded that the results were satisfactory, considering what would have otherwise been achieved in the majority of patients lacking suitable autologous vein. Similar results have been reported by others.[8-10] Perioperative and late graft thrombosis as well as nonoperative graft failure caused by infection, aneurysm formation, or progressive foot gangrene were also described in 87 grafts (8%). The overall infection

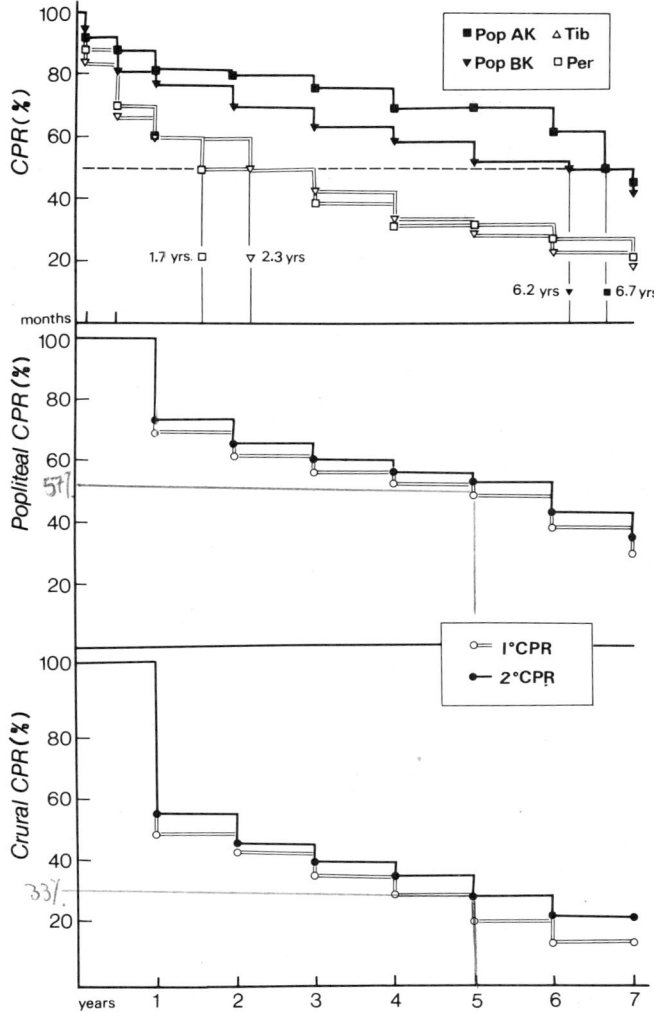

Figure 1 Cumulative graft patencies and half-life determinants during the first decade of experience (1975–1985) for popliteal and crural reconstructions using the umbilical vein graft. CPR = cumulative patency rate.

rate was 4.3%. The incidence of graft dilation and aneurysm development after 5 years was 36% aneurysms and 21% dilation. However, the overall clinical impact of graft degeneration remained minimal, 6% after 5 years.

Since 1986, the number of UV reconstructions performed at the Englewood Hospital and Medical Center has decreased significantly because of our commitment to primary autologous vein (Fig. 2). Nevertheless, approximately 20% of reconstructions require UV for the indications cited previously.

Since the first decade of UV experience, we have implanted an additional 167 UV grafts in 143 patients (153 limbs). During this interval (November 1985 to June 1993), several significant changes occurred that dealt primarily with procurement of the crude material, processing and manufacture, and quality-control mechanisms prior to distribution. On this basis, we have elected to analyze our current UV experience in groups using the current product (UV-2A), which we have implanted 71 times since January 1990 in 67 patients (4 patients had repeat or additional ipsilateral UV implants). Only three (4%) of the reconstructions were at the above-knee level (Table 1). Below-knee popliteal, posterior tibial, and peroneal sites accounted for more than 80% of the total number of bypasses. Of all the bypasses, 59% were infrapopliteal.

Cumulative graft patency rates had no significant differences between primary and secondary patency rates of a particular reconstruction (Fig. 3). Although these results with UV-2A are better than those achieved with prior grafts, this is a function of an increasing experience with this type of graft material, improved patient selection, perioperative and postoperative surveillance, and attentive management of the coagulation profile. Three year primary cumulative patency for UV grafts in the infrageniculate popliteal position was 58%, corrected to 64% with secondary procedures. Primary and secondary cumulative patency rates for crural reconstructions were 36% and 41%, respectively, which are statistically insignificant differences.

The current study also has lower rates of infection (2.8%) and stenosis (1.4%). There were no false aneurysms and no documented instances of biodegradation in the form of graft dilation or aneurysm formation (Table 2). The latter observation is significant in relation to our earlier experience, but longer periods of observation are essential. We have also documented the number of patients who expired with functioning grafts (withdrawal category in calculating life tables) and the total number of deaths, which includes patients with patent grafts and patients who died after graft complications (failure category in life table analysis). All major limb amputations in this series account for 10% of failed popliteal bypasses and 24% of crural bypass failures. Limb salvage rates by actuarial life table analysis are good (Figure 4).

The concern and fear of many surgeons regarding biodegradation with aneurysm formation leading to disastrous consequences are exaggerated. Those who have studied this phenomenon have noted that, although morphologic changes do occur with some frequency after several years of implantation, the actual clinical impact is low. The incidence of aneurysms requiring reoperation 5 years postoperatively is approximately 6%. Recent observations suggest a decreasing incidence of biodegradation with very few reconstructions required over the last 5 years. No aneurysms have been noted in the UV-2A grafts. Biodegradation is anticipated but at a decreased incidence and more remote from the date of operation.

Throughout the two decades of its existence, the UV graft has evolved into a clinically useful prosthesis. With an appreciation of its "negatives," that is, requirement for faultless technique and long-term (greater than 5 years) biodegradation in 50% of survivors, although clinically significant in only 6%, the assets of the UV graft include superior patency rates compared to alternative prosthetics and complication rates similar to those

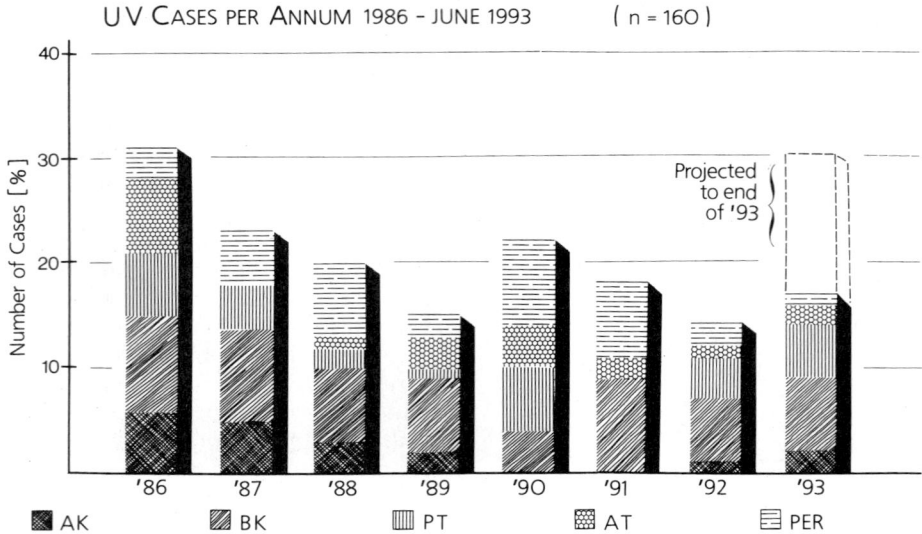

Figure 2 Number of umbilical vein reconstructions performed each year at the Englewood Hospital and Medical Center from 1986 through June 1993. The decrease from the prior decade reflects commitment to autologous vein. The recent increase represents a larger number of referred patients without autologous vein.

Table 1 Patient Data (January 1990–June 1993)

Group	Number (%)	Age (Range)	Male : Female	Diabetes	Smokers	Prior Limb Bypass
Popliteal above-knee	3 (4)	71 (55–86)	1 : 2	67%	67%	33%
Popliteal below-knee	26 (37)	69 (51–84)	1.2 : 1	42%	46%	31%
Posterior tibial	15 (21)	66 (53–78)	2 : 1	47%	53%	53%
Anterior tibial	9 (13)	67 (37–83)	1.3 : 1	56%	56%	67%
Peroneal	18 (25)	67 (48–81)	2.6 : 1	67%	83%	44%
Total	71	68 (37–86)	1.5 : 1	51%	59%	42%

*Includes two dorsalis pedis reconstructions.

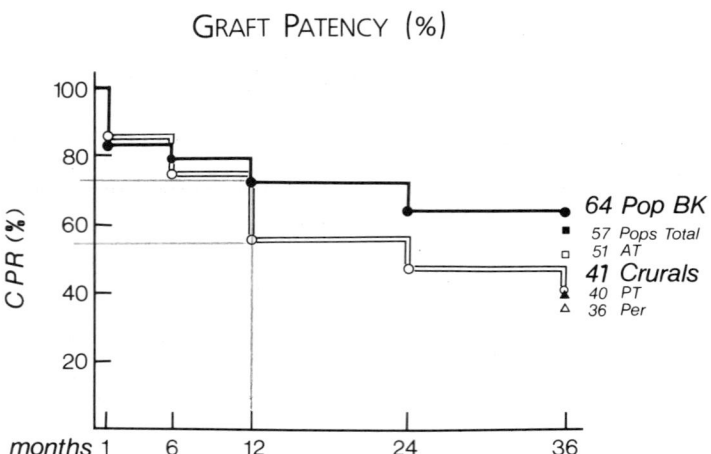

Figure 3 Current experience with below-knee popliteal and crural umbilical vein reconstructions since 1990. Although these curves are not significantly better from prior analysis, these groups, small in numbers and short in duration, show the trend of improved patency rates. Patency rates for each type of reconstruction is depicted at right with the exception of above-knee popliteals, in that only three were performed during this time interval.

Table 2 Complications (January 1990–June 1993)

Group	Number	Expired Open (%)	Total Expired (%)	Infection (%)	Stenosis (%)	False Aneurysm	Dilation and Aneurysm	Amputations (%)
Popliteal above-knee	3	0	0	0	0	0	0	1
Popliteal below-knee	26	5 (19)	11 (42)	0	0	0	0	2
Posterior tibial	15	0	2 (13)	2 (13)	0	0	0	4
Anterior tibial	9	0	0	0	0	0	0	2
Peroneal	18	0	0	0	1 (6)	0	0	4
Total	71	5 (7)	13 (18.3)	2 (2.8)	1 (1.4)	0	0	13 (18.3)

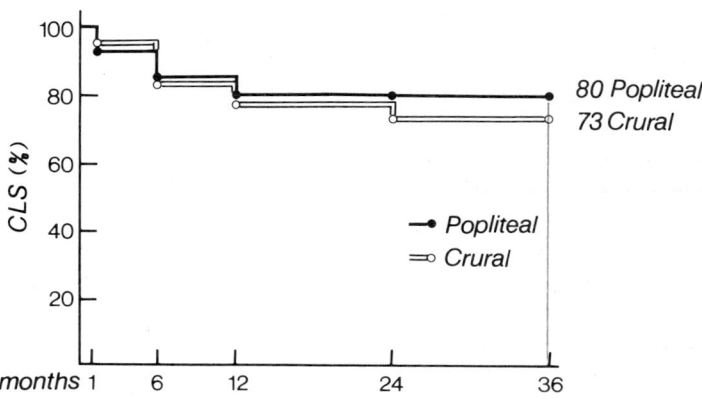

Figure 4 Limb salvage results for umbilical vein popliteal and crural reconstructions since 1990. These results closely approximate those with autologous vein and are superior to those obtained with other prosthetic materials.

associated with autologous vein. Curiously, most detractors of the UV graft have had no experience with it. Excellent patency and limb salvage rates are, in fact, attainable with the UV graft when autologous vein is unavailable or unsuitable.

REFERENCES

1. Veith FJ, Gupta SK, Ascer E, et al. Six year prospective multicenter randomized comparison of autologous saphenous vein and expanded polytetrafluoroethylene grafts in infrainguinal arterial reconstructions. J Vasc Surg 1986; 3:104–314.
2. Eickhoff JH, Buchardt Hansen HJ, Broome A, et al. A randomized clinical trial of PTFE versus human umbilical vein for femoropopliteal bypass surgery: Preliminary results. Br J Surg 1983; 70:85–88.
3. McCollum C, Kenchington G, Alexander C, et al. PTFE or HUV for femoro-popliteal bypass: A multi-centre trial. Eur J Vasc Surg 1991; 5 435–443.
4. Aalders GJ, van Vroonhoven TJ. Polytetrafluoroethylene versus human umbilical vein in above knee femoropopliteal bypass: Six year results of a randomized clinical trial. J Vasc Surg 1992; 16:816–824.
5. Johnson WC. Comparative evaluation of PTFE, HUV and saphenous vein bypasses in fem pop AK vascular reconstruction. Presented at the North American Chapter of the International Society for Cardiovascular Surgery, June 19, 1992, Chicago.
6. Quinones-Baldrich WJ, Busuttil RW, Baker JD, et al. Is the preferential use of polytetrafluoroethylene grafts for femoropopliteal bypass justified? J Vasc Surg 1988; 8:219–228.
7. Dardik H, Miller N, Dardik A, et al. A decade of experience with the glutaraldehyde tanned human umbilical cord vein graft for revascularization of the lower limb. J Vasc Surg 1988; 7:336–346.
8. Nevelsteen A, D'Hallewin MA, Deleersnijder J, et al. The human umbilical vein graft in below knee femoropopliteal and femorotibial surgery: An eight year experience. Ann Vasc Surg 1986; 1:328–334.
9. Raithel D, Schweiger H, Geutsch HH. Late results with Dardik-biograft in peripheral arterial surgery. J Cardiovasc Surg 1984; 25:222–224.
10. Hirsch SA, Jarrett F. The use of stabilized human umbilical vein for femoropopliteal bypass. Ann Surg 1984; 200:147–151.

SHORT VEIN GRAFTS FROM THE DISTAL SUPERFICIAL FEMORAL, POPLITEAL, OR INFRAPOPLITEAL ARTERIES TO MORE DISTAL ARTERIES FOR LIMB SALVAGE

ENRICO ASCER, M.D.
ROBERT M. POLLINA, M.D.

The superficial femoral artery (SFA) is the infrainguinal vessel most commonly involved with severe arteriosclerotic occlusive disease. Thus, it is not surprising that vascular surgeons have been reluctant to accept the concept of preferentially using an inflow site distal to the common femoral artery (CFA). Moreover, the CFA is usually a large, easily approachable vessel that has been repeatedly shown to be an acceptable donor site for infrainguinal reconstructions. Nevertheless, in some situations the use of the CFA may not be safe or feasible and a more distal donor site must be considered if limb salvage is to be achieved. These situations include patients presenting with dense groin scarring caused by previous operations or with groin infection. Also, increasingly, patients are found to have an insufficient length of autogenous veins to reach the CFA due to previous cardiac or infrainguinal bypass procedures.

Because of a surprisingly low incidence of short vein graft failure due to progression of proximal arteriosclerosis (6%), and because these bypasses have had better outcomes in restricted outflow situations, we are currently utilizing the distal, most continuously patent portion of the arterial tree as our choice for inflow in bypass procedures to the infrapopliteal arteries. This approach has also evolved from previously published experiences demonstrating the efficacy and durability of shorter arterial bypasses originating from the proximal or distal SFA, the popliteal artery, and even the tibial arteries.[1-9] Although we recognize that the superiority of the short vein approach, in terms of graft patency and limb salvage, has not conclusively been demonstrated, it offers several real and potential advantages.

GENERAL CONSIDERATIONS

Critical ischemia continues to be the only clear indication for arterial bypasses below the popliteal artery in patients with advanced arteriosclerosis. Approximately 70% of our patients present with tissue loss, and the remaining patients complain of severe rest pain.

Despite recent improvements in duplex scanning and magnetic resonance imaging of the peripheral vascular system, we rely primarily on standard contrast arteriography. In over 95% of patients, these images have documented a patent distal artery even in the presence of multisegmental disease. Selective catheterization, delayed filming, injection of intra-arterial vasodilators, and occasionally digital subtraction arteriography help identify suitable arteries for a distal bypass. Biplanar visualization of proximal inflow arteries, in particular, the bifurcation of the common iliac and femoral arteries, may unmask stenoses that are not evident in only one view.

The hemodynamic significance of arterial stenoses should be documented by intra-arterial blood pressure measurements with liberal use of vasodilators. If a significant blood pressure gradient is measured proximal to the elected bypass inflow site, we favor preoperative or operative balloon angioplasty to diminish the magnitude of the operation or to shorten the length of the vein graft required for the arterial reconstruction. In fact, we have not hesitated to perform a proximal angioplasty of the SFA or the popliteal artery in tandem with a short distal vein bypass.[10,11] Thus far, this combined approach has been limited to patients who lack a sufficiently long saphenous vein or have groin infection or a disadvantaged outflow tract.

Clearly, many patients with extensive occlusive disease of the SFA require an inflow from the CFA. In a recent review of our last 300 infrapopliteal bypasses, we noted that only 72 (24%) bypasses originated from the CFA. Because of a policy of using the shortest possible segment of vein for our infrainguinal reconstructions, we believe this to be an accurate representation of how often an adequate arterial segment distal to the CFA can be encountered in this patient population. However, it is important to emphasize that our high utilization of distal inflow sites may be due in part to the fact that almost half of these patients were diabetics and that we have accepted up to 40% stenosis of the inflow arteries.

IMPROVED GRAFT PATENCY RATES

In 1981, Veith and associates compared the patency results of 290 popliteal bypasses originating from the CFA to 60 popliteal bypasses originating from the SFA or above-knee popliteal artery.[1] At 4 years, the cumulative patency rates were 66% for the former group and 81% for the latter. Although this difference was not statistically significant, it attested to the durability of these nonstandard inflow sites. Similarly, the 4 year patency rate for 79 infrapopliteal bypasses originating from the CFA was 50%, and for 129 bypasses originating from the SFA or the popliteal artery it was 58% at comparable intervals.[1] More recently, an increased experience with 153 popliteal-to-infrapopliteal bypasses published by the Montefiore surgeons generated an acceptable primary bypass patency rate of 55% at 5 years.[8]

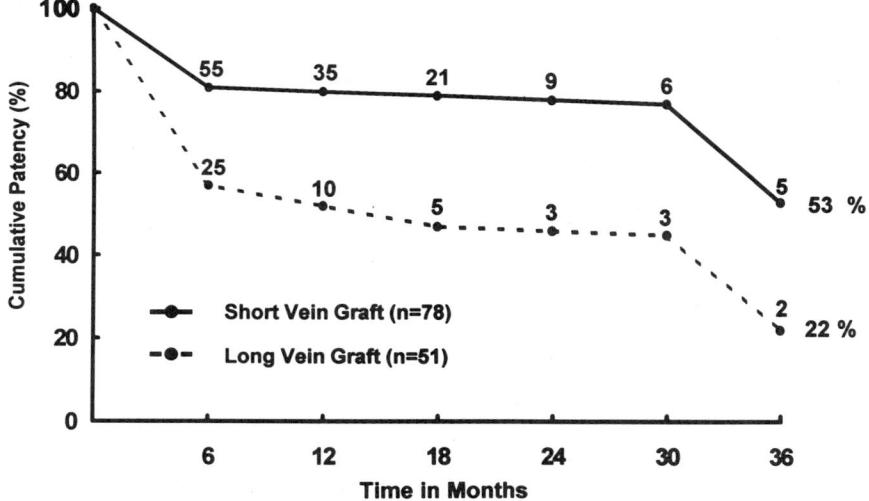

Figure 1 Cumulative life table primary patency rates for short vein bypasses (78) and long vein bypasses (51) in presence of poor runoff. Number of patients at risk are shown at 6 month intervals ($p < 0.01$).

Other investigators have published equally acceptable results with the use of inflow sites from the distal SFA and popliteal artery (Table 1). However, they were unable to document the superiority of short vein bypasses when compared to the ones constructed from the CFA.

In our study, we measured the length of the vein graft in infrapopliteal bypasses rather than the site of inflow, and only then was it possible to document the superiority of the shorter grafts in terms of patency.[2] This was a retrospective review of 237 infrapopliteal vein bypasses performed in 215 patients in which we arbitrarily divided these bypasses into two groups according to the length of the vein. In the long vein graft group (117 bypasses), the vein varied from 42 to 92 cm with a mean of 60.9 ± 9 cm, and in the short vein group (120 bypasses) the vein length varied from 6 to 40 cm with a mean of 24.7 ± 8 cm. Both groups were comparable for diabetic status, indication for operation, and site of the distal anastomosis. Poor runoff was more prevalent in the short vein group. Despite this important variable, the short vein group had significantly better patency rate at 3 years (45% long veins versus 63% short veins) ($p < 0.05$). When the 3 year graft patency rates for bypasses performed in presence of good runoff were compared for the short and long veins the differences were found to be statistically insignificant. Conversely, in poor or disadvantaged outflow situations, superior patency results were achieved by the short vein bypasses (Figs. 1 and 2). In addition, the 2 year graft patency for the 44 longest vein bypasses from the CFA to distal third of the infrapopliteal arteries were compared to 24 shortest tibiotibial vein bypasses. The results obtained were even more pronounced in favor of the short vein group (45% versus 86%) (Figs. 3 and 4).[3]

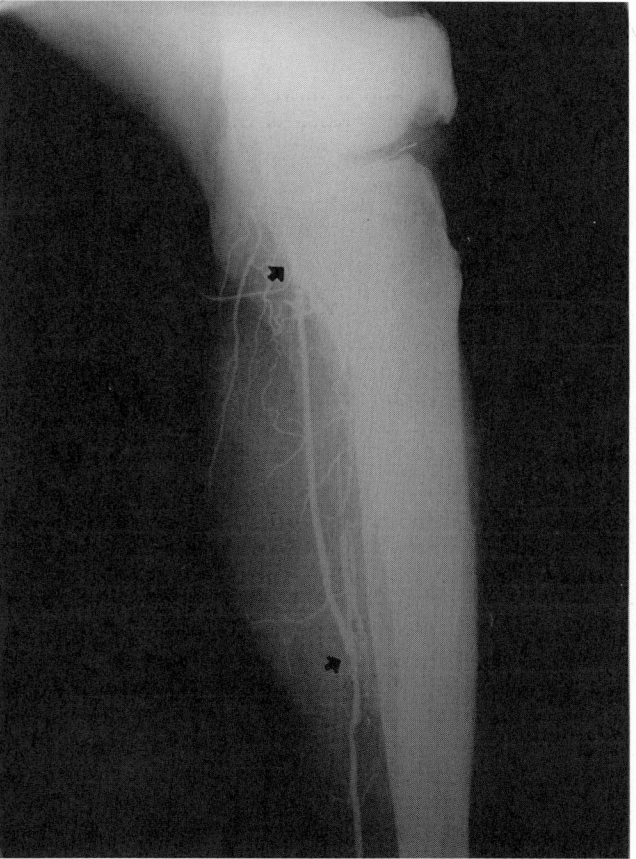

Figure 2 Operative arteriogram after a bypass from the distal popliteal artery to the posterior tibial artery in a patient with unimpeded flow to the popliteal artery. This bypass configuration is the most commonly performed in those patients amenable to short vein bypasses.

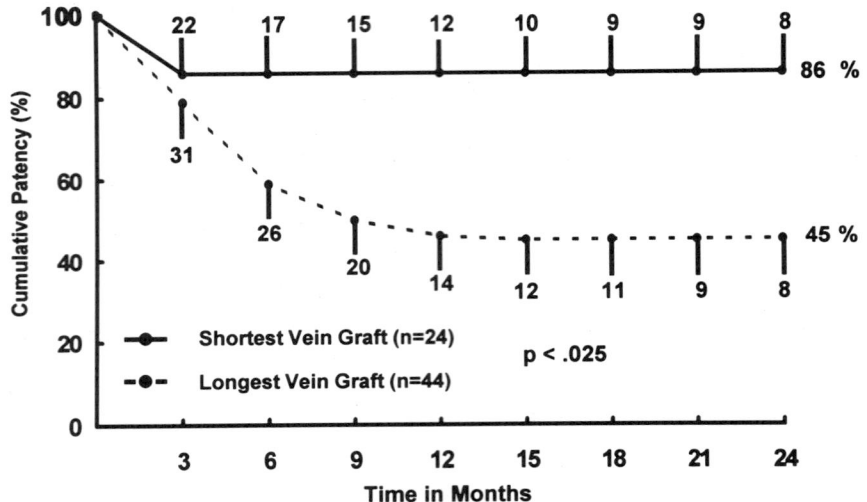

Figure 3 Cumulative life table primary patency rates for the 44 longest vein bypasses (from the common femoral to distal third of the infrapopliteal arteries) and for the 24 shortest vein bypasses (tibiotibial). Number of patients at risk are shown at 3 month intervals ($p < 0.025$).

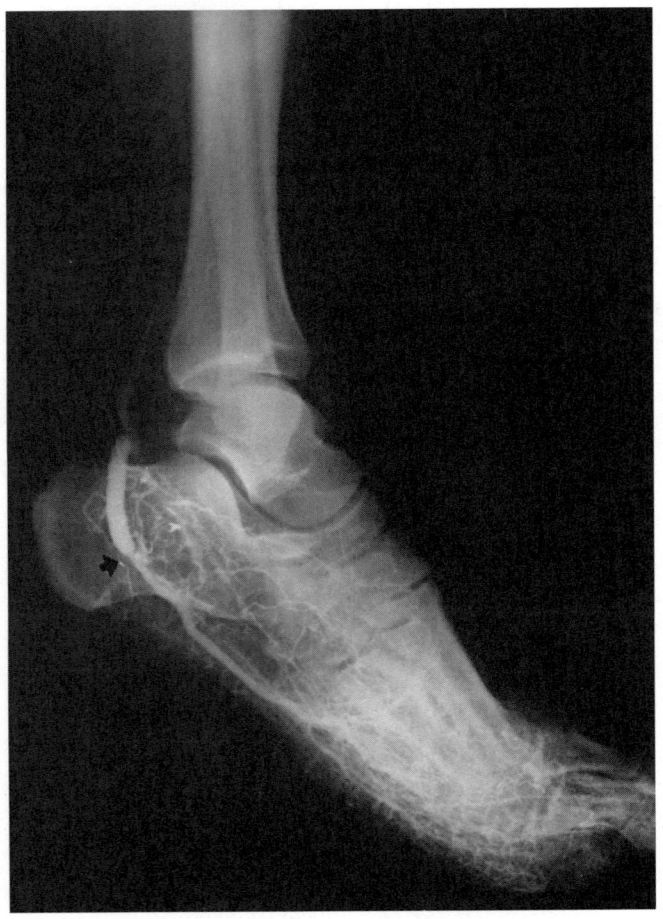

Figure 4 Operative arteriogram after one of the ultrashort vein bypasses from the inframalleolar posterior tibial artery to the lateral plantar artery in a patient with ischemic tissue loss in the foot and unimpeded flow to the posterior tibial artery.

DECREASED INCIDENCE OF VEIN GRAFT STENOSES

The superiority of short vein grafts may be directly related to a lesser susceptibility to the development of fibrotic stenoses. In our experience, frequent noninvasive graft surveillance revealed four times more high-grade stenoses in long vein grafts than in shorter grafts. Although at first glance this difference may appear to be related solely to the length of the graft, other mechanisms may be involved in causing this difference. Certainly, more optimal segments of vein may be selected for procedures requiring shorter conduit. Regions of vein that are questionable in gross appearance may be avoided, and shorter grafts have less potential for intimal injury during preparation.

INCREASED VEIN UTILIZATION

Approximately one-third of our patients had an ipsilateral saphenous vein that was either unavailable because of prior cardiac or lower extremity operations or was found to be inadequate because of small diameter, short usable length, previous phlebitis, or overlying infection. The combination of the use of a short segment of vein as well as the ability to harvest it from either the ipsilateral or contralateral greater saphenous vein, lesser saphenous vein, or arm veins have increased our vein utilization rate from 68% to 86%. Although these ectopic venous conduits have not conclusively been demonstrated as having the durability of the ipsilateral greater saphenous vein, their results are clearly superior to prosthetic infrapopliteal bypasses. Thus, absolute vein utilization is increased with the use of these shorter bypasses, and the need to resort to prosthetic conduit is lessened.

Table 1 Results of Short Vein Bypasses: Cumulative Patency and Limb Salvage Rates

Author, Date	Number	Inflow Site	Outflow Site	Patency (Years)	Limb Salvage
Veith et al, 1981	129	Distal superficial femoral and popliteal	Popliteal and tibial	73% (5)	N/A
Schuler et al, 1983	23	Distal superficial femoral and popliteal	Tibial	84% (2.5)	70%
Veith et al, 1985	14	Tibial	Tibial	79% (0.5–4)	79%
Cantelmo et al, 1986	32	Distal superficial femoral and popliteal	Tibial	79% (3)	82%
Sidaway et al, 1986	29	Distal superficial femoral and popliteal	Tibial	81% (6)	89%
Ascer et al, 1988	120	Distal superficial femoral and popliteal	Tibial	63% (3)	86%
Rosenbloom et al, 1988	46	Distal superficial femoral and popliteal	Popliteal and tibial	41% (5)	69%
Wengerter et al, 1992	153	Popliteal	Tibial	55% (5)	76%
Marks et al, 1992	32	Popliteal	Tibial	63.5% (4)	79%

FEWER VEIN HARVEST COMPLICATIONS

Vein harvest complications can be minimized by avoiding long incisions or by averting excessively obese or scarred areas. The wound harvest complications rate for long vein bypasses was 16%, yet it was only 6% for short vein bypasses ($p < 0.05$). This observation is likely a reflection of the avoidance of the groin as a potential source for infection and a decrease in the interruption of lymphatic and superficial collateral circulation inherent in using shorter harvest incisions.

OTHER ADVANTAGES

There are several other real and potential advantages of short veins. One relates to the ability to circumvent groin problems, such as infection and scar tissue, that are quite common, particularly when one subscribes to an aggressive reoperative approach. In these situations, the use of an unobstructed distal SFA may represent a safer and quicker alternative to the CFA. Conversely, when a short vein bypass failed or became infected, the option of having the unused ipsilateral CFA as an inflow still existed, thereby reducing the risk and complexity of a reoperative procedure.

Another advantage of using a short vein bypass is the possibility of discarding imperfect vein segments rather than attempting to repair them, which increases the operating time and risks of technical failures. The possibility of graft twisting or kinking with passage through tunnels and across joints is minimized when a shorter vein graft is utilized. These advantages become more obvious when a below-knee popliteal artery segment or one of the infrapopliteal arteries is chosen as a donor vessel.

DISADVANTAGES

Despite our enthusiasm for the preferential use of short vein bypasses whenever possible, some shortcomings should be mentioned. Progression of proximal disease in the intervening segment from the CFA to the chosen bypass site has been shown to account for approximately 5% of short vein graft failures.[8] Calcified arterial segments are encountered more frequently in the more distal arterial tree, particularly in this largely diabetic population. This may add to the difficulty of constructing the proximal anastomosis, particularly when smaller tibial arteries are used as inflow sources.

REFERENCES

1. Veith FJ, Gupta SK, Samson RH, et al. Superficial femoral and popliteal arteries as inflow sites for distal bypasses. Surgery 1981; 90:980–990.
2. Ascer E, Veith FJ, Gupta SK, et al. Short vein grafts: A superior option for arterial reconstructions to poor or compromised outflow tracts? J Vasc Surg 1988; 7:370–378.
3. Veith FJ, Ascer E, Gupta SK, et al. Tibiotibial vein bypass grafts: A new operation for limb salvage. J Vasc Surg 1985; 2:552–557.
4. Schuler JJ, Flanigan DP, Williams LR, et al. Early experience with popliteal to infrapopliteal bypass for limb salvage. Arch Surg 1983; 118:472–476.
5. Sidaway AN, Menzoian JO, Cantelmo NL, LoGerfo FW. Effect of inflow and outflow sites on the results of tibioperoneal vein grafts. Am J Surg 1986; 153:211–214.
6. Cantelmo NL, Snow R, Menzoian JO, LoGerfo FW. Successful vein bypass in patients with an ischemic limb and a palpable popliteal pulse. Arch Surg 1986; 121:217–220.
7. Rosenbloom MS, Walsh JJ, Schuler JJ, et al. Long term results of infragenicular bypasses with autogenous vein originating from the distal superficial femoral and popliteal arteries. J Vasc Surg 1988; 7:691–696.
8. Wengerter KR, Yang PM, Veith FJ, et al. A twelve year experience with the popliteal-to-distal artery bypass: The significance and management of proximal disease. J Vasc Surg 1992; 15:143–151.
9. Marks J, King TA, Baele H, et al. Popliteal to distal bypass for limb threatening ischemia. J Vasc Surg 1992; 15:755–759.
10. Peterkin GA, Belkin M, Cantelmo NL, et al. Combined transluminal angioplasty and infrainguinal reconstruction in multilevel atherosclerotic disease. Am J Surg 1990; 160:277–279.
11. Brewster DC, Cambria RP, Darling C, et al. Long term results of combined iliac balloon angioplasty and distal surgical revascularization. Ann Surg 1989; 210:324–331.

SURVEILLANCE OF LOWER EXTREMITY BYPASS GRAFTS

DENNIS F. BANDYK, M.D.

Table 1 Lesions That Can Precipitate Graft Failure

Technical errors
    Retained or scarred valve cusps
    Errors in graft tunneling (graft entrapment)
    Injured vein segments
    Sclerosed veins
    Runoff artery thrombosis
    Platelet aggregation
    Anastomotic stricture
    Intimal flaps
Postimplantation lesions
    Myointimal hyperplasia
    Atherosclerosis
    Aneurysmal degeneration

Surveillance of infrainguinal bypass graft function has evolved to a recommended standard of arterial reconstructive surgery.[1] The rationale for patient follow-up is based on the progressive nature of atherosclerosis and the propensity of both autologous vein and prosthetic conduits to develop postimplantation lesions that can progress to produce a low-flow state in the graft and result in thrombosis. Infrainguinal vein bypasses, constructed by either reversed or in situ grafting techniques, tend to form occlusive lesions within the conduit or at anastomotic sites during the first several months to years following implantation into the arterial circulation.[2-4] The origin of these lesions has not been determined with certainty, but most are felt to develop at sites of vein injury, to result from pre-existing vein disease, or to arise de novo in response to arterialization and the atherosclerotic environment (Table 1). By comparison, lower limb polytetrafluoroethylene (PTFE) grafts demonstrate a steady attrition rate (approximately 10%/year) as a result of progressive inflow and outflow occlusive disease. The location and appearance time of lesions are different from those of vein grafts, and intragraft and anastomotic lesions are uncommon (5% to 7%), with most stenoses developing in the graft outflow (58%) or inflow (30%) arteries.[5] Thus, to identify the lesions of the hemodynamically failing bypass, surveillance methods must differ relative to graft type.

Clinical examination detects only the most severe postimplantation lesions. Furthermore, less than half of patients admit to symptoms of limb ischemia; thus, detection of graft lesions prior to thrombosis requires objective vascular testing methods. Before duplex scanning became available, most surgeons opted to monitor lower limb bypass grafts using Doppler-derived ankle systolic blood pressures, pulse volume plethysmography, and arteriography. Surveillance studies based on duplex scanning have confirmed that strictures develop in 20% to 30% of infrainguinal vein bypasses during the first year. These lesions, typically the result of myointimal hyperplasia, were associated with a threefold increase in graft occlusion and accounted for 80% of graft failures within 5 years of operation. The efficacy of graft surveillance depends on the scanning protocol used, the expertise of the vascular laboratory, and the willingness of the surgeon and patient to intervene when vascular laboratory studies identify an abnormal graft.

The goal of graft surveillance is not only to detect lesions with a potential for precipitating graft thrombosis but also to provide hemodynamic criteria to aid in the timing of graft revision. The data that link severe graft stricture detected by either angiography or duplex scanning to an increased risk of graft occlusion are persuasive. Grigg and associates[6] and Moody and colleagues[7] observed a 21% to 23% incidence of thrombosis in stenotic vein bypasses when a conservative no revision policy was followed. Idu and co-workers reported all infrainguinal vein grafts identified to have a stenosis greater than 70% diameter reduction eventually occluded, compared to 10% of grafts with similar lesions but revised (p less than .004).[8] Mattos and associates also reported infrainguinal grafts identified to have stenosis by color duplex scanning (velocity ratio greater than 2) had a significantly lower 4 year patency of 57% compared to 83% observed in normal grafts.[9] Intervention, based on a duplex surveillance protocol, has resulted in 5 year assisted-primary patency rates of 82% to 93%, significantly higher than the 30% to 50% secondary patency rates of thrombosed vein grafts. Clinical studies indicate that routine infrainguinal bypass surveillance can enhance long-term patency by at least 15% to 20%.[2,9,10]

MECHANISMS AND HEMODYNAMICS OF GRAFT FAILURE

A successful surveillance program requires a thorough understanding of the mechanisms and hemodynamics of graft failure. Graft failure can occur by one of three mechanisms: occlusion by thrombosis or embolization, hemodynamic failure, and structural failure associated with aneurysmal degeneration or infection. The incidence of vein graft failure is highest during the first several postoperative days (4% to 10%), decreasing to approximately 1% per month during the first year, and then is approximately 2% to 4% per year thereafter. Perioperative (within 30 days) graft failure accounts for one quarter of all failures and may be due to technical errors in bypass construction (suture stenosis, intimal flaps, retained thrombus, graft entrapment and torsion), inadequate outflow, infection, or unrecognized hypercoagulable states. Failure between 30 days and 2 years is the result of focal myointimal hyperplasia within the vein conduit or at anastomotic sites; rarely, diffuse stricture of the venous conduit occurs. Late graft failure is most often the result of atherosclerotic disease progression. Graft failure as a result of aneurysmal degeneration, anastomotic false aneurysm, or thromboembolism can occur at any time after implantation but is uncommon and accounts for less than 10% of all failures.

The incidence of early graft failure can be minimized by careful operative assessment, but conditions such as hypercoagulable states, use of marginal, sclerotic venous conduits, low cardiac output, or poor outflow can produce graft thrombosis despite a technically perfect reconstruction. Infrainguinal bypasses, especially prosthetic grafts, with poor runoff can demonstrate a blood flow velocity near the thrombotic threshold velocity of the conduit and be prone to thrombosis with slight decreases in blood flow. The measurement of operative graft hemodynamics is an underemphasized principle of surveillance, despite studies that document a 5% to 10% incidence of vascular defects when quantitative Doppler spectral analysis was performed.[10] Surprisingly, duplex scanning, a technique with proven accuracy for graft surveillance, has been adopted by few surgeons as an operative aid. Reluctance to employ duplex scanning at operation has been attributed to its complexity, instrument availability, and the erroneous assumption that arteriography is superior.

A number of abnormalities can persist unsuspected after infrainguinal bypass grafting, especially when the in situ saphenous vein grafting technique is used. Retained valve cusps, errors in tunneling, vein conduit injury, or partial anastomotic occlusion can initiate thrombus formation and precipitate occlusion. Residual lesions can also be the origin of myointimal hyperplasia, a lesion known to cause graft failure during the first 2 years after operation. Atherosclerosis can also develop in grafts or adjacent native arteries to produce graft failure. This mechanism of graft failure tends to occur after postoperative year 2 in autologous vein bypasses but has been observed earlier in PTFE bypasses. Structural failure is an uncommon cause of graft failure and is manifest late as aneurysmal degeneration. The mechanism of graft thrombosis involves accumulation of mural thrombus within the aneurysmal segment leading to occlusion or distal embolization. This mode of failure should be suspected when thrombosis occurs in the setting of normal graft surveillance studies.

Occlusive lesions, including technical errors, myointimal graft stenosis, or atherosclerotic disease, produce graft thrombosis by decreasing blood flow velocity below a minimal velocity at which thrombus formation can ensue. Duplex scanning can, by providing objective data on hemodynamics, identify the subgroup of grafts with low-flow hemodynamics and, with imaging of the entire bypass, identify the focal flow abnormalities associated with stenosis (peak systolic velocity [V_p] greater than 150 cm/second, velocity ratio across the stenosis [V_r] greater than 2). Grafts demonstrating both a high-grade focal stenosis and low-flow state (V_p less than 45 cm/second) in a normal-diameter graft segment are at increased risk for thrombosis.

Based on the varied mechanisms of graft failure and the propensity of lower limb grafts both to harbor residual lesions and to develop de novo lesions, duplex scanning is recommended to assess graft anatomy and hemodynamics both at operation and for postoperative surveillance. Using an algorithm based on the severity of velocity spectra changes and abnormalities within the color-coded B-mode image, the information necessary to implement graft revision can be provided. High-grade (greater than 70% diameter reduction) stenoses are associated with a V_p greater than 250 cm/second, an end-diastolic velocity greater than 100 cm/second, or a V_r of greater than 4 across the stenosis. Grafts that develop these lesions also demonstrate a low-flow velocity in normal-sized (3.5 to 4.5 mm diameter) graft segments. A decrease in ankle brachial index (ABI) is also predictive of an acquired graft lesion but is associated with a low positive predictive value for graft thrombosis. A significant (greater than 30 cm/second) decrease in V_p on serial duplex scans has correlated with the development of a graft stenosis and should prompt complete imaging of the lower limb arterial circulation to delineate sites of stenosis. In selected patients, such as those with a high-grade stenosis identified in the body of the graft or at an anastomosis and a low graft flow velocity or ABI, duplex scanning can supplant arteriography for clinical decision making and the need for graft revision. The concept of serial duplex testing, beginning at operation, repeated before discharge from the hospital, and then at 3 to 6 month intervals offers several advantages. It gauges initial technical success, identifies deterioration in graft functional patency at a time when developing occlusive lesions may be easily managed by elective surgical revision or percutaneous transluminal angioplasty, and, equally important, documents the hemodynamic benefit of graft revision with normalization of graft flow velocity.

A wide range of duplex-derived blood flow velocities can be measured in infrainguinal grafts after successful bypass grafting. In general, V_p in the mid-distal graft segments exceeds 40 to 45 cm per second unless the conduit diameter is greater than 6 mm or the graft runoff is limited to an isolated tibial artery segment or dorsalis pedis artery. The V_p varies with luminal diameter, and it is recommended that duplex surveillance be performed using diameter-specific criteria. Belkin and colleagues found graft flow velocity was lower (p less than .04) in inframalleolar grafts (59 cm/second) compared to tibial (77 cm/second) and popliteal (71 cm/second) grafts.[11] Only 4 of 72 grafts, all to inframalleolar arteries, had a measured V_p below 45 cm/second. Use of arm vein or varicose saphenous segments was also associated with low graft conduit flow velocity. Thus, this hemodynamic parameter by itself does not predict impending thrombosis but may guide decision making regarding the potential benefit of instituting postoperative oral anticoagulation. When normal-sized (3 to 5 mm lumen diameter) venous conduits are utilized, identification of a graft flow velocity below 40 to 45 cm per second is uncommon, during or after operation, and in the authors experience has correlated with a residual graft lesion if measured perioperatively, or an acquired lesion if measured during follow-up. A low graft flow velocity because of poor runoff has been an infrequent finding, but when it occurred, arteriography confirmed severely diseased runoff vessels. When low flow is identified, a prompt and thorough graft evaluation should ensue, especially if the ABI is also abnormal (less than 0.9). Management of low-flow grafts due to poor runoff is controversial, but options include anticoagulation, sequential bypass grafting, or adjunctive distal arteriovenous fistulas, the latter two modalities being constructed to augment graft flow.

The velocity spectra used to monitor vascular grafts can be classified into two normal and three abnormal categories (Table 2). In limbs revascularized for critical ischemia, the normal graft blood flow pattern is one of antegrade flow throughout the pulse cycle, which reflects low peripheral vascular resistance associated with revascularization hyperemia. Within days to several weeks, hyperemic graft blood flow dissipates, and the velocity waveform gradually changes to a triphasic configuration, typical of normal peripheral artery blood flow and a normalization of the ABI. Transformation of the normal triphasic graft velocity waveform to a biphasic or monophasic configuration, coupled with a decrease in Vp, is highly diagnostic of a "remote" (proximal or distal to recording site) occlusive lesion. Three waveform configurations have been observed with the development of a pressure-reducing stenosis (Fig. 1). At the time of graft revision, all were associated with a low (less than 45 cm/second) or decreased (greater than 30 cm/second) Vp compared to prior testing. Type I, the most common abnormal graft waveform, present in approximately half of patients, was biphasic in configuration and associated with a resting ABI of 0.4 to 0.7. The reduction in waveform pulsatility and presence of a diastolic blood flow component is indicative of a pressure-reducing stenosis and compensatory arteriolar dilatation. The site of graft stenosis may be proximal or distal to the recording site. Type II, a monophasic waveform with low Vp, has been observed in approximately 40% of grafts with stenosis. All patients were asymptomatic and resting ABI varied from 0.7 to 0.9. Typically, the severity of stenosis was classified in the 50% to 75% diameter reduction (DR) category by both duplex scanning and arteriography. Type III, an uncommon (6% of abnormal grafts) but ominous waveform demonstrated a staccato velocity spectral pattern representing to-and-fro motion of blood within the compliant venous conduit with each pulse cycle. This waveform was always associated with a high-grade distal stenosis and was a harbinger of graft thrombosis. The minimal antegrade blood flow in these grafts complicates angiographic visualization of the distal graft and anastomosis, causing some clinicians to refer to this condition as "pseudoocclusive graft failure."

ESSENTIALS OF GRAFT SURVEILLANCE

The intensity of graft surveillance varies with graft type, runoff, likelihood of residual postimplantation

Table 2 Categories of Graft Blood Flow Patterns

Duplex Category	Velocity Spectra (Waveform) Characteristics
Normal	
Normal PVR	Triphasic configuration, Vp > 45 cm/second at mid-distal graft recording site; applicable for vein diameter 3-5 mm
Low PVR	Biphasic configuration, end-diastolic flow velocity > 0, Vp > 45 cm/second; an expected waveform at operation and in early postoperative period
Abnormal, low graft flow velocity	
High PVR	Monophasic configuration, no diastolic forward flow, Vp < 45 cm/second; ABI typically between 0.7 and 0.9
	Staccato Doppler signal with flow reversal during diastole, Vp < 45 cm/second, minimum antegrade flow due to high-grade distal stenosis
Low PVR	Biphasic waveform with Vp < 45 cm/second; greater than 30 cm/second decrease compared to prior level. Compensatory diastolic flow due to low ABI (0.4-0.7)

PVR = Peripheral vascular resistance; Vp = peak systolic velocity; ABI = ankle brachial index.

lesions, and whether limb blood pressures were normalized. Grafts should be examined by duplex scanning with determination of graft blood flow velocity and measurement of resting ankle pressure. The measurement of ABIs before and after exercise may also uncover a significant stenosis not causing a decrease in ABI at rest. Although most patients who develop a graft stenosis are asymptomatic, recurrent symptoms of limb ischemia should prompt complete duplex imaging of the graft or arteriography to identify a correctable lesion.

Other criteria for further diagnostic testing include loss of a previously palpable pulse, decrease in ABI of greater than 0.2 below the highest postoperative value, and development of a duplex-derived graft blood flow velocity less than 45 cm/second. Resting ABI measurement alone should not be used for surveillance. In the author's experience, approximately one-third of graft stenoses that were corrected after infrainguinal saphenous vein bypass grafting were not apparent from serial measurements of resting ABI. Limb edema and incompressibility of tibial arteries made the measurement unreliable in most patients. In contrast, all the patients had abnormal duplex examinations based on changes in the magnitude and configuration of graft blood flow velocity waveforms. In approximately 90% of patients, duplex scanning of the entire bypass ascertained the location and severity of the stenosis. Occlusive lesions produce characteristic real-time color Doppler images that eliminate the need for detailed center-stream sampling to locate the site of maximum diameter reduction. Accurate graft assessment using color duplex imaging requires the examiner be knowledgeable of the pitfalls of color Doppler imaging, as well as of normal and abnormal bypass graft anatomy. At sites of stenosis, color-flow imaging typically demonstrates aliasing of the color map and a color-coded "flow jet," a hemodynamic

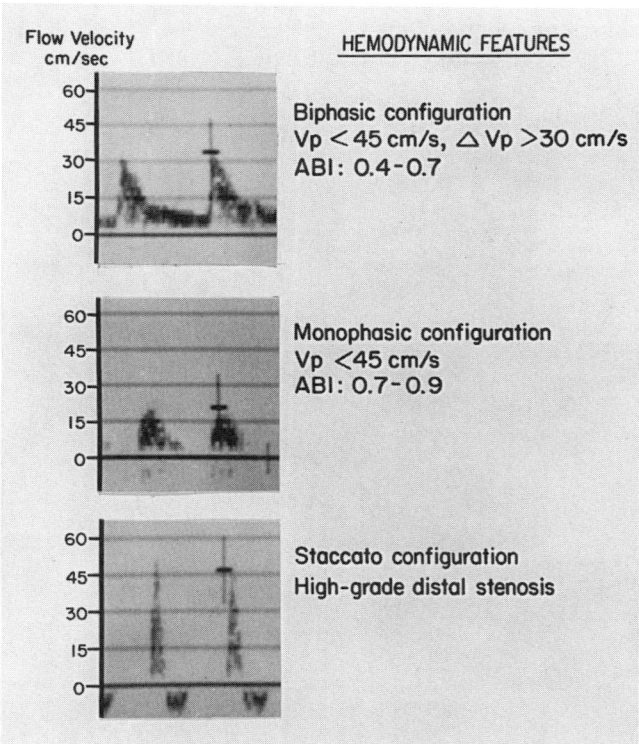

Figure 1 Three types of abnormal graft velocity waveforms recorded from hemodynamically failing bypasses with stenosis. Type I: biphasic waveform; peak systolic velocity (Vp) less than 45 cm/second; ABI 0.4-0.7. Type II: monophasic waveform, Vp less than 45 cm/second; ABI 0.7-0.9. Type III: staccato waveform, minimal antegrade flow in graft due to high-grade distal stenosis. Vp, Peak systolic flow velocity; ABI, ankle-brachial pressure index.

characteristic of greater than 50% DR lesions. Peak systolic velocities greater than 150 to 180 cm/second, spectral broadening throughout the pulse cycle, including reversed flow components in systole, and a Vr greater than 2 are accepted duplex criteria of greater than 50% DR stenosis. Grading of stenosis severity and measurements of Vp from normal graft segments must be performed using appropriate techniques, including Doppler-corrected angles of 60° or less.

Categories of Graft Stenosis

Sites of stenosis are apparent on duplex scanning by a lumen reduction, a localized increase in blood-flow velocity, and velocity spectra broadening. On the basis of the velocity spectra recorded proximal and distal to the stenosis, severity can be classified into four categories: wall irregularity of less than 20% DR, 20% to 49% DR, 50% to 75% DR, and greater than 75% DR (Table 3). In the two categories of greater than 50% DR stenosis, a pressure gradient normally exists across the stenosis at the basal blood flow rates, and a reduction in ankle pressure can be measured. The finding of a lesion with

Table 3 Classification of Graft Stenosis

Diameter Reduction	Velocity Ratio (Vr) and Velocity Spectra
<20% stenosis	Vr <1.5, mild spectral broadening in systole, peak systolic velocity <150 cm/second
20-50% stenosis	Vr 1.5-2.5, spectral broadening throughout systole, no change in waveform configuration across stenosis, peak systolic velocity <150 cm/second
50-75% stenosis	Vr >2.5, severe spectral broadening in systole with reversed flow components, peak systolic velocity >150 cm/second
>75% stenosis	Vr >3.5, end-diastolic flow velocity in "flow jet" >100 cm/second, peak systolic flow velocity >300 cm/second

the velocity spectrum of stenosis greater than 75% has uniformly correlated with an arteriographically detected lesion that warranted correction. Figure 2 shows velocity data recorded from a femoroposterior tibial in situ saphenous vein bypass that developed a greater than 75% stenosis in the below-knee graft segment 6 months after operation. Development of the high-grade stenosis was associated with a decrease in Vp in normal, nonstenotic graft segments to less than 40 cm/second.

After in situ bypass grafting, lesions with velocity spectra of 50% to 75% stenosis have been recorded at valve sites and thought to represent residual valve cusps. These lesions, typically with peak systolic velocities in the range of 180 to 250 cm/second, can be followed if graft flow velocity is normal (greater than 45 cm/second) and ABI is greater than 0.9. High-grade stenoses (Vp greater than 250 cm/second, Vr greater than 3.5, end-diastolic velocity greater than 100 cm/second) should be corrected. The method of secondary graft revision varies, depending on the extent and morphology of the lesion.

POSTOPERATIVE DUPLEX SCANNING PROTOCOL

Patients are placed in the supine position with the lower limb externally rotated and the knee bent slightly. With the patient in this position, the arterial system from the aorta to the tibial arteries can be imaged. The examiner should have available a complete description of the bypass graft procedure, the type and location of the conduit, sites of anastomoses, and any technical difficulties encountered at the primary operation. The bypass graft is imaged in the upper thigh and traced cephalad to the proximal anastomosis, typically the common femoral artery. The presence of a triphasic waveform in the femoral artery correlates with a hemodynamically normal aortoiliac segment. In the presence of a patent graft, a common femoral artery pulsatility index greater than 4 also confirms the absence of inflow occlusive disease. In questionable cases, the aortoiliac segment can be imaged directly for diameter

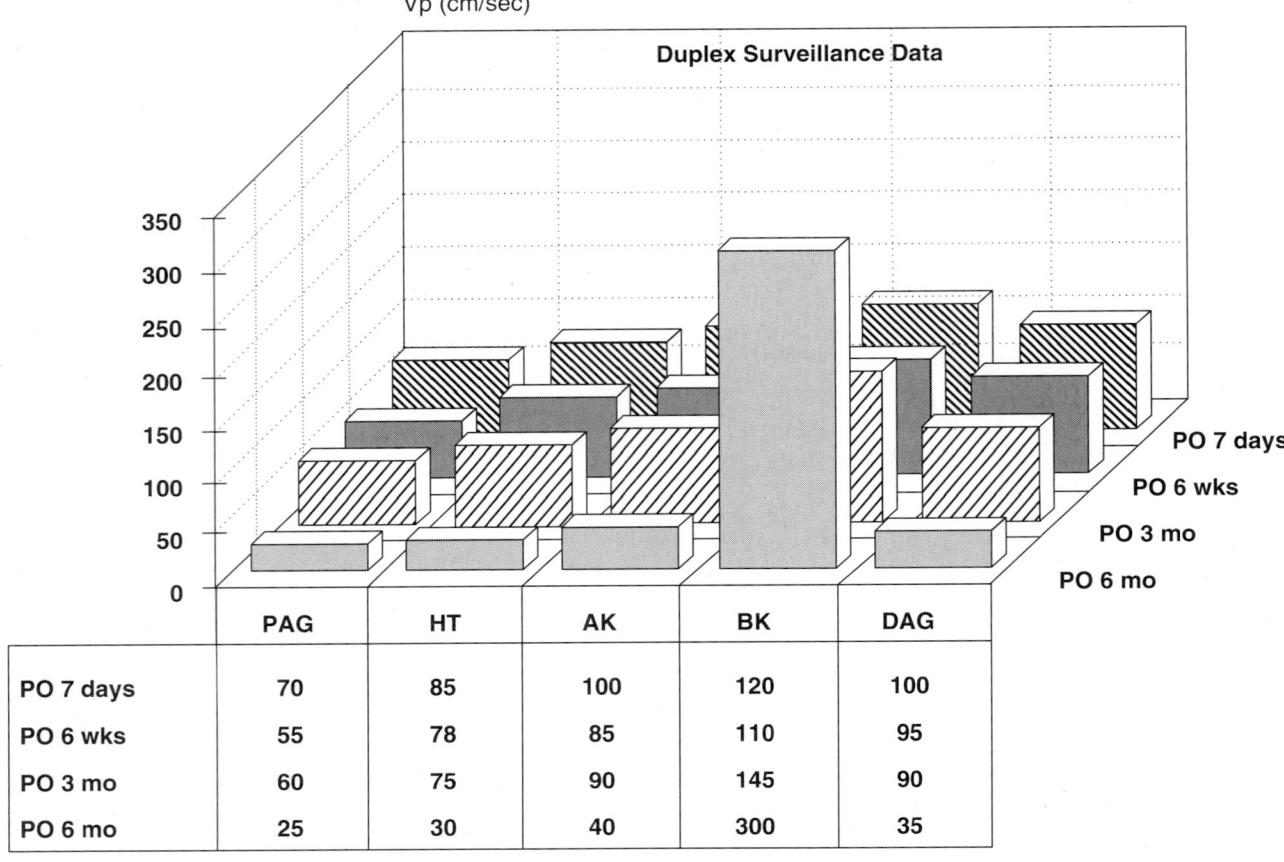

Figure 2 Bar graph depiction of peak systolic velocity data of a femoral posterior tibial in situ saphenous vein bypass that developed a graft stenosis in the below-knee (BK) segment 6 months following operation. Note decrease in graft flow velocity with development of stenosis and localized Vp increase at site of stenosis. PAG, Proximal anastomotic graft; HT, high thigh; AK, above-knee; DAG, distal anastomotic graft; PO, postoperative time interval; Vp, peak systolic velocity.

reduction and blood flow abnormalities indicative of a stenosis.

After assessment of graft inflow, anastomotic sites and the graft are mapped for structural abnormalities and for sites of blood flow disturbance. In situ vein bypasses lie superficial to the muscle fascia and are easily imaged throughout their length. The in situ saphenous vein bypass has a tapered configuration, with the largest vein diameter located in the thigh. Abrupt reductions in venous diameter typically occur at branch points and in duplicated venous segments. Reversed vein and prosthetic grafts, although commonly placed through deep tunnels adjacent to the native vessels, can be satisfactorily imaged. Graft anastomoses to the below-knee popliteal artery are best imaged using a posterior approach with the patient prone. Anastomotic sites on the peroneal artery are the most difficult to examine because of their deep location and position behind the tibia. Distal graft anastomoses typically are made in an end-to-side fashion to the native artery, thereby permitting blood to flow in both caudal and cephalad directions. When distal anastomotic sites cannot be imaged directly for analysis of the blood flow pattern, the functional resistance to flow of the anastomosis and outflow vessels can be estimated from the magnitude and configuration of velocity waveforms recorded in the distal graft.

After the graft is imaged, center-stream velocity waveforms are recorded from several above-knee and below-knee graft segments, where diameter does not vary and accurate assignment of the Doppler beam angle is possible. The magnitude and configuration of the velocity waveforms are used for comparison with previous or subsequent studies obtained at the same recording sites. It is not necessary to image the entire arterial system of the lower limb and the entire graft at each postoperative examination. Values of graft blood flow velocities and ABIs can be graphed at each postoperative visit to identify significant changes compared with prior values. Only grafts that develop a low flow state Vp

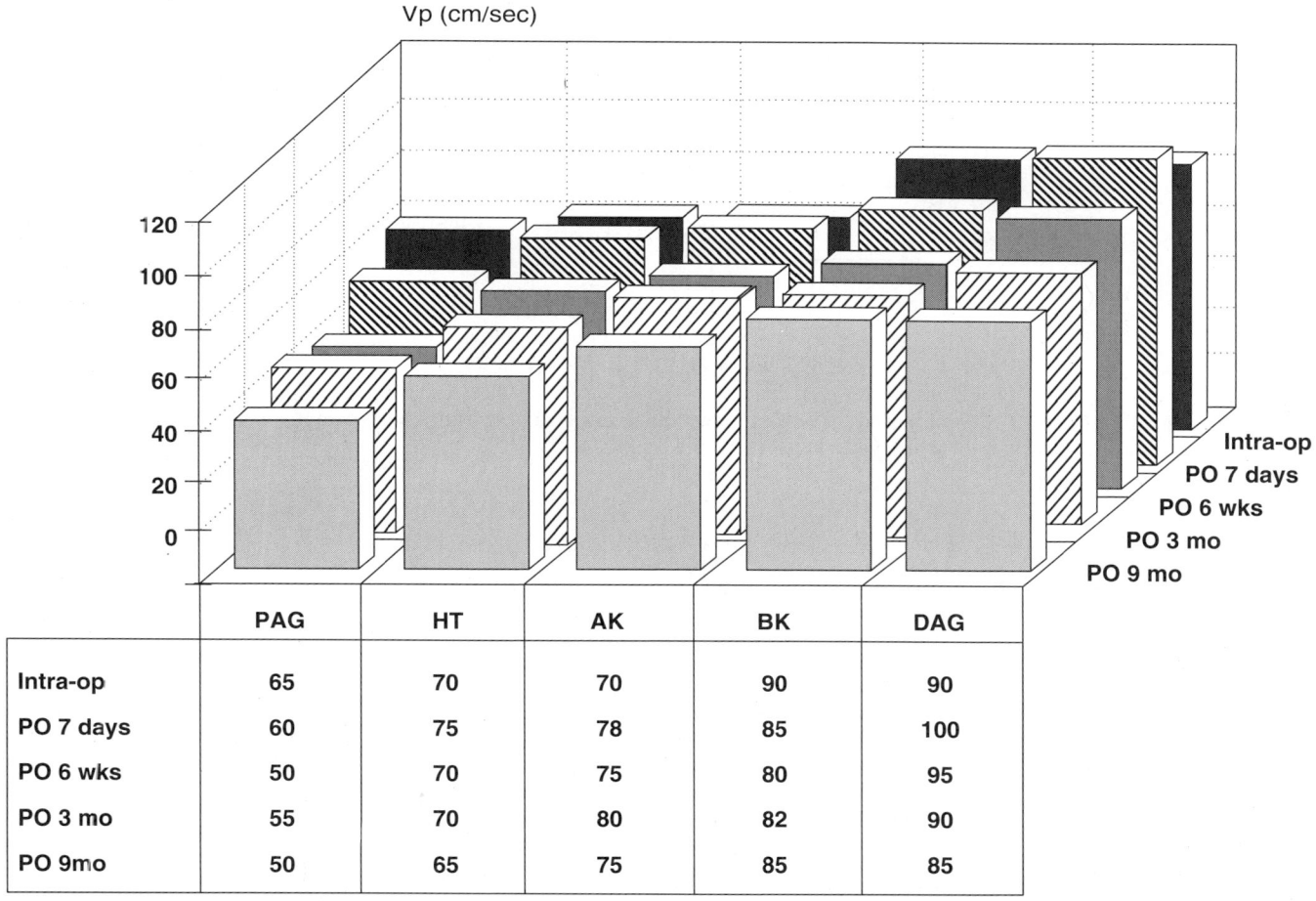

	PAG	HT	AK	BK	DAG
Intra-op	65	70	70	90	90
PO 7 days	60	75	78	85	100
PO 6 wks	50	70	75	80	95
PO 3 mo	55	70	80	82	90
PO 9mo	50	65	75	85	85

Recording Site

Figure 3 Bar graph depiction of peak systolic velocity (Vp) data recorded from various graft segments following femoropopliteal in situ saphenous vein bypass grafting. Increase in Vp along graft length is due to tapered in situ saphenous vein. Data are typical of normal graft surveillance studies with Vp measurements remaining stable during follow-up and no localized increase in Vp identified (i.e., graft stenosis). PAG, Proximal anastomotic graft; HT, high thigh; AK, above-knee; BK, below-knee; DAG, distal anastomotic graft; PO, postoperative time interval.

of less than 45 cm/second or a decrease (more than 30 cm/second) in blood-flow velocity require complete duplex scanning. When velocity measurements are used for predicting graft patency, the highest blood-flow velocity measured within the graft is chosen. For in situ bypasses, this corresponds to blood-flow velocity in the distal graft segment, whereas for reversed vein bypasses, the proximal graft segment should have the highest blood-flow velocity. Sites of blood flow disturbance are examined in detail to delineate the morphology of the lesion and to assess hemodynamic significance on the basis of changes in peak velocity and spectral content as compared to the normal proximal arterial segment.

Graft monitoring should ideally be instituted in the operating room and repeated before discharge from the hospital. Postoperative studies are performed in conjunction with measurement of resting limb blood pressures. Wound edema, hematoma, and incision tenderness may preclude detailed assessment of anastomotic sites in approximately 20% of patients for 2 to 3 weeks after operation. After discharge from the hospital, graft surveillance should be repeated at 6 weeks, then at 3 month intervals for 2 years, and every 6 months thereafter. Figure 3 shows velocity data recorded from a femoropopliteal in situ saphenous vein bypass with normal surveillance examinations. The protocol outlined appears adequate to detect the occasional rapid progression of a proliferative myointimal lesions at a site of moderate (less than 50%) residual stenosis. A normal duplex scan at 3 months appears to be a good predictor of graft patency and a low risk for the development of de novo graft stenosis.

In a series of 132 infrainguinal saphenous vein grafts (68 reversed, 56 in situ, and 8 nonreversed), early postoperative duplex scans were normal in 90 grafts (68%). Only two grafts developed de novo stenoses at 6 and 8 months, and one graft occluded after repetitive attempts to treat an external iliac artery occlusion. All

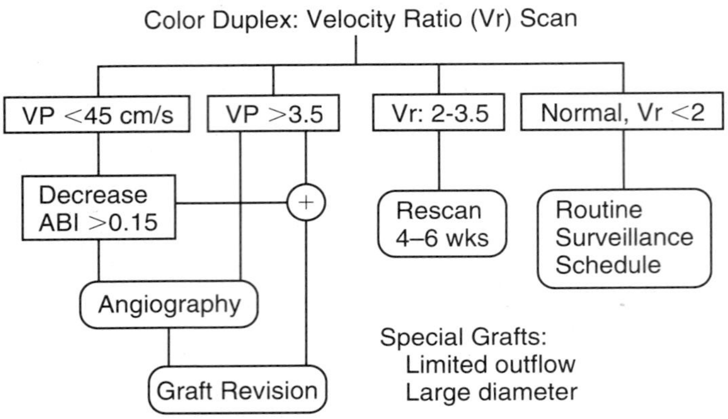

Figure 4 Algorithm for graft revision based on duplex surveillance using velocity ratio (Vr) scanning, changes graft flow velocity (Vp), and measurement of ankle-brachial systolic pressure index (ABI).

three grafts were successfully revised. Forty-two grafts had abnormal duplex scans with focal blood flow abnormalities (Vp greater than 150 cm/second; Vr greater than 1.5) In 12 grafts, the duplex abnormality normalized, but progression of the lesion was documented by duplex scanning in 18 grafts. When the lesions progressed to a high-grade lesion (Vp 205-620 cm/second; Vr 3.4-19), graft revision was performed. Lesions that progressed to a severe stenosis were apparent by duplex scanning at operation or by 6 weeks. In this series, 4 of 18 grafts with persistent, unrepaired stenosis (Vp 150-249 cm/second; Vr 1.7-3.4) lesions occluded between follow-up surveillance appointments.

OUTCOME OF GRAFT SURVEILLANCE

The ability of duplex ultrasonography to identify graft lesions in their preocclusive phase, its low potential for complication, and its high frequency of interpretable studies make it the preferred technique for monitoring lower limb bypass grafts. A carefully conducted surveillance program should identify bypasses at risk for thrombosis, clarify the mechanism of graft failure, and reduce unexpected infrainguinal vein bypass failure to less than 2% per year. Since initiating a vein graft surveillance program in our vascular section, a cumulative assisted primary patency of 96% at 1 year and 85% at 5 years was achieved in patients undergoing in situ saphenous vein femorodistal bypass grafting. Common to all reports dealing with graft surveillance is a caveat stating that symptomatic limb ischemia should not be a requisite criterion for graft revision. Because graft type, luminal diameter, configuration, and runoff vary widely, the surveillance protocol should not be based on rigid criteria applied at a single point in time, but rather be designed to detect changes from baseline graft and limb hemodynamics measured either at operation or in the perioperative period once an initially successful bypass is apparent. The combined velocity and pressure changes allow detection of low-flow, abnormal grafts, a hemodynamic state that commonly precedes graft failure (positive predictive value, 60% to 70%; negative predictive value, 95%). Interpreters of graft surveillance studies must remember that the magnitude and configuration of the graft velocity waveform depend on several factors, including the recording site, the time interval after operation, and outflow resistance. A single velocity criterion cannot be used to predict the likelihood of graft thrombosis. In the setting of serial testing, however, the author has observed an increased failure rate, especially for prosthetic grafts, when the maximum graft systolic velocity was less than 40 cm per second and no diastolic forward blood flow was present.

The indications for graft revision have not been clearly defined, except when patients have recurrent symptoms of claudication or develop ischemic lesions. In general, if arteriograms document a stenotic lesion of greater than 60% DR, elective repair should be performed to prevent graft thrombosis. Duplex criteria for graft revision have not been developed with certainty, but focal stenotic lesions demonstrating a Vp greater than 300 cm/second or end-diastolic velocity greater than 100 cm/second and/or a Vr of 3.5 or greater should be considered for revision, especially if graft flow velocity has decreased from maximum postoperative levels (Fig. 4). The clinical and hemodynamic features of lesions identified and corrected by a duplex surveillance program are listed in Table 4.

An effective graft surveillance protocol should be applicable to all patients; practical in terms of time, effort, and cost; reliable; and able to detect, grade, and assess the progression of discovered lesions. The combination of Doppler-derived pressure measurements and color duplex imaging is currently the most accurate surveillance technique for monitoring infrainguinal arterial reconstructions. The accuracy of duplex scanning for detection of occlusive and aneurysmal lesions is comparable to arteriography, and graft revision can be recommended and implemented based on noninvasive

Table 4 Clinical and Hemodynamic Features of Vein Graft Stenosis

Time Interval After Operation	Etiology	Incidence
0-30 days	Technical error	3-5%
	Abnormal duplex scan	22%
1-6 months	Residual lesion progression	10%
7-24 months	Myointimal hyperplasia	1%/month
>2 years	Atherosclerosis	2%/year
*Presenting symptoms**		
None, asymptomatic		60%
Claudication		30%
Critical ischemia		10%
Hemodynamic features of repaired stenoses		
Mean decrease in ABI of 0.28		
Peak systolic velocity in representative normal graft: 36 cm/second		
Mean maximum peak systolic velocity at stenosis: 350 cm/second		
Mean velocity ratio at stenosis: 6.5		

*Identified by surveillance program using duplex scanning and Doppler-derived pressure measurements.

testing alone. The fate of a distal arterial reconstruction depends on graft and patient risk factors and also on the philosophy and commitment of the surgeon to graft surveillance. A premium must be placed on detection of the failing vein graft before thrombosis occurs. Secondary procedures are safe, effective, and associated with excellent late graft patency (85% at 5 years following revision).

REFERENCES

1. DeWeese JA, Leather R, Porter J. Practice guidelines: Lower extremity revascularization. J Vasc Surg 1993; 17:280–294.
2. Bandyk DF, Schmitt DD, Seabrook GR, et al. Monitoring functional patency of in situ saphenous vein bypasses: The impact of a surveillance protocol and elective revision. J Vasc Surg 1989; 9:284–296.
3. Sladen JG, Reid JDS, Cooperberg PL. Color flow duplex screening of infrainguinal grafts combining low- and high-velocity criteria. Am J Surg 1989; 158:107–112.
4. Mills JL, Harris EJ, Taylor LM, Beckett WC. The importance of routine surveillance of distal bypass grafts with duplex scanning: A study of 379 reversed vein grafts. J Vasc Surg 1990; 12:379–389.
5. Sanchez LA, Suggs WD, Vieth FJ, et al. Is surveillance to detect failing polytetrafluoroethylene bypass worthwhile? Twelve-year experience with ninety-one grafts. J Vasc Surg 1993; 18:981–990.
6. Grigg MJ, Nicolaides AN, Wolfe JHN. Femorodistal graft stenoses. Br J Surg 1988; 75:737–740.
7. Moody AP, Gould DA, Harris PL. Vein graft surveillance improves patency in femoropopliteal bypass. Eur J Vasc Surg 1990; 4:117–121.
8. Idu MM, Blankenstein JD, de Gier P, et al. Impact of a color-flow duplex surveillance program on infrainguinal vein graft patency: A five-year experience. J Vasc Surg 1993; 17:42–53.
9. Mattos MA, van Bemmelen PS, Hodgson KJ, et al. Does correction of stenoses identified with color duplex scanning improve infrainguinal graft patency? J Vasc Surg 1993; 17:54–66.
10. Bandyk DF, Kaebnick, Bergamini TM, et al. Hemodynamics of in situ saphenous vein arterial bypass. Arch Surg 1988; 123:477–482.
11. Belkin M, Mackey WC, McLaughlin R, et al. The variation in vein graft flow velocity with luminal diameter and outflow level. J Vasc Surg 1992; 15:991–999.

PERSISTENT SCIATIC ARTERY

VIKROM S. SOTTIURAI, M.D., PH.D.

Since the recognition of persistent sciatic artery by Green in 1832[1] as an aberrant blood supply to the lower extremity, there have been approximately 129 cases of persistent sciatic artery documented in the literature. The early reports were focused on describing the embryologic development of the arterial vasculature in the lower extremities, whereas the recent reports have emphasized the clinical presentations and management of this anomaly.[2-10]

EMBRYOLOGY OF THE ARTERIAL GENESIS IN THE LOWER EXTREMITY

The sciatic artery arises as a branch from the umbilical artery near the root of the developing limb bud. It is recognized at the 6 mm stage, becomes well developed by the 9 mm stage, and regresses after 22 mm stage. Synonyms of the sciatic artery (axis artery, ischiadic artery) carries certain embryologic and developmental connotations. Customarily, in the adult, the main channel of the sciatic artery becomes rudimentary or involuted, and its residual segment extends dorsally and juxtaposed to the sciatic nerve. After exiting from the pelvis through the sciatic foramen, the residual remnants of sciatic artery persist as the inferior gluteal, popliteal, and peroneal arteries (Fig. 1). The persistent

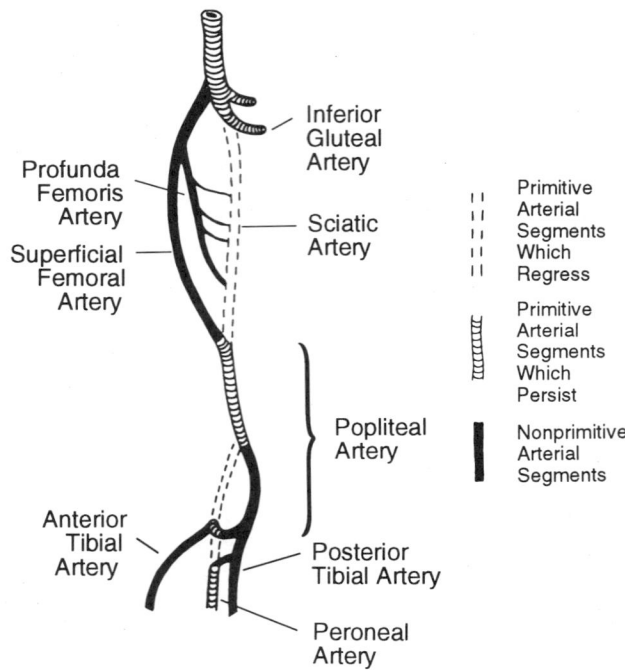

Figure 1 Diagrammatic presentation of the sciatic artery demonstrating the primitive arterial segments: regressed segment (*dash line*), primitive arterial segments (*shaded*), nonprimitive arterial segments (*solid*).

sciatic artery often occurs in two forms: (1) the complete persistent sciatic artery, which gives rise to the superior gluteal, inferior gluteal, and internal pudendal and then runs parallel and posterior to the sciatic nerve to become the popliteal and peroneal artery, and (2) the incomplete persistent sciatic artery that has the identical proximal course but terminates in the posterior thigh in small branches without a direct connection to the popliteal artery (Fig. 2). The external iliac artery arises from the umbilical artery more proximally. It becomes the femoral and posterior tibial arteries. The anterior tibial artery is derived from a series of longitudinal anastomoses of small vessels connecting to the popliteal artery.

HISTOLOGY OF THE PERSISTENT SCIATIC ARTERY

The transmural histology of the persistent sciatic artery differs from the morphology of a large artery in lacking the distinct trilaminar features (intima, media, and adventitia) and has a different pattern of cellular organization in the media. The intima accounts for 30% to 50% (normal 10% to 15%) of the wall thickness, the media 35% (normal 60% to 70%), and adventitia 15% (normal 15% to 20%) (Fig. 3).

The intima is often covered with laminated thrombi, and there is a paucity of cellular elements in the subintima. The media is composed of columns of smooth

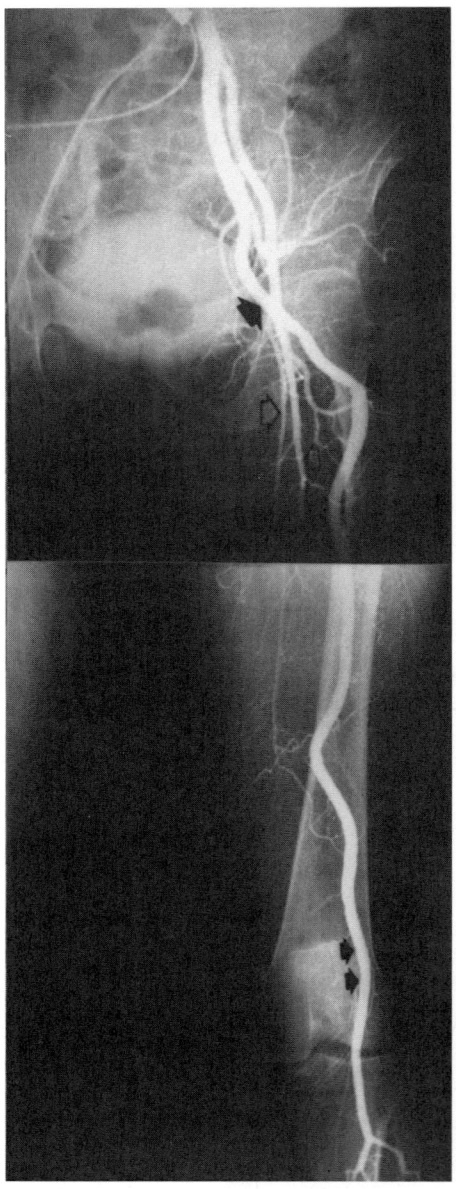

Figure 2 Arteriogram depicting the course of the persistent sciatic artery (*large solid arrow*) in continuity with the popliteal artery (*double solid arrow*). Note the characteristic tortuosity of the sciatic-popliteal artery. The superficial femoral artery is rudimentary (*large open arrow*); the deep femoral artery is normal in caliber (*small open arrow*).

muscle cells that are organized into bundles resembling skeletal muscle. Within the columns are clusters of smooth muscle cells with intervening fibrocollagenous septae (Fig. 4). The smooth muscle cells are functionally active, with numerous rough endoplasmic reticula, mitochondria, golgi complexes, and ribosomes. Myofilaments are found only in the periphery of these active smooth muscle cells (Fig. 5). These subcellular features

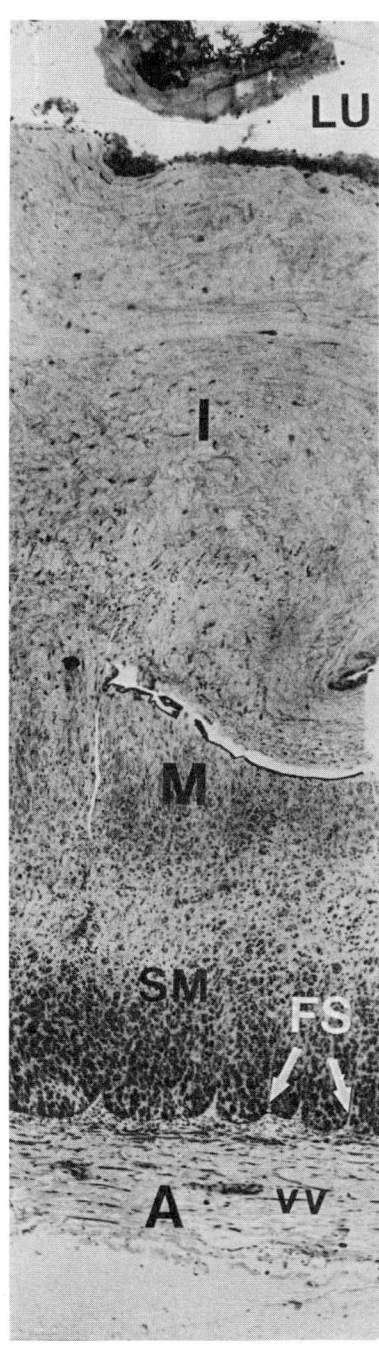

Figure 3 Light micrograph depicting the transmural morphology of the sciatic artery. Note the thick fibrocollagenous intima (I) containing randomly distributed fibrocollagen with a paucity of cellular elements. Smooth muscle cells (SM) of the media (M) are organized into columns surrounded by fibrous septae (FS). The smooth muscle tissue cell columns are oriented perpendicular to the intima and adventitia (A). The adventitia contains vasa vasorum (VV), fibroblasts (F), and collagen bundles.($\times 57$.)

characterize the protein synthetic phase of the smooth muscle cells.

CLINICAL MANIFESTATION OF PERSISTENT SCIATIC ARTERY

The persistent sciatic artery is most frequently encountered in middle-aged patients. Although it is distributed through all age groups, certain relevant facts emerged from tabulating data in the literature reporting gender and right or left distribution of persistent sciatic artery. Persistent sciatic artery is more frequent in males than in females (63 male, 42 female), and is bilateral in approximately one-third (33/96) of patients. When unilateral, the right leg is involved more frequently (right 33, left 27). The complete persistent sciatic artery is more prevalent, accounting for 71% of the cases without significant right or left preponderance and is usually bilateral (74%).

The most common clinical symptoms and findings in persistent sciatic artery are thigh and calf pain that improves with ambulation and worsens with sitting, rest pain, and gangrene (44%); pulsatile gluteal mass (31%); nonpulsatile gluteal mass (10%); and gluteal pain (7%). Other nonspecific complaints are limb hypertrophy, amenorrhea, varicosity, capillary hemangioma, neurofibromatosis, renal agenesis, and arteriovenous fistula (Fig. 6). There is no correlation between the persistent sciatic artery and diabetes mellitus, hypertension, hyperlipidemia, smoking, or cardiac or coronary artery disease.

DIAGNOSTIC EVALUATION

Doppler ultrasonography, duplex imaging, arteriography, and digital subtraction angiography are the established diagnostic modalities. Magnetic resonance angiography has also been utilized with some success. Nerve conduction studies may be needed to assess sciatic neuropathy secondary to aneurysmal compression. Coagulopathy evaluation (protein C, protein S, antithrombin III) has been proven useful in differentiating the cause of peripheral embolization versus thrombotic events. The typical clinical presentation—of ambulation relieving thigh-leg pain, while sitting enhances the pain—is helpful in making the correct diagnosis. A pulsatile gluteal mass occasionally referred to as "throbbing buttocks syndrome" is also a valuable finding in making the diagnosis of persistent sciatic artery.

THERAPY

There is unequivocal agreement that surgical correction is required for all persistent sciatic arteries with aneurysmal degeneration or signs of thromboembolism. However, there is no established single treatment per se

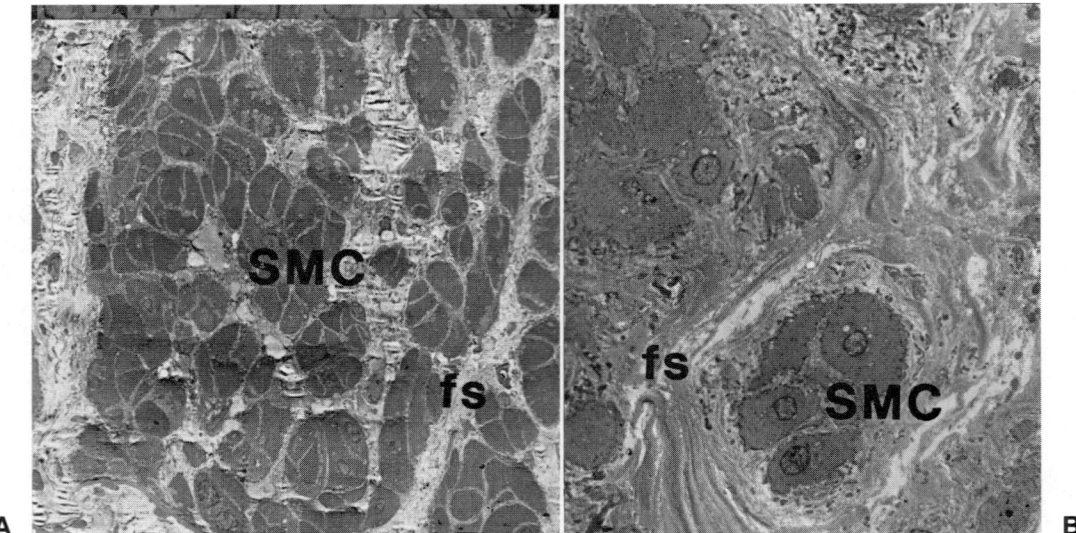

Figure 4 *A*, Low-magnification electron micrographs sampled from the intima and media. Clusters of smooth muscle cells from the subunits of smooth muscle cell column (*SMC*). The latter is oriented perpendicular to the adventitia, with the base of the smooth muscle cell columns abutting the adventitia. Note fibrous septae (*fs*). *B*, Smooth muscle cell clusters (*SMC*) are surrounded by laminated fibrous septum (*fs*). (Transverse section. × 2000.)

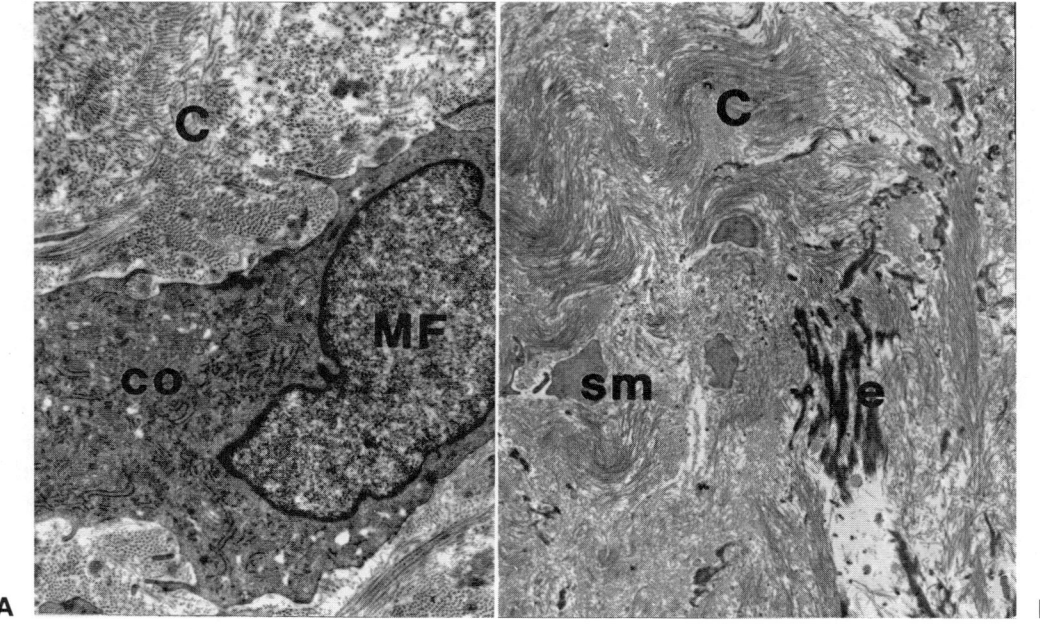

Figure 5 *A*, Electron micrographs sampled from the media of the sciatic arterial wall. Myofibroblast (*MF*) with indented nucleus and abundant cellular organelles in the cytoplasm (mitochondria, rough endoplasmic reticula, golgi complexes, and ribosomes are the principal organelles) represents the active synthetic phase of the smooth muscle cell. Collagen bundles (*C*) often surround the myofibroblasts (× 9230.). *B*, Smooth muscle cells (*sm*) were isolated and surrounded by collagen (*C*). Elastic tissue (*e*) in intima and media was fragmented. (× 3750.)

in the literature. This may be ascribed to a lack of long-term surveillance of this entity or not enough data for a sound, logical therapeutic approach to be formulated. Four operations have been employed in 34 cases of symptomatic persistent sciatic artery with aneurysm or thromboembolism: (1) sciatic artery ligation and jump graft to replace the aneurysmal portion of the artery, (2) sciatic artery excision and femoropopliteal bypass, (3) sciatic artery ligation and femoropopliteal bypass, and (4) ligation, endovascular occlusion, or embolization of

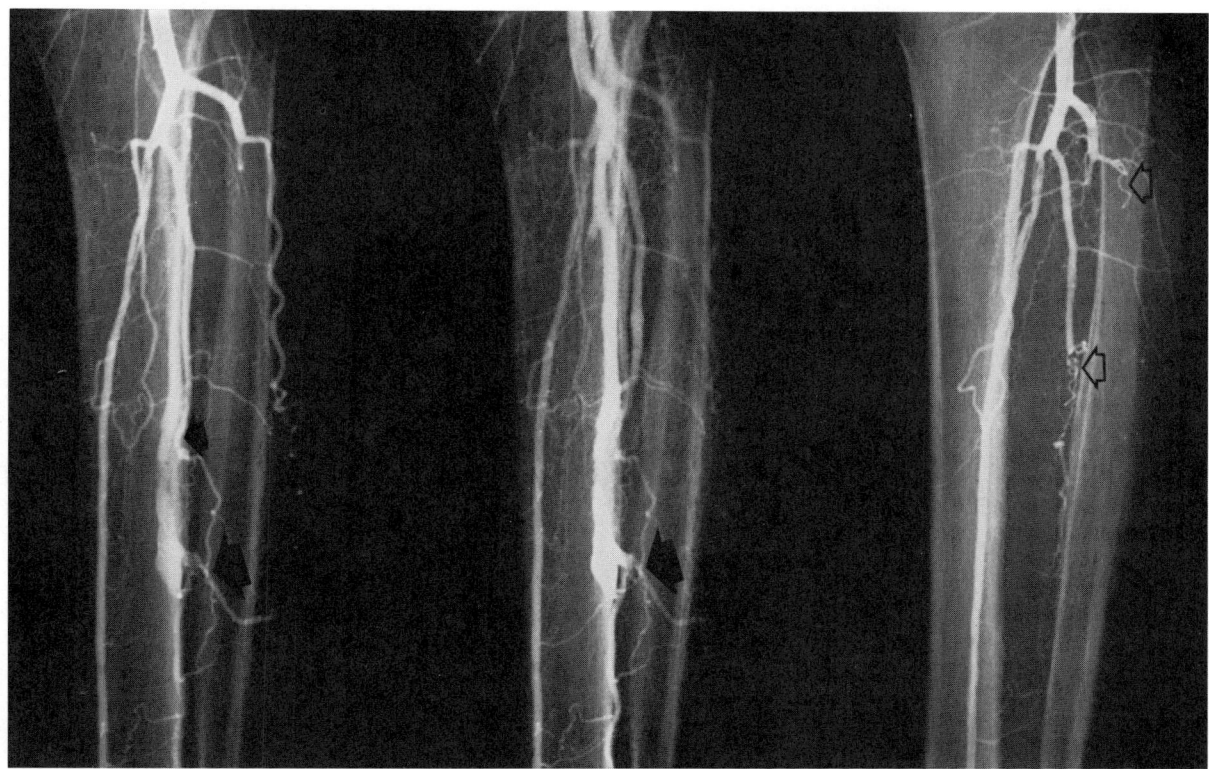

Figure 6 *A* and *B,* Arteriogram demonstrating the presence of AV fistula (*arrows*) in multiple views. *C,* Arteriogram of eliminated AV fistula (*arrows*) following embolization.

the sciatic artery aneurysm. The paraoperative amputation rate was 16%. Long-term follow-up of the 34 cases was nonexistent. Recognized complications include bleeding, sciatic nerve injury, and leg ischemia. These complications were more prevalent with endovascular repair and ligation without bypass.

It is generally agreed that for treatment of nonaneurysmal sciatic artery with embolic events, ligation or excision with femoropopliteal bypass is appropriate.

The natural history of the persistent sciatic artery is such that there is a high incidence of aneurysmal degeneration and thromboembolism. However, progression of the disease is very unpredictable.

Although the sciatic artery provides the major blood supply to the lower limb in the embryo in the 8 to 9 mm stage, regression is near complete by the 22 to 24 mm stage. The external iliac artery that arises from the umbilical artery more proximally continues distally to become the femoral artery and is connected to the sciatic artery by the ramus communicans superior. Unlike reptile and avian vessels, only remnants of the sciatic artery remain in the adult human vasculature. Branches distal to the sciatic foramen are the inferior gluteal, popliteal, and peroneal arteries, a portion of the anterior tibial artery, and perhaps remnants of the perforating arteries.

Extensive reviews of persistent sciatic artery are meager in the literature except for Shultze and co-workers, who reviewed 93 cases and gave a comprehensive account of the subject.[9] Sottiurai and Omlie, after reviewing 129 cases, produced a detailed account of the surgical and nonsurgical management and specific distribution in gender and each lower extremity.[10] They also provided an original detailed description of the light and electron microscopic histomorphology of the persistent sciatic artery. The unique and specific morphologic organization of the smooth muscle cells into bundles and columns with intervening fibrocollagenous septae, like skeletal muscles, led these authors to suggest that such a morphologic pattern may be a reflection of cellular adaptation following compression of the aberrant artery by the ischial tuberosity. The frequent observation of myofibroblasts and extracellular elements (collagen, elastin, and fibroreticular substances) may exemplify the active synthetic phase of the myoblast, also referred to as myofibroblasts.

REFERENCES

1. Green PH. On a new variety of the femoral artery. Lancet 1832; 1:730–731.
2. Martin KW, Hyde GL, McReady RA, et al. Sciatic artery aneurysms: Report of three cases and review of the literature. J Vasc Surg 1986; 4:365–371.
3. Freeman MP, Tisnado J, Cho SR. Persistent sciatic artery: Report of three cases and literature review. Br J Radiol 1986; 59:217–223.

4. Thomas ML, Blakeney CF, Browse NL. Arteriomegaly of persistent sciatic arteries. Radiology 1978; 128:55–56.
5. Donovan DL, Sharp WV. Persistent sciatic artery: Two case reports with emphasis on embryologic development. Surgery 1984; 95:363–365.
6. Noblet D, Gasmi T, Mikati A, et al. Persistent sciatic artery: Case report, anatomy, and review of the literature. Ann Vasc Surg 1988; 2:390–396.
7. Wolf YG, Gibbs BFM, Guzzetta VJ, Bernstein EF. Surgical treatment of aneurysm of the persistent sciatic artery. J Vasc Surg 1993; 17:218–221.
8. Mayschak DT, Flye MW. Treatment of the persistent sciatic artery. Ann Surg 1984; 199:69–74.
9. Shultze WP, Garrett WV, Smith BL. Persistent sciatic artery: Collective review and management. Ann Vasc Surg 1993; 7:303–310.
10. Sottiurai VS, Omlie W. Femoral artery hypoplasia and persistent sciatic artery with blue toe syndrome: A case report, histologic analysis and review of the literature. Int Angiol (in press).

POPLITEAL VASCULAR ENTRAPMENT SYNDROME

WILLIAM D. TURNIPSEED, M.D.

The term popliteal entrapment syndrome was initially coined by Love and Whelan in 1965.[1] Awareness of the condition dates back to the nineteenth century and was first described by Stuart in 1879.[2] The anatomic basis of popliteal entrapment is an abnormal relationship between the popliteal artery and the medial head of the gastrocnemius muscle.

The most cogent description of the variant congenital abnormalities associated with this condition was perhaps made by Insua and colleagues.[3] They described four anatomic variations, the first of which is the most prevalent and is characterized by medial deviation of the popliteal artery around the medial head of the gastrocnemius muscle. The second most common variation involves abnormal attachments of the medial head of the gastrocnemius muscle, with the popliteal artery passing medially but with less deviation than the type one entrapment. The third type involves aberrant slips of muscle from the medial head of the gastrocnemius that entrap the popliteal artery. Type four entrapment is associated with fibrous bands originating from the popliteus muscle, causing arterial impingement. Rich and associates have described another variant in which both artery and vein follow a deviant course around the medial head of the gastrocnemius muscle (Fig. 1).[4]

Popliteal entrapment most commonly affects men and usually becomes clinically evident before the age of 40 years. The most common presentation, in the absence of arterial occlusion or thrombosis, is that of mild, intermittent claudication. Claudication in young adults is uncommon. The differential diagnosis for this complaint includes premature atherosclerosis associated with malignant forms of hyperlipidemia or type I diabetes, medial cystic degenerative occlusive disease, vasculitis associated with underlying collagen vascular disorders, chronic exertional compartment syndrome, or popliteal entrapment. A history and physical examination may help distinguish individuals who have popliteal entrapment from those with other unusual causes of claudication. Patients with symptomatic popliteal entrapment often notice that claudication is aggravated by walking but not by running. On physical examination, tibial pulses may fade or disappear when the foot is placed in forced plantar flexion or the knee in fixed extension. This explains the paradox of "walker's" claudication because the knee is fixed in extension and plantar flexion of the foot is exaggerated in walking but not in running.

Noninvasive tests including pulse volume recordings (PVR), duplex imaging, computed tomography (CT), and magnetic resonance imaging (MRI) may be employed to confirm the etiology of claudication in these patients.[5,6] Symptomatic patients with normal resting and postexercise PVR studies should have positional stress testing performed to rule out popliteal entrapment.[7] The PVR technique is used to monitor plethysmographic change in the posterior and anterior tibial arteries with the foot in neutral and in forced plantar flexion and dorsiflexion. Blunting of the plethysmographic wave form and depression in the ankle-brachial index (ABI) provide objective confirmation of popliteal artery compression (Fig. 2).

Similar information can be derived by simply placing a Doppler probe over the posterior tibial artery and monitoring waveform changes that occur with the foot neutral or in forced plantar flexion while the patient is lying supine with the knee in full extension. Patients with positive PVR or Doppler entrapment screening tests should have duplex or MRI of the popliteal artery. Duplex imaging makes it possible to document dynamic compression of the popliteal artery while the patient is put through the stress maneuvers and can identify arterial occlusive or aneurysmal changes sometimes associated with this syndrome.

Perhaps the best method for characterizing popliteal entrapment is MRI. It can be used to analyze musculotendinous structures in the popliteal fossa and to document dynamic changes in their relationship with the popliteal vessels. Although CT has been used for this purpose, it is not as accurate or informative as MRI. Contemporary noninvasive diagnostic methods make

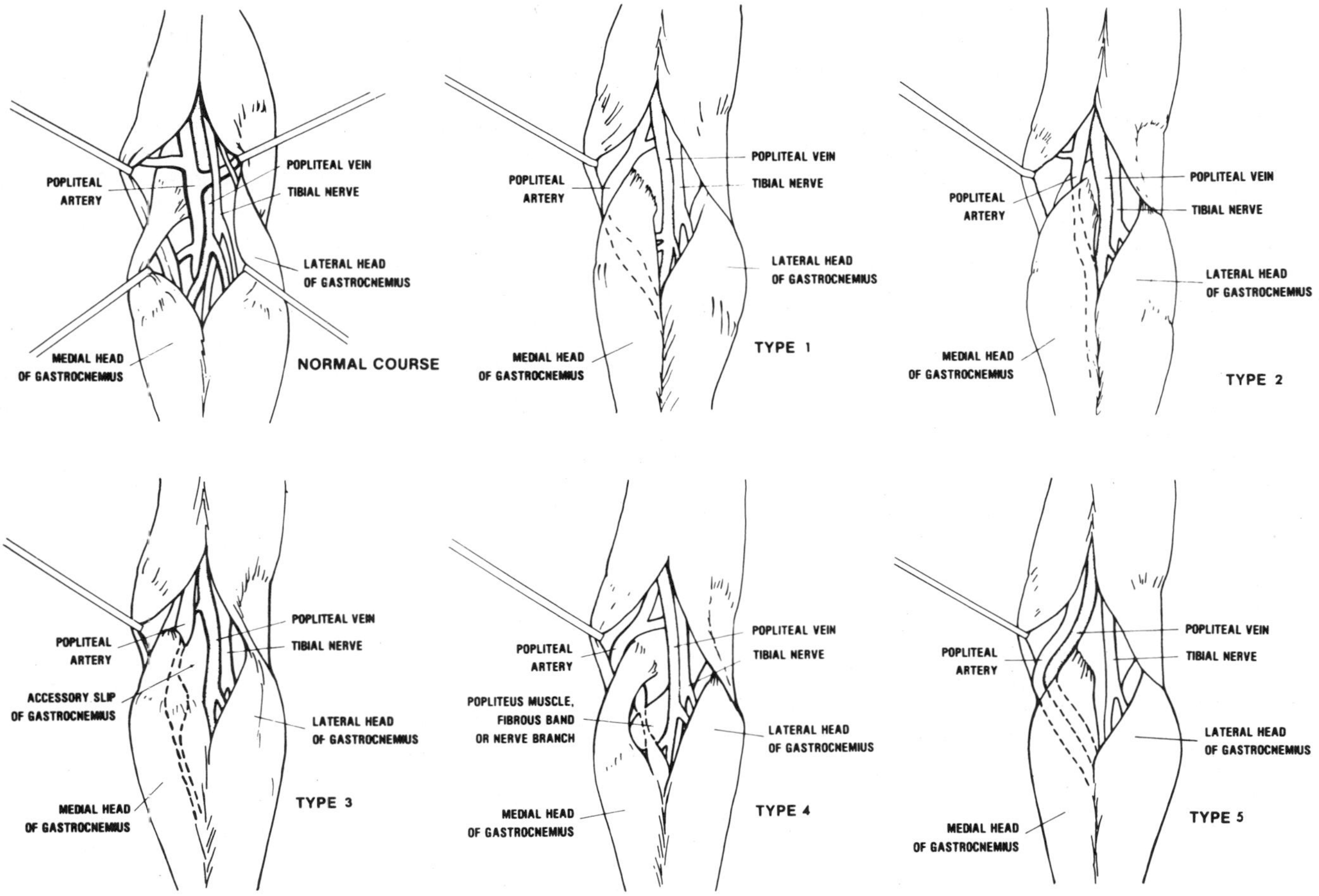

Figure 1 The five most common anatomic configurations for popliteal entrapment (From Rich NM, Collins GJ, McDonald PT, et al. Popliteal vascular entrapment: Its increasing interest. Arch Surg 1979; 114:1377–1384; with permission.)

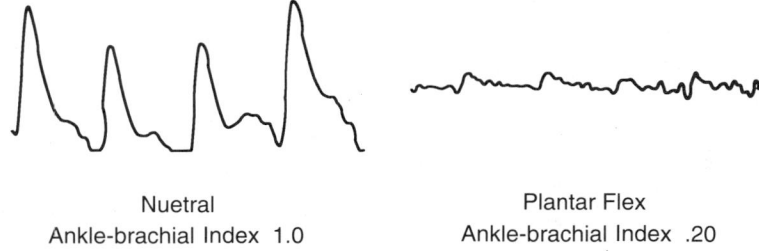

Nuetral
Ankle-brachial Index 1.0

Plantar Flex
Ankle-brachial Index .20

Figure 2 Patients with popliteal entrapment may have normal plethysmographic wave forms and ankle-brachial indices with the foot in neutral position, but when the foot is placed in forced plantar flexion, marked attenuation of both occurs.

arteriographic confirmation unnecessary except in individuals with weak or absent tibial pulses, or when scan evidence suggests aneurysmal change in the popliteal artery.

Young patients with palpable pulses, normal post-exercise PVRs, and negative screening tests for popliteal entrapment may have a chronic compartment syndrome. This condition commonly affects well-conditioned athletes and is usually associated with overuse injuries. Unlike other exertional injuries such as periostitis, stress fracture, or tendonitis, chronic compartment syndrome does not respond to anti-inflammatory medications or physical therapy and, much like the popliteal entrapment syndrome, is not effectively treated without surgical intervention. The symptoms often can be confused with those originating from popliteal entrapment. They include severe muscle cramping and tightness and occasional paresthesias that can affect athletic levels of performance and in some circumstances progress to acute neuromuscular injury. The diagnosis of chronic compartment syndrome can be confirmed by measuring muscle compartment pressures. In my experience, normal resting compartment pressures in the lower leg are less than 15 mm Hg. Borderline pressures are between 16 and 20 mm Hg, and pressures above 25 mm Hg, at rest, are abnormal and uniformly consistent with chronic compartment syndrome. Although abnormally elevated resting compartment pressures occur in most patients with chronic compartment syndrome (85%), some may have borderline pressure elevations and must be stressed until they become symptomatic and then remeasured. In normal patients, compartment pressures can increase to three or four times over baseline after vigorous activity but pressures rapidly return to normal levels within a few minutes. Patients with chronic compartment syndrome may triple or quadruple resting pressures after strenuous exercise and often have a prolonged postexercise interval before returning to baseline.

A functional form of popliteal entrapment has recently been identified that also tends to occur in well-conditioned athletes and may coexist with a symptomatic chronic compartment syndrome.[7] Symptoms associated with this functional form of popliteal entrapment include deep calf muscle cramping (soleus), rapid limb fatigue, and occasional paresthesias on the plantar surface of the foot. These symptoms are most predictably aggravated by running up inclines or by repetitive jumping and commonly affect athletes participating in sports such as cross country, basketball, and volleyball. Similar complaints have been identified in military personnel.

Over the past 4 years, we have reported on 120 patients who were referred to us from our Sports Medicine Clinic with a tentative diagnosis of chronic compartment syndrome. Twelve patients (10%) presented with symptoms of calf cramping and plantar anesthesia, and all had plethysmographic screening tests that were positive for popliteal entrapment. Thirteen patients with anterior compartment syndrome were also identified as having asymptomatic positive popliteal entrapment studies. Eleven of the 12 symptomatic patients had unilateral symptoms despite bilaterally positive compression studies. Duplex imaging or Doppler color flow analysis of the 12 patients with suspected popliteal entrapment confirmed popliteal artery compression with obliteration of arterial flow across the popliteal segment (Fig. 3). Intravenous digital subtraction arteriography (IVDSA) was performed with the foot in neutral and in active forced plantar flexion.[8] No arteriographic evidence of medial displacement or aberrant positioning of the popliteal artery could be demonstrated at rest. With forced plantar flexion, lateral compression of the popliteal artery against the condyle of the femur was observed (Fig. 4).

MRI of the popliteal vessels and calf muscles suggests that the neurovascular bundle is forced laterally against the femoral condyle proximally and laterally against the lateral angle of the fibrous soleus muscle sling by simultaneous contractions of the medial head of the gastrocnemius and plantaris muscles (Fig. 5). No evidence of intrinsic stenosis, thrombosis, or aneurysmal dilation of the popliteal artery has been documented in any of these patients. No abnormal muscle attachments, fibrous bands, or aberrant positioning of the popliteal vessels has been documented by MRI with the foot in neutral or in the forced plantar flexion positions.

Operation is the only effective method of treating patients with intermittent claudication caused by popliteal entrapment. Preoperative arteriograms should be performed when symptoms are associated with weak or absent resting pulses and when CT or MRI tests document anomalous positioning of the popliteal artery or abnormal musculotendinous structures in the popliteal fossa. A posterior surgical approach enables a detailed examination of the entire popliteal fossa and allows the surgeon to resect or to excise tendinous bands

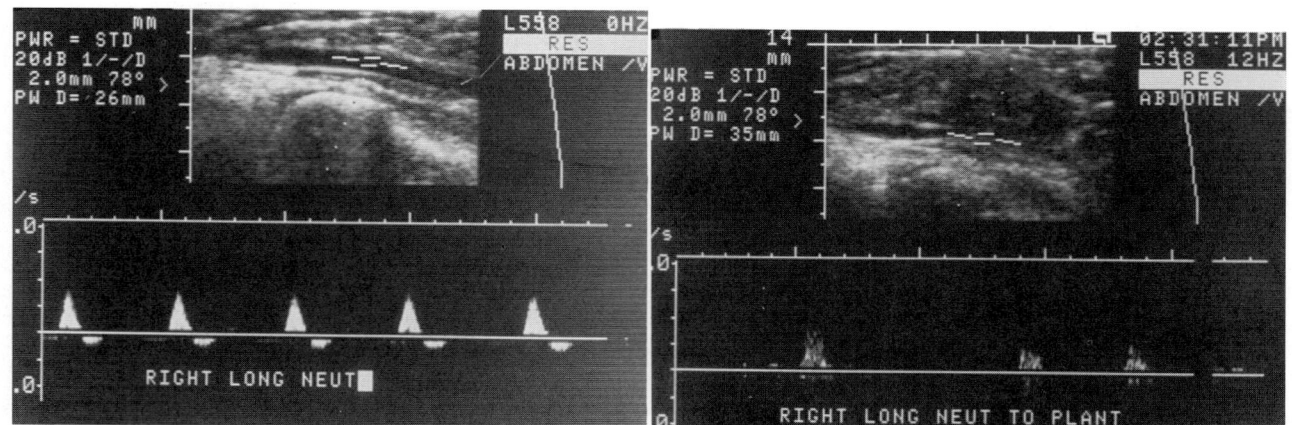

Figure 3 *A*, Duplex imaging of the popliteal fossa in a patient with popliteal entrapment demonstrates a widely patent vessel and normal flow with the foot in neutral position. *B*, With active forced plantar flexion, the popliteal artery is compressed, and Doppler flow signals obliterated.

and muscle segments that cause neurovascular impingement. Arterial reconstruction may be necessary when stenotic or aneurysmal lesions are identified in the popliteal artery. Resection of the medial head of the gastrocnemius muscle or offending fibrous bands is satisfactory treatment when no obstructive or aneurysmal vascular changes can be identified. Asymptomatic popliteal entrapment associated with anatomic impingement of the popliteal artery should be surgically corrected when identified in order to prevent the development of secondary vascular complications.

The treatment of patients with functional entrapment is somewhat different from the treatment of patients with anatomic abnormalities in the popliteal fossa. Symptoms are less common with functional impingement, and there have been no documented episodes of arterial occlusion, embolization, or aneurysm formation with this condition. In my experience, less than 25% of patients with positive screening studies have complaints of intermittent claudication. The functional entrapment syndrome becomes symptomatic with repetitive activities such as jumping or running on inclines. Many of these patients are professional or scholarship athletes. Operation in these patients is designed to allow maximum recovery of function and minimum rehabilitation. Exploration of popliteal fossa is performed using the medial approach. The incision is made just below the knee at the level of the upper midcalf. Insertions of the sartorius, the gracilis, the semimembranous, and semitendinous muscles should be left intact. Examination of the popliteal artery confirms normal positioning of the vessels and ensures that there are no anomalous muscular bands. Unlike the anatomic forms of entrapment, patients with functional entrapment have a dense fibrous band of fascia that extends along the upper edge of the soleus muscle and acts as a compression point for the neurovascular bundle. Resection of this fascial band requires that the medial attachments of the soleus muscle be taken down from the posterior surface of the tibia. This is done by placing the index finger into the soleal canal and using electrocautery. These attachments are divided, a technique commonly used to expose the distal tibial vessels. Once tibial attachments of the soleus muscle have been released, the neurovascular bundle can be easily identified. The anterior fascia of the soleus forms a fibrous sling that crosses the lower border of the popliteal fossa and attaches laterally to the proximal fibula. This fibrous fascial sling is sharply excised, including its lateral attachments. The posterior fascia of the popliteus muscle is also excised. Excision of the fascia from opposing surfaces of the popliteus and soleus muscles make it less likely for scar formation to re-entrap the neurovascular bundle. Once the soleal release has been completed, the plantaris muscle, which is often very large and hypertrophic in these patients, is resected.

The classic description of popliteal entrapment includes an anomalous relationship among the popliteal artery, the medial head of the gastrocnemius muscle, and

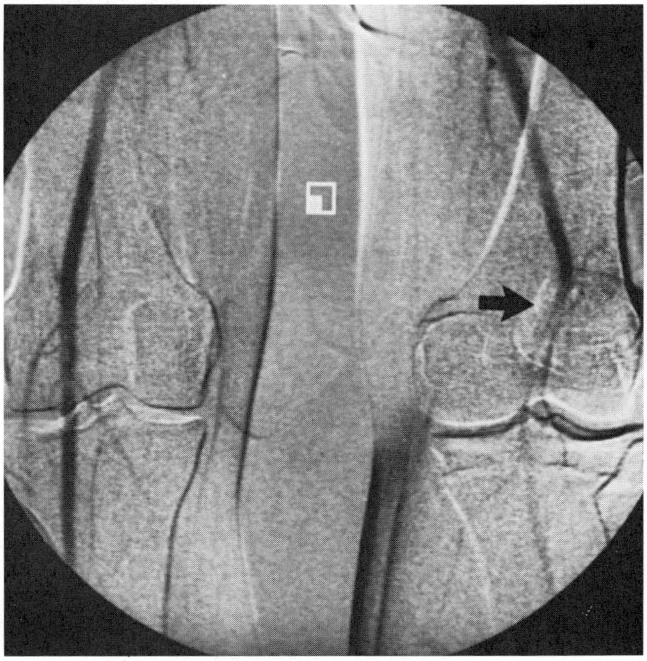

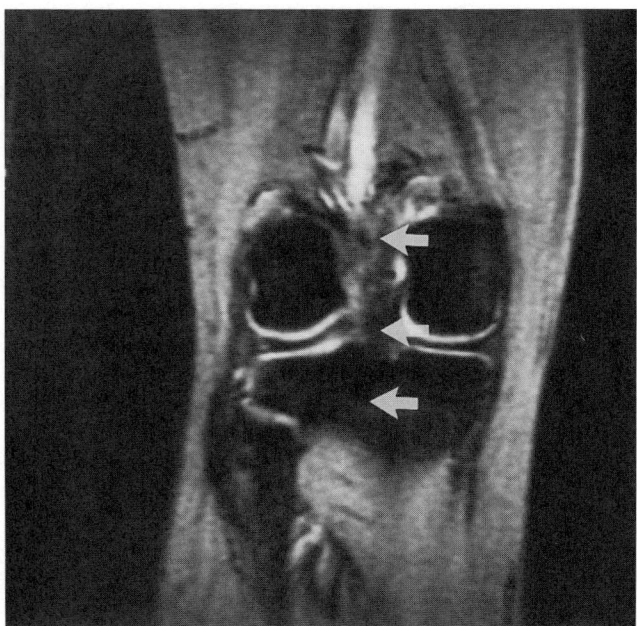

Figure 4 Intravenous digital subtraction arteriography demonstrates normal positioning of the popliteal artery on the right side and lateral deviation with compression of the popliteal artery (*arrow*) when forced plantar flexion of the foot occurs in a patient with functional entrapment.

Figure 5 Magnetic resonance imaging of the popliteal fossa performed on a patient with functional entrapment demonstrates lateral compression of the neurovascular bundle against the lateral condyle of the femur proximally and against the lateral angle of the soleal sling distally (*arrows*).

other musculotendinous elements in the popliteal fossa. Attempts to rigidly classify the anatomic forms of this disease have not accurately described all developmental variants associated with this condition. The most common anatomic abnormalities, however, involve passage of the popliteal artery medial to the head of the gastrocnemius muscle or normal positioning of the popliteal artery with compression by aberrant origins of the gastrocnemius and plantaris muscles.

As screening techniques are more widely used, it appears that functional forms of popliteal entrapment may occur in the absence of any musculotendinous developmental abnormalities, and that this form of neurovascular compression may represent a normal physiologic variant in well-trained and physically over-developed athletes or soldiers.[9] It also appears that there are significant differences in the morbidity associated with anatomic and functional forms of popliteal entrapment. Historical accounts suggest that arterial compression associated with deviations in the anatomic course of the popliteal artery or by anomalous musculotendinous bands may cause acute arterial occlusions or chronic aneurysmal degeneration. No clinical evidence exists to support the concept that functional entrapment, in the absence of any clinical symptoms, requires surgical intervention. Symptoms associated with the functional type of entrapment are uncommon and occur in only approximately 25% of those individuals with positive plantar flexion screening. No clear-cut evidence exists that compression of the popliteal artery in these patients actually causes soleal cramping or paresthesias. Physiologic and anatomic information derived from duplex imaging and MRI of the popliteal fossa suggests that the lateral displacement of the neurovascular bundle may compress the popliteal nerve as well as the vein and artery against the lateral angle of the soleal sling and the lateral condyle of the femur. Repeated trauma to the popliteal nerve with repetitive plantar flexion may cause a neuromuscular form of claudication and explain the intermittent paresthesias that are commonly associated with this condition.

Functional popliteal entrapment has many clinical similarities to the thoracic outlet syndrome. In both conditions, primary arterial ischemia is uncommon. Although complications from arterial or venous compression are possible, they rarely occur. In both instances, symptoms commonly develop when repetitive activity patterns result in neurovascular compression. Furthermore, in both conditions the only clinical beneficiaries from surgical intervention appear to be the symptomatic patients. Experience suggests that noninvasive testing such as duplex imaging and plethysmographic screening maybe incapable of distinguishing between anatomic and functional forms of the disease. Dynamic stress arteriography, (my preference is IVDSA) or MRI studies are more helpful in analyzing patients with popliteal entrapment and in distinguishing anatomic from functional forms of this disorder. Abnormal medial deviations in the course of the popliteal artery associated with segmental occlusion or aneurysmal formation are common arteriographic characteristics of the anatomic form of the disease. Patients with functional entrapment have no resting abnormalities, and with plantar flexion there is a lateral instead of medial displacement of the popliteal artery with compression against the soleal sling and lateral condyle of the femur.

The surgeon must be aware of several potential causes for popliteal entrapment. The decision to operate, the kind of operation, and the surgical approach should be tailored by information derived from clinical history and preoperative testing. The posterior approach with gastrocnemius muscle transection and artery repair may be quite appropriate in patients with threatened limbs resulting from anatomic entrapment. However, the medial approach, with resection of the plantaris muscle, proximal release of the soleus muscle, and excision of its fascial band, is effective for functional forms of the disease and minimizes rehabilitation efforts in the competitive athlete.

In summary, functional popliteal entrapment syndrome is more prevalent than anatomic entrapment. Symptoms associated with functional entrapment are uncommon and aggravated by specific physical activities in well-conditioned athletes. Operation is indicated for symptomatic patients with anatomic or functional forms of entrapment. Prophylactic correction of anatomic entrapment in asymptomatic patients should be considered because of associated vascular complications. Prophylactic operation is not indicated in asymptomatic patients with functional entrapment.

REFERENCES

1. Love JW, Whelan TJ. Popliteal artery entrapment syndrome. Am J Surg 1965; 109:620.
2. Stuart TPA. Note on a variation in the course of the popliteal artery. J Anat Physiol 1879; 13:162.
3. Insua JA, Young JR, Humphries AW. Popliteal artery entrapment syndrome. Arch Surg 1970; 101:771–775.
4. Rich NM, Collins GJ, McDonald PT, et al. Popliteal vascular entrapment: Its increasing interest. Arch Surg 1979; 114:1377–1384.
5. Turnipseed WD, Pozniak M. Popliteal entrapment as a result of neurovascular compression by the soleus and plantaris muscles. J Vasc Surg 1992; 15:285–294.
6. Williams LR, Flinn WR, McCarthy WJ, et al. Popliteal artery entrapment: Diagnosis by computed tomography. J Vasc Surg 1986; 3:360–363.
7. Turnipseed WD, Detmer DE, Girdley F. Chronic compartment syndrome: An unusual cause for claudication. Ann Surg 1989; 210:557–563.
8. Greenwood LH, Yrizarry JM, Hallett JW. Popliteal artery entrapment: Importance of the stress runoff for diagnosis. Cardiovasc Intervent Radiol 1986; 9:93–99.
9. Rignault DP, Pailler JL, Lunel F. The "functional" popliteal entrapment syndrome. Int Angiol 1985; 4:341–343.

POPLITEAL ARTERY ADVENTITIAL CYSTIC DISEASE

LOIS A. KILLEWICH, M.D., PH.D.
MICHAEL P. LILLY, M.D.
WILLIAM R. FLINN, M.D.

Adventitial cystic disease of the popliteal artery is a relatively rare cause of vascular insufficiency of the lower extremity in which single or multiloculated cysts develop within the adventitial layer of the wall of the popliteal artery. As the typical gelatinous secretions of the intramural adventitial cyst accumulate, the cyst produces progressive obliteration of the adjacent arterial lumen. The reduction of arterial flow leads to the subsequent development of ischemic symptoms, most often intermittent claudication.

The term *adventitial cystic disease* has been almost universally associated with the popliteal artery, but the first case of adventitial cystic disease was discovered in the external iliac artery by Atkins and Key in 1947.[1] They characterized the 7 cm lesion as reminiscent of a sausage and thought it to be a myxomatous tumor of the adventitia. The first description of adventitial cystic disease of the popliteal artery was that of Ejrup and Heirtonn in 1954.[2] They reported the incision of a mass filled with gelatinous material in a thickened area of the popliteal artery, which they believed at the time to represent mucoid degeneration of the media. Subsequently, adventitial cystic disease has been described in the radial, ulnar, and femoral arteries, but the majority of cases have involved the popliteal artery. A report by Flanigan and colleagues summarized the accumulated data from 115 worldwide cases of adventitial cystic disease of the popliteal artery to clarify understanding of the diagnosis and management of this problem.[3]

ETIOLOGY

The precise cause of popliteal artery adventitial cystic disease remains uncertain. Disparate reports of the findings from surgical exploration and from pathologic examination of cysts removed have resulted in several different theories. The first is the theory of microtrauma, in which repetitive stretch injury to the arterial wall or injury from surrounding musculotendinous structures is thought to cause cystic myxomatous degeneration of the adventitia. Past reports have noted that the young men afflicted were frequently heavy laborers or were athletically active. However, if trauma alone were the cause, the condition should be more frequent. Additionally, cases of adventitial cystic disease have been reported in children in whom chronic trauma would be unlikely.

The second theory proposes an extra-arterial origin for the adventitial cysts. Adventitial cysts closely resemble ganglion cysts and may originate from pericapsular joint tissue and then extend outward to involve the arterial wall. Advocates of this theory have noted that adventitial cystic disease has always been found adjacent to joint spaces and never in the mid-thigh or mid-calf. A ganglion arising from the tibiofibular joint has been reported to extend to and compress the lateral popliteal nerve, indicating the potential for these articular lesions to involve anatomically proximate structures. Further, some cases of adventitial disease of the popliteal artery have been reported to have a communication to the knee joint documented by an arthrogram or discovered at the time of surgical exploration. Others have reported a synovial cell lining in the cyst seen on microscopic examination, which would also suggest an articular origin.

There is little disagreement that the cyst contents in adventitial cystic disease of the popliteal artery are essentially identical to that of typical ganglion cysts. The viscid, gel-like material is rich in mucopolysaccharides with a high content of hyaluronic acid and is markedly dissimilar to synovial fluid.[4] Additionally, in most reported cases, microscopic examination has not identified a lining of synovial cells in the adventitial cyst. This has led many investigators to doubt an extra-arterial origin of adventitial cysts from adjacent joint tissue. This final theory suggests that adventitial cysts develop because of spontaneous ganglionic degeneration of the intrinsic connective tissue within the adventitia of the artery itself.

Whatever the precise origin of these unusual lesions, they appear to have a relatively benign clinical course overall. Once accurately diagnosed, most have been successfully treated. Resection of the cyst wall can be performed in most patients. When involvement of the artery is extensive or arterial thrombosis has occurred, resection with vein graft interposition has been successful. Recurrence of these cysts is infrequent, and limb loss or other serious morbidity is rare.

CLINICAL PRESENTATION

Adventitial cystic disease of the popliteal artery characteristically occurs in young, healthy, nonsmoking males without evidence of other vascular disease. Previous reviews of this disorder have noted a 5 to 1 predominance of men over women and a mean age of approximately 40 years in patients afflicted. The typical patient has a sudden onset of intermittent claudication in the calf of the affected leg. Severe, limb-threatening ischemia has been rare. Patients usually report symptoms of claudication early because of the abrupt onset and relatively disabling nature in these young men who have previously been very active in work or athletics. However, because of their young age and the absence of other risk factors, symptoms are often initially interpreted to be neurogenic or musculoskeletal, which may delay definitive diagnosis. The clinical picture may be further confused by the spontaneous resolution of symptoms and the disappearance of abnormal physical findings in some patients.[5] It should be re-emphasized that in young adults with intermittent claudication, or symptoms suggestive of claudication, adventitial cystic disease should be considered because there are now reliable noninvasive methods available to confirm the diagnosis in most patients.

DIAGNOSIS

Physical examination of patients with symptomatic adventitial cystic disease of the popliteal artery reveals reduced or absent pedal pulses on the affected side with a normal ipsilateral femoral pulse and normal pedal pulses in the asymptomatic leg. In contrast, patients with popliteal entrapment typically have normal pedal pulses at rest. Also, adventitial cystic disease is usually unilateral in contrast to popliteal entrapment, which is often bilateral. Distal pulses in patients with adventitial cystic disease may be obliterated by sharp flexion of the knee. This too could help differentiate this condition from popliteal entrapment, where pedal pulses are obliterated by knee extension and contraction of the gastrocnemius muscle. A bruit over the popliteal fossa may help establish the diagnosis of adventitial cystic disease in young patients with claudication.

In the past, the definitive diagnosis of adventitial cystic disease required standard contrast arteriography. If the adventitial cystic disease does not cause occlusion of the popliteal artery, the intramural cyst produces a focal, eccentric, smooth stenosis, the "scimitar sign," on arteriography (Fig. 1). If the cyst compresses the arterial lumen circumfrentially, an hourglass deformity is seen. Both anteroposterior and lateral arteriographic images should be obtained to ensure that such a lesion is not overlooked. When adventitial cystic disease of the popliteal artery has produced occlusion, accurate diagnosis by arteriography alone has been challenging. Helpful findings include the location of the occlusion distal to the adductor hiatus, the lack of other evidence of atherosclerotic arterial occlusive disease, and the young age of the patient. Patients with popliteal arterial thrombosis produced by adventitial cystic disease may be treated initially with thrombolytic therapy, after which the characteristic arteriographic deformity may be documented.[6]

Duplex ultrasound scanning combines arterial imaging with simultaneous detection of flow abnormalities and seems uniquely suited to a condition such as adventitial cystic disease in which a mass lesion produces an arterial stenosis. In the report by Kaufman and colleagues, the diagnosis of adventitial cystic disease was established by the B-mode image, but no flow disturbance was identifiable.[7] However, in other reports duplex scanning demonstrated no anatomic or flow abnormalities in a patient with adventitial cystic disease, and the diagnosis was established by magnetic resonance imaging (MRI).[5]

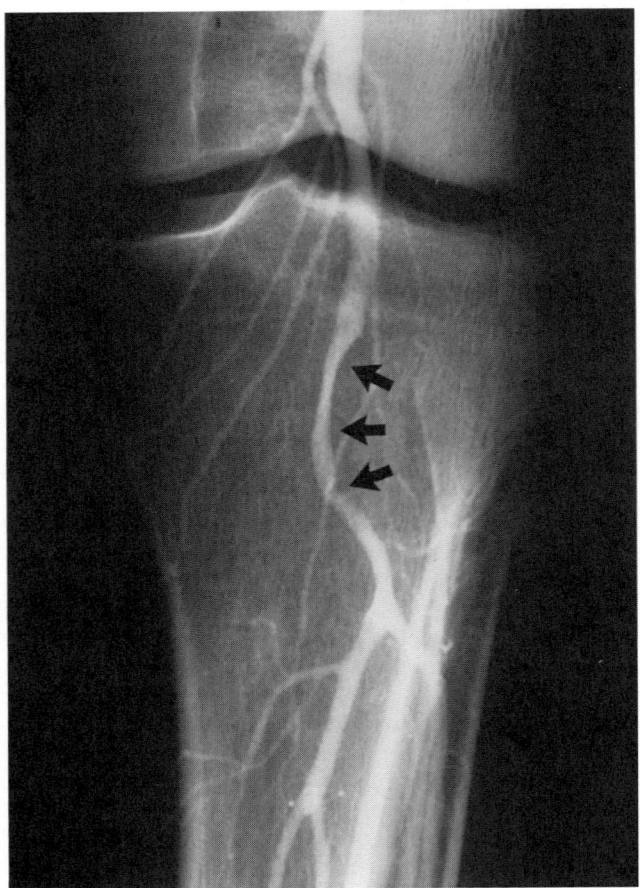

Figure 1 Arteriogram in a young athlete with calf claudication demonstrates a classic "scimitar sign" *(arrows)*, which is virtually diagnostic of adventitial cystic disease in a patient with no evidence of atherosclerosis.

Computed tomography (CT) has also been used to diagnose adventitial cystic disease of the popliteal artery and other uncommon popliteal arteriopathies.[8] Unlike arteriography, which is limited to opacification of the arterial lumen, CT provides examination of periarterial anatomy. This direct imaging is a significant benefit for evaluating rare disorders like popliteal entrapment or adventitial cystic disease (Fig. 2). Moreover, MRI scanning can also be diagnostic and requires no contrast media or ionizing radiation but is more expensive and less accessible than CT. Both CT and MRI may be particularly helpful to establish the accurate diagnosis of adventitial cystic disease if the lesion has produced occlusion of the popliteal artery and the "classic" arteriographic signs are absent.

TREATMENT

When diagnosis and treatment are initiated before cystic disease has produced arterial thrombosis, the operative procedure is simplified. With the expanding

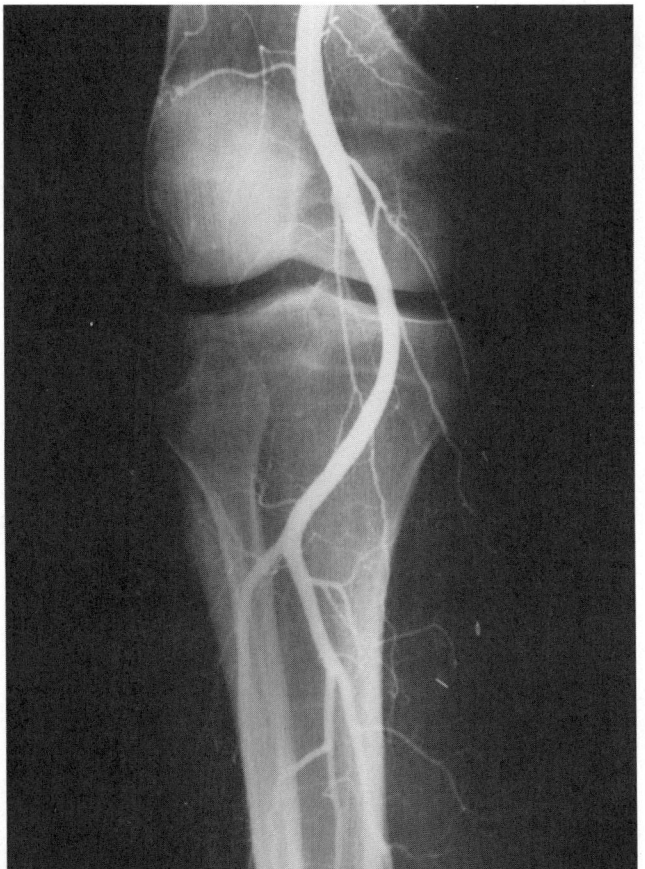

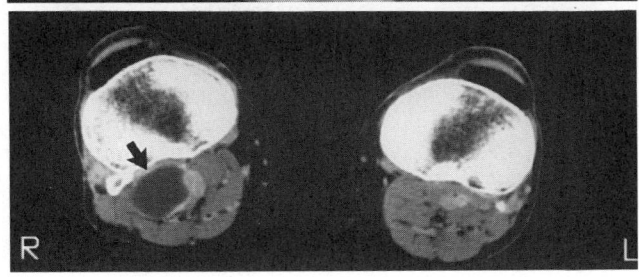

Figure 2 *A,* Arteriogram in a patient who demonstrated no significant occlusive lesion but had marked medial deviation of the popliteal artery, which might be suggestive of an entrapment syndrome. *B,* Imaging of the popliteal fossa by CT demonstrated that the medial deviation in this case was produced by an adventitial cyst of the popliteal artery *(arrow).*

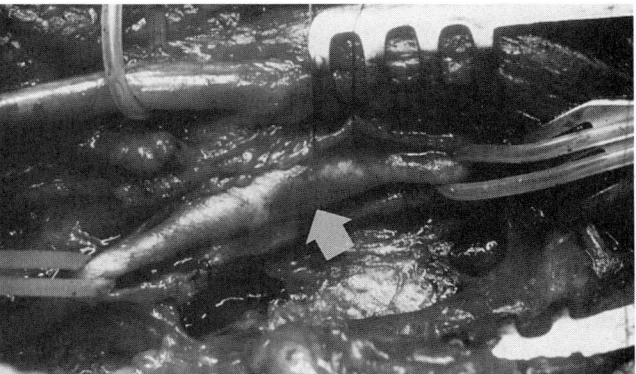

Figure 3 The posterior surgical approach allows exposure of mid-portion of the popliteal artery containing a small adventitial cyst *(arrow).* In this case, evacuation of the cyst contents and resection of the cyst wall resulted in a return of normal distal arterial flow without grafting.

application of invasive nonsurgical or endovascular procedures, it has become almost routine to consider percutaneous transluminal angioplasty (PTA) for treatment of a focal arterial stenosis in a patient with disabling claudication. However, PTA in cases of adventitial cystic disease of the popliteal artery has not been durable.[9] Initial success may be achieved by a forceful but temporary redistribution of the cyst contents within the wall of the artery. The response to this trauma may be the production of more cystic fluid and prompt return of symptoms.

Needle aspiration of cyst contents under ultrasound or CT guidance has been reported but has not provided definitive restoration of distal arterial perfusion or permanent relief of symptoms. It would appear that as long as the cyst wall remains intact there is a high likelihood that cyst contents will reaccumulate and produce a recurrence of ischemic symptoms.

Operation is the treatment of choice for adventitial cystic disease of the popliteal artery. Accurate diagnosis is even more important when surgical treatment of these lesions is planned. If classic arteriographic findings are documented or imaging of the cystic lesion has been successful by duplex, CT, or MRI, a posterior approach to the popliteal fossa is preferred over the standard medial approach used for femoropopliteal bypass. The posterior approach is performed with the patient prone and an S-shaped incision extends from medially above to laterally below the crease of the knee joint. This allows exposure of the involved area, which is behind the knee joint, an area that is relatively inaccessible using a medial approach unless extensive musculotendinous division is employed (Fig. 3). Because the uninvolved arterial segments are normal, surgical treatment can be easily accomplished in most patients with the somewhat more limited arterial exposure afforded by the posterior approach. With careful attention to the tibial and peroneal nerves, the morbidity should be minimal and recovery shortened with this approach.

The small number of patients in any single experience and the variety of treatments employed to date make it difficult to espouse a definitive surgical treatment for adventitial cystic disease. However, in most patients the cyst contents can be evacuated and the wall of the cyst can be resected. This restores normal luminal diameter to the popliteal artery and maintains an intact native arterial wall and endothelium. Resection of the cyst necessitates resection of at least part of the adventitia, but this does not appear to predispose to aneurysm formation. Arteriograms have been normal in patients so treated more than 9 years postoperatively.[10] Cyst resection is logically the most direct and effective surgical treatment and is recommended whenever anatomically possible.

When arterial thrombosis has occurred, restoration of normal arterial morphology and biology is probably not possible with thrombectomy combined with cyst evacuation or cyst wall resection. Resection of the involved popliteal artery with interposition graft replacement is recommended under these circumstances. Autogenous vein is the preferred graft material. Prosthetic grafts have been used successfully but are probably imprudent in young individuals.

REFERENCES

1. Atkins HJB, Key JA. A case of myxomatous tumour arising in the adventitia of the left iliac artery. Br J Surg 1947; 34:426.
2. Ejrup B, Heirtonn T. Intermittent claudication: Three cases treated by free vein grafts. Acta Chir Scand 1954; 108:217–230.
3. Flanigan DP, Burnham SJ, Goodreau MD, Bergan JJ Jr. Summary of cases of adventitial cystic disease of the popliteal artery. Ann Surg 1979; 189:165–175.
4. Jay GD, Ross FL, Mason RA, Giron F. Clinical and chemical characterization of an adventitial popliteal cyst. J Vasc Surg 1989; 9:448–451.
5. Crolla RMPH, Steyling JH, Hennipman A, et al. A case of cytic adventitial disease of the popliteal artery demonstrated by magnetic resonance imaging. J Vasc Surg 1993; 18:1052–1055.
6. Samson RH, Willis PD. Popliteal artery occlusion caused by cystic adventitial disease: Successful treatment by urokinase followed by nonresectional cystotomy. J Vasc Surg 1990; 12:591–593.
7. Kaufman JL, Kupinski AM, Shah DM, Leather RP. The diagnosis of adventitial cystic disease of the popliteal artery by duplex scanning. J Vasc Technol 1987; 11:132–135.
8. Rizzo RJ, Flinn WR, Yao JST, et al. Computed tomography for evaluation of arterial disease in the popliteal fossa. J Vasc Surg 1990; 11:112–119.
9. Fox RL, Kahn M, Adler J, et al. Adventitial cystic disease of the popliteal artery: Failure of percutaneous transluminal angioplasty as a therapeutic modality. J Vasc Surg 1985; 2:464–467.
10. Melliere D, Ecollan P, Kassab M, Becqemin JP. Adventitial cystic disease of the popliteal artery: Treatment by cyst removal. J Vasc Surg 1988; 8:638–642.

PERCUTANEOUS ARTERIAL DILATATION FOR ATHEROSCLEROTIC LOWER EXTREMITY OCCLUSIVE DISEASE

K. WAYNE JOHNSTON, M.D., F.R.C.S.C.

The results of the University of Toronto study of percutaneous transluminal balloon angioplasty (PTA) of the femoral and popliteal arteries allowed determination of variables that were predictive of early and late success of this procedure. In this study, symptomatic patients undergoing PTA for treatment of peripheral arterial occlusive disease were evaluated prospectively and were followed after PTA.[1,2] The methods overcome many of the limitations inherent in other reports, including definitions for success or patency that were not clearly stated, only arteriography used as the end point although it does not allow continuous regular follow-up, a nonconsecutive analysis of all patients having PTA, incomplete follow-up on all the patients in the study, lack of appropriate statistical methods, and consideration of only patients who have been a technical success in the analysis.

Logistic regression analysis was used to determine the multiple variables associated with early success for the defined variables. For individual variables, the Kaplan-Meier method was used to calculate the cumulative percent success rate of PTA versus time of follow-up. The statistical difference between Kaplan-Meier curves was determined using the log-rank test. For multivariate analysis, the Cox proportional hazards model was used to determine the factors that were associated with late success of PTA.

The PTA was considered a success if both the clinical grade and the noninvasive vascular laboratory measurements improved.[1] Even if a procedure fails, the patient may be partially or completely relieved of the original symptoms. Consequently, in addition to clinical criteria, it is important to use objective criteria of patency or hemodynamic improvement. Noninvasive measurements are ideal in providing objective hemodynamic data. Success is defined as improvement in the clinical grade by at least one level (i.e., asymptomatic, mild claudication, disabling claudication, ischemic pain or rest pain, or ulceration or gangrene) and in one or more of the following vascular laboratory measurements: ankle-brachial systolic pressure ratio increased by at least 0.1, monophasic Doppler frequency analysis recordings became biphasic or triphasic, the Doppler pulsatility index increased by more than 20%, or the treadmill exercise distance at least doubled. Our criteria for defining success are stricter than those used by many other authors but represent an appropriate approach for continuing follow-up.

RESULTS

Femoral popliteal PTAs represented 26% of the 984 procedures in the University of Toronto PTA study. The 254 femoral popliteal PTAs were performed in 236 patients. Their average age was 63 ± 10 years, and 67% were male patients.

Technical Failures

The technical failure rate was 4%, which is comparable to or better than most contemporary reports.[3-5]

Early Success Rate (1 Month)

Technical failures (4%) were included in the subsequent analysis. When evaluated 1 month after PTA, 89% of the procedures were defined as successful. Two variables proved to be predictors of success at 1 month: PTA of a stenosis was successful in 94%, whereas PTA of an occlusion was successful in 81% ($p = 0.002$); PTA for claudication was successful in 93%, whereas only 72% of PTAs were successful for limb salvage ($p < 0.001$). Other variables that were not related to early success were the site of the PTA, runoff, diabetes mellitus, age, sex, limb, number of lesions dilated, and predilation ankle-brachial blood pressure ratio.

These early success rates are similar to those reported by others;[4,6,7] however, it is possible that our results could be improved by the use of better modern imaging techniques, guide wires, and catheters or by the use of fibrinolytic agents to convert an occlusion to a stenosis before the PTA.

Complications

Complications were frequent following femoral and popliteal PTA. Although 13% of patients had complications, 6.6% were of no consequence. However, 6.3% were significant and caused death in 0.4%, required operation in 1.2% and transfusion in 1.6%, and delayed hospital discharge in 3.2%. The details of all complications are death during the hospitalization 0.4%, small hematoma 3.4%, large hematoma 3.2%, bleeding necessitating operation 0.4%, bleeding requiring transfusion 1.6%, false aneurysm 0.4%, ischemia necessitating emergency operation 0.4%, and other minor complications 3.2%.

Our incidence of complications is representative of other reports. In the review by Adar and co-workers,[6] 2.5% of patients required operation for the correction of complications, compared with 1.2% in our study. A similar low complication rate of 1.2% requiring operation was reported by Belli and co-workers,[8] but this included PTA at all sites. Gallino and colleagues reported that surgical intervention was required in 2% of patients.[9] Capek and associates noted complications in 10%: 1.4% died in hospital, 3.2% required operation because of arterial thrombosis or an arteriovenous fistula, and 1.2% had prolonged hospitalization because of ischemia.[4] In our study, the use of modern low-profile (5 Fr) angioplasty balloon catheters may have reduced the incidence of puncture site complications.

Late Success Rate

Cumulative percent success rates versus time of follow-up for all 254 PTAs of the femoral or popliteal arteries calculated by the Kaplan-Meier method were 63% at 1 year, 53% at 2 years, 51% at 3 years, 44% at 4 years, 38% at 5 years, and 36% at 6 years (Fig. 1).

In some reports, the authors excluded their early failures in calculating the results. When our data were recalculated excluding the 28 failures within 1 month of PTA, the overall success rates were 5% to 8% higher: 70% at 1 year, 59% at 2 years, 57% at 3 years, 50% at 4 years, 43% at 5 years, and 40% at 6 years.

As expected, when early failures are excluded, the calculated success rates are somewhat higher; however, data that exclude early failures are less applicable to clinical practice because they do not allow the clinician to predict a success rate prior to the PTA, only after the procedure has been successful.

A comparison of the results from the University of Toronto study with other published reports in the literature is noteworthy (Table 1).

Effects of Individual Variables on Results

Indication. Intermittent claudication was the indication for the procedure in 80% of patients, and critical ischemia in 20%. At 5 years the success rate was 40% for claudicators and 28% for patients undergoing PTA for salvage (Table 2).

Ankle-Brachial Systolic Pressure Ratio. Patients with an ankle-brachial blood pressure ratio of less than 0.57 had a 5 year success rate of 36%; those with a higher ratio had a 52% success rate (Table 3).

Type of Lesion (Stenosis Versus Occlusion). The artery was stenosed in 62% and occluded in 38% of patients. Stenoses were associated with a 5 year success

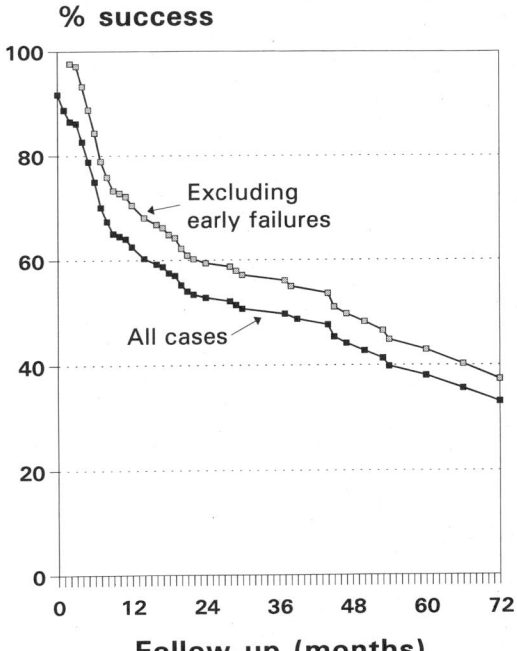

Figure 1 Results of 254 femoral and popliteal PTAs calculated by the Kaplan-Meier method. Also, the results recalculated excluding the early failures are plotted.

Table 1 Comparison of Early and Late Results of University of Toronto and Other Reports in Literature

Author	Cases Included	Technical Failure %	Early Success %	1 Year Success %	2 Year Success %	3 Year Success %	4 Year Success %	5 Year Success %	6 Year Success %
Johnston[2]	All cases	4	89	63	53	51	44	38	36
	If early success			70	59	57	50	43	40
Capek, et al[4]	Stenosis	7							
	Occlusion	18							
	If early success			81		61		58	
Jorgensen, et al[3]	Stenosis	2				68			
Jeans, et al[10]	Stenosis, good runoff					78			
	Occlusion, poor runoff					25			
Adar, et al[6]	Claudication		89			62			
	Salvage		77			43			
Wilson, et al[7]		16							
Blair, et al[11]	Salvage				18				
Henriksen, et al[12]					41				
Hewes, et al[5]								65	
Krepel, et al[13]			84					70	
Gallino, et al[9]								58	

Table 2 Effect of Indication on Late Results of PTA ($p = 0.005$); Cumulative Percent Success Calculated by the Kaplan-Meier Method

Time (Months)	Claudication Success %	Standard Error %	Salvage Success %	Standard Error %
3	91	2		
4	87	2		
5	83	3	62	7
6	80	3	55	7
7	74	3		
8	72	3	50	8
9	69	3		
10	68	3		
11	68	3		
12	66	4	47	8
14	64	4		
16	62	4		
17	62	4		
18	60	4		
19	60	4		
20	58	4	42	8
21	57	4		
22	56	4		
24	55	4		
28	55	4		
29	54	4		
30			37	9
37	53	4		
39	51	4		
44	50	4		
45	49	4	28	1
47	47	4		
50	46	5		
53	44	5		
54	42	5		
60	40	5		
66	38	5		
72	35	6	28	1

Table 3 Effect of Ankle/Brachial Systolic Blood Pressure Ratio on Late Results of PTA ($p = 0.004$); Cumulative Percent Success Calculated by the Kaplan-Meier Method

Time (Months)	Pressure Ratio < 0.57 Success %	Standard Error %	Pressure Ratio ≥ 0.57 Success %	Standard Error %
3			95	2
4	83	4	91	3
5	77	4	89	3
6	74	4	86	4
7	66	5	84	4
8	63	5	83	4
9	61	5	78	4
10	60	5		
11	59	5		
12	57	5	77	4
14	53	5		
16			74	5
17	51	5		
18	50	5	73	5
19	49	5		
20	47	5	70	5
21			68	5
22	46	5		
24			66	5
28			65	6
29			63	6
30			61	6
37	44	6		
44	42	6		
45	39	6		
47			57	7
50	36	6		
54			52	8
60			46	9
66	32	7		

Table 4 Effect of Type of Lesion (Stenosis or Occlusion) on Late Results of PTA ($p = 0.006$); Cumulative Percent Success Calculated by the Kaplan-Meier Method

Time (Months)	Stenosis Success %	Standard Error %	Occlusion Success %	Standard Error %
3	92	2		
4	89	3	72	5
5	86	3	67	5
6	83	3	61	5
7	77	4	58	5
8	74	4	57	5
9	71	4	56	5
10			54	5
11	70	4		
12	68	4	53	5
14	66	4	51	5
16	65	4	49	5
17			48	5
18	64	4		
19			46	5
20	62	4	45	6
21	60	4		
22			43	6
24	59	4		
28			42	6
29	57	5		
30	56	5		
37			39	6
39	55	5		
44	53	5		
45	51	5	35	6
47	50	5		
50			32	7
53	47	5		
54	45	6		
60	43	6		
66	39	6		
72	36	7	32	7

Table 5 Effect of Runoff on Late Results of PTA ($p = 0.001$); Cumulative Percent Success Calculated by the Kaplan-Meier Method

Time (Months)	Good Runoff Success %	Standard Error %	Poor Runoff Success %	Standard Error %
0.1	94	2	89	3
1	91	2	85	4
2	90	2	80	4
3			79	5
4	86	3	76	5
5	83	3	71	5
6	80	3	66	5
7	75	4	62	5
8	73	4	58	6
9	70	4	56	6
10			55	6
11	70	4		
12	69	4	52	6
14	66	4		
16			49	6
17	65	4		
18	64	4	47	6
19	64	4		
20	62	4	45	6
21	61	4	43	6
22	60	4		
24	59	4		
28	58	4		
29			41	6
30			40	6
37	56	5		
39	54	5		
44	53	5		
45			34	6
47			31	6
50			28	6
53	50	5		
54	47	6		
60			24	7
66			19	7
72	47	576	14	7

rate of 43%, whereas occlusions were only 32% successful (Table 4).

Runoff. The runoff was good with two or three tibial arteries patent in 64% of patients and poor with no or one tibial artery patent in 36%. The 5 year success rate was 47% for patients with good runoff and 28% for patients with poor runoff (Table 5).

Site of PTA. A PTA of the arterial segment above the knee was performed in 83% of patients and below the knee in 17%. There was no significant difference between above-knee PTA and below-knee PTA (Table 6).

Diabetes. Diabetes was present in 25% of the patients, but this variable did not have an effect on the long-term results.

PTA at One Site Versus Two or More Sites. The number of sites dilated was not related to the late results.

Pressure Gradient Across Stenosis. The pressure gradient measured across the stenosis at the time of the procedure was not a predictor of the late success rate.

Other Variables. Long-term results were not related to the patient's age or gender.

Effects of Multiple Variables on Results

The Cox proportional hazards model was used to determine which combination of these significant variables was associated with long-term success of femoral and popliteal PTA. Two variables proved to be significant ($p < 0.01$): the type of lesion (i.e., stenosis or occlusion) and the runoff (i.e., good or poor). Figure 2 illustrates the predicted 5 year success rates for the different combinations of type of lesion and type of runoff.

Note that if the early failures are excluded, only the runoff was a significant predictor of success as calculated by the Cox proportional hazards model. Thus, the major determinant of early success appears to be the type of

Table 6 Effect of Site of PTA on Late Results ($p = 0.1$); Cumulative Percent Success Calculated by the Kaplan-Meier Method

Time (Months)	Above-Knee PTA		Below-Knee PTA	
	Success %	Standard Error %	Success %	Standard Error %
3	88	2		
4	84	3	77	7
5	81	3	69	7
6	77	3	64	8
7	72	3	61	8
8	70	3	56	8
9	68	3	53	8
10	67	3		
11	66	3		
12	64	4		
14	62	4		
16	61	4		
17			50	8
18	59	4		
19	59	4		
20	56	4		
21	56	4	46	8
22			43	8
24	55	4		
28	54	4		
29	53	4		
30	52	4		
37	51	4		
39	50	4		
44	49	4		
45	46	4		
47	45	5		
50	43	5		
53			34	1
54	41	5		
60	39	5		
66			17	13
72	36	6	17	13

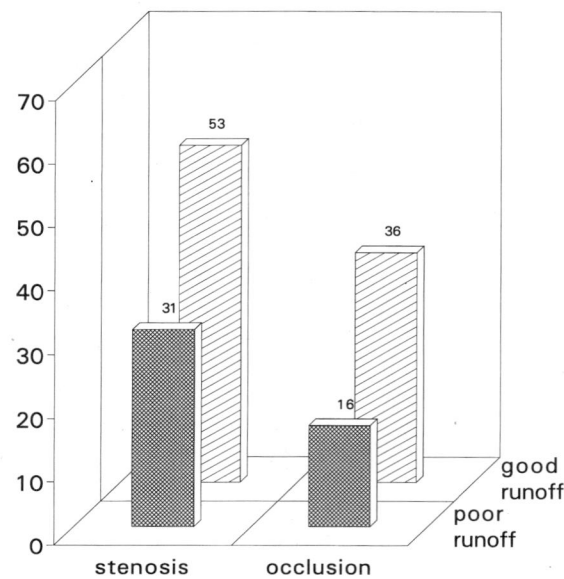

Figure 2 Predicted 5 year success rates based on type of lesion (stenosis or occlusion) and runoff (good or poor) as calculated by Cox proportional hazards method.

lesion, and the major determinant of late success appears to be the runoff.

ROLE OF PTA IN FEMORAL AND POPLITEAL ARTERIES

For the treatment of patients with femoral popliteal occlusive disease, PTA is a satisfactory option when the artery is stenosed and the runoff is good because the 5 year success rate is 53%. However, most patients with a femoral popliteal stenosis and good runoff usually complain of only intermittent claudication, and consequently most can be managed conservatively without interventional treatment. The results of PTA are less satisfactory for a stenosis with poor runoff (31% 5 year success), an occlusion with good runoff (36% 5 year success), and an occlusion with poor runoff (16% 5 year success). In these circumstances, an attempt at PTA seems justified if the patient has critical ischemia or very severe intermittent claudication and arterial reconstruction does not seem applicable because the patient is a high risk, the patient has a limited life expectancy, or autogenous bypass material is not available.

REFERENCES

1. Johnston KW, Rae M, Hogg-Johnston SA, et al. 5-year results of a prospective study of percutaneous transluminal angioplasty. Ann Surg 1987; 206:403–413.
2. Johnston KW. Reanalysis of the results of balloon angioplasty of the femoral and popliteal arteries. Radiology 1992; 183:767–771.
3. Jorgensen B, Tonnesen KH, Holstein P. Late hemodynamic failure following percutaneous transluminal angioplasty for long and multifocal femoropopliteal stenoses. Cardiovasc Intervent Radiol 1991; 14:290–292.
4. Capek P, McLean GK, Berkowitz HD. Femoropopliteal angioplasty: Factors influencing long-term success. Circulation 1991; 83(Supp 1):70–80.
5. Hewes RC, White RI Jr, Murray RR, et al. Long-term results of superficial femoral artery angioplasty. Am J Roentgenol 1986; 156:1025–1029.
6. Adar R, Critchfield GC, Eddy DM. A confidence profile analysis of the results of femoropopliteal percutaneous transluminal angioplasty in the treatment of lower-extremity ischemia. J Vasc Surg 1989; 10:57–67.
7. Wilson SE, Wolf GL, Cross AP. Percutaneous transluminal angioplasty versus operation for peripheral arteriosclerosis: Report of a prospective randomized trial in a selected group of patients. J Vasc Surg 1989; 9:1–9.
8. Belli AM, Cumberland DC, Knox AM, et al. The complications rate of percutaneous peripheral balloon angioplasty. Clin Radiol 1990; 41:380–383.
9. Gallino A, Mahler F, Probst P, Nachbur B. Percutaneous transluminal angioplasty of the arteries of the lower limbs: A 5 year follow-up. Circulation 1984; 70:619–623.

10. Jeans WD, Armstrong S, Cole SEA, et al. Fate of patients undergoing transluminal angioplasty for lower limb ischemia. Radiology 1990; 177:559–564.
11. Blair JM, Gewert BL, Moosa H, et al. Percutaneous transluminal angioplasty versus surgery for limb-threatening ischemia. J Vasc Surg 1989; 9:698–703.
12. Henrikson LO, Jorgensen B, Holstein PE, et al. Percutaneous transluminal angioplasty of infrarenal arteries in intermittent claudication. Acta Chir Scand 1988; 154:573–576.
13. Krepel VW, van Andel GJ, van Erp WF, Breslau PJ. Percutaneous transluminal angioplasty of the femoropopliteal artery: Initial and long-term results. Radiology 1985; 156:325–328.

ATHERECTOMY DEVICES IN THE MANAGEMENT OF INFRAINGUINAL OCCLUSIVE DISEASE

SAMUEL S. AHN, M.D.

Mechanical atherectomy is the selective removal of atheroma from stenotic or occluded vessels, which can be performed percutaneously or through a small arteriotomy remote from the diseased site. During the developmental stage, three theoretical advantages of atherectomy over balloon angioplasty were proposed: (1) a higher immediate success rate with less subintimal dissection and subsequent occlusion; (2) greater therapeutic options for lesions currently not amenable to angioplasty alone, such as diffusely diseased vessels, occlusive lesions, or eccentric stenoses; and (3) reduction of the restenosis rate due to the debulking of the atheromatous mass.[1] A variety of atherectomy catheters have been devised, and each offers unique advantages as well as disadvantages. However, only three have produced any significant results: the Simpson Atherocath, the Theratek catheter, and the Auth Rotablator. A critical evaluation of their usage in the management of infrainguinal occlusive disease follows.

ATHERECTOMY DEVICES

Simpson Atherocath

Description

The Simpson peripheral atherectomy catheter (Devices for Vascular Intervention, Redwood City, California) is a flexible 7 Fr to 11 Fr catheter that has a small circular cutter spinning at about 2,000 rpm inside a metal housing with a 15 or 20 mm window as its cutting element. The plaque is forced through the window into the housing by inflating a balloon (20 to 40 lb/in^2; PSI) on the opposite side of the housing. Advancing the rotating cutter in the housing cuts the plaque, and the distal collection chamber traps the pieces. An ultrasound chip in the cutting window has been developed in some of the newer models to guide correct alignment of the window with the lesion prior to cutting and to evaluate the result after a cut is made.

Indication

The Simpson Atherocath can optimally treat short, discrete, eccentrically placed atheroma (Table 1). Stenoses are amenable to treatment, whereas occlusions are generally avoided unless the housing can penetrate the lesion. It can also be utilized in treating ulcerative atherosclerotic plaques and intimal hyperplasia lesions. Heavily calcified lesions can create some difficulties for the cutter but can be managed. The Simpson Atherocath has also been used as an adjunct to balloon angioplasty to debulk calcific eccentric stenoses not normally receptive to dilation.

Technique

The atherectomy catheter is advanced through the stenotic lesion and torques appropriately to position the cutting window toward the plaque by fluoroscopy. With the catheter properly positioned, the balloon in inflated to 20 to 40 PSI to push the open chamber against the arterial lesion, thereby wedging the atheroma into the window. The motor drive of the cutter is activated, and the rotating circular blade slices and pushes the atheroma into the distal collecting chamber. The collecting chamber rotates, and the entire process is repeated. Multiple cuts and passages are required to complete the atherectomy. When the collecting chamber is full, the catheter is withdrawn, and the slices of atheroma are removed. The procedure is repeated until recanalization is complete.[1]

Results

Polnitz and co-workers reported an initial angiographic success rate of 90% and a clinical success rate of 82% in treating 63 stenoses and 31 occlusions with the Simpson Atherocath.[2] At 1 year among 25 patients with the initial success, 72% maintained clinical patency, 15% required repeated atherectomy, and 8% required operation for restenosis or occlusion.

Hinohara and co-workers also achieved a 90% initial success rate in treating 195 lesions, and 83% of patients continued clinical improvement at 6 months.[3] The failures were primarily due to the inability to cross the lesions or to remove enough atheroma. Overall, the restenosis rate was 36%.

Table 1 Current Application of Atherectomy Devices

	Ideal Lesions	Site	Limitations
Simpson	Short Eccentric Stenotic, < 4 cm	Iliac Femoral Popliteal	Restenosis Bulky device Lengthy procedure
Theratek	Occluded Stenotic	Femoral Popliteal	Perforation Restenosis
Auth Rotablator	Calcified Stenotic	Femoral Popliteal Tibial	Thromboemboli Restenosis

Graor and Whitlow reported 100% and 93% initial success rate in patients with lesions shorter than 5 cm and longer than 5 cm, respectively.[4] However, unlike other groups who defined their initial success rate as stenosis less than 50% after atherectomy, Graor and Whitlow achieved less than 20% stenosis among their initially successful patients. At 12 months, the patency rates were 93% and 83%, respectively.

Vroegindeweij and co-workers recently reported clinical improvement in 15 of 16 atherectomy procedures; however, the 1 year patency rate was only 25%.[5] Furthermore, they preferred the intraoperative technique to the percutaneous approach.

Complications and Limitations

The Simpson Atherocath has a relatively low complication rate (Table 2). Hematoma due to bleeding at the site of atherectomy entry has been the primary complication.[2-4] Graor and Whitlow, for instance, reported seven instances of severe hematoma that required surgical intervention.[4] A few episodes of distal embolization were also noted by the Polnitz and Hinohara groups.[2,3]

Restenosis is the main long-term limitation, with the reported rates ranging from 11% to 47%. This appears to be lower for eccentric lesions, which are especially suited for the Simpson Atherocath.[1,2] For example, Polnitz and associates reported 24% and 11% restenosis rates for concentric and eccentric lesions, respectively.[2]

The Simpson Atherocath is also relatively ineffective in long, diffusely diseased segments and long occluded lesions (Table 1). Using the atherocath under these circumstances usually results in a lengthy procedure, and restenosis rates are much higher in these lesions. Furthermore, the bulkiness and stiffness of the catheter contraindicate its use in the tibial arteries or tortuous vessels.

Theratek Catheter

Description

Once known as the Kensey atherectomy device, the Theratek catheter (Theratek, Miami, Florida) is a flexible device with a distal cam-tip attached to a central drive shaft. The cam rotates at 100,000 rpm and ventures into the path of least resistance. A high-pressure irrigating system dilates the artery while the rotating cam pulverizes the atherosclerotic intima. The rotating tip selectively pulverizes fibrous or firm atheromatous tissue while leaving viscoelastic tissue uninjured. Originally, the catheter was available only in the 8 Fr size, requiring adjunctive balloon angioplasty to adequately dilate the artery. The device is currently under modification, with both 5 and 10 Fr calibers available in the near future. It is made more flexible, and a guide wire is being added.

Indication

The Theratek catheter is ideally suited for occlusive lesions, especially of the superficial femoral artery (Table 1). There is no need for a coaxial central guide wire to cross the lesion first. Similar to the Simpson Atherocath, the catheter is not effective on long lesions.

Technique

The Theratek atherectomy procedure can be performed percutaneously or through a small open arteriotomy in the common femoral artery. A 9 Fr introducer sheath is first placed and then followed by the catheter into the artery being treated. The catheter tip is positioned directly against the occluded site in the artery under fluoroscopic guidance. Through the irrigation channel, contrast medium dye mixed with urokinase, dextran, and heparin sodium is infused at a rate of 30 ml/minute. Then, the electric motor drive is activated to rotate at approximately 100,000 rpm. The catheter is advanced slowly and gently under direct fluoroscopic control in a to-and-fro manner, allowing time for the rotating cam to pulverize the atheroma. After the catheter has recanalized the occluded lesion, standard balloon angioplasty techniques are conducted to dilate any residual stenosis.[1]

Results

In a study performed by Snyder and co-workers, atherectomy with the Theratek catheter was technically successful in 67% of the 46 superficial femoral artery occlusions; however, only 59% (27 of 46) had hemodynamic improvement.[6] The primary patency rate at 1 year was 63.9% among the initial hemodynamically successful patients.

In contrast, Debrosse and co-workers reported a success rate of 87% (40 of 46) in recanalizing femoropopliteal occlusions. However, 13% (5 of 40) reoccluded within 48 hours.[7] Using intravenous angiographic studies the primary patency rate obtained at 1 year was 70% (14 of 20). Furthermore, it is critical to note that these success rates by the Snyder and Debrosse groups were achieved with the use of adjunctive balloon angioplasty, postoperative antiplatelet therapy, and, in Debrosse's study, "antivitamin K" therapy.

Lukes and co-workers achieved a technical success of 64% among 11 patients treated with the Theratek

Table 2 Simpson Atherocath: Complications

	Hinohara, et al	Polnitz, et al	Graor and Whitlow
Number of patients	134	60	112
Arterial thrombosis	1	—	—
Distal embolization	2	1	—
Cardiorespiratory complications	—	—	1†
Hematoma	1	2	7
Others	3*		
Total	7/134 (5%)	3/60 (5%)	8/112 (7%)
Death	—	—	1†

*One occlusion, one emergency bypass, and one surgical repair at the access site.
†Cardiogenic shock after atherectomy.

Table 3 Theratek Catheter: Complications

	Snyder, et al	Debrosse, et al
Number of patients	46	46
Arterial thrombosis	—	5
Distal embolization	—	3
Perforation	11	4
Total	11 (24%)	12 (26%)

catheter. However, only 36% (4 of 11) had clinical improvement.[8] All of the initial technically successful lesions remained patent at 1 year.

Complications and Limitations

The major complication is perforation induced by the rotating cam (Table 3). Snyder and colleagues reported a perforation rate of 23% (11 of 46),[6] and Debrosse a 9% (4 of 46) rate.[7] One of the perforations in the Snyder group's study required surgical intervention. Furthermore, Debrosse and associates noted all four of their perforations had calcified lesions. This may have been caused by the catheter, which often follows the path of least resistance away from hard, calcified atherosclerotic lesions, making it difficult for the Theratek catheter to treat. The high perforation rate and difficulty in recanalizing calcified plaque limit the use of the Theratek catheter.

Distal embolization has also been documented by Debrosse and associates in three patients (Table 3).[7] Thus, the Theratek catheter can cause distal embolization in spite of the micropulverization of atherosclerotic plaques to the particle size of red blood cells.

Auth Rotablator

Description

The Auth Rotablator (Heart Technology, Bellevue, Washington) is a flexible, catheter-deliverable atherectomy device with a variable-sized, football-shaped metal burr on the distal tip. Multiple 22 to 45 µm diamond chips in the burr function as microblades. The size of the burr ranges from 1.25 to 6 mm in diameter to fit the size of the artery being treated. Arteries can be dilated by using progressively larger burrs. The burr rotates at 100,000 to 200,000 rpm and tacks along a central guide wire required to cross the lesion before the rotational atherectomy can proceed. The high-speed rotation allows the diamond microchips to remove hard, calcified atheroma, preferentially while leaving the surrounding elastic soft tissue of normal arterial wall intact. The device is designed to leave a smooth, polished luminal surface with no intimal flaps.

Indication

The Auth Rotablator is designed for hard, calcified atheroma, especially in patients with diabetes mellitus (Table 1). Stenotic lesions are preferred because a central guide wire must first traverse the lesion. Eccentric lesions can also be treated with the Auth Rotablator because the burr preferentially attacks rigid atheroma.

Technique

Atherectomy is performed preferentially through an open arteriotomy. A 9, 12, or 14 Fr introducer sheath is inserted into the artery through the arteriotomy. Under angioscopic or fluoroscopic guidance, a small atraumatic guide wire is passed through the lesion, followed by an exchange guide catheter. The exchange guide catheter is a 0.009 inch atherectomy guide wire that is stiffer and more rigid than others. The burr is then passed over the stiff atherectomy guide wire to the site of the obstructive lesion. The turbine drive is activated to maintain a rotating speed of 100,000 to 200,000 rpm. In a vibrato-like, to-and-from manner, the rotating atherectomy is advanced slowly over the guide wire. After the initial atherectomy, the burr is removed, leaving the guide wire in place. The next-sized burr is placed, and atherectomy is repeated until a satisfactory-sized lumen is obtained. The patient undergoes anticoagulation therapy for 24 hours postoperatively to prevent early thrombosis. Aspirin is also administered postoperatively.[1]

Results

In a multicenter trial using the Auth Rotablator, the operative arteriographic and in-hospital success rates were 89% (70 of 79) and 77% (61 of 79), respectively.[9] The resulting cumulative primary patency was 69% at 1 month, 47% at 6 months, only 31% at 12 months, and 18.6% at 2 years. The length of lesion, indications for atherectomy, use of heparin sodium, and/or type of lesion (stenosis versus occlusion) did not significantly influence the patency rates. No significant difference was noted in patency rates between the percutaneous and open surgical methods.

Table 4 Auth Rotablator: University of California, Los Angeles; Stanford; and Albert Einstein: Complications for 79 Patients

Complication	Number
Hemoglobinuria	10
Pseudo-aneurysm	1
Hematoma	4
Infection	1
Major emboli	4
Minor emboli	4
Limb loss	2
Total	26 (32.5%)
Death	0

Complications and Limitations

Ahn and associates reported that 9 of 79 limbs had initial arteriographic failure. Dissection and perforation were the primary reasons for failure.[9] Nine limbs developed in-hospital thrombosis, and four of them had an associated hypercoagulable state. Furthermore, multiple other complications occurred within 30 days (Table 4). Four instances of clinically significant emboli also developed during atherectomy; three resulted in cutaneous necrosis and one in toe amputation.

The main long-term limitation of the Auth Rotablator is restenosis or reocclusion within 12 months. Arteriographic, angioscopic, or surgical findings of these intermediate-term recurrent lesions suggested intimal hyperplasia in 13 patients.

COMMENT

Each atherectomy device is designed to serve a different role in treating peripheral arterial lesions. The Simpson Atherocath is used for short, discrete, eccentric lesions; the Theratek catheter for occlusive lesions; and the Auth Rotablator for hard, calcified atheroma. Each has promised to surpass balloon angioplasty in its application. However, all atherectomy devices have failed to achieve this promise because of a high restenosis rate. Despite actual removal, debulking, and even polishing of the atherosclerotic intima, these atherectomy devices seem to incite intimal hyperplasia. Until the problem of restenosis can be solved, atherectomy has a limited application.

REFERENCES

1. Ahn SS. Status of peripheral atherectomy. Surg Clin North Am 1992; 72:869–878.
2. Polnitz A, Nerlich A, Berger H, et al. Percutaneous peripheral atherectomy: Angiographic and clinical follow-up of 60 patients. J Am Coll Cardiol 1990; 15:682–688.
3. Hinohara T, Robertson G, Selmon M: Directional atherectomy: The Simpson atherectomy catheter. In: Ahn SS, Moore WS, eds. Endovascular surgery. Philadelphia: WB Saunders, 1992; 275.
4. Graor RA, Whitlow PL. Transluminal atherectomy for occlusive peripheral vascular disease. J Am Coll Cardiol 1990; 15:1551–1558.
5. Vroegindeweij D, Demper FJM, Buth T, et al. Recurrence of stenoses following balloon angioplasty and Simpson atherectomy of the femoropopliteal segment. Eur J Vasc Surg 1992; 6:164–171.
6. Snyder S, Wheeler J, Gregory RT, et al. The Trac-Wright atherectomy device. In: Ahn SS, Moore WS, eds. Endovascular surgery. Philadelphia: WB Saunders, 1989; 299.
7. Debrosse D, Petet H, Torres E, et al. Percutaneous atherectomy with the Kensey catheter: Early and midterm results in femoropopliteal occlusions unsuitable for conventional angioplasty. Ann Vasc Surg 1990; 4:550–552.
8. Lukes P, Wihed G, Tidebrant G, et al. Combined angioplasty with the Kensey catheter and balloon angioplasty in occlusive arterial disease. Acta Radiol 1992; 33:230–233.
9. Ahn SS, Mehigan JT, Gupta SK, et al. Peripheral atherectomy with the Rotablator: A multicenter report. J Vasc Surg 1994; 19:509–515.

BALLOON ANGIOPLASTY IN THE MANAGEMENT OF FAILING INFRAINGUINAL BYPASS GRAFTS

ANTHONY D. WHITTEMORE, M.D.

Despite numerous advances in the field of infrainguinal vascular reconstruction, 20% to 30% of all bypasses fail within 5 years for a variety of reasons. Approximately 10% fail within 1 year from stenotic lesions resulting primarily from fibrous intimal hyperplasia. It has been repeatedly documented that surgical treatment for these vein graft lesions proves successful most often when the lesions are detected prior to graft occlusion.[1] Several studies have since attested to the durability of surgical patch angioplasty for vein graft stenoses occurring within the graft itself or at the anastomosis, and patency rates of 60% to 80% 5 years after revision have been reported.[1-3] In contrast, the same procedure after initial thrombectomy required for an occluded vein graft provides a limited 25% to 30% patency. The need for some form of intervention for failing vein grafts has therefore become well established, and various graft surveillance protocols have become integral parts of the management.

Simultaneously with the emergence of percutaneous transluminal angioplasty for arterial stenoses, balloon angioplasty was postulated to provide a more expeditious approach to the failing vein graft that would obviate the necessity for operation altogether.[4-6] In an effort to clarify the role of balloon angioplasty, several centers have recently reviewed experiences of the past decade with conflicting results. Perler and associates documented the characteristically high initial success rate (96%) of balloon dilation but also documented a disappointing patency rate of only 22% after 3 years and confirmed the superior durability of surgical revision.[2]

Our experience at Brigham & Women's Hospital consisted of 54 balloon angioplasties carried out in 30 patients for stenotic lesions with a mean stenosis of 80%.[7] These stenoses occurred in 30 in situ, 12 reversed, 9 nonreversed, 2 composite grafts, and a single arm vein conduit. Recurrent symptoms included intermittent claudication in 57% of limbs, rest pain in 22%, and tissue necrosis in 21%. Lesions were identified after a mean interval of 18 months after initial reconstruction and were documented earlier in our experience with arteriography indicated by the recurrence of symptoms and a significantly diminished ankle-brachial index. More recently, lesions were identified with color-assisted duplex imaging. Hemodynamic significance was determined using high-flow criteria characterized by peak systolic flow velocities in excess of twice that observed in the adjacent segment. Eleven (20%) grafts were thrombosed and therefore required thrombolytic therapy prior to balloon angioplasty. Twenty-four lesions (44%) were defined as focal, involving no more than a 1 cm segment of graft, and 30 (56%) were diffuse lesions involving longer segments of the graft as determined arteriographically.

Balloon angioplasty was carried out in the radiologic angiography suite with intravenous sedation following routine diagnostic survey (Fig. 1A). Access for distal lesions was through the ipsilateral common femoral artery; more proximal lesions required a contralateral retrograde approach. The lesion was initially traversed with a soft guide wire, and subsequently smaller caliber catheters were serially exchanged for the balloon angioplasty catheter. Inflation to a maximum of 10 atmospheres was sustained for 45 to 60 seconds, and simultaneous anticoagulation with heparin sodium was routinely utilized. Of the 54 angioplasties, 18 were single, isolated angioplasties in individual grafts in 17 patients. The remaining angioplasties were repetitive procedures in 13 additional patients who required either sequential or simultaneous angioplasties of multiple lesions within the same graft. Most lesions were located near the distal anastomosis, but 20% were located near the proximal anastomosis and 15% were located within the midportion of the graft. The mean degree of stenosis caused by these hyperplastic lesions was 78 ± 18%.

All stenotic lesions were dilated to less than 30% residual stenosis and were therefore considered technically successful dilations in all 54 instances (Fig. 1B). Recently, hemodynamic confirmation of the technical success was obtained with immediate color-assisted duplex imaging. Patients were subsequently maintained in the hospital for 24 hours on systemic heparin sodium and were discharged on aspirin. Follow-up consisted of symptomatic and hemodynamic assessment at intervals of 4 months. Routine color-assisted duplex imaging has been used more recently. There were no deaths during the 30 days following the procedure, and 11% of patients sustained minor morbidity consisting of groin hematomas or puncture site oozing. The 5-year survival rate for this group of patients was 82%.

The overall 4-year patency rate, however, was a disappointing 18% (Fig. 2), comparable to the 3-year patency rate of 22% found by Perler.[2] Whereas the Perler group's studies specifically excluded grafts initially treated with thrombolytic therapy, 11 of our 54 grafts required lytic therapy prior to dilation. Whether a graft required initial lysis, however, proved statistically insignificant. Three-year patency rates achieved with angioplasty undertaken for recurrent claudication (25%) proved no better than for limb salvage (24%). Neither the location of the lesion within the vein graft nor the length of segment involved (greater or less than 1 cm) reached statistical significance. The only variable of significance was the number of dilations required. Grafts that required a single dilation for a single lesion, most of which were focal, had a 59% 3-year patency rate, significantly higher than the 6% 3-year patency rate associated with grafts requiring multiple dilations (Fig. 3).

Since these initial studies of relatively heteroge-

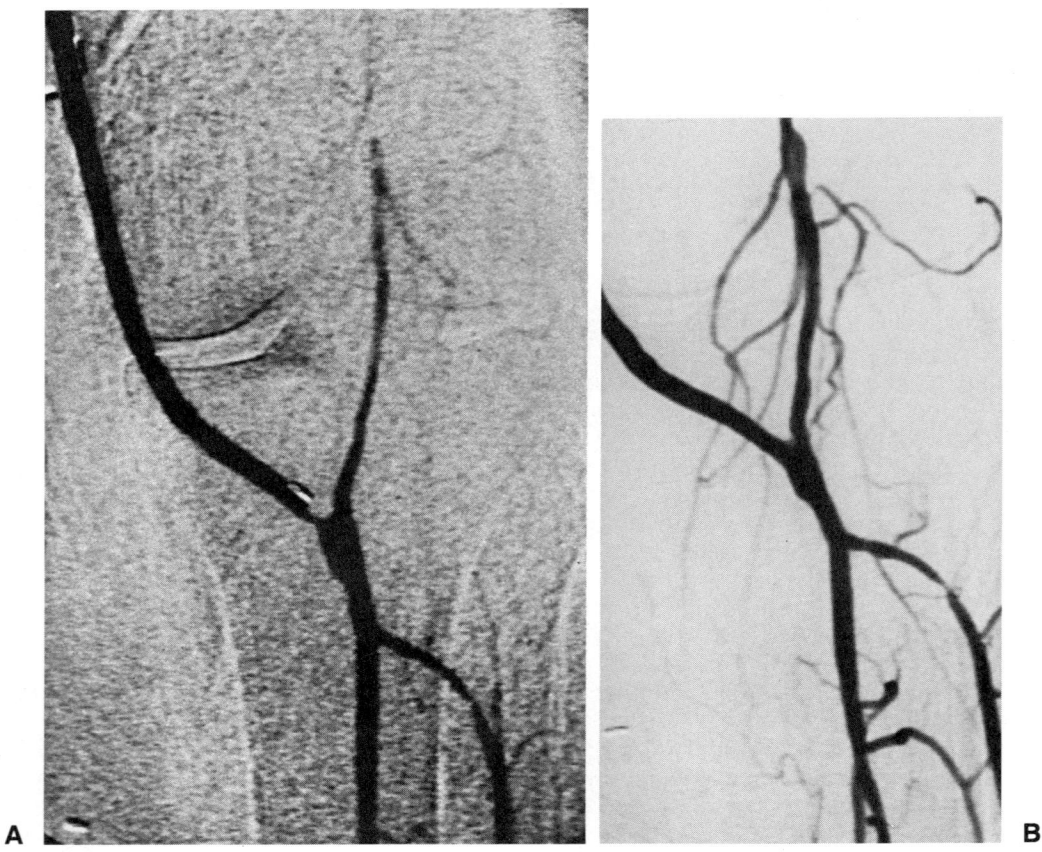

Figure 1 *A,* Routine arteriographic diagnostic survey detects near occlusion of bypass graft. *B,* Following balloon angioplasty with balloon inflated to a maximum of 10 atmospheres for 45 to 60 seconds, lesion was dilated to less than 30% residual stenosis.

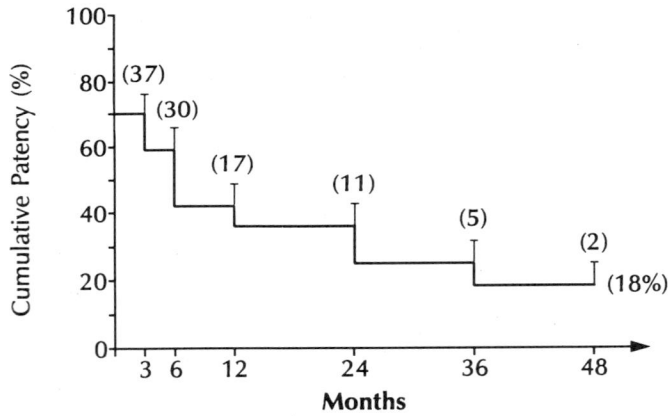

Figure 2 Four-year cumulative patency rate is a disappointing 18%.

neous populations, more recent information continues to define the particular subset of individuals who may benefit from balloon angioplasty. Taylor and co-workers reported a 73% 2-year patency rate for vein graft lesions less than 1 cm in length,[8] similar to the 76% patency rate documented by Sanchez and colleagues for lesions less than 1.5 cm in length located within vein grafts greater than 3 mm in diameter.[3] Berkowitz and colleagues reported an overall 5-year patency rate of 58% following balloon angioplasty, but a higher rate of 66% was achieved for lesions located in the most proximal aspect of the graft.[9] They were unable, however, to find a significant difference in 5-year patency rates between focal (less than 2 cm) stenoses and longer, more diffuse

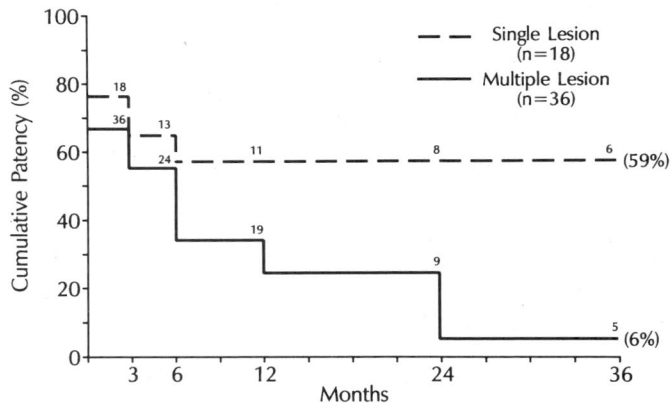

Figure 3 Three-year patency rate shows that the number of dilations required is a significant variable. Grafts that required a single dilation for a single lesion had a 59% 3-year patency rate; the 3-year patency rate for grafts requiring multiple dilations was only 6%.

lesions but noted that the small number of longer lesions included in their patient population may well have introduced significant bias.

Marin and colleagues have recently examined the histopathology of 15 vein graft lesions excised from 14 patients with failing infrainguinal reconstructions.[10] Each lesion was focal with a mean length of 2 cm, yet neointimal thickness differed dramatically. After ex vivo angioplasty, luminal dilation varied with the initial thickness of the intimal lesions. In addition, the more cellular lesions, which initially responded favorably to angioplasty, consistently developed multiple intimal flaps that might have compromised the ultimate result. These ex vivo studies document yet an additional subset that, on the basis of qualitative morphologic differences, may respond differently and explain some of the disparate findings in currently available reports.

The role of balloon angioplasty in the management of vein graft stenoses continues to be controversial. It appears that short-segment focal lesions within vein grafts, particularly in grafts of moderate to large caliber, may benefit from a single attempt at dilation. For longer-segment lesions, especially those in small-caliber grafts, or for recurrent lesions after an initial attempt at angioplasty, surgical revision remains the best alternative.

REFERENCES

1. Whittemore AD, Clowes AW, Couch, NP, Mannick JA. Secondary femoropopliteal reconstruction. Ann Surg 1981; 193:35–42.
2. Perler BA, Osterman FA, Mitchell SE, et al. Balloon dilatation versus surgical revision of infrainguinal autogenous vein graft stenoses: Long-term follow-up. J Cardiovasc Surg (Torino) 1990; 31:656–661.
3. Sanchez LA, Gupta SK, Veith FJ, et al. A ten-year experience with one hundred fifty failing or threatened vein and polytetrafluoroethylene arterial bypass grafts. J Vasc Surg 1991; 14:729–738.
4. Alpert JR, Ring EJ, Berkowitz HD, et al. Treatment of vein graft stenoses by balloon catheter dilatation. JAMA 1979; 242:2769–2771.
5. Ring EJ, Alpert JR, Freiman DB, et al. Early experience with percutaneous transluminal angioplasty using a vinyl balloon catheter. Ann Surg 1980; 191:438–442.
6. Spraygen S, Veith FJ. Vein graft angioplasty with non-balloon catheters. Radiology 1983; 146:224–225.
7. Whittemore AD, Donaldson MC, Polak JF, Mannick JA. Limitations of balloon angioplasty for vein graft stenosis. J Vasc Surg 1991; 14:340–345.
8. Taylor PR, Gould D, Harris P, et al. Balloon dilatation of graft stenoses: Reasons for failure. Br J Surg 1991; 78:371.
9. Berkowitz HD, Fox AD, Deaton DH. Reversed vein graft stenosis: Early diagnosis and management. J Vasc Surg 1992; 15:130–142.
10. Marin ML, Veith FJ, Gordon RF, et al. Analysis of balloon dilatation of human vein graft stenoses. Ann Vasc Surg 1993; 7:2–7.

ANGIOSCOPY IN THE MANAGEMENT OF INFRAINGUINAL OCCLUSIVE ARTERIAL DISEASE

FRANK W. LoGERFO, M.D.
CHRISTOPHER J. KWOLEK, M.D.

The earliest reports of vascular endoscopy are in the cardiac surgery literature, describing the use of rigid scopes with or without distensible balloons attached distally to try to allow visualization of intracardiac structures by displacing blood. However, many of these devices were poorly tolerated from a hemodynamic standpoint.

In the mid-1960s, several groups began to experiment with more flexible scopes in the peripheral vascular system. These scopes were essentially variations of the currently available flexible fiberoptic choledochoscopes, but sacrificed optical quality in exchange for flexibility, allowing further visualization into the more tortuous peripheral vascular system.

Additional reports of clinical series began appearing in the mid-1970s and included Towne and Bernhard's description of vascular endoscopy to evaluate the outcome of 91 arterial reconstructive procedures.[1] Endoscopic abnormalities were discovered in 65% of the vessels examined; however, fewer than half of these findings were considered clinically significant. Finally, no comparison in outcome was made between patients undergoing and not undergoing endoscopy. Thus, the utility of these procedures needed to be evaluated in a prospective randomized fashion.

CURRENT STATUS

The development of small-diameter, high-resolution, flexible endoscopes has allowed the more extensive application of endoscopy in the peripheral vascular system. Most current systems consist of an angioscope with a usable working length of 70 to 120 cm, the greater length being more important for assistance in bypass grafts to the tibial or pedal vessels. The outer diameters of the scopes vary from 0.5 mm to 3 mm. In general, as the size of the scope increases, the size and visual quality of the image improve, along with the ability to add unidirectional deflection of the scope tip or separate irrigation ports or working channels. We have found that an assortment of several scope sizes is useful, depending on the types of procedures being performed. We prefer the 1.4 mm angioscope for almost all distal bypass graft examination, including grafts to the tibial and pedal level. The 2.2 mm angioscope is useful for preparation of arm vein graft segments and bypasses to the popliteal vessels.

With the advent of endoscopic procedures in many different areas of surgery, high-intensity xenon or quartz-halogen light sources have become widely available. These light sources in conjunction with the fiberoptic light systems within the angioscopes have made it possible to obtain high-quality images from scopes less than 3 mm in diameter.

In addition, a miniature video camera and a high-resolution videomonitor are important to enhance the picture transmitted by the angioscope. This setup also eliminates the problems with contamination encountered in earlier systems when the surgeon had to look directly into the eyepiece of the angioscope. A videorecording system is also useful to document the procedure and review the operation later.

Selection of a good irrigation method is critical when performing angioscopy. Larger scopes may have an irrigation port within the scope itself. Unfortunately, we have found that these scopes tend to be too wide for distal bypass procedures. Coaxial irrigation through a 20 gauge angiocath placed through the same side branch as the angioscope, or the use of a 7 Fr irrigation sheath inserted in the end of the vein or through a large side branch work well. The use of a specifically designed irrigation pump allows the surgeon to control the flow of irrigation solution by using a foot pedal with both high and low flow settings. We have found that this system allows us to rapidly clear any blood from the field with the high-flow pedal and then maintain a clear visual field with the low-flow pedal, while limiting the volume of fluid used.[2]

ADVANTAGES AND DISADVANTAGES

The angioscope has several advantages over other methods for monitoring grafts and blood vessels. First, the angioscope provides a direct picture of the luminal surface of the graft or vessel with the equivalent of a three-dimensional view. This can be used for either therapeutic or diagnostic procedures. Therapeutically, the angioscope has been used for many applications including preparation of in situ and nonreversed vein grafts with angioscopically assisted valve lysis and identification of unligated tributaries and retained valve cusps, preparation of arm vein bypass grafts, monitoring endovascular procedures such as atherectomy and laser-assisted angioplasty, the management of intimal flaps secondary to trauma, and assisting in the management of balloon catheter thrombectomy.[3,4] The angioscope has been used for completion studies to evaluate arterial bypass grafts and the distal anastomoses and to evaluate occluded grafts after thrombolytic therapy to identify the reason for graft failure.

Other advantages of the angioscope are that it allows observation of the effect of irrigation on the treated artery or vein segment and allows correction of any defects prior to re-establishing arterial flow in the system. Additionally, it provides an alternative method for visualizing the vascular system in patients with renal failure or a history of contrast media allergy, while requiring no radiation exposure to either the patient or the surgical team.

The ability to monitor directly procedures such as valve lysis helps minimize trauma to the endothelium of the vein graft and obviates the need for entering the vein multiple times to recut missed or poorly cut valves. Finally, visualization of the lumen provides immediate feedback on the technical adequacy and patency of the distal anastomosis.

Several significant disadvantages also should be recognized for angioscopy. First, temporary occlusion of proximal blood flow is necessary, usually through the use of a proximal vascular clamp or an occluding balloon. Second, all blood in the lumen needs to be replaced with a transparent medium, usually a crystalloid solution, and maintained under pressure to prevent backflow from collateral branches or the distal runoff bed.

The ideal angioscope would be durable, reusable, and easy to sterilize, have excellent optical quality, be flexible enough to be passed into the peripheral vascular system without causing endothelial trauma, be steerable with an irrigation port and a port for endovascular intervention, and be small enough and long enough to reach into the lumen of the most distal vessel in the lower extremity. Unfortunately, no ideal angioscope exists. However, we have found that using a combination of different types of scopes allows the surgeon to choose those that are the most important for the procedure being performed.

A concern expressed by some has been the potential for fluid overload in the high-risk population undergoing vascular surgical procedures. Although this concern is valid, we have found through a prospective randomized study performed at our own institution that the average amount of fluid required for most studies can be limited to less than 400 ml. In addition, the overall cardiac morbidity and mortality are no greater in patients undergoing angioscopy. It should be noted, however, that these results have been achieved by developing a close working relationship with the anesthesiologists with respect to perioperative fluid management and the aggressive use of hemodynamic monitoring techniques.[5]

With angioscopy, there is the potential for injury of the vessel lumen by either direct trauma from the scope or from distention of the vessel from intraluminal irrigation. These problems can be compounded by scopes without an attached steering mechanism. We have found that by carefully distending all grafts prior to inserting the scope, and by choosing an angioscope that is small enough to fit easily within the lumen of the vessel, we have not encountered any significant problems with injury to the vessel wall. The careful use of the irrigation pump allows us to minimize the total volume of fluid required while keeping the pressure inside the lumen within a physiologic range. In addition, even nonsteerable scopes can be manipulated by gently torquing the scope and carefully applying external pressure to the vessel wall with minimal apparent trauma to the lumen.

Another potential drawback to the use of angioscopy is its sensitivity in identifying irregularities within the vessel lumen. A recent prospective randomized trial from the group at Dartmouth evaluated the use of duplex scanning, angioscopy, and arteriography during the course of in situ saphenous vein bypass grafting.[6] This study documented that angioscopy was more sensitive in detecting residual unligated side branches and in identifying residual or partially cut valve cusps than either duplex scanning or arteriography. In addition, angioscopy was able to correctly evaluate the adequacy of the distal anastomosis without any of the false-positive findings that occurred with arteriography. We have had similar results with angioscopically assisted distal bypasses.[7] Whereas the angioscope was found to be very sensitive in identifying abnormalities, more than 85% of the findings were related to potential problems with the conduit, and a small percentage were related to the distal anastomosis or runoff vessel. This increased sensitivity has led some to question the clinical significance of these findings because the majority of the abnormalities in the conduit are related to identifying unligated tributaries or partially cut valve cusps.

CURRENT TECHNIQUE

Our current technique of angioscopic evaluation and valve lysis has been previously described; however, several points are worth reviewing. Angioscopically directed valve lysis for nonreversed saphenous vein and arm vein segments should be performed ex vivo to eliminate the possibility of the patient receiving fluid during the course of vein graft preparation. When performing valve lysis for the in situ bypass grafts, we have found it useful to expose the saphenous vein completely and ligate any major venous side branches prior to performing valve lysis. This helps to minimize the volume of fluid the patient receives. We have not found the technique of exposing individual side branches to be useful in those patients with long in situ grafts with multiple side branches because of the large amounts of fluid often required to maintain a clear visual field. Once the largest branches have been ligated, a flexible valvulotome with interchangeable cutting heads can be introduced through the distal end of the vein graft to perform valve lysis with minimal trauma to the endothelium.

Completion angioscopic studies can also be performed to evaluate the conduit and the distal anastomosis once the graft is in place. For reversed vein bypass grafts, we perform angioscopy after the distal anastomosis has been completed and the graft has been placed in the proper anatomic position. The angioscope can then be inserted through a small sheath introduced into the open proximal end of the distended vein graft. This allows the surgeon to evaluate the distal anastomosis and the lie of the graft itself. For in situ and nonreversed grafts, both anastomoses are completed and the angioscope is inserted through a proximal vein side branch. An irrigation catheter or small needle is inserted in the same or an adjacent side branch, and the angioscope is advanced to the distal anastomosis with flow still in the graft. The inflow is then occluded, and the vein graft is flushed until all of the blood has been removed. Angioscopic inspection is then performed on withdrawal of the scope to minimize the amount of fluid that the patient receives. Using this technique, we have effectively visualized the distal artery, anastomosis, and vein graft in more than 90% of patients.

We routinely use a pH-balanced electrolyte solution, such as Normasol, for irrigation without the addition of heparin sodium and have not experienced any problems with graft thrombosis. However, we routinely heparinize patients prior to occluding any vessels with 50 to 75 units/kg of intravenous heparin sodium. All grafts are initially distended and irrigated with normosal plus heparin sodium and papaverine to eliminate venospasm.

When using the angioscope for the evaluation of thrombolytic therapy in occluded grafts, we insert the scope directly into the lumen of the occluded vessel through a cut-down site. Irrigation can be performed through an angiocath or an irrigation sheath placed directly into the vessel lumen.

At present, the value of angioscopy is in the improved preparation of autogenous venous conduits. Although blind valve lysis is successful, direct visualization of valve lysis is advantageous. Most surgeons, upon directly viewing valve lysis and confirming incompetency of the cut leaflets, are convinced that this is advantageous. This is especially true with arm vein conduits where pre-existing intraluminal defects are frequently present.[8] These are usually a result of venipunctures or introduction of catheters and are manifested by scar formation, webs, and bands across the lumen. Also, at times the vein may appear abnormal on external inspection but have a clear lumen with a smooth endothelial surface. In complex arm vein preparation using the basilic-antecubital-cephalic conduit, angioscopy is especially helpful.[9] Here the valves are cut in the basilic portion, the cephalic segment is not reversed, and the antecubital segment is left in continuity.

Complex redo vein grafting often involves translocated nonreversed segments, sometimes as composite grafts with reversed segments. Angioscopy provides a superb method for evaluating the status of the completed conduit. Additional benefits of angioscopy, such as identification of untied tributaries with in situ grafts and inspection of the distal anastomosis, are probably of less importance. Inspection of the distal anastomosis by angioscopy is highly effective, but it is probably not significantly advantageous to routine completion angiography.[10]

REFERENCES

1. Towne JB, Bernhard VM. Vascular endoscopy: Useful tool or interesting toy. Surgery 1977; 82:415–419.
2. Miller A, Campbell DR, Gibbons GW, et al. Routine intraoperative angioscopy in lower extremity revascularization. Arch Surg 1989; 124:604–608.
3. Fleisher HM, Thompson BW, McGowan TC, et al. Angioscopically monitored saphenous vein valvulotomy. J Vasc Surg 1986; 4:360–364.
4. White GH, White RA, Kopchok GE, et al. Endoscopic intravascular surgery removes intraluminal flaps, dissections, and thrombus. J Vasc Surg 1990; 11:280–288.
5. Kwolek CJ, Miller A, Stonebridge PA, et al. Safety of saline irrigation for angioscopy: Results of a prospective randomized trial. Ann Vasc Surg 1992; 6:62–68.
6. Gilbertson JJ, Walsh DB, Zwolak RM, et al. A blinded comparison of angiography, angioscopy, and duplex scanning in the intraoperative evaluation of in situ saphenous vein bypass grafts. J Vasc Surg 1992; 15:121–129.
7. Miller A, Stonebridge PA, Jepsen SJ, et al. Continued experience with intraoperative angioscopy for monitoring infrainguinal bypass grafting. Surgery 1991; 109:286–293.
8. Stonebridge PA, Miller A, Tsoukas A, et al. Angioscopy of arm vein infrainguinal bypass grafts. Ann Vasc Surg 1991; 5:170–175.
9. LoGerfo FW, Paniszyn C, Menzoian JO. A new arm vein graft for distal bypass. J Vasc Surg 1987; 5:889–891.
10. Miller A, Marcaccio EJ, Tannenbaum GA, et al. Comparison of angioscopy and angiography for monitoring infrainguinal bypass vein grafts: Results of a prospective randomized trial. J Vasc Surg 1993; 17:382–398.

INTRAVASCULAR ULTRASOUND FOR IMAGING OF DISEASED ARTERIES

RODNEY A. WHITE, M.D.

Intravascular ultrasound (IVUS) imaging has developed in the last 5 years and provides a new perspective from which to view cardiovascular disease. High-resolution transmural images of the vessel allow investigation of pathology and the effects of interventions in a unique way. The thrust of current IVUS development is to incorporate it as an adjunct to coronary and peripheral angioplasty procedures, providing both endovascular device guidance and accurate assessment of the intervention.

COMPARISON WITH OTHER CATHETER IMAGING MODALITIES

Various invasive catheter-based techniques to image vascular pathology and to provide angioplasty guidance are being utilized, including contrast angiography, angioscopy, spectroscopy, and IVUS. Each method provides unique information regarding vascular diseases.

Contrast arteriography is considered the standard for imaging the distribution and severity of vascular lesions. Uniplanar arteriography is accurate in defining vessel luminal dimensions and cross-sectional area if the luminal profile is circular, as it is in most normal or mildly diseased arteries. In advanced disease, however, arteriography provides limited information regarding the morphology and extent of disease in the arterial wall, aside from documenting visible calcification and the topography of the luminal surface. In instances where the lumen is elliptical or eccentric, biplanar arteriograms may be required to more accurately define luminal cross-sectional areas and calculate percent-area stenosis. It has been shown that arteriography is restricted in imaging vessels with substantial luminal ellipticity, usually overestimating the luminal cross-sectional areas and underestimating the degrees of stenosis.[1]

Angioscopy is useful in determining the diagnosis and etiology of vascular diseases, evaluating the technical success of vascular interventions, and visualizing intraluminal instrumentation.[2] Studies have documented that angioscopy reveals clinically important information that is not apparent by extraluminal inspection or arteriography in 20% to 30% of vascular procedures and that this information frequently alters the therapeutic approach. During angioplasty, the most valuable applications of angioscopy may be in preprocedure and postprocedure assessment of arterial morphology, rather than in directly monitoring the procedure. Of special benefit is the capability of immediately examining the vessel for complications and gaining a three-dimensional representation of the vessel lumen and the adequacy of recanalization.

Spectroscopic analysis is a developing method of intraluminal guidance that relies on the principle that tissues not only absorb laser energy but also re-emit the energy at different wavelengths. Because normal blood vessel constituents have different spectroscopic patterns from atherosclerotic tissue, spectroscopic analysis has been useful in enhancing the target specificity of laser energy. Target-specific laser angioplasty has been investigated extensively using emitted fluororescent patterns, but complications such as vessel perforation and dissection have not been significantly reduced with this technology.

INTRAVASCULAR ULTRASOUND IMAGING

In the early 1970s, 360° cross-sectional intraluminal ultrasound imaging of vascular structures became available. This was achieved by scanning the ultrasound beam through a full circle and synchronizing the beam direction and deflection on the display, either by mechanically rotating the imaging elements or by electronically switching a transducer array (Fig. 1).

Electronically switched array devices use frequencies of 10 to 30 MHz in 4 to 12 Fr catheters to produce cross-sectional images of the vascular segment being examined. The catheters are flexible, and image resolution is excellent; however, a bright circumferential artifact known as the ring down surrounds the catheter and prevents imaging of structures in the area immediately surrounding the catheter. Mechanical transducers use one of two basic configurations, either the transducer itself or an acoustic mirror that is rotated at the tip of the catheter using a flexible, high-torque cable that extends the length of the device.

Several studies have reported that IVUS is accurate in determining the luminal and vessel wall morphology of normal or minimally diseased arteries both in vitro and in vivo[3] (Fig. 2). In muscular arteries, distinct sonographic layers are visible with the media appearing as an echolucent layer between the more echodense intima and adventitia. Even small intimal lesions such as flaps or tears are well visualized because of their high fibrous tissue content and the difference in echoic properties of these structures when compared with surrounding blood. The three-layer appearance of muscular arteries is not readily seen in larger vessels such as the aorta because of the increased elastin content in the media.

Intravascular ultrasound devices are sensitive in differentiating calcified and noncalcified vascular lesions. Because the ultrasound energy is strongly reflected by calcific plaque, it appears as a bright image with dense acoustic shadowing behind it. Gussenhoven and colleagues described four plaque components that can be distinguished using 40 MHz IVUS in vitro:[4] (1)

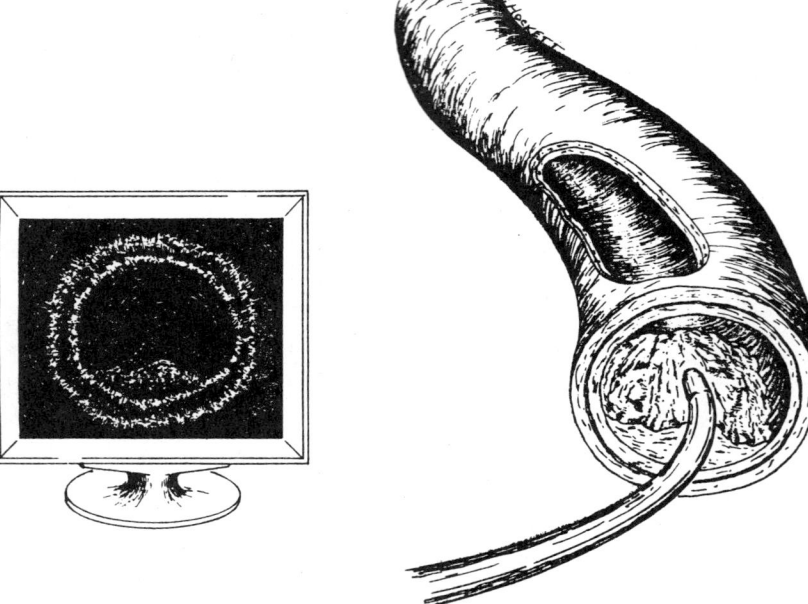

Figure 1 Schematic of intravascular ultrasound (IVUS) catheter imaging. The IVUS catheter is advanced through the vessel lumen *(right)* and displays a real-time cross-sectional vessel image on a gray scale monitor *(left)*. (From Cavaye DM, White RA. Intravascular ultrasound: Basic principles, techniques and applications. In: Cavaye DM, White RA, eds. Arterial imaging: Modern and developing technology. London: Chapman & Hall, 1993:109, with permission.)

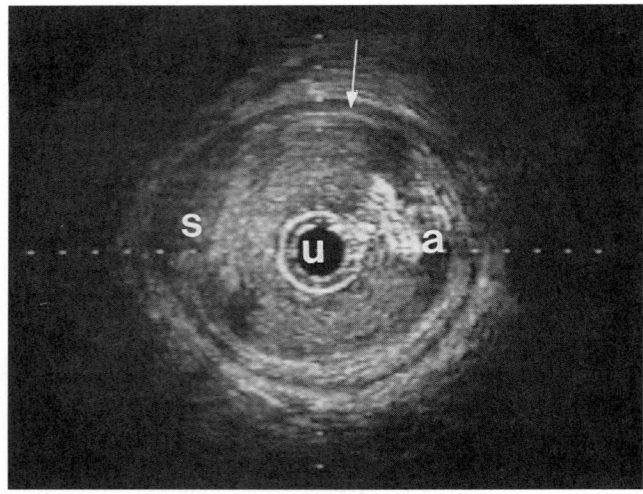

Figure 2 Intravascular ultrasound image of a human iliac artery. *U,* Ultrasound probe; *arrow,* normal vessel wall demonstrating a three-layered appearance of a muscular artery wall; *s,* soft plaque; *a,* artifact produced by a thin metalic wire along the axis of the catheter.

echolucent, which is lipid; (2) soft echoes, fibromuscular tissue and intimal proliferation, including varying amounts of lipid; (3) bright echoes, collagen-rich fibrous tissue; and (4) bright echoes with acoustic shadowing, calcified tissue.

Recent advances in echographic image processing and computer technology have resulted in the availability of on-line three-dimensional IVUS image construction, using a personal computer–based system. Computerized reconstruction produces a solid, surface-tracked model of the vessel by "stacking" a longitudinally aligned set (up to 300 images per set) of consecutive two-dimensional IVUS images. Three-dimensional IVUS has a unique potential to display vascular pathology and atherosclerotic lesion volume, distribution, and tissue characteristics, which are particularly relevant to evaluating the severity of lesions and for determining therapy (Fig. 3).

Clinical Utility

Intravascular ultrasound imaging displays vascular pathology and documents the immediate results of interventions in a unique way. Its advantages over other vascular imaging modalities include defining the transmural distribution of disease within the vessel, characterizing plaques and intimal lesions, and providing accurate cross-sectional information regarding luminal and vessel wall morphology before and after endovascular interventions.

An example of the potential of IVUS is emphasized by recent studies comparing 2D and 3D IVUS to arteriography and 3D computed tomography for imaging abdominal aortic aneurysms.[5] Each modality provides unique information regarding the anatomy of the aorta and the distribution of components of the aneurysm (Fig. 4).

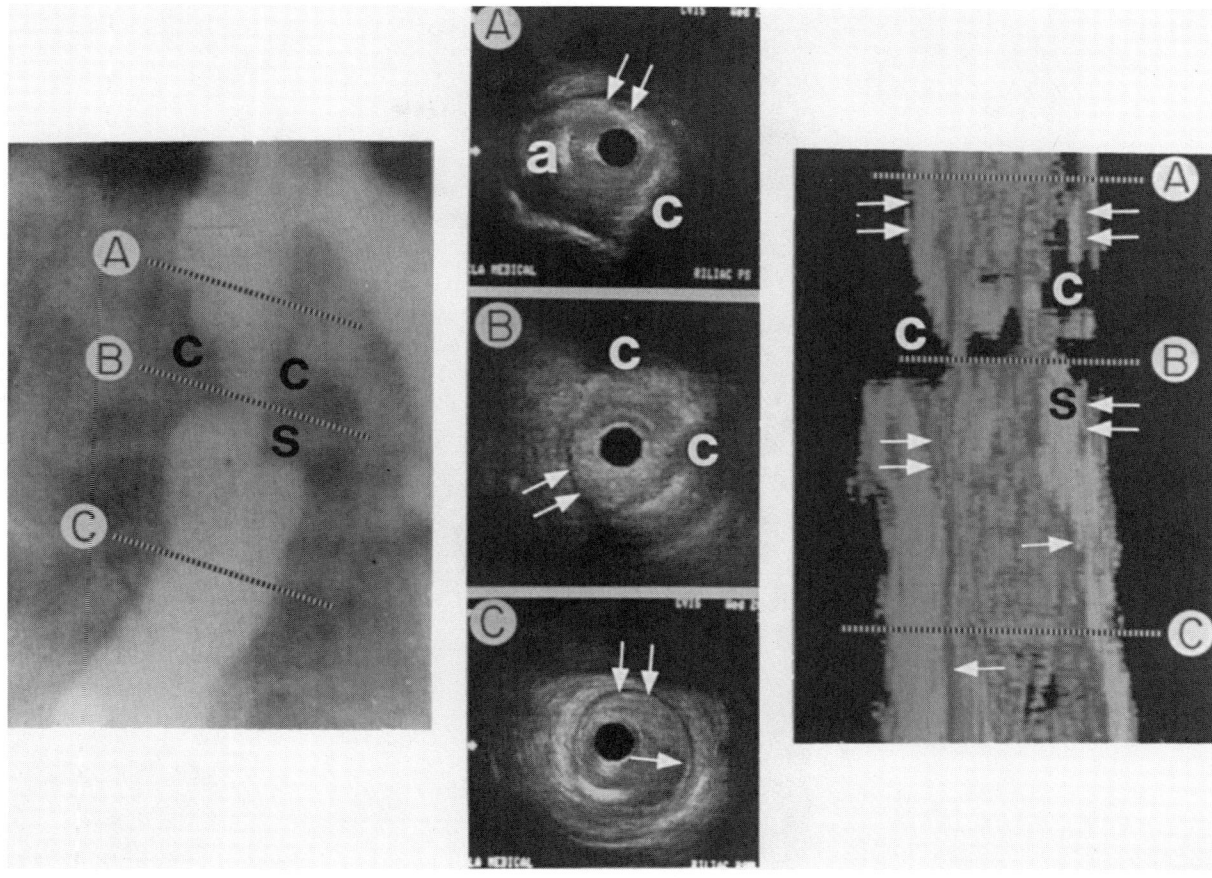

Figure 3 Arteriogram *(left)*, two-dimensional intravascular ultrasound, IVUS *(center)*, and three-dimensional IVUS *(right)* of an atherosclerotic human iliac artery. The labels *A, B,* and *C* correspond to same sites on the arteriogram and the three-dimensional ultrasound reconstruction. In the ultrasound images, double arrows mark the hypoechoic media in this muscular artery, and the single arrows mark the luminal surface in relatively normal segments of the artery. Calcified areas *(c)* in the lesion are differentiated from soft plaque *(s)* by attenuation of the image beyond the calcification *(a)* wire artifact in image *A*. (From Cavaye DM, White RA. Intravascular ultrasound: Redefining vascular imaging using 2-D & 3-D reconstruction. J Vasc Surg 1992; 15:1081 (letter); with permission.)

During cardiovascular procedures, conventional arteriography has been unable to provide adequately sensitive data regarding the effects of interventions. For meaningful critical assessment of endoluminal procedures, plaque consistency and distribution of residual lesions following an intervention must be known. Intravascular ultrasound imaging provides the ability to accurately measure percent stenoses produced by a lesion by displaying the transmural pathology, whereas arteriography is limited to assessment of percent stenoses by comparing luminal dimensions to normal-appearing adjacent reference vessels.

IVUS is useful in the investigation of arterial wall dissections by determining the size, location, and extent of intimal flaps. Because IVUS is a dynamic, real-time imaging modality, the movement of artery wall segments with systolic-diastolic blood flow can be seen. The precise location and orientation of a flap is important because it may determine the need for excision and grafting or repair by intraluminal stents.[6,7] Three-dimensional IVUS imaging is especially useful because aortic dissection commonly results in a spiral or complex flap that is difficult to appreciate on arteriograms alone. Three-dimensional reconstructions allow identification of the dissection entry site, extent of the flap, and relation of the false lumen to major visceral branches.

Recent studies have documented that percutaneous transluminal balloon angioplasty balloon size is often underestimated when selection is made by using quantitative arteriography and that optimal balloon size is more accurately determined by IVUS. Additional IVUS findings suggest that arteriographic success of balloon angioplasty is more likely when hard lesions are disrupted with dissections extending into the media of the vessel, whereas failure is seen in lesions that are nondisplaceable or when circumferential dissections or intimal flaps occur. Arteriographic success in soft lesions is associated with superficial fissures or fractures of the luminal surface, whereas vessel recoil and luminal disruption or thrombosis at sites of plaque rupture lead

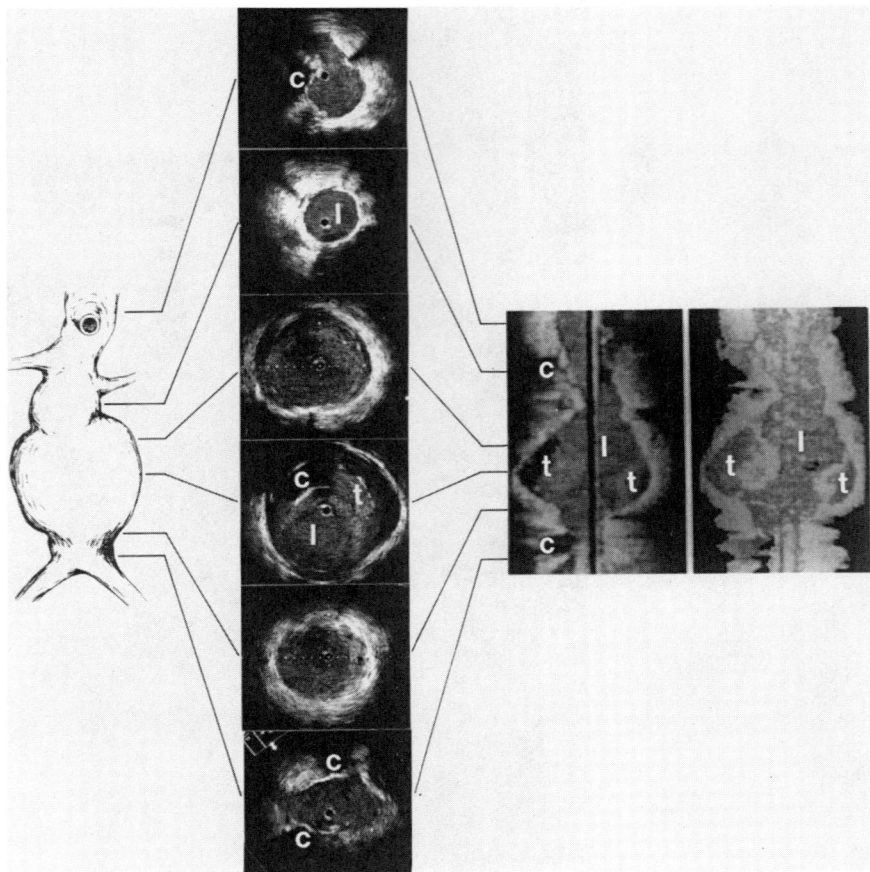

Figure 4 Selected cross-sectional images of the aorta and aneurysm at various levels *(center)* compared to a schematic diagram of the lesion *(left)* and the longitudinal gray scale and three-dimensional intravascular ultrasound images *(right)* of the aneurysm. Note the evidence of thrombus *(t)* and calcification *(c)* at several levels throughout the length of the vessel *(l)*. Lumen. (From White RA, Scoccianti M, Back M, et al. Innovations in vascular imaging: Angiography, 3D CT and 2D and 3D intravascular ultrasound of an abdominal aortic aneurysm, Ann Vasc Surg 1994; 8:285–289; with permission.)

to failure. For these reasons, IVUS may be valuable in providing information that will be used to choose lesions suitable for balloon dilation therapy.[8,9]

Intravascular ultrasound also provides a method to guide deployment and assess the effect of intravascular stents in peripheral vessels. It allows selection of the correct stent size and is useful in identifying the most appropriate site for stenting. The decision to place a stent and guidance for the deployment are based on two- and three-dimensional image reconstruction. Also, adequacy of deployment and changes in morphology produced by the stent can be seen.

Future angioplasty guidance devices may combine the benefits of arteriography, angioscopy, and IVUS in delivery systems suitable for guided assessment and recanalization of lesions (Fig. 5). Angioscopy would allow visual inspection of the lumen with ultrasound determining the vessel wall characteristics and dimensions. Arteriography would allow assessment of smaller, distal vessels, providing an objective assessment of vascular outflow. An added benefit of IVUS-based guidance of devices would be the ability to select an appropriate

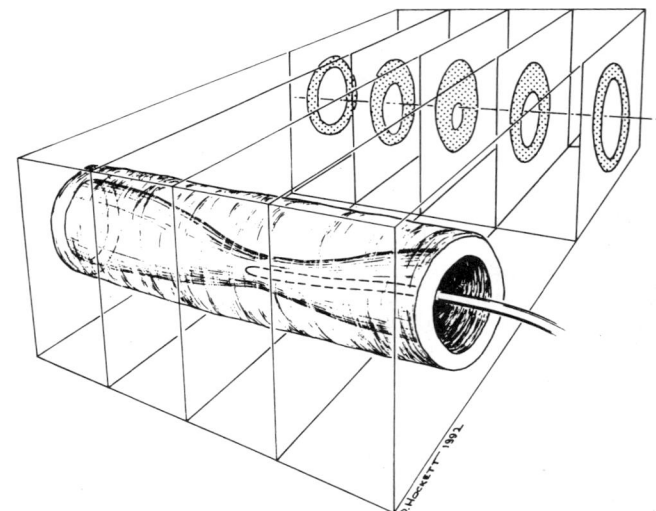

Figure 5 Schematic of the guidance provided by intravascular ultrasound for a catheter-based interventional device through the lumen of an atherosclerotic artery.

ablation method for particular plaque types or volumes. Recent advances in IVUS technology also provide forward-look imaging that may be useful in treating occluded arteries. In the future, IVUS will also provide opportunities in vascular research, including the investigation of blood vessel dynamics caused by disease or intervention and the natural history of atherosclerosis.

REFERENCES

1. Tabbara MR, White RA, Cavaye DM, Kopchok GE. In vivo human comparison of intravascular ultrasound and angiography. J Vasc Surg 1991; 14:496–502.
2. White GH, White RA, eds. Angioscopy: Vascular and coronary applications. St Louis: Mosby–Year Book, 1989.
3. Gussenhoven WJ, Essed CE, Lancee CT. Arterial wall characteristics determined by intravascular ultrasound imaging: An in vitro study. J Am Coll Cardiol 1989; 14:947–952.
4. Gussenhoven WJ, Essed CE, Frietman P, et al. Intravascular echographic assessment of vessel wall characteristics: A correlation with histology. Int J Card Imaging 1989; 4:105–116.
5. White RA, Scoccianti M, Back M, et al. Innovations in vascular imaging: Angiography, 3D CT and 2D and 3D intravascular ultrasound of an abdominal aortic aneurysm. Ann Vasc Surg 1994; 8:285–289.
6. Cavaye DM, French WJ, White RA, et al. Intravascular ultrasound imaging of an acute dissecting aortic aneurysm: A case report. J Vasc Surg 1991; 13:510–512.
7. Cavaye DM, White RA, Lerman RD, et al. Usefulness of intravascular ultrasound for detecting experimentally induced aortic dissection in dogs and for determining the effectiveness of endoluminal stenting. Am J Cardiol 1992; 69:705–707.
8. Hoyne J, Mahon DJ, Jain A, et al. Morphological effects of coronary balloon angioplasty in vivo assessed by intravascular ultrasound. Circulation 1992; 85:1012–1025.
9. Gerritsen GP, Gussenhoven EJ, The SHK, et al. Intravascular ultrasonography before and after intervention: In vivo comparison with angiography J Vasc Surg 1993; 18:31–40.

NONOPERATIVE, NONPHARMACOLOGIC MANAGEMENT OF LOWER EXTREMITY OCCLUSIVE DISEASE

ROBERT A. GRAOR, M.D.

Whether or not an operation to treat lower extremity ischemia is needed, a program of nonpharmacologic treatment should be prescribed. A well-performed operation does not affect the atherogenic process, either in the region of the operation or elsewhere. Although operation may bypass the disease, it is hardly an optimal path to health.

Three important tenets of nonpharmacologic treatment of lower extremity disease are (1) prevent the progression of atherosclerotic disease, (2) improve the blood supply to the limb by stimulating the development of collateral circulation, and (3) protect the leg from injury. This chapter explores treatment options and reviews common risk factors and risk factor control, as well as other beneficial nonpharmacologic measures to treat lower extremity occlusive disease.

PREVENTION OF ATHEROSCLEROTIC DISEASE PROGRESSION

Diet

Although coronary artery disease (CAD) remains the leading cause of mortality in patients with peripheral vascular disease, it is strictly an illness of Western civilization and those of other cultures who have adopted the Western lifestyle. Diet is considered to be an important lifestyle factor. Americans consume 135 pounds of fat per year, 1 ton every 15 years, and 4 tons of fat and oils by the age of 60. If it is agreed that fat and oils are directly related to the development of atherosclerotic plaque, it is not surprising that we develop this progressive disease. Roberts reported that there is but one true risk factor for coronary artery disease, namely, the lifetime presence of a serum cholesterol level over 150 mg/dl.[1] In some patients, a low cholesterol level has been shown to reverse the process of atherosclerosis, and in many situations it has been demonstrated to arrest the process.

Although creative nutritional therapy—that is, aggressive and strict dietary cholesterol restriction—in conjunction with other standard medical therapy has not been compared with surgical therapy, it seems by nonparallel evaluations that equivalent results may be able to be achieved. A wealth of epidemiologic, clinical, and laboratory data now link elements of the diet, specifically dietary saturated fat and cholesterol, to the incidence of CAD and atherogenesis. Those who deal with peripheral vascular disease need to accept that coronary atherogenesis may be similar, albeit not necessarily identical, to the development of peripheral vascular disease. Indirect, interventional studies have indicated that alterations in serum cholesterol may affect disease progression involving the superficial femoral artery.

Dietary interventional studies have shown some evidence that this is true. Two studies have documented a decline in CAD rates associated with decreasing saturated fat and serum cholesterol levels.[2,3] Another study, examining the effects of both diet-induced cholesterol reduction and smoking cessation, documented a substantial initial decline (47%) in first-time coronary events and, after more than 8 years of follow-up, a significantly lower (33%) total mortality in the treated group compared with subjects having unchanged dietary and smoking habits.[4] The major differences between the two groups appear to be largely due to dietary cholesterol lowering because the difference in smoking rates between the two groups was only marginal. Although these studies do not directly reflect progression or regression of peripheral vascular disease, it is clear that these patients die from coronary disease and, therefore, we need to control risk factors associated with their major cause of death.

The effect of dietary cholesterol on blood cholesterol has been a subject of debate. Without engaging in this debate, it is probably safe to make the following statements: First, both dietary cholesterol and saturated fat can raise circulating levels of total cholesterol and low-density lipoprotein (LDL); however, saturated dietary fat is three to four times as potent as dietary cholesterol in raising blood cholesterol levels. Second, in large population studies, dietary cholesterol and saturated fat predict average circulating cholesterol levels with some individual variability, but this is of little relevance to public health recommendations. Third, there is growing evidence that dietary cholesterol and saturated fat each may predict coronary risk independent of its effects on circulating cholesterol levels. Thus, the observed effects of these factors on circulating total and LDL cholesterol levels may reflect only a portion of their atherogenic capability. This may in part explain why interrelationships among dietary fat, blood cholesterol, and coronary heart disease rates have been difficult to demonstrate within populations.

Circulating lipoprotein levels also seem to be influenced by other dietary fats, including so-called omega-6-polyunsaturated fats, found primarily in temperate zone vegetable oils (corn, cotton seed, soybean, and safflower) and omega-3-fatty acids found in deep sea and cold water fish. Omega-6-polyunsaturated fats appear to lower total and LDL cholesterol levels with about half of the potency with which saturated fats raise those levels. However, when these vegetable fats are consumed, the levels of high-density lipoprotein (HDL cholesterol) may fall; moreover, the effects of these fats on coronary heart disease rates in populations are not well understood because no population naturally takes in large amounts of omega-6 fats.

The observation that omega-3-fatty acids lowered CAD rates was stimulated by the lack of this disease among Eskimos, Japanese, Dutch, and some U.S. populations that ingest large or moderate amounts of fish. Whether this effect was directly related to fish oils is unclear, although omega-3 oils do reduce blood levels of both fasting and postprandial triglyceride-carrying lipoproteins and interfere with platelet aggregation. Conversely, fish oils have been repeatedly shown to raise the blood level of LDL cholesterol. The LDL-raising effect has been demonstrated in individuals with diabetes mellitus and isolated hypertriglyceridemia and in those with combined elevations of cholesterol and triglycerides.

Ultimately, one can make a case that the major benefit of polyunsaturates in fish oils is that they serve as dietary substitutes for calories that otherwise would be derived from saturated fat. Therefore, the LDL-lowering effects may be simply a consequence of saturated fat calories that are not ingested.

Alcohol

Epidemiologic and clinical studies have shown moderate alcohol intake to be associated with lower rates in CAD in men and women and higher plasma levels of HDL cholesterol and the major HDL apolipoproteins, AI and AII. On balance, there seems to be little reason to encourage alcohol ingestion as a cardioprotective mechanism because the presumed benefits are very modest, and it is well known that alcohol aggravates obesity, hypertension, and hypertriglyceridemia, it tends to promote antisocial behavior, and there is a significant risk of addiction.

Dietary Guidelines

Based on the preceding data, several health care agencies have made public recommendations for healthy dietary intake. These prominent programs and societies have all endorsed the consumption of a low-cholesterol, low-saturated fat diet by all adult Americans.

The saturated fat intake of U.S. citizens is estimated to be about 15% of total daily calories, and daily cholesterol intake is about 300 to 500 mg. All published guidelines advocate that saturated fat intake be limited to 10% or less of total calories and cholesterol intake to less than 300 mg/day. These recommendations generally stipulate that less than 30% of calories come from total fat intake, with 10% provided by polyunsaturated fat and 10% by monosaturated fat. The remaining caloric needs are to be made up by carbohydrate (50% to 60%) and protein (10% to 20%).

Smoking

A recent report published by the U.S. Surgeon General clearly stated, "Cigarette smoking is the single, most powerful risk factor for peripheral vascular disease." In fact, multivariant analyses suggest that smoking has an independent effect greater than other risk factors, and it also appears to be a more important risk factor for the development of peripheral arterial disease than for ischemic heart disease.[5] The extent to which smoking contributes to the development of disease has also been calculated from cross-sectional studies, where current smoking is an independent risk factor and appears to contribute to between 14% and 53% of disease. In the Framingham Study, 16 years of follow-up suggested that 78% of cases of intermittent claudication could be attributed to smoking.

The possible pathogenic mechanisms of smoking are

many. Cigarette smoking transiently enhances adhesiveness of platelets, raises blood pressure, accelerates heart rate, and lowers the ventricular fibrillation threshold. At the same time, the oxygen-carrying capacity of the blood is reduced by the accumulation of carboxyhemoglobin, and tissue utilization of myoglobin is impaired. These effects, coupled with the acute stimulation of catecholamine release and increased myocardial oxygen demand probably account for only part of the effects of smoking. Therefore, smoking is one of the strongest predictors of cardiovascular disease and, in particular, the progression of peripheral arterial disease.

STIMULATION OF COLLATERAL DEVELOPMENT

Because a common manifestation of peripheral arterial disease is intermittent claudication, understanding the mechanism of intermittent claudication and improving the deficits that produce this symptom are integral to the overall treatment. Intermittent claudication results from muscle ischemia due to blood flow inadequate to meet the muscle oxygen demand during exercise. The primary outcome of peripheral bypass reconstruction is to relieve claudication and improve blood flow to the lower extremity and to produce limb salvage. It has been noted that changes in an ankle-brachial index (ABI) or calf blood flow may not adequately reflect or predict the effects of operation on the ability to walk without claudication pain. Similarly, exercise performance in these patients has been shown to correlate poorly with peripheral arterial hemodynamics. Additionally, extremity revascularization for the treatment of disabling intermittent claudication significantly improves treadmill performance, but the degree of improvement is not predicted from the location or extent of surgical reconstruction or from the change of the ABI.[6] However, it is true that when control subjects are placed on an exercise program and followed over time, there is no spontaneous improvement in treadmill exercise performance or self-reported walking ability. Therefore, in patients who have had bypass operations and improved their walking capability or functional status, these changes can be attributed only to the bypass operation.

It was noted in the study by Regensteiner and colleagues that patients who underwent bypass operations for claudication had an increase in muscle oxygen consumption postoperatively. Their subjects had an entry peak oxygen consumption ($\dot{V}O_2$) of 15.5 ml/kg/minute, which indicated an ability to perform only very light activity such as driving a car, sitting at a desk, or self-care. Six weeks after operation, an increase in the $\dot{V}O_2$ to 19.1 ml/kg/minute allowed patients to perform activities requiring moderate energy expenditure such as vigorous walking, bicycling, or gardening. However, the lack of further increase in $\dot{V}O_2$ at 12 weeks and the stagnation of $\dot{V}O_2$ values at levels lower than those of normal age-matched values, suggested that additional factors such as deconditioning continued to limit the ability to attain higher age-matched $\dot{V}O_2$ values. These investigations found no relationship between the initial ABI or the change in ABI and the improvement in exercise ability resulting from operation. They also disclosed that neither the anatomic location of the arterial occlusive disease nor the number of diseased segments operated on predicted functional outcome.

Studies of patients with peripheral arterial occlusive disease who have undergone exercise conditioning reported an increase in treadmill exercise performance and less severe claudication pain during exercise. This consistent finding demonstrates that exercise training programs can have a clinically important impact on functional capacity in patients for whom other treatment options are limited and for whom spontaneous recovery does not occur. It is clear from studies that training with constant load treadmill protocols can result in improvement of walking distance and walking with less claudication pain. In studies that employ graded exercise protocols, at a given submaximal workload, exercise training leads to decreases in heart rate, ventilation, and oxygen consumption. These changes may contribute to the ability to sustain walking exercise for a longer time before claudication pain limits the activity. It is also noted from these studies that the severity of arterial disease does not appear to affect the training response. In one study, patients with ischemic rest pain improved as much as those who were only mildly or moderately affected by claudication. Other studies confirm this observation in that the ankle-arm index at rest could predict only 10% of the increased walking distance on the treadmill after an exercise program. Also, disease location and associated condition, such as CAD, do not limit the ability to receive benefit from a training program. Therefore, patients should not be excluded from consideration for a training program simply on the basis of the severity of their illness or other confounding illnesses.

Methods of Exercise Rehabilitation

A formal supervised exercise program should be individualized and most commonly uses a treadmill. Generally, the patient exercises three times a week for approximately 1 hour each time, and a 3 month period of training is customary. A 5 minute warmup precedes every session, and a 5 minute cool down follows to minimize the risk of injury. The warmup period is designed to increase the heart rate slowly and promote flexibility; it should involve the use of large muscle groups, especially the muscles used for walking. The cool-down period is designed to return the heart rate to baseline value and primarily involves stretching the large muscle groups, particularly those in the legs. Gait abnormalities can be treated through the attention of a physical therapist who works with the patient to normalize gait. Muscular weakness can be treated by strengthening exercises and the help of a physical therapist.

If exercise programs are not available, the patient

should be encouraged to warm up and cool down and aim for a goal of at least 1 hour of walking exercise daily. The patient should not stop walking at the first sign of claudication, but should continue as far as possible until the discomfort requires stopping. However, the patient should be warned not to continue walking if chest pain develops. Other forms of exercise for the legs include jogging, cycling, and swimming. The use of a stationary bike can also be encouraged but should not replace walking, if walking is possible.

MEASURES TO PROTECT LEGS AND FEET

Prevention of trauma from mechanical, chemical, or thermal injuries is a very important step in all patients with critically ischemic limbs. Gangrenous changes from trauma are potentially preventable in half of the patients who develop these changes if proper precautions are exercised in caring for the feet.

Mild soap and water should be used to clean the feet, which should then be rinsed with clear water. Water temperatures should not exceed 35 to 37.7°C. Lanolin creams should be applied to the skin to prevent cracking and chafing from skin dryness. Footwear should be tailored to the individual patient, accommodating abnormalities in the foot and avoiding pressure areas. Current available tennis shoes seem to be practical footwear for patients with ischemic lower extremities.

Nail care has to be rendered cautiously by the physician or podiatrist when arterial insufficiency is present.

In general, protective pads, bandages, and bulky footwear are reserved for only those patients with severe arterial insufficiency. These patients with severe ischemic rest pain can be improved with elevation of the head of the bed 4 to 6 inches. Prolonged dependency of the feet by sitting should be avoided because this posture favors the development of orthostatic edema that can further impair capillary circulation.

REFERENCES

1. Roberts WC. Atherosclerosis risk factors: are there ten or is there only one? Am J Cardiol 1989; 64:552–554.
2. Dayton S, Pearce ML, Hashimoto S, et al. A controlled clinical trial of a diet high in unsaturated fat in preventing complications of atherosclerosis. Circulation 1969; 39–40(suppl 20):1–63.
3. Leren P. The Oslo Diet/Heart Study eleven-year report. Circulation 1970; 42:835–942.
4. Holme I, Hjermann I, Helgeland I, Wren P. The Oslo Study: Diet and anti-smoking advice; additional results from a five-year primary prevention trial in middle-aged men. Prev Med 1985; 14:279–292.
5. Gordon T, Kannel WB. Predisposition to atherosclerosis in the head, heart and legs. JAMA 1972; 221:661–666.
6. Regensteiner JG, Hargarten ME, Rutherford RB, Hiatt WR. Functional benefits of peripheral vascular bypass surgery for patients with intermittent claudication. J Vasc Surg 1993; 17:437–446.

PHARMACOLOGIC TREATMENT OF LOWER EXTREMITY ARTERIAL OCCLUSIVE DISEASE

JAY D. COFFMAN, M.D.

In the past two decades, pharmacologic treatment of lower extremity arterial occlusive disease has evolved from the use of vasodilator drugs to agents that improve ischemic muscle metabolism, counteract the accumulation of toxic factors, or improve blood rheology (Table 1). This development came about due to the inadequacy of vasodilator drug therapy. Unfortunately, it is still difficult to evaluate the clinical usefulness of drugs in arterial occlusive disease. We must still rely on treadmill testing of initial claudication distance (ICD) and maximum walking distance (MWD). The objective tests of the ankle systolic blood pressure or the ankle-brachial systolic blood pressure ratio (ankle-brachial index) do not correlate with the patients' improvement in walking distance. Transcutaneous Po_2 has also not proved to be helpful.

It is difficult to envision that any agent would have dramatic effects in patients with intermittent claudication or ischemic rest pain, ulcers, or gangrene. The distal blood pressure in a limb with an obstructed or stenosed artery is lower than the arm blood pressure. The collateral vessels that supply the limb distal to the obstruction arise from the proximal arteries, are of small caliber, and offer a high resistance to blood flow. Limb blood flow in most patients with intermittent claudication is normal at rest. During exercise, the blood pressure distal to the obstruction decreases further, and blood flow may fall or even cease because of the external pressure of the contracting muscles on the low-pressure blood vessels. Agents that would improve patients must dilate the collateral vessels, stimulate their growth, or raise systemic blood pressure besides improving muscle metabolism and blood rheology. Otherwise, a meaningful improvement in the patient's symptoms does not occur.

VASODILATOR DRUGS

Several vasodilator agents with different modes of action have been used in patients with lower extremity arterial occlusive disease.[1] Nylidrin increases muscle

Table 1 Pharmacologic Agents in the Treatment of Lower Extremity Arterial Occlusive Disease

>Vasodilator drugs
>>Nylidrin
>>Isoxsuprine
>>Tolazoline
>>Niacin and derivatives
>>Cyclandelate
>>Papaverine and derivatives
>
>Rheological drugs
>>Pentoxifylline
>>Hydroxyethyl starch, dextran
>
>Antiplatelet drugs
>>Aspirin and dipyridamole
>>Ticlopidine
>
>Chelation therapy
>>Ethylenediamine-tetracetic acid
>
>Metabolic and rheological agents
>>(Not available in United States)
>>L-carnitine and L-propionylcarnitine
>>Defibrotide
>>Naftidrofuryl
>>Prostaglandins

blood flow by stimulation of beta-adrenoceptors. Isoxsuprine was fashioned to stimulate beta-adrenoceptors but probably has a direct relaxing action on blood vessels. Tolazoline has multiple actions but is primarily an alpha-adrenoceptor antagonist that increases cutaneous blood flow. Other drugs that relax vascular smooth muscle are niacin and its derivatives, cyclandelate, and papaverine and its derivatives. Almost all these drugs increase limb blood flow in animals, and some increase blood flow in normal human subjects. In my studies of patients with aortoiliac or femoropopliteal occlusive disease, tolazoline, nylidrin, and isoxsuprine did not increase resting foot blood flow. Resting calf blood flow was significantly increased only by nylidrin in patients with femoropopliteal disease. Nylidrin, isoxsuprine, and nicotinyl alcohol failed to increase exercising muscle blood flow in the same patients.

Isoxsuprine was given to patients with intermittent claudication for 4 weeks in a placebo-controlled study. No effect was seen in the systolic blood pressure gradient of the diseased limb, postexercise ankle systolic blood pressure, or maximum treadmill walking time. In another study, isoxsuprine did not increase the claudication time on a treadmill or limb blood flow. Well-controlled studies with nylidrin have documented no beneficial effect in patients with intermittent claudication. Oral papaverine and its derivatives also have not benefited patients. Nicotinic acid or its analogs have no benefit or slight symptomatic improvement in long-term studies. Cyclandelate has been reported to increase walking distance in about 50% of patients in uncontrolled studies. Tolazoline was found to increase foot blood flow in patients with obstructive arterial disease but only in the absence of rest pain. In some studies, variable changes and even a decrease in blood flow to ischemic feet was found. It can be concluded that vasodilator drugs are without value for patients with intermittent claudication or rest pain.

RHEOLOGICAL AGENTS

Pentoxifylline

Pentoxifylline is a xanthine derivative that inhibits adenosine 3,5 monophosphate diesterase, leading to an increase in red blood cell cyclic adenosine monophosphate. This effect leads to vascular smooth muscle relaxation. It has been claimed to reduce whole-blood viscosity, decrease fibrinogen concentration, increase white or red blood cell filterability, decrease platelet adhesiveness, and reduce the generation of oxygen free radicals by leukocytes in ischemic legs. However, there are negative studies for each of these actions. Therefore, its mode of action in patients with intermittent claudication remains uncertain. The increased walking distance with pentoxifylline has not been found to correlate with a decrease in blood viscosity.

There are many small studies with the use of pentoxifylline in patients with intermittent claudication. Most found a beneficial effect. Two large studies reported an increased maximum walking distance for patients on the drug compared to placebo, and one large study showed no benefit.[2] Only one of the studies found a significant increase in pain-free walking distance. The increases in walking distance were small but could be clinically important for patients with moderately severe disease who can cover only small distances. In one of the large studies, patients did not report subjective improvement, and in an uncontrolled study only 5% of patients reported satisfaction with their treatment.[3] Continuous use of pentoxifylline for 120 days was reported to reduce the incidence of invasive therapeutic and diagnostic procedures in the first year of follow-up in a historical cohort study of health maintenance organization patients.[4] However, no difference was found in the risk of arterial obstructive disease–related hospitalization or cost of related care. The conclusion was that the drug may reduce the risk of vascular reconstruction while not decreasing the total cost of care. One meta-analysis of the controlled studies with pentoxifylline concluded that there was a significant improvement in walking distance with the drug compared with placebo.[5] However, a more critical meta-analysis documented that the limited amount and quality of reported data did not allow an overall, reliable estimate of pentoxifylline's efficacy.[2] A further problem is that a negative correlation between sample size and response occurred in these studies, with the larger studies having the least benefit of the drug.

Hemodilution

Hemodilution (isovolemic) with a colloidal solution of hydroxyethyl starch (HES) or low-molecular-weight dextran (LMWD) has been advocated for the treatment of patients with intermittent claudication for several years. The hemodilution may decrease the hematocrit, plasma viscocity, and erythrocyte aggregation and increase resting blood flow. Ankle blood pressures do not change. The HES was superior to Ringer's lactate solution and an exercise regimen in increasing the ICD in one study. Another study found no difference between 10% HES and dextran 40 infusions. One report found LMWD more beneficial in increasing the MWD than pentoxifylline. These are small studies, and patients usually had a high hematocrit before hemodilution. Blood must be removed and replacement solutions given once or twice a week for several weeks. The inconvenience and discomfort associated with this treatment in unlikely to be acceptable to patients in view of the small benefit.

ANTIPLATELET DRUGS

Aspirin and ticlopidine have not been extensively studied for intermittent claudication, although they have been investigated for the prevention of cardiovascular events and death. In a study of 296 patients with intermittent claudication, both aspirin with dipyridamole and ticlopidine decreased platelet aggregation, beta-thromboglobulin, platelet factor IV, and fibrinopeptide A concentration, as well as increased antithrombin III concentrations and erythrocyte filterability. In this 6 month study, the ankle-brachial index improved by a small amount in patients on aspirin plus dipyridamole and ticlopidine but not with xanthinol nicotinate. Walking distances were not reported. In one study of 240 patients, 330 mg of aspirin plus 75 mg of dipyridamole three times a day delayed progression of arteriographically followed peripheral arteriosclerotic lesions significantly better than placebo or aspirin alone over a 2 year period.[6] Another small study of 54 patients found that aspirin plus dipyridamole was significantly better than aspirin alone in increasing ICD and resting limb blood flow. In the U.S. Physicians' Health Study, the risk of peripheral artery reconstruction was significantly reduced in those who took 325 mg of aspirin every other day over an average period of 5 years.[7] However, there was no decrease in the development of intermittent claudication with aspirin among these 22,071 physicians.

Ticlopidine is a potent inhibitor of platelet aggregation with a different action on platelets than aspirin. In several studies, ticlopidine increased the walking distance in patients with intermittent claudication, although one study reported no benefit. In one study of 151 patients, the ankle-brachial index was improved at rest and after exercise.[8] When studies up to 1988 were analyzed together, there was a significant improvement in walking distance and patients' status with ticlopidine compared with placebo. Patients must be observed carefully on ticlopidine because leukopenia may occur. Antiplatelet drugs deserve further study in patients with intermittent claudication.

CHELATION THERAPY

A study of 153 patients with intermittent claudication has shown chelation therapy with ethylenediaminetetraacetate (EDTA) to be of no benefit. It was a randomized, double-blind, controlled study comparing 20 intravenous infusions of Na_2EDTA with saline infusions over 5 to 10 weeks. There was no change in ICD, MWD, ankle-brachial index, or subjective symptoms over 3 to 6 months of follow-up. Arteriograms in 30 patients before, during, and after treatment were unchanged.

NEW THERAPIES (UNAVAILABLE IN UNITED STATES)

L-Carnitine and L-Propionylcarnitine

Biopsies of ischemic muscles have shown abnormalities in carnitine metabolism and carnitine acetyltransferase. At rest, the diseased legs have a higher content of long-chain acylcarnitines than controls, and with exercise there is a large increase in muscle short-chain acylcarnitine. Other investigators found only abnormalities of short-chain acylcarnitine in some patients. Administration or either carnitine or L-propionylcarnitine corrected the abnormalities but not the enzyme deficiency. A few studies have reported that L-carnitine or its analog increased the ICD and MWD in patients with intermittent claudication.[9] A small study of diabetic patients found that the ankle-brachial index at rest and walking distances improved with the oral analog. In a large, multicenter study of propionylcarnitine, the increases in ICD and MWD were small, about 50 and 90 m, respectively, compared to 18 and 35 m in the placebo group. Carnitine and its analog provide an interesting approach to the treatment of arterial obstructive disease. Further studies need to be done.

Defibrotide

Defibrotide is a polydeoxyribonucleotide that activates fibrinolysis. It stimulates endothelial cells to release tissue plasminogen activator, prostacyclin, and $PGF_{1-\alpha}$, and reduces plasminogen activator inhibitor. A large double-blind, multicenter, placebo-controlled study reported that oral defibrotide significantly increased the MWD over a 6 month period compared with placebo. The ankle-brachial index was also improved, but there was a decrease in systemic blood pressure, which makes this finding difficult to evaluate. In a small study in which defibrotide was administered intravenously to patients with arterial occlusive disease, beta-thromboglobulin decreased, indicating the drug may have an antiaggregating effect on platelets. Walking distance and rest pain were improved in this uncontrolled study. Defibrotide is an interesting compound deserving further study because increases in MWD were more than 100 m compared with 40 m for placebo in the multicenter study.

Naftidrofuryl

Naftidrofuryl, an acid ester of diethylaminoethanol, has been advocated for the treatment of arterial occlusive disease. In normal subjects, it decreases the lactate-pyruvate ratio following exercise, probably by activating succinic dehydrogenase, promoting cellular glucose uptake, and increasing ATP. It also inhibits $5-HT_2$ receptors. In a meta-analysis of four trials involving 452 patients, it significantly increased ICD over a 3 to 6 month period.[10] The increase was 55.1% for the drug and 24.8% for placebo. Best results occurred in patients who had a greater than 150 m ICD at the start of treatment. There is some indication that naftidrofuryl may be of more benefit to patients over 60 years of age. This is another interesting agent that deserves further study.

Prostaglandins

Some prostaglandins are powerful vasodilators but also have platelet antiaggregatory activity. Prostaglandin E_1 and iloprost, a stable analog of prostaglandin I_2, have been given to patients intravenously for rest pain, ulcers, or gangrene and also for intermittent claudication. Small studies have reported good results with both agents, but some studies found no benefit. However, the infusions must be given for several days, up to 28 days, and the adverse effects during the infusions are numerous. Much more information about the benefit of these drugs is needed before they can be recommended.

COMMENT

Currently, no pharmacologic therapy is more beneficial than an exercise regimen for patients with intermittent claudication. Our approach to patients with intermittent claudication is to institute an exercise regimen and interdict tobacco usage. Hygienic care of the feet is emphasized. A daily 325 mg aspirin is prescribed for patients with no previous problems with it. If there is no improvement in 3 months, pentoxifylline might be tried in patients with moderately severe claudication. If there is still no improvement and the symptoms are interfering with the patient's employment or lifestyle, angioplasty or vascular reconstruction is considered. Patients with rest pain, ulcers, or gangrene are immediately considered for invasive interventions.

REFERENCES

1. Coffman JD. Vasodilator drugs in peripheral vascular disease. N Engl J Med 1979; 300:713–717.
2. Radack K, Wyderski RJ. Conservative management of intermittent claudication. Ann Intern Med 1990; 113:135–146.
3. Abrahma AF, Woodruff BA. Effects and limitations of pentoxifylline therapy in various stages of peripheral vascular disease of the lower extremity. Am J Surg 1990; 160:266–270.
4. Stergachis A, Sheingold S, Luce BR, et al. Medical care and cost outcomes after pentoxifylline treatment for peripheral arterial disease. Arch Intern Med 1992; 152:1220–1224.
5. Rössner M, Müller R. On the assessment of the efficacy of pentoxifylline (Trental). J Med 1987; 18:1–15.
6. Hess H, Mietaschk A, Deichsel G. Drug-induced inhibition of platelet function delays progression of peripheral occlusive arterial disease. Lancet 1985; 1:415–419.
7. Goldhaber SZ, Manson JE, Stampfer MJ, et al. Low-dose aspirin and subsequent peripheral artery surgery in the Physicians' Health Study. Lancet 1992; 340:143–145.
8. Balsano F, Coccheri S, Libretti A, et al. Ticlopidine in the treatment of intermittent claudication: A 21 month double-blind trial. J Lab Clin Med 1989; 114:84–91.
9. Brevetti G, Chiariello M, Ferulano G, et al. Increases in walking distance in patients with peripheral vascular disease treated with L-carnitine: A double-blind cross-over study. Circulation 1988; 77:767–773.
10. Lehert P, Riphagen FE, Garnand S. The effect of naftidrofuryl on intermittent claudication: A meta-analysis. J Cardiovasc Pharm 1990; 16(suppl 3):581–586.

OPERATIVE MANAGEMENT OF ACUTE THROMBOSIS OF LOWER EXTREMITY BYPASS GRAFTS

LAKSHMIKUMAR PILLAI, M.D.
JOHN J. RICOTTA, M.D.

Maintaining graft patency depends on a program of rigorous graft surveillance with early intervention if needed. Despite best efforts, however, graft thrombosis occurs. The early failure rate of infrainguinal bypass grafts remains approximately 5%,[1-3] with late failure rates ranging from 20% to 30%, depending on the level of distal anastomosis, length of follow-up, and definition of patency (primary, assisted primary, or secondary).

Operative management of acute thrombosis of lower extremity bypass grafts must begin with a thorough preoperative evaluation. The patient's overall condition, risk of amputation, and the likelihood of success of the proposed secondary, tertiary, or even quaternary procedure must be assessed before the appropriate treatment of the failed graft is selected. Assessment of the various risks and benefits as well as the potential for successful outcome is imperative. These should be considered in conjunction with the patient's opinion regarding revascularization, especially a patient who has had multiple previous revascularization attempts and has now "come to the end of the road" with no available autogenous conduit and poor distal outflow. In general, secondary reconstructions are reserved for patients with limb-threatening ischemia in whom some autogenous conduit or composite graft is available. Under rare circumstances, distal bypass with nonautogenous tissue is undertaken in patients with limited life expectancy (less than 2 years).

The operative management of acute thrombosis of infrainguinal bypass grafts is based on the severity of lower extremity ischemia as set forth in the SVS/ISCVS criteria. According to the SVS/ISCVS Committee on Reporting Standards, the clinical classes of acute limb ischemia are:

1. Viable: Not immediately threatened, no ischemic pain, no neurologic deficit, skin capillary circulation adequate; clearly audible Doppler pulsatile flow signal, and pedal arteries or ankle pressure above 30 mm Hg.
2. Threatened viability: Implies reversible ischemia and a limb salvageable without major amputation if arterial obstruction properly relieved; ischemic pain and/or mild and incomplete neurologic deficit present (e.g., sensory loss involving only vibration, touch composition, or weakness of toe/foot dorsal flexion); "pulsatile flow" in pedal arteries not audible with Doppler instrumentation but venous patency demonstrable.
3. Major, irreversible ischemic change: Will require major amputation regardless of therapy; profound sensory loss and muscle paralysis, absent capillary skin flow or evidence of more advanced ischemia (e.g., muscle rigor or skin marbling); neither arterial nor venous flow signals audible distally.

If the limb has been judged to manifest class 3 ischemia, the patient should be advised to have a primary amputation. Patients with class 1 or class 2 ischemia may be considered for revascularization. Unless there are serious contraindications, all patients with class 1 and class 2 ischemia should undergo systemic heparinization as soon as the initial diagnosis is made in order to protect against further clot propagation and to protect the patency of collaterals. Following this, the decision of whether to proceed with preoperative arteriography is made based on the severity of ischemia, expected delay associated with obtaining arteriography, and coexisting medical conditions.

Arteriography is favored in all patients with class 1 limb ischemia and in any class 2 patients when the procedure does not cause delay of more than 2 to 3 hours in operation. The benefits of preoperative arteriography cannot be overemphasized in planning secondary reconstructions. This is at variance with our approach to patients with acute embolic ischemia, where arteriography can often be deferred preoperatively.

Arteriography should consist of visualization of the aortoiliofemoral segment with distal runoff to the level of the ankle-foot. A detailed history is taken. The number of prior reconstructions, type of graft, duration of bypass patency, and vein graft configuration are all important factors in investigating the causes of graft failure and estimating the possibilities of a successful revision. Information on whether the graft has undergone duplex surveillance and results of surveillance can provide information on potential mechanisms of failure. If possible, the presence of suitable residual autogenous vein should be ascertained. We prefer duplex vein mapping to accomplish this. If the operative report and the completion arteriogram from the initial graft placement are available, they are reviewed for clues about the mechanisms of graft failure. Also, prior to heparinization, blood samples are drawn in order to evaluate possible congenital or acquired causes of hypercoagulability including protein C and protein S levels, antithrombin III level, lupus anticoagulant, and anticardiolipin antibody, as well as studies for heparin-induced platelet aggregation.

OPERATIVE APPROACH

The three basic operative approaches to the treatment of failed infrainguinal bypass grafts are (1) placement of a new bypass, (2) thrombectomy and revision of the existing bypass, and (3) lytic therapy with graft revision or extension to a distal outflow site. Sometimes this can also be to a more proximal outflow site, especially in the case of a failed vein bypass to a tibial artery below an open isolated popliteal segment.

The operative approach is dictated by the cause of thrombosis. Early graft failures (less than 30 days) due to technical reasons and focal conduit problems can be treated by thrombectomy with correction of the underlying lesions. Generalized conduit problems are treated by graft replacement. On occasion, this requires replacement of an inadequate vein or substitution of an autogenous conduit for a prosthetic. Graft failure within the intermediate period (3 to 18 months) can be treated with thrombolytic therapy and revision if a focal underlying abnormality can be identified. We try to identify this in autogenous veins by a vigorous duplex surveillance program. Patients with prosthetic conduits are subjected to lysis only when autogenous vein is in limited supply and prosthetic is to be used as an inflow for an autogenous bypass extension that would otherwise be impossible. Occasionally, late hemodynamic failure "pseudo-occlusion," occurs with a patent conduit. Under these circumstances, proximal or distal extension is all that is required. However, patients with late graft thrombosis almost always require placement of a new conduit. Distal extension is virtually always required, and in our experience this precludes the use of prosthetic material.

Adjunctive thrombolytic therapy may be of use in grafts that have failed in the intermediate period if it can be determined that the graft failure was due to a discrete lesion, such as an intrinsic vein graft stenosis, that may be amenable to operative angioplasty or segmental graft replacement. We have been disappointed with transluminal angioplasty as a method to correct these lesions and use it only in exceptional circumstances.

In performing a new bypass graft, we attempt to use all autogenous tissue whenever possible, employing, in order, ipsilateral lesser saphenous or contralateral greater saphenous and lesser saphenous veins. We have not had extensive experience with arm veins, although good results have been reported by others.[4,5] Dissection in previously undissected anatomic planes above and below the sites of previous graft placement is recommended if graft replacement is chosen. The suprainguinal approach to the external iliac artery may be used to access inflow, and alternate approaches to the popliteal and infrapopliteal vessels may be used to access outflow.[6-8]

If graft replacement cannot be performed with all autogenous tissue, we prefer composite polytetrafluoroethylene (PTFE) autogenous vein jump graft as opposed to utilizing arm vein. In rare cases where no autogenous vein is available in tibial reconstruction, PTFE with or without adjunctive arteriovenous fistula or Taylor patch may be considered. We have occasionally used cryopreserved veins as conduits, although the long-term results of each of the nonautogenous alternatives is poor.

The role for thrombectomy and revision of thrombosed vein grafts is limited in our experience. Technical rather than structural problems with the vein graft and graft failure due to hypercoagulability are probably the most common situations amenable to thrombectomy and revision. This technique will probably not succeed in grafts that have been occluded for longer than 7 days. It has been shown that results of intermediate or late graft thrombectomy of both prosthetic and saphenous vein grafts are poor.[9] Therefore, attempts at thrombolysis are preferred to operative thrombectomy except in cases of early graft failure.

Extension grafts may be done for progression of inflow or outflow disease and when graft thrombosis occurs, requiring preoperative lytic therapy, and arteriography documents inflow or outflow disease progression. Distal extension grafts are preferentially constructed from autogenous tissue, whereas prostheses are usually used for proximal extensions.

Intraoperative lytic therapy may be used during any of these operative approaches. In our experience, catheter thrombectomy is initially performed in order to establish inflow and outflow followed by infusion of 500,000 units of urokinase dissolved in 100 ml of the patient's own blood over 10 to 20 minutes with inflow occlusion. Intraoperative lytic therapy is done if there is a suggestion of residual thrombus in the outflow vessels based on Doppler flow signals or completion angiography.

Postoperatively, the patient is maintained on heparin sodium and converted to warfarin, especially when the original conduit is reused and in those with limited runoff. Chronic anticoagulation is indicated if graft failure was due to hypercoagulability or a disadvantaged outflow tract. Chronic anticoagulation is usually not required in patients with graft failure due to a conduit problem with good inflow and outflow and when a satisfactory secondary reconstruction using autogenous tissue is performed. The patient can be maintained perioperatively on an infusion of low-molecular-weight dextran while aspirin therapy (325 mg daily) is started if there are contraindications to postoperative systemic anticoagulation.

Some authors have advocated the use of mannitol in addition to postoperative anticoagulation in order to minimize the local and systemic effects of ischemia and reperfusion injury. Four-compartment fasciotomy is done routinely in patients with class 2 limb ischemia and selectively in those with class 1 limb ischemia when the ischemia interval exceeds 6 hours. All grafts that are successfully salvaged and all successful secondary, tertiary, or quaternary reconstructions undergo graft surveillance. Our protocol includes complete graft duplex examination with measurement of ankle-brachial indices prior to discharge, at 3 month intervals for the first 2 years, then every 6 months thereafter for the next year, and then on a yearly basis.

REFERENCES

1. Bandyk DF, Kaebnick HW, Stewart GW, et al. Durability of the in situ saphenous vein arterial bypass: A comparison of primary and secondary patency. J Vasc Surg 1987; 5:256–268.
2. Taylor LM Jr, Phinney ES, Porter JM. Present status of reversed vein bypass for lower extremity revascularization. J Vasc Surg 1986; 3:288–297.
3. Mills JL, Fujitani RM, Taylor SM. Contribution of routine intraoperative completion arteriography to early infrainguinal bypass patency. Am J Surg 1992; 164:506–511.
4. Harris RW, Andros G, Dulana B, et al. Successful long-term limb salvage using cephalic vein bypass grafts. Ann Surg 1984; 200:785–794.
5. Marcaccio EJ, Miller A, Tarnenbaum GA, et al. Angioscopically directed interventions improve arm vein bypass grafts. J Vasc Surg 1993; 17:994–1004.
6. Veith FJ, Ascer E, Nunez A, et al. Unusual approaches to infrainguinal arteries. J Cardiovasc Surg 1987; 28:58.
7. Nunez A, Veith FJ, Collier P, et al. Direct approach to the distal portions of the deep femoral artery for limb salvage bypasses. J Vasc Surg 1988; 8:576–581.
8. Veith FJ, Ascer E, Gupta SK, Wengerter KR. Lateral approach to the popliteal artery. J Vasc Surg 1987; 6:119–123.
9. Green RM, Ouriel K, Ricotta JJ, DeWeese JA. Revision of failed infrainguinal bypass grafts: Principles of management. Surgery 1986; 100:646–654.

FIBRINOLYTIC THERAPY FOR ACUTELY THROMBOSED LOWER EXTREMITY ARTERIES AND GRAFTS

BRUCE A. PERLER, M.D.

Acute limb ischemia has traditionally been a surgical problem. The first successful embolectomy was performed more than 80 years ago, and operative management was substantially enhanced with the introduction of the Fogarty embolectomy catheter in the 1960s. Although there has been considerable improvement in outcome among patients operated upon for acute limb ischemia over the past 3 decades, amputation rates remain considerable. For example, in a study of patients undergoing emergency operation for acute limb ischemia, excluding limbs that were deemed irreversible at presentation, the major amputation rate was 13%.[1]

Some have suggested that such results argue for alternative approaches such as fibrinolytic therapy. Although fibrinolytic drugs were first administered intravenously nearly 30 years ago, it has been only over the past decade that intraarterial fibrinolytic therapy has been widely used, and it remains somewhat controversial.

PHARMACOLOGIC AND THERAPEUTIC CONSIDERATIONS

All first- and second-generation fibrinolytic drugs act by directly or indirectly stimulating the conversion of plasminogen, a circulating proenzyme, into plasmin, the primary fibrinolytic enzyme (Table 1).[2] To date, streptokinase (SK) and urokinase (UK) have been the most frequently administered drugs for peripheral arterial and graft fibrinolysis, with only limited clinical experience reported for tissue plasminogen activator (rt-PA).[3] The anticipated clinical benefits and limitations of these agents are predicated upon their documented pharmacologic properties (Table 2).

SK is relatively inexpensive and has been widely used. This experience has emphasized several inherent limitations of the drug. For example, SK is a bacterial protein and therefore is antigenic. Not only do allergic reactions occur, but circulating antistreptococcal antibodies may inhibit its fibrinolytic efficacy. UK, on the other hand, is nonantigenic. Furthermore, SK has less affinity for thrombus-bound plasminogen than UK, which in part explains the greater proteolytic states with SK (Table 2). As a result of these and other factors successful thrombolysis has been reported more frequently and bleeding complications less often in association with the intra-arterial administration of UK than SK. Rt-PA is more specific than UK or SK for fibrin-bound plasminogen, but it is associated with occasional bleeding complications, since like all fibrinolytic agents, it cannot differentiate pathologic thrombus from thrombus-sealing invaded sites.[3]

Irrespective of the agent used, several recent refinements in the method of drug administration have improved overall therapeutic results (Table 3). For example, it is important to embed the infusion catheter directly in the clot, both to activate thrombus-bound plasminogen more reliably and effectively and to reduce systemic washout of the drug with the development of systemic fibrinolysis. Newer multihole catheters allow rapid drug delivery. Passage of a guide wire across the occlusion before instituting the infusion is a useful prognostic test, since it usually indicates that the occlusion is a relatively fresh thrombus. Conversely, if the guide wire cannot be completely advanced across the occlusion, it may reflect more chronic disease in that artery or graft, and one may choose not to begin the infusion or at least not to persist with it without significant lysis on early follow-up arteriogram. Furthermore, it now appears that the success rate of intra-arterial fibrinolysis is inversely correlated and the complication rate directly correlated with the duration of infusion. Therefore, rather than a relatively low dose of a particular drug over a protracted period, as was customary with intravenous therapy, one should administer a high dose to complete fibrinolysis in as brief a period as possible is recommended. For example, when treating a patient with UK, use a stepped-down regimen

Table 1 Fibrinolytic Agents

Streptokinase (SK)
Urokinase (UK)
Acylated plasminogen-streptokinase activator complex (APSAC)
Recombinant single-chain urokinase plasminogen activator (SCU-PA)
Recombinant tissue-type plasminogen activator (rt-PA)

Table 2 Pharmacologic and Clinical Properties of Fibrinolytic Agents

	SK	UK	rt-PA
Half-life (min)	23	16	5
Plasma proteolytic state	4+	3+	1+
Antigenicity	Yes	No	No
Allergic side effects	Yes	No	No
Expense	1+	3+	4+

Table 3 Recent Refinements in Intra-Arterial Fibrinolysis

Catheter in clot
Multihole catheter
Guide wire test
Stepped-down dosage
Adjunctive heparin sodium
Follow-up angiography

of 240,000 units/hour for 1 to 2 hours, 120,000 units/hour for the next 1 to 2 hours, and a follow-up arteriogram. If significant lysis has occurred, reduce the dosage to 60,000 units/hour until completion of therapy. However, if no significant lysis appears after the first 2 to 4 hours of therapy and if the guide wire did not pass through the occlusion, terminating therapy is suggested.[4]

In addition to frequent clinical examinations of the affected extremity, periodic arteriography should be performed to assess ongoing lysis. Be prepared to stop the infusion if peripheral ischemia worsens and/or evidence of arteriographic improvement is minimal, especially after 12 to 24 hours of treatment. Finally, most recent data suggest that the adjunctive administration of heparin sodium will reduce the formation of embologenic pericatheter thrombus, which can be an important cause of worsening distal ischemia.

In view of the need for close clinical follow-up, the indwelling arterial catheter, and the risk of bleeding, the patient is best managed in a monitored nursing unit during therapy. Hematologic parameters, including prothrombin time, partial thromboplastin time, fibrinogen level, and the level of fibrinogen degradation products, are measured prior to treatment and serially during the infusion. Some have suggested that the incidence of bleeding complications rises when the fibrinogen level falls below 100 mg/dl, although this finding is challenged by others.

SELECTION OF PATIENTS

A fundamental consideration in selecting patients for fibrinolysis is the level of ischemia in the affected extremity. Specifically, neuromuscular function should be intact to allow several hours for diagnostic arteriography and fibrinolytic infusion. Other absolute and relative contraindications to fibrinolytic therapy have been well established in recent years (Table 4).

Although there is considerable variability in results reported, in part because of differences among drugs and dosage regimens, selection of patients, and definitions of a successful outcome, it is possible to draw some general conclusions regarding outcome as it relates to clinical indications.[4-6] Successful fibrinolysis is more likely in native arteries than in grafts, and results have generally been better in treating synthetic than autogenous vein grafts in the infrainguinal position. Embolic arterial occlusions appear more amenable to successful fibrinolysis than thrombotic occlusions. Not surprisingly, the older the occlusion, the less likely is fibrinolysis to be successful, although some chronic arterial and graft occlusions have been successfully treated with these drugs.

Native Arterial Occlusions

Besides restoring perfusion and reducing the urgency of surgical intervention, the major benefit of fibrinolysis in treating the patient with a native arterial

Table 4 Contraindications to Intra-Arterial Fibrinolysis

Absolute	Relative
Active bleeding	Surgery within 10 days
CVA within less than 2 months	Organ biopsy within 10 days
Intracranial or intraspinal surgery within 2 months	Recent GI bleeding
	Puncture noncompressible vessels
Intracranial tumor or aneurysm	Severe hypertension
Known hypersensitivity to drug	Recent trauma
	Left heart thrombus
	Liver dysfunction
	Bleeding diathesis

thrombosis is as an adjunct to diagnosis. Successful fibrinolysis allows a complete biplane arteriogram, which usually reveals the anatomic cause of the thrombosis and the most appropriate method of definitive correction. In as many as one-third of patients, complete fibrinolysis will reveal no anatomic cause for the occlusion, so that the infusion spared the patient an operation. However, most patients have underlying arteriosclerotic occlusive disease that may be amenable to endovascular treatment, which obviates the need for operation. If operation is required, fibrinolysis buys time to prepare the patient and to obtain information necessary to formulate an appropriate revascularization plan. In addition, fibrinolytic therapy lyses clot in the relatively inaccessible distal vessels and microvasculature of the extremity, improving outflow and maximizing the chance of successful surgical reconstruction. Recent studies have documented successful arterial fibrinolysis in more than 75% of patients using high-dose UK and employing other recent refinements in technique (Table 3).[4,7] Furthermore, in a recent study all patients who required a surgical procedure following successful fibrinolysis had a successful surgical outcome.[4] This approach is particularly appropriate, for example, in the patient with an acutely thrombosed popliteal artery aneurysm, since many of these patients also have thrombosis of the outflow tract at presentation (Fig. 1).

Although most workers have reported somewhat better results with treatment of embolic occlusions, fibrinolysis as primary treatment is reserved for the patient whose the clinical examination suggests a very distal embolus, generally distal to the popliteal trifurcation. Since most peripheral emboli originate from mural thrombus in the heart, even though the risk of systemic fibrinolysis is relatively low when the drug is administered intra-arterially, there nevertheless remains a small risk of inducing a cerebral embolus during treatment. Furthermore, surgical thromboembolectomy can usually be performed easily, under local anesthesia, with rapid restoration of perfusion. Nevertheless, fibrinolytic therapy may have an adjunctive role in selected patients, since there are limitations to surgical thromboembolectomy. In a significant percentage of patients, for example, clot removal from the large vessels by the balloon catheter is incomplete. Also, even when the named

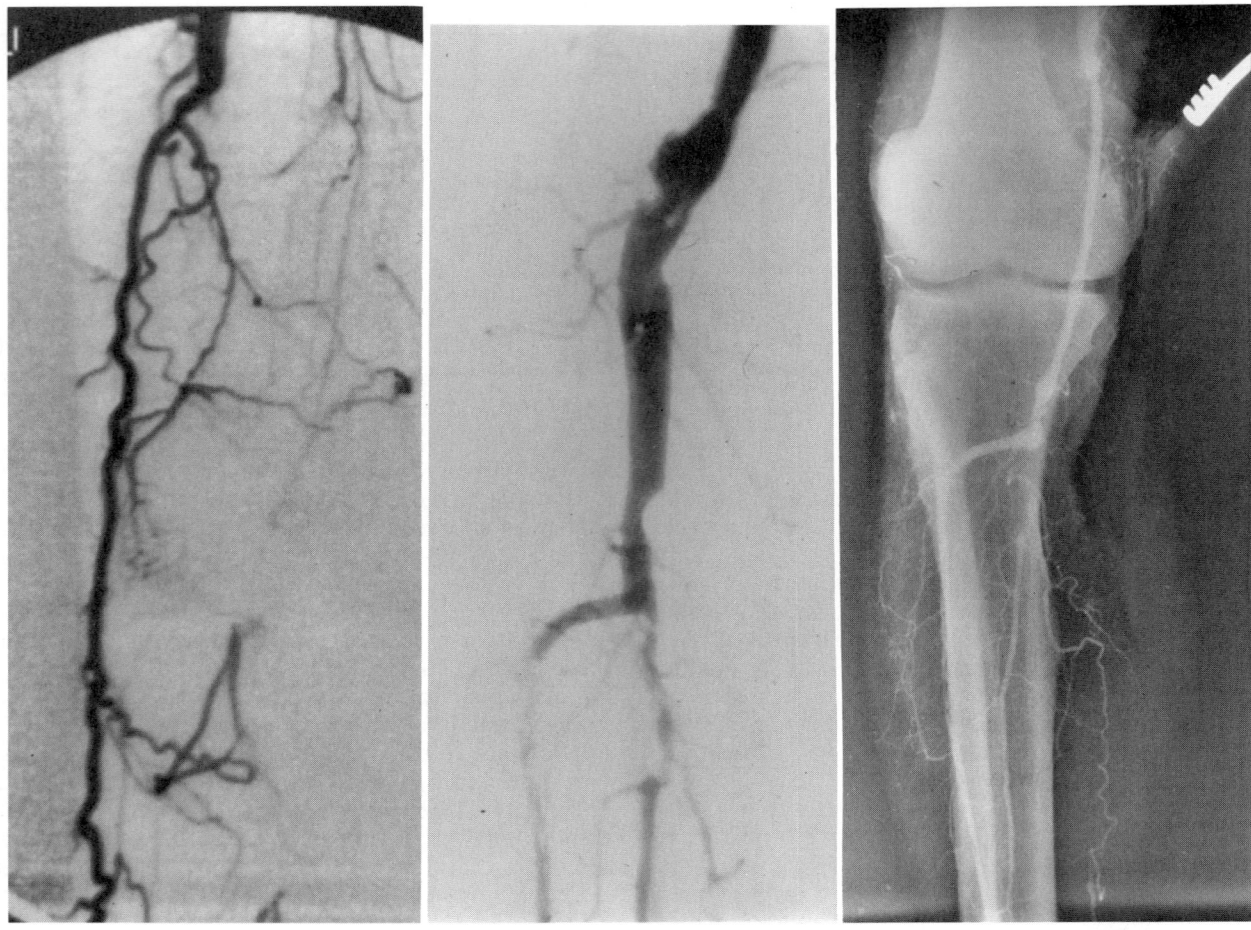

Figure 1 *A,* Arteriogram in patient with acute thrombosis of popliteal aneurysm. Note significant collaterals around knee but no reconstitution of distal vessels. *B,* Follow-up arteriogram after UK infusion demonstrates reconstitution of popliteal artery, apparent chronic occlusion of tibioperoneal trunk, and runoff via the anterior tibial artery. *C,* Operative completion arteriogram demonstrating patent saphenous vein graft.

vessels are completely cleared of clot, the branches of those vessels and the microvasculature of the limb may remain thrombosed. Recent clinical experience has documented that the operative infusion of high-dose fibrinolytic drugs can address these limitations and improve the outcome associated with surgical thromboembolectomy.[8] In fact, the judicious administration of a fibrinolytic agent during the immediate postoperative period may salvage a limb that has developed extensive distal small-vessel thrombosis not accessible to surgical removal.[9]

Graft Occlusion

A primary benefit of fibrinolytic therapy is its aid to diagnosis. Since early postoperative graft thrombosis should almost always be managed by immediate reoperation, the primary role of fibrinolytic therapy is in treating late graft failure. The cause of late graft occlusion depends upon the anatomic site of the graft and—when the graft is infrainguinal—the graft material. For example, late occlusion of an aortofemoral bypass graft (ABF) limb in most patients results from progressive infrainguinal arteriosclerosis. In most of these patients, after the graft limb is recanalized, patency is maintained by extending the graft as a profundaplasty. In as many as 25% to 30%, however, it may be necessary to construct a new infrainguinal bypass to provide adequate outflow to maintain graft limb patency. Preoperative arteriographic delineation of the infrainguinal arterial tree can be invaluable in planning operative repair. Unfortunately, in the patient with a thrombosed ABF graft limb arteriography may not provide much anatomic information (Fig. 2, *A*). After successful fibrinolysis of the graft limb, however, follow-up arteriography will provide valuable information for selection of the most appropriate definitive procedure (Figure 2, *B*).

On the other hand, most late infrainguinal saphenous vein graft thromboses result from intrinsic vein graft hyperplastic lesions, much more frequently than from progressive arteriosclerotic disease. Surgical thrombectomy with repair of thrombosed saphenous vein grafts

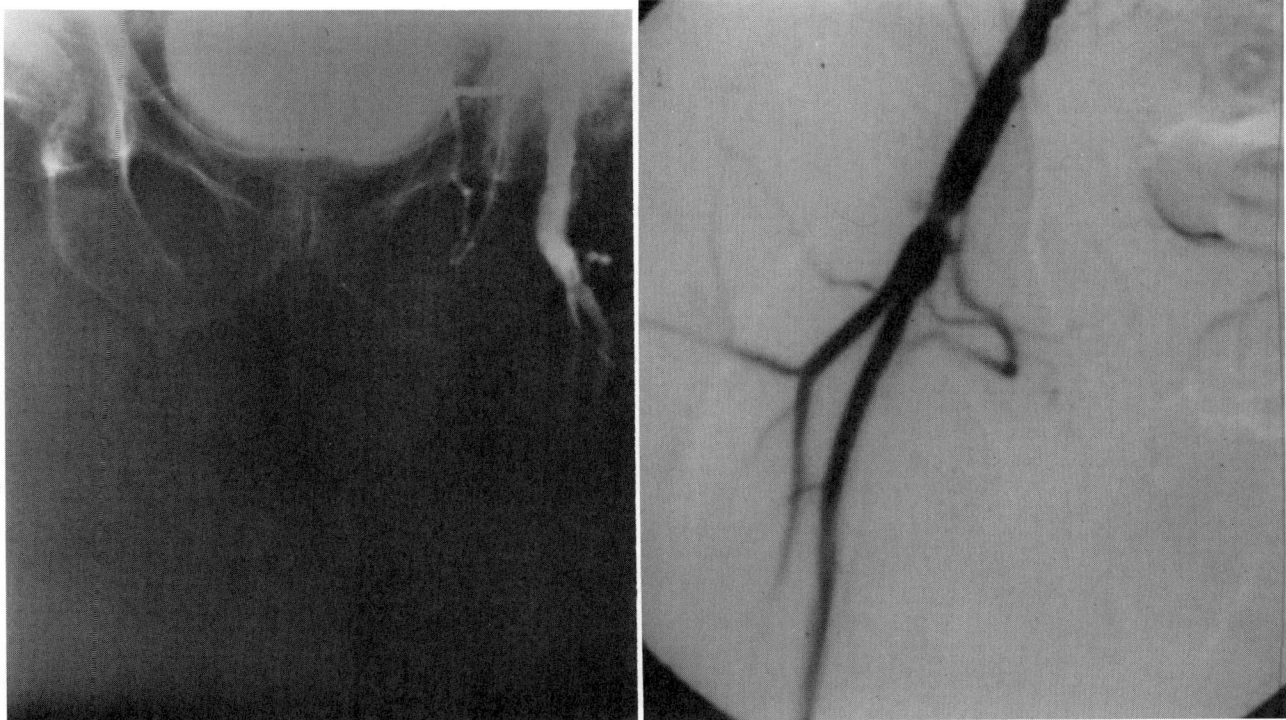

Figure 2 *A*, Arteriogram in patient with acute occlusion of right limb of aortofemoral graft. Note nonvisualization of infrainguinal arterial tree. *B*, Arteriogram following UK infusion, demonstrating nearly complete recanalization of graft limb and distal anastomotic stenosis.

Table 5 Limitations of Thrombectomy of Saphenous Vein Grafts

Mechanical damage to vein intima
Residual mural thrombus
Distal microvascular thrombosis
Residual graft stenoses

has several drawbacks that may explain the relatively disappointing long-term patency associated with this approach (Table 5). Graft fibrinolysis avoids balloon catheter damage to the veins and may yield more complete clot removal, both within the graft and in the outflow tract. Also, after the clot has been lysed, it allows a biplane arteriogram from which the cause of graft occlusion can be diagnosed and the most appropriate method of revision determined. Although successful graft fibrinolysis is being reported today in from 70% to 90% of patients, long-term vein graft patency after successful fibrinolysis has been relatively disappointing. These results may be explained in part by the fact that in most centers graft fibrinolysis is followed by percutaneous transluminal angioplasty (PTA) of the responsible lesions. Growing experience suggests that long-term results of surgical revision of vein graft lesions are superior to those of PTA. Therefore, not only does graft fibrinolysis not preclude surgical repair of the underlying pathology, but there is reason to believe that surgical revision of the lesions following fibrinolysis may yield superior long-term patency.

Although thrombosed infrainguinal bypass grafts of prosthetic materials such as polytetrafluoroethylene are easily thrombectomized and almost always result from anastomotic stenoses, the observation that extensive thrombosis of the outflow tract occurs at the time of graft occlusion is an important indication for initial treatment of such grafts with fibrinolytic drugs. Should surgical revision of the graft be necessary, maximizing outflow prior to operation and minimizing the necessity for passage of balloon catheters into the infrapopliteal vessels at the time of repair should improve the chance for a successful outcome and minimize operative morbidity. Finally, irrespective of the graft material, failure to identify a correctable lesion after successful fibrinolysis portends a relatively poor prognosis.

COMPLICATIONS

The incidence of complications associated with fibrinolytic therapy depends upon the agent, method of drug administration, condition being treated, duration of infusion, and other factors. The most frequent complication is bleeding, although modern techniques and better selection of patients have substantially reduced the incidence of bleeding complications. For example, in one of the largest recent series of patients receiving intra-arterial UK, major hemorrhagic complications occurred in fewer than 3%. Furthermore, in many studies the risk of bleeding has not been predictable on the basis of hematologic parameters.[7] Stroke resulting from intracerebral hemorrhage or cerebral embolus is perhaps the most devastating complication, although it is reported in less than 3% of patients in recent reports. The risk of peripheral embolization, often due to pericatheter thrombus formation, can be reduced by the adjunctive administration of heparin sodium during fibrinolysis, although this may increase the risk of bleeding complications.

REFERENCES

1. Yeager RA, Moneta GL, Taylor LM Jr, et al. Surgical management of severe acute lower extremity ischemia. J Vasc Surg 1992; 15:385–393.
2. Marder VJ, Sherry S. Thrombolytic therapy: Current status. N Engl J Med 1988; 318:1512–1520;1585–1595.
3. Graor RA, Risius B, Geisinger MA, et al. Thrombolysis with recombinant human tissue-type plasminogen activator in patients with peripheral artery and bypass graft occlusions. Circulation 1986; 74(suppl 1):1–15.
4. McNamara TO, Bomberger RA, Merchant RF. Intra-arterial urokinase as initial therapy for acutely ischemic lower limbs. Circulation 1991; 83(suppl):I106–I119.
5. Towne JB, Bandyk DF. Application of thrombolytic therapy in vascular occlusive disease: A surgical view. Am J Surg 1987; 154:548–559.
6. Earnshaw JJ. Thrombolytic therapy in the management of acute limb ischemia. Br J Surg 1991; 78:261–269.
7. McNamara TO, Fischer JR. Thrombolysis of peripheral arterial and graft occlusions. Improving results using high-dose Urokinase. Am J Roentgenol 1985; 144:769–775.
8. Comerata AJ, White JV, Grosh JD. Intraoperative intraarterial thrombolytic therapy for salvage of limbs in patients with distal arterial thrombosis. Surg Gynecol Obstet 1989; 169:283–289.
9. Perler BA, Osterman FA. Immediate post-operative urokinase infusion: Extending the limits of limb salvage surgery. J Cardiovasc Surg 1990; 31:184–188.

ROLE OF ANTITHROMBOTIC DRUGS IN MAINTAINING GRAFT PATENCY

TED R. KOHLER, M.D.

Graft thrombosis usually results from a systemic or local hypercoagulable state, most commonly at the highly thrombotic surface of a prosthetic graft or injured vein graft, in conjunction with decreased flow caused by atherosclerotic plaque or intimal hyperplasia.

SEQUENCE OF EVENTS IN CLINICAL THROMBOSIS

The first step in thrombosis is the adherence of platelets to the graft surface. Normal endothelium protects against thrombosis by production of a number of factors that reduce platelet aggregation (PGI_2), interfere with the action of coagulation factors (thrombomodulin, heparin sulfate), promote lysis of fibrin (tissue-type plasminogen activator and urokinase), and cause vasodilatation (endothelium derived relaxation factor and PGI_2). Endothelial cells also produce promoters of coagulation, including tissue factor, plasminogen activator inhibitor, and various coagulation factors. While normally the balance is in favor of inhibition, after injury damaged endothelium may produce more activators than inhibitors. Furthermore, in denuded regions the blood is exposed to highly thrombogenic factors in the subendothelium and underlying media such as collagen, disrupted cell membranes, and tissue thromboplastin. Adhesion of platelets to the damaged wall occurs within minutes but is remarkably brief. In animal models, very little platelet accumulation persists beyond the first 24 hours following injury. However, this may be one of the primary differences between injury of normal arteries in animal models and treatment of human atherosclerosis. Thrombosis can be a significant and persistent component of restenosis when the highly thrombogenic material in atherosclerotic plaque is exposed to blood. Following adhesion to the damaged surface, platelets become activated by a number of factors including thrombin, adenosine diphosphate (ADP), serotonin, and epinephrine. They then change their shape, release granules containing mitogens and vasoactive components, and aggregate.

The next step in thrombosis is activation of the coagulation system with formation of active factors VII and X and production of thrombin (Fig. 1). Thrombin converts fibrinogen to fibrin, which forms the framework of the thrombus and is a potent activator of platelets, stimulating them to release thromboxane A_2, serotonin, and ADP, which further enhance platelet aggregation.[1] Fibrinogen binds to the platelet receptor glycoprotein IIb-IIIa, linking aggregating platelets.

PHASES OF GRAFT FAILURE

There are three distinct phases of graft failure. The early phase is the first 30 days. During it failure is caused largely by technical factors. The second phase is the first year. Its failures are most commonly caused by intimal hyperplasia. The final phase begins after a year has passed. Its failures are caused by advanced intimal hyperplasia or progressive atherosclerosis in the graft or

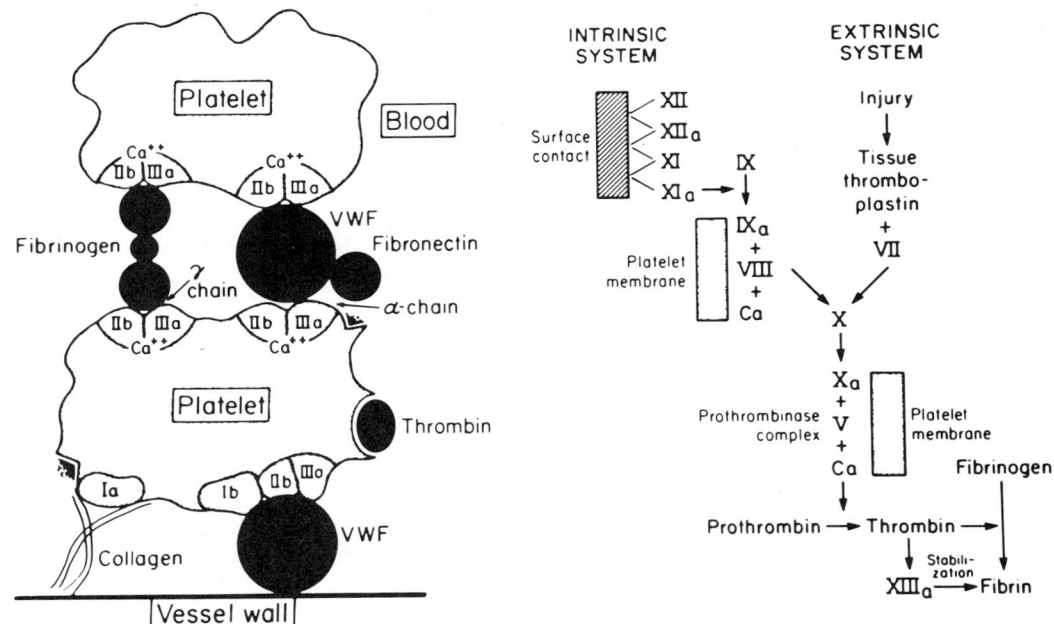

Figure 1 Interactions between platelets, the damaged vessel wall, and the coagulation system. Vascular injury results in thrombus formation both through the intrinsic (surface-activated) and extrinsic (tissue factor–dependent) pathways. Interactions between coagulation factors are facilitated by the platelet membranes. (Modified from Stein B, Fuster V, Halperin JL, Chesebro JH: Antithrombotic therapy in cardiac disease. Circulation 80:1501, 1989; with permission.)

runoff vessels. The role of antithrombotic therapy varies among these three phases.

Phase One: The First 30 Days

Graft failure in the first days to weeks after operation is usually a primary thrombotic process. Early graft thrombosis is generally the result of inadequate flow due to poor outflow or anastomotic stenosis; lacking normal endothelium, the graft surface has inadequate resistance to thrombosis. Low flow is usually caused by a technical problem such as inadequate inflow or outflow vessels, poor surgical technique resulting in graft or anastomotic stenosis, poor quality of vein, or inappropriate use of prosthetic material in poor runoff situations. Antithrombotic treatment has been shown to improve graft patency in this period. Its main role may be to prevent platelet aggregation for the first days or weeks until graft surface becomes less thrombogenic. Because platelet deposition occurs immediately after blood flow is restored to the graft, antiplatelet agents must be present at the time of operation to be effective.

Phase Two: The First Year

During the intermediate phase (a month to a year) intimal hyperplasia is the primary cause of graft failure. Thrombosis appears to be less important in this phase than in early graft failure, and the benefit of antithrombotic therapy is less clear. Lesions of restenosis obtained from retrieved human vein grafts or atherectomy specimens have a thickened intima with abundant smooth muscle cells (SMCs) and matrix (collagen, elastin, and proteoglycans). Platelet-derived growth factor (PDGF) released from degranulating platelets is a potent mitogen for SMCs in culture and has been implicated as a cause of SMC proliferation in atherogenesis and following injury. Intimal hyperplasia consists of two distinct SMC responses, proliferation and migration from the media across the internal elastic lamina into the intima. Recent animal studies suggest that PDGF is more important in stimulating SMC migration, and proliferation is stimulated primarily by basic fibroblast growth factor released from damaged SMCs.

Phase Three: After a Year

Late graft failure is generally caused by progression of distal atherosclerotic disease or graft stenosis. Late lesions in grafts often have characteristics of atherosclerotic plaques. Antiplatelet agents appear to have little ability to prevent this process, although some experimental models suggest that antiplatelet agents can reduce vein graft wall thickening in fat-fed animals. Other studies suggest that aspirin may help prevent progression of atherosclerosis in arteries and in vein grafts, yet most data are unconvincing. Lipid-lowering drugs may be more effective in this regard. Recent evidence suggests that increased levels of low density lipoproteins and apolipoprotein B are major risk factors for atherosclerosis in vein grafts. However, thrombosis may also contribute to late stenosis. A study of vein grafts removed during reoperative coronary artery bypass documented that two-thirds of the grafts had mural or occlusive thrombus. Grafts that had evidence of atherosclerotic changes or aneurysmal dilatation were particularly prone to developing thrombus.

ROLE OF ANTITHROMBOTIC AGENTS IN PREVENTING GRAFT FAILURE

Antiplatelet Agents

Aspirin

Aspirin is the least expensive and most widely used antiplatelet agent now in clinical use. It reduces the production of thromboxane A_2 from arachidonic acid by acetylating and thus irreversibly blocking cyclooxygenase in the platelet. This inhibits the production of thromboxane A_2. Platelet aggregation induced by ADP, collagen, or thrombin is only partially inhibited. Aspirin does not prevent a monolayer of platelets from forming on the subendothelium, nor does it prevent the release of granule contents.[2] It does prevent platelet aggregate formation. Other nonsteroidal anti-inflammatory drugs act in a similar fashion.

Because platelets lack a nucleus and cannot synthesize enzyme, the effect of aspirin continues until new platelets are created. A dose of 1 mg/kg/day is effective.[2] Higher doses of aspirin can also block endothelial production of the prostacyclin (PGI_2), a prostaglandin that inhibits platelet aggregation. The endothelium can regenerate cyclo-oxygenase, so this effect of aspirin is reversible. Theoretically, low-dose aspirin can block the harmful effects of thromboxane while not blocking generation of PGI_2 by the endothelium, but drug trials with high and low doses of aspirin have failed to support this concept. Adverse reactions to aspirin even at low doses are very common, but generalized bleeding rarely occurs unless aspirin is combined with anticoagulant therapy. A dose of 160 to 325 mg/day of aspirin avoids most of the toxic side effects while maintaining the benefit of platelet cyclooxygenase inhibition.

Some clinical and experimental data suggest that measurement of platelet aggregability can identify individuals who are prone to graft thrombosis. Antiplatelet agents such as aspirin and ticlopidine reduce platelet aggregability in vitro and improve graft patency in animals with high aggregability. In other experimental models, aspirin alone or in combination with dipyridamole has been found to reduce platelet accumulation on prosthetic grafts and to inhibit intimal thickening in vein and polytetrafluoroethylene (PTFE) grafts. Studies using indium labeling have documented that platelet deposition is decreased at sites of carotid endarterectomy (CEA) in patients treated with aspirin and dipyridamole. Both Dacron and PTFE grafts in man accumulate platelets for as long as a decade after implantation, with Dacron being more thrombogenic than PTFE. Aspirin and low-molecular-weight dextran decrease platelet adherence to both Dacron and PTFE in the baboon ex vivo shunt model. Platelet accumulation on prosthetic grafts in humans also can be reduced with antiplatelet therapy or by endothelial cell seeding. In one study this reduction was associated with a trend toward increased patency of PTFE grafts. On the other hand, femoropopliteal vein grafts accumulate very little indium-labeled platelets by 7 days following operation, and this is not affected by antiplatelet agents. This may explain why antiplatelet agents seem to affect patency of prosthetic grafts more than vein grafts.

Several studies of coronary artery bypass vein graft failure suggest that aspirin and perhaps ticlopidine when given in the immediate perioperative period can improve short-term patency rates, probably by reducing early thrombosis.[3] Preoperative use of aspirin increases the risk of bleeding and reoperation. Dipyridamole does not appear to add substantially to the effects of aspirin; however, this drug has the theoretic advantage of reducing platelet activation by the extracorporeal pump and maintaining the platelet count during operation. Some investigators have used dipyridamole preoperatively followed by aspirin in the immediate postoperative period with good results and no increase in the incidence of bleeding complications. Antiplatelet therapy is not effective if begun more than 48 hours after operation. Several studies have documented continued benefit of antiplatelet therapy as long as one year after operation (Fig. 2).

Similar studies of lower-extremity bypass grafts have had mixed results.[4] The group from the University of Rochester randomized 49 patients with infrainguinal PTFE grafts to placebo, aspirin, or aspirin plus dipyridamole.[5] A year later both treatment groups had significantly improved patency of above-knee bypasses. No other significant differences were found, including aspirin alone versus aspirin plus dipyridamole. In a subsequent trial involving 100 patients receiving placebo or aspirin and dipyridamole begun in the immediate postoperative period, there was no benefit of antiplatelet therapy in a mixed group of vein and prosthetic femoropopliteal and femorotibial grafts.[6] However, there was a trend toward increased patency in the small group of femorotibial grafts (70% versus 35%). In a more recent prospective randomized trial, dipyridamole (200 mg twice a day) begun 48 hours preoperatively followed by dipyridamole plus aspirin (300 mg daily) for 6 weeks significantly improved patency of femorotibial bypass grafts.[7] The benefit arose at 1 month, persisted at 1 year, and was entirely due to improved patency in prosthetic grafts (85% treatment versus 53% control; $p < .01$). A larger study involving 549 patients randomized to placebo or aspirin and dipyridamole started preoperatively and continued indefinitely failed to show any benefit in patency of femoropopliteal vein grafts.[8] However, the treatment group did have significantly

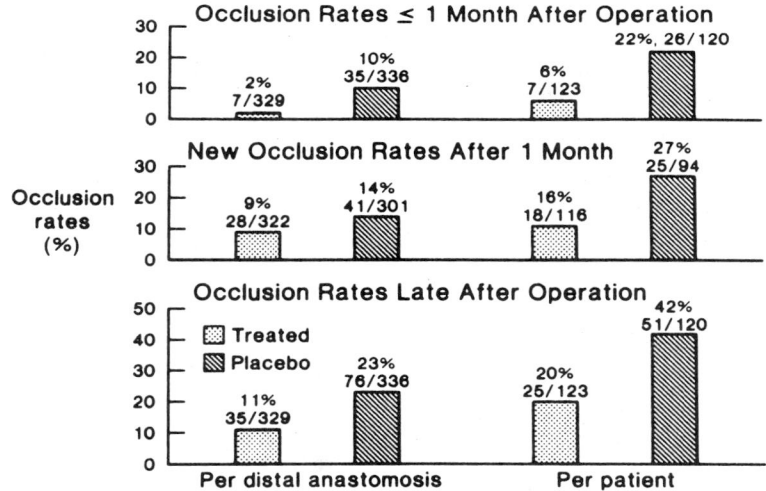

Figure 2 Early, intermediate, and late patency in coronary artery bypass grafts from 343 patients treated with placebo or aspirin plus dipyridamole, with the later drugs started 48 hours preoperatively. Results are demonstrated both per distal anastomosis and per patient and represent patency as determined by angiography. Treatment continued to be effective in preventing vein-graft occlusion as long as one year following operation. (Modified from Chesebro JH, Fuster V, Elveback LR, et al: Effect of dipyridamole and aspirin on late vein-graft patency after coronary bypass operations. N Engl J Med 310:209, 1984; with permission.)

fewer cardiovascular events, including myocardial infarction and strokes.

Although some experimental work has suggested that aspirin and dipyridamole can decrease intimal hyperplasia in vein grafts, these agents appear to have little effect on the long-term problem of intimal hyperplasia. This may be because they do not prevent platelet adhesion to injured surfaces. In a prospective randomized trial, aspirin plus dipyridamole failed to reduce the incidence of restenosis after CEA. In fact, the treatment group had a slightly higher incidence of restenosis. Aspirin with or without dipyridamole is not effective in preventing restenosis after percutaneous transluminal coronary angioplasty (PTCA), but there is some suggestion that these drugs may reduce the severity of this recurrent lesion.

Hirudin

Hirudin is one of several peptide blockers of thrombin-mediated platelet activation. This molecule is the anticoagulant of the European leech.[1] It binds 1:1 with thrombin, inactivating this potent activator of platelets. In animal models of arterial injury hirudin reduces fibrin deposition and at high does can eliminate mural thrombosis and most platelet deposition.[1] Hirudin, unlike heparin sodium, is a small molecule and can penetrate thrombus and inhibit thrombin bound to fibrin. Antithrombin therapy may play an important role in treatment of acute coronary occlusion or in preventing thrombus formation at sites of angioplasty or after lytic therapy. Thrombin inhibitors and ticlopidine have been shown to decrease platelet deposition on prosthetic grafts in animal models, but heparin, aspirin, and dipyridamole have not.

Sulfinpyrazone

Sulfinpyrazone is a competitive inhibitor of platelet cyclo-oxygenase. The exact mechanism of its antiplatelet activity is not fully understood. It has been shown to have some efficacy in decreasing thrombosis in arteriovenous cannulas and artificial heart valves. In the Veterans Administration Cooperative Study on early saphenous vein graft patency after coronary artery bypass, sulfinpyrazone increased early saphenous vein graft patency almost as much as aspirin, but its effect did not quite reach statistical significance. Its use resulted in less perioperative bleeding than regimens that included aspirin. In another study sulfinpyrazone was effective in increasing graft patency only in grafts that had flow rates greater than 30 ml/minute, suggesting that antiplatelet therapy cannot improve patency in grafts with inadequate flow.

Ticlopidine

Ticlopidine inhibits platelet function by an unknown mechanism. It may block the interaction of platelets with fibrinogen and von Willebrand factor.[2] Ticlopidine may be effective in prevention of myocardial infarction in patients with unstable angina and in reducing acute occlusion after coronary angioplasty. Recent studies demonstrate that ticlopidine is slightly more effective than aspirin in preventing stroke, myocardial infarction, and death in patients with transient ischemic attacks.

There has been some suggestion that this drug can improve early (3 month) patency rates of coronary artery bypass grafts, but there was no effect on late patency. There have been no large, convincing clinical trials documenting the efficacy of ticlopidine in preventing lower-extremity graft failure. It is more costly than aspirin and has more significant side effects, including a 0.6% incidence of reversible neutropenia.

Dextran

Dextran improves hemodynamics, reduces platelet aggregation, perhaps by interference with the factor VIII–von Willebrand factor complex, alters fibrin formation and enhances thrombus lysis. It has failed to improve results following coronary angioplasty and can cause anaphylactoid reactions in 0.6% of patients.[2] In one study dextran reduced platelet deposition on synthetic PTFE grafts. In a prospective multicenter randomized trial dextran 40 administered preoperatively and for 3 days following operation improved immediate patency rates (less than 30 days) of difficult lower-extremity bypass grafts.[9] These included femoropopliteal grafts using vein if the runoff was poor, femoropopliteal bypass grafts that did not use vein, infrapopliteal grafts, and any bypass associated with endarterectomy, thrombectomy, angioplasty, or transluminal dilatation. However, by 1 month the difference between the dextran and control groups was no longer statistically significant.

Other Platelet Inhibitors

Agents that may reduce the effects of thromboxane include imidazole analogs that inhibit thromboxane synthase and blockers of thromboxane and prostaglandin endoperoxide receptors. In human studies the specific thromboxane A_2 receptor blocking drug AH23848 reduced radio-labeled platelet deposition in mature Dacron aortobifemoral grafts. It is possible that the synthetase inhibitors both suppress thromboxane A_2 synthesis and enhance prostacyclin production. However, none of these agents have yet proven beneficial in clinical trials. Prostacyclin analogs such as iloprost and ciprostene can increase platelet cyclic adenosine monophosphate and inhibit platelet aggregation. Unlike prostacyclin, these agents are pharmacologically useful because they are stable at neutral pH.[2] They may have some benefit in treatment of thromboembolic disease and prevention of restenosis, but solid clinical data are lacking.

Newer and more potent agents that interfere with platelet adherence, such as monoclonal antibodies to the glycoprotein IIb-IIIa receptor for fibrinogen and von Willebrand factor, may be more effective than traditional antiplatelet agents in preventing platelet adhesion to prosthetic grafts. However, these may not be practical because of their greater effects on hemostasis.

Anticoagulants

Heparin Sodium

Heparin sodium reduces intimal hyperplasia following arterial injury and vein graft hyperplasia in some animal models. Its principal effect is inhibition of SMC proliferation, although it also limits migration. Heparin sodium exerts its effect early in the cell cycle and has to be present for only 24 to 72 hours after the injury to be effective. It is possible that this agent acts by binding basic FGF and releasing it from the matrix. Heparin sodium decreases the expression of tissue-type plasminogen activator and displaces urokinase from the cell layer. These effects may interfere with the ability of SMCs to degrade their surrounding matrix, which is necessary for their migration and proliferation. The effects of heparin sodium are not related to its anticoagulant properties, since some nonanticoagulant fractions that do not bind antithrombin III are equally effective. Nonanticoagulant fractions of heparin sodium are particularly promising for clinical use, and clinical trials with these agents are under way. So far, clinical trials using heparin sodium have been disappointing. For example, heparin sodium given for 12 to 24 hours did not reduce restenosis after PTCA.

Sodium Warfarin

Oral anticoagulants work by inhibiting vitamin K epoxide reductase and thereby limiting γ/carboxylation of prothrombin and factors VII, IX, and X. Carboxylation of protein C and S is also inhibited.[10] Since the half-life of these anticoagulants is shorter than that of most of the coagulation factors that are affected, a temporary hypercoagulable state may appear in the first 2 days of warfarin therapy. This is particularly true in patients with hereditary deficiencies in protein C or S and may account for the occasional case of warfarin-induced skin necrosis. This hypercoagulable state can be eliminated by heparin sodium therapy during the first two days of warfarin treatment. It has been recommended that the standard prothrombin time (PT) be abandoned because variability in commercially available thromboplastin reagents makes it unreliable. This variability is eliminated by using the standardized international ratio, which compares the PT with a reference standard. Long-term anticoagulation with warfarin is more attractive now that lower doses than traditionally used are proved equally effective. Sodium warfarin at a dose that produces an international normalized ratio (INR) of 2 to 3 rather than the higher traditional dose produces fewer bleeding complications yet is adequate for treatment of deep venous thrombosis, atrial fibrillation, and prevention of stroke and death in patients who have peripheral arterial disease or have suffered a myocardial infarction. It does not necessarily follow that the same dose of sodium warfarin will be effective in reducing graft surface thrombosis, since prevention of emboli from mechanical heart valves requires higher doses (INR 2.5 to 3.5).

Some authors have advocated the perioperative use of heparin sodium followed by chronic warfarin therapy with or without aspirin to improve the patency rates of femorotibial bypass grafts, composite grafts, below-knee PTFE femoropopliteal grafts, and axillopopliteal grafts following thrombectomy and have reported apparent success in retrospective, uncontrolled studies. One prospective study of 130 patients receiving saphenous vein femoropopliteal bypass grafts found improved late patency in patients randomized to receive warfarin therapy starting in the second postoperative week.[11] This effect appeared to be restricted to patients operated upon for limb salvage rather than claudication. In this study patient survival was also increased in the treatment group.

Sodium warfarin treatment is also indicated in patients who have certain hypercoagulable states such as deficiency in antithrombin III (ATIII), protein C, or protein S. In one study 18% of patients undergoing femorotibial bypass were found to have a deficiency in ATIII. The risk for early graft thrombosis was doubled in these patients. Even patients with normal coagulation systems are in a relative hypercoagulable state for the first week following operation, with increased platelet responsiveness to collagen and a fall in ATIII levels. Aspirin administration abolished the platelet abnormality.

SECONDARY PREVENTION OF VASCULAR DISEASE

The ability of anticoagulants and antiplatelet agents to prevent myocardial events may be more important than any beneficial effect on graft patency. Studies by Hertzer at the Cleveland Clinic documented that more than 90% of patients undergoing lower-extremity revascularization for chronic occlusive disease have coronary artery disease. While the benefits of long-term antiplatelet therapy for extending graft patency are not fully known, this treatment does appear to have a secondary benefit of reducing adverse vascular events. The Antiplatelet Trialists' Collaboration reviewed the results of 31 randomized trials using antiplatelet treatment in patients with coronary or cerebrovascular disease. Antiplatelet therapy reduced the risk of vascular mortality by 15% and the risk of stroke or myocardial infarction by 30%. Risk reduction was independent of the dose of aspirin used and whether or not dipyridamole was added. Since most patients who have bypass grafts placed for atherosclerotic peripheral arterial occlusive disease also have coronary or cerebrovascular disease, antiplatelet therapy is likely to reduce the incidence of serious vascular events in this group. It has been recommended that men older than 50 years who have significant coronary risk factors such as a strong family history of coronary artery disease, hyperlipidemia, or diabetes should take 325 mg of aspirin daily or every other day for primary prevention of myocardial infarction.[3] While women in this age group with comparable risk profiles may also benefit from aspirin treatment, there are no good clinical trials to substantiate this. Clinical data do suggest that treatment with aspirin or aspirin and dipyridamole can decrease the progression of lower-extremity arterial occlusive disease and that anticoagulant therapy can improve patient survival following femoropopliteal bypass. While other antiplatelet agents may be equally effective, aspirin in a dose of 160 to 325 mg daily is the best studied, least expensive, and least toxic agent.[2]

RECOMMENDATIONS

Most of our understanding of the role of antithrombotic agents comes from clinical studies of saphenous vein coronary artery bypass grafts. It is clear from these studies that antiplatelet agents begun in the perioperative period can increase early graft patency. Aspirin is the best studied, least toxic, and least costly of these agents. Increased bleeding caused by preoperative administration of aspirin can be eliminated by substituting dipyridamole preoperatively. Anticoagulation with warfarin may produce similar results, although possibly with greater morbidity. Although large series with follow-up for many years is lacking, several studies have found a continued benefit of antithrombotic therapy as long as 1 year postoperatively. Data for lower-extremity bypass grafts are not as clear; however, aspirin, dextran, and warfarin treatment have all been found to increase function, particularly early patency, in several studies. Particular benefit has been noted in patients with high-risk grafts, including prosthetic and infrapopliteal grafts and grafts placed in association with ancillary procedures such as endarterectomy or angioplasty. Little benefit has been found in saphenous vein femoropopliteal grafts. Routine use of low-dose aspirin, 160 mg to 325 mg daily, by patients undergoing lower-extremity revascularization seems justified. This recommendation is further supported by the finding that this treatment can improve life expectancy of these patients, who are at high risk for stroke or death from cardiovascular events.

REFERENCES

1. Chesebro JH, Webster MW, Zoldhelyi P, et al. Antithrombotic therapy and progression of coronary artery disease. Antiplatelet versus antithrombins. Circulation 86:III 100–110, 1992.
2. Stein B, Fuster V, Israel DH, et al. Platelet inhibitor agents in cardiovascular disease: An update. J Am Coll Cardiol 14:813–836, 1989.
3. Goodnight SH, Coull BM, McAnulty JH, Taylor LM. Antiplatelet therapy: Part 1. West J Med 158:385–392, 1993.
4. Goodnight SH, Coull BM, McAnulty JH, Taylor LM. Antiplatelet therapy: Part 2. West J Med 158:506–514, 1993.
5. Green RM, Roedersheimer LR, DeWeese JA. Effects of aspirin and dipyridamole on expanded polytetrafluoroethylene graft patency. Surgery 92:1016–1026, 1982.

6. Kohler TR, Kaufman JL, Kacoyanis G, et al. Effect of aspirin and dipyridamole on the patency of lower extremity bypass grafts. Surgery 96:462–466, 1984.
7. Clyne CA, Archer TJ, Atuhaire LK, et al. Random control trial of a short course of aspirin and dipyridamole (Persantin) for femorodistal grafts. Br J Surg 74:246–248, 1987.
8. McCollum C, Alexander C, Kenchington G, et al. Antiplatelet drugs in femoropopliteal vein bypasses: A multicenter trial. J Vasc Surg 13:150–161, 1991.
9. Rutherford RB, Jones DN, Bergentz SE, et al. The efficacy of dextran 40 in preventing early postoperative thrombosis following difficult lower extremity bypass. J Vasc Surg 1:765–773, 1984.
10. Hirsh J, Dalen JE, Deykin D, Poller L. Oral anticoagulants: Mechanism of action, clinical effectiveness, and optimal therapeutic range. Chest 102:312S–326S, 1992.
11. Kretschmer G, Herbst F, Prager M, et al. A decade of oral anticoagulant treatment to maintain autologous vein grafts for femoropopliteal atherosclerosis. Arch Surg 127:1112–1115, 1992.

PROTHROMBOTIC STATES AND VASCULAR THROMBOSES

MICHAEL SOBEL, M.D.

The balance between thrombosis and hemorrhage is nowhere more delicate than in vascular surgery patients. It is not surprising that repetitive thromboses of vascular grafts have been the stimulus to recognition of a number of now well-characterized thrombotic disorders. These syndromes have been called the hypercoagulable state, the prethrombotic state, and prothrombotic diathesis. Perhaps the best conceptualization of these disorders is a paraphrase of Wessler: a perturbed but partially compensated system that has not yet progressed to clot formation; an unperturbed system in which the threshold to clot formation is lower than normal.[1]

Clinical recognition of these patients is not always obvious, especially when the thrombotic event is clearly related to a specific vascular insult. The clinical and laboratory diagnosis can be confounded by the chicken-and-egg conundrum: did the initial vascular injury give rise to the pathologic clotting and consequent laboratory abnormalities, or was there an underlying pathologic predisposition to thrombosis? The clinical characteristics of a thrombotic episode that may help distinguish patients who are most likely to have an underlying hypercoagulable state can help determine when a detailed laboratory evaluation is indicated (Table 1).

Hypercoagulable states can be classified under a variety of rubrics: inherited versus acquired, natural anticoagulants versus procoagulants, and so on. It is perhaps better to consider the conditions according to their frequency of occurrence. Few prospective comprehensive surveys on this subject have been done in vascular patients. It is likely that 10% of the elective vascular surgery population has a clearly definable predisposition to thrombosis. The percentage is probably higher if emergencies and less well defined syndromes are included.

COMMON DISORDERS

Antiphospholipid Antibodies

Antiphospholipid antibodies (APA) is the preferred term to describe the lupus anticoagulant, or anticardiolipin antibodies. These acquired antibodies are directed against the negatively charged phospholipids of endothelial cell membranes. Coincidentally, the antibodies interfere with the thromboplastin reagent of the activated partial thromboplastin time. They were first encountered in lupus patients; hence the misnomer *lupus anticoagulant.* Immune injury to the endothelium, activation of platelets, and interference with natural anticoagulants have all been hypothesized as mechanisms for thrombosis. Venous thromboembolism and fetal loss are common presentations.[2] Compared with antithrombin III or protein C/S deficiencies, the antiphospholipid syndrome seems more frequently associated with spontaneous thromboses in the arterial circulation. Among patients with arterial occlusion, APA should be suspected in young patients with stroke, those with unusual sites of thrombosis such as the upper

Table 1 Clinical Characteristics That May Distinguish Hypercoagulable States

Characteristic	High Probability	Low Probability
Family history of thrombosis	Yes	No
Frequency of thrombosis	Multiple episodes	Single episode
Site(s) of thrombosis	Unusual locations, multiple sites and multiple clots	Typical site, single thrombosis
Provocative factors and response	Spontaneous thrombosis or exaggerated response to minor injury	Usually associated with a provocative insult, to which the extent of thrombosis is appropriate
Age, risk factors	Young age, no apparent risk factors	Characteristic age and risk factors for the type of thrombosis

extremity, and generally in young patients, women, and nonsmokers.[3] After vascular reconstruction, high rates of early graft failure and recurrent graft thromboses can be expected in these patients.

The diagnosis should be suspected by the clinical presentation or an unexplained prolongation of the partial thromboplastin time. Specific laboratory tests are the lupus anticoagulant test, a clotting assay, and a serologic test for APA. The serologic test is unaffected by anticoagulant therapy and can be positive even if the clotting assays are normal. Treatment for APA, not yet standardized, depends on the nature and severity of the thrombotic condition. The use of corticosteroids remains controversial. The consensus suggests that intense anticoagulation with sodium warfarin (international normalized ratio of 3 to 3.5) is indicated after a serious thrombosis or vascular reconstruction.[2]

Deficiencies of Proteins C and S

Proteins C and S are part of a natural anticoagulant pathway that retards thrombosis and enhances fibrinolysis. When free thrombin binds to thrombomodulin on the endothelial surface, it forms a complex that activates protein C. Protein S binds protein C, forming a circulating complex that neutralizes activated factor V and enhances fibrinolysis. Patients with congenital heterozygous deficiencies of protein C or S commonly have recurrent venous thromboembolism beginning in early adulthood.[4] Spontaneous arterial thromboses are rarer but may be precipitated by arterial interventions or operations. Acquired deficiencies have also been described. As both proteins depend on vitamin K for synthesis, sodium warfarin therapy induces a deficiency. But there is no predisposition to thrombosis, because factors II, VII, IX and X are also depressed. If a large loading dose of sodium warfarin is given, protein C levels will fall much faster because of its short plasma half-life, and warfarin skin necrosis may occur. Three-fifths of protein S circulates bound to the C4b binding protein of the complement system, and only the free two-fifths is functional. Thus, infection, inflammation, and thrombosis may increase C4b levels, which is an acute phase reactant, and induce a relative functional deficiency of protein S. Free protein S may also be deficient in liver disease and the nephrotic syndrome.

Protein C and S levels should be measured in patients with repeated episodes of venous thromboembolism and in vascular patients with recurrent graft thromboses, especially lacking technical factors that might contribute to premature graft failure. Heparin sodium therapy will not affect protein levels, but chronic sodium warfarin will reduce levels to the range of 30% to 50% of normal. Ideally, levels should be measured when the patient is off warfarin. Assay can detect either the antigen or the activity of the protein. For protein S, both the absolute concentration and the biologic activity should be measured. Values for both types of assays are expressed as a percentage, and normal values can range from 75% to 120%, depending on the laboratory.

Both heparin and sodium warfarin can effectively counteract the thrombotic tendency in these deficiency states. For patients undergoing vascular reconstruction, heparin anticoagulation should be gently converted to chronic warfarin therapy using initially low doses of sodium warfarin. Indefinite warfarin therapy is also indicated for patients with confirmed deficiencies and repeated episodes of venous thromboembolism. The optimal intensity of anticoagulation is not known.

Antithrombin III Deficiency

Antithrombin III (ATIII) is the most important of the natural anticoagulant proteins. It inhibits the enzymatic activities of thrombin and other activated clotting factors. Naturally occurring heparin-like molecules lining the endothelium accelerate ATIII's anticoagulant activity, as does pharmacologic heparin. The classic heterozygous genetic deficiency may affect one in 2,000 people, although not all will manifest a thrombotic tendency. Recurrent venous thromboembolism is the typical clinical problem, although thrombi may develop in unusual sites such as the renal veins. Deficient surgical patients are prone to deep venous thrombosis or arterial thrombosis at sites of vascular injury. A number of mutant variants of ATIII have also been identified. The protein is synthesized in normal quantities but lacks function. This emphasizes the importance of functional assays for diagnosis. With classic deficiency, levels may be 25% to 60% of normal, lower with some mutant antithrombins. Acquired deficiencies of ATIII occur with protein loss in the nephrotic syndrome, with impaired synthetic function in liver disease, and with rapid consumption in sepsis and disseminated intravascular coagulation.

When thrombotic complications occur, intravenous heparin and ATIII concentrates are the treatment of choice. Without ATIII supplementation, some patients may require unusually high doses of heparin to achieve therapeutic effects. In the perioperative period blood levels of ATIII should be monitored and maintained near normal with the infusion of ATIII concentrates. In emergencies fresh frozen plasma can substitute. After vascular reconstruction or the acute treatment of a thrombotic complication the patient should be maintained on chronic warfarin therapy.

Heparin-Associated Thrombocytopenia and Thrombosis

Approximately 5% of patients exposed to an extended course of intravenous heparin will develop drug-induced immune thrombocytopenia.[5] Sensitization may also develop after several brief exposures to heparin or rarely after the minimal doses used to flush vascular catheters. The thrombocytopenia is caused by an acquired antibody directed at a combination of constituents of the platelet membrane and heparin. In contrast to other immune thrombocytopenias, these antibodies activate the platelets by way of the platelet Fc receptor.

Continued or recurrent exposure to heparin can cause pathologic arterial or venous thromboemboli. The whitish appearance of these platelet-rich thrombi invoked the name *white clot syndrome*. Typical manifestations of the syndrome include a platelet count below 100,000/µl while receiving heparin, heparin resistance, and a prompt rise in the platelet count within 3 to 5 days after stopping heparin. If pathologic thrombosis occurs in conjunction with thrombocytopenia during heparin therapy, the diagnosis is very likely. Specialized platelet aggregation testing is essential to confirm the diagnosis.

Who should be screened for heparin sensitivity? If the patient has never before received heparin, screening is unnecessary. However, it is such a ubiquitous drug for hospitalized patients that many have received it without their knowledge. Some patients become sensitized to it during previous vascular procedures although the thrombocytopenia goes unnoticed. In such patients, re-exposure to heparin for subsequent procedures can incite the anamnestic immune response and result in graft thrombosis. When possible preoperatively, it is wise to review the laboratory records of anyone who has had previous heparin therapy. Some surgeons preoperatively screen all patients who have had heparin, but this remains controversial. Certainly any patient who has suffered an unexplained thrombosis of previous vascular reconstruction should be screened.

If the diagnosis is made preoperatively, operation should be delayed until alternative management strategies can be developed.[5] If the syndrome is suspected in the perioperative period, all heparin must be stopped and the diagnosis confirmed by in vitro testing. A platelet inhibitor such as aspirin or low-molecule dextran is usually helpful in abating the generalized platelet activation. Sodium warfarin is a good choice when continued anticoagulation is indicated. Patients with this syndrome may demonstrate a predisposition to thrombosis for several months after vascular reconstruction. Chronic aspirin plus low-dose sodium warfarin therapy may reduce the risks of graft failure during this period.

Conditions Associated with Activation of Platelets and Plasma Coagulation

Malignancy

Disseminated malignancy and some myeloproliferative disorders can cause a low-grade disseminated intravascular coagulation (DIC) the principal manifestations of which are thrombotic. Thromboplastic substances and tumor cells leak into the circulation, chronically activating the coagulation cascade. ATIII levels may be depressed. Mucin-producing adenocarcinomas are the worst offenders, as exemplified by the migratory phlebitis of Trousseau's syndrome. In the asymptomatic patient the added thrombotic stimulus of vascular injury can easily tip the balance to pathologic thrombosis. This syndrome exemplifies Wessler's first definition of hypercoagulability, namely a perturbed system that has not yet progressed to clot formation.

It is important to maintain a high index of suspicion to diagnose a thrombotic diathesis in the cancer patient. Compensatory production of clotting factors and platelets may match or exceed consumption. Plasma fibrinogen and platelet counts may be normal or even elevated. The presence of elevated fibrin or fibrinogen degradation products indicates intravascular clotting. Frequently the thrombin time is abnormal, reflecting hypofibrinogenemia or impairment of fibrin polymerization by circulating degradation products.

Heparin remains the most effective treatment for frank thromboses, and antithrombin concentrates can be considered when ATIII levels are low. When vascular intervention is required, heparin should be used as liberally as can be done safely. There is also an increased risk of postoperative venous thromboembolism, so effective methods of prophylaxis should be used when indicated.

Pregnancy, Estrogens

Pregnancy and childbirth are associated with an increased risk of venous thrombosis and pulmonary embolism. Anatomic and mechanical factors undoubtedly contribute, but physiologic changes in the levels of clotting factors and natural inhibitors tilt the balance toward a prothrombotic state.[4] Estrogen therapy is also associated with an increased risk of both venous and arterial thrombosis, although the mechanisms are still unclear. The newer low-estrogen contraceptives do not carry a higher thrombotic risk except in smokers. From this it is possible to predict that other cardiovascular risk factors may compound the prothrombotic effects of estrogen.

Systemic Diseases

There is a well-known association between the nephrotic syndrome and pathologic thrombosis, probably due to low levels of ATIII and free protein S. A number of systemic disorders related to cardiovascular disease have been loosely associated with a predisposition to thrombosis. Researchers have observed evidence of platelet hyperactivity or increased platelet activation in patients with diabetes mellitus, familial type II hyperlipidemia, and myocardial infarction. The adaptive responses to the stress of operation include many subtle but measurable changes in platelet function and plasma coagulation that favor clotting. In the vascular surgical patient with diabetes, peripheral atherosclerosis, gangrene, and infection, these independent stimuli can yield a hypercoagulable state that may be as clinically significant as the better-defined disorders. Useful markers for this ill-defined type of hypercoagulability are an elevated platelet count and plasma fibrinogen level. Large epidemiologic studies have shown that the fibrinogen level is a strong independent risk factor for arterial thrombosis.

UNCOMMON DISORDERS

Derangements of Fibrinolytic Pathways

Because the fibrinolytic system naturally delimits and dissolves clot, derangements of this system will frequently result in a thrombotic tendency. This exemplifies Wessler's second definition of hypercoagulability, in which the system is unperturbed but the threshold to clot formation is lowered.

With the advent of improved biochemical techniques to measure the quantity and biologic activities of plasminogen, tissue-type plasminogen activator, and plasminogen activator inhibitor 1, a number of fibrinolytic derangements have been identified.[6] Congenitally dysfunctional variants of plasminogen have been associated with recurrent thromboses.[7] Abnormal fibrinogens have been identified with thrombi that are extremely resistant to lysis. Excessively high levels of activator inhibitors have also been found.

The patient with a thrombotic disorder of fibrinolysis may not be clinically distinguishable from one with other plasma protein–based disorders, and recurrent venous thromboembolism is typical, although arterial complications can also occur. A useful screening test is the euglobulin lysis time. If it is excessively prolonged, a fibrinolytic disorder should be sought with more specific assays for plasminogen and its activators and inhibitors.

Primary Endothelial Disorders

In addition to its contributions to fibrinolytic pathways, the endothelium plays other critical roles in thromboregulation. Endothelial injury impairs the synthesis of prostacyclin and endothelial-derived relaxing factor, leading to vasoconstriction and disinhibition of platelets. Denudation of the endothelium releases tissue factor and exposes subendothelial collagen and von Willebrand factor, to which platelets adhere. Thus, intrinsic inflammatory conditions of the arteries can predispose to thrombosis.[8] Collagen vascular diseases (especially scleroderma), inflammatory vasculitides (giant cell arteritis, Takayasu's), and Behcet's disease may all present with pathologic arterial thrombosis. The cause of thrombosis in homocystinuria is not as well understood, but it is related in part to biochemical injury to the endothelium. Most of these patients have other features that are clinically distinctive of their primary diseases.

LABORATORY DIAGNOSIS

In this era of cost-consciousness the selection of patients for in-depth screening is perhaps the most controversial area of all. Routine coagulation screening tests are not helpful except for the partial thromboplastin time, which may reveal antiphospholipid antibodies. Clinical presentations cannot easily distinguish between diagnoses, so an initial battery of possibly expensive tests is necessary. On the other hand, screening should be extremely cost effective if it can obviate the expenses of major thrombotic complications and reoperation. Selection criteria can help in choosing which patients should be screened (Table 1). A basic panel of tests can evaluate the common disorders (Table 2). Some tests can be excluded on the basis of clinical presentation. Ideally, blood should be obtained when the patient is free of anticoagulants. Heparin can interfere with functional assays of protein C, and both protein C and S are depressed by sodium warfarin. Laboratory tests cannot replace the advice and consultation of an individual

Table 2 Laboratory Assessment of Hypercoagulable States

Suspected Disorder	Testing Method	Interpretation
Antiphospholipid antibodies	Lupus anticoagulant: a modified partial thromboplastin time. Anticardiolipin antibodies: a serology test that directly detects the antibodies.	Clotting assays are usually interpreted as positive or negative. Antibody titers are reported against a normal range.
Protein C deficiency Protein S deficiency Antithrombin deficiency	Immunologic methods measure the total concentration of protein present. Functional assays measure the biologic activity of the proteins.	Values are reported as a percentage (100% being ideal). The range of normal is wide and laboratory dependent (60%–140%). Generally below 50%–60% is abnormal.
Heparin-induced thrombocytopenia and thrombosis	Specialized platelet aggregation testing or serotonin release studies are performed using patient's platelets and plasma or patient's plasma mixed with normal platelets when thrombocytopenia is present.	Normally, platelets do not aggregate or secrete serotonin in response to low concentrations of heparin (0.1-1 U/ml).
Disorders of fibrinolysis	Euglobulin lysis time: a subfraction of plasma containing the fibrinolytic enzymes is clotted and the time for dissolution recorded.	A prolonged lysis time indicates impaired fibrinolytic activity.
Disseminated intravascular coagulation	A semiquantitative assay for fibrin or fibrinogen degradation products (FDP) based on the agglutination of latex particles coated with antibody.	Normally FDP are very low. Intermediate levels are found after major thromboses or surgery. High levels (>40 μg/dl) suggest DIC.
Plasma fibrinogen	A variety of clot-based and other assays.	Elevated levels of fibrinogen are an independent risk factor for thrombosis.

experienced in the diagnosis and treatment of thrombotic disorders. Once abnormalities in these screening tests are detected, advice regarding more detailed testing and management of the patient can be very helpful.

Molecular markers for pathologic thrombosis are rapidly approaching clinical applicability. Peptide fragments of proenzymes of the coagulation cascade circulate when the cascade is activated, and these can be detected in nanogram quantities. Elevated blood levels of fibrinopeptide A, prothrombin fragments 1+2, and β-thromboglobulin, a platelet release protein, have all been observed in patients with pathologic thrombosis or hypercoagulable states. Soon it may be possible to predict a patient's susceptibility to thrombotic complications based solely on one or two of these biochemical markers.[9]

Meanwhile, the principal tools for the vascular surgeon are a heightened awareness of these defined syndromes and an understanding of their diagnosis and pathobiology. For these patients the final recourse is frequently chronic anticoagulation with sodium warfarin, for want of a better or more specific remedy. The optimal antithrombotic regimen after vascular surgery, with or without a hypercoagulable state, remains controversial.[10] Novel and specific antithrombotic agents and recombinant protein drugs are under development. With precise diagnosis, these agents may also permit precise treatment.

REFERENCES

1. Wessler S. Thrombosis and sex hormones: A perplexing liaison. J Lab Clin Med 1980; 96:757–761.
2. Triplett DA. Antiphospholipid antibodies and thrombosis: A consequence, coincidence, or cause? Arch Pathol Lab Med 1993; 117:78–88.
3. Shortell CK, Ouriel K, Green RM, et al. Vascular disease in the antiphospholipid syndrome: A comparison with the patient population with atherosclerosis. J Vasc Surg 1992; 15:158–166.
4. Schafer AI. The hypercoagulable states. Ann Intern Med 1985; 102:814–828.
5. Sobel M. Heparin-induced thrombocytopenia. Perspect Vasc Surg 1992; 5:1–30.
6. Bick RL, Ucar K. Hypercoagulability and thrombosis. Hematol Oncol Clin North Am 1992; 6:1421–1431.
7. Robbins KC. Dysplasminogenemias. Prog Cardiovasc Dis 1992; 34:295–308.
8. Nachman RL, Silverstein R. Hypercoagulable states. Ann Intern Med 1993; 119:819–827.
9. Gershlick AH. Are there markers of the blood-vessel wall interaction and of thrombus formation that can be used clinically? Circulation 1990; 81:I28–34.
10. Clagett GP, Graor RA, Salzman EW. Antithrombotic therapy in peripheral arterial occlusive disease. Chest 1992; 104:516s–528s.

COMPLICATIONS OF HEPARIN THERAPY

MICHAEL J. ROHRER, M.D.
H. BROWNELL WHEELER, M.D.

Heparin sodium is widely used for the treatment and prophylaxis of venous thromboembolism. It is also used for the prevention of arterial thrombosis and embolization during arterial reconstructive procedures and for the routine irrigation of arterial and venous catheters. This widespread use exposes many patients to the drug. An awareness of its potential complications, some of which are idiosyncratic, is therefore essential for contemporary practice.

HEMORRHAGIC COMPLICATIONS

Bleeding is the most common complication of heparin therapy. The most common sites of bleeding are operative wounds and areas of pre-existing pathology such as peptic ulceration and cancer; however, bleeding may occur from many sites. Intracranial bleeding or retroperitoneal hemorrhage may be life threatening. Major bleeding after administration of heparin sodium is usually due to an overdose of heparin sodium or to an underlying pathologic condition that predisposes the patient to hemorrhage.

Overdosage

An overdose of heparin sodium usually results from failure to adjust the amount administered in response to the results of laboratory tests. Optimal therapeutic serum concentrations of heparin sodium are about 0.2 to 0.4 units/ml, but a direct assay of heparin concentration is not available in many hospitals. Most surgeons therefore rely on the activated partial thromboplastin time (aPTT) to guide their therapy. In many hospitals the aPTT is expressed as a ratio, using a normal control as a reference, with the clinical objective being to achieve an aPTT elevation of 2 to 2.5 times normal. However, there are practical problems with this guideline. The responsiveness of the particular reagents used in the assay is critical in determining the laboratory result. The relationship between the aPTT and serum heparin level with different reagents may not be parallel, and therefore, expressing aPTT as a normalized ratio has inherent inaccuracies.[1] These practical limitations in the laboratory assessment of dosage may contribute to bleeding complications with heparin therapy. Nevertheless, it is critical to monitor the anticoagulant effect of heparin sodium with the best laboratory method available, which in most hospitals is the aPTT.

Once heparin treatment is instituted, its effect on the clotting mechanism must be monitored at least daily. Heparin sodium requirements may change dramatically and unpredictably with the patient's condition, and the dosage of heparin sodium may require substantial adjustment. The dose should be reduced when the aPTT exceeds 2.5 times the normal control level. Bleeding complications are clearly correlated with the intensity of anticoagulation, and high elevations of aPTT are associated with an increased incidence of hemorrhage.[2,3]

Bleeding due to heparin overdosage will often stop when an elevated aPTT is brought back to the therapeutic range. If blood loss is substantial, or if it occurs in a critical location such as the central nervous system, heparin sodium must be stopped immediately and consideration given to reversing its anticoagulant effect with protamine sulfate.

Most bleeding complications of heparin therapy occur within the first 5 days of therapy, with the peak risk on the third day.[4] Many observers have noted that bleeding complications are relatively rare at the onset of therapy. Patients with venous thromboembolic disease have been treated with 60,000 to 90,000 units of heparin sodium per day for the first 48 hours without any increase in the risk of bleeding.[5] Patients undergoing coronary angioplasty have received high doses of heparin sodium, with an aPTT more than three times the control value, for 1 or 2 days without any increase in bleeding complications.[6] Massive heparin sodium doses during cardiopulmonary bypass also have a low incidence of bleeding other than in the operative field. At the time of the initiation of treatment it is important to use an adequate dose to achieve the therapeutic objective; but it is also important to monitor dosage by laboratory assessment thereafter.

Underlying Coagulation Disorders

Severe bleeding may occur during heparin anticoagulation in a patient with an underlying coagulation disorder, even with a usual and customary dose of heparin sodium. A history of bleeding complications is the best clue to an underlying congenital coagulation disorder. Most acquired coagulation disorders can also be suspected from the medical history. It is important to inquire about underlying diseases such as liver disease that may affect the coagulation mechanism as well as the use of medications that may affect the coagulation system such as sodium warfarin or aspirin. When there is any suspicion of a bleeding tendency from the patient's medical or family history, a coagulation profile should be obtained and should include prothrombin time, aPTT, platelet count, and bleeding time.

Other Pathologic Conditions

Patients on heparin treatment may also be predisposed to hemorrhage by underlying disease. It is not uncommon for an occult cancer of the colon, uterus, or kidney to manifest itself first by bleeding when the patient is anticoagulated. Acid peptic ulcer disease and severe hypertension also may give rise to bleeding during treatment with heparin sodium. When unexpected bleeding is observed in an anticoagulated patient, the physician should suspect occult underlying disease, particularly when the aPTT is not prolonged excessively or the heparin dosage is relatively small, as in prophylaxis for deep venous thrombosis (DVT). Any patient with unexplained bleeding while taking heparin sodium should receive an appropriate diagnostic evaluation for underlying disease, even if the bleeding is relatively minor and stops promptly.

Other risk factors for bleeding complications during heparin treatment include chronic renal failure,[1,2] liver disease,[2] aspirin use,[4] and heavy alcohol consumption.[4] Advanced age and female sex, especially in combination, have been consistently identified as risk factors for hemorrhage associated with the therapeutic administration of heparin sodium.[1-4] (Table 1).

THROMBOTIC COMPLICATIONS

Underdosage

Although hemorrhagic complications can result from overaggressive use of heparin sodium, the patient

Table 1 Ways to Reduce the Hemorrhagic Complications of Heparin Anticoagulation

Cause	Warning Signs	Management
1. Overdosage	aPTT greater than 2.5 × control, or serum heparin level greater than 0.4 units/ml	Reduce or stop heparin sodium, possibly administer protamine sulfate
2. Underlying coagulopathy	History of pathologic bleeding	Coagulation profile prior to initiation of anticoagulation
3. Associated pathology	History of recent peptic ulcer, severe hypertension, cancer, renal failure, liver disease	Reduce dosage of heparin sodium, frequent monitoring
4. Patient's characteristics	Heavy alcohol use, aspirin or sodium warfarin use, advanced age, female sex	Reduce dosage of heparin sodium, frequent monitoring

can also be exposed to thrombotic or embolic complications from overcautious use of it. Patients who have had a pulmonary embolus are 10 to 15 times as likely to sustain a recurrent pulmonary embolus if the aPTT is subtherapeutic, and patients with a recent myocardial infarction are 22 times as likely to develop a left ventricular mural thrombus if anticoagulants are not administered.[1] Audits of routine hospital practice indicate that heparin doses are often too conservative, especially at the onset of treatment, and that a substantial delay frequently occurs before reaching therapeutic levels of anticoagulation, which results in an unnecessary risk of subsequent thromboembolic events.[7]

Antithrombin III Deficiency

The hypercoagulable state associated with congenital deficiency of antithrombin III (ATIII) is not effectively treated with heparin sodium, since ATIII is a necessary cofactor for heparin's anticoagulant action. An ATIII deficiency should be suspected in any young patient with deep venous thrombosis without known risk factors, especially if the patient requires unusually large doses of heparin sodium to increase the aPTT. Blood for ATIII levels should be drawn prior to the administration of heparin sodium. If ATIII deficiency is documented, the patient can be treated with an exogenous source of ATIII (either fresh frozen plasma or the commercially available preparation), which will enhance the effectiveness of heparin until anticoagulation with warfarin can be achieved.

Thrombocytopenia Associated with Heparin Sodium

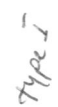

Thrombocytopenia associated with the administration of heparin sodium occurs in two distinct forms. The first involves a transient and relatively mild fall in the platelet count within the first few days of administration of heparin sodium. Although it is found in 15% to 33% of patients, its pathophysiology is unknown. This form of thrombocytopenia improves spontaneously and is of no clinical significance.

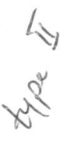

A second less common but more serious type of heparin-associated thrombocytopenia (HAT) is an immune-mediated idiosyncratic reation in which thrombocytopenia can occur in association with pathologic thrombosis. This threatening type of HAT can occur not only during the administration of therapeutic concentrations of heparin sodium but also during heparin prophylaxis for DVT. Even the minute amounts of heparin sodium administered as a flush solution for the maintenance of arterial lines can precipitate this syndrome, as can the heparin sodium present on heparin-bonded catheters. Clinically, this second form of HAT is characterized by a falling platelet count and an increasing resistance to anticoagulation with heparin sodium, followed by pathologic thrombosis in spite of the continued administration of heparin sodium and the presence of thrombocytopenia.

Incidence

The second form of HAT occurs in 2% to 6% of patients undergoing treatment with therapeutic concentrations of heparin sodium. Pathologic thrombosis occurs in 0.4%, with an associated high morbidity and mortality.[1]

Pathophysiology

The pathologic form of HAT is caused by an immune mechanism mediated by heparin-associated antiplatelet antibodies (HAAPA). In the presence of heparin sodium these antibodies fix complement to the platelet membrane, initiating prostaglandin synthesis with the production of endoperoxidases and thromboxane A_2. The resulting platelet release reaction liberates serotonin and adenosine diphosphate, which together with endoperoxidase and thromboxane A_2 induce platelet activation and aggregation and cause simultaneous thrombosis and thrombocytopenia.[8]

Clinical Presentation

The thrombocytopenia that develops as a result of HAAPA is typically seen after 3 to 15 days of heparin therapy. However, patients who have previously received heparin sodium and become sensitized may develop a more rapid immunologic response. Thrombocytopenia and thrombosis may occur within the first day of treatment.[8]

HAT may present first as an asymptomatic fall in the platelet count, or it may become manifest initially as arterial or venous thrombosis. Occasionally it presents clinically as localized skin necrosis secondary to thrombosis of the capillaries and veins of the fat and overlying skin, either at the site of subcutaneous heparin sodium injection or at remote sites. Rarely, HAT may present as a hemorrhagic complication due to the associated thrombocytopenia.

Management

Patients undergoing treatment with heparin sodium should have periodic screening platelet counts to detect thrombocytopenia before they develop thrombotic complications. If the platelet count falls below 100,000/mm³ or if a sudden drop in the platelet count is noted, heparin sodium administration should be stopped and screening for HAAPA should be performed.

Several methodologies have been employed to test for the presence of HAAPA, but the most convenient and widely used technique is platelet aggregometry. A positive test is suggested by the ability of serum or plasma from the patient to cause spontaneous aggregation of platelets from a normal donor in the presence of heparin sodium.

When thrombocytopenia develops during treatment with heparin sodium and HAAPA testing is positive, heparin sodium must be stopped and alternative methods of anticoagulation considered. Patients being

Table 2 Ways to Reduce the Thrombotic Complications of Heparin Therapy

Cause	Warning Signs	Management
1. Underdosage	aPTT less than 2 × control or recurrent thrombosis or embolization	Increase dosage to maintain aPTT 2–2.5 × control
2. ATIII deficiency	Unexplained thrombosis, especially in a young patient, with subtherapeutic aPTT in spite of large doses of heparin sodium	Check ATIII levels before giving heparin sodium and fresh frozen plasma (FFP); administer FFP and heparin sodium if ATIII levels low; start warfarin early
3. Heparin-associated thrombocytopenia	Platelet count <100,000 mm³, skin necrosis, or recurrent thrombotic episodes	Stop heparin sodium, check for heparin-associated antiplatelet antibodies; if present, administer alternative anticoagulant (warfarin, low-molecular-weight heparin, ancrod, iloprost, antiplatelet agents)

treated for venous thrombosis or pulmonary embolism may require a vena cava filter if therapeutic levels of sodium warfarin have not yet been achieved. Low-molecular-weight heparin has been successfully administered as an alternative to unfractionated heparin sodium in the presence of HAAPA, but HAT has also been shown to persist in some cases.[8,9]

Difficult problems in clinical management may occur when patients with a history of HAAPA must undergo cardiopulmonary bypass or vascular reconstructions that require anticoagulation. Ideally, such procedures should be postponed until platelet aggregation studies become negative, which typically occurs in approximately 6 weeks. Alternative methods of anticoagulation have been employed for patients who must be anticoagulated sooner. Ancrod, a derivative of Malayan pit viper venom, is an effective and selective defibrinogenating agent. Therapeutic anticoagulation can be achieved by lowering the fibrinogen levels to 20 to 40 mg/dl in 6 to 12 hours.[10] Not only does this provide therapeutic anticoagulation, but the depletion of fibrinogen further inhibits platelet aggregation, since fibrinogen is the platelet-to-platelet cross-linking agent. Other strategies to allow safe anticoagulation have employed antiplatelet agents to prevent platelet aggregation and thereby allow the continued use of heparin sodium as an anticoagulant. There are case reports of patients who have safely undergone cardiopulmonary bypass or hemodialysis with heparin sodium after treatment with aspirin or aspirin and dipyridamole. There have also been reports of the successful use of iloprost, a short-acting, stable prostacyclin analog that inhibits platelet aggregation even in the presence of HAAPA and heparin sodium. Plasmapheresis and thrombin inhibitors have also been used successfully in the management of HAT (Table 2).

OTHER HEPARIN-RELATED COMPLICATIONS

Other idiosyncratic complications are related to heparin therapy. Immediate hypersensitivity reactions associated with heparin sodium administration have been reported but are rare. Osteoporosis occurs in 1% to 20% of individuals treated with doses of heparin sodium greater than 20,000 units/day for more than 6 months.[11] This heparin-related loss of bone mass is probably reversible upon cessation of treatment. Alopecia has also been associated with the administration of heparin sodium. When heparin sodium is required for the treatment of venous thrombosis in pregnant women, vaginal bleeding has been noted. In spite of this problem, heparin sodium is preferred to sodium warfarin for the treatment of venous thrombosis during pregnancy, since heparin sodium does not cross the placenta and is therefore less likely to cause fetal complications.[1,11]

REFERENCES

1. Hirsh J. Heparin. N Engl J Med 1991; 324:1565–1574.
2. Landfeld CS, Cook EF, Flatley M, et al. Identification and preliminary validation of predictors of major bleeding in hospitalized patients starting anticoagulant therapy. Am J Med 1987; 82:703–713.
3. Kelton JG, Hirsh J. Bleeding associated with antithrombotic therapy. Semin Hematol 1980; 17:259–291.
4. Walker AM, Jick H. Predictors of bleeding during heparin therapy. JAMA 1980; 244:1209–1212.
5. Conti S, Daschbach M, Blaisdell FW. A comparison of high-dose versus conventional-dose heparin therapy for deep venous thrombosis. Surgery 1982; 92:972–980.
6. McGarry TF, Gottlieb RS, Morganroth J, et al. The relationship of anticoagulation level and complications after successful coronary angioplasty. Am Heart J 1992; 123:1445–1451.
7. Anderson FA Jr, Wheeler HB. Physician practices in the management of venous thromboembolism: A community-wide survey. J Vasc Surg 1992; 15:707–714.
8. Warkentin TE, Kelton JG. Heparin-induced thrombocytopenia. Prog Hemost Thromb 1991; 10:1–34.
9. Chong BH, Ismail F, Cade J, et al. Heparin-induced thrombocytopenia: Studies with a new low molecular weight heparinoid, Org 10172. Blood 1989; 73:1592–1596.
10. Demers C, Ginsberg JS, Brill-Edwards P, et al. Rapid anticoagulation using ancrod for heparin-induced thrombocytopenia. Blood 1991; 78:2194–2197.
11. Ginsberg JS, Hirsh J. Use of anticoagulants during pregnancy. Chest 1989; 95:156S–160S.

CUTANEOUS ULCERS IN THE ISCHEMIC DIABETIC FOOT

JOHN M. MAREK, M.D.
WILLIAM C. KRUPSKI, M.D.

Cutaneous foot ulcers are one of the most frequent and devastating problems facing patients with diabetes mellitus. There are approximately 12 million diabetics in the United States, 25% of whom will seek medical attention for foot disorders in their lifetime. Each year, 6 of every 1,000 diabetics will undergo amputation at various levels in their lower extremities. At least half of all nontraumatic amputations occur in diabetics—over 60,000 major amputations annually. Complications of diabetic foot ulcers account for more hospital days than all other complications of diabetes combined.

PATHOPHYSIOLOGY

Foot problems in diabetics are complex and multifactorial. Diabetic foot ulcers have been divided into two main categories, ischemic and neurotrophic. These categories are not mutually exclusive, and most diabetic patients have components of both types.

Complications of diabetes mellitus begin to appear roughly 10 years after onset of the disease. Peripheral neuropathy, a common complication, frequently causes the foot lesions that ultimately lead to amputations. After 20 years of diabetes approximately 45% of patients will develop some evidence of peripheral neuropathy.

The cause of diabetic neuropathy is not completely understood, but both vascular and metabolic factors have been implicated. Chronic hyperglycemia is thought to be the major factor in the development of peripheral neuropathy. Neuropathy affects the foot in three different ways: loss of sensation, degeneration of motor fibers, and deterioration of the sympathetic nervous system. Sensory neuropathy leads to a decrease in perception of light touch, proprioception, and recognition of pain, and it thereby facilitates recurrent trauma to the foot. Motor neuropathy changes the biomechanics of the foot. Alterations in weight distribution to the metatarsals increase pressure over the first and fifth metatarsal heads. Decreased motor function of the intrinsic muscles of the foot results in extension of the metatarsalphalangeal joint with flexion of the proximal interphalangeal joint (hammer toe deformity) that in turn produces excessive pressure over the metatarsal head and subsequent ulceration and necrosis. Autonomic neuropathy contributes to the development of foot ulcers. Loss of sweat gland activity leads to dry, cracked skin, and vasomotor dysfunction leads to diversion of blood away from the skin by arteriovenous shunts.

Severe peripheral neuropathy ultimately may lead to Charcot deformity with mid-foot collapse, or rocker-bottom foot. This process results from motor nerve dysfunction, loss of lumbrical muscle tone, and repeated stress applied to an insensate foot. In a Charcot foot the abnormal contact on the plantar surface leads to ulceration (Fig. 1A).

Neuropathic ulcers over the metatarsal heads are called *mal perforans* ulcers. Typically, mal perforans ulcers occur on the plantar surface of the foot over the first, second, or fifth metatarsal head. They usually have a deep punched-out appearance with a surrounding heavy callus (Fig. 1B). Neuropathic ulcers are usually painless, but they often become secondarily infected.

Approximately 50% of diabetics develop peripheral vascular disease, usually beginning 10 years after onset of diabetes. Atherosclerosis occurs at an earlier age, proceeds more rapidly, and portends a worse prognosis in diabetics than nondiabetics. Macroscopically and microscopically, the disease process is similar to that found in nondiabetic patients with advanced atherosclerosis; however, the pattern of arterial occlusive disease in the diabetic patient is unique, consisting of tibiperoneal stenosis or occlusion with sparing of the pedal vessels. In general, vessels proximal to the popliteal trifurcation have nonocclusive lesions.

Numerous authors, particularly endocrinologists, have attributed vascular disease in diabetics to small-vessel disease, meaning diminished blood flow in the microcirculation. This process consists of intimal thickening involving mainly the basement membrane. The term small-vessel disease is the subject of major controversy. Microvascular disease is known to occur in the retina (diabetic retinopathy) and the kidney (diabetic nephrosclerosis), but the clinical significance of microvascular disease in the diabetic foot is debated.

Ischemic arterial ulcers typically occur on the digits or heel rather than beneath the metatarsal heads. Ulceration develops when the ischemic foot is subjected to trauma, during clipping nails, pressure from ill-fitting shoes, bed rest, immobilization, thermal injury, or striking the foot while walking barefoot. In contrast to the neurotrophic ulcer, ischemic ulcers are usually painful, although pain may be blunted by coexistent neuropathy.

FOOT ULCERATION WITH SECONDARY INFECTION

Ulceration sets the stage for secondary infection in the ischemic foot. An infected ulcer can predispose to additional tissue loss by increasing metabolism, which exceeds the blood supply in many diabetic patients. Moreover, inflammatory cells and some bacteria secrete substances that act as procoagulants and cause small-vessel thrombosis, further increasing ischemia. Diabetics have difficulty combating infections because of their impaired immune status. Dysfunction of leukocytes, including decreased adherence, chemotaxis, phagocytosis and killing ability, occur in diabetics. In general these

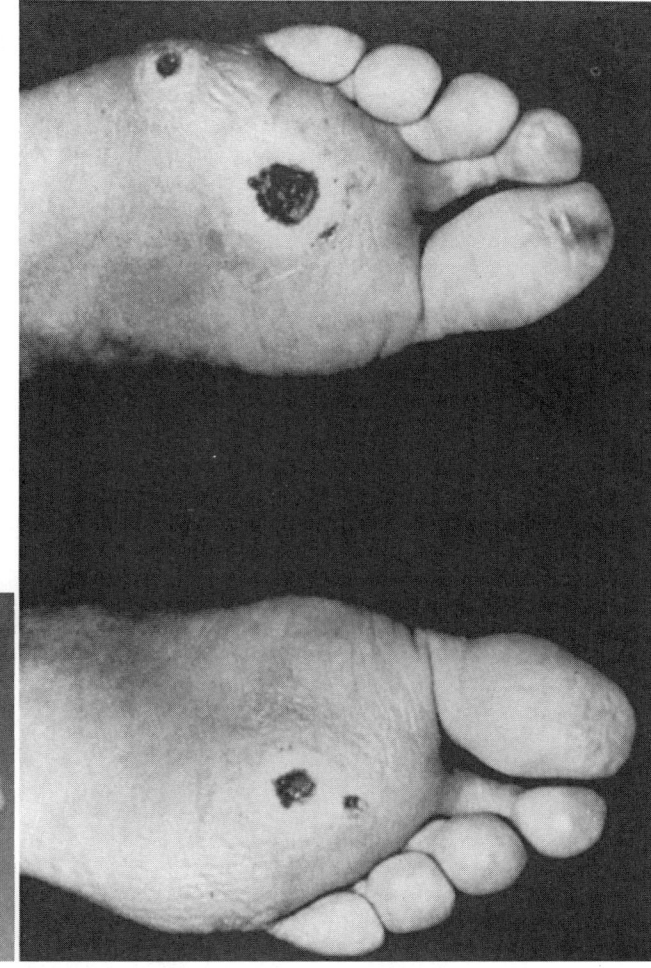

Figure 1 *A,* Charcot foot with plantar ulcer. *B,* Mal perforans ulcers. (From Levin ME, O'Neal LW, Bowker JH, eds. The diabetic foot. St. Louis: Mosby–Year Book, 1993; with permission.)

defects are aggravated or produced by hyperglycemia. Whether these disorders are due to impaired energy use by the cell or qualitative modification of cell adherence molecules is speculative.

OSTEOMYELITIS

Osteomyelitis is a particularly serious and common problem in the diabetic. Establishment or exclusion of bone infection may be difficult. Most patients with presumptive evidence of osteomyelitis have a history of a longstanding ulcer associated with local swelling and surrounding erythema. Some patients have systemic manifestations of infection, although this is uncommon.

Plain foot roentgenograms, which should be the first study for evaluation of osteomyelitis, may document osteomyelitis. However, films must be interpreted carefully, because diabetic osteopathy, a bone resorptive process due to autonomic neuropathy, closely resembles osteomyelitis on x-ray film. Osteopathy requires no intervention. It is important to remember that 10 to 14 days are required for osteomyelitis to become apparent on x-ray film. Useful hematologic tests include white blood cell count and sedimentation rate. Erythrocyte sedimentation rate greater than 70 with a clinically noninflamed ulcer correlates very well with osteomyelitis, but determination of inflammation is subjective. In some studies communication of a sterile probe from the ulcer to the bone or joint space and ulcer size wider than 2 cm both correlated with osteomyelitis.[1] A three-phase technetium-99m radionuclide bone scan with or without a gallium scan may not differentiate osteomyelitis and other causes of increased bone metabolism or increased vascularity such as cellulitis, neuropathic osteoarthropathy, and abscess, and it is costly.

Magnetic resonance imaging (MRI) is the newest of the radiographic techniques for evaluating osteomyelitis. A growing literature suggests that this technique may be more sensitive for detecting both osteomyelitis and deeper soft tissue infections in the diabetic foot. Although series are small, it has been observed that MRI findings of diabetic osteoarthropathy (low T1 and T2WI signal intensity in marrow space) differ from the findings with osteomyelitis (high signal intensity in marrow space on T2WI).[2] The cost of an MRI of the foot is high. Therefore, this test should be reserved for treatment failures. It should be emphasized that neither clinical, radiographic, nor radionuclide studies can definitively distinguish between osteomyelitis and diabetic osteoarthropathy. In many patients the definitive diagnosis can be confirmed only by bone cultures.

Osteomyelitis in the diabetic foot carries a poor prognosis, and even with long-term medical therapy most patients eventually require amputation of the infected bone.

EVALUATION OF THE ISCHEMIC ULCER

A small cutaneous ulcer may represent only the tip of the iceberg. Signs of limb- or life-threating ischemia or infection should be sought, including signs of systemic illness, necrosis, gangrene, and crepitus of the extremity. X-ray film should be obtained to observe for gas, foreign body, and osteomyelitis. Pulses should be palpated, and other signs of ischemia should be evaluated, including dependent rubor, pallor on elevation, loss of integumentary structures, and so on.

The diabetic patient may harbor a severe plantar space infection while remaining relatively asymptomatic. Fluctuance or tenderness over the arch indicates plantar space infection that requires immediate operative drainage. Edema of the extremity from congestive heart failure or venous insufficiency may obscure the diagnosis and diminish healing potential.

PREDICTION OF HEALING

It is important to ascertain whether perfusion is adequate to effect healing with local wound care. A number of studies provide an algorithm for prediction of healing (Figure 2).

Noninvasive Vascular Studies

Special considerations apply to evaluating noninvasive tests in diabetics. It is well known that medial calcification commonly present in the vessels of the diabetic patient may artifactually elevate segmental limb pressures. Several studies have shown an inability to predict healing in the diabetic despite ankle pressures associated with excellent healing in the nondiabetic, greater than 70 to 90 mm Hg. On the other hand, Apelqvist and co-workers[3] noted that only 8% of extremity wounds healed in diabetic patients with absolute ankle pressures less than 40 mm Hg, and none healed with pressures less than 30 mm Hg. This suggests that while absolute ankle pressures do not accurately predict healing, they do reliably predict nonhealing in the diabetic.

Diabetics may have occlusive lesions distal to the ankle that make the ankle pressures even more difficult to interpret. However, calcification of the digital arteries is rare even in diabetics. Thus, measurement of toe pressures is especially useful. In general 85% to 100% of foot lesions will heal when toe pressures are greater than 40 mm Hg, whereas fewer than 10% will heal if the toe pressure is less than 20 mm Hg. Toe pressures between 20 and 40 are indeterminate with respect to healing potential. Unfortunately, the great toe is the only

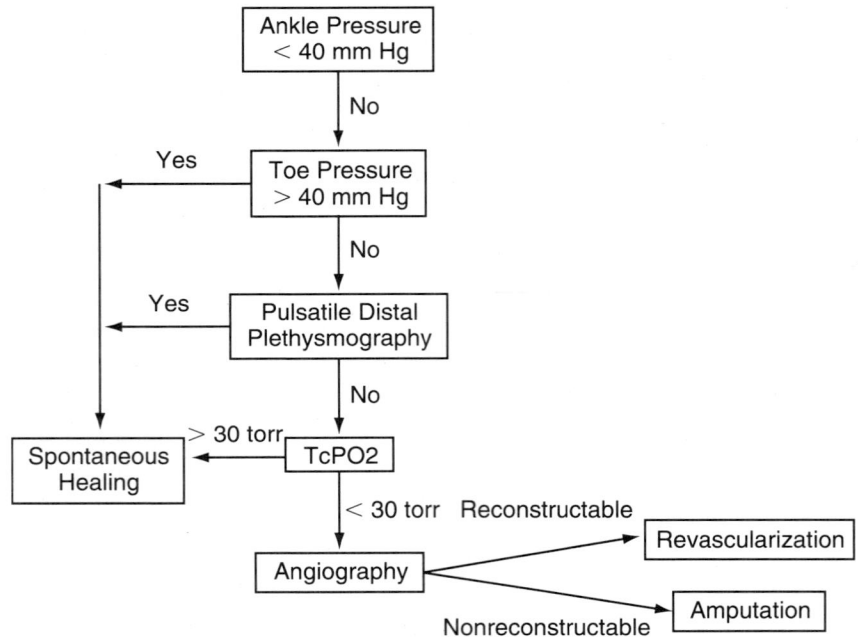

Figure 2 Algorithm for vascular assessment of wound healing potential in diabetic foot lesions.

consistently reliable site for accurate digital pressures, and many diabetics may have already lost this toe.

Plethysmographic waveforms are also useful in predicting healing. Raines and associates[4] found that 27 patients, all with pulsatile ankle plethysmographic tracings, healed a below-knee amputation. In addition 90% of patients with pulsatile transmetatarsal tracings healed foot lesions. Whereas most investigators have corroborated the high positive predictive value of pulsatile plethysmographic tracings, others have shown that more than 50% of foot lesions will heal even with poor or absent waveforms, so the negative predictive value is marginal.

Transcutaneous Oxygen Pressures

Transcutaneous oxygen pressure ($TcPo_2$) is widely applied for assessing wound healing potential. When $TcPo_2$ in the region of the ulcer is less than 10 mm Hg, wounds fail to heal. A $TcPo_2$ greater than 30 mm Hg correlates well with healing. A number of caveats pertain to $TcPo_2$ measurements. The test is time consuming and should be performed by an experienced technician. Because cutaneous vasoconstriction adversely affects $TcPo_2$, the patient should be placed in a warm room with time for temperature equilibration. Likewise, sufficient time must be allowed for the $TcPo_2$ probe to equilibrate, and a reference value must be obtained, most commonly on the chest wall. Hauser and co-workers[5] derived a regional perfusion index for each limb calculated as (foot $TcPo_2$/chest $TcPo_2$) × 100. They found this index superior to standard ankle-brachial pressure index and pulse volume recording in diagnosing degree of ischemia in diabetics. Some have advocated warming the affected extremity or assessing the increase in $TcPo_2$ produced by inhalation of supplementary oxygen; both techniques have been reported to improve sensitivity. It is important to place the probe on the dorsum of the foot, because thick skin on the sole interferes with oxygen diffusion and produces erroneously low values.

Radionuclide Studies

Skin perfusion clearance with xenon-133 and other radioisotopes are complex and rarely used. Xenon-133 washout studies are based on the direct relationship between the disappearance of xenon-133 from the skin after subcutaneous injection and cutaneous blood flow. Additional techniques include the use of intravenous thallium-201 or intra-arterial technetium-99m-labeled albumin microspheres to document perfusion or relative hyperemia at the ulcer site. Although studies have suggested these tests to be helpful in the prediction of healing, few laboratories are equiped to perform them.

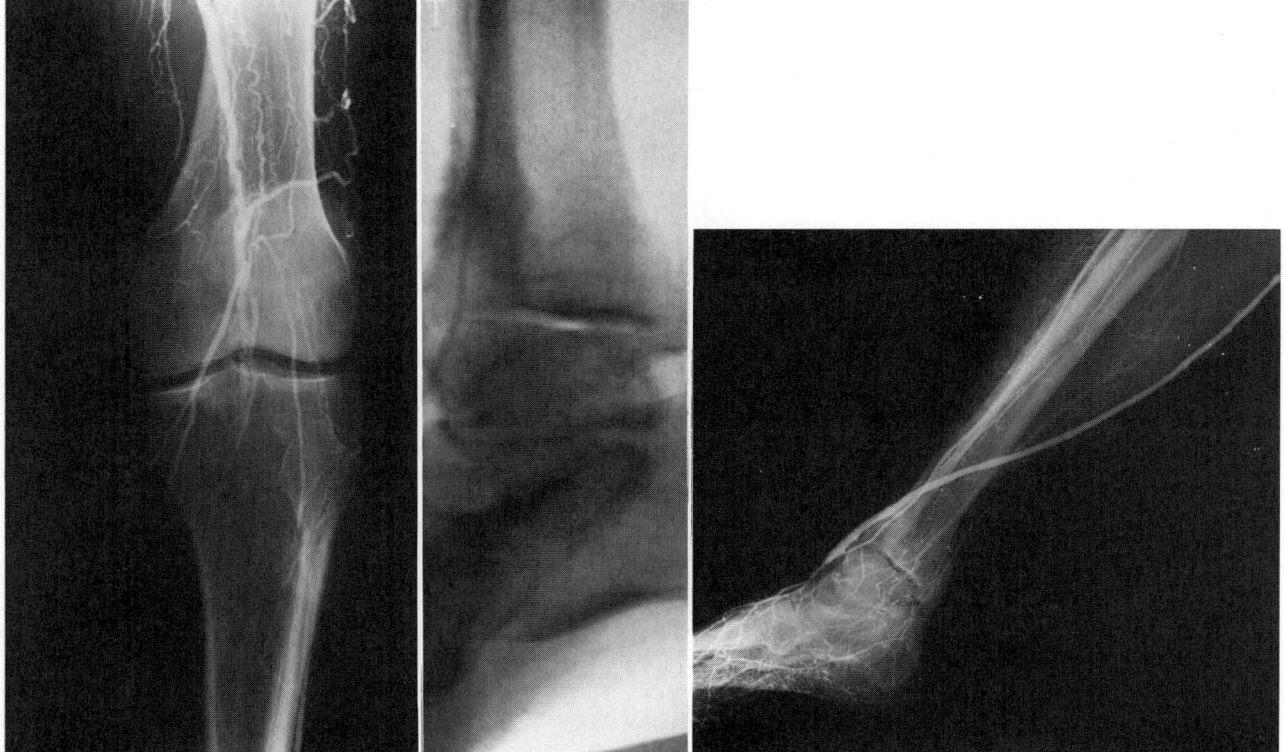

Figure 3 Preoperative and postoperative arteriograms of diabetic foot vessels. *A,* Severe infrapopliteal occlusion. *B,* Delayed digital subtraction films show patent dorsalis pedis vessel, which proved to be an excellent conduit for bypass *(C)*.

Arteriography

Patients in whom ulcer healing is doubtful by clinical or noninvasive assessment should undergo arteriography to assess the potential for revascularization. Of added importance in the diabetic patient is visualization of the pedal vessels for planning distal bypasses (Fig. 3). Intra-arterial digital subtraction angiography is advisable to obtain optimal views of pedal vessels. Additional techniques to visualize the distal vasculature include induction of reactive hyperemia by inflation and deflation of a proximal blood pressure cuff, administration of vasodilators, and temporary inflow occlusion by means of a percutaneous balloon occlusion catheter.

Caution should be observed in diabetic patients with underlying renal disease to avoid contrast-induced renal insufficiency, because they are more susceptible to this complication than nondiabetic patients. Judicious intravenous hydration with or without administration of mannitol is useful to avoid contrast induced renal insufficiency.

Magnetic Resonance Imaging

Magnetic resonance angiography has recently been evaluated for visualization of distal runoff vessels. MRA is becoming widely available, and with special software good representations of the pedal vessels can be obtained (Fig. 4). Unfortunately, when arterial flow is very low, confusion between arteries and veins can occur and is worsened by administration of enhancing agents like gadolinium.

TREATMENT

Conservative

Basic management of the diabetic foot ulcer includes evaluation of the degree of infection, debridement, immobilization, metabolic control, nutritional supplementation, systemic or local antibiotics, and assessment of the vascular status of the foot. Most diabetic patients with a foot ulcer and evidence of

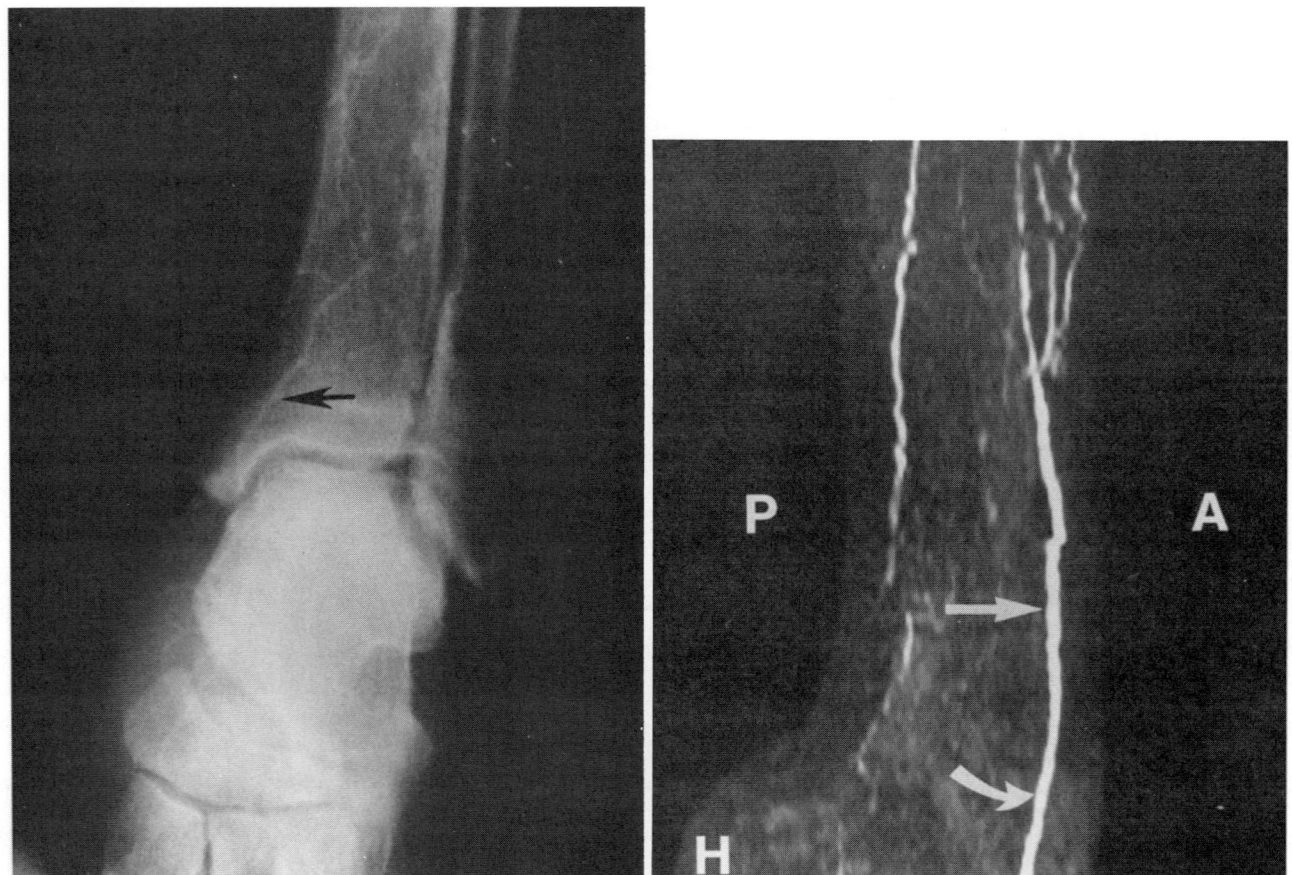

Figure 4 MRI of distal runoff vessels. *A*, Small collateral on standard angiography. *B*, MRA of dorsalis pedis vessel later found to be suitable for bypass (A-anterior; P-posterior; H-heel). (From Owen RS, Carpenter JP, Baum RA, et al. N Engl J Med 1992; 326:1577–1581; with permission.)

infection should be admitted to the hospital for aggressive debridement, metabolic control, and intravenous antibiotics. Strict non–weight bearing of the involved extremity is mandatory, especially if the ulcer occurs over a weight-bearing surface.

Most diabetic foot infections are polymicrobial, with an average of 3 to 5 species per culture. *Staphyloccus aureus, Staphylococcus epidermidis,* and Streptococcus species are the most common organisms recovered. Anaerobes and gram-negative bacilli are also frequently cultured. Despite numerous anecdotal reports, there is a conspicious absence of controlled studies regarding specific antibiotics, length of treatment, and which ulcers should be treated. Broad-spectrum antibiotics are generally advisable, given for at least 7 to 10 days.

Superficial cultures or swabs are usually of little value and may be misleading. If a deep wound specimen, curettage, or aspirate through unbroken skin can be obtained, the relevant bacteria are more likely to be discovered.

Growth Factors

Platelets and macrophages are the dominant cells in the initial stages of wound healing. These cells produce a plethora of biologically active compounds that influence the response to injury. At least five growth factors have been identified in platelet granules, and even more factors are present in macrophages. These growth factors are being applied topically in many wound care centers in an attempt to promote healing. However, to date, despite extensive use, there has been little conclusive evidence of efficacy. Most studies of platelet-derived wound healing factors (PDWHF) have been retrospective. A small prospective controlled trial in 12 patients from two institutions has shown favorable results, but to date no large multicenter trial has been reported. We have seen no benefit of PDWHF treatment compared with placebo in a pilot study of 18 patients with lower extremity ulcers.[6] The treatment is expensive, cumbersome, and in our opinion unproven.

Operation Therapy

Foremost in the management of the ischemic diabetic foot ulcer is early and aggressive debridement of all necrotic or devitalized tissue. Diabetics frequently require urgent or emergency surgical therapy for infection and ischemia of the foot. Immediate two-stage major lower extremity amputation offers a definitive solution to the problem. The obvious disadvantage of this strategy is the long-term disability for these patients posed by possible loss of the remaining limb, shortened survival, and failure to regain independent ambulation and maintain employment.

Aggressive debridement, drainage, and limited open phalangeal or forefoot amputations are preferable to major lower extremity amputation. When amputation of the foot is required due to extensive tissue loss, a two-stage approach with initial guillotine amputation offers the optimal results. Fisher and associates[7] in a prospective study randomized 47 patients (25 diabetic) with wet gangrene to one- or two-stage amputations. They documented a significantly increased incidence of wound complications (21% versus none) and increased hospital stay (52 days versus 37 days) in the one-stage group compared with the two-stage group.

Advances in revascularization techniques have improved results of distal reversed or in situ saphenous vein bypasses. Many recent studies have documented equal or superior graft patency and limb salvage in diabetic compared with nondiabetic patients. Hurley and associates[8] in a review of 259 distal arterial bypasses (57% in diabetics) noted improved graft patency and limb salvage in diabetics at 6-year follow-up. Saphenous vein grafts to the pedal vessels in diabetics have patency rates equal to those of more proximal infrageniculate arteries. We prefer to use the common femoral artery as our inflow vessel; however, if the vein is too short, the distal femoral or popliteal artery may be used. Even in the presence of infection, arterial bypasses are often advantageous. A recent study of 56 dorsal pedal vein bypasses documented graft patency and limb salvage rates of 92% and 98%, respectively, at 3 years in diabetic patients presenting with ischemic foot lesions complicated by infection.[9] Not surprisingly, results are less favorable with proximal bypasses to tibial vessels not in continuity with the pedal vessels, especially when extensive ischemic tissue loss or infection is present.

Metatarsal Head Resection

Several treatments for chronic mal perforans ulcers have been described, including ray amputation, bed rest, and total contact casting. Each of these methods may be successful, but all have disadvantages, and they usually involve prolonged healing time and hospitalization. Several recent series have documented good results with metatarsal head resection. The technique consists of resection of the incriminated metatarsal head using a dorsal incision with or without resection and closure of the plantar ulcer. Martin and associates[10] described 40 diabetic patients with longstanding mal perforans ulcers who underwent metatarsal head resection. Three patients required revascularization prior to the procedure. All 40 patients had primary healing of their ulcer with no amputations and no readmissions for forefoot sepsis during a 38-month follow-up.

Ulcer Recurrence

When healing of diabetic foot ulcers is successful, close follow-up is mandatory. Readmission to the hospital for ulcer recurrence or further revisions of partial amputations may be required. In patients in whom a diabetic foot ulcer heals, recurrence of the ulcer remains a distressing problem. Recurrence rates are high, largely due to uncorrectable neuropathy despite adequate vascular supply. Most recurrences occur within 2 months, and ulcers are likeliest to recur if present for a long period prior to healing. Compliance with therapy, education, alleviation of risk factors, and aggressive preventive measures such as frequent visits to a specialized foot care clinic are important aspects of care.

PREVENTIVE MEASURES

Education regarding foot care has long been recognized as essential for patients with diabetes. Several large clinical centers have reduced the rate of amputations in diabetics by 44% to 85% after the implementation of educational and improved foot-care programs. Guidelines and information booklets such as *Diabetic Foot Care* produced by the American Diabetes Association are readily available. In particular, patients must be educated on proper foot hygiene and footwear, avoidance of trauma, the need to stop smoking, the importance of daily foot inspections, and when to contact a health professional regarding foot problems.

Adequate foot care plays an important role in the early detection and prevention of minor foot problems that left undetected would lead to amputation. Although it is recommended that the feet of the high-risk diabetic patient be examined at every clinic visit, studies show that such examinations are performed as infrequently as 10% of the time, even in clinics exclusively caring for diabetics. Specific foot care that includes removal of calluses, skin and nail care, proper footwear, and early detection of foot lesions are paramount in prevention of severe ulceration and amputation.

The frequency of visits to the foot care clinic depends on the patient's history and compliance, but in the high-risk patient with previous ulcers upward of every 1 to 2 months is reasonable for optimal preventive care. Whether it is removal of a callus, admission to the hospital for intravenous antibiotics, or surgical debridement, the earlier the intervention, the better the outcome.

REFERENCES

1. Levin S. Digest of Current Literature. Infect Dis Clin Pract 1992; 1:49–50.
2. Wang A, Weinstein D, Greenfield L et al. MRI and diabetic foot infections. Magn Reson Imaging 1990; 8(6):805–809.
3. Apelqvist J, Castenfors J, Larsson J, et al. Prognostic value of systolic ankle and toe blood pressure levels in outcome of diabetic foot ulcer. Diabetes Care 1989; 12:373–378.
4. Raines JK, Darling RC, Buth J, et al. Vascular laboratory criteria for the management of peripheral vascular disease of the lower extremities. Surgery 1976; 79:21–29.
5. Hauser CJ, Klein SR, Mehringer CM, et al. Superiority of transcutaneous oximetry in noninvasive vascular diagnosis in patients with diabetes. Arch Surg 1984; 119:690–694.
6. Krupski WC, Reilly LM, Perez S, et al. A prospective randomized trial of autologous platelet-derived wound healing factors for treatment of chronic nonhealing wounds: A preliminary report. J Vasc Surg 1991; 14:526–536.
7. Fisher DF, Clagett GP, Fry RE, et al. One-stage versus two-stage amputation for wet gangrene of the lower extremity: A randomized study. J Vasc Surg 1988; 8:428–433.
8. Hurley JJ, Auer AI, Hershey FB, et al. Distal arterial reconstruction: Patency and limb salvage in diabetics. J Vasc Surg 1987; 5:796–800.
9. Tannenbaum GA, Pomposelli FB, Maracaccio EJ, et al. Safety of vein bypass grafting to the dorsal pedal artery in diabetic patients with foot infections. J Vasc Surg 1992; 15:982–990.
10. Martin JD, Delbridge L, Reeve TS, Clagett GP. Radical treatment of mal perforans in diabetic patients with arterial insufficiency. J Vasc Surg 1990; 12:264–68.

TREATMENT OF INFECTED VASCULAR GRAFTS IN THE GROIN

ALAN M. GRAHAM, M.D.

Vascular graft infection is one of the most feared complications to the vascular surgeon. Occurring in 1% to 2% of aortic graft replacements and up to 6% of femoropopliteal grafts, it leads to unacceptable mortality rates and major morbidity including amputation. Sources of contamination include breaks in surgical technique with resultant contamination of the graft and direct contamination of the graft in superficial areas such as the groin. Late graft infections are secondary to hematogenous spread of bacteria to the graft from a remote site.

The clinical presentation and timing of the initial operation of a femoral graft infection depend not only on the cause of the infection but also on the infecting organism. Risk factors for groin wound infections include age, obesity, length of operation, length of hospital stay, diabetes mellitus, and loss of skin integrity in the affected limb. Gram-positive organisms are often associated with a more indolent course than gram-negative organisms, especially *Pseudomonas*, which produce a much more virulent infection.

Recent advances in understanding of the microbiology investigative techniques and surgical procedures, including an in situ replacement policy, allow an up-to-date analysis of the problem of graft infections in the groin.

DIAGNOSIS

Unlike grafts in the aortic position, which are often difficult to diagnose as infected, the femoral graft, whether the distal end of an aortofemoral graft or proximal end of a femoropopliteal bypass, is much easier to diagnose as infected. A tender or pulsatile mass in the groin, cellulitis, abscess, or a draining sinus in a patient with a groin prosthesis should be treated as an infected graft unless proven otherwise.

Laboratory Tests. These include a white blood cell (WBC) count with differential, erythrocyte sedimentation rate, and blood cultures. A large number of special tests have been devised to confirm the diagnosis in patients without an obvious graft infection who have fever of unknown origin or other subclinical signs following a prosthetic graft placement.

Arteriography. The findings of an anastomotic aneurysm in a patient suspected of a graft infection should be assumed to confirm the diagnosis.

Computed Tomography and Magnetic Resonance Imaging. Anastomotic aneurysms often are associated with a perigraft fluid collection. If both of these findings are present, this is pathognomonic for graft infection. Although the infection is usually obvious clinically, the computed tomography (CT) scan or magnetic resonance imaging (MRI) scan is helpful in the obese patient or to determine whether the rest of the graft is involved.

Indium-111 WBC Scan. Labeled WBC with indium-111 is very sensitive for infected grafts.[1] It is, however, not accurate in the early postoperative period because of the perigraft reaction in the wound healing phase.

Sinogram. A persistent draining sinus in the groin is often the result of a graft infection. The extent of the infectious process and how proximal or distal to the sinus area it extends can often be determined by the gentle injection of contrast medium into the sinus tract.

Aspiration of Perigraft Fluid. This relatively easy test can often differentiate between a graft infection and a benign lymph collection. Organisms seen on Gram's stain will both confirm the diagnosis and allow appropriate preoperative antibiotics prior to definitive surgical therapy.

MICROBIOLOGY

Virtually any organism can cause vascular graft infection. The most common organism is *Staphylococcus aureus*—in up to 50% of patients. Gram-negative organisms including *Pseudomonas aeruginosa*, *Escherichia coli* and *Klebsiella* species are also frequently encountered, especially in early appearing graft infections.

Coagulase-negative infections with *Staphylococcus epidermidis* are being identified more often. This slime-producing organism, which secretes an impervious glycocalyx is especially seen in graft infections delayed more than 6 months after operation. These organisms are often associated with a benign clinical course in conjunction with graft-healing complications such as poor tissue incorporation of the graft, false aneurysms, and graft-cutaneous sinuses.[2] The organisms adhere to the graft within the biofilm but are not often cultured from the perigraft fluid. Mechanical dislodgement from the graft fabric facilitates a positive culture.

TREATMENT

The management of infected grafts in the groin is changing. It depends on the extent of the infection, the site of the graft—aortofemoral versus femoropopliteal—the organism involved, and associated medical problems (Fig. 1).

Historically, a number of general principles have been followed. For this discussion these general principles include (1) removal of the entire infected prosthesis, (2) debridement and drainage of the area after graft removal, (3) antibiotic therapy, and (4) revascularization by extra-anatomic bypass.

The therapeutic options have broadened for graft infections in the groin to include (1) local wound irrigations and povidine iodine dressings, (2) in situ graft replacement with antibiotic coverage, (3) in situ graft replacement with or without vascularized pedicle muscle flap closure, and (4) antibiotic-coated grafts in conjunction with the other options. Proper selection of patients for these less traditional treatments requires appropriate clinical judgment, accurate assessment of the extent of the graft infection, and sensitive microbiologic cultures to identify the organism. Appropriate systemic antibiotics remain a constant despite the selected treatment regime.

Graft Excision, Debridement and Extra-Anatomic Replacement

Grossly infected grafts in the groin with involvement of the suture line cannot be treated with local wound care. If the infection is caused by an aggressive organism such as *Pseudomonas* or other gram-negative organisms, standard surgical principles should be applied. Removing the entire infected graft, debriding the area, and treating with broad-spectrum antibiotics often leaves the patient with an ischemic lower extremity. Revascularization via extra-anatomic routes is required to minimize limb loss. These options include rerouting a graft to the distal profunda femoris artery from the axillary artery or contralateral femoral artery or via an obturator bypass.[3] The prosthesis of choice is autogenous vein, but most often this is not available, so polytetrafluoroethylene (PTFE) is recommended because of the anecdotal findings of relatively less infectivity of this material.

Local Wound Irrigation

Grafts in the groin can be exposed by the breakdown of the tissues that accompanies groin wound infections. Such a graft is usually contaminated by mixed flora but of itself is not an infected prosthesis. If there is no suture line involvement, this complication may respond to local wound treatment with providine iodine dressings in conjunction with long-term antibiotics. The disadvan-

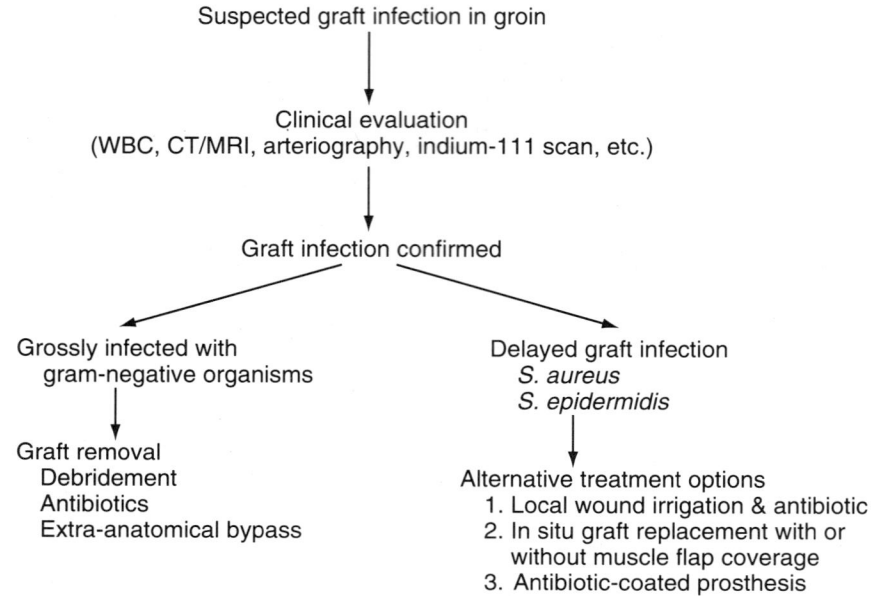

Figure 1 Algorithm for the management of graft infection in the groin.

tages of this form of therapy are risk of late recurrence of infection and the high cost of long-term hospital care. For these reasons local wound care for the benign-appearing groin infection is commonly used in conjunction with muscle flap closure. Mixter and associates[4] have treated established groin infections with local wound care followed by a rotational muscle flap coverage. The muscles used included the rectus femoris, rectus abdominis, tensor fasciae latae, vastus lateralis, gracilis, and rarely the sartorius. These vascularized pedicle flaps deliver high oxygen content to the contaminated area and allow high levels of antibiotics to be delivered to the perigraft tissues.

In Situ Graft Replacement

Due to the high risk of limb ischemia with total graft excision, some surgeons are replacing the infected groin graft with an in situ graft, usually of PTFE. Once the graft has been replaced, further treatment with muscle pedicle flaps has been advocated.

In a swine model, in situ graft replacement of an aortic graft infected with *S. aureus* and treated with a vascularized pedicle wrap of either rectus abdominis muscle or seromuscular jejunum minimized recurrent graft infection (1 of 20 infected) and maintained patency (3 of 20 thrombosed) compared with controls or treating the infected graft only by a muscle flap.[5]

Towne and co-workers[6] suggested that in situ graft replacement with gracilis or sartorius muscle flap coverage was appropriate if the infecting organism is *S. epidermidis*. Among 21 patients treated in this manner all grafts remained patent with no limb loss after a mean follow-up of 4.5 years.

However, this is not appropriate therapy for an advanced and aggressive infection caused by organisms such as *Pseudomonas*. Appropriate surgical judgment must be used with this difficult clinical problem.

Antibiotic-Coated Grafts: Are They Useful?

An additional adjunct in the patient with a graft infection may be an antibiotic-coated prosthesis. Scattered reports are appearing regarding the use of these grafts. The most important aspect of this technology is in selecting an antibiotic with broad-spectrum coverage to the *Staphylococcus* species, both nonslime and slime producers, and gram-negative organisms. Recently rifampin has been used on Dacron grafts with some early promising results. In vitro and in vivo tests confirm a decrease in infectivity of these grafts compared with controls.[7,8,9] Work in our laboratory with rifampin-impregnated gelatin-sealed Dacron grafts evaluated the pharmokinetics of these grafts and also their ability to combat infection in the aortic position in a swine model following *S. aureus* contamination. Rifampin was present in the grafts for up to 72 hours postoperatively and in the perigraft fluid for 24 hours but was never detected in the serum. The grafts had inhibitory activity in vitro against *S. aureus* and the biofilm phase of *S. epidermidis* for up to 3 days and against *E. coli* for 2 days. The pigs receiving the rifampin graft had a lower infection rate than either the controls ($p < .001$) or those given intravenous rifampin ($p = .04$).[10]

REFERENCES

1. McDougall IR, Baumert JE, Lantieri RL. Evaluation of 111 Indium leukocyte whole body scanning. Am J Roentgenol 1979; 133:849.

2. Bandyk DF, Bergamini TM, Kinney EV, et al. In situ replacement of vascular prosthesis infected by bacterial biofilms. J Vasc Surg 1991; 13:575–583.
3. Pearce WH, Ricco JB, Yao JST, et al. Modified technique of obturator bypass in failed or infected grafts. Ann Surg 1983; 197:344–347.
4. Mixter RC, Turnipseed WD, Smith DJ, et al. Rotational muscle flaps: A new technique for covering infected vascular grafts. J Vasc Surg 1989; 9:472–478.
5. Mehran RJ, Graham AM, Ricci MA, Symes JF. Evaluation of muscle flaps in the treatment of infected aortic grafts. J Vasc Surg 1992; 15:487–494.
6. Towne JB, Seabrook GR, Bandyk D, et al. In situ replacement of arterial prosthesis infected by bacterial biofilms: Long-term follow-up. J Vasc Surg 1994;19:226–235.
7. Strachan CJL, Newsom SWB, Ashton TR. The clinical use of an antibiotic-bonded graft. Eur J Vasc Surg 1991; 5:627–632.
8. Powell TW, Burnham SJ, Johnson G. A passive system using rifampin to create an infection-resistant vascular prosthesis. Surgery 1983; 94:765–769.
9. Torsello G, Sandmann W, Gehrt A, Jungblut RM. In situ replacement of infected vascular prostheses with rifampin-soaked vascular grafts: Early results. J Vasc Surg 1994; 19:675–682.
10. Lachapelle K, Graham AM, Symes JF. Antibacterial activity, antibiotic retention and infection resistance of a rifampin impregnated gelatine-sealed dacron graft. J Vasc Surg 1994; 19:675-682.

EMBOLIC DISEASE OF THE EXTREMITIES

SPONTANEOUS ATHEROEMBOLISM

RALPH G. DePALMA, M.D.

Atheroembolism is a protean syndrome caused by embolization of atherosclerotic debris into small arteries and arterioles. This entity was first described in 1862,[1] and 221 histologically verified cases had been described by 1987.[2] This phenomenon is probably more common when clinically diagnosed cases are considered. While best known to vascular surgeons as blue toe syndrome, spontaneous atheroembolism's clinical spectrum ranges from peripheral gangrene to progressive multiorgan failure. As with any diffuse vascular disease, its manifestations can involve virtually any organ or tissue. This chapter reviews diagnosis and treatment of spontaneous atheroembolism, emphasizing several characteristic pictures related to segmental aortic and peripheral arterial involvement. Embolization from carotid artery ulceration is a form of this syndrome, as is postoperative trash foot. Special instances, particularly postoperative embolization, are usually not spontaneous and quite clearly relate temporally to surgical interventions.

PATHOGENESIS

Atherosclerotic plaques contain porridge-like material within their center cores. With ulceration or plaque rupture, the contained debris, largely acicular cholesterol crystals and also fibrinoplatelet debris, can embolize distally. With plaque rupture there may be only a single episode. A unique facet of spontaneous atheroembolism is that while ulcerated plaques are common in the aorta and other vessels, embolization occurs rather infrequently. In spontaneous atheroembolism there are recurrent microembolic showers.

The central core of a typical ulcerated plaque is confined by a fibrin layer separating underlying atheromatous debris from the bloodstream. For unknown reasons, in spontaneous atheroembolism this fibrin layer becomes unstable, leading to repeated episodes of microembolization consisting mainly of cholesterol crystals, fibrin, and platelets. Characteristically, the microdebris traverses the large and medium-sized vessels, ultimately lodging in small arteries, arterioles, and precapillary arterioles. Atherosclerotic aneurysms also cause microemboli consisting of typical cholesterol crystals and atherosclerotic debris. Such microemboli have been documented in renal and muscle biopsies, the skin, the urinary tract, bone marrow, lymph nodes, larynx, and virtually the entire gastrointestinal tract. The acicular cholesterol crystals cause an intense inflammatory reaction within the vessel wall, patchy ischemia of the affected organs or tissues, and finally scarring, fibrosis, and infarction.

The clinical picture of atheroembolism is determined by the arterial location of the ulcerative or aneurysmal atheromatous disease. Usually the aorta, sometimes in its entirety, is involved. Less commonly, the iliac and femoral popliteal segments are affected. Another form of this syndrome is due to mobile polypoid atheromas of the ascending aorta. Here atheroembolism affects the brain or upper extremity. This entity is a particular problem in cardiac surgery.[3] In contrast to the diffuse form of shaggy thoracoabdominal aortic involvement, atherosclerotic polyps in the ascending aorta can sometimes be quite discrete. It is useful to classify spontaneous atheroembolism syndrome based on intensity and distribution of the proximal lesions. These include the ascending thoracic aorta, the suprarenal thoracoabdominal aorta, the infrarenal abdominal aorta, and above knee lower extremity arteries. Each gives rise to a typical clinical picture, and differing approaches to diagnosis and therapy are needed.

CLINICAL SYNDROMES

Although spontaneous atheroembolism is characterized as a great masquerader, several distinct clinical pictures or syndromes emerge. The classic blue toe syndrome is due to ulcerated atheromas, usually involving the infrarenal aorta and sometimes the iliac or femoropopliteal segments. Patients are seen with sudden onset and repeated episodes of painful cyanotic toe or toes with scattered areas of petechiae or cyanosis of the soles of the feet or less frequently proximally on the

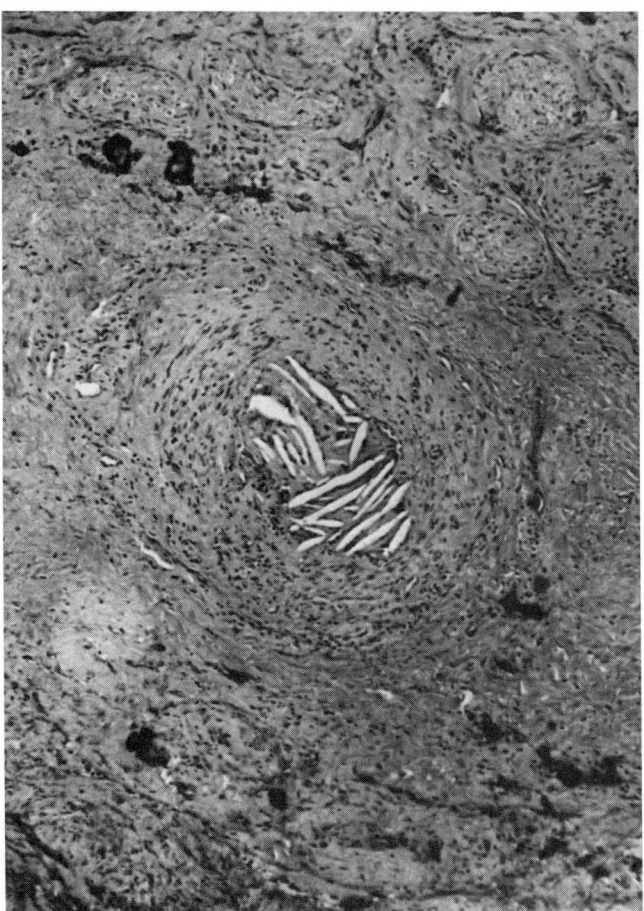

Figure 1 Systemic atheroembolism with typical acicular cholesterol embolus: occlusion of dorsal penile artery resulting in a painful skin slough of the glans penis. (From Kaufman JL, Stark K and Brolin RE. Surgery 1987; 102:63; with permission.)

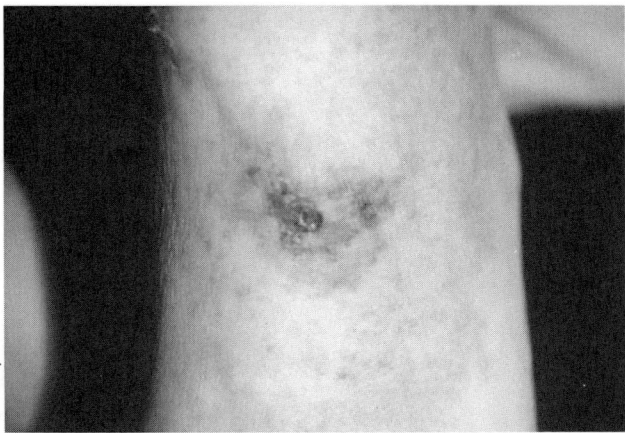

Figure 2 Skin infarction in the infracrural area due to emboli from ulcerated and aneurysmal disease involving the femoropopliteal segment. Note central biopsy site.

lower extremity. There is often accompanying livedo reticularis extending to the thigh or buttocks, calf muscle tenderness, and skin infarcts. The picture usually occurs in the presence of palpable pedal pulses. Untreated, the recurrent showers of emboli lead to soft-tissue necrosis and often to amputation.

With extensive thoracoabdominal involvement, microemboli occur in virtually every organ supplied by the aortic branches. An interesting example involved the penile vessels (Fig. 1) in a lethal case described by Kaufman and associates.[4] The visceral form is usually but not necessarily accompanied by blue toe syndrome. The kidneys can be affected due to atheromas located in the suprarenal aortic segment or near the orifices of the renal arteries. The clinical picture is of sudden renal failure, hypertension, and peculiarly, profound eosinophilia. The diagnosis can sometimes be made upon renal biopsy, but more frequently it must be suspected on clinical grounds alone.

Cholesterol emboli from atheromas of the ascending aorta will affect the arms and brain. Systemic cholesterol embolization has caused pleural effusion, and microscopically documented atheroemboli to the colon and rectum have caused gastrointestinal bleeding.[5] When atheroembolism produces sudden failure of one or more organ systems, peripheral involvement must be actively sought. The clinical picture of low-grade fever, eosinophilia, multisystem involvement, and an elevated sedimentation rate suggests connective tissue disease or arteritis. However, petechiae or infarcts of the skin of the lower extremities provide important diagnostic clues. Biopsy findings of typical acicular cholesterol emboli are diagnostic of spontaneous atheroembolism and rule out systemic vasculitis. In examination of amputated toes it is important to section the most distal portions to detect the characteristic arteriolar involvement.

PRECIPITATING FACTORS

In contrast to patients with connective tissue disease or vasculitis, virtually all of these individuals exhibit stigmata of atherosclerosis. These include an intense risk factor history, usually cigarette smoking, hypertension, and present or past hyperlipidemias. The author has not seen atheroembolism in diabetics with peripheral involvement. While the diagnosis of spontaneous atheroembolism is usually made on clinical findings, a definitive diagnosis requires biopsy with microscopic inspection of small vessels.

A few brief case reports are illuminating. Infracrural atheroembolism can lead to skin infarction (Fig. 2). This is related to a small popliteal aneurysm along with ulcerated plaques involving the femoral artery. The central lesion is a cutaneous biopsy site inasmuch as vasculitis had been suspected by the dermatology service prior to vascular consultation. Blue toe syndrome is notable on the right sole and toes but not on the left (Fig. 3). This patient had patent arteries and bounding pedal pulses on the right but not on the left. The responsible

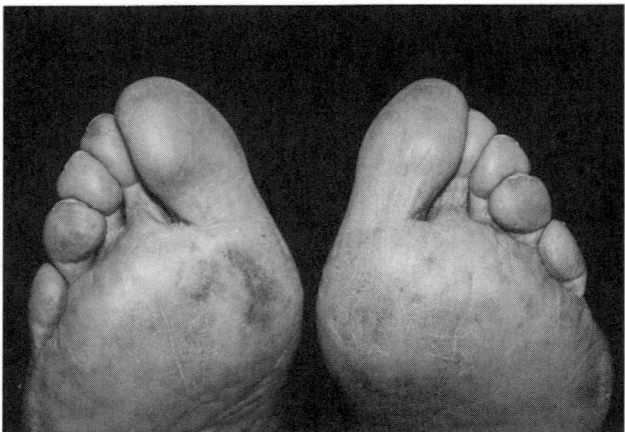

Figure 3 Blue toe syndrome in a 64-year-old man manifested after heparin-tissue plasminogen activator treatment for acute myocardial infarction. Pulses present on right, absent on left; femoropopliteal occlusion present on left, femoral artery was patent on right.

ulcerated aortic lesions were delineated on lateral aortography (Fig. 4). This 64-year-old man manifested his atheroemboli over 2 weeks along with an episode of renal failure that gradually resolved. The entire episode was precipitated by 24 hours of treatment with heparin sodium and tissue plasminogen activator (TPA) for acute myocardial infarction. The time sequence of such precipitating episodes demonstrates the important role of the fibrin laminar layer overlying and presumably stabilizing an ulcerating atheroma. An instability in this fibrin layer is sometimes also brought about by sodium warfarin treatment and more rarely after uncomplicated arteriographic studies. Another precipitating factor can be dialysis in elderly uremic patients.[4] In this situation sudden multiple organ failure is associated with a poor prognosis, in sharp contrast to the prognosis when atheroembolism affects lower extremities alone. An ominous note has been sounded in France, where spontaneous atheroembolism has been noted in HIV-positive men. This has not been reported in the Western Hemisphere.

EVALUATION OF THE PATIENT

Evaluation must be prompt and aggressive. With signs of peripheral atheroembolism, even when the blue toe component is minor, arteriography offers the only opportunity to localize and document the sites of arterial ulceration. Noninvasive studies are useful in assessing the relative contributions of proximal and distal arterial disease to the severity of ischemia. Not all blue toes are due to emboli; many are due to occlusive disease. An important point, emphasized by Karmody and associates,[6] Kempczinski,[7] and others is the importance of proceeding to arteriography, even when distal pulses are present and Doppler pressures

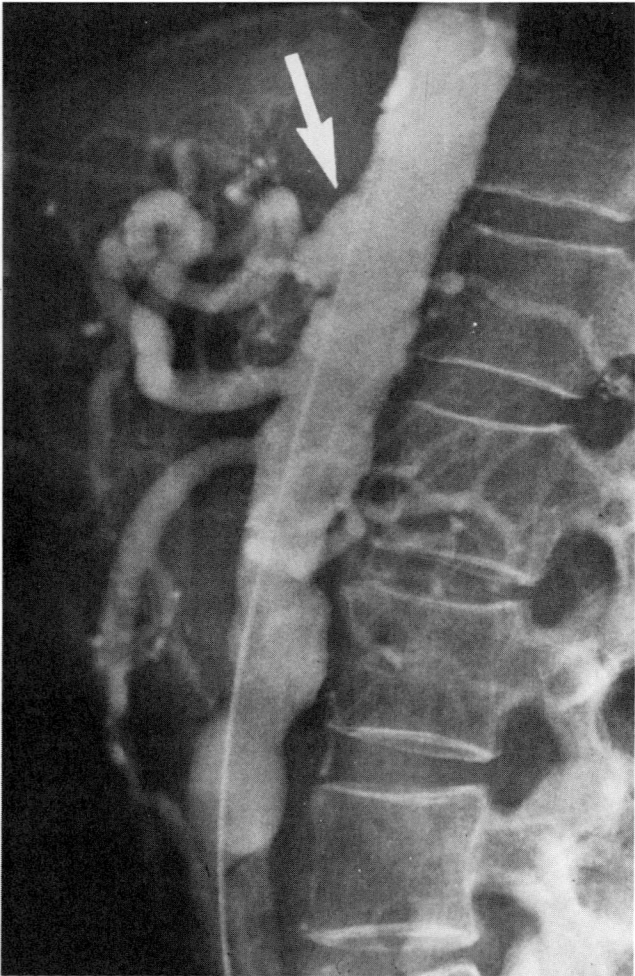

Figure 4 Lateral view of aorta in same 64-year-old man. Infrarenal segment was replaced 3 years earlier for aneurysmal disease. Note thoracoabdominal ulcerated area *(arrow)*. Transient renal failure also occurred. Patient was treated with aspirin alone.

are normal. This point has been underscored repeatedly in every surgeon's experience. For example, arteriography was denied to an active 59-year-old woman with unilateral blue toe syndrome for over 2 years because of the presence of distal pulses. Ultimately segmental resection of a small common iliac aneurysm and ulcerated plaque resulted in complete relief of her atheroembolism without further sequelae for a 10-year follow-up. With systemic or visceral involvement, the risks and benefits of arteriography will be weighed against the practicality of major aortic reconstruction. However, once dialysis is required for renal failure, there is little to be lost and much to be gained by aortic visualization. In the ascending aorta, transesophageal ultrasound has been useful in detecting polypoid atheromatous involvement.[3]

TREATMENT

Complete exclusion and bypass or replacement of the aortoiliac segment or the involved peripheral segment are required to prevent continuing lower extremity atheroembolism. Gratifying results have been noted with aortobifemoral bypass and exclusion or interposition grafts for aneurysms or ulcerated lesions of the iliac artery and similar results with involvement of the femoropopliteal segment. A recent interesting approach has been that of Kaufman and co-workers,[8] who described six patients with disseminated atheroembolism complicated by severe unremitting pain from bilateral foot lesions. These patients were not considered candidates for thoracoabdominal resection and were treated with exclusion ligation of the external iliac arteries and axillobifemoral grafts. Kaufman and associates did note continuing presence of disseminated visceral atheroembolism while foot pain was relieved and gangrenous peripheral changes arrested.

No specific medical treatment has been developed for this condition. Based on pathogenesis, the uncovering of lesions with anticoagulant therapy, anticoagulant therapy appears to be contraindicated. A possible exception might be a single polypoid lesion of the ascending aorta, where emboli would consist largely of fibrin and clot. Some favorable information does exist regarding antiplatelet therapy. In 1980 Morris-Jones and colleagues[9] described reversal of signs and symptoms in more than 50% of 35 patients with gangrene or pregangrene of the feet with palpable pulses who were treated with aspirin and dipyridamole. There has not been a systematic approach to antiplatelet therapy, and notably, in visceral embolism all the patients operated upon by Kaufman and associates[8] failed to respond to antiplatelet therapy. The author has seen cessation of blue toe syndrome due to a lesion of the left common iliac artery in a 42-year-old man who ceased smoking and received aspirin 640 mg twice daily for 6 weeks. A left iliac lesion cleared as documented by serial arteriography, as did all distal clinical manifestations. Aortoiliac endarterectomy was not subsequently required.[10] The patient illustrated was also treated with aspirin 640 mg daily, and was followed for 2 years (Figs. 3 and 4). He did not require thoracoabdominal resection. Finally, sympathectomy has been suggested as an adjunct to improve blood flow to the skin after atheroembolism. Its role appears to be secondary to exclusion of the source of microemboli whenever possible.

REFERENCES

1. Panum PL. Experimentelle Beitrage zur Lehre von den Embolie. Virchow's Arch Pathol Anat 1862; 25:308.
2. Lie JT. Cholesterol atheromatous embolism: The great masquerader revisited. Pathol Ann 1992; 27(pt 2):17–50.
3. Ribakove HG, Katz ES, Galloway AC, et al. Surgical implications of transesophageal echocardiography to grade the atheromatous aortic arch. Ann Thorac Surg 1992; 53:758–763.
4. Kaufman FL, Stark K, Bralin RE. Disseminated atheroembolism from extensive degenerative atherosclerosis of the aorta. Surgery 1987; 202:63–70.
5. O'Brian DS, Jeffers M, Kay EW et al. Bleeding due to colorectal atheroembolism: Diagnosis by biopsy of adenomatous polyps or of ischemic ulcer. Am J Surg Path, 1991; 15:1078–1082.
6. Karmody AM, Powers SR, Monaco VJ et al. "Blue toe" syndrome, an indication for limb salvage surgery. Arch Surg 1976; 3:1263–1268.
7. Kempczinski RF. Lower extremity arterial emboli from ulcerating atherosclerotic plaques. JAMA 1979; 241:807–810.
8. Kaufman JL, Saifi J, Chang BB, et al. The role of extra-anatomic exclusion bypass in the treatment of disseminated atheroembolism syndrome. Ann Vasc Surg 1990; 4:260–263.
9. Morris-Jones W, Preston EF, Greaney M, et al. Gangrene of the toes with palpable peripheral pulses: Response to platelet suppressive therapy. Ann Surg 1981; 193:462–466.
10. DePalma RG. Regression - arrest of atherosclerosis: Does it happen? In: Greenhalgh RM, ed. Hormones and vascular disease. London: Pitman Books, 1981:71–92.

ANTICOAGULANT AND LYTIC THERAPY FOR ARTERIAL MACROEMBOLISM IN THE EXTREMITIES

ROBERT J. PITSCH, M.D.
PETER F. LAWRENCE, M.D.

ANTICOAGULATION

Heparin sodium is a negatively charged mucopolysaccharide that occurs naturally. It forms complexes with positively charged plasma proteins to inhibit the formation of fibrin at several points in the clotting cascade. Small amounts of heparin sodium potentiate antithrombin III's ability to interfere with activated factor X, the result of which is to inhibit the conversion of prothrombin to thrombin. Larger amounts of heparin sodium can inhibit active thrombosis by inactivating thrombin, which prevents the conversion of fibrinogen to fibrin. It also inhibits the activation of fibrin-stabilizing factor, which prevents the formation of a stable fibrin clot. Heparin sodium does not have fibrinolytic activity. It can be given intravenously with rapid onset of action or subcutaneously to reach peak plasma levels in 2 to 4 hours. Treatment can be monitored through the partial thromboplastin time (PTT). The half-life is approximately 90 minutes after intravenous injection. Rapid reversal of activity can be obtained with protamine sulfate 1% solution, 1 mg for every 100 units of heparin sodium, administered slowly while monitoring the patient for hypotension and anaphylactoid reactions.

Other anticoagulants include sodium warfarin, aspirin, and dipyridamole. Sodium warfarin competes with vitamin K to interfere with the hepatic synthesis of factors II, VII, IX and X. Sodium warfarin must be given orally, and the onset of action varies from 36 to 72 hours because of the long half-lives of several of the vitamin K–dependent factors. Consequently, sodium warfarin is rarely if ever used to treat acute emboli. It can take up to 7 days to reverse naturally, or it can be reversed with vitamin K or fresh frozen plasma. Aspirin and dipyridamole interfere with platelet plug formation and prolong bleeding time. However, they are not major anticoagulants. Unlike heparin sodium, these agents are not appropriate when rapid anticoagulation is required.

Preoperative Heparin Anticoagulation

The patient with symptomatic arterial macroemboli needs removal or dissolution of the embolus, but while awaiting this procedure the vessels distal to the emboli have sluggish blood flow and may be in spasm. The goal of preoperative heparinization is fast therapeutic anticoagulation and prevention of distal propagation of thrombus beyond the embolus. This can usually be achieved by administration of an intravenous heparin sodium bolus of 7,000 to 10,000 units followed by initiation of an intravenous heparin infusion at 1,000 to 1,500 units per hour. The dose should be adjusted to maintain a PTT at 2 to 2.5 times normal. A larger dose of heparin sodium than what is used for routine perioperative prophalaxis is necessary because these patients already have an activated clotting cascade. Once therapeutic anticoagulation is achieved, it is not unusual for maintenance requirements to decrease gradually.

Heparin sodium should be administered in the emergency room as soon as a brief history and physical examination confirm the diagnosis. A common error is to delay administration of heparin sodium because the diagnosis is in doubt or an arteriogram is anticipated. If the patient subsequently does require arteriography or immediate operation, anticoagulation with heparin sodium will rarely cause significant bleeding, while failure to heparinize at once allows thrombus to propagate into nutrient vessels that supply calf muscles.

Postoperative Heparin Anticoagulation

There are two reasons to anticoagulate a patient in the postoperative period: to prevent rethrombosis of the damaged artery and for treatment of the source of the emboli. Administration of heparin sodium in the immediate postoperative period is controversial. During embolectomy the arterial intima is injured by the balloon catheter, resulting in a thrombogenic surface. Some investigators advocate restarting the continuous heparin infusion as early as 1 hour postoperatively, believing that the benefits of preventing thrombosis of the damaged artery outweigh the risk of bleeding. Other investigators have reported an increased rate of postoperative bleeding and hematomas.[1,2] Eventually heparin therapy should be resumed in the postoperative period to prevent recurrent embolization from the primary source.

Patients who have cardiac sources of emboli will require conversion from heparin sodium to sodium warfarin for chronic anticoagulation. An unacceptably high rate of recurrent embolism can be expected in patients who are not adequately anticoagulated. Green and associates[3] reported a 9% incidence of recurrent emboli in hospitalized patients adequately anticoagulated postoperatively, and those not receiving treatment had a 31% recurrence. We usually restart a continuous heparin infusion approximately 12 hours postoperatively. This avoids the risk of wound hematomas, and we have not seen recurrent embolic events. Patients are started on sodium warfarin on the second postoperative day, when the likelihood of further operation is minimal.

Anticoagulation and Nonoperative Management

Nonoperative management of arterial macroemboli using only high-dose heparin therapy has been reported as an alternative to operative management. Based on observations that historical mortality rates were significantly higher in patients with advanced ischemia, Blaisdell and associates[4] avoided thromboembolectomy in patients without paralysis or anesthesia 8 hours after embolization. Patients with ischemic but viable limbs were treated with high-dose heparin therapy followed by delayed elective revascularization. Using this approach, they reported a significant decrease in mortality (7.5% compared with historical controls ranging from 15% to 48%), no increase in limb loss, and a limb salvage rate of 67%.[4]

While this approach yielded good results, few surgeons have been willing to use only anticoagulation, since recent studies following balloon embolectomy have reported improved limb salvage (85% to 95%) with mortality rates in the range of 10% to 20%. Furthermore, experience with thrombolytic drugs in the past 10 years has provided an acceptable alternative for some high-risk patients. Thrombolytic agents also have the potential to reopen thrombosed distal arteries not accessible by balloon catheters, and may restore perfusion to areas that would have been lost if only heparin sodium were used.

THROMBOLYSIS

The most commonly used thrombolytic agents are streptokinase (SK), urokinase (UK), and tissue plasminogen activator. SK was the first agent used clinically. It acts by combining in equimolar amounts with plasminogen to form an active complex that converts the plasminogen molecule to active plasmin, which is capable of clot lysis. SK can degrade fibrinogen and fibrin in thrombus or elsewhere. The longer SK is infused, the greater the risk of developing systemic fibrinolysis and bleeding complications. SK is inexpensive and readily available. However, it is antigenic, and in people with prior exposure there is a risk of allergic reactions. UK is a direct activator of plasminogen and is not antigenic. It is the most commonly used thrombolytic agent for peripheral artery emboli and thrombi. The major disadvantage of UK is expense. Recombinant tissue–type plasminogen activator (rt-PA) is a more powerful and expensive thrombolytic than either SK or UK. However, there is less clinical experience with this agent in peripheral vascular disease. Theoretically, rt-PA is a more site-specific activator of plasminogen found in thrombus than is UK or SK. Clinical studies on rt-PA have not documented a therapeutic advantage over UK.[5]

The goal of thrombolysis is to dissolve the clot and recanalize the native vessel lumen. Generally, the more recent the occlusion, the more likely are thrombolytic agents to be successful. As fibrin organizes, cross-linking occurs. Cross-linked fibrin is not as susceptible to lysis by thrombolytic agents. The aging of the embolism begins at the time of its formation, which precedes the embolic event. This may explain why success varies with lysis of emboli from the heart. Thromboemboli in a patient with a recent myocardial infarction are more likely to be fresh than emboli that develop in a patient with chronic atrial fibrillation. Likewise, emboli from an aortic aneurysm may be relatively disorganized compared with material from an atherosclerotic aorta.[6] However, it is impossible to predict in any of these situations whether emboli are mature or relatively fresh.

Dotter and associates[7] reported that the best results after thrombolysis were obtained if the occlusion was less than 72 hours in duration. Many authors have reported increased failure rate of fibrinolysis if the event was greater than 10 to 21 days; however, Katzen and associates[2] reported clot lysis in arterial occlusions of up to 4 months' duration. Most investigators agree that patients with old emboli are unlikely to benefit from thrombolytic therapy.

Nonoperative Thrombolytic Management

Nonoperative thrombolytic management of embolic events is indicated in poor-risk patients and in patients with emboli that are difficult to reach operatively. Patients selected for this approach must have viable limbs and be able to tolerate at least an additional 24 hours of ischemia. Consequently, this approach is contraindicated in patients with advanced signs of ischemia such as paralysis, paresthesias, mottling, or a nonviable limb (Fig. 1).

The major drawback to nonoperative thrombolytic therapy is the time required for treatment. Patients must be able to tolerate the ischemia without further endangering the limb from the time they go to the angiographic suite until the thrombolytic agents reestablish perfusion. This interval is often 24 to 48 hours.[1,8]

Other contraindications to thrombolysis are relative. They include a history of gastrointestinal bleeding, intracardiac thrombus, recent major operation or trauma, recent stroke, severe hypertension or proliferative diabetic retinopathy, and an acquired or hereditary coagulation disorder.

Rarely, a fully anticoagulated patient on sodium warfarin may present with an embolic event. If a trial of thrombolytic therapy is desired, it may be unwise to proceed immediately, because if systemic fibrinolysis develops, fatal hemorrhage is possible. We recommend at least partial reversal of the warfarin effect (International Normalized Ratio less than or equal to 1.5) with either fresh frozen plasma (FFP) or vitamin K. FFP works quickly, but disadvantages include cost, possible volume overload if the patient has a history of congestive heart failure, and the use of blood products. Vitamin K is less expensive, but it has a slower onset of action (12 to 24 hours). Also, reanticoagulation with heparin sodium may take longer after the use of vitamin K. After the warfarin effect is partially reversed and heparin therapy is initiated, thrombolytic agents may be used with less risk of hemorrhage. Any bleeding can usually be controlled by stopping the infusions, because both heparin sodium and lytic agents have relatively short half-lives.

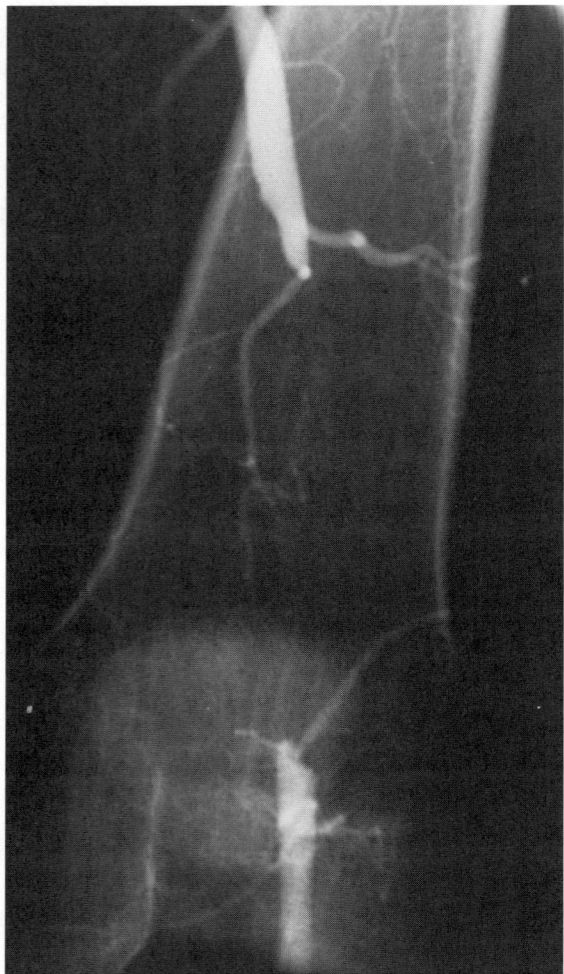

Figure 1 This arteriogram demonstrates an acutely occluded popliteal artery secondary to an embolus prior to treatment with urokinase. The patient does not have any significant collateral flow or history to suggest chronic peripheral vascular disease.

Technique

Thrombolytic therapy can be performed by percutaneous placement of a fluroscopically guided arterial catheter. The catheter often can be advanced over a guide wire through the area of obstruction. If the occlusion cannot be transversed with a guide wire, only 10% of patients will obtain successful recanalization. The thrombolytic agent is then infused via an intravenous pump for several hours with concurrent heparin therapy to prevent thrombus formation on the infusion catheter.[8] The initial rate of infusion is usually 4,000 IU/minute of UK for 1 to 2 hours; then the dose is usually decreased to 1,000 IU/minute.[9] After 6 to 12 hours repeat arteriography is performed to check for residual embolus and thrombus. It is not unusual for complete resolution to require 18 to 48 hours or more of therapy (Fig. 2).

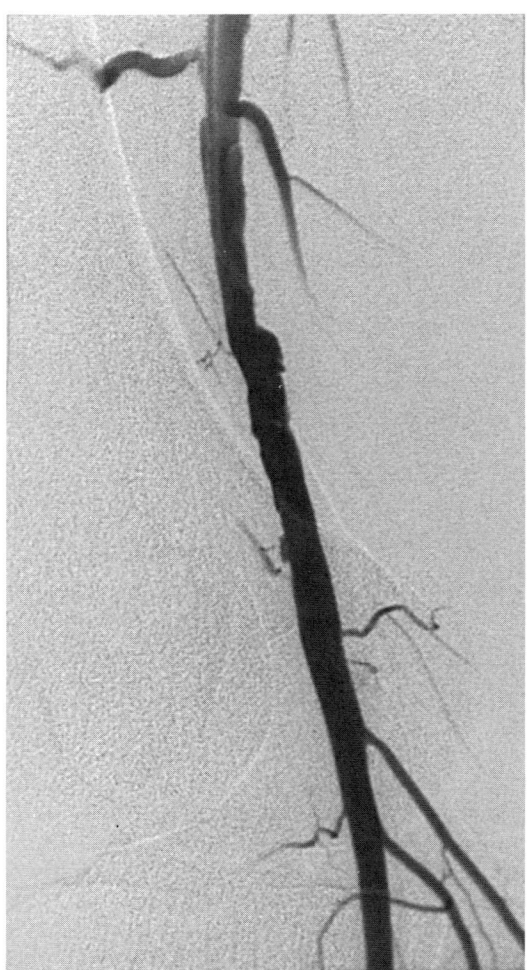

Figure 2 After treatment with a urokinase infusion, the embolus and distal thrombus cleared, leaving a mildly diseased popliteal artery. There is no critical stenosis in this vessel; therefore, thrombosis was unlikely.

Results

Taylor and associates[6] reported on thrombolysis of embolic occlusion of the popliteal artery in three patients and the tibial arteries in one. All four patients were treated with SK infusion for up to 48 hours. Arterial patency was restored in all. However, one patient with chronic atrial fibrillation needed an operation to remove residual embolic debris. Berni and associates[1] reported successful lysis of arterial emboli in 5 of 6 patients compared with successful lysis of thrombotic occlusion in seven of ten patients. They concluded that the cause of the occlusion did not significantly influence the ability to achieve effective thrombolysis. Using high-dose UK infusions, McNamara and associates[9] reported successful lysis in 94% of patients with embolic ischemia versus 82% with ischemia secondary to local thromboses. They concluded that the combination of the clinical degree of ischemia and the arteriographic pattern is a better predictor of outcome

Table 1 Nonoperative Trials with Lytic Agents after Embolic Occlusions

	Patients	Agent	Success	Ave. Time	Surgery	Hemorrhage
Berni et al. 1983[1]	6	SK	80%	37.5 hr	0.0%	25.0%
Katzen et al. 1984[2]	6	SK	50	26	—	9.1
Taylor et al. 1984[6]	4	SK	75	48	25.0	0.0
McNamara et al. 1991[9]	16	UK	94	18	1.6	2.8
Decrinis et al. 1993[10]	60	rt-PA	88	12	2.0	2.0

than whether the lesion was embolus or thrombus. Using rt-PA, Decrinis and associates[10] reported recanalization success rates of 88% in occluded vessels secondary to an embolus compared with 59% in occluded vessels secondary to thrombosis (Table 1). Thus, several authors have reported successful lysis of embolic material, often with results that are similar to or better than the results obtained in patients with thrombosis.

Perioperative Use of Thrombolytic Agents

Preoperative Thrombolytic Therapy

Generally there is no indication to delay operation in a patient if embolectomy is indicated. Occasionally the decision is made to try to avoid a surgical procedure in a high-risk patient using thrombolytic infusions. However, after lysis, residual embolic material may persist and require surgical removal. Thus, lytic agents may have been used preoperatively, but the patient with an embolus who undergoes operation following lytic therapy does so by default.

In contrast to the limited preoperative role for thrombolysis in patients with emboli, there is a well-defined role in patients with spontaneous thrombosis and ischemia. Under these circumstances preoperative thrombolytic therapy followed by definitive bypass procedure is a reasonable option if the patient can tolerate the additional time for lytic therapy.

Intraoperative Thrombolytic Therapy

The most common indications for intraoperative thrombolysis are failed balloon catheter embolectomy and persistent ischemia or residual filling defects on completion arteriography. Operative arteriography has documented residual thrombus after catheter embolectomy in 40% of patients. Inaccessible thrombus is often in the anterior and posterior tibial arteries. If embolectomy fails to remove all thromboembolic material, lytic therapy should be considered.

The advantages of intraoperative thrombolytic therapy include a reduction in the total amount of embolus that must be lysed, since much has been removed by the balloon catheter, decreased amounts of thrombolytic agents that must be used, decreased overall time to re-establish extremity perfusion, and decreased washout of thrombolytic agents, which minimizes the activation of systemic fibrinolysis and risk of hemorrhagic complications. Also, repeat use of the embolectomy catheter after thrombolytic therapy removes additional thrombus that was either missed on earlier passes or was freed by thrombolysis. Lastly, the proximal clamp makes it unnecessary to place the infusion catheter adjacent to or within the thrombus, as is required by the percutaneous technique.[11]

Technique. Removal of as much of the embolic material and proximal thrombus as possible with a balloon catheter is performed. With the inflow vessel occluded, an irrigation catheter is introduced into the artery and the thrombolytic agent administered by one of three techniques. The most commonly used technique is administration by slow bolus over several minutes. Other techniques include administration by gravity infusion over approximately 30 minutes. This technique has gained favor because of concern that bolus injection tends to leach out of the distal arterial tree and into the systemic circulation. The third approach adapts the tourniquet isolated limb technique. Using this technique, the extremity is isolated before the infusion of thrombolytic agents. This allows infusion of larger doses of lytic agents in higher concentrations. Isolated limb perfusion prevents washout, decreasing the risk of systemic fibrinolysis and the incidence of hemorrhage. Patients with absolute contraindications to conventional thrombolytic therapy may be candidates for thrombolysis using this technique.[5]

Bolus administration of 50,000 to 100,000 units of UK has been used, with the total dose depending on the location of the thrombus and the size of the limb. Using the infusion technique, doses of 100,000 to 375,000 units of UK over 30 minutes have been reported. Infusions as high as 650,000 units of UK have been reported over 60 minutes during limb-isolation procedures.[5] Arteriography or angioscopy is used to determine the completeness of clot lysis. The infusion is repeated if there is no improvement. Repeat transfemoral embolectomy after fibrinolytic therapy may be successful, since the thrombotic material may loosen after lysis.[11]

Results. Bolus therapy was successful at removing residual thrombus or establishing a clinically viable limb in 64% to 100% of patients. Infusion therapy was successful in 74% to 100%. Less clinical experience has been reported with limb isolation techniques, although Lawrence and Goodman[12] reported re-establishment of blood flow in seven of their patients. Bleeding complications occurred in 5% to 28% of patients. Bleeding was less common with UK than with SK.[5]

Postoperative Thrombolytic Therapy

The use of thrombolytic agents in the postoperative patient has a higher risk of hemorrhagic complications. Lower-extremity limb-isolation perfusion technique has been used intraoperatively with success on patients who have undergone recent major operations including coronary bypass. Lytic therapy has been used postoperatively with infusion distal to skin incisions. However, there are no reports of thrombolytic agents being used for recurrent embolic episodes after operation. At least 7 to 10 days should elapse between a major surgical procedure and thrombolytic therapy.

REFERENCES

1. Berni GA, Bandyk DF, Zierler RE. Streptokinase treatment of acute arterial occlusion. Ann Surg 1983; 198:185–191.
2. Katzen BT, Edwards KC, Albert AS, Breda AV. Low-dose direct fibrinolysis in peripheral vascular disease. J Vasc Surg 1984; 1:718–722.
3. Green RM, DeWeese JA, Rob CG. Arterial embolectomy before and after the Fogarty catheter. Surgery 1975; 77:24.
4. Blaisdell FW, Steele M, Allen RE. Management of acute lower extremity arterial ischemia due to embolism and thrombosis. Surgery 1978; 84:822–834.
5. Pitsch RJ, Lawrence PF. Intraoperative thrombolytic therapy in the ischemic extremity: A review of methods, applications, and results. Vascular Forum 1993; 1:260–267.
6. Taylor LM, Porter JM, Baur GM. Intraarterial streptokinase infusion for acute popliteal and tibial artery occlusion. Am J Surg 1984; 147:538–588.
7. Dotter CT, Rosch J, Seaman AJ. Selective clot lysis with low-dose streptokinase. Radiology 1974; 111:31–37.
8. McNamara TO, Fischer JR. Thrombolysis of peripheral arterial and graft occlusions: Improved results using high-dose urokinase. Am J Roentgenol 1985; 144:769–775.
9. McNamara TO, Bomberger RA, Merchant RF. Intra-arterial urokinase as the initial therapy for acutely ischemic lower limbs. Circulation 1991; 83(suppl 1):I106–I119.
10. Decrinis M, Pilger E, Stark G et al. A simplified procedure for intra-arterial thrombolysis with tissue-type plasminogen activator in peripheral arterial occlusive disease: primary and long-term results. Eur Heart J 1993; 14:297–305.
11. Quinones-Baldrich WJ, Zierler RE, Hiatt JC. Intraoperative fibrinolytic therapy: An adjunct to catheter thromboembolectomy. J Vasc Surg 1985; 2:319–326.
12. Lawrence PF, Goodman GR. Thrombolytic therapy. Surg Clin North Am 1992; 4:899–918.

BALLOON CATHETER EMBOLECTOMY FOR MACROEMBOLISM IN THE EXTREMITIES

ROY L. TAWES Jr. M.D.

A milestone in modern vascular surgery was the development of the thromboembolectomy catheter in 1963 by Fogarty and colleagues.[1] This ingenious device allowed mechanical retrieval of clot under local anesthesia without multiple surgical exposures. Despite this simple and straightforward technical advancement, however, complications were usually high until 1978, averaging a mortality of 25% with a 40% amputation rate due to the coexistence of severe cardiac disease in these patients.[2] The value of postoperative heparin sodium therapy following catheter thromboembolectomy was reported in 1983, with vastly improved limb salvage rates of 95% and a decrease in the mortality to 7.6%.[3] With the recognition that the etiology of emboli shifted to atherosclerosis from rheumatic heart disease in the early 1960s, surgeons were confronted with a more complex group of patients, one-fourth of whom had severe pre-existing peripheral vascular disease, as well as advanced heart disease.[4] Despite advanced technology and techniques, these patients were a sicker, more complex group, requiring not only judicious selection but also aggressive multimodal therapy during operation.[5]

Although the basics of therapy remain much the same since our 1987 report, there have been some new, innovative improvements in the treatment of thromboembolism. Now, managed anesthetic care agents may augment local anesthesia and facilitate the procedure for both the patient and the surgeon. New technology, such as angioscopy, and newer embolectomy catheters should result in a further decrease in morbidity and mortality, as should the implementation of lytic agents, such as urokinase or tissue plasminogen activator (TPA). In an earlier report the importance of secondary reconstructive operations was emphasized not only to salvage the leg but also to maximize its functional performance.[4] We noted the necessity of corrective cardiac operations in a small but significant proportion of patients following embolectomy.

PREOPERATIVE DIAGNOSIS AND MANAGEMENT

About 90% of the time the diagnosis can be made from a careful clinical history and physical examination. A history of heart disease, particularly arrhythmias, or use of medications to treat cardiac conditions is the first clue to a cardiac etiology. History of claudication or leg cramps alerts the surgeon to pre-existing peripheral vascular disease (PVD) and probably a diagnosis of thrombosis. On physical examination the finding of normal pulses on the contralateral leg favors an embolic occlusion. The affected leg with compromised circulation usually presents with the classic findings of the four Ps: pulselessness, pallor, paresthesia, and paralysis. With acute arterial occlusion, the leg is cool or cold with mottling. The calf muscles may be firm and tender. With a saddle embolus, occurring in less than 10% of patients, both legs may appear similar, with absent bilateral femoral pulses.

With an early presentation in a patient who has spontaneously converted to a normal cardiac rhythm, the diagnosis of embolism may be a bit tricky. Doppler examination is helpful in these circumstances in differentiating embolism from thrombosis.

Once the diagnosis is established, 10,000 units of heparin sodium are administered intravenously. Unless the diagnosis is unclear, a preoperative arteriogram is rarely performed, with intraoperative arteriography preferred. Although rigid time frames are often inappropriate,[4] one usually proceeds without delay to operation unless the underlying cardiac condition or medical problems preclude prompt embolectomy. Severe, previously undiagnosed or untreated congestive heart failure (CHF) or atrial fibrillation should receive some form of preoperative therapy, such as an initial dose of furosemide, digitalis, or blocking agents, which actually requires very little time. In the quest to save the leg, these severely ill cardiac patients can die if not managed judiciously. Unequivocally, patients with a long history of ischemia with clinical findings of irreversible ischemia, including loss of motor function and sensation to light touch, should not undergo embolectomy. This is a singularly unrewarding exercise in futility in these particular patients and may result in their demise. Recent interest has focused on the use of lytic agents in this subgroup of patients.[6]

OPERATIVE MANAGEMENT

Anesthesia

Invasive monitoring is required in many of these critically ill patients. A central venous or Swan Ganz catheter is placed in the internal jugular or subclavian position, and an arterial line is inserted for systemic blood pressure and pH monitoring. In most patients, local xylocaine anesthesia is sufficient. In some, managed anesthetic care with propofol, a new pharmologic agent, is helpful. Only in rare circumstances is a general anesthetic necessary.

Incision

The ischemic leg is fully prepped with an iodine compound, and a Betadine-impregnated skin drape employed. With suspected saddle or iliofemoral thromboemboli, the contralateral groin and leg are prepped. For exposure, a vertical incision is preferred with isolation of the femoral vessels with vessel loops.

Arteriotomy

A longitudinal incision over the common femoral artery is used in most patients, exposing it to the bifurcation. A 4 Fr or 3 Fr Fogarty balloon catheter is used for the embolectomy. A 4 Fr catheter is passed first as far distally as possible several times until the clot is retrieved. The initial catheter usually goes down the peroneal or posterior tibial arteries. A second 3 Fr catheter passed alongside often enters the anterior tibial artery. Liberal systemic and local heparin sodium is used, and the activated clotting time is monitored to maintain anticoagulation levels between 200 to 300 seconds. A significant proportion of heparin sodium is taken up by the endothelium, where it acts as a cofactor with antithrombin III to prevent local thrombosis. The arteriotomy is closed with interrupted 5-0 or 6-0 monofilament sutures after completion of intraoperative arteriography and/or angioscopy. Clinical and Doppler assessment of distal perfusion usually indicates whether further or additional exposure of the popliteal or tibial-peroneal vessels is necessary to accomplish a functionally adequate embolectomy. Although arteriography is the gold standard in this operation, it is sometimes wise to restrict the contrast medium load because these patients are prone to CHF and renal failure. Angioscopy has been a positive contribution in this respect but is limited to the larger vessels. The runoff is best assessed with an arteriogram. In determining the success of the embolectomy, back-bleeding may be an unreliable indicator.

The systemic heparin effect is not reversed. If satisfactory hemostasis in the wound is not obtained, a drain is placed, and the patient placed on prophylactic antibiotics. Wound hematomas occur in only about 20% of patients.[4]

THE DIFFICULT EMBOLECTOMY: HELPFUL HINTS

The primary concern of the surgeon during embolectomy should be directed toward not jeopardizing the

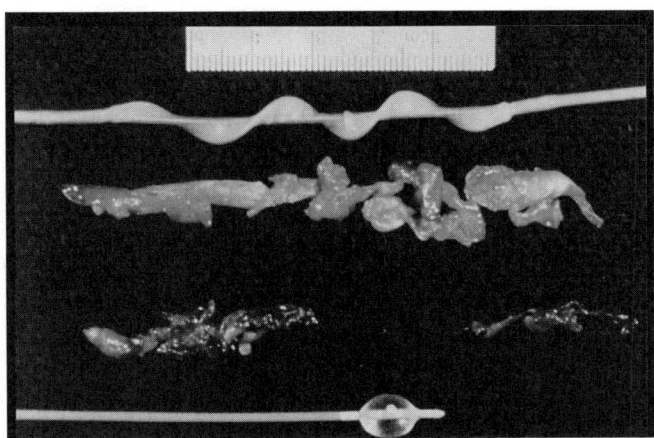

Figure 1 Fogarty adherent clot catheter.

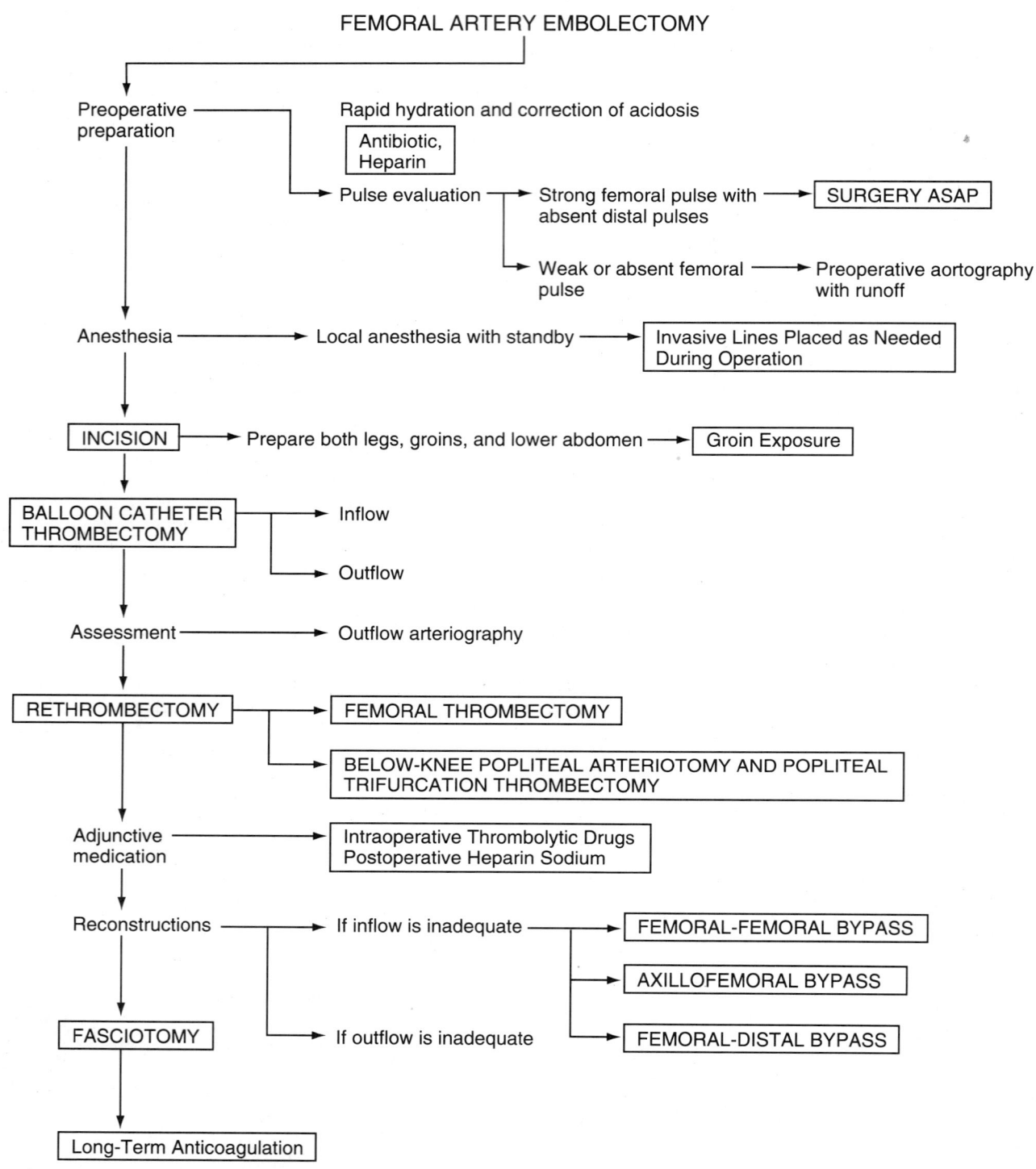

Figure 2 Algorithm for femoral artery embolectomy.

patient's life in an overzealous attempt to salvage the limb. Foremost is the consideration of the adverse effects of the reperfusion syndrome on the heart, lungs, and kidneys. The potentially harmful washout of venous effluent high in potassium, microaggregates, and myoglobin can lead to death from myocardial irritability, adult respiratory distress syndrome, and renal failure, respectively. To avoid these potentially fatal complications, the patient's central venous blood pressure or pulmonary arterial blood pressure, potassium, pH, and urine output are carefully monitored. Prior to restoration of blood flow to the extremity, sodium bicarbonate is administered, as well as mannitol and furosemide. In advanced cases of ischemia, 300 to 500 ml of the initial femoral venous return is removed from the femoral vein and washed in a Cell-Saver; the red blood cells are reinfused, if needed. Adverse systemic effects of reperfusion are ameliorated by this approach.

When retained thrombus causes poor initial results following catheter embolectomy, as judged by arteriography, angioscopy and clinical assessment, several options exist that were not available at the time of some earlier publications. As alternatives to popliteal and ankle incisions for further retrieval of retained or inaccessible clot, surgeons now have at their disposal lytic agents and a new adherent clot thromboembolectomy catheter developed by Fogarty. Both of these relatively new approaches have resulted in improved limb salvage in the most difficult cases.

The author has a modest experience in more than 50 patients with the use of intraoperative urokinase. After the embolectomy and identification of retained clot or inaccessible clot, 250,000 units of urokinase is flushed distally through the common femoral arteriotomy with proximal occlusion for 20 to 30 minutes. Blood flow is then restored and the arteriogram and/or angioscopy repeated. It is amazing how many collateral branches open up with this lytic technique. No adverse systemic bleeding effects have been noted thus far.

Recently, Fogarty introduced the adherent clot catheter, which the author has tried in a few patients with long-standing adherent clot, recalcitrant to standard embolectomy techniques (Fig. 1). Although experience has been limited, the device seems more suitable and promising in the setting of prosthetic graft thrombosis.

Another consideration in the difficult patient is the management of concomitant PVD that coexists in about 25% of patients.[3] Occasionally, a lesion may be discovered after embolectomy that is amenable to balloon angioplasty during the same operation. In general it is best to treat these secondary lesions after the patient has been stabilized.[4,5] Fasciotomy is performed liberally in advanced cases of ischemia to avoid a compartment syndrome that could compromise an otherwise successful embolectomy.

Practice has been not to reverse the heparin effect, and, in fact, to continue heparin sodium therapy postoperatively to prevent rethrombosis or recurrent

Table 1 Thromboembolism: Summary of Results, 1963 to 1983

Therapy	Number of Patients	Deaths No.	Deaths %	Amputations No.	Amputations %
Heparin	38	3	8	4	11
Embolectomy	61	4	7	9	16
Embolectomy and heparin					
Tawes Group	280	22	8	12	5
Fogarty Group	360	54	15	18	6
Total	640	76	12	30	5

From Tawes RL, Harris EJ, Brown WH, et al. Arterial thromboembolism: A 20-year perspective. Arch Surg 1985; 120:596; with permission.

Table 2 Secondary Peripheral Operations

Type	No. Performed
Reconstruction	105
Deep and common femoral thromboendarterectomy/angioplasty	37
Femoral-popliteal-tibial bypass	19
Femoral-femoral bypass	24
Aortofemoral graft	11
Proximal endarterectomy	14
Sympathectomy (lumbar)	24
Repeat thromboembolectomy	15
Adjunctive dilation	9
Popliteal exploration (angioplasty)	8
Total	161

From Tawes RL, Harris EJ, Brown WH, et al. Arterial thromboembolism: A 20-year perspective. Arch Surg 1985; 120:596; with permission.

Table 3 Types of Operations

Type	No. Performed
Resection of ventricular aneurysm and/or coronary artery bypass graft	14
Replacement of mitral valve	
Ruptured papillary	2
Rheumatic	12
Replacement of prosthetic valve	
Aortic	2
Mitral	6
Resection of mural infarct	5
Repair of infarct ventricular septal defect	2
Triple valve	1
Total	44

From Tawes RL, Harris EJ, Brown WH, et al. Arterial thromboembolism: A 20-year perspective. Arch Surg 1985; 120:596; with permission.

Table 4 Cause of Death

Therapy	No. of Deaths	Causes
Heparin	3	Cardiac (CHF and MI)
Embolectomy	4	Cardiopulmonary (2)
		Cardiac (2)
Embolectomy and Heparin	74	Cardiac (MI, 37)
		Cardiopulmonary (CHF, 23)
		CVA (6)
		Pulmonary embolus (5)
		Renal failure (3)

CHF = Congestive heart failure; MI = Myocardial infarction; CVA = Cardiovascular accident.

From Tawes RL, Harris EJ, Brown WH, et al. Arterial thromboembolism: A 20-year perspective. Arch Surg 1985; 120:596; with permission.

emboli.[3-5] All patients are placed on long-term anticoagulation with sodium warfarin.

An algorithm summarizing an approach to macroembolism (Fig. 2)[7] presents the many options available. Good clinical judgment is paramount to achieve optimal results (Tables 1 to 4).

COMMENT

Based on an experience with 739 patients with lower extremity thromboembolism since the advent of the balloon catheter in 1963, the author has several important observations. First, with the etiologic shift from rheumatic to atherosclerotic disease, a more complex group of patients, one-fourth of whom have severe, pre-existing peripheral arterial occlusive disease are being treated. Second, early diagnosis and treatment are essential to decrease the mortality and morbidity, which prior to 1978 ranged about 25% ± 10%. Third, to attain optimal results, anticoagulation must be continued in the postoperative period, accepting wound hematomas as a fair trade-off to prevent recurrent emboli and distal thrombosis in areas inaccessible to the catheter. Fourth, postoperative use of heparin sodium helps to further assess marginal results of embolectomy by allowing arteriography and careful planning of secondary operations if required. It is noteworthy that there were 162 secondary operations in 135 patients following embolectomy, consisting of repeated thromboembolectomy, popliteal exploration, sympathectomy, bypass graft(s), angioplasty, and endarterectomy. Additionally, 44 patients underwent operation to correct the cardiac source of their embolism. An overall mortality (12%) and limb salvage (95%) show marked improvement over earlier reports. Therefore, combined embolectomy and heparin sodium therapy as the primary choice of therapy is recommended.

The positive impact of lytic agents and new technology, such as angioscopy, balloon angioplasty, and adherent clot catheters, on improved morbidity and mortality is yet to be documented in clinical studies with controlled observations and statistical evaluation. All appear promising.

REFERENCES

1. Fogarty TJ, Cranley JJ, Krause RJ. A method for extraction of arterial emboli and thrombi. Surg Gynecol Obstet 1963; 116: 241–244.
2. Blaisdell FW, Steele M, Allen RE. Management of acute lower extremity arterial ischemia due to embolism and thrombosis. Surgery 1978; 84:822–834.
3. Tawes RL Jr, Beare JP, Scribner RG, Value of postoperative heparin therapy in peripheral arterial thromboembolism. Am J Surg 1983; 146:213–215.
4. Tawes RL, Harris EJ, Brown WH. Arterial throboembolism: A 20-year perspective. Arch Surg 1985; 120:595–599.
5. Tawes RL Jr, Harris EJ, Brown WH, Acute limb ischemia: Thromboembolism. J Vasc Surg 1987; 5:901–902, 913–916.
6. O'Donnell TF. Arterial thrombosis and management of acute thrombosis of the lower extremity. Can J Surg, 1993; 36:349–353.
7. Rosenman, JE, Tawes RL. Femoral artery embolectomy. In: Scribner RG, Brown WH, Tawes RL, eds. Decision making in vascular surgery. Toronto: BC Decker, 1987:144.

PERCUTANEOUS ASPIRATION THROMBOEMBOLECTOMY

PETER G. KALMAN, M.D.
KENNETH W. SNIDERMAN, M.D.

Embolic occlusion of the peripheral arterial circulation is most often managed surgically. Similarly, a surgical approach is indicated in selected individuals for massive, life-threatening pulmonary arterial emboli with cardiovascular collapse; the operation is performed through a sternotomy and on cardiopulmonary bypass. The first successful report describing a percutaneous aspiration technique for retrieval of thrombus from the circulation was by Greenfield and associates[1] for the management of pulmonary emboli. This procedure is performed using local anesthesia by introducing a steerable catheter with a suction cup at its tip through the femoral vein.[2] The catheter is then guided through the right heart and into the pulmonary circulation up to the embolus under fluoroscopic control. Subsequent reports describe successful percutaneous aspiration thromboembolectomy (PAT) for peripheral arterial emboli, although extensive individual experience with these techniques is not available.[3-6]

TECHNIQUE FOR PERCUTANEOUS ARTERIAL ASPIRATION THROMBOEMBOLECTOMY

Aspiration thromboembolectomy involves arterial catheterization through an intravascular sheath to the level of obstruction, wedging of the catheter into the thrombus, suction on the catheter tip to bind the thrombus to the catheter temporarily, and withdrawal of the catheter and thrombus through the sheath. Although initially successful, the early equipment was not suited for widespread embolectomy. First, the thrombus had the potential to be dislodged from the catheter tip during withdrawal, resulting in drop emboli and necessitating further catheter insertions. Second, the standard vascular sheath did not permit withdrawal of thrombus

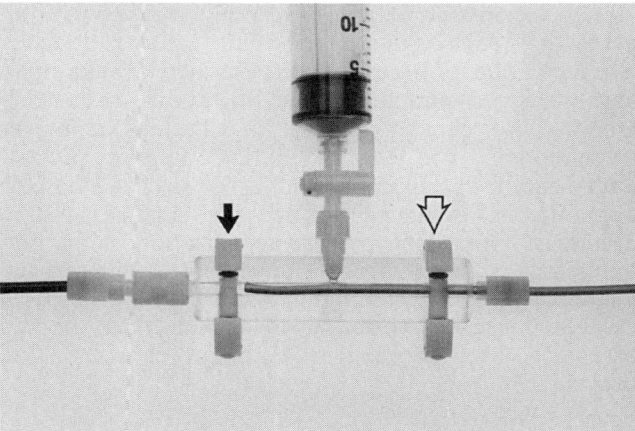

Figure 1 The one-handed clot aspiration valve set system (OCAVS) comprises an 80-cm 8.5-Fr nontapered catheter available with a curved or straight tip, a 40-cm 9-Fr sheath, and a clear acrylic clot reception chamber with an 8.5-Fr internal lumen for catheter passage. This device Luer-loks onto the sheath and has proximal *(open arrow)* and distal *(closed arrow)* valves, with a side port for flushing with a syringe.

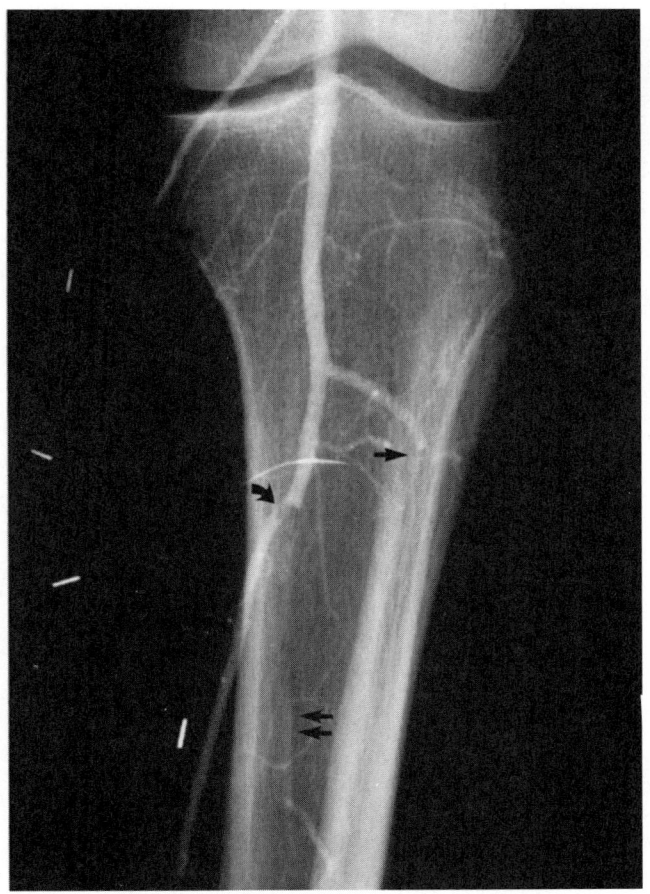

Figure 2 Arteriogram with embolic occlusion of the anterior tibial artery *(single arrow)* and peroneal artery *(double arrow)*, and non-occlusive embolus in the posterior tibial artery *(curved arrow)*.

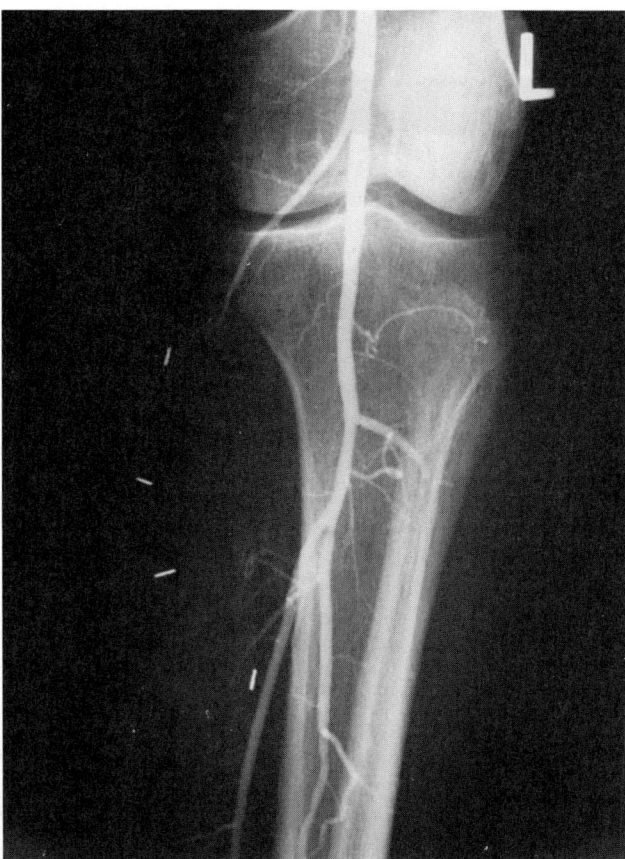

Figure 3 After aspiration embolectomy, the peroneal and posterior tibial arteries are patent and the anterior tibial artery remains occluded.

through the proximal diaphragm, which necessitated a clumsy sheath exchange each time the catheter was withdrawn, sometimes causing recurrent embolization.

The technical difficulties with the earlier equipment[3] led to development of a one-handed clot aspiration valve set catheter system (OCAVS) (Fig. 1).[4] This apparatus permits PAT with a reduced potential for drop emboli, and sheath exchange after catheter withdrawal is not necessary. After insertion of the 9-Fr chamber sheath assembly, an 8.5-Fr nontapered catheter is advanced through the chamber and into the artery to the level of obstruction. The catheter is wedged into the thrombus, and the catheter and attached thrombus are withdrawn through the sheath into the chamber during continuous suction by an attached syringe. Drop emboli do not occur, since they remain within the long sheath. The distal valve on the chamber is closed and the catheter is removed. A syringe attached to the chamber side port is used to flush the chamber clear of debris through the proximal valve, and then the latter is closed. The distal valve is opened, and the chamber sheath is aspirated with the side port syringe to further remove any debris within the sheath. These steps have allowed chamber sheath clearing of debris without sheath removal. Arteriography can be performed by injection through the sheath side port and the embolectomy repeated if necessary for residual debris (Figs. 2 and 3).

DISCUSSION

Peripheral arterial emboli are most often spontaneous and usually from a cardiac source, secondary to myocardial infarct with development of mural thrombus, valvular disease, or atrial fibrillation. Emboli may also occur during endovascular procedures such as percutaneous balloon angioplasty (PTA) and atherectomy. Regardless of the cause, clinically significant emboli are usually treated surgically by balloon catheter embolectomy. The incidence of peripheral arterial emboli has increased because of our aging population and high prevalence of cardiac disease as well as the frequency of invasive endovascular procedures. Large saddle emboli to the aortic bifurcation were at one time more frequent, but at present smaller emboli to the distal circulation are encountered with increased frequency. Embolization occurs during PTA in up to 4% to 5% of patients and is more common after PTA of an occlusion than a stenosis.[3,5]

Immediate percutaneous aspiration thromboembolectomy is a valuable alternative to operation for selected patients with small emboli to the distal circulation, particularly after an endovascular procedure. Several passes can be performed through a single puncture.

Access to embolic debris in arterial branches with an acute angle such as the anterior tibial artery is possible. The technique for PAT that was described by Sniderman and associates[3] and later revised by Starck and associates[5] requires changing the sheath-catheter system over a guide wire for each aspiration pass to prevent embolization of debris trapped in the sheath. The new apparatus is an advance, since the chamber system minimizes blood loss, permits visualization of the embolus as it is removed, and allows safe flushing of the system to remove residual debris. The curved steerable catheter permits aspiration of emboli from branch arteries, while the long sheath protects the side branches.

REFERENCES

1. Greenfield LJ, Bruce TA, Nichols NB. Transvenous pulmonary embolectomy by catheter device. Ann Surg 1971; 174:881–886.
2. Stewart JR, Greenfield LJ. Transvenous vena caval filtration. Surg Clin North Am 1982; 62:411–430.
3. Sniderman KW, Bodner L, Saddekni S, et al. Percutaneous embolectomy by transcatheter aspiration. Radiology 1984; 150:357–361.
4. Sniderman KW, Kalman PG, Quigley MJ. Percutaneous aspiration embolectomy. J Cardiovasc Surg 1993; 34:255–257.
5. Starck EE, McDermott JC, Crummy AB, et al. Percutaneous aspiration thromboembolectomy. Radiology 1985; 156:61–66.
6. Turnipseed WD, Starck EE, McDermott JC, et al. Percutaneous aspiration thromboembolectomy: An alternative to surgical balloon techniques for clot retrieval. J Vasc Surg 1986; 3:437–441.

OXYGEN FREE RADICAL SCAVENGERS IN ACUTE ISCHEMIA AND REPERFUSION SYNDROME

PAUL M. WALKER, M.D., Ph.D.
ALEXANDER ROMASCHIN, Ph.D.

Among patients treated by vascular surgeons the clinical syndrome of tissue ischemia followed by restoration of blood flow most commonly affects the lower extremity. Despite a technically successful operation, enough muscle necrosis may occur that limb dysfunction or even amputation may result. The final degree of necrosis is a combination of direct ischemic damage and the additional cellular injury that occurs during the period of reperfusion. Only this latter portion of the injurious cycle is often clinically open to therapeutic interventions. Understanding the multiple mechanisms contributing to cell injury may lead to treatment modalities to reduce the extent of muscle cell necrosis.

Our studies have delineated injurious pathways initiated during the ischemia and reperfusion syndrome, including adenine nucleotide depletion,[1,2] decreased intracellular substrate stores,[3] calcium influx,[4] complement activation,[5] enhanced neutrophil adherence and activation,[5] phospholipase A_2 activation, and oxidant-dependent phospholipid peroxidation.[6]

SOURCE OF OXYGEN FREE RADICALS

The absence of a terminal electron acceptor during the period of ischemia sets the stage for aberrant oxygen metabolism during reperfusion and reoxygenation. Normally oxygen is reduced tetravalently in the electron transport chain, producing carbon dioxide and water. If nontetravalent reduction occurs, however, oxidizing species, including superoxide anion, hydrogen peroxide, and hydroxyl radicals, are formed. An oxygen free radical species possesses an unpaired electron in its outer bonding orbit and is chemically more reactive than oxygen as an oxidant. Oxygen is a biradical species but is chemically a slow molecular oxidant due to a kinetic spin restriction barrier imposed by the improbability of two electrons of parallel spin being donated to molecular oxygen during a collision. Other oxygen-containing radicals such as superoxide anion and hydroxyl radicals are variably reactive depending upon their environment. Superoxide radicals can act as either reductants or oxidants, depending largely upon the presence of solvent accessible redox cycling transition state metals such as iron and copper and spontaneous dismutation to hydrogen peroxide. Superoxide anions can be transported across biological membranes by anionic carriers such as the chloride transporters. Conversely, hydroxyl radicals are extremely potent oxidants and react with virtually the first molecules with which they collide. Although hydrogen peroxide is not a radical species, it is a potent oxidant, less reactive than hydroxyl radicals but more reactive than superoxide anion, that is membrane permeable and capable of diffusing substantial distances before serving as an electron acceptor.

After a long period of ischemia the mitochondrial electron transport chain, which accumulates reducing equivalents, is overwhelmed by the sudden reintroduction of molecular oxygen. The normal small degree of nontetravalent oxygen reduction can be enhanced beyond the point of control by intracellular scavenger pathways, which include superoxide dismutases, catalases, and peroxidases. The protection of membrane bilayers against peroxidative injury depends upon the content of intramembrane chain breaking antioxidant (d-alpha-tocopherol, or vitamin E). Protein oxidation of essential thiol, methionyl, and phenolic groups is likely the most sensitive target of free radical and oxidant attack, resulting in enzyme and transport protein inactivation. This early protein oxidative injury is reversible, but combined with substantial membrane phospholipid oxidation, it progresses to irreversible changes in osmotic regulation and metabolic compartmentalization.

Another source of oxygen free radical production is the xanthine–xanthine oxidase system.[7] During ischemia there is a gradual breakdown of the adenine nucleotides ATP, ADP, and AMP to the nonphosphorylated nucleoside bases. In many tissues such as gut and livers, there is concomitant proteolytic conversion of the enzyme xanthine dehydrogenase to xanthine oxidase mediated by calcium-activated proteases such as calpain. This enzyme catalyzes the conversion of hypoxanthine and xanthine to uric acid, but with the by-product of O_2^- rather than NADH, which is the usual dehydrogenase electron acceptor. In the ischemia-reperfusion cascade in skeletal muscle there is abundant production of the substrate precursors of this reaction, namely xanthine and hypoxanthine. In comparison with intestine, however, the ischemia-induced conversion of this enzyme occurs only to a very limited degree, and in our studies xanthine oxidase activity was barely detectable in canine skeletal muscle. Conversely, Granger and associates[8] documented a rapid and extensive enzyme conversion induced by ischemia of the small intestine.

A further source of superoxide anion and oxidant production is from the NADPH-oxidase system found in the plasma membrane of neutrophils.[9] This cytotoxic enzymatic hardware normally participates in the phagocytic activity of stimulated leukocytes. We have shown an early and extensive accumulation of neutrophils in skeletal muscle following ischemic challenge.[5] The sequestration continues for up to 48 hours as demonstrated by a significant increase in tissue myeloperoxidase. The trigger for this cellular adherence is multifactorial and likely involves local complement activation, local upregulation of ICAM-1 on the endothelial surface, release of PMN chemotoxins and activators, and interaction of endothelium and myocytes with activated integrin ligands on the neutrophil surface. The process of PMN adhesion to endothelium and possibly underlying myocytes by this ICAM-1–integrin binding stimulates oxidant production. The hydrogen peroxide produced by this respiratory burst reacts with halogen anions via the enzyme myeloperoxidase, released during azurophil degranulation, to form hypohalous acids or chlorine bleach. The large number of white blood cells recruited by this response creates a high capacity for production of potent cytotoxic oxidants by these concerted reactions.

Oxygen free radical generation results in significant structural injury in tissues which translates into tissue necrosis and loss of motor function and destruction to surrounding tissues. Particularly highly reactive species such as the hydroxyl radical have been shown to degrade most types of biomolecules, including nucleic acids, proteoglycans, proteins, most lipid species, and complex carbohydrates. Iron, which can be mobilized by superoxide anions from its sequestered sites bound to apoferritin, can play a major role in the generation of hydroxyl radicals via redox cycling known as the Haber-Weiss reaction. In this reaction sequence superoxide anions transfer single electrons to iron $= +++$ resulting in the iron $= ++$ ion, which subsequently reduces hydrogen peroxide to a hydroxyl radical and regenerates the oxidized iron. Hydroxyl radicals and other oxidants can readily attack the cisallylic carbon-hydrogen bond of polyunsaturated fatty acyl groups at the SN2 position of membrane phospholipid. This reaction results in a carbon-centered radical that rapidly rearranges and adds molecular oxygen to form a hydroperoxy radical. The rearranged fatty acyl structure now contains a conjugated double bond, and the resulting hydroperoxy radical can abstract electrons from adjacent phospholipid fatty acyl groups to propagate a chain reaction that if left unabated can oxidate thousands of molecules. The physicochemical effects of this process on membrane structure include changes in membrane fluidity, ion and solvent permeability, and membrane protein structure. Free radical effects on proteins include oxidation of methionyl sulfide groups to sulfoxides and formation of tyrosine dimers. Numerous proteins are highly sensitive to free radical attack, including alpha$_1$-antitrypsin, glutamate dehydrogenase, sodium-potassium ATPase, and sarcoplasmic reticulum calcium ATPase, to name a few. Chemical modifications of peptide residues by free radicals not only affect protein conformation and function but also make proteins more susceptible to proteolytic degradation and disposal by the reticuloendothelial system and other pathways. The combined effects of oxygen free radicals and oxidants on lipid and protein structure and function translate into physiological derangements in ion homeostasis, nonproductive ATP use, poisoning of mitochondria, and ultimately cell lysis and death.

IDENTIFICATION OF OXYGEN FREE RADICAL DAMAGE

Conjugated diene bonds in membrane phospholipids are a chemical signature of free radical–mediated damage, and an accumulation of these by-products provides evidence for the production of free radicals. We believe that substantial and persistent membrane lipid peroxidation constitutes a major mechanism of injury for the progression of cells from reversible to irreversible injury.

We have studied free radical damage in the canine gracilis muscle model and compared the effects of 3 hours versus 5 hours of ischemia.[10] Biopsies were taken prior to ischemia, during ischemia, and during the reperfusion phase. No conjugated dienes were produced during the period of ischemia, but with the reintroduction of oxygen a significant accumulation of conjugated dienes was identified. A cumulative burden of significant conjugated diene products was identified following both 3 and 5 hours of ischemia. Although these studies confirmed that oxygen free radical–mediated lipid peroxidation had occurred, they did not identify the specific source of free radical production.

In further studies we established a relationship between lipid peroxidation and neutrophil accumulation.[6] In one gracilis muscle we allowed normal reperfusion to occur, and in the other muscle neutrophils and plasma proteins were removed for the first 45 minutes of reperfusion. In the muscle that received neutropenic reperfusion there was no increase in lipid-conjugated dienes during the period of early reperfusion, in contrast to the contralateral ischemic-reperfused control. This demonstrated a significant increase in phospholipid conjugated diene levels. As soon as the neutrophil-containing blood was reintroduced, however, conjugated dienes were formed, and peroxidation products increased to levels indistinguishable from those of the contralateral ischemic-reperfused control muscle. These observations suggested that neutrophils constitute a major source of oxidant production in the ischemic-reperfused muscle.

THERAPEUTIC INTERVENTIONS

While oxygen free radical damage may be only a portion of the entire spectrum of ischemia-reperfusion injury, a number of successful therapeutic interventions have been aimed at reducing free radical damage in the gut and myocardium. In skeletal muscle there have been several direct attempts at free radical scavenging. Korthuis and associates,[11] in an in vitro model of perfused gracilis muscle, attenuated the increase in the vascular permeability reflection coefficient by pretreatment of the muscle with free radical scavenger enzymes and the antioxidants superoxide dismutase, catalase, allopurinol, and dimethyl sulfoxide.[11,12] This attenuation of increased vascular permeability could translate into a decrease in muscle necrosis due to prevention of intracellular osmotic overload and calcium influx.

We have examined the role of the free radical scavengers in preventing muscle necrosis in the in vivo canine gracilis hindlimb model. Our strategies were adapted after those of Lucchesi, who first reported success in myocardial experiments. They identified the need for a reduction in the rate of delivery of oxygen to the tissues in addition to supplementation of the reperfusate with free radical scavenging compounds. Controlled oxygen delivery was accomplished by creating a critical stenosis in the arterial inflow to the coronary tissue.

Our parallel strategy was to control the rate of oxygen delivery to the skeletal muscle in addition to providing compounds capable of scavenging free radicals. We reduced the rate of arterial inflow to prevent the reactive hyperemia that normally accompanies the return of circulation and reduced the rate of oxygen delivery by removing red blood cells and then gradually returning autologous red blood cells in three stages to increase the hematocrit level to normal. In addition, we added superoxide dismutase, catalase, and mannitol to the reperfusate buffer solution (Modified Krebs-Henseleit) to enhance radical scavenging capacity.

This intervention strategy resulted in a reduction in the extent of necrosis from 78% ± 8% to 53% ± 7%. This study was the first to demonstrate in vivo the beneficial effects of anti–free radical intervention in the reperfusion phase with significant reduction in skeletal muscle necrosis following ischemia.[13] In further studies we established that the removal of white blood cells using a leukocyte filter could not only reduce muscle necrosis by approximately 50% but also had a significant effect on muscle lipid peroxidation.[5] In the control experiments lipid peroxidation increased between 1 and 48 hours of reperfusion. This evidence of continuing leukocyte accumulation and lipid peroxidation during the first 48 hours of reperfusion suggested that free radical–mediated injury in skeletal muscle was a protracted process, and more effective reperfusion-based intervention strategies were likely to address this prolonged course of injury. During this reperfusion phase, in addition to the evidence of lipid peroxidation, we have demonstrated evidence of remodeling of the phospholipid bilayer. There was a significant phospholipid deacylation-reacylation cycle in the reperfused muscle that was likely triggered by phospholipase A_2 activation. This cycle resulted in a selective increase in phospholipid stearic acid content but had no significant effect on total phospholipid content and likely reflects the activation of repair processes that excise oxidized fatty acyl groups from the membrane.

In a search for strategies for long-term protection of muscle from oxidant-mediated reperfusion injury, we have investigated monoclonal antibodies that block neutrophil adhesion to sites of inflammation and tissue injury. This approach is based on the premise that neutrophils, despite their beneficial actions related to digestion of necrotic tissue in preparation for fibrosis, also have the capacity to injure innocent bystander tissue or to injure damaged but viable cells irreversibly. To test this approach we have used a monoclonal antibody directed against the common beta subunit of the CD11-CD18 family of leukocyte integrin receptors. The murine monoclonal antibody (IB4, supplied by Dr. K. Arfors courtesy of Pharmacia) was tested in a rabbit model of skeletal muscle injury. The antibody was administered just prior to reperfusion of the posterior leg muscles, which were ischemic for 5 hours.[14] The antibody therapy alone reduced muscle necrosis, but this strategy alone did not achieve statistical significance. When anti-CD18 monoclonal antibody therapy was combined with decompressive fasciotomy, however, a significantly better protective effect was achieved than with fasciotomy or antibody therapy alone. The combined strategy of decompressive fasciotomy and anti-CD18 monoclonal antibody therapy reduced muscle necrosis by 75% compared with the control group, which was reperfused without any therapeutic intervention. Further studies have revealed that a release of mediators from the ischemic muscle bed results in the activation of naive heterologous neutrophils and promotes their CD11-CD18 dependent surface adhesion and respiratory burst activity.[15] The release of these systemic mediators peaks after 24 hours of reperfusion and contributes to the prolonged leukosequestration and activation that characterize many models of skeletal muscle ischemia-reperfusion injury. Two important therapeutic tangents have emerged from our recent animal studies. First, early controlled reperfusion strategies that exclude PMNs and complement plasma proteins from the reperfusion for the first 45 minutes of reperfusion have a lasting effect on muscle salvage. Second, a long-term strategy that controls intracompartmental pressure and white cell sequestration and activation further enhances the reclamation of viable muscle tissue.

Our clinical view is that leg morbidity following acute ischemic insult is not likely to be altered by improvements in surgical techniques. Rather, reductions in morbidity are due to our ability to modify perioperatively and postoperatively the deleterious reactions that occur during the reperfusion and reoxygenation phase, when nutrient blood flow is re-established.

REFERENCES

1. Lindsay T, Liauw S, Romaschin A, Walker P. The effect of ischemia/reperfusion on adenine nucleotide metabolism and xanthine oxidase production in skeletal muscle. J Vasc Surg 1990; 12:8–15.
2. Rubin B, Liauw S, Tittley J, et al. Prolonged adenine nucleotide resynthesis and reperfusion injury in post ischemic skeletal muscle. Am J Physiol 1992; 262:H1538–H1547.
3. Harris K, Walker P, Mickle D, Romaschin A. Metabolic response of skeletal muscle to ischemia. Am J Physiol 1986; 250:H213–H220.
4. Smith A, Hayes G, Walker P, Romaschin A. The role of extracellular calcium in ischemia/reperfusion injury in skeletal muscle. J Surg Res 1990; 49:153–156.
5. Rubin B, Smith A, Liauw S, et al. Complement activation and white cell sequestration in post ischemic skeletal muscle. Am J Physiol 1990; 259:H525–H531.
6. Rubin B, Chang G, Liauw S, et al. Phospholipid peroxidation deacylation and remodeling in post ischemic skeletal muscle. Am J Physiol 1992; 263:H1695–H1702.
7. McCord J. Oxygen-derived free radicals in post ischemic tissue injury. N Engl J Med 1985; 312:159–163.
8. Granger N, Rutili G, McCord J. Superoxide radicals in feline intestinal ischemia. Gastroenterology 1981; 81:22–27.
9. Babior B. Oxygen dependent microbial killing by phagocytes. N Engl J Med 1978; 298:659–668.
10. Lindsay T, Walker P, Mickle D, Romaschin A. Measurement of hydroxy conjugated dienes after ischemia reperfusion in canine skeletal muscle. Am J Physiol 1988; 254:H578–H583.
11. Korthuis R, Grisham M, Granger N. Leukocyte depletion attenuates vascular injury in post ischemic skeletal muscle. Am J Physiol 1988; 254:H823–H827.
12. Carden D, Smith J, Korthuis R. Neutrophil mediated microvascular dysfunction in post ischemic canine skeletal muscle: role of granulocyte adherence. Circ Res 1990; 66:1436–1444.
13. Walker P, Lindsay T, Labbe R, et al. Salvage of skeletal muscle with free radical scavengers. J Vasc Surg 1987; 5:68–75.
14. Petrasek P, Liauw S, Romaschin A, Walker P. Salvage of post ischemic skeletal muscle by monoclonal antibody blockade of neutrophil adhesion molecule CD18. Surgery (in press).
15. Petrasek P, Lindsay T, Romaschin A, Walker P. Delayed activation of neutrophil CD18 after acute skeletal muscle ischemia: Evidence for a mechanism of late systemic injury. J Vasc Surg (in press).

NONINVASIVE METHODS OF DIAGNOSING CARDIAC SOURCES OF MACROEMBOLI

BRIAN G. RUBIN, M.D.
GREGORIO A. SICARD, M.D.

ETIOLOGY OF CARDIAC EMBOLI

Arterial embolism is associated with mortality rates of up to 25%, despite advances in the techniques of embolectomy and peripheral vascular reconstruction. This mortality reflects comorbid factors, particularly advanced cardiac disease, present in the majority of these patients. Approximately 85% of peripheral emboli are of cardiac origin (Table 1). This percentage has remained unchanged for the past several decades. The advancing age of patients presenting with arterial emboli has resulted in a redistribution of etiology away from rheumatic valvular disease and toward complications of atherosclerotic cardiac disease.

Atrial fibrillation is associated with two-thirds to three-quarters of all peripheral arterial emboli which usually originate from clot in the left atrial appendage. One convenient scheme of describing the etiology of atrial fibrillation is the presence or absence of associated cardiac valvular disease. For patients with rheumatic mitral valvular disease and atrial fibrillation, the minimum lifetime risk of an arterial embolic event is 20%. Eighty-two percent of emboli occur while the patient is in atrial fibrillation.[1] Nonvalvular atrial fibrillation due to hypertensive or ischemic coronary artery disease is much more prevalent than rheumatic heart disease, but the event rate of arterial emboli in nonvalvular atrial fibrillation is low. Thus, the typical elderly patient with ischemic heart disease and atrial fibrillation has a fivefold to sixfold increased embolic risk versus a control population, with a 3% to 5% annual risk and a 35% lifetime risk for clinically significant arterial emboli.[2]

Myocardial infarction (MI), particularly transmural anterior wall MI, is associated with a 40% chance of developing left ventricular apical clot. Thrombus has been noted in 30% of patients with transmural MI and 44% of patients following fatal MI.[2] The thrombus generally begins to form within the first 14 days after MI, and this early period represents the time of greatest risk for peripheral embolization. The embolic risk associated with ventricular thrombus following transmural MI peaks late in the first week, then diminishes rapidly so that by 2 months the risk is 0.35 events per 100 patient years.[2]

Late development of ventricular aneurysm formation in an akinetic portion of the ventricular apex is associated with a 50% chance of developing thrombus and a 5% long-term risk of arterial embolization. Several risk factors increase the likelihood of an embolic event in the peri-infarction period. Plasma fibrinogen concentration peaks 4 to 6 days following MI, and in one study all 10 patients with peripheral emboli had fibrinogen levels above 650 mg/dl.[2] Infarctions associated with large akinetic ventricular segments and, in particular, anterior wall MIs are associated with a greater risk of emboli. Although anticoagulation does not uniformly decrease the incidence of postinfarction ventricular thrombus formation, it is associated with a decreased embolic risk.

Prosthetic cardiac valve replacement is also associated with an increased risk of embolization. The prosthetic device may be prone to clot formation along the thrombogenic surface of the sewing ring or in areas of low flow such as at the hinge points in tilting disk valves. A previous problem with escape of a fragment or the entire ball (poppet) from a ball-cage type of prosthetic valve is now extremely rare. Finally, inadequate anticoagulation, particularly with a mitral valvular prosthesis, increases the risk of intracardiac thrombus formation and subsequent peripheral emboli. We have also noted thrombus formation on native valve leaflets and have reported a case that occurred subsequent to valvular injury during cardiac catheterization.[3]

Valvular vegetations from endocarditis occur occasionally; slower growing organisms such as *Aspergillus* and *Candida* or carbon dioxide–requiring organisms such as *Haemophilus* generally result in large vegetation size.[2] Vegetation size seems to correlate with embolic risk. In one recent study, the development of a vegetation diameter greater than 10 mm resulted in embolic events in 22 of 47 patients (47%), whereas vegetations less than 10 mm in diameter were associated with a lower embolic rate (11 of 58 patients, 19%).[4] Although uncommon, primary or metastatic intracardiac tumors also may be an embolic source. Of the primary tumors, atrial myxoma is the most common. Dilated cardiomyopathy, particularly alcoholic cardiomyopathy, is associated with essentially 100% chance of development of intracardiac thrombus. This risk persists throughout the remainder of the

Table 1 Cardiac Sources of Peripheral Arterial Emboli

Atrial fibrillation
    Valvular (rheumatic or arteriosclerotic heart disease)
    Nonvalvular
Myocardial infarction
    Early postinfarction intracardiac thrombus
    Late postinfarction intracardiac thrombus (usually associated with left ventricular aneurysm formation)
Prosthetic valves
    Thrombus formation on thrombogenic surfaces (sewing ring, hinge points)
    Prosthetic material emboli (e.g., poppet escape)
    Inadequate anticoagulation
Intracardiac tumors
    Primary
    Metastatic
Valvular vegetations (endocarditis)
Native valvular thrombi (noninfected)
Dilated cardiomyopathy (alcoholic, peripartum, hypereosinophilic)
Intracardiac right-to-left shunt with paradoxic embolism

patient's life. Thus, these patients benefit from lifetime anticoagulation.

Finally, a right-to-left intracardiac shunt permits venous emboli to enter the arterial circulation. Several anatomic conditions allow paradoxic embolization, including a patent foramen ovale, atrial septal defect, ventricular septal defect, pulmonary arteriovenous malformation, and some congenital cardiac anomalies. The most common of these conditions is a patent foramen ovale, which occurs in 27% to 35% of the population.

NONINVASIVE METHODS OF DIAGNOSIS

Because atrial fibrillation, regardless of its etiology, is associated with the majority of peripheral embolic events, the electrocardiogram (ECG) should be carefully reviewed. In addition to providing important information about the cardiac rhythm, the ECG should be compared with previous ECGs for the presence of a new MI. A clinically significant arterial embolus may be the presenting sign of a recent silent MI.

In the 1970s and early 1980s, left ventriculography at the time of cardiac catheterization was the diagnostic gold standard, but it has subsequently been shown to have a sensitivity of only 31% and a specificity of 75%. Nuclear medicine studies with technetium-99m–labeled red blood cells have been used to identify abnormalities on nucleotide ventriculographic images that correlate with the presence of ventricular thrombus. Finding a discrete filling defect attached to the cardiac border or an abnormality at the left ventricular apex was associated with sensitivities of 62% to 77% and specificities of 88% to 100%.[1] Indium-111–labeled platelet imaging studies have also been utilized to gain information about the biologic activity of intracardiac thrombus. The time-consuming nature of this study, which often takes 3 to 5 days to complete, as well as its lack of widespread availability, discouraged its routine use, despite its high specificity.[1] All of these techniques have now been replaced by echocardiography.

Echocardiography utilizes identical principles and instrumentation as the duplex scanner in the vascular laboratory. Pulsed Doppler-derived velocity information, B-mode imaging, and color flow mapping are routinely used to perform an echocardiographic examination. A "bubble" study is incorporated into the examination in all patients who are being evaluated for potential right-to-left shunt. The standard two-dimensional transthoracic echocardiogram is the most widely utilized initial diagnostic evaluation. Its low cost and widespread availability, as well as accuracy rates of 90%,[1] have helped establish it as the initial diagnostic modality of choice.

Sonographic findings predictive of increased risk of embolism are thrombus protrusion and thrombus mobility. Thrombus protrusion, occuring in 35% to 55% of patients, is associated with 22% to 56% chance of emboli, whereas flat thrombi embolize in 3% to 13% of patients. Immobile thrombi are present 73% to 85% of the time, with 5% to 16% of patients suffering systemic embolism. In contrast, mobile thrombi embolize in 35% to 83% of patients.[1] The primary limitation of transthoracic echocardiography remains the inability of ultrasound to penetrate adequately, which is particularly problematic in patients with chronic obstructive pulmonary disease, prosthetic valves, or obesity. Importantly, much of the posterior aspect of the heart is inaccessible to transthoracic echocardiography, particularly the left atrial appendage, which can be identified in only about 20% of patients. The left atrial appendage may be the only site of intracardiac thrombus in 40% of patients with valvular disease and peripheral emboli. However, transthoracic echocardiography excels in detection of left ventricular apical thrombi and may outperform transesophageal echocardiography in this application.

Because the left atrium and left atrial appendage are the typical sites for thrombi in patients in atrial fibrillation, an inability to reliably visualize these portions of the heart is a substantial shortcoming of transthoracic echocardiography. For this reason, transesophageal echocardiography (TEE) has gained popularity. The current technique of TEE, utilizing an ultrasound transducer mounted on the end of a flexible gastroscope, was introduced in 1980. From a vantage point in the esophagus behind the left atrium, the entire heart, particularly the left atrium and left atrial appendage, can be carefully evaluated. Because of the short distance between the transducer and heart, higher frequency transducers can be utilized that result in improved image resolution. The recently introduced technique of biplanar TEE offers an opportunity to insonate in both the transverse and longitudinal planes. It can be performed in the awake or sedated patient, and its safety, even with critically ill patients, has been extensively documented. It also demonstrates the phenomenon of "spontaneous echocardiographic contrast," which reflects sludging of red blood cells or platelet aggregates. This finding is associated with an increased risk of peripheral embolization. Several clinical studies report better sensitivity with TEE than with transthoracic echocardiography. A large European multicenter study of patients with cerebral ischemic events or arterial embolism documented potential sources for arterial emboli in 176 of 479 patients (37%) with transthoracic imaging. However, TEE identified 310 (65%) with potential cardiac sources of their arterial emboli. TEE more frequently identified mitral valve prolapse, patent foramen ovale, left atrial and left atrial appendage thrombi, spontaneous echo contrast, atrial septal aneurysm, and valvular vegetations.[5] Its ability to identify small valvular vegetations consistently has been reported,[6] and our clinical experience confirms it (Figs. 1 and 2).[3] Another advantage of TEE is its ability to image a significant portion of the descending thoracic aorta which has increasingly been recognized as a potential site of origin for embolic debris.[7] We currently reserve the role of TEE for patients whose previous evaluation, including electrocardiogram and transthoracic echocar-

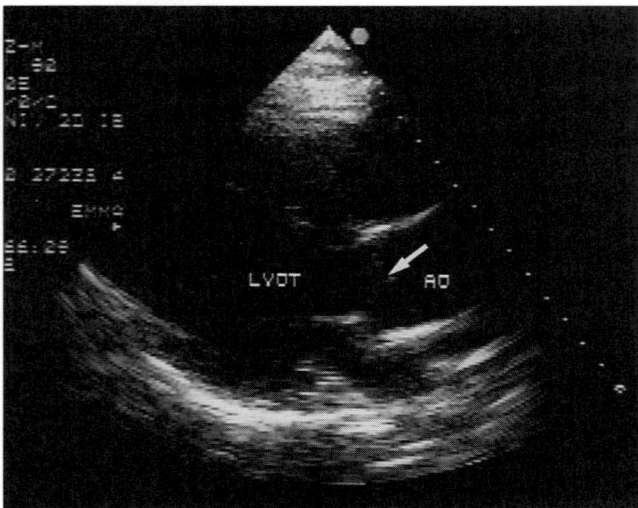

Figure 1 Transthoracic echocardiogram showing the region of the aortic valve. The aorta (AO) and left ventricular outflow tract (LVOT) are labeled. The solid white arrow points to the aortic valve leaflets. No abnormalities of the aortic valve were reported on this examination. (From Rubin BG, Barzilai B, Allen BT, et al. Detection of the source of arterial emboli by transesophageal echocardiography. J Vasc Surg 1992; 15: 573–577; with permission.)

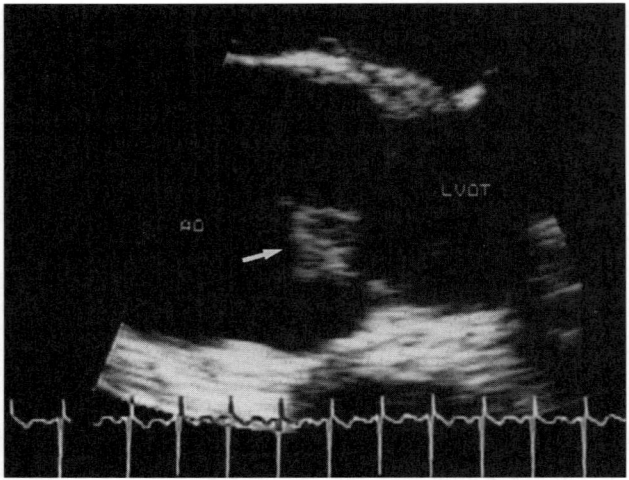

Figure 2 A transesophageal echocardiogram of the aortic valve on the same patient as Figure 1. The aortogram (AO) and left ventricular outflow tract (LVOT) are labeled. A large mass is clearly seen hanging on the aortic valve cusp in the flow lumen. Transthoracic echocardiogram of this same region was reported to be normal. The patient underwent successful aortic valve replacement with resolution of his embolic problems. (From Rubin BG, Barzilai B, Allen BT, et al. Detection of the source of arterial emboli by transesophageal echocardiography. J Vasc Surg 1992; 15:573–577; with permission.)

diography, failed to detect a cardiac source of suspected arterial emboli.

Magnetic resonance imaging (MRI) and computed tomography (CT) have also been utilized to identify cardiac sources of arterial emboli. The CT imaging results in better spatial resolution than MRI, and CT's faster acquisition time, widespread availability, and lower cost than MRI are all positive attributes. However, the significant motion artifact that is created by the beating heart has been difficult to overcome. In addition, the need to inject intravenous contrast material and the need to carefully time the image acquisition to contrast injection are significant shortcomings of CT. Ultrafast CT or spiral CT may overcome several of the former shortcomings. However, the exact role of these newer, albeit more rapid and costly, imaging techniques awaits clinical evaluation of their sensitivity and specificity.

In contrast to CT imaging, MRI sacrifices spatial resolution for better soft tissue contrast, and it allows multiple planes of image reconstruction. For cardiac imaging, the slice acquisition can be ECG gaited, allowing either multiple images of a single section at different points in the cardiac cycle or multiple images of the entire heart at a single point in the cardiac cycle. The T1-weighted images provide good contrast between cardiac tissues (long T1) and mediastinal fat (short T1);[8] the T2-weighted images result in enhanced contrast between myocardium (short T2) and tumor (long T2). The signal intensity of intracardiac thrombus is variable and probably related to the age of the thrombus.[9] On spin echo images, the rapidly flowing nature of blood within the cardiac chambers usually results in a signal void and in a high degree of contrast between the intracardiac blood pool and the myocardium. Sluggish blood flow may result in a signal that mimics intraluminal thrombus. This can occur in pathologic low flow states as well as occur normally in the left ventricle during diastole and occasionally in the left atrium in late systole.[9] Perhaps the current role of MRI is to complement echocardiography. In a recent report, 34 patients with echocardiographically detected cardiac lesions underwent MRI. In 15 of these patients, MRI confirmed the echocardiographic findings, in 7 an anatomic abnormality explained the abnormal sonographic findings, and in the remainder the MRI was normal. All patients have continued to do well in 1- to 2-year follow-up.[8]

REFERENCES

1. Stratton JR. Common causes of cardiac emboli: Left ventricular thrombi and atrial fibrillation (specialty conference). West J Med 1989; 151:172–179.
2. Adams PC, Cohen M, Chesebro JH, Fuster V. Thrombosis and embolism from cardiac chambers and infected valves. J Am Coll Cardiol 1986; 8:76–87.
3. Rubin BG, Barzilai B, Allen BT, Detection of the source of arterial emboli by transesophageal echocardiography: A case report. J Vasc Surg 1992; 15:573–577.
4. Mügge A, Daniel WG, Günter F, Lichtlen PR. Echocardiography in infective endocarditis: Reassessment of prognostic implications of vegetation size determined by the transthoracic and the transesophageal approach. J Am Coll Cardiol 1989; 14:631–638.
5. Daniel WG, Angermann C, Engberding R, et al. Transesophageal echocardiography in patients with cerebral ischemic events and

arterial embolism: A European multicenter study. Circulation 1989; 80 (suppl 2):273.
6. Erbel R, Rohmann S, Drexel M. Improved diagnostic value of echocardiography in patients with infective endocarditis by transesophageal approach: A prospective study. Eur Heart J 1988; 9:43–53.
7. Rubin BG, Allen BT, Anderson CB, et al. An embolizing lesion in a minimally diseased aorta. Surgery 1992; 112:607–610.
8. Brown JJ, Barakos JA, Higgins CB. Magnetic resonance imaging of cardiac and paracardiac masses. J Thorac Imaging 1989; 4:58–64.
9. Siegel MJ, Weber CK. Cardiac and paracardiac masses. In: Gutierrez FR, Brown JJ, Mirowitz SA, eds. Cardiovascular magnetic resonance imaging. St Louis: Mosby–Year Book, 1991:112.

PARADOXICAL EMBOLISM

TIMOTHY F. KRESOWIK, M.D.

Paradoxical embolism denotes an arterial embolic event with the embolic material originating in the venous system or right heart and passing into the arterial system through a right-to-left shunt. The term paradoxical embolism is usually associated with the embolization of venous thrombus into the arterial system through a patent foramen ovale. However, embolization of other material, including air, tumor, fat, catheters, and bacteria, through any right-to-left shunt, such as a ventricular septal defect, pulmonary arteriovenous fistula, or patent ductus arteriosum, is also correctly referred to as paradoxical embolism.

Paradoxical embolization is a relatively uncommon cause of an embolic arterial ischemic event but should be considered in any patient who presents with simultaneous pulmonary embolism or deep venous thrombosis (DVT) and acute arterial ischemia. Current echocardiographic technology has made the noninvasive diagnosis of right-to-left cardiac shunts relatively straightforward. The ease of diagnosis of the relatively common patent foramen ovale has led to renewed enthusiasm for implicating paradoxical embolism as the cause of many otherwise unexplained embolic events. However, the diagnosis remains presumptive rather than definitive in most cases, a fact relevant to consideration of invasive treatment strategies. The rarity of documented paradoxical embolism has resulted in most treatment recommendations being based on anecdotal reports or clinical supposition.

PATHOPHYSIOLOGY

Any congenital or acquired communication between the right heart or pulmonary arteries and the left heart or systemic arteries can be the route through which a paradoxical embolus bypasses the lung. The most common potential communication is a patent foramen ovale (Fig. 1). The foramen ovale is the normal valvelike communication between the right and left atria that allows the physiologic right-to-left shunt of the fetal

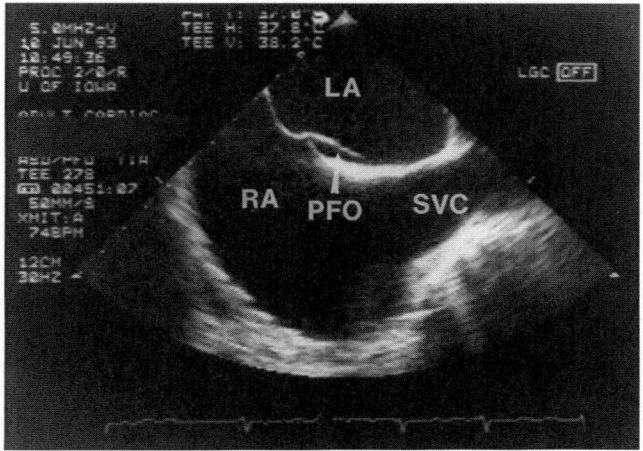

Figure 1 Transesophageal echocardiogram in a patient with a patent foramen ovale clearly demonstrating the flap that allows right-to-left but not left-to-right flow. LA, left atrium; RA, right atrium; PFO patent foramen ovale; SVC, superior vena cava.

circulation. After birth the rise in left atrial pressure causes the valve to close, and the communication is sealed in most adults. Autopsy studies have demonstrated that the potential communication persists in 25% to 30% of normal adults, with a decreasing incidence with age.[1] Any pathologic condition leading to pulmonary hypertension or right heart failure could cause enough elevation in right atrial pressure to allow shunting of blood and, thus, the potential for embolization through a patent foramen ovale. Pulmonary embolism can be the cause of elevated right heart pressures and is commonly present in reported cases of paradoxical embolism.[2] In addition to pathologic states, echocardiographic studies have documented that transient right-to-left shunting can occur through a patent foramen ovale in association with a Valsalva maneuver, coughing, or even as a normal part of the cardiac cycle.[3,4]

DIAGNOSIS

Paradoxical embolization should be suspected in any patient who presents with acute arterial ischemia suggestive of an embolic etiology when no obvious source of emboli is identified. Suspicion should obviously be heightened in patients with pre-existing or concomitant pulmonary embolism or DVT. The absence of a history or definitive documentation of lower extremity DVT does not exclude the possibility of paradoxical embolism. Studies of patients with documented pulmonary emboli have shown that DVT is frequently clinically silent and that diagnostic evaluation for a lower extremity deep venous source following pulmonary emboli may be negative. Still, paradoxical embolization remains an uncommon cause of embolic events. More common causes of arterial embolization, such as myocardial infarction or cardiomyopathy, are also predisposing factors for DVT. In some patients with the triad of arterial embolism, venous thrombosis, and a patent foramen ovale, paradoxical embolism is likely not to be the mechanism of embolization. The arterial embolism and DVT will have been independent events, and the patent foramen ovale an unrelated chance occurrence. Definitive confirmation of paradoxical embolism—echocardiographic observation of an embolus trapped or passing through a patent foramen ovale[5]—is often lacking; thus the diagnosis remains presumptive in many cases. An example of this diagnostic dilemma is the controversy about the role of paradoxical embolism as a mechanism of unexplained stroke in young patients. Studies in this group of patients have shown a relatively high incidence of patent foramen ovale, approximately 50%, yet most of these patients do not have a documented venous source of emboli.[6] Because the incidence of patent foramen ovale in normal young adults is approximately 35%, the documentation of a patent foramen ovale in itself should not be considered proof that paradoxical embolization was the cause of the stroke.

Diagnosis of right-to-left shunting has become relatively straightforward with current echocardiographic techniques. Any patient with an unexplained embolic event should undergo echocardiography. A transthoracic study is less sensitive than a transesophageal study but is less invasive, and a positive transthoracic study may preclude the need for a transesophageal examination. Color Doppler studies may provide documentation of shunting.

In addition, echocardiographic "contrast" studies with microbubbles can be performed[3,4] (Fig. 2). Contrast is obtained by agitating saline or another intravenous solution between two syringes connected by a stopcock and then rapidly injecting the solution into a peripheral vein. The injected solution fills the right atrium with echo-reflecting microbubbles. Early appearance of the bubbles in the left atrium suggests a right-to-left communication. In addition to studies at rest, the contrast study can be combined with provocative maneuvers such as Valsalva or coughing to increase the sensitivity in detecting patent foramen ovale. Contrast transesophageal echocardiography studies with provocative maneuvers done in normal volunteers document an incidence of patent foramen ovale similar to the autopsy incidence, suggesting a high sensitivity for this study.[3] Similar microbubble studies have also been done with a transcranial Doppler to detect microbubbles entering the cerebral circulation after venous injection.[7] The transcranial Doppler microbubble examination documents the presence of any right-to-left shunt, including noncardiac shunts such as pulmonary arteriovenous fistulas, but cannot identify the location of the shunt.

TREATMENT

Treatment of paradoxical embolism depends on the clinical presentation, cause of the right-to-left shunt, and the location of the arterial embolus. Anticoagulation is an essential component of therapy and in some patients the only treatment required. The purpose of the anticoagulation is to prevent further propagation of thrombus in both the venous and arterial circulation, prevent further embolization, and tip the normal

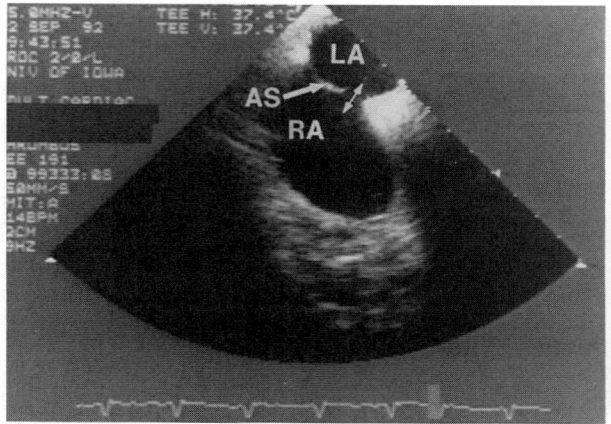 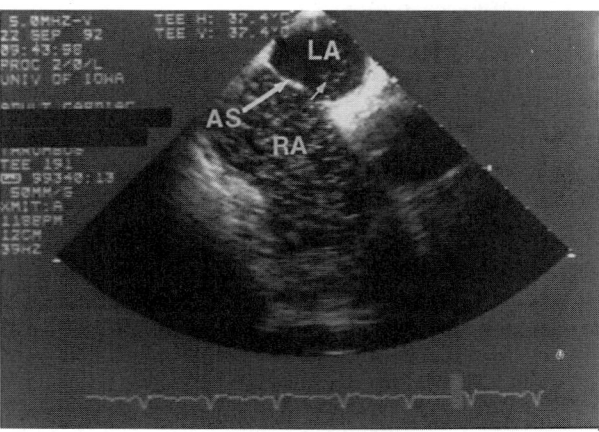

Figure 2 Transesophageal echocardiogram in a 39-year-old man who presented with lower extremity deep venous thrombosis, pulmonary embolism, and a femoral artery embolus that was presumed to be paradoxical after this study revealed an atrial septal defect (*arrow*). *A,* B-mode image demonstrating the atrial septal defect (*arrow*). *B,* Microbubble contrast study demonstrating right-to-left communication. RA, Right atrium; LA, left atrium; AS, atrial septum.

thrombotic-thrombolytic balance toward a thrombolytic state. This treatment remains important for the patient whose embolic presentation is stroke, as long as cerebral hemorrhage has been excluded on CT scan. In the absence of contraindications such as active bleeding or a hemorrhagic stroke, patients with paradoxical embolism should initially receive full anticoagulation with heparin sodium. In most cases, after the acute episode has been treated, the patient requires further anticoagulant treatment with warfarin for 3 to 6 months. Long-term or permanent anticoagulant therapy may be necessary for a patient with a hypercoagulable state or recurrent thromboembolic episodes.

The arterial embolism may require immediate attention if it is life- or limb-threatening. Preoperative arteriography is avoided in patients in whom the diagnosis of embolism rather than thrombosis of a diseased vessel is relatively certain or in the presence of severe, immediately limb-threatening ischemia. Intraoperative digital fluoroscopy can be extremely helpful, as it allows diagnostic evaluation of both inflow and outflow vessels. Fluoroscopy can be used to direct catheters into distal vessels from a proximal arteriotomy, along with allowing direct visualization of balloon inflation and withdrawal by using contrast in the balloon. The direct catheter visualization allows almost all extremity embolectomy procedures to be performed from proximal vessel exposure, for example, femoral, with local anesthesia. Real-time fluoroscopic arteriography allows monitoring of the progress of thromboembolectomy and avoids both unnecessary catheter passages and retained thrombus.

Thrombolytic therapy has been used in the treatment of all three processes—DVT, pulmonary embolism, and arterial embolism—that are usually present with paradoxical embolism. At first glance, thrombolysis therefore seems to be an ideal approach. However, the simplicity, effectiveness, and low complication rate of embolectomy for typical extremity embolization are hard to improve. Systemic thrombolytic therapy is not as effective as direct intra-arterial therapy in the treatment of arterial emboli, and acute embolic stroke must still be considered a contraindication to systemic thrombolysis. The primary role for systemic thrombolytic therapy appears to be in patients with noncerebral paradoxical emboli who are candidates for thrombolysis because of

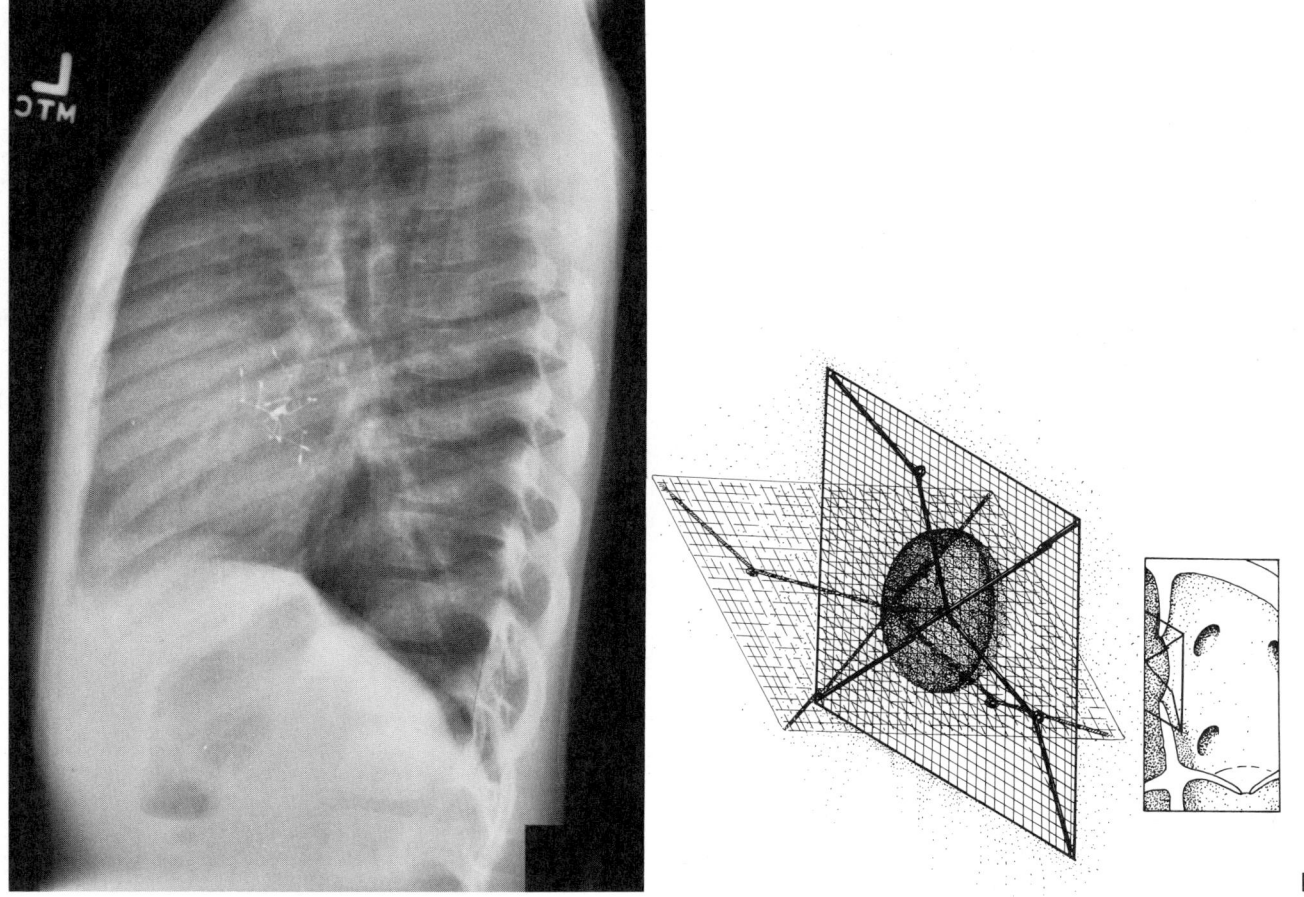

Figure 3 Clamshell septal umbrella for transcatheter closure of atrial septal defects or patent foramen ovale. *A,* Lateral chest film in a 4-year-old girl who underwent transcatheter closure of an atrial septal defect. *B,* Schematic of clamshell septal umbrella.

simultaneous pulmonary embolism causing hemodynamic compromise. Intra-arterial thrombolytic therapy may be of benefit in the treatment of emboli to sites that are more difficult to approach surgically or as an intraoperative adjunct to embolectomy when concomitant small vessel thrombosis has occurred distal to the embolus.

The role of caval filtering devices such as the Greenfield filter in the treatment of paradoxical embolism is unclear. The Greenfield filter seems intuitively an attractive solution because of its well-documented low complication rate and high effectiveness in treating pulmonary embolism. The problem lies in the different consequences of emboli in the pulmonary circulation versus those in the systemic circulation. The Greenfield filter traps large emboli but does allow passage of small emboli that have minimal consequences in the pulmonary circulation but may have devastating effects in the cerebral or other systemic arterial beds.[8] If Greenfield filters are used in patients with paradoxical emboli, the patients should also be anticoagulated unless the indication for filter placement was an absolute contraindication to anticoagulation. A caval filter should be placed in a patient with paradoxical embolus from a lower extremity source and contraindications to anticoagulation in order to prevent major pulmonary emboli, even if prevention of arterial embolism is not assured.

An obvious approach to paradoxical embolism is closure of the right-to-left shunt by correction of the cardiac defect or resection of a pulmonary arteriovenous fistula. In patients in whom the physiologic consequences of the shunt indicate correction or in whom emboli have recurred despite anticoagulation and/or caval filter placement, the decision to eliminate the shunt is relatively straightforward. In treating an initial episode of paradoxical embolism, a decision to recommend operative correction of a patent foramen ovale is more problematic because anticoagulation alone may be sufficient treatment. The development of endovascular techniques for shunt closure may impact on the therapeutic approach. Successful treatment of pulmonary arteriovenous fistulas have been carried out with obliterative embolotherapy.[9] Devices designed for endovascular closure of atrial septal defects or a patent foramen ovale have also been employed[10] (Fig. 3). Enthusiasm for the seemingly attractive endovascular approach must be tempered by the realization that any prosthetic material in a cardiac chamber poses a risk for thromboembolic complications. The cure should not present a higher embolic risk than the disease.

REFERENCES

1. Hagen PT, Scholz DG, Edwards WD. Incidence and size of patent foramen ovale during the first 10 decades of life: An autopsy study of 965 normal hearts. Mayo Clin Proc 1984; 59:17–20.
2. Loscalzo J. Paradoxical embolism: Clinical presentation, diagnostic strategies, and therapeutic options. Am Heart J 1986; 112:141–145.
3. Movsowitz C, Podolsky LA, Meyerowitz CB, et al. Patent foramen ovale: A nonfunctional embryological remnant or a potential cause of significant pathology? J Am Soc Echocardiogr 1992; 5:259–270.
4. Langholz D, Louie EK, Konstadt SN, et al. Transesophageal echocardiographic demonstration of distinct mechanisms for right to left shunting across a patent foramen ovale in the absence of pulmonary hypertension. J Am Coll Cardiol 1991; 18:1112–1117.
5. Nelson CW, Snow FR, Barnett M, et al. Impending paradoxical embolism: Echocardiographic diagnosis of an intracardiac thrombus crossing a patent foramen ovale. Am Heart J 1991; 122:859–862.
6. Ranoux D, Cohen A, Cabanes L, et al. Patent foramen ovale: Is stroke due to paradoxical embolism? Stroke 1993; 24:31–34.
7. Teague SM, Sharma MK. Detection of paradoxical cerebral echo contrast embolization by transcranial Doppler ultrasound. Stroke 1991; 22:740–745.
8. Dalman R, Kohler TR. Cerebrovascular accident after Greenfield filter placement for paradoxical embolism. J Vasc Surg 1989; 9:452–454.
9. Pennington DW, Gold WM, Gordon RL, et al. Treatment of pulmonary arteriovenous malformations by therapeutic embolization: Rest and exercise physiology in eight patients. Am Rev Respir Dis 1992; 145:1047–1051.
10. Bridges ND, Hellenbrand W, Latson L, et al. Transcatheter closure of patent foramen ovale after presumed paradoxical embolism. Circulation 1992; 86:1902–1908.

VASCULAR TRAUMA

NONARTERIOGRAPHIC ASSESSMENT OF PENETRATING VASCULAR INJURIES

KAJ JOHANSEN, M.D., PH.D.

The trauma victim who has suffered an extremity arterial injury—with a physical examination characterized by loss of arterial pulses, a rapidly expanding hematoma, or an arteriovenous (AV) fistula—requires urgent operation, and arteriography or other diagnostic modalities are required only rarely. The latter generally occurs in the distinctly unusual circumstance of tandem arterial lesions or when the precise site of the arterial injury is otherwise unclear. More commonly, however, the clinician is confronted by a patient who manifests "soft" signs of arterial injury—neurologic changes, diminished pulses, a history of arterial bleeding, hypovolemic shock—or no basis for concern at all, other than proximity of a wound to a major artery. In such a circumstance, an occult major vascular injury must be identified or ruled out.

Historically, the apparent lack of sensitivity and specificity of physical examination for occult arterial injury led to a policy of mandatory operative exploration of worrisome extremity wounds so that occult arterial damage could be ruled out by direct visual examination of the vessel in question. This policy fell into disfavor with the observation that its yield was low. In addition, emergency contrast arteriography had been found to be highly sensitive and specific, at levels greater than 95% in the diagnosis of occult arterial damage. Contrast arteriography as a "screening" or "exclusion" technique became the standard of practice, even at centers that had previously disparaged it.

Recently, however, there has been re-evaluation of the proper diagnostic approach to be adopted toward trauma victims with few or no signs of arterial injury, but in whom such damage must be ruled out. This has taken two forms: (1) a resurrection of the serial physical examination and (2) the introduction of two noninvasive diagnostic techniques well established in the evaluation of chronic arterial disease—Doppler arterial pressure measurement and duplex sonography—as substitutes for arteriography in the diagnosis of acute arterial damage.

COSTS OF ARTERIOGRAPHY

Its accuracy notwithstanding, several features of contrast arteriography make it a poor choice as a screening examination for patients potentially harboring an occult arterial injury. First, arteriography has a small but nontrivial incidence of complications including bleeding, pseudoaneurysm, contrast medium reactions, and nephrotoxicity, that are potential risks to the patient. Second, because it is an invasive test requiring substantial outlays in equipment and personnel, arteriography is costly. Single-limb emergency contrast arteriograms may cost from $800 to as much as $4,000. Third, arteriography may consume unacceptable amounts of time. In a study of patients managed in a prominent trauma center by an acknowledged expert in trauma arteriography, the mean period of time required to perform a screening extremity arteriogram was 2.4 hours.[1] Such an obligatory delay for the performance of a screening study, which is rarely positive and even less frequently useful in changing the trauma victim's course, may be unacceptable, especially in the polytrauma victim in whom other significant problems may require urgent resolution. Fourth, contrast arteriography generally requires moving the patient to the angiography suite, which may pose monitoring and resuscitation problems in an unstable trauma victim.

Finally, all large studies of arteriograms performed to rule out extremity arterial damage document a 2% to 7% incidence of false-negative and false-positive examinations, the former resulting in the failure to diagnose potentially important vascular injuries, and the latter causing further fruitless evaluation or even unnecessary operative exploration. Given these shortcomings of "screening" or "exclusion" contrast arteriography for extremity arterial trauma, a series of clinical studies was initiated in the late 1980s to re-evaluate old practices and new technologies in a search of an accurate, cost-effective substitute.

THE PHYSICAL EXAMINATION REVISITED

Physical examination originally fell into disfavor in patients potentially harboring arterial injuries because of the occasional observation of intact distal pulses, despite the subsequent documentation of significant arterial damage. Further, findings on physical examination may be altered or masked by hematoma or edema, dressings or splints, hypotension or intoxication, or central or peripheral neurologic damage. Finally, physical examination clearly may be unhelpful in cases of venous trauma or of relatively minor but potentially significant arterial damage, such as with nonocclusive arterial intimal flaps or AV communications.

Recently, however, clinical investigators at several institutions have revisited the concept of careful, systematic, serial physical examination of patients whose injuries place them at risk for occult arterial injury. Studies by Francis[2] and Dennis[3] and their colleagues clearly suggest that the sensitivity and specificity of serial physical examinations performed by an experienced clinician are excellent. These and other workers concede that physical examination may not be helpful in diagnosing nonocclusive arterial injuries, a point emphasized by Perry.[4] Interestingly, however, this may not matter. Several prospective studies suggest that the vast majority of arterial intimal flaps, pseudoaneurysms, and AV fistulas follow a benign course and may, in fact, never require intervention.[5,6] Accordingly, current data suggest that serial physical examinations by an experienced clinician may provide satisfactory diagnostic accuracy in the patient who may be harboring an occult arterial injury.

DOPPLER ARTERIAL BLOOD PRESSURE MEASUREMENTS

Use of the hand-held Doppler instrument to measure ankle systolic arterial blood pressure is the objective mainstay in the evaluation of chronic arterial occlusive disease. The possibility that significant acute arterial occlusive lesions, especially those following blunt or penetrating trauma, could be diagnosed by the same technique seemed reasonable. In an arteriography-controlled study of 100 consecutive extremity injuries, Lynch and Johansen documented that an arterial pressure index (API; systolic blood pressure in the injured extremity divided by systolic blood pressure in an uninjured arm) had an 87% sensitivity and 95% specificity for arterial disruption.[7] Because of two false-positive arteriograms (2%) in this study, the sensitivity and specificity of API as compared to clinical outcome were even better: 95% and 97.5%, respectively.[1]

These investigators then tested the hypothesis that Doppler API could be used as an accurate screening test for occult extremity arterial injury (Fig. 1). In another series of 100 consecutive extremity injuries, arteriography was performed only when API was found to be less than 0.9. In these 100 limbs 17 had an API less than 0.9; arteriography was positive in 16 (94%), and 7 (46%)

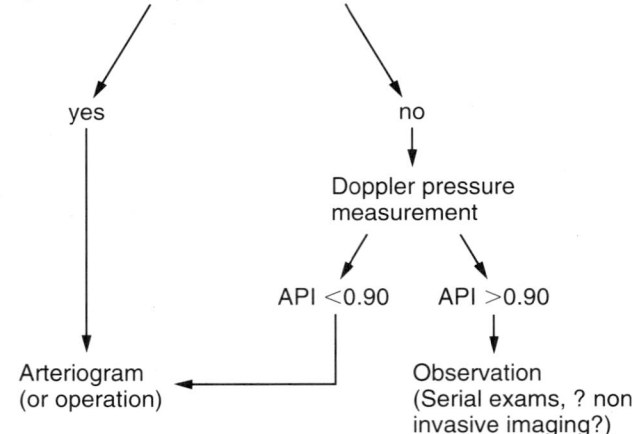

Figure 1 A diagnostic algorithm for potential extremity arterial injury based on Doppler-derived arterial pressure indices (From Lynch K, Johansen KH. Can Doppler pressure measurements replace "exclusion" arteriography in extremity trauma? Ann Surg 1991; 214:737–741; with permission.)

underwent arterial reconstruction. In contrast, among 83 limbs with API greater than 0.9 and followed up clinically, only 4 were ultimately found to have arterial lesions; 3 pseudoaneurysms resolved without intervention, and a profunda femoris AV fistula following a right groin gunshot wound was repaired uneventfully.[7]

Other studies have suggested the value of initial screening by Doppler blood pressure measurements to rule out major occult arterial injury of the extremities. Use of a threshold value of API greater than or equal to 1.0 appears more sensitive but results in a higher likelihood of negative arteriogram results.

The Seattle group validated Doppler arterial blood pressure measurements only for extremity arterial injuries distal to the inguinal and axillary crease. More proximal injuries (for example, to the iliac or axillosubclavian arteries) continue to require contrast arteriography as a primary screening examination.[7] The technique also is inaccurate for venous injuries, for damage to nonaxial vessels such as the profunda femoris artery, and for certain nonocclusive arterial injuries.[7] However, as is clinically evident and also suggested by several studies, failure to detect such injuries may have no clinical import.[5,6]

DUPLEX SCANNING

Duplex scanning has become a state of the art diagnostic technology for the evaluation of chronic arterial and venous diseases. Several groups have embarked upon clinical studies designed to assess the accuracy and reproducibility of duplex sonography in the trauma victim.

Meissner, Paun, and Johansen evaluated 89 trauma victims with potential injuries to extremity or cervical arteries.[8] This group had previously used duplex sonography for secondary surveillance in their prospective

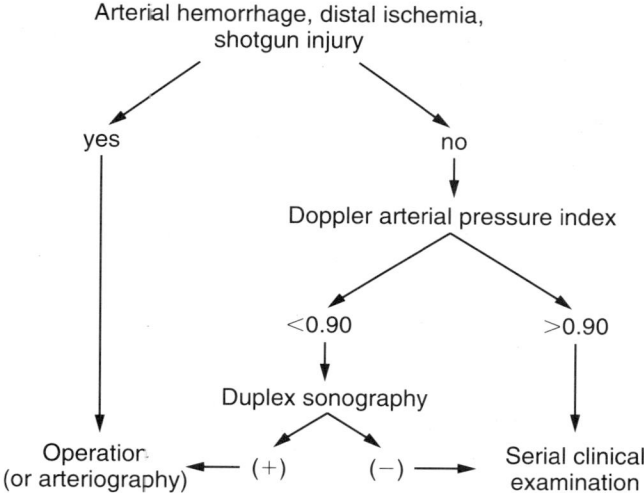

Figure 2 A contemporary diagnostic algorithm for potential extremity arterial injury based on Doppler-derived arterial pressure indices and duplex sonography.

study of Doppler arterial pressure measurements. In fact, duplex scanning had documented the three pseudoaneurysms and one profunda AV fistula discovered during follow-up in patients not undergoing arteriography in that study. In their 89 patients Meissner and colleagues documented 25 arterial injuries by duplex scan. There were four false-negative duplex scans and no false-positive studies.[8]

Bynoe and colleagues, in an even larger study from the University of South Carolina, evaluated 198 patients with 319 potential sites of arterial injury in the extremities and neck. Duplex scanning documented 23 injuries, with one false-positive and two false-negative studies. Sensitivity of duplex sonography was calculated to be 95%, specificity 99%, and overall accuracy 98%.[9]

In a study of experimental canine arterial injuries (occlusion, intimal flap, arterial laceration, AV fistula, extrinsic compression, pseudoaneurysm), Panetta and co-workers compared duplex scans and contrast arteriography. This evaluation documented that duplex scanning was more sensitive overall than arteriography (90.1% versus 80.2%, $p < .002$) and that arteriography had a higher specificity (94.7% versus 68.4%, $p < .04$). Duplex scanning documented arterial lacerations much more accurately (88% versus 56%, $p < .02$) and had the capability of delineating arterial wall morphology.[10]

Duplex scanning costs an average of $250, and an extremity arterial examination consumes approximately 20 minutes. Unlike arteriography, the technique is portable; it can readily be performed at the bedside in the trauma center. As suggested by the experimental canine study of Panetta and associates,[10] duplex scanning has, besides its rapidity, portability, low cost, and accuracy, as an advantage its ability to document venous injury and extraluminal lesions such as pseudoaneurysms and hematomas.

Occasionally, duplex scanning may miss arterial injuries later documented by other techniques. This technique's utility for assessing more centrally placed vessels of the thorax, abdomen, and pelvis remains unproven. These reservations notwithstanding, duplex scanning appears well validated as a screening test for potential vascular injuries of the extremities.

OTHER NONARTERIOGRAPHIC DIAGNOSTIC TECHNIQUES

Occasional efforts at utilizing other imaging techniques in obvious or suspected extremity trauma have been made. Magnetic resonance imaging and radioisotope scintiangiography have shown some promise in this setting. Unfortunately, consumption of time and resources, the need to move the trauma victim to another site, and the absence of proper prospective validation trials make conclusions from these reports little more than speculative at this time.

A PROPOSED MANAGEMENT ALGORITHM

A management plan has evolved from an arteriographically controlled study of Doppler arterial blood pressure measurements in patients possibly harboring occult extremity arterial injuries.[1] The algorithm itself was validated prospectively.[7] Subsequent demonstration of duplex sonography's ability to detect occult extremity arterial injuries permits presentation of a rational contemporary management algorithm for the trauma victim at risk for an extremity vascular injury[8,9] (Fig. 2).

REFERENCES

1. Lynch K, Johansen KH. Can Doppler pressure measurements replace "exclusion" arteriography in extremity trauma? Ann Surg 1991; 214:737–741.
2. Francis H, Thal ER, Weigelt JA, et al. Vascular proximity: Is it a valid indication for arteriography in the asymptomatic patient? J Trauma 1991; 31:512–514.
3. Dennis JW, Frykberg ER, Crump JM, et al. New perspectives in the management of penetrating trauma in proximity to major limb arteries. J Vasc Surg 1990; 11:85–93.
4. Perry MO. Complications of missed arterial injuries. J Vasc Surg 993; 17:399–407.
5. Frykberg ER, Crump JM, Dennis JW, et al. Nonoperative observation of clinically occult arterial injuries: A prospective evaluation. Surgery 1991; 109:85–96.
6. Stain SC, Yellin AE, Weaver FA, et al. Selective management of nonocclusive arterial injuries. Arch Surg 1989; 124:1136–1142.
7. Johansen K, Lynch K, Paun M, Copass MK. Non-invasive vascular tests reliably exclude occult arterial trauma in injured extremities. J Trauma 1991; 31:515–522.
8. Meissner M, Paun M, Johansen K. Duplex scanning for arterial trauma. Am J Surg 1991; 161:552–555.
9. Bynoe RP, Miles WS, Ben RM, et al. Noninvasive diagnosis of vascular trauma by duplex ultrasonography. J Vasc Surg 1991; 14:346–352.
10. Panetta TF, Hunt JP, Buechter KJ, et al. Duplex ultrasonography versus arteriography in the diagnosis of arterial injury: An experimental study. J Trauma 1992; 33:627–635.

ROLE OF ARTERIOGRAPHY IN PENETRATING VASCULAR INJURIES

MALCOLM O. PERRY, M.D.

Arteriograms are usually obtained for one of three reasons in the management of patients with suspected major arterial injuries: (1) to detect injuries that might otherwise not be apparent despite a careful history and physical examination, (2) to plan the operative management of complex injuries, and (3) to exclude the need for surgical exploration in patients who have no other indications for operation.[1,2]

Several studies have concluded that many injuries of major arteries of the extremities are easily detected by a careful physical examination, and in most of these patients arteriograms were not necessary.[3,4] The damage inflicted by stab wounds and low-velocity bullets is usually confined to the wound tract, and thus the diagnosis is relatively straightforward in most patients. If there is a discrepancy in distal pulses, active arterial bleeding, large hematomas that may or may not be pulsatile, or a history of serious arterial bleeding, the decision to operate is relatively easy. Moreover, some of these patients show other indications for operation related to damage to contiguous structures, and the arterial exploration would be a part of that procedure. Arteriography is rarely needed in such patients. A few patients may have occult injuries of the deep femoral or the deep brachial arteries or one of the three tibial arteries, and in such situations arteriograms may be helpful.

Arteriography performed solely for suspected proximity of the wound tract to the vessels has a low yield, varying from 5% to 20%, depending on the trauma centers supplying the data.[5,6] Furthermore, the definition of proximity is vague and imprecise. It is often related to the experience of an examining surgeon, who should have an accurate interpretation of three-dimensional anatomy.

ARTERIOGRAPHY

Although some surgeons favor two-dimensional biplane arteriography for all injuries, others have successfully used single-plane, one-injection arteriography to exclude vascular injuries in patients who had no other indications of such an injury.[6] Controversy continues to surround the actual method, but if arteriograms are to be performed, clearly the vessel must be visualized both proximal and distal to the area of suspected injury, and sequential films are recommended rather than single digital studies. Markers should be placed at entrance and exit wounds for better orientation, and the studies should not be terminated until the surgeon has an opportunity to review the films.

Varying interpretations have also clouded the picture because in some studies spasm or displacement of the artery has been interpreted as an injury, whereas in reality it is arguable. Solid signs of arterial injury include extravasation of contrast medium, the detection of a false aneurysm, an arteriovenous (AV) fistula, and arterial disruption with or without obstruction. Minor defects in the intima may or may not represent a significant arterial injury. It has been documented that some of these lesions are not seen on delayed studies, and some may heal without sequelae.[4] Obviously, until standardized methods of study and interpretation are employed, comparison of various reports is likely to be inaccurate.

NATURAL HISTORY OF ARTERIAL WOUNDS

Recent studies have suggested that the natural history of occult arterial wounds of the extremities can be benign.[3,4] Although this is certainly true for some injuries, long-term follow-up studies have not been done, and one cannot be certain about the outcome of all these injuries. There is an inappropriate tendency to equate iatrogenic arterial injuries occurring under controlled circumstances with traumatic arterial wounds. The natural history of traumatic arterial injuries has been

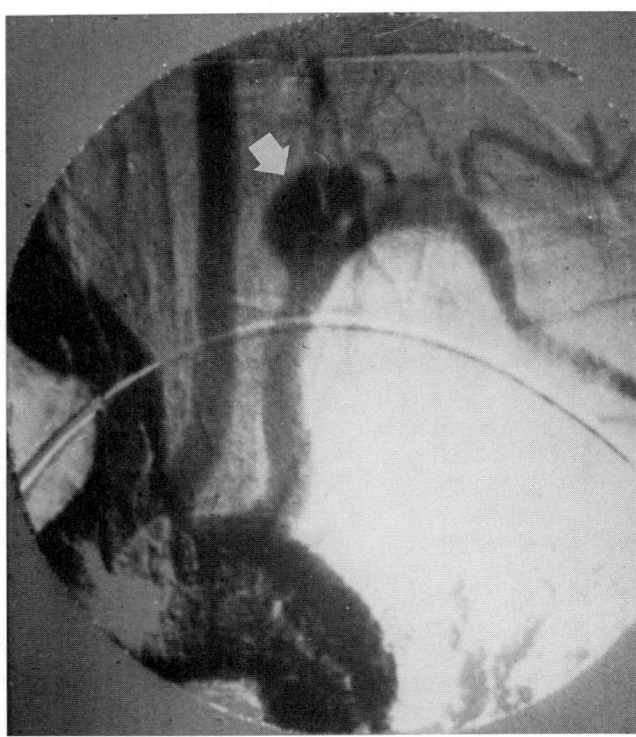

Figure 1 This false aneurysm of the subclavian artery was discovered several months after the patient had a stab wound.

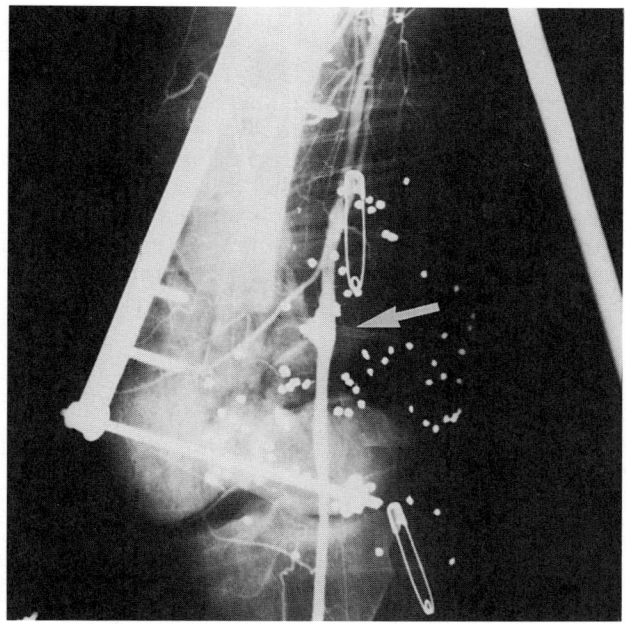

Figure 2 Despite this injury of the femoral artery, the patient had normal distal pulses and blood pressures.

carefully studied by Shumacker and Wayson.[7] In following up 245 post-traumatic arterial AV fistulas and 122 false aneurysms, they found that spontaneous cure occurred in 6.6% of the false aneurysms and 2.2% of the AV fistulas. This outcome is in marked contrast to what is seen with iatrogenic arterial wounds from needles and catheters, although some of these wounds also have caused serious delayed complications.[8]

The natural history of occult arterial injuries in the neck and the trunk is likely to be more serious than that of arterial wounds in the extremities. No prospective studies of such injuries has been done, and very few long-term studies have been reported. In none of them have the patients been followed with independent objective studies to detect or rule out delayed complications. The true natural history and risk in these patients await further definition.

ADJUNCTIVE DIAGNOSTIC METHODS

It has been clearly established that patients can have proximal arterial injuries of major arteries in the extremities and yet have what appear to be normal distal

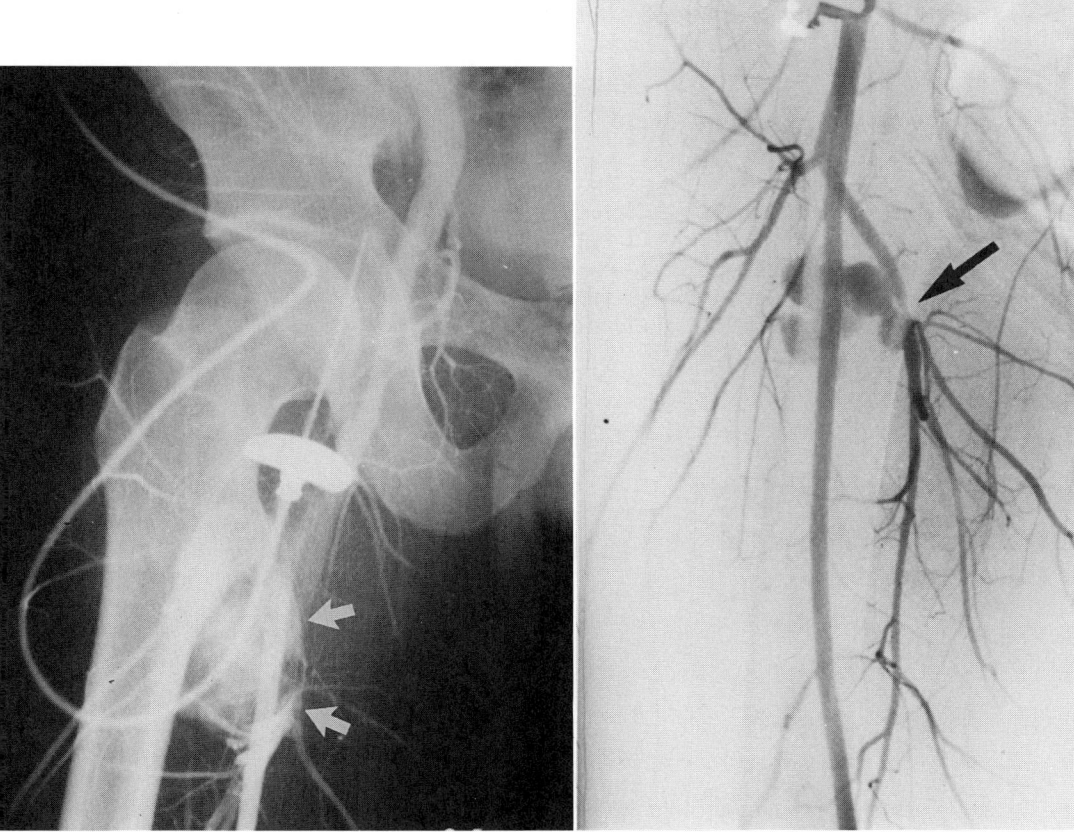

Figure 3 These two patients each had an injury of the profunda femoral artery (*arrow*), but both had normal distal pulses and blood pressures.

pulses (Fig. 1). The report from Drapanas and associates from Charity Hospital documented that 27% of patients with operatively proven proximal arterial injuries had normal pulses, and others have confirmed these findings.[1,5,9] The pulse wave is a pressure wave that reaches velocities of 13 m/second, and it can be transmitted beyond intimal flaps, through collaterals, or even past areas of soft thrombus (Fig. 2). Moreover, injuries of a profunda femoral, a profunda brachial, or one of three tibial arteries may not result in distal pulse deficits (Fig. 3). Although the ankle-brachial index is useful as part of the physical examination, it is not totally reliable because of these hemodynamic discrepancies. There are numerous reports in the literature of patients with normal ankle-brachial indices and normal distal pulses who had operatively proven major arterial injuries. The method is useful, but it is not infallible.

Recent studies using duplex imaging suggest that this modality may be helpful in the evaluation of possible arterial injuries in asymptomatic patients.[10] Although many hospitals are likely not to have a vascular laboratory and trained technologists available 24 hours a day, 7 days a week, these adjunctive methods may be useful in evaluating these patients. With a thorough history, a careful physical examination, the use of ankle-brachial indices, and, if available, duplex imaging, it would appear that most of the patients can be treated satisfactorily without arteriography. The dependability of these studies needs to be validated by independent objective methods and by careful long-term follow-up.

CURRENT RECOMMENDATIONS

The weight of evidence in the literature suggests that most arterial injuries in the extremities can be detected with a careful history and physical examination and that patients can be managed without arteriography. Arteriograms are obtained usually for one of three reasons, but in patients who have penetrating trauma to the neck and the trunk, arteriography may be required more liberally because of the inability to expose these injuries. Secondary issues include the ability to evaluate and treat minor arterial injuries with endovascular methods. The newer techniques require some form of active visualization of the vessels. Experienced trauma surgeons for many years have identified and treated patients with vascular injuries in the extremities without arteriography or other adjunctive diagnostic methods, and it appears that newer diagnostic techniques will permit an extension of these practices.[1-3]

REFERENCES

1. Perry MO. Complications of missed arterial injuries. J Vasc Surg 1991; 17:399–407.
2. Turcotte JK, Towne JB, Bernhard VM. Is arteriography necessary in the management of vascular trauma of the extremities? Surgery 1978; 84:55–62.
3. Schwartz MR, Weaver FA, Bauer M, et al. Refining the indications for arteriography in penetrating extremity trauma: A prospective analysis. J Vasc Surg 1993; 17:116–124.
4. Frykberg ER, Crump JM, Dennis JW, et al. Nonoperative observation of clinically occult arterial injuries. A prospective evaluation. Surgery 1991; 109:85–96.
5. Feliciano DV, Bitondo CG, Mattox KL, et al. Civilian trauma in the 1980's. Ann Surg 1984; 199:717–724.
6. Francis H III, Thal ER, Weigelt JA, et al. Vascular proximity: Is it a valid indication for arteriography in asymptomatic patients? J Trauma 1991; 11:512–514.
7. Shumacker HB, Wayson EE. Spontaneous cure of aneurysms and arteriovenous fistulas, with some notes on intravascular thrombosis. Am J Surg 1950; 79:532–544.
8. Kent KC, McArdle CR, Kennedy RJMS, et al. A prospective study of the clinical outcome of femoral pseudoaneurysms and arteriovenous fistulas caused by arterial puncture. J Vasc Surg 1993; 17:125–133.
9. Drapanas T, Hewitt RL, Weichert RF, et al. Civilian vascular injuries: A critical appraisal of three decades of management. Ann Surg 1970; 172:351–360.
10. Bynoe RP, Miles WS, Bell RM, et al. Non-invasive diagnosis of vascular trauma by duplex ultrasonography. J Vasc Surg 1991; 14:346–352.

PENETRATING AND BLUNT EXTRACRANIAL CAROTID ARTERY INJURIES

MICHAEL P. BYRNE, M.D.
RICHARD E. WELLING, M.D.

Extracranial carotid arterial trauma continues to be a challenge to the surgeon, in both its early diagnosis and its preferred treatment strategies. Definitive studies to address controversial areas of carotid trauma face several confounding obstacles. First is the infrequent nature of carotid injuries. In most large series, carotid trauma comprises 5% of all vascular injuries, with 95% being penetrating in origin.[1] This prevents any one institution from gaining extensive experience with carotid trauma. The relative infrequency of injury to the carotid artery is due to its limited anatomic exposure and the lethality of severe carotid injuries, from either exsanguination or asphyxiation. Second, patients with carotid trauma present with a wide range of concomitant neurologic deficits, degrees of shock, and other life-threatening injuries that preclude clear-cut categorization of patient groups. Finally, only 20% of the population has a normal circle of Willis. In patients with an abnormal circle of Willis, half have a developmental anomaly that hinders effective collateral blood flow.[1] Therefore, the status of collateral blood flow in the patient with carotid trauma is "predictably unpredictable" and not readily defined in the clinical setting.

PENETRATING CAROTID TRAUMA

Epidemiology and Etiology

Penetrating carotid trauma is usually caused by stab wounds or low-velocity missiles. The typical patient is male, age 20 to 40 years, and often under the influence of alcohol or drugs. Twenty-five percent of patients present with hemorrhagic shock. Most can be resuscitated and stabilized prior to surgical exploration. Neurologic deficits are present in 20% to 45% of patients.[2,3] The common carotid artery is most commonly injured (70% to 90%).[3,4] Because of the proximity of many other anatomic structures, associated injuries are quite common. The most frequent concomitant injury, occurring in 15% to 30% of patients, is to the internal jugular vein. Other structures injured include the vertebral, subclavian, and innominate arteries in 12%; tracheal and laryngeal injuries in 9%; pharynx and esophageal injuries in 4%; and spinal cord and brachial plexus injuries in 2%.[4]

Initial Management

The first priority in management is to recognize a compromised airway and secure access. Airway compromise from a rapidly expanding hematoma, intratracheal bleeding, or neurologic deficit requires endotracheal intubation. Prophylactic intubation should always be considered in the patient with a penetrating neck injury and a stable but significant hematoma. In distal internal carotid artery injuries, occult bleeding may cause intraoral airway compromise with no evidence of external swelling. If exposure of the distal internal carotid artery (ICA) might be needed, nasotracheal intubation is preferred to allow easier manipulation of the mandible.

The second management priority is correction of hypovolemia. Bleeding can usually be controlled with digital pressure or packing. Two large-bore intravenous lines should be placed with at least one in the lower extremity if large veins in zone I may have been injured. Blind clamping or digital probing of wounds is contraindicated because it may cause injury to adjacent structures or aggravate an existing vascular injury. Vigorous resuscitation of shock is mandatory. Resolution of shock not only re-establishes blood flow to an already compromised brain but also often improves the neurologic deficit. If the patient is unresponsive to initial resuscitative efforts, immediate surgical exploration for control of injury is necessary.

A third management priority is as thorough a neurologic examination as circumstances allow. Neurologic deficits may have a variety of etiologies and should not be assumed to be from the carotid injury. Other

Table 1 Etiology of Neurologic Deficit

Hypoxia
Hypotension
Alcohol or drugs
Direct central nervous system injury
Spinal cord injury
Peripheral nerve injury
Carotid trauma

etiologies include direct central nervous system (CNS) trauma; shock and ischemia; spinal cord, cranial nerve, or brachial plexus injuries; and altered mental status from alcohol or drugs (Table 1). In stable patients, a cervical spine series and chest x-ray are both mandatory. Up to one-fourth of patients with a zone I injury have a concomitant intrathoracic injury.

Diagnostic Evaluation

Significant injury can be ruled out if, on local exploration of the wound, there is no evidence or suspicion of platysma penetration. Significant vascular injury is strongly suggested by the presence of a pulsatile or expanding hematoma, significant or pulsatile bleeding, presence of a pulse deficit, distal neurologic deficit, or the presence of a thrill or bruit. Intraoral palpation of the peritonsillar fossa may reveal a pulsatile hematoma indicating significant injury to the distal ICA. In the stable patient with no signs of obvious vascular injury, controversy still exists regarding mandatory or selective exploration of penetrating neck wounds. If a policy of mandatory exploration is followed, there is a 40% to 60% negative exploration rate. In several recent prospective studies, the morbidity and mortality were equal for selective versus mandatory exploration.

The role of arteriography also remains controversial. Most studies document that the accuracy of four-vessel arteriography is 95% to 100% in diagnosing carotid injury. Arteriovenous (AV) fistulas have been missed presumably because of a rapid clearing of contrast. Using the divisions proposed by Monson and co-workers,[5] the indications for arteriography can be better defined. Zone I extends from 1 cm above the clavicle inferiorly to include the base of the neck and the thoracic outlet, zone II extends from 1 cm above the clavicle to the angle of the mandible, and zone III extends from the angle of the mandible to the base of the skull. Clinical assessment often fails to detect injuries in zones I and III. Knowing preoperatively that there is a zone I or III injury would allow the surgeon to plan incisions, facilitate proximal and distal arterial control, and minimize blood loss. The strong consensus is that arteriography is desirable in all stable suspected zone I and III injuries. There is considerable disagreement about whether arteriography is useful or necessary for zone II injuries. Arguments for arteriography include the following: (1) The trajectory may go from zone II to either other zone; (2) preoperative localization facilitates where to dissect to gain proximal and distal control;

(3) therapeutic embolization can be performed at the same time; (4) other unsuspected vascular injuries may be recognized, especially vertebral artery injuries; (5) the cerebral vasculature can be assessed prior to possible arterial ligation of the injured vessel; and (6) gunshot wounds can be assessed because of the potential for multiple sites of injury. Contraindications to arteriography include hemodynamic instability from bleeding or a compromised airway.

Computed tomography (CT) scanning of the head is seldom indicated except in patients with severe neurologic deficits. In the comatose patient with an occluded carotid artery, a CT scan documenting a large hemorrhagic infarction or bilateral cerebral edema would be best treated by ligation.

Treatment

Medical

In several clinical situations medical management has been successful. Anticoagulation or simple observation have both been used successfully in patients with small arteriographic intimal defects. These injuries are thought to be similar to those following direct carotid puncture for arteriography.[6] Cautious observation should be followed, as several surgeons have noted that what were thought to be small intimal defects on the arteriogram were lacerations at the time of exploration. Serial duplex scans are useful in following these patients if the point of injury can be insonated.

Surgical

Virtually all penetrating injuries to the extracranial carotid arteries require operation consisting of either primary repair, interposition grafting, or ligation. The choice of procedure is dictated by the nature of the injury to the carotid and the neurologic status of the patient. In the subset of patients with a normal neurologic examination and carotid injury with prograde blood flow, repair has been successful in maintaining neurologic status in almost 100%. In patients with a normal examination and carotid occlusion, there has been some concern with distal embolization if repair is attempted. Fry and Fry[1] cautioned that, if left unattended, there may be propagation of the thrombus into the circle of Willis, resulting in neurologic deficits 36 to 48 hours later. Most studies document a low morbidity with re-establishment of blood flow in the occluded artery and successful maintenance of a normal neurologic status long term. Liekweg and Greenfield[3] reviewed 223 patients and concluded that if a patient had any neurologic deficit less than coma, repair yielded a good outcome in 85%, whereas ligation had a good outcome in only 50% of patients. This and subsequent reports[2,4] strongly support the recommendation that, in patients with mild neurologic deficits, repair should be performed whether or not there is prograde blood flow at the time of operation.

The most controversial area is the comatose patient with carotid injury. Bradley cautioned against repair in the setting of coma.[7] He reported two patients who died after revascularization and who had hemorrhagic cerebral infarction at autopsy. Later studies refuted this with autopsy data documenting that after revascularization in carotid injury cerebral edema and ischemic infarct and not hemorrhagic infarct were the cause of death.[4,8] Data from several recent reports suggest that the prognosis is abysmal in comatose patients with carotid injury undergoing ligation.[2,4,8-10] Of 28 patients treated by ligation, 14% were reported normal, and there was a 61% mortality rate. From these same reports, 42 comatose patients underwent revascularization. Overall 50% of these patients were normal or greatly improved, 24% had a permanent deficit, and the overall mortality was 26%. A final argument for revascularization in the comatose patient is to avoid excluding those patients who were in coma from shock, alcohol, or drugs.

Ligation is the best surgical option in certain situations. If there is a concomitant, severe, direct cerebral injury, diffuse cerebral edema, or large hemorrhagic infarction, it would be prudent to ligate an injured carotid artery rather than undertake a repair. A complex carotid injury along with ongoing life-threatening hemorrhage from associated injuries would best be treated expeditiously with ligation or detachable balloon embolic occlusion. If after careful thrombectomy there is no significant backbleeding from the distal carotid, chances of re-establishing prograde blood flow are minimal and ligation is the best option. Injuries of the external carotid artery (ECA) are best treated by ligation. Injuries of branches of the ECA must be treated by individual ligation and not ligation of the ECA itself because persistent bleeding may occur or there may be subsequent development of an arteriovenous (AV) fistula or pseudoaneurysm.

Operative Approach

The operative field should include the lower face and scalp, neck, and anterolateral chest because occasional median sternotomy or left thoracotomy is necessary for proximal arterial control. The usual surgical approach is an oblique incision paralleling the anterior border of the sternocleidomastoid muscle. Initially, proximal and distal control of the injury site is accomplished but is often the most difficult aspect, especially in zone I and III injuries.

The clinical indications for shunts have not been determined. Among patients with no neurologic deficit, shunts are rarely used with almost universal success. In patients with neurologic deficits with prograde blood flow, the use of a shunt seems reasonable, especially in complex injuries. A stronger case can be made for using a shunt in the patient with an occluded carotid artery with a neurologic deficit. This may represent a functional failure of the collateral circulation, and shunting could afford cerebral protection.

When a vein graft interposition is necessary, shunts provide protection during a prolonged procedure and additionally act as a stent during repair. In very distal ICA lesions where distal control is difficult, the intraluminal balloon occlusion shunt can provide both prograde blood flow and distal control of backbleeding.

Many surgeons use systemic heparin sodium during repair unless concomitant injuries contradict such. However, use of heparin sodium does not seem to improve overall results over studies in which it was not used. We have not found systemic heparin sodium therapy to be beneficial.

In 5% to 10% of patients, primary repair cannot be performed, and an interposition graft is necessary. Choices include internal jugular vein, saphenous vein, or polytetrafluoroethylene (PTFE). The use of internal jugular vein is discouraged because of long-term problems with aneurysmal dilation. Several surgeons have anecdotal reports of acute thrombosis following use of PTFE grafts, whereas this does not appear to be a significant problem with saphenous vein grafts.[6] Therefore, the choice of most surgeons is a saphenous vein graft. Another option is to reconstruct the proximal ICA by resection and transposition of the ECA over to the distal ICA.

Occasionally, significant thrombosis of the injured carotid necessitates balloon thrombectomy. This must be done with minimal inflation of the balloon to minimize the risk of injury to the intracranial portion of the ICA. Carotid cavernous fistula formation secondary to vigorous balloon catheter thrombectomy is possible in these circumstances.

Zone III injuries of the distal ICA pose several unique challenges. Initial maneuvers that improve access to the distal ICA include division of the posterior belly of the digastric muscle, ligation of the occipital artery, division of the ansa cervicalis nerve, mobilization of the hypoglossal nerve, and division of the stylohyoid muscle. A final practical maneuver is manipulation of the mandible by either subluxation or division and retraction. Our experience would favor stepped division of the mandible with replating. If adequate exposure for safe repair of ICA cannot be accomplished, then most authors advocate ligation, which prevents future problems with pseudoaneurysm or AV fistula. There are a few reports of ligation with extracranial-intracranial (EC-IC) bypass. The average EC-IC bypass is capable of 25 to 50 ml/minute of blood flow and is not enough to maintain a cerebral hemisphere. Nevertheless, the argument made is that it might be adequate to prevent further injury.[1] Completion arteriography is recommended to validate adequate repair and rule out distal thromboembolism.

Prognosis

The prognosis of penetrating carotid trauma is closely related to the patient's neurologic status at the time of admission. In the most recent studies, the mortality of carotid injury is 5% to 20%,[4,9] and most deaths are due to concomitant injuries, especially central nervous system (CNS) trauma and shock.

BLUNT CAROTID TRAUMA

Epidemiology

Blunt trauma to the carotid arteries is infrequent, representing only 3% to 10% of all carotid artery injuries. Increasing awareness has identified more patients, with one study recording 37% of all carotid injuries due to blunt trauma.[6] Many injuries go unrecognized because they are asymptomatic or symptoms are attributed to other injuries, particularly concomitant head injury or shock.

Pathophysiology

Blunt injuries begin as a disruption of the intima or media resulting in dissection or intramural hematoma. The initial site of injury is the distal ICA or carotid bifurcation in 90% of patients. Usually over a period of hours, these lesions progress, causing extensive dissection, intimal flaps, occlusion, AV fistula, or pseudoaneurysm. Only after these complications do symptoms appear.

There are four main mechanisms of blunt carotid

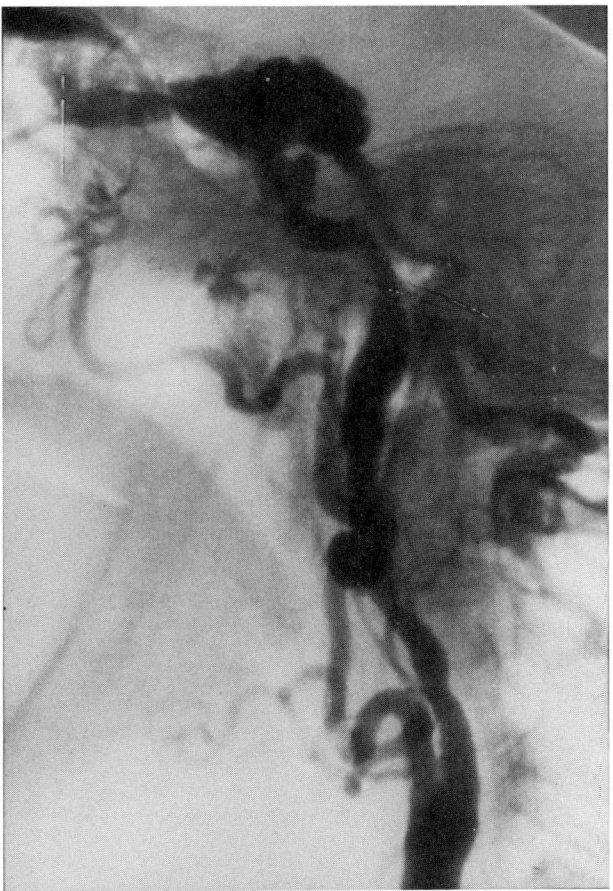

Figure 1 Arteriogram of a carotid cavernous fistula secondary to a basilar skull fracture.

injury that result in four characteristic patient profiles. The first is a direct blow to the neck that causes injury to the common carotid artery or proximal ICA. These patients often have a hematoma at the base of the neck and usually do not have an associated cerebral injury. The second and most commonly recognized mechanism is rapid hyperextension of the neck with contralateral rotation of the head, which causes the distal ICA to be stretched and compressed over the transverse processes of C2 and C3. Occasionally, there is bilateral ICA injury, which is typical of a rapid deceleration injury, such as a motor vehicle accident. The third mechanism is from intraoral trauma, commonly seen in children falling with objects in their mouths and impaling the region of the peritonsillar fossa. The fourth mechanism occurs with basilar skull fractures. Disruption of the cavernous portion of the carotid artery and cavernous sinus creates an abnormal communication between the high-pressure arterial system and the low-pressure venous system, resulting in a carotid cavernous fistula (Fig. 1).

Table 2 Signs Suggesting Blunt Carotid Trauma

Lucid interval followed by focal neurologic deficit
Focal neurologic deficit with normal sensorium
Altered mental status with normal head CT scan
Ipsilateral Horner's syndrome
Lateral neck hematoma
Carotidynia
Posterior displacement of mandibular fracture

Clinical Presentation

The typical patient is involved in a motor vehicle accident and often has other severe associated injuries, including CNS trauma, cervical spine fractures, long bone fractures, and abdominal injuries. More than half of the patients have no external signs of cervical trauma. Only half have neurologic deficits at the time of presentation. The other half have a delayed onset of focal neurologic deficits, often with a normal sensorium. By the first 24 hours, 57% to 73% have the onset of neurologic symptoms.[6] A significant minority may present days to years later with neurologic symptoms. The most common clinical scenario is the patient with a lucid interval after an injury, followed by a delayed focal neurologic deficit. Other signs suggesting possible blunt carotid trauma include lateral neck hematoma, ipsilateral Horner's syndrome, carotidynia, transient ischemic attack (TIA), progressive limb paresis in an alert patient, altered mental status with a normal head CT scan, and mandibular fracture with posterior displacement of the mandible (Table 2).

Signs suggesting a carotid cavernous fistula are an audible bruit, pulsation of the orbit, chemosis, diplopia, visual disturbances, headache, and exophthalmos. Pseudoaneurysms of the extracranial carotid manifest with embolic symptoms (Fig. 2). Physical examination may reveal a palpable pulsatile mass in the neck or peritonsillar fossa. Symptoms usually appear days to months after the injury.

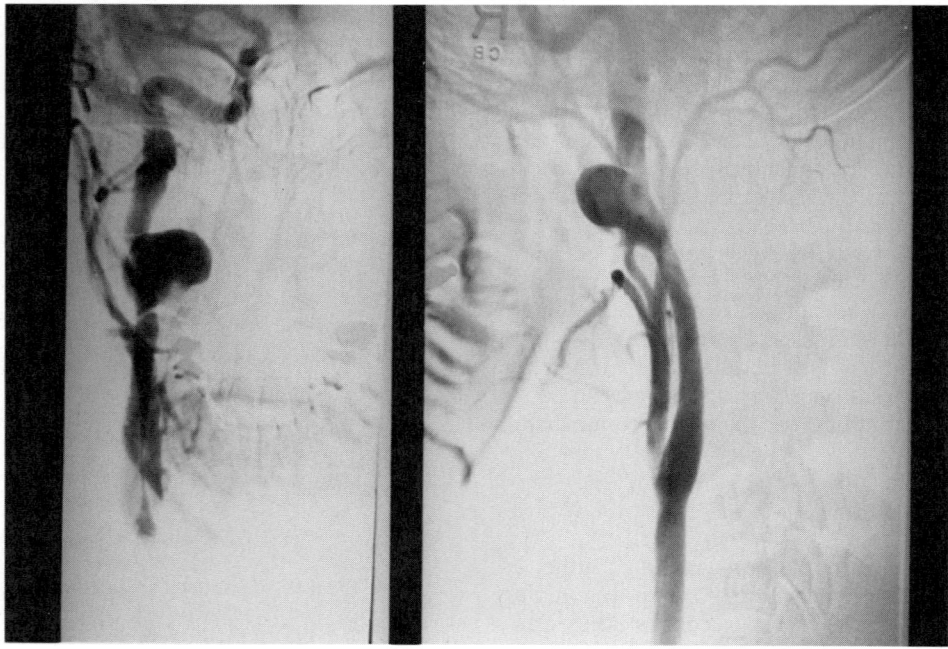

Figure 2 Arteriogram of an extracranial distal internal carotid artery pseudoaneurysm that was discovered by intraoral examination.

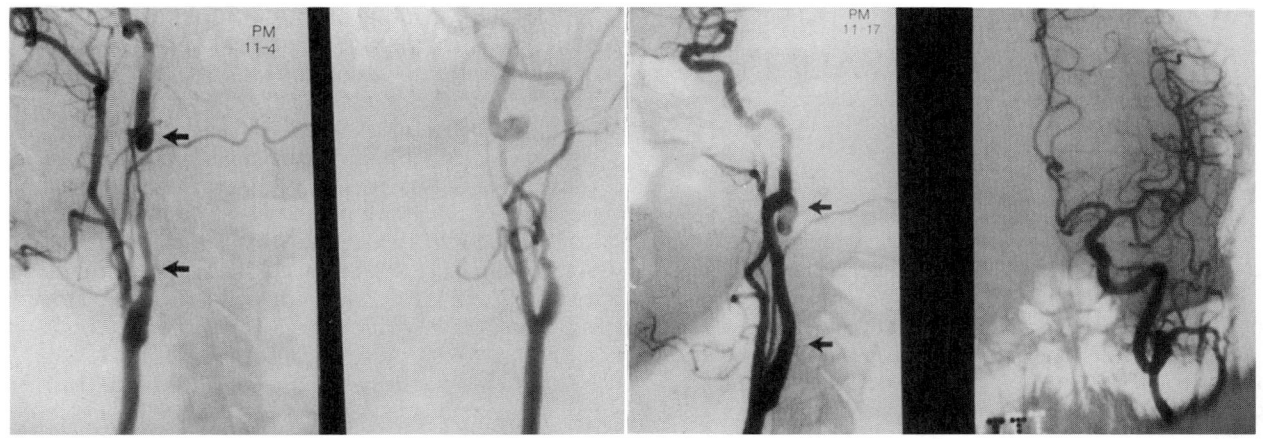

Figure 3 *A*, Arteriogram of internal carotid artery showing internal dissection (*between arrows*). *B*, Arteriogram of patent artery 13 days after treatment with intravenous heparin sodium and oral sodium warfarin.

Diagnosis

Once suspected, the diagnosis should be confirmed with biplanar arteriography, which is highly accurate and also gives information on the status of collateral circulation. The role of duplex scanning is yet to be defined. In many of these multiply injured patients, access to the neck is limited. Because many of the injuries are intimal lesions of the distal ICA, visualization may be quite difficult. Finally, the quality of duplex scanning is technician-dependent and its availability during off hours may be inconsistent. Duplex scanning may be more appropriate for long-term follow-up of patients with intimal flaps or dissection.

Treatment

Surgical repair is indicated for an accessible localized defect of the carotid with prograde blood flow in patients with TIAs, stroke in evolution, or mild neurologic deficits. The majority of blunt carotid injuries are discovered late with dissections up to the base of the skull or occlusion with concomitant severe neurologic deficits. Thrombosis extending up into the intracranial portion of the carotid is best treated by anticoagulation to prevent further propagation or embolization (Fig. 3). Controversy exists as to the best management of a localized thrombus in a surgically accessible carotid lesion with a significant neurologic deficit. The extent of the neurologic deficit, severity of the injured carotid, and the suspected time of onset are important determinants of whether surgical or medical management should be utilized. Small intimal flaps from blunt injury are treated by heparinization, with operation reserved for neurologic symptoms. In all blunt injuries treated by heparinization, anticoagulation with sodium warfarin is continued for 3 to 6 months and either duplex scan or arteriogram is used to re-evaluate the injured carotid.

The treatment of carotid cavernous fistula is detachable balloon occlusion or embolization with thrombogenic agents.[10] Pseudoaneurysms are best treated with resection and interposition grafting, assuming extracranial distal ICA control is possible.

Prognosis

The prognosis following blunt carotid injury is poor. Mortality is 10% to 40%, and the incidence of permanent neurologic deficit is 40% to 80%. With earlier recognition and prompt repair or anticoagulation, the outlook may be greatly improved. Fabian and co-workers reported a 10% mortality with the use of anticoagulation.[6] Recognition of the high-risk patient and aggressive use of arteriography or duplex scanning may result in more lesions recognized early enough for either successful surgical intervention or initiation of sodium heparin therapy to prevent propagation of thrombus.

REFERENCES

1. Fry WJ, Fry RE. Management of carotid artery injury. In: Bergan JJ, Yao JST, eds. Vascular surgical emergencies. Orlando: Grune & Stratton, 1987:587.
2. Robbs JV, Human RR, Rajaruthnam P, et al. Neurologic deficit and injuries involving the neck arteries. Br J Surg 1983; 70:220–222.
3. Liekweg WG, Greenfield LJ. Management of penetrating carotid arterial injury. Am Surg 1978; 188:587–592.
4. Brown MF, Graham JM, Feliciano DV, et al. Carotid artery injuries. Am J Surg 1982; 144:748–753.
5. Monson DO, Saletta JD, Freeark RJ. Carotid vertebral trauma. J Trauma 1969; 9:987–999.
6. Fabian TC, George SM, Croe MA, et al. Carotid artery trauma: Management based on mechanism of injury. J Trauma 1990; 30:953–963.
7. Bradley EL. Management of penetrating carotid injuries: An alternative approach. J Trauma 1973; 13:248–255.
8. Ledgerwood AM, Mullins RJ, Lucas CE. Primary repair versus ligation for carotid artery injuries. Arch Surg 1980; 115:488–493.
9. Jebara V, Tabet GS, Ashoush R, et al. Penetrating carotid injuries: A wartime experience. J Vasc Surg 1991; 14:117–120.
10. Welling R, Saul TG, Tew JM, et al. Management of blunt injury to the internal carotid artery. J Trauma 1987; 27:1221–1226.

PENETRATING AND BLUNT VERTEBRAL ARTERY TRAUMA

THOMAS H. WEBB, M.D.
BRUCE L. GEWERTZ, M.D.

The vertebral arteries are less frequently affected by blunt and penetrating cervical trauma than are the extracranial carotid arteries. This is due, in part, to their smaller size as well as their deeper location beneath the cervical musculature and course in the foramina of the cervical vertebrae. Nevertheless, in recent years there has been an increased recognition of vertebral artery injuries, which reflects a trend toward a more aggressive diagnostic approach in patients with cervical injuries, as well as the continued escalation of urban violence. Although clinical experience has grown, controversy still exists as to the optimum management of patients with vertebral artery injuries; in particular, the specific indications for operative therapy, radiologically guided interventions, and more conservative management remain controversial.

ANATOMY

The vertebral artery is the first and usually the largest branch of the subclavian artery. It can be conveniently divided into four segments. The first segment of the vertebral artery courses upward and backward from its origin to the sixth cervical foramen. It is crossed anteriorly by the vertebral vein, the inferior thyroid artery, and, on the left side, the thoracic duct. Posteriorly, the sympathetic trunk and cervicothoracic (stellate) ganglion are in close proximity. The second segment of the vertebral artery ascends almost vertically within the foramina of the cervical vertebrae. A dense network of sympathetic fibers and a plexus of veins accompany the second portion of the vertebral artery in its bony canal. A variable number of branches originate from the second portion of the artery to supply the deep cervical musculature as well as the spinal cord. The distal portion of the second segment, within the foramina of the atlas and axis, is very tortuous, coursing posteriorly and circling over the atlas laterally. The third segment of the vertebral artery exits the foramen of the atlas and enters the vertebral canal by passing under the margin of the atlanto-occipital membrane. Finally, the fourth segment of the artery pierces the dura mater and travels medially to join with the opposite vertebral artery to form the basilar artery.

In most individuals the right and left vertebral arteries unite to form a common basilar artery. However, in approximately 15% of patients an anatomic variant exists in the posterior circulation. The most common abnormalities are hypoplastic right (10%) and hypoplastic left (5%) vertebral arteries. More important, approximately 3% of left and 2% of right vertebral arteries are atretic and do not communicate with the basilar artery. These anomalies are clinically relevant because ligation or balloon occlusion of a dominant vertebral artery contralateral to a hypoplastic vessel may result in critical reductions in basilar artery blood flow. Further, in the rare circumstance that the posterior inferior cerebellar artery originates from the distal portion of a vertebral artery, which does not then communicate with the basilar artery, proximal ligation can lead to lateral medullary ischemia and Wallenberg's syndrome (contralateral sensory deficits; dysfunction of cranial nerves V, IX, X, XII; Horner's syndrome; ataxia; and dysmetria).

PENETRATING INJURIES

The majority of vertebral artery injuries are the result of penetrating cervical trauma. In most large clinical experiences, gunshot wounds account for more than two-thirds of these injuries. The proximity of the other brachiocephalic vessels, the spinal cord, and accompanying nerve roots account for the fact that isolated injuries to the vertebral arteries are relatively rare. Recent reports document concomitant cervical injuries in more than half of patients with penetrating vertebral artery trauma.[1-3] Unfortunately, the recognition of associated injuries is not particularly helpful in identifying patients with vertebral artery injuries. In one large study, 32 of 43 (72%) patients with documented vertebral artery injuries had no findings suggestive of arterial trauma on physical examination.[3] Moreover, in most patients those neurologic deficits that are present are usually attributable to nerve or spinal cord injury. Less than 10% of patients demonstrate symptoms specifically referrable to vertebrobasilar ischemia.

The occult nature of these injuries mandates four-vessel extracranial arteriography for optimum diagnosis and treatment (Fig. 1). At the University of Chicago, our policy is to perform arteriography on all hemodynamically stable patients with zone I (thoracic outlet) and zone III (angle of mandible to skull base) penetrating cervical injuries. Arteriography is particularly helpful in these circumstances because clinical assessment is often misleading and surgical exposure is limited by anatomic restraints. We also prefer angiography in hemodynamically stable patients with zone II penetrating injuries (cricoid cartilage to angle of mandible) in whom a nonoperative approach is contemplated. Arteriography should begin with an aortic arch injection, and selective catheterization of each vessel may be added, depending on the initial images and the level of clinical suspicion. Identification of any vertebral artery injury should prompt complete imaging of the posterior circulation and contralateral vertebral vessel. Whereas duplex imaging of the vertebral arteries is occasionally useful in documenting patency and the direction of blood flow, such studies cannot be relied on to exclude injury.

In most urban trauma experiences, the location of

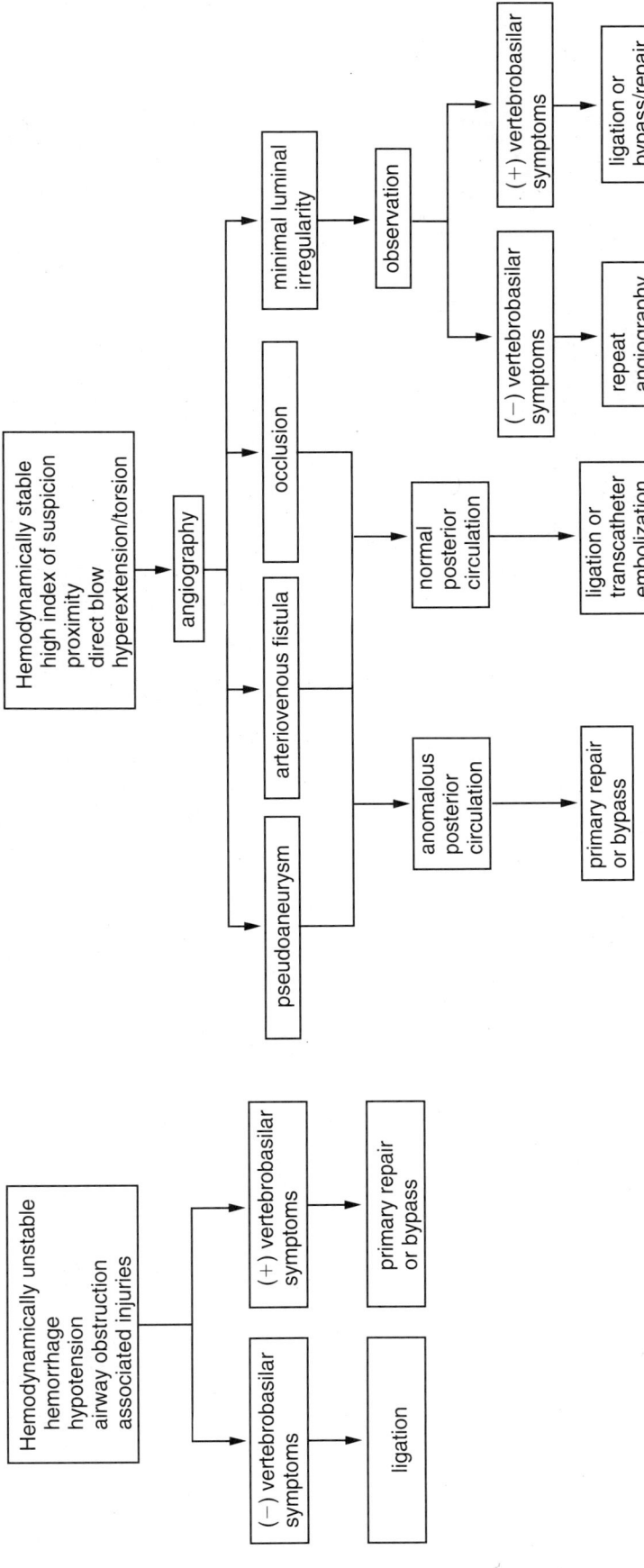

Figure 1 Algorithm for management of vertebral artery injuries.

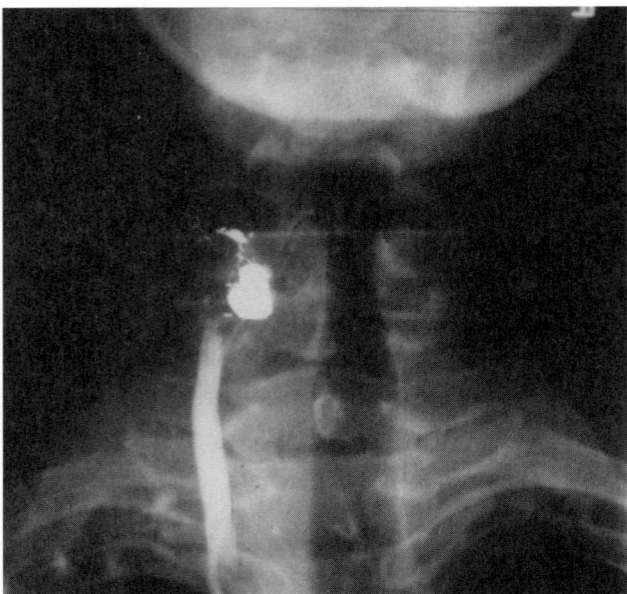

Figure 2 Large-caliber bullet causing occlusion of right vertebral artery. (From Malago M, Gewertz BL. Vertebral artery injuries. In: Berguer R, Caplan L, eds. Vertebral artery disease. St Louis: Quality Medical Publishing, 1991:193; with permission.)

vertebral artery injuries resulting from penetrating trauma is evenly distributed among all three extracranial anatomic segments of the vessel. The acute and chronic sequelae of vertebral artery injuries are similar and include hemorrhage, sudden or delayed occlusion, arteriovenous fistula formation, pseudoaneurysm formation, and dissection (Figs. 2 and 3).

Whereas arteriography is helpful in detecting the presence of vertebral artery damage after penetrating injuries, it is less accurate in determining the nature of the injury. This fact is well illustrated in the Parkland Hospital experience in which 34 of 35 injuries determined by positive arteriograms were confirmed at the time of surgical exploration (accuracy of 97%).[3] However, in only 50% of patients did the operative findings correlate with the specific preoperative arteriographic findings. The predominant arteriographic findings were occlusion (57%), disruption (16%), intimal injury (9%), and arteriovenous fistula formation (5%). In contrast, the most common operative findings were disruption (64%), occlusion (24%), intimal injury (6%), and arteriovenous fistula formation (6%).

BLUNT INJURIES

Blunt injuries to the vertebral artery are relatively rare. Mechanisms of injury include direct powerful blows to the posterolateral neck, hyperextension, rotation, blunt intraoral trauma, and basilar skull fractures. Less obvious activities, as diverse as painting a ceiling, swimming, driving an automobile, and chiropractic manipulation, have also been reported to cause vertebral artery injury. The anatomic basis for these injuries may be reflected in the less morbid syndrome of "stretch syncope" in adolescents, in which loss of consciousness occurs after neck hyperextension and torsion, presumably because of atlantoaxial compression of both vertebral arteries.

Direct blows most commonly lead to injury of the interforaminal vertebral artery (second segment), usually with cervical vertebra fracture or dislocation. The most common sequela of such injuries is immediate or delayed occlusion due to transmural contusion. More violent trauma can lead to vessel transection with hematoma, pseudoaneurysm, or arteriovenous fistula formation.

Torsion and deceleration may also lead to vertebral artery injury, usually manifested by intramural dissection. Remarkably, axial vessel patency is maintained in many instances. Ischemic symptoms may develop from subsequent embolic events or delayed vessel occlusion.

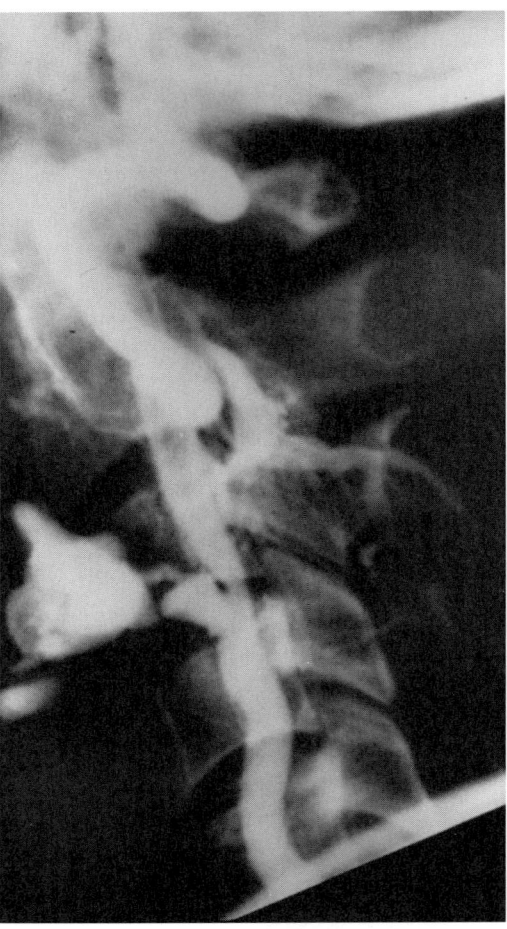

Figure 3 Gunshot wound of interosseous portion of vertebral artery with pseudoaneurysm and persistent patency of vessel. (from Malago M, Gewertz BL. Vertebral artery injuries. In: Berguer R, Caplan L, eds. Vertebral artery disease. St Louis: Quality Medical Publishing, 1991:193, with permission.)

These injuries usually occur in the more mobile first and third segments of the vertebral artery because the second and fourth segments are relatively fixed by bony attachments.

Blunt vertebral artery injuries, like penetrating trauma, are frequently occult. Although some patients may have a bruit (20% to 30%) or cervical hematoma (10%), approximately 50% of patients have no objective evidence of cervical injury.[4] Horner's syndrome from stellate ganglion trauma and vertebrobasilar ischemia are uncommon. Even in these rare patients, the majority display a lucid interval of several hours prior to the onset of neurologic deficits. The importance of serial neurologic examination is self-evident.

Arteriography is indicated in all patients suffering blunt cervical trauma who present with focal vertebrobasilar deficits in the absence of intracranial pathology. This diagnostic paradigm is particularly important in patients developing a deficit after an initial lucid interval. As with victims of penetrating cervical injuries, the history of a mechanism of cervical trauma compatible with blunt vertebral trauma (hyperextension, acceleration-deceleration) should increase clinical suspicion of such an injury.

TREATMENT

Only 10% to 15% of patients with vertebral artery injuries present with clinically important cervical hemorrhage. In these patients an expeditious direct surgical approach with ligation of the involved vertebral artery is indicated. We prefer an anterior approach to the first segment of the vertebral artery, very similar to Henry's classic descriptions. An oblique skin incision is made along the anterior border of the sternocleidomastoid muscle. The carotid artery and internal jugular vein are retracted medially, and the phrenic nerve is identified and mobilized to allow division of the underlying anterior scalene muscle. Careful dissection is necessary to avoid injury to the sympathetic ganglia and to the thoracic duct in the left neck. In addition, iatrogenic injury to the large and thin-walled vertebral vein overlying the proximal portion of the artery must be avoided. This vein services as an excellent landmark for identification of the vertebral artery. Bleeding and tissue staining from injury to the vein can obscure distinctions between neural fibers and other less vital structures.

In the unusual circumstance in which bleeding continues despite occlusion of the proximal vertebral artery, it may be necessary to expose and ligate the distal portion of the second segment at the level of C1–C2. Alternative approaches include balloon catheter occlusion of the distal vessel and exploration through the injury tract to the interosseous portion of the vessel. This latter approach is not recommended except in extraordinary circumstances because dissection within the vertebral canal can be associated with profuse bleeding, not only from the arterial injury but also from the dense plexus of surrounding veins. Intraoperative catheter occlusion, well described by Buscaglia and Crowhurst, requires cannulation through a proximal vertebral arteriotomy and successful passage of a small balloon catheter through the injury site.[5] The catheter is subsequently occluded with a large hemoclip or No. 28 wire that obstructs the lumen and maintains balloon inflation. The catheter is transected and the wound closed, leaving the remnant in the vessel. In a preliminary experience in five patients, the authors report no wound complications, neurologic sequelae, or rebleeding episodes.

Exposure for distal ligation is most expeditiously obtained at the C1–C2 level. This approach has been well described.[6] Briefly, the oblique midcervical skin incision is extended to the mastoid process superiorly. The sternocleidomastoid muscle is rotated laterally or transected from the mastoid process to allow palpation of the key landmark, the transverse process of C1 behind the digastric muscle. The spinal accessory nerve should be identified and protected. Incision of the prevertebral fascia with detachment of the levator scapulae muscle and tendon of the thinner splenius cervicis exposes the intertransverse space between C1 and C2 in which the vertebral artery lies. The anterior ramus of C2 nerve root crosses the artery in this interspace and serves as an excellent guide for the unroofing of the overlying musculature. The intraoperative use of a Doppler probe can be helpful in determining the exact location of the distal vertebral artery.

In patients undergoing less urgent procedures for a vertebral artery arteriovenous fistula, dissection, or pseudoaneurysm, ligation is the preferred management. Preoperatively, the patency of the contralateral vertebral artery and continuity of the basilar artery with the ipsilateral posterior inferior cerebellar artery must be documented. If one of these conditions is not met, as occurs in less than 15% of patients, reconstruction or bypass of the injured vertebral artery is necessary. When the injury involves the first segment of the vertebral, local vein bypass or reimplantation of the distal segment into the side of the carotid artery is technically quite simple. If the intraosseous portion (second segment) of the vessel is injured in conjunction with an anomalous posterior circulation, vein graft bypass to the C1–C2 segment is required. It is usually not possible to primarily repair this segment of the vessel.

The most important development in the management of vertebral artery trauma has been the success of nonoperative occlusive devices in treating a wide range of injuries. Controlled embolization of pseudoaneurysms and arteriovenous fistulas with various types of thrombosis-inducing coils and detachable balloons has been reported with increasing frequency.[7] These techniques require considerable interventional experience and careful delineation of the anatomy of the posterior circulation. In addition, current techniques are limited in obtaining distal control of the C1–C2 segment because of the tortuous path of this portion of the vessel. As a consequence, most transluminal embolizations and induced thromboses are the anatomic equivalent of proximal ligation alone. Further, because these therapies are associated with persistent pseudoaneurysms in approximately 15% of patients, close follow-up is essential. We recommend repeat arteriography in 1 week to evaluate the need for further adjunctive procedures. Even with these limitations, the anatomic considerations involved in exposure of the intraosseous and distal portions of the vertebral artery and the overall effectiveness of interventional techniques make it likely that such nonoperative approaches will play an even greater role in the treatment of these injuries in the future. The continued development of smaller steerable catheters and more reliable detachable balloons should further enhance utilization.

Some experienced clinicians have recently advocated observation in the management of carefully selected vertebral artery injuries.[1] Twelve patients with vertebral artery injuries (nine with occlusion and three with minimal injuries) were successfully managed with observation alone without significant neurologic or vascular sequelae. At the time of the report, only two of these patients had been re-evaluated with follow-up arteriography; confirmation of the effectiveness of this approach is therefore difficult.

In fact, the inaccuracy of arteriography in defining the specific nature of the arterial injury would argue against expectant management in the majority of these patients. At the University of Chicago we treat most injuries with catheter ablation or operative intervention.[8] Observation is employed only in instances of minor luminal irregularity and other segmental narrowing suggestive of spasm or the incidental discovery of an occluded vertebral artery in the presence of other life-threatening injuries. In the latter circumstances, repeat arteriography is performed when the patients are stable, and elective therapy is considered, if appropriate.

As a final option, a recent report describes duplex-directed manual occlusion of a traumatic pseudoaneurysm of the distal vertebral artery.[9] Satisfactory thrombosis of the pseudoaneurysm was obtained with maintenance of vessel patency and no luminal defect on follow-up arteriography. The importance of this technique remains to be determined because anatomic considerations would appear to limit its applicability.

REFERENCES

1. Blickenstaff KL, Weaver FA, Yellin AE, et al. Trends in the management of traumatic vertebral artery injury. Am J Surg 1989; 158:101–106.
2. Golueke P, Scafani S, Phillips T, et al. Vertebral artery injury: Diagnosis and management. J Trauma 1987; 27:856–865.
3. Reid JDS, Weigelt JA. Forty-three cases of vertebral artery trauma. J Trauma 1988; 28:1007–1012.
4. Dragon R, Saranchak H, Lakin P, et al. Blunt injuries to the carotid and vertebral arteries. Am J Surg 1981; 141:497–500.
5. Buscaglia LC, Crowhurst HD. Vertebral artery trauma. Am J Surg 1975; 138:269–272.
6. Berguer R. Distal vertebral artery bypass: Technique, the "occipital connection," and potential uses. J Vasc Surg 1985; 2:621–626.
7. Ben-Menachem Y, Fields WS, Cadavid G, et al. Vertebral artery trauma: Transcatheter embolization. AJNR 1987; 8:501–507.
8. Malago M, Gewertz BL. Vertebral artery injuries. In: Berguer R, Caplan L, eds. Vertebral artery disease. St Louis: Quality Medical Publishing, 1991:193.
9. Feinberg RL, Sorrell K, Wheeler JR, et al. Successful management of traumatic false aneurysm of the extracranial vertebral artery by duplex-directed manual occlusion: A case report. J Vasc Surg 1993; 18:889–894.

PENETRATING TRAUMA TO THE AORTIC ARCH, INNOMINATE, AND SUBCLAVIAN ARTERIES

ROBERT F. WILSON, M.D.
JAMES G. TYBURSKI, M.D.

Injury to thoracic great vessels is uncommon. Although in-hospital mortality rates have been reported as between 8% and 30%, the prehospital mortality resulting from such injuries has been estimated at about 50% to 60%.[1]

At Detroit Receiving Hospital in the period July 1980 through June 1992, 89 patients were seen with penetrating wounds of thoracic great vessels (Table 1). Among the 28 patients who had a total of 33 penetrating vessel injuries to major thoracic vessels, 8 (29%) died. Half of the deaths occurred in patients who had an emergency department (ED) thoracotomy for a cardiac arrest. One patient died in the ED, four died in the operating room (OR), and three died postoperatively.

ANATOMIC ANOMALIES

There is considerable variation in the configuration of the aortic arch branches. The common three branch pattern—innominate, left common carotid, and left subclavian arteries—is present in 65% to 75% of patients. Two branches—a left subclavian and an innominate artery—are seen in 10% to 27%, and two innominate arteries are seen in 0.5% to 2.5%. In 0.5% to 2.5%, four vessels—both carotid and both subclavian arteries—come off the aortic arch, and in 0.5% to 1.2% of patients the left vertebral artery arises from the aortic arch just proximal to the left subclavian artery. A right aortic arch is present in 0.1% to 0.14% of the population.

Table 1 Mortality Rates for 118 Thoracic Great Vessel Injuries in 89 Patients

Vessel Injured	Number	Mortality Rate
Arteries		
Subclavian	25	24%
Aorta	21	86%
Pulmonary	14	79%
Common carotid	5	20%
Innominate	4	50%
Subtotal	69 (58 patients)	57%
Veins		
Subclavian	19	16%
Superior vena cava	9	78%
Inferior vena cava	6	100%
Pulmonary	5	80%
Innominate	5	80%
Internal jugular	5	20%
Subtotal	49 (41 patients)	54%
Total	118	55%

DIAGNOSIS

History

Signs of life or vital signs at the scene and in transit are important in considering whether to perform a resuscitative ED thoracotomy, if the patient arrives in cardiac arrest. The size of a knife and its depth and angle of penetration may indicate the organs most likely to be injured. With bullets, it is helpful to know the trajectory and if the bullet was a high-velocity missile (greater than 2,000 feet/second) that damages much more tissue.

Physical Examination

Up to a third of patients with major vascular injuries at the thoracic inlet may have none of the usual diagnostic signs.[2] Presence or absence of pulses can be particularly unreliable. The excellent collateral circulation about the shoulder may provide a palpable distal pulse when a proximal vascular injury occurs, and occasionally severe vascular spasm may cause loss of a pulse because of trauma to adjacent tissues. In a recent study by Calhoon and colleagues, 14 (64%) of 22 patients with proximal thoracic vascular injuries had normal peripheral pulses.[3] Nevertheless, if pulse loss is accompanied by a bruit or expanding hematoma, arterial injury is present in at least 80% of patients.[4] Occasionally, an upper mediastinal hematoma may cause superior vena caval syndrome or respiratory distress.

One should auscultate the entire chest, back, and neck for bruits after injury. A systolic bruit suggests a false aneurysm, and a continuous bruit suggests an arteriovenous fistula. A careful neurologic examination is also indicated with injuries near the thoracic inlet because a neurologic deficit may be present in up to a third of these patients.[3]

Radiography

The initial chest film is the single most important radiographic study. If possible, an upright posterior-anterior (PA) film should be obtained. With penetrating injury to thoracic great vessels, a hemothorax is generally present. However, if the patient is supine up to 1,000 ml of blood may cause only a slightly increased haziness on the involved side. On an upright film, subpulmonic blood can be mistaken for an elevated diaphragm. A decubitus film is usually diagnostic in this instance. Other findings suggesting great vessel injury include presence of mediastinal widening or an apical density. However, in one study, the initial chest radiograph was read as normal in 18% of patients with great vessel injuries.[3]

Arteriography remains the gold standard for major thoracic vascular injury and should be employed in stable patients who would not otherwise require operation, as it usually provides accurate localizing information. Occasionally, however, the injured vessel may have become sealed, causing a falsely negative study.

Computed tomography (CT) and magnetic resonance imaging are generally not as diagnostic as arteriography, but they can identify localized hematomas, and occasionally one may see an irregular vessel outline, divided lumen, or intimal flap.

INITIAL TREATMENT

Emergency Department Resuscitation

Early endotracheal intubation should be performed for any respiratory distress with suspected vessel injuries in the upper chest or thoracic outlet. Tracheostomy should be avoided because of the possibility of precipitating massive bleeding from an otherwise contained hematoma.

If the patient is in shock, two or three veins not likely to drain into injured veins are cannulated with large-gauge needles or catheters. Patients with severe shock (systolic blood pressure less than 50 mm Hg) are taken to the OR. With mild to moderate shock (systolic blood pressure 50 to 89 mm Hg), 2,000 to 3,000 ml of balanced electrolyte solution is infused in 5 to 10 minutes. If the shock is persistent or recurs, the patient is taken to the OR.

Occasionally, external hemorrhage may be the sole source of blood loss, and insertion of a finger or pack into such a wound, especially at the thoracic inlet, may control the hemorrhage.

Chest Tube (Thoracostomy) Drainage

Blood in the pleural cavity should generally be removed as completely and rapidly as possible. However, if the patient needs an immediate thoracotomy because of massive bleeding, insertion of a chest tube delays operation and can greatly increase the blood loss.

When the chest tube is initially inserted, blood may come out at a rapid rate. If the patient's vital signs deteriorate as blood is removed, the chest tube should be clamped, and the patient taken immediately to the OR. The corollary is that a chest tube may not evacuate all the blood secondary to its position, previous pleural scarring, or clot in the tube.

Emergency Department (Resuscitative) Thoracotomy

Although ED thoracotomies can be lifesaving, especially in patients with penetrating wounds of the chest, if the patient can be treated in the OR, the results are generally much better. In our study, of 33 patients having an ED thoracotomy, 32 (97%) died. Of the 56 patients who had an OR thoracotomy, only 12 (21%) died (p less than .001).

Antibiotics

Antibiotics to cover *staphylococcal* and *streptococcal* contamination should be given just prior to performing a thoracotomy. If there has been much operative blood loss, the antibiotics should be readministered after the bleeding has been controlled.

OPERATING ROOM THORACOTOMY

Indications

Unstable vital signs, especially if unresponsive to a fluid challenge, are a major indication for urgent thoracotomy. Their importance cannot be overemphasized, as delays from obtaining further radiographic evaluations or placement of invasive monitor catheters may be disastrous. Even if the patient's vital signs are stable, one should perform a thoracotomy for blood loss exceeding 1,500 to 2,000 ml in the first 4 to 8 hours, continuing blood loss from the chest tubes exceeding 300 ml/hour for 2 or more hours, or evidence of a substantial retained hemothorax in spite of properly inserted and functioning chest tubes.

Only 9% of our patients admitted with penetrating chest injuries have required a thoracotomy for continuing hemorrhage.[5]

Incisions

Posterolateral Thoracotomy

The standard posterolateral thoracotomy provides excellent exposure to almost all areas of the hemithorax. However, the lateral decubitus position of the patient tends to reduce venous return and can cause a precipitous drop in blood pressure if the patient is hypovolemic. In addition, the dependent lung is at risk to be flooded from bleeding into the tracheobronchial tree. This incision provides limited access to the abdomen if celiotomy is required.

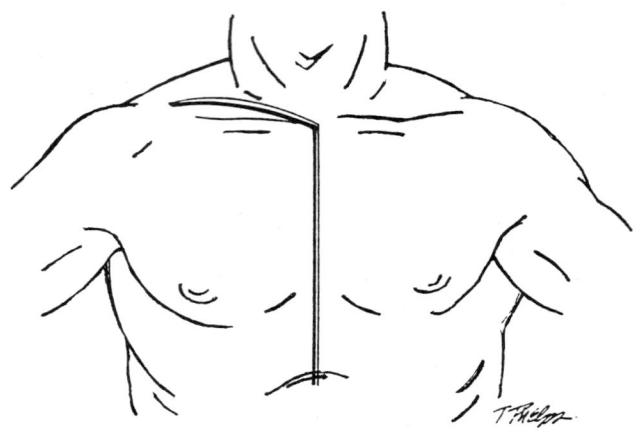

Figure 1 Median sternotomy with right supraclavicular extension is usually performed for complete exposure of the right subclavian artery and vein. When combined with subperiosteal resection or complete removal of the right clavicle and division of the scalenus anterior muscle, all three portions of the right subclavian artery and the entire right subclavian vein are easily visualized. (From Feliciano DV, Graham JM. Major thoracic vascular injury. In Champion HR, Robbs JV, Trunkey DD (eds): Operative Surgery. Boston, Butterworths, 1989, pp 288.)

Median Sternotomy

A median sternotomy incision is usually ideal for penetrating wounds involving the innominate artery or proximal portions of the carotid or right subclavian arteries (Fig. 1). Extension of the median sternotomy into the neck along the upper border of the clavicle provides excellent exposure to the right subclavian and middle and distal left subclavian arteries (Fig. 1). Exposure of the proximal left subclavian artery can be improved by placing a vertical sheet roll between the shoulder blades so that the shoulders can be pulled back. If posterior structures, such as the esophagus or azygous or hemizygous veins, are also injured, it may be difficult to get adequate exposure without an additional incision along one of the intercostal spaces. Such an incision does necessitate some surgical expertise, and, in emergency situations, it has a higher incidence of wound complications.

Anterolateral Thoracotomy

If the patient is in severe shock, has moderate to severe hemoptysis, or requires internal cardiac massage with or without aortic cross-clamping, the patient is kept supine, and an anterolateral thoracotomy is performed. The incision in the fourth intercostal space should start about 2 cm lateral to the sternum to miss the internal mammary artery and continue into the axilla. Cutting the costal cartilages of one or two ribs above and below the incision can also help with the exposure. However,

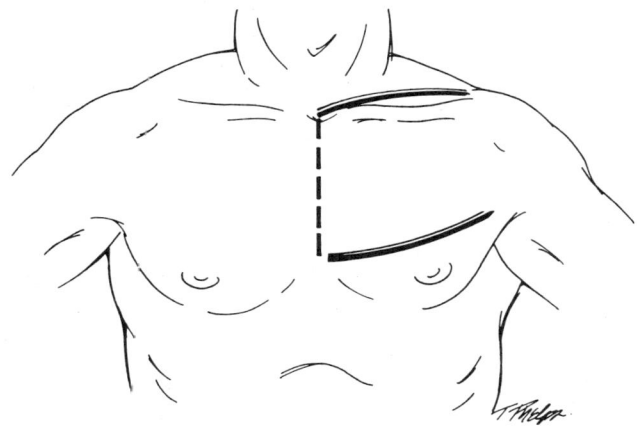

Figure 2 A transverse supraclavicular incision connected to a median sternotomy, in turn connected to an anterior thoracotomy in the third intercostal space to expose the proximal left subclavian vessels. (From Feliciano DV, Graham JM. Major thoracic vascular injury. In: Rob & Smith's operative surgery. Trauma surgery, part 1. Boston: Butterworths, 1989:286, with permission.)

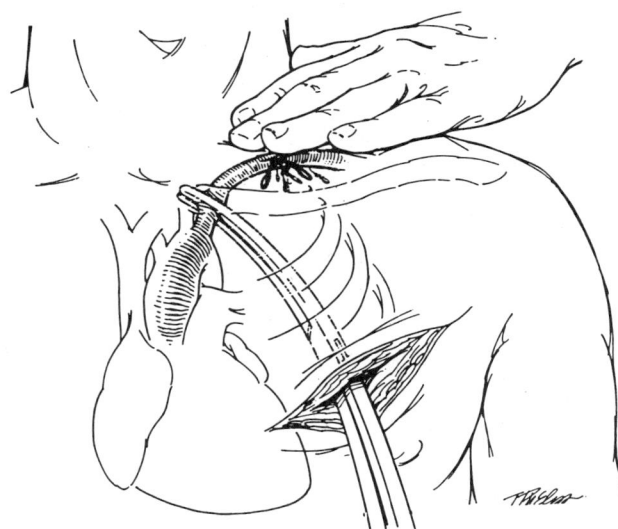

Figure 3 To obtain rapid control of bleeding from the subclavian arteries, one can perform a third interspace anterior thoracotomy incision to clamp the innominate artery or proximal left subclavian artery near its origin. (From Feliciano DV, Graham JM. Major thoracic vascular injury. In: Rob & Smith's operative surgery. Trauma surgery, part 1. Boston: Butterworths, 1989:289, with permission.)

exposure to posterior thoracic structures is relatively poor through this incision.

Bilateral Thoracotomy

An anterolateral thoracotomy can be extended into a bilateral anterolateral thoracotomy (clamshell incision) quite rapidly by cutting the sternum transversely with rib shears or a Lebschke knife. Exposure of both pleural cavities and the mediastinum can thus be quickly attained without the need for a sternal saw. If the incision is extended laterally into both axillas, one has excellent exposure to virtually all organs in the chest. An upper median sternotomy and cervical extension can be added if greater exposure is needed.

Trapdoor Incisions

A transverse supraclavicular incision connected to a median sternotomy that in turn is connected to an anterior thoracotomy in the third intercostal space may be used to expose the proximal left subclavian vessels (Fig. 2). Problems with this incision include difficulty in folding back the chest wall, iatrogenic injury to subclavian or innominate veins, difficulty in wound closure, and postoperative paradoxical ventilation and causalgia pain.

High Anterior Thoracotomy

A high anterolateral thoracotomy at the level of the third intercostal space above the nipple can be performed to obtain proximal innominate or subclavian control (Fig. 3).

Clavicular Incisions

If subperiosteal or complete removal of the medial portion of the clavicle is combined with division of the scalenus anticus muscle, all three portions of the right subclavian artery and most of the middle and distal left subclavian artery are exposed. Iatrogenic injury to the subclavian vein can be avoided by performing an anterior subperiosteal resection of the clavicle.

Intraoperative Resuscitation

Once bleeding sites are controlled with packs or vascular clamps, further dissection should be delayed until the anesthesiologist can resuscitate the patient adequately. If control of the bleeding sites and aggressive fluid therapy does not raise the systolic blood pressure to at least 90 mm Hg, one can consider temporarily compressing or clamping the descending thoracic aorta.

Surgical Exploration

It is important to explore all hematomas over all major arteries and the larger veins. We are aware of at least three aortic injuries and two major venous injuries that bled later that were missed at various hospitals because only the obvious great vessel injuries that were bleeding were treated. If at all possible, one should have proximal and distal control of vessels before an overlying hematoma is explored.

Techniques of Thoracic Aortic Clamping

Most repairs for penetrating injury can be achieved with direct suture without the clamping of the aorta. The next most common scenario is the aortic injury that can be controlled with a side-biting vascular clamp and then sutured. More extensive injuries and those at the junction of major vessels may require complete aortic clamping.

Clamping the thoracic aorta in the distal arch or isthmus may cause severe central hypertension and left heart failure. Clamping for more than 30 minutes without a shunt or bypass graft increases the risk of paraplegia. Therefore, we believe that this clamp and sew technique for complex penetrating wounds of the aorta should be avoided by surgeons who do not have special expertise and experience with these types of operations.[6]

Aortic shunting techniques include cardiopulmonary bypass, external shunts, and partial bypass without an oxygenator. This latter bypass technique is attractive because utilizing heparin sodium–bonded cannulas and a centrifugal pump without an oxygenator requires little or no heparin sodium, and improved results have been obtained.[7]

Aortic Repairs

Exposure of the Injured Area

If the distal aortic arch is involved, proximal control is generally obtained after incision of the pericardium by cross-clamping the aortic arch between the left common carotid and left subclavian arteries and by clamping the left subclavian artery proximal to its branches. The distal aorta is cross-clamped below the hematoma.

If exposure of the concavity or posterior surface of the aorta is necessary, the pulmonary artery and aorta are separated by sharp dissection. Dissection of the concave and posterior surfaces of the aortic arch from outside the pericardium is hazardous because the fibrous layer of the pericardium blends into the aortic adventitia, and extrapericardial dissection can easily penetrate the aortic wall.

Vessel Repair

In most instances, the hole in the aorta is rather small, and lateral aortorrhaphy is often easily accomplished by suturing under a finger or a side-biting vascular clamp.

Aortic sutures should be pledgeted. Large-diameter sutures are also less apt to tear through the vessel. If a 2 to 3 inch long aortic tear must be repaired, the best technique that we have found is a running horizontal mattress suture that everts about 2 to 3 mm of vessel wall on each side, followed by a running simple suture over the everted wound edges.

Whenever possible, sutures in the aorta should be tied while the intraluminal pressure is low. This can be accomplished by digital compression above and below the injury or by applying a side clamp around the injury.

Digital compression of both vena cavae combined with pharmacologic reduction of blood pressure may also be used but must be employed with caution. The safe time for inflow occlusion is thought to be about 1.5 minutes, but it can be repeated after a recovery period of 3 minutes.[8]

Innominate Artery Repairs

With severe injuries to the innominate artery, it is prudent to bypass the injury before entering the surrounding hematoma.[6] The proximal ascending aorta is exposed, and an 8 mm knitted Dacron bypass graft can be sewn onto it by using a partial occlusion clamp. The hematoma around the proximal innominate artery is not entered until both the aortic arch at the origin of the artery and the innominate bifurcation or the origins of the right subclavian and common carotid arteries have been dissected free and clamped separately. The previously inserted Dacron bypass graft may then be sewn end to end to the distal innominate artery. If the distal innominate artery and the origins of both the right common carotid artery and right subclavian artery must be replaced, a bifurcation graft can be used.

If the stump blood pressure of the right common carotid artery distal to the cross-clamp on the innominate artery is less than 50 mm Hg or cannot be measured, a temporary external or internal shunt is prudent to ensure adequate blood flow to brain. Systemic heparinization is usually not advised if there are other injuries, particularly ones involving the central nervous system.

Subclavian Artery Repairs

For injuries involving the proximal left subclavian artery, many recommend a standard left thoracotomy or a small left anterior thoracotomy in the second or third intercostal space. More distal injuries can be reached via a standard supraclavicular incision with partial resection of the clavicle. However, this approach may take some time, and a thoracotomy may be required for initial proximal control.

The subclavian artery is often quite thin and fragile, and it can be easily torn by vascular clamps or any tension on the sutures. Tension on end-to-end anastomoses can be avoided by sacrificing the vertebral, internal mammary, or thyrocervical branches, as well as by inserting a prosthetic graft.

Schimpf and associates have documented that up to 7.5 cm of the subclavian artery can be resected and a primary anastomosis still achieved by mobilizing the axillary artery and passing it through the first intercostal space.[9]

Although distal gangrene of the upper extremity is unusual with ligation of the subclavian artery, ligation should be avoided whenever possible. Exercise ischemia of the arm may occur, and if the ligation is proximal to the vertebral artery, a subclavian steal syndrome may develop.

Associated Injuries

In our own series of 28 patients with penetrating injuries of the aortic arch or innominate or subclavian arteries, associated injuries included 17 major veins in 11 patients (39%), the lungs in 7 (25%), other major arteries in 4 (14%), thoracic duct in 3 (11%), and brachial plexus in 2 (7%).

Venous Injuries

Associated venous injuries can usually be ligated, but the superior vena cava and one innominate vein should be repaired if possible to reduce the likelihood of a superior vena caval syndrome. Injuries of the subclavian vein can be particularly difficult to repair because of numerous small venous branches that are easily avulsed during rapid dissection.

Nerve Injuries

Injuries to the brachial plexus are particularly common if the second or third portion of a subclavian artery is involved. However, many of these injuries are due to contusions or stretching and eventually resolve. Bullet injury to the spinal cord can also occur.

Tracheobronchial or Esophageal Injuries

Injuries to the trachea, major bronchi, or esophagus are present in about 5% to 10% of patients. These should be considered a source of contamination so that a prosthetic graft should be avoided, if possible. Repairs of these organs and any vessel should be separated and buttressed with normal tissue.

POSTOPERATIVE CARE

The chest tubes used to drain the chest should be connected to an autotransfusion collection device so that shed red cells can be washed and returned to the patient, if necessary. Hypothermia is prevented or reversed with heating blankets, warmed fluids, and heated ventilator gases. Coagulopathies are corrected by making the patient normothermic and giving fresh frozen plasma or cryoprecipitate and platelets, as necessary. In critically ill patients who have prolonged shock, we place a pulmonary artery catheter and attempt to obtain an oxygen delivery and oxygen consumption of at least 600 ml/minute/m^2 and 150 ml/minute/m^2, respectively.

REFERENCES

1. Bladergroen M, Brockman R, Luna G, et al. A twelve year survey of cervicothoracic vascular injuries. Am J Surg 1989; 157:483–486.
2. Flint LM, Snyder WH, Perry MO, et al. Management of major vascular injuries in the base of the neck. Arch Surg 1973; 106:407.
3. Calhoon JH, Grover FL, Trinkle JT. Chest trauma: Approach and management. Clin Chest Med 1992; 13:55–67.
4. McCready RA, Procter CD, Hyde GL. Subclavian-axillary vascular trauma. J Vasc Surg 1986; 3:24–31.
5. Washington B, Wilson RF, Steiger Z. Emergency thoracotomies for penetrating trauma. Curr Surg 1984; 41:14–17.
6. Mattox KL. Thoracic great vessel injury. Surg Clin North Am 1988; 68:693–703.
7. Hess PJ, Howe HR, Robiesek F, et al. Traumatic tears of the thoracic aorta: Improved results using the biomedicus pump. Ann Thorac Surg 1989; 48:6–9.
8. Vosloo SM, Reichart BA. Inflow occlusion in the surgical management of a penetrating aortic injury: Case report. J Trauma 1990; 30:514–515.
9. Schimpf P, Burt D, Wagner R. Left subclavian artery trauma: In situ vs rib interspace mobilization for primary anastomosis. J Trauma 1985; 25:1069–1073.

BLUNT ARTERIAL INJURIES OF THE SHOULDER AND ELBOW

ERIC D. ENDEAN, M.D.

BLUNT ARTERIAL INJURIES OF THE SHOULDER

The major vessels injured with shoulder girdle trauma are the axillary and subclavian arteries. The muscle and bones of the shoulder girdle, which surround these arteries, provide considerable protection against injury. Thus, axillary and subclavian vascular injuries are unusual. Most studies of axillary or subclavian artery injuries report that the majority are caused by penetrating trauma, whereas blunt trauma accounts for only 5% to 7% of all axillary and subclavian artery injuries.[1-3]

Types of blunt trauma that result in axillary and subclavian artery injury include hyperabduction of the arm, shoulder dislocation, scapulothoracic dissociation, and fracture of the first rib or clavicle. Hyperabduction of the arm may avulse arterial branches of the axillary and subclavian arteries, transect the arteries, or disrupt intima by stretch injury. Intimal injury, or disruption of the vessel wall may result in vessel thrombosis, embolism, or pseudoaneurysm formation.

Shoulder dislocations typically do not result in arterial injury. When arterial injury does occur, it is most often associated with anterior dislocations in elderly individuals. Such patients likely have advanced atherosclerosis and lack elasticity of the vessel. Consequently, the artery cannot accommodate the stretch caused by the dislocation. Axillary artery injury can also occur during reduction of chronic shoulder dislocations. Under these circumstances, scarring and atherosclerosis act to fix the vessel, and the axillary artery cannot accommodate the additional stretch needed during the traction required to reduce the dislocation.[4] Scapulothoracic dissociation occurs after severe crush or traction injury to the shoulder and is associated with subclavian and/or axillary artery injury. First rib and clavicular fractures occasionally impinge on the underlying subclavian artery.

The branches of the subclavian and axillary arteries provide an extensive arterial collateral network around the shoulder. As a result, signs and symptoms of ischemia may not be evident even if the axillary or subclavian arteries are occluded or transected. Because the brachial plexus is in close proximity to the distal subclavian and the axillary arteries, blunt shoulder trauma often results in injury to these nerves. The axillary vessels and the brachial plexus are surrounded by an extension of the prevertebral layer of the deep cervical fascia in the arm. Bleeding into this sheath can cause significant compression of the brachial plexus, another mechanism that can result in brachial plexus damage.

Presentation and Diagnosis

Patients with shoulder trauma may present with signs and symptoms of arterial insufficiency of the upper extremity, an expanding hematoma, a pulsatile mass, signs of ongoing hemorrhage, or hemothorax. However, because of the rich collateral circulation around the shoulder joint, some patients with significant arterial injuries present with minimal or no signs of upper extremity ischemia. They may even have palpable wrist pulses. Signs of hemorrhage are more difficult to appreciate, especially in muscular or obese patients. Therefore, clinicians must have a high index of suspicion to make an early diagnosis of a vascular injury.

The presence of associated shoulder injuries often provides a clue regarding the presence of an underlying vascular injury. Clavicular fracture, shoulder dislocation, first rib fracture, brachial plexus injury, scapular fracture, or proximal humeral fracture raise the likelihood of an associated major arterial injury. Frequently, nerve root avulsion causes a devastating brachial plexus injury when the arm is forcibly hyperabducted. In addition, compression of the brachial plexus by hematoma within the neurovascular sheath can also cause substantial neurologic impairment. In all cases, prompt exploration is indicated.[5]

Arteriography is the cornerstone for diagnosis of arterial injury associated with blunt shoulder trauma. Liberal indications for arteriography should be used to rule out the diagnosis of axillary or subclavian artery injury. All patients who are hemodynamically stable and present with signs of upper extremity arterial insufficiency should undergo arteriography. Arteriography is useful to plan the best operative approach, especially when a proximal subclavian artery injury is identified. Arteriography is also helpful to exclude the presence of vascular trauma in patients without clear signs of arterial injury. However, patients with obvious arterial disruption or those with hemodynamic instability should have emergent operative exploration and repair. Expedient operations are usually required for penetrating trauma. Blunt trauma is less likely to result in hemodynamic instability.

Operative Management

The type of incision and exposure needed for control of the subclavian or axillary arteries must be individualized and depends on the location, severity, and extent of the injury. In general, patients should be positioned and prepared so that, if needed, the proximal subclavian artery can be quickly exposed for control. Injuries to the distal two-thirds of the subclavian artery can be successfully approached with a supraclavicular incision. Furthermore, a portion of the clavicle can be resected to improve exposure. When the proximal third of the subclavian artery is injured, obtaining control of the artery is more difficult. If the injury involves the right subclavian artery, exposure of the brachiocephalic trunk is usually required. A median sternotomy, with supraclavicular extension, offers the best exposure. Because the left subclavian artery arises posteriorly from the aortic arch, an anterolateral thoracotomy, through the third or fourth intercostal space, provides the best access to the vessel. Additional exposure can be obtained with a supraclavicular incision on the left. The supraclavicular incision and the thoracotomy can be joined medially by incising the sternum. This creates a trap door that provides exposure of the entire left subclavian artery.

The axillary artery is exposed through an infraclavicular incision extended into the deltopectoral groove.[1] The fibers of the pectoralis major or minor muscles may be split or the tendons transected if additional exposure of the injured portion of the vessel is needed. The pectoralis major muscle tendon should be reapproximated at the completion of the operation. In some patients, proximal exposure of the subclavian artery through a separate supraclavicular incision may be useful. Care should always be taken to preserve the major branches of these axial vessels, which serve as important collateral pathways.

Patients with axillary or subclavian artery injuries frequently have other concomitant injuries. Treatment priorities for the other injuries need to be established. Because of the excellent arterial collateral circulation around the shoulder, the upper extremity is often at less risk for ischemic sequelae. Therefore, treatment of other life-threatening injuries can be given priority over arterial repair. However, vascular reconstruction should not be excessively delayed.

Technique

When the vascular injury is localized to a short segment of the artery, resection and end-to-end primary repair is preferred. This is frequently not possible because blunt trauma often affects a long segment of the artery, and the numerous branches do not allow for sufficient mobilization of the artery to create a tension-free anastomosis. In such cases, resection of the injured segment of artery and an interposition graft are often needed. Autogenous tissue is the conduit of choice, the most accessible conduit being the saphenous vein. Because the subclavian and axillary arteries are large vessels, a size mismatch between these vessels and saphenous vein may make the use of this conduit less than ideal. A spiral graft or a panel graft can be created from the saphenous vein, or a prosthetic graft can be used. Both Dacron and polytetrafluoroethylene have been implanted successfully in these situations. Polytetrafluoroethylene may be more resistant to graft infection, a rationale that indicates at least some theoretical advantage for its use.

Systemic anticoagulation with heparin sodium should not be used in patients with concomitant injuries. Arterial thrombus formation can be retarded by injecting saline containing heparin sodium (10 IU/ml) into the artery locally after proximal and distal control have been obtained. The brachial plexus should always be evaluated. Unless a severed nerve is sharply and cleanly transected, which is unusual in blunt trauma, the nerve ends should be tagged with nonabsorbable suture for future repair. Venous injuries are commonly associated with the arterial injury. Such injuries can be difficult to control because of the large size of the vessel, thin wall, and the rapid bleeding. Attempts to repair veins are appropriate in otherwise stable patients. However, in some situations, injured veins may require ligation. Upper extremity edema and venous hypertension may occur as the result of proximal vein ligation.

The long-term outcome for repair of axillary and subclavian injuries secondary to blunt trauma has not been well defined. Injury to these vessels is unusual, and most series do not differentiate between blunt and penetrating trauma. Patency of repair is usually reported to be greater than 90% and even 100% in some series.[2,3,5] Mortality is usually related to associated injuries, especially those that involve the heart or origin of the great vessels. Significant morbidity results from associated brachial plexus injuries.[5-7] Patients with avulsion injuries of the brachial plexus have a poor prognosis for recovery of upper extremity function, regardless of a patent vascular repair. Arm amputation may be indicated in some patients with these injuries to control intractable pain.

BLUNT ARTERIAL INJURIES OF THE ELBOW

Elbow dislocation, which is virtually always due to blunt trauma, is a relatively common orthopedic injury. It is the third most common joint dislocation, following glenohumeral and patellar-femoral dislocations.[8] However, arterial injury with elbow dislocation is uncommon. Most descriptions of these injuries in the literature appear as case reports. The characteristics of elbow dislocation that have been implicated as factors associated with arterial injury include open or closed dislocation, anterior or posterior dislocation, and associated upper extremity fractures.

In a series of 63 elbow dislocations, identified in 62 patients, eight arterial injuries (13%) were found.[9] Three factors were shown to be statistically associated with arterial injury: (1) open dislocation, (2) absence of a radial pulse before reduction of the dislocation, and (3) other associated injuries. Absence of an upper extremity pulse is an obvious predictor of arterial injury. The other two significant factors—open dislocation and associated injuries—are indicative of greater magnitude of force transmitted to the patient during trauma. Any patient with an elbow dislocation should have a careful and accurate vascular examination before the elbow is reduced. Concern for the presence of a concomitant vascular injury should be raised in patients who have associated systemic injuries or open dislocations, both which serve as evidence that a force of significant intensity was transmitted to the patient. Arteriography is the diagnostic procedure of choice to identify or exclude an arterial injury.

Arterial injuries associated with elbow dislocation include intimal damage with or without subsequent thrombosis, laceration, transection, or formation of an intimal flap. Repair of these arterial injuries is indicated in most patients. Normally the elbow has an extensive arterial collateral network comprised of four main pathways, two anterior and two posterior to the elbow joint.[10] The anterior collateral pathways are the inferior ulnar collateral artery, which anastomoses with the anterior ulnar recurrent branch of the ulnar artery, and the profunda brachii artery, which anastomoses with the radial recurrent artery. The collateral pathways posterior to the joint are the superior ulnar collateral artery, which anastomoses with the posterior ulnar recurrent artery, and the interosseous recurrent artery, which anastomoses with the profunda brachii artery. In patients with brachial artery thrombosis or transection, these collateral pathways are needed for maintenance of hand and forearm viability. In a study by Louis, and associates, posterior elbow dislocation was produced in cadaver upper extremities by forceful hyperextension.[10] The inferior ulnar collateral to anterior ulnar recurrent pathways were disrupted in 13 of 14 specimens. Because of the high incidence of injury to elbow collateral vessels with elbow dislocation, it has been concluded that the collateral network should not be relied on to maintain forearm and hand viability when the brachial artery is injured. This underscores the need for reconstruction of brachial artery injuries associated with elbow dislocation. A long segment of artery is often injured because of the magnitude of the force required to cause both elbow dislocation and arterial injury. Thus, an interposition graft is usually necessary. The saphenous vein closely approximates the size of the brachial artery and is the ideal conduit for repair. Repair of brachial artery injuries with prosthetic vascular grafts is not recommended.

When an arterial injury is associated with elbow dislocation, the orthopedic and vascular injuries need simultaneous attention. The proper sequence of repair, however, may be debated. A stabilized joint can simplify the vascular repair and eliminate the concern of excess tension on the anastomosis during orthopedic manipulation. In addition, graft length can be better determined when the elbow is reduced, preventing redundant or short grafts. Vascular repair should take precedence in a severely ischemic extremity, especially patients with prolonged preoperative ischemia. When the vascular repair is done prior to orthopedic manipulation of the elbow joint, a member of the vascular team should be present in the operating room to assure that excess tension is not placed on the vascular repair.

Forearm fasciotomy may be needed when treating arterial injuries associated with elbow dislocation. Standard indications of fasciotomy such as prolonged ischemia, increased compartment pressure, or evidence of severe soft tissue swelling are used to determine the need for fasciotomy. In a recent report of elbow dislocations, forearm fasciotomy was done in 5 of 8 (63%) patients who had arterial injury and in only 1 of 55 (2%) patients without an arterial injury.[9] The volar aspect of the forearm is most often involved with compartment syndrome, and both the superficial and deep flexor compartments should be released through a long curvilinear skin incision. The dorsal compartment can be opened through multiple small incisions or one long skin incision.

Outcome of patients with blunt arterial injury of the elbow joint is generally good. In a report of elbow dislocations,[9] one patient required an amputation 6 days after injury to treat a life-threatening forearm infection, associated with extensive soft tissue damage. At the time of amputation, the brachial artery, which had been repaired with a vein graft, was patent. Of the remaining seven limbs that had a vascular injury, six had normal neurologic function at follow-up. Fifty-three of the 55 extremities that had an elbow dislocation without arterial injury were also normal neurologically at the time of follow-up examination. Mortality associated with this injury is most often the result of associated injuries.

REFERENCES

1. Graham JM, Mattox KL, Feliciano DV, DeBakey ME. Vascular injuries of the axilla. Ann Surg 1982; 195:232–238.
2. Orcutt MB, Levine BA, Gaskill HV, Sirinek KR. Civilian vascular trauma of the upper extremity. J Trauma 1986; 26:63–67.
3. Borman KR, Snyder WH, Weigelt JA. Civilian arterial trauma of the upper extremity: An 11 year experience in 267 patients. Am J Surg 1984; 148:796–799.
4. Raskin KB. Acute vascular injuries of the upper extremity. Hand Clin 1993; 9:115–130.
5. McCready RA, Procter CD, Hyde GL. Subclavian-axillary vascular trauma. J Vasc Surg 1986; 3:24–31.
6. Sturm JT, Strate RG, Mowlem A, et al. Blunt trauma to the subclavian artery. Surg Gynecol Obstet 1974; 138:915–918.
7. Klein SR, Bongard FS, White RA. Neurovascular injuries of the thoracic outlet and axilla. Am J Surg 1988; 156:115–118.
8. Bennett JB, Tullos HS. Elbow instability. In: Evarts CM, ed. Surgery of the musculoskeletal system. 2nd ed. New York: Churchill Livingstone, 1990:1683.
9. Endean ED, Veldenz HC, Schwarcz TH, Hyde GL. Recognition of arterial injury in elbow dislocation. J Vasc Surg 1992; 16:402–406.
10. Louis DS, Ricciardi JE, Spengler DM. Arterial injury: A complication of posterior elbow dislocation. J Bone Joint Surg [Am] 1974; 56:1631–1636.

PENETRATING ARTERIAL INJURIES IN THE EXTREMITIES

NORMAN M. RICH, M.D.

The widely acknowledged first documented successful vascular repair in 1759 involved an extremity artery.[1] Hollowell, as described in a letter by Lambert from Newcastle-upon-Tyne, had used a farrier's stitch to close a simple laceration caused by a blood leading instrument injuring the brachial artery. Although there were few additional reports of successful vascular repairs over the next 150 years, there were scattered anecdotal reports of managing vascular injuries, usually of the extremities. Most reports with representative references cited over the last century, whether civilian or military, emphasize the predominance of extremity vascular injuries.[1-10]

Continuing warfare in many areas of the world, combined with crime, high-speed transportation, and an increasing utilization of invasive diagnostic and therapeutic techniques, contribute to an increasing incidence of vascular trauma. Until very recently, 80% to 90% of all vascular injuries involved extremity arterial and venous trauma. The retrospective epidemiologic report in 1989 by Mattox and colleagues, however, documented the less frequent occurrence of extremity vascular injuries. Prior to their experience, those who sustained vascular injuries associated with penetrating trauma to the neck and torso essentially exsanguinated prior to successful resuscitation and transport to a surgical center.[7]

There have been differences between civilian and military experiences, with the former having a predominance of vascular injuries in the upper extremities and latter having the majority of the vascular injuries in the lower extremities.[1] Antipersonnel devices ("booby traps") utilized by the military have an impact on the type of injuries, whereas civilian hostilities are directed more frequently toward the chest and upper extremities. Although the emphasis is on penetrating trauma, blunt trauma to the extremities resulting in vascular injury has significant challenges and associated complications.

The World War II classic report by DeBakey and Simeone outlined the management of 2,471 acute arterial injuries in the European theater among American troops, with the vast majority treated by ligation.[3] Hughes and Bowers, during the Korean conflict, were among the first surgeons to document that successful arterial and venous repairs could be accomplished even on the battlefield.[4]

PATHOPHYSIOLOGY

Penetrating injuries are usually caused by bullets and knives. Although direct injury is usual, there may be additional injury with high-velocity missiles. These wounds, relegated originally to the battlefield, are being seen with increasing frequency in urban trauma. Associated displaced fractures can also compress or injure arteries. Diagnostic and therapeutic procedures have a relatively low incidence of associated arterial trauma.

DIAGNOSIS

Bright red pulsatile bleeding from an extremity penetrating wound signals acute arterial injury. This may cease after a few minutes because of retraction and spasm of the severed artery; however, a partially severed artery may continue to bleed to the point of exsanguination of the patient if control of hemorrhage is not instituted. Therefore, the patient may present in hypovolemic shock. Signs and symptoms of the presence or absence of distal pulses, skin color and temperature, extremity pain, and neurologic changes from loss of sensation to motor loss may or may not be present. The type and location of the wound are particularly appropriate for evaluation. Associated surrounding hematoma and the presence or absence of a thrill or bruit are important to include in the evaluation. Concomitant injuries to bone, nerve, and veins are important to evaluate and are frequently present.

PATIENT MANAGEMENT

Complete and rapid patient evaluation and supportive care of multiple injuries must be effected as soon as possible. Care must include establishment of a patent airway, ensuring adequate ventilation, and providing appropriate circulatory support. The adage "life over limb" must always be considered. Control of external bleeding with digital pressure or compressive bandages can be helpful. Tourniquet use must be appropriate and observed closely with temporary and intermittent application.

Proximity of the penetration to an artery that may have questionable injury involves the debated role of preoperative arteriography. With obviously severed arteries, repair may be performed in an urgent manner without any consideration for preliminary arteriography. Preoperative arteriography can be valuable in identifying the location and magnitude of the vascular injury. The extent of thrombosis determined by arteriography can assist in planning the appropriate operation. It is possible, even in the emergency room, to obtain arteriograms through direct proximal arterial percutaneous puncture.

The goal of management of arterial injuries is rapid operative intervention with restoration of distal arterial blood flow as soon as possible and in less than 6 hours. Coverage with broad-spectrum antibiotics, continued for 3 to 5 days, helps eliminate the threat of infection. After adequate preparation of the extremity, the vascular injury can be approached rapidly through standard incisions. The goal is rapid proximal and distal arterial control. If the injury is in the lower extremity, both extremities should be prepped and draped from the groins to the toes to allow for the possible excision of a segment of saphenous vein from the uninjured lower extremity for arterial repair if required. Cephalic vein can be used as an alternate conduit to the saphenous vein. Simple lateral suture may be possible in limited clean lacerations of major-caliber arteries. Resection of a segment of the superficial femoral artery up to 1.5 cm with end-to-end anastomosis without sacrifice of collaterals or without undue tension may also be possible. If an interposition conduit is required, the autogenous greater saphenous vein is preferred. Synthetic conduits from Dacron to polytetrafluoroethylene have been used with varying degrees of success. Atraumatic vascular clamps and forceps, as well as fine synthetic monofilament sutures on small, atraumatic needles, helps to ensure success. Vascular optical loops and/or the operating microscope may be helpful in elective arterial repair, particularly in stable situations. Intraluminal Fogarty balloon catheters can be used to control arterial hemorrhage both distally and proximally as well as in the extraction of distal thrombus prior to repair. Regional or systemic heparinization can help prevent propagation of thrombus in the extremity; however, the overall patient situation must be considered.

Appropriate immobilization of associated fractures adds challenge to these injuries. Bivalved plaster casts, suspension-traction devices, or external fixation devices are best utilized. Earlier in this century, civilian circumstances allowed internal fixation devices such as intramedullary nails or plates and screws to be used more successfully than in the combat situation; however, there is increasing acceptance of external fixation of associated fractures. Concomitant venous repair, particularly by lateral suture, may be rapid and prevent troublesome bleeding prior to arterial repair.

Completion arteriography is of paramount importance after extremity vascular repairs in ensuring adequate repair and the absence of additional injuries. Identity of residual thrombus distal to the arterial repair can also be noted.

The wound should be irrigated copiously with saline and antibiotic solutions after removal of all devitalized and foreign material from the wound. The arterial repair must be covered with viable muscle, and drains should never be placed adjacent to arterial repairs. Temporary biologic dressing may be utilized where there has been massive loss of tissue.

Although the role of fasciotomy remains controversial, the experience as early as that in the Korean conflict emphasized the value of adequate fasciotomy of both the skin and the fascia to release pressure in musculofascial compartments, particularly in the lower extremities. With delay of repair or concomitant venous injuries, there is increasing rationale for liberal utilization of fasciotomy. The techniques that have been used include fibulectomy and four-compartment decompression in the lower extremities; however, the penetrating injury may also contribute to the "decompression."

If there is a significant delay in arterial repair, utilization of intraluminal shunts has been of value. Extra-anatomic bypasses, particularly if there are large soft tissue defects, may be indicated in rare circumstances for limb salvage in isolated extremity wounds. In equally rare situations, there may be value in considering the use of sympathectomy.

POSTOPERATIVE CARE

The patient must be observed carefully in the early postoperative period, with elevation of the extremity to reduce edema. Elastic bandages, support stockings, intermittent compression, and other measures may assist. Temporary splints for the extremities can be helpful in preventing sudden movements and in relieving stress on vascular repairs. Heparin sodium should be avoided in the postoperative period, particularly with multiple injuries; however, antibiotics should be continued for several days as noted earlier.

OUTCOME

Successful repair of injured extremity arteries is anticipated and usually achieved. Amputation rates from World War I and World War II that averaged 50% after ligation of injured extremity arteries fell to approximately 13% in the Vietnam War, where widespread arterial repair was effected promptly, and have fallen to less than 10% in most civilian series. An exception is repair of the popliteal artery, where amputation rates in many civilian and combat series continue as high as 30%. The ideal conduit for replacement of missing arterial segments remains to be identified; however, the autogenous greater saphenous vein continues to be a durable interposition graft in repairing injured extremity arteries, including those associated with contaminated wounds.

REFERENCES

1. Rich NM, Spencer FC. Vascular trauma. Philadelphia: WB Saunders, 1978.
2. Makins GH. Gunshot injuries to the blood vessels. Bristol, England: John Wright, 1919.
3. DeBakey ME, Simeone FA. Battle injuries of the arteries in World War II: An analysis of 2,471 cases. Ann Surg 1946; 123:534–578.
4. Hughes CW, Bowers WF. Traumatic lesions of peripheral vessels. Springfield, Ill: Charles C Thomas, 1961.
5. Perry MO. The management of acute vascular injuries. Baltimore: Williams & Wilkins, 1981.
6. Hobson RW 2d, Rich NM, Wright CB, eds. Venous trauma: Pathophysiology, diagnosis and surgical management. Mount Kisco, NY: Futura Publishing, 1983.

7. Mattox KL, Feliciano DV, Burch J, et al. Five thousand seven hundred sixty cardiovascular injuries in 4459 patients: Epidemiologic evolution 1958 to 1987. Ann Surg 1989; 209:698–707.
8. Bongard FS, Wilson SE, Perry MO, eds. Vascular injuries in surgical practice. Norwalk, Conn: Appleton & Lange, 1991.
9. Flanigan DP, Schuler JJ, Mayer JP, eds. Civilian vascular trauma. Philadelphia: Lea & Febiger, 1992.
10. Rich NM. Military vascular injuries in Croatia. Cardiovasc Surg 1993; 1:2 (editorial).

BLUNT AND PENETRATING ABDOMINAL VASCULAR INJURIES

ASHER HIRSHBERG, M.D.
KENNETH L. MATTOX, M.D.
MATTHEW J. WALL Jr., M.D.

Abdominal vascular trauma presents clinically as either a free intraperitoneal hemorrhage or a contained retroperitoneal hematoma. The patient with a free hemorrhage usually presents in profound shock. More often than not, the patient with a contained or partially contained retroperitoneal hematoma is also hemodynamically unstable from either vascular injury or associated visceral damage. Although some clinical signs, such as absent femoral pulses or a bullet trajectory across the abdominal midline, may suggest a vascular injury, in most patients the indication for urgent celiotomy is clear, and diagnosis is made at operation. The only exception is deceleration injury to the renal pedicle in an otherwise stable patient, which requires arteriography for diagnosis.

Time must not be wasted on unnecessary diagnostic tests or futile attempts at stabilization. In fact, no scientific evidence validates the benefits of massive fluid resuscitation in the hypotensive trauma patient. It may actually adversely affect outcome.[1]

OPERATIVE PRINCIPLES

The usual scenario encountered at celiotomy is vigorous bleeding or an expanding hematoma in a relatively inaccessible site, combined with other visceral injuries. Under these adverse circumstances, it is important to maintain priorities and avoid pitfalls.

The first priority is control of bleeding. If the obvious origin of profuse bleeding is the vascular injury, it must be addressed. If, however, the presumed vascular injury is contained within a stable retroperitoneal hematoma and there is bleeding from another source or gross spillage of bowel content, these injuries are addressed first. Whereas control of bleeding usually can be quickly obtained, vascular reconstruction is time-consuming and not always necessary. The surgeon's first priority is to save life; although complex vascular reconstructions in the critically wounded make elegant textbook drawings, they may also result in a dead patient. The operating room is a physiologically hostile environment for the critically injured patient. Prolonged operation and massive blood replacement result in a triad of hypothermia, acidosis, and coagulopathy that is self-propagating and lethal. Currently in trauma surgery the goal is to avoid crossing the physiologic limits by employing rapid temporary measures to control bleeding and spillage of bowel content, such as packing and closure of bowel without resection (Fig. 1). The operation is then terminated and the skin is rapidly closed, followed by stabilization and rewarming in the surgical intensive care unit. The patient is later returned to the operating room for a planned reoperation and definitive repair.[2] This philosophy of abbreviated celiotomy is particularly relevant to the patient with abdominal vascular injury. Even after obtaining control of a major bleeding vessel, the surgeon still must race against time. After 1 hour of operation and replacement of 10 units of blood, the patient with a temperature of 33°C and a pH of 7.2 is rapidly approaching phsysiologic limits.

Several options preclude lengthy vascular reconstructions in these patients. Many intra-abdominal vessels are amenable to ligation with no or reasonably acceptable consequences. The inferior vena cava, iliac veins, celiac axis, and renal arteries with nephrectomy are but some examples.[3-5] Intraluminal stents are sometimes useful in maintaining blood flow without reconstruction in the iliac vessels, and packing is a useful hemostatic maneuver for inaccessible bleeding from deep pelvic veins. The common denominators of all these bail-out techniques are simplicity and speed.

The use of synthetic grafts in the injured abdomen is a subject of controversy.[6] Primary vascular repair should be attempted whenever feasible, but use of prosthetic material in a potentially contaminated operative field is sometimes unavoidable. Copious irrigation follows repair of intestinal injuries; after gloves and instruments are changed, vascular repair is performed.

INITIAL CONTROL AND EXPOSURE

Celiotomy is performed through a midline incision. Rapid evisceration of the small bowel and evacuation of

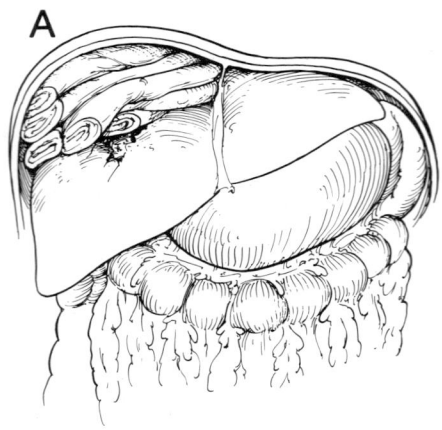

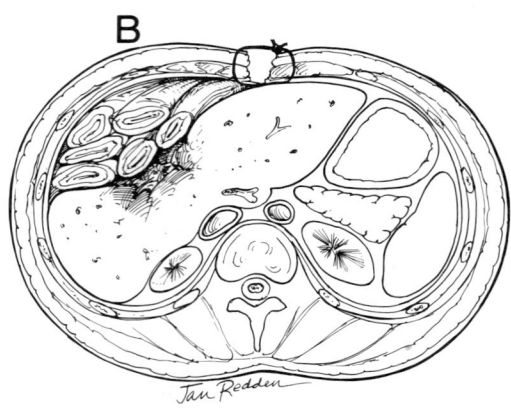

Figure 1 Drawing of packed liver injury, a desperate bail out maneuver. Other such maneuvers include towel clip closure of the abdominal wall and application of the "Bogota bag." (Copyright Baylor College of Medicine.)

blood enables a quick assessment of the site and type of vascular injury. Free bleeding must be controlled, usually initially by direct digital pressure. A Foley catheter or a Fogarty balloon catheter, when inserted into a bleeding cavity, is a useful adjunct. Blind groping in an attempt to clamp a large bleeding vessel usually fails. Once bleeding is temporarily controlled, stop. Take time to make necessary preparations to optimize the surgical approach to the injured vessel. Assure availability of an autotransfusion device, a full range of vascular instruments, blood, and additional help. Use this time also to determine approach and exposure techniques. A contained retroperitoneal hematoma is a less dramatic facet of the same problem, which, nevertheless, presents a classic surgical pitfall.[2-7] The surgeon should resist the urge to address the hematoma directly, concentrating on proximal and distal control and optimizing operative conditions prior to opening the hematoma. Gastrointestinal repairs may also be addressed, if the hematoma is stable.

Aortic cross-clamping is a time-honored maneuver traditionally used as both an adjunct to resuscitation and a means of reducing torrential arterial hemorrhage. The aorta may be clamped in the following locations.

1. The supradiaphragmatic descending aorta is cross-clamped via a left thoracotomy. Used mainly as one of the steps in a resuscitative thoracotomy, it is also a technique for controlling the aorta prior to celiotomy, especially in the presence of a tense hemoperitoneum.
2. The supraceliac aorta may be clamped at the diaphragmatic hiatus through the lesser sac. The peritoneum over the esophagus is opened, and the esophagus is encircled and reflected, with blunt opening of the left diaphragmatic crus to the left of the esophagus. The same site may also be approached through medial rotation of the left-sided abdominal viscera (Fig. 2).[3,7]
3. The suprarenal aorta is clamped or compressed directly through an opening in the lesser sac.
4. The infrarenal aorta is clamped beneath the left renal vein by rightward reflection of the small bowel, division of the ligament of Treitz, and

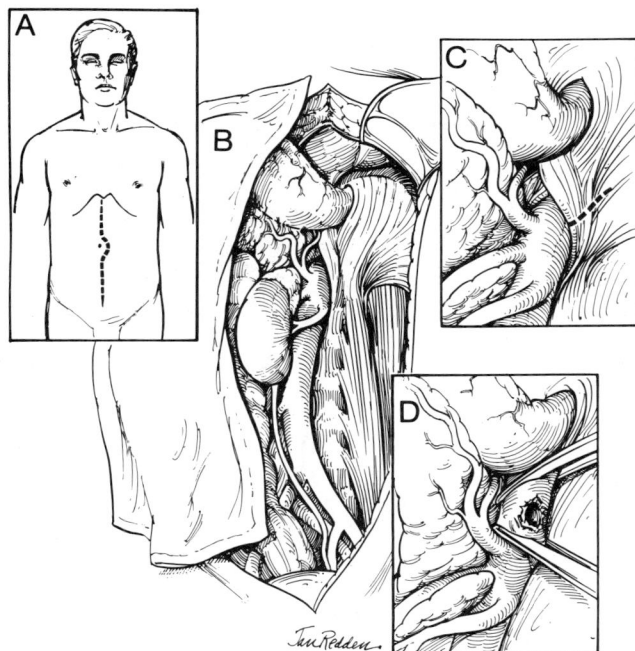

Figure 2 Drawing of a left medial visceral rotation to expose the abdominal aorta behind the kidney, anterior to the psoas muscle. Repair of injuries to the supraceliac and mesenteric abdominal aorta are aided by using this maneuver. (Copyright Baylor College of Medicine.)

opening of the posterior parietal peritoneum between the duodenum and the inferior mesenteric vein.
5. Retrograde transfemoral aortic occluding balloons are currently being investigated (Fig. 3).

Two major problems with aortic clamping are disregarded in the literature but acknowledged by experienced surgeons. First, clamping the aorta through the lesser sac is not always quick and easy, especially in a pool of blood. Meticulous dissection is often impossible, and iatrogenic injury to the celiac axis, esophagus, left gastric artery, or even the aorta itself is a real concern. The second problem is the physiologic effect of clamping. Although it dramatically improves the data on the monitor screen, the sudden afterload augmentation and visceral and peripheral ischemia are detrimental to the patient's already borderline physiologic reserves. Although at times a lifesaving maneuver in a rapidly deteriorating patient and certainly necessary for control of aortic injuries, aortic clamping should be used judiciously and not reflexively. Furthermore, manual compression of the aorta through the lesser sac is less likely to cause iatrogenic damage than blunt dissection and clamping, and it achieves the same effect.

Experience with several basic exposure and control techniques is vital for accomplishing adequate exposure of abdominal vascular injuries. Selection of the appropriate technique hinges on correct identification of the type of retroperitoneal hematoma or site of bleeding.

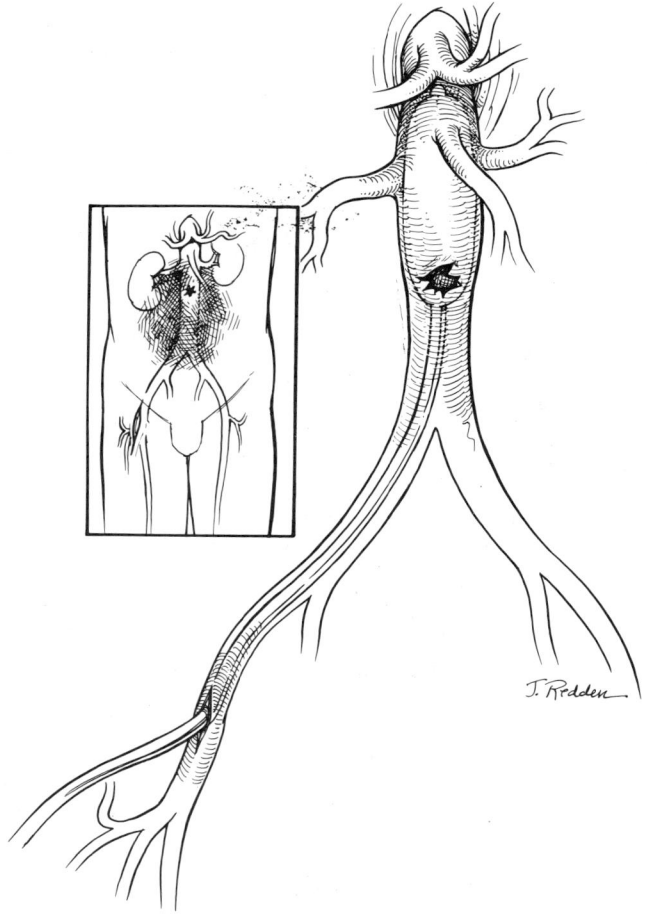

Figure 3 Drawing of an alternate desperate maneuver to control bleeding from an abdominal aortic injury. A large intra-aortic occluding balloon is inserted retrograde via the femoral artery and inflated for temporary control. This technique is still under investigation. (Copyright Baylor College of Medicine.)

Proximal control of midline supramesocolic central retroperitoneal hematoma or hemorrhage is obtained by clamping or compressing the aorta at the diaphragmatic hiatus, and exposure is provided by medial rotation of the left-sided abdominal viscera. Medial visceral rotation affords quick and easy access to the entire intra-abdominal aorta and its branches, except the right renal artery. The lateral peritoneal attachment of the left colon is incised, and the incision is carried upward lateral to the spleen. Blunt digital dissection behind the kidney and on the posterior abdominal wall muscles brings the left-sided viscera to the midline and is easily performed because part of the dissection has already been done by the hematoma itself.

A central inframesocolic hematoma is the result of injury to the aorta, inferior vena cava, or their infrarenal branches. Bleeding or a contained hematoma in this area is approached in much the same way as the elective resection of an aortic aneurysm.

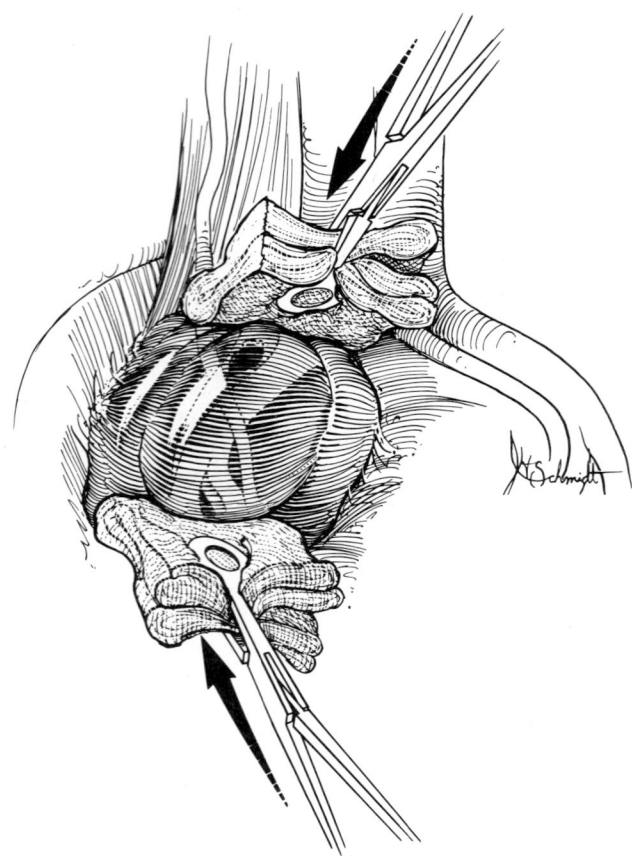

Figure 4 Drawing of one maneuver to use direct compression to control bleeding from injured iliac vessels. Once controlled, exposure and repair can be attempted. (Copyright Baylor College of Medicine.)

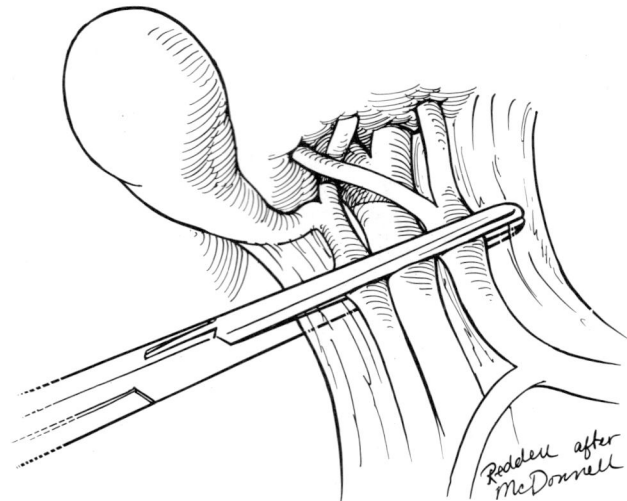

Figure 5 Drawing of the Pringle maneuver used to temporarily occlude the porta hepatis. It is imperative that a noncrushing vascular clamp be used for this maneuver. (Copyright Baylor College of Medicine.)

Control of right iliac artery and vein injuries as well as exposure of the infrarenal inferior vena cava are accomplished through an extended Kocher maneuver. The right colon and duodenum are reflected medially by incising the peritoneum immediately lateral to them (Fig. 4). The dissection is then carried on to detach the posterior attachments of the small bowel mesentery so that the bowel is reflected onto the lower chest. When performed to its full extent, this maneuver provides exposure of the infrarenal inferior vena cava, distal aorta, and their bifurcations. The entire length of the right iliac vessels is exposed, as is the proximal part of the left iliac vessels. However, mobilization of the sigmoid colon is required to provide more distal exposure of the left iliac vessels.[4]

Traditional teaching advocates cautiously approaching a lateral perinephric hematoma. Prior to opening the hematoma, midline looping of the ipsilateral artery and vein in juxtaposition to the aorta and inferior vena cava is recommended as a safe precaution. However, this dissection is time-consuming and often unnecessary. Especially when active bleeding is present or when speed is important, the injured kidney is rapidly mobilized by incising the posterior peritoneum and Gerota's fascia lateral to it, elevating the kidney medially, and clamping the hilar vessels in a manner similar to a rapid splenectomy.

Bleeding from the hepatoduodenal ligament usually originates from an injured portal vein or hepatic artery. Initial control is obtained with digital pressure, followed by a Pringle maneuver (Fig. 5). A double Pringle with clamping of the portal triad above and below the site of bleeding may be required to control backbleeding from the liver. Bleeding from an injured mesenteric artery or vein is best initially controlled by compressing the entire base of the mesentery between the thumb and forefinger.[3,5]

Distal vascular control can be difficult, especially in several inaccessible sites such as the suprarenal aorta, inferior vena cava, or the iliac vessels. If direct distal clamping is impossible, balloon occlusion of the lumen, further dissection and mobilization of the vessel to improve exposure, and accepting some backbleeding are the three major options.

SPECIAL PROBLEMS AND CONTROVERSIES

Exploration of Retroperitoneal Hematoma

As a general rule, a retroperitoneal hematoma following penetrating abdominal trauma is explored because major vascular injury must be ruled out, even in stable, nonexpanding hematomas. Exceptions to this rule include, for example, the patient with a stable perinephric hematoma in whom the extent of renal parenchymal damage is known from preoperative imaging studies. If there is no major urine extravasation, the hematoma may be left unexplored. Similarly, the same hematoma in a critically injured patient who undergoes an abbreviated celiotomy and planned reoperation should not be explored at the initial procedure. Most experienced trauma surgeons do not explore a stable nonbleeding retrohepatic hematoma because attempted surgical repair is associated with a very high mortality.

The approach to a retroperitoneal hematoma following blunt trauma depends on the location of the hematoma. Central supramesocolic and inframesocolic hematomas are explored routinely. Every effort should be made to avoid exploring a pelvic hematoma, especially one associated with a pelvic fracture. Thus, a hematoma should be opened only if a major vascular injury is suspected within it, if access is required to repair an injured bladder, or if the patient is exsanguinating.

Renal Pedicle Injury

Blunt renovascular deceleration trauma is usually asymptomatic and is discovered when a kidney fails to opacify on excretory urography or computed tomography. Arteriography is required for diagnosis and may document a spectrum of injuries ranging from minimal intimal tear to complete renal artery thrombosis. Because blunt renovascular trauma is characteristically associated with more life-threatening injuries, a significant diagnostic delay is almost inevitable. This has raised the controversial issue of delayed renal revascularization. In most patients with multiple injuries, attempted renal salvage by major vascular reconstruction is not a viable option. In those who are suitable candidates for such an undertaking, opinions differ regarding the time limit that precludes a successful revascularization. If 4 to 6 hours have elapsed since injury and the renal artery is occluded, repair should not be undertaken.

Iliac Vessels

Trauma to the iliac arteries and veins is probably the most underrated of all abdominal vascular injuries. The mortality rate is around 30%, and the leading cause of death is uncontrollable hemorrhage.[5] The difficulties in obtaining vascular control are compounded by the relative inaccessibility of the iliac veins and the internal iliac arteries. Often the pelvic hematoma is so large it is difficult to ascertain which side is injured. Thus, the iliac vessels should initially be controlled away from the site of injury, in combination with direct pressure on the source of bleeding—digitally, with laparotomy pads, or with sponge sticks (Fig. 4). As the dissection proceeds toward the bleeding site, clamps are sequentially advanced closer to the injury until all backbleeding is eliminated. Occasionally an overlying common iliac artery must be divided to provide access to a venous injury lying behind it.

A special problem arises when iliac artery reconstruction is required in the presence of gross fecal contamination. Use of a synthetic graft cannot always be avoided. Although several ingenious methods of arterial transposition have been described, a femorofemoral bypass is a more practical course of action if the patient's

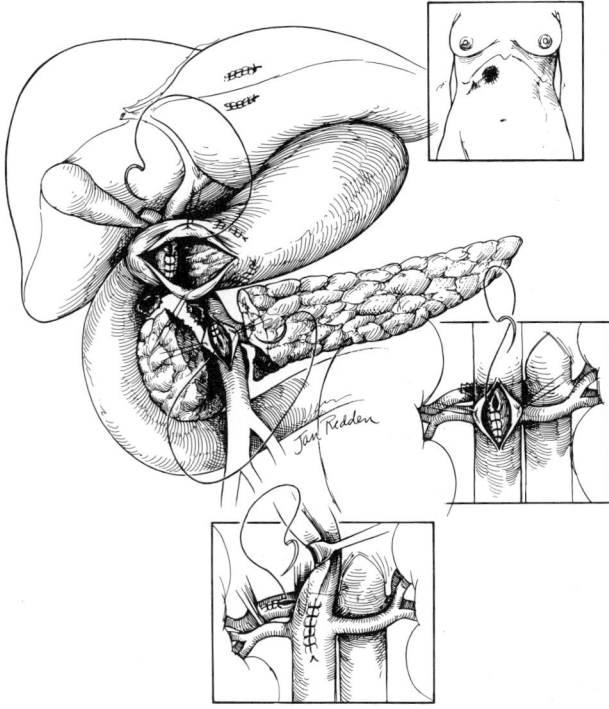

Figure 6 Drawing of deliberate division of the neck of the pancreas for exposure of the proximal portal vein. Note that this patient also had a double injury to the inferior vena cava. (Copyright Baylor College of Medicine.)

condition allows for the additional time in the operating room.

Mesenteric and Portal Circulation

Trauma to the superior mesenteric artery is uncommon and carries a high mortality because of associated injuries. The origin of the artery can be approached through a medial visceral rotation, whereas the infrapancreatic superior mesenteric artery can be approached directly through the root of the mesentery after pulling the small bowel down and to the left. Most injuries are amenable to lateral repair or direct end-to-end anastomosis. Clinical evidence is not available to support or refute the view that the suprapancreatic superior mesenteric artery can be safely ligated with bowel viability maintained by collateral circulation. Thus, blood flow in the superior mesenteric artery should be reconstituted whenever feasible, but ligation at the origin of the artery may occasionally be an unavoidable necessity.

The most important principle of graft interposition for superior mesenteric artery injuries is keeping the proximal suture line away from associated pancreatic or duodenal injuries. The graft takeoff should be placed in the lower aorta just above the bifurcation, away from the upper abdominal injuries and well covered with posterior peritoneum. A planned reoperation to ascertain bowel viability is employed by some surgeons.

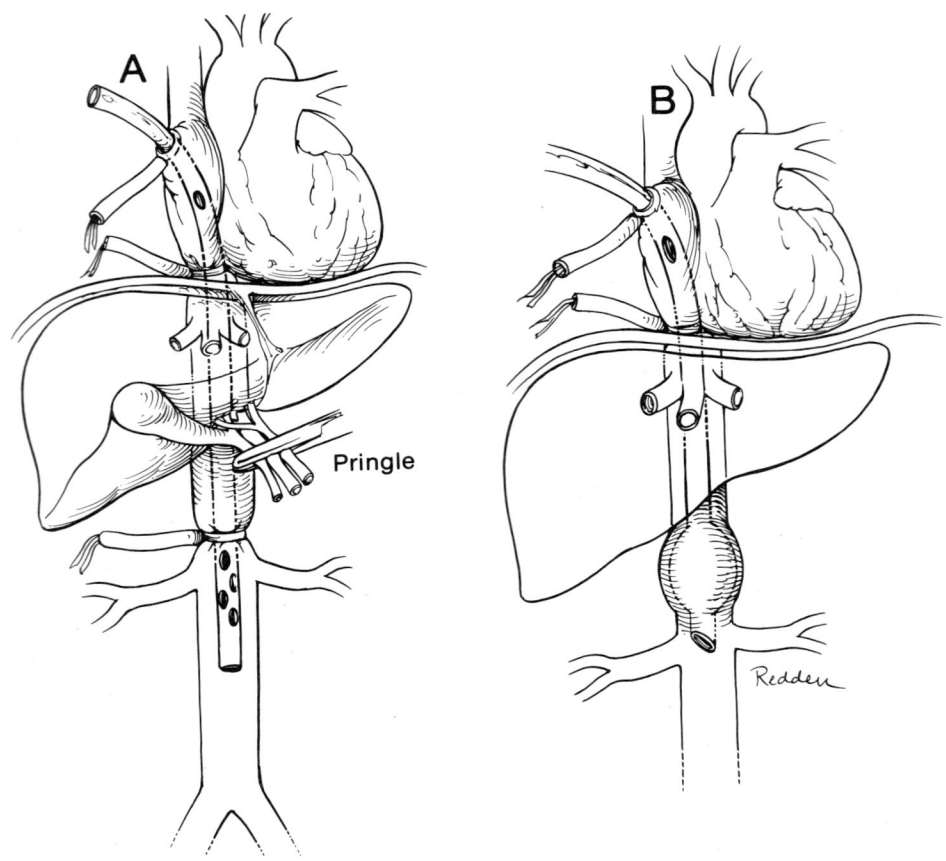

Figure 7 Drawing of the atriocaval shunt inserted for hemorrhage following a retrohepatic inferior vena cava or hepatic vein injury. Note that an extra hole is cut in the proximal end of the shunt to allow venous return to the heart via the shunt. (Copyright Baylor College of Medicine.)

Although superior mesenteric and portal venous injuries are usually amenable to lateral repair, both veins present accessibility problems. Access to the proximal superior mesenteric artery may require pancreatic transection over a finger insinuated from the root of the mesentery toward the portal triad, between the pancreas and the superior mesenteric vessel. Exposure of the portal vein is complicated by its posterior location and overlying structures (Fig. 6). In the presence of multiple injuries, ligation of the superior mesenteric artery or portal vein is an option but requires aggressive postoperative fluid resuscitation to replace the resulting massive splanchnic sequestration.

Retrohepatic Inferior Vena Cava

Injuries to the retrohepatic inferior vena cava and hepatic veins are perhaps the least accessible of all abdominal vascular injuries. Often associated with high-grade hepatic parenchymal trauma, these injuries present as vigorous bleeding from behind the liver. This bleeding characteristically continues despite a Pringle maneuver.

Several techniques have been described to approach the retrohepatic inferior vena cava, including direct exposure by full mobilization and medial rotation of the right hepatic lobe, hepatic vascular isolation by a Pringle maneuver combined with infrahepatic and suprahepatic transdiaphragmatic caval clamping, and hepatic transection in the principal plane to expose the inferior vena cava directly from within the liver. The most widely discussed technique is the atriocaval shunt, a conceptually elegant solution that employs an intracaval shunt placed through the right atrial appendage (Fig. 7). A drawing of this shunt appears in almost every publication on abdominal vascular or hepatic trauma, and successful placement is generally applauded as a major feat.[8] However, rapid placement usually requires two teams—one working in the chest and the other in the abdomen—and a degree of experience to avoid pitfalls. Because these injuries are rare, the decision to insert the shunt is almost invariably made for a critical patient who has already lost a vast amount of blood. It is therefore not surprising that the mortality rate of retrohepatic caval injuries continues to be extremely high.[9] At the Ben Taub General Hospital, only one long-term survivor was reported from 18 atriocaval shunt insertions during the last 2 years. Clearly, a more effective solution is needed. Packing may be an effective solution to retrohepatic caval injuries, and it may ultimately prove a more feasible approach to these lethal injuries.

REFERENCES

1. Mattox KL, Feliciano DV, Beall AC, et al. Five thousand seven hundred sixty cardiovascular injuries in 4459 patients: Epidemiologic evolution 1958–1988. Ann Surg 1989; 209:698–705.
2. Burch JM, Ortiz VB, Richardson RJ, et al. Abbreviated laparotomy and planned reoperation for critically injured patients. Ann Surg 1992; 215:476–484.
3. Accola KD, Feliciano DV, Mattox KL, et al. Management of injuries to the superior mesenteric artery. J Trauma 1986; 26:313–317.
4. Burch JM, Richardson RJ, Martin RR, Mattox KL. Penetrating iliac vascular injuries: Recent experience with 233 consecutive patients. J Trauma 1990; 30:1450–1459.
5. Graham JM, Mattox KL. The wounded soul. Tex Med 1982; 78:51–54.
6. Lau JM, Mattox KL, Beall AC Jr, DeBakey ME. Use of substitute conduits in traumatic vascular injury. J Trauma 1977; 17:541–546.
7. Mattox KL, McCollum WB, Beall AC Jr, et al. Management of penetrating injuries of the suprarenal aorta. J Trauma 1975; 15:808–815.
8. Burch JM, Feliciano DV, Mattox KL. The atriocaval shunt:Facts and fiction. Ann Surg 1988; 207:555–568.
9. Beal SL. Fatal hepatic hemorrhage: An unresolved problem in the management of complex liver injuries. J Trauma 1990; 30:163–169.

IATROGENIC UPPER EXTREMITY ARTERIAL CATHETER INJURY

RICHARD J. FOWL, M.D.
RICHARD F. KEMPCZINSKI, M.D.

The widespread use of coronary and peripheral arteriography has resulted in extensive transarterial catheterization. The most common vessel used for arteriography is the femoral artery. However, the upper extremity arteries are still frequently used as alternative sites, especially in patients with severe aortoiliac occlusive disease. Paralleling this increased arterial access, there has been a concomitant increase in the number of iatrogenic upper extremity arterial injuries.

INCIDENCE

The true incidence of iatrogenic upper extremity arterial injury is unknown. However, one can obtain an estimation based on reports from centers performing a large volume of cardiac and peripheral arteriography. The brachial artery is the most commonly utilized upper extremity artery for cardiac catheterization. At Baylor University, there was a 0.9% incidence of known brachial arterial injuries over a 3-year period in which 12,158 cardiac catheterizations were performed.[1] At the Cleveland Clinic from 1980 to 1988, there were 34,291 transbrachial cardiac catheterization studies performed, 1.5% of which resulted in a known brachial artery injury.[2]

Although the radial artery is not used for arteriography, it is the most common vessel used for arterial blood pressure monitoring. The incidence of postcatheterization radial artery thrombosis ranges from 2.5% to 25%.[3,4] Radial artery thrombosis is usually asymptomatic. However, severe hand ischemia is estimated to occur in 0.2% to 0.5% of patients following radial artery cannulation.[3] The axillary artery is less commonly utilized for both coronary and peripheral arteriography. The incidence of major axillary artery complications ranges from 0.8% to 2.1%, with a less than 1% incidence of brachial plexus injury.[5,6]

ETIOLOGY

Multiple mechanisms for arterial injury follow catheterization procedures (Fig. 1). First, the vessel may become narrowed after improper suture closure of the arteriotomy. Second, intimal disruption or dissection with a resulting intimal flap may lead to thrombosis of the artery. Third, intimal erosion of the posterior wall of the artery by the catheter may produce a thrombogenic arterial luminal surface that can lead to thrombosis. Fourth, thrombus may form around the indwelling catheter, and, when the catheter is removed, the thrombus is stripped off and results in arterial emboli or thrombosis.[1,7]

Several risk factors predispose an artery to thrombosis.[1,3] Repeated catheterization of the same artery is an important risk factor that can increase the amount of local trauma to the vessel, if multiple catheters have been inserted. If the catheter remains in place for a prolonged period, risk for pericatheter thrombus formation increases. Multiple exchanges of catheters through a vessel also increases the risk of trauma and can result in arterial thrombosis. Small arteries, often in women, are predisposed to thrombus formation. Inadequate anticoagulation with heparin sodium during catheterization promotes increased thrombus formation. Physicians inexperienced with using the brachial artery have higher complication rates. Pre-existing atherosclerotic disease results in an increased risk for intimal flap formation.

In patients with indwelling radial artery cannulas, several other factors may predispose to arterial occlusion. Prolonged cannulation over several days is one of the most important risk factors leading to thrombosis.

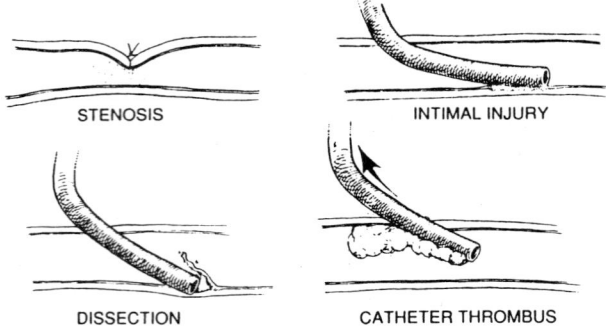

Figure 1 Mechanisms of catheter arterial injury.

Because many patients requiring continuous blood pressure monitoring are hemodynamically unstable, prolonged hypotension that results in intense peripheral vasoconstriction may lead to thrombus formation. Excessive external pressure following catheter removal to prevent hematoma formation may lead to arterial thrombosis.

The best method for preventing radial artery occlusion with subsequent severe hand ischemia is to assess the collateral circulation prior to insertion of the cannula. In awake patients, an Allen's test should be performed to determine if there is adequate ulnar collateral circulation of the hand. Approximately 1.6% of patients have incomplete palmar arches, and cannulating and occluding the radial artery in them could lead to severe hand ischemia.[3] However, the Allen's test cannot be used in patients who are unconscious or anesthetized. Therefore, an alternative method for assessing the circulation is to occlude the radial artery manually while monitoring Doppler signals in the digital vessels. If the Doppler signals disappear with radial artery compression, there is inadequate collateral circulation via the ulnar artery and the radial artery should not be cannulated. If the hand becomes pale or cyanotic following radial artery cannulation, the cannula should be promptly removed, and the hand should be gently warmed and carefully observed. If the ischemic signs do not promptly resolve, urgent radial artery repair should be performed.

Because the axillary artery is a large vessel, occlusion is much less common than hematoma formation. A major risk of hematoma formation is compression of the cords of the brachial plexus, which can result in temporary or even permanent neurologic dysfunction of the upper extremity. Immobilization of the arm and careful observation of the axilla following removal of an axillary artery catheter are important in minimizing serious complications. The most likely cause of an axillary hematoma is inadequate external pressure after removal of the cannula. Some authors recommend that external compression should be performed by the physician rather than a subordinate.[5] A small catheter also reduces the incidence of hematoma formation.

OPERATIVE TREATMENT

Arterial Repair

Once arterial thrombosis has occurred, prompt and effective treatment is essential to ensure a satisfactory outcome. The patient should be transferred expeditiously from the catheterization laboratory or the radiology suite to the operating room, where better light and instruments are available to undertake repair of the injured artery. The patient should be prepped from the shoulder to the fingertips to permit examination of the distal pulses following repair of the injured vessel. The upper thigh or the ankle should also be included in the surgical preparation to permit removal of the saphenous vein in case a bypass graft is needed. Arm vein is also acceptable as a replacement graft, if it is of adequate caliber. Most repairs of the brachial artery can be undertaken with local anesthesia. However, for proximal axillary artery repairs, a general anesthetic is usually advisable because wide exposure of the vessel may be required, including proximal control of the axillary artery through an infraclavicular incision in the case of a rapidly expanding hematoma following an axillary artery puncture.

Once the extremity is properly prepared and draped, the first surgical objective is to obtain adequate exposure of the site of injury. If the artery was closed with sutures, they should be removed. A transverse or longitudinal incision can be made in the vessel to inspect the area of injury. We prefer a longitudinal incision because we feel it allows better exposure of the injury and can be extended as needed. A Fogarty catheter can be passed proximally and distally to remove all thrombus. Once inflow and retrograde backbleeding have been obtained, the vessel is carefully inspected to determine the extent of injury. If only an intimal flap is present, it can be excised or tacked. If the vessel is extensively damaged, it may need to be resected and replaced. If the area of injury is 2 cm or less, then an end-to-end anastomosis with interrupted 6-0 polyprolene sutures is usually possible. If the extent of injury is greater than 2 cm, then an interposition vein graft is required. If a longitudinal arteriotomy has been used, closure with a small vein patch of either cephalic or saphenous vein is preferred.

An axillary artery injury can usually be repaired by correcting the intimal flap and closing the arteriotomy with a vein patch. If the artery is severely injured, then a vein graft repair is usually the preferred treatment. If a hematoma develops after axillary artery puncture, very careful observation for the earliest signs of neurologic impairment is essential to prevent permanent injury to the brachial plexus. If a deficit develops, prompt operative evacuation of the hematoma is mandatory.

Radial artery thrombosis usually does not require surgical repair unless symptoms of severe hand ischemia develop. Then thrombectomy and vein patch closure or a vein interposition graft is usually required to restore adequate perfusion.

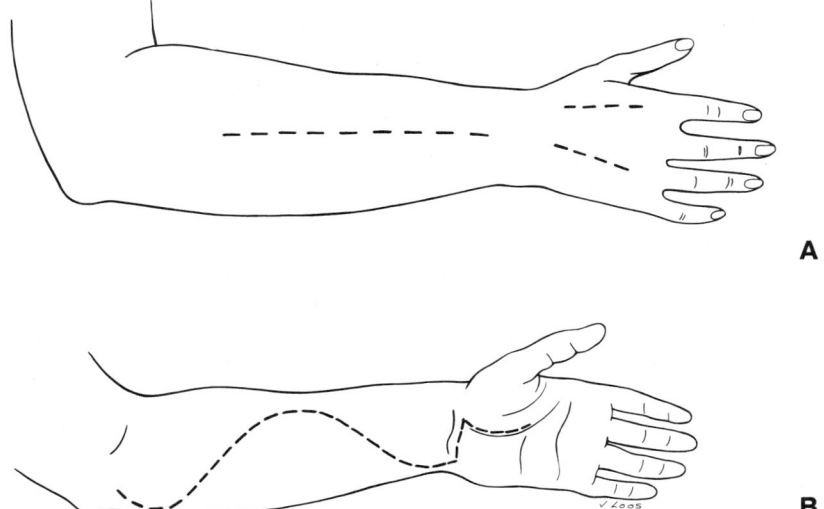

Figure 2 *A*, Incisions for dorsal arm fasciotomy. *B*, Incision for volar arm fasciotomy.

Fasciotomy

Fasciotomy is rarely necessary when dealing with catheter-induced arterial injury to the upper extremity, especially when it results in brachial artery thrombosis. However, if acute axillary artery occlusion occurs and either is unrecognized or there is a significant (usually greater than 6 hours) delay in restoring circulation, compartment pressures should be measured in both the dorsal and volar compartments of the arm. If intracompartmental pressure approaches or exceeds 40 mm Hg, prompt and adequate decompression is essential (Fig. 2). Note that the volar incision should cross the carpal ligament and extend into the hand.

RESULTS

In two recent large studies of brachial artery injuries following cardiac catheterization, the incidence of early brachial rethrombosis was 3% to 5%.[1,2] Other complications include incisional hematomas (2.6%) and neurologic dysfunction such as dysesthesia, causalgia, or paresis (0.8%).[2] In both of these reports, 95% to 97% of patients obtained an excellent result when the artery was repaired promptly following diagnosis of the injury.

In patients who do not undergo early repair, approximately one-third develop late symptoms of arm exercise ischemia. In these patients a more complicated repair, such as a vein graft bypass, is usually required to correct the chronic arterial occlusion. Axillary hematomas with neurologic deficits should be operatively explored urgently. Patients who are operated upon within 24 hours are significantly more likely to obtain complete recovery compared to those patients who undergo operation beyond 24 hours.[8] Therefore, all iatrogenic upper extremity injuries should be repaired promptly following diagnosis except in instances in which the patient's overall medical condition is critical and any operation may pose excessive risk to the patient's life.[2]

REFERENCES

1. McCollum CH, Mavor E. Brachial artery injury after cardiac catheterization. J Vasc Surg 1986; 4:355–359.
2. Kline RM, Hertzer NR, Beven EG, et al. Surgical treatment of brachial artery injuries after cardiac catheterization. J Vasc Surg 1990; 12:20–24.
3. Baker RJ, Chunprapaph B, Nyhus LM. Severe ischemia of the hand following radial artery catheterization. Surgery 1976; 80:449–457.
4. Weiss BM, Gattiker RI. Complications during and following radial artery cannulation: A prospective study. Intensive Care Med 1986; 12:424–428.
5. Westcott JL, Taylor PT. Transaxillary selective four-vessel arteriography. Radiology 1972; 104:277–281.
6. McIvor J, Rhymer JC. Two hundred forty-five transaxillary arteriograms in arteriopathic patients: Success rate and complications. Clin Radiol 1992; 45:390–394.
7. Karmody AM, Lempert N, Jarmolych J. The pathology of post-catheterization brachial artery occlusion. J Surg Res 1976; 20:601–606.
8. O'Keefe DM. Brachial plexus injury following axillary arteriography. J Neurosurg 1980; 53:853–857.
9. Page CP, Hagood CT, Kemmerer WT. Management of postcatherization: Brachial artery thrombosis. Surgery 1972; 72:619–623.

COMPLICATIONS OF THE LOWER EXTREMITIES AFTER PERCUTANEOUS ARTERIAL PUNCTURE

RICHARD L. McCANN, M.D.

The past decade has witnessed an explosion in the use of minimally invasive techniques for the management of surgical problems. The broad field of endovascular surgery has increased in scope since the introduction of coaxial dilation by Dotter in 1964 and balloon dilation by Grüntzig in 1974. During the last decade technical advances include development of several types of arterial dilating catheters, temporary reperfusion catheters, atherectomy devices, and placement of intraluminal stents, as well as intravascular placement of circulatory assist devices. With the future prospect of intraluminal grafting, various types of embolotherapy, and potential use of percutaneous thromboembolism-treating strategies, the increase in diagnostic and therapeutic arterial punctures is likely to continue. Even though these endoluminal therapies have been largely successful and useful, they have resulted in an increase in the occurrence of local access site arterial injuries. It is not uncommon for large tertiary care institutions to perform 5,000 or more of these procedures annually. Even though the reported incidence of significant local complications is low, this large number of procedures results in a substantial number of limb- and life-threatening complications that require careful and expert management by experienced vascular surgeons to minimize morbidity and mortality.

INCIDENCE AND RISK FACTORS

In a series of more than 24,000 cardiac catheterizations at Duke University, the incidence of vascular injury requiring repair was 0.9%.[1] Other large series have suggested incidences between 0.8% and 3%.[2,3] The incidence seems to be changing favorably over time, which may be attributed to continued efforts at miniaturization and the use of smaller and smaller access ports for intraluminal devices.

A number of clinical factors influence complication rates. Large studies have reported that catheterizations for therapeutic procedures result in complications requiring surgical intervention at a rate two or three times that of simple diagnostic procedures.[4] Several factors contribute to this increase. Among them are the larger catheter required for therapeutic procedures and these patients' greater severity of illness. Therapeutic procedures also require a longer time, and the increased amount of catheter manipulation may be significant.

Finally, the more frequent use of anticoagulants and fibrinolytic drugs in association with such interventional procedures may predispose to occurrence of vascular complications. Other factors that may play a role include the presence of congestive heart failure and both excessive and diminutive body size. Importantly, the degree of peripheral vascular disease present at the access site and distally in the affected limb also contributes significantly to the incidence and long-term outcome of peripheral vascular complications.

SPECIFIC COMPLICATIONS

Hematoma, Hemorrhage, and Pseudoaneurysm

Percutaneous arterial interventions by definition require puncture of the arterial wall and entry into the arterial lumen. Upon withdrawal of the catheter, closure of the puncture site occurs by several mechanisms. The arterial wall elasticity contracts to minimize the size of the defect. Blood is prevented from escaping through the residual defect by appropriate external manual compression of local tissues by the operator. The technique of external compression is critical if complications are to be minimized. Compression should adequately seal the anterior puncture site without completely obliterating flow in the vessel. Compression that completely obliterates all flow in the lumen predisposes to vessel thrombosis. Compression is most effective if the puncture occurs in the common femoral artery so that the vessel can be compressed against the femoral head. Punctures above or below this location or in the deep femoral artery are subject to inadequate occlusion of the puncture site and extravasation of blood. Punctures above the inguinal ligament especially are to be avoided. A seal is difficult to achieve with an arterial defect in the pelvis, and a large amount of blood can extravasate into the pelvis and retroperitoneal space before becoming clinically apparent. Compression may also be ineffective in the very obese or as a result of a failure of the hemostatic mechanisms of platelet aggregation and fibrin formation that are due to hematologic disease or intentional anticoagulant or fibrinolytic therapy. Vessels affected with severe atherosclerotic disease may have stiff walls, which minimize the effect of elastic recoil. The simple extravasation of blood into the perivascular tissues results in a hematoma. If a large mass of blood accumulates, a palpable mass may occur; when severe, it may cause enough pressure to compromise the overlying skin viability. If the thigh becomes tense and painful or if blisters appear on the skin, then operative evacuation should be considered. If there is evidence of continued blood loss and transfusion is required, then operative intervention should also be considered.

In some cases when the puncture site fails to seal, a liquid cavity forms. The walls of this cavity include thrombus and the local tissue of the thigh. It is often referred to as a pseudoaneurysm because the aneurysmal sac lacks a true vascular wall. It is the persistence of fluid blood in the center of the lesion that distinguishes a pseudoaneurysm from an uncomplicated hematoma. Most of these lesions are discovered shortly after catheterization, although some may be found months or even years later. Pseudoaneurysms, because they are acute expansions, are often moderately tender. The classic physical finding includes a palpable, pulsatile mass. It is often possible for an experienced examiner to distinguish this lesion on physical examination from a bland, simple hematoma through which a normal femoral pulse is transmitted, in that the pseudoaneurysm is pulsatile in a radial fashion when the lateral edges of the lesion are palpated between the fingers. A more accurate and definitive diagnosis can be obtained by ultrasound imaging.[5] Arteriography is almost never required. In these circumstances, with the widespread availability and relative portability of Doppler color flow and two-dimensional ultrasonographic imaging units, any suspicion of vascular complications after catheterization of the femoral artery should prompt an ultrasound examination (Fig. 1).

Treatment of hematomas and pseudoaneurysms should be individualized according to the characteristics and severity of the lesion as well as the patient's status. Patients with severe heart disease, for example, may not tolerate even small amounts of blood loss; therefore, a hematoma or false aneurysm with even a small potential to rupture might be more aggressively treated in the patient who is severely compromised than in a patient who is healthy. Hematomas that continue to enlarge or are so large as to create a definite cavity with or without potential pressure necrosis of the overlying skin should be evacuated. At the time of evacuation, consideration should be given to identifying the femoral artery puncture site and, if found, suturing it even if it is not actively bleeding at the time of examination. It would not be prudent to rely on a recently formed fibrin plug that might dislodge and require return to the operating room at a later time.

False aneurysms, when small, may be observed initially.[6] Because the cavity is lined with thrombus material, subsequent complete thrombosis of the cavity occurs in a high percentage of patients. This occurs more frequently if there is a relatively long neck between the cavity and the open puncture site. Alternatively, thrombosis is encouraged by external compression of the lesion, particularly if performed under ultrasound guidance to avoid complete compression of the femoral

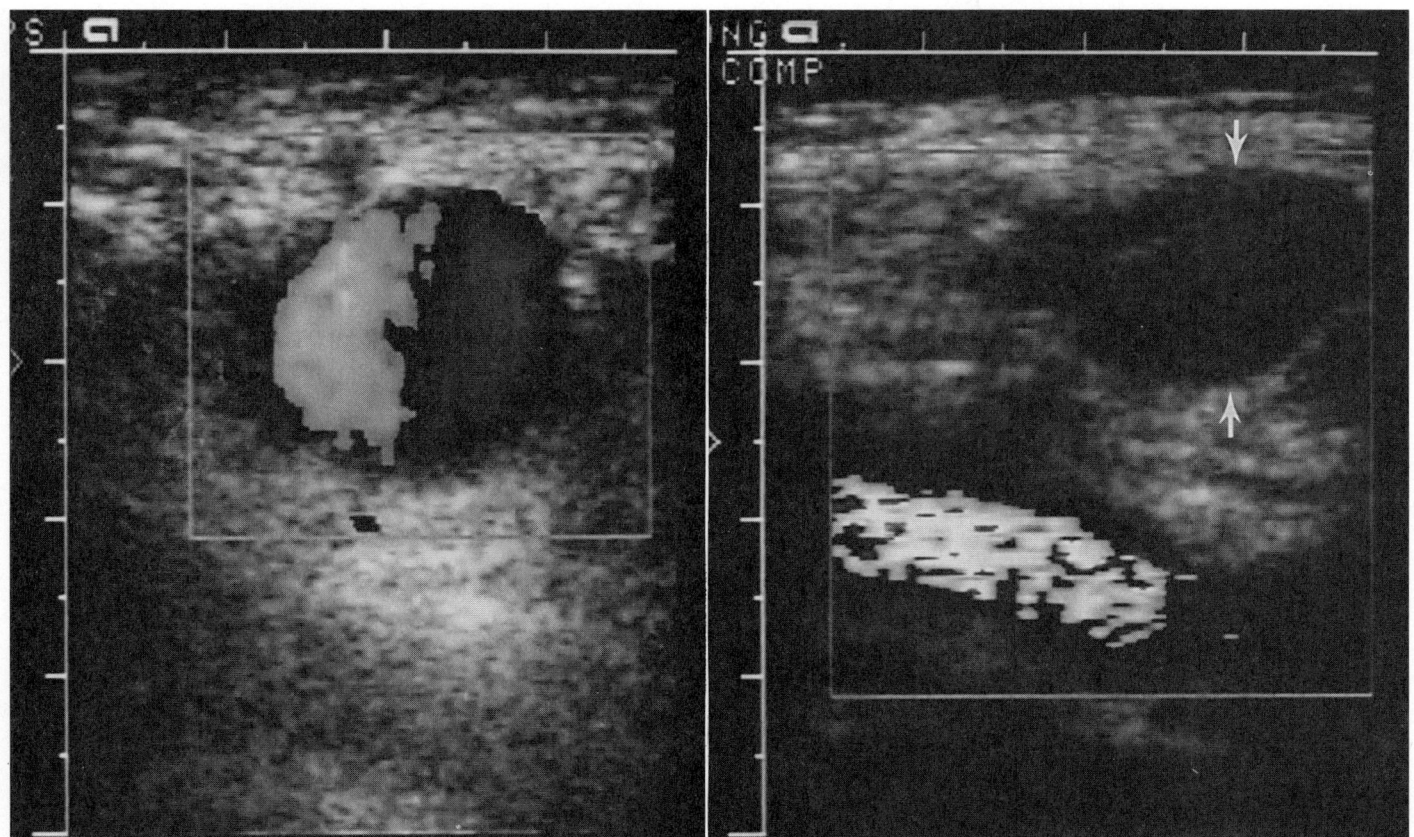

Figure 1 *A,* a 72-year-old woman, 4 days following cardiac catheterization, with a pulsatile hematoma at the groin puncture site. Doppler ultrasound demonstrates a pseudoaneurysm. Note the swirling pattern, termed the "ying-yang" sign. The pseudoaneurysm neck is not seen on this view. *B,* After 30 minutes of ultrasound-guided compression, the pseudoaneurysm thrombosed. There is no flow demonstrated within the pseudoaneurysm *(arrows).*

artery but only compression of the pseudoaneurysm cavity.[7] Mechanical devices are available that can be used to apply groin pressure for long periods of time. It is important not to release pressure and allow accumulated local thrombus to wash away. With experience, as many as 95% of pseudoaneurysms can be thrombosed by this method. Aneurysms that are tender, that fail compression therapy, or for which compression therapy is impractical because of the pain involved should be considered for surgical repair. Left untreated, these lesions may rupture into the thigh or retroperitoneum and result in severe and potentially fatal hemorrhage.

There is considerable debate regarding appropriate surgical techniques for closure of acute femoral false aneurysms. Except for the smallest of lesions, we prefer regional or general anesthesia. An incision is first made in the inguinal region and the feeding external iliac artery exposed extraperitoneally and controlled with a vascular clamp. This allows a second incision in the groin with direct entry into the cavity. Backbleeding from the profunda femoris and superficial femoral arteries can be controlled digitally while the surface of the femoral artery is exposed. It is important to dissect the artery completely to conclusively identify the arterial wall. Sutures in the false aneurysm wall rather than in the vessel wall may only temporarily control the bleeding. With subsequent thrombolysis, recurrent aneurysm or hemorrhage may occur. The defect is identified and sutured with interrupted vascular sutures. The proximal clamp minimizes blood loss, which may be poorly tolerated, particularly in patients with severe cardiac disease as the indication for the interventional procedure in the first place. We have experienced no difficulties with the proximal incision, which uniformly heals well and does not substantially increase perioperative morbidity. When there has been extensive extravasation of blood into the tissues of the groin, wound healing may be less than ideal. Obviously nonviable skin and subcutaneous tissue should be debrided at the original operation, even if it requires open packing of the groin wound.

Thromboembolism

A second category of catheter-related vascular complication is limb ischemia due to thrombosis or embolism. Thrombosis may occur at the puncture site because the catheter occludes blood flow in the vessel, stasis results, and local thrombosis is promoted. Alternatively, major or minor injury to the intima by the catheter may promote intravascular thrombus formation. Embolism may occur from thrombi that adhere to the catheter and become dislodged during catheter manipulation. Also, pre-existing mural thrombi may be dislodged by passage of a catheter or intravascular device and result in distal embolism. These complications are more common in patients with severe atherosclerotic vascular disease affecting the access vessels.

This complication is recognized by the onset of acute ischemia in the limb or an exacerbation of chronic ischemic changes. The clinical manifestations depend on the pre-existing vascular status prior to the catheterization. On the one hand, occlusion of the iliac artery may be subtle if the distal circulation is normal and may be manifest in the patient at bedrest only as absence of a distal pulse that was present before the procedure. On the other hand, distal thromboembolism or occlusion of the femoral artery, particularly in the setting of pre-existing superficial femoral artery disease, may result in an acute ischemic syndrome requiring emergency treatment. In any event, worsening of lower extremity ischemia following catheterization must never be ascribed to spasm but must be considered due to local thrombosis or intimal injury until proven otherwise. We advocate aggressive early exploration for ischemia. In contrast to bleeding, these procedures often can conveniently be carried out using local anesthesia. Generous exploration of the affected vessels should be carried out, particularly if there is significant femoral artery disease. Not infrequently, repair requires local endarterectomy and often vein or fabric patch angioplasty.

The morbidity and mortality from acute peripheral ischemia following catheterization is significant. Complications, which may occur in as many as 30% of patients, include hematoma, wound infection, deep vein thrombosis, myocardial infarction, sepsis, and multisystem organ failure. Amputation may be required in up to 5% of patients, mostly because of either extensive thrombosis or delay in recognition of ischemia. Mortality has often been reported but is usually due to the underlying cardiac disease that was the indication for the original catheterization.

Femoral artery thrombosis in infants and young children, in contrast, is usually well tolerated, and the foot and leg remain viable in the absence of multilevel embolic disease. The results of surgical therapy for thrombosis in very small infants is poor, so alternative approaches have been devised. In this age group, thrombolytic therapy with or without peripheral angioplasty has been utilized with success.

Arteriovenous Fistula

When simultaneous catheterizations of the artery and ipsilateral vein are performed, there is a significant incidence of iatrogenic arteriovenous fistula. Fistula formation is more common after inadvertent low puncture in the superficial femoral or profunda femoris arteries. Fistulas usually become apparent by the appearance of a new bruit or thrill in the groin. The diagnosis is easily confirmed by Doppler color flow ultrasonography, and arteriography is not necessary. Fistula blood flow is usually modest initially and increases quite slowly. Furthermore, many arteriovenous fistulas close spontaneously in the first weeks after formation. Therefore, fistulas discovered in the early postcatheterization period, in the absence of arterial, venous, or cardiac insufficiency, may be initially managed expectantly. Fistulas that have not closed after 6 weeks are unlikely to do so spontaneously, and surgical repair should be considered to prevent subsequent hemodynamic and infectious sequelae. Fistula takedown may usually be performed with local anesthesia. All four poles of the fistula should be identified and controlled prior to dividing the fistula. Primary repair of the artery and vein are then performed unless the vein is not a major trunk. Small veins may be safely ligated. Results are excellent and recurrence is rare.

MINIMIZING VASCULAR COMPLICATIONS

Optimum patient care can occur only if invasive cardiologists, interventional radiologists, and vascular surgeons maintain close cooperation to rapidly identify and treat vascular complications of femoral artery diagnostic and interventional catheterization. Patients undergoing catheterization should have recorded a thorough and accurate peripheral vascular examination by an experienced examiner for comparison, should suspicion of a vascular complication arise after the procedure. Femoral catheterization should be carried out as expeditiously and atraumatically as possible. Technically expert mechanical hemostasis following catheter withdrawal cannot be overemphasized. The mechanical compression can be performed either by a skilled operator or by carefully applied and monitored mechanical C clamp. It must be emphasized that the choice of method is not as important as the technique. Steady and evenly applied pressure that occludes the arterial defect but allows luminal flow is essential. Any lapse leads to disruption of the primary clot and failure of the hemostatic process.

REFERENCES

1. McCann RL, Schwartz LB, Pieper KS. Vascular complications of cardiac catheterization. J Vasc Surg 1991; 14:375–381.
2. Messina LM, Brothers TE, Wakefield TW, et al. Clinical characteristics and surgical management of vascular complications in patients undergoing cardiac catheterization: Interventional versus diagnostic procedures. J Vasc Surg 1991; 13:593–600.
3. Oweida SW, Roubin GS, Smith RB III, Salam AA. Postcatheterization vascular complications associated with percutaneous transluminal coronary angioplasty. J Vasc Surg 1990; 12:310–315.
4. Muller DWM, Shamir KJ, Ellis SG, Topol EJ. Peripheral vascular complications after conventional and complex percutaneous coronary interventional procedures. Am J Cardiol 1992; 69:63–68.
5. Sheikh KH, Adams DB, McCann R, et al. Utility of Doppler color flow imaging for identification of femoral arterial complications of cardiac catheterization. Am Heart J 1989; 117:623–628.
6. Rivers SP, Lee ES, Lyon RT, et al. Successful conservative management of iatrogenic femoral arterial trauma. Ann Vasc Surg 1992; 6:45–49.
7. Agrawal SK, Pinheiro L, Roubin GS, et al. Nonsurgical closure of femoral pseudoaneurysms complicating cardiac catheterization and percutaneous transluminal coronary angioplasty. J Am Coll Cardiol 1992; 20:610–615.

ARTERIAL INJURIES ASSOCIATED WITH FRACTURES AND EXTENSIVE SOFT TISSUE TRAUMA

J. DAVID RICHARDSON, M.D.
DAVID A. SPAIN, M.D.

Prior to the Korean War, amputation rates for extremity trauma with associated vascular injury exceeded 50%. With development of modern techniques of vascular surgery, amputation rates for penetrating injuries fell during the Korean and Vietnam conflicts. Despite these advances in military care, amputation rates for lower extremity trauma with associated vascular injury in civilian series still range from 10% to 45%.[1] Two major factors are responsible: delay in recognition of vascular injury, especially at or below the popliteal artery; and extensive nerve and soft tissue damage associated with blunt civilian trauma.

MECHANISM

The mechanism of injury can be divided into three categories: blunt trauma, penetrating trauma, and industrial accidents. Angulation of the fractured segments, especially around the knee, leads to laceration or transection of the artery and vein. These patients present with an acutely ischemic limb with no distal pulses or Doppler signals. A small number have a partial arterial transection or an intimal injury and may present with intact pulses, only to have a subsequent thrombosis with delayed diagnosis.

Penetrating trauma causes injury by three means. The missile may directly injure the vessel or fracture long bones and lead to injury by angulation. Additionally, a close-range shotgun wound or high-velocity missile may produce a blast effect with intimal injury, pseudoaneurysm, or arteriovenous fistula.

INITIAL EVALUATION

Severe lower extremity injuries are very dramatic on presentation to the emergency department; however, many of these patients have other life-threatening injuries, and they must be resuscitated according to advanced trauma life support guidelines. During the survey, obvious dislocations and fractures should be immobilized and reduced, if possible. A thorough and accurate vascular and neurologic examination must be performed. If pulses are not palpable, Doppler ultrasound is used to detect arterial flow. When possible, the ankle:brachial index should be determined.

If a vascular injury is confirmed or suspected, extremity biplanar arteriography is usually necessary. The decision of whether to perform it in the radiology suite or operating room is based on patient and institutional factors. Active hemorrhage requiring immediate surgical control, prolonged ischemia, or lack of immediately available vascular radiology necessitates operative arteriography. In the lower extremity, this is done via a femoral cutdown with temporary inflow occlusion; in the upper extremity, axillary or brachial artery cutdown is used, depending on the level of injury. In our experience, this is usually sufficient to direct surgical exploration.

Patients with suspected or possible arterial injuries without ischemia or active hemorrhage are evaluated with biplanar arteriography in the radiology department. Most commonly these are patients with knee dislocations, intermittently palpable pulses before or after reduction, or proximity shotgun injuries. Based on a retrospective review of 37 patients, Dennis and associates have argued against routine arteriography in patients with posterior knee dislocations.[2] Half of their patients were excluded from arteriography based on physical examination alone; therefore, some of these patients may have had undiagnosed injuries. Follow-up averaged only 9 months, and delayed complications due to missed injuries may occur. Additionally, all seven injuries identified (three intimal defects and four narrowings) were treated nonoperatively. This approach is not widely accepted and is not practiced in our unit. Although arteriograms are often negative, orthopedic and soft tissue injuries often make it difficult to detect delayed thrombosis and ischemia. The cost of missed injuries—in terms of both limb function and medicolegal liability—is great. Therefore, we continue to recommend arteriography for patients with posterior knee dislocations.

Injuries to the infrapopliteal vessels are managed selectively. If at least one vessel is patent to the foot by arteriography and the ankle:brachial index exceeds 0.5, the patient is managed nonoperatively with frequent reassessment. If the ankle:brachial index is less than 0.5, fasciotomies are performed. If no vessels are patent, then surgical exploration is undertaken.[1] In a patient who has multiple injuries (including a lower extremity injury) that require treatment, we may choose to defer arteriography if there is a good Doppler signal at the ankle and a clearly viable foot. Arteriography can then be performed after other injuries are treated. In many trauma situations, the goal should be to return the patient to as normal a condition as possible. However, we do not attempt a bypass to the ankle if one trifurcation vessel is open. It is not needed and usually will thrombose, presumably secondary to competitive flow.

OPERATIVE MANAGEMENT

Patients must be prepared for combined vascular and orthopedic procedures. This includes use of an operating table compatible with x-rays and preparation of the entire involved extremity as well as of vein conduit harvest sites. The most commonly used vein is the saphenous from the uninjured extremity, although cephalic and internal jugular veins have to be used on occasion. The first operative priority is complete assessment of all injuries. Arteriography should be considered at this time if it was not done preoperatively. Occasionally, the arterial injury may be seen in the depth of the wound and can be directly approached without an arteriogram. The wound is explored to determine the nature and extent of arterial injuries and associated venous injuries. Nerve injury and type, contusion or transection, and soft tissue loss should be assessed.

Most vascular injuries associated with closed humeral or femoral fractures are relatively straightforward to repair. The bone should be stabilized and the vessel repaired. Occasionally, the surgeon is tempted to delay vascular repair because the extremity is viable. We discourage this approach and recommend immediate repair of these vascular injuries. Complex injuries with associated fractures, vessel injuries, and nerve and soft tissue loss are vexing problems.

Once all injuries have been assessed, the first operative decision is whether to attempt limb salvage. A variety of grading scales have been proposed to establish objective guidelines for predicting the unsalvageable extremity; however, most are subjective and too complex to be easily applied in the operating room.[3]

At the University of Louisville Hospital, we have developed a team approach to determine when primary amputation is warranted. All of these patients are evaluated operatively by experienced senior trauma and orthopedic surgeons. First, the patient's general condition and extent of other injuries, especially head injuries, must be considered. If the patient has other severe injuries, prolonged attempts at limb salvage may be detrimental, and primary amputation should be strongly considered. The more common and difficult scenario is the hemodynamically stable patient with moderate, but not immediately life-threatening, injuries. We believe the decision to amputate the lower limb should be based on the level of injury and the degree of nerve injury associated with the vascular injury. Complete sciatic nerve avulsion mandates amputation. Posterior tibial nerve transection results in an insensate foot and a 50% to 70% limb disability rate, and therefore should lower the threshold for primary amputation.[4] Most trauma patients are young males who do well with a below-knee prosthesis.[5] Therefore, if the injury is devastating and can be treated in one or two stages with below-knee amputation, this should be considered. Patients with amputations above the knee do not fare as well, and more aggressive attempts at limb salvage should be made in this situation. The decision to amputate an upper extremity is much more difficult and emotional. Because of psychological factors and prosthesis performance, more heroic attempts are made at upper extremity salvage.

If the senior surgeons involved believe a primary amputation is appropriate, we discuss this prospect clearly with the patient, if possible, and with the family. If we believe an amputation is the preferred treatment, then we strongly recommend this procedure. Patients or their surrogates invariably choose an option other than amputation if given a choice, even when that option is clearly less desirable. We believe that two senior surgeons, preferably from different disciplines, should clearly document the reason for primary amputation. These cases often undergo legal review retrospectively, and a clearly documented chart has many obvious advantages.

Once the decision has been made to attempt limb salvage, operative strategy must be determined. The sequence of orthopedic stabilization and revascularization is tailored to the patient. Patients with active hemorrhage or prolonged ischemia for longer than 4 to 6 hours should have vascular repair prior to orthopedic fixation. Additionally, patients in whom stabilization will prevent adequate exposure, especially of the popliteal artery, should have their vascular injuries addressed first. In the remaining patients, orthopedic stabilization may precede vascular repair. This allows adequate estimation of vessel loss, provides a stable framework for the repair, and prevents kinking and occlusion of the graft during subsequent stabilization. With severe bony instability or shortening, orthopedic fixation may be necessary before vascular repair, and it may take several hours to obtain. In these patients, use of a shunt to temporarily reestablish blood flow allows fixation without prolonging ischemic time. Several types of shunts can be used, but we generally prefer shunts used for carotid endarterectomy because they are readily available. If heparin sodium–bonded tubing is available in the proper size, it is excellent. All shunts require continuous attention by the vascular surgeon during the orthopedic procedure, as they may dislodge, kink, or occlude if unattended.

The injured artery is exposed and resected back to normal vessel. Many times this process precludes primary anastomosis. The favored conduit for most extremity arterial injuries is the reversed saphenous vein, harvested from the uninjured extremity. We perform extra-anatomic bypass in the following situations. First, if heavy contamination is present in the operative field, infection may occur in the graft. Second, when extensive bone injury may lead to delayed thrombosis because of luxuriant callus formation. Third, when questionable, nonviable muscle may lead to an exposed graft after later muscle debridement. Fourth, if there is insufficient soft tissue to cover the graft in its anatomic position, then extra-anatomic bypass is considered. If systemic anticoagulation is contraindicated, the distal vascular tree is filled with a dilute heparin-saline solution (20 units/ml).

Venous injuries should be repaired, if it is easily accomplished and does not significantly prolong operative time. Repair of the popliteal vein is especially important and should be attempted under most circumstances. However, most of these patients have extensive venous injuries, and ligation may often be necessary. The extremity should be elevated postoperatively to reduce edema. Yelon and Scalea reported on 48 patients with lower extremity or pelvic venous injuries treated with ligation. There was no increase in postoperative morbidity, need for fasciotomy, or leg edema in short-term follow-up.[6] In our experience, ligation of major venous wounds in the leg increases the need for fasciotomy and compartment pressures should be measured.

Necrotic muscle and fascia are debrided, and all muscle compartments are decompressed. We have used fasciotomy liberally. In our experience it contributes little to the long-term morbidity of these patients.[7] When the soft tissue defect is large, the first priority is given to coverage of the vascular graft with viable muscle. Inexperienced surgeons often do not realize the absolute necessity to have exposed grafts covered with viable tissue. Failure to ensure graft coverage has resulted in hemorrhage in 100% of the patients we have treated. The use of a muscle or skin flap to cover the repair is essential. We have occasionally covered short areas of exposed saphenous vein with a thin split-thickness skin graft, which may prevent breakdown of the conduit. Soft tissue wounds are treated with dressing changes and, if necessary, frequent debridement under general anesthesia. Recent improvements in free tissue transfer has allowed coverage of wounds with extensive soft tissue loss.[8]

POSTOPERATIVE CARE

Postoperative care must include careful monitoring of the vascular repair. Any change in the vascular examination must be promptly investigated with either surgical exploration or arteriogram. Attributing postoperative change in pulses or Doppler signals to spasm is a frequent mistake, leading to ischemia and delayed limb loss. Postoperative anticoagulation is not routinely used. Broad-spectrum antibiotics are begun preoperatively and continued for at least 5 days after operation, or longer if clinical course or culture results dictate.

After attempting limb salvage, the surgeon must objectively assess whether the limb is compromising the patient. This can be very difficult, as the patient and family often become emotionally attached to the salvaged limb postoperatively. The surgeon may fall prey to a similar attachment after having invested an enormous amount of effort toward saving the limb. Roessler and colleagues attempted to identify objective data to determine when the salvaged limb was compromising the patient and thereby provide guidelines for the decision to amputate postoperatively.[9] They reviewed their experience in 80 patients with isolated lower extremity injuries. Although the overall mortality was only 4%, all 3 deaths occurred in the 14 patients who presented without a pulse or Doppler signal in whom limb salvage was attempted. This represents a 21% mortality for this group of patients with isolated lower extremity injuries. All three of these patients had markedly positive (greater than 3 L) fluid balance in the first 24 hours after operation. The Roessler group recommended amputation postoperatively if the patient is systemically compromised as measured by fluid balance studies. If infection or systemic signs of tissue necrosis are present, amputation should generally be performed. The surgical dictum of not losing a life while trying to save a limb still applies.

OUTCOME

Long-term functional outcome data for these injuries are scarce. Most reports on complex extremity injuries have short-term follow-up on a small percentage of patients. Of those limbs salvaged, 40% to 50% of patients have a good result, and 20% to 30% are permanently disabled. Between 25% and 33% of salvaged limbs come to delayed amputation, usually because of nonunion, chronic osteomyelitis, or neuropathic ulcers.

Traumatic amputation in our experience is associated with acceptable functional results. In a review of 37 patients from our institution who suffered traumatic amputations, 19 of 26 (73%) patients with lower extremity amputations were wearing a prosthesis at long-term follow-up.[5] Drost and co-workers reported that seven of eight (88%) patients with primary amputation were found to be ambulatory and either working or attending school at follow-up.[10] If the patient is a candidate for a below-knee prosthesis, the results are generally excellent, and the patient can often be rapidly rehabilitated, compared to the months spent attempting to salvage a mangled lower leg.

REFERENCES

1. Flint LM, Richardson JD. Arterial injuries with lower extremity fracture. Surgery 1983; 93:5–8.
2. Dennis JW, Jagger C, Butcher C, et al. Reassessing the role of arteriograms in the management of posterior knee dislocations. J Trauma 1992; 32:955.
3. Bonanni F, Rhodes M, Lucke JF. The futility of predictive scoring of mangled extremities. J Trauma 1993; 34:99–104.
4. Aldea PA, Shaw WW. Management of acute lower extremity nerve injuries. Foot Ankle 1986; 7:82–94.
5. Seiler JG, Richardson JD. Amputation after extremity injury. Am J Surg 1986; 152:260–264.
6. Yelon JA, Scalea TM. Venous injuries of the lower extremity and pelvis: repair versus ligation. J Trauma 1992; 33:532–538.
7. Vitale GC, Richardson JD, George SM et al. Fasciotomy for severe, blunt and penetrating trauma of the extremity. Surg Gynecol Obstet 1988:397–401.
8. Gorman PW, Barnes CL, Fischer TJ, et al. Soft-tissue reconstruction in severe lower extremity trauma. Clin Orthop 1989; 243: 57–64.
9. Roessler MS, Wisner DH, Holcroft JW. The mangled extremity: When to amputate. Arch Surg 1991; 126:1243–1249.
10. Drost TF, Rosemurgy AS, Proctor D, et al. Outcome of treatment of combined orthopedic and arterial trauma to the lower extremity. J Trauma 1989; 29:1331–1334.

BLUNT ARTERIAL INJURIES TO THE KNEE

ALLAN R. DOWNS, M.D.

Popliteal artery injury associated with blunt trauma about the knee joint continues to be complicated by delayed diagnosis, severe ischemia, and amputation. In 1986 the author reported on 53 blunt injuries with an amputation rate of 30%.[1] In 1988 Wagner and colleagues reported an amputation rate of 15% in 100 consecutive patients with blunt popliteal artery injuries.[2] When preoperative ischemia was present, their amputation rate was 23%.[2]

A high index of suspicion for arterial injury in the emergency room must exist for all patients suffering blunt injury to the lower extremity. Most of these patients are motor vehicle accident victims, either pedestrians or occupants, and many have multiple injuries. Upper tibial fractures and unrecognized knee dislocations are most often associated with popliteal artery injuries. These skeletal injuries result from a hyperextension force applied at the knee. This hyperextension creates traction on the popliteal artery that may cause intimal disruption with thrombosis or complete transection, which often does not bleed because the adventitia is pulled over the ends of the retracted artery. The popliteal vein and nerves are often injured by the traction, although nerve disruption is rare. Additional soft tissue trauma interferes with the collateral circulation and accentuates the ischemia.

DIAGNOSIS

Popliteal artery injuries must be suspected in all patients with lower extremity trauma, particularly with knee dislocation, upper tibial fractures, and supracondylar femoral fractures. Closed knee dislocations may not be recognized as the reduction of the dislocation may be accomplished at the scene of the accident or during transportation. Combined femoral shaft and upper tibial fractures may have an associated unrecognized knee disruption. The presence of clinical signs of ischemia such as a cool, pale or cyanosed, pulseless foot makes immediate vascular assessment mandatory. On occasion, assessment is complicated by associated multiple injuries in an unstable patient. Comparison with the opposite extremity, if uninjured, is usually helpful. A Doppler examination by an experienced observer allows assessment of the adequacy of the circulation. The absence of a Doppler signal at the ankle demands further urgent assessment. The presence of a signal does not exclude a popliteal injury. In the uncooperative or unconscious patient, assessment of sensory and motor function may not be reliable.

The most common cause of delay in treatment is failure to recognize the severity of the ischemia. Frequently, pulses are documented as present preoperatively, but a completely disrupted popliteal artery is found. Capillary return as a sign of adequate blood flow is not reliable. X-rays are necessary to assess the associated skeletal injury and, if time permits, arteriography can be performed at this time. In the presence of severe ischemia, it is preferable to perform arteriography in the operating room or to explore the artery directly. In multiple fractures of the extremity, the arterial injury is not always at the site of the obvious fracture, and for that reason arteriography may be helpful. In the presence of severe ischemia, undue delay to obtain arteriograms in the radiology suite is not desirable.

MANAGEMENT

The priorities of treatment must be determined. Life-threatening injuries take precedence over management of the limb injury, but complete muscle ischemia beyond 6 hours causes irreversible muscle necrosis.[3] The patient should be stabilized rapidly. After adequate assessment, if a popliteal injury is suspected, the objective should be to restore circulation as soon as possible. If the ischemia is critical and there will be an undue delay in obtaining arteriography, the patient should be taken directly to the operating room for popliteal exploration. If associated abdominal or chest injuries require surgical management, two operating teams should be available to keep the period of limb ischemia at a minimum. The 6 hour time frame from onset of ischemia to restoration of blood flow should be constantly reviewed. In isolated popliteal injuries, heparinization is indicated, if the patient is stable. Both legs should be prepared from the groin to the foot with plastic foot drapes to allow assessment of the distal circulation and access for fasciotomy when indicated.

Vascular Repair

When ischemia is present, arterial repair should be performed before skeletal fixation. Rarely is the limb so unstable that fixation is necessary prior to arterial repair. If the limb is flail because of multiple fractures of the femoral shaft and tibia, arterial blood flow can be re-established with a temporary shunt while the femoral fracture is stabilized. The patient should be heparinized, if it is not contraindicated by other injuries. We do not use a tourniquet as bleeding is rarely a problem.

The popliteal artery is exposed with a medial incision. To gain access to the full length of the popliteal artery, it is necessary to divide the gracilis, semitendinosis, sartorius, and semimembranosis tendons as well as the medial head of the gastrocnemius muscle. This exposure allows complete assessment of the popliteal artery and vein. It allows mobilization of the popliteal artery with ligation of geniculate branches on the proximal segment to permit a primary end-to-end anastomosis in almost half the patients treated.[1]

There may be more than one injury in the popliteal artery, and for that reason it should be visualized down to the anterior tibial origin. Occasionally the anterior tibial artery is avulsed, and the tibial peroneal trunk is injured, which then mandates a segmental vein graft replacement or bypass to the tibioperoneal trunk or posterior tibial artery.

Full mobilization of the proximal popliteal artery allows 2 cm of artery to be excised without compromising a tension-free end-to-end anastomosis. The ends of the artery are spatulated, triangulation stitches are placed, and then the anastomosis is completed with interrupted or continuous polypropylene sutures between the stay stitches. In small arteries, the anastomosis is completed with interrupted sutures. When the injury is more extensive with complete disruption of the artery, a reversed saphenous vein graft is used for replacement. The ipsilateral or contralateral saphenous vein from the thigh is used. We have generally used the ipsilateral saphenous vein when the popliteal vein is not injured, as it is more convenient. This practice has not contributed to any significant problem with venous drainage. When a vein graft is used, the proximal anastomosis is done first to allow better assessment of the appropriate length of the graft to avoid kinking. The ends of the vein are spatulated to allow a large anastomosis. Backflow should be assessed, and the distal artery should be irrigated with heparin saline. A Fogarty catheter should be carefully passed proximally and distally to extract any thrombus. In severe ischemia there may be little or no backflow. Completion arteriography is essential to assess the adequacy of the repair and determine the status of the outflow. Frequently spasm is present in the distal arterial tree, and intra-arterial papaverine may be helpful. The arteriogram may document extravasation of contrast medium into the tissue, indicating fluid leak and poor muscle perfusion. Both findings suggest the need for fasciotomy.

If the popliteal vein is disrupted, it should be repaired if possible, but vein grafting for popliteal vein injury is not advocated. When the popliteal vein is injured, the contralateral saphenous vein should be used, if required for arterial repair. We have used a segment of the injured popliteal vein for arterial repair, with an arteriogram 25 later documenting a functioning graft. The patient has small varicosities but no evidence of chronic venous insufficiency. Recent experience reported by Timberlake and colleagues suggests that concomitant venous repair is not as critical as was previously thought.[4]

Orthopedic Management

Except in the presence of a flail limb, the skeletal fixation is usually not necessary until the arterial repair has been performed. Internal fixation is usually not necessary immediately, and definitive knee reconstruction is not advocated in the presence of arterial injury. Usually, adequate stabilization can be attained with external fixation devices that allow access to the limb for postoperative assessment and wound care. Delayed internal fixation may be desirable. Immobilization in traction when indicated is acceptable but is usually supplemented by external fixation devices.

It is essential that the arterial repair be reassessed after the orthopedic procedures. On only one occasion have we found it necessary to revise the arterial repair after the fracture stabilization. No attempt is made to determine the presence of nerve injury, which is nearly always due to neuropraxia and ischemia. In the acute stage it is difficult to ascertain the cause of the neurologic deficit. Every attempt should be made to obtain viable soft tissue coverage over the arterial repair. This is usually not a problem, but in massive soft tissue injury a consultation with a plastic surgeon may be desirable.

Compartment Syndrome and Reperfusion Injury

Muscle compartments should be assessed before, during, and after arterial reconstruction. If ischemia has been prolonged beyond 6 hours and if the compartments are tense preoperatively, four-compartment fasciotomy with two full-length medial and lateral incisions should be performed. If the compartments become tense after revascularization, fasciotomy should be performed. We have used clinical assessment to determine the need for fasciotomy. Compartment pressure measurements may be useful, and it is suggested that a tissue pressure greater than 40 mm Hg dictates fasciotomy.[5] We do not think fasciotomy should be done routinely. When fasciotomy is not performed at the time of revascularization, close postoperative assessment of the muscle compartments is necessary, and pressure measurements may then be useful. Frequently, a preoperative associated nerve injury precludes the use of neurologic examination as an indication for decompression. Fasciotomy predisposes to infection, and early skin coverage is desirable. Mannitol may be helpful in the prevention and management of the reperfusion injury.[6] Mannitol is given preoperatively and continued postoperatively in the presence of severe ischemia.

POSTOPERATIVE CARE

Careful frequent monitoring with Doppler ultrasound is essential to determine the patency of the repair. Any suspicion of failure with recurrence of ischemia demands arteriography for reassessment. Occlusion of the repair requires immediate revision. Distal pulses are often not present early postoperatively so their absence is not a reliable sign of occlusion.

The limb is often insensate because of the neuropraxia, and care is necessary to avoid pressure necrosis of the skin. This is particularly applicable to the heel pad and Achilles tendon area, which are often weight-bearing sites in bed or in a sling. We have found it helpful to put a Steinman pin through the calcaneus to maintain limb suspension without heel pressure.

The amputation rate remains high for blunt popliteal artery injuries, mainly because of delay in diagnosis and treatment. In our experience there were no amputations in patients with ischemia of less than 6 hours when a primary anastomosis of the popliteal artery could be accomplished.[1] Amputation rates are higher with vein graft repair, reflecting the presence of more extensive injuries and greater probability of occlusions of the repair. In ischemia present for more than 12 hours, the amputation rate is higher than 50%.[1] Even though the amputation rate has been greatly reduced, the long-term morbidity of the ischemia remains high because of irreversible muscle and nerve injury.

REFERENCES

1. Downs AR, MacDonald P. Popliteal artery injuries: Civilian experience with sixty-three patients during a twenty-four year period (1960–1984). J Vasc Surg 1986; 4:55–62.
2. Wagner WW, Culkins ER, Weaver FA, et al. Blunt popliteal artery trauma: One hundred consecutive injuries. J Vasc Surg 1988; 7:736–748.
3. Miller HH, Welch CS. Quantitative studies of the time factor in arterial injuries. Ann Surg 1949; 130:428–438.
4. Timberlake GA, O'Connell RC, Kerstein MD. Venous Injury: To repair or ligate, the dilemma. J Vasc Surg 1986; 4:553–558.
5. Whiteside TE, Haney TC, Harada H, et al. A simple method for tissue pressure determination. Arch Surg 1975; 110:1311–1313.
6. Buchbinder D, Karmody AM, Leather RP, Shah DM. Hypertonic mannitol: Its use in the prevention of revascularization syndrome after acute arterial ischemia. Arch Surg 1981; 46:725–729.

VASCULAR INJURY SECONDARY TO DRUG ABUSE

ALBERT E. YELLIN, M.D.
JOSEPH H. FRANKHOUSE, M.D.
FRED A. WEAVER, M.D.

The 1960s spawned a marked increase in intravenous drug abuse (IVDA) with a concomitant increase in vascular complications. Previously, most drug-related vascular injuries were due to inadvertent intra-arterial injections of barbiturates by anesthesiologists. Regardless of etiology, there can be injuries to arteries, veins, and lymphatics. The range of problems includes soft tissue abscesses, septic phlebitis, deep venous thrombosis, mycotic aneurysms, and accidental intra-arterial injection with arterial occlusion. Therefore, treatment of these patients requires a basic understanding of the principles of antibiotic therapy, wound debridement, anticoagulation, revascularization, amputation, and rehabilitation. It is imperative that the treating physician recognize when therapeutic intervention may be effective in limiting tissue or limb loss.

Vascular injuries, whether iatrogenic or due to IVDA, can be caused by several mechanisms. There are three common etiologies: direct trauma caused by the needle during intravascular injection, an inflammatory response to the injected materials or to a bacterial inoculation and toxic effect of the drug, the diluents, or impurities in the drug mixture.

In both arterial and venous injections, direct needle trauma is rarely the sole cause of vascular injury unless repetitive to the same site. Rather, it incites the inflammatory response responsible for healing and coagulation. Needle puncture in combination with local sepsis can contribute to destruction of the vascular wall with resultant mycotic aneurysm formation or septic phlebitis. Cytotoxic impurities are a major component of illicit drugs, particularly street drugs, which are self-made with fillers and diluents in contaminated environments. Many of these additives have been shown to initiate thrombosis either directly or via inflammatory mediators. With an intravenous (IV) injection, the drug and its impurities are progressively diluted in the venous circulation. This reduces but does not eliminate the likelihood of an immediate inflammatory or thrombotic event. Following an intra-arterial injection, the mixture of drug and impurities becomes progressively more concentrated as the arterial tree divides distally, thus increasing the possibility of inciting an inflammatory reaction and subsequent thrombosis. Rarely does the vascular injury result from a single etiology. Most are multifactorial and vary from patient to patient.

The drugs used most often are those most in vogue or available. They are limited only by the imagination of the user and the marketplace. There are numerous additives and diluents (Table 1).[1,2] Heroin, cocaine, methamphetamine, and meperidine are among the most commonly abused drugs. In most cases the preparations are self-made, often from crushed oral medications, and therefore have a multiplicity of impurities. Magnesium silicate (talc) is an important component of oral tablets, thereby making it the most frequently cited additive associated with complications. Lactose and starch are two other commonly used additives associated with street drugs. Iatrogenic injuries usually occur with intra-arterial injections of chemically pure barbiturates and sedatives designed for parenteral use.

Table 1 Commonly Injected Substances

Drugs	Additives
Bismuth	Betose
Chlorpromazine (Thorazine)	Caffeine
Cocaine	Colloidal silica
Codeine	Cornstarch
Dextroamphetamine	Dibasic calcium phosphate
Diazepam	Gelatin
Hydromorphone (Dilaudid)	Lactose
Hydroxyzine (Vistaril)	Magnesium silicate (talc)
Lorazepam	Magnesium stearate
Meperidine	Procaine
Mephenesin (Myonesin)	Psyllium
Methylphenidate (Ritalin)	Quinine
Pentobarbital	Sodium bicarbonate
Pentazocine (Talwin)	Starch
Phenylcyclidine (PCP)	Sucrose
Phenytoin (Dilantin)	
Promazine (Sparine)	
Propoxyphene (Darvon)	
Secobarbital	
Thiopental (Pentothal)	

SYSTEMIC COMPLICATIONS

Systemically, IVDA may have several manifestations. Most systemic sequelae rarely come to the attention of the vascular surgeon but are important considerations in the overall care of the patient. Bacterial endocarditis due to bacteremia has been well described. These valvular vegetations, usually on the tricuspid valve, are associated with a significant cardiac morbidity and require up to 6 weeks of antibiotic therapy or, in advanced resistant cases, require valve excision.

Necrotizing angiitis, indistinguishable from periarteritis nodosa, has also been reported. It is most prevalent in individuals injecting methamphetamines. This entity may manifest itself clinically with hypertension, renal failure, and pulmonary edema, involving small arteries of the kidneys, heart, brain, and gastrointestinal tract.[3] Treatment is supportive.

SOFT TISSUE COMPLICATIONS

Soft tissue infections constitute a major cause of hospital admissions for IV drug abusers. The use of unsterile needles and syringes results in repeated bouts of cellulitis. These infections lead to fibrosis and eventual loss of the dermal and deep lymphatics. This effect is most notable in addicts who "skin pop," that is, inject their drugs subcutaneously. As the extremity loses lymphatic channels, the risk of cellulitis and further lymphatic destruction increases. In this setting, simple cases of cellulitis, which ordinarily could be treated with antibiotics, often progress to frank subcutaneous abscesses.[1] Occasionally, necrotizing fasciitis may develop.

Abscesses occur at the sites most frequently injected, and the groin is a common location. The antecubital fossa, axilla, neck, and lower leg may also be involved. Neck abscesses may result from cervical injection and if untreated, they could lead to airway compromise. Any abscess in juxtaposition to an artery, regardless of whether it is pulsatile, could represent a mycotic aneurysm.

Although most cases of superficial cellulitis do not come to the attention of the surgeon, the more advanced cases of septic phlebitis and soft tissue abscess usually do. Many cases of superficial septic phlebitis result in an abscess, and therapy is similar. The microbiologic profile of these patients reflects the mouth contact many drug addicts use in the preparation of their drugs and needles. *Staphylococcus aureus* is a common pathogen, and over 40% are methicillin resistant. However, the more common oral flora, such as streptococcal species and anaerobic species, like *Peptostreptococcus* and *Bacteroides*, are also often found in cultures of these abscesses. The mainstay of therapy for the soft tissue abscess is operative incision and drainage. In many patients a thrombosed vein, with or without purulence, is identified. The involved vein must be removed in its entirety. The skin is left open to heal either by secondary intention or by delayed primary closure 4 to 5 days later. In necrotizing soft tissue infection, it is essential that all devitalized tissue be widely debrided.

As a cautionary note, a radiograph of the involved area should be taken preoperatively because the broken needle tips that are often encountered could place the unwary surgeon at risk for a needle stick. Many IV drug abusers are infected with hepatitis or human immunodeficiency virus and place the treating surgical team at risk. Universal precautions for infection should be followed.

VENOUS COMPLICATIONS

Typically, venous injuries are the result of chronic or repetitive trauma and usually do not require surgical intervention. The local irritation to the venous endothelium results in sclerosis and subsequent thrombosis. Gradually the superficial veins are lost, and the extremity relies on deep veins for drainage. The sclerotic process may extend to the deep veins and the fibrosis to the surrounding soft tissue. These patients are at high risk for deep vein thrombosis (DVT) due to the compression caused by fibrosis. Drug addicts occasionally lose consciousness after injecting and leave on a tourniquet for extended periods of time. This practice may lead to DVT. Thrombosis of the deep veins is frequently seen in the larger draining veins cephalad to the injection sites, and is therefore not due to direct needle trauma. Many of these patients present with the insidious onset of a swollen, painful extremity due to their chronic DVT. Others have nonspecific systemic complaints such as arthralgias and myalgias. Septic phlebitis of the deep venous system must be considered when the presentation includes fever, leukocytosis, and positive blood cultures. The organism most commonly recovered from secondarily infected thrombi is *S. aureus,* often methicillin resistant.

The groin veins are most readily accessible; therefore, lower extremity DVT is more common than upper extremity DVT. Nonetheless, brachial, axillary, and subclavian vein thromboses have all been reported in drug addicts who do not have any other known risk factors for DVT. Central vein thrombosis and sepsis have also been reported in drug abusers who have an indwelling central venous catheter. Although most cases of central vein thrombosis respond to catheter removal, antibiotic or antifungal therapy, and anticoagulation, resistant cases may require surgical thrombectomy.[4]

The sequelae of DVT in IV drug abusers are not unique to this population. Pulmonary embolism remains the most lethal risk, and although more frequently caused by lower extremity DVT, the source can be from upper extremity veins. The initial presentation may be that of pulmonary embolism, and in addicts these may be septic emboli, thereby adding bacterial endocarditis and lung abscesses as potential secondary complications.

Classically, physical examination in patients with DVT is notoriously insensitive, with a false negative rate greater than 50%. Findings such as edema, erythema, pain, Homans' sign, or phlegmasia may be present, but the absence of such signs does not rule out the diagnosis. Confirmatory tests such as color flow duplex or phlebography are usually diagnostic.

Anticoagulant therapy remains the cornerstone of treatment for any patient with DVT. Intravenous infusion of heparin sodium should be started with an initial IV bolus of 5,000 to 10,000 IU, followed by a continuous infusion of approximately 1000 IU/hour. The goal of therapy is to maintain the partial thromboplastin time at 2 to 2.5 times control, hoping to prevent clot propagation and mitigate symptoms. Sodium warfarin can be instituted concurrently and continued on an outpatient basis with close monitoring to maintain a prothrombin time of 2 to 3 times control. The length of therapy ranges from 6 to 12 weeks. Long-term therapy is difficult because of the unreliability of the drug addict population. It should be noted that vancomycin, often needed in the treatment of septic DVT, is inactivated by heparin sodium when the two are mixed together in the same IV line.

Although aneurysms are traditionally thought of as

involving arteries, the common femoral vein can become pseudoaneurysmal after repeated injection. These are similar to an arterial mycotic aneurysm. Such patients usually present with a painful groin mass, half of which are associated with cellulitis but usually are not pulsatile. An unwary incision and drainage of suspected groin abscesses without needle aspiration or duplex examination can result in major hemorrhage. Treatment entails complete excision of the affected vein, proximal, and distal ligation.

ARTERIAL COMPLICATIONS

Mycotic Aneurysm

Sir William Osler, in 1885, first described mycotic aneurysms. They were manifested by arterial wall destruction and aneurysm formation caused by emboli from endocarditis. This term has come to include any aneurysm or pseudoaneurysm caused by an embolic or local infectious process.[5] In the drug abuser with a painful inguinal or antecubital mass, the differential diagnosis must include, in addition to soft tissue abscess, femoral or brachial artery mycotic aneurysm.

The pathogenesis of mycotic aneurysms entails repetitive needle trauma of the artery or vein and bacterial inoculation of the area surrounding the vessel. The local sepsis, combined with trauma, leads to eventual destruction of the vessel wall and subsequent pseudoaneurysm formation. The arterial wall may become aneurysmal without direct arterial needle trauma if the infection extends from an adjacent site or if bacterial emboli lodge in the vasa vasora of the vessel wall and cause destruction.[5]

Careful pretreatment evaluation of any soft tissue mass in juxtaposition to an artery is critically important to avoid the potential complication of massive hemorrhage during casual incision and drainage of a presumed abscess that is, in reality, a mycotic aneurysm. Arterial mycotic aneurysms are pulsatile in only half the patients and are inconsistently associated with bruits or loss of distal pulses. Therefore, the clinical diagnosis is frequently difficult. Additionally, unsuspected arteriovenous fistulas are encountered in approximately 5% of patients with mycotic aneurysms. Arteriograms have been the gold standard for confirming the diagnosis of mycotic aneurysm. Recently, ultrasonography has been used reliably to diagnose the presence of a mycotic aneurysm, to differentiate not only the degree of tissue involvement but also the structures involved (artery or vein) and document the presence of thrombus.[6] It is prudent to enlist one of these diagnostic tools prior to embarking on any exploration of a groin mass and to explore them only in the operating room.

The complications of mycotic aneurysms include rupture, thrombosis, or distal embolization with resultant gangrene. These complications can develop rapidly and require urgent treatment. The basis of treatment is parenteral antibiotics, wide debridement of all infected tissue, proximal and distal ligation of the aneurysmal vessel, and removal of the entire infected arterial segment. If diseased artery remains, delayed rupture can occur.

The issue of revascularization, whether immediate or delayed, is controversial. Brachial mycotic aneurysms can almost uniformly be excised and ligated without ischemic sequelae. In the groin, severe ischemia following ligation of the superficial or deep femoral arteries is uncommon. Surprisingly, severe ischemic complications occur in less than half of those undergoing ligation of the common femoral artery. Routine revascularization is complicated by the fact that autogenous venous conduits are usually not available in the drug abuser. There is a 50% incidence of bacteremia, and a high septic complication rate in those undergoing bypass with a synthetic graft. Postoperative graft infection, hemorrhage, and amputation frequently occur. Therefore, many surgeons employ revascularization only when absolutely necessary. There is no consensus regarding selective immediate revascularization or selective delayed revascularization.

Our approach is similar to that of Padberg and associates, who advocated performing immediate bypass only if postligation operative Doppler blood flow was unobtainable.[7] Autogenous conduits should be used when possible, infected tissue planes should be avoided, and anastomoses made only to noninvolved segments of artery. In the groin, obturator bypass and lateral circumflex bypass have been employed. For patients not requiring immediate revascularization, the decision to perform a delayed bypass is based on the postoperative development of ischemic symptoms. Subsequent revascularization is usually unnecessary because these patients are relatively young with excellent collateral blood flow. If clinically important ischemia develops, delayed revascularization can be accomplished after the tissues have healed and the infection cleared, thereby permitting in-line reconstruction.

Neck injections can result in carotid mycotic aneurysms. A painful neck mass near a major blood vessel should alert the physician to the possibility of a mycotic aneurysm. Ultrasonography can be used as a diagnostic or screening tool, and arteriography may also be required to delineate the anatomy. In these patients, the common carotid artery is usually involved and carotid ligation can be safely done. There have been no neurologic sequelae in the cases reported.

Septic emboli from heart valve vegetations may result in mycotic aneurysms anywhere in the body. Pulmonary artery mycotic aneurysms result from right heart valvular vegetations. These have been noted on autopsy and have also been associated with lung abscesses. They do not require surgical intervention but are treated with appropriate antibiotic therapy. Left heart vegetations may result in septic emboli to the systemic arteries, most commonly involving intracerebral, renal, adrenal, splenic, and mesenteric vessels.

Of importance to the vascular surgeon are mycotic aneurysms involving the superior mesenteric artery (SMA). The clinical presentation usually includes bacterial endocarditis combined with chronic or acute abdominal pain due to ischemic or gangrenous bowel. Visceral mycotic aneurysms are usually not palpable and are rarely diagnosed prior to rupture. The microbiology reflects the cardiac source of the emboli and usually involves *S. aureus*. If gut ischemia is suspected, visceral arteriography to localize the aneurysm is recommended, followed by antibiotics and arterial excision. Revascularization is recommended only if bowel ischemia develops after SMA ligation. It is rarely necessary because adequate collateral blood flow usually develops in response to gradual occlusion of the visceral vessels.[8] Operative Doppler evaluation of the mesenteric vessels can establish the presence of adequate blood flow.

Intra-arterial Injection

Chronic IV drug abuse leads to sclerosis of the veins and the loss of readily accessible surface veins. As the addict searches for deeper veins, the likelihood of an accidental intra-arterial drug injection (IADI) is more likely. Whereas many complications of IVDA are chronic or indolent, IADI is possibly the most devastating and emergent injury facing the vascular surgeon. Acute limb ischemia involving small vessels invariably results, and tissue loss is a frequent occurrence. As yet, an ideal, universally effective treatment regimen has yet to be agreed upon.

In 1942, Van der Post reported the first case of iatrogenic IADI with pentothal.[9] Most early cases reported were secondary to inadvertent injections by anesthesiologists. As illicit recreational drug abuse became more common, the frequency of IADI rose. The additives and impurities of homemade preparations are an important mechanism in causing the arterial injury. Of equal or greater importance, these patients often delay seeking medical attention and may not be capable of providing adequate histories.

Vascular anatomy is an important factor in both iatrogenic and drug abuser IADI. The antecubital fossa is the most common site of injection for both. Anesthesiologists and drug addicts preferentially search this area for IV access. The left antecubital fossa is more commonly used in addicts, who use the dominant right hand to inject. Distal to the elbow, the brachial artery lies superficially and medial to the biceps tendon, immediately prior to bifurcating. It is most frequently injected at this location. The radial artery is anatomically the more superficial of the two branches, and in some patients the radial artery runs just deep to the fascia, making it an easy inadvertent target. For these reasons, more than 80% of IADI involve either the radial or brachial arteries.[2,10] Although the brachial artery usually divides below the elbow, in 10% of patients the bifurcation lies proximally. In that scenario the ulnar artery, which usually runs deep, comes to lie superficially and is involved in IADI. The incidence of IADI is increased in patients with aberrant arterial anatomy.

Small series and case reports of IADI have been published but, because of the low incidence of this problem, no prospective randomized treatment protocols have been done. In 1972, at the Los Angeles County–University of Southern California (LAC + USC) Medical Center, Gaspar and Hare[10] reported our early experience with 20 drug abusers with IADI treated over 3 years. In 1990, Treiman and colleagues reported another 48 patients. Since that time, we have seen only one patient on the Vascular Service. This clinical problem may be becoming less common, possibly due to a downward trend in IV drug abuse. However, additional cases of both iatrogenic IADI and drug addicts' IADI are reported, indicating that this clinical entity is still important. It is important to understand the pathophysiology of the injury and the principles of treatment.

A variety of theories have been suggested to explain the resultant limb ischemia in IADI. Early reports sought to implicate arterial spasm as the sole cause. It was thought that there was an immediate direct toxic effect of the injected material on the endothelium. Other theories included embolization of particulate matter, pH alteration with drug crystallization, platelet aggregation, release of thromboxane, and sympathetic release with concomitant vasospasm.

Nonetheless, the end result of IADI seems to be both arterial and venous endothelial injury, leading to venospasm and venous thrombosis. The drug itself or the impurities can be cytotoxic to the endothelium, leading to intimal disruption and vessel wall necrosis. The venous thrombosis then propagates to the arteriolar system, where further endothelial damage and coagulation occur. Lazarus and co-workers made these experimental observations and proposed that norepinephrine release, due to IADI, acts directly or via mediators on venous endothelium leading to venoconstriction. They alternatively hypothesized that acid crystals formed by pH changes may pass through arteriovenous fistulas, leading to venous occlusion and thrombosis.[11] The initial injury, even with IADI, is to the small veins (Fig. 1). The injury seen in IADI is in the small vessels which may extend, albeit rarely, to larger arteries (Fig. 2). The resultant ischemia, therefore, involves mostly digits, and the rest of the limb is less commonly affected.

Therefore, the initial vascular insult from IADI may be a venous injury followed secondarily by arterial injury and ischemia. Outflow obstruction from the venous thrombosis slows capillary blood flow and increases capillary pressure. As this capillary pressure exceeds plasma oncotic pressure, fluid transudation into the interstitium occurs. With increased interstitial pressure, soft tissue perfusion is impaired and tissue ischemia develops. Secondary arterial insufficiency may develop and, combined with venous stasis, often results in ischemic necrosis. Clinically, this sequence of events presents as edema, which can be strikingly severe, followed by stagnation of blood flow with cyanosis.

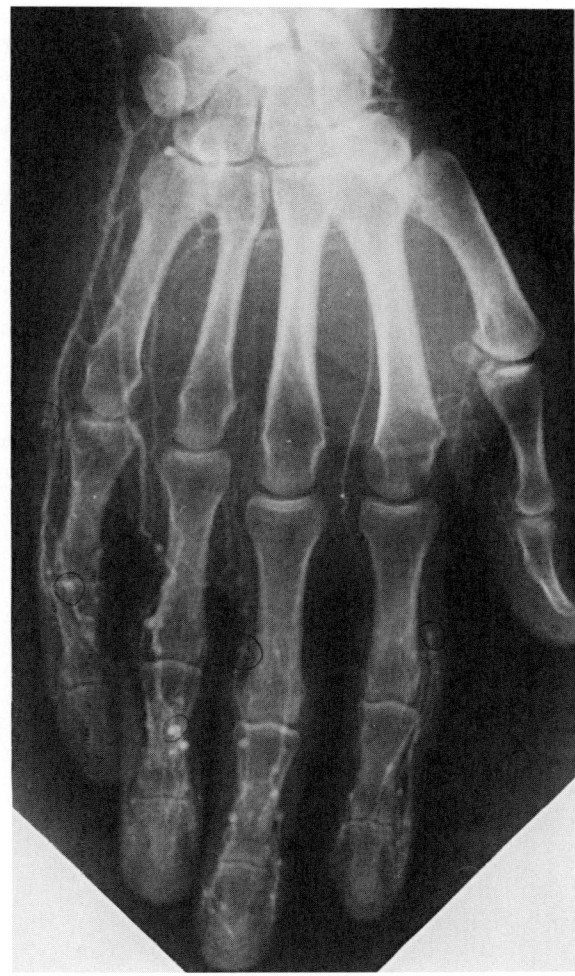

Figure 1 Venous phase of an arteriogram documents sequential venous thrombosis and venous microaneurysms.

Secondary arterial insufficiency and tissue hypoxia result in a cool extremity with progressive neurologic deterioration and, ultimately, gangrene. In these patients emergent intervention is imperative to prevent the ischemia from progressing to necrosis and loss of tissue or function.

The patient's history is usually helpful. Typically the patient describes an intense pain immediately after injection, without the usual drug-induced high. Often these patients are writhing in pain and holding the affected extremity. Narcotic pain relief may be required simply to obtain a history. If pulsation was used to identify an injection site, if the aspirated blood was redder than usual, or if weakness, numbness, or swelling rapidly ensued, the diagnosis is evident. Pain, however, is the most frequent symptom and often it overshadows all others.

Physical examination should attempt to assess the degree of tissue injury. An injection puncture wound might be evident (Fig. 3). The most immediately obvious finding is edema. The fingers and wrist are often fixed in a flexed clawlike position. The swelling can appear so extreme as to question the need for emergent fasciotomy for compartment syndrome. Few patients, however, ever develop compartment syndrome. Compartment pressures can be obtained. Fasciotomy is ordinarily required for pressures exceeding 40 mm Hg. Although reports cite the need for fasciotomy, we believe that it is rarely indicated and have yet to perform one in any of the 69 patients seen at LAC + USC.

Mottling, cyanosis, or outright gangrenous changes are most prominent in the digits, reflecting the small vessel thrombosis. Sensory loss is often present and should be documented by a careful neurologic examination. Further examination should assess the distal pulses. However, normal pulses do not lessen the risk of distal ischemia. The distal pulse is often normal or accentuated, owing to the degree of outflow obstruction. Strong pulsation only helps differentiate IADI from other forms of injury causing limb ischemia.

In our experience, the severity of the injury correlates with the clinical signs. All patients have edema, and most have cyanosis. These are early changes and not invariably associated with irreversible injury. The development of temperature loss and sensory deficit represents more significant injury that is more likely to result in permanent neurologic dysfunction or tissue loss.

The use of arteriography to assess the extent of arterial occlusion is controversial. Some use it routinely, some not at all, and some selectively. Arteriography has been used not only to document the initial damage but also to follow the response to treatment.[12] Others use it only in a pulseless extremity where there is a suspicion of a thrombus in a major artery. These studies generally document thrombosis of the digital arteries. Arteriograms do not assist in planning therapy or operation because revascularization is not an option. Rarely, large-vessel thrombosis occurs due to the trauma of the arterial puncture. If this is suspected, arteriography is performed and thrombectomy carried out. We believe that arteriography may aggravate the ischemic injury, infrequently assists in the treatment, and should be used very selectively.

Beginning in 1972, a treatment regimen was developed using heparin sodium, dextran, dexamethasone, and elevation. Active and passive range-of-motion therapy was begun as soon as tolerated. Analgesics were used to control pain. This therapy resulted in 30% of patients losing one or more digits but no major limb loss.

Treiman and colleagues, in 1990, reported our results in a subsequent group of 48 patients treated similarly between 1972 and 1988.[2] The treatment protocol is essentially similar and that which we currently recommend. This regimen includes heparin sodium 10,000 units intravenously, followed by a continuous infusion to keep the partial thromboplastin time 1.5 to 2.5 times control; dexamethasone 4 mg IV every 6 hours; low-molecular-weight dextran (Dextran 40) intravenous infusion at 20 cc/hour; opiates or other analgesics for pain control; extremity elevation in an Osborne sling; and early use of passive and active range-of-motion exercises. Patients are treated until all acute symptoms resolve and there is return to a normal extremity, necrosis ensues, or a stable functional deficit results. This typically requires a minimum of 72 hours of treatment, ranging up to 8 days. Physical therapy may be required for several months. Debridement of ischemic tissue is delayed until there is frank demarcation in order to preserve the maximum amount of tissue.

Our treatment protocol was designed to minimize the various pathologic events that lead to tissue hypoxia and gangrene, namely, stasis, thrombosis, inflammation, and edema. Heparin sodium is used to prevent thrombosis or propagation of clot in small veins and the capillary microcirculation, thereby preventing outflow obstruction, stasis, and occlusion of the arteries. Dexamethasone is used to protect cellular integrity, limit edema, and control the release of inflammatory mediators in response to tissue ischemia. Dextran minimizes platelet aggregation and sludging in small vessels. Elevation serves to reduce edema and alleviate stasis. Early mobilization with active and passive range-of-motion exercises minimizes contracture development and residual motor deficit.

We previously developed a tissue ischemia score (TIS) to assign prognostic significance to the findings present on initial presentation.[2] This score records as normal or abnormal the four clinical parameters of color, capillary refill, sensory function, and limb temperature. Specifically, the limb may appear cyanotic, with capillary refill more than 3 seconds, a motor or sensory deficit, or cool to touch, all of which indicate significant abnormal findings. Generally, patients with one or two abnormal

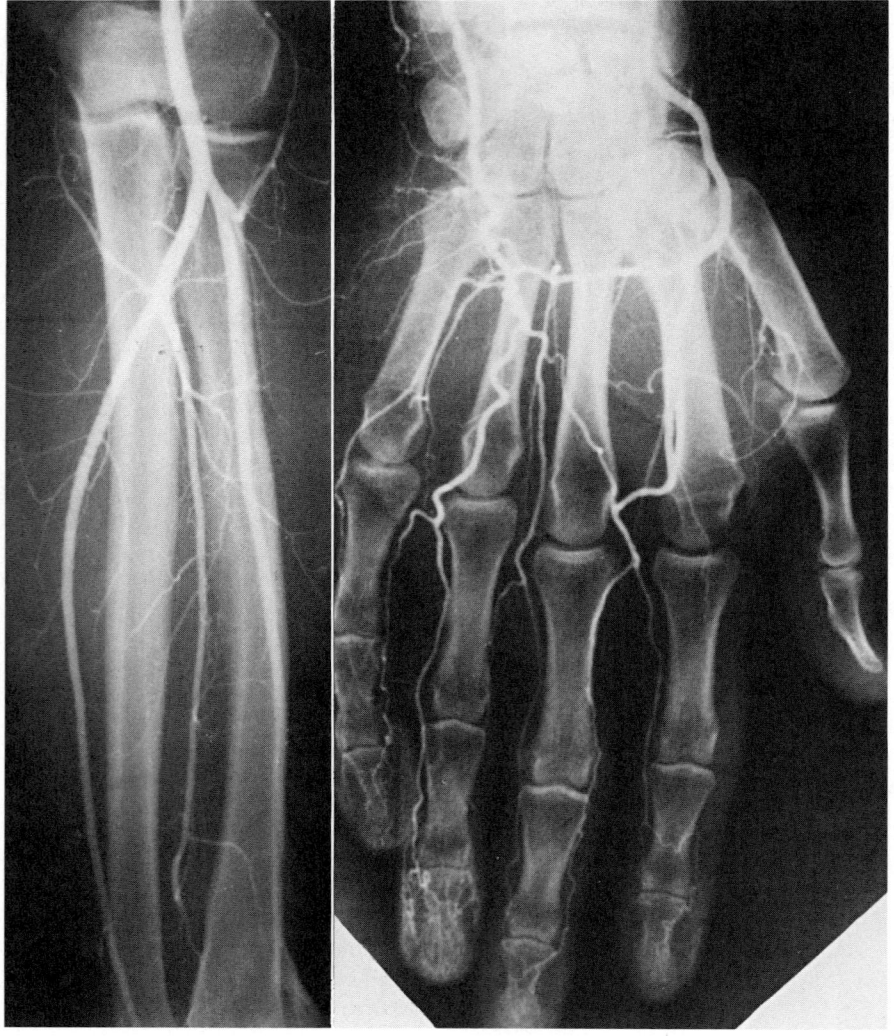

Figure 2 *A*, Brachial, radial, and ulnar arteries are patent. *B*, The palmar arch is patent but there are multiple occlusions of digital arteries. The tips of four fingers required amputation.

findings have a minimal injury and tend to do well regardless of the timing or type of treatment. In contrast, patients with more severe injuries, indicated by three or more abnormalities, have a worse prognosis if there is a delay prior to onset of therapy. The promptness with which therapy is begun is of importance in limiting the extent of ischemia. Therapy cannot reverse pre-existing gangrene, but it can limit the progression of the ischemic process and preserve borderline viable tissue. We believe that, regardless of the degree of ischemia or time to presentation, these patients benefit from this protocol, which addresses each of the presumed pathophysiologic consequences of IADI.

Other treatment regimens have been reported. Nerve blocks, intra-arterial and systemic vasodilators, and intra-arterial tolazoline have been used with varying degrees of success. Because of the anecdotal nature of the reports and the small numbers of patients, comparison to the therapeutic regimen used at LAC + USC is difficult.

Accidental intra-arterial injections administered by physicians still occur. Compared to IADI in drug addicts, iatrogenic injections are quickly recognized; they are limited to a single, pure substance manufactured for parenteral use; and treatment is rendered promptly, prior to the onset of irreversible ischemia. Early iatrogenic IADI was due to 10% thiopentone, and subsequent animal studies showed the concentration of the drug significantly affected the amount of necrosis. Currently, only 2.5% thiopentone is available, which results in less severe injury when administered intra-arterially. Reports of gangrenous complications continue to appear, even at this dilute concentration.

Other medications that have been reported in iatrogenic incidents include diazepam, vecuronium, epinephrine, ampicillin, and phenytoin. A variety of therapeutic regimens have been proposed. Again, these are limited to small numbers of patients. Dilution of the medication with saline, stellate ganglion block, intra-arterial dexamethasone or phentolamine, and thrombolytic therapy have all been reported as leading to a successful outcome.

Because of the rarity of IADI, our knowledge has been gained largely through anecdotal reports, small series, and the experience at LAC + USC, which is perhaps the largest retrospective series to date (Table 2). A prospective trial has never been done, owing to the very low incidence of this problem. Based on case reports, it would seem that intra-arterial thrombolytic therapy may hold promise if the clot occluding arterioles

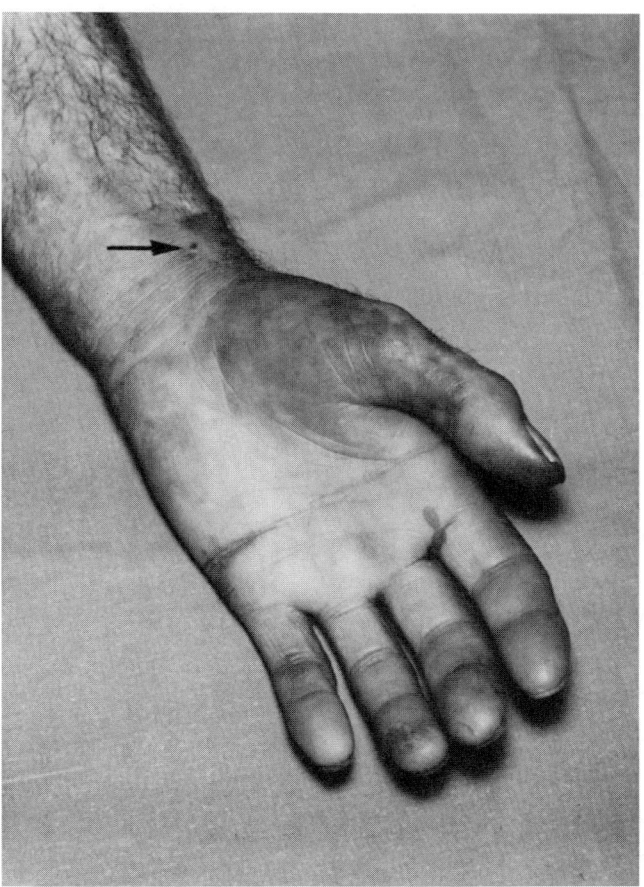

Figure 3 Ritalin was injected into the radial artery (*arrow*). Despite severe pain, mottling, cyanosis, and edema, there was full recovery.

Table 2 Experience at LAC + USC with Intra-Arterial Drug Injections, 1972–1993

Artery Injected	Patients	Outcome		
		Normal	Tissue Loss	Neurologic Deficit
Brachial	16	10	4	1
Radial	23	15	6	3
Ulnar	6	4	2	0
Dorsalis pedis	2	1	1	0
Posterior tibial	1	0	1	0
Digital	1	0	1	0
Total	49	30	15	4

and venules can be lysed and blood flow restored prior to the onset of irreversible ischemia. However, thrombosis at the level of the microcirculation suggests that this injury is not amenable to thrombolysis. The risks of intra-arterial catheters, the potential for further endothelial damage, and thrombosis of these small distal vessels as a complication of thrombolytic therapy must be considered. We have not yet employed thrombolysis in our patients. Our experience indicates that prompt intervention with our regimen, especially in those with severe injuries, can slow the ischemic process and act to prevent the gangrenous changes and subsequent amputation that can result from IADI.

REFERENCES

1. Saroyan RM, Senkowsky J, Kerstein MD. Vascular injury secondary to drug abuse. In: Ernst CB, Stanley JC, eds. Current therapy in vascular surgery, 2nd ed. Philadelphia: BC Decker, 1991:649.
2. Treiman GS, Yellin AE, Weaver FA, et al. An effective treatment protocol for intra-arterial drug injection. J Vasc Surg 1990; 12:456–465.
3. Citron BP, Halpern M, McCarron M. Necrotizing angiitis associated with drug abuse. N Engl J Med 1970; 283:1003–1011.
4. Kelly R, Yellin AE, Weaver FA: Candida thrombosis of the innominate vein with septic pulmonary emboli. Ann Vasc Surg 1993; 7:343–346.
5. Yellin AE. Ruptured mycotic aneurysm. Arch Surg 1977; 112: 981–986.
6. Sandler MA, Alpern MB, Madrazo BL, et al. Inflammatory lesions of the groin: Ultrasonic evaluation. Radiology 1984; 151:747–750.
7. Padberg F, Hobson R, Lee B, et al. Femoral pseudoaneurysm from drugs of abuse: Ligation or reconstruction? J Vasc Surg 1992; 15:642–648.
8. Friedman SG, Pogo GJ, Moccio CG. Mycotic aneurysm of the superior mesenteric artery. J Vasc Surg 1987; 6:87–90.
9. Van der Post CWM. Report of case of mistaken injection of pentothal sodium into an aberrant ulnar artery. S Afr Med J 1942; 16:182.
10. Gaspar MR, Hare RR. Gangrene due to intra-arterial injection of drugs by drug addicts. Surgery 1972; 72:573–577.
11. Lazarus HM, Hutto W, Ellerston DG. Therapeutic prevention of ischemia following intra-arterial barbiturate injection. J Surg Res 1977; 22:46–53.
12. Silverman SH, Turner WW. Intra-arterial drug abuse: New treatment options. J Vasc Surg 1991; 14:111–116.

FASCIOTOMY IN VASCULAR TRAUMA AND COMPARTMENT SYNDROME

JOSEPH L. MILLS, M.D.

Fasciotomy is an important limb-saving adjunct in the management of trauma, acute ischemia, and compartment syndrome of the upper and lower extremities. Unfortunately, significant clinical confusion has arisen over the indications, timing, and technique of fasciotomy because of controversies concerning the accuracy of clinical diagnostic criteria and the critical level of compartment pressure necessary for development of compartment syndrome. Nevertheless, compartment syndrome is a surgical disease requiring early recognition and prompt operative decompression. A thorough knowledge of the pathophysiology, diagnosis, and pertinent anatomy of extremity compartment syndrome, as well as a familiarity with proven techniques of compartment decompression, is essential to minimize morbidity and improve patient outcome.

COMPARTMENT SYNDROME

Definition and Mechanisms

Compartment syndrome has been defined as a condition in which "increased pressure within a limited space compromises the circulation and function of the tissues within that space."[1] There are thus only two prerequisites necessary for compartment syndrome to develop: an enclosed space surrounded by a limiting envelope and elevated pressure. The osteofascial compartments of the forearm and leg are clinically the most important anatomic regions at risk for the development of compartment syndrome. A number of mechanisms may result in elevated compartment pressure. Mubarak and others[2,3] have described a useful classification of compartment syndromes based on whether the elevated pressure is caused by decreased compartmental size or increased compartmental contents (Table 1).

In practice, crush injury or blunt trauma with associated fracture, especially of the tibia, and vascular injury has been the most frequent condition requiring fasciotomy for compartment syndrome. Ischemia and reperfusion of extremities following arterial embolization or bypass graft thrombosis, especially in patients with delayed diagnosis, has been the next most common predisposing condition. A recent literature review indicated that 8% to 10% of patients require fasciotomy following arterial embolectomy for acute arterial occlusion.[4] In contrast, clinically significant compartment syndrome is extremely uncommon following elective extremity revascularization for chronic arterial occlusive disease; Patman and Thompson reported an incidence of fasciotomy in such patients of only 0.45%.[5]

Several less commonly encountered mechanisms associated with the development of compartment syndrome may present more subtly and tax the diagnostic skills of the clinician. Limb compression and prolonged immobilization in patients with drug overdose or in patients following general anesthesia and operation in the lithotomy or knee-chest position may also lead to compartment syndrome. Careful observation and examination of the extremities of such patients are critical to avoid delayed recognition and treatment with the attendant risks of muscle necrosis and rhabdomyoglobinuric renal failure. Residual central nervous system depression from drug overdose or anesthetic agents may mask the usual clinical symptoms.

Treatment: Historical Background

Fasciotomy is a relatively recent development in the history of surgery (Table 2). Von Volkmann first described post-traumatic contracture deformities of the extremity, which he attributed to skeletal muscle ischemia.[6] In 1926, Jepson demonstrated experimentally that the muscle ischemia resulted from increased pressure and that early decompression of the affected extremity could prevent subsequent contracture.[7] The first widespread clinical use of fasciotomy occurred in the 1940s, particularly during World War II[8] for the treatment of battlefield injuries. The liberal and timely use of fasciotomy for extremity trauma was further emphasized by Rich, based on extensive experience in Vietnam.

Over the ensuing decades, further study of the pathophysiology of compartment syndrome and efforts to prompt, improved, and earlier diagnosis led to the evolution of several techniques for the direct measurement of intracompartmental pressures.[9,10] Unfortunately, these attempts to add science to the clinical diagnosis of compartment syndrome have confused the issue. In particular, the search for the critical pressure necessary for the development of compartment syndrome—and therefore the pressure that mandates fasciotomy—has engendered controversy.

In animal studies, 30 mm Hg for an 8 hour period is the lowest pressure documented to cause muscle necrosis.[3] Rorabeck and Clarke, in 1978, documented critical pressures of 40 to 50 mm Hg in an experimental model of anterior tibial compartment syndrome.[9] In a series of 30 patients at risk for the development of compartment syndrome, Matsen and associates performed continuous compartmental pressure monitoring by an infusion catheter technique. No patient with maximum compartment pressures of less than 45 mm Hg required fasciotomy or developed neuromuscular deficits. All patients with peak pressures exceeding 55 mm Hg developed significant neuromuscular sequelae of compartment syndrome.[1]

The accumulated data on compartment pressures would suggest that duration of compartment hypertension, as well as the absolute level of pressure elevation,

Table 1 Mechanisms Associated with the Development of Compartment Syndrome

Decreased compartmental size
 External constriction or compression
  Casts
  Circumferential dressings
  Military antishock trousers (MAST)
  Eschar (burn injury)
  Surgical closure of fascial defects
Increased compartmental contents
 Blood
  Trauma (fracture, vascular injury)
  Bleeding disorders (hemophilia)
  Anticoagulant therapy (warfarin, heparin, thrombolytic agents)
 Edema
  Ischemia/reperfusion (arterial injury, embolus, thrombosis, tourniquet)
  Limb compression, immobilization
   Drug overdose
   General anesthesia, position (lithotomy, knee-chest)
  Venous thrombosis (phlegmasia cerulea dolens)
  After open cardiac surgery
  Shock
  Eclampsia
  Nephrosis
 Fluid (exogenous)
  Intravenous infiltration

Table 2 Fasciotomy: A Historical Perspective

Year	Surgeon	Contribution
1881	von Volkmann	Muscular ischemia leads to contracture deformity
1926	Jepson	Early decompression prevents contracture
1941	Bywaters and Beall	Extremity crush syndrome in London bombing victims
1945	Horn	Acute ischemia of anterior compartment muscles
1945	Debakey and Simeone	Fasciotomy for battlefield injuries (WWII)
1966	Howse and Seddon	Re-emphasized role of local pressure as the cause of subsequent muscle contracture
1967	Kelly and Whitesides	Transfibular fasciotomy first described
1969	Rich	Fasciotomy for battlefield injuries (Vietnam)
1970	Patman and Thompson	Use of fasciotomy in peripheral vascular surgery
1971	Ernst	Technique of fibulectomy-fasciotomy
1975	Whitesides	Manometric measurement of compartment pressures
1976	Mubarak	Wick catheter measurement of compartment pressures
1976	Matsen	Infusion catheter measurement of compartment pressures
1977	Mubarak and Owen	Double-incision fasciotomy
1978	Rorabeck and Clarke	Critical closing pressures of 40 to 50 mm Hg in experimental model of anterior tibial compartment syndrome
1980	Nghiem and Boland	Single incision parafibular fasciotomy

is important in the pathogenesis of compartment syndrome. In addition, individual patients vary with respect to their tolerance for increased tissue pressure. A multitude of factors such as patient position, blood volume status, the presence of shock, and the duration of pressure elevation are clinically relevant determinants that may not always be available to or quantifiable by the clinician. In addition, as Matsen and associates have emphasized, the concept of a critical intracompartmental pressure that mandates surgical decompression is of limited clinical utility.[1] If a critical value at the lower end of the spectrum is selected to increase diagnostic sensitivity, then many patients will be subjected to unnecessary fasciotomy. If the critical value selected is too high, then some patients will develop permanent neuromuscular deficits that would have been avoidable by earlier fasciotomy. Compartment pressure measurement is most prudently applied to patients at risk in whom physical findings are equivocal or who have other associated conditions that obscure the signs and symptoms of compartment syndrome. Such patients would include multiple-trauma victims undergoing general anesthesia for the repair of other injuries and patients with head injury, drug overdose, or any other condition that impairs the patient's ability to express subjective symptoms of pain and paresthesia. Limb injury or swelling in such patients should raise the suspicion of compartment syndrome and prompt the measurement of compartment pressures. Four-compartment fasciotomy should be performed if pressures exceed 30 mm Hg, because the duration of pressure elevation is usually unknown, and the patient's altered mental status prohibits evaluation and monitoring on clinical grounds alone.

Pathophysiology

Multiple events may trigger the development of compartment syndrome. Once the cycle of increased tissue pressure, muscle edema, closure of the capillary bed, increased capillary permeability, further tissue swelling, and muscle edema begins, muscle necrosis and permanent nerve injury occur unless relieved by decompressive fasciotomy. Both partial and complete ischemic events can precipitate compartment syndrome. Perry documented that 3 hours of partial limb ischemia (mean arterial pressure of 50 mm Hg) caused significantly greater cell membrane dysfunction than 3 hours of total limb ischemia induced by tourniquet application.[3] This mechanism may account for the development of compartment syndrome in patients without direct limb injury or arterial occlusion, such as following shock or open heart surgery.

Reperfusion events may compound the initial ischemic insult. Abundant experimental evidence shows that cell membrane dysfunction and increased capillary permeability are mediated by oxygen free radicals (O_2^-, OH^-).[11] These observations are the basis for the use of free-radical scavengers such as mannitol, allopurinol, and superoxide dismutase to ameliorate the increased cell membrane and capillary permeability that perpetuates compartment syndrome.

Despite these improvements in our understanding at the cellular level of the mechanisms of ischemia-reperfusion events, prompt fasciotomy remains the treatment of choice for extremity compartment syndrome. The ultimate function of the limb is determined primarily by the promptness and adequacy of compartmental decompression. Sheridan and Matsen,[12] in a classic clinical study of fasciotomy in the treatment of 44 patients, emphasized the adverse outcomes obtained because of delays in performing fasciotomy: "Fasciotomy performed early, that is, less than twelve hours after the onset of compartment syndrome, resulted in normal function in 68% of extremities. Only 8% of those having late fasciotomy had normal function." The incidence of complications, including infection, amputation, renal failure, and death, was twelvefold greater in the group of patients undergoing late fasciotomy (54% versus only 4.5%). These data underscore the adverse clinical—and potentially medicolegal—consequences of delay in surgical decompression of patients with compartment syndrome. Concern over the development of wound-healing problems and infection often leads to delay in recommending fasciotomy. It would appear undeniable, however, that delayed fasciotomy is much more likely to lead to such complications than early fasciotomy carried out prior to irreversible muscle ischemia or necrosis. Significant wound problems are rare if fasciotomy is performed promptly and meticulous postoperative wound care is provided.

Clinical Signs and Symptoms

In an alert, responsive patient, the most common sign is a deep, throbbing pain out of proportion to that expected from the underlying extremity injury alone. This important clinical indicator obviously is lacking in patients with diminished levels of consciousness. In these patients, the wary clinician needs to be especially alert to the possibility of compartment syndrome.

The second useful clinical sign is pain induced by passive stretch of the muscles in the involved compartment. A working knowledge of compartmental anatomy (Table 3) is needed to elicit this finding. In the leg, the anterior compartment is most frequently affected by compartment syndrome. The deep peroneal nerve courses through this compartment. Two major muscles, the extensor digitorum longus and the extensor hallucis longus, serve to extend the toes. Painful passive movement would be elicited by toe flexion. Pain with passive stretch can be tested for each of the compartments in the leg and the forearm by applying knowledge of the functional anatomy of each compartment.

The remaining clinical findings associated with compartment syndrome include paralysis or paresis of the affected muscles, paresthesia or hypesthesia in the cutaneous distribution of the nerves coursing through the affected compartments, palpable tenseness of the involved musculature, and diminished or absent distal

Table 3 Compartmental Anatomy

Compartment	Nerve	Muscles	Muscle Function	Sensory Innervation
Leg				
Anterior	Deep peroneal	Tibialis anterior	Toe extension	Webspace between great and second toe
		Extensor digitorum longus	Foot inversion and dorsiflexion	
		Extensor hallucis longus		
		Peroneus tertius		
Lateral	Superficial peroneal	Peroneus longus	Foot dorsiflexion	Dorsal foot
		Peroneus brevis	Foot eversion	
Superficial posterior	Sural	Gastrocnemius	Foot	Lateral foot
		Soleus	Plantar flexion	
			Knee flexion	
Deep posterior	Tibial	Tibialis posterior	Toe flexion	Sole of foot
		Flexor digitorum longus	Foot plantar flexion and inversion	
		Flexor hallucis longus		
Forearm				
Volar	Median ulnar	Pronator teres	Forearm flexion and pronation	Palm of hand
		Flexor digitorum profundus	Wrist and digit flexion	
		Flexor carpi ulnaris		
		Flexor pollicis longus		
		Flexor carpi radialis		
		Flexor digitorum superficialis		
		Palmaris longus		
Mobile wad		Extensor carpi radialis	Wrist extension and supination	
		Brachioradialis		
Dorsal	Radial	Extensor digitorum	Wrist and digit extension	Dorsum of hand
		Extensor carpi ulnaris		
		Abductor pollicis longus		

pulses. The latter two findings usually occur late in the course of compartment syndrome. It should be emphasized that compartment syndrome often exists in the presence of palpable pulses.

In equivocal cases, or when limb swelling occurs in an obtunded patient, measurement of compartment pressures may be extremely useful. Although multiple methods of obtaining such measurements exist, the recent development of a solid-state transducer (STIC) within a catheter tip has simplified determination of intracompartmental pressures (Fig. 1). This device permits repetitive, reproducible pressure measurements.[3] In the presence of any clinical findings or in patients with a diminished level of consciousness, fasciotomy should be performed if compartment pressures exceed 30 mm Hg. Alert, cooperative patients who remain asymptomatic may be followed if pressures lie between 30 and 45 mm Hg. In light of Matsen's clinical data, the finding of compartment pressures in excess of 45 mm Hg is a relative indication for fasciotomy.[1,12]

Fasciotomy should be promptly performed whenever there are clear findings of symptomatic compartmental hypertension. Clinical findings and compartment pressure measurements should be used in a complementary fashion in patients with equivocal presentations. The concept of prophylactic fasciotomy has been controversial. Certain settings are associated with such a high incidence of compartment syndrome that prophylactic fasciotomy should be considered. These situations include combined arterial and venous injuries (especially of the popliteal vessels), crush injuries, and grade III-C limb fractures (combined fracture, soft tissue, and vascular injury). Prolonged (greater than 6 hours)

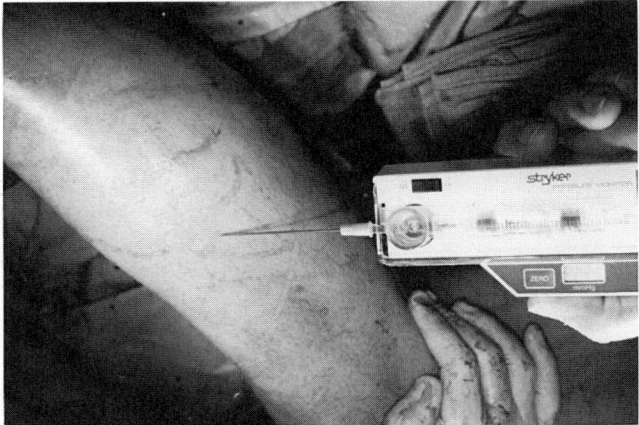

Figure 1 When clinically indicated, compartment pressures can be simply and reproducibly measured with a solid-state transducer (STIC) within a needle catheter tip.

ischemia prior to revascularization is a relative indication for fasciotomy. If decompressive fasciotomy is not carried out at the initial operation, close clinical follow-up with consideration of compartment pressure monitoring is required. It should be remembered that the major complications of compartment syndrome arise from delayed rather than premature fasciotomy.

TECHNIQUES OF FASCIOTOMY

A useful technique of fasciotomy should adequately and completely decompress all involved compartments, relieve compartmental hypertension, prevent muscle necrosis, and result in minimal wound complications. Three techniques serve these purposes for compartment syndrome of the leg: fibulectomy-fasciotomy, single-incision parafibular fasciotomy, and double-incision fasciotomy.

For the mechanisms of compartment syndrome likely to be encountered by the vascular or trauma surgeon, it is prudent to routinely decompress all four compartments of the leg by fasciotomy (Fig. 2). Whereas fibulectomy adequately accomplishes this goal, this technique is rarely used today.[13] It has been supplanted by simpler techniques without bony excision that use either single or double incisions.

Four-compartment fasciotomy may be performed through one incision using a parafibular approach, as first described by Nghiem and Boland.[14] A long skin incision is made laterally over the length of the fibula. Skin flaps are elevated, and the anterior and lateral compartments are decompressed after carefully identifying the intermuscular septum. Care must be taken proximally to prevent injury to the common peroneal nerve as it crosses the neck of the fibula. The superficial peroneal nerve is also vulnerable to injury in the distal third of the leg when the lateral compartment is opened. The posterior skin flap is then elevated, and the superficial posterior compartment entered and decompressed. The deep compartment is then decompressed by retracting the gastrocnemius and soleus muscles posteriorly and taking the fascial attachments down along the length of the fibula. This technique has the advantage of using only one incision, but it requires careful application, particularly to be certain that the deep posterior compartment is completely released.

The double-incision technique is preferred.[2] It is simple, expedient, and the easiest to teach general surgical housestaff. In addition, because most vascular injuries are repaired from a medial approach, the medial incision allowing access to the superficial and deep posterior compartments has already been made. Long skin incisions are also preferred to make certain that the skin and subcutaneous tissue do not limit the complete release of compartmental pressure. Long skin incisions also ensure adequate identification of the anatomy so that the surgeon may be confident that all four compartments have been identified and adequately decompressed.

Through the medial incision, the superficial and deep posterior compartments are released from the knee

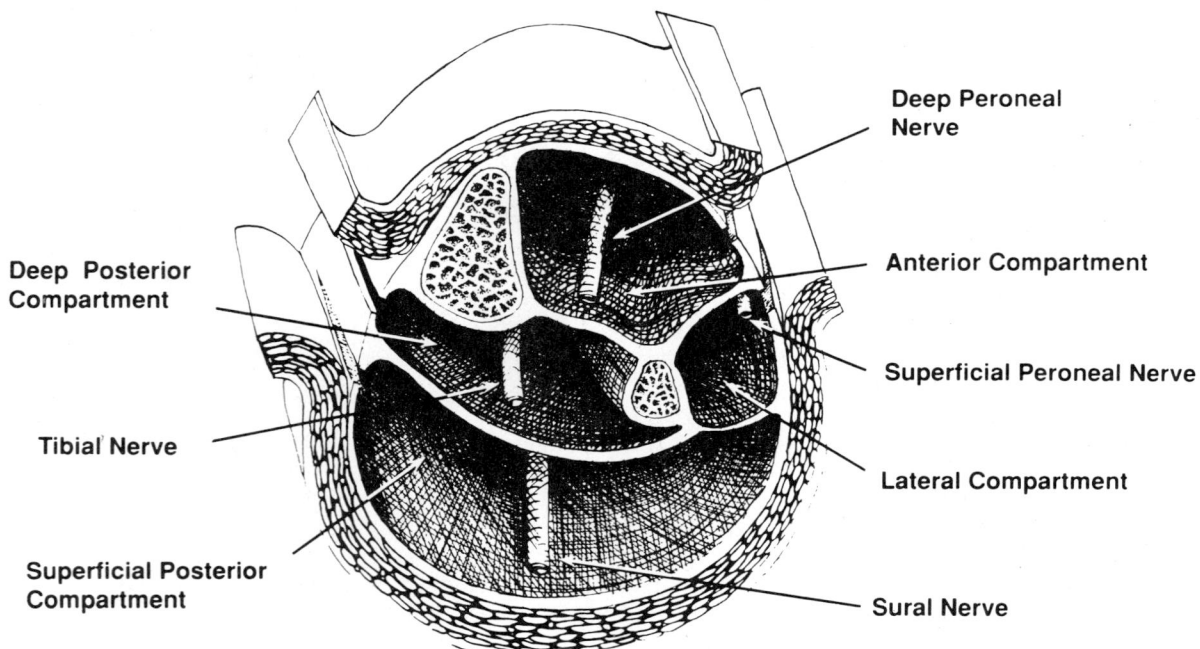

Figure 2 Cross-section through the mid-leg indicating the four osteofascial compartments and the major nerve coursing within each. Medial and lateral skin incisions yield easy access for decompression of all four compartments.

to the ankle. The saphenous vein and nerve should be spared. By elevating the anterior skin flap, the deep compartment may be entered along the posterior margin of the tibia. A second anterolateral incision serves to decompress the anterior and lateral compartments. After the skin is incised longitudinally, a small transverse fascial incision may be made to locate the intermuscular septum with certainty. The anterior and lateral compartments can then be decompressed through separate, longitudinal fascial incisions with scissors.

Skin incisions are not closed. Epigard, a synthetic skin substitute, is placed over the open wound, trimmed to fit the defect loosely, and stapled to the skin edges. The biologic dressing is covered with a loosely applied gauze roll. The use of this dressing protocol markedly reduces fluid losses associated with standard, bulky, wet-to-dry gauze dressings and simplifies postoperative wound care. If all muscle is viable, the Epigard dressing is left intact until the third or fourth postoperative day. The patient is then returned to the operating room for fasciotomy closure. The muscle beneath the Epigard nearly always remains clean and moist during this interval. If the skin can be closed primarily without undue tension, this is accomplished with simple, interrupted, 2-0 or 3-0 nylon sutures. With the double-incision technique, usually the lateral incision is primarily closed and a split-thickness skin graft is harvested, meshed, and placed over the medial incision.

If the initial fasciotomy was delayed and necrotic muscle encountered, all obviously necrotic muscle should be sharply debrided. Epigard dressing may still be used, but re-exploration, debridement, and pulsatile irrigation should be carried out in 24 to 48 hours to prevent infection and eliminate systemic complications of myonecrosis. Multiple reoperations may be required, particularly in patients with crush injury or grade III-C tibia fractures, who may develop myonecrosis despite revascularization and prompt fasciotomy because of the delayed effects and magnitude of the initial soft tissue and muscle injury. Significant wound complications are uncommon in patients subjected to early fasciotomy before muscle necrosis has developed.

If a compartment syndrome is recognized in a patient with limb trauma or prolonged arterial ischemia, fasciotomy is performed at the beginning of the procedure, prior to revascularization. This decompresses the compartments promptly, avoiding the potentially hazardous effects of ongoing compartmental hypertension. Mannitol, 25 g by intravenous infusion, should be given prior to fasciotomy. If any ischemic or frankly necrotic muscle is encountered, brisk diuresis should be ensured perioperatively with adequate hydration, and the urine should be alkalinized.

Fasciotomy of the forearm is occasionally required after repair of traumatic injuries or reconstruction for critical ischemia. Forearm fasciotomy may be accomplished through volar and dorsal incisions. The volar incision is begun proximal to the antecubital skin crease and extends across the wrist crease to allow decompression of the carpal tunnel.

COMPLICATIONS

The most serious local and systemic complications of fasciotomy result from delays in recognition and decompression of compartment syndrome, as well as inadequate decompression. Limited skin incisions may result in inadequate decompression of severely edematous muscle. Serious wound infections are unusual if fasciotomy is performed promptly before the development of muscle necrosis. Incomplete debridement of necrotic muscle may also result in infection. Although some degree of disability is unavoidable if extensive muscle debridement is necessary, proper physical therapy and appropriate use of orthotic appliances postoperatively often yield an acceptable functional result.

Nerve injury may occur during the performance of fasciotomy. The incidence of this complication can be minimized by the use of sufficiently long skin incisions to permit adequate visualization and by precise knowledge of the anatomic characteristics of each compartment.

If the patient has any evidence of myonecrosis at the time of fasciotomy or if significantly elevated creatine phosphokinase levels are detected postoperatively, a brisk diuresis should be initiated and maintained with adequate intravenous hydration, mannitol administration, and alkalinization of the urine to prevent myoglobin precipitation within the renal tubules. All necrotic muscle should be debrided, and frequent second-look procedures may be required postoperatively to prevent both the serious local and systemic complications of myonecrosis.

REFERENCES

1. Matsen FA, Winquist RA, Krugmire RB. Diagnosis and management of compartmental syndromes. J Bone Joint Surg [Am] 1980; 62:286–291.
2. Mubarak SJ, Owen C. Double-incision fasciotomy of the leg for decompression in compartment syndromes. J Bone Joint Surg [Am] 1977; 59:184–187.
3. Perry MO. Compartment syndromes and reperfusion injury. Surg Clin North Am 1988; 68:853–864.
4. Mills JL, Porter JM. Basic data related to clinical decision-making in acute limb ischemia. Ann Vasc Surg 1991; 5:96–98.
5. Patman RD, Thompson JE. Fasciotomy in peripheral vascular surgery. Arch Surg 1970, 101:663–672.
6. Von Volkmann R. Die ischaemischen muskellahmungen und Kontrakturen. Zentralbl Chir 1881; 8:801. (Translated by Bick, EM. Ischemic muscle paralyses and contractures. Clin Orthop 1967; 50:5.)
7. Jepson PN. Ischemic contracture: Experimental study. Ann Surg 1926; 84:785–795.
8. Bywaters EGL, Beall D. Crush injuries with impairment of renal function. Br J Med 1941; 1:427.
9. Rorabeck CH, Clark KM. The pathophysiology of the anterior tibial compartment syndrome: An experimental investigation. J Trauma 1978; 18:299–304.
10. Whitesides TE Jr, Haney TC, Morimoto K, Harada H. Tissue pressure measurements as a determinant for the need of fasciotomy. Clin Orthop 1975; 113:43–51.
11. Odeh M. The role of reperfusion-induced injury in the pathogenesis of the crush syndrome. N Engl J Med 1991; 324:1417–1422.
12. Sheridan GW, Matsen FA. Fasciotomy in the treatment of the

… 13. Ernst CB, Kaufer H. Fibulectomy-fasciotomy. An important adjunct in the management of lower extremity arterial trauma. J Trauma 1971: 11:365–380.

14. Nghiem DD, Boland JP. Four-compartment fasciotomy of the lower extremity without fibulectomy: A new approach. Am Surg 1980; 46:414–417.

ISCHEMIA-INDUCED MYONECROSIS, MYOGLOBINURIA, AND SECONDARY RENAL FAILURE (REPERFUSION SYNDROME)

F. WILLIAM BLAISDELL, M.D.

In 1960 Haimovici defined the myonephropathic-metabolic syndrome, which, in his original case report, followed reperfusion of a severely ischemic lower limb.[1] The patient, a 64-year-old man, had developed thrombosis of the right common iliac artery shortly following an abdominoperineal resection:

> Following extraction of the thrombus, the previously cyanotic mottled lower limb that had been anesthetic and paralyzed improved, although stiffness of the toes, ankle, and knee persisted. Within 24 hours, the limb became massively swollen and extremely hard, with nonpitting edema. The patient's urine was cherry red and the pigment was identified as myoglobin. On the third day, renal shutdown was complete and there was early gangrene of the right foot, although the femoral pulse was still palpable. The patient died of renal failure on the 10th postoperative day. At autopsy, histologic sections of the kidneys revealed myoglobin in necrotic renal tubules.

Many patients undergoing arterial embolectomy have similar problems to those described by Haimovici. In 1969 we analyzed 16 patients who had 12 or more hours of circulatory compromise. All presented with signs of advanced arterial ischemia manifested by paralyzed, blue, mottled limbs. The mortality following attempts at revascularization was 85% in this group. When saline was flushed through the distal arterial tree following embolectomy, large amounts of fresh thrombus emerged from a femoral venotomy, focusing attention on the coagulation system. Following reperfusion were systemic acidosis and marked elevation of the serum potassium. When these patients died acutely of heart failure or respiratory failure, thrombotic material could be seen in the lungs.

In an experimental model in a dog, we were able to reproduce the syndrome seen in humans by temporarily occluding the infrarenal aorta and simultaneously ligating all collateral blood flow so as to drop the distal blood pressures in the lower extremities to negligible levels. Following 4 hours of arterial occlusion and restoration of blood flow to the extremities, 90% of the animals died of pulmonary failure within 24 hours, and the lung pathology resembled what we had seen clinically: atelectasis; pulmonary, venous, and capillary congestion; interstitial edema; intra-alveolar hemorrhage; and pulmonary capillaries filled with degenerating platelets, leukocytes, and erythrocytes. Injection of the pulmonary arteries with radiopaque material revealed numerous filling defects throughout. When the vena cava blood was sampled immediately after removal of the aortic occluding clamps, fibrin-platelet aggregates were documented in the blood returning from the ischemic extremities. The degree of morbidity and mortality appeared to be directly related to the duration and severity of ischemia.

A series of experiments was then done to assess the hypothesis that pulmonary pathologic changes involving ischemia of the lower extremities were caused by procoagulants and inflammatory mediators released by the ischemic tissues. The right lung was isolated from the inferior vena cava by superior vena cava–to–right pulmonary shunt (Glenn procedure). Following 4 hours of cross-clamping and reperfusion, pathologic changes developed in the left lung that received infrarenal venous return, whereas the right lung receiving superior vena cava blood flow was not damaged. When inferior vena cava blood was directed through the liver prior to reaching the lung by portacaval transposition, no pulmonary changes occurred. This suggested that the liver was a potent filtering and detoxifying site for the by-products of ischemia coming from the extremities.

Following this experience, we instituted the principle that the treatment of choice for lower extremity embolic occlusion in patients with advanced ischemia was anticoagulation.[2] Whereas the mortality rate had been more than 25% in surgical group, in this subsequent anticoagulation-treated group, the mortality was 7.5%. Of the 54 patients in the latter series, 4 died; of the remaining 50 patients, only 6 required amputation.

As part of this review, the English-language literature was surveyed from 1963, the advent of the Fogarty embolectomy catheter, to 1978, the time of our report.[2] Of 35 embolectomy studies surveyed, the average mortality rate was in excess of 25%, even though most of the operations were done using local anesthesia through a simple femoral incision. On a review of our experience, as well as the combined series, the cause of death in more than 80% of patients appeared to be either cardiopulmonary or embolic in nature; 53% died from cardiopulmonary problems, 11% from pulmonary embolism, 8% from strokes, 4% from multiple recurrent emboli, 4% from renal failure, and 2% from mesentery infarction; 5% of the deaths were due to sepsis, and 12% were due to miscellaneous causes.

This 4% incidence of death from renal failure found on literature survey is grossly at odds with the original experience described by Haimovici, in which the primary course of death following lower extremity ischemia was related to myoglobinuria and renal failure.[3] Because limbs with advanced ischemia still are being revascularized and devitalized muscle is being reperfused, it is appropriate to raise the issue regarding the significance of myoglobinemia and the etiology of the uropathy.

Nerves and muscles are the most sensitive tissues in the extremities to ischemia (Table 1). Death of muscle, as documented by numerous tourniquet experiments, occurs within 3 to 5 hours of circulatory deprivation.[4] Labbe and associates assessed the extent and distribution of skeletal muscle necrosis in experimental animals after graded periods of complete ischemia.[5] They found 2% necrosis at 3 hours and 90% by 5 hours (the enveloping fascia had been removed). Thus, 6 to 8 hours of ischemia should result in extensive muscle death, and revascularization should produce a large renal myoglobin load. If myoglobin were directly toxic to the kidney, there should be consistent renal failure. Current reports indicate that there is no correlation between the degree of myoglobinemia and renal failure.[4,6] In fact, our experience and that of the current literature indicate that renal failure is rare, whereas pulmonary failure is far more common and the principal cause of morbidity and death.[2,7]

Even though myoglobin released from skeletal muscle is probably toxic, multiple factors undoubtedly are involved, including breakdown products from dead and dying tissue, such as lysozymes and fatty acids (Table 2). These are capable of activating inflammatory mediators such as oxygen radicals that produce diffuse vascular permeability alterations. Breakdown products of tissue also act as procoagulants that induce clotting in the corresponding venous system and result in a systemic clotting tendency.[2] In the ischemic limb, clot is present not only on the arterial side of the system but in the venous system as well. With restoration of blood flow, this fresh clot in the venous system is flushed back into systemic circulation and ends up in the pulmonary microvessels. The systemic clotting tendency also stimulates thrombosis of vessels in other organs such as heart, kidney, and mesenter.[2]

Our contention has been that damaged tissue, most particularly muscle because it constitutes the primary vulnerable tissue in the extremity, activates intravascular coagulation—the degree dependent upon the mass of tissue injured—and parallel stimulation to clotting by tissue factors, shock, and acidosis. Subsequently, inflammatory mediators are activated secondary to activation of the intrinsic clotting system (factor XII) (Table 3). Factor XII not only activates the clotting cascade but also activates in parallel other inflammatory components including kinins, complement, and prostaglandins. This inflammatory process also can produce diffuse endothelial damage and alterations in systemic vascular permeability.[7,8] This leads to third spacing as fluid and protein leak from this permeable vascular system resulting in parallel hypovolemia. If vascular volume is maintained, this third spacing results in systemic edema that is primarily manifested in the lung as compromised pulmonary function or the respiratory distress syndrome. If patients are not monitored and vascular volume not maintained, vital organ function including renal cortical perfusion is compromised, and renal cortical necrosis develops. Myoglobin present in the urine precipitates in the renal tubule, implying direct myoglobin toxicity.[1]

The reperfusion syndrome is not necessarily limited to the lower extremities, but the severity of the reperfusion syndrome correlates with the mass of ischemic tissue and the duration and severity of the ischemia. Major mesenteric vascular ischemia results in similar lethality, not only because of extensive injury to the gastrointestinal tract but to the other vital organs in the mesenteric circulation.[8]

The severity of the problem depends on the length of time a given tissue can go without circulation (Table

Table 1 Tissue Critical Ischemic Time

Tissue	Time
Muscle	4 hours
Nerve	8 hours
Fat	13 hours
Skin	24 hours
Bone	4 days

From Steinau H-U. Major limb replantation and postischemia syndrome: Investigation of acute ischemia-induced myopathy and reperfusion injury. New York: Springer-Verlag, 1988; by permission.

Table 2 Reperfusion-Venous Efflux

Acid phosphatase
Amino acid, purine bases, nucleotides
Enzymes SGOT, LDH, and isoenzymes, CPU
Histamine-like mediators and proteolytic enzymes
Inorganic phosphate
Lactate
Myoglobin
Platelet and fibrin aggregates
Potassium
Procoagulants

Table 3 Inflammatory Mediators

Oxygen radicals
Histamine-like mediators
Complement
Kinins
Thromboxane
Serotonin
Tumor necrosis factor
Leukotrines

1). When the ischemia involves an extremity, skeletal muscle is the critical tissue. Morbidity and mortality develop primarily when reperfusion of nonviable limbs is carried out, the manifestation of nonviability being paralysis and anesthesia. When paralysis and anesthesia are present for 4 hours or more, death of muscle is inevitably present. Reperfusion of the limb at this point results in the systemic manifestations described.

In a young patient, reperfusion of an ischemic lower leg results in severe morbidity; in an aged patient, death. Reperfusion of an ischemic thigh and lower leg results in severe morbidity and death in even a young patient.[4]

The best treatment for the reperfusion syndrome is prevention. When lower limbs have been nonviable for 6 to 8 hours, as manifested by limb paralysis and anesthesia, no attempt should be made to revascularize a limb. The patient should be treated with heparin sodium anticoagulation, and amputation should be carried out as necessary.[2] When the decision to reperfuse marginal limbs is made, careful monitoring of the patient is critical. This usually involves placement of a central line and a Swan-Ganz catheter. Sufficient fluid volume should be given to maintain normal circulation, ensuring perfusion of vital organs. Urinary output should be assessed hourly, and sufficient fluid administered to maintain urinary output in excess of 50 ml per hour.

Mannitol may be of value; it has the theoretical advantage of being an antioxidant and also a diuretic.[1] It is also osmotically active and helps maintain renal tubular urine flow. Elevated potassium levels can be treated by maintaining urinary output and, if necessary, administering glucose and diuretics. Acidosis is best treated by maximizing cardiac output and ensuring good tissue perfusion. Fasciotomy is controversial. Even though it may increase the salvage of muscle, there is no question that it increases the severity of the reperfusion syndrome by augmenting the systemic infusion of the breakdown products of ischemic tissue and compromises the physician's ability to anticoagulate the patient.[2,7,9,10]

Anticoagulation, particularly if started prior to reperfusion, is of unquestionable benefit. It decreases the risk of further thromboembolism in the ischemic extremity, decreases vascular permeability and edema in the reperfused limb, decreases the incidence and severity of pulmonary failure, and decreases systemic thrombotic problems.[2,4]

REFERENCES

1. Haimovici H. Arterial embolism with acute massive ischemic myopathy and myoglobinuria. Surgery 1960; 47:739–745.
2. Blaisdell FW, Steele M, Allen RE. Management of lower extremity arterial ischemia due to embolism and thrombosis. Surgery 1978; 84:822–830.
3. Haimovici H. Myopathic-nephrotic-metabolic syndrome associated with massive arterial occlusions. J Cardiovasc Surg 1973; 14:589–600.
4. Steinau H-U. Major limb replantation and postischemia syndrome: Investigation of acute ischemia-induced myopathy and reperfusion injury. New York: Springer-Verlag, 1988.
5. Labbe R, Lindsay T, Walker TM. The extent and distribution of skeletal muscle necrosis after graded periods of complete ischemia. J Vasc Surg 1987; 6:152–157.
6. Adiseshiah M, Round JM, Jones DA. Reperfusion injury in skeletal muscle: A prospective study in patients with acute limb ischemia and claudicants treated by revascularization. Br J Surg 1992; 79:1026–1029.
7. Anner HM, Kaufman RP, Valeri CR, et al. Reperfusion of ischemic lower limbs increases pulmonary microvascular permeability. J Trauma 1988; 28:607–616.
8. Kubes P, Suzuki M, Granger DN. Platelet-activating factor-induced microvascular dysfunction: Role of adherent leukocytes. Am J Physiol 1990; Suppl G:158–163.
9. Rush DS, Fraine SB, Bell RM, et al. Does open fasciotomy contribute to morbidity and mortality after acute lower extremity ischemia and revascularization. J Vasc Surg 1989; 10:343–350.
10. Michaelson M. Crush injury and crush syndrome. World J Surg 1992; 16:899–903.

CONCOMITANT VENOUS REPAIR IN THE MANAGEMENT OF EXTREMITY ARTERIAL INJURIES

JAMES J. SCHULER, M.D.

Although much has been learned about the management of major venous injuries over the past 15 to 20 years, the optimal management of these injuries remains somewhat controversial. Prior to the Vietnam Conflict, the vast majority of major venous injuries encountered in both civilian and military practice were treated by ligation. Based upon reports generated from the Vietnam Vascular Registry,[1,2] as well as large series of venous injuries reported from civilian experience[3-6] during the 1970s and early 1980s, the repair of major venous injuries in the extremities has been shown to be feasible, with acceptable short-term and long-term patency rates. In general, repair produces less short- and long-term morbidity than venous ligation.

LIGATION VERSUS REPAIR

The primary goal of treating major venous injuries is to control and prevent exsanguinating hemorrhage by either ligation or repair. The only proven advantage of venous ligation is a shortened operative time. The only postulated, but unproven, advantage of venous ligation is a decreased postoperative incidence of pulmonary embolism. The disadvantages of ligation of major extremity veins are an increased incidence of postoperative edema and swelling in both the upper and lower extremities and, in the lower extremities, an increased incidence of postphlebitic syndrome and chronic venous stasis ulceration. In contrast, the documented advantages of repairing major venous injuries are a decreased incidence of short- as well as long-term extremity swelling and edema, as well as a decreased incidence of late development of postphlebitic syndrome and venous stasis ulceration in the lower extremities.[7-9]

In lower extremity combined arterial and venous injuries, the major advantage of venous repair is an increased limb salvage rate, presumably due to an increased arterial repair patency rate. The reasons for this increased rate of limb salvage in combined arterial and venous injuries of the femoral and especially popliteal vessels are not clear but appear to be due in part to the presumed maintenance of normal peripheral vascular resistance in the vascular bed distal to the repaired vein that occurs with successful venous repair as opposed to the dramatic increases in peripheral vascular resistance and concomitant decreases in femoral arterial blood flow, which persists for 24 to 48 hours after venous ligation.[10] The major disadvantage of venous repair is the increased operating time needed to repair major venous injuries. This increase can vary from as little as 10 to 15 minutes for repairs that can be accomplished by simple lateral venorrhaphy to as much as 90 minutes for repairs requiring paneled vein grafts used as interposition grafts. The postulated and as yet unproven disadvantage of venous repair is a presumed increase in the incidence of pulmonary embolism following thrombosis of the repaired vein.

Most controversy surrounding the management of major venous injuries that prevailed in the 1970s and early 1980s has abated, and most authors now agree that major venous injuries should be repaired if the repair can be accomplished safely and expeditiously without prolonged hemodynamic instability or delaying the treatment of other associated injuries.

Much of the remaining controversy stems from the lack of a clear definition of the long-term natural history of repair versus ligation. Many disabling aspects of the postphlebitic syndrome, such as chronic venous stasis dermatitis and recurrent venous stasis ulceration, may not become clinically important problems for as much as 10 to 15 years after deep venous thrombosis. If one accepts a similarly late development of disability after thrombosis of a repaired vein or venous ligation, then it follows that the presumed long-term benefits of venous repair versus ligation will not be proven or disproven until long-term follow-up studies extending 10 to 15 years have been performed. To date such studies do not exist. In view of what is known about the relative merits of major venous repair as opposed to ligation and accepting the probability that the long-term natural history of repair versus ligation will probably never be clearly defined, most surgeons have adopted a policy of repairing major upper and lower extremity venous injuries when the repair can be accomplished without jeopardizing patient safety. When one considers the increasing frequency of combined arterial and venous injuries in the extremities resulting from urban street violence as well as an increasing number of extremity vascular injuries in patients surviving high-speed motor vehicle accidents, the importance of a safe and effective management policy for these combined injuries becomes apparent. The management guidelines described here are safe and effective in terms of both patient survival and salvage of functional extremities.

MANAGEMENT GUIDELINES

Approximately a third to a half of patients with arterial injuries to the extremities have associated injuries to the adjacent veins, and approximately half of these injured veins have been repaired. The pertinent points in management include (1) liberal use of preoperative arteriography in stable patients without severe ongoing hemorrhage, ischemia, or associated thoracic or abdominal injuries; (2) immediate operative exploration for all patients with severe ischemia, ongoing hemorrhage, or expanding hematoma; (3) liberal use of fasciotomy at the earliest sign of any degree of compartmental hypertension; (4) orthopedic fixation and stabilization of associated fractures or dislocations prior to vascular repair whenever possible; (5) ligation of brachial vein or distal venous injuries in the upper extremities; (6) repair of axillary vein and proximal major venous injuries in the upper extremities; (7) ligation of isolated profunda femoris and tibial vein injuries or distal venous injuries in the lower extremity; (8) repair of popliteal and proximal major venous injuries in the lower extremity; (9) use of autogenous vein grafts, usually greater saphenous vein from the uninjured contralateral extremity, for all venous repairs; (10) enforced postoperative elevation of the extremity after either ligation or venous repair for at least 3 to 5 days postoperatively; (11) repair of venous injuries before arterial injuries unless severe arterial ischemia is present; and (12) full therapeutic anticoagulation for 3 to 4 months for patients with documented occlusion of repaired major veins.

We have not employed preoperative phlebography and do not routinely employ anticoagulation in the immediate postoperative period. Although the general guidelines for veins that should be repaired versus those that can be ligated have been established, the fundamental surgical dictum of "life before limb" must be followed at all times. Experience has shown that any vein distal to the vena cava can be ligated without an increase in mortality over what would be expected from the associated nonvenous injuries alone. Only popliteal vein ligation and, to a lesser extent, femoral vein ligation have been shown to increase amputation rates over what would be expected from comparable arterial injuries alone; this increased amputation rate is modest but significant. In patients who are hemodynamically unstable from ongoing hemorrhage or inadequate resuscitation or in whom associated head, thoracic, or abdominal injuries require urgent treatment, injured extremity veins should be ligated.

Technique

A wide variety of techniques have been used in repairing injured extremity veins: simple lateral repair, vein patch angioplasty, interposition vein graft conduits, and, infrequently, paneled or spiral vein graft conduits placed as interposition grafts. Most lacerations of veins caused by knife or glass wounds can be repaired with simple lateral repair or end-to-end repair. The majority of venous injuries caused by gunshot wounds, shotgun wounds, and avulsion or traction injuries, such as those popliteal vein injuries secondary to knee dislocations, require resection of such lengths of injured vein that end-to-end repair without excessive tension is impossible. In these latter circumstances, interposition grafts of greater saphenous vein or occasionally lesser saphenous vein or brachial veins inserted in a nonreversed direction have served well and are an acceptable size match for most injuries distal to the mid-superficial femoral veins in the leg and distal to the mid-subclavian vein in the upper extremity. Repair of some common femoral vein injuries and most iliac vein injuries requires paneled vein grafts to avoid major size discrepancies between the interposition grafts and the native veins. In the upper extremity, paneled vein grafts have been required only for proximal subclavian and/or innominate vein injuries.

In children and adolescents, all vein repairs are performed with simple interrupted suture technique to avoid the pursestringing effect and subsequent venous stenosis as that would occur with a continuous running suture as the child grows. In adults, most simple lateral repairs and vein patch angioplasty repairs are performed with continuous running suture technique. We have utilized a technique in which approximately half the circumference of the anastomosis (usually the back wall) is done with continuous running suture and the remaining half (usually the anterior wall) is done with simple interrupted sutures for all end-to-end anastomoses with interposition grafts. This technique, in conjunction with applying only as much tension as is needed to gently approximate the edges of the vein and the graft, has effectively prevented stenosis secondary to pursestringing. We have used primarily 5-0 and 6-0 polypropylene suture for most venous repairs. The caliber of 7-0 polypropylene is so small and the walls of some deep veins, especially those of the upper extremity, are so thin that 7-0 suture material slices through and pulls out of the vein walls, whereas the larger 5-0 and 6-0 material does not.

All repairs are performed under full anticoagulation with heparin sodium given at a dose of 100 IU/kg body weight except in patients with contraindications to systemic anticoagulation, such as those with associated head, spinal cord, or ocular injuries or extensive thoracic and abdominal injuries. In those rare instances in which the decision to repair rather than ligate injured veins in patients with the associated injuries, regional anticoagulation, using 100 to 200 ml of normal saline with 100 units of heparin sodium/ml instilled into the injured veins proximal and distal to the site of the injury, is employed.

Except in patients in whom severe distal ischemia is present, we usually repair the vein before repairing the adjacent injured artery. It has been our general impression that in patients who have arterial blood flow restored prior to re-establishing venous continuity there is an increased need for fasciotomy. Another reason for repairing the venous injury first is the experimental data of Wright and Swan,[11] which documented transient but dramatic decreases in arterial blood flow occurring shortly after venous interruption. A repaired and patent venous outflow system should, therefore, allow for maximum blood flow velocity through the repaired artery and thus minimize the chances of the arterial repair occluding secondary to low flow velocities caused by increased distal resistance.

Preoperative Preparation

Because phlebography is not performed preoperatively and very few major venous injuries are identified on preoperative arteriography, it follows that most venous injuries are discovered during operative exploration for control and repair of known or suspected major arterial injuries.

Because intraoperative blood loss is much greater with combined arterial and venous injuries than with comparable arterial injuries alone, we have utilized intraoperative autotransfusion devices whenever combined arterial and venous injuries in the extremities are known or suspected. We have found that intraoperative autotransfusion decreases both the need for banked blood transfusions and the incidence of coagulopathy after massive transfusion of banked blood.

Because all venous repairs are best performed with autogenous greater saphenous vein, the uninjured contralateral leg should be included in the operative field to allow vein harvest in all cases of unilateral lower extremity vascular injury as well as all unilateral or bilateral upper extremity vascular injuries. The reason for not using the saphenous vein from the injured extremities is that, should the deep venous repair thrombose, as occurs in approximately 40% of venous repairs in our experience, the intact ipsilateral saphenous vein serves as an important source of venous outflow from the lower extremity. In patients with known or suspected bilateral lower extremity combined arterial and venous injuries, at least one upper extremity should be prepped to permit harvest of cephalic, basilic, or occasionally brachial vein for lower extremity repair of arterial and venous injuries.

Some patients with combined vascular injuries have a long history of intravenous drug abuse. In these patients, the greater saphenous vein and most upper extremity veins are chronically scarred or thrombosed and thus not suitable for use in the repair of either venous or arterial injuries. However, the lesser saphenous vein is frequently normal and can be used for vascular repair.

When only a small amount of vein is needed for vein patch angioplasty, another source is the lateral femoral cutaneous vein in the proximal thigh. This vein originates from the anteromedial aspect of the greater saphenous vein approximately 4 to 6 cm distal to the saphenofemoral junction and courses anterolaterally. In most patients the proximal 5 to 10 cm of the lateral femoral cutaneous vein is 3 to 4 mm in diameter and serves well either for a source of vein patch material or as a short-segment interposition graft when the greater saphenous vein is unavailable.

Repair of Upper Extremity Venous Injuries

There is no benefit from repairing upper extremity veins distal to the axillary vein. Ligation of these veins produces little or no edema or swelling in the hand or forearm. On the rare occasion when edema or swelling does occur, it resolves completely within a few days of venous ligation. The only exception is in those patients who have incurred circumferential or nearly circumferential, very deep lacerations of the arm that have transected all arteries and veins and major muscle groups. These rare injuries are usually encountered in patients who have fallen through or been pushed through glass doors or windows. In these circumferential injuries, we have repaired at least two and preferably more major veins as well as all major arteries.

Axillary and subclavian venous injuries should be repaired whenever such can be done safely. In axillary vein injuries, transection of the pectoralis minor muscle or tendon facilitates exposure for control of hemorrhage as well as performance of the venous repair and causes little if any postoperative morbidity in the vast majority of patients. Likewise, resection of the proximal and midportions of the clavicle is useful in gaining control of and repairing injuries to the middle and distal portions of the subclavian vessels.

In the majority of axillary and distal subclavian vein injuries that cannot be treated by lateral repair or vein patch angioplasty, the proximal greater saphenous vein can be used as an interposition graft. For repair of the middle and proximal segments of the subclavian vein, the saphenous vein is usually too small. In this situation, we have employed paneled saphenous vein grafts. However, because construction of a paneled saphenous vein graft requires 30 to 60 minutes, depending on length, we have employed such grafts only in patients who are hemodynamically stable and have no associated injuries requiring urgent treatment. In patients with hemodynamic instability, the axillary vein and proximal veins can be ligated without increasing the risk of upper extremity amputation and in most patients with little short- or long-term morbidity. The upper extremity edema and swelling that follows axillary or subclavian vein ligation is usually moderate and resolves spontaneously in a few weeks to a few months with no specific treatment. In 15 years of experience, only one of our patients has experienced long-term upper extremity edema secondary to axillary vein ligation.

Repair of Lower Extremity Venous Injuries

Injuries to the tibial and peroneal veins can be treated by ligation with very little short-term morbidity. Ligation of these veins usually produces a modest amount of calf and foot edema, which can be minimized by elevation of the extremity and usually resolves completely and without specific treatment in a few weeks to a few months. Ligation of tibial or peroneal vein injuries has not led to any increased risk of lower extremity amputation. Isolated profunda femoris vein injuries in which the common and superficial femoral veins are uninjured can be ligated with no adverse short-term sequelae. We have repaired profunda femoris vein injuries only when there are associated injuries to the common or superficial femoral vein that have been repaired. Reasons for repairing the profunda femoris vein are (1) that approximately 40% of repaired veins will thrombose within a week of repair[4] and (2), should the superficial femoral vein repair thrombose, the patent profunda femoris vein functions as an important source of venous return.

Popliteal, superficial femoral, and common femoral venous injuries should be repaired whenever this can be done safely. Ligation of these veins as compared to repair has been shown to lead to an increased amputation rate as well as an increased rate of edema, postphlebitic syndrome, and venous ulceration. These sequelae of venous ligation are most likely to occur after popliteal vein ligation.[3,6,7,9]

In most patients in whom popliteal vein repair cannot be accomplished by simple lateral venorrhaphy or vein patch angioplasty, the proximal greater saphenous vein from the contralateral uninjured extremity is a good size match and serves well as an interposition graft. In many superficial femoral vein injuries and most common femoral vein injuries, a paneled saphenous vein graft used as an interposition graft is required to avoid a major size match discrepancy.

In patients who have had prolonged periods of severe lower extremity ischemia secondary to combined venous and arterial disruption, the tissue beds distal to the injury have been undergoing mainly anaerobic metabolism with an attendant increase in lactic acid production. Such prolonged ischemia can also lead to temporary cell membrane dysfunction and an accumulation of potassium ions in the extracellular space. The sudden restoration of arterial flow can lead to a washout acidosis and hyperkalemia, which can induce or exacerbate hemodynamic instability and cardiac arrhythmias. In such circumstances, we have employed the following technique: The venous repair is performed first, but the last two to three stitches needed to complete the venous repair are not placed, thus leaving a vent hole from which venous effluent blood can be flushed and collected. After completion of the repair of the associated arterial injuries, the proximal and distal arterial clamps as well as the distal venous clamps are released while the proximal venous control clamp is left in place, allowing the venous effluent blood with its high concentration of lactic acid and potassium to be flushed, collected, and sent through the autotransfusion apparatus, where the blood is washed, centrifuged, and returned to the patient as packed red blood cells without an excessive amount of acid or potassium. The volume of blood collected in this manner is usually 300 to 500 ml. Concurrent with this flushing, collecting, and washing sequence, the anesthesiologists are instructed to give crystalloid solution rapidly in such volume as is needed to prevent hemodynamic instability on the basis of hypovolemia. It has been our clinical impression that use of this technique has decreased the incidence of declamp hypotension in patients with prolonged and severe extremity ischemia.

Fasciotomy is required much more frequently in combined lower extremity venous and arterial injuries than in isolated lower extremity arterial injuries.[6] In regard to the need for fasciotomy, we have not found the measurement of intracompartmental pressures to be useful but have relied upon sequential physical examination and palpation to determine the need for fasciotomy. We perform lower extremity fasciotomy early and extensively at the first signs of the development of any degree of compartmental hypertension and accept the possibility that rarely a fasciotomy may not have been required. However, it is impossible to determine this prospectively and because the morbidity of fasciotomy is only cosmetic, whereas a delay in the performance of fasciotomy frequently leads to limb loss or a minimally functional extremity, we feel that the liberal and early use of fasciotomy is justified.

RESULTS OF VENOUS REPAIR AND RECOMMENDATIONS

Adherence to the general guidelines and principles described here has led to a high rate of limb salvage and a lower incidence of short-term minor morbidity after repair of major extremity venous injuries.[1-4] The short-term patency of these repairs as assessed by contrast phlebography has recently been documented. The overall patency rate of venous repairs at 1 week was 61%. However, the patency rate varied with the type of repair employed. Those few veins repaired with end-to-end anastomosis technique had 100% patency, whereas those repaired with either lateral repair or vein patch angioplasty had patency rates of 83% and 67%, respectively. Interposition vein grafts and paneled vein grafts had 1 week patency rates of 40% and 50%, respectively.[4] There were no perioperative deaths, and 100% limb salvage was achieved in all patients. Although this relatively low rate of vein repair patency for veins repaired with interposition or paneled vein grafts appears discouragingly low, it does not seem to adversely affect overall limb salvage or short-term limb function. Furthermore, in a report[5] dealing with the long-term results of venous reconstruction, eight of nine repaired veins that had been documented to be occluded by phlebography 7 days after repair were documented to be patent and nonstenotic as assessed by color flow duplex imaging performed at a mean follow-up of 49 months, with follow-up ranging from 6 to 108 months. It therefore appears that a vein repair that thromboses in the immediate postoperative period usually undergoes recanalization similar to that which occurs following deep venous thrombosis in the lower extremities. This high incidence of recanalization of previously thrombosed vein repairs seems to account for the decreased incidence of postphlebitic morbidity in patients who have undergone lower extremity vein repair as compared to lower extremity vein ligation.

In our entire experience with repair of approximately 200 major venous injuries of the upper and lower extremities, we have encountered only one clinically apparent pulmonary embolus. This occurred approximately 1 week after the lateral repair of an innominate vein injury and was fatal. In patients in whom thrombosis of a venous repair in the extremities was documented in the postoperative period, we used full therapeutic anticoagulation with sodium warfarin for 3 to 4 months.

REFERENCES

1. Rich NM, Hughes CW, Baugh JH. Management of venous injuries. Ann Surg 1970; 171:724–730.
2. Rich NM, Collins GJ Jr, Anderson CA, et al. Autogenous venous interposition grafts in repair of major venous injuries. J Trauma 1977; 17:512–520.
3. Pasch AR, Bishara RA, Schuler JJ, et al. Results of venous reconstruction after civilian vascular trauma. Arch Surg 1986; 121:607–611.
4. Meyer J, Walsh J, Schuler J, et al. The early fate of venous repair after civilian vascular trauma. Ann Surg 1987; 206:458–464.
5. Nypaver TJ, Schuler JJ, McDonnell P, et al. Long-term results of venous reconstruction after vascular trauma in civilian practice. J Vasc Surg 1992; 16:762–768.
6. Pasch AR, Bishara RA, Lim LT, et al. Optimal limb salvage in penetrating civilian vascular trauma. J Vasc Surg 1986; 3:189–195.
7. Rich NM, Hobson RW, Collins GJ Jr et al. The effect of acute popliteal venous interruption. Ann Surg 1976; 183:365–368.
8. Agarwal N, Shah PM, Clauss RH et al. Experience with 115 civilian venous injuries. J Trauma 1982; 22:827–832.
9. Blumoff RL, Powell T, Johnson G Jr. Femoral venous trauma in a university referral center. J Trauma 1982; 22:703–705.
10. Hobson RW, Wright CB, Swan KG, et al. Current status of venous injury and reconstruction in the lower extremities. In Bergan JJ, Yao JST, eds. Venous problems. Chicago: Year Book, 1978:469.
11. Wright CB, Swan KG. Hemodynamics of venous occlusion in the canine hind limb. Surgery 1973; 73:141–146.

BLUNT AND PENETRATING RENAL VASCULAR INJURIES

GERALD B. ZELENOCK, M.D.

Vascular surgeons encounter injuries to the renal artery and vein in the context of overt trauma, either penetrating or blunt, or as an iatrogenic complication.[1-4] Initially, the usual trauma resuscitation priorities are followed. The airway is secured, volume and blood restoration are accomplished, and more immediately life-threatening injuries are treated. Attention is then focused on the diagnosis and management of the renal vascular injury (Table 1). A high index of suspicion is necessary to suspect and confirm some injuries, which may be subtle, such as a stretch-traction injury producing an intimal flap during the course of medial visceral rotation or an iatrogenic intimal injury during diagnostic arteriogram. Occasionally, an obvious iatrogenic injury is produced, such as arterial disruption during an operation or a balloon angioplasty.

Traumatic injuries are usually classified as blunt or penetrating. Diagnosis in the latter is straightforward, and wounds of entrance and exit, along with an anticipated trajectory, may indicate a high likelihood of renal vascular pedicle injury. Knife injuries usually create a localized wound with little likelihood of a remote injury. Injury from a high-velocity projectile may cause damage by means of direct transsection or laceration, whereas a relatively remote injury may result from cavitation, ricochet, or tumbling with an erratic intracavitary pathway. If the patient is stable and a retroperitoneal or renal vascular injury is suspected, and if time and facilities allow, an arteriogram is highly specific and sensitive for confirming a renal vascular injury. If the patient is unstable or other injuries require immediate operative intervention, a renal vascular injury may become suspect in the presence of a large or pulsating zone II retroperitoneal hematoma. Proximal and distal aortic control as well as proximal and distal renal pedicle control usually allows safe exploration of such hematomas. In the presence of a small, nonpulsatile hematoma secondary to a knife wound, many would feel comfortable not exploring the retroperitoneum, whereas with a high-velocity missile injury even such small hematomas should be explored.

Nonpenetrating injuries due to blunt abdominal trauma or rapid deceleration are more difficult to diagnose and often occur in a context in which the diagnosis is delayed and appropriate management of more immediately life-threatening injuries takes priority. Securing the airway, stabilization of the cervical spine, volume resuscitation, and treatment of hemopneumothorax, pericardial tamponade, associated head injuries, thoracic aortic disruption, and severe intraperitoneal hemorrhage usually require more immediate diagnostic and therapeutic efforts, relegating the investigation of renal vascular injuries to a secondary role. If the patient can be stabilized and a renal parenchymal injury is suspected, an intravenous pyelogram (IVP) is often obtained. A single-shot IVP is relatively insensitive and usually serves only to establish the presence or absence of both kidneys. A more detailed IVP, utilizing multiple films or nephrotomograms, is more sensitive for documenting a renal parenchymal injury but remains relatively insensitive and nonspecific for a renal vascular injury. Computed tomographic (CT) scans are frequently performed for the evaluation of abdominal and retroperitoneal trauma and are sensitive indicators of renal parenchymal injury and major vascular disruptions. If time allows and excess contrast has not been required for various CT scans and arch aortograms, a flush aortogram at the level of the renal arteries provides more adequate detail to assess the renal vasculature. This latter study is both sensitive and specific.

Often, other injuries such as intraperitoneal hemorrhage from a lacerated spleen or liver require immediate operative intervention, and detailed renovascular diagnostic studies are not possible. Under such circumstances, a renal vascular injury may be discovered intraoperatively. A large, enlarging, or pulsatile hematoma in zone II of the retroperitoneum is strongly suggestive of a renal vascular injury. Control of the proximal and distal aorta as well as the renal hilum is essential, except for the most simple and straightforward lacerations that can be treated with simple closure. Most renal vascular injuries require grafting procedures for repair, and autogenous saphenous vein remains the conduit of choice for both renal arterial or venous reconstruction. For this reason, one or both lower extremities should be prepped whenever renovascular repair might be required. For venous injuries close to the vena cava, it may be possible to simply oversew the proximal and distal renal vein, with adequate egress of venous blood occurring through the central adrenal, gonadal, and second lumbar veins. With severe renal hilar injuries or those involving most of the renal

Table 1 Renal and Renal Vascular Injury Paradigms

- Overall likelihood of renal injury with blunt trauma is 12% (6%–15%); with penetrating trauma it is 6% (4%–8%).
- Hematuria is sensitive but not specific.
- For blunt trauma, shock, gross hematuria, and major associated injuries (pelvic or spine fractures and other major intra-abdominal injuries) indicate high likelihood of renal injury; absent any one of these, significant injury is unlikely.
- Penetrating injuries are more difficult to characterize and require liberal indications for imaging.
- Renal contusions and minor parenchymal lacerations may be treated expectantly.
- In patients undergoing urgent trauma celiotomy for other indications, an expanding or pulsatile perinephric hematoma is an indication for renal exploration.
- Control of the proximal and distal aorta, control of the proximal and distal renal artery and vein, and mobilization of the right or left colon allow optimal exposure, assessment, and repair.

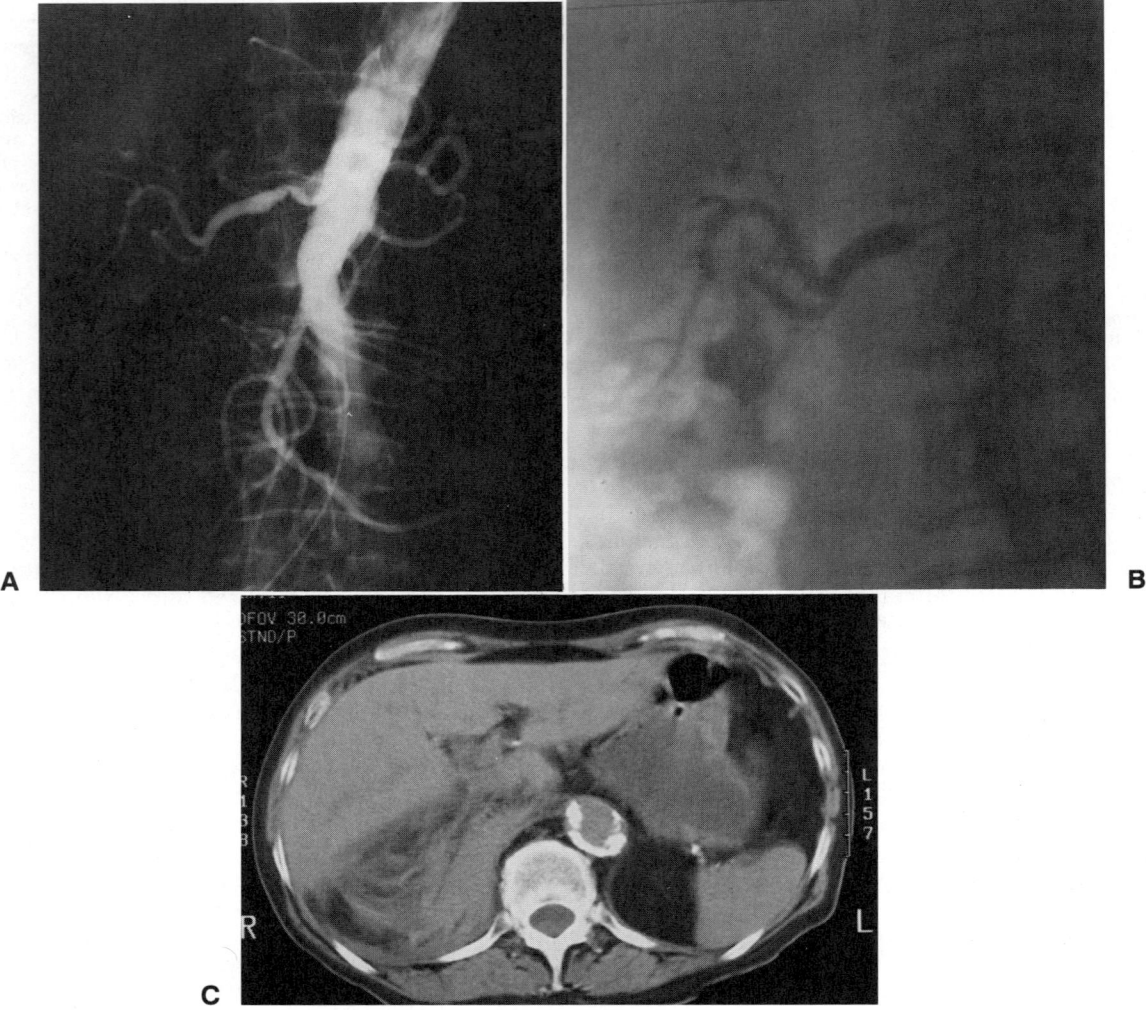

Figure 1 *A,* Moderate atherosclerotic stenosis in right renal artery associated with labile 4 drug hypertension and a serum creatinine of 1.8 mg/dl. *B,* Balloon dilation of stenosis with excellent anatomic result. *C,* Thirty-six hours later, unstable vital signs and a drop in hematocrit prompted this CT scan demonstrating a right perinephric hematoma. Exploration of the perinephric hematoma did not demonstrate active bleeding. Following recovery, blood pressure has remained well controlled with no medications, and serum creatinine is 1.5 mg/dl at 10 months.

parenchyma, nephrectomy may be required. If the injury is confined to the kidney at one or the other pole, heminephrectomy may suffice.

IATROGENIC TRAUMA

Iatrogenic injury to the renal vasculature is not common but can and does occur in the setting of diagnostic and therapeutic arteriography and other interventional techniques. A close working relationship between vascular surgeons and interventional radiologists lessens the sequelae of such injuries. Occasionally during diagnostic arteriography, small intimal flaps may be raised. Most of these are self-limited and need no special treatment. Large flaps may be stented or repaired operatively.

An aggressive approach to occlusive lesions of the main renal artery often results in better control of hypertension and preservation of renal function. Both surgical and interventional angiographic techniques are appropriate. The latter is safe in select patients but may occasionally result in significant complications such as thrombosis or hemorrhage from arterial wall disruption. Following balloon angioplasty, certain arterial disruptions are immediately recognized. Some can be definitively treated with intravascular stents. Others require stabilization with an inflated balloon and immediate operation for control of exsanguinating hemorrhage. Inflation of a balloon with tamponade of the bleeding is a useful step, albeit at the cost of a more significant ischemic injury. Delayed recognition of vascular injury due to balloon angioplasty is also possible (Fig. 1).

At present there is enthusiasm for placement of

intravascular aortic stents to deal with aortic aneurysms. Clearly, the potential to compromise renal blood flow by thrombosis or inadvertent covering of a renal arterial orifice is real, but sufficient experience has not yet accumulated to allow appropriate treatment algorithms to be developed for this complication.

Iatrogenic injury also may occur during medial visceral rotation to expose the midabdominal or visceral aorta. On two occasions we have seen mid-renal artery intimal fracture that required operative repair during the course of a thoracoabdominal aneurysmectomy. We believe the mechanism of injury to be stretch-traction, which fractures the relatively less elastic intima and leaves the media and adventitia intact. Both such injuries were recognized by a diminished pulse that was confirmed by Doppler interrogation. Each was easily repaired by incising the renal artery and performing a localized intimectomy and tacking the residual intima. Closure of the renal artery was then accomplished with a patch.

With any blunt, penetrating, or iatrogenic renal vascular injury requiring operative repair, it is important to have the lower extremities prepped in order to obtain saphenous vein if required. Adjunctive measures to ensure optimal renal preservation from the threat of renal ischemic injury include vigorous and precise volume resuscitation, the use of mannitol, heparin sodium (either systemic or local) during the period of vessel clamping, and flushing of the kidney with cold, heparinized preservation fluid, as well as an expeditious and precise repair. Warm renal ischemia of even 1 hour's duration results in significant parenchymal injury, and total interruption of blood flow may produce irreparable injury within 4 hours. Nevertheless, in a clinical context arbitrary time limits that would limit an otherwise feasible repair should not be imposed. Pre-existing collateral vessels or partial ischemia may allow marginal but organ-sustaining perfusion. Further, in the setting of trauma, hypothermia is common, which greatly extends tolerable ischemic times. Renal salvage 12 to 24 hours following injury has been noted.[5]

REFERENCES

1. Holcroft JW, Blaisdell FW. Trauma to the torso. American College of Surgeons/Scientific American. Care of the surgical patient, pp 51–56, New York.
2. MacKersie RC. Trauma definitive care phase: Retroperitoneal injuries. In: Greenfield LJ, Mulholland MW, Oldham KT, Zelenock GB, eds. Surgery: Scientific principles and practice. Philadelphia: JB Lippincott, 1993; 311.
3. Rich NM, Spencer FC. Injuries of miscellaneous intra-abdominal arteries. In: Rich NM, Spencer FC, eds. Vascular trauma. Philadelphia: WB Saunders, 1978; 457.
4. Trunkey DD. Torso trauma. Curr Probl Surg 1987; 4:259–264.
5. Stanley JC. Renal vascular emergencies. In: Haimovici H, ed. Vascular emergencies. New York: Appleton-Century-Crofts, 1982; 541.

IATROGENIC PEDIATRIC VASCULAR INJURIES

PHILIPPE A. MASSER, M.D.
LLOYD M. TAYLOR JR., M.D.
GREGORY L. MONETA, M.D.
JOHN M. PORTER, M.D.

Vascular injuries in infants and young children require substantially different management than such injuries in older children and adults. Most arterial injuries in infants and children under age 5 years are iatrogenic, resulting from arteriography, umbilical artery catheters, or extracorporeal membrane oxygenation catheters. In this section we address the diagnosis and management of these specific injuries. Vascular injuries in children over 5 years of age are more likely to result from blunt or penetrating trauma and are generally managed using conventional techniques like those in adults.

GENERAL PRINCIPLES OF ARTERIAL REPAIR IN INFANTS

Two important facts guide the repair of arterial injury in infants and small children: (1) These patients have a remarkable capacity to develop collateral circulation in response to arterial occlusion, greatly exceeding that found in older children and adults, and (2) the small size of vessels found in infants and small children means that operative repairs are technically difficult and less likely to be successful than in older patients.

Limb arterial injuries producing occlusion that would frequently result in limb loss in adults rarely do so in infants. Indeed, development of sufficient collaterals to rapidly restore palpable pulses is the rule. Similarly, reports of successful arterial repairs in infants documented by restoration of palpable pulses must be viewed with skepticism, because this appears to also be the natural history in patients not undergoing operation.[1]

These features suggest that arterial repairs in infants be undertaken only rarely and that most injuries can be successfully and optimally managed without operation. In our practice, repair of arterial injuries in infants and children is performed only when limb viability is clearly and persistently threatened or when life-threatening hemorrhage or other complications are present.

If operative repair is essential in infants and small children, optimal management of fluid status, oxygenation, and underlying medical conditions is imperative. Temperature regulation is limited in infants, and hypothermia must be prevented with warming devices and an elevated operating room temperature. General anesthesia and prophylactic antibiotics are routinely used. Loupe magnification is helpful. Vascular control is obtained with use of vessel loops or Heifitz clamps. A 2 Fr balloon catheter usually does not pass beyond the common femoral artery in neonates. The routine use of vein patch angioplasty rather than direct closure of femoral arteriotomy is recommended in small children. If grafting is necessary, the internal iliac artery has been used with success in small children, and saphenous vein in larger children. To accommodate for later growth of vessel anastomoses, we use generous spatulation and interrupted 6-0 to 8-0 suture. Anastomoses ideally should be approximately three times arterial diameter. Vasospasm complicating arterial repairs can be treated with gentle mechanical dilation with a 2 Fr Fogarty balloon or pharmacologically with topical or intra-arterial papaverine, 1% lidocaine, or nitroglycerin. Care is required to avoid ligation of collateral vessels, on which limb viability may depend in case of failure of the arterial repair. End-to-side rather than end-to-end anastomoses are preferred on this account.

Vasospasm accompanying arterial trauma is a much more frequent and important phenomenon in infants and children than in adults, and it may mimic or contribute to arterial thrombosis. Cyanotic heart disease, low blood flow states, and the hypercoagulability of polycythemia are frequently present in critically ill infants and may contribute to arterial thrombosis in the presence of iatrogenic arterial trauma. Specific treatment of these associated conditions is frequently required to optimize arterial blood flow.

FEMORAL ARTERY INJURY

Many iatrogenic vascular complications of femoral artery catheterization in adults, including bleeding, hematoma formation, and pseudoaneurysm, are rarely encountered in young children and infants because of small arterial size and the effectiveness of direct postcatheterization compression. The early practice of superficial femoral artery ligation following open arteriography in infants vividly demonstrated the adequacy of the usually excellent collateral flow in maintaining limb viability. Such did not always support normal limb growth, however, and for this reason some authorities advocate aggressive surgical therapy for iatrogenic arterial thrombosis. We disagree and believe this approach unjustified. It is important to be aware that common femoral artery thrombosis occurs in more than a third of infants undergoing diagnostic catheterization.[1] Most such thromboses are not clinically evident and only a few produce symptoms.

Initial management of postangiography common femoral artery thrombosis in infants and young children includes assessment of limb viability and immediate initiation of heparin sodium anticoagulation, unless contraindicated. The usual clinical signs of limb ischemia, including pallor, coolness, and lack of pulses, are reliable in infants and children. Clinical assessment should be supplemented by Doppler pressure measurement at the ankle. Arteriography is contraindicated to document postcatheterization injuries in infants and small children because of the obvious additional risk of further arterial injury.

In our experience, iatrogenic femoral artery thromboses in infants rarely cause truly limb-threatening ischemia. Rehydration of the patient accompanied by heparin anticoagulation results in rapid improvement in limb perfusion in an overwhelming majority of patients. Frequent clinical reassessment of limb ischemia is mandatory. Observation over 4 to 6 hours from the onset of ischemia is generally sufficient to detect obvious improvement in the clinical signs of ischemia resulting from the cumulative effects of hydration, anticoagulation, and resolution of vasospasm, if present. Ischemia that persists beyond 4 to 6 hours is rarely caused by vasospasm, but is almost uniformly the result of proximal arterial thrombosis.[2] If the limb remains severely ischemic, as indicated by the absence of distal Doppler signals or neurologic impairment, surgical repair is appropriate. As long as the limb remains viable and develops audible ankle Doppler signals, we recommend continued anticoagulation and observation for expected improvement.

At the Oregon Health Sciences University, occurrence of significant long-term symptoms from femoral arterial thrombosis in children younger than age 5 years is extremely unusual.[1] Advocates of early repair of postangiographic femoral artery thrombosis have never convincingly demonstrated that most of these repairs remain patent. It is well established that the development of excellent collaterals may allow young patients to regain normal ankle pulses and pressures despite permanent femoral occlusion. Given the unpredictable patency of attempted acute femoral artery repair in infants and small children, we do not feel repair is justified in the presence of limb viability as previously above.

If detectable ischemia persists at 1 month, these children should be enrolled in a long-term observational program to assess diminished limb growth leading to leg length discrepancy. Abnormal ankle:brachial indices (ABIs) correlate well with leg length discrepancy resulting from femoral thrombosis. If an abnormal ABI persists at age 5 years, we recommend radiographic monitoring of bone length. Those with limb length discrepancies of 1 cm or more should have yearly follow-up. Because leg length discrepancy of greater than 2 cm is generally accepted as the smallest that is clinically significant, we recommend late arterial repair a year or so before puberty if this degree of discrepancy is detected or predicted during follow-up.[3] Arteriography is essential for surgical planning in patients with chronic limb ischemia and impaired leg growth. Delayed reconstruction generally allows repair of a relatively short occluded arterial segment in a older, larger patient and appears to be preferable to a repair attempted acutely. Correction of chronic ischemia has been shown anecdotally to improve leg length discrepancy,[4,5] although insufficient cases have been reported to permit a reliable prediction of improvement.

EXTRACORPOREAL MEMBRANE OXYGENATION

Extracorporeal membrane oxygenation is a well-established although infrequently applied adjunct in the care of critically ill neonates with respiratory failure. The long-term vascular and neurologic consequences of right carotid artery ligation, as usually performed after removal of the cannulae, are not clear. Although not widely practiced, recent reports suggest carotid reconstruction at the time of cannula removal with debridement of damaged arterial wall and primary closure is feasible in most patients. This repair appears associated with satisfactory patency and minimal complications[6,7] and seems reasonable, given the need for operation to remove the catheters.

UMBILICAL ARTERY CATHETER INJURIES

Umbilical artery catheters (UAC) are used frequently in critically ill neonates. Hypertonic solutions, catheter manipulation, prolonged catheter use, type of catheter material, dehydration, and hypercoagulability all appear to contribute to the arterial complications of UAC. These arterial complications include vasospasm, partial or total aortic or iliac artery thrombosis, and embolism to peripheral or visceral vessels. Hypertension and congestive heart failure (CHF) may accompany aortic thrombosis. Management of UAC-induced aortic thrombosis is dictated by the nature and severity of the symptoms resulting from the thrombosis.

In infants with lower extremity arterial emboli in otherwise viable limbs, the UAC should be removed, heparin anticoagulation started unless contraindicated, and the patient observed. The same treatment should be used in the presence of moderate peripheral ischemia due to partial thrombotic occlusion of the aorta or iliac arteries. Duplex ultrasound is invaluable in assessing aortic patency and serially determining the progression or regression of the aortic thrombus (Fig. 1). Diagnostic aortography may be performed initially with the UAC in place but is otherwise technically difficult and potentially harmful. The percentage of occlusion of the aorta is a reasonable predictor of both symptomatic ischemic severity and outcome.[8] Many neonates have only mild

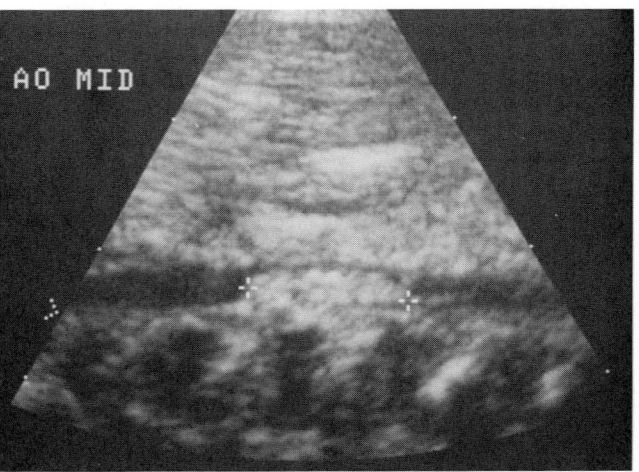

Figure 1 Ultrasound documenting aortic thrombus due to umbilical artery catheter.

symptoms with a partially occlusive aortic thrombus, whereas aortic occlusion as determined by duplex scanning is usually associated with more severe symptoms. Partial occlusion presenting with hypertension or CHF is also treated initially by UAC removal, anticoagulation, and hydration as indicated. The natural history is generally one of improvement (Fig. 2). Neonates with extremity ischemia following UAC-induced thrombosis should be treated and followed as previously described.

Operative thrombectomy is reserved for infants with aortic occlusion who deteriorate with appropriate medical management as shown by the development of severe and worsening hypertension, CHF, lower extremity ischemia, intestinal ischemia, renal failure, coagulopathy, or multisystem organ failure.[9] The presence of aortic thrombosis can usually be established reliably and noninvasively by duplex examination, although detection of accompanying visceral and renal arterial occlusion may require aortography. Operative thrombectomy is indicated in infants with severely symptomatic aortic thrombosis because nonoperative management has generally proven unsuccessful.

Although operative thrombectomy, once elected, must not be unduly delayed, adequate attention must be directed to fluid resuscitation and prevention of hypothermia. Therapeutic anticoagulation should be initiated if not already started. Either a transperitoneal or a retroperitoneal approach to the thrombosed aorta can be used. The transabdominal route allows inspection of ischemic bowel and resection if necessary. Vessel loops are used for vascular control. A transverse aortotomy in the distal aorta above the bifurcation allows extraction of clot from the iliac arteries with a 3 Fr balloon catheter and from the femoral arteries with a 2 Fr balloon catheter. A longitudinal arteriotomy and temporary suprarenal aortic control may be necessary for access to the renal artery orifices. Interrupted CV-8 polytetrafluo-

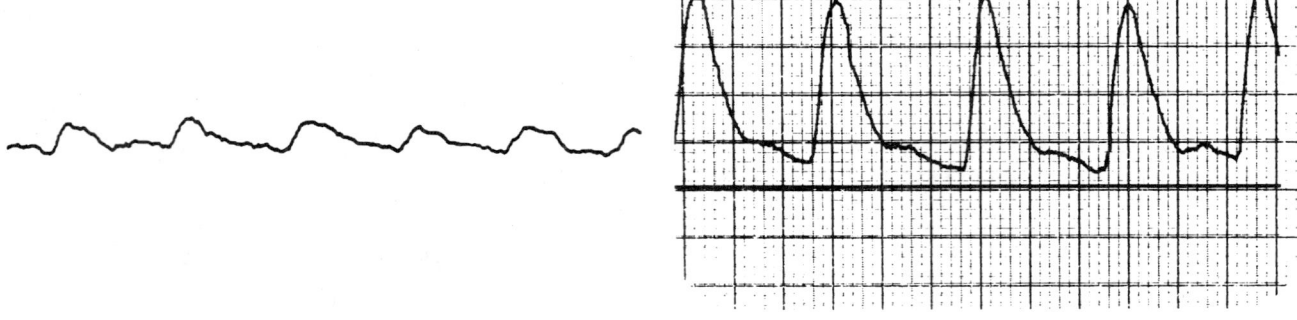

Figure 2 Common femoral artery Doppler waveforms at 1 month (*a*) and 14 months (*b*) after umbilical artery catheter–induced aortic thrombosis causing lower extremity ischemia; treated nonoperatively.

roethylene suture is used to close the aortotomy. Limb fasciotomies may be required after relief of prolonged ischemia.

THROMBOLYTIC THERAPY

It is well established that continuous heparin infusion during diagnostic arteriography decreases the incidence of thrombotic complications. Heparin anticoagulation also improves outcome in patients with thrombosis treated nonoperatively. Although thrombolytic therapy has found occasional use in adults, its place in the treatment of iatrogenic pediatric arterial thromboses is undetermined. The use of these drugs has been reported in the treatment of both iatrogenic postarteriographic femoral artery thrombosis as well as UAC-associated aortic thrombosis. Neonates present an added difficulty in the effective use of thrombolytics because of their reduced levels of plasminogen. Giacoia recently reviewed the available literature on the use of thrombolytics in neonates.[10] He found that thrombolysis was more likely to be successful if high doses of urokinase were used and suggested doses up to 40,000 U/kg/hour to compensate for the diminished levels of plasminogen in neonates. He also found no convincing benefit resulting from thrombolytics.

Whereas thrombolytics may have a role in accelerating the resolution of aortic thrombosis responding inadequately to anticoagulation, an accurate assessment of the usefulness of these drugs is impossible in that the available publications report widely varying indications for thrombolysis, drugs used, doses used, lack of controls, and lack of objective assessment of therapeutic success. In addition to these reporting problems, these reports have also uniformly failed to indicate the extent of thrombotic obstruction before thrombolysis. Thus, it is impossible to predict the anticipated natural history without the use of thrombolytics. Additionally, many infants with aortic thrombosis have significant hypertension and appear at increased risk for intraventricular hemorrhage. We have not routinely used thrombolytic therapy in neonates and note that the few published series generally report success rates of 50% or less, no better than a well-performed operation.

REFERENCES

1. Taylor LM, Troutman R, Feliciano P, et al. Late complications after femoral artery catheterization in children less than five years of age. J Vasc Surg 1990; 11:297–306.
2. Mansfield PB, Gazzania AB, Litwin SB. Management of arterial injuries related to cardiac catheterization in children and young adults. Circulation 1970; 42:501–507.
3. Mosely C. A straight line graph for leg length discrepancies. Clin Orthop 1978; 136:33–40.
4. Bloom JD, Mozersky DJ, Buckley CF, Hagood CO. Defective limb growth as a complication of catheterization of the femoral artery. Surg Gynecol Obstet 1974; 138:524–526.
5. Rubinstein RA, Taylor LM, Porter JM, Beals RK. Limb growth after late bypass graft for occlusion of the femoral artery. J Bone Joint Surg [Am] 1990; 72-A:935–937.
6. Crombleholme TM, Adzick S, deLorimier AA, et al. Carotid artery reconstruction following extracorporeal membrane oxygenation. Am J Dis Child 1990; 144:872–874.
7. Spector ML, Wiznitzer M, Walsh-Sukys MC, Stork EK. Carotid reconstruction in the neonate following ECMO. J Pediatr Surg 1991; 26:357–361.
8. Vailas GN, Brouillette RT, Scott JP, et al. Neonatal aortic thrombosis: Recent experience. J Pediatr 1986; 109:101–108.
9. Colburn MD, Gelabert HA, Quiñones-Baldrich W. Neonatal aortic thrombosis. Surgery 1992; 111:21–28.
10. Giacoia G. High-dose urokinase therapy in newborn infants with major vessel thrombosis. Clin Pediatr (Phila) 1993; 32:231–237.

COLD INJURY

RACHEL PODRAZIK BAER, M.D.

The documentation and study of cold injury have paralleled the history of armed conflict in human civilization dating from the conquests of Alexander the Great to the World Wars and the Korean Conflict of this century. Cold injury is a problem of everyday relevance, however, affecting those who work outdoors or enjoy winter sports as well as the increasing population of the elderly and homeless who frequently face cold exposure without adequate protection.

Although prevention of cold injury is most desirable, rapid treatment of such injury can limit the degree of physiologic insult, tissue damage, and long-term disability. Hypothermia refers to generalized cooling of the body, whereas frostbite encompasses local cold injury resulting from skin and peripheral tissue exposure to reduced ambient or freezing temperatures.

HYPOTHERMIA

Accidental hypothermia in humans is an unintentional drop in core body temperature below 35°C (95°F), generally occurring in otherwise healthy people exposed to a cold environment. Hypothermia is classified as mild, moderate, or severe (Table 1). Accidental hypothermia develops in a number of settings. Frequently, victims are winter sports participants, accident victims trapped in the cold, or victims of cold water immersion. An increased susceptibility to hypothermia is well recognized among the elderly, newborn, and those with severe illnesses. In recent years, increasing attention has focused on hypothermia in urban settings among the elderly, the homeless, the destitute, and those suffering from drug and alcohol addiction. Hypothermia is an underreported cause of death in the United States. Frequently, death is attributed to other factors, and hypothermia is considered a secondary cause. Fewer than 19% of severely hypothermic patients survive to reach the hospital. Among hypothermic patients who are hospitalized, mortality rates range widely from 0 to 65%, depending on treatment, population risk factors, and data collection methods. The best outcomes reported are among patients with mild hypothermia who do not sustain cardiac arrest.

The human body functions best within a narrow range of core temperature. The normal diurnal variation is only 1°C, and, in general, cold acclimatization in humans is poor. Without protection from the environment, heat is lost primarily by radiation (60%). Conduction, convection, and evaporation together account for the remaining 40%. Wet clothing and water immersion increase conductive loss markedly.

Whereas multiple mechanisms rapidly dissipate heat, humans must rely, in large part, on adaptive behavior for heat conservation.

In regard to thermoregulatory mechanisms,[1] a human may be physiologically divided into a homiothermic core, which includes the deep muscles and internal organs, and a poikilothermic shell, which includes the skin, the subcutaneous tissue, and the superficial muscles. The shell subserves the core in an attempt to maintain central temperature. Ambient temperature change is detected by thermal receptors in the skin. Afferent spinal cord pathways transmit this information to the anterior hypothalamus. The posterior hypothalamus then coordinates a well-defined response to prevent heat loss and augment heat production. Muscle tone is increased, which leads to shivering and an associated fivefold increase in heat production. Shivering increases the rate of heat loss, however. Metabolic mechanisms of heat generation include increases in epinephrine, norepinephrine, and thyroxine secretion, leading to a rise in basal metabolic rate. Another important heat regulatory mechanism is blood flow to the skin. During cold stress, marked vasoconstriction leads to virtual cessation of blood flow to the integument. Finally, and most important, decreases in ambient temperature initiate conscious responses to seek shelter, increase physical activity, and apply protective clothing. Diminished perception of cooler temperature, interruption of sensory signals to the central nervous system, altered processing of these neural inputs, or diminished metabolic or behavioral responses predispose to hypothermia.

The extent of pathophysiologic change that accompanies hypothermia depends on the severity of the insult, the causal factors, and the patient's premorbid state of health. The pathophysiologic changes for each organ system are well described.

Hypothermia results in progressive depression of the central nervous system. Normal mentation gives way to confusion and combativeness, then a semiconscious state, and finally coma, as the severity of hypothermia increases.

The heart responds to hypothermia with an initial increase in cardiac output; a progressive decline then occurs with worsening hypothermia and a concomitant decrease in blood pressure. In severe hypothermia, the QRS and ST segments lengthen as electrical conduction slows. The J wave, a characteristic positive-negative deflection immediately following the QRS complex, is noted in approximately one-third of patients. As temperature declines below 29°C, bradycardia and atrial and ventricular arrhythmias are common. Spontaneous ventricular fibrillation occurs at temperatures lower than 25°C, and cardiac standstill occurs at 21°C.

In the pulmonary system, respiratory rate usually increases after sudden cold water immersion. The medullary respiratory center is increasingly depressed, however, as hypothermia worsens. Atelectasis, pneumonia, and aspiration after rewarming are explained by a depressed cough reflex, cold-induced slowing of the tracheobronchial cilia, excessive production of tenacious secretions, and, frequently, a diminished level of con-

Table 1 Classification of Hypothermia

Definition	Temperature	Signs and Symptoms
Mild	Less than 35° C	Shivering
		Complaint of cold
		Usually conscious
		Sometimes confused
		Normal blood pressure
Moderate	Less than 32° C	Semiconscious, combative
		Shivering ceases
		Muscle rigidity
		Dilated pupils
		Ventricular fibrillation with agitation
		Decreased ventilatory rate
		Blood pressure difficult to obtain
Severe	Less than 26.5° C	Comatose
		Flaccid
		Apnea
		Spontaneous ventricular fibrillation

Adapted from Britt LD, Dascombe WH, Rodriguez A. New horizons in management of hypothermia and frostbite. Surg Clin North Am 1991; 71:345–370; with permission.

sciousness. Pulmonary edema is frequently observed after rewarming.

The kidneys respond with cold-induced diuresis despite decreases in glomerular filtration rate and renal blood flow. Hepatic function is also depressed with a concomitant reduction in the detoxification of drugs. Gastric stress ulcers and hemorrhagic pancreatitis have been reported at temperatures below 27°C.

Metabolic effects include a shift in the oxyhemoglobin dissociation curve to the left, increasing the affinity of hemoglobin for oxygen. This change is offset by an increase in the diffusion of oxygen and by a reduction of oxygen consumption by 50% at 30°C. The metabolic rate is reduced by 50% for every 10°C fall in temperature. Other metabolic effects include the impairment of insulin action contributing to hyperglycemia. Elevated potassium levels result from an alteration in the sodium-potassium pump during hypothermia, and hypokalemia frequently develops after rewarming. Metabolic acidosis is present in a significant number of patients secondary to respiratory depression, lactic acid generation from shivering, the increase in CO_2 diffusibility, and the decreased hepatic metabolism of organic acids.

Hematologic changes include an increase in blood viscosity due to hemoconcentration. Impaired coagulation and disseminated intravascular coagulation may be present with severe hypothermia. These changes are thought to be caused by the release of tissue thromboplastin from ischemic tissue and resolve promptly with rewarming. A temporary thrombocytopenia has also been noted with hypothermia.

Hypothermia is a true medical emergency. Emergency care should be handled in a timely but disciplined fashion to avoid untoward treatment effects. Therapy should take advantage of hypothermic protection that prevents continued rapid deterioration of certain core organs and that may allow time to correct the body's homeostatic milieu. Goals of care are to recognize the condition as soon as possible, prevent further heat loss, rewarm the victim as rapidly and safely as possible, and recognize and rapidly treat ventricular fibrillation.

The treatment of hypothermia frequently begins outside the hospital. Only essential measures are performed in the field. Extent and duration of cold exposure and a history of past medical problems are determined. The victim is removed from the cold environment. Wet clothing is removed, and warm blankets applied. Thereafter, the patient is moved as little as possible to reduce the risk of arrhythmias. Peripheral intravenous access is obtained, and intravenous saline with 5% dextrose is administered because effective circulatory volume is diminished. Lactated Ringer's solution should be avoided to prevent worsening lactic acidosis in the face of the hypothermic liver's lowered efficiency for metabolizing lactate. Patients with altered mental status are given intravenous thiamine (100 mg), naloxone (0.8 mg) and 50% dextrose. Patients with spontaneous respirations receive oxygen by mask warmed to 40°C to 45°C. Those with no respirations are intubated and ventilated. Ventilation should be at modest rates in that data suggest that mild alkalosis may be physiologically advantageous, but excessive alkalosis may further compromise the heart. Patients with a core temperature, lower than 28°C should receive intravenous bretylium, 5 mg/kg, to prevent ventricular fibrillation. In severe hypothermia, detection of spontaneous respiration or pulses may be quite difficult, and several minutes of monitoring are required before deciding to initiate cardiopulmonary resuscitation (CPR). Defibrillation, if available in the field, is indicated to correct ventricular fibrillation. Bretylium is an effective adjunct to managing hypothermia-induced ventricular fibrillation. Defibrillation attempts are rarely successful when the core temperature is lower than 30°C. In fact, field CPR is unlikely to succeed without timely transport to the emergency department. Defibrillation attempts should be repeated for every 2°C to 3°C rise in the patient's temperature.

The first challenge in the emergency department is the proper measurement of core temperature. Most standard thermometers do not record temperatures below 34°C. Measurement of core temperatures below this level requires special equipment such as cold-recording rectal thermometers, ear probes, esophageal probes, or high-rectal thermistors. Rectal temperatures are generally most practical. Baseline studies include a complete blood count, serum electrolytes, glucose, an arterial blood gas, coagulation parameters, blood cultures, a chest radiograph, and an electrocardiogram (ECG). Bladder catheterization is performed. Continuous monitoring of the ECG and vital signs, measurement of central venous pressure and urine output, and serial electrolyte and arterial blood gas determinations are conducted during rewarming.

A variety of rewarming techniques have been described. Passive techniques include a warm environment and blanket insulation. Active external warming uses heating pads, warm water immersion, hot water bottles, and environmental heaters. Active internal or core warming techniques include warmed intravenous solutions, peritoneal lavage with warm fluids, gastric or colonic lavage, airway rewarming, mediastinal lavage, and extracorporeal blood rewarming. In most cases of mild hypothermia, passive external warming is sufficient for healthy adults. In general, several active rewarming techniques should be used for moderate to severe hypothermia, for example, heating pad application, delivery of warm O_2, infusion of warmed intravenous solutions, and warm peritoneal lavage.

The best way to warm the patient has not been identified, however. Success with all modalities has been reported in experimental models and in limited human studies. Unfortunately, a paucity of prospective clinical trials does not permit conclusions about the advantages of one technique over another. There is consensus that patients rewarmed at a rate of less than 0.5°C/hour have a poorer prognosis than patients warmed at a rate of 1°C to 2°C/hour. There is no evidence that rewarming at a faster rate improves survival.

One purported disadvantage of active external rewarming techniques is the "afterdrop" phenomenon—a paradoxic decrease in core temperature after the start of rewarming. This complication was thought to be caused by active external rewarming-induced peripheral vasodilation with shunting of cold, acidotic blood trapped in the periphery to the relatively warmer core. An acute drop in core temperature of 2°C to 3°C after the onset of rewarming may cause further myocardial compromise, aggravate hypotension, and precipitate arrhythmias. Recent studies, however, challenge peripheral vasodilation as the stimulus for this phenomenon.

The role of extracorporeal rewarming deserves special note. Most clinicians accept the superiority of extracorporeal bypass for rewarming hypothermic, hemodynamically unstable patients. With the expanded availability of emergency portable bypass systems, it has been suggested that all patients receive the direct hemodynamic support of extracorporeal bypass when rewarming from temperatures lower than 32°C. A multi-institutional trial is required to resolve this issue. Certainly recovery without this measure, even among unstable patients receiving CPR and other warming techniques, has been reported. Experimental work in dogs documented an equal return of myocardial function and similar survival rates with cardiac arrest, at temperatures between 25°C and 28°C, whether partial cardiac bypass or external chest compressions were used.[2] Success of CPR in conjunction with other rewarming modalities points to the relative cytoprotection of hypothermia and tolerance of lower cardiac output because of the decreased basal metabolism associated with hypothermia. At present, it is reasonable to use extracorporeal rewarming in the unstable, hypothermic patient, when available, but successful recovery from a hypothermic event with hemodynamic instability does not require this technology.

FROSTBITE

The second major form of cold injury, frostbite, relates to local tissue injuries resulting from freezing temperature exposure. Frostbite is injury caused when tissue freezes. Not all local cold injuries are caused by freezing tissue conditions, however. Milder forms of local cold injury are considered here first.

Frostnip is the mildest form of cold injury. It is the only reversible cold injury, and this injury represents ice crystal formation on the skin, usually developing slowly and painlessly. Simple blanching of the skin is frequently detected by a companion first. Numbness of the skin and a frosted appearance of the skin develop, and, thus, frostnip may resemble frostbite. However, frostnip does not involve damage to the dermal or subcutaneous tissue if rewarming is promptly instituted. Treatment is by firm, steady contact of the affected part with a warm hand, blowing hot breath over the injured area, or holding the frostnipped fingers or toes in the axilla or crotch. A tingling sensation may be experienced in the affected area as warmth and color return. The injured skin may be erythematous and flake for several days. Prevention includes adequate protection of the normally exposed portions of the body.

Chilblains, also known as pernio, is also caused by nonfreezing cold conditions. This clinical entity is characterized by the recurrent, cold-induced appearance of red, raised lesions on unprotected extremities. These lesions classically occur after prolonged exposure to cold, dry, nonfreezing weather. Typically lesions start acutely as single or multiple, red or purple swellings. They may itch, burn, or cause pain. In severe cases there may be purpura, blistering, or ulceration. Lesions resolve spontaneously, usually within several weeks. The extremities are most often affected, especially the dorsum of the proximal phalanges of fingers and toes, the plantar surfaces of toes and heels, and the ears and nose.

Chilblains commonly affects young and middle-aged women. Differential diagnosis includes the dermatologic manifestations of systemic lupus erythematosis, cutaneous vasculitis, lupus pernio (a manifestation of sarcoidosis), or lesions seen in elderly men with monocytic leukemia. Patients with severe, recalcitrant chilblains should have a complete blood count and a rheumatologic evaluation. In most patients, chilblains can be controlled with reassurance, warm housing, and warm clothing. In patients with severe recurrent chilblains, nifedipine has been shown to be effective in a prospective, double-blind, clinical trial.[3]

Trenchfoot, or immersion foot, is another entity in the spectrum of cold injury. Trenchfoot has been extensively studied by the military because it has contributed significantly to troop morbidity and attrition during war. The syndrome is appearing with greater frequency among the homeless population.[4] The condition results from prolonged exposure to wet, cold conditions at temperatures usually less than 50°F. Classically, feet have been submerged for periods of 4 hours or more. The pathophysiology is waterlogging of the stratum corneum of the soles of the feet. Biopsy specimens show thickening, swelling, and fragmentation of the stratum corneum with variable amounts of upper dermal edema. The clinical presentation of these patients is usually bilateral, painful edema of the feet. The soles of the feet are typically white, wrinkled, and painful. More severe cases may progress to involve the dorsum of the foot, but deep injury and progression to gangrene are rare. Drying and elevation of the feet are usually adequate initial therapy. Prevention is the best long-term therapy. Adequate foot care with at least 8 hours each day to dry the feet is optimal. Heavy boots are better than tennis shoes for prevention because of their greater impenetrability to water.

Frostbite develops when tissue freezes. In the absence of wind, tissue freezes at $-2°C$. Wind chill significantly increases the rate of tissue freezing. Frostbite injuries usually involve the extremities or exposed areas such as the cheek, nose, or ears. The extent and severity of the injury is directly related to the rate of heat loss, tissue temperature, intensity of the initial exposure, and the length of time before adequate circulation can be restored. In addition, the underlying peripheral circulation of an individual plays an important role in determining the severity of frostbite. Pre-existing arterial disease and local ischemia of the extremity, as well as constrictive clothing, contribute to increased tissue freezing. Smoking and other causes of hypoxia, such as exposure to high altitudes, are factors in frostbite injury. Cold acclimatization seems to have an influence on the degree of cold injury sustained. Such acclimatization has been observed in as little as 6 weeks.

Although the most serious consequence of frostbite is cellular injury with resultant cell death, the mechanism by which it occurs is not precisely defined. Whether this process is the result of the direct effect of freezing of the cell at the time of cold exposure, the result of inadequate tissue perfusion secondary to microvascular occlusion, or results from a combination of these mechanisms has not been fully elucidated.

In the pathophysiology of frostbite, an initial generalized constriction of all blood vessels occurs during cold exposure. Following vasoconstriction, the temperature of the extremity falls rapidly and plateaus at the freezing point ($-2°C$). At the cellular level, ice crystals begin to form within the interstitium and then within the intravascular and intracellular compartments. Because crystallization is an exothermic process, the temperature of the limb may plateau at $-2°C$ for a time. After this, the limb temperature falls rapidly to reach ambient temperature. Freezing and crystallization produce cell injury and death by three mechanisms: first, interstitial crystallization causes a hyperosmolar environment and draws water from the intracellular compartment to cause cellular dehydration. Second, mechanical disruption of cells by growing crystals occurs. Third, structural damage to the cell wall itself occurs with freezing. Once rewarming begins, a reversal of the freezing process occurs. The extremity temperature rises rapidly as interstitial crystals melt, with reversed fluid flux into cells. Morphologic characterization by Marzella and colleagues documented that endothelial cells, particularly within the arterioles, are the initial cells injured following rewarming.[5] Within the first hour, the microvasculature sustains extensive damage. Platelet aggregation parallels this injury. Reperfused capillaries are highly permeable, resulting in immediate interstitial edema with extravasation of erythrocytes beginning at about 6 hours. Further, the Marzella group noted that parenchymal elements of the skin appeared to be free of damage during this time. Continued tissue injury may follow reperfusion by a variety of mechanisms, including free radical–mediated injury and the pathologic effects of prostaglandins, specifically thromboxane A_2 and prostaglandin $F_{2\alpha}$. The exact timing and extent to which prostaglandins contribute to injury are not known.

Frostbite has traditionally been classified as first-, second-, third-, and fourth-degree injury. An additional modification of this classification considers injury as superficial or deep (Table 2). This system classifies injury not only on the basis of depth of tissue injury but also clinical findings and subsequent course, allowing some assessment of prognosis.

When frostbite is suspected, the victim should be transported to an emergency facility rapidly. During transport, the affected body parts should not be allowed to thaw and refreeze. Wet clothing is removed and replaced by soft, dry garments.

In the emergency department, core temperature should be measured and hypothermia treated prior to rewarming the frostbitten limb. Rapid effective rewarming of the affected parts is performed by immersion in warm water at 40°C to 42°C for 15 to 30 minutes. Rapid rather than slow rewarming decreases the time of tissue exposure to cold injury, enhances cutaneous vasodilation, and more rapidly restores blood flow to affected

Table 2 Classification of Frostbite Injury

Classification	Symptoms
Superficial	
First degree: partial skin freezing	
Erythema, edema, hyperemia	Transient stinging and burning
No blisters or necrosis	Throbbing and aching possible
Occasional skin desquamation (5–10 days later)	May have hyperhidrosis
Second degree: full-thickness skin freezing	
Erythema, substantial edema	Numbness; vasomotor disturbances in severe cases
Vesicles with clear fluid	
Blisters that desquamate and form blackened eschar	
Deep	
Third degree: full-thickness skin and subcutaneous tissue freezing	Initially no sensation
Violaceous/hemorrhagic blisters	Involved tissue feels like "block of wood"
Skin necrosis	Later, shooting pains, burning, aching
Fourth degree: full-thickness skin, subcutaneous tissue, muscle, tendon and bone freezing	Possible joint discomfort
Little edema	
Initially mottled, deep red or cyanotic	
Eventually dry, black, mummified	

Adapted from Britt LD, Dascombe WH, Rodriguez A. New horizons in management of hypothermia and frostbite. Surg Clin North Am 1991; 71:345–370; with permission.

tissue. Dry heat should not be used because it is difficult to regulate and risks burn injury to the already insensitive tissue. Analgesics are administered because thawing is frequently accompanied by intense pain. Tetanus prophylaxis is given.

On completion of rewarming, treatment goals are to preserve viable tissue and prevent infection. No consensus exists for the best methods of treating these injuries. Some debride all blisters, whereas others leave blisters intact unless signs of infection are present. Prophylactic antibiotics are used routinely by some, but not by others. Based on experimental work, McCauley and colleagues have described a protocol to reduce the potentially injurious role of prostaglandin mediators in frostbite injury:[6] White blisters, known to contain high concentrations of prostaglandins, are debrided, and aloe vera ointment, a specific thromboxane inhibitor, applied every 6 hours. Hemorrhagic blisters, representing structural damage to the subdermal plexus, are left intact to prevent further microvascular injury, and topical aloe vera is applied every 6 hours. Oral ibuprofen and intravenous prophylactic penicillin are administered. Daily hydrotherapy in water at 38°C is used to gently debride nonviable tissue. In a nonrandomized clinical trial, McCauley and associates have reported a lower amputation rate and shorter hospital stays among 56 patients treated by this regimen compared with 96 patients treated with warm saline and Silvadene dressings.

Early surgical therapy of frostbite is not indicated unless fasciotomy is necessary to reduce ischemia due to a compartment syndrome or escharotomy is required to improve the circulation or movement of an affected digit. Late surgical management may be necessary if gangrene ensues. In such patients, amputation with primary wound closure is carried out weeks after injury. Autoamputation of digits involved with deep injury may obviate the need for surgical amputation.

Considerable experimental work has been performed to identify adjuvant agents that might limit frostbite injury. Agents studied include thrombolytic agents, heparin sodium, low-molecular-weight dextran, reserpine, peripheral vasodilators, calmodulin antagonists, and sympathectomy. To date, limited benefit has been documented in animal models. Far less information and only anecdotal reports of benefit have been reported in clinical settings. Thus, no treatment has been shown to be superior to rewarming in clinical trials. Further study, involving the therapeutic modulation of prostaglandin mediators and free radical–mediated injury, may be efficacious in reducing the ultimate extent of injury.

The resolution of frostbite injury may proceed along three paths: complete healing without sequelae; healing, but with a variety of postinjury sequelae; or frank tissue necrosis and gangrene. In many patients, a combination of these outcomes is seen. Ervasti's review of 812 patients with frostbite documented that healed extremity frostbite injuries were characterized by cold sensitivity (82%), persistent skin color changes (73%), hyperhidrosis (59%), and pain with extremity use (40%).[7] In addition, intrinsic muscle atrophy and bone growth retardation in children has been reported.

REFERENCES

1. Britt LD, Dascombe WH, Rodriguez A. New horizons in management of hypothermia and frostbite. Surg Clin North Am 1991; 71:345–370.
2. Moss JF, Haklin M, Southwick HW, et al. A model for severe accidental hypothermia. J Trauma 1986; 26:68–74.

3. Rustin MHA, Newton JA, Smith NP, et al. The treatment of chilblains with nifedipine: The results of a pilot study, a double-blind placebo-controlled randomized study and a long-term open trial. Br J Dermatol 1989; 120:267–275.
4. Wrenn K. Immersion foot: A problem of the homeless in the 1990s. Arch Intern Med 1991; 151:785–788.
5. Marzella L, Jesudass RR, Manson PN, et al. Morphologic characterization of acute injury to vascular endothelium of skin after frostbite. Plast Reconstr Surg 1989; 83:67–75.
6. McCauley RL, Hing DN, Robson MC, et al. Frostbite injuries: A rational approach based on the pathophysiology. J Trauma 1983; 23:143–147.
7. Ervasti E. Frostbites of the extremities and their sequelae. Acta Chir Scand 1962; 299(suppl):7.

AMPUTATION

NONINVASIVE METHODS OF DETERMINING AMPUTATION LEVELS

JOHN L. PROVAN, B.Sc., M.B., M.S.

There is nothing worse than the complication of "creeping amputation" for vascular surgeons performing amputations on patients with peripheral arterial insufficiency. A toe amputation in a diabetic patient that remains unhealed, leading to a below-the-knee (BK) amputation and occasionally after that to an above-the-knee (AK) amputation, is not likely to instill confidence in the unfortunate patient or the patient's relatives, yet all surgeons come across situations where an apparently clinically appropriate level of selection for amputation fails to achieve the desired result of primary healing.

When the conflicting desires of the surgeon, the patient, and the prosthetist for the most conservative amputation are balanced against the greater likelihood of achieving primary healing with a more proximal amputation, the dilemma that faces the surgeon is real. Many studies have shown the enormous advantage for those patients whose knee joint can be preserved, with regard to mobility and oxygen consumption. Similarly, the presence of a portion of the foot enables elderly patients to reach the bathroom at night without crutches or a prosthesis.

The surgical challenge, therefore, is to determine how to achieve the most distal possible leg amputation with the least surgical morbidity in relation to reliable healing. This is best done by means of an objective evaluation of skin blood flow. Because general conditions such as poor nutrition, chronic cardiac failure, and infection may adversely affect primary healing of an amputation stump, improvement of these should be undertaken if time permits. There has also been much discussion regarding the effect that a previous reconstructive operation may have on amputation level. Whereas some have suggested that a higher amputation results after failure of arterial reconstruction, most believe that a failed reconstructive procedure has little impact on the eventual level of amputation.

METHODS OF NONINVASIVE ASSESSMENT

It must be stated at the outset that there is no single method of noninvasive assessment of skin blood flow that reliably, consistently, and unequivocally determines the appropriate level of amputation. In addition, excessive reliance on a particular noninvasive method must be tempered by clinical judgment, particularly if the noninvasive method in use indicates a higher level of amputation than clinical judgment would suggest. Too great a reliance on such a finding may, given the unpredictability of healing of amputations, lead to a reduced number of lower level amputations with the associated disadvantages noted previously.

Clinical Judgment

In general, the presence of a normally palpable pulse above the limb segment where an amputation is contemplated leads to reliable healing in most patients. However, the reverse is not true, and increasingly surgeons have been able to achieve successful BK amputations in as many as 85% of patients, many in the absence of a palpable popliteal pulse. Palpation of pedal, popliteal, and femoral pulses is, therefore, a very important part of the noninvasive assessment. It should, however, be accompanied by clinical assessment of skin temperature at the proposed incision levels, venous filling, and the presence or absence of dependent rubor. Particularly in diabetic patients, the presence or absence of infection adjacent to the proposed lines of incision must also be determined. Particular care must be taken to ensure the absence of infection in the deep plantar spaces as shown by swelling or tenderness in the sole of the foot. Radiologic investigation may also be required to exclude infection by gas-forming organisms when foot amputations in diabetics are being considered.

The skin temperature, despite earlier writings to the contrary, is best assessed by the palm of the hand. Laying the whole hand across the surface to be examined provides more sensitivity to temperature than the use of the back of the knuckles. Venous filling with the foot in the supine position, again compared with the opposite limb, is also useful. Examination of the foot after dependency for 2 to 3 minutes indicates dependent rubor in the distal limb in those with severe peripheral ischemia. This sign is only of value in that a distal amputation of toe or forefoot will never heal if incisions are made through areas of dependent rubor.

Our own study of the role of transcutaneous oxygen tension ($PtcO_2$) measurements as a predictor of healing indicated the lack of reliability of clinical findings in selecting BK compared to AK amputations.[1] The difficulty associated with clinical evaluation as a predictor of amputation level is much greater in the selection of amputations below the ankle, where failure rates of 60% have been reported with use of clinical criteria alone.

Segmental Doppler Systolic Blood Pressure Measurements

Although this method has been used to predict healing for various levels of amputation for nearly 15 years, its predictive value declines when foot and toe amputations are considered, probably as a result of errors in pressure determination due to calcific changes in the vessels of some patients. It cannot be recommended as useful for BK amputations because popliteal artery occlusion pressures with a cuff have been inconsistent in defining a blood pressure below which BK amputations do not heal. Some have noted that most BK amputations heal with a popliteal artery pressure above 50 mm Hg. Other authors have noted successful amputations below this blood pressure, and similar findings have been noted when the systolic blood pressure level predicting successful amputation has been 60 or 70 mm Hg. Several studies have been unable to determine a statistically significant difference in systolic blood pressure level in amputations that healed compared to those that did not.

Skin Blood Flow Techniques

Techniques using radioactive xenon or iodothyronine were extensively investigated in the 1980s, again without providing evidence that would unequivocally predict successful healing of BK amputations compared to those above the knee. Both techniques involve the intradermal injection of a radioisotope, clearance of which from the skin should, in theory, be related to the blood flow in the area of the injection. Unfortunately, the clearance of the radioisotope is heavily dependent on the precise site of the injection, readings that are falsely low or falsely high being possible if the injection is subcutaneous or too superficial in the epidermis. These techniques are also heavily dependent on other factors that may affect skin blood flow, including ambient temperature, body temperature, cardiac function, and anxiety. It may be impossible to produce standardized situations for these tests, even though they are theoretically very attractive. Both techniques have a large overlap between the skin blood flow of patients with successful and unsuccessful amputations. No study has indicated a predictable cutoff level for skin blood flow based on the clearance of these isotopes.

A variant of this technique involves the measurement of skin perfusion pressure by using an intradermal injection of a radioactive tracer whose clearance from the skin is measured with the skin blood flow techniques defined earlier. In this technique the skin perfusion pressure is determined by repeated inflation of a blood pressure cuff, which is applied over the injection site at gradually increasing pressures until the clearance of isotope from the area stops. The pressure at which this occurs is the skin perfusion pressure. This technique is uncomfortable, tends to be time-consuming, and has not indicated a cutoff level of skin perfusion pressure that can reliably predict below-knee healing. In general, a perfusion pressure of 20 mm Hg or more at the distal site suggests a higher likelihood of healing, but not all authors concur, and in some a cutoff figure of 30 mm Hg seemed to prove more reliable.

Laser Doppler flowmetry and fluorescein uptake techniques are other methods of measuring skin blood flow. The value of the former seemed to be greater when skin hyperemia was produced by heating the skin, although this still provided unpredictable results. The fluorescein uptake technique is much simpler to perform and requires only the intravenous injection of sodium fluorescein, whose fluorescence in the skin following exposure to ultraviolet light can be quantified. However, this technique may be risky in that cardiac arrest has been described following fluorescein injection, and both false-positive and false-negative results have occurred.

Transcutaneous Oxygen Pressure Measurements

This technique, which has been investigated in our laboratory,[2] provides an alternative means of measuring skin perfusion that is simple to perform with relatively inexpensive equipment. Skin hyperemia using a heated Clark electrode attached to the skin overcomes the variability in skin perfusion that may be produced by some of the factors mentioned before, such as changes in ambient temperature or hypertension. Early experiments indicated a close correlation between $PtcO_2$ measurements in patients with intermittent claudication and ischemic rest pain and gangrene compared to normals. In addition, the fall in $PtcO_2$ occurring after exercise in patients with claudication and the rise in $PtcO_2$ produced by dependency after the legs were supine have all indicated the value of this method of assessing skin blood flow. In relation to amputation, we showed that $PtcO_2$ measurements of 25 mm Hg or above successfully predicted below-knee amputations more effectively than clinical evaluation. Although $PtcO_2$ measurements in the foot did not differ significantly in patients undergoing AK or BK amputations, there was a statistically significant difference in $PtcO_2$ measurements below the knee (34.92 ± 10.84 mm Hg) compared to those undergoing AK amputation (9.5 ± 5.6 mm Hg).

These findings were very similar whether the $PtcO_2$ measurements were made anteriorly or posteriorly below the knee. In our study, comparison was made with clinical evaluation. In 38 amputations $PtcO_2$ measurements and clinical judgment differed on 5 occasions, a lower amputation being indicated by $PtcO_2$ twice and by clinical selection three times. Amputation was performed at the most distal level indicated by either technique and in the two patients where an AK amputation was selected on clinical grounds and the $PtcO_2$ measurements favored a BK amputation, primary healing occurred at the BK level. In the three patients in whom clinical impression suggested a BK amputation and the $PtcO_2$ values were less than 24 mm Hg, primary healing did not occur.

Similar results have been obtained by other workers, but the level of $PtcO_2$ that appeared to predict primary healing has varied widely. The study by Burgess and co-workers indicated a cutoff level of 40 mm Hg,[3] whereas others have suggested a level of 35 mm Hg. Although our earlier results suggested that $PtcO_2$ readings successfully predicted 100% healing, subsequent use of this technique has not confirmed its absolute reliability. It has been suggested that, using the long posterior myoplastic flap for below-knee amputation, it might be advisable to measure the $PtcO_2$ level lower in the calf than with our study. However, it is usually the anterior portion of the incision on the proximal flap that fails to heal, and this failure to heal is probably more dependent on technical factors during the course of the operation, such as forcible elevation of the skin from the anterior surface of the tibia, than on the actual blood flow at that site.

Measurement of $PtcO_2$ probably provides the easiest and most effective noninvasive technique in use at present. However, as with other methods of noninvasive assessment, there appears to be no absolutely reliable cutoff value. The limitations of the use of $PtcO_2$ measurements relate to the fact that a profound fall in skin perfusion pressure is probably necessary before $PtcO_2$ measurements decline significantly, although the use of skin hyperemia may better define skin perfusion by maximizing capillary vasodilation. It is not clear how this technique is affected by changes in cardiac output or systemic blood pressure. Some of our results have surprisingly indicated little effect on $PtcO_2$ measurements as a result of changes in either cardiac output or systemic blood pressure.[4] The discriminant value of $PtcO_2$ also seems not to be affected by breathing oxygen or by the use of hyperbaric oxygen, although another of our studies did show that a failure to increase $PtcO_2$ in the foot on standing from the recumbent position was predictive that primary revascularization would be unsuccessful in patients with advanced lower limb ischemia.[5]

Thermography and Capillary Microscopy

Little work has been done to evaluate these techniques, although their use does seem to increase the rate of BK amputation when compared with clinical judgment alone. It is possible that all of these techniques merely serve to refine clinical judgment and do nothing to mitigate the bad results of poor surgical technique in patients where a BK amputation might have been expected to heal.

There is virtually no work using noninvasive techniques to predict healing in Symes, forefoot, transmetatarsal, or toe amputations, for which clinical judgment and the nature of the ischemic lesion often define the only possible amputation. In patients in whom forefoot amputation is considered, pedal pulses are often present, and infection may be the final determining factor in suggesting a proximal rather than a more distal amputation in the lower leg or foot, usually in diabetic patients.

The excellent review by Sarin and associates described the relative advantages and disadvantages of the tests used to assess the level of amputation.[6] Certainly $PtcO_2$ has received the most widespread attention as a predictor of amputation level. Sarin and colleagues suggest that its predictive power is only fair, reporting ankle:brachial pressure indices and segmental blood pressures as having the best predictive powers. Although this has not been our experience, the ready availability and low cost of segmental blood pressure measurement equipment may make it the most useful technique. It is also possible that combinations of techniques may add to the sensitivity of the tests, although most studies using more than one technique have done so only to compare the value of techniques. In contrast to the Sarin group's findings, Lantsberg and Goldman, who compared laser Doppler flowmetry, $PtcO_2$ measurements, and Doppler pressures, found that Doppler pressures showed poor discrimination, that $PtcO_2$ confirmed some of the data from our early study, and that laser Doppler flowmetry appeared to be the best discriminator of skin flap perfusion.[7] In this study of 24 patients, 100% primary healing was obtained with clinical assessment only. It seems hard to improve on this result with any of the noninvasive tests. The conclusion must therefore be that at present no single noninvasive technique can confidently predict primary healing, particularly of below-knee amputations.

REFERENCES

1. Ameli FM, Byrne P, Provan JL. Selection of amputation level and prediction of healing using transcutaneous tissue oxygen tension (Ptc O_2). J Cardiovasc Surg (Torino) 1989; 30:220–224.
2. Byrne P, Provan JL, Ameli FM, Jones DP. The use of transcutaneous oxygen tension measurements in the diagnosis of peripheral vascular insufficiency. Ann Surg 1984; 200:159–165.
3. Burgess EM, Matsen FA, Wyss CR, Simmons CW. Segmental transcutaneous measurements of PO_2 in patients requiring below-the-knee amputation for peripheral vascular insufficiency. J Bone Joint Surg [Am] 1982; 64:378–382.
4. Joyce WP, Provan JL, Ameli FM. The influence of central haemodynamics on transcutaneous oxygen measurements. Eur J Vasc Surg 1990; 4:375–377.
5. Oh PJ, Provan JL, Ameli FM. The predictability of the success of

TOE AND FOOT AMPUTATION

DANIEL F. FISHER Jr., M.D.

Any surgical specialist performing toe and foot amputations has to ask two questions prior to operation. First, is there enough circulation in the foot to heal the amputation? Second, can the remaining foot be accommodated by prosthetic shoe modification to prevent neuropathic ulceration and further amputation? The former question can be answered by feeling for pedal pulses. If they are absent, arteriography should almost always precede the amputation. The chances for a successful amputation can generally be improved with a bypass prior to amputation that hopefully can restore palpable pedal pulses.

The second answer may be more difficult and may vary from area to area, depending on the experience and training of the prosthetist. If the surgeon is planning to perform some of the more unusual foot amputations, such as Chopart, Lisfranc, and Syme, prior consultation with a prosthetist is advisable to make sure that the resultant foot can be adequately fitted with a shoe that prevents ulceration and further amputation.

GENERAL PRINCIPLES

End-stage vascular disease often results in dry or wet gangrene. It is crucial for the treating physician to be able to differentiate these two conditions. Although dry gangrene may be an urgent problem, wet gangrene is a true emergency. Evaluation of both groups of patients starts with an estimation of the degree of impaired circulation in the involved foot. The standard pulse examination, ankle:brachial indices, toe blood pressures, and tissue oximetry may all be helpful in deciding whether a toe or forefoot amputation is likely to heal without prior vascular reconstruction.[1]

Dry Gangrene

Dry gangrene is more likely in atherosclerotic patients than in diabetics. It frequently results from embolization to the toe or forefoot. The patient often has only one or two toes involved. The patient may have palpable femoral pulses but no distal pulses, suggesting femoropopliteal occlusive disease, or absent leg pulses, suggesting aortoiliac disease. Most of these patients do not have enough circulation to the foot to heal a digital or transmetatarsal amputation. The patient should be admitted to a hospital to undergo an aortogram with long leg runoff to evaluate the possibilities for vascular reconstruction prior to foot amputation. If the patient's cardiac status permits the proposed operation, a bypass procedure to try to restore a pulse in the foot should be done before any digital or transmetarsal amputation. Once the bypass is completed, the surgeon can either perform a simultaneous amputation, or observe the foot in hopes that the toe will auto-amputate with improved circulation.

Wet Gangrene

Wet gangrene is more likely in diabetic patients who are not diligent about caring for their sensory and motor neuropathy. Wet gangrene may involve only one toe, or it may encompass the entire foot. The responsible surgeon needs to make an experienced decision about whether the foot can be salvaged. If only one or two toes are involved, it is preferable to start broad-spectrum antibiotic therapy and proceed with an open toe amputation on the day of admission. If the patient has one or two palpable pedal pulses, the foot should be observed for signs of healing. This type of patient generally receives 7 days of antibiotics. If the patient does not have a palpable pulse, arteriography within 24 to 36 hours after amputation is recommended to evaluate the limb for an urgent bypass.

If wet gangrene involves so much of the forefoot or foot that an extensive debridement procedure would result in a mangled and useless foot, an ankle guillotine amputation on the day of admission should be performed under the cover of broad-spectrum antibiotics.[2] This limb is revised into a below-knee or above-knee amputation approximately 72 hours after the guillotine amputation. Antibiotics are stopped 24 hours after the below-knee amputation because this operation is now a clean-contaminated procedure.

GENERAL TECHNIQUES IN AMPUTATION

Ischemic tissue demands the utmost in meticulous technique. Forceps should be used sparingly, if at all. The skin should be cut straight and perpendicular. Tendons are cut as short as possible. Bones are cut cleanly with small oscillating saws to prevent splintering. Bone wax is avoided to prevent a foreign body reaction and possible infection. Grossly infected tissues must be left open. Clean tissues are always closed without tension with nonabsorbable suture.

Phalangeal Amputation

Phalangeal amputations are not very practical in atherosclerotic and diabetic patients. Phalangeal amputations require reasonable circulation for healing at the very end of the toe; because this circulation is rarely present, this procedure is rarely utilized unless there is a distal crush injury to a toe with excellent circulation.

Toe Disarticulation

If the surgeon feels that the patient has enough skin around the base of the toe to heal a toe disarticulation, this amputation is easy to perform and has excellent functional results. The metatarsal head is not removed, so foot balance is preserved. This is especially important in dealing with the great toe. There is a controversy about whether to remove the relatively ischemic cartilage from the metatarsal head. If the skin over the amputation heals, the remaining cartilage is rarely a problem. Toe disarticulation is usually done by making a racquet-shaped incision around the base of the toe, leaving as much plantar skin as possible.

Metatarsal (Ray) Amputation

The difference in being able to perform a toe disarticulation and a ray (transmetarsal) amputation is usually the viability of the skin at the base of the toe. If viable skin is deficient, resection of the metatarsal head and part of the metatarsal shaft may allow primary skin closure. In addition, removal of a metatarsal head that is responsible for neuropathic ulceration may cure the problem. It does decrease the resultant surface area of the foot, possibly allowing for other areas to ulcerate. Foot imbalance may become a major problem if the great toe or fifth toe requires this amputation, and shoe modification is needed. Transmetatarsal amputation with small oscillating saws designed for hand surgery avoids splintered bone edges, which may occur with other crushing instruments.

Transmetatarsal Amputation

If more than the great toe medially, or the fourth and fifth toes laterally, need to be amputated, the surgeon might better perform a transmetatarsal amputation.[3] This procedure requires more plantar skin for a posterior flap than dorsal skin. This procedure removes all the metatarsal heads in the foot, and it may be an excellent amputation for some diabetics with multiple areas of neuropathic ulceration. It may also be a good amputation for forefoot necrosis in patients treated with vasoconstrictive agents for low cardiac output states. Shoe modification is mandatory, but these patients have a very functional foot, considering the amount of forefoot removed.

Chopart, Lisfranc, and Pirogoff Amputations

In general, Chopart, Lisfranc, and Pirogoff amputations have not been popular or successful, although recently there seems to be a rising popularity.[4] Equinus deformity is the major complication with the Chopart and Lisfranc amputations. Recurrent pressure and ulceration problems have occurred because of the difficulty in fitting these amputated feet with prosthetic shoes. The problem of equinus deformity may be avoided by dividing the Achilles tendon at the time of operation.

The biggest problem with the Pirogoff amputation is the necessity for bone union. Many experts think that the Pirogoff amputation offers very little advantage over the Syme amputation for the adult. It is not an amputation to offer a patient with an active infection.

Syme Amputation

The Syme amputation is controversial for two reasons. Authors debate about its ease of prosthetic fitting, and the healing potential ranges from 40% to 70%. With newer prosthetic innovations and better prosthetist training, the former objection should not deter performance of this amputation in well-selected patients. This amputation generally requires a palpable posterior tibial pulse for the posterior flap to heal.[5] If this operation is offered to patients with a palpable posterior tibial pulse, regardless of age or diabetic status, healing in the range of 70% to 75% can be expected. Shoe modification is mandatory for this to be an effective weight-bearing stump. The complete length of the tibia is maintained, although the extremity is 2 to 3 cm shorter because the calcaneus is removed. The two-stage technique, not performing resection of the malleoli is preferred at the time of disarticulation.

POSTOPERATIVE MANAGEMENT

Weight-bearing ambulation is not allowed for 4 to 6 weeks. Professional podiatric shoe fitting is important for the foot with a recent amputation and for the contralateral foot to prevent later problems with sensory ulceration.

REFERENCES

1. Dwars BJ, van den Broek TAA, Rauwerda JA, Bakker FC. Criteria for reliable selection of the lowest level of amputation in peripheral vascular disease. J Vasc Surg 1992; 15:536–542.

2. Fisher DF, Clagett GP, Fry RE, et al. One-stage versus two-stage amputation for wet gangrene of the lower extremity: A randomized study. J Vasc Surg 1988; 8:428–433.
3. Effeney DJ, Lim RC, Schecter WP. Transmetatarsal amputation. Arch Surg 1977; 112:1366–1370.
4. Roach JJ, Deutsch A, McFarlane DS. Resurrection of the amputations of Lisfranc and Chopart for diabetic gangrene. Arch Surg 1987; 122:931–934.
5. Francis H, Roberts JR, Clagett GP, et al. The Syme amputation: Success in elderly diabetic patients with palpable ankle pulses. J Vasc Surg 1990; 12:237–240.

BELOW-THE-KNEE AMPUTATION

LLOYD A. JACOBS, M.D.
PAUL W. DURANCE, Ph.D.

Lower extremity amputation constitutes an important aspect of the practice of vascular surgery. Amputation may be indicated where arterial reconstruction has failed or when such an operation is contraindicated. Failure of arterial reconstruction should be acknowledged when early graft occlusion and subsequent attempts to attain a patent reconstruction are fruitless. Occasionally, a successful arterial reconstruction is attained, only to encounter failure of the extremity to heal. Patient conditions that may preclude vascular reconstruction include generalized problems such as advanced congestive failure or dementia, or local problems such as gangrene to an extent that would not permit the salvage of a useful extremity even if arterial reconstruction was successful.

In circumstances indicating lower extremity amputation, it is important for the primary surgeon to resist the temptation to disengage. Such disengagement may be purely emotional on the part of the surgeon or may be manifested by delegation of these operations to junior members of the team. The final successful rehabilitation of patients requiring amputation depends on the primary surgeon's continued involvement.

The most common major lower extremity amputation is that performed in the classical below-the-knee (BK) position. This amputation eliminates rest pain or gangrenous tissue and has excellent rehabilitative potential. It should be selected over above-the-knee (AK) or through-the-knee (TK) amputations in virtually every feasible instance. The ultimate success of rehabilitating patients with BK amputations depends not only on surgical expertise and attention, but also on the patient's muscle strength, ability to learn, and social support systems.

REHABILITATIVE POTENTIAL

The ultimate goal of amputation should be bipedal ambulation, and BK amputation is excellently suited to this goal. Analysis of energy expenditure by ambulatory amputees support the use of BK amputation over other major amputations. Whereas energy expenditure for walking on a BK prosthesis is distinctly increased over normal, it is considerably less than that required for ambulation on an AK prosthesis.[1]

If otherwise healthy, a unilateral BK amputee with good muscle strength can expect to be ambulating within 4 to 6 weeks and to ambulate with a barely perceptible gait alteration within months. The likelihood of reaching this potential depends on a number of factors on which the surgeon has potential impact. The length of the BK stump is important in this regard. The presence of adequate tibial length allows weight to be borne on the patellar tendon surface and to some degree upon the condyles. This precludes the need for a hip harness as is necessary in AK amputations. Adequate tibial length allows the prosthesis to be propelled forward by the quadriceps mechanism, thus greatly facilitating the development of a nearly normal gait. Ideal tibial length should be in the range of 12 to 15 cm below the tibial tuberosity.

Many methods have been proposed to determine whether a BK amputation will heal or a higher amputation is inevitable.[2] These have included determination of muscle pO_2, laser Doppler flowmetry, determination of transcutaneous oxygen tension, and use of noninvasive vascular laboratory criteria. At present, most surgeons agree that clinical assessment is as reliable as any of these methods. Finally, it seems wise to attempt a BK amputation even in marginal cases in view of the improved rehabilitative potential for BK amputation over TK or AK amputation.

The attainment of adequate stump length may not always be possible due to the extent of ischemic gangrene. In such patients, it is better to compromise on stump length than to risk wound edge necrosis and infection, the latter of which invariably results in an AK amputation. Stump lengths shorter than 10 cm usually require special attention from the prosthetist, but still are to be considered superior to TK or AK amputations. The shortest possible stump length allowing satisfactory rehabilitation is approximately 2 cm distal to the tibial tuberosity.

Advances in materials engineering have improved the fabrication of strong and lightweight prostheses. Furthermore, modern plastics are easily molded to produce an excellent fit and avoid pressure necrosis of the skin of the amputation stump. In spite of these advances, patient age, muscle strength, and athletic ability have considerable impact on ultimate rehabilitation. The surgeon who works closely with a multidisciplinary rehabilitation team more frequently attains the goal of full rehabilitation, particularly in older patients. Severe dementia, however, has proven to be a nearly insurmountable obstacle to full rehabilitation. In fact, patients with severe dementia who are already nonambulatory may be best served by a TK or AK amputation in that knee flexion contractures almost invariably occur with decubiti ultimately developing on the end of the below-knee stump. This complication usually eventuates in AK amputation.

Bilateral amputation greatly reduces rehabilitative potential.[3] Most elderly or debilitated bilateral BK amputees require long-term institutional care. Even in younger, healthier persons, bilateral amputations require a prolonged period of rehabilitation, and normal gait is rarely achieved.

COST AND SOCIETAL IMPACT

The ultimate cost of vascular reconstruction for limb-threatening ischemia has repeatedly been shown to be less than the cost of amputation.[4] Amputation invariably requires relatively long hospitalization and a prolonged period of rehabilitation. Both are cost intensive. Furthermore, a sizable percentage of patients undergoing amputation, particularly elderly bilateral amputees, subsequently are institutionalized for long periods, often for the remainder of the patient's life. Successful vascular reconstruction avoids these requirements and clearly results in less cost to society as well as a more optimal patient outcome. In spite of these observations, multiple and repeated attempts at arterial reconstruction should be avoided. Cost escalates rapidly, and ultimate outcome becomes less certain with each subsequent procedure. Appropriate judgment is required to determine at what point further attempts at arterial reconstruction become futile and amputation is inevitable. This decision should be made as promptly as possible. A prolonged waiting period increases cost and greatly increases the likelihood of postoperative difficulties at the amputation site. Finally, immediately upon the need for amputation becoming clear, the vascular surgeon should consult with experts in geriatrics and in social work, as appropriate; many aged patients require institutionalization or prolonged follow-up.

PATIENT PREPARATION

Whenever arterial reconstruction is discussed with the patient, the possibility of amputation should be mentioned. Furthermore, in patients who appear to have gangrenous changes that may preclude reconstruction, amputation should be discussed early. Patients undergoing amputations experience a sequence of grieving similar to that of patients facing death. Anticipatory grieving is clearly helpful in this situation, and early introduction of the possibility of amputation appears to assist patients in coming to terms with such loss.[5] Amputation should be discussed in the context of the patient's continuing care, with rehabilitation as the ultimate goal. Patient and surgeon alike should see amputation as a step to full rehabilitation, instead of as the ultimate failure.

CONTROL OF INFECTION

The avoidance of a wound infection in the amputation stump is of great importance. This complication frequently eventuates in AK amputation. This complication, therefore, greatly reduces the patient's rehabilitative potential, increases the length of hospital stay, and, in fact, is occasionally life-threatening.

Intrinsic infection from infected gangrene or infection of wounds used for previous reconstructive procedures are more common than extrinsic infection. All wounds should be cultured prior to amputation. If time permits, the antibiotic regimen should be selected, based on the bacterial culture results. In any case, the culture results may be used in adjusting antibiotic regimens postoperatively. Preliminary debridement or incision and drainage, as appropriate, may assist in bringing infections of the forefoot under control. If forefoot infection has extended into the deep spaces of the foot or infection involves the entire foot, preliminary guillotine amputation at the level of the malleoli is efficacious in reducing BK amputation site infection and improving the ultimate outcome.[6] Such preliminary amputations should be carried out not higher than a few centimeters above the malleoli, even when cellulitis extends above this level. Open amputation with no flaps allows adequate drainage and usually allows infection to be brought under control. More proximal guillotine amputation results in muscle contraction and compromises the likelihood of subsequent successful BK amputation.

When guillotine amputation is used as a preliminary step, the subsequent BK amputation should be delayed for approximately 1 week. During that time, antibiotics and dressing changes should be utilized to bring sepsis under control.

OPERATIVE TECHNIQUE

The soft tissue:bone ratio is an important determinant of successful outcome for BK amputation. A tight amputation closure, particularly in ischemic tissue, almost certainly fails. The most common soft tissue flaps at present are a very short anterior flap and a long posterior flap. This lengthy posterior flap is based on the collateral circulation of the skin, which originates from the geniculate arteries. The anterior skin incision should be approximately 1 cm distal to the site of tibial transection. The posterior flap should be approximately 8 to 10 cm long and should be debulked so that it folds forward easily. The soft tissue should fit loosely over the residual bone, and soft tissue dog ears should be left in place. Even if rehabilitation requires a prolonged period of stump shrinkage, avoidance of ischemia from tension is of great importance. Occasionally, extensive gangrene dictates the use of side-to-side or other flaps for adequate bony coverage.[7]

The tibia has traditionally been divided using a Gigli saw. This technique should be replaced with the use of air-driven or electrical saws, which provide much greater control and avoid trauma to the surrounding soft tissue and skin. The fibula may be transected with a double-lever-action bonecutter and should be transected approximately 4 cm above the end of the tibia. The anterior aspect of the tibia should be beveled at approximately 45° for 1 cm. The electric cautery should be used sparingly, and care should be taken to avoid trauma to the skin. The use of a tourniquet to control bleeding is not indicated, as it may increase ischemic injury to the area of the stump.

In many situations, the popliteal artery is occluded. If it is not, double ligatures are in order to avoid bleeding. The posterior tibial nerve should be dissected carefully and transected sharply to avoid neuralgic pain postoperatively. Careful hemostasis is important. Wound hematomas, even if sterile, represent a significant complication that may eventuate in AK amputation. Flaps should be approximated with deep sutures of absorbable material, such as polyglycolic acid. The skin should be closed with widely separated, loosely tied nylon sutures. Nylon sutures cause fewer instances of necrosis of the skin edges than staples. If staples are used, they should be placed widely apart, and care should be taken to avoid crushing tissue within the staple line.

POSTOPERATIVE CARE

The use of bulky, rigid, or semirigid dressings in the immediate postoperative period is helpful in the avoidance of wound complications. In addition to wound complications, the single most important complication of BK amputation is the development of flexion contracture at the knee. This complication also may be avoided by a rigid or semirigid dressing. Such dressings should be applied in the operating room. Many surgeons have described and advocated the use of a pylon and foot attached to a rigid dressing, which allows rehabilitation from the outset. Our own belief, however, is that the application of a pylon and foot in the operating room is time-consuming and may inhibit the patient's movement in bed during the initial hours of recovery.

Avoidance of injury to the BK stump is important. Many patients awaken at night somewhat disoriented and may attempt to get out of bed to go to the bathroom. Occasionally, the more disoriented patient may attempt to get up for other unclear reasons. It may sometimes be necessary to place a loose cloth restraint on the patient's opposite wrist, more as a reminder than as a true barrier to ambulation. The need for such restraint usually passes within 2 to 3 nights.

Pain control is important during the initial postoperative days and greatly facilitates early rehabilitation. The pain of a BK amputation can invariably be controlled with moderate doses of morphine or droperidol.

Rehabilitation in the form of physical therapy should begin on the first postoperative day. The patient should be helped out of bed and encouraged to take meals in a chair, and weight bearing on the intact extremity should be encouraged. This can be facilitated with a portable walker as well as by attendants who can help the patient balance. The maintenance of upper extremity strength as well as strength of the proximal muscles of the lower extremities is important. Prolonged bed rest leads not only to atrophy of these muscle groups but also to an increased incidence of pulmonary complications such as atelectasis and embolism. By postoperative day 4 or 5, most patients should be prepared to visit the physical therapy department to begin rehabilitation. Work on the parallel bars as well as early gate training with a pylon and foot attached to the dressing should begin at this time. With aggressive management, most patients should be ready for the fitting of a prosthesis by 30 days after operation.

RESULTS

Below-knee amputation is accompanied by high mortality and complication rates, more because of the intrinsic disease of most patients undergoing this procedure than because of the physiologic impact of the procedure itself. Still, the period of immobilization, frequently begun many weeks before amputation, is an important contributor to this complication rate. In 1991, 1,735 BK amputations were performed in Department of Veterans Affairs Hospitals. Among these patients, 202 died during that hospitalization for mortality of approximately 11.6%, which compares favorably to most published reports.[8] In 253 patients (14.5%), the BK amputation was preceded within 90 days by one or more vascular reconstructive procedures. Approximately 471 (27.2%) patients underwent one or more foot debridements or guillotine amputations during the same hospitalization. Operations to control sepsis were, therefore, an important part of the spectrum of this disease. Of all patients undergoing amputation who were admitted from their homes, only 67.7% were discharged back to their homes. Approximately 20% were discharged to other institutions, presumably for prolonged care.

REFERENCES

1. Czerniecki JM, Gitter A. Insights into amputee running. A muscle work analysis. Am J Phys Med Rehabil 1992; 71:209–218.
2. Sarin S, Shami S, Shields DA, et al. Selection of amputation level: A review. Eur J Vasc Surg 1991; 5:611–620.

3. Datta D, Nair PN, Payne J. Outcome of prosthetic management of bilateral lower-limb amputees. Disabil Rehabil 1992; 14:98–102.
4. Raviola CA, Nichtert LS, Baker JD, et al. Cost of treating advanced leg ischemia. Bypass graft vs primary amputation. Arch Surg 1988; 123:495–496.
5. Rando TA. Loss and anticipatory grief. Lexington, Mass: Lexington Books, 1986.
6. McIntyre KE Jr, Bailey SA, Malone JM, Goldstone J. Guillotine amputation in the treatment of nonsalvageable lower-extremity infections. Arch Surg 1984; 119:450–453.
7. Ruckley CV, Stonebridge PA, Prescott RJ. Skewflap versus long posterior flap in below-knee amputations: Multicenter trial. J Vasc Surg 1991; 13:423–427.
8. Greant P, Van Den Brande P. Amputation in elderly and high-risk vascular patients. Ann Vasc Surg 1990; 4:288–290.

ABOVE-THE-KNEE AMPUTATION AND HIP DISARTICULATION

ERIC D. ENDEAN, M.D.

ABOVE-THE-KNEE AMPUTATION

Major limb amputation is often considered to be a failure of vascular intervention. This may be true in some cases, but other conditions arise in which amputation is the most appropriate therapy. Almost always, an amputation either is lifesaving or offers significant relief from pain and discomfort. Historically, above-the-knee (AK) amputation has been the preferred level because greater than 90% healing success can be anticipated.[1] However, with recognition of the importance of the knee joint for subsequent prosthetic ambulation, below-the-knee (BK) amputation should generally be considered the procedure of choice if it is feasible.

Most patients who undergo AK amputation for an ischemic extremity are elderly and have other medical problems, such as diabetes mellitus, as well as cardiac, pulmonary, renal, and neurologic impairment. These conditions must be recognized and appropriately managed perioperatively to minimize operative morbidity and mortality. The same care and attention to technical detail that are given to major vascular reconstructive procedures must also be applied to amputations for successful outcomes. Too often an amputation is considered a minor operation and delegated to the most junior member of the surgical team. It is important that the surgeon consider an amputation to be a significant procedure that substantially affects that patient's quality of life.

Indications and Contraindications

The most frequent indication for AK amputation is advanced ischemia, of an acute or chronic nature. Patients who have had a delay in diagnosis or treatment of acute limb ischemia may sustain irreversible muscle injury, manifested by rigor of the knee joint, failure of the muscles to contract when stimulated, and a gray appearance of the muscle tissue. Open AK amputation through viable-appearing tissue is the most prudent operation because determination of tissue viability may be difficult. Performance of an open amputation allows for inspection and debridement of the tissue as needed.

Most often, patients require AK amputation for sequelae of chronic ischemia. It should be performed in individuals who have severe flexion contractures of the knee or who have tissue ischemia in an area that precludes a BK amputation. Patients with dry gangrene or severe rest pain, who because of underlying medical conditions do not ambulate and are not expected to walk again, should undergo AK amputation, even if a BK amputation could be done. The conditions that result in the bedridden state include severe dementia, terminal cancer, end-stage pulmonary or cardiac dysfunction, and multiple or severe strokes. These patients are at risk for developing knee flexion contractures after BK amputations with the subsequent development of pressure ulcers on the end of the stump. Treatment of this problem ultimately requires revision to an AK amputation.

Few absolute contraindications exist to AK amputation. Patients with life-threatening infections that involve the soft tissues of the proximal thigh or hip are not candidates for AK amputation and need a hip disarticulation. Inadequate blood flow that would compromise wound healing is a contraindication to AK amputation. Bunt has identified three clinical situations that represent relative contraindications to AK amputation: (1) absent femoral pulse to palpation and thrombosis of both the inflow and outflow grafts from a prior revascularization procedure, (2) combined superficial femoral artery occlusion with a high-grade stenosis or occlusion of the profunda femoris artery, and (3) no detectable pulse volume recordings at the high thigh level.[2] In these situations, a revascularization procedure should be done prior to amputation, unless other objective evidence suggests that blood flow to the thigh would support wound healing. Finally, any patient who has reasonable potential for ambulation should first be considered for a BK amputation.

Technique

General, spinal, or epidural anesthesia can be used. In some patients, local nerve block (femoral, sciatic, and obturator nerves) can provide adequate anesthesia. An AK amputation is generally done at one of three levels: distal thigh, just proximal to the knee joint; mid thigh; or proximal thigh. Amputations that leave a long stump are preferred because a long femoral shaft provides a better lever for ambulation with a prosthesis. Bedridden patients also benefit from long above-knee amputation stumps. Because these patients have a tendency to develop hip flexion contractures after AK amputation, a long stump that weighs more tends to prevent this problem.

A fishmouth incision, forming equal anterior and posterior flaps, is made 2 to 3 cm below the anticipated level of bone transection. A circular incision can also be employed. The incision is carried through the skin, subcutaneous tissue, and fascia circumferentially. The muscles of the anterior flap are sharply divided. Strict maintenance of hemostasis is required, although a tourniquet is usually not necessary. Electrocautery is used by some to divide the muscle, but ligation of individual bleeding vessels with absorbable suture is preferred because electrocautery causes coagulation necrosis of surrounding tissue. The periosteum of the femur is incised and elevated to the level where the bone will be divided. The femur is transected with a handsaw, Gigli saw, or air-driven reciprocating saw. Attention must be directed to protecting the surrounding soft tissue and skin. The superficial femoral artery and veins are individually suture ligated. The posterior muscle flap is sharply incised, which can be done with an amputation knife. The sciatic nerve is identified and gently pulled into the wound. A heavy ligature is used to control the small artery that accompanies the nerve. The nerve is then transected and allowed to retract within the muscles. The wound is copiously irrigated. Persistent bleeding from the cut end of the bone can be controlled with bone wax or a hemostatic agent such as a slurry made of absorbable gelatin and thrombin. Drains are not usually necessary if strict attention to hemostasis is employed. The anterior and posterior fascia are approximated with interrupted absorbable sutures, and the skin is closed with interrupted vertical mattress monofilament suture material. A soft, bulky dressing is placed on the wound and is typically left in place for 3 to 5 days. Unexplained fever or incisional pain out of proportion to the usual postoperative discomfort requires immediate inspection of the wound. An Ace wrap to assist stump molding can be applied over the dressing at the time of amputation or later, when wound healing has been established. Immediate postoperative prostheses are not used with AK amputations.[3]

All patients undergoing major lower extremity amputations should have prophylaxis for deep venous thrombosis using leg elevation, subcutaneous low-dose heparin sodium, or venous sequential compression devices, alone or in combination with each other. Patients should be encouraged to begin rehabilitation soon after operation to help maintain upper extremity strength and muscle tone, prevent development of atelectasis and pneumonia, and offer a psychological boost to the patient. Positioning the patient in the prone position each shift helps prevent hip flexion contracture.

Results

Healing should be expected in more than 90% of patients undergoing AK amputation.[1] This excellent success rate constitutes the major advantage of this operation. However, fewer than 50% of patients eventually achieve prosthetic ambulation as opposed to 66% or more of patients who have undergone a BK amputation. In part, this low incidence of ambulation after AK amputation may be due to the selection of patients who have decreased potential for ambulation. However, the energy expenditure required for ambulation with an AK prosthesis is much greater than that of normal walking and also greater than that required for ambulation with a BK prosthesis. Other concomitant medical conditions, such as limited cardiac and pulmonary reserve, also contribute to the inability for postoperative ambulation. Newer prostheses that use lightweight plastic materials may increase the number of patients who will become ambulatory after AK amputation.

Up to 50% of patients who survive for at least 2 years after amputation require a contralateral limb amputation, especially patients with diabetes mellitus.[4] For this reason, patients must be closely followed for evidence of ischemia or infection in the remaining extremity. Early intervention may prevent contralateral amputation.

Complications

A number of early and late complications have been identified. The death rate for AK amputation (20% to 40%) is greater than that of BK amputation (3% to 10%).[3,5] This finding may be related to the severity of the underlying diseases resulting in the need for amputation, and also to the fact that AK amputation is selected for patients who have debilitating or terminal conditions. The majority of deaths are due to cardiovascular complications, including myocardial infarction, stroke, and congestive heart failure. Atelectasis and pneumonia pose significant postoperative problems. Patients who undergo AK amputation are often bedridden and especially prone to respiratory morbidity. It has been stated that amputees are at increased risk for development of deep venous thrombosis and pulmonary embolism. Prolonged bed rest, division of deep veins, and prior vascular reconstructions that could have injured adjacent deep veins have been implicated as factors leading to venous stasis.[3] Prophylaxis against deep venous thrombosis and early ambulation should be employed to decrease this risk. Failure of the wound to heal and wound infection are serious complications that may require revision of the amputation to a higher level. Most patients experience some degree of phantom pain after amputation. Although this pain usually improves over time, in some patients it can be a major cause of disability. Late complications include hip flexion contracture, stump breakdown, erosion of the bone through the stump, stump trauma from a poorly fitting prosthesis, and excessive soft tissue at the end of the stump, making prosthetic fitting difficult. These problems often require operative correction, especially in patients who have achieved prosthetic ambulation. Meticulous attention to detail in performing the amputation should minimize these complications.

HIP DISARTICULATION

Hip disarticulation is an operation rarely performed in a vascular surgery practice. Because of the increased morbidity of hip disarticulation, AK amputation is preferred. Most lower extremity ischemic problems requiring amputation can be successfully managed with a high AK amputation. However, some circumstances necessitate hip disarticulation.

Indications and Contraindications

The indications for hip disarticulation are similar to those for AK amputation, except that the proximal extent of the disease process precludes AK amputation. Indications include proximal lower extremity musculoskeletal malignancies, severe lower extremity trauma involving the hip joint, life-threatening infection that has ascended to the hip joint, or proximal ischemia with tissue necrosis or gangrene that would preclude an AK amputation. Some patients have more than one indication for hip disarticulation, such as an ischemic extremity complicated by infection. Few contraindications exist to hip disarticulation. Life-threatening infectious processes, such as gas gangrene, that extend proximal to the hip joint and involve the trunk can be seen in premorbid patients, and any treatment may be futile. However, even in cases of extensive soft tissue infection, hip disarticulation associated with extensive soft tissue debridement may be lifesaving.

When performing a hip disarticulation, the status of the blood supply to the pelvis must be considered. Some patients may have poor blood flow to the hip and pelvis, as could occur with bilateral internal iliac artery occlusions. In such a patient, healing of a hip disarticulation could be compromised. Concomitant revascularization of an internal iliac artery should be entertained.

Technique

The surgical technique for hip disarticulation, which has been well described by Sugarbaker and Chretien,[6] involves control of the femoral vessels and creation of a gluteal muscle flap. The patient is positioned on the operating table on the contralateral side, with the affected leg up. A bean bag is useful to maintain position. A circumferential incision is made to create a posteriorly based gluteal muscle flap. The incision is begun 1 to 2 cm medial to the anterior superior iliac spine and extended toward the pubic tubercle. The incision is continued medially to a point 3 to 4 cm distal to the ischial tuberosity. The posterior portion of the incision is begun 3 to 4 cm anterior to the greater trochanter and then extended around the back of the leg in the gluteal crease. As the anterior incision is deepened, the superficial epigastric artery and pudendal branches require division and ligation. The common femoral artery and vein are exposed, divided, and ligated under the inguinal ligament. The femoral nerve is likewise identified and placed on gentle traction. The nerve is ligated and divided, allowing it to retract under the inguinal ligament. The sartorius muscle is transected from the anterior superior iliac spine, and the tissue posterior to the femoral sheath is incised to expose the anterior surface of the hip joint. The iliopsoas muscle is then divided at its attachment to the lesser trochanter. The pectineus muscle is transected at its origin from the pelvis. The obturator externus is divided through its tendinous insertion on the lesser trochanter. The remaining adductor muscles (gracilis, adductor longus, adductor brevis, adductor magnus) are divided at their origins on the pubis. The obturator artery and vein, which lie on the obturator externus, are securely ligated. Laterally, the tensor fascia lata and gluteus maximus muscles are divided in the plane of the incision. These are the only two muscles that are not divided either at their points of insertion or origin. The rectus femoris muscle is transected at its origin from the anterior inferior iliac spine. Finally, the muscles inserting onto the greater trochanter are divided at their insertion points. These muscles include the gluteus medius, gluteus minimus, piriformis, superior gemellus, obturator internus, inferior gemellus, and quadratus femoris. The joint capsule is then incised, and the leg is removed. After irrigation of the wound, the quadratus femoris and the iliopsoas muscles are approximated to cover the joint capsule. Likewise, the obturator externus and gluteus medius muscles are joined to cover the acetabulum. The gluteus maximus fascia is approximated to the inguinal ligament with interrupted absorbable sutures. The skin is closed with interrupted vertical mattress sutures. A drain is frequently required and is placed beneath the gluteus maximus muscle. In patients who undergo hip disarticulation for infection, the skin should be left open. Delayed closure or skin grafts can be utilized to provide coverage after the infection has resolved. The open technique also allows for wound debridement in those situations when there is a question of tissue viability.

Results

In a recent review of hip disarticulation, overall wound complications such as infection, dehiscence, and necrosis affected 60% of patients.[7] The urgency of the operation (elective versus urgent or emergent) was the only factor identified that predicted the likelihood of wound complications. In a life-threatening situation, marginally viable tissue or retained residual infection may be left in the wound, accounting for the higher complication rate. The overall mortality rate was 21%. The highest incidence of death occurred in patients with ischemia; there were no perioperative deaths in patients undergoing hip disarticulation for tumor. Unruh and co-workers reported a perioperative mortality rate of 44%, highest in patients treated for trauma and followed next by patients with ischemia.[8] They also reported a similar wound infection rate of 65%.

REFERENCES

1. Keagy BA, Schwartz JA, Kotb M, et al. Lower extremity amputation: The control series. J Vasc Surg 1986; 4:321–326.
2. Bunt TJ. Gangrene of the immediate postoperative above-knee amputation stump: Role of emergency revascularization in preventing death. J Vasc Surg 1985; 2:874–877.
3. Malone JM, Goldstone J. Lower extremity amputation. In: Moore WS, ed. Vascular surgery. 2nd ed. Orlando: Grune & Stratton, 1986:1139.
4. Bodily KC, Burgess EM. Contralateral limb and patient survival after leg amputation. Am J Surg 1983; 146:280–282.
5. Porter JM. Baur GM, Taylor LM. Lower-extremity amputations for ischemia. Arch Surg 1981; 116:89–92.
6. Sugarbaker PH, Chretien PB. A surgical technique for hip disarticulation. Surgery 1981; 90:546–553.
7. Endean ED, Schwarcz TH, Barker DE, et al. Hip disarticulation: Factors affecting outcome. J Vasc Surg 1991; 14:398–404.
8. Unruh T, Fisher DF, Unruh TA, et al. Hip disarticulation: An 11-year experience. Arch Surg 1990; 125:791–793.

UPPER EXTREMITY AMPUTATION

JOHN GRAY SEILER III, M.D.
FRANK D. ELLIS, M.D.
LAMAR L. FLEMING, M.D.

Acute and chronic vascular conditions occasionally result in the need for upper extremity amputation to salvage remaining hand or upper limb function. Their management may be complex.[1-11] Critical to the decision in such situations is a thorough knowledge of the patient's needs, including vocation, avocation, handedness, cultural and social background, and sense of body image, as well as knowledge of the various amputation levels and the functional outcome that is reasonable to expect at each amputation level.

Most frequently, upper extremity amputations are necessitated by irreparable upper extremity vascular injury, chronic vascular disease, or tumors. Less frequently, amputations are required following upper extremity thermal injury, extravasation injuries, ischemia from the administration of vasopressor agents and cannulation injuries, injection injuries, or congenital disorders. More challenging are patients with acute unreconstructible arterial insufficiency or arm sepsis who require amputations to preserve life. The overwhelming majority of these patients are best treated with traditional amputations and early prosthetic fitting. The ultimate goal of amputation surgery is to return the patient to a maximal functional level of activity as quickly as possible. This goal is most easily accomplished through the coordinated efforts of physician, nurse, therapist, and prosthetist.

GENERAL PRINCIPLES

Prior to an elective surgical procedure, a clear preoperative plan should be established that includes a decision on the proposed level of amputation and the anticipated prosthetic requirements for the patient. Individual patients may have strong personal reasons for preferring certain amputation types. Many patients prefer not to have a Krukenberg type of procedure, although it is fairly functional, for example, because of the cosmetic appearance of the limb.

With the exception of proximal shoulder amputations, upper extremity amputations are most easily done with the patient positioned supine and the arm placed on a hand table. Either regional or general anesthesia is satisfactory for these procedures. A brachial tourniquet is applied and used when necessary to facilitate dissection. In our practice, we prefer setting the tourniquet pressure to 100 mm Hg above the patient's systolic blood pressure. One gram of an intravenous first-generation cephalosporin antibiotic is administered approximately 30 minutes prior to the anticipated time of insufflation of the tourniquet and continued perioperatively for 24 hours.

The most utilitarian incisions for amputations of the upper extremity are the fishmouth type of incisions. These incisions should be made to allow tension-free closure of the wound following osteotomy of the bone and completion of the amputation. For some procedures, creation of a longer volar flap allows the line of closure to be placed away from areas of weight bearing or pinch. On the hand, zigzag incisions are useful as they allow exposure of adjacent structures important to the reconstruction phase of the procedure.

Muscles are beveled as they are divided to allow for later closure. Neurovascular structures should be isolated early in the surgical procedure. All major arteries should be isolated, divided, and ligated. Nerves are dissected proximally and divided in a location where they will be unlikely to cause a painful neuroma. Osteotomy is performed after all other structures have been divided and is most easily done with an oscillating saw. Rough or sharp bone ends should be smoothed with a rasp to prevent soft tissue complications. Amputations done in children can often be done through joints to limit the appositional deposition of new bone on the amputated limb, a common reason for stump revision in the pediatric population. Prior to closure, the tourniquet should be deflated to ensure that satisfactory hemostasis has been obtained. For clean wounds, a layered closure allows the musculotendinous units to be reapproximated separately covering and protecting the bone ends. To minimize fluid collections within the stump, a hemovac drain is inserted. Soft dressings are sufficient in most patients. Range-of-motion exercises should be started within 24 hours of operation.

Patients with septic limbs or digits should initially undergo a guillotine type of amputation and be returned to the operating room 48 to 72 hours later for second debridement and possible wound closure. Central to the management plan for these patients is intensive local wound care, intravenous antibiotics, and tetanus prophylaxis.

Occasionally, additional attempts at preservation of limb length are necessary. In these patients, inadequate soft tissue coverage usually limits wound closure. Local rotation flaps or free microsurgical tissue transfer may be indicated to preserve the desired extremity length.

OPERATIVE TECHNIQUE

Terminal Symes Amputation

This procedure can be done to treat distal digital necrosis, selected cases of distal phalangeal osteomyelitis, and chronic nailbed problems. Usually done under digital anesthesia and with a finger tourniquet, a dorsal incision is made around the area of the nailbed. Both the sterile and the germinal matrix (dorsal and volar) are excised, allowing the distal phalanx to be debrided as necessary. The distal flap is then folded proximally, trimmed, and sewn into place with monofilament, nonabsorbable sutures. The important technical considerations during this procedure are to preserve the digital arteries to the distal flap and to excise the entire nail matrix.

Digital Amputation

Digital amputations are frequently indicated for both chronic and acute arterial problems. For amputations done distal to the insertion of the flexor digitorum superficialis, patients retain satisfactory flexion of the proximal interphalangeal joint and can be expected to use the finger actively. The flexor digitorum profundus should be divided and allowed to retract proximally. Any effort to advance the flexor digitorum profundus tendon may result in quadriga and limit the function of adjacent normal fingers. Amputations done proximal to the flexor digitorum superficialis insertion may result in a short finger with little mobility. Although amputations through the proximal phalanx preserve the metacarpal and therefore the breadth of the palm, digits of this kind may become a nuisance to the patient for handling small objects or writing. Often patients bypass their foreshortened digit in favor of using a more normal finger for these tasks. When disarticulation through the distal or proximal joints is necessary, the condyles should be contoured to allow skin closure.

Distal digital amputations may be done with digital (amputations distal to the proximal interphalangeal joint) or wrist block (digital amputations proximal to the proximal interphalangeal joint) anesthesia. We prefer 1% lidocaine without epinephrine with the use of a finger tourniquet. Digital and wrist nerve blocks should be done with an agent containing no epinephrine.

Circumferential incisions, made with the apices at the midlateral line of the digit, allow exposure of the neurovascular bundles, flexor and extensor apparatus (Fig. 1). A critical step in minimizing the pain in fingers following digital amputation is isolation and division of each digital nerve well proximal to the line of incision. The tendons are divided just proximal to the line of incision and allowed to retract. The phalanx is cut with an oscillating saw and the bone ends smoothed with a small rasp. The skin is reapproximated with a 5-0 monofilament suture. Prior to closure, the tourniquet should be removed or deflated, and the viability of the skin margins examined. If the capillary refill is poor or if the wound cannot be closed without tension, then a more proximal level of amputation should be considered.

Ray Amputation

Ray amputation, or amputation of a digit at the base of the metacarpal, is a useful procedure for eliminating devitalized tissue and preserving hand function (Figs. 2 and 3). By removing the digit through the base of the metacarpal, the surgeon has the opportunity to narrow the hand by reconstruction of the interpalmar plate ligament or osteotomy and translocation of adjacent metacarpals; such a change improves postoperative grasp and the handling of small objects. Patients

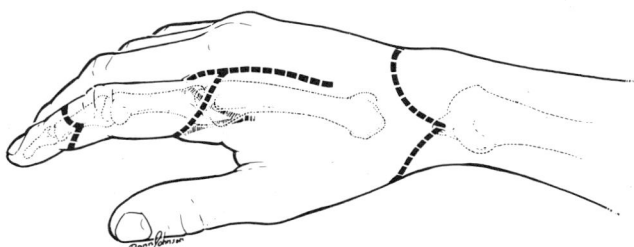

Figure 1 Preferred incisions for digital amputation, ray amputation, and wrist disarticulation.

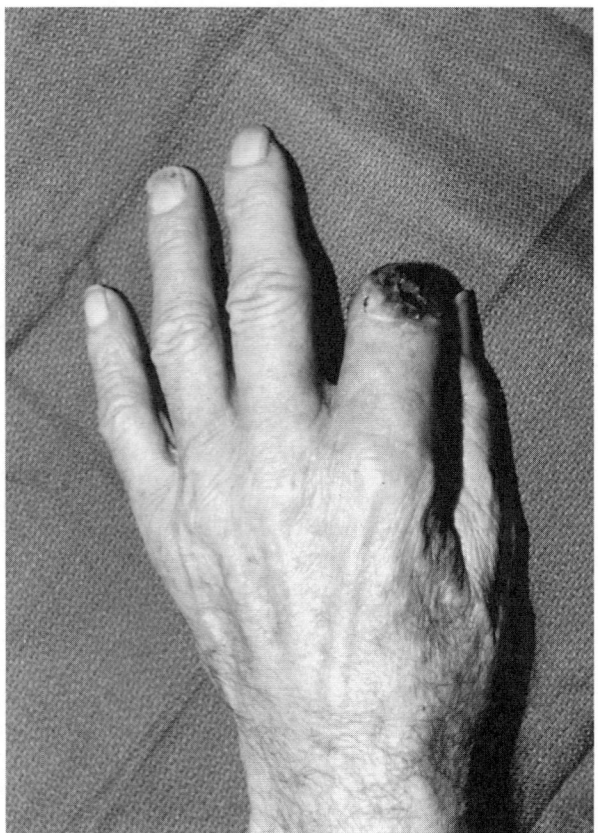

Figure 2 A patient with digital gangrene secondary to chronic arterial occlusive disease. A previous distal fingertip amputation failed to heal.

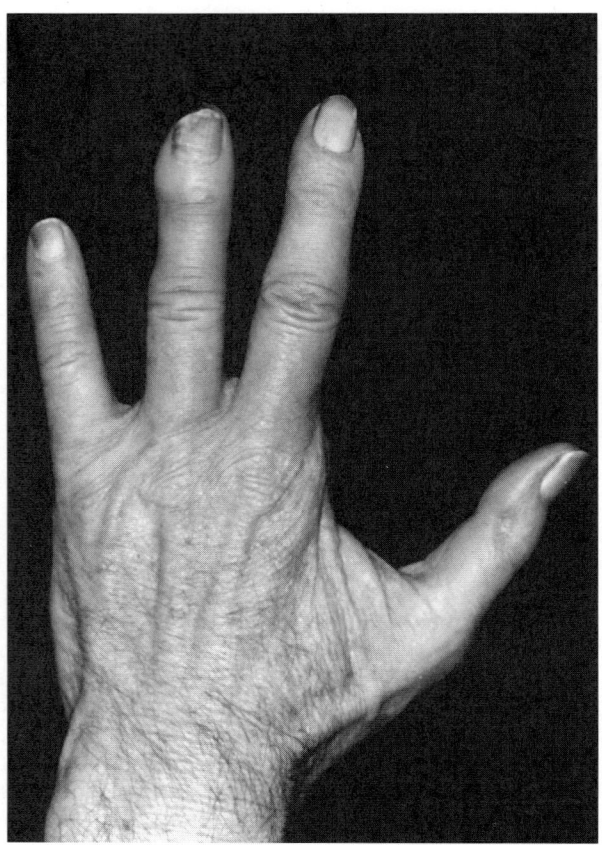

Figure 3 Following ray amputation, the hand retained good appearance and function.

experience a 20% decrease in grip power and key pinch following this procedure. This procedure may be done using regional anesthesia. A brachial tourniquet is applied and inflated if necessary.

Dorsally, a zigzag incision over the metacarpal allows broad exposure of the adjacent metacarpals. A second incision on the palmar surface is made to expose the flexor apparatus and neurovascular bundles. The neurovascular bundles should be divided well proximal to the line of incision to avoid the formation of painful neuromas. Osteotomy of the base of the metacarpal, division of the flexor and extensor mechanisms, and subperiosteal dissection of the interosseous muscles allows the amputation to be completed. Closure of the wound should include reconstruction of the interpalmar plate ligament with 2-0 nonabsorbable braided Dacron sutures. Percutaneous pinning of the adjacent metacarpals or metacarpal translocation is occasionally required to close the gap between the digits.

Following closure, the wounds are dressed with a compressive soft dressing for 7 to 10 days. Digital range-of-motion exercises are encouraged on the first postoperative day. No prosthetic care is necessary.

Metacarpal Amputations

Transmetacarpal amputations are uncommon procedures usually indicated for post-traumatic conditions and unusual vascular complications. Preservation of as much metacarpal length as possible aids in performing bimanual tasks by preserving a hand paddle and maintaining wrist motion.

The procedure is done with regional or general anesthesia and a brachial tourniquet. When the skin flaps are constructed, a long palmar flap is developed that can be advanced to cover the ends of the metacarpals. The metacarpals are easily identified through the dorsal incision and are divided, obliquely on the border metacarpals and transversely on the central metacarpals, with an oscillating saw. Through the palmar incision, each digital nerve should be identified and divided proximal to the line of closure. The wound is repaired with a monofilament nonabsorbable suture.

Wrist Disarticulation

Wrist disarticulation, once a procedure out of favor because of the limitations of prosthetic fitting, has emerged again because of newer prosthetic fitting methods. This procedure has the advantage of preserving the distal radio-ulnar-joint, which allows full forearm pronation and supination postoperatively. In children, this procedure allows full forearm development and prevents problems with stump overgrowth.

Incisions are made with the apices at the radial styloid and the ulnar styloid. The palmar flap is made slightly longer than the dorsal flap. The flexor and extensor tendons are divided and allowed to retract. The median, palmar cutaneous, ulnar, and superficial radial nerves should be identified individually and resected at a more proximal level. This can be done through the same incision or through separate proximal incisions. The radial and ulnar arteries should be identified and ligated. While completing the amputation through the radio-carpal joint, attention should be given to preserving the triangular fibrocartilage complex. The triangular fibrocartilage complex is critical to stabilization of the distal radio-ulnar joint and preservation of normal forearm pronation and supination. Occasionally, the radial and ulnar styloid prominences must be smoothed with a rasp.

Below-Elbow Amputation

One of the most common of upper extremity amputation procedures, below-elbow amputation is done with the goal of preserving elbow flexion. As little as 5 cm of ulna distal to the coronoid allows the fitting of a standard prosthesis. Forearm rotation and strength increase with more distal levels of amputation. Proximal levels of amputation provide better muscle flaps for stump coverage and heal quickly because of the improved proximal vascularity.

This operation can be done using regional or general anesthesia and a brachial tourniquet. Skin incisions are made proximal to the level of devitalized tissue (Fig. 4). The median, ulnar, radial, medial antebrachial cutaneous, and lateral antebrachial cutaneous nerves should be individually identified and divided well proximal in the forearm. Some authors have concluded that it is easier to make separate proximal incisions to ensure an appropriate point of nerve division. The radial and ulnar arteries are ligated. The radius and ulna are transversely divided at the same level with an oscillating saw. When practical, a myofascial closure is done as part of a layered wound repair. A closed suction drain is used for 24 hours, and a soft dressing applied.

Elbow Disarticulation

Preservation of the entire humerus has the advantage of maintaining humeral rotation postoperatively. Following operation, a properly fitted prosthesis is molded to the humeral condyles so that the improved humeral rotation can be transmitted to the prosthesis and used to improve function. In the pediatric population, the preservation of the distal humeral epiphysis allows the development of a normal length brachium and prevents stump overgrowth.

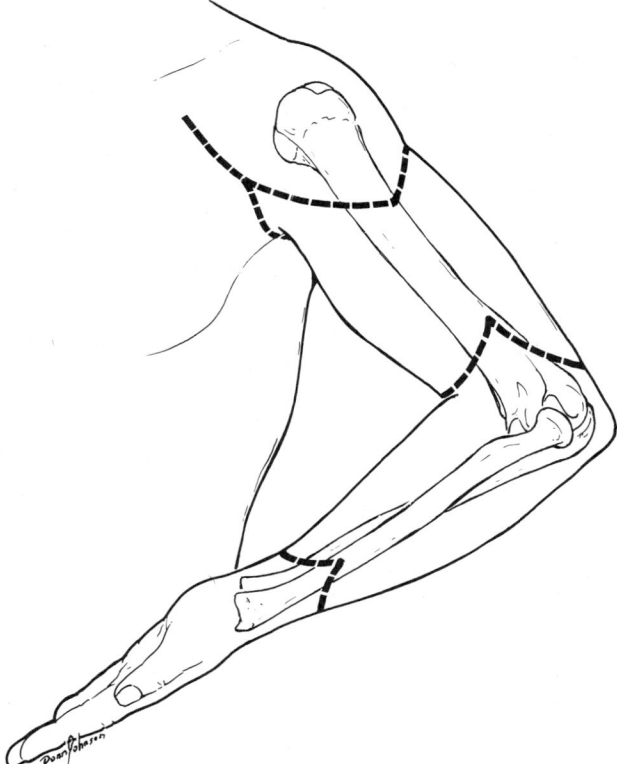

Figure 4 Preferred incisions for below-elbow amputation, above-elbow amputation, and shoulder disarticulation.

This procedure may be done with regional or general anesthesia and a brachial tourniquet. Skin incisions are made with the distal margin on the forearm to ensure sufficient soft tissue length to cover the humerus. The median nerve, brachial artery, and vena comitantes are easily identified 4 cm proximal and 4 cm medial to the medial epicondyle. The ulnar nerve is identified behind the medial intermuscular septum and medial epicondyle. The medial brachial and antebrachial cutaneous nerves should also be identified on the medial side of the arm. Most superficial on the lateral side is the terminal branch of the musculocutaneous nerve, the lateral antebrachial cutaneous nerve, which is identified exiting beneath the biceps. Also laterally, the radial nerve and profunda brachii artery are identified between the brachialis and brachioradialis. After division of the nerves proximally and ligation of the arteries, the biceps, brachialis, and triceps are divided distally to allow exposure of the distal humerus. The amputation is completed by subperiosteal medial and lateral collateral ligament excision, release of the flexor-pronator group of muscles medially and the wrist extensors laterally.

A myofascial closure can be done, reapproximating the anterior fascia of the biceps and brachialis to the posterior fascia of the triceps with large, absorbable sutures. A deep, closed suction drain is placed, and a soft tissue dressing applied.

Above-Elbow Amputation

Maintenance of length is especially important in above-elbow amputations for rotational arm control and arm strength. For extremely proximal above-elbow amputations, the humeral head and proximal 4 cm of humerus should be preserved to improve shoulder contour and the stability of prosthetic fit. For distal above-elbow amputations, the site of osteotomy should be approximately 4 cm from the elbow joint to allow the use of a standard elbow hinge in the prosthesis.

A tourniquet may not be used for this procedure because of the level of amputation that is required. For very proximal above-elbow amputations, the deltopectoral interval needs to be opened to isolate the neurovascular structures. For more distal levels, anterior and posterior flaps are developed distal to the line of intended bone section. The median, ulnar, and radial nerves are isolated and divided proximal to the incision line. The brachial artery is isolated medially and ligated. The biceps, brachialis, and triceps muscles should be divided several centimeters distal to the level of bone section and beveled to facilitate closure. After division of the humerus with an oscillating saw, the biceps fascia may be reapproximated to the triceps fascia with absorbable sutures. A closed suction drainage tube is placed beneath the layer of muscular closure. The skin is reapproximated, and a sterile dressing applied.

Shoulder Disarticulation

Whenever this procedure is necessary, consideration should be given to preserving the humeral head. If the humeral head can be preserved, the patient's shoulder retains a more normal contour, and prosthetic suspension is facilitated.

The patient should be positioned supine with a rolled towel under the ipsilateral scapula. The arm may be placed on a hand table or at the patient's side. The entire forequarter should be prepped and draped. An anterior incision is made beginning at the inferior margin of the clavicle extending to a distal racquet incision extending through the axilla and around the lateral surface of the humerus (Fig. 4). Anteriorly, the deltopectoral interval is opened, the short head of the biceps is released from its origin on the coracoid process, and the pectoralis major muscle is released from its insertion on the humerus. Lateral retraction of the deltoid muscle and medial retraction of the pectoralis major muscle allow exposure of the neurovascular structures in the infraclavicular area. The axillary artery and vein should be individually ligated. The terminal branches of the brachial plexus (radial, median, ulnar, axillary, musculocutaneous, medial brachial, and antebrachial cutaneous nerves) and the intercostobrachial nerve are identified and divided beneath the pectoralis minor muscle so that they are protected from the line of closure.

The deltoid muscle is released from its insertion on the humerus and reflected proximally to expose the glenohumeral joint. The amputation is completed by dividing the biceps, triceps, subscapularis, supraspinatus, infraspinatus, and teres minor muscles. Division of the subscapularis muscle is facilitated by external arm rotation. Division of the supraspinatus, infraspinatus, and teres minor muscles is facilitated by internal rotation of the arm and distal longitudinal traction. The deltoid muscle may be tailored and sutured over the glenoid rim protecting the scapula. If the proximal humerus can be retained, then the biceps and triceps muscles are sutured together with nonabsorbable suture, covering the end of the humerus. The skin is reapproximated with nonabsorbable sutures.

Forequarter Amputation

This uncommon operation removes the entire shoulder girdle with the arm from the thoracic wall and is most commonly used for excision of malignant tumors. Although it has been described from both anterior and posterior approaches, the posterior approach is technically simplest to perform. Details of the procedure are available in the excellent article by Littlewood.[4]

The patient should be positioned in the lateral decubitus position, and the forequarter draped free. Posteriorly, a large, medially based, U-shaped flap is made to extend transversely along the entire posterior surface of the clavicle, vertically along the lateral border of the scapula, and then transversely again at the inferior angle of the scapula to within 5 cm of the spinous processes. Subcutaneous dissection medially exposes the vertebral border of the scapula. The trapezius, latissimus dorsi, serratus anterior, rhomboid major, rhomboid minor, levator scapulae, and omohyoid muscles are then divided. The clavicle is identified through the posterior incision and divided near its medial end. Forward retraction on the arm facilitates exposure of the subclavian artery, vein, and brachial plexus. The artery and vein are ligated and the brachial plexus divided. An anterior incision is made lateral to the deltopectoral interval and continued into the axilla, rather than onto the brachium. Division of the pectoralis major and pectoralis minor muscles allow completion of the amputation. The skin should be trimmed and closed with nonabsorbable monofilament suture. A closed suction drainage tube is placed.

AFTERCARE

Upper extremity amputations should be dressed initially so that adjacent joint range of motion can be done. Rigid postoperative dressings provide excellent wound protection and limit perioperative complications. However, rigid dressings may impair joint mobilization or cause additional skin problems, if they are heavy or inappropriately applied. Unless immediate prosthetic fitting is being done, we prefer a soft dressing to allow easy wound inspection and to facilitate range-of-motion and strengthening exercises. We prefer the wound to be covered by a sterile, nonadherent material, which is then covered by an initial layer of sterile gauze sponges and followed by a generous amount of Dacron padding. A gauze wrap is used to secure the dressing, which is finally covered by a stockinette and an elastic wrap

Early range-of-motion exercises are encouraged for adjacent or proximal joints beginning on the first postoperative day. Although these exercises can usually be initiated and carried out by a well-informed and motivated patient, often patients require the supervision of an occupational therapist to ensure maintenance of range of motion. At the time of suture removal, patients are instructed in the care of the amputation stump, including methods to diminish stump swelling and techniques in preventing incisional hypersensitivity. During the first month following operation, patients should visit with a certified prosthetist to obtain information about the various types of prosthetic limbs available for their level of amputation. With this information, patients can participate in the selection of the device that will be most useful to them.

For patients with chronic vascular occlusive disease, prosthetic fitting and training in prosthetic use is usually done between 4 and 6 weeks after amputation. For younger patients with traumatic amputations or patients with little chance of wound complications, early prosthetic fitting should be done. Begun as early as the day of operation, this method of prosthetic management allows early reinstitution of bimanual tasks, facilitates rehabilitation, and shortens the overall period of disability. Following prosthetic fitting, patients should be examined periodically to ensure that the device fits properly and works effectively.

PROSTHETICS

Some understanding of the available prosthetic devices and their use by patients is critical to the planning of upper extremity amputations. Because of the significant improvements in prosthetic design and newer materials, almost any level of upper extremity amputation can be fitted with a functioning prosthesis. The patient's use of a prosthesis decreases with more proximal levels of amputation because of the complexity of the devices and their weight. Long-term prosthetic usage rates are highly variable, ranging between 40% and 90%.

The conventional below-elbow prosthesis consists of a figure-of-eight shoulder harness, a forearm shell, a cable for activation of the terminal device, and the terminal device. In addition, above-elbow prostheses have a brachial shell and uniaxial locking elbow, activated by shoulder depression and extension. Specialized hinges are available for patients undergoing below-elbow amputation and elbow disarticulation.

Terminal Devices

The most commonly prescribed terminal device is the voluntary opening hook. By initiating voluntary shoulder abduction and flexion, the patient uses the shoulder harness to tense the cable, causing the hook to open and allow objects to be placed within its jaws. Muscular relaxation allows the hook to close, firmly gripping the object. The closing power of these devices is proportional to the number of elastic bands placed at the base of the hook. These durable devices come in a variety of sizes, shapes, and weights and have variable closing strengths to accommodate variations in individual muscle strength. Single-purpose terminal devices can be constructed for individuals who have specific needs.

Battery-powered myoelectric hands, although an attractive theoretic option, have not yet replaced standard terminal devices. Whereas initial studies suggested that patients with a choice in prosthesis wear preferred myoelectric devices more than 60% of the time, longer-term studies of use have documented that the rate of repair is high, the time to accomplish individual tasks is slow, the rate of disuse increases with time, and most people with a requirement for heavy lifting or manipulation prefer standard terminal devices. Myoelectric hands are cosmetically appealing, are usable without a harness power system, can be used for overhead tasks, and are effective for light tasks. With improvements in microelectronics and biomaterials, the use of myoelectric hands will increase in popularity. Cosmetic hands are valuable additional devices for individuals who are concerned about image following amputation, and they can be ordered at the time of initial prosthetic fitting.

REFERENCES

1. Aitken GT, Frantz CH. The juvenile amputee. J Bone Joint Surgery [Am] 1953; 35:659.
2. Burkhalter WE, Mayfield G, Caramona LS. The upper extremity amputee: Early and immediate post-surgical prosthetic fitting. J Bone Joint Surg [Am] 1976; 58:46.
3. Lambert CN. Amputation surgery in the child. Orthop Clin North Am 1972; 3:473.
4. Littlewood H. Amputations at the shoulder and at the hip. Br Med J 1922; 1:381.
5. Louis DS. Amputations. In: Green DP, ed. Operative hand surgery. New York: Churchill Livingstone, 1982:811.
6. Mooney V, et al. Comparison of postoperative stump management: Plaster vs soft dressings. J Bone Joint Surg [Am] 1971; 53:241.
7. Pillet J. The aesthetic hand prosthesis. Orthop Clin North Am 1981; 12:961.
8. Rooks MD, Fleming LL. Upper extremity amputations. In: Rutherford RB, ed. Vascular surgery. 3rd ed. Philadelphia: WB Saunders, 1989:1741.
9. Silcox DH, Rooks MD, Vogel RD, Fleming LL. Myoelectric prostheses: A long term follow-up study of the use of alternate prostheses. J Bone Joint Surg [Am] 1993; 75:1781–1789.
10. Tooms RE. Amputation surgery in the upper extremity. Orthop Clin North Am 1972; 3:383.
11. Tooms RE. Upper extremity amputation surgery. In Campbell's operative orthopaedics. 7th ed. St. Louis: Mosby–Year Book, 1987:637.

MESENTERIC VASCULAR DISEASE

DUPLEX SCANNING IN THE DIAGNOSIS OF SPLANCHNIC ARTERY OCCLUSIVE DISEASE

D. EUGENE STRANDNESS JR., M.D.

Although the prevalence of chronic mesenteric ischemia is low, the diagnostic problems in evaluating the elderly patient with abdominal discomfort and weight loss can often be formidable. In patients in whom the diagnosis of chronic mesenteric ischemia is entertained, duplex scanning can be an excellent screening method. Before considering the use of duplex scanning for this purpose, it is necessary to review the clinical syndrome because knowledge of its pathogenesis and pathophysiology are essential to our understanding of its detection and of how it can be treated.

PATHOGENESIS AND PATHOPHYSIOLOGY

The disease leading to this problem is most commonly atherosclerosis, which tends to involve branch points and bifurcations in the arterial system. Its localization in patients with the "fear of food syndrome" is to the orifices and first 2 cm of the major visceral arteries. One of the remarkable aspects of the blood supply to the gut is the prodigious collateral circulation that is available to provide blood flow when a major arterial trunk is significantly narrowed or occluded. This great capacity is what makes the incidence of the clinical syndrome so low.

It is well known that a single visceral artery—celiac, superior mesenteric, or inferior mesenteric—is capable of supplying the entire small bowel in a normal fashion with no symptoms as long as the occlusive process develops slowly. This fact is remarkable, given that the gut, much like the legs, demands marked increases in the amount of blood flow during digestion.

It is now well established that all three of the major arteries supplying the small bowel must have a lesion that produces a reduction in blood pressure and flow that restricts circulatory needs for digestion. This is the key factor to remember when the results of duplex scanning are reviewed in its role as a diagnostic test.

Under fasting circumstances, the small bowel can be likened to an intermediate- to high-resistance vascular bed. During fasting, the arterial velocity patterns in the superior mesenteric artery are similar to those observed in the arteries supplying the lower extremity.[1-3] The velocity patterns are triphasic with forward flow, reverse flow, and late forward flow components. The reverse flow component and the end-diastolic velocity distinguish the vascular beds with a high resistance from those whose resistance to flow is minimal regardless of the time of day or level of activity.

When food is ingested, the increases in blood flow to the small bowel are to a degree dependent upon the nature of the ingested meal. In our evaluation of this response, we found the greatest increase to occur with the ingestion of a mixed meal.[4] The time of onset for the blood flow increase is within the first 20 minutes after food ingestion with the maximum levels reached in approximately 30 to 60 minutes. After peak blood flow is reached, blood flow begins to decrease but remains elevated 90 to 100 minutes after eating.

Recently, we have also been able to study the colonic blood flow response to a meal by interrogating the velocity changes in the inferior mesenteric artery after a patient ingests a mixed meal and after a meal that is destined to be handled entirely by the colon itself.[5] The colon normally does not increase its blood flow in response to the foodstuffs that are handled by the small bowel but does so when a material such as lactulose is taken by mouth. When this material reaches the colon, the blood flow velocity in the inferior mesenteric artery increases.

DUPLEX SCANNING

Because the arteries supplying the small bowel originate in the posterior abdomen from the aorta, they may be difficult to reach unless a low-frequency scanhead is employed (2 to 3.5 mHz). It must also be remembered that at such depths, image quality is not optimal so the observer has to depend entirely upon the detected flow velocity patterns to assess the status of the visceral arteries.

Normally, the peak systolic velocity in the abdominal aorta adjacent to the celiac and superior mesenteric arteries is in the range of 100 ± 20 cm/second. As the sample volume is moved to the orifice and first portion of the celiac and superior mesenteric arteries, the peak systolic velocity increases. What is needed is to determine the range of normal velocity values that will permit the selection of patients who may have chronic mesenteric ischemia.

Moneta and associates studied 34 patients who had both arteriography and duplex scans to determine the range of velocities that were associated with a greater than 70% diameter-reducing stenosis of the celiac and superior mesenteric arteries.[6] They postulated that peak systolic velocities of greater than 200 cm/second for the celiac and greater than 275 cm/second for the superior mesenteric were sufficient for the detection of a greater than 70% diameter-reducing stenosis. To test this hypothesis, lateral aortograms were performed in 100 patients undergoing diagnostic peripheral arterial studies who had also undergone duplex studies of these two arteries.

The arteriograms were read independently of the duplex studies. The peak systolic velocities and end-diastolic velocities were measured for those arteries with a less than 70% diameter reduction as compared to those with tighter lesions. It was found that normal velocities or values less than 275 cm/second for the celiac and less than 200 cm/second for the superior mesenteric artery were sufficiently accurate to rule out the presence of greater than 70% diameter-reducing stenosis, which they considered necessary for the production of ischemic symptoms.

Clinical Applications

Because of its rarity, no single group of surgeons has a large clinical experience with chronic mesenteric ischemia. We have studied seven patients with this syndrome who had it verified by arteriography and operation. In each of these patients, the diagnosis, with the help of duplex scanning, was relatively simple. For the diagnosis to be made, however, knowledge concerning the extent of disease that must exist is critical. The collateral circulation that is available in most patients with chronic occlusive disease is extensive.

Most of our efforts have been confined to examination of the celiac and superior mesenteric arteries. Theoretically, we should also examine the inferior mesenteric artery as well because it can be the entire source of blood supply for the small bowel. In fact, Moneta and co-workers have published a case in which the small bowel was entirely supplied by the inferior mesenteric artery.[7] Even more remarkable was that the blood flow response to a food challenge was entirely normal.

At present, we use the following guidelines in making the diagnosis of chronic mesenteric ischemia:

1. The patient must satisfy the clinical criteria, with particular emphasis on the weight loss, which is a key part of the symptomatology.
2. The duplex study must document that both the celiac and superior mesenteric arteries are severely diseased, with the findings of very high grade stenoses or occlusions.
3. An attempt is made to study the inferior mesenteric artery. If it is found to be normal, the food challenge may be necessary to test its ability to increase blood flow to the ingestion of a mixed meal.
4. Lateral aortography is performed to document the location and extent of the disease, which is essential in planning operative therapy.

Another advantage of duplex scanning is its value as a method of following the patient after operation. Because the site of the arterial reconstruction is known, it is a relatively simple matter to reassess the operative site to document the result. Even though our overall experience is limited, the following three examples document the value of duplex scanning in the postoperative period.

Patient 1. This 49-year-old white female presented with a history of postprandial cramping abdominal pain, diarrhea, and weight loss. Duplex scanning confirmed high-grade lesions of both the celiac and superior mesenteric arteries. A vein graft was placed from the supraceliac aorta to the superior mesenteric artery. This was initially successful, but within 9 months her symptoms reappeared. A repeat duplex study documented an occluded graft that was confirmed by repeat arteriography. Fortunately, it was possible to dilate the stenosis in the superior mesenteric artery with complete relief of her symptoms.

Patient 2. This 65-year-old white female presented with classic symptoms of chronic gut ischemia. A duplex study confirmed lesions in the celiac and superior mesenteric arteries, which were found to be occluded. The arteriogram confirmed the duplex findings. Because her superior mesenteric artery was occluded, we placed a vein graft from the left common iliac artery to the mid-superior mesenteric artery. She did well for about 9 months but returned with recurrent symptoms. A repeat duplex scan documented that the vein graft was patent, but there was a high-grade stenosis in the vein just beyond its origin from the iliac artery (Fig. 1). Because of the location of the vein graft, a balloon angioplasty was a relatively simple matter, with return of nearly normal flow to the small bowel. This completely relieved her symptoms. She did have some return in symptoms at a later date associated with a recurrence of the lesion in

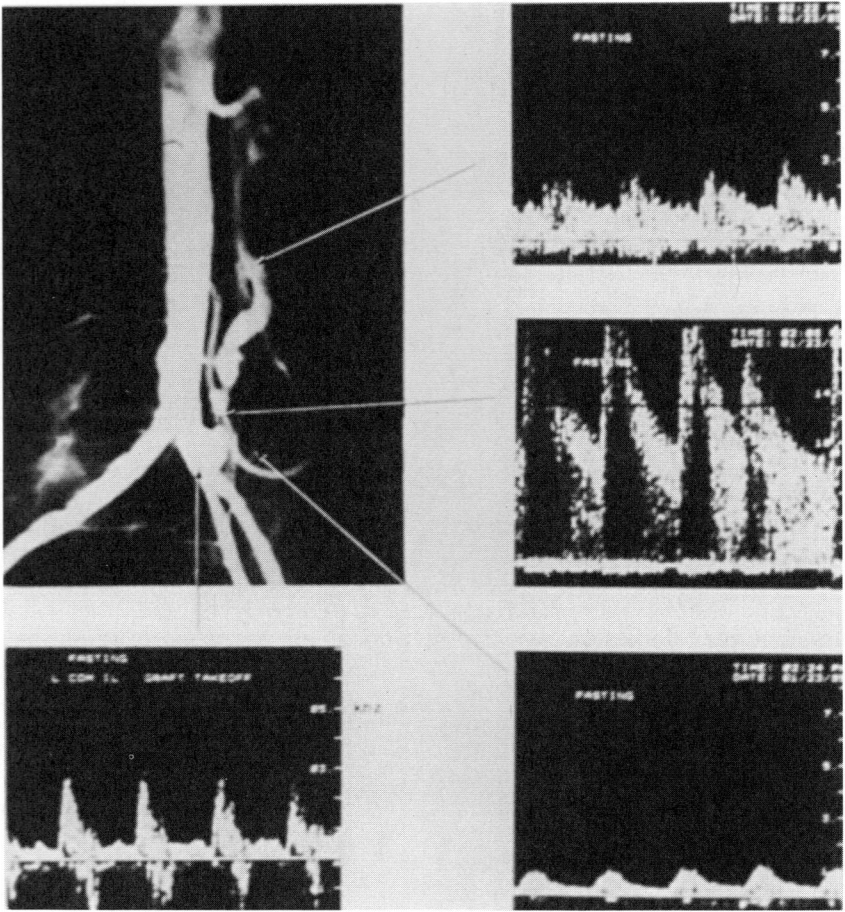

Figure 1 The stenosis in the vein graft near its origin from the iliac artery is accompanied by a large increase in peak systolic velocity. This was treated by angioplasty with return of velocities to a normal range. The patient's current symptoms were relieved. (From Strandness, DE Jr: Duplex scanning in vascular disorders. 2nd ed. New York: Raven Press, 1993; with permission)

the vein graft, but the symptoms were not severe and she declined further study. She remains well 4 years after the original procedure.

Patient 3. This 60-year-old white female presented with symptoms and signs compatible with the diagnosis of chronic mesenteric ischemia. She was found to have an occlusion of the celiac artery and a high-grade stenosis of the superior mesenteric artery. A bifurcated Dacron graft was placed from the supraceliac aorta to the midportion of the common hepatic and the superior mesenteric arteries. Her postoperative course was relatively benign, but she developed an ileus that did not respond to nasogastric suction. A postoperative duplex scan revealed that the prosthetic graft was occluded. A thrombectomy was required, along with a patch applied to the junction of the bifurcation with the two limbs. The early results of this second operation were successful.

Clearly a duplex study is not necessary to document failure of a bypass procedure, but it does permit the documentation of both early and late results. This is important in correcting problems that may develop after reconstruction.

At present, duplex scanning should be the first test for those patients who present with symptoms and signs suggestive of chronic mesenteric ischemia. The duplex findings are often definitive in ruling in or ruling out the diagnosis. If one or both of the major inputs to the small bowel are normal, there is no need to further implicate the involvement of the first portions of the celiac and superior mesenteric arteries as the cause of the problem. However, in rare instances the occlusions that lead to problems may be beyond the origin of the superior mesenteric artery. When the diagnosis remains likely in this setting, it may be necessary to resort to arteriography to confirm the diagnosis. After therapy, be it angioplasty or operation, repeat studies will establish the extent to which the procedure has been successful in restoring intestinal blood flow to normal.

REFERENCES

1. Nicholls SC, Kohler TR, Martin RL, Strandness DE Jr. Use of hemodynamic parameters in the diagnosis of mesenteric insufficiency. J Vasc Surg 1986; 3:507–510.
2. Jager KA. Measurement of mesenteric blood flow by duplex scanning. J Vasc Surg 1986; 3:462–469.
3. Jager KA, Fortner GS, Thiele BL, Strandness DE Jr. Noninvasive diagnosis of intestinal angina. J Clin Ultrasound 1984; 12:588–591.
4. Moneta GL, Taylor DC, Helton WS. Duplex ultrasound measurement of postprandial intestinal blood flow: Effect of meal composition. Gastroenterology 1988; 95:1294–12301.
5. Verlato F, Zaccardi M, Beach KW, Strandness DE Jr. Inferior mesenteric artery blood flow response to ingestion of lactulose: A preliminary study. Unpublished data.
6. Moneta GL, Lee RW, Yeager RA, et al. Mesenteric duplex scanning: A blinded prospective study. J Vasc Surg 1993; 17:79–86.
7. Moneta GL, Cummings C, Castor J, Porter JM. Duplex ultrasound demonstration of postprandial mesenteric hyperemia in splanchnic circulation collateral vessels. J Vasc Tech 1991; 15:37–39.

PERCUTANEOUS TRANSCATHETER THERAPY OF VISCERAL ISCHEMIA

CHARLES J. TEGTMEYER, M.D.
ALAN H. MATSUMOTO, M.D.
J. FRITZ ANGLE, M.D.

CHRONIC MESENTERIC ISCHEMIA

Chronic mesenteric ischemia is an entity amenable to transcatheter therapy. However, percutaneous transluminal angioplasty (PTA) has not been widely utilized in the mesenteric vessels,[1-9] probably because the syndrome of chronic intestinal ischemia is relatively uncommon and the diagnosis has been marked by controversy since its inception. The rich collateral network in the mesenteric system prompted a difference of opinion as to the degree of mesenteric vascular compromise necessary to cause intestinal angina. Many authors felt that severe disease in at least two of the three main vessels (Fig. 1) was necessary to produce symptoms. However, isolated significant stenoses (Fig. 2) or occlusions have been proven to cause symptoms in some patients. It is now accepted that obstruction of a single artery or a combination of the three main vessels supplying the viscera can cause symptoms. Conversely, the patient may be asymptomatic when several of these vessels are involved. In symptomatic patients an arteriogram is necessary for a definitive answer as to the vascular disease present. A biplane abdominal aortogram is required for thorough evaluation of the origins and complete extent of the celiac, superior mesenteric, and inferior mesenteric arteries. Oblique and selective filming may be necessary.

Patients with documented intestinal angina and a stenosis of 70% or greater in a visceral artery are candidates for angioplasty. Stenoses of 50% to 70% may not be critical; however, a peak-to-peak systolic blood pressure gradient greater than 10 mm Hg is significant. Stenoses of less than 50% are usually not the cause of the patient's symptoms.

Percutaneous Transluminal Angioplasty

Percutaneous transluminal angioplasty is indicated in the treatment of atherosclerotic and fibromuscular lesions. Arteritis may respond to balloon dilation, but the response of these lesions is variable, and these patients need to be evaluated on a case-by-case basis. Stenoses in bypass grafts are usually amenable to PTA. These stenoses are usually located at the distal anastomosis.

The technique for mesenteric angioplasty is similar to that used in the renal arteries. The femoral approach is employed when possible. However, in patients with severe weight loss, the arteries often originate at a steep caudad angle, and the axillary approach is utilized. The axillary approach is in reality a high brachial artery puncture. The left brachial artery is preferred because it offers a more direct route to the abdominal aorta and mesenteric vessels. With the standard over-the-wire balloon system, approaching the vessel from above provides greater control for crossing the stenosis with the guide wire. Passing the balloon catheter over the wire and through the stenosis is also easier because this approach allows a more directed force to be applied. The high brachial approach may achieve a better result in resistant lesions because the balloon lies flat and does not kink at the origin of the vessels as it does in an approach from below. The drawback to the high brachial approach is the increased risk of a hematoma around the brachial plexus and a resultant brachial plexus injury.

The lesion is selected with Bentson wire and a preshaped 5 Fr catheter. A shepherd's crook catheter is usually preferred for the femoral approach, and a multipurpose or cobra catheter is employed for the high brachial approach. Once the lesion has been crossed, 2,000 to 3,000 units of heparin sodium are injected through the catheter. The catheter is exchanged for the balloon catheter over a 200 cm Rosen wire. After dilation, the result is checked by placing a 0.018 inch guide wire in the vessel. Contrast is injected through the catheter by using a Tuohy Borst adaptor. The end point is complete ablation of the lesion, when possible. A

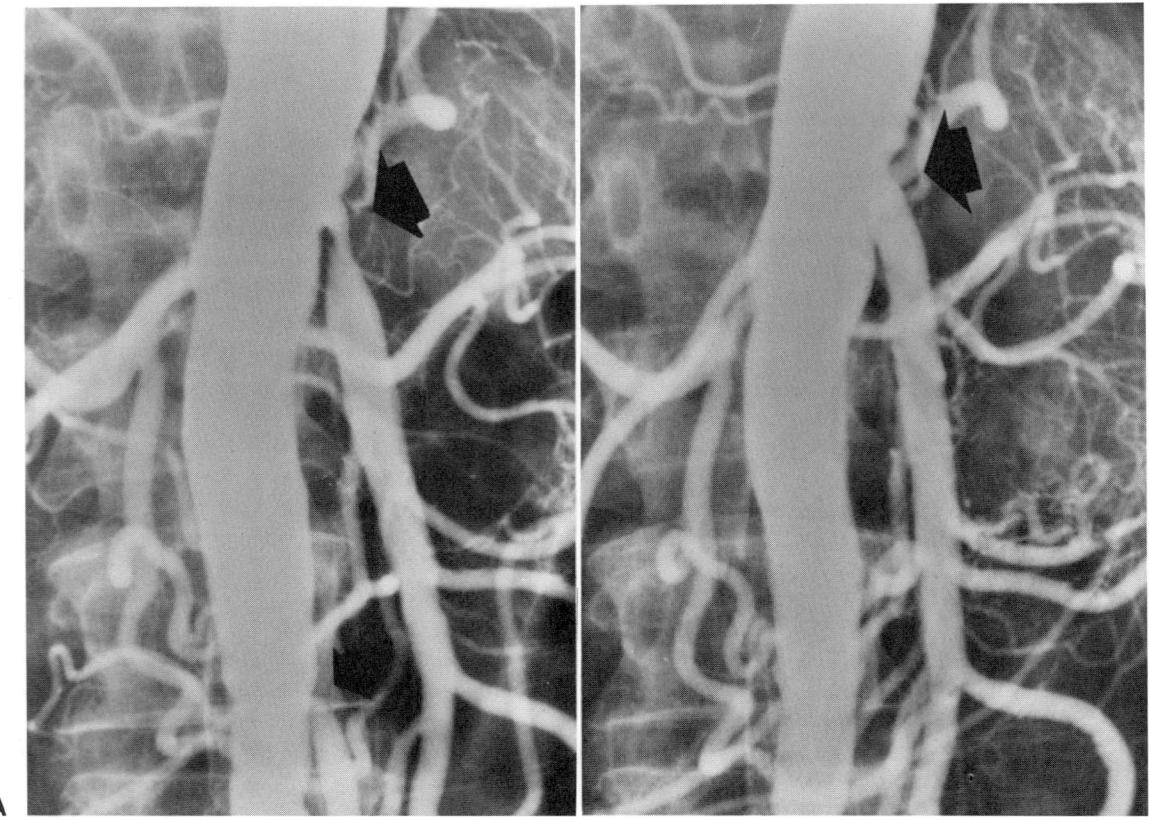

Figure 1 Fifty-nine-year-old woman with chronic mesenteric ischemia. *A,* There is a tight stenosis at the origin of the superior mesenteric artery *(arrow).* The celiac artery is occluded, and there is a tight stenosis in her inferior mesenteric artery. *B,* Follow-up arteriogram 16 months after operation demonstrates a widely patent superior mesenteric artery *(arrow).* The inferior mesenteric artery is now occluded.

residual stenosis of greater than 30% has an increased rate of early recurrence.

An alternative technique employs the coaxial Tegwire system. A sheath is placed in the femoral artery, and the appropriate 7 Fr guiding catheter is placed in the abdominal aorta. The balloon on a wire, Tegwire, is placed in the guiding catheter.[10] The vessel to be dilated is selected with the guiding catheter and the Tegwire balloon, which has a 0.014 inch tip, is advanced across the lesion. The lesion is dilated and the results are easily checked by injecting contrast material through the guiding catheter.

Results

Since Furrer and co-workers' initial description of superior mesenteric artery (SMA) angioplasty in 1980,[1] there have been only scattered reports (Table 1). Analysis of the literature reveals that PTA for the treatment of mesenteric ischemia has a technical success rate of 88%, an initial clinical success rate of 92%, and a long-term secondary success rate of 93%. We recently analyzed the results in 19 patients at the University of Virginia.[9] Four patients were initial technical failures. All the failures were in lesions associated with extrinsic compression of the artery. The median arcuate ligament was responsible for three of the failures. Median arcuate ligament syndrome does not respond favorably to PTA. The fourth patient had carcinoma of the pancreas encasing the SMA. Fifteen patients had a technically successful result, and 12 (80%) of this group had immediate relief of their symptoms. One patient with successful dilation of the SMA and celiac arteries had persistent symptoms and was found to have diffuse metastatic adenocarcinoma. The other two patients who were technical successes but did not have relief of their symptoms had occlusions of their other two visceral arteries. Surgical revascularization of one additional vessel was required in each patient to provide relief of symptoms. Eleven (93%) of the 12 clinically successful angioplasties are asymptomatic at 4 to 73 months (mean 25 months) of follow-up, although one patient needed repeat angioplasty.

The symptoms of occult abdominal malignancy may mimic the symptoms of chronic mesenteric ischemia. Therefore, it is important to be alert to the possibility of malignancy in these patients.

The complications from mesenteric PTA are similar to those encountered in patients with diffuse vascular disease who are undergoing peripheral angioplasty. We

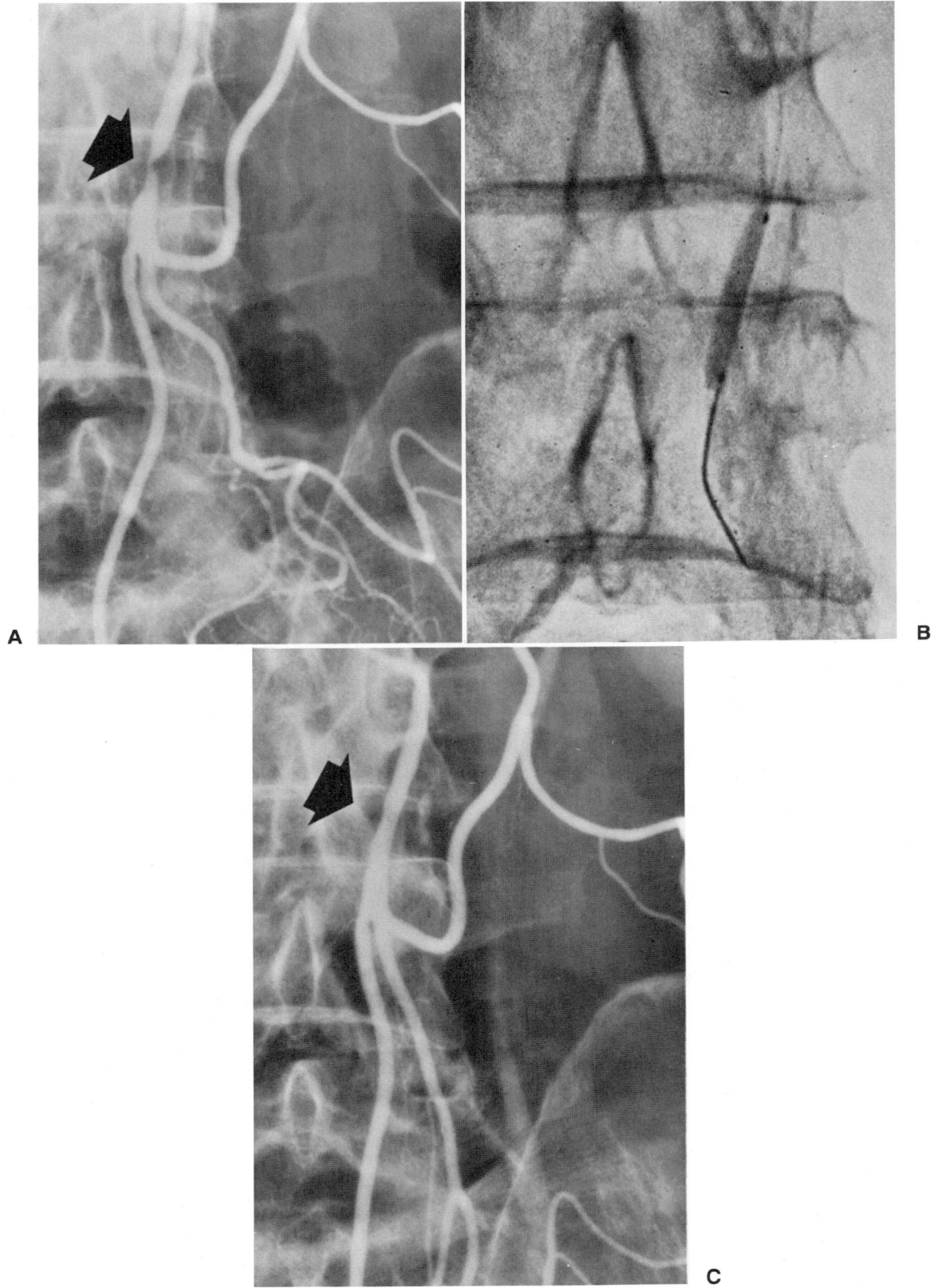

Figure 2 Sixty-one-year-old man with ischemic colitis. *A*, The patient has a short, tight stenosis of the inferior mesenteric artery *(arrow)*. *B*, The 3 mm Tegwire balloon is in place. *C*, Follow-up film after dilation shows a good result *(arrow)*.

Table 1 Results of Mesentery Angioplasty

Study	No. Patients Treated	Initial Technical Success (Patients)	Initial Clinical Success	Primary Long-Term Clinical Success	Secondary Long-Term Clinical Success	Follow-Up Range in Months (Mean)
University of Virginia[9]	19	15/19 (79%)	12/15 (80%)	10/12 (83%)	11/12 (92%)	4–73 (25)
Sniderman[8]	13	11/13 (85%)	11/11 (100%)	6/11 (55%)	9/11 (82%)	1–96 (N/A)
Simonetti (Chronic mesenteric ischemia patients only) et al[7]	22	21/22 (90%)	18/21 (100%)	16/18 (88%)	18/18 (100%)	24–36 (N/A)
McShane et al[6]	6	5/6 (83%)	5/5 (100%)	2/5 (40%)	4/5 (80%)	7–24 (16)
Levy et al[5]	4	4/4 (100%)	4/4 (100%)	2/4 (50%)	4/4 (100%)	8–42 (25)
Wilms and Baert[4]	8	7/8 (88%)	7/7 (100%)	7/7 (100%)	—	1–15 (N/A)
Roberts et al[3]	4	4/4 (100%)	4/4 (100%)	2/4 (50%)	4/4 (100%)	16–28 (22)
Golden et al[2]	7	6/7 (86%)	6/6 (100%)	6/6 (100%)	—	up to 28 (N/A)
Total	83	73/83 (88%)	67/73 (92%)	51/67 (76%)	50/54 (93%)	N/A

had three major complications, but only one required operation. One limb of a previous aortobifemoral graft occluded at the access site in the femoral artery, and this resulted in a below-the-knee amputation. There were no deaths. However, two deaths were reported in the literature in the 81 patients treated with mesenteric angioplasty.

ACUTE MESENTERIC ISCHEMIA

Fibrinolytic Therapy

There are few indications for interventional catheter therapy in acute mesenteric ischemia. The role of arteriography is mainly diagnostic. Although catheter-directed fibrinolytic therapy has enjoyed success in the peripheral vessels, there are few indications for its use in the splanchnic bed. Thrombolytic therapy usually requires 12 to 36 hours for success. Acute mesenteric ischemia frequently requires urgent revascularization to prevent bowel infarction, and it is often difficult to ascertain whether infarction has already occurred in these patients. Cautious use of thrombolytic therapy may be indicated in patients with short vascular occlusions due to thrombus if there are adequate distal collateral vessels to protect the bowel.[11] The role of thrombolytic therapy is limited. It may be attempted in select patients without peritoneal signs if the patients have adequate collaterals.

Nonocclusive Mesenteric Ischemia

Nonocclusive mesenteric ischemia is characterized by severe vasoconstriction of the arteries supplying the viscera, and it is the most common cause of acute mesenteric ischemia. The condition is the result of low cardiac output due to cardiogenic or hemorrhagic shock, cardiac arrhythmias, or congestive heart failure. Digitalis has been implicated as a predisposing factor of the condition. Mesenteric ischemia occurs because the splanchnic vasoconstriction may persist after the patient's hemodynamic status has been stabilized.

The patients present with abdominal pain out of proportion to their physical findings. Usually, rebound tenderness is absent. If untreated, the condition can progress to bowel infarction. The angiographic pattern is one of multiple short segmental vasoconstrictions at the origins of mesenteric branches. There is reduced blood flow to the peripheral arcades. The condition may be localized or diffuse. In the absence of peritoneal signs, pharmacoangiographic therapy may be attempted. A test infusion of papaverine, 45 mg over 15 minutes, may be administered through the superior mesenteric catheter. If the vasospasm is reversed, a prolonged infusion of papaverine may be given at a rate of 30 to 60 mg/hour through the mesenteric catheter. If signs of peritoneal irritation appear during the infusion, prompt surgical exploration is indicated. The infusion is continued during operation, and the nonviable bowel is resected. In questionable circumstances, a second-look operation may be necessary. The papaverine infusion is continued postoperatively until all angiographic and clinical signs of vasoconstriction have resolved. When no peritoneal signs are present, the infusion is continued for 24 hours. The infusion therapy will not be successful if the patient's underlying hemodynamic instability cannot be corrected.

REFERENCES

1. Furrer J, Gruntzig A, Kugelmeier J, Goebel N. Treatment of abdominal angina with percutaneous dilatation of an arteria mesenterica superior stenosis. Cardiovasc Intervent Radiol 1980; 3:43–44.
2. Golden DA, Ring EJ, McLean GK, Freiman DB. Percutaneous angioplasty in the treatment of abdominal angina. Am J Roentgenol 1982; 139:247–249.
3. Roberts L, Wertman DA, Mills SR, et al. Transluminal angioplasty of the superior mesenteric artery: An alternative to surgical revascularization. Am J Roentgenol 1983; 141:1039–1042.
4. Wilms G, Baert AL. Transluminal angioplasty of superior mesenteric artery and celiac trunk. Ann Radiol (Paris) 1986; 29:535–538.
5. Levy PJ, Haskell L, Gordon RL. Percutaneous transluminal angioplasty of splanchnic arteries: An alternative method to elective revascularisation in chronic visceral ischaemia. Eur J Radiol 1987; 7:239–242.
6. McShane MD, Proctor A, Spencer P, et al. Mesenteric angioplasty for chronic intestinal ischaemia. Eur J Vasc Surg 1992; 6:333–336.
7. Simonetti G, Lupattelli L, Urigo F, et al. Interventional radiology in the treatment of acute and chronic mesenteric ischemia. Radiol Med (Torino) 1992; 84:98–105.
8. Sniderman KW. Transluminal angioplasty in the management of chronic intestinal ischemia. In: Strandness DE, van Breda A, eds. Vascular diseases: Surgical and interventional therapy. New York: Churchill Livingstone, 1994:803.
9. Fitzcharles EK, Matsumoto AH, Tegtmeyer CJ, et al. Balloon angioplasty for the treatment of mesenteric ischemia: Results and clinical follow-up. JVIR 1994; 5:47.
10. Tegtmeyer CJ. Guide wire angioplasty balloon catheter: Preliminary report. Radiology 1988; 169:253–254.
11. Vujic I, Stanely J, Gobien RP. Treatment of acute embolus of the superior mesenteric artery by topical infusion streptokinase. Cardiovasc Intervent Radiol 1984; 7:94–96.

ACUTE EMBOLIC AND THROMBOTIC MESENTERIC ISCHEMIA

DANIEL S. RUSH, M.D.
PAVEL J. LEVY, M.D.
JAMES L. HAYNES, M.D.

Despite considerable progress in the diagnosis and management of acute mesenteric ischemia, reported mortality rates from embolic and thrombotic mesenteric arterial occlusion remain greater than 50%.[1] Patients at risk for mesenteric ischemia are often elderly and debilitated and have other cardiovascular problems. Delay in diagnosis continues to be the primary factor contributing to high mortality, and the number of reported patients successfully revascularized for acute mesenteric ischemia is surprisingly small.[1] Aggressive use of diagnostic mesenteric arteriography and mesenteric revascularization, conservative intestinal resection, and planned re-exploration have been proposed as the best means of improving overall survival.[2]

PATHOPHYSIOLOGY

Mesenteric Arterial Anatomy

An understanding of the arterial distribution to the gastrointestinal (GI) tract is required to appreciate the patterns of bowel ischemia produced by acute embolic and thrombotic mesenteric occlusion. Three aortic branches—the celiac, superior mesenteric, and inferior mesenteric arteries—provide the major blood supply to the intestinal tract and communicate via collaterals. All three vessels play an important role in chronic mesenteric ischemia, but arterial reconstruction in acute mesenteric ischemia is directed primarily at the superior mesenteric artery (SMA). The SMA arises from the aorta, just distal to the celiac and proximal to the origin of the renal arteries, and supplies the distal duodenum, the entire small intestine, and the colon to the splenic flexure. The SMA first branches into the middle colic artery, then into jejunal and ileal branches, and terminates as the ileocolic artery. A collateral network connects the celiac and SMA via pancreaticoduodenal branches and may be sufficient to limit ischemia of the distal duodenum and proximal jejunum following acute SMA occlusion. The inferior mesenteric artery (IMA) branches ventrally from the aorta and supplies the left and sigmoid colon. A major collateral, the meandering mesenteric artery, connects the middle colic branch of the SMA with the proximal IMA. The meandering mesenteric artery becomes especially prominent—and may be easily documented arteriographically—after gradual atherosclerotic narrowing of either SMA or IMA origins. Acute occlusion of either the celiac artery or the IMA in normal individuals may be well tolerated because of collaterals, but acute occlusion of the SMA generally produces infarction throughout its small bowel and colonic distribution. Distal SMA occlusion produces segmental intestinal and colon ischemia because of its middle colic, jejunal, and ileal branches.

Intestinal Ischemic Injury and Mesenteric Vasospasm

Intestinal ischemia progresses transmurally from the mucosa to the serosa. The extent of injury to the bowel wall following acute arterial occlusion is dependent on the duration of ischemia, the pattern of mesenteric arterial occlusion, and collateral blood supply. Over time, mesenteric ischemia produces marked epithelial and endothelial damage, which increases vulnerability to lysosomal and digestive enzymes, lowers mucosal barriers to bacterial invasion, and results in microcirculatory stagnation with edema from increased vascular permeability. Bacterial toxins and products of intestinal cellular necrosis become released into the portal venous circulation and produce profound systemic effects. Adverse hemodynamics explain the high frequency of acidosis, sepsis, and shock found in patients with delayed diagnosis of acute mesenteric ischemia and are associated with mortality.[1] Liver and pulmonary dysfunction have been observed after SMA revascularization and may progress to multisystem organ failure.[1,3]

Acute insult to the intestinal wall may not end after mesenteric revascularization. Volume depletion and toxicity may continue postoperatively and produce persistent mesenteric hypoperfusion unless corrected. Many patients with acute occlusive mesenteric ischemia have pre-existing cardiovascular compromise; thus, use of hemodynamic monitoring in the management of volume status and optimal cardiac performance is a necessity. Digitalis is known to have an adverse effect on the mesenteric microcirculation. Experimental work in animal models of occlusive intestinal ischemia provides insight into treatment options that have not yet been established by prospective clinical trials. Studies indicate that mesenteric arterial vasospasm plays a major role in splanchnic hypoperfusion; it may persist independently of other adverse systemic hemodynamics following revascularization and establishes a physiologic basis for the adjunctive use of vasodilators in the treatment of mesenteric ischemia.[4] Papaverine and tolazoline produce vascular smooth muscle relaxation and can be injected directly into the SMA. These vasodilators are nonspecific and ineffective if given systemically but can be infused by transfemoral arterial catheter selectively into the SMA. Glucagon is a potent and specific splanchnic vasodilator that can be given directly into the SMA or infused systemically by peripheral vein.[4] Effective use of vasodilators requires blood volume restoration to prevent mesenteric pooling and hypotension. Other experimental studies indicate that gut reperfusion injury may be caused by oxygen-derived free radicals. Consideration should be given to the adjunctive use of free-radical scavengers and pentoxifyllin, which have been shown to reduce systemic toxicity.[5]

CLINICAL FEATURES

Acute Embolic Mesenteric Arterial Ischemia

Superior mesenteric artery thromboembolism is the most common etiology of acute occlusive mesenteric ischemia and represents 76% of reported cases.[1] Acute SMA embolism produces a characteristic syndrome of abrupt abdominal pain followed by gastrointestinal emptying by vomiting, diarrhea, or both. Symptoms suggesting chronic mesenteric ischemia are absent because the intestinal circulation was intact prior to the acute embolic event. In contrast, associated cardiac diseases known to be thromboembolic sources are common and include chronic atrial fibrillation, myocardial infarction or left ventricular aneurysm with mural thrombus, congestive heart failure, and mitral stenosis. More than a third of patients with acute SMA embolism have a past history of peripheral arterial embolism, and a cardiac source is most frequently found.[1] Occasional patients have concurrent SMA and peripheral arterial emboli. Bowel sounds may be initially hyperactive, with evacuation of the GI tract, but later become hypoactive. Signs of peritonitis—abdominal tenderness, rebound, and guarding—do not occur until after bowel has become infarcted. Fever, leukocytosis, acidosis, shock, and sepsis are late signs of bowel infarction indicating systemic toxicity, and they have a very poor prognosis.

Location of emboli within the SMA determines the subsequent pattern of intestinal ischemia. Most SMA emboli lodge at or near the origin of the middle colic artery and produce ischemia from proximal jejunum to the splenic flexure of the colon. Smaller emboli may lodge in distal SMA branches and produce segmental bowel ischemia. Biplane arteriography is the best preoperative method to localize SMA emboli, but the sterile Doppler probe can be a useful operative technique to identify the location of SMA emboli and assess the adequacy of embolectomy. Treatment of the embolic source and anticoagulation are recommended to prevent recurrence.

Acute Thrombotic Mesenteric Arterial Ischemia

Acute intestinal ischemia associated with atherosclerotic mesenteric arterial occlusive disease is much less common than SMA embolism, with fewer than 60 revascularized cases published.[1] Acute SMA thrombosis does not follow a characteristic clinical syndrome. Acute thrombotic mesenteric occlusion usually involves the SMA and at least one other mesenteric artery, but the pattern of intestinal infarction may vary depending on the collateral blood supply. Symptoms of unrecognized chronic mesenteric ischemia, nonspecific abdominal pain, and weight loss may precede the onset of acute intestinal ischemia by weeks or months.[6] Although such symptoms may not be classic for intestinal angina, patients with chronic mesenteric ischemia are at high risk for acute intestinal infarction. In several recent studies, 25% of hospitalized patients awaiting operation for chronic mesenteric ischemia developed acute intestinal ischemia.[3,7] Such patients may have already undergone evaluation and treatment for problems such as occult gastrointestinal malignancy or peptic ulcer disease. Given the difficulty of early diagnosis for intestinal ischemia generally, the correct diagnosis of acute thrombotic mesenteric ischemia is often further delayed because of the gradual, rather than abrupt, transition from chronic to acute symptoms and the confusion with other presumed gastrointestinal problems. Because of the better results with surgical treatment for chronic mesenteric ischemia, aggressive and preventive revascularization in such patients is preferred to management of acute thrombotic intestinal ischemia.

DIAGNOSIS

Acute intestinal ischemia can be one of the most difficult surgical diagnoses. It requires a high index of clinical suspicion in elderly patients with otherwise nonspecific abdominal pain and associated cardiovascular risk factors. Signs of peritonitis do not occur until after intestinal infarction and, thus, do not appear until late in the course of the disease. Standard teaching states that patients with acute mesenteric ischemia have abdominal pain out of proportion to their physical examination. Actually, few patients with acute occlusive mesenteric ischemia have this clinical picture, but when present it could be an important clue to the diagnosis. Acute SMA embolism is generally easier to diagnose than acute SMA thrombosis because of the characteristic abrupt onset of symptoms. Acute SMA thrombosis is often preceded by a history of gastrointestinal complaints that may be indistinguishable from the acute event until after intestinal infarction. Unfortunately, delay in the diagnosis of acute occlusive mesenteric ischemia is frequent and has a major adverse impact upon patient survival.

Although a number of serum and radionuclide tests for acute mesenteric ischemia have been investigated, none has become widely adopted or routinely available as diagnostic tests.[8] Abdominal x-rays and computed tomography are usually nondiagnostic in early acute mesenteric ischemia but may demonstrate pneumatosis intestinalis or gas in the portal system as late and ominous findings. Duplex mesenteric arterial ultrasonography has become widely accepted as a screening test for chronic visceral ischemia but has not been shown reliable under conditions present in unprepared patients with acute symptoms. Only biplane arteriography, with delayed films to demonstrate the venous phase, has sufficient diagnostic specificity in patients with suspected acute intestinal ischemia for use preoperatively to evaluate the mesenteric arterial and venous systems.[9] In early acute mesenteric ischemia, diagnostic arteriography facilitates rather than delays surgical intervention and defines the etiology and anatomy for revascularization. In patients with undiagnosed abdominal pain and an arteriographically documented SMA occlusion, it must be assumed that mesenteric ischemia is the cause of the acute symptoms.

For patients in whom the diagnosis of acute intestinal ischemia is made during surgical exploration, the etiology and anatomy of mesenteric arterial occlusion may be very difficult to determine. In this situation, intraoperative arteriography should be used if available, but physical assessment and sterile Doppler insonation of the mesenteric vessels may be sufficient to permit revascularization. Postoperative arteriography to evaluate the adequacy of revascularization and for selective SMA vasodilator infusion is recommended. Intestinal viability cannot currently be determined preoperatively, but diagnostic laparoscopy has been reported and may have an established role in the near future.

COMBINED SURGICAL TREATMENT

As soon as the diagnosis of acute occlusive mesenteric ischemia is made, whether preoperatively or operatively, the patient should be systemically anticoagulated with heparin sodium to prevent thrombus propagation. Upon exploration of the abdomen through a midline incision, obviously gangrenous or perforated bowel should be immediately resected to reduce soilage and systemic toxicity. Initially, it may be difficult to determine intestinal viability; thus, bowel resection should be conservative. Ischemic or marginally viable bowel should be revascularized first and then objectively evaluated before resection. The proximal SMA can be exposed by reflecting the transverse colon superiorly and the small bowel to the right. This exposure is the same as that commonly used for the infrarenal aorta. The ligament of Treitz is divided, and the root of the small bowel mesentery incised. The SMA is encountered, along with many lymphatics, to the left of the superior mesenteric vein, and it can be followed cephalad into the transverse mesocolon to its origin from the aorta. Fortunately, the space between the left renal vein and the origin of the SMA is devoid of other structures, which allows adequate exposure. Palpation and sterile Doppler assessment of the SMA at this point can identify the location of occlusion intraoperatively.

In acute SMA thromboembolism, Doppler assessment is helpful to localize the embolus with or without a preoperative arteriogram. A transverse arteriotomy can be made at the site of SMA occlusion or proximal to the middle colic artery, where the SMA is larger. The embolus is then removed by balloon catheter, although care should be taken because the lining of the SMA is often friable, and its jejunal and ileal branches are delicate and easily disrupted. Vasodilators and heparin saline solution can be irrigated directly into the SMA through the arteriotomy. The transverse arteriotomy is then closed by interrupted sutures. If the SMA is small or proximal occlusive disease is suspected, the SMA can be explored through a longitudinal arteriotomy that allows either SMA embolectomy or SMA bypass. If only an embolectomy is required, the longitudinal SMA arteriotomy can be closed with a vein patch angioplasty.

In acute SMA thrombosis, mesenteric revascularization can be accomplished by either aortomesenteric bypass or SMA thromboendarterectomy. Contrary to the elective management of chronic mesenteric ischemia, in which as many mesenteric arteries are reconstructed as possible, the primary goal in acute SMA thrombosis is to reconstruct the SMA. In these critically ill patients, it is impractical, under emergent conditions, to attempt extensive multiarterial reconstructions. In patients with peritoneal spillage from necrotic bowel, it is preferable to reconstruct the SMA with autologous material.

Ironically, prosthetic mesenteric grafts have been shown to have better long-term patency than autologous vein in chronic mesenteric ischemia, but no advantage in acute mesenteric ischemia has been established. In patients without bowel infarction, prosthetic aortomesenteric grafts are preferable.

No data support the view that antegrade grafts originating from the aorta proximally function better in acute mesenteric ischemia than retrograde grafts originating distally from the infrarenal aorta or iliac arteries. A suprarenal aortic anastomosis should be used only if no other inflow site is available, but in emergent situations clamping the aorta may have adverse effects upon systemic hemodynamics, cardiopulmonary function, and renal perfusion. An iliac inflow anastomosis avoids these untoward effects and is technically a much simpler surgical procedure. Opinion is divided as to whether the SMA anastomosis should be constructed end to end or end to side, and neither has proven superiority in acute ischemia. Technically, the end-to-side SMA anastomosis is easier to perform and less inclined to kinking. An omental pedicle can be brought down through the transverse mesocolon to cover and protect the SMA bypass.

An SMA thromboendarterectomy with vein patch angioplasty has appeal for atherosclerotic SMA occlusive disease confined to its origin, but results from this procedure are inferior to aorto-SMA bypass in acute mesenteric ischemia.[1] Direct SMA endarterectomy through a longitudinal SMA arteriotomy extended onto the side of the aorta can be closed with a vein patch. Transaortic mesenteric endarterectomy via a thoracoabdominal approach may be difficult under emergent conditions, especially the management of infarcted bowel. An SMA endarterectomy can be performed but at present is not recommended if aorto-SMA bypass is equally feasible.

Recent reports suggest that percutaneous transluminal balloon angioplasty of the SMA and thrombolytic therapy have been used to treat acute intestinal ischemia. These reports are difficult to place in perspective because many of the patients did not undergo surgical exploration to verify the severity of bowel ischemia. At present, no criteria define which patients with symptoms of acute occlusive mesenteric ischemia might be candidates for less than standard surgical management. Although some patients may be successfully treated by interventional techniques, surgical exploration is recommended to evaluate intestinal viability.

Once mesenteric revascularization is completed, clinical assessment of bowel viability becomes critical. Color change in the intestinal serosa and return of peristalsis or sterile Doppler examination of the mesenteric vessels may be important indicators of bowel viability. Physical appearance of the bowel may be misleading if the patient has not been fully resuscitated. Also, mesenteric Doppler examination requires some experience and may not be reliable if an arterial flow signal is absent, especially in the colon. Uniform bowel fluorescence under Wood's lamp examination after intravenous fluorescein infusion is probably the best means of determining viability intraoperatively.[9] At this point injection of vasodilators into the SMA or systemic infusion of glucagon may be of benefit. At least 30 minutes of intestinal reperfusion should be allowed after arterial blood flow restoration before intestinal viability is determined and any bowel resected.

Once it has been determined that an intestinal segment is nonviable, it is best to resect conservatively at the first operation. Massive bowel resection despite successful SMA revascularization has a low survival rate, and the few patients who survive often develop short-gut syndrome. Small intestinal reanastomosis can be performed, but it is sometimes preferable to create stomas, which prevent intraperitoneal soilage and can be observed externally. It is especially important to bring out an ostomy when ischemic or gangrenous colon is resected, rather than risk the complications of anastomotic failure. If questions regarding intestinal viability remain, it is best to re-evaluate the situation at a planned second exploration within 24 to 36 hours. The decision to perform a second exploration should be made at the initial operation based on objective criteria and should be performed regardless of subsequent clinical improvement. Conversely, clinical deterioration should prompt earlier re-exploration. The time between these procedures should be spent by further resuscitation and maintenance of optimal hemodynamics. Planned re-exploration is not mandatory if all the GI tract is viable, no bowel has been resected, and the patient responds well to postoperative treatment.

Patients undergoing surgical treatment of acute occlusive mesenteric ischemia require intensive postoperative care. These patients generally have existing cardiovascular compromise and need continuous invasive monitoring of blood volume status, cardiac performance, and systemic hemodynamics. Some degree of multiple-system organ failure, especially involving the liver and lungs, can usually be detected.[1,3] Postoperative infusion of vasodilators to improve the mesenteric microcirculation, heparin sodium anticoagulation to prevent recurrent emboli or rethrombosis, follow-up mesenteric arteriography to assess the adequacy of SMA revascularization, and second-look procedures to evaluate bowel viability are all strongly recommended adjuncts to the successful treatment of acute occlusive mesenteric ischemia.

REFERENCES

1. Levy PJ, Rush DS, Hornung CA, et al. Determinants of survival and intestinal salvage following superior mesenteric artery revascularization in patients with acute mesenteric ischemia. Unpublished data.
2. Levy PJ, Krausz MM, Manny J. Acute mesenteric ischemia: Improved results, a retrospective analysis of 92 patients. Surgery 1990; 107:372–380.
3. Harward TRS, Brooks DL, Flynn TC, Seeger JM. Multiple organ dysfunction after mesenteric artery revascularization. J Vasc Surg 1993; 18:459–469.

4. Kazmers A, Zwolak R, Appleman HD, et al. Pharmacologic interventions in acute mesenteric ischemia: Improved survival with intravenous glucagon, methylprednisolone, and prostacyclin. J Vasc Surg 1984; 1:472–481.
5. Horton JW, White DJ. Free radical scavengers prevent intestinal ischemia-reperfusion-mediated cardiac dysfunction. J Surg Res 1993; 55:282–289.
6. Kwaan JHM, Connoly JE. Prevention of intestinal infarction resulting from mesenteric arterial occlusive disease. Surg Gynecol Obstet 1983; 157:321–324.
7. Rheudasil JM, Stewart MT, Schellack JV, et al. Surgical treatment of chronic mesenteric arterial insufficiency. J Vasc Surg 1988; 8:495–500.
8. Rush DS, Jordon JA, Zarins CK, Rosenberg IH. Noninvasive detection of experimental intestinal ischemia. J Surg Res 1983; 35:315–318.
9. Boley SJ, Sprayregan S, Siegelman SS, Veith FJ. Initial results from an aggressive roentgenological and surgical approach to acute mesenteric ischemia. Surgery 1977; 52:848–855.

TRANSAORTIC SPLANCHNIC ENDARTERECTOMY FOR CHRONIC MESENTERIC ISCHEMIA

LOUIS M. MESSINA, M.D.
RAJABRATA SARKAR, M.D.

Chronic mesenteric ischemia is a relatively uncommon but challenging clinical syndrome manifested by postprandial epigastric abdominal pain and severe weight loss. The abdominal pain can progress to near total abstinence from eating due to fear of this pain. Unfortunately, in some patients chronic occlusive disease of the splanchnic arteries can also progress silently and present after intestinal infarction.

Although atherosclerotic occlusive lesions of the splanchnic arteries are not rare, symptomatic chronic mesenteric ischemia is relatively uncommon because of the rich collateral network that exists between the splanchnic arteries. The central collateral network between the celiac artery and the superior mesenteric arteries (SMA) is through collaterals between the superior pancreaticoduodenal arcade of the celiac artery and the inferior pancreaticoduodenal arcade of the SMA. The central collateral network between the SMA and the inferior mesenteric artery (IMA) is formed through the meandering mesenteric artery, which is comprised of the middle colic artery branch of the SMA and the ascending colic branch of the IMA. Finally, a rich collateral network exists between the IMA and the internal iliac arteries through branches of the superior and inferior hemorrhoidal arteries. Because of this extensive collateral network between the mesenteric arteries, at least two of the three mesenteric arteries must have stenoses or occlusions for chronic mesenteric ischemia to develop.

Management of chronic mesenteric ischemia remains a challenge because of the technical requirements of a successful mesenteric revascularization and the relative infrequency of this disease. Adequate exposure of the celiac artery and SMA, which arise from the midaorta at the junction of the abdominal and thoracic cavities, requires an extensive dissection. In addition, mesenteric revascularizations must be accomplished within a relatively short time frame to avoid complications secondary to foregut ischemia.

The syndrome of chronic mesenteric ischemia was first clinically recognized by Dunphy in 1936, who reviewed the autopsy results of patients dying of gut infarction and documented that most patients had a prodrome of abdominal pain and weight loss prior to the development of gut infarction.[1] Recognition of this clinical syndrome suggested the potential for identification of patients prior to gut infarction, a critical observation because attempts at splanchnic revascularization for acute mesenteric ischemia continue to be accompanied by a very high operative mortality rate. In 1958, Shaw and Maynard reported the first successful mesenteric revascularization by the technique of transarterial endarterectomy of the SMA.[2] Subsequent to this report, in 1961 Morris and colleagues reported the use of retrograde aortomesenteric bypasses using synthetic Dacron grafts.[3] Although this technique avoided the technical challenges of exposing the mid-aorta, it was sometimes complicated by tortuosity and kinking of the retrograde grafts. These complications of tortuosity and kinking of retrograde grafts led others to develop techniques of antegrade aortomesenteric bypass, originating the graft from the usually disease-free supraceliac aorta.[3-6]

In parallel to the development of these techniques, Stoney, Ehrenfeld, and Wylie developed the alternative approach of transaortic mesenteric artery endarterectomy.[4,5,7] This technique evolved from their experience in transaortic renal endarterectomy and was facilitated by development of the thoracoretroperitoneal aortic exposure. Transaortic mesenteric artery endarterectomy was accomplished through a trap door aortotomy and eversion endarterectomy of the mesenteric vessels (Fig. 1). This technique has been subsequently modified to avoid the complications of the thoracic incision by substituting medial visceral rotation to expose the midaorta through an abdominal incision.[8]

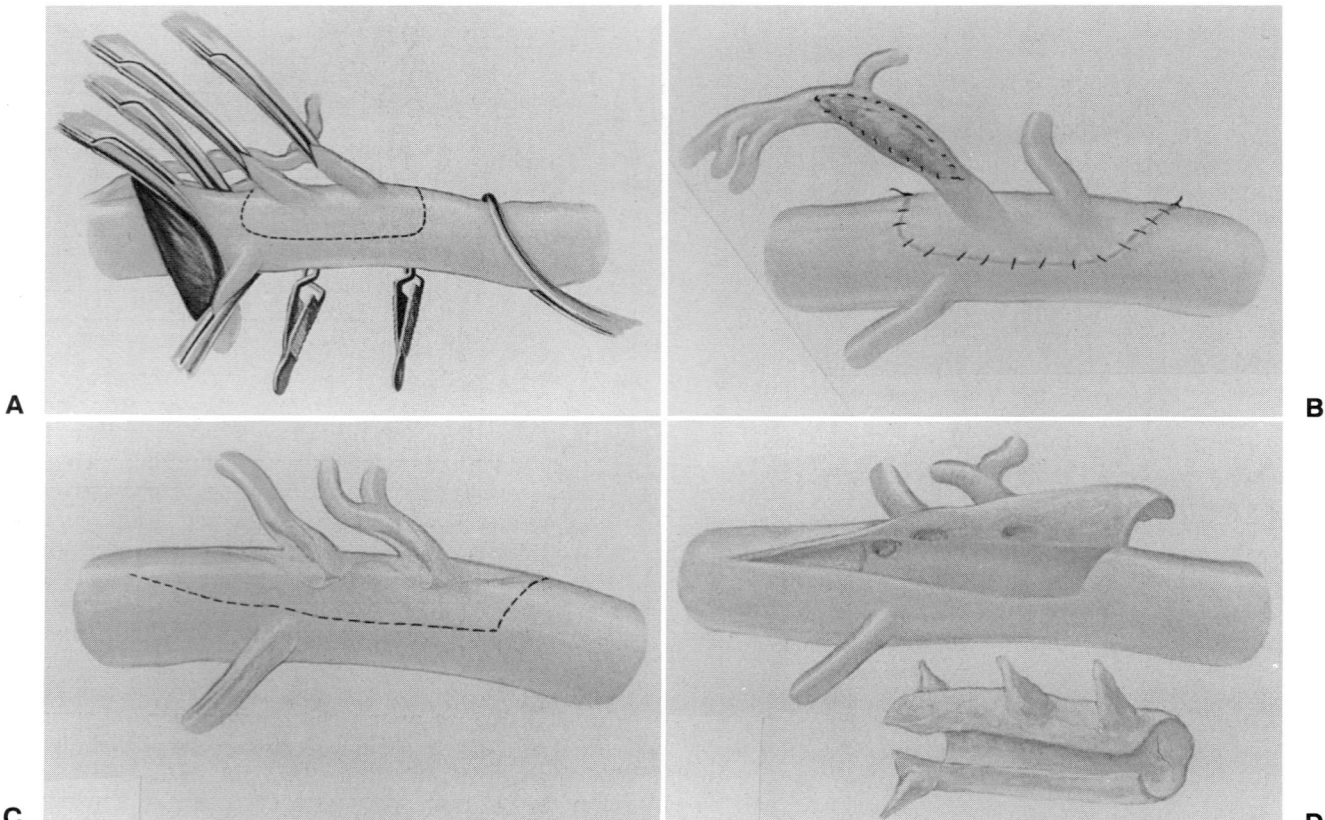

Figure 1 *A,* Trapdoor aortotomy. *B,* Completed transaortic endarterectomy with vein patch closure of superior mesenteric artery. Combined splanchnic and renal endarterectomy. *C,* Aortomy incision, and *D,* endarterectomy specimen. (From Wylie EJ, Stoney RJ, Ehrenfeld WK. Visceral endarterectomy. In: Wylie EJ, Stoney RJ, Ehrenfeld WK, eds. Manual of vascular surgery. New York: Springer-Verlag, 1980:214; with permission.)

DIAGNOSIS

Because chronic mesenteric ischemia is an uncommon clinical entity, often a long delay occurs between the onset of symptoms and clinical recognition of this syndrome. Unlike extremity arterial occlusive disease or carotid artery occlusive disease, symptomatic mesenteric artery occlusive disease is seen more commonly in women than in men. Virtually every patient who presents with mesenteric ischemia continues to smoke and have manifestations of advanced systemic atherosclerosis despite a relatively young age (sixth or seventh decade).

Chronic mesenteric ischemia is diagnosed only after exclusion of all alternative diagnoses. Most typically, these patients describe epigastric postprandial pain that usually occurs within 15 to 30 minutes of ingestion of a meal. Diarrhea or other manifestations of malabsorption are distinctly uncommon. The severity and chronicity of the postprandial pain often leads to a fear of eating and subsequent weight loss. Once the diagnosis of chronic mesenteric ischemia is entertained in a particular patient, an extensive evaluation is begun to exclude alternative diagnoses, most commonly a gastrointestinal malignancy. A not uncommon feature of chronic mesenteric ischemia is the development of gastric ulcers, which are often multiple small ulcers of irregular shapes with whitish sclerotic bases located in the antrum.[9] These ulcers often fail to heal with conservative therapy and are themselves a manifestation of ischemia. Delays in treatment often result from either attributing the patient's symptoms to these gastric ulcers or attempting to persist with medical therapy beyond a reasonable time. It is important to recognize that these ulcers will heal rapidly after gut revascularization.

In the absence of a pathognomonic test for chronic mesenteric ischemia, most patients undergo extensive gastrointestinal x-rays, upper and lower gastrointestinal endoscopy, and computed tomographic examination of the abdominal cavity. Once the clinical syndrome of postprandial pain and weight loss is recognized and evaluation for other potential causes of these symptoms, including a gastrointestinal malignancy, have been excluded, the patient should undergo lateral aortography. More than 90% of patients with chronic mesenteric ischemia have severe stenoses or occlusions of the celiac and mesenteric arteries. Characteristically, the atherosclerotic plaque is confined largely to the ventral aspect of the aorta.

TRANSAORTIC SPLANCHNIC ENDARTERECTOMY

Transaortic splanchnic endarterectomy is an effective and durable technique to manage patients with symptoms of chronic mesenteric ischemia.[9] This technique is particularly applicable to good-risk patients who require, in addition to the management of their mesenteric occlusive disease, treatment of renal and infrarenal aortic occlusive disease. Transaortic endarterectomy of all the splanchnic arteries, including the renal arteries, can be accomplished during a relatively short period of aortic occlusion and avoids multiple proximal and distal anastomoses required by the use of bypass grafts. An additional advantage of transaortic splanchnic endarterectomy is that the repair is entirely autogenous, which may be particularly important in patients who have subacute ischemia. Antegrade aortosplanchnic bypass is a more appropriate procedure in high-risk patients who cannot tolerate aortic clamp occlusion or the systemic consequences of liver and gut ischemia.

Prior to undergoing transaortic splanchnic endarterectomy, the patient's overall condition should be maximally improved. A period of parenteral hyperalimentation sufficient to reverse a longstanding catabolic state may reduce the rate of postoperative complications in the patient who is malnourished and anergic.

Optimal exposure of the midaorta can be accomplished through a transabdominal incision and medial visceral rotation. A roll is placed beneath the patient at the level of L2, with the patient lying on the operating room table in the supine position. A bilateral subcostal incision is used, which originates and ends at the midaxillary lines, midway between the costal margin and the iliac crest. Exposure is optimized by the use of a self-retaining retractor.

Medial visceral rotation is accomplished by first incising the lateral peritoneal attachments of the sigmoid and descending colon. The plane in the retroperitoneum is developed so that the left kidney is left in situ. The retroperitoneal plane is developed with blunt dissection until the aorta is encountered. This plane is extended proximally beneath the pancreas and spleen. At this point the exposure is adjusted so that the fascia overlying the esophagus and midaorta is incised and the esophagus may be retracted to the right. After the plane beneath the pancreas and spleen has been developed fully from below, the lateral peritoneal attachments of the spleen are incised first along the abdominal wall and then along the left diaphragm. This sequence of exposure minimizes unintentional injury to the spleen. The spleen, pancreas, stomach, and small bowel are all rotated medially and appropriately covered with moistened laparotomy sponges. Particular care is taken to protect both the spleen and the pancreas from retraction injury. Constant vigilance throughout the procedure must be maintained in order to avoid unnecessary trauma to the pancreas and spleen, which may result in either postoperative pancreatitis or splanchnic injury requiring splenectomy.

The dissection of the distal aorta is commenced at the appropriate level, depending on the extent of the planned procedure. After incising the soft tissue over the infrarenal aorta, the left renal vein is dissected fully. Dissection of the renal vein is completed from its junction with the vena cava to the renal hilum. Full mobilization of the renal vein is necessary to expose the pararenal and paramesenteric aorta. Mobilization is facilitated by transecting both the adrenal and gonadal veins so that the left renal vein can be retracted inferiorly without the risk of injury. After completion of the dissection of the renal vein, the plane on the aorta is continued proximally. This requires incising the neural tissues surrounding the SMA and celiac artery. The median arcuate ligament and diaphragmatic crura are incised in order to expose sufficient supraceliac aorta.

In the region of the proposed endarterectomy, the aorta should be mobilized circumferentially so that all the lumbar arteries may be clamped to prevent back-bleeding during the period of aortic occlusion. Particular care is taken to avoid injury to the right-sided lumbar arteries at the level of the celiac artery and SMA, as these may be torn during blunt dissection of the aorta in that region. After full mobilization of the aorta, the celiac artery and SMA are then dissected sharply. The celiac trunk is dissected sufficiently so that all of the primary branches of the celiac artery can be clamped individually prior to the endarterectomy. Similarly, the SMA is exposed at least to the level of the first branch, either the inferior pancreaticoduodenal or the middle colic artery. The SMA is palpated to determine the distal extent of the atherosclerotic plaque. Alternatively, if the SMA is occluded, usually a long piece of chronic thrombus can be palpated to extend to the level of the first patent branch of this artery.

Prior to aortic cross-clamping, the patient is given heparin sodium intravenously, sufficient to prolong the activated clotting time to twice that of the control level. The distal SMA as well as the branches of the celiac artery are clamped individually. The aorta is then clamped first distally and then proximally. The proximal clamp must leave enough aorta free for the aortotomy to be opened and closed without tension. A trapdoor aortotomy incision is made (Fig. 1). This incision is first made perpendicular to the long axis of the aorta proximal to the orifice of the celiac artery and extended to a level lateral to the orifice of the celiac artery and then continued in the aorta along the long axis to below the orifice of the SMA, where the incision then is continued perpendicular to this plane of the aorta, avoiding the orifice of the left renal artery.

The endarterectomy plane is developed within the deep media at the thickest portion of the plaque in the flap of aortic wall containing the orifices of the splanchnic arteries. Critical to the success of any endarterectomy is that the appropriate tissue plane in the deep media is identified. The endarterectomy plane around the orifices of the celiac and mesenteric arteries is developed by maintaining traction on the aortic plaque and sweeping the aortic wall away from the plaque. After circumferential mobilization of this plaque, eversion

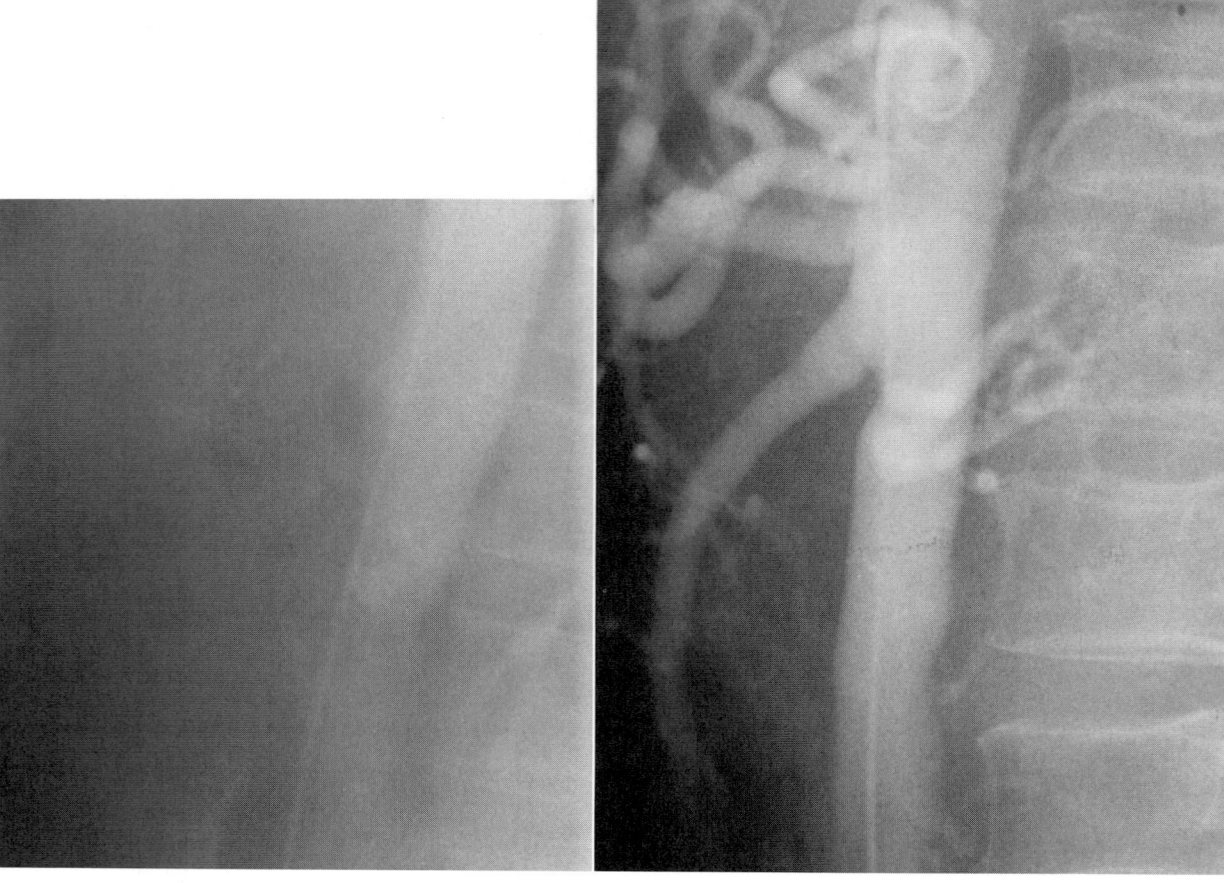

Figure 2 *A,* Preoperative lateral aortogram showing occlusions of the celiac, superior mesenteric, and inferior mesenteric arteries in patients with symptomatic chronic mesenteric ischemia. *B,* Postoperative lateral aortogram after transaortic celiac and superior mesenteric artery endarterectomy.

endarterectomies, first of the celiac artery and then of the SMA, are undertaken. When an SMA occlusion is present preoperatively, a long tail of chronic thrombus needs to be included within the specimen. This is best accomplished by avoiding fracturing the plaque or chronic thrombus during eversion endarterectomy of the SMA. Eversion endarterectomy of the SMA is facilitated by pushing the clamp on the SMA toward the aorta, thereby allowing the SMA to be everted into the aortic lumen. The remaining portion of the aortic plaque is removed. Care is taken to inspect both the celiac artery and the SMA for any residual flaps of tissue. After ascertaining the adequacy of the backbleeding, both vessels are flushed with heparinized saline. The aortotomy is closed with 3-0 or 4-0 continuous suture. Prior to completion of the closure, the aorta is first backbled and then forward flushed. Aortic flow is restored slowly to avoid unnecessary, sudden declamp hypotension. After removing the clamps from the celiac artery and SMA, the adequacy of blood flow is determined by using either a directional continuous wave Doppler probe or intraoperative duplex scanning.

Transaortic visceral endarterectomy can be compli-

cated by a significant residual intimal flap within the celiac artery or SMA or by bleeding through the aorta or branch artery wall secondary to too deep an endarterectomy plane. Most commonly, a distal flap may occur in the SMA, particularly in arteries that are occluded preoperatively. Such flaps can be removed through longitudinal arteriotomy, which may require patch closure if the vessel diameter is small (Fig. 1). Bleeding through the wall of the endarterectomized aorta can occur, particularly in patients who have transmural calcification of their plaque. The presence of transmural calcification may make it difficult to maintain the proper endarterectomy plane within the deep media. When such defects in the aortic wall occur, they can usually be managed by either multiple "darning" stitches or, if the wall is particularly thin, use of a skeletal muscle or synthetic pledget.

Postoperatively, patients may develop evidence of multisystem organ failure 48 to 72 hours after uncomplicated mesenteric revascularization.[10] Elevation of the liver enzymes usually peaks between the second and fourth postoperative days. The multisystem organ failure is characterized largely by a short period of pulmonary insufficiency that may require reintubation of the patient for a short period of mechanical ventilation. After the patient has recovered, a postoperative aortogram is obtained prior to discharge (Fig. 2).

OUTCOME

Transaortic celiac and SMA endarterectomy is effective in managing chronic mesenteric ischemia in more than 90% of the patients. Operative mortality rates for patients undergoing splanchnic revascularization range from 5% to 15%.[9] Such mortality rates are not unexpected, in view of the poor condition of many of these patients preoperatively as well as the complexity of the surgical procedure. Although long-term follow-up studies have not been performed in a large number of patients, approximately 85% to 95% of patients remain symptom-free.

The results of surgical management of chronic mesenteric ischemia have evolved considerably over the last two decades. Both antegrade aortomesenteric bypass and transaortic splanchnic endarterectomy offer effective and durable methods for managing symptomatic patients. Unfortunately, long delays prior to accurate diagnosis of this condition remain common. Nonetheless, once patients are identified, the appropriate choice of splanchnic revascularization should be based on the skill and experience of the surgeon because both antegrade aortomesenteric bypass and transaortic endarterectomy are effective techniques of surgical therapy. Transaortic splanchnic endarterectomy is most appropriately applied in the good-risk patient who may require, in addition to splanchnic artery revascularization, renal and infrarenal aortic reconstruction.

REFERENCES

1. Dunphy JE. Abdominal pains of vascular origins. Am J Med Sci 1936; 192:109–113.
2. Shaw RS, Maynard EP. Acute and chronic thrombosis of the mesenteric arteries associated with malabsorption. N Engl J Med 1958; 258:874–878.
3. Morris GC, Crawford ES, Copoley DA, DeBakey MA. Revascularization of the celiac and superior mesenteric arteries. Arch Surg 1962; 84:95–107.
4. Stoney RJ, Ehrenfeld WK, Wylie EJ. Revascularization methods in chronic visceral ischemia caused by atherosclerosis. Ann Surg 1977; 186:468–476.
5. Rapp JH, Reilly LM, Qvarfordt PG, et al. Durability of endarterectomy and antegrade grafts in the treatment of chronic visceral ischemia. J Vasc Surg 1986; 3:799–806.
6. Zelenock GB, Graham LM, Whitehouse WM Jr, et al. Splanchnic arteriosclerotic disease and intestinal angina. Arch Surg 1980; 115:497–501.
7. Stoney RJ, Wylie EJ. Surgical management of arterial lesions of the thoracoabdominal aorta. Am J Surg 1973; 126:157–163.
8. Stoney RJ, Schneider PA. Technical aspects of visceral artery revascularization. In: Bergan JJ, Yao JST, eds. Techniques in arterial surgery. Philadelphia: WB Saunders, 1990:271.
9. Cherry RD, Jabbari M, Goresky CA, et al. Chronic mesenteric vascular insufficiency with gastric ulceration. Gastroenterology 1986; 91:1548–1552.
10. Harwood TRS, Brooks DL, Flynn TC, Seeger JM. Multiple organ dysfunction after mesenteric artery revascularization. J Vasc Surg 1993; 18:459.

BYPASS PROCEDURES FOR CHRONIC MESENTERIC ISCHEMIA

JOSE MENA, M.D.
LARRY H. HOLLIER, M.D.

Chronic obstruction of the mesenteric vessels may be completely asymptomatic or may present as an uncommon syndrome manifested by symptoms that span the gamut from mild abdominal pain to the devastating complication of intestinal infarction and death. The diagnosis requires a high index of suspicion on the part of the clinician dealing with patients at high risk for this disease. Patients with symptomatic chronic mesenteric ischemia are frequently seen by the general practitioner or the gastroenterologist and are subjected to a wide variety of diagnostic tests in an effort to elucidate the underlying pathology responsible for the individual's ailments. Unfortunately, for some patients the diagnosis is not made for a significant period while they continue to experience severe symptoms, whereas in others the diagnosis is made at celiotomy with the findings of infarcted bowel or at postmortem examination. Baur and associates noted that the time from onset of symptoms to diagnosis was as long as 24 months, with an average of 9 months.[1] The most common cause of chronic intestinal ischemia is atherosclerotic occlusive disease.[2,3] Other causes include fibromuscular dysplasia, arteritis, compression by fibrous bands, and neurofibromatosis.

Chronic mesenteric ischemia is most common in the sixth and seventh decades but may occur in younger individuals; some patients are as young as 24 years old.[3] It occurs more commonly in women than in men,[1-3] although the reason for this is not clear. Symptomatic occlusive disease of the mesenteric circulation usually occurs when multiple vessels are involved, probably because chronic occlusion of one vessel is compensated by the development of collateral channels from the other patent vessels, which provide adequate perfusion to the region of the occluded vessel. Once the blood supply to the intestine has been decreased to the point where the demand is greater than the supply, the patient becomes symptomatic. Ingestion of food is normally followed by increased blood flow to the gut. Mesenteric occlusive disease does not permit the needed augmentation of blood flow for digestion. Pain is the result of this supply and demand mismatch. The term abdominal angina has been used to describe the pain that characterizes this syndrome. Typically, the pain occurs 20 to 30 minutes after the ingestion of a meal and subsides 1 to 2 hours later. It varies from a dull ache to a severe colicky pain and is usually located in the epigastrium but may become diffuse, with radiation to the back. As the disease progresses, the pain may become constant. Because of the association between meals and pain, these patients develop a fear of food that leads to weight loss. In one study this weight loss varied between 10 and 100 pounds, with an average of 35 pounds;[1] in another, it varied from 5 to 109 pounds, with an average of 32.5 pounds.[2] Although malabsorption has been implicated as a cause, the generally accepted reason for the patient's weight loss is fear of food, with decrease in the size and frequency of meals. Other symptoms include nausea, vomiting, and diarrhea or constipation. An epigastric bruit is present in about 75% of affected patients.[2,3] Although a bruit is not diagnostic, its presence in a patient with evidence of diffuse atherosclerotic disease who is also experiencing intestinal angina and weight loss should alert one to the possibility of chronic intestinal ischemia.

OPERATIVE MANAGEMENT

Except in patients with arteritis, mesenteric arterial reconstruction is indicated in an effort to relieve symptoms, reverse the weight loss and malnutrition, and prevent bowel infarction. Since the first mesenteric revascularization, a variety of procedures have been employed to manage this problem, including bypass to the mesenteric arteries, patch angioplasty of the vessel origins, reimplantation of the vessels, endarterectomy, and balloon angioplasty. Considerable debate continues with regard to which operation is best and, in the case of bypass, whether an antegrade bypass from the supraceliac aorta is superior to a retrograde bypass originating from the infrarenal aorta, as well as whether prosthetic material or autogenous vein or artery is better.

Although there are no large studies comparing graft material, it seems that a Dacron prosthetic is superior to vein for bypass. Veins seem to have a greater tendency to kink, and patency rates may be less than that of Dacron.

Antegrade revascularization from the supraceliac aorta is preferred because this region is usually free of disease, and anastomatic turbulence is generally avoided because of the direction of blood flow. Anastomatic turbulence may be significant with retrograde perfusion, and this can be a stimulus for neointimal hyperplasia, which would decrease the longevity of the graft. The Oregon group advocates taking the graft in a retrograde fashion from the infrarenal aorta, making a wide loop, and performing the anastomosis in an end-to-side fashion to provide prograde flow, thereby minimizing turbulence.[1]

We believe that all diseased mesenteric vessels should be reconstructed. Patients may experience relief of symptoms with single vessel revascularization, but the late recurrence is significantly higher with incomplete arterial reconstructions. Hollier and colleagues reported that patients who underwent revascularization of one of three or one of two diseased arteries had a 50% recurrence rate. Patients with reconstruction of two of three diseased vessels had a 29% recurrence, whereas those who underwent complete revascularization had only an 11% recurrence rate.[2] McAfee and associates reported the experience at the Mayo Clinic from 1981 to 1988.[3] They concluded that increased graft patency and survival in patients with three-vessel disease was highest in those patients who had complete revascularization.

Consideration should be given to three groups of patients: (1) those with mesenteric occlusive disease detected on diagnostic tests performed for other reasons, (2) symptomatic patients who have no concomitant aortic or renal arterial disease, and (3) symptomatic patients with concomitant abdominal aortic aneurysm, or renal and/or aortoiliac occlusive disease.

The incidental finding of mesenteric arterial occlusion should be managed expectantly. We see no reason to subject a patient to a very taxing operation fraught with risks when they have no symptoms or signs of mesenteric ischemia.

In symptomatic patients without concomitant renal or aortic disease, our preference is to perform an antegrade bypass using a bifurcated 14 by 7 mm or 12 by 6 mm Dacron graft originating at the supraceliac aorta in an end-to-side fashion. One limb is anastomosed to the celiac artery in an end-to-end manner or to one of its branches in an end-to-side configuration. The other limb is passed through a retropancreatic tunnel and anastomosed end to side to the superior mesenteric artery. If the inferior mesenteric artery (IMA) is also diseased, one may either do a patch angioplasty, endarterectomy with reimplantation, or bypass from the infrarenal aorta to the IMA.

If there is an infrarenal abdominal aortic aneurysm or occlusive disease of the aortoiliac segment with mesenteric ischemic symptoms, a bifurcated knitted Dacron graft would be placed from the infrarenal aorta to the iliac or femoral arteries, and then a bypass to the celiac and superior mesenteric arteries is performed in a retrograde fashion from the infrarenal aortic graft. When there is concomitant renal artery stenosis or occlusion, transaortic endarterectomy of the visceral and renal vessels using a medial visceral rotation is preferred. If the infrarenal aorta is severely diseased or occluded, an aortobiiliac or aortobifemoral bypass would be added to the transaortic endarterectomy, utilizing a bifurcated knitted Dacron graft.

The mortality rate for mesenteric revascularization operations is between 5% and 10%. The true incidence of graft occlusion is underestimated because one of multiple grafts may occlude and the patient remains asymptomatic. It is, however, more common for symptoms to recur if graft occlusion occurs in a patient who had single-vessel reconstruction. Of note is that patients whose grafts occlude in the early postoperative period usually experience bowel infarction.

REFERENCES

1. Baur GM, Millay DJ, Taylor LM Jr, Porter JM. Treatment of chronic visceral ischemia. Am J Surg 1984; 148:138–140.
2. Hollier LH, Bernatz PE, Pairolero PC, et al. Surgical management of chronic intestinal ischemia: A reappraisal. Surgery 1981; 90:940–946.
3. McAfee MK, Cherry KJ Jr, Naessens JM, et al. Influence of complete revascularization on chronic mesenteric ischemia. Am J Surg 1992; 164:220–222.

CELIAC COMPRESSION SYNDROME

DOUGLAS L. JICHA, M.D.
RONALD J. STONEY, M.D.

In 1965, Dunbar and colleagues described a syndrome of abdominal pain caused by compression of the celiac axis by the median arcuate ligament.[1] This syndrome has been variously called celiac compression syndrome, celiac band syndrome, and median arcuate syndrome. The significance of compression of the celiac axis either by the median arcuate ligament or with dense perivascular tissue remains controversial. Celiac axis compression commonly occurs in completely asymptomatic patients. Further, varied clinical presentations of the patients who are thought to be symptomatic have been a consistent finding. However, symptoms with celiac artery compression mimic the symptoms produced by impaired splanchnic blood flow that is caused by atherosclerosis.

ETIOLOGY

The celiac artery arises from the ventral midline aorta, usually opposite the the distal third of the twelfth thoracic vertebra and the proximal third of the first lumbar vertebra. Covered anteriorly by a variable amount of periarterial and neural ganglion tissue, it originates inferior to the crossing median arcuate ligament. Celiac compression may occur from impingement of the median arcuate ligament and encasement by periarterial neural tissue. A high origin of the celiac artery has been associated with compression in some patients, yet others may have caudad displacement of the fibrous median arcuate ligament as the etiology of the compression. Prolonged compression of the celiac artery causes intimal fibrosis leading to luminal stenosis and poststenotic dilation.

The pathologic mechanism of symptom production in the celiac axis compression syndrome remains controversial. Whereas visceral symptoms associated with atherosclerosis are nearly always produced by at least two major visceral artery occlusive lesions, this has been rarely observed with the celiac compression syndrome. When only the celiac axis blood flow is impaired, ischemia has been presumed to result from inadequate collaterals[1] or mesenteric steal.

A neurogenic mechanism of symptom production has also been considered. Carey and associates observed that celiac decompression procedures result in denervation of the celiac ganglion and perivascular sympathectomy.[2] They proposed that sympathectomy is a major reason for symptomatic relief in surgically treated patients. Alternatively, the neural tissue surrounding the celiac artery may be directly traumatized by the arterial pulsations of the vessel. Corroboration of either neurogenic mechanism for symptom production is lacking, yet persistence of abdominal pain is well described following operative procedures that produce a splanchnic sympathectomy but fail to relieve the luminal stenosis that impairs celiac blood flow.[3]

CLINICAL PRESENTATION

The presentation of patients with celiac compression syndrome is variable, with most reports describing a small number of patients with incomplete characterization. Female patients predominate, with most presenting in their fourth or fifth decade of life. Abdominal pain from chronic visceral ischemia is characteristically cramping, epigastric pain occurring 20 to 30 minutes after eating. The duration and severity of pain are related to the size of the meal and generally last for 1 to 3 hours. This pain pattern occurs in patients with symptomatic celiac compression, but the atypical types of pain have perturbed patient selection for operation and led to poor responses following surgical intervention. Weight loss from decreased food intake generally accompanies the pain and should be greater than 10% of normal body weight. Symptoms of nausea, vomiting, and altered intestinal motility are often present. Occasionally, patients may report a positional response to their postprandial pain, with the supine position exacerbating the postprandial symptoms.

Physical examination typically reveals an asthenic ectomorphic female. The majority have an epigastric bruit that is accentuated on expiration, a classic finding in celiac compression syndrome. Abdominal tenderness is variable, with epigastric or generalized tenderness observed in some patients.

DIAGNOSIS

A careful history should characterize the abdominal pain, including its relationship to meals, duration, and periods of remission. The duration and amount of weight loss are important. The history and subsequent evaluation should exclude other conditions that might mimic the symptoms. Evaluation should include ultrasound, contrast gastrointestinal (GI) studies, oral cholecystography, computed tomographic scan, malabsorption studies, and possible upper GI endoscopy with or without retrograde choledochopancreatography.

If evaluation is negative for other conditions and the history, physical, and clinical findings suggest visceral ischemia, aortography is necessary to document celiac compression. Anteroposterior views document collateral flow via the gastroduodenal artery from the superior mesenteric artery, whereas lateral views display the typical deformity of celiac compression and poststenotic dilation. Superior mesenteric artery compression may be seen in a small number of patients in conjunction with celiac artery compression. Lateral aortograms document the extrinsic celiac artery compression caused by the arcuate ligament of the diaphragm which is worse on expiration (Fig. 1).

TREATMENT

The preferred surgical approach is transabdominal through the gastrohepatic omentum unless prior operations dictate an alternative approach. Excellent exposure of the celiac axis is afforded by left medial visceral rotation. The abdomen should be thoroughly examined for other lesions prior to exposing the subdiaphragmatic area. The transcrural exposure of the aorta is facilitated by using a self-retaining retractor.

The left lobe of the liver is retracted to the right and the esophagus and lesser curve of the stomach to the left; the thickened median arcuate ligament is identified and elevated with a hemostat (Fig. 2A). The median arcuate ligament and the dense perivascular neural tissue are

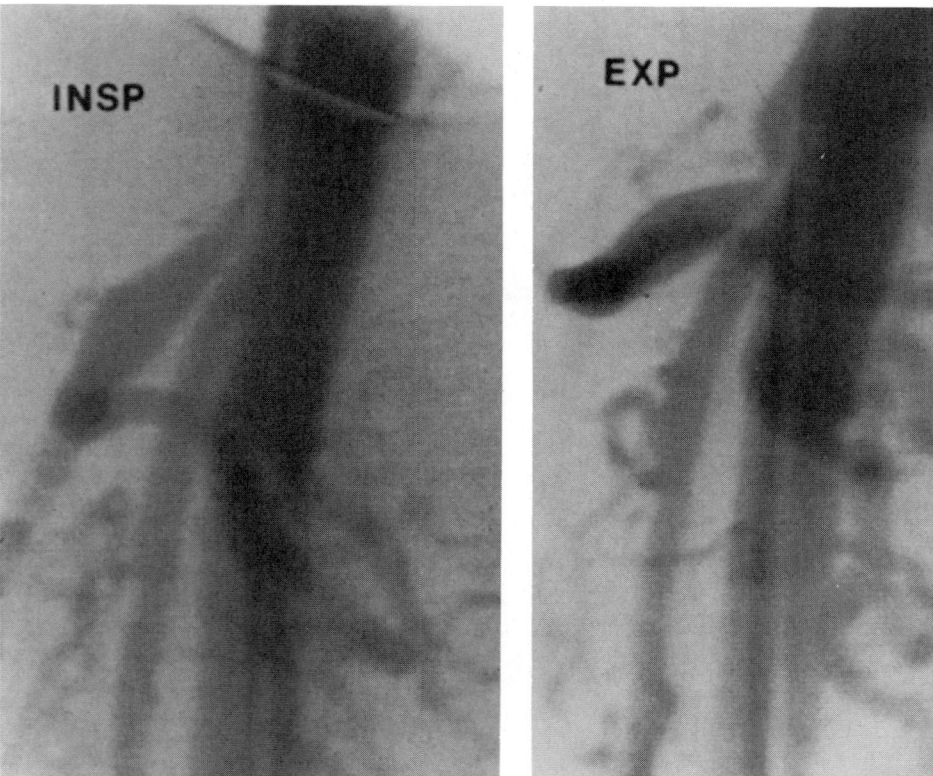

Figure 1 Lateral aortogram displaying inspiratory *(left)* and expiratory *(right)* views of celiac artery compression by the median arcuate ligament. (From Wylie EJ, Stoney RJ, Ehrenfeld WK. Manual of vascular surgery. Vol 1. New York: Springer-Verlag, 1980; with permission.)

resected, and the celiac axis is mobilized near its origin (Fig. 2B). Next, fibers of the left crus of the diaphragm are divided to expose and mobilize the lower thoracic aorta for clamping (Fig. 2C). The celiac arterial branches are mobilized for several centimeters, and the investing aortic fascia between the celiac axis and superior mesenteric artery is cleared. Supraceliac and infraceliac aortic clamps are then applied, along with clamping of the hepatic and splenic vessels. A temporary clip is used to control the left gastric artery. Dilators up to 5 mm are passed retrograde from a transverse splenic arteriotomy through the celiac artery into the aorta in order to restore a normal lumen (Fig. 2D). Following closure of the splenic arteriotomy with interrupted sutures, blood flow is restored. Intraoperative duplex scanning is employed to document the luminal enlargement.[4] Blood pressure measurements to assess gradient ablation have been abandoned.[3] In patients in whom the celiac deformity persists or operative duplex scanning suggests a deformity following dilation, celiac artery reconstruction with either resection and primary anastomosis or antegrade aortoceliac bypass is effective.

RESULTS

Reports of operation for celiac compression syndrome have been characterized by small numbers of patients, incomplete treatment of the patients' symptoms, and nonstandard surgical techniques without operative confirmation of luminal enlargement. Short-term follow-up without postoperative arteriographic verification of operative results has also made evaluation of results difficult.

Lord and Tracy summarized short-term results in 238 patients reported in the literature.[5] They noted that 83% of patients were asymptomatic following celiac decompression by any method. Their report highlights the favorable results reported at short-term follow-up.

The long-term results, mean of 9 years follow-up, of treatment of 51 patients operated upon for celiac compression syndrome at our institution have been reported.[3] No operative deaths occurred, and 44 (86%) patients were available for long-term evaluation. Improvement from operative intervention favored those who had characteristic postprandial abdominal pain

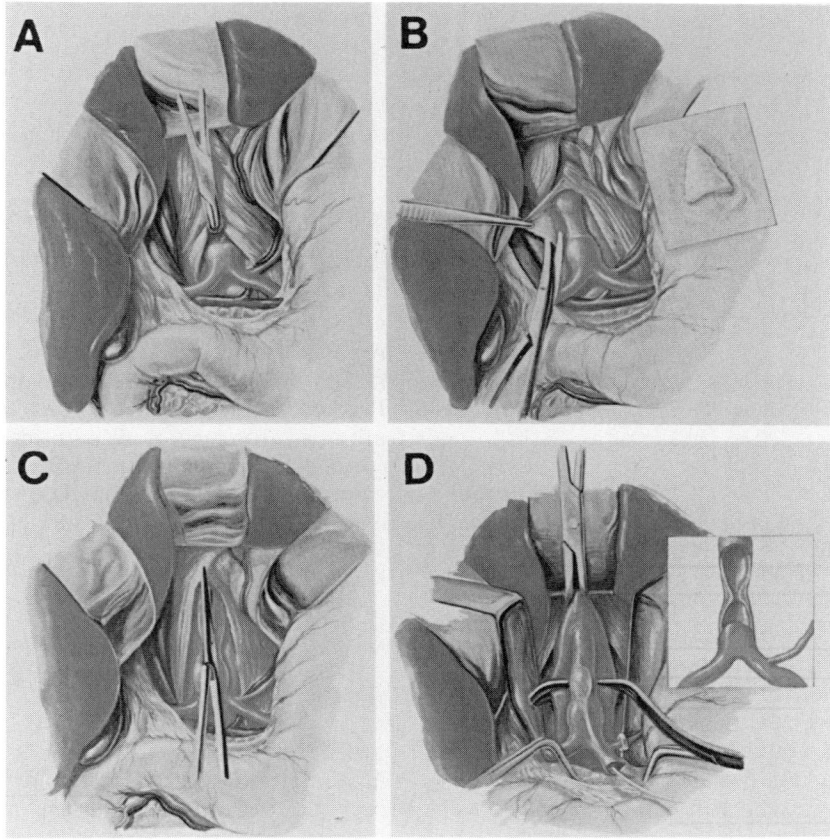

Figure 2 The surgical technique for celiac decompression. *A*, The identification of the thickened median arcuate ligament and elevation with a hemostat is followed by resection of the perivascular tissue *(B)*. The aorta is further mobilized with division of the left crus of the diaphragm *(C)* to allow for aortic clamping. *D*, Subsequent dilation of the celiac axis is performed through a transverse arteriotomy in the splenic artery. (From Wylie EJ, Stoney RJ, Ehrenfeld WK. Manual of vascular surgery. Vol 1. New York: Springer-Verlag, 1980; with permission.)

resembling visceral angina, were female between 40 and 60 years of age, and had lost greater than 15% of body weight. Negative clinical response was correlated with atypical pain, periods of remission of pain without treatment, a history of ethanol abuse or psychiatric disorder, and inconsistent or no weight loss. This highlights the importance of careful patient selection and is reinforced by Williams and colleagues, who found that satisfactory long-term results occurred in patients with food-related pain and a paucity of other nongastrointestinal symptoms.[6] Currently, we favor operative intervention when a classic clinical history exists and significant stenosis of the celiac axis typical of compression is documented by aortography. Patients with atypical symptoms should be observed for the development of more overt symptoms or the appearance of another clinical disorder.

Reilly and co-workers also documented the importance of the surgical procedure selected to treat patients.[3] In this study, 16 patients underwent celiac decompression alone, 17 underwent decompression with celiac artery dilation, and 18 underwent decompression with reconstruction. In long-term follow-up, only 53% of the patients who only had celiac decompression were asymptomatic, compared to 76% who had either dilation or reconstruction following the decompression. Evans employed only celiac decompression in his report of 59 patients followed long term, and only 41% were asymptomatic at late follow-up.[7] This result further supports the view that symptom relief is best achieved with operative strategies that restore normal blood flow through the celiac axis.

Acknowledgment. Supported in part by the Pacific Vascular Research Foundation.

REFERENCES

1. Dunbar JD, Molnar W, Beman FF, et al. Compression of the celiac trunk and abdominal angina. Am J Roentgenol 1965; 95:731–744.
2. Carey JP, Stemmer EA, Connolly JE. Median arcuate ligament syndrome. Arch Surg 1969; 99:441–446.
3. Reilly LM, Ammar AD, Stoney RJ, et al. Late results following operative repair for celiac artery compression syndrome. J Vasc Surg 1985; 2:79–91.
4. Stoney RJ, Effeney DJ. Thoracoabdominal aorta and its branches. Philadelphia: JB Lippincott, 1992;212.
5. Lord RA, Tracy GD. Coeliac artery compression. Br J Surg 1980; 67:590–593.
6. Williams S, Gillespie P, Little JM. Celiac axis compression syndrome: Factors predicting a favorable outcome. Surgery 1985; 98:879–886.
7. Evans EE. Long-term evaluation of the celiac band syndrome. Surgery 1974; 76:867–871.

NONOCCLUSIVE MESENTERIC ISCHEMIA

ELIZABETH T. CLARK, M.D.
BRUCE L. GEWERTZ, M.D.

Intestinal ischemia may result from arterial embolus, arterial or venous thrombosis, or vasospasm. The outcome of an ischemic episode is determined by many factors, including the mechanism of flow interruption, the vessel involved, the rapidity of onset and duration of the insult, and the length of bowel affected. With the more frequent utilization of diagnostic arteriography in recent years, recognition of the nonocclusive form of mesenteric ischemia (NOMI) has increased. This entity has been estimated to account for approximately 25% of all acute mesenteric ischemic events.

Although mortality rates with this syndrome have been high, often exceeding 50%, current results have improved substantially because of earlier diagnosis and more effective nonoperative therapies. Nonetheless, the patient population at risk for this disorder continues to grow and the prognosis remains grim, if even a single segment of bowel infarcts prior to treatment.

RISK FACTORS AND PATHOPHYSIOLOGY

Nonocclusive mesenteric ischemia was first described by Ende in 1958 and more extensively characterized by Boley and associates.[1-3] These and subsequent reports have identified multiple risk factors for acute mesenteric ischemia in general and NOMI in particular. Predictors include age older than 50 years, severe atherosclerotic heart disease, congestive heart failure, cardiac arrhythmias, recent myocardial infarction, hypovolemia, and hypotension. The syndrome is often associated with infusions of alpha-adrenergic and other vasopressors in treatment of life-threatening conditions such as trauma, burns, pancreatitis, or gastrointestinal hemorrhage. Finally, there have been reports of NOMI following elective mesenteric revascularization procedures, especially antegrade prosthetic bypasses to the superior mesenteric artery (SMA).[4]

Clinically important NOMI is usually limited to the SMA distribution. The onset is often predated by an acute deterioration in cardiac function with a reduction in systemic perfusion pressure and increases in portal venous pressure. These events are associated with a failure of splanchnic blood flow autoregulation; this paradoxic vasoconstriction is the essential pathophysiologic mechanism of NOMI.[5] Endogenous secretion of catecholemines may further increase the vasoconstrictive process. Because the majority of patients with nonocclusive mesenteric ischemia have histories of digitalis use, the effects of this drug on the mesenteric vasculature have been studied. Digitalis compounds have been shown to induce contraction of arterial and venous smooth muscle in vitro and in vivo and to accentuate the myogenic vasoconstriction of arterioles in response to acute venous hypertension.[5,6]

CLINICAL PRESENTATION

Whereas acute mesenteric embolic or thrombotic events classically present with severe abdominal pain, significant NOMI may occur in the absence of such complaints.[2] Some degree of abdominal pain is usually present, but, on occasion, clinical signs may be limited to shock, acidosis, hemoconcentration, and sepsis of unknown etiology.

The clinician's single greatest tool for successful diagnosis of this syndrome is a high index of suspicion in patients with multiple risk factors. Early diagnosis and institution of therapeutic measures prior to bowel infarction are essential to decrease mortality. If diagnosis occurs within 24 hours, 60% of patients survive; survival decreases to less than 30% if more than 24 hours pass between onset of symptoms and diagnosis. Although many laboratory abnormalities occur with mesenteric ischemia and infarction—hemoconcentration, leukocytosis with a significant left shift, metabolic acidosis, hyperamylasemia, and hyperphosphatemia—most are nonspecific and thus not diagnostic. The serum glutamic-oxaloacetic transaminase, lactate dehydrogenase, and creatine phosphokinase may be elevated, but they often do not rise until 6 to 12 hours after infarction occurs.

Abdominal plain films are useful in excluding other causes of abdominal pain such as mechanical small bowel obstruction, perforation of a hollow viscus, or appendicitis with fecalith. Most patients with mesenteric ischemia have at least one of the following signs on abdominal film: ileus, ascites, small bowel dilation, thickening of valvulae conniventes, and separation of small bowel loops. On occasion, a gasless abdomen is seen due to fluid accumulation within the bowel lumen. A grave roentgenographic sign is the presence of intramural or portal air, indicative of infarction and colonization with gas-forming organisms.

Barium studies are contraindicated because barium in the bowel interferes with arteriography, the essential diagnostic study. In fact, diagnostic arteriography should be performed even if indications for operation are evident at the initial patient presentation because preoperative knowledge of the specific etiology of intestinal ischemia expedites appropriate surgical treatment. Successful arteriography mandates hemodynamic stabilization of the patient because hypotension alone may cause significant splanchnic vasoconstriction and preclude an adequate study. Any vasoactive drugs with splanchnic vasoconstriction properties should be stopped if at all possible. A complete arteriogram,

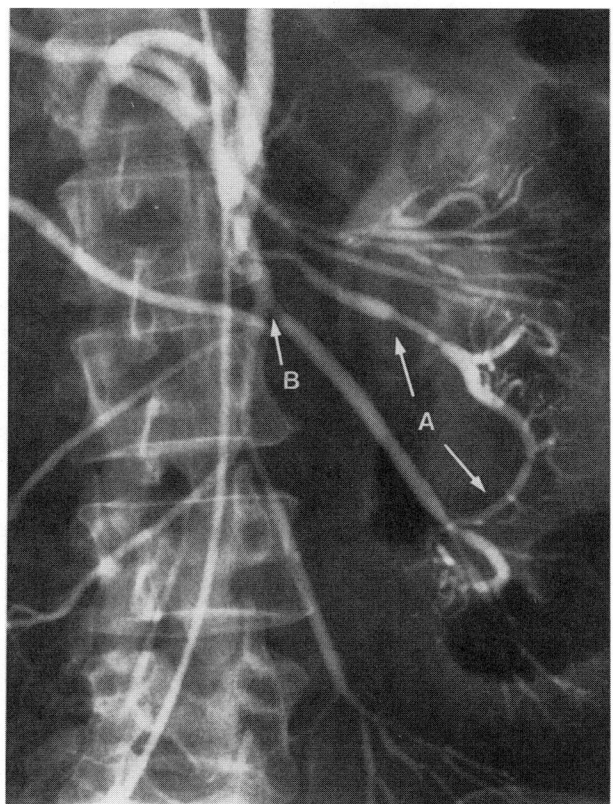

Figure 1 Classic radiologic findings of nonocclusive mesenteric ischemia include *(A)* string of sausages sign and *(B)* segmental vasospasm at branch points. In this case, nonocclusive mesenteric ischemia occurred after mesenteric revascularization. (From Gewertz BL, Zarins CK. Postoperative vasospasm after antegrade mesenteric revascularization: A report of three cases. J Vasc Surg 1991; 4:382–385; with permission.)

including both anterior-posterior (AP) and lateral views of the aorta, is required. The AP view best documents collateral vessels, whereas lateral aortography better documents the origins of major visceral arteries that overlie the aorta in the AP plane.

Arteriographic signs of nonocclusive ischemia include multiple areas of narrowing and irregularity of major branches of the SMA, which has been termed the string of sausages sign (Fig. 1). The capillary blush of small and medium intramural vessels is absent or much reduced. Importantly, other causes for intestinal ischemia should be excluded. The origin and first 5 cm of the SMA should be carefully scrutinized for emboli, which usually lodge just proximal or distal to the origin of the middle colic artery. Evidence of thrombotic occlusion of pre-existent stenotic lesions and generalized aortic atherosclerosis and the presence of extensive collaterals should be minimal or absent. Perhaps the most difficult diagnosis to exclude is mesenteric venous thrombosis. This uncommon syndrome is suggested by a generalized slowing of arterial blood flow without

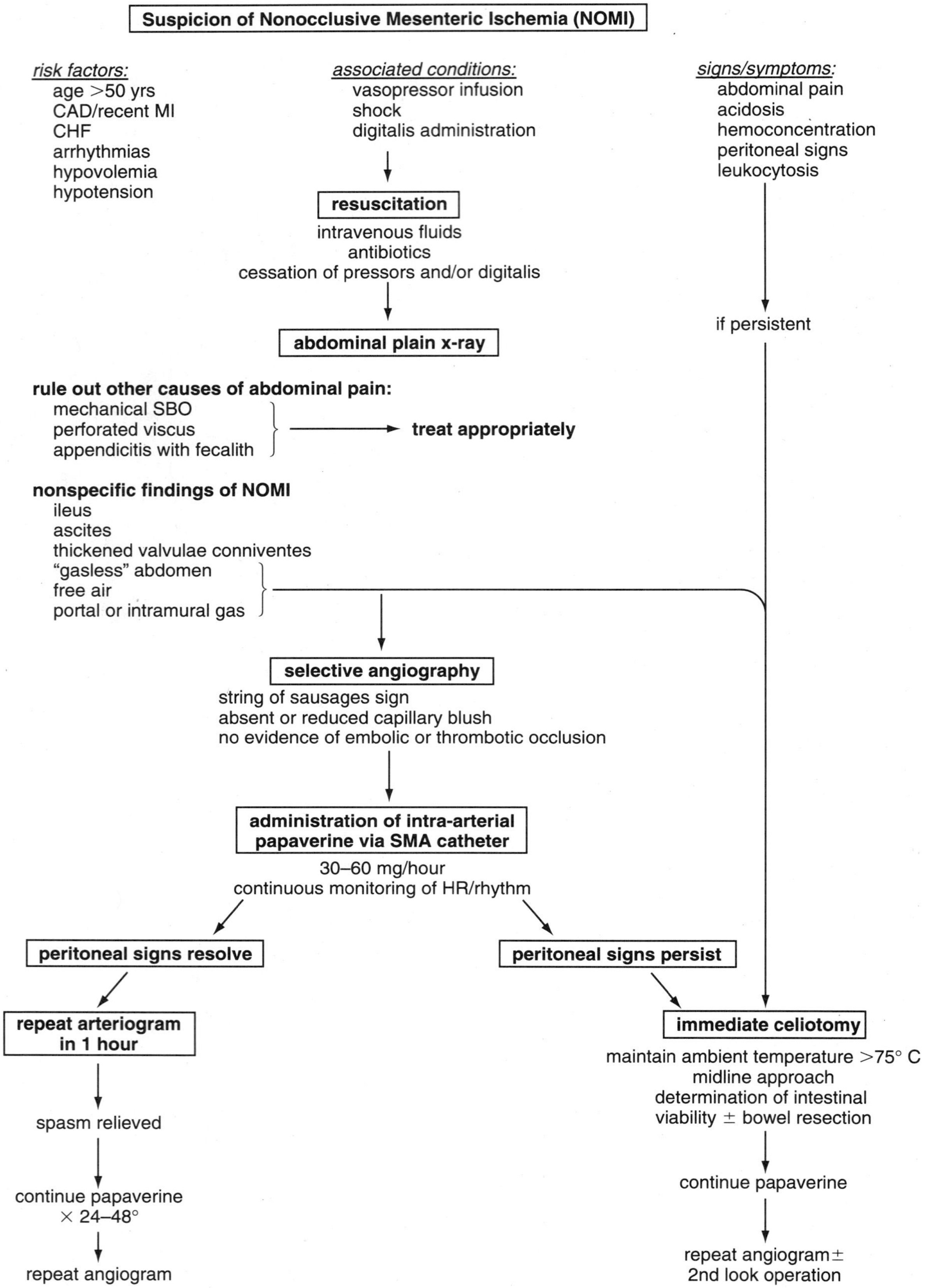

Suspicion of Nonocclusive Mesenteric Ischemia (NOMI)

risk factors:
- age >50 yrs
- CAD/recent MI
- CHF
- arrhythmias
- hypovolemia
- hypotension

associated conditions:
- vasopressor infusion
- shock
- digitalis administration

↓

resuscitation
intravenous fluids
antibiotics
cessation of pressors and/or digitalis

signs/symptoms:
- abdominal pain
- acidosis
- hemoconcentration
- peritoneal signs
- leukocytosis

↓

abdominal plain x-ray

rule out other causes of abdominal pain:
- mechanical SBO
- perforated viscus
- appendicitis with fecalith

→ **treat appropriately**

nonspecific findings of NOMI
- ileus
- ascites
- thickened valvulae conniventes
- "gasless" abdomen
- free air
- portal or intramural gas

if persistent

↓

selective angiography
string of sausages sign
absent or reduced capillary blush
no evidence of embolic or thrombotic occlusion

↓

administration of intra-arterial papaverine via SMA catheter
30–60 mg/hour
continuous monitoring of HR/rhythm

↙ ↘

peritoneal signs resolve | **peritoneal signs persist**

↓ | ↓

repeat arteriogram in 1 hour | **immediate celiotomy**
 | maintain ambient temperature >75° C
 | midline approach
 | determination of intestinal
 | viability ± bowel resection

↓ | ↓

spasm relieved | continue papaverine

↓ | ↓

continue papaverine × 24–48° | repeat angiogram ± 2nd look operation

↓

repeat angiogram

Figure 2 Algorithm for the diagnosis and treatment of nonocclusive mesenteric ischemia.

evidence of spasm, in conjunction with nonopacification of the corresponding mesenteric or portal veins.

TREATMENT

When the diagnosis of NOMI is considered, a specific treatment plan should be considered (Fig. 2). Every effort should be made to discontinue the administration of vasoactive drugs with significant alpha-adrenergic effects. Intra-arterial infusion of papaverine into the SMA should be considered the primary mode of therapy. Papaverine should be administered as a constant infusion at a rate of 30 to 60 mg/hour for at least 24 to 48 hours. Because papaverine is primarily metabolized by the liver, persistent hypotension is unusual. Nonetheless, careful monitoring of mean arterial blood pressure, heart rate, and rhythm is desirable in that the drug may occasionally have systemic effects. If a sudden decrease in blood pressure is noted, the position of the catheter should be checked to ensure that the drug is not being infused systemically. Because heparin sodium is incompatible with papaverine, it should not be added to the infusion but administered through a separate intravenous infusion site, if necessary.

It is prudent to repeat an arteriogram approximately 1 hour after institution of papaverine therapy to ensure that spasm has been relieved. Arteriograms should then be repeated prior to the discontinuation of the papaverine. Most patients should be treated for at least 24 hours, and a small number require infusions for more than 48 hours. Because many of these patients are at substantial risk for renal dysfunction, it is important to perform an adequate but minimal arteriographic study, thereby limiting the total amount of contrast medium.

Operation may be avoided in patients with nonocclusive ischemia if the diagnosis is confirmed on arteriography and if abdominal signs and symptoms totally resolve with papaverine infusion. Specific indications for operation include: (1) continued abdominal pain or rebound tenderness, (2) free intraperitoneal air, (3) persistent or increasing leukocytosis, and (4) grossly bloody stools. In fact, operation should be considered if stool becomes hematest-positive at any point in the therapy.

Although most patients with nonocclusive ischemia can be treated nonoperatively if the diagnosis is made promptly, operation should not be delayed if clear indications are present. During celiotomy, the operating room should be maintained at a higher temperature than normal (75°F) to avoid exacerbating vasospasm. A midline incision is usually preferred. Bowel affected by NOMI is often edematous, gray, and distended without peristalsis. If arteriography has excluded SMA occlusive disease or embolization, the primary purpose of the operation is to excise obviously infarcted segments of bowel while additional papaverine is infused to enhance the viability of the remaining tissue. Another supportive maneuver that may be useful is lavage of the peritoneal cavity with warm saline.

Intraoperative determination of intestinal viability may be performed using a variety of techniques. Clinical judgments are often based on the return of normal bowel color, mesenteric arterial pulsations, and visible peristalsis. By experienced examiners, these assessments are fairly accurate, but on occasion may be too conservative, resulting in unnecessary bowel resection, or, worse, too optimistic, leaving ischemic or infarcted bowel in place. Hence, more objective methods for determining viability—detection of pulsatile mural blood flow by intraoperative Doppler ultrasound or fluorescein injection and inspection with a Wood's light—have been developed.[7]

Once intestinal viability is determined and bowel resection completed, a decision must be made regarding restoration of intestinal continuity. If there is any question of viability at the resected margins, exteriorization with cutaneous enterostomies may prevent a second look celiotomy at 24 hours. It should be cautioned that the decision for repeat celiotomy should be based on findings at the time of the initial operation and must not be affected by apparent clinical improvement in the immediate perioperative period.

Careful attention to fluid management in the perioperative period is essential. Antibiotic coverage with broad-spectrum agents should be continued for at least 5 days. If the diagnosis of NOMI is unequivocal, heparin sodium and/or warfarin therapy is not essential.

REFERENCES

1. Ende N. Infarction of the bowel in cardiac failure. N Engl J Med 1958; 258:879–892.
2. Boley SJ, Brandt LJ, Veith FJ: Ischemic disorders of the intestines. Curr Probl Surg 1978; 15:6–85.
3. Boley SJ, Feinstein FR, Sammartano R, et al. New concepts in the management of emboli of the superior mesenteric artery. Surg Gynecol Obstet 1981; 153:561–569.
4. Gewertz BL, Zarins CK. Postoperative vasospasm after antegrade mesenteric revascularization: A report of three cases. J Vasc Surg 1991; 4:382–385.
5. Kim EH, Gewertz BL. Chronic digitalis administration altes mesenteric vascular reactivity. J Vasc Surg 1987; 5:382–389.
6. Mikkelsen E, Andersson DK, Pedersen OL. Effects of digoxin on isolated human mesenteric vessels. Acta Pharmacol Toxicol (Copenhagen) 1979; 45:249–256.
7. Bulkley GB, Zuidema GD, Hamilton SR, et al. Intraoperative determination of small intestinal viability following ischemic injury. Ann Surg 1981; 193:628–637.

MESENTERIC VENOUS THROMBOSIS

TIMOTHY R. S. HARWARD, M.D.
JAMES M. SEEGER, M.D.

Mesenteric venous thrombosis (MVT) is an uncommon but important cause of intestinal ischemia that is responsible for 5% to 15% of mesenteric vascular events.[1] It can occur at any age, although it is most common in the sixth and seventh decades of life. This disease process was first described in 1895 by Elliot,[1] but only since the report of Warren and Eberhart in 1935 has it been recognized as a clinical entity distinct from mesenteric arterial occlusion.[1] Over the last several decades, MVT has been a more frequently identified problem, primarily because of improved diagnostic techniques and a better understanding of its unique pathophysiology. As a result, improved treatment strategies have been developed that have led to increased survival of patients with this disease.

Early reports uniformly described bowel infarction in association with MVT, and the mortality of extensive MVT approached 100%.[2] Fortunately, recent studies using new diagnostic techniques have documented that intestinal ischemia is absent in many patients with MVT until late in its clinical course. Left untreated, however, bowel infarction and peritonitis eventually occur in most patients, and even prompt operative intervention in this late stage is associated with an operative mortality of up to 80% and recurrent bowel infarction in up to 30% of patients.[3] Thus, survival of patients with MVT depends on early recognition and prompt treatment of the problem.

ETIOLOGY

Like other types of venous thrombosis, factors associated with MVT can generally be understood in terms of Virchow's triad of stasis, endothelial damage, and a hypercoagulable state (Table 1). Low flow states in the mesenteric venous system may be produced by disorders such as liver cirrhosis, portal hypertension, or congestive heart failure.[1,4] Abdominal visceral infections such as appendicitis, pancreatitis, diverticulitis, pelvic abscess, or visceral perforation can damage mesenteric venous endothelium from local inflammatory reaction and/or release of chemical toxins from bacterial overgrowth in organs drained by the mesenteric venous system.[1,4] Other associated conditions likely to predispose to MVT by producing a hypercoagulable state include malignancy, most commonly colonic or pancreatic,[1] trauma,[1,4] oral contraceptive use,[1,3,4] polycythemia vera,[1] and recent operation,

Table 1 Etiologies of Mesenteric Venous Thrombosis

Portal hypertension
Visceral infections
    Appendicitis
    Diverticulitis
    Pelvic Abscess
    Perforated viscus
Acute pancreatitis
Inflammatory bowel disease
Abdominal trauma
Malignancy
Splenectomy with thrombocytosis
Polycythemia vera
Oral contraceptive pills
Coagulation disorders
    Antithrombin III deficiency
    Protein C deficiency
    Protein S deficiency
    Dysfibrinogenemia
Pregnancy

particularly splenectomy with its attendant thrombocytosis.[1,3]

Previously, MVT has been described as either secondary, occurring in association with another underlying pathologic process, or primary, occurring without a predisposing condition. However, recent studies have identified underlying coagulation disorders producing a hypercoagulable state in almost 90% of patients thought to have primary MVT. Underlying coagulation disorders are important in the pathogenesis of MVT, regardless of other predisposing factors. A hypercoagulable state is found in 87% of patients with MVT[5] and a previous history of DVT in 15% to 44%.[4,5] The hypercoagulable state in patients with MVT has been shown to be caused by (1) a flaw in the fibrinolytic process such as a protein C or protein S deficiency, (2) a deficiency in the intrinsic control of the thrombotic process such as an antithrombin III deficiency, or (3) an exuberant thrombotic process.[5] Although no abnormality in platelet function has yet been found to cause MVT, this may also be a possibility.

PATHOPHYSIOLOGY

Acute mesenteric venous occlusion in dogs produces massive influx of fluid into the bowel wall and bowel lumen (greater than 100 ml/kg/hour for the first hour), which leads to hypovolemia, hemoconcentration, leukocytosis, and eventually cardiovascular collapse, provided a significant portion of the small bowel is involved.[6] Sludge forms in the capillaries within minutes of venous occlusion and hemorrhage (greatest in the submucosal and subserosal regions) due to capillary distention, and rupture occurs after 5 to 10 minutes.[6,7] Progressive thrombosis then leads to venous dilation, bleeding into the mesentery with bowel wall cyanosis, spasm, and congestion, which produces blood-tinged ascites. On gross inspection, the bowel and mesentery are edematous, thick, and rubbery, and the bowel lumen is filled with bloody fluid.[4] Proximal small bowel dilation may also occur secondary to a functional partial small bowel obstruction. Thrombus extrudes from cut ends of mesenteric veins while mesenteric arteries are usually patent but in spasm.[2,4]

Bowel infarction is reported in clinical studies in 38% of patients.[5] The location and degree of MVT determine the severity and location of bowel injury.[2,4] Thrombus in the major venous channels including the superior mesenteric vein and portal vein does not commonly lead to bowel infarction because of good venous collateral channels within the mesentery and bowel wall. In addition, thrombosis of the inferior mesenteric vein is infrequently associated with bowel ischemia because of the extensive retroperitoneal collaterals from the colonic venous system to the renal, splenic, and hemiazygos veins. In contrast, thrombotic occlusion of tributaries of the mesenteric veins, such as vasa recti, venous arcades, and intramural collaterals, has been reported to be associated with significant intestinal injury. Of 57 patients with bowel infarction due to MVT reported by Johnson and Baggenstoss, 55 had this pattern of thrombosis.[8]

CLINICAL MANIFESTATIONS

Mesenteric venous thrombosis produces two general patterns of symptoms. One is the readily recognized acute surgical abdomen when MVT is associated with early bowel infarction; however, this presentation is uncommon. The second pattern, which is more frequent but more difficult to recognize, is the insidious development of benign abdominal signs and symptoms. In patients with MVT who do not present with an acute surgical abdomen, the most common complaint is vague abdominal pain. The pain is poorly localized but constant with intermittent episodes of increased intensity. Rarely, the pain has a sudden onset,[4] but more common is a days to weeks prodromal period of progressively increasing pain.[1,2,4] Most patients also complain of a change in bowel habits and nausea with or without vomiting.[1,2,4] Complaints of hematochezia and hematemesis are rare.[2] Finally, patients may continue to eat normally without complaints of postprandial pain,[1,4] although this is unusual.

Physical examination of patients who have had the insidious onset of abdominal symptoms may reveal a low-grade fever (less than 101°F), abdominal distention, and active bowel sounds. Tenderness to palpation of the abdomen is generalized but mild, and complaints of abdominal pain appear to be out of proportion to the physical findings. Signs of peritoneal inflammation including guarding and rebound are absent unless intestinal infarction has occurred.[1] Stool from the rectal examination is positive for hemoglobin in 80% to 100% of patients.[1] Signs of hypovolemia may also be present, but overt shock is rare.[1]

DIAGNOSTIC STUDIES

Laboratory and standard radiologic evaluation in patients with MVT are seldom helpful. An elevated hematocrit indicating hemoconcentration, and leukocytosis of 15 to 30,000/mm^3 are common,[1] and a left shift in the differential white cell count may also be noted. Paracentesis may occasionally be helpful, producing serosanguineous fluid if intestinal ischemia or infarction have occurred.[2] Elevated serum phosphate has also been proposed as a marker of acute intestinal ischemia with infarction, but this observation has not been confirmed. Supine and upright abdominal x-rays are abnormal but nonspecific in 50% to 75% of patients. Marked bowel wall thickening is the most common finding; combined with mucosal irregularity, it may be suggestive of intestinal ischemia.[1,2,4] A dilated, fixed, gas-filled small bowel with a surrounding ground-glass appearance may be seen, but this pattern is difficult to differentiate from a nonspecific ileus, ascites, or both. Gas in the portal venous system or in the wall of the bowel may be seen, but only long after intestinal infarction has occurred.[1] Finally, small bowel barium studies are frequently positive but usually nonspecific.

Selective mesenteric arteriography can provide definitive evidence of MVT, although this examination is not without risks. Characteristic arteriography findings of MVT include (1) reflux of contrast back into the aorta during contrast injection, (2) intense spasm of the arterial branches supplying the involved ischemic bowel, (3) a prolonged arterial phase and prolonged opacification of the thickened bowel wall, (4) contrast extravasation into the lumen of the bowel, and (5) visualization of venous thrombus (Fig. 1) and/or nonvisualization of the venous phase. With the exception of visualization of venous thrombus, these findings are all indirect evidence of MVT. However, any or all of these findings in a patient suspected of having MVT strongly suggest the diagnosis.

Over the past decade, computed tomographic (CT) scanning has also proved to be a valuable diagnostic tool (Figs. 2 and 3). A waterlogged appearance of the mesentery and a rim of fat around the mesenteric vasculature were initially identified as baseline characteristic CT findings in patients with thrombosis of the superior mesenteric vein.[1,4,5] In addition, using intravenous contrast enhanced CT scanning, mesenteric vein enlargement and increased density of the venous wall, with a central area of decreased density representing luminal thrombus can be readily seen.[1,4,5] Using CT scanning, Vogelzang and co-workers correctly identified 14 patients with MVT,[9] whereas Harward and associates correctly diagnosed MVT in 10 of 11 patients (91%).[5] In retrospect, the one missed diagnosis in the Harward group's study had subtle but definite evidence of MVT when the CT scans were re-examined.[5]

Other noninvasive diagnostic techniques, including abdominal duplex ultrasound and magnetic resonance imaging (MRI), have also been investigated. Miller and Berland noted that abdominal duplex examination was

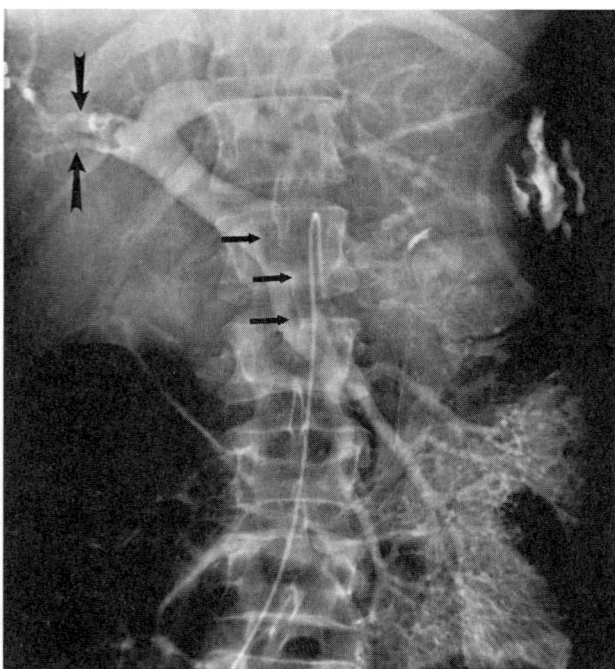

Figure 1 Venous phase image following a superior mesenteric artery selective arteriogram demonstrating thrombus in the superior mesenteric vein *(small arrows)* with a separate thrombus in the right branch of the portal vein *(large arrows)*.

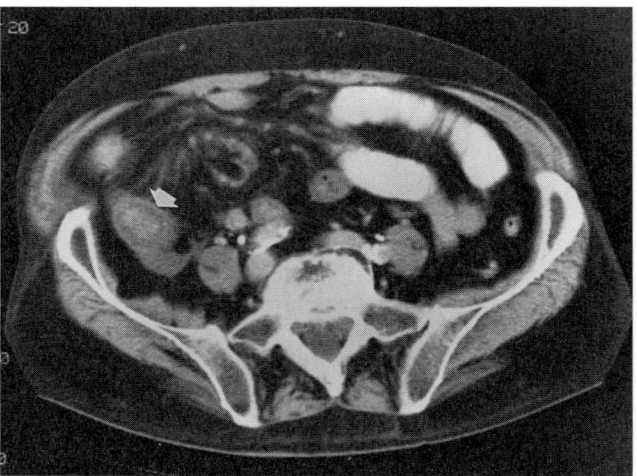

Figure 3 Abdominal CT scan of the patient in Figure 2 demonstrating extensive edema of both the small bowel mesentery and bowel wall *(arrow)* due to venous hypertension caused by mesenteric vein occlusion. (From Harward TRS, Coe D, Flinn WR. Mesenteric venous thrombosis. In: Strandness WE, van Breda, eds. Vascular diseases: Surgical and interventional therapy. New York: Churchill Livingstone, 1993, with permission.)

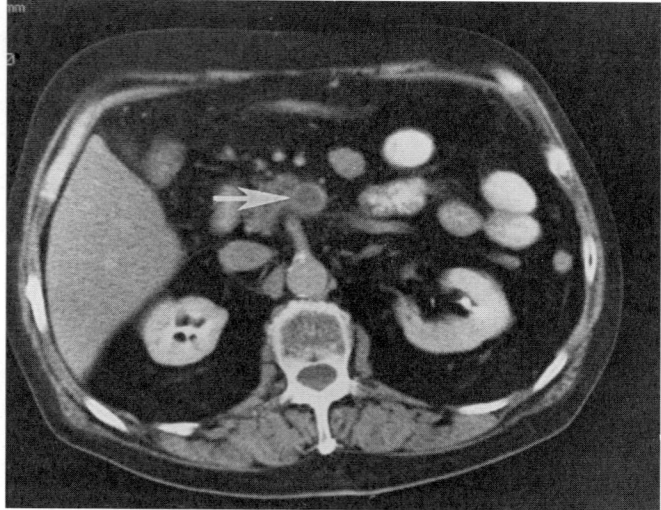

Figure 2 Abdominal CT scan from a patient with angiographically proven mesenteric venous thrombosis demonstrating a dilated superior mesenteric vein *(arrow)* with an intraluminal filling defect and a contrast-enhanced venous wall due to arterial filling of the vein wall vasa vasorum. (From Harward TRS, Coe D, Flinn WR. Mesenteric venous thrombosis. In: Strandness WE, van Breda, eds. Vascular diseases: Surgical and interventional therapy. New York: Churchill Livingstone, 1993, with permission.)

equivalent to CT scanning in visualization of the major mesenteric veins and accurate identification of thrombus in the superior mesenteric vein.[10] However, abdominal duplex scanning can be technically difficult, especially if significant bowel gas is present. Gehl and co-workers[11] compared MRI to CT scanning and, using MRI, correctly identified 15 abdominal venous obstructions in 15 patients, 5 of which involved the mesenteric veins. Whereas MRI has the advantages of allowing multiplanar images and of not requiring ionizing radiation or contrast media, its expense and limited availability currently restrict the value of MRI in the evaluation of patients suspected of having MVT.

In the past, MVT has been considered an uncommon entity, but this concept has been challenged by several recent reports in which CT scanning and MRI were used.[5] In addition, older reports documented that MVT was a surgical emergency because of the possibility of associated bowel infarction. However, in more recent studies in which CT scanning was used, less than one-third of the patients required operation. Thus, newer diagnostic techniques that allow early, accurate detection of MVT have documented that MVT is not rare, is commonly benign, and does not require immediate surgical intervention if discovered early in its clinical course.

TREATMENT

The first step in treatment of MVT is fluid resuscitation.[2,3] Systemic anticoagulation with intravenous heparin sodium prevents further propagation of thrombus and subsequent intestinal necrosis. Then, if physical examination shows no evidence of bowel ischemia or peritonitis, observation with continuing anticoagulation and serial physical examination is appropriate.

If signs of bowel ischemia develop during observation or are present when the patient is initially evaluated, immediate operation with resection of necrotic bowel is mandatory because, without surgical intervention, mortality approaches 100%.[1,4] Wide resection of the bowel accompanied by restoration of intestinal continuity should be done. Niatove and Weismann suggest that exploration of the bowel mesentery to define the extent of the thrombosis should also be done, hypothesizing that if all thrombi are not removed, further thrombus extension and intestinal necrosis will occur;[2] however, the value of this approach has not been documented. Regardless, in reported series, 22% to 29% of patients developed recurrent thrombosis after initial bowel resection, and 60% of the recurrences involved the intestinal anastomosis, suggesting inadequate bowel resection or thrombus removal at the initial exploration.[4]

When intestinal compromise is found at operation, several authors have also advocated venous thrombectomy.[1] In three reported patients in whom this was done, bowel color and peristaltic activity immediately improved. However, animal studies have documented that thrombectomy more than 2 hours after occlusion does not improve the overall prognosis.[7] Thus, despite these anecdotal reports of the value of venous thrombectomy, this procedure is generally not recommended in that the thrombus almost certainly has been present for more than 2 hours at the time of abdominal exploration, and underlying problems such as a coagulopathy are likely to lead to recurrence. In contrast, if thrombosis of a major splanchnic vein occurs during an intra-abdominal procedure, venous thrombectomy may be considered.[4]

Postoperative care consists of vigorous multisystem therapy, along with systemic anticoagulation using heparin sodium.[1,3,4] In addition, when significant bowel injury has occurred and extensive bowel resection has been required, a planned second-look procedure should be done to assess whether ongoing thrombosis and bowel necrosis have occurred.[1,3,4] Re-exploration should also be done if the diagnosis of recurrent thrombosis is entertained, regardless of the status of the bowel at the initial exploration. Recurrent thrombosis occurs in up to 29% of patients,[3] usually early in the postoperative period, and is associated with a mortality of 35% to 40%.[1,3,4] Prevention of recurrent thrombosis or propagation of existing thrombus appears essential in preventing late intestinal necrosis, with its high associated mortality. Niatove and Weismann reported the risk of recurrent thrombosis to be significantly lower (14%) in patients with MVT who were anticoagulated compared to patients who are not anticoagulated (22%). They found a 50% mortality rate in patients not anticoagulated postoperatively compared to no mortality when anticoagulation was used.[2] Lifelong anticoagulation with sodium warfarin is also essential for patients with familial or congenital coagulopathies, such as a protein S, protein C, or antithrombin III deficiencies. In addition, long-term anticoagulation with sodium warfarin should be used in patients with recurrent MVT in whom an underlying etiology has not been found.

REFERENCES

1. Grendell JH, Ockner RK. Mesenteric venous thrombosis. Gastroenterology 1982; 82:358–372.
2. Niatove A, Weismann RE. Primary mesenteric venous thrombosis. Ann Surg 1965; 161:516–523.
3. Khodadadi J, Rozencwajg J, Nacasch N, et al. Mesenteric vein thrombosis: The importance of a second-look operation. Arch Surg 1980; 115:315–317.
4. Abdu RA, Zakhour BJ, Dallis DJ. Mesenteric venous thrombosis: 1911 to 1984. Surgery 1987; 101:383–388.
5. Harward TRS, Green D, Bergan JJ, et al. Mesenteric venous thrombosis. J Vasc Surg 1989; 9:328–333.
6. Polk HC. Studies in experimental mesenteric venous occlusion. Part I: The experimental system and its parameters. Am J Surg 1964; 88:693–698.
7. Freidenberg MJ, Polk HC, McAlister WH, Shochat SJ. Superior mesenteric arteriography in experimental mesenteric venous thrombosis. Radiology 1965; 85:38–45.
8. Johnson CC, Baggenstoss AH. Mesenteric vascular occlusion. I: Study of 99 cases of occlusion of veins. Mayo Clin Proc 1949; 24:628–635.
9. Vogelzang RL, Gore RM, Anschnetz SL, Blei AT. Thrombosis of the splanchnic veins: CT diagnoses. Am J Roentgenol 1988; 150:93–96.
10. Miller VE, Berland LL. Pulsed doppler duplex sonography and CT of portal vein thrombosis. Am J Roentgenol 1985; 145:73.
11. Gehl HB, Bohndorf K, Klose KC, et al. Two-dimensional MR angiography in the evaluation of abdominal veins with gradients refocused sequences. J Comput Assist Tomogr 1990; 14:619.

CELIAC, HEPATIC, AND SPLENIC ARTERY ANEURYSMS

LINDA M. GRAHAM, M.D.
CHARLES L. MESH, M.D.

Visceral artery aneurysms are uncommon lesions often encountered as incidental findings during radiologic studies. Their importance lies in the potential for rupture and life-threatening hemorrhage. Splenic artery aneurysms are the most commonly encountered visceral aneurysm, followed in frequency by hepatic, superior mesenteric, and celiac artery aneurysms.[1] Multiple splanchnic and somatic artery aneurysms are encountered in 36% of patients with visceral artery aneurysms.[2]

The etiology of visceral aneurysms has changed distinctly since they were first recognized centuries ago. At that time most were mycotic, syphilitic, or traumatic in origin. Today most true aneurysms are secondary to arteriosclerosis or abnormalities of the media, whereas false aneurysms usually follow trauma. The presentation of visceral artery aneurysms has also evolved. In the past they were rarely recognized clinically, and most were identified at autopsy following death due to aneurysm rupture. Now, asymptomatic lesions are often identified as an incidental finding on radiologic procedures undertaken for other disease processes. Nonetheless, presentation with abdominal pain, due to aneurysm enlargement or to pressure on adjacent structures, is not unusual. Less commonly, patients develop gastrointestinal or intra-abdominal hemorrhage due to rupture of the aneurysm. Because the etiology, presentation, and treatment of splenic, hepatic, and celiac aneurysms differ, they are considered separately.

CELIAC ARTERY ANEURYSMS

Celiac artery aneurysms account for approximately 4% of visceral artery aneurysms and are discovered in only 1 of 8,000 to 19,300 autopsies.[3] The natural history appears to be one of expansion and eventual rupture. In the past most celiac aneurysms were not diagnosed until after rupture; however, in more recent reports nearly 90% of aneurysms were diagnosed while still intact. Although the risk of rupture is not well defined, aggressive surgical therapy is recommended for all reasonable-risk patients because of the catastrophic consequences of rupture.

Etiology

The etiology of celiac artery aneurysms changed in the mid-twentieth century.[3] Prior to 1950 most celiac artery aneurysms were syphilitic. Since 1950, most appear to be secondary to atherosclerosis or medial defects. However, the difficulty of distinguishing between atherosclerosis as a primary cause rather than a secondary event often makes assigning an etiology impossible. Less common causes of celiac artery aneurysms are poststenotic dilatation, trauma, re-entry of aortic dissection, and septicemia-related mycotic lesions.

Concomitant with the change in etiology has been a change in the typical patient with a celiac artery aneurysm. In the early twentieth century, celiac artery aneurysms were found predominantly in males (9:1). Today, males and females are affected with equal frequency. The average age has increased from approximately 40 years to 52 years. Nearly 20% of patients have an abdominal aortic aneurysm, and approximately 40% have other splanchnic aneurysms.[3]

Diagnosis

The clinical manifestations of celiac artery aneurysms are protean, ranging from asymptomatic to life-threatening hemorrhage. Approximately three-quarters of patients reported since 1950 have been symptomatic at the time of diagnosis. Abdominal pain is a frequent complaint. Epigastric discomfort radiating to the back or vague abdominal discomfort accompanied by nausea and vomiting is often described. Intense pain may occur with aneurysm expansion. Occasionally, the pain is increased with meals, suggesting intestinal angina. Gastrointestinal bleeding is uncommon but may be the only sign of the aneurysm.

A palpable mass is present in nearly 30% of patients, and a prominent pulse or bruit is present in 37%. However, neither sign is diagnostic.[3] Evidence of a coexisting splanchnic or peripheral aneurysm may be found because associated aneurysmal disease is common.

A celiac artery aneurysm may be suggested by a curvilinear calcification on roentgenograms of the abdomen or by a vascular mass on ultrasonography or computed tomographic (CT) scan. However, arteriography is essential to establish the diagnosis. Most asymptomatic celiac artery aneurysms are discovered on arteriography undertaken for other disease processes. Visceral arteriography also defines the extent of the lesion, the anatomy of the celiac axis, and distal vasculature, and it is critical to planning appropriate therapy. It is best accomplished with biplanar aortography and selective injections of the celiac axis and superior mesenteric artery.

Treatment

Operative treatment is indicated for all celiac artery aneurysms except for an asymptomatic lesion in the high-risk patient. Operative technique must be individualized because celiac aneurysms are often associated with aneurysms of other intra-abdominal vessels, and surgical therapy may require complex reconstructions. Many small, isolated aneurysms can be approached through the abdomen, with control of the aorta obtained at the level of the diaphragmatic hiatus. However, in other situations a thoracoabdominal approach is necessary. The preferred treatment for small celiac artery aneurysms is aneurysmectomy with arterial reconstruction of the celiac trunk. If the size or extent of the aneurysm does not permit end-to-end reanastomosis of the celiac axis, a graft is inserted from the lower thoracic or upper abdominal aorta to the distal celiac axis or hepatic artery. In this configuration with a short, high-flow conduit, the saphenous vein has no proven patency benefit over prosthetic material. As such, the selection of graft, saphenous vein, or prosthesis depends on other concomitant operative interventions as well as the size of the recipient artery.

Celiac artery ligation alone is considered safe if adequate collateral circulation to the foregut can be documented and preserved. However, hepatic necrosis is a risk, and occurred in 2 of 4 cases where all branches of the celiac artery were ligated.[3] Similarly, transcatheter occlusion techniques are not indicated except the high-risk patient with favorable vascular anatomy.

Results of elective surgical therapy for intact aneurysms are good, with operative mortality rates of approximately 5%. The patency rates of primary reconstructions and bypasses are high, and long-term results are excellent. In contrast, mortality for ruptured aneurysms remains significantly higher in spite of improved surgical therapy.

HEPATIC ARTERY ANEURYSMS

Hepatic artery aneurysms are the second most common visceral artery aneurysms and account for approximately one-fifth of all such lesions. Approximately 80% of these lesions are extrahepatic and 20% intrahepatic. The common hepatic artery is involved in 63% of patients, the right hepatic in 28%, the left hepatic in 5%, and both the right and left hepatic arteries in 7%.[4] The male to female ratio is 2:1.[1] When lesions secondary to trauma are excluded, the usual patient is in the sixth decade of life. Approximately 20% of hepatic artery aneurysms progress to rupture, an event accompanied by death in 35% of cases.[1]

Etiology

As with other mesenteric aneurysms, in the past, infection was the most common cause of hepatic artery aneurysms. Today, the etiology is atherosclerosis in 32% of lesions, medial degeneration in 24%, trauma in 22%, and infection in only 10%.[1] Although atherosclerosis is a frequent histologic finding, it often represents a secondary rather than a primary process. Most intrahepatic lesions are traumatic and result from deep fractures of the liver parenchyma. Arteriopathies and periarterial inflammation associated with cholecystitis or pancreatitis are responsible for an occasional hepatic artery aneurysm.

Diagnosis

The diagnosis of hepatic artery aneurysms is difficult, and most intact lesions are unexpected findings during an evaluation for abdominal pain. Although hepatic artery aneurysms may be asymptomatic, many patients present with a variety of vague and nonspecific complaints. Patients may describe diffuse pain in the right upper quadrant or epigastrium that radiates to the back or right shoulder and is unrelated to meals. Jaundice may result from bile duct compression by a large hepatic artery aneurysm. Erosion of aneurysms into nearby structures, including the stomach, duodenum, portal vein, and pancreatic duct, occurs but is uncommon. Extrahepatic lesions may rupture into the peritoneal cavity, causing vascular collapse from sudden exsanguination. Intrahepatic aneurysms can rupture into the hepatobiliary tree, causing hematobilia. Following biliary erosion, the classic symptom triad of pain suggestive of biliary colic, hematobilia, and obstructive jaundice occurs in only one-third of patients.[5]

Physical examination seldom suggests the presence of a hepatic artery aneurysm because intact lesions are rarely palpable. An abdominal bruit may be present but is not diagnostic. Both duplex scanning and CT imaging with intravenous contrast can distinguish an aneurysm from a cystic hepatic mass or from adjacent structures. Arteriography is essential to establish the diagnosis (Fig. 1). Furthermore, it can document the precise location of the aneurysm and define the vascular anatomy of the foregut and midgut. Because the hepatic artery and its branches can arise from either the celiac axis or the superior mesenteric artery, selective arteriography of these vessels is particularly important in the evaluation of hepatic artery aneurysms.

Treatment

Because of the risk of rupture, all hepatic artery aneurysms should be treated unless the patient is in extremely poor medical condition. The treatment modality most appropriate for a hepatic artery aneurysm depends on the location of the lesion, the vascular anatomy, and the fitness of the patient.

Extrahepatic aneurysms should be excluded or excised and hepatic arterial blood flow preserved or restored. Simple exclusion is appropriate for aneurysms of the common hepatic artery in which continuity of the gastroduodenal and right gastric arteries provide adequate hepatic blood flow. This may be accomplished either by radiologic occlusion with coils or with proximal and distal ligation. If vascular abnormalities or occlusive disease limit collateral blood flow, common hepatic artery ligation or occlusion is inappropriate and risks hepatic necrosis. In these patients aneurysmorrhaphy or arterial reconstruction is necessary. Aneurysms of the proper hepatic artery always require arterial reconstruction because of the risk of hepatic necrosis, if arterial continuity is interrupted. Autogenous saphenous vein or prosthetic grafts may be used for arterial reconstruction. Saphenous vein is usually

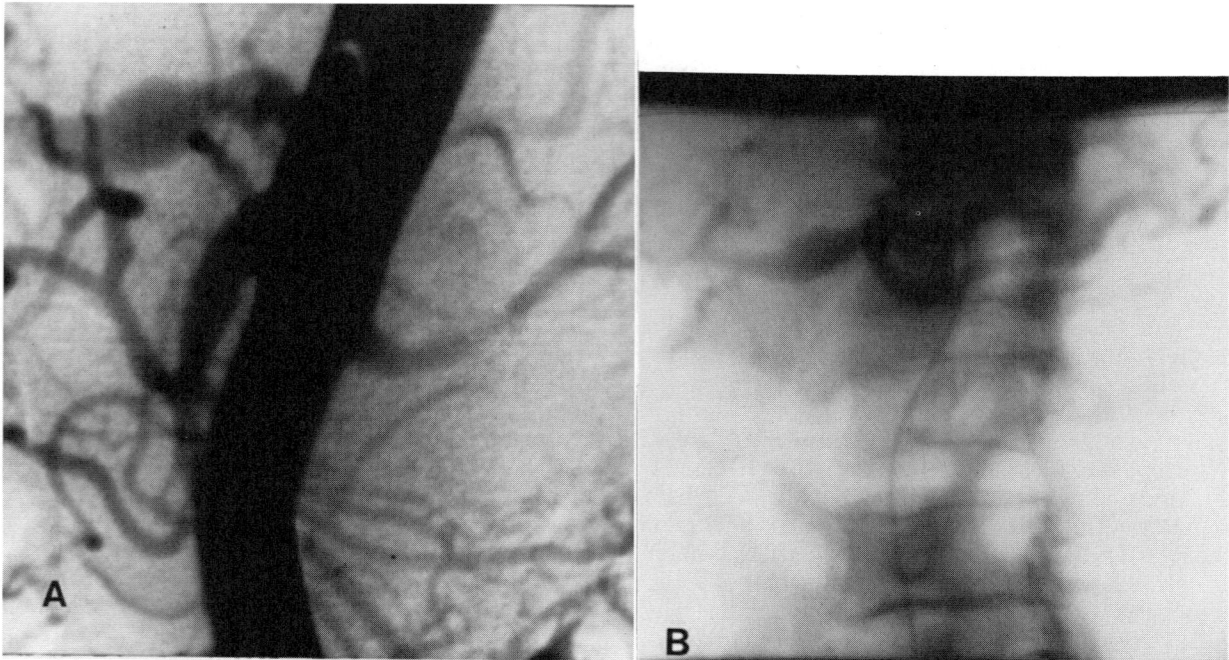

Figure 1 *A,* Aortogram performed on a patient with suspected renovascular hypertension suggesting an aneurysm in the upper abdomen. *B,* Selective celiac arteriogram on the same patient confirming the presence of an aneurysm of the common hepatic artery.

chosen for the reconstruction of smaller vessels such as the proper hepatic artery.

Embolization or coil occlusion is useful for the treatment of intrahepatic aneurysms. This reliable, relatively safe method avoids the surgical alternative, which is an anatomic liver resection.[6] Transcatheter embolization is not without risks such as hepatobiliary necrosis with sepsis and abscess formation. Inadvertent occlusion of the cystic artery with gallbladder ischemia and fibrosis may occur.[7]

Results of elective therapy for intact aneurysms are excellent. Treatment of ruptured aneurysms has much higher morbidity and a mortality rate of at least 35%.

SPLENIC ARTERY ANEURYSMS

Splenic artery aneurysms are the most common, accounting for approximately 60%, of all splanchnic aneurysms.[4] The incidence of these aneurysms is not well defined, but they are incidental findings on 0.78% of arteriograms.[1] Depending on the age of patients studied and the care with which lesions are sought, splenic artery aneurysms are noted in 0.098% to 10.4% of autopsies.[1] Approximately two-thirds of splenic artery aneurysms are solitary lesions, and nearly 80% are located in the distal third of the artery, with most of the rest in the middle third.[8] Splenic artery aneurysms are more frequent in women than in men, with more than 80% of patients being women.[8,9]

Aneurysm rupture represents the most serious complication of splenic artery aneurysms but is rare. It occurs in approximately 2% of nonpregnant patients with splenic artery aneurysms,[8] and in this setting is associated with a 25% mortality. In contrast, splenic artery aneurysm rupture is reported to complicate 98% of aneurysms diagnosed during pregnancy and carries maternal and fetal mortalities of nearly 70% and 95%, respectively.[8,9]

Etiology

Most splenic artery aneurysms are secondary to abnormalities of the media of the artery and are located at arterial bifurcations, where most developmental lesions occur.[8] Pregnancies, fibromuscular dysplasia, portal hypertension, and pancreatitis contribute to the development of these aneurysms.[9] Multiple pregnancies are an important etiologic factor, and in one report 92% of the women had been pregnant an average of 4.5 times.[8] The altered hemodynamics in the splenic artery during pregnancy may contribute to aneurysm formation. In addition, the hormonal changes, especially during the last trimester, may cause alterations in the media of the arterial wall. Fibromuscular dysplasia is the etiology of 13% of splenic artery aneurysms. Four percent of patients with renal artery fibromuscular dysplasia also have splenic artery aneurysms. Splenic artery aneurysms are found in 7% of patients with portal hypertension, and 10% of patients with splenic artery aneurysms have portal hypertension as the probable cause.[9] The altered hemodynamics in the splenic vessels caused by portal hypertension are believed to be a causative factor. Pancreatitis may cause aneurysm formation when the inflammatory process erodes the vessel wall. Evidence of atherosclerosis is found in many aneurysms but represents secondary changes in most. A few splenic artery aneurysms may be due to atherosclerosis. Finally, blunt or penetrating abdominal trauma can cause splenic artery aneurysms.

Diagnosis

Most patients with splenic artery aneurysms are asymptomatic, but as many as one-quarter have symptoms of vague left upper quadrant or epigastric pain. Acute expansion or rupture of the aneurysm may be accompanied by intense pain, diaphragmatic irritation, diaphoresis, and hypotension. Occasionally, patients present with gastrointestinal hemorrhage after rupture of the aneurysm into the gastrointestinal tract or, in an aneurysm resulting from pancreatitis, into the pancreatic duct. In some cases of rupture, hemorrhage may be confined to the lesser sac initially and then escape into the peritoneal cavity through the foramen of Winslow. This double rupture phenomenon may provide an opportunity for urgent surgical intervention during lesser sac tamponade prior to exsanguinating hemorrhage.

Findings on physical examination suggestive of a splenic artery aneurysm are rare. Because most splenic aneurysms are less than 2 cm in diameter, the presence of a palpable pulsatile abdominal mass is distinctly unusual. Left upper quadrant discomfort or an abdominal bruit may be present.

The diagnosis of a splenic artery aneurysm may be suspected during radiologic studies for unrelated diseases. Identification of a curvilinear or signet ring calcification in the left upper quadrant on an abdominal roentgenogram suggests the presence of a splenic artery aneurysm. Duplex scanning or CT imaging with intravenous contrast material may help differentiate a vascular lesion from a cystic lesion of an adjacent structure, but the diagnosis of a splenic artery aneurysm is made on arteriographic studies (Fig. 2). In addition, arteriography is necessary to define the location of the aneurysm and identify other aneurysms.

Treatment

In view of the high incidence of rupture during pregnancy, treatment of splenic artery aneurysms is indicated for all women of childbearing age. In addition, all patients with symptomatic or enlarging lesions should undergo intervention. An asymptomatic aneurysm greater than 2 cm in diameter should be treated unless the patient is at high risk. In that the reported incidence of rupture is less than 2% and the reported mortality rate following rupture is less than 25% in nonpregnant patients,[8,9] elective operations for splenic artery aneurysms should be undertaken only when the surgical

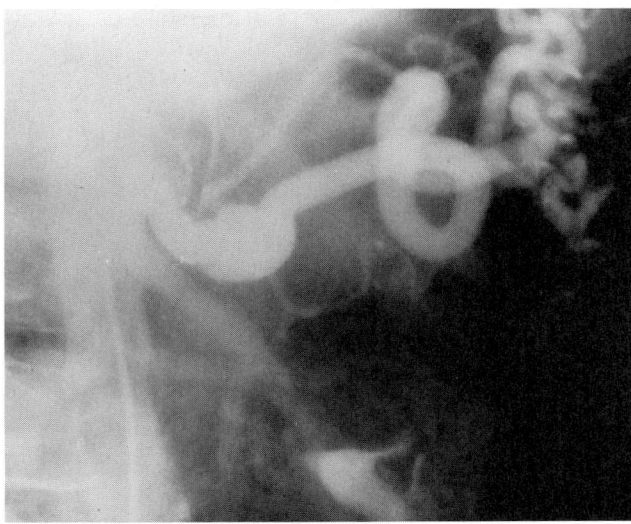

Figure 2 Arteriogram demonstrating a splenic artery aneurysm.

mortality is less than 1%. Small asymptomatic lesions in high risk patients are best followed.

Surgical therapy is dictated by the location and number of aneurysms. Aneurysms in the splenic hilum are usually treated by splenectomy and removal of that portion of the splenic artery containing the aneurysm. Pseudoaneurysms of the distal splenic artery associated with pancreatitis are treated by distal pancreatectomy, splenectomy, and excision of the aneurysm. For aneurysms involving the proximal and midportion of the splenic artery, aneurysmectomy with proximal and distal artery ligation without splenectomy is appropriate. When excessive dissection of the pancreas is required for excision of the aneurysm, aneurysm exclusion by ligation of contributing vessels from within the aneurysmal sac is preferred. Arterial reconstruction to restore splenic flow is usually not necessary, but in all patients the splenic artery must be examined for other aneurysms. When surgical therapy is undertaken for a ruptured aneurysm, the proximal splenic artery should be controlled prior to approaching the area of the aneurysm.

Percutaneous transcatheter occlusion of splenic artery aneurysms is a relatively safe alternative to operation and has the advantage of splenic preservation. It is particularly applicable to patients with portal hypertension or patients in poor health in whom treatment of the aneurysm is otherwise indicated. However, transcatheter embolization is not without risk. Massive splenic infarction and abscess formation can occur after transcatheter embolization or coil placement, but this is uncommon.[10] Localized infarction in the spleen may occur following occlusion of the splenic artery, but this is limited by the abundant collateral circulation to the spleen. Previous surgical procedures, which have compromised collateral circulation, increase the likelihood of massive splenic infarction and pose a relative contraindication to transcatheter occlusion of the splenic artery.

The results of therapy of splenic artery aneurysms vary dramatically between elective operation on an intact lesion and emergency operation for ruptured aneurysms. For elective operations results are excellent and operative mortality is rare. However, for ruptured aneurysms, operative mortality is approximately 25%. Ruptured aneurysms during pregnancy carry an even less favorable prognosis, with maternal mortality close to 70% and fetal mortality of 95%.[8,9]

REFERENCES

1. Stanley JC, Wakefield TW, Graham LM, et al. Clinical importance and management of splanchnic artery aneurysms. J Vasc Surg 1986; 3:836–840.
2. Busuttil RW, Brin BJ. The diagnosis and management of visceral artery aneurysms. Surgery 1980; 88:619–624.
3. Graham LM, Stanley JC, Whitehouse WM Jr, et al. Celiac artery aneurysms: historic (1745–1949) versus contemporary (1950–1984) differences in etiology and clinical importance. J Vasc Surg 1985; 2:757–764.
4. Stanley JC, Thompson NW, Fry WJ. Splanchnic artery aneurysms. Arch Surg 1970; 101:689–697.
5. Countryman D, Norwood S, Register D, et al. Hepatic artery aneurysm. Report of an unusual case and review of the literature. Am Surg 1983; 49:51–54.
6. Mathisen DJ, Athanasoulis CA, Malt RA. Preservation of arterial flow to the liver. Goal in treatment of extrahepatic and post-traumatic intrahepatic aneurysms of the hepatic artery. Ann Surg 1982; 196:400–411.
7. Wagner WH, Lundell CJ, Donovan AJ. Percutaneous angiographic embolization for hepatic arterial hemorrhage. Arch Surg 1985; 120:1241–1249.
8. Trastek VF, Pairolero PC, Joyce JW, et al. Splenic artery aneurysms. Surgery 1982; 91:694–699.
9. Stanley JC, Fry WJ. Pathogenesis and clinical significance of splenic artery aneurysms. Surgery 1974; 76:898–909.
10. Tihansky DP, Lluncor E. Transcatheter embolization of multiple mycotic splenic artery aneurysms: A case report. Angiology 1986; 37:530–534.

VASCULAR MALFORMATIONS OF THE SPLANCHNIC CIRCULATION

ASHBY C. MONCURE, M.D.

The important vascular malformations in the splanchnic circulation are angiodysplasia, mesenteric varices, telangiectasias associated with the hereditary hemorrhagic telangiectasia (Rendu-Osler-Weber syndrome), and hemangiomas.

ANGIODYSPLASIA

Angiodysplasia is the most common vascular malformation of the gastrointestinal tract and is also termed an arteriovenous malformation or vascular ectasia. It is postulated that the more frequent acquired form the angiodysplastic lesion is a consequence of chronic low-grade venule obstruction at the point where a vein passes through the muscularis of the bowel wall. With venous distention, the capillary network and its associated sphincters are disrupted, leading to the formation of minute arteriovenous shunts.[1] In the less frequent congenital form, the lesion contains thick-walled arteries and veins that communicate directly with each other.

These lesions may produce gastrointestinal bleeding, typically intermittent and chronic but occasionally acute or intermittently acute. Chronic intermittent gastrointestinal hemorrhage is a clinical problem encountered frequently. The usual diagnostic approach is initially guided by the presence of symptoms or signs suggesting the diagnosis, and the most likely site of hemorrhage is first investigated. If there are no directing symptoms or signs and the source for hemorrhage remains obscure, endoscopic examination of the large bowel, esophagus, and stomach, plus as much of the small bowel as possible, is undertaken. If the site of hemorrhage remains unknown and the presentation of gastrointestinal hemorrhage is strident, arteriography of the splanchnic circulation is urgently undertaken. If the clinical presentation is that of chronic low-grade hemorrhage, a contrast examination of the small bowel is performed; if it is negative, it is followed by splanchnic arteriography.

It should be emphasized that the initial responsibility of the managing physician pertains to the life-threatening aspects of the hemorrhage. The earliest possible estimate of quantity and rate of blood loss, rather than the exact diagnosis, is the key to initial management of massive hemorrhage, with efforts directed toward preventing hypovolemia and its complications. Determination of the origin of hemorrhage in the gastrointestinal tract is necessary to direct definitive treatment. Diagnostic and therapeutic procedures in many instances must proceed simultaneously, each giving way to the other under appropriate circumstances. Because of the dual considerations of diagnosis and therapy, the overall responsibility for management of the patient must be delegated to one person.

Two separate populations of patients are encountered with angiodysplasia. More rarely, it is encountered in otherwise healthy young patients and hence felt to be congenital. Such lesions are found throughout the gastrointestinal tract from stomach to rectum. They are found more frequently in the small intestine, and usually no significant family history can be obtained. Much more frequently, angiodysplastic lesions are encountered in the aged, with distribution primarily in the right colon and rarely in the small intestine. The lesions are associated in many instances with acquired aortic or mitral valvular disease or chronic renal failure.[2,3]

The definitive diagnosis may be obtained with use of selective mesenteric arteriography or, if the lesion is within the colon, occasionally by colonoscopy. Findings suggesting the arteriographic diagnosis include a localized vascular blush or tuft, a slightly dilated feeding artery with early drainage of contrast from the area through a dilated vein, or, in the late venous phase, a delayed-draining enlarged vein. The venous findings are nonspecific and may occasionally be associated with carcinoma of the colon.[4]

Colonoscopy, with excellent bowel preparation, has been reported to allow visualization of the colonic lesions in up to 80% of patients, with distinct red mucosal patches and dilated, tortuous associated vessels. If the colonic lesions can be visualized, endoscopic electrocoagulation or laser photoablation have been reported effective in over 60% of patients.[5]

Surgical resection, the definitive treatment in all noncolonic and many colonic lesions, relies on accurate preoperative localization in that the lesions usually cannot be visualized, transilluminated, or palpated intraoperatively. Accurate localization is more easily obtained in colonic lesions because of the embryonic rotation and fixation of the large intestine, which permits accurate arteriographic estimation of the area of colon involved. Arteriographic localization of the small intestine angiodysplastic lesion is more difficult because the small bowel is not fixed, and the small bowel segment involved cannot be precisely identified (Fig. 1). Superselective mesenteric arterial catheter placement with angiographic techniques, following the diagnostic arteriogram, has been developed (Fig. 2). Through a preoperatively positioned angiographic catheter in the appropriate mesenteric arterial feeding vessel, methylene blue injection into the catheter at celiotomy may allow accurate identification of the involved segment of small intestine. This technique has been helpful in both allowing definitive resection of the lesion and limiting the amount of small intestine resected (Fig. 3).[6]

Angiodysplasia may also occur and cause hemorrhage in the upper gastrointestinal tract, the most common site being the stomach, followed by the duodenum. Heretofore it has been considered rare, but at present it is recognized with much greater frequency. In 676 patients who underwent endoscopy at Barnes Hospital for upper gastrointestinal tract bleeding, angiodysplasia was diagnosed in 4% of the patients.[3] There was a strong correlation with age (mean age 63 years), with renal failure, and with renal dialysis. Brief episodes of overt bleeding had been noted in 23 of the 30 patients. The lesions were flat and bright red, ranged from 2 to 10 mm, and occurred in both the stomach and duodenum. Typical pathologic findings were reported in the excised specimens. They tended to appear in other areas after

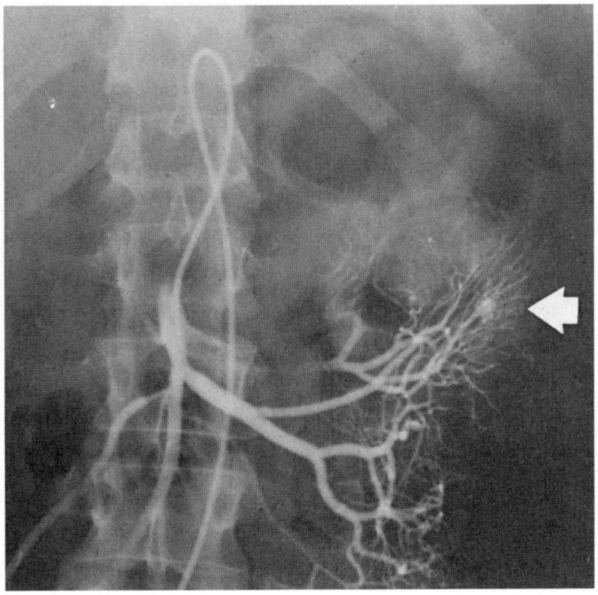

Figure 1 Superior mesenteric arteriogram of an arteriovenous malformation of jejunum. The arrow points to the malformation.

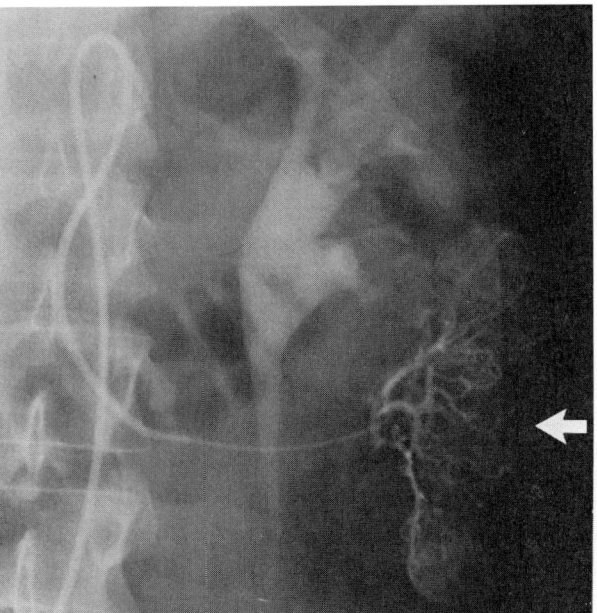

Figure 2 Superior mesenteric arterogram demonstrating a coaxial catheter system that has been placed superselectively in the jejunal artery supplying the lesions *(arrow)*. The catheter is injected intraoperatively with methylene blue to identify the involved segment of jejunum and allow conservative resection.

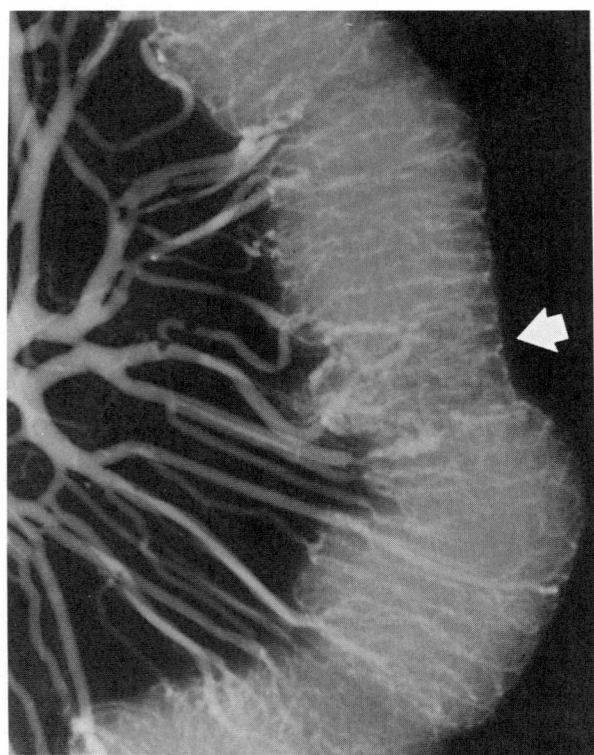

Figure 3 Radiograph of the resected jejunal segment with vessels injected with radiopaque silicone rubber. The arrow points to the arteriovenous malformation.

endoscopic cauterization or, in a few patients, after gastric resection.

The ectatic vessels may collapse upon interruption of the blood supply. In the absence of a mucosal lesion to direct the pathologist, vascular injection techniques such as silicone-rubber injection and clearing may be necessary to allow definitive diagnosis within the resected specimen. Upon resection of the involved segment of bowel, the vessels are injected immediately with radiopaque silicone rubber. A radiograph of the injected specimen is obtained, and the presence of the lesion within the resected segment can be confirmed prior to abdominal closure (Fig. 3). By immersing the specimen in increasing concentrations of alcohol, then 100% alcohol, and finally in a solution of methyl salicylate, the vessels of the optically clear specimen can be examined and photographed under the dissecting microscope. This dehydration process subsequently can be reversed and the specimen submitted for histologic examination.[6]

Between 5% and 37% of patients have recurrent gastrointestinal hemorrhage following operation. Repeat arteriography should be obtained in those patients with recurrent hemorrhage.

MESENTERIC VARICES

Varices within the small or large bowel may be secondary to generalized portal hypertension from prehepatic, intrahepatic, or posthepatic venous blockage or from more localized mesenteric venous obstruction from malignancies, the most common being carcinoma of the head of the pancreas. It is also seen from a portal-systemic venous shunt within postoperative adhesions in patients with generalized portal hypertension, the affected bowel being adherent to the adhesions or old suture lines.[7]

Gastrointestinal hemorrhage may ensue. The diagnosis may be achieved by endoscopy, if the affected bowel is accessible to the endoscope, or by late venous phase splanchnic arteriography.

The treatment of active hemorrhage from these mesenteric varices ranges from bowel resection to portal-systemic shunting, or both.

TELANGIECTASIA

Clinically important telangiectasias are usually associated with hereditary hemorrhagic telangiectasia (Rendu-Osler-Weber syndrome), an autosomal dominant inherited disease.[8] They are most common about the head, extremities, and chest and also occur in all parts of the gastrointestinal tract, with gastrointestinal bleeding occurring in up to 44% of patients. There is frequently a positive family history and variable presence of skin and mucosal lesions.

The diagnosis is suggested by the family history and associated findings. The site of hemorrhage may be documented by endoscopy or arteriography. Massive hemorrhage may force operation. Multiple or newly emerging lesions unfortunately lead to variable degrees of success in long-term management, in that these lesions have sclerotic vessel walls and intervascular fibrosis.

HEMANGIOMA

Hemangiomas, arising from a submucosal vascular plexus and exhibiting histologically large blood-filled sinuses within a connective tissue framework, are a rare cause of gastrointestinal bleeding. They may occur in the rectum, colon, or small intestine. Either endoscopy or arteriography may suggest the diagnosis. Treatment involves local excision of the tumor or resection of the segment of bowel containing the lesion.[9]

REFERENCES

1. Boley SJ, Sammartano R, Adams A, et al. On the nature and etiology of vascular ectasias of the colon. Gastroenterology 1977; 72:650–660.
2. Meyer CT, Troncale FJ, Galloway S, Sheahan DG. Arteriovenous malformations of the bowel. Medicine 1981; 60:36–48.
3. Clouse RE, Costigan DJ, Mills BA, Zuckerman GR. Angiodysplasia as a cause of upper gastrointestinal bleeding. Arch Intern Med 1985; 145:458–461.
4. Baum S, Athanasoulis CA, Waltman AC, et al. Angiodysplasia of the right colon: A cause of gastrointestinal bleeding. Am J Roentgenol 1977; 129:789–794.

5. Trudel JL, Fazio VW, Sivak MV. Colonoscopic diagnosis and treatment of arteriovenous malformations in chronic lower gastrointestinal bleeding. Dis Colon Rectum 1988; 31:107–110.
6. Athanasoulis CA, Moncure AC, Greenfield AJ, et al. Intraoperative localization of small bowel bleeding sites with combined use of angiographic methods and methylene blue injection. Surgery 1980; 87:77–84.
7. Moncure AC, Waltman AC, Vandersalm TJ, et al. Gastrointestinal hemorrhage from adhesion-related mesenteric varices. Ann Surg 1976; 183:24–29.
8. Reilly PH, Nostrant TT, Clinical manifestations of hereditary hemorrhagic telangiectasia. Am J Gastroent 1984; 79:363–367.
9. Abrahamson J, Shandling B. Intestinal hemangiomata in childhood and a syndrome for diagnosis: A collective review. J Pediatr Surg 1973; 8:487–495.

SPLANCHNIC AND PORTAL ARTERIOVENOUS FISTULAS

THOMAS E. BROTHERS, M.D.

Portal hypertension most commonly results from mechanical obstruction causing impedance to portal blood flow at the presinusoidal, sinusoidal, or postsinusoidal levels. In fewer than 1% of patients the culprit is not increased impedance, but increased portal blood flow due to an arteriovenous connection located within the splanchnic circulation.[1-3] These arteriovenous fistulas (AVF) represent potentially curable causes of portal hypertension distinguished by the preservation of normal liver function when diagnosed early. Nearly 300 cases of portal AVF have been reported in the literature, with 75% being acquired in origin. Since the advent and widespread application of new transhepatic interventional radiologic techniques, approximately 60% of acquired fistulas are now iatrogenic.

PATHOPHYSIOLOGY

The severity of the portal hypertension is a function of the volume of blood flow across the fistula, the capacitance of the portal venous system, and the impedance offered by the hepatic sinusoids.[4] Two impedance beds acting in series occur within the portal venous circulation. The primary bed consists of the intestine and spleen. The intrahepatic portal and hepatic veins and sinusoids comprise the secondary bed. Circumvention of the primary impedance bed by a portal AVF immediately increases the portal venous pressure toward systemic levels. As the total impedance of the portal circuit decreases with this fistula, the total portal blood flow increases. Because impedance correlates directly with blood flow rate, the relative impedance contributed by the liver further increases. The portal vein pressures may exceed 55 mm Hg in patients with portal AVF, pressures significantly higher than those seen in cirrhotic patients.

Chronic unprotected exposure of the liver to increased portal blood flow and pressure leads to irreversible portal hepatosclerosis.[5] Following fistula interruption, elevated portal blood pressures return to normal only about 70% of the time because of the development of persistent obstruction to portal flow. Exposure of the canine portal circulation to arterial blood pressures leads to progressive increases in fibrous tissue in the portal triads, muscular hypertrophy of portal vein radicals, and thickening of the vein walls.[6] Sinusoidal dilation, increased hemosiderin deposition, and decreased hepatic microsomal enzyme activity also occur. Dilated portal venous radicals are present in nearly half of all biopsies in patients with portal AVF. Although the presence of normal liver function may differentiate portal AVF from other causes of portal hypertension, these liver function tests may also be abnormal in up to a third of patients.

During the first 6 to 9 months after development of a portal AVF, massive gastrointestinal bleeding or acute enteritis with abdominal colic and diarrhea may develop.[7] Both symptom complexes result from mucosal hyperemia and portal congestion scattered diffusely throughout the bowel, although such hyperemia may also remain localized to the region of the fistula. This portal congestion regresses slightly over a period of years as collateral circulation develops. Eventually gastrointestinal complications of chronic portal hypertension evolve secondary to hepatoportal sclerosis.

SIGNS AND SYMPTOMS

The demographic data and relative incidence of the most common symptoms of portal AVF are reported according to fistula site (Tables 1 and 2). Fistulas arising postoperatively or following trauma are most likely to produce a pathognomonic bruit, whereas bruits are least commonly described in association with congenital lesions. In contrast, esophageal and gastric variceal bleeding most often occurs in association with congenital lesions, perhaps reflecting the longer duration of systemic arterial-portal flow. Local compression of surrounding structures and acute mucosal congestion both cause pain acutely, but chronic pain often relates to a vascular steal phenomenon, particularly in the presence of underlying arterial occlusive disease.[8] Nonspecific abdominal pain typically localizes to the left upper quadrant with splenic AVF and right upper quadrant with hepatic AVF, although pain may also be referred to

Table 1 Demographics of Portal Arteriovenous Fistulas

Demographics	Splenic	Hepatic	Other Splanchnic
Age (mean ± S.D.)	43 ± 16	44 ± 18	35 ± 16
Male-female ratio	0.56:1	1.9:1	3.8:1
Operative mortality*	9%	20%	13%

*Prior to angiographic embolization techniques.

Table 2 Signs and Symptoms of Portal Arteriovenous Fistulas

Sign/Symptom	Splenic	Hepatic	Other Splanchnic
Portal hypertension	62%	29%	20%
Abdominal bruit	47%	86%	80%
Gastrointestinal hemorrhage	48%	43%	20%
Abdominal pain	40%	43%	67%
Ascites	33%	0%	13%
Congestive heart failure	11%	—	—

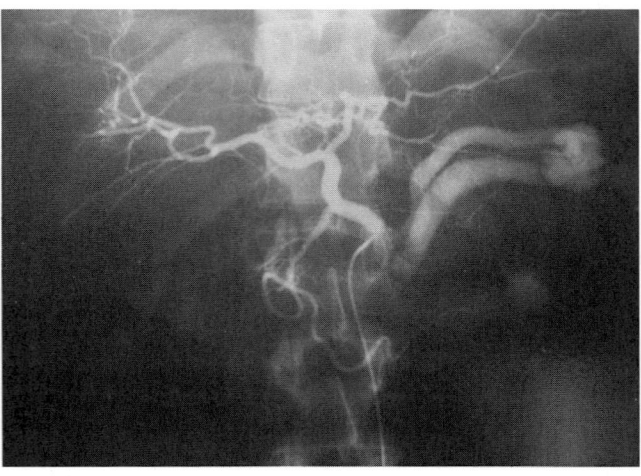

Figure 1 Celiac injection study demonstrating pseudoaneurysmal arteriovenous communication arising approximately 3 cm proximal to the ligated distal splenic artery and confirmed by early visualization of the splenic vein.

the epigastrium with either condition. The combination of hepatic congestion and a chronic disturbance of hepatic function, usually accompanied by fibrosis and fatty infiltration, appears necessary for the development of ascites. Ascites develops in a third of patients with splenic AVF but rarely in patients with hepatic or intestinal AVF or in patients with AVF of congenital origin. Congestive heart failure occurs uncommonly in adults with portal AVF due to the inherent impedance of the liver. Therefore, acute presentation with congestive heart failure suggests either compromise of cardiac reserve or spontaneous development of portosystemic shunts.

DIAGNOSIS AND MANAGEMENT

Timely diagnosis is essential to the appropriate management of portal AVF. Unfortunately, the correct diagnosis is made preoperatively in only about 60% of patients. Barium swallow and esophagogastroscopy document the presence of esophageal or gastric varices but do not specifically implicate portal AVF as the cause. Roentgenographic detection of calcification from an arteriosclerotic aneurysm may suggest splenic artery involvement. Duplex abdominal ultrasound shows promise but has been infrequently utilized to date. Computed tomography in association with arterial portography may document collateral pathways and arteriovenous shunts with a sensitivity (85%) approaching that of arteriography. Magnetic resonance imaging with time-of-flight phase techniques successfully images the portal venous system and should prove to be a superior diagnostic modality in the future. Despite these technologic advancements, arteriography continues to play a crucial role for diagnosis and planning of intervention. Arteriography documents early portal venous filling in the area of the fistula and identifies the relevant anatomy to determine the necessity of revascularization after fistula ligation or excision, especially in the splanchnic circulation (Fig. 1). Arteriography is also critical for assessing the feasibility of nonoperative interventional techniques. Transjugular intrahepatic portosystemic shunting (TIPS) in the presence of a portal AVF creates a high-output shunt, so routine use of pre-TIPS arteriography seems imperative.

Existence of a hemodynamically significant portal AVF should be regarded as sufficient indication for intervention. If the diagnosis is delayed, liver failure may ensue and become irreversible, despite subsequent fistula division. Treatment must always be directed at the fistula because procedures designed to address the portal hypertension alone are doomed to failure. However, if the primary symptom related to the AVF is variceal hemorrhage, portal decompression may be a reasonable therapeutic addition to fistula interruption, especially if secondary changes of hepatoportal sclerosis can be demonstrated.

Procedures that ligate, excise, or exclude the fistula are preferable to simple truncal ligation. Noncritical vessels may be proximally and distally ligated if accessible, whereas revascularization is necessary in the absence of sufficient collateral perfusion. The morbidity of operative intervention primarily originates from major intraperitoneal (8%) and gastrointestinal (3%) hemorrhage. Severe portal hypertension, high-pressure arterial collaterals, and associated inflammatory reaction contribute to potentially difficult operative management. Modern techniques of rapid intravenous infusion, autotransfusion of shed blood, and hypothermia with or without cardiopulmonary bypass may be useful. Although the overall mortality in one early series of portal AVF was 26%, with the availability of these techniques,

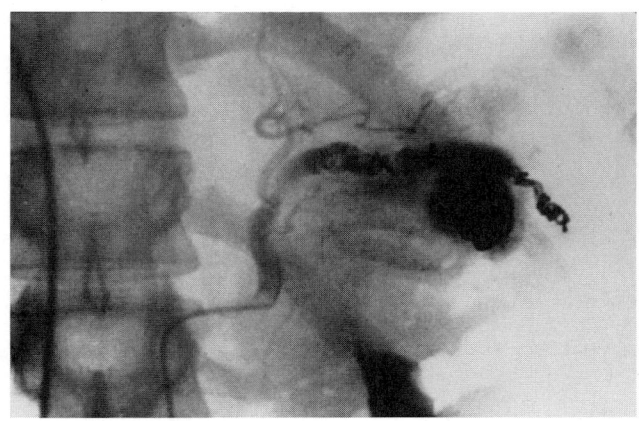

Figure 2 Repeat injection study following angiographic embolization reveals Gianturco coils lodged within, the fistula, as well as proximal and distal to the fistula, with resultant thrombosis.

no perioperative mortality has been described among 24 case reports published since 1977.[7] Absence of primary liver disease should facilitate cure for many of these patients.

Percutaneous management with transluminal embolization is rapidly becoming popular and useful, especially in unstable patients, either as a sole therapy or preoperatively to diminish vascular inflow.[8] Embolization may be accomplished with ethanol or isobutylcyanoacrylate infusion, Gianturco coils, gelatin sponges, or balloon occlusion (Fig. 2). Coils are most appropriate for larger-caliber fistulas but have a risk of distal migration to the liver parenchyma if the fistula diameter is larger than 8 mm. Embolization may not be appropriate for proximal control of larger vessels because of resultant ischemia. Loss of high blood flow through an enlarged portal vein may cause portal vein occlusion and cavernous transformation. Embolization therapy has proven to be quite useful, especially for lesions not readily amenable to surgical ligation or resection.

Splenic Fistulas

Rupture of splenic artery aneurysms account for 44% of splenic AVF. They are found primarily in women (86%). Free hemorrhage may be preceded in 12% of patients by incomplete extravasation into the bursa omentalis such that local erosion into the splenic vein precludes catastrophic intraperitoneal extension of the rupture. Various congenital arteriovenous malformations (20%) constitute the next most common etiology of splenic AVF. Splenic AVF arising in the vascular pedicle following splenectomy (13%) are associated with mass ligature, use of transfixion sutures, and enzymatic necrosis of the vessel wall from trauma to the pancreatic tail. Blunt and penetrating abdominal trauma, percutaneous splenoportography, mycotic aneurysm, and diffuse capillary hemangiomatosis of the spleen are responsible for the remainder. Splenic AVF occur exclusively in the main arterial trunk in 41% of patients, splenic hilum in 37%, and splenic parenchyma in 9%, with the rest occurring at multiple locations. Preoperative portal and/or splenic vein thrombosis complicates 8% of splenic AVF secondary to propagation of thrombus within the dilated venous side of the fistula or by compression of the vein by the aneurysm or surrounding inflammatory reaction. The majority of splenic AVF are single (75%), although congenital lesions tend to be multiple (73%).

Resection is most appropriate for AVF in the parenchyma or hilum of the spleen. In approximately 10% of splenic AVF, pancreatectomy may also be necessary because of the difficult dissection, surrounding inflammatory reaction, or involvement of small pancreatic branches within the fistula. Four-quadrant ligation and oversewing of the fistula with occasional splenic preservation may be considered, if technically feasible. Whenever possible, ectatic afferent and efferent vessels should be removed completely up to the nearest large bifurcation. Significant postoperative mesenteric or portal vein thrombosis has occurred in a few patients and is thought to result from thrombosis of a large, collapsed residual splenic vein stump extending to the portal vein.

Hepatic Fistulas

Congenital hepatic arteriovenous malformations include hemangiomas and the hereditary telangiectasia of Osler-Weber-Rendu syndrome. Although most fistulas in children involute with time, simultaneous occurrence of high-output cardiac failure in infancy has a mortality of 31% to 68%, if untreated. Most acquired hepatic AVF originate following abdominal trauma, more typically penetrating than blunt. Percutaneous liver biopsy and transhepatic biliary catheterization or drainage are increasing in frequency among causes of hepatic AVF, now estimated to occur after 5%, 4%, and 26% of these procedures, respectively. Fortunately, such fistulas typically tend to be small and unassociated with portal hypertension; often they spontaneously close. Hepatic artery aneurysms may also rupture into the portal vein to cause a fistula. Arteriographic evidence of transvasal hepatic arterioportal shunting develops in 2% to 10% of patients with hepatocellular cancer but rarely with cholangiocarcinomas or metastatic tumors. The majority of hepatic AVF reside within the parenchyma of the liver. As with other portal AVF, they tend to be inaccessible and involve multiple collaterals. Intrahepatic fistulas seem to remain more hemodynamically stable than their extrahepatic counterparts.

Many iatrogenic hepatic AVF close spontaneously if they are uncomplicated, have low blood flow, and are not associated with a bruit. Resection by partial hepatectomy may be performed for extensive lesions, but the rich collateral network within the liver increases the risk of recurrence. Hepatic artery ligation may be most appropriate in the setting of hepatocellular carcinoma. Percutaneous transluminal embolism has proven to be increasingly reliable for management of hepatic AVF that require intervention.

Other Splanchnic Fistulas

Other splanchnic AVF most commonly occur after gastric or intestinal resection and usually result from mass ligature or use of transfixion sutures. Traumatic splanchnic AVF are less common, with fewer than 20 reported cases.[9] Such AVF may be missed at the time of operation, if the fistulas are small or if routine exploration of central hematomas is not performed. Fistulas may also occur secondary to erosion of a splanchnic aneurysm into a neighboring vein. Occasional reports of AVF associated with pancreatic tumors or ileocecocolic angiodysplasia have appeared. Involvement of an AVF with central mesenteric vessels poses a special problem with regard to preserving intestinal blood supply while interrupting the fistula, and often it mandates concomitant visceral arterial bypass.

Proximal control of most central AVF usually requires clamping of the celiac or superior mesenteric artery and may require access to the supraceliac aorta along with medial visceral rotation or thoracoabdominal extension of the incision. Ligation of the superior mesenteric artery appears to be well tolerated if it is proximal to the origin of the middle colic artery. Arterial reconstruction with use of a saphenous vein or prosthetic interposition graft has also been utilized in about 20% of patients to preserve visceral flow after ligation of such an AVF.

REFERENCES

1. Van Way CW 3rd, Crane JM, Riddell DH, Foster JH. Arteriovenous fistula in the portal circulation. Surgery 1971; 70:876–890.
2. Pietri J, Remond A, Reix T, et al. Arterioportal fistulas: Twelve cases. Ann Vasc Surg 1990; 4:533–539.
3. Thiele BL, Royle JP, Thomas D. Splenic arteriovenous fistula: A report of two cases. Vasc Surg 1980; 14:4–8.
4. Williams DB, Payne WS, Foulk WT, Johnson CM. Splenic arteriovenous fistula. Mayo Clin Proc 1980; 55:383–386.
5. Pasternak BM, Cohen H. Arteriovenous fistula and forward hypertension in the portal circulation. Angiology 1978; 29:367–373.
6. Zuidema G, Gaisford W, Abell M, et al. Segmental portal arterialization of canine liver. Surgery 1963; 53:689–698.
7. Stone HH, Jordan WD, Acker JJ, Martin JD Jr. Portal arteriovenous fistulas. Review and case report. Am J Surg 1965; 109:191–196.
8. Strodel WE, Eckhauser FE, Lemmer JH, et al. Presentation and perioperative management of arterioportal fistulas. Arch Surg 1987; 122:563–571.
9. Dietrick J, McNeill P, Posner MP, et al. Traumatic superior mesenteric artery–portal vein fistula. Ann Vasc Surg 1990; 4:72–76.

PORTAL HYPERTENSION

ANATOMIC BASIS OF PORTAL HYPERTENSION

FREDERIC E. ECKHAUSER, M.D.
LISA COLLETTI, M.D.
JAMES A. KNOL, M.D.

Esophageal varices are dilated, thin-walled collateral veins that develop in the submucosa of the lower esophagus and gastric cardia in response to portal hypertension. Portal hypertension that is clinically silent does not require treatment. However, the development of complications such as encephalopathy, ascites, and variceal hemorrhage has significant potential consequences for the patient and society alike. Regardless of the ultimate clinical manifestations, the etiology and pathophysiology of portal hypertension have a significant bearing on the development of these complications and their management. Improved understanding has aided the development of clinical and hemodynamic criteria to help clarify the respective roles of nonselective and selective portosystemic shunt procedures as well as the role of nonshunt operations in patients with unsuitable portal venous anatomy or severely compromised liver function that would preclude a portosystemic shunt.

PATHOGENESIS

Extensive collaterals form between the portal and systemic venous circulations in response to portal hypertension (Fig. 1). Communications that develop at the gastroesophageal junction are complex and consist of four interconnected anatomic zones.[1] The gastric zone consists of a band of longitudinally oriented veins located within the submucosa of the proximal stomach. At the distal end of this zone, veins within the submucosa coalesce to form larger trunks that ultimately communicate with the portal vein through the left gastric or coronary vein and with the splenic vein via the short gastric veins. More proximally, veins of the gastric zone extend several centimeters above the gastroesophageal junction to penetrate the muscularis mucosa and network with veins that lie within the lamina propria of the palisade zone. Above the palisade zone, vessels again penetrate the muscularis mucosa to lie within the submucosa. The perforating zone lies 3 to 5 cm proximal to the gastroesophageal junction and consists of longitudinal trunks formed by the confluence of veins from the palisade zone. These vessels perforate the esophageal wall to form an extramural plexus and larger external esophageal veins. Ultimately they coalesce into larger trunks and repenetrate the wall at irregular intervals to form submucosal venous trunks that comprise the truncal zone.

Portal hypertension is defined as a pathological, sustained increase in blood pressure in one or more compartments of the portal circulation. In patients with portal hypertension, this circulation accommodates a marked increase in venous blood flow, redirecting as much as 400 to 500 ml/minute of portal blood. The area of maximum resistance to increased blood flow occurs within the gastroesophageal venous plexus at the level of the palisade zone. Increased back pressure results in formation of gastric varices. Continued dilation of poorly supported, high-resistance, thin-walled vessels within the lamina propria of the palisade zone may predispose to acutely increased wall tension and rupture, giving rise to what Conn described as the "exploding volcano" phenomenon.[2]

Elevated portal blood pressure is implicated in the pathogenesis of acute variceal bleeding, but the specific factors that contribute to varix rupture remain undefined. There is a fairly good correlation between the extent of varices documented with endoscopy or radiologic studies and the degree of portal blood pressure elevation. However, there is not a clear relationship between the degree of portal hypertension and the risk of variceal bleeding. Unlike arterial pressure, portal blood pressure is not static and levels vary widely. The normal portal blood pressure measured in the supine position at rest and expressed as the corrected sinusoidal pressure (CSP)—that is, the difference between wedge hepatic vein pressure (WHVP) or free portal pressure (PVP) and systemic venous pressure measured in the infrahepatic portion of the inferior vena cava—ranges from 3 to 6 mm Hg. There is also an excellent correlation between wedge hepatic vein blood pressure and free portal blood pressure, except when the etiology of portal

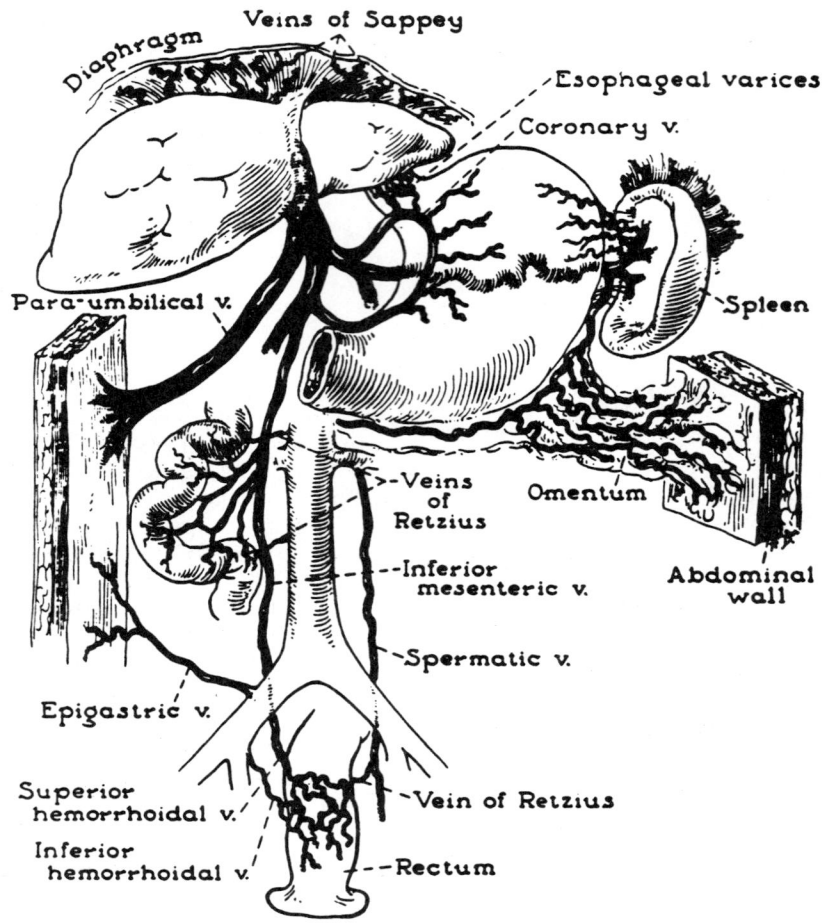

Figure 1 Collateral venous channels that may develop in obstruction of the portal system. (From Gray HR, Whitsell FB Jr. Hemorrhage from esophageal varices: Surgical management. Ann Surg 1950; 132:798–810; with permission.)

hypertension is presinusoidal or extrahepatic in origin (Fig. 2). The greatest benefit of the percutaneous WHVP measurement is the ability to obtain serial in situ measurements of portal blood pressure and thereby gauge the patient's response to pharmacologic therapy. Based on repeated measurements in patients with cirrhosis, bleeding related to and probably originating from esophageal varices is unlikely if the CSP is less than 12 mm Hg.

CLASSIFICATION OF PORTAL HYPERTENSION

Sustained portal hypertension generally develops from obstruction to portal venous blood flow and may give rise to diverse clinical syndromes. To better understand the relationship between physiologic and anatomic alterations in the portal circulation, a unifying classification was developed based on the hepatic sinusoid (presinusoidal, sinusoidal, postsinusoidal). Hepatic sinusoids are spiderlike microcirculatory networks that receive blood from portal venules and hepatic arterioles and flow into collecting venules that join to form terminal hepatic venules. The endothelial lining of sinusoids is thin and fenestrated, permitting rapid passage of fluids and nutrients into the space of Disse. This is a vulnerable site where collagen deposition or scarring can lead to significant impairment of nutrient transport and exchange. This classification is useful for prognosis and therapy because presinusoidal etiologies are generally not associated with impaired hepatic reserve. Conversely, obstruction of portal flow at or distal to the level of the sinusoid is commonly associated with impaired hepatic function.

Presinusoidal extrahepatic portal hypertension is due primarily to pylephlebitis with portal pyemia, pyogenic liver abscess, and portal vein thrombosis. A variety of intra-abdominal infections are implicated including appendicitis, diverticulitis, pyelonephritis with perinephric abscess, and gynecologic conditions. Portal vein thrombosis can also result from splenectomy performed for trauma, Hodgkin's or lymphoma staging, and hematologic disorders. Thrombus occurring in a long splenic vein stump can propagate distally, involving the portal or mesenteric veins and resulting in either partial or complete thrombosis.

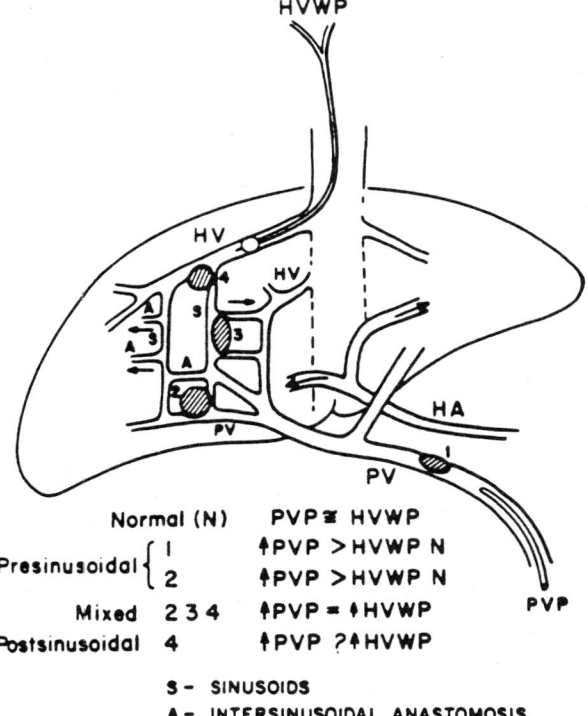

Figure 2 Diagrammatic representation of the relationship between wedge hepatic vein pressure and free portal pressure with obstruction of the portal circulation at different levels. Sinusoids (S) and intersinusoidal anastomoses (A) are depicted. A unifying classification divides sites of portal obstruction into presinusoidal (1,2), sinusoidal or mixed 2-4), and postsinusoidal (4). (From Conn HO, Groszmann RJ. The pathophysiology of portal hypertension. In: Arias I, Popper H, Schachter D, Slafritz DA, eds. The liver: biology and pathobiology. New York, Raven Press, 1982:821–848; with permission.)

Schistosomiasis, an endemic disease in many parts of the world including Africa and the Middle East, is the paradigm of presinusoidal intrahepatic portal vein obstruction. Ova are released by the parasite, *Schistomsoma mansoni* and *S. japonicum*, into the portal circulation, where they evoke an inflammatory response that ultimately causes obstruction to portal blood flow. The veno-occlusive effects of the ova are proportional to the severity of the schistosomal infestation. In all forms of presinusoidal portal vein obstruction, portal blood pressure is elevated, but WHVP remains normal. The reduction in portal venous blood flow is accompanied by a compensatory increase in hepatic arterial blood flow that maintains estimated total liver blood flow at near normal levels. Parenchymal function is generally well preserved, and portal decompressive procedures to control variceal bleeding are usually well tolerated.

Other causes of presinusoidal intrahepatic portal hypertension are uncommon. Nodular regeneration of the liver is considered an immunopathologic disorder associated with little intrahepatic fibrosis in which formation of minute nodules throughout the liver distorts intrahepatic portal venules. Congenital hepatic fibrosis is an autosomal recessive disorder associated with formation of microscopic intrahepatic cysts and pericystic fibrosis that develop predominantly in the portal tracts, distort portal venules, and give rise to portal hypertension. Idiopathic portal hypertension or noncirrhotic portal fibrosis occurs primarily in Asia and is characterized histologically by varying degrees of portal fibrosis. It is postulated that microthrombi developing in the intrahepatic portal venules lead to progressive obliteration of middle-order portal veins, resulting in portal hypertension. As with other forms of presinusoidal portal hypertension, the PVP is elevated and the WHVP is generally normal.

Cirrhosis is the most common cause of sinusoidal portal hypertension. Alcoholic liver disease is most common among Western patients and is characterized morphologically by regenerating pseudolobules of liver parenchyma surrounded by diffuse fibrosis. The resulting distortion of the intrahepatic vascular anatomy causes increased resistance to portal blood flow and portal hypertension. Cirrhosis is a chronic and progressive disorder that ultimately results in impaired hepatic parenchymal function. Other causes of cirrhosis include postnecrotic as well as primary and secondary forms of biliary cirrhosis. In sinusoidal obstruction, all measurements of portal pressure are elevated, and the PVP and WHVP are approximately equal.

Postsinusoidal causes of portal hypertension are uncommon but interesting from a pathophysiologic standpoint. With this group of disorders, resistance to blood flow occurs at the level of either the intrahepatic venules or extrahepatic veins, depending on the nature of the process. Intrahepatic veno-occlusive disease results most commonly from endophlebitis of centrilobular and intraparenchymal hepatic veins caused by chronic ingestion of plants containing pyrrolidizine (Senecio) alkaloids but is also seen in patients undergoing chemotherapy or hepatic irradiation. Hemodynamic data are scarce, but theoretically sinusoidal and portal vein pressures should be elevated and approximately equal. The major clinical manifestation of this form of postsinusoidal obstruction is ascites, although portosystemic collaterals can develop and result in variceal hemorrhage.

Hepatic vein thrombosis (Budd-Chiari syndrome) was described originally in the mid-nineteenth century and is characterized by hepatic vein thrombosis resulting in hepatomegaly, right upper quadrant discomfort, and the rapid or insidious onset of ascites, which is often intractable. This disorder is associated with trauma, myeloproliferative syndromes, tumors arising in organs adjacent to the liver and vena cava, pregnancy, and the use of oral contraceptives. Early operative intervention should be considered to prevent irreversible fibrosis and parenchymal atrophy. Operative approaches are usually governed by the underlying venous anatomy, that is, patency of the portal vein and/or inferior vena cava.

DEVELOPMENT OF PORTOSYSTEMIC COLLATERALS

The collateral patterns that develop in response to portal hypertension are determined by the site of obstruction in the portal circulation. Each type of obstruction results in its own unique pattern of collaterals, which in turn dictates therapeutic options. With splenic vein occlusion, localized splenic venous hypertension develops, resulting in splenomegaly and distention of perisplenic collaterals. The short gastric veins enlarge in an effort to establish collateral blood flow into the systemic circulation via the azygous vein. The left gastroepiploic vein also enlarges with the formation of splenorenal and adrenal collaterals.

Extrahepatic portal vein occlusion is associated with a variety of unusual hematologic, inflammatory, and neoplastic disorders, but for the most part is considered idiopathic in origin. Collaterals develop upstream from the site of obstruction and are especially prominent in the splenorenal area. Engorgement of the inferior mesenteric vein causes venous stasis in the descending colon and ultimately development of a hemorrhoidal venous plexus. The coronary vein dilates with eventual formation of gastroesophageal varices (Fig. 1). Collaterals in the abdominal wall become progressively more prominent and may reanastomose with a recanalized umbilical vein, thereby returning blood to the left branch of the portal vein. Partial recanalization of the portal vein (cavernous transformation) and progressive development of portal collaterals re-establish significant hepatopedal flow, resulting in normal hepatic parenchymal and synthetic function. The stigmata of liver disease are generally absent; if present, variceal bleeding is unanticipated and occurs in an otherwise healthy patient. Operative treatment is warranted only if complications such as variceal hemorrhage cannot be controlled with nonoperative techniques such as endoscopic therapy or rubber band ligation. Because of well-preserved liver function, these patients tolerate repeated hemorrhage, and emergency operations are rarely necessary. Death from exsanguination is rare and occurs in fewer than 5% to 10% of patients followed for long periods of time.[3]

ANATOMIC BASIS OF SURGICAL TREATMENT FOR PORTAL HYPERTENSION

Obstruction of the portal circulation can occur at many levels. The site of obstruction and resulting hemodynamic consequences, as well as the coexistence or absence of hepatic parenchymal disease, determine the role of nonoperative or operative treatment. Diagnosis in all patients should include endoscopic or radiologic documentation of esophageal and/or gastric varices, biochemical measures of liver function, and, if necessary, histologic confirmation of the presence or absence of liver disease and thorough angiographic assessment of the portal, mesenteric, and splenic venous circulations, including measurement of portal and systemic blood pressures.

PRESINUSOIDAL PORTAL OBSTRUCTION

Splenic Vein Occlusion

Occlusion of the splenic vein causes sinistral or left-sided portal hypertension with formation of gastric varices. In this condition, hypertension is confined to the splenic venous compartment of the portal circulation. Coronary, short gastric, and gastroepiploic veins dilate to accommodate increased blood flow and serve as a bridge between the high-pressure splenic venous compartment and the normotensive mesenteric and portal venous compartments (Fig. 3). Characteristic angiographic findings include failure to visualize the splenic vein, marked dilation of the gastroepiploic veins, and serial opacification of the coronary and portal veins. Hemodynamic measurements show normal WHVP and PVP. However, splenic pulp pressure can be measured percutaneously and is elevated in virtually all patients. In addition, splenoportography can be used to visualize the portal system and may be the only means other than operation for directly measuring blood pressure upstream from the obstruction. Establishing a correct diagnosis of this form of compartmental portal hypertension is important, because splenectomy is curative. It is imperative to distinguish this condition from generalized portal hypertension in order to avoid inadequate variceal decompression or needless exposure to encephalopathy or accelerated liver failure.

Portal Vein Occlusion

The classic clinical presentation of extrahepatic portal vein occlusion is unanticipated variceal hemorrhage in an otherwise healthy adult. Stigmata of liver disease are absent, and the liver is functionally and histologically normal. Venous phase angiography is diagnostic and must be interpreted carefully with regard to the patency and availability of venous tributaries, should a portal decompressive shunt become necessary. It is also important to document vascular continuity between the esophagogastric variceal watershed and the proposed venous tributary to be used for the shunt to ensure satisfactory decompression and afford protection from variceal rebleeding.

When considering operative treatment, a number of procedures, including splenectomy alone and transgastric or transesophageal varix ligation, are clearly contraindicated. One must be especially careful because the initial procedure, if properly selected and performed, has the greatest chance of success. When feasible, a portosystemic shunt is most likely to confer long-term protection against variceal rebleeding.

Splenorenal shunts provide satisfactory results but the end-to-side variant is associated with late thrombosis and postsplenectomy sepsis, especially in children. The most successful shunt for this condition has been the mesocaval shunt. The original Marion-Clatworthy direct mesocaval shunt, which entails dividing the vena cava and anastomosing the divided proximal end of the vena cava to the side of the superior mesenteric vein, affords adequate portal decompression but, in adults, is accompanied by a 10% incidence of lower extremity venous insufficiency (Fig. 4). Interposition mesocaval shunts avoid this problem, but an autologous venous conduit using either a single large-caliber vein or a baffle graft should be used in preference to prosthetic materials to reduce the risk of late thrombosis.

Up to 40% of patients with portal vein occlusion have venous anatomy that precludes a standard portosystemic shunt. In this setting, esophagogastrectomy, total esophagectomy with cervical esophagogastric anastomosis, and colonic interposition have all been used with some success. Extensive esophagogastric devascularization with splenectomy and esophageal transection with reanastomosis (Sugiura procedure) is another alternative. Major complications of the Sugiura procedure including esophageal leak and anastomotic stricture, develop in 8% to 10% of patients, but most esophageal leaks resolve with nonoperative treatment. Although varices recur in the majority of patients, bleeding is relatively uncommon and can usually be controlled with injection sclerotherapy or rubber band ligation.

Generalized Portal Hypertension

Construction of a portosystemic shunt in a cirrhotic patient can be associated with prohibitive mortality and morbidity from accelerated liver failure and encephalopathy. Several clinical and hemodynamic selection criteria have been adopted to minimize these potential risks. In 1964 Child and Turcotte introduced a classification system based on three clinical findings and two liver function tests.[4] These criteria define three risk groups, accurately predict operative mortality, and approximate long-term survival as well.[5] Despite its popularity, the Child-Turcotte classification has been criti-

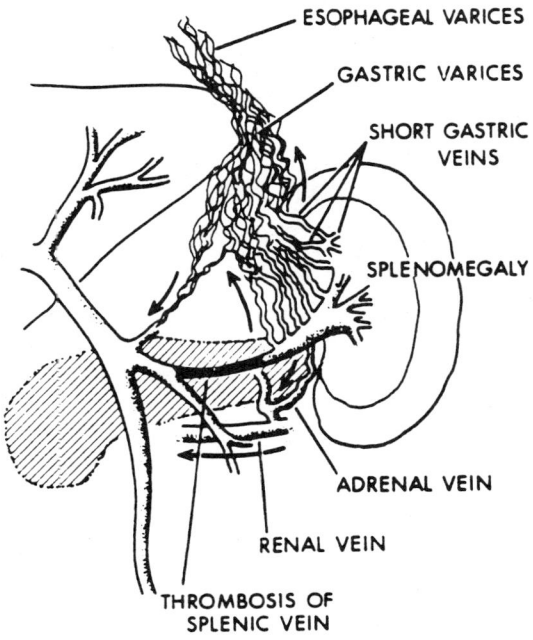

Figure 3 Diagram of the patterns of collateral flow in splenic vein thrombosis. (From Conn HO, Grozmann RJ: The pathophysiology of portal hypertension. In: Arias I, Popper H, Schachter D, Shafritz DA, eds. The liver: Biology and pathophysiology. New York: Raven Press, 1982:821–848; with permission.)

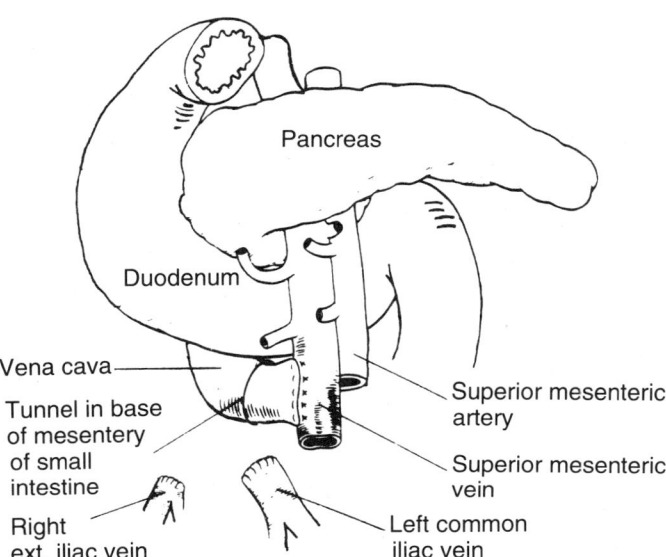

Figure 4 Diagram of direct mesocaval shunt showing relationship of anastomosis to the duodenum and pancreas. (From Zuidema GD, Ebert PA. Mesenteric caval anastomosis for portal decompression. Johns Hopkins Med J 1967; 120:201–209; with permission.)

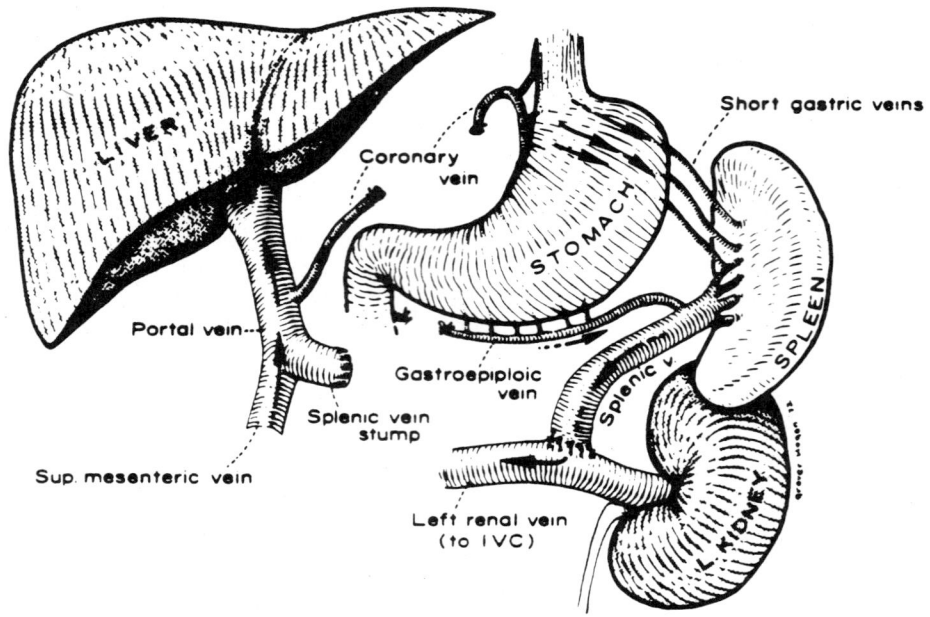

Figure 5 The distal splenorenal (Warren) shunt, which selectively decompresses the gastroesophageal watershed yet partially maintains prograde portal flow and mesenteric venous hypertension. The coronary, gastroepiploic, and inferior mesenteric veins are divided to discourage diversion of portal flow through these potential collaterals. (From Salam AA, Warren WD: Anatomic basis of the surgical treatment of portal hypertension. Surg Clin North Am 1974: 54:1251–1257; with permission.)

cized because assignment of patient risk may be somewhat arbitrary. In spite of its inherent limitations, efforts to develop more objective criteria by assigning point values to evaluation parameters do not provide better predictive value than the original Child-Turcotte classification.

Clinical criteria are useful in predicting operative mortality but are less helpful in predicting the likelihood of long-term survival, encephalopathy, or late liver failure. The hemodynamic thesis was promulgated in the late 1950s and elaborated further by Warren and associates in 1963.[6] This hypothesis suggests that patients with normal portal blood flow poorly tolerate complete diversion of portal blood that results from construction of a portosystemic shunt. By comparison, cirrhosis may protect patients from the portoprival effects of complete portal decompression because the process itself causes progressive diversion of prograde portal blood flow through collaterals and greater dependence on hepatic arterial inflow. The entire concept of "selective" shunts was based on this hemodynamic premise, and most shunt surgeons approach the management of portal hypertension with the belief that blood flow to the liver should be maintained whenever possible.

Nonselective versus Selective Shunts

Nonselective portosystemic shunts theoretically divert all portal blood flow away from the liver into the systemic venous circulation. Excluding the end-to-side portocaval shunt, which precludes any possibility of sinusoidal perfusion with portal blood and does not decompress the hepatic sinusoid, all other shunts are functionally side-to-side shunts. Collectively they convert the hepatic limb of the portal vein into an outflow tract and thereby may deprive the liver of nutrients and/or hepatotrophic factors contained in portal blood.

The efficacy of nonselective shunts has been questioned by the results of several prospective randomized therapeutic shunt trials. The majority of these studies have documented that early (1 year) and late (5 years) survival is better for the surgical patients than for the medical patients. However, the differences are not statistically significant. In addition, the incidence of encephalopathy after randomization is almost equal between the two groups. Based on these studies, some investigators believe that total shunts are indicated only in urgent or emergency situations to prevent exsanguinating hemorrhage.

The selective shunt was designed to lower blood pressure in the gastroesophageal watershed while maintaining partial prograde portal blood flow and mesenteric venous hypertension. The prototype operation described by Warren and co-workers in 1967 consists of dividing the splenic vein near its confluence with the mesenteric vein and anastomosing the divided end of the splenic vein with the side or end of the left renal vein (Fig. 5).[7] The distal splenorenal shunt is combined with ligation of the coronary, gastroepiploic, and inferior mesenteric veins to discourage diversion of portal blood flow through these preformed collaterals.

Selective shunts are recommended for portal decompression whenever feasible but with certain qualifi-

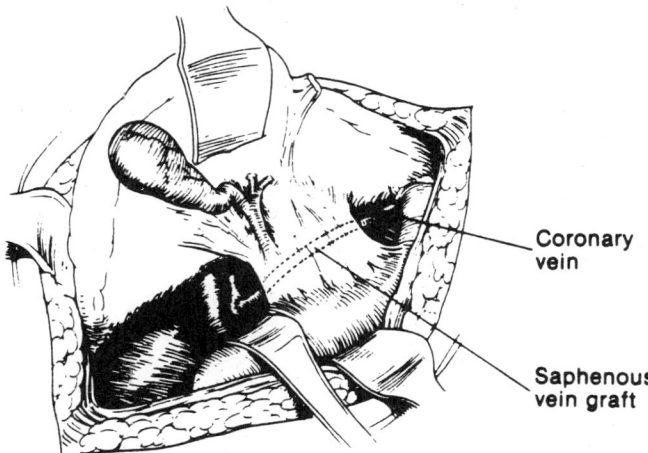

Figure 6 Diagram of the coronary caval (Inokuchi) shunt for selective variceal decompression. It is frequently necessary to interpose a segment of saphenous vein to bridge the distance between the divided end of the coronary vein and the inferior vena cava. (From Smith G. Portal hypertension. In: Zuidema GD, ed. Schackleford's surgery of the alimentary tract. Philadelphia: WB Saunders, 1991:324–394; with permission.)

cations. The extensive retroperitoneal dissection interrupts lymphatics and may aggravate pre-existing acites that may become intractable. This may be compounded by the fact that partially maintaining mesenteric venous hypertension is a prescribed goal of the operation. These procedures are also technically demanding and therefore less expedient than total shunts in urgent or emergent situations. Finally, certain anatomic factors, including prior splenectomy, splenic vein thrombosis, a splenic vein diameter of less than 10 mm, and the presence of a retroaortic or structurally abnormal left renal vein, preclude a selective shunt. That selective shunts preserve prograde portal flow makes them ideal for patients with presinusoidal etiologies of portal obstruction and normal liver function. The other selective shunt is the coronary-caval shunt described by Inokuchi and colleagues (Fig. 6).[8] This procedure usually requires interposition of a segment of saphenous vein between the central end of the coronary vein and the side of the vena cava. Despite the optimistic clinical results published by the Inokuchi group, the technical difficulty of the procedure and growing experience with the distal splenorenal shunt have limited its popularity in Western countries.

The results of selective shunts include an overall mortality rate of 7% and postoperative complications that are similar to those following other portosystemic shunts. The major early complications include ascites, which usually responds to medical management, and portal vein thrombosis, which occurs in approximately 10% of patients and may be fatal. Late complications include rebleeding and encephalopathy. It was originally anticipated that selective shunts would provide protection against encephalopathy by maintaining prograde portal flow. However, over time, new collaterals form between the portal and systemic venous circulations and progressively divert portal flow away from the liver. This phenomenon abrogates the beneficial effect of the selective shunt and results in an increased incidence of encephalopathy beyond 2 years.

Recurrent bleeding after a selective shunt is relatively uncommon, with an overall rate of 10% to 15%. Early postoperative bleeding may be due to shunt dysfunction or thrombosis and to nonvariceal sources of bleeding such as gastritis or peptic ulcer disease. Based on the results of several controlled therapeutic trials, selective shunts do not appear to confer any early or long-term survival benefit over nonselective shunts. The operative mortality rate for the two procedures is comparable. The incidence of early postoperative encephalopathy is lower following a selective shunt, but this advantage disappears somewhat over time. However, the quality of life for selective shunt patients may be improved because they require fewer hospitalizations for recurrent encephalopathy. Despite these limitations, the selective shunt remains the operation of choice for patients with presinusoidal portal obstruction. For rehabilitated alcoholic patients who fail injection sclerotherapy alone or combined with pharmacologic treatment, the selective shunt is a reasonable therapeutic choice in the absence of anatomic contraindications or severe ascites.

REFERENCES

1. Vianna A, Hayes PC, Moscoso G, et al. Normal venous circulation of the gastroesophageal junction: A route to understanding varices. Gastroenterology 1987; 93:876–889.
2. Conn HO. The volcan varix connection. Gastroenterology 1980; 79:1333–1337 (editorial).
3. Voorhees AP Jr, and Price JB Jr. Extrahepatic portal hypertension: A retrospective analysis of 127 cases and associated clinical implications. Arch Surg 1974; 108:338–341.
4. Child CG III, Turcotte JG. Surgery and portal hypertension. In: Child CG III, ed. The liver and portal hypertension. Philadelphia: WB Saunders, 1964:49–51.
5. Wantz GE, Payne MA. Experience with portocaval shunt for portal hypertension. N Engl J Med 1961; 265:721–728.
6. Warren WD, Restrepo JE, Respass JC, et al. The importance of hemodynamic studies in management of portal hypertension. Ann Surg 1963; 158:387–404.
7. Warren WD, Zeppa R, Fomon JJ. Selective transsplenic decompression of gastroesophageal varices by distal splenorenal shunt. Ann Surg 1967; 166:437–455.
8. Inokuchi K, Kobayashi M, Kusaba A, et al. New selective decompression of esophageal varices by a left gastric venous–caval shunt. Arch Surg 1970; 100:157–162.

PHARMACOLOGIC INTERVENTION, BALLOON TAMPONADE, AND CATHETER EMBOLIZATION FOR VARICEAL HEMORRHAGE

B. TIMOTHY BAXTER, M.D.
LAYTON F. RIKKERS, M.D

Esophageal varices are only one of a number of collateral venous channels that develop in response to an increased blood pressure gradient between the portal and systemic venous systems. Varices of the distal esophagus have clinical significance because of their propensity to bleed. Bleeding varices represent the most acute, life-threatening problem in end-stage liver disease. Variceal hemorrhage is directly responsible for death in a third of patients with cirrhosis. This increase in portal vein blood pressure can result from both intrahepatic and extrahepatic lesions.

Local anatomic factors in the distal esophagus are probably responsible for the great propensity of esophageal varices to bleed in comparison to other portal-systemic venous collaterals. The superficial veins in the distal esophagus are in the lamina propria and have less surrounding connective tissue support than varices at other sites. This allows for dilation, which results in attenuation of the venous wall. The relationship between changes in tangential wall stress (τ), internal radius (r_i), and wall thickness (d) within a cylinder are best described by the following equation:

$$\tau = P \times r_i/d$$

At a constant pressure (P), a threefold increase in the radius without a change in the mass of the wall increases tangential stress per unit area by a factor of 12.[1] Lebrec and colleagues have documented that increasing varix size is associated with increased bleeding risk.[2] They found that patients with large varices (greater than 5 mm) are more likely to have a history of bleeding than those with small or medium-sized varices (38% versus 10%) and are more likely to bleed within 1 year than those with small or medium-sized varices (20% versus none). Furthermore, by direct measurement of variceal blood pressure, calculated wall tension was significantly increased in bleeding versus nonbleeding varices. Although chemical injury from gastroesophageal reflux has also been suggested to contribute to variceal erosion and bleeding, this is unlikely because there is no evidence of inflammation in esophageal biopsies and prophylactic treatment with H2 blockers is ineffective in reducing bleeding episodes.[3]

The management of variceal bleeding requires a purposeful approach (Fig. 1). As with all hemorrhage regardless of the source, fluid resuscitation of the patient assumes the highest priority. Through large-bore intravenous catheters, red cells, fresh frozen plasma, and platelets are administered to maintain adequate oxygen-carrying capacity, replete coagulation factors, and correct thrombocytopenia, respectively. The remainder of the volume deficit is replaced with isotonic crystalloid solutions, accepting that these may contribute to ascites following successful resuscitation.

Once resuscitation is begun, determining the bleeding site becomes the next priority. Hematemesis or melena with a positive nasogastric (NG) aspirate confirms an upper gastrointestinal (GI) source. Gastric lavage with a large-bore Ewald tube helps to clear the stomach of clots and facilitates accurate endoscopic evaluation. If there is no evidence of continued bleeding, the timing of endoscopy (immediate versus delayed) is controversial but we recommend it be done early in the cirrhotic. With ongoing bleeding, the source must be sought expeditiously. Although clinical evidence of liver disease suggests variceal bleeding, endoscopic confirmation is important because other sources of upper GI bleeding are not uncommon in patients with cirrhosis.

After upper GI endoscopy has established that acute bleeding is from varices, the appropriate intervention must be chosen. Sclerotherapy is effective in controlling acute hemorrhage in 60% to 90% of patients and is the only nonsurgical technique that has been shown to reduce the frequency of early rebleeding. For these reasons, it is the method of choice for initial control of variceal hemorrhage. Because of the high prevalence of cirrhosis in the United States, the small proportion of individuals in whom sclerotherapy fails to control bleeding (10% to 30%) represents a large number of patients. Furthermore, the success of esophageal sclerotherapy has led to an increased incidence of bleeding from gastric varices and portal hypertensive gastropathy. Although emergent surgical decompression of the portal system is effective in controlling hemorrhage, the morbidity and mortality rates are especially formidable in the setting of uncontrolled bleeding. Thus, it is imperative that both surgeon and physician be aware of the indications for and efficacy of other nonsurgical approaches to control acute variceal bleeding, including pharmacologic therapy, balloon tamponade, catheter embolization, and transjugular intrahepatic portosystemic shunt (TIPS).

PHARMACOLOGIC THERAPY

Despite the lack of a high degree of correlation between the risk of variceal bleeding and the gradient between systemic and portal blood pressures, there is a threshold of 12 mm Hg, above which varices develop and may bleed. The experience with surgical portal-systemic shunts clearly demonstrates that reduction of this blood pressure gradient stops active bleeding and prevents

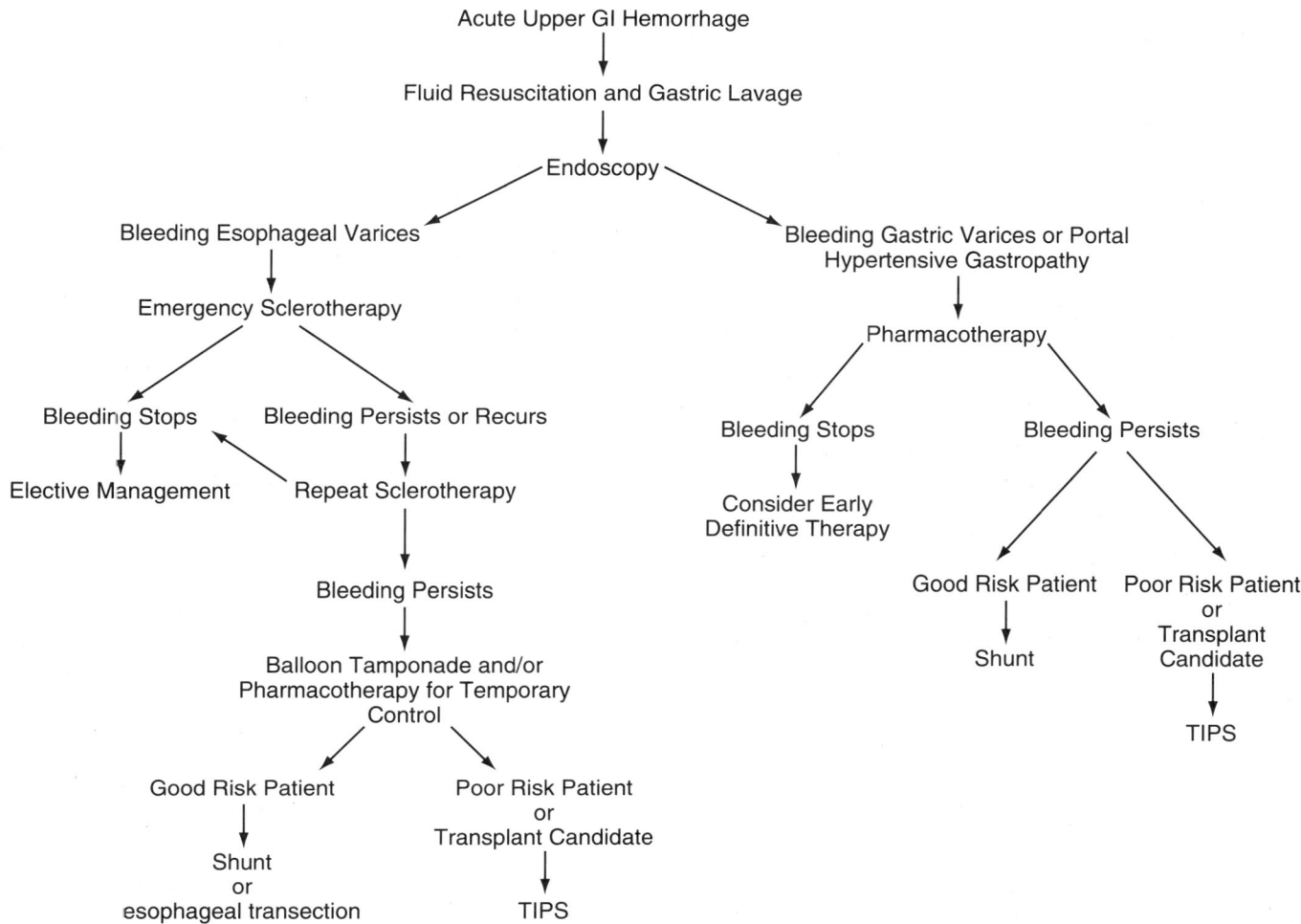

Figure 1 Algorithm for the management of bleeding varices.

subsequent bleeding. Achieving this reduction in the blood pressure gradient through pharmacologic means is an appealing concept. It might be accomplished by selectively reducing mesenteric blood flow or reducing resistance in the portal venous bed. The first objective could be accomplished with vasoconstrictors, preferably those that selectively target mesenteric blood flow. Although the resistance in the portal system is largely fixed at an increased level by the underlying liver fibrosis, the portal venous bed appears to retain some degree of vascular motor tone that can be inhibited.

Vasoconstrictors that have been used most extensively in clinical trials to reduce splanchnic blood flow include vasopressin, its analog terlipressin, and somatostatin. Although randomized trials comparing vasopressin to placebo have not consistently found vasopressin superior, meta-analysis of these studies suggests that vasopressin is effective in controlling acute variceal hemorrhage.[4] Unfortunately, its vasoactive effects are not limited to the splanchnic circulation, and both myocardial and extremity ischemia are common, life-threatening side effects. Vasodilators, especially the nitrates, when used in combination with vasopressin, significantly decrease these side effects and augment a reduction in portal venous pressure. Although only one of three randomized studies comparing vasopressin to vasopressin plus nitroglycerin found the combination therapy to be more effective at controlling hemorrhage, all three documented a marked reduction in side effects, regardless of the route of administration of the nitrates (sublingual, intravenous, or transdermal). The success rate of vasopressin and nitroglycerin in controlling acute hemorrhage in trials comparing it to sclerotherapy or vasopressin alone was 65% and 68%, respectively.[5,6]

Terlipressin is an inactive form of vasopressin that is slowly cleaved in vivo, resulting in gradual release of vasopressin. The theoretical advantage terlipressin offers is ease of administration (bolus infusion versus continuous IV infusion). The potential drawback is that ischemic side effects cannot be as easily reversed as with intravenous vasopressin. There has been little experience with terlipressin in the United States, but it has been evaluated in randomized trials in Europe. In the two randomized studies that have compared vasopressin to terlipressin, terlipressin was found to be superior in controlling variceal hemorrhage. These results, however, are somewhat counterintuitive because the active agent is vasopressin in both cases. Furthermore, the studies have some flaws, including small sample sizes and a remarkably low 9% rate of control of hemorrhage in the vasopressin group in one study and the concomitant use of balloon tamponade in both groups. If, in subsequent studies conducted in the United States, terlipressin proves to be as effective as vasopressin without increased side effects, it could become a cost-effective alternative to intravenous vasopressin.

Somatostatin and its synthetic analog, octreotide, are vasoconstrictors that appear to be more specific for the mesenteric circulation. In randomized studies, somatostatin has been shown to be more effective than placebo and equivalent to balloon tamponade in its ability to stop acute variceal bleeding. Among randomized trials comparing vasopressin to somatostatin, two studies found somatostatin to be superior in controlling acute hemorrhage.[7,8] In both studies, however, the success of vasopressin in controlling hemorrhage was surprisingly low (33% and 28%). Thus, although somatostatin may yet prove to be more effective than vasopressin and nitroglycerin, our assessment is that they are comparable in their ability to control acute bleeding. One consistent finding in studies of somatostatin has been a low incidence of side effects. Less information is available about octreotide, but, as one would expect, it too appears to be effective in controlling variceal hemorrhage.

Although several of the randomized studies suggest a benefit to using a single agent such as somatostatin to control acute variceal bleeding, our assessment is that none of these agents has yet demonstrated consistent superiority over the combination of vasopressin and nitroglycerin. Furthermore, considering both the cost of the drug and its administration, somatostatin is approximately ten times more expensive than vasopressin alone and three to four times more costly than the combination of intravenous vasopressin and nitroglycerin. These cost differences would be offset if one drug eventually proves more effective in controlling hemorrhage. When pharmacotherapy is indicated, we continue to use vasopressin and nitroglycerin. We prefer intravenous nitroglycerin to the sublingual or transdermal route because it allows for more rapid withdrawal of the drug, if the patient becomes hypotensive. The initial dose of vasopressin we use is a 20 unit bolus given over 20 minutes, followed by an infusion rate of 0.2 units/minute. Intravenous nitroglycerin is started at a rate of $0.3\mu g/kg/minute$. The dose of vasopressin is increased to 0.6 to 0.8 units/minute as needed to control bleeding, which is monitored by NG aspiration. To minimize the side effects of vasopressin, we increase nitroglycerin to levels in the range of 0.5 to $1\mu g/kg/minute$, as the patient's blood pressure allows.

BALLOON TAMPONADE

Balloon tamponade is a temporizing maneuver designed to mechanically reduce variceal blood flow and directly apply pressure to bleeding varices. The simplest device, the Linton-Nachlas tube, uses a large gastric balloon that is inflated in the stomach and pulled up against the gastroesophageal (GE) junction. The Sengstaken-Blakemore tube has a second balloon that is inflated in the esophagus to directly compress varices. Although this latter device conceptually would seem to provide more complete tamponade, there is no proven superiority of one device over the other, suggesting that reduction of variceal flow through traction at the GE junction is the most important component of this therapy. Although one of the most feared complications of balloon tamponade, rupture of the esophagus, has occurred, it is rare. The more common serious complications relate to aspiration and airway compromise. Attention to several important details minimizes this risk. First, strong consideration should be given to elective intubation prior to balloon placement, which is especially important if the patient is obtunded, as is often the case. Second, although both available tubes for balloon tamponade have lumina for aspiration of gastric contents, some do not have a port for aspiration of esophageal contents proximal to the inflated balloon. In this case a sump type of suction catheter should be positioned in the esophagus and placed on continuous suction. Finally, too much traction on the balloon, as might occur if the patient suddenly attempted to remove it, may result in migration up the esophagus and compression of the airway. A scissors must be kept nearby to cut the tube, should this occur.

Balloon tamponade has been reported in one randomized trial to control acute hemorrhage in 87% of patients, but this level of success has not been approached by any other randomized trial. In four of the five randomized trials comparing sclerotherapy to balloon tamponade, sclerotherapy was found to be significantly more effective. In a randomized trial comparing balloon tamponade with vasopressin and nitroglycerin, balloon tamponade proved more effective at controlling acute hemorrhage (87% versus 66%).

Although the reported success rate of balloon tamponade varies widely among randomized studies (42% to 87%), taken together these data suggest that balloon tamponade stops acute bleeding in the majority of patients. Its major drawback has been the high rate of rebleeding with deflation. Balloon tamponade does not appear to result in thrombosis or have any prolonged effect on varices, as evidenced by the fact that the rate of rebleeding after balloon deflation equals the rate of rebleeding without treatment. Despite this inability to favorably affect the natural history of the bleeding varices, we find this technique to be a valuable adjunct in the management of acute variceal hemorrhage not controlled by sclerotherapy. It allows time for stabilization, resuscitation, and further radiographic evaluation in preparation for more definitive intervention.

CATHETER EMBOLIZATION

The ability to access the portal vein and its branches percutaneously, in combination with techniques for angiographic occlusion of arteries and veins, offers a theoretically attractive approach to controlling acute variceal hemorrhage. The growing experience with percutaneous catheter embolization includes several uncontrolled trials. The procedure, which is technically successful in the majority of patients (71% to 94%), has been associated in some series with a relatively high incidence of complications, including intra-abdominal hemorrhage, pleural effusion, portal vein thrombosis, and death. Acute bleeding was controlled in the majority of individuals (76% to 83%), but the rates of rebleeding were high through new or recanalized variceal channels. The only randomized comparison of percutaneous embolization to a control group receiving vasopressin and balloon tamponade found no differences in control of acute hemorrhage, the rate of rebleeding, or mortality. In an effort to reduce complications and rebleeding, percutaneous angiographic occlusion of arterial splenic and gastric blood flow has been combined with variceal embolization through the superior mesenteric vein, which was accessed at celiotomy.[9] The complication rates of this approach were higher, in some cases, than those reported using the percutaneous technique. Addition of arteriographic devascularization does not appreciably improve results over variceal embolization alone. One innovative way in which variceal embolization has been used recently is in association with TIPS.[10] If, after successfully establishing a transhepatic shunt, bleeding continues, the shunt can be used to access the portal vein and embolize the varices.

These uncontrolled studies and the single randomized trial suggest that variceal embolization is effective in controlling acute bleeding. This approach, even when combined with angiographic arterial devascularization, appears to have no long-term impact on mortality or rates of rebleeding and no demonstrable benefit over pharmacotherapy and balloon tamponade.

REFERENCES

1. Sumner DS. Hemodynamics and diagnosis of arterial disease: Basic techniques and applications. In: Rutherford RB, ed. Vascular surgery. Philadelphia: WB Saunders, 1989:17.
2. Lebrec D, DeFleury P, Rueff B, et al. Portal hypertension, size of esophageal varices and risks of gastrointestinal bleeding in alcoholic cirrhosis. Gastroenterology 1980; 79:1139–1144.
3. Rector WG, Reynolds TB. Risk factors for hemorrhage from esophageal varices and acute gastric erosions. Clin Gastroenterol 1985; 14:139–153.
4. Grace ND. Variceal hemorrhage: Pharmacologic approach. In: McDermott WV, Bothe A, eds. Surgery of the liver. Boston: Blackwell Scientific, 1988:303.
5. Westaby D, Hayes PC, Gimson AES, et al. Controlled clinical trial of injection sclerotherapy for active variceal bleeding. Hepatology 1989; 9:274–277.
6. Gimson AE, Westaby D, Hegarty J, et al. A randomized trial of vasopressin and vasopressin plus nitroglycerin in the control of acute variceal hemorrhage. Hepatology 1986; 6:410–413.
7. Jenkins SA, Baxter JN, Corbett W, et al. A prospective randomized controlled clinical trial comparing somatostatin and vasopressin in controlling acute variceal haemorrhage. Br Med J 1985; 290:275–278.
8. Bagarani M, Albertini V, Anza M, et al. Effect of somatostatin in controlling bleeding from esophageal varices. Ital J Surg Sci 1987; 17:21–26.
9. Berman HL, DelGuercio LRM, Katz SG, et al. Minimally invasive devascularization for variceal bleeding that could not be controlled with sclerotherapy. Surgery 1988; 104:500–506.
10. LaBerge JM, Ring EJ, Gordon RL, et al. Creation of transjugular intrahepatic portosystemic shunts with the Wallstent endoprosthesis: Results in 100 patients. Radiology 1993; 187:413–420.

ENDOSCOPIC SCLEROTHERAPY AND LIGATION OF ESOPHAGEAL VARICES

THOMAS N. ZWENG, M.D.
WILLIAM E. STRODEL, M.D.

Hemorrhage from varices caused by portal hypertension may occur throughout the gastrointestinal (GI) tract, but most bleeding varices occur in the distal esophagus within 5 cm of the esophagogastric junction. Bleeding from varices in the gastric fundus accounts for only 10% of cases of variceal hemorrhage.

In patients with portal hypertension, all the veins of the distal esophagus become dilated. The deep submucosal veins become giant varices, and the dilated intraepithelial and superficial subepithelial vessels, lying directly over the giant varices, may be pushed toward the esophageal lumen. These superficial vessels account for the findings of cherry red spots and red wale markings on large varices, as varices on varices.

For many years, the only reliable and durable method for controlling hemorrhage from esophageal varices was operative portosystemic shunting. In the last two decades, several new modalities have been described and tested. With the exception of liver transplantation, all of these therapeutic maneuvers are palliative, in that they do not deal with the underlying obstruction in the portal system. Nonoperative attempts have been made to decrease the blood pressure in the portal system, and therefore to stop hemorrhage and decrease the likelihood that bleeding will recur. Other strategies have been directed toward obliteration of the bleeding varices, particularly varices located in the esophagus. The Japanese popularized a direct operative approach to varices by describing a technique that included variceal ligation, esophageal transection, and devascularization of the distal esophagus and proximal stomach.

A nonoperative but direct approach to esophageal varices was first described in 1928 by Crafoord and Frenckner, who injected the bleeding varices of a 19-year-old with quinine-uretan solution.[1] The procedure was performed with rigid esophagoscopy and required general anesthesia. Repeated injections were required, but the patient had a satisfactory outcome. Increased risk of general anesthesia in the patient with compromised liver function and the risk of perforation with the rigid endoscope resulted in minimal enthusiasm for this technique. The technique continued to be practiced by investigators abroad, but shunt operations became the primary mode of treatment. Interest in sclerotherapy increased in the 1970s, when dissatisfaction with shunts began to develop. European endoscopists showed that endoscopic sclerotherapy was an excellent option for the treatment of variceal bleeding. Interest in sclerotherapy increased further in the 1980s, when the therapeutic frontiers of flexible fiberoptic endoscopy were being defined. The procedure could now be done under intravenous sedation by using the fiberscope.

In 1986, endoscopic variceal ligation, a technique that is similar to the concept of band ligation of internal hemorrhoids was described. Variceal ligation avoids the injection of sclerosants, and therefore should eliminate many of the complications associated with sclerotherapy.

ENDOSCOPIC SCLEROTHERAPY

For the initial treatment of upper GI hemorrhage, it is important to establish the diagnosis quickly. Patients with stigmata of portal hypertension may have a variety of causes of upper GI hemorrhage other than varices. More than one lesion may also be present. Conversely, extrahepatic portal hypertension may not be associated with liver dysfunction; therefore, varices may not be suspected in this group of patients. No attempt is made initially to determine a cause of the portal hypertension, although patients who have arterioportal venous fistulas are less likely to respond to sclerotherapy and more likely to develop recurrent massive bleeding.

Patients who initially are candidates for sclerotherapy usually present with massive upper GI hemorrhage and may be hemodynamically unstable. It is important to resuscitate the patient before embarking on any endoscopic examination. Many patients require only crystalloid resuscitation and supplemental oxygen before safely undergoing intravenous sedation and endoscopic examination. Others require airway control with an endotracheal tube, transfusion with packed red blood cells and fresh frozen plasma, and initiation of an infusion of intravenous vasopressin. If the patient presents to the Emergency Department early in the course of the hemorrhage, an attempt to clear the stomach of blood is made with lavage through a large-bore orogastric tube.

A dual-channel or large single-channel therapeutic gastroscope is used for the procedure. The patient is placed in the left lateral decubitus position for the endoscopic examination. If no endotracheal tube is present, careful monitoring of the airway is requisite, with frequent oral suctioning. A general survey of the upper GI tract is performed to find a source of bleeding. The position of the patient may need to be changed to move any clot remaining in the stomach after lavage and thereby expose the entire mucosal surface. If esophageal varices are not actively bleeding, a diagnostic survey of the duodenum, stomach, and esophagus is conducted, including retroflexion of the endoscope to view the proximal stomach and esophagogastric junction. The esophageal varices are carefully viewed for any signs of recent hemorrhage or findings suggesting a high likelihood of bleeding, such as a red wale sign or cherry red spots. If varices are actively bleeding, sclerotherapy is frequently performed before surveying the remainder of the upper GI tract. If no other lesions are found, but the varices have stigmata of high risk for bleeding, sclerotherapy is performed after evaluating the duodenum and stomach.

We do not routinely use an overtube for sclerotherapy. Occasionally, the endoscope must be withdrawn to permit removal of an adherent clot that obstructs the viewing lens.

A variety of sclerosants have been used alone or in combination, including alcohol, cefazolin, thrombin, tetradecyl sodium, ethanolamine oleate, polidocanol, sodium morrhuate, hypertonic glucose, and hypertonic saline. The most commonly used sclerosants in the United States are 1% to 3% tetradecyl sodium and 5% sodium morrhuate solutions. In clinical trials, no survival advantage has been documented for any single sclerosant or combination of agents. Using a less concentrated (1.5%) solution of sodium morrhuate may be as efficacious for controlling hemorrhage but reduce the number and degree of mucosal ulcerations. We use 5% sodium morrhuate and restrict the volume injected per variceal column and total volume per session.

The sclerosant is delivered via a disposable syringe attached to a catheter with a retractable needle passing through a polyethylene sheath. The needle protrudes from the tip of the sheath a distance of 4 to 6 mm.

Two injection techniques have been used: (1) the paravariceal and (2) the intravariceal techniques. In the former, multiple injections of small volumes of sclerosant are made along the variceal columns in the distal esophagus for a distance of 5 to 10 cm proximally in the esophagus. The result of paravariceal injection is the production of a fibrotic, protective covering to the varix without disrupting the collateral pathway function of the venous channels. Although the paravariceal technique of sclerotherapy has been popular in Europe, the technique is not widely practiced in the United

States and has been mainly superseded by the obliterative technique.

Intravariceal injection is performed by most American endoscopists. From 1 to 3 ml of sclerosant are injected directly into the variceal lumen. Injections are started at the level of the esophagogastric junction and proceed proximally for a distance of only 5 cm. The goal is thrombosis of the varix at the site of injection. The pH of sodium morrhuate is 9 to 10. Contact of this agent with vascular endothelium produces a prompt inflammatory reaction. When the injection is performed, the endoscopist should observe distention and blanching of the varix. Submucosal hemorrhage may also be noted. A slight degree of oozing may be present at the conclusion of the session. Irrigation of the esophageal lumen through the endoscope may be necessary to distinguish persistent bleeding from regurgitated blood. The total volume of sclerosant injected at the initial session is usually 20 ml. On occasion, this total may be exceeded, but increasing the volume injected per varix or the number of injection sites increases the likelihood of stricture formation or the severity of ulceration.

Combination intravariceal and paravariceal therapy frequently occur, not by intention, but by accident. Even in the cooperative patient, respiratory, cardiac, esophageal, and sometimes gastric motion interferes with the precise insertion of the sclerotherapy needle. The injection that is intended to be paravariceal may be introduced into the variceal lumen. In addition, it is sometimes advantageous to perform a subendothelial injection to raise a wheal in that layer. Subendothelial injections above and below the level of the bleeding site produce compression of the hole in the varix and decrease the rate of bleeding while the inflammatory response to the sclerosant is developing.

The endoscope is frequently passed into the stomach to decompress the trapped air that accumulates secondary to insufflation. The endoscope may also tamponade the varices while the tip remains in the stomach. Some endoscopists have advocated the use of an overtube or a balloon to provide tamponade after injections. The senior author used both these devises early in his experience but was not impressed that either one provided any advantage by reducing the rate of bleeding or hastening thrombosis of the varices. We do not routinely place a nasogastric tube after the procedure.

Complications of sclerotherapy may result from the endoscopic procedure (pulmonary aspiration, reaction to sedation, perforation) or from the systemic or local effects of the injected sclerosant. Mechanical perforation of the esophagus is less likely to occur with the use of the flexible fiberoptic endoscope compared to the rigid endoscope.

Precipitation of hemorrhage from laceration of a varix by the injector needle has been reported but is usually treated by sclerotherapy or balloon tamponade. Pulmonary effects have been reported in as many as 80% of patients with chest x-ray as an indicator. Aspiration can be minimized by endotracheal intubation and careful attention to the patient's airway during the procedure. Most of the radiographic changes demonstrated clear spontaneously without active treatment.

The systemic effects of the sclerosant depend on the agent. Transient decrease in pulmonary function has been reported with ethanolamine oleate but not with tetradecyl sodium or sodium morrhuate. Other systemic effects include bacteremia, distant venous thrombosis, and fever. The fever is usually self-limited. The potential of developing bacteremia suggests the use of prophylactic antibiotics in patients who have previously implanted prosthetic materials or ascites. Thrombosis of the portal vein and the mesenteric veins has been reported infrequently. The presumed mechanism is direct contact with the venous endothelium in those instances where there is reversal of flow through the venous collaterals toward the liver.

Substernal pain is frequently noted immediately after injection of the sclerosant. The pain may be due to local effects of the sclerosant or esophageal spasm and usually resolves spontaneously without specific treatment. Transient dysphagia is also observed in a majority of patients after a sclerotherapy session.

Ulceration at the site of injection occurs in the vast majority of patients within 1 week of treatment. The degree and extent of ulceration depend on the volume of sclerosant injected per varix and the distribution of the injections with the esophagus. Care should be taken not to inject deeply into the esophageal wall in order to decrease the likelihood of perforation. When we first started performing sclerotherapy, we injected columns at several levels and used large volumes of sclerosant. The ulcerations that developed involved a significant length of the esophagus, and many of the ulcers were deep. One perforation that was contained was documented with water-soluble contrast and treated expectantly with antibiotics. Ulceration also appears to be exacerbated by prolonged balloon tamponade either before or after sclerotherapy. The combination of pressure and sclerosant is particularly injurious to the esophageal mucosa.

Occurrence of ulceration raises concern for rebleeding when the eschar sloughs into the esophageal lumen. If the underlying varix has thrombosed, bleeding is minimal. Rebleeding from ulcer slough occurs in 2% to 13% of patients. Because all the varices are unlikely to be occluded after the first treatment with sclerotherapy, other varices may bleed before complete obliteration is achieved; they account for most of the reports of rebleeding. We use acid-suppression therapy to reduce the degree of acid reflux into the distal esophagus. In addition, we use sucralfate to provide a protective layer to the ulcer once it forms.

Extensive or deep ulceration may result in esophageal stricture in nearly 10% of patients undergoing sclerotherapy. Usually the stricture is short in length and easily managed by esophageal dilation with a wire-guided dilator. We recommend waiting until the varices are obliterated before performing the dilation. We have not had to dilate the stricture more than twice in any patient. Esophageal motility seems not to be impaired in

Table 1 Comparison of Sclerotherapy Versus Medical Therapy for Variceal Hemorrhage Prospective Studies

Author	Year	EIS/Med Rx†	Rebleeding	Rebleeding Episodes	% Survival
Barsoum et al.[2]	1982	50/50	13/29*	—	70/48*
Paquet and Feussner[3]	1985	21/22	4/7	—	67/33*
Soderlund and Ihre[4]	1985	57/50	32/33	50/99*	49/34
Terblanche et al.[5]	1983	37/38	14/20	43/73*	38/37
Westaby et al.[6]	1985	56/60	31/49	66/125*	68/47*

*Significant difference.
†EIS = endoscopic injection sclerosis.

Table 2 Comparison of Sclerotherapy Versus Shunt Operation for Variceal Hemorrhage Prospective Studies

Author	Year	Shunt/EIS	% Rebleeding	% Salvage Operations	% Survival
Cello et al.[7]	1987	24/28	21/50	11	17/32
Warren et al.[8]	1987	35/36	3/53	31	51/75
Rikkers et al.[9]	1987	27/30	19/57	7	65/61
Teres et al.[10]	1987	42/48	14/38	6	71/68

studies that have been performed 2 weeks after treatment.

After the initial sclerotherapy treatment, additional sessions are required to achieve obliteration. The timing of the repeat sessions must be balanced between a desire to obliterate the varices as soon as possible and the development of mucosal ulceration. Most endoscopists use a 7 to 21 day cycle for treatments. Once the varices are obliterated, the patient usually undergoes an examination at 6 and 12 months to ensure persistent obliteration. Small varices may not be injected at these times, if they appear in the mid-esophagus and are not columnar.

Results

Summary results of five prospective controlled studies comparing sclerotherapy and medical therapy are revealing (Table 1). The incidence of rebleeding was less in the sclerotherapy groups, and the survival rates were also significantly better in the patients treated with sclerotherapy. Combined data from several trials subjected to meta-analysis suggest that sclerotherapy reduces the likelihood of death from variceal hemorrhage by 25%.

Summary data from four prospective clinical trials comparing sclerotherapy to shunt operations are revealing (Table 2). Cello and co-workers' study was the only one to use portacaval shunt;[7] the others used splenorenal shunts. Only Warren and associates' study documented a survival advantage for sclerotherapy, although 31% of patients who were initially treated with sclerotherapy required a shunt operation.[8] In the other studies there is no difference in survival between the two types of treatment.

The Veterans Administration Cooperative Trial documented greater mortality in patients who were receiving prophylactic sclerotherapy than in a group receiving medical therapy. Unless a good method is devised for identifying patients at high risk for bleeding from varices—two-thirds of all patients with varices do not bleed—prophylactic sclerotherapy is not indicated.

LIGATION OF ESOPHAGEAL VARICES

Endoscopic ligation of esophageal varices is performed in a similar fashion to sclerotherapy. The patient undergoes resuscitation and survey of the upper gastrointestinal tract for other lesions. An overtube is used because the endoscope must be withdrawn after each banding in order to mount a new band and cylinder. The banding begins with the varix that is bleeding or, if no varices are actively bleeding but variceal bleeding is suspected, the most distal varix is banded first. The banding then proceeds proximally for a distance of 5 cm. Re-entering the stomach with the endoscope is avoided to prevent dislodging of the bands on ligated varices.

A target varix is identified and suction is applied through the endoscope channel to draw the varix into the cylinder mounted on the tip of the endoscope. Once the varix is within the cylinder opening, the trip wire is pulled and the band is released around the mucosa and varix. The cylinder impedes the view through the endoscope so that the survey of the gastrointestinal tract should be done before fitting the endoscope for banding. A recent improvement in the cylinder uses clear plastic and produces an expanded view of the esophageal lumen.

Initial control of variceal bleeding is accomplished equally well with sclerotherapy and band ligation. Repeat ligation is usually required to achieve obliteration of varices. Additional sessions are performed every two weeks. Rebleeding occurs at a rate similar to

Table 3 Comparison of Sclerotherapy Versus Ligation for Variceal Hemorrhage Prospective Studies

Author	Year	EIS/EVL*	No. Sessions to Obliteration	Stricture (%)	Ulceration (%)	Rebleeding (%)
Laine et al.[11]	1993	39/38	6.2/4.1	33/0	15/2.6	26/44
Young et al.[12]	1993	13/10	6.2/3.6	—	83/100	8/10
Gimson et al.[13]	1993	49/54	4.9/3.4	0/0	57/67	53/30
Stiegmann et al.[14]	1992	65/64	5/4	12/0	—	48/36

*EVL = endoscopic variceal ligation.

sclerotherapy until the varices are eradicated. After obliteration, rebleeding is unusual.

Complications after band ligation are significantly fewer than after sclerotherapy. Although nearly all patients who undergo band ligation develop ulceration, the ulcers are small and superficial. Conversely, 25% of patients undergoing sclerotherapy develop deep ulcers. The bands remain in place for 5 to 7 days, until the resultant coagulative necrosis begins to slough. The inflammation appears confined to the superficial submucosa. Stricture rarely occurs with band ligation. Bacteremia has been reported with band ligation, but the incidence was lower than with sclerotherapy.

Laine and associates documented that there was no difference between band ligation and sclerotherapy with regard to recurrent bleeding, volume of blood transfused, length of hospitalization, and survival[11] (Table 3). The studies by Young,[12] Gimson,[13] and their colleagues documented a decreased time to obliteration but no survival advantage to either technique. In the study by Stiegmann and co-workers, there was a survival advantage for band ligation.[14]

Massive variceal hemorrhage from insertion of the overtube, esophageal perforation from the overtube, and acute obstruction of the esophageal lumen have been recorded as isolated case reports. It has been suggested that the overtube be introduced over a tapered esophageal dilator to avoid the pinching effect of advancing the larger overtube over a smaller-diameter endoscope. With another technique, the endoscope is advanced more rapidly than the overtube when the overtube reaches the level of the cricopharygeous. Some studies document an additional advantage to the use of the overtube, less pulmonary aspiration. Complications from the band ligation remain unusual.

Sclerotherapy and band ligation are not mutually exclusive treatments for esophageal varices. Hashizume and colleagues have described in a controlled clinical trial the use of band ligation followed by sclerotherapy with ethanolamine oleate.[15] Patients required less sclerosant to obliterate varices and had fewer complications than patients treated with sclerotherapy alone. Using the two techniques at the same session has also been described in preliminary reports. The number of sessions required to achieve obliteration is reduced from an average of 4.4 for sclerotherapy to 1.2 for the combination therapy. Band ligation may also be used if sclerotherapy fails because of rebleeding.

The role of transjugular intrahepatic portosystemic shunts (TIPS) in the management of acute variceal bleeding is currently being defined. In addition, how sclerotherapy, band ligation, and TIPS will be integrated remains undetermined. Algorithms must be developed, tested, and proven before the best method for managing variceal hemorrhage can be recommended. In addition to the traditional aspects of morbidity and mortality, the economic aspects of the different modalities will play a major role in defining the correct mix of techniques. Some combination of these methods will probably emerge to bridge many of the patients to liver transplantation, the most definitive treatment for portal hypertension due to hepatic causes.

REFERENCES

1. Crafoord C, Frenckner P. New surgical treatment of varicous veins of the oesophagus. Acta Otolaryngol (Stockh) 1928; 27:422–429.
2. Barsoum M, Bolous F, El-Rooby A, et al. Tamponade and injection sclerotherapy in the management of bleeding oesophageal varices. Br J Surg 1982; 69:76–78.
3. Paquet KJ, Feussner H. Endoscopic sclerosis and esophageal balloon tamponade in acute hemorrhage from esophagogastric varices: A prospective controlled randomized trial. Hepatology 1985; 5:580–585.
4. Soderland C, Ihre T. Endoscopic sclerotherapy v. conservative management of bleeding esophageal varices: A 5 year prospective controlled trial of emergency and long term treatment. Acta Chir Scand 1985; 151:449–453.
5. Terblanche J, Bornman P, Kahn D, et al. Failure of repeated injection sclerotherapy to improve long-term survival after oesophageal variceal bleeding: A five year prospective controlled clinical trial. Lancet 1983; 2:1328–1330.
6. Westaby D, Macdougall B, Williams R. Improved survival following injection sclerotherapy for esophageal varices: Final analysis of a controlled trial. Hepatology 1985; 5:827–831.
7. Cello J, Grendell J, Crass R, et al. Endoscopic sclerotherapy versus portacaval shunt in patients with severe cirrhosis and acute variceal hemorrhage: Long-term follow-up. N Engl J Med 1987; 316:11–15.
8. Warren WD, Henderson JM, Millikan JW, et al. Distal splenorenal shunt versus endoscopic sclerotherapy for long-term management of variceal bleeding: Preliminary report of a prospective, randomized trial. Ann Surg 1987; 203:454–459.
9. Rikkers LF, Burnett DA, Volentine GD, et al. Shunt surgery versus endoscopic sclerotherapy for long-term treatment of variceal bleeding: Early results of a randomized trial Ann Surg 1987; 206:261–267.
10. Teres J, Bordas JM, Bravo D, et al. Sclerotherapy vs. distal splenorenal shunt in the elective treatment of variceal hemorrhage: A randomized controlled trial. Hepatology 1987; 7:430–436.

11. Laine L, El-Newihi H, Migikovsky B, et al. Endoscopic ligation compared with sclerotherapy for the treatment of bleeding esophageal varices. Ann Intern Med 1993; 119:1–7.
12. Young MF, Sanowski RA, Rasche R. Comparison and characterization of ulcerations induced by endoscopic ligation of esophageal varices versus endoscopic sclerotherapy. Gastrointest Endosc 1993; 39:119–122.
13. Gimson AES, Harrison PM, Hayllar K, et al. Randomised trial of variceal banding ligation versus injection sclerotherapy for bleeding oesophageal varices. Lancet 1993; 342:391–394.
14. Stiegmann GV, Goff JS, Michaletz-Onody PA, et al. Endoscopic sclerotherapy as compared with endoscopic ligation for bleeding esophageal varices. N Engl J Med 1992; 326:1527–1532.
15. Hashizume M, Ohta M, Uero K, et al. Endoscopic ligation of esophageal varices compared with injection sclerotherapy: a prospective randomized trial. Gastrointest Endosc 1993; 39: 123–126.

OPERATIVE VARICEAL LIGATION AND GASTROESOPHAGEAL DEVASCULARIZATION FOR VARICEAL HEMORRHAGE

ROBERT C. GORMAN, M.D.
ERNEST F. ROSATO, M.D.

The treatment of bleeding esophageal varices has stimulated the development of multiple therapeutic options, including medical, endoscopic, and surgical approaches. The goals common to all include control of acute hemorrhage, prevention of recurrent hemorrhage, and preservation of hepatic function. Currently, the consensus is that acute hemorrhage should be treated initially with endoscopic sclerotherapy. The optimal treatment of sclerotherapy failures and prevention of recurrent hemorrhage remain an area of debate. The relatively recent introduction of two new treatment modalities, liver transplantation and transjugular intrahepatic portosystemic shunts, has made therapeutic decision making even more complex. Nonselective shunts—portocaval, mesocaval, and central splenorenal shunts—had long been considered the standard surgical therapy for bleeding varices. These operations effectively stop bleeding; however, associated encephalopathy and accelerated liver failure resulting from the loss of hepatic portal perfusion have led to dissatisfaction with these shunts.

Warren and associates subsequently developed the distal splenorenal shunt (DSRS) in an attempt to reduce the incidence of encephalopathy and liver failure. The theoretic goal of this procedure is to decompress varices while maintaining hepatic portal perfusion. Several randomized trials have proven the efficacy of the DSRS in preventing recurrent hemorrhage. Extended follow-up, however, has documented a tendency for loss of prograde venous flow. The incidence of clinical or subclinical encephalopathy was reported by Warren and co-workers to occur in up to 30% of their patients over a mean follow-up period of 7 years.[1]

The desire to prevent the encephalopathy and hepatic failure associated with shunt operations has led to the development of procedures designed to ablate varices directly while maintaining portal flow. This type of procedure also provides an alternative for patients in whom a DSRS is contraindicated (Table 1). These alternative procedures employ varying combinations of esophagogastric devascularization, esophageal transection, and direct variceal ligation (Table 2). The introduction of easy-to-use automatic stapling devices for esophageal transection and reanastomosis has helped to stimulate renewed interest in these nonshunting procedures.

VARICEAL LIGATION

In most patients, surgical control of gastrointestinal hemorrhage consists of a direct approach to the bleeding site. Boerema and Crile, applying this concept, employed direct suture ligation of bleeding submucosal esophageal varices.[2] Others have recommended direct ligation as a temporizing procedure prior to a definitive shunt. The

Table 1 Contraindications to Distal Splenorenal Shunting

Severe ascites
Renal vein hypertension
Aberrant splenic vein anatomy
Previous splenectomy
Extrahepatic portal vein thrombosis
Previous failed shunt

Table 2 Nonshunting Operations for Bleeding Varices

Procedure	Indication
Variceal ligation	None
Splenectomy	Gastric varices due to splenic vein thrombosis
Esophageal transection	Acute sclerotherapy failures
Devascularization without transection (Hassab)	Bilharzial cirrhosis
Devascularization and transection (Sugiura, Rosato)	Distal splenorenal shunt contraindicated or surgeon's preference

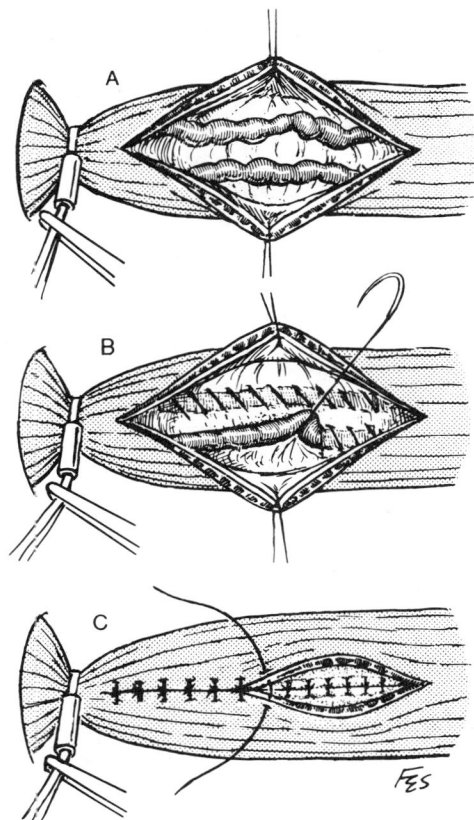

Figure 1 Variceal ligation. *A,* An esophagotomy is performed for 6 to 8 cm proximal to the gastroesophageal junction. *B,* Variceal columns are identified and oversewn with a running suture. *C,* The esophagotomy is closed in two layers. (From Rossi RL, Jenkins RL, Nielsen-Whitcomb FF. Management of complications of portal hypertension. Surg Clin N Am 1985; 65:231–262; with permission.)

procedure is performed via a left seventh interspace thoracotomy. The esophagus is isolated and periesophageal veins are ligated. An esophagotomy is then performed at the gastroesophageal junction and extended proximally 6 to 8 cm. Columns of varices are identified and oversewn with running sutures. The esophagus is closed in two layers (Fig. 1). The theoretical advantage of this operation is that it provides rapid control of bleeding while preserving hepatic perfusion. However, recurrent bleeding is commonplace, as varices recur with the development of new portal-azygos collaterals.

Transthoracic suture ligation of varices requires a major operation, usually on debilitated patients, and often does not provide definitive long-term control of bleeding. Endoscopic sclerotherapy, because of its effectiveness, relative safety, and widespread availability, has largely supplanted direct suture ligation as a method for arresting hemorrhage from acutely bleeding esophageal varices.

SPLENECTOMY

Splenectomy alone is ineffective in stopping esophageal variceal hemorrhage. This procedure is, however, efficacious in stopping bleeding from isolated gastric varices that results from sinistral portal hypertension secondary to splenic vein thrombosis. In this situation, splenectomy serves to interrupt the collateral flow from the pancreas and spleen through the upper stomach and thence to the coronary vein.

DEVASCULARIZATION WITHOUT ESOPHAGEAL TRANSECTION

Hassab has described an extensive gastric devascularization procedure without esophageal or gastric transection for the treatment of bleeding varices in patients with schistosomiasis.[3] Patients with bilharzial portal hypertension are usually young, have normal liver function, and are particularly likely to develop encephalopathy after shunting procedures. Encephalopathy occurs in 60% of patients after nonselective shunts and up to 30% after DSRS.[4] Use of an effective nonshunting procedure is therefore highly desirable in this patient population. Hassab's procedure involves ligation of the left gastric, gastroepiploic, and short gastric vessels, as well as any intra-abdominal periesophageal veins. A splenectomy is also performed. In 355 patients, the reported operative mortality was 12%, with a late rebleeding rate of 3%. No patient developed encephalopathy. It is difficult to extrapolate the excellent results of this procedure in the typically young patient with normal liver function and schistosomiasis to the patients commonly requiring treatment in the United States. Nevertheless, excellent results continue to be reported by Hassab and others using this procedure in bilharzial cirrhosis and should be reproducible in good-risk patients with varying etiologies for their portal hypertension.

ESOPHAGEAL TRANSECTION

Esophageal transection with subsequent reanastomosis obliterates esophageal varices and is conceptually similar to endoscopic sclerotherapy and direct ligation. Renewed interest in this procedure resulted from the development of easy-to-use circular stapling devices that are capable of transection and reanastomosis with a single application of the device. This operation is performed most effectively and with the least morbidity via a transabdominal approach. Through an anterior gastrotomy, an EEA stapling device is introduced into the esophagus. A ligature is tied around the esophagus between the anvil and cartridge of the stapler approximately 2 cm above the gastroesophageal junction, and the stapler is fired (Fig. 2). Some authors recommend adding coronary vein ligation to decrease the incidence of recurrent varices.[2,5]

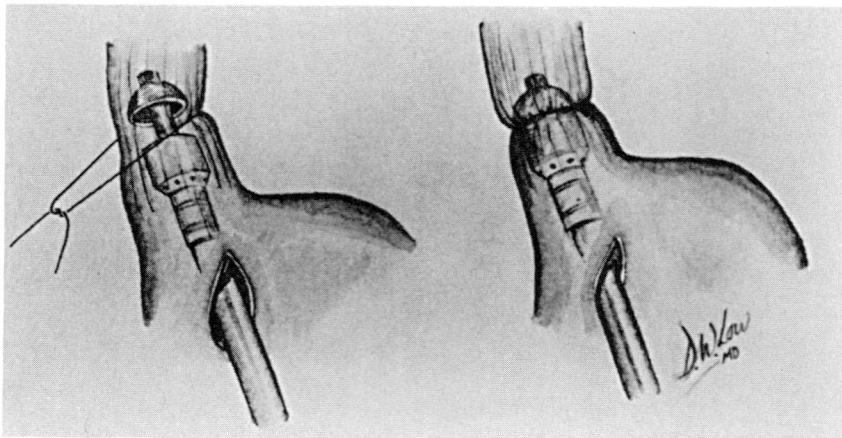

Figure 2 Esophageal transection. An EEA stapling device is introduced via an anterior gastrotomy. A tie is then placed around the esophagus between the cartridge and the anvil prior to firing the stapler.

A recent randomized prospective study comparing emergent esophageal transection with endoscopic sclerotherapy has documented that transection is equal to or better than the sclerotherapy for arresting acute hemorrhage.[6] The authors of this study recommend esophageal transection in the acutely bleeding patient who has failed two attempts at sclerotherapy. Whereas esophageal transection is effective in stopping acute hemorrhage, late rebleeding rates approach 33%, even with the addition of coronary vein ligation.[2] As with other direct approaches to variceal hemorrhage, esophageal transection results in suboptimal long-term control of bleeding.

COMBINED DEVASCULARIZATION AND TRANSECTION PROCEDURES

McIndoe in 1928 documented the importance of the coronary vein in development of periesophageal and submucosal collaterals to the azygos system in patients with portal hypertension.[7] Understanding the significance of this pathologic shunting has led to the development of several procedures designed to sever the portal-azygos connections responsible for esophageal varices. This approach involves varying combinations of esophagogastric devascularization and esophageal or gastric transection.

Sugiura and Futagawa in 1973 introduced a procedure designed to obliterate the submucosal component of the portal-azygos collaterals but at the same time maintain the periesophageal connections. The theoretic advantage was that preservation of the extra esophageal venous channels would prevent variceal recurrence. In their hands, the procedure has had unparalleled success, with an operative mortality of 4.3%, a late rebleeding rate of 1.5%, and no encephalopathy in 671 patients.[8] The operation as described by Sugiura and Futagawa includes first esophagogastric devascularization from the inferior pulmonary vein to the angularis incisuria. Care is taken to ligate vessels close to the walls of the esophagus and stomach to preserve periesophageal portal-azygos connections. Second, transection and reanastomosis of the esophagus are performed to obliterate submucosal and intramural collaterals. Third, splenectomy is performed to decrease portal venous flow. Fourth, pyloroplasty is necessitated by the vagotomy effect produced by devascularization. The procedure is accomplished in one operation or by staged thoracic and abdominal incisions as the patient's condition dictates (Fig. 3). The exceptional results reported by Sugiura and Futagawa have not been reproduced in studies from Western societies. Perhaps this reflects a difference in the patient population and the etiology of portal hypertension. In the Japanese series, 25% of the patients were noncirrhotic, only 10% were alcoholic, and 30% of the operations were done prophylactically.

Over the past 15 years, the senior author has developed a modified version of the Sugiura procedure for the treatment of esophageal varices secondary to hepatic cirrhosis. The current operation has evolved as experience was gained from operating upon 40 unselected cirrhotic patients with recent or ongoing hemorrhage due to varices.[9] The operation is performed through a left eighth interspace thoracotomy with access to the abdominal cavity by a circumferencial diaphragmatic incision. Devascularization along the lesser curvature of the stomach is accomplished by ligating vessels within the lesser omentum rather than at the gastric wall to lessen the potential for ischemic necrosis of the upper stomach. Ligation of the right gastric artery at the angularis incisura is performed to discourage recanalization of the left gastric artery. The procedure has been further modified to include truncal vagotomy and ligation of the collateral azygos veins. These steps serve to simplify the procedure technically. Azygos preservation is unnecessary after ligation of the coronary vein in the lesser omentum. The esophageal venous ligation is extended up to the inferior pulmonary vein or even higher, if large collaterals extend above that area.

In patients who have not undergone previous

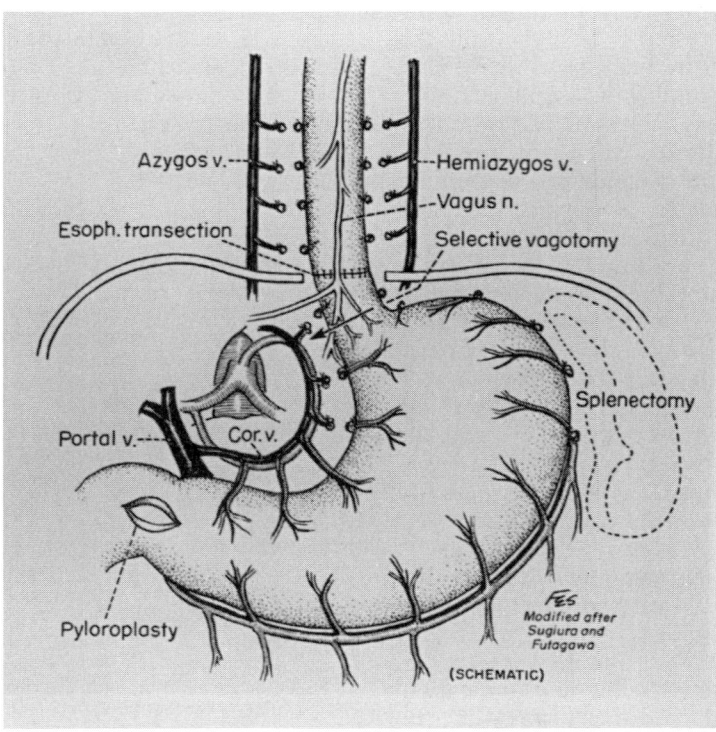

Figure 3 Schematic of the Sugiura procedure. Note that devascularization is performed at the stomach and esophageal walls to preserve coronary-azygos collaterals. (From Rossi RL, Jenkins RL, Nielsen-Whitcomb FF. Management of complications of portal hypertension. Surg Clin N Am 1985; 65:231–262; with permission.)

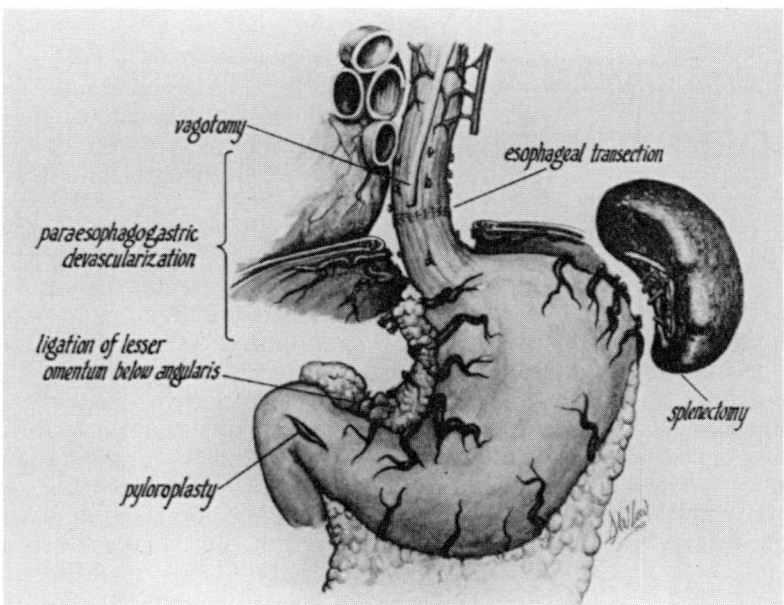

Figure 4 Modified Sugiura procedure. Devascularization is performed at the omental level, and collateral azygos veins are ligated in the chest.

sclerotherapy, esophageal transection may be performed using an EEA stapler. Transection is omitted in patients who have undergone previous sclerotherapy. Esophageal transection after sclerotherapy is technically difficult and hazardous to perform because of the intense inflammatory response surrounding the esophagus. Sclerotherapy in these patients has been sufficient to control bleeding from submucosal varices when it is combined with the devascularization and splenectomy components of the procedure. Pyloroplasty is performed in all patients. In patients undergoing transection, a fundoplication around the staple line may be added to reduce the incidence of anastomotic leak (Fig. 4). In the last several years, esophageal transection has been omitted because of the effectiveness of endoscopic techniques for obliteration of submucosal esophageal varices. Results with this procedure have been excellent in Child's class A and B patients, with an operative mortality of 14% and late rebleeding rate of 17%. Mortality in Child's class C patients, however, approaches 60%. In these patients, other techniques should be utilized because of the high operative mortality.

The choice between a portosystemic shunt and a devascularization procedure in cases of elective operation must consider the hepatic reserve of the patient, the skill of the surgeon, and the potential effects of encephalopathy on the life and livelihood of the patient and the patient's family. Both procedures can be difficult technically; they are best applied in good-risk patients and in elective situations. Child's class C patients are probably best served by liver transplantation.

Finally, transabdominal staple transection of the esophagus is effective for immediate control of bleeding. The long-term efficacy of this operation is questionable, but it should be considered in the management of acute failures of repeated sclerotherapy and for the immediate control of refractory bleeding in poor-risk patients.

REFERENCES

1. Warren WD, Millikan MD, Henderson JM, et al. Ten years of portal hypertension surgery at Emory. Ann Surg 1982; 195:530–542.
2. Wexler MJ, Stein BL. Nonshunting operations for variceal hemorrhage. Surg Clin North Am 1990; 70:425–448.
3. Hassab MA. Gastroesophageal decongestion and splenectomy in the treatment of esophageal varices in bilharzial cirrhosis: Further studies with a report of 355 operations. Surgery 1967; 61:169–176.
4. Raia S, Mies S, Macedo AL. Surgical treatment of portal hypertension in schistomsomiasis. World J Surg 1984; 8:738–752.
5. Wexler MJ. Treatment of bleeding esophageal varices by transabdominal esophageal transection with the EEA stapling instrument. Surgery 1980; 88:406–411.
6. Burroughs AK, Hamilton G, Phillips A, et al. A comparison of sclerotherapy with staple transection of the esophagus for the emergency control of bleeding esophageal varices. N Engl J Med 1989; 321:857–862.
7. Chandler JG. The history of the surgical treatment of portal hypertension. Arch Surg 1993; 128:925–940.
8. Sugiura M, Futagawa S. Esophageal transection with paraesophagogastric devascularization (the Sugiura procedure) in the treatment of esophageal varices. World J Surg 1984; 8:673–680.
9. Barbot DJ, Rosato EF. Experience with the esophagogastric devascularization procedure. Surgery 1987; 101:685–689.

DECOMPRESSIVE SHUNTS FOR VARICEAL HEMORRHAGE

ATEF A. SALAM, M.D.

The definition of a total shunt is a portasystemic anastomosis designed to decompress the entire portal circulatory bed. Examples include portacaval, mesocaval, and central splenorenal shunts. The definition of a selective shunt is a portasystemic anastomosis designed to decompress the variceal bed while maintaining portal blood flow to the liver. Examples include the distal splenorenal and coronocaval shunts.

TOTAL SHUNTS

The portacaval shunt is the oldest and most extensively evaluated total shunt. Its efficacy in the control of variceal bleeding has been well established. However, randomized trials to evaluate the procedure—first in the prevention of variceal bleeding as a prophylactic shunt and then in the prevention of recurrence of bleeding as a therapeutic shunt—have documented no difference in survival between patients who are medically managed and those who receive operation.[1] According to these studies, the benefit realized by 95% control of bleeding in surgically treated patients is offset by death from postshunt liver failure. In addition, hepatic encephalopathy has been shown to be a major cause of morbidity in portacaval shunt patients.

The portacaval shunt is the most durable shunt in terms of long-term patency. The classic technique consists of an end-to-side portacaval anastomosis. More recently, Sarfeh and associates have proposed a small (8 mm) interposition H-graft to achieve partial decompression of the portal system, which is sufficient to control bleeding but not to divert all prograde portal flow.[2] Further evaluation of this procedure is needed to determine whether partial portal decompression can be achieved without an undue rise in shunt occlusion rate.

In the 1970s, the H-graft interposition mesocaval shunt became increasingly popular because it was perceived by many as a technically easier operation than the conventional portacaval shunt. Consequently, the procedure became the operation of choice in an emergency situation. One drawback for using a prosthetic graft is the increased risk of delayed shunt occlusion.

The central splenorenal shunt is currently rarely used. Splenectomy in the setting of portal hypertension adds to the complexity of the operation. The procedure has no physiologic advantage over the portacaval shunt, and there is evidence that it has a higher incidence of failure due to shunt thrombosis.

SELECTIVE SHUNTS

The object of selective shunting is to achieve variceal decompression without interfering with antegrade flow of portal blood to the liver. Preservation of this important component of liver blood supply is designed to prevent the two most serious complications of portasystemic shunting, namely, postshunt encephalopathy and progressive liver deterioration. The distal splenorenal or Warren shunt (DSRS) is designed to achieve these objectives (Fig. 1).[3,4] In this procedure the splenic vein is divided. Its splenic end is anastomosed end-to-side to the left renal vein. The other end of the splenic vein is oversewn. The low pressure system thus constructed consists of the short gastric and the left gastroepiploic veins, the splenic pulp, and the splenic vein. Venous return from the stomach is diverted to this low pressure system, across the anastomosis, to the left renal vein. With relief of gastric venous congestion, the variceal bed is decompressed, and the objective of prevention of rebleeding is achieved. By design, the DSRS does not lower the blood pressure in the superior mesenteric or the portal veins. High portal venous perfusion pressure is essential to maintaining antegrade portal blood flow in the presence of cirrhosis. It is important in this procedure to interrupt collateral venous channels between the high-pressure mesoportal venous system and the decompressed branches of the splenic vein. Otherwise, with time, these collaterals will enlarge and result in significant diversion of portal blood away from the liver from a high-pressure zone to a low-pressure zone.

PATIENT SELECTION AND PREOPERATIVE PATIENT PREPARATION

Varices that have never bled do not warrant sclerotherapy or surgical intervention. In acute variceal bleeding, injection treatment is highly successful. For long-term treatment, sclerotherapy is used until the variceal bed has been eradicated. The selective shunt is indicated for patients who fail to respond to chronic sclerotherapy. Our studies have documented that better results are obtained by this approach than by the selective shunt as the primary treatment (Fig. 2).[5] Shunt operations should be avoided in patients with poor liver reserve (Child's C class patients). Preoperative preparation for selective shunting includes correction of existing ascites and malnutrition. Preoperative angiographic studies include selective splenic and superior mesenteric arterial injections with serial radiographic evaluation of the portal system during the venous phase. Phlebography of the left renal vein is also obtained to confirm its suitability for splenorenal shunt construction.

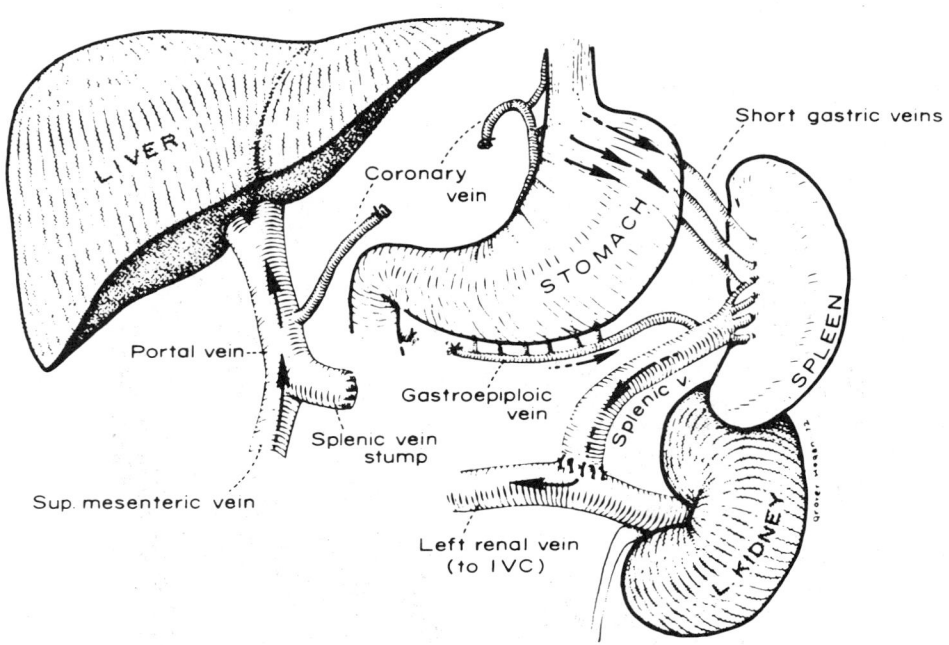

Figure 1 Diagrammatic representation of the distal splenorenal shunt.

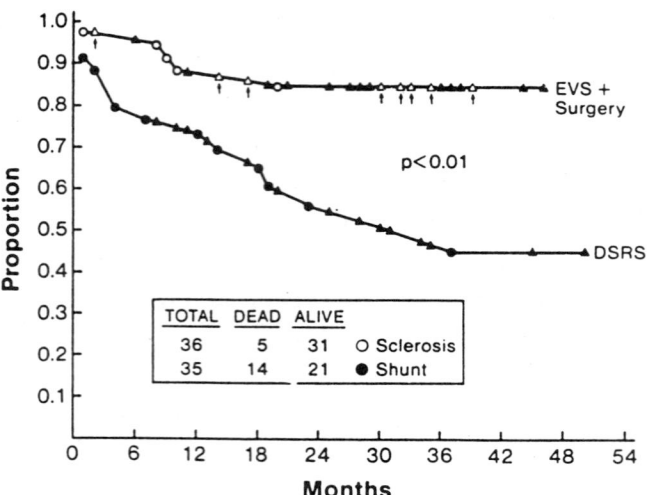

Figure 2 Kaplan-Meier plot of survival curve for sclerosis *(open circles)* and distal splenorenal shunt (DSRS; *black circles*). The randomized sclerosis group, with adjuvant surgery for 31% of patients, has significantly improved survival compared to DSRS. Black triangles represent censored observations: data are analyzed on a monthly basis; hence some points are duplicated. Arrows pointing to open triangles represent censored sclerosis patients who have required surgery and are still alive. (From Warren WD, Henderson JM, Millikan WJ, et al. Distal splenorenal versus endoscopic sclerotherapy for long term management of variceal bleeding. Preliminary report of a prospective randomized trial. Ann Surg 1986; 203:454–462; with permission.)

The diameter of the splenic vein and the distance between it and the left renal vein are assessed radiographically. It is rare that the distance between the two vessels is so great as to require modification of the procedure. There is a higher risk of shunt occlusion with splenic veins less than 1 cm in diameter in patients with coexistent pancreatic inflammation.

Traditionally, the DSRS is performed through a left subcostal incision starting from the left midaxillary line to the right border of the right rectus muscle. In patients who have had previous abdominal operations through a vertical incision, the author's preference is to use the same incision to avoid undue weakening of the abdominal wall.

The greater curvature of the stomach is mobilized by dividing its peritoneal attachment from the pylorus to the point of origin of the first short gastric vein. The lesser sac is entered, and dissection is started at the lower border of the pancreas to expose the splenic vein. A search for the splenic vein is begun medially, where it is more accessible, and once the vessel is identified, it is carefully mobilized in the retropancreatic plane. The most technically demanding aspect of this procedure is the isolation of numerous pancreatic tributaries, which requires delicate dissection because of their tendency to bleed. After the splenic vein is adequately mobilized, the left renal vein is exposed. The splenic vein is then divided and its central end oversewn. With proper orientation, the splenic end of the splenic vein is anastomosed to the side of the left renal vein by using standard vascular techniques. The shunt should not be under any tension, and there should be no redundancy of the splenic vein. The operation is completed by ligating the coronary vein.

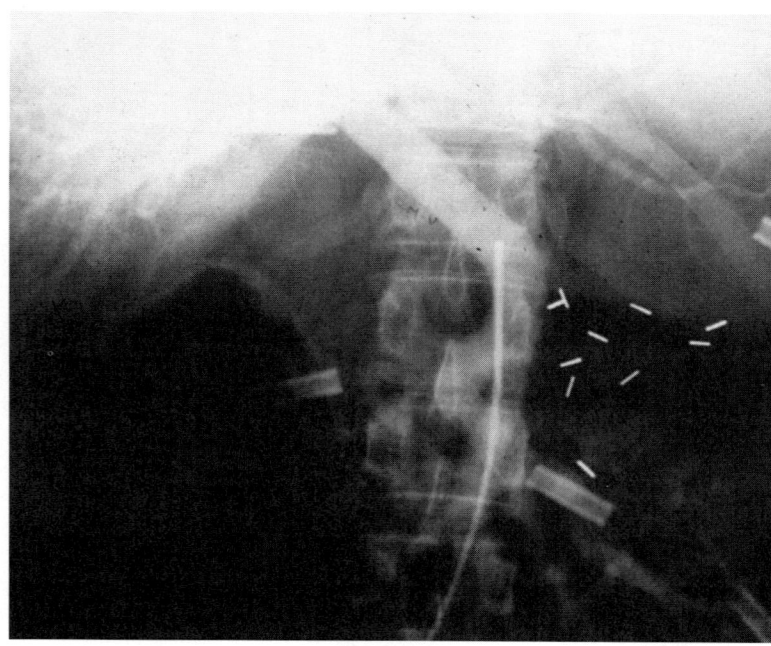

Figure 3 Venous phase of superior mesenteric arterial injection showing prograde portal blood flow to the liver after DSRS.

POSTOPERATIVE MANAGEMENT

Proper fluid and electrolyte management is of special importance in the postoperative care of selective shunt patients. Because of the tendency to accumulate ascites after this procedure, intravenous fluid and sodium intake should not exceed the calculated volume for daily maintenance and for replacement of abnormal losses, even if the urinary output is in the 30 to 50 ml range. Half of the daily fluid requirement is administered as 5% albumin in the first 48 hours, and diuretic therapy is started on the second or third postoperative day. By the end of the first week, ascites usually begins to abate, as evidenced by decreasing abdominal girth, decreasing body weight, and increased urine output. Chylous ascites should be suspected if the ascites persists. The milky appearance of the ascitic fluid readily confirms this diagnosis. Chylous ascites is treated by repeated abdominal paracenteses and total parenteral hyperalimentation.

RESULTS

This evaluation is based on our experience with the selective shunt over more than 25 years. The operative mortality in patients with good liver reserve, Child's class A and B, is less than 5%, but the rate rises in Child's class C patients. The shunt patency rate is 90% to 95%, with early occlusion almost always the result of a technical error. Late occlusion is extremely rare.

Postshunt encephalopathy is significantly less common after selective shunting than after total shunting operations. In our randomized study, the incidence of encephalopathy 3 years after operation was 12% in the selective shunt group versus 52% in the total shunt group. Using routine angiographic evaluation before hospital discharge, we have found that portal perfusion is retained in more than 90% of the selective shunt patients (Fig. 3). Late angiographic studies, however, have documented progressive development of collateral venous channels between the high-pressure portal and superior mesenteric veins and the decompressed tributaries of the splenic vein, with loss of prograde portal blood flow in one-third of the patients.

DISTAL SPLENORENAL SHUNT IN BILHARZIAL PORTAL HYPERTENSION

Worldwide, bilharziasis is the most common cause of portal hypertension. In a study cosponsored by the author and conducted in Egypt, the DSRS was evaluated in the treatment of this entity. The results were similar in bilharzial and nonbilharzial patients in terms of operative mortality, shunt patency, and postoperative portal venous perfusion. More favorable long-term survival was noted in the bilharzial patients, mostly because of their superior liver functions as compared with cirrhotic patients (Fig. 4).[6] Massive splenomegaly is often found in patients with schistosomiasis. In these instances, temporary clamping of the splenic artery is used to prevent overengorgement of the spleen during construction of the shunt and to facilitate dissection of the splenic vein. Tortuosity of the splenic vein is another complicating factor in patients with schistosomiasis. In extreme cases, the author resorts to splenocaval instead of splenorenal anastomosis. The inferior vena cava lies

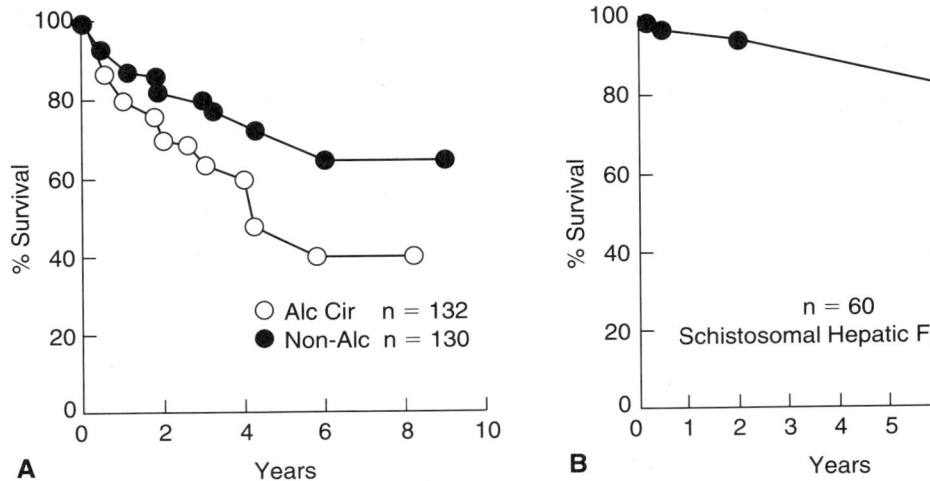

Figure 4 Kaplan-Meier survival plot for survival after selective shunt in alcoholic and nonalcoholic cirrhosis versus schistosomal hepatic fibrosis. Five-year survival is 88% in schistosomal patients *(B)*, 70% in nonalcoholic cirrhotic patients, and 40% in alcoholic cirrhotic patients *(A)*. Data plotted in A from Warren WD, Henderson JM, Millikan WJ, et al. Distal splenorenal versus endoscopic sclerotherapy for long term management of variceal bleeding. Preliminary report of a prospective randomized trial. Ann Surg 1986; 203:454–462. From Ezzat FA, Abu-Elmagd KM, Aly IY, et al. Distal splenorenal shunt for management of variceal bleeding in patients with schistosomal hepatic fibrosis. Ann Surg 1986; 204:566–573; with permission.)

at a more anterior plane than the left renal vein. Hence, excessive angulation or kinking of the splenic vein is less likely to occur with a splenocaval anastomosis.

REFERENCES

1. Jackson FC, Perrin EB, Felix WR, et al. A clinical investigation of the portacaval shunt. Ann Surg 1972; 174:672–701.
2. Sarfeh IJ, Rypins EB, Mason GR. A systemic appraisal of portacaval H-graft diameters: Clinical and hemodynamic perspectives. Ann Surg 1986; 204:356–363.
3. Warren WD, Zeppa R, Fomon JJ. Selective transsplenic decompression of gastroesophageal varices by distal splenorenal shunt. Ann Surg 1967; 166:437–455.
4. Salam AA, Warren WD, Lapage JR, et al. Hemodynamic contrasts between selective and total portasystemic decompression. Ann Surg 1971; 173:827–844.
5. Warren WD, Henderson JM, Millikan WJ, et al. Distal splenorenal versus endoscopic sclerotherapy for long term management of variceal bleeding. Preliminary report of a prospective randomized trial. Ann Surg 1986; 203:454–462.
6. Ezzat FA, Abu-Elmagd KM, Aly IY, et al. Distal splenorenal shunt for management of variceal bleeding in patients with schistosomal hepatic fibrosis. Ann Surg 1986; 204:566–573.

BUDD-CHIARI SYNDROME

DARRELL A. CAMPBELL Jr., M.D.
FREDERIC E. ECKHAUSER, M.D.

The Budd-Chiari syndrome is an unusual disorder produced by occlusion of the hepatic veins. The result is a classic triad of intractable ascites, abdominal pain, and hepatosplenomegaly. In Western cultures, the disorder most often involves primary thrombosis of the hepatic veins. In this setting the inferior vena cava (IVC) and portal vein may become thrombosed secondarily. In Eastern cultures, the Budd-Chiari syndrome is most often the result of caval obstruction above the level of the hepatic vein outflow, with or without thrombosis of the hepatic veins. Caval obstruction in this setting is most often the result of a congenital diaphragmatic web. Budd-Chiari syndrome must be distinguished from veno-occlusive disease of the liver, which does not involve thrombosis of the hepatic veins, but rather of sublobular veins and terminal hepatic venules. Veno-occlusive disease of the liver results in a clinical picture similar to Budd-Chiari syndrome but occurs in a different clinical setting, usually involving high-dose chemotherapy or graft-versus-host disease associated with bone marrow transplantation.

CLINICAL CLASSIFICATION AND ETIOLOGY

The clinical presentation of patients with the Budd-Chiari syndrome varies according to the number of hepatic veins involved, the degree of obstruction of the hepatic veins, and the rapidity of the process. The varied clinical presentations that result from interaction of these factors have been described as the fulminant, acute, subacute, and chronic forms of the disease.[1] We have found this clinical classification helpful in making treatment decisions. In the fulminant phase, liver cell failure develops rapidly, resulting in encephalopathy and multiorgan failure. This condition is the result of rapid and complete thrombosis of all major hepatic veins. In the acute and subacute phases, which occur over a period of months, the patient develops impressive ascites and abdominal pain. In the acute phase, transaminases are typically elevated fourfold to fivefold above normal, whereas transaminases are not elevated at presentation in the subacute form. The acute phase presents generally 2 to 3 months after hepatic vein occlusion; the subacute phase typically presents 12 to 18 months after the initial thrombotic event. In the acute or subacute phases, most patients experience problems related to portal hypertension and ascites control. A smaller group of patients show signs of hepatic decompensation, however, with encephalopathy and progressive abnormalities of synthetic function. In the chronic phase, the patient develops significant cirrhosis, and the clinical difficulties encountered are not different from patients with other types of cirrhotic liver disease. The development of cirrhosis may be particularly rapid in Budd-Chiari syndrome, occurring over a period of months.

Temporary improvement in the patient's condition usually occurs shortly after the initial thrombotic event. Abdominal pain diminishes in severity and ascites is controlled with diuretics. The clinical improvement is related to hypertrophy of the caudate lobe, which occurs by virtue of this lobe's independent venous drainage into the IVC, an area uninvolved by the thrombotic process. Improvement is only transient, and progressive deterioration is inevitable in the absence of treatment. The hypertrophied caudate lobe may be mistaken for a hepatic neoplasm at celiotomy or during laparoscopy. Radionuclide imaging occasionally documents a central area of increased uptake, a "hot spot" representing the hypertrophied caudate lobe.

The etiology of Budd-Chiari syndrome is not well understood, but there is a clear association with exogenous estrogen administration. This may partially explain the predominance of the disease in young women. Other significant associations include polycythemia vera, essential thrombocytosis, paroxysmal nocturnal hemoglobinuria, various malignancies, hepatic infections, and prior history of hepatitis. In most large series, up to 30%

of patients will be labeled idiopathic at presentation. Many of these patients develop clinically apparent myeloproliferative disorders years after successful treatment of Budd-Chiari syndrome.

DIAGNOSIS

Budd-Chiari syndrome should be suspected in any patient who develops ascites rapidly. Abdominal pain may or may not be present. The two most important diagnostic tests are angiography and liver biopsy. Angiography consists of evaluation of the vena cava and hepatic veins with IVC and wedged hepatic vein pressure determinations as well. Selective mesenteric arteriography is also done routinely, primarily to evaluate the patency of the portal and superior mesenteric veins. Obtaining an accurate IVC blood pressure determination is critical, as the gradient between the wedged hepatic blood pressure and IVC blood pressure must be sufficiently large to promote long-term patency of a portacaval or mesocaval shunt. Liver biopsy is important to confirm the diagnosis and also to assess the degree of cirrhosis that might have occurred. Typical findings on liver biopsy include central lobular congestion with necrosis. Most patients with Budd-Chiari syndrome have developed mild to moderate fibrosis as well, but some patients occasionally present with established cirrhosis. The latter group are better candidates for liver transplantation than for the more traditional portosystemic shunting procedures. Liver biopsy is contraindicated in patients with uncorrectable coagulopathy.

Noninvasive tests such as hepatic Doppler duplex ultrasound and magnetic resonance imaging are helpful when the clinical presentation is unclear and other diagnoses are being entertained. At our institution, findings suggestive of Budd-Chiari syndrome by either of these modalities are always confirmed angiographically.

NONOPERATIVE MANAGEMENT

An occasional patient with a history suggestive of Budd-Chiari syndrome is found to have thrombosis of only one hepatic vein, or partial thrombosis of more than one vein. In such patients, a conservative approach consisting of long-term anticoagulation may be beneficial.

Thrombolytic therapy has proved to be of little benefit in the management of Budd-Chiari syndrome because the occluding thrombus is usually several weeks old by the time of diagnosis and is no longer responsive to thrombolytic agents.

Various interventional radiologic techniques have been applied to the treatment of Budd-Chiari syndrome. Patients with Budd-Chiari syndrome resulting from a membranous web obstructing the IVC above the level of the hepatic veins are most likely to benefit from percutaneous transluminal angioplasty (PTA). This technique has replaced operative membranotomy as the treatment of choice for this condition. It has also been applied to cases of Budd-Chiari syndrome resulting from stenosis but not thrombosis of the right hepatic vein and segmental narrowing of the IVC.[2] Repeated dilations may be necessary, but the procedure appears to be safe and is indicated in patients with stenosis or weblike membranes resulting in Budd-Chiari syndrome. It may also be helpful to patients in whom segmental narrowing of the retrohepatic IVC results in high IVC pressure, precluding portosystemic shunting procedures. In these patients, PTA with or without placement of an expandable intravascular stent may allow reduction in caval pressures and successful construction of a portosystemic anastomosis.

We are less enthusiastic about transluminal angioplasty in instances involving complete obstruction of the vena cava because of the risk of pulmonary embolization and a lack of follow-up data concerning long-term caval patency with this approach.

OPERATIVE MANAGEMENT

Portosystemic decompression is the treatment of choice for the acute and subacute forms of Budd-Chiari syndrome, providing that hepatic decompensation has not occurred. In the latter, transplantation is preferred, as it is in the fulminant and chronic phases of the disease.

Side-to-side portacaval or interposition mesocaval shunts convert the portal vein into an outflow tract, decompress the portal venous system, and prevent further hepatic injury. In contrast to other circumstances in which such procedures are done, postoperative encephalopathy is rare, providing that cirrhosis is not present. Controversy exists as to the best procedure to achieve portal decompression. We prefer the interposition mesocaval shunt procedure, using either autologous jugular vein or 16 to 18 mm externally reinforced polytetrafluoroethylene (PTFE) graft. This approach avoids the occasional technical difficulty encountered in constructing the side-to-side portacaval anastomosis when the caudate lobe is greatly hypertrophied and avoids dissection in the portal triad, preserving the portal vein for possible subsequent transplantation. Other groups have had success with standard side-to-side portacaval shunts. The long-term results of portosystemic decompression for Budd-Chiari syndrome are excellent. In one report, 20 of 21 patients treated with various portosystemic decompressive operations were alive a mean of 5.1 years postoperative and were free of ascites.[1] Of 13 patients treated by side-to-side portacaval shunt, 12 survived from 3 to 16 years postoperatively with excellent rehabilitation.[3]

An important question involves the procedure of choice in the patient with a patent IVC but elevated caval blood pressures. The retrohepatic vena cava is often narrowed in the patient with Budd-Chiari syndrome as the result of pressure from the hypertrophied caudate lobe. The resulting caval compression worsens ascites formation and results in elevated caval blood pressure measurements. Past a certain point, portosystemic shunting in this situation is unwise, as the small blood pressure gradient between the portal and systemic circulations does not adequately decompress the portal circulation. This critical blood pressure difference is not entirely known, and the strategy in this situation depends on personal preference. An attempt to alleviate retrohepatic vena caval stenosis with an expandable intravascular stent is not unreasonable. If the caval blood pressure gradient is less than 20 mm Hg, a mesocaval shunt should be performed using reinforced PTFE graft material. If the pressure gradient is higher than 20 mm Hg, consideration should be given to construction of a mesoatrial shunt.[4]

The patient with a completely obstructed IVC is a surgical challenge, in that no form of portosystemic anastomosis alone will provide relief to the obstructed liver. Mesoatrial shunting has been used most extensively in this setting, using 16 mm ring-reinforced prosthetic graft material. An important technical feature of the procedure is the use of an additional silicone rubber cuff to protect the graft as it passes through the diaphragm.[4] When performed by an experienced surgical team, long-term results have been excellent. Graft strictures, a not uncommon occurrence, may be treated with percutaneous balloon angioplasty.[5] The simultaneous construction of a side-to-side portacaval anastomosis with cavoatrial bypass, using externally supported prosthetic graft material, has been described as an alternative to this problem.[6] Such an approach might lessen the incidence of thrombosis because the flow in the graft would be augmented by caval blood as well as portal blood. If neither procedure is considered feasible, liver transplantation is an acceptable alternative.

Whether patients treated for Budd-Chiari syndrome by creation of a portasystemic shunt should be chronically anticoagulated is controversial. In our center such patients are anticoagulated only if intraoperative measurements or postoperative Doppler ultrasound investigations suggest sluggish flow across the anastomosis.

LIVER TRANSPLANTATION

Two clear indications for liver transplantation in patients with Budd-Chiari syndrome are fulminant hepatic failure and evidence for established cirrhosis. Patients with the acute or subacute phases and encephalopathy or progressive deterioration of hepatic synthetic function should also be considered for transplantation. The decision to proceed with transplantation is, however, something of a trade-off. On the one hand, rapid resolution of abnormalities in liver function and normalization of portal pressure are very desirable; on the other, the burden of a lifetime of immunosuppression and the constant risk of allograft rejection are a heavy price to pay. Despite the potential disadvantages, it is important to emphasize that the recent results of liver transplantation for this indication have been excellent. In the Cambridge–Kings College series, 3 year actuarial patient survival for 17 transplanted patients was 88%.[7] In the UCLA experience, 14 patients with Budd-Chiari

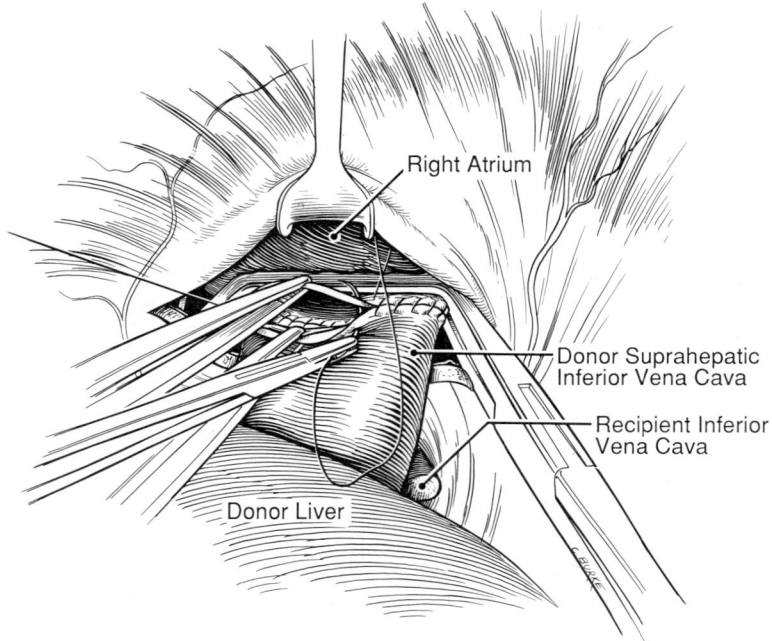

Figure 1 The donor suprahepatic inferior vena cava is anastomosed directly to the recipient's right atrium with continuous polypropylene suture material. Upon completion of the transplant, the diaphragmatic incision is closed and a mediastinal drainage tube is placed. (From Burtch GD, Merion RM. Transdiaphragmatic exposure for direct atrial-caval anastomosis in liver transplantation for Budd-Chiari syndrome. Transplantation 1989; 47:161–163; with permission.)

syndrome undergoing transplantation had a 76% 3 year survival.[8] Rehabilitation of the transplanted patients was excellent. Outstanding results are related to continued refinements in patient selection, immunosuppressive management, and operative technique. With regard to the latter, the standard infradiaphragmatic suprahepatic caval anastomosis is often impossible in this setting, as the result of the thrombotic process and surrounding inflammation. This finding requires that the suprahepatic vena caval anastomosis be performed in the pericardium at the level of the right atrium, which is accomplished by entering the pericardium inferiorly, without the need for median sternotomy (Fig. 1).[9]

The patient with Budd-Chiari syndrome who undergoes liver transplantation is at risk for recurrent hepatic vein thrombosis unless permanently anticoagulated. Several cases of recurrent hepatic vein thrombosis have been reported in which either the patients were inadvertently underanticoagulated or anticoagulation was temporarily discontinued for the purposes of liver biopsy. In our center, patients with Budd-Chiari syndrome who undergo liver transplantation are treated with heparin sodium as soon as feasible in the postoperative period, with subsequent conversion to chronic dicumarol therapy. An occasional patient with essential thrombocytosis has been treated with urea and salicylates.

REFERENCES

1. Bismuth H, Sherlock DJ. Portasystemic shunting versus liver transplantation for the Budd-Chiari syndrome. Ann Surg 1991; 214:581–589.
2. Sparano J, Chang J, Trasi S, et al. Treatment of the Budd-Chiari syndrome with percutaneous transluminal angioplasty. Am J Med 1987; 82:821–828.
3. Orloff MJ, Girard B. Long term results of treatment of Budd-Chiari syndrome by side to side portacaval shunt. Surg Gynecol Obstet 1989; 168:33–41.
4. Klein AS, Sitzmann JV, Coleman J, et al. Current management of the Budd-Chiari syndrome. Ann Surg 1990; 212:144–149.
5. Savader SJ, Venbrux AC, Klein AS, et al. Percutaneous intervention in the portosystemic shunts in Budd-Chiari syndrome. JVIR 1991; 2:489–495.
6. Orloff MJ, Daily PO, Girard B. Treatment of Budd-Chiari syndrome due to inferior vena cava occlusion by combined portal and vena caval decompression. Am J Surg 1992; 163:137–143.
7. Campbell DA Jr, Rolles K, Jamieson N, et al. Hepatic transplantation with perioperative and long term anticoagulation as treatment for Budd-Chiari syndrome. Surg Gynecol Obstet 1988; 166:511–518.
8. Shaked A, Goldstein RM, Klintmalm GB, et al. Portosystemic shunt versus orthotopic liver transplantation for the Budd-Chiari syndrome. Surg Gynecol Obstet 1992; 174:453–459.
9. Burtch GD, Merion RM. Transdiaphragmatic exposure for direct atrial-caval anastomosis in liver transplantation for Budd-Chiari syndrome. Transplantation 1989; 47:161–163.

TRANSJUGULAR PORTOSYSTEMIC SHUNTS

ROBERT K. KERLAN Jr., M.D.
ZIV J. HASKAL, M.D.
ERNEST J. RING, M.D.

Management of acute variceal hemorrhage has traditionally focused on pharmacologic agents, mechanical compression with tamponading balloons, and endoscopic techniques, including sclerotherapy and variceal banding. The role of operative portosystemic shunting has diminished over the past several years because of unpredictable postoperative morbidity from hepatic failure or encephalopathy. Although orthotopic liver transplantation provides a unique and effective solution to these problems, it is often impractical in the emergent setting and may not be necessary if the hemorrhage can be reliably controlled by other means. The transjugular intrahepatic portosystemic shunt (TIPS) was conceived as a way to relieve portal hypertension without the need for an open operative procedure.

HISTORY

In 1982, Colapinto and colleagues reported the first clinical use of TIPS in a cirrhotic patient who was bleeding from varices.[1] A 12 mm angioplasty balloon was left inflated for 12 hours across the parenchyma between the hepatic and portal veins. When the balloon was deflated, a tract persisted and portal pressure dropped by 20%. In a follow-up study in 1983 that included five additional patients, Colapinto and co-workers inflated a 9 mm balloon in the tract for 10 to 15 minutes.[2] All of these shunts were found to be patent by repeat angiography performed 12 hours after the procedure. Although the patients all died within 6 months, the shunts were patent in three of four patients who underwent autopsy.

In 1989, Richter and associates reported the first clinical use of the Palmaz stent to perform TIPS.[3] The patient was a 49-year-old man with end-stage cirrhosis. The procedure was successful and resulted in a reduction of the portosystemic pressure gradient from 38 mm Hg to 18 mm Hg. The patient died 11 days later from respiratory failure, and an autopsy documented the shunt to be patent. A follow-up article published in 1990 documented the success of this technique.[4]

In 1992, we described our initial results using Wallstents to perform TIPS in 13 patients who developed intractable variceal bleeding while awaiting liver transplantation.[5] All of the patients had significant gastric or esophageal variceal bleeding despite multiple attempts at endoscopic sclerotherapy. We found that the TIPS could be safely performed in these high-risk patients and that it effectively lowered portal pressure and controlled bleeding until the transplant could be performed. Histologic examination of the explant specimens revealed a neoinitmal lining along the luminal surface of the stent within 3 weeks after placement. We have continued to evaluate the role of TIPS as a bridge to transplantation but have expanded the indications to include patients who are not transplant candidates.

TECHNIQUE

Preprocedural Evaluation and Medications

All patients undergo complete esophagogastroscopy prior to the procedure to confirm the diagnosis of variceal bleeding. Duplex ultrasound is performed to evaluate portal vein patency. Mesenteric arteriography is performed only when ultrasound fails to document portal blood flow or there is suspicion of hypervascular malignant tumor.

Preoperative laboratory assessment consists of a complete blood count with platelet count, prothrombin time (PT), partial thromboplastin time, serum total bilirubin, serum electrolytes, and serum creatinine. If the platelet count is below 50,000 mm^3, platelet transfusions are administered immediately prior to the procedure. If the PT is longer than 20 seconds, fresh frozen plasma or cryoprecipitate is administered.

All patients receive intravenous broad-spectrum antibiotics prior to the procedure. If the serum creatinine is elevated, mannitol (25 g) can also be administered.

Anesthesia

Although some investigators prefer attempting TIPS under general anesthesia, it is usually not necessary in adult patients. Conscious sedation with a combination of intravenous narcotic (meperidine or fentanyl), augmented by a hypnotic sedative (midazolam and droperidol), is usually sufficient.

Venous Access

The preferred approach for performing TIPS is the right internal jugular vein. If several passes are made without successful entry, ultrasound is used to confirm patency of the vein and to direct the puncture. Using standard Seldinger technique, a 9 Fr 40 cm angiographic sheath with a 30° angle at its distal tip is placed into the infrahepatic inferior vena cava (IVC). A pressure measurement is obtained at this location.

If the right internal jugular vein is occluded, the left internal jugular vein is punctured. If the left is also occluded, the procedure can be performed from the right external jugular vein, although the angles created from this approach may make the procedure more difficult. A successful TIPS from a femoral venous approach has been reported but requires aberrant portal venous anatomy and should not be attempted unless this anatomic variation is present.

Selecting the Hepatic Vein

The 9 Fr sheath is retracted to the atrial-caval junction and a curved angiographic catheter is manipulated under fluoroscopic guidance into a hepatic vein. Selection of an appropriate hepatic vein is critical. A vein of suitable diameter and appropriate angle greatly facilitates the procedure. The right hepatic vein is generally preferred, but TIPS can also be constructed from the middle and left hepatic veins. Significant overlap between the right and middle hepatic veins is present in the frontal projection. Visualization in an oblique view is usually required for accurate anatomic assessment of the selected hepatic vein.

Portal Venous Puncture

Once the appropriate hepatic vein has been selected, the catheter is removed and replaced with a transjugular hepatic puncture needle. Although several needles have been developed for this purpose, we prefer the Colapinto needle, which has two parts, a curved 16 gauge metal needle and an outer 9 Fr catheter. This device is actually a modification of the Ross transseptal needle, but the orientation of the bevel has been reversed to facilitate passage through the curved segment of the 9 French sheath to help negotiate the angle between the hepatic vein and the IVC–right atrial junction. Moreover, the stiffness of the Colapinto needle enables a controlled puncture even through hard, cirrhotic liver parenchyma. The internal lumen of the needle allows passage of a 0.035 inch guide wire.

The Rosch-Uchida transjugular needle was designed to be more flexible and have a leading tip of a smaller caliber than the Colapinto system. It consists of a 10 Fr 41 cm length introducer sheath, a 10 Fr 52 cm length Teflon catheter with a 30° bend at its distal tip, a 14 gauge 51 cm length curved metal cannula that fits inside the 10 Fr Teflon catheter, a 62 cm length 5 Fr catheter, and a 62 cm 0.038 inch flexible needle that extends through the tip of the 5 Fr catheter. The first three components are used to stabilize the system within the hepatic vein. The latter two components are used for transparenchymal puncture into the portal venous system.

The needle is rotated anteromedially and advanced caudally out of the right hepatic vein 4 to 5 cm into the hepatic parenchyma. A syringe is attached, and the needle is aspirated as it is slowly withdrawn. When blood returns, contrast medium is injected to determine which vascular structure has been entered. When a portal vein branch is identified, a guide wire is passed through the needle and manipulated down the main portal vein into the splenic or mesenteric vein. A 5 Fr catheter is advanced into the portal venous system. After the 5 Fr catheter has been advanced into the portal venous system, pressure measurements are made and portal phlebography performed. The portal phlebogram documents the anatomy, determines the direction of portal venous flow, and documents the variceal collaterals.

Targeting the portal vein for puncture remains a controversial area. We have had a high degree of success using fluoroscopy to guide the needle into the anticipated region of the hepatic hilum without additional imaging. Other investigators recommend various means of localizing the portal vein to guide the transhepatic puncture. In the early reported studies, a percutaneous transhepatic catheter or stone basket was placed in the portal vein to facilitate the puncture. However, serious bleeding complications caused the death of at least one patient, and this method has largely been abandoned. Other reported localization methods include real-time Doppler ultrasound guidance, placement of portal venous platinum tip guidewires, deposition of platinum microcoils adjacent to the portal vein, portal venous catheterization through paraumbilical venous collaterals, and using contrast that has been extravasated around the portal vein during the course of the procedure (tunnel sign).

Tract Dilation

The 5 Fr catheter is then exchanged for a 5 Fr balloon dilation catheter, which is positioned within the parenchymal tract extending from the hepatic vein to the portal vein and inflated. Several inflations may be required to fully dilate the portal vein entry site, the intervening hepatic parenchyma, and the hepatic vein entry site. Following the tract dilation, the balloon catheter is removed and the stent is deployed.

Stent Deployment

In the United States, most TIPS are performed using the Wallstent to stent the hepatic parenchymal tract. This wire mesh endoprosthesis currently has an unconstrained maximal diameter of 10 mm. The wire mesh of the Wallstent is composed of 100 μm stainless steel filaments. The stent is preloaded on a 7 Fr catheter and is deployed by pulling back a retractable plastic membrane. When the Wallstent is released from the catheter, it shortens as it expands. The amount it shortens is determined by the final diameter of the expanded stent.

The principal advantage of the Wallstent is its flexibility, which allows it to easily negotiate the angles of the hepatic vein and portal vein entries. Moreover, this stent is directly attached to the delivery catheter and does not require preliminary passage of a large introducer sheath. The delivery catheter is also relatively small (7 Fr) and quite flexible, so that it can be introduced from almost any point of entry into the portal venous system. Once expanded, the Wallstent maintains a cylindrical lumen even around sharp bends and follows the venous anatomy from small peripheral portal venous branches into more central veins that have a sufficient diameter to form an adequate shunt.

The Palmaz stent was the first stent used in TIPS, and significant experience is available with this device. The Gianturco-Rosch Z stent has also been employed. The Strecker stent has also been used on an experimental basis in swine with occlusion in seven of eight pigs 4 weeks after the procedure. This high occlusion rate may possibly be explained by the lack of portal hypertension in the experimental model.

Stent Dilation

We initially dilate the Wallstent to 8 mm, using an angioplasty balloon. The portal phlebogram is then repeated and the blood pressure remeasured. If the portal blood pressure gradient (difference between absolute portal blood pressure and IVC blood pressure) is 15 mm Hg or greater, or there continues to be prominent filling of varices on the portal phlebogram, the stent is further dilated with a 10 mm diameter balloon catheter. Following the dilation, the portal phlebogram is repeated and the blood pressure is reassessed. If varices are still filling briskly, they are selectively catheterized and embolized. In about 10% of patients, a 10 mm diameter shunt does not produce sufficient reduction in the portosystemic gradient to prevent recurrent bleeding (greater than 15 mm Hg residual gradient). In these patients, further reduction in portal blood pressure is obtained by performing a second parallel TIPS from a different hepatic vein to a portal vein branch in the opposite lobe of the liver. This can usually be obviated if a larger stent is used.

Postprocedural Management

At the completion of the shunt, the jugular vein catheter is exchanged for a shorter 8.5 Fr sheath through which fluid and blood can be administered, when necessary. All patients are then observed at least overnight in the intensive care unit. On the following day, duplex ultrasound of the liver and TIPS shunt are performed. If the shunt is patent and there is no suggestion of a technical problem, the jugular sheath is removed. If a problem is detected, the patient is returned to the angiography suite for TIPS phlebography, which is performed prior to removal of the jugular sheath.

RESULTS

The results of TIPS have been reported in several large series.[4,6-8] Technical success ranges from 95% to 100% with a residual portal blood pressure gradient of

9 to 15 mm Hg. In our own series of 250 patients, the procedure was successful in 97%; absolute portal blood pressure diminished from 35.8 mm ± 6.8 Hg before TIPS to 26.3 ± 6.4 mm Hg following the shunt. The average portal-systemic gradient dropped from 22.7 ± 6.8 mm Hg to 10.5 ± 4.9 mm Hg.

Thirty day mortality rates following TIPS are 5% to 15%.[4,6-8] However, few deaths are related to the procedure, and most of the patients who die are very critically ill before attempting the TIPS, as evidenced by a mean APACHE II score of over 25 in the patients in our series who died within 30 days. Procedural deaths can occur from intraperitoneal hemorrhage if the liver capsule is traversed during the procedure. Central venous blood pressure routinely rises after TIPS and this can lead to heart failure if fluid administration is not carefully monitored. One patient in our series who had severe pre-existing pulmonary hypertension died following TIPS placement from acute cor pulmonale. Although not encountered in our series, two procedurally related deaths due to hepatic arterial injury have been reported.[9]

Nonfatal procedure-related complications included self-limited intraperitoneal hemorrhage (1% to 6%), hemobilia (1% to 4%), sepsis (up to 10%), transient oliguric renal failure, and atrial arrhythmias. Increases in serum bilirubin, transaminases, PT, and ammonia that peak within the first week after TIPS and subsequently resolve occur in 10% to 20% of patients.[10,11] Although we have not encountered stent migration or marked stent misplacement during the course of a TIPS procedure, these complications and their management have been reported.[9] Encephalopathy occurs in about 25% of patients after TIPS. In most patients the symptoms are mild and can usually be readily managed with dietary protein restriction and lactulose therapy. Uncontrolled encephalopathy pose a major clinical problem in less than 5% of patients.[10]

STENOSIS AND OCCLUSIONS

Shunt occlusion during the first week after TIPS from technical problems such as tract tortuosity or inadequate stent length occur less often with experience. Delayed shunt malfunction develops in 25% to 40% of patients 1 to 6 months following TIPS. The histologic appearance of patent, stenotic, and occluded shunts has been observed in explant specimens from patients undergoing liver transplantation.[10] After 4 days the shunt has an irregular luminal surface with liver parenchyma protruding between the stent wires. A patchy layer of endothelial cells is already beginning to line the shunt surface. By 3 weeks, the lumen has become round and smooth as the stent wires are covered by a pseudointimal surface composed of granulation tissue and a contiguous layer of endothelial cells.

In stenotic shunts, pseudointimal hyperplasia appears to be the causative lesion, as opposed to ingrowth of hepatic parenchyma. This pseudointimal hyperplasia varies in thickness from 0.5 mm to 5 mm and becomes more cellular near the luminal surface. Subjacent transected bile ducts were noted in three of six malfunctioning stents, and it has been postulated that in some patients bile intravasation within the pseudointima may be a stimulus for the proliferative reaction.[11] Because TIPS stenosis can be easily treated with balloon dilation or restenting, with careful surveillance, primary assisted and secondary patency rates approach 100%.[7]

REFERENCES

1. Colapinto RF, Stronell RD, Birch SJ. Creation of an intrahepatic portosystemic shunt with a Gruntzig balloon catheter. Can Med Assoc J 1982; 126:267–268.
2. Colapinto RF, Stronell RD, Gildiner M, et al. Formation of intrahepatic portosystemic shunts using a balloon dilation catheter. Preliminary clinical experience. Am J Roentgenol 1983; 140:709–714.
3. Richter GM, Palmaz JC, Noeldge G, et al. The transjugular intrahepatic portosystemic stent-shunt. A new nonsurgical percutaneous method. Radiology 1989; 29:406–411.
4. Richter GM, Noeldge G, Palmaz JC, et al. Transjugular intrahepatic portacaval stent shunt: Preliminary clinical results. Radiology 1990; 174:1027–1030.
5. Ring EJ, Lake JR, Roberts JP, et al. Using transjugular intrahepatic portosystemic shunts to control variceal bleeding before liver transplantation. Ann Intern Med 1992; 116:304–309.
6. LaBerge JM, Ring EJ, Gordon, et al. Creation of transjugular intrahepatic portosystemic shunts with the Wallstent endoprosthesis: Results in 100 patients. Radiology 1993; 187:413–420.
7. Rossle M, Haag K, Ochs A, et al. The transjugular intra-hepatic portosystemic stent-shunt procedure for variceal bleeding. N Engl J Med 1993; 330:165–171.
8. Freedman AM, Sanyal AJ, Tisnado J, et al. Results with percutaneous transjugular intrahepatic protosystemic stent-shunts for control of variceal hemorrhage in patients awaiting liver transplantation. Transplant Proc 1993; 25:1087–1089.
9. Haskal ZJ, Pentecost MJ, Rubin RA. Hepatic arterial injury after transjugular intrahepatic portosystemic shunt placement: Report of two cases. Radiology 1993; 188:85–88.
10. Somberg, KA, Riegler JL, Doherty M, et al. Hepatic encephalopathy following transjugular intahepatic portosystemic shunts (TIPS): Incidence and risk factors. Hepatology 1992; 16:122A.
11. Sellinger M, Haag K, Ochs A, et al. Factors influencing the incidence of hepatic encephalopathy in patients with transjugular intrahepatic portosystemic stent-shunts (TIPSS). Hepatology 1992; 16:122A.

LIVER TRANSPLANTATION IN THE MANAGEMENT OF PORTAL HYPERTENSION

KIM M. OLTHOFF, M.D.
RONALD W. BUSUTTIL, M.D., Ph.D.

Portal venous hypertension is present in most patients who are candidates for orthotopic liver transplantation (OLT) and is often the primary indication for transplantation when coupled with other manifestations of end-stage liver disease (ESLD). Many of these patients present with life-threatening variceal hemorrhages or severe, intractable ascites. With survival rates for transplanted Child's C patients exceeding those of sclerotherapy and shunting, OLT has emerged as an important alternative for treatment of portal hypertension in patients with ESLD. However, in patients whose only manifestation of liver disease is symptomatic portal hypertension, transplantation may not be required.

ETIOLOGY OF PORTAL HYPERTENSION

The most common form of portal hypertension in the United States is a combination of intrasinusoidal and postsinusoidal hypertension usually caused by alcoholic liver disease, postnecrotic cirrhosis, or, less frequently, hemochromatosis. These patients develop marked portal hypertension from mechanical obstruction of the portal blood flow by regenerating hepatic nodules and cirrhotic bands. They also develop increased splanchnic perfusion from the formation of multiple arteriovenous shunts and collaterals. Patients often have poor hepatic reserve because the hepatocytes are already impaired by the disease process and may decompensate rapidly with each bleeding episode or after any surgical procedure such as cholecystectomy or umbilical hernia repair. It is the patient with this form of portal hypertension who is most frequently referred for consideration for OLT.

The other forms of portal hypertension are seen less frequently by the transplant surgeon. Extrahepatic presinusoidal obstruction is usually due to portal vein thrombosis, most commonly in children secondary to infection, but also in adults from pancreatitis, tumor, hypercoagulable states, or mechanical obstruction. These patients usually do not require transplantation because the hepatocytes and hepatic function are normal.

Intrahepatic presinusoidal obstruction is caused by fibrosis and compression of portal venules as seen in congenital hepatic fibrosis, Wilson's disease, primary biliary cirrhosis, biliary atresia, sarcoidosis, hepatoportal sclerosis, schistosomiasis, and myeloproliferative disorders. Hepatic function is usually preserved in the early stages of these diseases, but significant impairment may result from progressive cirrhosis. Liver transplantation is frequently performed for end-stage primary biliary cirrhosis and biliary atresia and less commonly for Wilson's disease and congenital hepatic fibrosis.

Extrahepatic postsinusoidal obstruction is the result of thrombosis in the hepatic veins. Budd-Chiari syndrome exemplifies this type of portal hypertension and is characterized by massive ascites, esophageal varices and hemorrhage, and hepatic failure. The presentation of Budd-Chiari syndrome may be fulminant or gradual. Patients are treated initially with anticoagulation, although this form of treatment is rarely successful. Shunting or transplantation is the definitive treatment for Budd-Chiari syndrome, and the choice of therapy is determined by the hepatic reserve.[1]

TREATMENT OPTIONS

The management of the patient with portal hypertension requires specialized care. The physician needs to be able to manage the acute complications of variceal hemorrhage, as well as the chronic sequelae of ESLD including malnutrition, fluid and electrolyte imbalance, ascites, and coagulopathy, which may precipitate additional bleeding episodes. The decision to refer a patient for shunting or transplantation is not always easy and requires knowledge of all treatment options.

In patients who present with acute variceal hemorrhage, the most important initial therapy is volume resuscitation, followed by determination of the source of bleeding with upper endoscopy. Medical therapy can be initiated with vasopressin and propranolol, and emergent sclerotherapy can be performed at the time of endoscopy. Balloon tamponade may be necessary for temporary control. Patients who bleed massively often require additional advanced intervention such as angiographic embolization, a transjugular intrahepatic portosystemic shunt (TIPS) procedure, or emergency surgical shunting. Emergency OLT is not an appropriate intervention for massive acute variceal bleeding because temporizing measures are successful in more than 95% of patients.

In patients who have been stabilized from their acute bleeding episodes, one must consider what options are available to prevent further hemorrhage. Besides chronic medical management with agents such as propranolol, there are four main therapeutic interventions: sclerotherapy, TIPS, surgical shunting, and transplantation.

Transplantation versus Shunt

Liver transplantation is a well-established modality in the care of patients with portal hypertension and ESLD and has been called the ultimate shunt. With the increasing popularity and success of OLT, the role of surgical shunting and other nontransplant procedures has been the subject of considerable debate. Most published survivals for liver transplantation exceed those for shunt operations. Iwatsuki and colleagues at the University of Pittsburgh compared 302 Child's C patients who underwent OLT to shunt survivals in the literature and found OLT patients to have significantly higher survival.[2]

Our experience at UCLA has also documented that superior survival is afforded to Child's C patients by transplantation (Table 1). In a series of 761 patients operated upon between January 1986 and December 1991, 77 underwent portosystemic shunting as their initial procedure, and 684 underwent hepatic transplantation. Of those transplanted, 86% were Child's C patients, whereas only 16% of the shunt patients were Child's C. Fifteen percent of the shunt patients eventually required liver transplantation for progressive hepatic deterioration, and the 5 year survival of the shunt group was 64% in contrast to a 73% 5 year survival for the transplanted patients. This supports the impression that Child's class C patients who are deemed appropriate transplant candidates are best managed by liver transplantation.

The essential features of any consideration of the role of shunting versus liver transplantation is the underlying cause of the hepatic disease, the current stage of hepatic dysfunction, and the expected progression of the disease. Patients who are Child's class A and some Child's class B should be considered for a distal splenorenal shunt unless other factors related to the disease process or quality of life are significant enough to warrant transplantation. A shunt may allow these patients to live for several more years without any problems and can afford them additional time before a transplant may be required. For others, assuming that the patients are reasonable transplant candidates and that the liver disease is approaching end stage, transplantation should be strongly considered. This recommendation needs to be weighed against the limitations of liver transplantation: the high expense of the procedure, the limited supply of donors, and the requirement of lifelong immunosuppression. If the patient is not a transplant candidate, then he or she should be treated with the best therapy available: sclerotherapy, TIPS, or shunting.

Patient Selection

Recipient selection remains one of the most important considerations for successful outcome after OLT. Patients are considered for transplant if they have proven irreversible ESLD manifested by portal hypertension, poor hepatic synthetic function, hyperbilirubinemia, hepatic encephalopathy, or severe lifestyle limitation secondary to intractable ascites, fatigue, or pruritus. Most patients have a combination of these indications. Although the specific diseases for which transplantation is performed have changed little in the past decade, we have broadly extended our acceptability standards for recipients, including more older patients, status 4 patients, and patients with portal vein thrombosis. Strict contraindications still exist. Extrahepatic malignancy, advanced disease of other organ systems, patient noncompliance, active ongoing substance abuse, and the human immunodeficiency virus are considered absolute contraindications to OLT.

Table 1 University of California at Los Angeles Experience: Results of Portosystemic Shunting and Liver Transplantation from January 1986 to December 1991

	Number Patients	Child's C (%)	5 Year Survival
Portosystemic shunt*	77	16	64
Liver transplant	684	87	73
Total	761		

*Of shunt operations 50% were distal splenorenal shunts; 15% of shunt patients eventually underwent liver transplantation.

Meticulous screening of potential candidates is essential to ensure excellent results. Patients are evaluated by surgeons, hepatologists, and multiple consultants. Preoperative liver biopsies can be beneficial but certainly are not mandatory and in fact may be risky in patients with severe coagulopathy or massive ascites. Ultrasound and duplex scanning of the liver and its vasculature are routinely performed during transplant evaluations to identify possible masses and determine the patency and direction of blood flow in the portal vein. This study is especially important in the patient with a prior shunt to determine if the shunt is still functioning. With the current technology of color flow duplex imaging, angiography is rarely, if ever, needed.

OPERATIVE CONSIDERATIONS

In many instances, dissection and removal of the recipient liver is the most demanding part of liver transplantation. Marked portal hypertension with massive collaterals, severe coagulopathy, and previous abdominal operations and shunts create technically demanding conditions. We have found that careful dissection using the electrocautery exclusively and the venovenous bypass routinely allows successful hepatectomy in the face of difficult surgical situations.

Venovenous Bypass

The development of venovenous bypass has greatly facilitated the recipient hepatectomy and subsequent graft implantation. Many centers, including our own, use venovenous bypass almost exclusively in adults. Systemic bypass is accomplished via the femoral and axillary veins, and splanchnic decompression is accomplished through the portal vein (Fig. 1). If portal vein thrombosis is present, the inferior mesenteric vein can be used for splanchnic decompression. When venovenous bypass is used early in the hepatectomy prior to the retrohepatic dissection, it allows splanchnic and systemic venous decompression during what can be the bloodiest part of

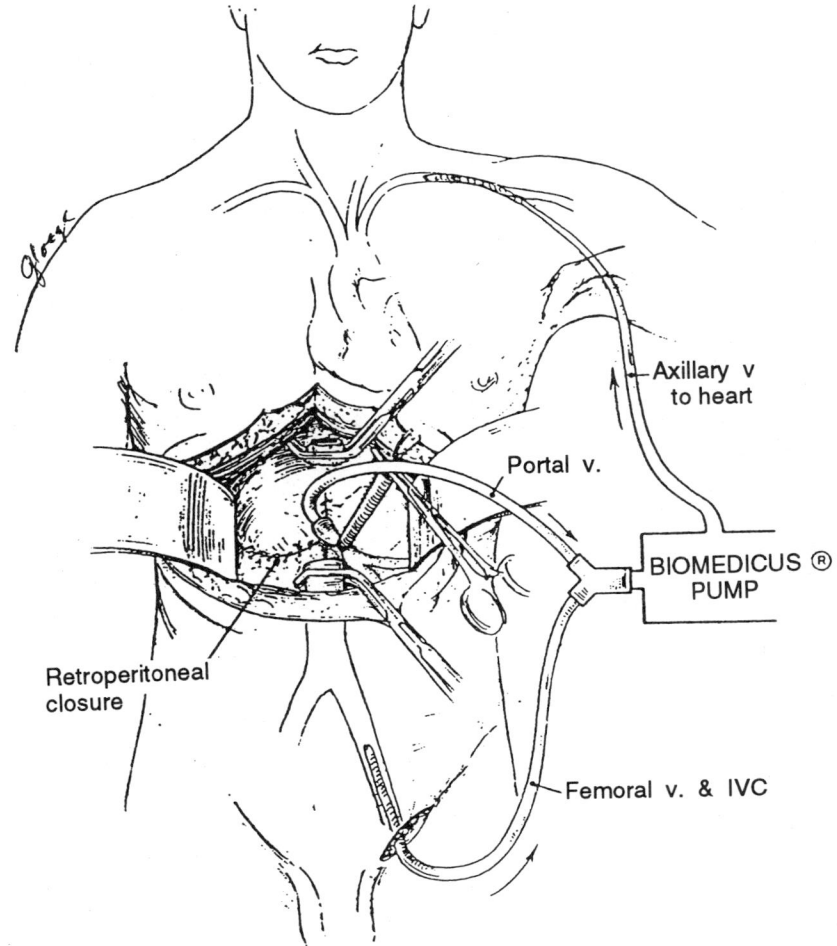

Figure 1 Venous-venous bypass for circulatory support during the anhepatic phase.

the operation. With the portal vein on bypass, the infrahepatic dissection and circumferential control of the inferior vena cava are greatly facilitated. Venovenous bypass also affords hemodynamic stability during the anhepatic phase so that implantation of the liver can be done in a controlled fashion.

Previous Shunt Procedures

Many patients with advanced liver disease and portal hypertension who have been treated with a shunt procedure are later considered for transplantation. Because the portal vein may become small and sclerotic after shunting, preoperative evaluation by duplex imaging to determine portal vein patency and size is important for preoperative planning. Central shunts in the form of end-to-side or side-to-side portocaval shunts require dismantling during liver implantation and increase the complexity of the portal anastomosis. The inferior vena cava and portal vein are isolated above and below the shunt prior to removal of the explant. The shunt provides portal decompression during the anhepatic phase, allowing caval blood return alone to be used for venovenous bypass. The shunt is then taken down after the suprahepatic caval anastomosis (Figs. 2 and 3). The dismantling of these central shunts is associated with greater blood loss, increased incidence of primary nonfunction, and longer hospitalization.[3] The most facile shunt to dismantle is the mesocaval H-graft, which requires simple ligation. In addition, we have now ligated three side-to-side portocaval shunts after reperfusion with minimal dissection. Distal splenorenal shunts do not require takedown after implantation. There does not appear to be any difference in survival following OLT between those who had prior portosystemic shunts and those who did not, but Mazzaferro and associates did document that the type of previous shunt had a significant impact on survival; end-to-end portocaval shunts and end-to-side portocaval shunts had much worse survival.[4]

Portal Vein Thrombosis

Once considered a contraindication to OLT, the presence of portal vein thrombosis (PVT) now does not preclude graft implantation. Transplantation in the face

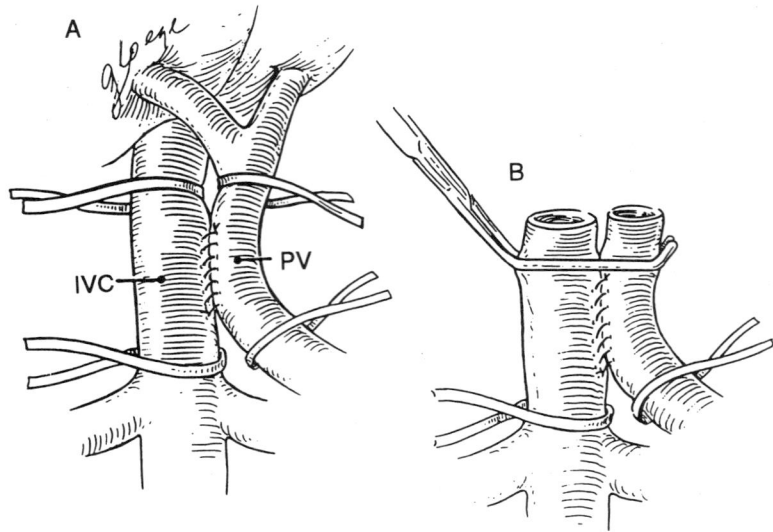

Figure 2 Technique for isolation of side-to-side portocaval shunt during an orthotopic liver transplant.

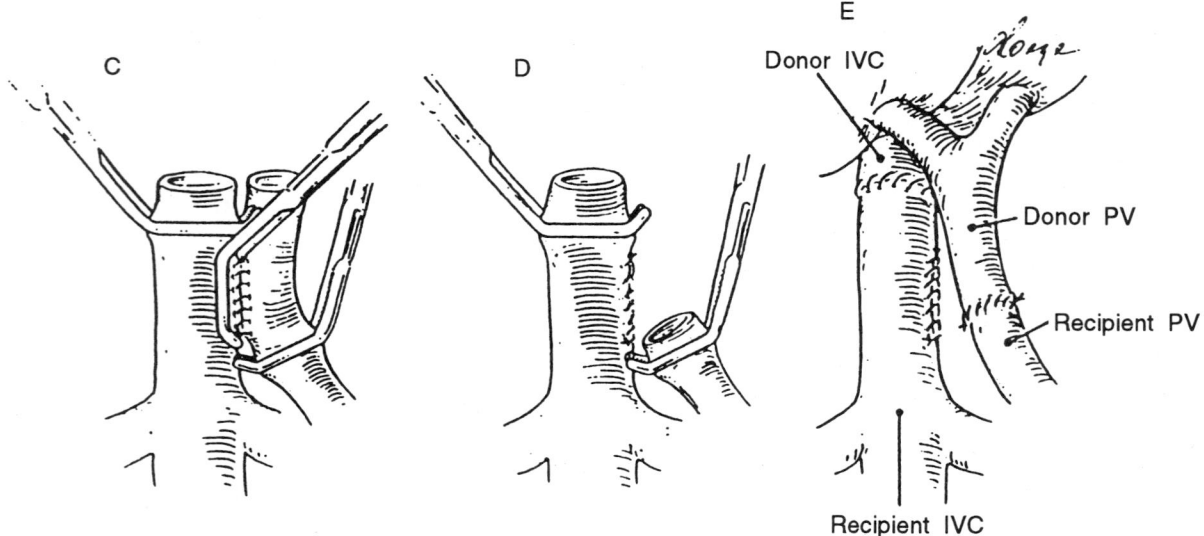

Figure 3 Dismantling of a side-to-side portocaval shunt during an orthotopic liver transplant.

of PVT has been accomplished by using operative techniques of thromboendarterectomy of the native vessel, retrograde dissection to the splenomesenteric junction, and the utilization of venous conduits from the portal vein and the superior mesenteric vein. In the review of our patients with PVT, rethrombosis of the portal vein was low, but hospital stays were longer and 90 day mortality was higher than for other transplanted patients.[5] In a more recent analysis of our experience, we transplanted significantly more patients with portal vein abnormalities with no impact on mortality, documenting that transplantation can succeed in patients with PVT, with better patient selection and surgical experience.[6]

RESULTS

Survival following liver transplantation continues to improve and is currently approximately 70% at 5 years in most reported series. The results achieved by liver transplantation far exceed those achieved by shunts when comparing patients with end-stage Child's C liver disease (Table 2).[2] At UCLA, 1 year graft and patient survival for all transplants is now 79% and 88%, respectively. In comparing our first 100 liver transplants to our most recent 200, we found we had transplanted more older patients and higher risk candidates with improved results, substantially shorter operative times,

Table 2 Survival Comparison Among Various Treatments for Bleeding Esophageal Varices (Child's Class C, Poor Liver Function)

Study	Number of Patients	Survival Rates (%)				
		1 year	2 years	3 years	4 years	5 years
Turcotte et al (1973)						
Nonselective shunt	50	36	32	22	20	17
Warren et al (1982)						
Selective shunt	?	60*	53*	45*	40*	35*
Nonselective shunt	?	50*	40*	37*	20*	15*
Rikkers et al (1984)						
Shunt and nonshunt operations†	24	45*	35*	30*	20*	17*
Chandler et al (1985)						
Shunt‡	30	36*	30*	25*	20*	13*
Iwatsuki et al (1988)						
Liver transplantation	302	79	74	71	71	71

*Value estimated from survival curve.
†Fifteen nonselective shunts, seven selective shunts, and two nonshunt operations.
‡Both selective and nonselective operations.
From Mazzaferro V, Iwatsuki S, Starzl TE. Liver transplantation in the management of portal hypertension. In: Ernst CB, Stanley JC, eds. Current therapy in vascular surgery. 2nd ed. Philadelphia: BC Decker, 1991:807; with permission.

decreased transfusion requirements, and no intraoperative deaths. The improved survival was also coupled with an improved use of hospital resources, as reflected by less time in the intensive care unit and shorter hospital stays, resulting in a 31% decrease in the median cost of a liver transplant between these two periods.[6]

REFERENCES

1. Shaked A, Goldstein RM, Klintmalm GB, et al. Portosystemic shunt versus orthotopic liver transplantation for the Budd-Chiari syndrome. Surg Gynecol Obstet 1992; 174:453–459.
2. Iwatsuki s, Starzl T, Todo S, et al. Liver transplantation in the treatment of bleeding esophageal varices. Surgery 1988; 104:697–705.
3. Brems J, Hiatt J, Klein A, et al. Effect of prior portasystemic shunt on subsequent liver transplantation. Ann Surg 1989; 209:51–56.
4. Mazzafero V, Todo S, Tzakis AG, et al. Liver transplantation in patients with previous portosystemic shunt. Am J Surg 1990; 160:111–116.
5. Shaked A, Busuttil RW. Liver transplantation in patients with portal vein thrombosis and central portacaval shunts. Ann Surg 1991; 214:696–702.
6. Busuttil RW, Shaked A, Millis JM, et al. One thousand liver transplants, the lessons learned. Ann Surg 1994; 219:490–499.

PORTAL HYPERTENSION IN CHILDREN

FREDERICK M. KARRER, M.D.
JOHN R. LILLY, M.D.

The important clinical consequences of portal hypertension are the same in children as in adults, namely, esophageal variceal hemorrhage, ascites, and hypersplenism. The cause of portal hypertension in children, however, is quite different. In adults, cirrhosis of the liver, due most often to alcohol abuse, is the predominant cause. In children, about half of the instances of variceal bleeding occur with normal liver function in which portal hypertension is caused by portal vein thrombosis. In the remainder, portal hypertension is caused by intrahepatic disease, such as biliary atresia. The treatment of portal hypertension in children is therefore directly influenced by the natural history and prognosis of the underlying disease.

ETIOLOGY

Increased portal blood pressure is the product of both increased resistance to splanchnic blood flow through the liver and increased blood flow in the portal circuit. The restriction of splanchnic venous flow may be suprahepatic, as with hepatic vein obstruction; intrahepatic, as with cirrhosis; or prehepatic, as occurs with portal vein thrombosis. From a pathophysiologic standpoint, it is important to separate conditions in which the hepatic parenchyma itself is under pressure from those in which the increased pressure is presinusoidal. Examples of the latter are portal vein obstruction and congenital hepatic fibrosis. In presinusoidal portal hypertension, liver function is typically normal, ascites and coagulopathy are transient or absent altogether, bleeding episodes are mild, and the prognosis generally good. In those conditions, such as cirrhosis or hepatic veno-occlusive disease, in which the obstruction is at or downstream from the hepatic sinusoid, liver synthetic function is impaired, ascites is common, coagulopathy is worse, hemorrhage is difficult to control, and the prognosis is guarded.

Portal Vein Thrombosis

Thrombosis of the portal venous system may involve only the main portal vein or extend into the major tributaries, the superior mesenteric vein and splenic vein (Fig. 1). Occasionally, portal vein thrombosis can be traced back to neonatal umbilical vein catheterization, omphalitis, intra-abdominal sepsis, dehydration, or some hypercoagulable state, but many times no clear etiologic event can be discovered. Collaterals surrounding the obstructed portal vein and recanalization of the thrombosis result in so-called cavernous transformation of the portal vein.

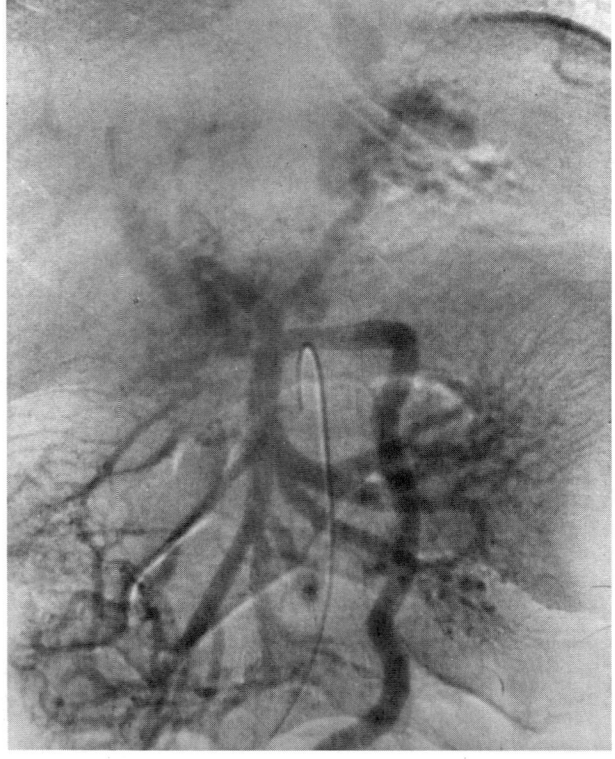

Figure 1 Venous phase of a mesenteric arteriogram showing severe partial obstruction of the portal vein (cavernous transformation) and a dilated, tortuous coronary vein draining into the esophageal varices.

Congenital Hepatic Fibrosis

Congenital hepatic fibrosis is at one end of a spectrum of polycystic diseases of the liver and kidneys. Portal hypertension is the result of linear fibrous bands in the portal space that causes a presinusoidal obstruction to portal venous flow. These children usually develop hepatomegaly and varices; however, hepatic synthetic function is preserved.

Biliary Atresia

Biliary atresia is the most common intrahepatic cause of portal hypertension in children. Even though bile flow can be re-established with Kasai's operation, progression of disease or incomplete decompression often results in biliary cirrhosis. Fibrosis and regenerative nodules impede portal venous flow through the sinusoid to cause a postsinusoidal obstruction. Consequently, many children have portal hypertension to varying degrees.[1]

Budd-Chiari Syndrome

Obstruction to hepatic venous outflow, Budd-Chiari syndrome, may be due to thrombosis, fibrous obliteration, congenital webs, or tumor obstructing the hepatic veins or the suprahepatic vena cava. It is a rare cause of portal hypertension in children. It is most often seen in association with blood dyscrasias, such as polycythemia. Because Budd-Chiari syndrome is a postsinusoidal obstruction, hepatocellular damage is extensive because of hepatic congestion of the liver.

CLINICAL MANIFESTATIONS

In portal hypertension, emphasis has been placed on the obstruction to portal blood flow, but an important accompaniment is increased splanchnic blood flow in the portal system. Unlike the passive stasis of congestive heart failure, most examples of portal hypertension are associated with a hyperdynamic splanchnic circulation, bounding peripheral pulses, increased cardiac output, and low systemic vascular resistance.[2] The exact mechanisms behind this hyperdynamic state are not well understood but are thought to be caused by either elevated levels of circulating vasodilators, such as glucagon, or reduced sensitivity to vasoconstrictors, such as catecholamines. The end result of this unusual combination of both increased resistance and increased blood flow is the development of portosystemic collaterals in an attempt to decompress the portal circuit.

Esophageal Varices

Clinically, the most important portosystemic collaterals, which develop to decompress the portal system, occur in the distal esophagus, the portal to azygous-hemiazygous system. In the distal esophagus, the veins are very superficial, existing in the lamina propria rather than being submucosal as in the rest of the esophagus and gut. As the esophageal vein becomes varicose, the vein wall thins and the propensity to rupture increases. Bleeding from esophageal varices typically presents suddenly with painless, massive hematemesis. Occasionally, melenic stools may be the initial manifestation. When the cause of variceal hemorrhage is portal vein thrombosis, the onset of bleeding occurs in a previously healthy child, between 3 and 6 years old. Stigmata of liver disease are absent except, perhaps, for an enlarged spleen. Conversely, most children with portal hypertension from cirrhosis are known to have liver disease for years and have typical physical findings of jaundice, ascites, splenomegaly, spider angioma, and poor growth.

The natural history of esophageal varices is an important factor in selection of therapy. In children with portal vein thrombosis, less dangerous spontaneous portosystemic collaterals develop over time. Varices become (1) more easily controlled by local endoscopic measures, (2) less prone to hemorrhage, and (3) more likely to regress. By contrast, varices associated with cirrhosis tend to become larger and more numerous over time and, because of progressive liver dysfunction, coagulopathy, and portal hypertension, are more likely to bleed and less likely to stop spontaneously.

Ascites

Ascitic fluid originates from the serosal surfaces of the gastrointestinal tract and in some instances from the liver surface. Ascites is rare in children with portal vein thrombosis but is common in patients with advanced decompensated liver disease. The obstruction to portal venous flow through the liver, combined with hypoalbuminemia, overwhelms the Starling forces, favoring ascites formation. Liver dysfunction is usually well recognized, and the development of ascites is a harbinger of further liver decompensation. The gradual increase in abdominal girth over months or years may go unnoticed until the ascites is of sufficient volume to permit detection of a fluid wave or shifting dullness by clinical examination. In the setting of sepsis, infection of the ascitic fluid or spontaneous bacterial peritonitis must be ruled out by paracentesis. Progressive ascites can also result in diaphragmatic elevation and respiratory embarrassment.

Hypersplenism

Enlargement of the spleen frequently accompanies portal hypertension, but spleen size correlates poorly with the level of portal blood pressure. By contrast, the degree of splenomegaly is closely correlated with splenic arterial blood flow. Paradoxically, rather than the splenic arterial blood flow being decreased as might be expected if splenomegaly were due simply to passive congestion, splenic arterial blood flow is usually increased. As splenic blood flow increases, more blood percolates through the splenic pulp, and more abnormal cells (and eventually normal cells) are sequestered by the reticuloendothelial system. Hypersplenism is a clinical syndrome in which there is a reduced platelet count or white blood cell count in the presence of splenomegaly. Significant anemia from destruction of red blood cells is rare. Typically, the thrombocytopenia is mild, and the reduction in platelets is not sufficient to cause petechiae, bruising, or spontaneous nonvariceal bleeding.

TREATMENT

Management of complications of pediatric portal hypertension must be individualized according to the underlying cause. In children with cirrhosis, the prognosis of the liver disease should impact the decision to perform high-risk operative procedures versus liver transplantation. Similarly, the good prognosis of children with portal vein obstruction should suggest the most effective but least invasive and risky treatment plan.

Variceal Hemorrhage

The therapeutic options to control pediatric esophageal variceal hemorrhage are (1) endoscopic techniques, (2) portosystemic shunts, and (3) devascularization procedures.

Endoscopic Techniques

The original description of endoscopic control of variceal hemorrhage by injection of sclerosant solutions was introduced years ago but only recently popularized by Terblanche and colleagues.[3] Endoscopic sclerosis can be performed with either rigid or flexible endoscopic equipment. We prefer intravariceal injection using 5% sodium morrhuate in up to three varices at each session (Fig. 2).[4] Initially, the sclerosis may be required every few days but the interval between treatments is gradually

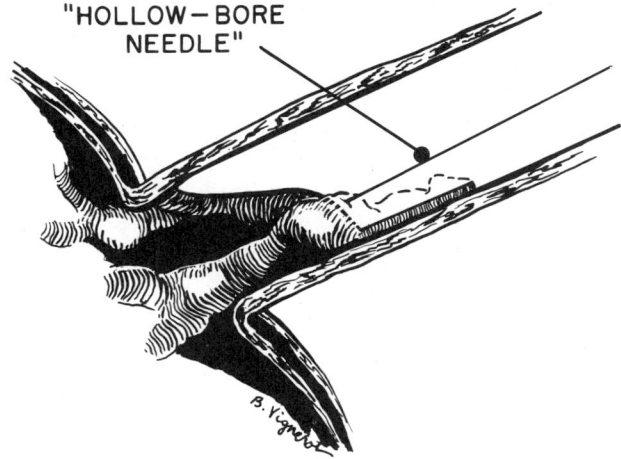

Figure 2 Artist's depiction of rigid endoscopic sclerosis. The varix is entrapped in the slot of the endoscope, where it can be injected intraluminally with sclerosant.

extended. Control of variceal hemorrhage has been quite good, especially hemorrhage caused by portal vein thrombosis.

Another novel technique is endoscopic variceal ligation, which uses an elastic band to strangle the varices at the gastroesophageal junction (Fig. 3).[5] The device used for this consists of two fitted cylinders that attach to the end of a standard flexible gastroscope. An elastic O-ring stretched over the tip of the inner cylinder can be released by retraction of the cylinder with a trip wire passed through the biopsy channel. The ring is placed on the base of a varix by gentle suction of the varix into the device. Results with this technique are promising in early reports.

Portosystemic Shunts

Procedures designed to decompress the portal system by diversion of portal venous blood into the systemic venous system were the mainstay of treatment for 30 years. Historically, mesocaval and central splenorenal shunts enjoyed the greatest popularity for children. They were chosen because neither requires patency of the portal vein that so often is not present in this age group. Recently, two large studies have been reported using side-to-side splenorenal anastomoses.[6,7] The technique eliminates the necessity of vena caval interruption required for mesocaval shunts and of splenectomy for central splenorenal shunts, both of which may have undesirable consequences for children. The complication of encephalopathy was not reported with the side-to-side splenorenal shunt.

Still, the use of portosystemic shunts has decreased significantly over the last 10 years. Several factors have influenced the decline. First, the small vein size in children increases the technical difficulty, which translates into a higher rate of shunt thrombosis, shunt failure, and rebleeding. Second, less invasive, less risky endoscopic techniques have proven successful. Third, the diversion of portal blood flow may result in encephalopathy or accelerate hepatic deterioration. Fourth, liver transplantation in children with cirrhosis as the preferred treatment for end-stage liver failure and portosystemic shunt procedures, particularly those that use the portal vein, make subsequent hepatic replacement significantly more difficult and complicated. Finally, the new nonoperative methods of transvenous intrahepatic portosystemic stent shunting (TIPSS) appear to provide

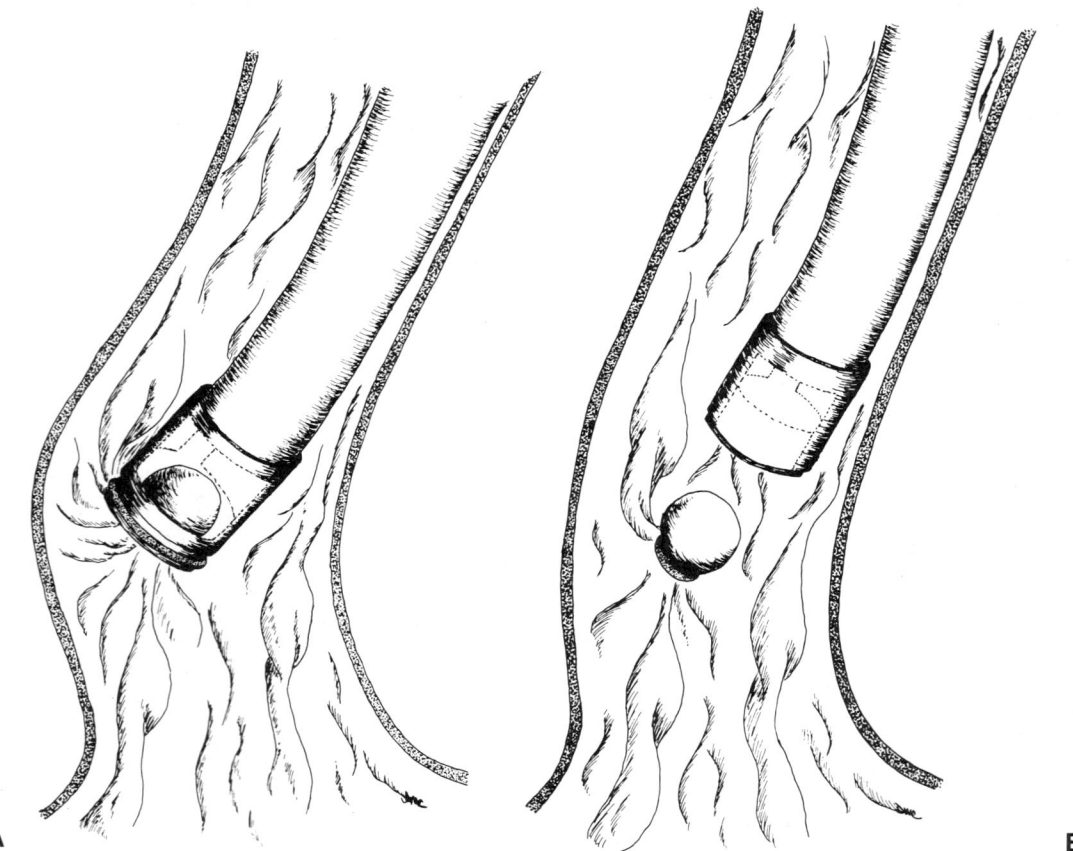

Figure 3 Artist's drawing of endoscopic variceal ligation. *A,* Using a flexible gastroscope with the ligating device affixed to the end, the varix is aspirated into the banding chamber. *B,* The trip wire is pulled, which releases the elastic ligature around the base of the varix, strangulating it.

a more acceptable alternative.[8] Use of this technique in children, however, is as yet very limited.

Nonshunting Procedures

A variety of nonshunting procedures have been offered to control variceal hemorrhage, including esophageal transection, direct ligation of esophageal varices, and Sugiura's procedure of gastric devascularization, esophageal transection, and splenectomy.[9] None has been used extensively in children. All require a major operation and are not infrequently associated with significant rebleeding rates. The situation in which these procedures may have a role is in the exceptional patient whose bleeding cannot be controlled endoscopically and who is not a candidate for liver replacement or portosystemic shunting.

Ascites

Conservative management of clinically significant ascites consists of dietary sodium and water restriction, diuresis with spironolactone and furosemide, and occasionally paracentesis. Peritoneovenous shunts can effectively treat respiratory complications, but because severe ascites usually accompanies significant hepatic synthetic deterioration with coagulopathy and hypoalbuminemia, consideration of liver transplantation should take precedence.

Hypersplenism

Clinically significant hypersplenism with pancytopenia is rare, even though massive splenomegaly is not. Treatment by splenectomy, although effective, has fallen out of favor because of the recognized hazard of overwhelming postsplenectomy sepsis. Partial splenic embolization is a nonoperative technique aimed at eliminating hypersplenism while preserving splenic immune function. Using small gel foam particles, 60% to 80% of the spleen is peripherally embolized via the splenic artery. The consequent splenic infarction is accompanied by transient fever and pain and frequently by ileus, pleural effusion, and atelectasis as well. At our center, 10 of 13 patients have had sustained resolution of thrombocytopenia and leukopenia following partial splenic embolization.[10]

Acknowledgment. Supported in part by a grant (RR-69) from the General Clinical Research Centers Program at the Division of Research Resources, National Institutes of Health and the Pediatric Liver Center, University of Colorado/The Children's Hospital, Denver, Colorado.

REFERENCES

1. Ohi R, Mochizuki I, Komatsu K, Kasai M. Portal hypertension after successful hepatic portoenterostomy in biliary atresia. J Pediatr Surg 1986; 21:271–274.
2. Benoit JN, Granger DN. Splanchnic hemodynamics in chronic portal hypertension. Semin Liver Dis 1986; 6:287–298.
3. Terblanche J, Northover JM, Bornman P, et al. A prospective evaluation of injection sclerotherapy in the treatment of acute bleeding from esophageal varices. Surgery 1979; 85:239–245.
4. Lilly JR. Endoscopic sclerosis of esophageal varices in children. Surg Gynecol Obstet 1981; 152:513–514.
5. Karrer FM, Holland RM, Allshouse MJ, Lilly JR. Portal vein thrombosis: Treatment of variceal hemorrhage by endoscopic variceal ligation. J Pediatr Surg 1994; 29:1149–1151.
6. Orloff MJ, Orloff MS, Rambotti M. Treatment of bleeding esophagogastric varices due to extrahepatic portal hypertension: Results of portal-systemic shunts during 35 years. J Pediatr Surg 1994; 29:142–154.
7. Mitra SK, Rao KLN, Narasimhan KL, et al. Side-to-side lienorenal shunts without splenectomy in noncirrhotic portal hypertension in children. J Pediatric Surg 1993; 28:398–402.
8. Simpson KJ, Chalmers N, Redhead DN, et al. Transjugular intrahepatic portasystemic stent shunting for control of acute and recurrent upper gastrointestinal haemorrhage related to portal hypertension. Gut 1993; 34:968–973.
9. Sugiura M, Futagawa S. A new technique for treating esophageal varices. J Thorac Cardiovasc Surg 1973; 66:677–685.
10. Brandt CJ, Rothbarth LJ, Kumpe DA, et al. Splenic embolization in children: Long-term efficacy. J Pediatr Surg 1989; 24:642–645.

RENOVASCULAR DISEASE

PATHOLOGY OF RENAL ARTERY OCCLUSIVE DISEASE

RAJABRATA SARKAR, M.D.
LOUIS M. MESSINA, M.D.

Although occlusive lesions of the renal arteries may develop from a variety of distinct pathologic processes, they have the similar hemodynamic and clinical consequences of reduced renal blood flow and the subsequent development of renovascular hypertension and loss of renal function. Pathologic identification of the etiology of occlusive lesions of the renal arteries is complicated by the generally late stage of disease at which excision and examination of occlusive lesions occurs; thus, there is superimposition of secondary artery wall changes onto the primary disease process. Nevertheless, several distinct renal artery occlusive disease processes have been identified, including atherosclerosis, fibromuscular disease, and developmental malformations. Rarer causes of renal artery occlusive disease are the inflammatory arteritidies including Takayasu's disease, radiation arteritis, and retroperitoneal fibrosis.

RENAL ARTERY ATHEROSCLEROSIS

Atherosclerosis of the renal artery is the most common cause of renal artery occlusive disease and usually becomes clinically evident in the elderly. Distribution of renal artery atherosclerosis between the sexes is similar to that of atherosclerotic lesions elsewhere in the arterial circulation. An initial male predominance diminishes with advancing age until an equal distribution is seen in those over 80 years of age. This late equalization of gender distribution may be due to the loss of the antiatherogenic effects of estrogen and progesterone on the artery wall that occurs in women after menopause.

Autopsy studies of renal artery atherosclerosis document significant stenoses in approximately half of normotensive and three-fourths of hypertensive individuals. Significant lesions are almost always located at the renal orifice or within the first one-third of the main renal artery. The systemic nature of atherosclerosis is highlighted in the renal arteries by the high incidence of bilateral lesions with a severe stenosis in one renal artery associated with a greater than 50% chance of a significant stenosis in the contralateral artery. No unique risk factors for renal artery atherosclerosis have been identified, but affected patients have the well-known risk factors for systemic atherosclerosis, including smoking, hypertension, diabetes, and lipid abnormalities.

The predilection of renal artery atherosclerosis to affect the orifice and proximal aspect of the renal artery most likely reflects the unique patterns of hemodynamic forces at these locations. For the purposes of treatment, including balloon angioplasty and transaortic endarterectomy, orificial and proximal lesions are considered as "aortic spillover" lesions. In the minority of patients with isolated renal artery atherosclerosis, it is possible that another primary disorder of the renal artery was initially present and became a nidus for secondary atherosclerotic changes over time. The advanced nature of atherosclerotic renal artery plaques at the time of excision and examination makes histologic documentation of such a hypothesis difficult.

The pathology of renal artery atherosclerosis is similar to that of complicated atherosclerotic plaques elsewhere in the vascular system. Atherosclerosis is a disease of the intima characterized by extracellular lipid deposition and smooth muscle migration and proliferation (Fig. 1). Features of complex lesions include a fibrous cap containing smooth muscle cells and inflammatory cells that overlie a central core of necrotic debris. These lesions can be further complicated by calcification, intraplaque hemorrhage, and luminal thrombus following cap rupture. Once a significant renal artery lesion has been established, progression of the plaque occurs in both transverse and longitudinal directions. Approximately 50% of hemodynamically significant lesions have progression detectable by arteriography within 1 year. This accelerated process may be due to positive feedback between development of hypertension and worsening of renal artery atherosclerosis, where each pathologic process accelerates the progression of the other.[1]

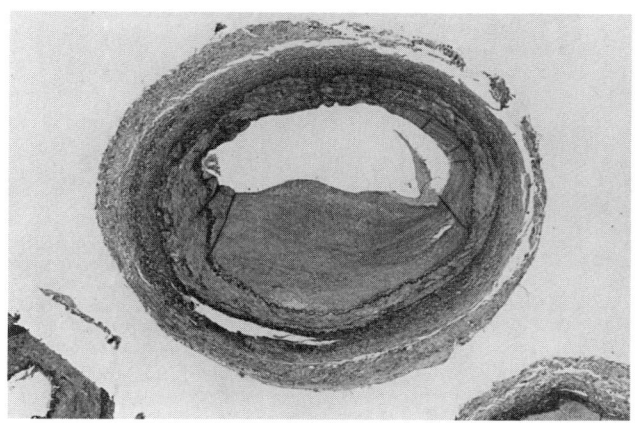

Figure 1 Atherosclerosis. Complex, eccentric plaque comprised of smooth muscle acculumation, extracellular lipid deposition, and inflammatory cells. (Movat stain × 60.)

RENAL ARTERY FIBROMUSCULAR DISEASE

Fibromuscular disease is the second most common cause of surgically correctable hypertension, yet it is an unusual disorder whose etiology and biology remain elusive. Fibromuscular disease is classified topographically by the pattern and extent of transmural involvement of the affected arterial wall. This classification has been noted to correlate in some cases with arteriographic findings.[2]

Intimal fibroplasia primarily affects children and young adults and does not display a gender predeliction. It is noted in approximately 5% of all fibromuscular lesions and occurs in the main renal artery as long, irregular, tubular stenoses in younger patients and as smooth, focal stenoses in older patients.[3] Intimal fibroplasia appears to progress at a slower rate than medial fibromuscular disease. Intimal fibroplasia, which is arteriographically indistinguishable from medial fibromuscular disease, can be subdivided into primary intimal fibroplasia, which is usually seen as a tapered focal stenosis in the main renal artery, and secondary intimal fibroplasia, which is associated with abnormalities in other layers of the artery wall. Secondary intimal fibroplasia also refers to reactive changes in the small intrarenal arteries in renal parenchymal disease,[4] but these are distinct from those lesions occurring in the main renal artery.

Histologic characteristics of intimal fibroplasia include preservation of the internal elastic lamina and leaflets of cellular intimal tissue protruding into the lumen. Clefts often separate these leaflets and may extend almost to the level of the internal elastic lamina. The intimal leaflets are composed of numerous disorganized cells with varying degrees of surrounding matrix. The media and adventitia are usually unaffected. Secondary intimal fibroplasia is distinguished from primary intimal fibroplasia by the presence of dysplastic changes in the other layers of the vessel wall, such as medial dysplasia or overall vessel hypoplasia.

The etiology of intimal fibroplasia is not well defined. Primary intimal fibroplasia may be due to pathologic proliferation of vestigial vascular structures such as fetal arterial musculoelastic cushions. Secondary intimal fibroplasia may be similar to diffuse intimal thickening noted in atherosclerotic vessels in that both may represent intimal reactions to alterations in local blood flow. Previous intraluminal pathology such as thrombosis, intimal fracture from trauma, or prior vessel wall inflammation from viral or immunologic causes have all been considered as potential etiologies of secondary intimal fibroplasia.

Medial hyperplasia is a rare pathologic finding that has been described as a separate disease by some investigators,[3] although others believe that it may represent an early stage of medial fibroplasia.[5] These lesions are arteriographically similar to intimal fibroplasia[3] and are seen most often in women aged 30 to 50 years. Lesions with increases in medial smooth muscle without significant extracellular matrix deposition are considered medial hyperplasia. Aneurysms are not seen in this subtype, and the media is usually intact without dissection or other disruption.[4] If one considers medial hyperplasia as a separate disorder, then it accounts for less than 1% of renal artery fibromuscular disease.

A factor that supports the classification of lesions with medial hyperplasia as early forms of a continuum of fibromuscular disease is the location of these potentially early lesions in the midportion of the main renal artery without involvement of segmental vessels. One study used the presence or absence of smooth muscle hyperplasia, as opposed to the extent of involvement of the vessel wall, to classify fibromuscular lesions.[5] The presence of smooth muscle hyperplasia was associated with a short history of hypertension, fewer aneurysms, and less extension of disease in branch vessels, suggesting that these hyperplastic lesions may be precursors of advanced and more widespread fibrotic lesions, rather than representing a distinct disease process.

Medial fibroplasia is the most common subtype of fibromuscular disease, comprising approximately 85% of all lesions (Fig. 2). Medial fibroplasia predominantly affects white women in the fourth decade of life. Although medial fibroplasia most frequently affects the renal arteries, reports of lesions in the extracranial internal carotid artery and external iliac artery with concurrent renal artery involvement suggest that this disorder can affect the arterial tree diffusely.

Medial fibroplasia most frequently affects the distal main renal artery with extension into branch vessels in approximately one-fourth of patients. The disease is bilateral in 55% of patients and, when unilateral, affects the right side in 80% of patients.[3] The arteriographic appearance of medial fibroplasia is the classic "string of beads" description associated with fibromuscular disease, and this appearance is due to aneurysms greater in size than the adjacent artery wall alternating with luminal weblike projections (Fig. 2A). Other arteriographic presentations are possible with medial fibroplasia, and pathologic studies of solitary, saccular renal

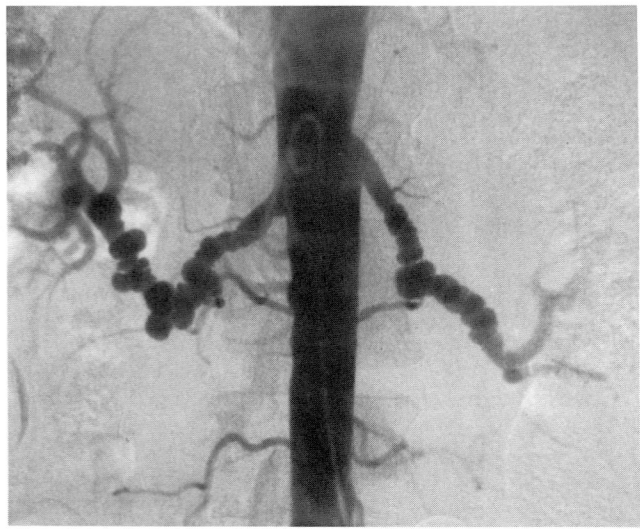
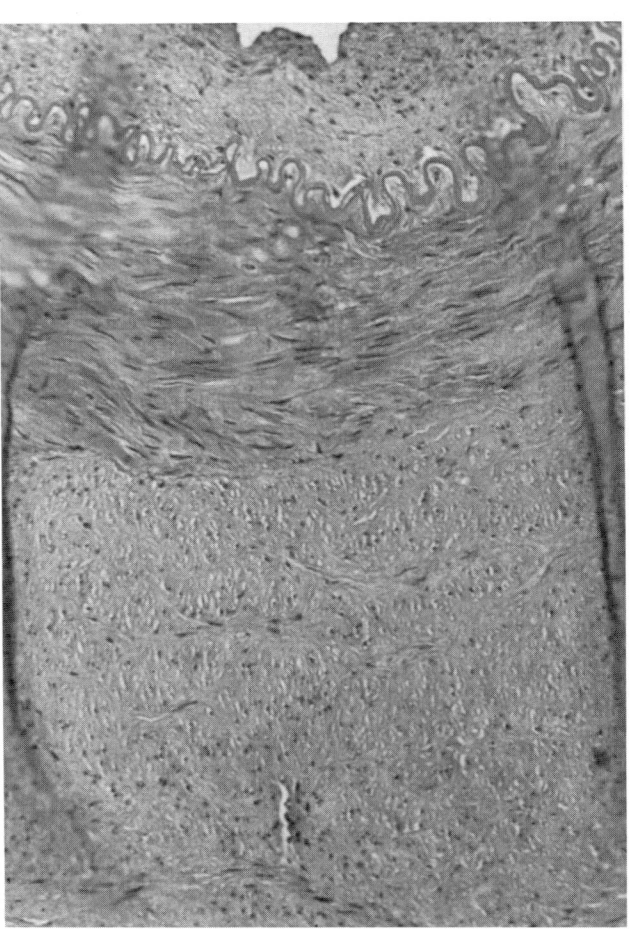

Figure 2 Medial fibrodysplasia. *A,* Arteriographic documentation of characteristic bilateral string of beads appearance. *B,* Histologic evidence of peripheral medial disorganization with excess ground substance and fibrous tissue accompanied by myofibroblasts. (Hematoxylin and eosin × 120.)

artery aneurysms documented that most have histologic evidence of fibromuscular disease, usually without a characteristic clinical presentation of renovascular hypertension. Progression of medial fibroplasia appears to be less frequent than perimedial dysplasia.[2]

Examination of medial fibroplasia reveals two variants—peripheral and diffuse medial fibroplasia—with intermediate examples and transitions from one type to another in a single specimen. In peripheral medial fibroplasia, which is the more common subtype in younger patients, the smooth muscle of the outer media is replaced by dense fibrous tissue and the inner media and internal elastic lamina are generally spared.[3] These lesions are sometimes confused with perimedial dysplasia, although they lack the characteristic collar of elastic fibers surrounding the external elastic lamina that defines the latter subtype.

Diffuse medial fibroplasia is seen more frequently than the peripheral variant and is characterized by fibrous replacement and disruption of normal architecture throughout the media (Fig. 2*B*). Diffuse medial fibroplasia was twice as common in one study[3] and was noted to have medial thinning alternating with dysplastic projections of connective tissue that corresponded to the string of beads radiologic appearance. Ultrastructural analysis of medial fibroplasia documents secretory changes in the cells of the lesion and excessive deposition of extracellular matrix.[6] Aneurysms were noted in 13% of arteries and dissections in less than 1% of arteries. Aneurysms and dissections of the renal artery occur secondary to medial thinning and disruption of elastic fibers and should not be considered as distinct pathologic processes but as complications of fibromuscular disease.

Perimedial dysplasia is characterized by accumulation of elastic tissue at the media-adventitia junction and is noted in 10% of fibromuscular lesions (Fig. 3). This subtype is seen in young women in whom arteriography documents either focal stenosis or multiple "beading" stenoses of the main renal artery but without the intervening aneurysmal dilations that characterize medial fibroplasia. Perimedial dysplasia frequently causes

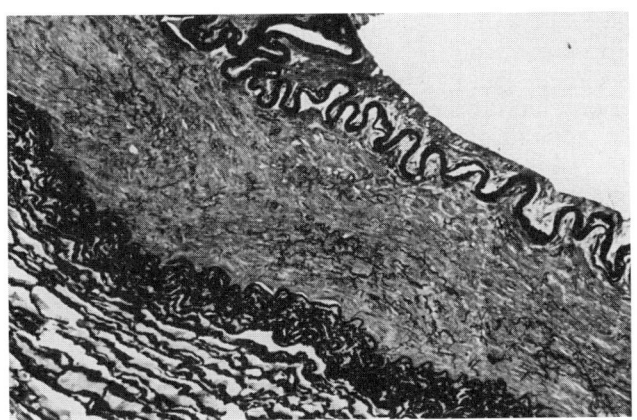

Figure 3 Perimedial dysplasia. Excessive accumulation of elastin fibers at medial-adventitial junction. (Verhoeff × 120.)

renovascular hypertension and progresses more frequently to renal artery occlusion than intimal or medial fibroplasia.[2] Perimedial dysplasia can be distinguished from periarterial fibrosis by several criteria. Periarterial fibrosis extends into the perirenal fat and often is part of a generalized fibrosis of the retroperitoneum, whereas perimedial dysplasia is limited to the vessel wall. The characteristic collar of elastic fibers surrounding the media is not seen in periarterial fibrosis. Further support for the classification of perimedial dysplasia as a primary disorder of the vessel wall is found in ultrastructural studies, which document modified smooth muscle cells but no fibroblasts in these lesions.[6]

The etiology of fibromuscular disease is the subject of much speculation; however, objective evidence to support the myriad proposed etiologies is lacking. Three factors that have received particular attention are hormonal influences, artery wall ischemia, and mechanical stresses.

The overwhelming predilection of fibromuscular disease for women is contrary to the known protective effects of estrogens against human atherosclerosis, another vasoproliferative disorders, as well as the experimental evidence at both the cellular level[7] and artery level,[8] documenting an antiproliferative effect of estrogen on vascular smooth muscle. Oral contraceptives and pregnancy, particularly multiparity, which has been associated with some degenerative vascular lesions such as splenic artery aneurysms, are not significant risk factors for fibromuscular disease.[3]

Ischemia of the vessel wall may play a role in the development of fibromuscular disease. Vasa vasora of muscular arteries originate from branch points of the artery and supply oxygen and nutrients to the artery wall. The arteries affected by fibromuscular dysplasia—the renal, internal carotid, and external iliac—have long arterial segments that are free of branches and thus have long segments with few vasa vasora. Fibromuscular disease may develop as a result of ischemia of the artery wall following an insult to the sparse vasa vasora of these vessels. Support for this theory is found in animal studies in which occlusion of the vasa vasora induces formation of a dysplastic lesion and the location of both perimedial dysplasia and peripheral medial fibroplasia at the medial-adventitial junction, where nutrient blood flow from the vasa vasora is most critical.

Mechanical forces may also play a role in the development of fibromuscular disease because of the unique stresses affecting the arteries in which this disorder occurs. The external iliac, internal carotid, and renal arteries may be subject to lifelong stretch forces not present on other arteries. In support of this concept is the predominance of right-sided lesions in fibromuscular disease. The right renal artery is longer than the left and may be subject to greater stretch, particularly if the kidneys are ptotic.

DEVELOPMENTAL RENAL ARTERY STENOSES

Developmental stenoses are a very rare form of renal artery occlusive disease. In the subset of children with renovascular hypertension, 40% had stenoses characterized as developmental in origin.[9] Developmental renal artery stenosis has been described in young adults with middle aortic syndrome, which consists of a long tubular stenosis of the abdominal aorta, often accompanied by renal and visceral artery stenoses.[10] A subset of adults with either secondary intimal fibroplasia or isolated renal artery atherosclerosis may have had a developmental stenosis that became secondarily affected by either intimal fibroplasia or conventional atherosclerosis; however, documentation of this chain of events is difficult.

Developmental stenosis of the renal artery usually is a hypoplastic lesion with a corresponding diminution of the external diameter of the artery corresponding to the luminal stenosis (Fig. 4). Intimal fibroplasia is usually present, and duplication of the internal elastic lamina is common. Medial thinning and excess perimedial elastic tissue may be present, and poststenotic dilation is not unusual.

The etiology of developmental renal artery stenoses may involve other vascular lesions or focal disruptions of renal artery development. Formation of the main renal artery occurs in the fourth week of gestational life, at which time the paired dorsal aortas fuse to form a single aorta. A single vessel is left following regression of the multiple vessels to the mesonephros, and this single vessel dominates, presumably because of a hemodynamic advantage over the adjacent vessels. Disruptions in blood flow during this critical period such as overfusion of the dorsal aortas with resulting aortic hypoplasia may result in persistence of multiple renal arteries or malformation of renal arteries. Support for this theory includes the 80% incidence of developmental renal artery stenoses in children with abdominal aortic coarctation or aortic hypoplasia.[9] Additional evidence is the presence of multiple renal arteries in 70% of children with congenital abdominal aortic malformations.[9] Intrauterine renal artery development

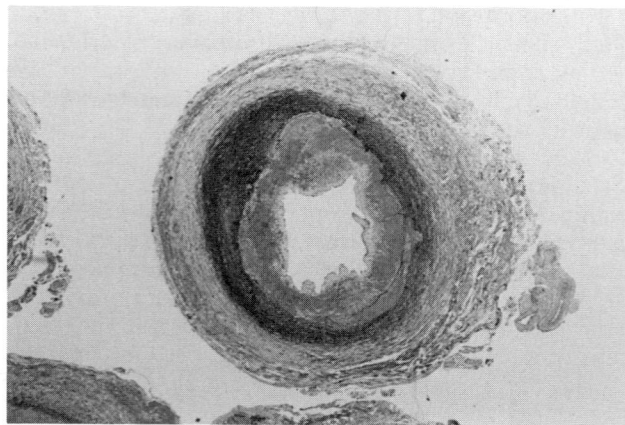

Figure 4 Developmental stenosis. Diminutive, hypoplastic artery exhibiting secondary intimal fibroplasia, irregular medial thinning, and excess accumulations of perimedial elastic tissue. (Movat × 80.)

can also be disrupted by cytocidal viral infections such as rubella, which has been associated with renal artery stenosis in children.

Other unusual causes of renal artery occlusive disease include Takayasu's arteritis and radiation arteritis. Takayasu's aortitis is an inflammatory disease of the aorta, principally the thoracic aorta. Renal artery involvement occurs in approximately one-third of patients and is secondary to ostial involvement from adjacent aortic inflammation. Radiation injury to the renal arteries is secondary to irradiation of abdominal malignancies and can manifest itself as accelerated atherosclerosis, relative arterial hypoplasia with resulting stenosis as a child grows, or pediatric renovascular hypertension.

A variety of diseases can cause occlusive lesions of the renal artery. The diverse etiologies and biologic processes involved in these disorders are difficult to elucidate from pathologic examination of the advanced lesions. Future improvements in our understanding of the cellular and molecular mechanisms involved in atherosclerosis, fibromuscular disease, and other disorders will allow correlation with the well-described histologic findings seen in renal artery occlusive disease.

REFERENCES

1. Wollenweber J, Sheps SG, Davis GD. Clinical course of atherosclerotic renovascular disease. Am J Cardiol 1968; 21:60–71.
2. Goncharenko V, Gerlock AJ, Shaff MI, Hollifield SW. Progression of renal artery fibromuscular dysplasia in 42 patients as seen on angiography 1981; 139:45–51.
3. Stanley JC, Gewertz BL, Bove EL, et al. Arterial fibrodysplasia: Histopathologic character and current etiologic concepts. Arch Surg 1975; 110:561–566.
4. Harrison EG, McCormack LJ. Pathologic classification of renal arterial disease in renovascular hypertension. Mayo Clin Proc 1971; 46:161–167.
5. Alimi Y, Mercier C, Pellissier JF, et al. Fibromuscular disease of the renal artery: A new histopathologic classification. Ann Vasc Surg 1992; 6:220–224.
6. Sottiurai VS, Fry WJ, Stanley JC. Ultrastructure of medial smooth muscle and myofibroblasts in human arterial dysplasia. Arch Surg 1978; 113:1280–1288.
7. Karas RH, Caur W, Tassi L, Mendelsohn ME. Inhibition of vascular smooth muscle cell growth by estrogen. Circulation 1993; 88:325.
8. Vargas R, Wroblewska B, Rego A, et al: Oestradiol inhibits smooth muscle cell proliferation of pig coronary artery. Br J Pharmacol 1993; 109:612–617.
9. Stanley JC, Fry WJ. Pediatric renal artery occlusive disease and renovascular hypertension: Etiology, diagnosis and operative treatment. Arch Surg 1981; 116:669–676.
10. Messina LM, Reilly LM, Goldstone J, et al: Middle aortic syndrome: Effectiveness and durability of complex arterial revascularization techniques. Ann Surg 1986; 204:331-339.

DUPLEX SCANNING FOR RENAL ARTERIAL OCCLUSIVE DISEASE

KIMBERLEY J. HANSEN, M.D.
SCOTT W. REAVIS, R.V.T.
RICHARD H. DEAN, M.D.

Evaluation for renovascular occlusive disease continues to evolve through several screening methods. In respective eras, rapid-sequence intravenous pyelography, peripheral plasma renin activity, infusion of angiotensin II antagonists, and radionuclide renography have been proposed as valuable screening tests to detect hemodynamically significant renovascular disease (RVD). In the past, none of these methods survived close scrutiny or sustained use owing to a lack of sensitivity, specificity, or both.

Among the currently applicable technologies, we have chosen renal duplex sonography (RDS) as our screening test of choice. Continuing improvements in probe design and color flow imaging have enhanced the usefulness of RDS over conventional arteriography and have decreased the time required for examination.[1-3] Consequently, we have evaluated the role of RDS as a surface study to initially screen for RVD, as well as a surveillance method to monitor the stability of renal artery balloon angioplasty and surgical reconstructions. Renal duplex sonography of sufficient accuracy to guide further management of correctable RVD requires proper equipment, as well as close collaboration between the vascular surgeon and a committed technologist. A low carrying frequency probe (2.5 to 3 mHz) with small footprint is required to obtain Doppler interrogation at the anatomic depth of the renal arteries. The small probe is necessary for subxiphoid and flank examination. Additionally, even an experienced sonographer must be allowed sufficient opportunity to perform studies in conjunction with the vascular surgeon. This interchange is important to establish and conduct validity analysis, which defines the overall accuracy of the examination for each vascular laboratory. Using this approach, we have performed more than 2,000 RDS studies to screen patients ranging from 2 to 90 years in age. Technically satisfactory studies, defined as complete main renal artery Doppler interrogation from aortic origin to renal hilum, have been obtained in 96% of renal arteries studied. Combining the results from initial and ongoing comparisons between RDS and conventional cut film arteriography in 156 patients, we have observed an overall accuracy of 96% (Table 1).

Patients for screening examination and examination following balloon angioplasty or surgical reconstruction are fasted overnight. Early in our experience, we routinely administered 10 mg biscodyl by mouth the evening before examination; however, we currently reserve biscodyl for patients requiring a repeat study due to bowel gas interference. The B-scan images and Doppler-shifted signals from the aorta, visceral, and renal arteries are first obtained in the supine position with either a 3 mHz mechanical long focus probe or a 2.25 mHz phase array probe with Doppler color flow capability. Positioned in the abdominal midline just below the xiphoid process, the sagittal B-scan image of the upper abdominal aorta defines the origins of the celiac and superior mesenteric arteries. At this level, a center stream aortic peak systolic velocity (PSV) may be obtained. Using the origin of the superior mesenteric artery and the left renal vein as visual references, the origin of each main renal artery can usually be defined in transverse projection during peak inspiration (Fig. 1).

For a complete examination, we require that sequential renal artery Doppler-shifted signals and calculated PSVs are obtained throughout the renal artery in

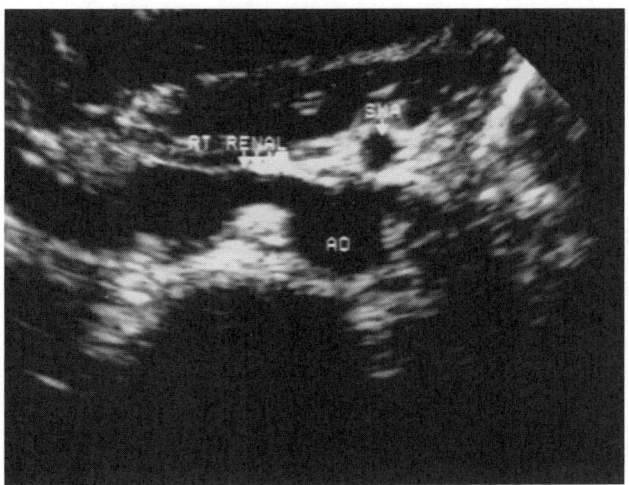

Figure 1 Transverse projection of aorta and renal arteries (From Hansen KJ, Reavis SW, Dean RH, et al. Use of duplex scanning in renovascular hypertension. In: Yao JST, Pearce WH, eds. Technologies in vascular surgery. Philadelphia: WB Saunders, 1991:174; with permission)

Table 1 Comparative Analysis of Parameter Estimates and Their 95 Percent Confidence Intervals

Group	Number	Measure	Estimate	95 Percent Confidence Interval
All kidneys	142 (kidneys)	Sensitivity	0.88	(0.84, 0.92)
		Specificity	0.99	(0.97, 1.00)
		PPV	0.98*	(0.96, 0.99)
		NPV	0.92*	(0.89, 0.95)
	148 (kidneys)	Accuracy	0.91	(0.87, 0.95)
Kidneys with single renal artery	122 (kidneys)	Sensitivity	0.93	(0.90, 0.96)
		Specificity	0.98*	(0.96, 1.00)
		PPV	0.98*	(0.96, 1.00)
		NPV	0.94	(0.91, 0.97)
	148 (kidneys)	Accuracy	0.91	(0.87, 0.95)
Kidneys with multiple renal arteries	21 (arteries)	Sensitivity	0.67	(0.53, 0.81)
		Specificity	1.00*	—
		PPV	1.00*	—
		NPV	0.79*	(0.68, 0.90)
		Accuracy	0.86	(0.76, 0.96)
All patients	74 (subjects)	Sensitivity	0.93	(0.87, 0.99)
		Specificity	1.00*	—
		PPV	1.00*	—
		NPV	0.91*	(0.84, 0.98)
		Accuracy	0.96	(0.91, 1.00)

*Estimated standard error is zero; confidence level is inestimable.
PPV, Positive predictive value; NPV, negative predictive value.
(From Hansen KJ, Tribble RW, Reavis SW, et al. Renal duplex sonography: Evaluation of clinical utility. J Vasc Surg 1990; 12:227–236; with permission.)

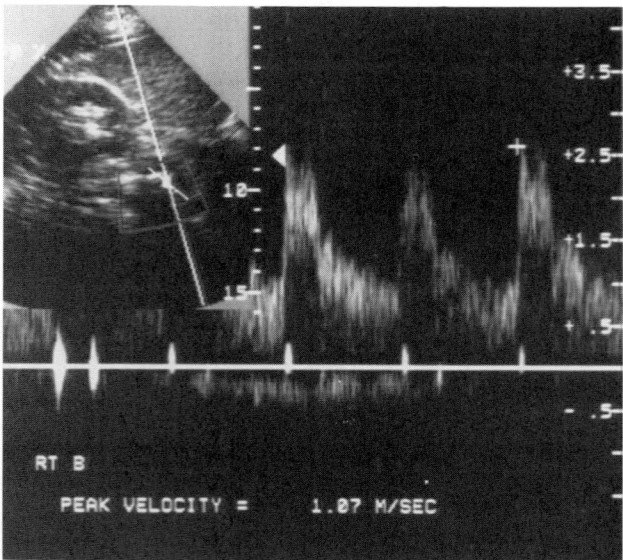

Figure 2 Normal Doppler spectral analysis during surface renal duplex sonography from undiseased right renal artery. (From Hansen KJ, Reavis SW, Dean RH, et al. Use of duplex scanning in renovascular hypertension. In: Yao JST, Pearce WH, eds. Technologies in vascular surgery. Philadelphia: WB Saunders, 1991:174; with permission)

continuity from aorta to renal hilum. Doppler color flow capability permits a more rapid identification of the renal artery origins and the anatomic course to the kidney (Fig. 2). In kidneys with normal parenchymal renovascular resistance, documentation of forward blood flow throughout diastole is consistent but not uniquely characteristic of the renal artery color flow signal. The celiac axis and its branches also have forward flow during diastole and may occasionally be confused with a renal artery signal. The B-scan identification and Doppler interrogation is then repeated using a flank approach with the patient in a decubitus position. This flank approach improves B-scan image quality and Doppler signal. From the flank, the liver and kidney provide solid organ acoustic windows free of bowel gas interference, and the surface transducer can be placed closer to the area of renal artery interrogation, improving image quality. Inherent errors in estimation of renal artery peak systolic velocity (RA-PSV) are reduced by minimizing the angle of insonation. Finally, the kidney length, width, and thickness are determined.

Doppler-shifted signals are obtained from regions of arcuate and interlobar arteries, and color flow parenchymal mapping are performed. Color flow Doppler from the flank approach helps to identify the intraparenchymal vascular anatomy. Several investigators have suggested that Doppler spectral analysis of the distal renal artery and parenchymal vessels alone may be sufficient to detect a critical renal artery stenosis. We have examined the utility of Doppler spectral waveform recognition and systolic acceleration times from these sites; however, we consider this information only a qualitative expression of renovascular and parenchymal disease.

Table 2 Doppler Criteria for Renal Artery Stenosis

Stenosis	Criteria
Less than 60% diameter-reducing renal artery (RA) stenosis	RA peak systolic velocity (PSV) from entire RA < 2 m/sec
60% or greater diameter-reducing RA stenosis	*Focal* RA-PSV ≥ 2 m/sec *and* distal turbulent velocity waveform
Occlusion	No Doppler-shifted signal from renal artery B-scan image
Inadequate study for interpretation	Failure to obtain Doppler samples from entire main renal artery

Table 2 depicts RDS criteria for critical renal artery stenoses. Assuming that RA-PSV varied with the degree of renal artery stenosis and aortic PSV, most authors have advocated the ratio of RA-PSV to aortic PSV (the renal-aortic ratio) to define a critical renal artery stenosis. In contrast, we have found no relationship between RA-PSV and aortic PSV in the presence or absence of disease. Focal RA-PSV 2 m/sec or more in combination with distal poststenotic turbulence has proved to correlate highly with the arteriographic presence of 60% or greater diameter-reducing renal artery stenosis (Table 1). In our first validity analysis of 122 kidneys with single renal arteries and renal arteriograms for comparison, RDS correctly identified 67 of 68 kidneys with normal and less than 60% renal artery stenosis, and 30 of 39 kidneys with 60 to 99% renal artery stenosis. All 15 renal artery occlusions were correctly identified by failure to obtain a Doppler-shifted signal from an imaged renal artery. Using these techniques and criteria for interpretation, RDS was 93% sensitive and 98% specific, with a positive predictive value of 98% and a negative predictive value of 94%. Overall accuracy was 96% when compared prospectively to cut film arteriography.

These results are superior to all alternative screening tests for RVD; however, strict attention to patient preparation, skilled performance of the scan, and adherence to these criteria are prerequisites for this level of success. We feel that interrogation of the entire renal artery is necessary to ensure these results because accelerated blood flow velocity secondary to stenosis may normalize two vessel diameters distal to the lesion. Furthermore, the increase in RA-PSV must be focal and accompanied by turbulent distal spectral waveforms (Fig. 3). Turbulent waveforms are characterized by delayed acceleration in early systole with mosaic Doppler color flow patterns. Of our patients screened for significant RVD, 4% had more than 2 m/sec RA-PSV uniformly throughout the renal artery. In general, these patients are younger than 50 years old, fail to demonstrate distal turbulent spectral waveforms, and fail to

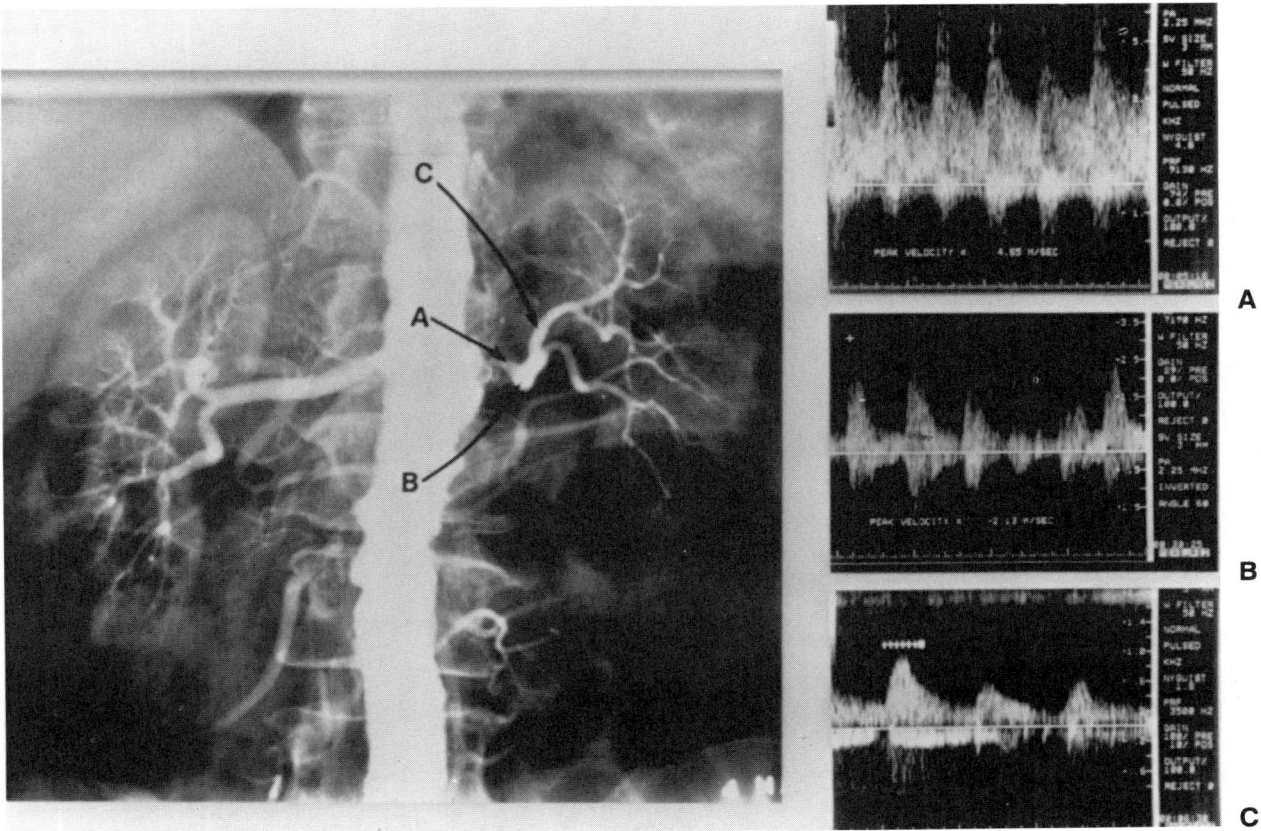

Figure 3 Cut-film aortogram demonstrating high-grade left renal artery stenosis. *A,* Doppler spectral analysis at the site of stenosis demonstrating focal increase in renal artery peak systolic velocity (RA-PSV) (4.6 m/sec). *B,* Distal spectral analysis demonstrating turbulent waveform—decreased RA-PSV with ragged spectral envelope and spontaneous bi-directional signals. *C,* Spectral analysis of several vessel diameters distal to stenosis demonstrating return of near-normal waveform. (From Hansen KJ, Reavis SW, Dean RH, et al. Use of duplex scanning in renovascular hypertension. In: Yao JST, Pearce WH, eds. Technologies in vascular surgery. Philadelphia: WB Saunders, 1991:174; with permission.)

demonstrate anatomic disease by conventional cut film arteriography. The lack of focality and distal turbulence distinguish this subgroup from those patients with anatomic disease. Finally, although not confirmed by prospective study, our experience with color flow mapping suggests that a mosaic parenchymal pattern coincides with grossly disturbed, poststenotic turbulence.

When used as an initial screening study for RVD causing hypertension, multiple or polar renal arteries, and branch renal artery disease, pose a potentially serious limitations of surface RDS. Of the patients presenting to our institution for evaluation of renovascular hypertension, 19% have had polar renal arteries documented by arteriography. Among these patients, 43% have had multiple vessels to both kidneys and 40% of all the multiple vessels have 60% or greater diameter-reducing stenoses or occlusions.

Because of variable polar vessel origin, small vessel size, and compromised image quality associated with low-frequency probes, identification of polar vessels and their associated disease is difficult. In our first validity analysis of surface RDS, we identified only 1 of 43 polar arteries. Although Doppler color flow has enhanced recognition of multiple renal arteries, failure to identify these polar vessels and their associated disease continues to comprise the largest single source of our false-negative studies.

Failure of RDS to identify polar vessel disease relates to the prevalence of such disease within the patient population examined and the clinical indication for surface RDS. Of our patients submitted to repair for unilateral RVD and presumed renovascular hypertension, 14% have had only polar branch disease. We believe this group constitutes a significant minority of patients. We therefore proceed with conventional arteriography in patients younger than 60 years of age with poorly controlled hypertension despite multidrug therapy, even in the presence of a negative surface RDS. When RDS is used to screen for ischemic nephropathy and renal insufficiency, however, a negative RDS effectively excludes significant RVD because polar vessel disease alone does not account for renal insufficiency.

Finally, the suggestion that diastolic features of the renal artery Doppler spectra might predict the clinical

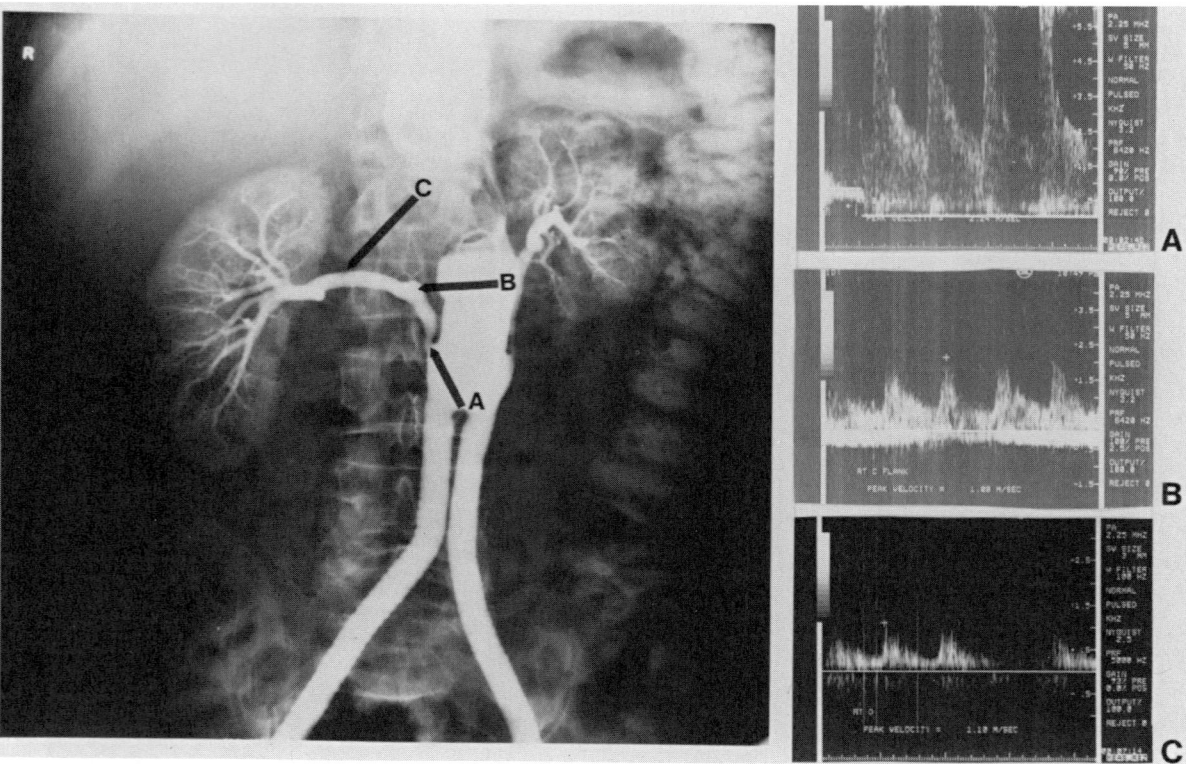

Figure 4 Tubular aortorenal saphenous vein graft stenosis 8 months after repair of inflammatory abdominal aortic aneurysm and bilateral renal artery (RA) bypass. Renal duplex sonography spectra from right RA bypass demonstrate increased RA-peak systolic velocity (PSV) (*A*, RA-PSV >2 m/sec) and poststenotic turbulence *(B)* with near normal distal RA spectra *(C)*. (From Hudspeth DA, Hansen KH, Reaves SW, et al. Renal duplex sonography after treatment of renovascular disease. J Vasc Surg 1993; 18:381–390; with permission.)

Table 3 Comparative Analysis of Parameter Estimates and Their 95% Confidence Intervals

Group	Number	Measure	Estimate	95% Confidence Interval
All procedures	61 kidneys	Sensitivity	0.69	(0.61, 0.77)
		Specificity	0.99	(0.96, 1.00)
		PPV	0.98	(0.85, 0.95)
		NPV	0.92	(0.88, 0.96)
		Accuracy	0.91	(0.88, 0.96)
Kidneys with main RA disease procedure	50 kidneys	Sensitivity	0.89	(0.82, 0.96)
		Specificity	0.98	(0.95, 1.00)
		PPV	0.89	(0.82, 0.96)
		NPV	0.98	(0.95, 1.00)
		Accuracy	0.96	(0.91, 1.00)
Kidneys with branch RA disease	11 kidneys	Sensitivity	0.25	(0.15, 0.35)
		Specificity	1.00*	—
		PPV	1.00*	—
		NPV	0.70	(0.59, 0.81)
		Accuracy	0.73	(0.63, 0.83)

PPV, Positive predictive value; NPV, negative predictive value; RA, renal artery.
*Confidence interval cannot be calculated as standard error of mean is zero.

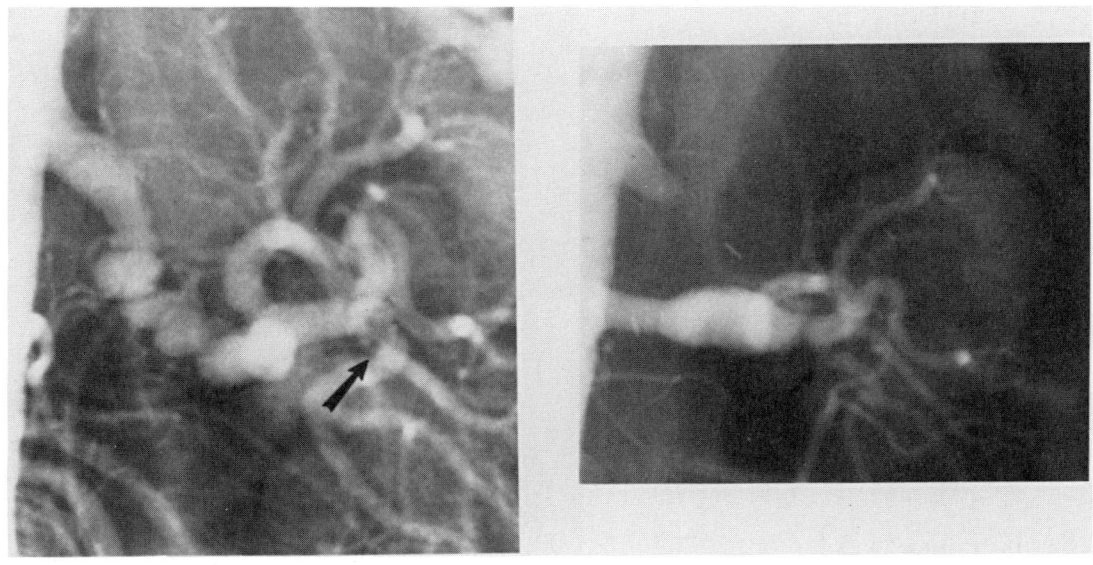

Figure 5 *A,* This 48-year-old woman had severe hypertension and bilateral renal artery fibromuscular dysplasia. She had branch-level disease noted in her left renal artery distribution *(arrow)* before bilateral saphenous vein aorto-renal bypass. *B,* Although she remains cured of hypertension, a persistent left renal artery lower pole branch lesion *(arrow)* is apparent on follow-up arteriography. This lesion was not detected by renal duplex sonography. (From Hudspeth DA, Hansen KH, Reaves SW, et al. Renal duplex sonography after treatment of renovascular disease. J Vasc Surg 1993; 18:381–390; with permission.)

success of renovascular reconstruction has not proved valid in our experience. A screening test that simultaneously determines the presence of anatomic renal artery disease and the clinical response to repair would have wide applicability. Although we have observed an inverse correlation between renal artery end-diastolic velocity (RA-EDV) and estimated creatinine clearance, RA-EDV has not correlated with hypertension response or change in serum creatinine following renovascular repair. Even though low RA-EDV is consistent with high intrarenal vascular resistance and intrinsic renal parenchymal disease, a low RA-EDV does not preclude a favorable clinical response after renovascular repair and should not be used to support any particular plan of management.

In addition to a useful screening test to define the presence or absence of significant renovascular disease, we utilize surface RDS after balloon angioplasty and operation to survey the anatomic result of intervention. Because favorable blood pressure response can occur after renal artery thrombosis and renal infarction, the equivalent of nephrectomy, we require anatomic assessment after renal revascularization to define the result of therapy. Although arteriography is routinely performed immediately after balloon angioplasty, the intimal disruption inherent to the dilation process may make accurate anatomic assessment impossible. Additionally, follow-up RDS provides a useful assessment of long-term results of intervention, as well as monitoring untreated renal artery disease.

We have retrospectively compared RDS with conventional arteriography after renovascular reconstruction (Fig. 4).[4] This analysis documented sensitivity and specificity for main renal artery repair and angioplasty equivalent to RDS as a surface screening test (Table 3). In contrast to reports from other centers, our completion rate RDS after intervention exceeds 98%. In our institution, preoperative and intraoperative RDS frequently precede the postprocedure study. These RDS studies are performed by a few technicians who often perform all three examinations. That experience, combined with a specific knowledge of the native arterial anatomy and the surgical reconstruction, has resulted in a high rate of technically complete studies.

Although RDS accurately defines the status of main renal artery reconstruction, the examination fails to define the result of complex branch renal artery repair. It does not accurately delineate persistent or recurrent branch renal artery disease (Fig. 5). For these reconstructions, we continue to require cut film arteriography prior to patient discharge. Otherwise, we use RDS frequently in the first year after reconstruction and annually thereafter, if a favorable clinical response is maintained. It is the first diagnostic study obtained, should hypertension or renal function worsen. The requirement for subsequent arteriography despite a negative RDS examination depends on the clinical indications for study. If RDS after intervention is obtained in the evaluation of hypertension in combination with renal insufficiency, arteriography is not required because main renal artery stenosis or occlusion is reliably excluded. For evaluation of severe hypertension alone, particularly after branch renal artery repair, arteriography is recommended because a negative RDS does not exclude critical disease at this level.

REFERENCES

1. Kohler TR, Zierler RE, Martin RL, et al. Noninvasive diagnosis of renal artery stenosis by ultrasonic duplex scanning. J Vasc Surg 1986; 4:450–456.
2. Taylor DC, Kettler MD, Moneta GL, et al. Duplex ultrasound scanning in the diagnosis of renal artery stenosis: A prospective evaluation. J Vasc Surg 1988; 7:363–369.
3. Hansen KJ, Tribble RW, Reavis SW, et al. Renal duplex sonography: Evaluation of clinical utility. J Vasc Surg 1990; 12:227–236.
4. Hudspeth DA, Hansen KH, Reavis SW, et al. Renal duplex sonography after treatment of renovascular disease. J Vasc Surg 1993; 18:381–390.

FUNCTIONAL SIGNIFICANCE OF RENAL ARTERIAL OCCLUSIVE DISEASE

THOMAS G. PICKERING, M.D., PH.D.

Occlusive disease of the renal arteries can occur from a number of causes, the most common of which are atherosclerosis and fibromuscular dysplasia. From a surgical point of view, the latter is of secondary importance, because it can be effectively treated by renal angioplasty and also because it rarely progresses to the extent of significantly impairing renal function. Thus, in a recently reported series of surgical operations for occlusive renal arterial disease, the underlying disease was atherosclerosis in 90% of patients.[1]

In contrast to fibromuscular disease, atherosclerosis is a diffuse process, involving not only one or both renal arteries but also other regional arterial beds. The major cardiovascular risk factors—smoking, hyperlipidemia, and hypertension—are presumed to accelerate the development of atherosclerotic plaques in the renal arteries as elsewhere. The distribution of these lesions is rarely symmetrical, and atherosclerotic renal arterial disease almost always begins as being functionally unilateral.

The major consequence of a unilateral renal artery stenosis is renovascular hypertension. In the case of atherosclerotic stenoses, hypertension may be of mixed origin, a renovascular component superimposed on essential hypertension. This explains why the cure rate of hypertension after successful revascularization is lower for atheromatous than for fibrodysplastic disease.

The resulting hypertension may further accelerate the development of atheroma, such that functionally significant bilateral renal artery stenoses develop. This leads to the second major consequence of the disease process, which is a progressive impairment of renal function, commonly referred to as ischemic nephropathy. A third consequence, which occurs in a subset of patients with bilateral renal arterial disease, is the occurrence of recurrent pulmonary edema.

PATHOPHYSIOLOGY

The demonstration of a renal artery stenosis in a hypertensive patient does not necessarily establish a diagnosis of renovascular hypertension because essential hypertension may accelerate the development of atheromatous plaques, which do not necessarily have any functional significance. Ideally, it is necessary to demonstrate that there is also renal ischemia, which is thought to be the stimulus that raises the blood pressure and leads to a decline of renal function.

The role of the renin-angiotensin system in the development of renovascular hypertension is paramount (Fig. 1). In experimental animals, two distinct models of renovascular hypertension can be produced. In the first, the one-clip, two-kidney model (analogous to unilateral renal artery stenosis in humans), the hypertension is renin-dependent. In the second, the one-clip, one-kidney model (analogous to renal artery stenosis in a solitary kidney or possibly to bilateral renal artery stenosis in humans), the hypertension is sodium and volume dependent, and blockade of the renin-angiotensin system has little effect on blood pressure unless the animal has been sodium depleted.

Pathophysiologic Differences Between Unilateral and Bilateral Stenoses

An important question is whether the pathophysiology of the two common human patterns can be equated with the two animal models. The resemblance between unilateral human renal artery stenosis and the one-clip, two-kidney model is close in that both are clearly dependent on increased secretion of renin by the ischemic kidney. What is much less clear is what occurs with bilateral stenoses. Relatively little information is available concerning peripheral renin levels, although peripheral renin has been reported to be high in patients with both unilateral and bilateral disease. Consistent with this finding, patients with bilateral renal artery stenosis are just as likely to show a decrease of blood pressure when given converting enzyme inhibitors. The pattern of renal vein renin activity is also indistinguishable, and in patients with bilateral renal artery stenoses the renins tend to lateralize to the most ischemic kidney.

In addition to this evidence of hypersecretion of

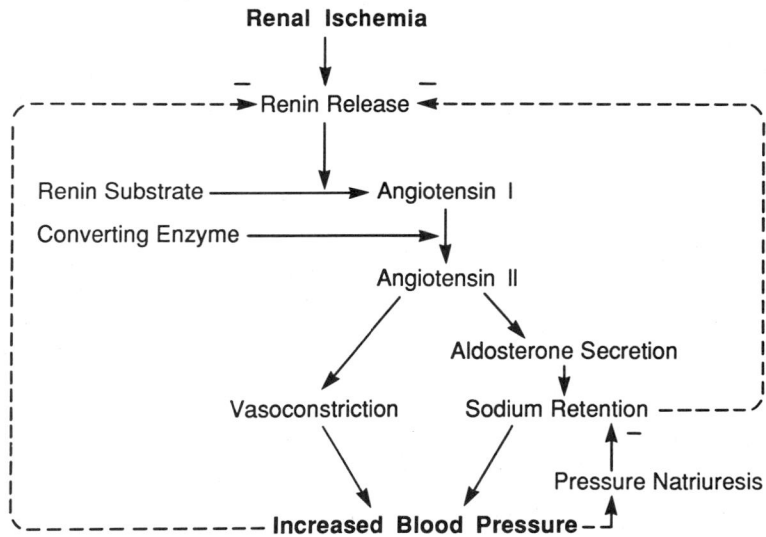

Figure 1 The effects of renal ischemia on the renin-angiotensin-aldosterone system in renovascular hypertension.

renin in patients with bilateral renovascular disease, circumstantial evidence suggests an increased effective blood volume. First, in patients with bilateral disease, the cardiac output is usually higher than in patients with unilateral disease. Second, recurrent pulmonary edema is more common in patients with bilateral than unilateral disease.[2] Third, successful revascularization by angioplasty in a patient with bilateral renal artery stenosis or a solitary kidney is frequently followed by diuresis, which is not seen in patients with unilateral disease (Fig. 2).[3]

The overall picture in patients with bilateral renal artery stenosis is, thus, a mixed one, with both renin and volume factors typically involved (Table 1). In this respect, bilateral involvement differs from the one-kidney animal model, which is more highly dependent on volume factors. The most likely reason is that bilateral disease almost never develops symmetrically in the two kidneys, as witnessed by the common finding of unequal kidney sizes and asymmetrical renal vein renin patterns. All bilateral cases presumably begin with unilateral disease. During the early stages of unilateral involvement, there may well be parenchymal disease developing in the contralateral kidney, which would impair the blood pressure natriuresis by which the contralateral kidney normally maintains the classic high renin–normal volume pattern of unilateral renal artery stenosis. This volume retention would be further exacerbated when the second stenosis develops in the contralateral renal artery.

Plasma catecholamines are usually normal in human renovascular hypertension, unless there is azotemia. The ischemic kidney produces increased amounts of prostaglandins (particularly E_2) as well as renin, and both may be suppressed by nonsteroidal anti-inflammatory drugs such as aspirin. These agents may lower blood pressure in patients with renovascular hypertension; in essential hypertensives, they tend to raise it.

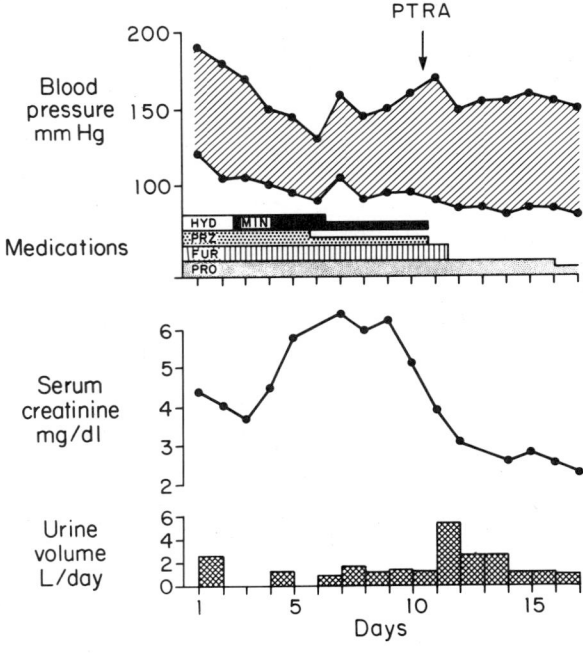

Figure 2 The effects of renal angioplasty in a patient with bilateral renal artery stenosis, showing an improvement in serum creatinine and a diuresis.

The Renin-Angiotensin System and the Control of Intrarenal Hemodynamics in Renovascular Hypertension

The clinical observation that converting enzyme inhibitors may cause a deterioration of renal function in some patients with renovascular hypertension can be accounted for by animal studies, which have documented the important effects of angiotensin on intrarenal

Table 1 Comparison of Animal and Human Models of Renovascular Hypertension

	Animal	Human
	Two-Kidney, One-Clip	Unilateral Stenosis
Renin	High	High
Plasma volume	Normal	Normal
BP response to ACEI	Decrease	Decrease
	One-Kidney, One-Clip	Bilateral Stenosis
Renin	Normal	Normal/high
Plasma volume	High	? High
BP response to ACEI	No change	Decrease

ACEI, Angiotensin converting enzyme inhibitor; BP, blood pressure.

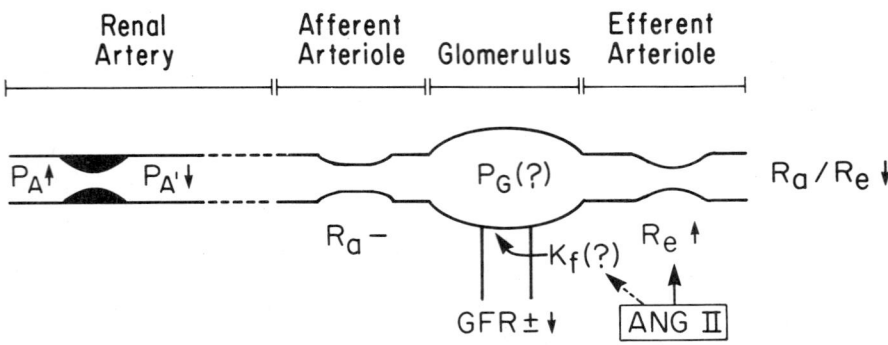

Figure 3 Hypothetical effects of angiotensin (ANG II), in the ischemic kidney with occlusive renal artery disease. P_A, blood pressure in renal artery proximal and distal (P_A^1) to a stenosis; R_a and R_e, afferent and efferent arteriolar resistance; PG, glomerular pressure.

hemodynamics.[4] One of the most important intrarenal effects of angiotensin II is to decrease renal blood flow, with a smaller decrease of glomerular filtration rate (GFR). Thus, the filtration fraction increases. It has been proposed that these changes are brought about by a vasoconstriction of both afferent and efferent arterioles, with the predominant effect being on the latter (Fig. 3). Thus, in the normal kidney, particularly when renin levels are high, angiotensin blockade increases renal blood flow, with less consistent changes of GFR. In the ischemic kidney, GFR is maintained by angiotensin II–mediated efferent vasoconstriction, so that angiotensin blockade lowers it. This effect provides the rationale for captopril renography.

CONSEQUENCES OF OCCLUSIVE RENAL ARTERIAL DISEASE

Renovascular Hypertension

The prevalence of renovascular hypertension is unknown but is probably between 0.2% and 5% of the general hypertensive population, although in patients with more severe hypertension it may be much higher. In patients with accelerated or malignant hypertension (grade III or IV retinopathy), a prevalence of 43% in white patients and 7% in blacks has been reported.[5]

These results were all based on clinical studies, which, with one exception,[5] did not utilize arteriography for the diagnosis. The prevalence rates are therefore almost certainly an underestimate. However, the situation is complicated by the fact that a stenosis in the renal artery of a hypertensive patient does not imply that the lesion is causing the hypertension because renal artery stenosis has been reported to occur not infrequently in normotensive subjects.[6]

The finding of hypertension in a middle-aged man with other evidence of atheromatous disease such as coronary artery disease should raise the possibility of atheromatous renovascular hypertension. In patients undergoing coronary arteriography, a significant and previously unsuspected renal artery stenosis was reported in 17% of hypertensives but was equally common in normotensives.[6] In patients referred for investigation of peripheral vascular disease, 59% had stenosis (of 50% or more) of at least one renal artery.[7] The presence or absence of a stenosis was unrelated to hypertension. These studies emphasize the importance of establishing the functional significance of a renal artery stenosis before proceeding to renal revascularization.

Renal Failure: Ischemic Nephropathy

Occlusive renal arterial disease that is either bilateral or present in a solitary kidney is becoming increasingly recognized as an important and potentially reversible cause of renal failure. It has been termed ischemic nephropathy. In a recently reported surgical series, 72% of operations for renal revascularization were undertaken primarily for the salvage of renal function; most of these patients had atheromatous renal arterial disease.[1]

A striking and unexplained epidemiologic trend has been the sixfold increase over the past 10 years in the proportion of new cases of end-stage renal disease (ESRD) attributable to hypertension, at a time when the medical treatment of hypertension has become not only more effective but also more widely utilized. The degree to which ischemic nephropathy has contributed to this is uncertain, although it has been estimated to be present in approximately 15% of new cases of ESRD.[8]

There are several clinical manifestations of ischemic nephropathy. One clue to its presence may be a sudden deterioration of renal function that follows the introduction of an angiotensin-converting enzyme (ACE) inhibitor to a patient's antihypertensive regimen. This has been attributed to the abolition of angiotensin-mediated vasoconstriction of the efferent glomerular arterioles, which helps to maintain glomerular filtration in this condition. It should be pointed out, however, that this is not a very specific diagnostic finding because not all patients whose renal function deteriorates with ACE inhibitors have ischemic nephropathy,[9] and other antihypertensives can induce it in patients who do have ischemic nephropathy.

Renal artery disease may also be suspected in azotemic patients who have evidence of atherosclerosis elsewhere in the body. In a small series of patients aged 45 to 75 years and serum creatinine levels above 2 mg/dl, ischemic nephropathy was detected in 15%.[10]

Finally, in patients with known renovascular disease, particularly when they are treated medically, progression of azotemia may also occur when ischemic nephropathy evolves.

Recurrent Pulmonary Edema

The relatively frequent occurrence of pulmonary edema in patients with advanced renovascular hypertension is impressive.[2] In a series of 55 consecutive patients who were also azotemic, pulmonary edema had occurred in 13 (23%). In 92%, renal artery stenoses were bilateral or there was a solitary kidney with a stenosed artery. Successful revascularization of even one of the ischemic kidneys prevented further occurrence of the pulmonary edema. The occurrence of pulmonary edema was not related to the severity of the hypertension or renal failure. Although it was more common in patients who had associated coronary heart disease, it could also occur in patients with normal coronary arteries.

Another series of 17 patients has been reported by Messina and co-workers that comprised 8.9% of their patients undergoing surgical revascularization.[11] All had severe hypertension and azotemia (mean serum creatinine 3.8 mg/dl), and 94% had bilateral renal artery disease. Renal revascularization was uniformly effective in controlling the episodes of pulmonary edema, over an average follow-up period of 2.4 years.

The pathophysiology of this syndrome appears to be related to a number of factors. The common features are severe hypertension, bilateral renal artery disease, azotemia, and a generally excellent blood pressure response to revascularization, which may indicate that the hypertension is truly renovascular. In an analogy with the one-clip, one-kidney animal model of renovascular hypertension, hypervolemia may be considered a factor. This is one of the physiologic features that distinguishes the condition from unilateral renal artery stenosis. When the disease is unilateral, hypervolemia may be prevented by a natriuresis operating via the normally functioning contralateral kidney, but when disease is bilateral, no renal tissue is exposed to the systemic level of blood pressure, so that the natriuresis is less.

The heart may also contribute to the pathogenesis of pulmonary edema. Although coronary artery disease is often present, it is usually not severe and in some patients may be absent. Myocardial function is good, as might be expected from the high blood pressure levels that are frequently generated. The most consistent finding is marked left ventricular hypertrophy, and the accompanying diminution of diastolic compliance may also be presumed to contribute to the increased pulmonary capillary pressure that results in pulmonary edema.

DIAGNOSIS

Renovascular hypertension is almost certainly underdiagnosed in clinical practice. Extensive screening of all hypertensive patients is impractical, but a number of clinical clues should increase the clinician's suspicion of its presence (Table 2).

There is no perfect screening test for its detection. The large number of tests proposed can be classified in two categories. First are those that can be done in a physician's office and are relatively simple to perform and inexpensive, but do not indicate which kidney is involved. Measurement of peripheral plasma renin activity and the captopril test are in this category. Second are tests that provide anatomic or functional information about each kidney. Ideally, one or more of these tests should be done following the first-stage test.

Captopril renography is currently one of the most popular noninvasive diagnostic tests and is performed by comparing renograms obtained before and after a single dose of captopril. The rationale is that the GFR of an ischemic kidney is dependent on the effects of angiotensin on the efferent glomerular arterioles and hence

Table 2 Testing for Renovascular Hypertension: Clinical Index of Suspicion as a Guide to Selecting Patients for Work-Up

Index of Clinical Suspicion

Low (should not be tested)
  Borderline, mild or moderate hypertension, in the absence of clinical clues
Moderate (noninvasive tests recommended)
  Severe hypertension (diastolic blood pressure greater than 120 mm Hg)
  Hypertension refractory to standard therapy
  Abrupt onset of sustained moderate to severe hypertension at age <20 or >50 years
  Hypertension with a suggestive abdominal bruit (long, high pitched and localized to the region of the renal artery)
  Moderate hypertension (diastolic blood pressure exceeding 105 mm Hg) in a smoker, a patient with evidence of occlusive vascular disease (cerebrovascular, coronary, peripheral vascular), or a patient with unexplained but stable elevation of serum creatinine
  Normalization of blood pressure by an angiotensin-converting enzyme inhibitor in a patient with moderate or severe hypertension (particularly a smoker or patient with recent onset of hypertension)
High (may consider proceeding directly to arteriography)
  Severe hypertension (diastolic blood pressure greater than 120 mm Hg) with either progressive renal insufficiency or refractoriness to aggressive treatment (particularly in a patient who has been a smoker or has other evidence of occlusive arterial disease)
  Accelerated or malignant hypertension (grade III or IV retinopathy)
  Hypertension with recent elevation of serum creatinine, either unexplained or reversibly induced by an angiotensin-converting enzyme inhibitor
  Moderate to severe hypertension with incidentally detected asymmetry of renal size

Table 3 Sensitivity and Specificity of Screening Tests for Renovascular Hypertension

Test	Sensitivity (%)	Specificity (%)
Office tests		
Plasma renin activity	60	65
Captopril test	75	90
Lateralization tests		
Intravenous pyelogram	75	85
Renal scan	75	75
Captopril scan	90	95
Renal vein renin	75	90
Duplex Doppler imaging	85	90

falls markedly with converting enzyme inhibition. There are also less pronounced changes in renal blood flow. Thus, the characteristic effect of captopril in a kidney with a renal artery stenosis is to cause a decreased uptake and delayed excretion of isotope, which may be diethylene-triamine-pentaacetic acid, hippuran, or technetium-99m-mercapto-acetyltriglycine (Mag_3). Captopril renography has been found to have a high sensitivity and specificity (Table 3).

Other diagnostic tests include renal vein renin measurement, which typically shows marked asymmetry in the renin concentrations of the two renal veins in patients with occlusive renal arterial disease, but cannot distinguish between unilateral and bilateral disease. Duplex ultrasound scanning has its advocates but requires a highly skilled operator.

Treatment Choices

There are three potential treatment choices for patients with occlusive renal arterial disease: medical, surgical, and angioplasty. Because the cure rate with either form of revascularization is relatively low in patients with advanced atheromatous disease,[8] medical treatment is almost always a component. Nevertheless, medical management is also rarely the treatment of choice, for three reasons. First, all of the three major manifestations of renal arterial disease—hypertension, azotemia, and pulmonary edema—can be improved by successful revascularization, whether by operation or angioplasty. Second, atherosclerotic lesions tend to progress to occlusion of the renal artery.[12] Third, there is a possibility that lowering blood pressure with medical therapy may exacerbate the renal ischemia, leading to further reduction of renal function.[13] For these reasons, the documentation of functionally significant occlusive renal arterial disease is generally an indication for revascularization, either by angioplasty or operation.

REFERENCES

1. Bredenberg CE, Sampson LN, Ray FS, et al. Changing patterns in surgery for chronic renal artery occlusive diseases. J Vasc Surg 1992; 15:1018–1024.
2. Pickering TG, Herman L, Sotelo JE, et al. Recurrent pulmonary edema as a manifestation of renovascular hypertension and its treatment by renal revascularization. Circulation 1987; 76(suppl 4):274.
3. Sutters M, Al-Kutoubi MA, Mathias CJ, Peart S. Diuresis and syncope after renal angioplasty in a patient with one functioning kidney. Br Med J 1987; 295:527–528.
4. Navar LG, Rosivall L. Contribution of the renin-angiotensin system to the control of intrarenal hemodynamics. Kidney Int 1984; 25:857–868.
5. Davis BA, Crook JE, Vestal RE, Oates JA. Prevalence of renovascular hypertension in patients with grade III or IV hypertensive retinopathy. N Engl J Med 1979; 301:1273–1276.
6. Harding MB, Smith LR, Himmelstein SI, et al. Renal artery stenosis: Prevalence and associated risk factors in patients undergoing routine cardiac catheterization. J Am Soc Nephrol 1992; 2:1608–1616.
7. Choudri AH, Cleland JGF, Rowlands PL, et al. Unsuspected renal artery stenosis in peripheral vascular disease. Br Med J 1990; 301:1197–1198.

8. Rimmer JM, Gennari FJ. Atherosclerotic renovascular disease and progressive renal failure. Ann Intern Med 1993; 118:712–719.
9. Toto RD, Mitchell HC, Lee HC, et al. Reversible renal insufficiency due to angiotensin converting enzyme inhibitors in hypertensive nephrosclerosis. Ann Intern Med 1991; 115:513–519.
10. O'Neil EA, Hansen KJ, Canzanello UL, et al. Prevalence of ischemic nephropathy in patients with renal insufficiency. Ann Surg 1992; 58:485–490.
11. Messina LM, Zelenock GB, Yao KA, Stanley JC. Renal revascularization for recurrent pulmonary edema in patients with poorly controlled hypertension and renal insufficiency: A distinct subgroup of patients with arteriosclerotic renal artery occlusive disease. J Vasc Surg 1992; 15:73–82.
12. Tollefson DFJ, Ernst CB. Natural history of atherosclerotic renal artery stenosis associated with aortic disease. J Vasc Surg 1991; 14:327–331.
13. Dean RH, Kieffer RW, Smith BW, et al. Renovascular hypertension. Anatomic and renal functional changes during drug therapy. Arch Surg 1981; 116:1408.

ARTERIOGRAPHIC DIAGNOSIS OF RENOVASCULAR HYPERTENSION

THOMAS A. SOS, M.D.

Intravenous digital subtraction angiography was a promising and attractive technology. If carefully performed with injections in the right atrium, the vast majority of studies can be technically adequate, but detection of branch renal artery disease and significant fibromuscular dysplasia is not reliable. For these reasons, especially with the advent of safer intra-arterial techniques, this technique has fallen into some disfavor.

ARTERIOGRAPHY

Advances in imaging, arteriographic techniques, and contrast media have made aortography and selective renal arteriography safe, quick, and simple. Catheters of 4 Fr and 5 Fr diameter can be safely introduced into the abdominal aorta on an outpatient basis.

In spite of the proliferation of multiple screening and diagnostic tests for renovascular hypertension, arteriography remains the gold standard for detection of anatomically significant renal artery stenoses. The arteries of all patients with suspected renovascular hypertension, especially those who are known or suspected to have other coexistent vascular disease, should be manipulated very carefully. Following arterial puncture, the guide wire should be gently and carefully advanced into the upper abdominal aorta and a 4 Fr aortic flush catheter introduced. The side holes of the catheter should be positioned at the upper end plate of the first lumbar vertebral body because the vast majority of renal arteries originate at this level. Catheters with minimal cephalad reflux are preferred. This avoids opacification of the branches of the celiac axis and superior mesenteric arteries, which may overlie the main renal artery or its branches and thereby make diagnosis of renal artery stenosis more difficult.

With intra-arterial digital subtraction techniques, satisfactory aortograms can be obtained with 15 to 20 ml of 30% conventional ionic contrast material injected at 15 to 20 ml per second and filmed at three to four images per second. An aortogram is first obtained in the frontal projection. If a renal artery stenosis is definitely identified, particularly if it is in the ostial or proximal portion of the renal artery, the diagnostic study should be terminated. If a proximal or ostial stenosis is suspected but not confirmed, oblique aortographic studies should be obtained.

It must be kept in mind that renal arteries, especially the right renal artery, originate ventrolaterally from the aorta. Therefore, to visualize the proximal portion of each renal artery, the ipsilateral anterior oblique projection should be obtained. This projection also better demonstrates the mid to distal portions of the contralateral renal artery. If a proximal or ostial stenosis is identified, selective catheterization should not be performed; in fact, it is contraindicated unless an angioplasty is to be attempted at the same time. This is because the most difficult part of an angioplasty is crossing the stenosis, and not infrequently inexperienced operators' attempts to obtain more selective diagnostic arteriograms have resulted in renal artery dissections or occlusions.

Conversely, branch renal artery lesions are more frequent in children and young women. If aortography is normal, selective-magnification renal arteriograms in multiple oblique views are mandatory. In patients with significant renal dysfunction, a single frontal aortogram is usually adequate to detect significant renal artery lesions that may be responsible for hypertension, azotemia, or both.

Fifteen milliliters of 30% contrast medium is rarely contributory to further decline in renal function. Unfortunately, the new generation of low osmolar contrast media, whether ionic or nonionic, has not been proven to have lesser nephrotoxicity. Use of carbon dioxide (CO_2) as a negative contrast agent for intra-arterial digital subtraction arteriography (IADSA) is promising but has not been widely evaluated. Carbon dioxide is non-nephrotoxic and nonallergenic and presents no osmolar load.

Microcholesterol embolization, another rare but much feared complication of arteriography, occurs in fewer than 0.1% of patients. Significant cholesterol microembolization occurs in approximately 1% of patients with atheromatous renal artery disease who undergo renal angioplasty.

Renal arteriography in patients with suspected renal artery stenosis should be undertaken only after a decision has been made as to whether a significant stenosis, if identified, will be treated by angioplasty or surgical reconstruction. A diagnostic arteriogram that is followed by a separate catheter study for treatment exposes the patient to a double jeopardy of catheterization that should be avoided.

We use the following arteriographic criteria to identify significant renal artery stenosis:

1. Renal artery stenosis greater than 75% of luminal diameter
2. The presence of collateral circulation
3. Diminished velocity of blood flow across the stenotic area
4. Poststenotic dilatation
5. Diminished ipsilateral renal size
6. A peak systolic blood pressure gradient greater than 20% of aortic systolic blood pressure; however, the catheter itself may contribute to the stenosis (trans-stenotic gradient measurements and selective catheterization of the renal artery should be performed only if an angioplasty is contemplated)

We do not believe that the additional time and risks of selective catheterization to perform "pharmacoangiography" with vasodilators or vasoconstrictors significantly improves the diagnostic accuracy of arteriography.

Before attempting a renal angioplasty, appropriate further arteriographic studies should be performed, depending on preferred surgical options. If the operation of choice is a bypass from branches of the celiac axis, then the blood pressure in the celiac axis must be measured. We believe that a lateral aortogram is not sufficient to evaluate the patency and significance of a stenosis in the celiac axis, and it requires a significant amount of additional contrast medium. For this reason, we prefer to catheterize the celiac axis selectively and to do a pullback blood pressure to establish whether a gradient is present. A small injection of 5 ml of 30% contrast medium with IADSA can also be performed to define the relationship of branches of the celiac axis to the renal arteries and to document the location of the catheter.

Patients for arteriography can arrive on the morning of the study as outpatients. If the diagnostic arteriogram is negative, they can remain as outpatients and, following a 6 hour stay, can be discharged. If a significant renal artery stenosis is identified, these outpatients can and should be admitted, and treated by renal angioplasty or surgical reconstruction. After angioplasty the patient should be followed for at least 24 hours after the procedure in hospital.

PERCUTANEOUS ARTERIAL DILATION FOR RENOVASCULAR HYPERTENSION

DAVID M. WILLIAMS, M.D.
MICHAEL D. DAKE, M.D.

PROCEDURAL CONSIDERATIONS

Indications

The indications for percutaneous transluminal renal angioplasty (PTRA) are uncontroversial and include renal artery stenoses causing or aggravating hypertension or compromising renal function. Controversy persists as to whether a given stenosis is hemodynamically significant and on the topic of identifying stenoses unsuitable for PTRA because of poor response to dilation or high risk of complications. The decision to proceed with PTRA is based on the clinical features of a patient's hypertension or poor renal function prior to arteriography, the etiology of the stenosis as determined from the clinical history and the arteriogram, the technical difficulty of the procedure as determined from the arteriographic appearance of the aorta and the renal artery, the risk of accumulating additional evidence of hemodynamic significance and of the angioplasty itself, and, last, the experience of the operator. For example, in a young woman who has classical arteriographic findings of uncomplicated medial fibroplasia, PTRA is a high-yield and low-risk procedure. Proceeding from the arteriographic documentation of tight stenoses involving a main renal artery to immediate PTRA without measuring blood pressures, obtaining selective renal vein renin studies, pharmacologically manipulating collateral blood flow, or consulting a vascular surgeon is widely accepted. In an elderly hypertensive patient with a solitary kidney, declining renal function, and arteriographic evidence of severe aortic and moderate proximal renal artery atherosclerotic disease, the angiographer might wish to measure the renal artery blood pressure gradient and consult with a vascular surgeon before undertaking PTRA.

Periprocedural Care

All patients have intravenous lines for administration of fluids and medications. Patients are mildly sedated during the procedure. Because renal artery rupture, a feared but uncommon complication of PTRA, is heralded by severe flank pain, it is advisable to have the patient conscious at the time of dilation. Medications commonly used to prevent arterial spasm and thrombosis associated with angioplasty include nifedipine, nitroglycerin, aspirin, and heparin sodium. We selectively administer 100 μg nitroglycerin into the renal artery before advancing the guide wire into it and then heparin sodium just after the catheter crosses the stenosis. Aspirin may be continued until the angioplasty site has healed, at approximately 1 month. After successful PTRA, close monitoring of blood pressure is necessary to guard against rebound hypotension due to residual effects of previously administered antihypertensive medication.

Results and Complications

Angioplasty is judged by the technical success of the procedure; short- and long-term patency of the renal artery; clinical response of the patient with respect to blood pressure, renal function, and medication requirements; and complications. A technical success in renal angioplasty is ablation of the stenosis without a major complication and with a small residual stenosis, which varies from 20% to 50%, depending on the authority. Patency is a straightforward concept and ideally should be documented by a clinical examination and an imaging study. Patency ceases when symptoms recur at the same magnitude as before angioplasty and blood flow is compromised in the treated segment. Clinical benefit includes cure, defined as a diastolic blood pressure less than 90 mm Hg when the patient is off all antihypertensives, and improvement, a diastolic blood pressure either (1) less than 90 or (2) between 90 and 110 with at least a 15 mm Hg diastolic blood pressure decrease following angioplasty, while the patient is on equal or reduced antihypertensive medication compared to the preangioplasty status; clinical failure is an absence of cure or improvement. Unfortunately, these definitions of technical and clinical success are not universally accepted. Measurements of percent stenosis are usually unvalidated; in general, published reports of large series contain insufficient data to allow the reader to analyze the outcomes of various authors' experiences using the standard definitions of results and complications.

Major complications may be classified as direct, involving the puncture site or the renal artery, and indirect or remote. Puncture site complications include a hematoma requiring transfusion or surgical evacuation or resulting in a neurologic deficit, arterial pseudoaneurysm, arterial thrombosis, or arteriovenous fistula. Major complications at the angioplasty site include renal artery rupture, thrombosis, occlusive dissection, spasm or embolism resulting in infarction, and loss of renal allograft. Remote or indirect complications include contrast medium–induced renal insufficiency or anaphylactoid reaction; low flow state resulting in significant mesenteric, coronary, or cerebral ischemia; and nonrenal atheroemboli. The rate of major complications is reported as 10% to 25%, depending on patient selection and the definition of major. They include puncture and angioplasty site arterial damage requiring urgent surgical repair (approximately 5%), cholesterol microemboli, irreversible renal failure, and cerebral and myocardial ischemia (1% to 2%). The mortality associated with angioplasty is 1% to 2%.

Experienced operators have fewer complications. The use of better preprocedural hydration, reduced contrast material, vascular sheaths at the puncture site, digital imaging, and newer techniques of crossing the stenosis were associated with fewer complications.

RESULTS

The technical success, clinical benefits, and restenosis rates of renal artery angioplasty vary with the etiology, location, and severity of occlusive disease. The blood pressure response to successful angioplasty is rapid, with maximum benefit evident within several days. In contrast, the improvement in renal function that occurs after ischemic nephropathy is ameliorated by angioplasty may not be fully realized for several months.

Fibrodysplastic Disease

Fibromuscular dysplasia accounts for approximately a third of adult renovascular hypertension in the United States. Uncomplicated medial fibroplasia involving the middle third of the main renal artery represents the ideal lesion for renal artery angioplasty, by consensus of surgeons as well as interventional radiologists.[1,2] Treatment of medial fibroplasia complicated by branch vessel involvement or a large aneurysm is difficult and prone to complications, and the patient is best served by close consultation between vascular surgeon and interventional radiologist. Lesions of intimal and subadventitial fibroplasia do not respond as well to angioplasty as those of medial fibroplasia, but the small number of these lesions treated even in large series makes it difficult to generalize. Short-term clinical benefit of angioplasty in fibromuscular dysplasia has been reported as 95% (40% cure and 55% improvement). Long-term benefit is sustained up to several years at 90% with cure (improvement) rates ranging from 39% (59%) to 66% (24%).[3,4] Tegtmeyer and co-workers have estimated the incidence of restenosis at 8% of lesions (10% of patients) at a mean of 15.7 months.[3]

Atherosclerotic Disease

Atherosclerotic narrowing of the renal artery accounts for approximately two-thirds of adult renovascular hypertension in the United States. Hypertensive patients with atherosclerotic stenoses are approximately 20 years older than those with fibromuscular dysplasia, and underlying the renovascular component of hypertension in these patients may be essential hypertension and glomerular disease, which confound analysis of the hemodynamic benefits of angioplasty. Technical success in several large series recently published ranges from 73% to 83%. Numerous series document that cure, as opposed to improvement, of hypertension following dilation of atherosclerotic lesions is uncommon. Six-month cure rates range from 3% to 11%, and improvement rates from 78% to 87%. As expected, benefit rates decline in follow-up at 2 to 5 years, with cure rates of 0 to 15% and improvement rates of 48% to 81%. The results of angioplasty at its best are comparable with results of contemporary surgical treatment of atherosclerotic renovascular lesions with an operative mortality of 3%, perioperative morbidity prolonging hospital stay of 17%, cure rate of 15% and an improvement rate of 75%.[5] However, the wide variation in clinical benefit following angioplasty of atherosclerotic lesions has stimulated attempts to stratify patients by anatomic and clinical features to identify lesions likely to respond to dilation. This variation has highlighted the need to standardize criteria of technical and clinical success and to validate measurements of stenoses and normal renal artery diameter and engendered controversy over whether angioplasty is even appropriate for atherosclerotic disease.[6,7]

Atherosclerotic stenoses have been classified as ostial or nonostial, depending on whether the renal atheroma is part of a bulky aortic lesion, and unilateral or bilateral. The apparent refractory nature of ostial lesions was recognized early in the experience of renal angioplasty, but recent experience has been mixed. Rodriguez-Perez and associates analyzed results according to lesion site and found significant decreases in systolic blood pressure 8 years after angioplasty in patients with bilateral or nonostial lesions.[4] They also found significant diastolic blood pressure benefit in all four groups of unilateral, bilateral, ostial, and nonostial disease, but no difference between groups.

It should be noted that, in severe atheromatous disease, arteriography does not distinguish ostial lesions created by large aortic atheromas from lesions confined to the proximal few millimeters of the renal artery. Furthermore, even in reports of large series of patients, long-term follow-up using arteriography is uncommon, and the clinical finding of recurrent hypertension does not distinguish between restenosis, progression of disease elsewhere in the renal artery, and nonrenovascular causes of hypertension. These ambiguities in lesion stratification and treatment follow-up make it difficult to reconcile apparently conflicting claims. However, a common theme is the recognition that a substantial fraction (60% to 80%) of patients with atherosclerotic renal artery stenosis experience improved blood pressure control and that many of the late failures can be salvaged with repeat angioplasty.

Renal Transplants

Renal artery stenosis complicates 5% to 10% of renal transplants. Most stenoses are evident within 6 months of the transplant operation, almost all within a year. Because there are many causes of hypertension and renal failure in the transplant patient, we request Doppler ultrasound as a noninvasive screen of renal artery stenosis, before proceeding with arteriography. Because most anastomoses are end to side to the external iliac artery, it is frequently difficult to visualize the arterial anastomosis in profile, and our threshold for measuring the blood pressure gradient across the anastomosis is low. A widely accepted anatomic criterion for transplant stenosis is a 50% diameter narrowing. Criteria for technical success vary and require, for example, a 10% reduction in diastolic blood pressure, a 15% reduction in serum creatinine, or a 20% improvement in arterial diameter with a residual narrowing of less than 50%. Published series of transplant renal artery angioplasty are retrospective and small, typically containing 15 to 50 patients. Technical success, clinical benefit, and complication rates vary with definition, the type of anastomosis, and the location of the stenosis. Technical success rates range from 60% to 90%. Clinical benefit rates in technically successful procedures range from 60% to 80% at 1 year. In longer term follow-up of blood pressure control, benefit rates of 40% at nearly 3 years have been reported, increasing to 50% if redilations of recurrent stenoses are included. Average numbers of antihypertensive medications are reduced. Reports of improvement in renal function are mixed. The consensus appears to be that transplant renal function stabilizes or improves following renal angioplasty. The complication rate is 10% to 30%, with loss of the graft or damage to the renal artery requiring surgical repair reported as 0 to 10%. In retrospective analyses, higher complication rates have been associated with angioplasty of anastomotic stenoses. Because uncomplicated but failed angioplasty does not preclude surgical revision of the transplant arterial conduit, transplant renal angioplasty remains, among surgeons and interventional radiologists, the primary method of treating renal artery narrowing.

Pediatric Renal Artery Stenosis

The most common causes of renovascular hypertension in children are fibromuscular disease, transplant renal artery stenosis, and hypoplastic narrowings due to developmental defects, including neurofibromatosis and aortic coarctation. For hypertension due to uncomplicated medial fibroplasia or to allograft renal artery stenosis, children appear to respond to angioplasty as well as adults.[8] Renal artery stenosis associated with neurofibromatosis usually fails to respond well to angioplasty. Furthermore, the proximal lesion easily accessible to a balloon catheter may be associated with branch stenoses. In typical thoracic aortic coarctation, surgical or balloon catheter therapy is directed at the thoracic lesion. In abdominal aortic coarctation of hypoplasia, the midabdominal aorta as well as visceral artery origins are narrowed, and the renal artery revascularization is a component of an extensive abdominal arterial reconstruction.

Miscellaneous

Other causes of renovascular hypertension potentially amenable to PTRA include arteritis, trauma, and aortic dissection. Renal artery stenoses due to nonspecific aortoarteritis or Takayasu disease are uncommon in the United States. Extensive experience with angioplasty of these lesions and associated aortic stenoses has been reported from Asia.[9] In addition to the usual hemodynamic criteria qualifying a patient for angioplasty, a normal erythrocyte sedimentation rate is necessary to document inactive disease. These stenoses are more resistant to dilation than those due to atherosclerosis and fibromuscular dysplasia and require high-pressure balloons. Technical success was 85% to 90%, with failures associated with coexisting aortic disease. Significant improvement in blood pressure was seen within several days in most patients, but in some it developed slowly over several weeks. Clinical benefit rates were 80% to 90% at 1 to 2 years follow-up. Long-term results are not available.

Aortic dissection has been reported to involve the renal arteries and cause renal ischemia in 8% of patients. Stenoses secondary to dissecting hematoma in the proximal renal artery have responded to angioplasty and deployment of endovascular stents.

RESTENOSIS

The durability of renal artery angioplasty is limited by immediate and long-term compromise of the dilated segment. Immediate collapse of the dilated segment may be due to elastic recoil, bulky atheromatous plaque near the renal artery origin that was not remolded by inflation of the balloon, spasm with local thrombosis, and renal artery dissection. Intravascular stents appear poised to raise the technical success rate of renal artery angioplasty in ostial atherosclerotic lesions to that of angioplasty in fibromuscular dysplasia. Long-term narrowing of the dilated renal artery is due to restenosis by progression of disease at the same or nearby segment or by intimal hyperplasia. The true restenosis rate requires anatomic imaging of a representative sample of treated renal arteries and an unambiguous definition and validated measure of stenosis; few such studies have been performed. In a follow-up study of 92 of 104 patients who underwent technically successful renal artery angioplasty, Plouin and colleagues found an overall 16% incidence of restenosis.[7] Restenosis was more frequent in patients with ostial or branch lesions than with main renal artery lesions (35% versus 12%) and in patients with atheromatous lesions, aortitis, or infrarenal aortic ectasia than without them (35% versus 8%).[7] Other estimates of restenosis range from 8% to 36% overall at 6 to 24 months mean follow-up, 15% to 22% in dysplastic lesions, and 40% to 45% in atherosclerotic lesions. Restenosis at the angioplasty site in inactive Takayasu disease was found in 6 (21%) of 28 lesions. Half of the stenoses are apparent within 6 months of initial angioplasty and three-quarters within 1 year. The relative fractions of restenoses due to progression of atherosclerosis and intimal hyperplasia are not known.

NEW DEVELOPMENTS

Noninvasive Vascular Imaging

Arteriography is the accepted standard for the diagnosis of renal artery stenosis. Because arteriography is accompanied by a modest risk of complications, there is an understandable reluctance to perform the procedure unless there is a prior commitment to surgical revascularization or percutaneous angioplasty if a significant lesion is found. Likewise, following successful angioplasty or revascularization, arteriography is generally performed only if recurrent hypertension or renal failure develops, not to document long-term results. Until recently, the absence of a noninvasive anatomic test that permits visualization of the renal arteries has precluded randomized trials of renal artery angioplasty and rigorous follow-up, the lack of which has been decried by many. Recent developments and technical refinements in renal duplex ultrasonography, spiral computed tomography, and magnetic resonance angiography offer encouragement that accurate noninvasive visualization of the renal arteries is imminent, and that sound clinical trials and follow-up are forthcoming.

Intravascular Stents

The relatively low technical success and clinical benefit rates of angioplasty for ostial atherosclerotic stenoses, as compared to fibromuscular dysplastic stenoses, are thought to be due primarily to the inability of the balloon in the renal artery to remold overflow atheroma from the aorta. It is hoped that intravascular stents can be used to buttress open the vascular channel compromised by bulky aortic atheroma. In addition, intravascular stents have been used to treat acute occlusions following angioplasty in the coronary, iliac, and renal arteries. Mechanisms of acute closure include spasm, thrombosis, and localized dissection compromising blood flow. Several preliminary reports have been published describing the use of stents to treat ostial renal artery stenoses, either to salvage a technical success by reversing elastic recoil immediately after angioplasty or to treat delayed restenosis (Fig. 1). Technical success (residual stenosis less than 30%) rates were 80% to 95%.

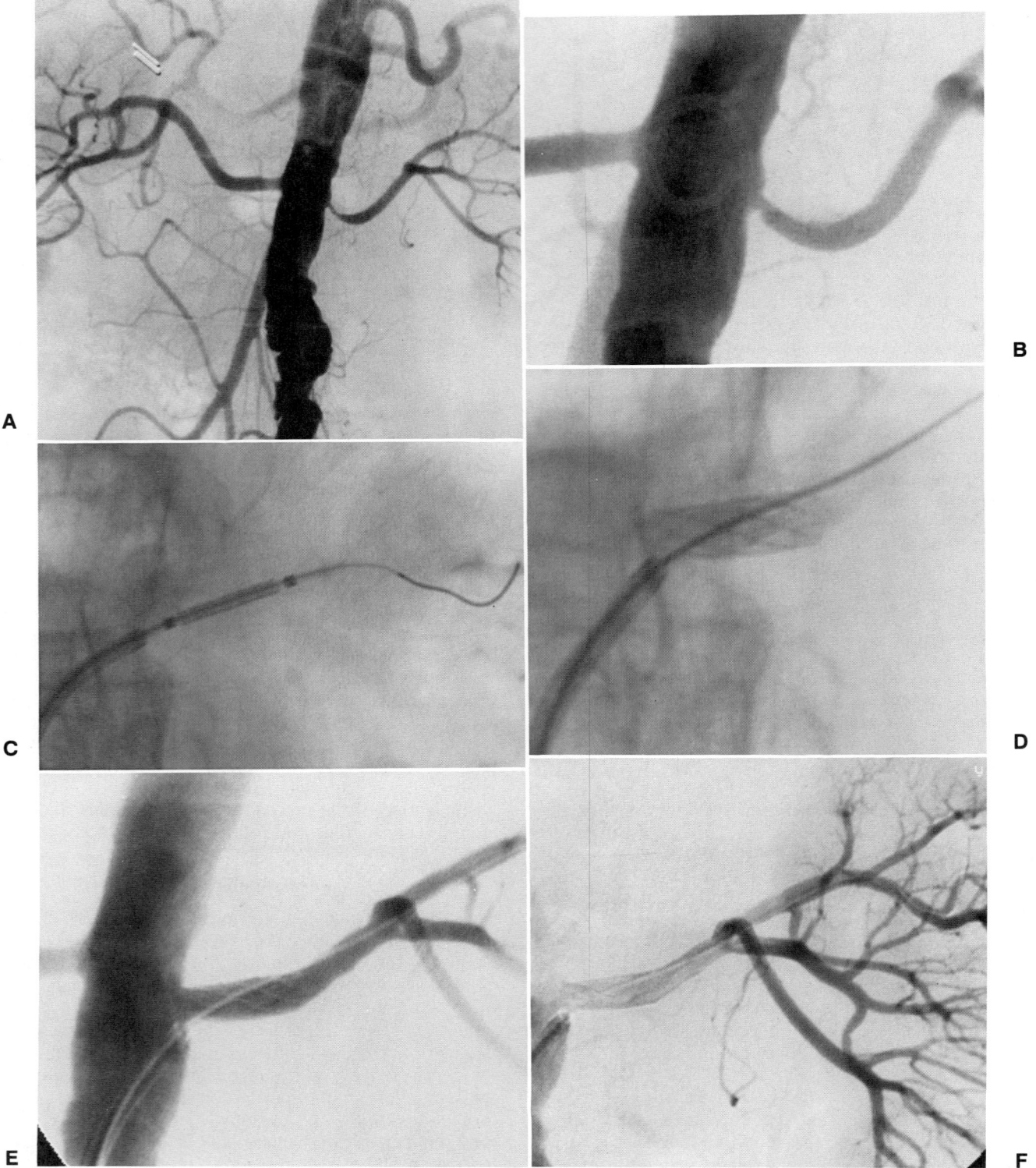

Figure 1 Use of an intravascular stent in the renal artery. Initial aortogram (*A*) shows tight proximal stenosis of the left renal artery; the right renal artery is normal. Despite angioplasty with a 6 mm balloon, a residual 75% cross-sectional stenosis persists at the angioplasty site, secondary to elastic recoil (*B*). A Palmaz balloon-expandable stent is poised in the proximal renal artery, between the radiopaque markers on the balloon catheter; the delivery sheath has been retracted into the aorta (*C*). The balloon is inflated, deflated, and removed over the guide wire, leaving the expanded stent in the proximal renal artery (*D*). Early (*E*) and late (*F*) images from a postdeployment aortogram show good position of the stent and perfusion of all renal branches.

Technical success of 95% with residual stenoses under 15% seems feasible with balloon-expanded and self-expanding stents. Short-term benefit rates for blood pressure response are 65% to 75% at 6 months, declining slowly thereafter. Angiographic restenosis appears in approximately one-third of patients in 6 months. In patients with renal insufficiency, renal function improves in a third, remains stable in a third, and deteriorates in a third. Further study is required before the appropriate indications, complication rates, and clinical benefit rates associated with renal artery stents are known.

REFERENCES

1. Standards of Practice Committee of the SCVIR. Guidelines for percutaneous transluminal angioplasty. J Vasc Interven Radiol 1990; 1:5–15.
2. Novick AC. Current concepts in the management of renovascular hypertension and ischemic renal failure. Am J Kidney Dis 1989; 18 (suppl 1):33–37.
3. Tegtmeyer CJ, Selby JB, Hartwell GD, et al. Results and complications of angioplasty in fibromuscular disease. Circulation 1991; 83(suppl I):I155–I161.
4. Rodriguez-Perez JC, Plaza C, Reyes R, et al. Treatment of renovascular hypertension with percutaneous transluminal angioplasty: Experience in Spain. J Vasc Interven Radiol 1994; 5:101–109.
5. Hansen KJ, Starr SM, Sands RE, et al. Contemporary surgical management of renovascular disease. J Vasc Surg 1992; 16:319–331.
6. Ramsay LE, Waller PC. Blood pressure response to percutaneous transluminal angioplasty for renovascular hypertension: An overview of published series. BMJ 1990; 300:569–572.
7. Plouin PF, Darne B, Chatellier G, et al. Restenosis after a first percutaneous transluminal renal angioplasty. Hypertension 1993; 21:89–96.
8. Norling LL, Chevalier RL, Gomez RA, Tegtmeyer CJ. Use of interventional radiology for hypertension due to renal artery stenosis in children. Child Nephrol Urol 1992; 12:162–166.
9. Tyagi S, Singh B, Kaul UA, et al. Balloon angioplasty for renovascular hypertension in Takayasu's arteritis. Am Heart J 1993; 125:1386–1393.

AORTORENAL BYPASS FOR RENOVASCULAR HYPERTENSION IN ADULTS

CALVIN B. ERNST, M.D.

Bypass procedures remain central to successful operative management of renovascular disease, even though percutaneous renal arterial dilation has assumed a place in the management of renovascular hypertension in adults. However, because of the expanded role of percutaneous arterial dilation (PAD) for both fibromuscular dysplasia (FMD) and atherosclerotic renal arterial lesions, surgical procedures are performed less often now than several years ago. Furthermore, because only the least complicated stenoses, such as main renal arterial FMD lesions and nonosteal atherosclerotic lesions, are managed by PAD, renal arterial lesions requiring bypass procedures are becoming increasingly complex.[1,2]

Over the past two to three decades, the distribution and extent of renal arterial disease referred for surgical therapy has changed so that aortorenal bypass is less frequently performed.[1] Many atherosclerotic lesions have progressed to occlusion in patients who are at high risk by the time they are referred to the vascular surgeon. Consequently, in an effort to avoid a major aortic operation in such high-risk individuals, use of alternative bypass procedures such as splenorenal and hepatorenal bypasses has increased.[3,4] Nonetheless, aortorenal bypass remains a useful and durable procedure, particularly for treating a complicated atherosclerotic lesion, an occluded renal artery with a salvageable kidney, PAD failures, and complex FMD lesions extending into primary renal artery branches. Also, the natural history of atherosclerotic renal arterial lesions suggests that aortorenal bypass adjunctive to aortic reconstruction has merit, particularly for preocclusive arterial stenoses.[5,6]

INDICATIONS

The major indications for aortorenal bypass are renovascular hypertension, ischemic nephropathy, and adjunctive to aortic reconstruction. Atherosclerosis and FMD account for practically all renal arterial stenoses requiring repair. Many such lesions, however, are amenable to PAD except osteal atherosclerotic lesions and FMD extending into the branches of the renal artery, both of which are best treated with arterial reconstructive procedures, primarily aortorenal bypass. Some FMD lesions are associated with renal arterial aneurysms that cannot be safely dilated and therefore require aortorenal bypass for successful repair (Fig. 1). Failures of PAD may also require aortorenal reconstruction, either emergently for the occasional renal arterial perforation or electively for lesions that recur or those that cannot be dilated for technical reasons.

Renovascular Hypertension

Renovascular hypertension, especially in patients under 55 years of age who have been hypertensive for less than 5 years, responds very well to renal revascu-

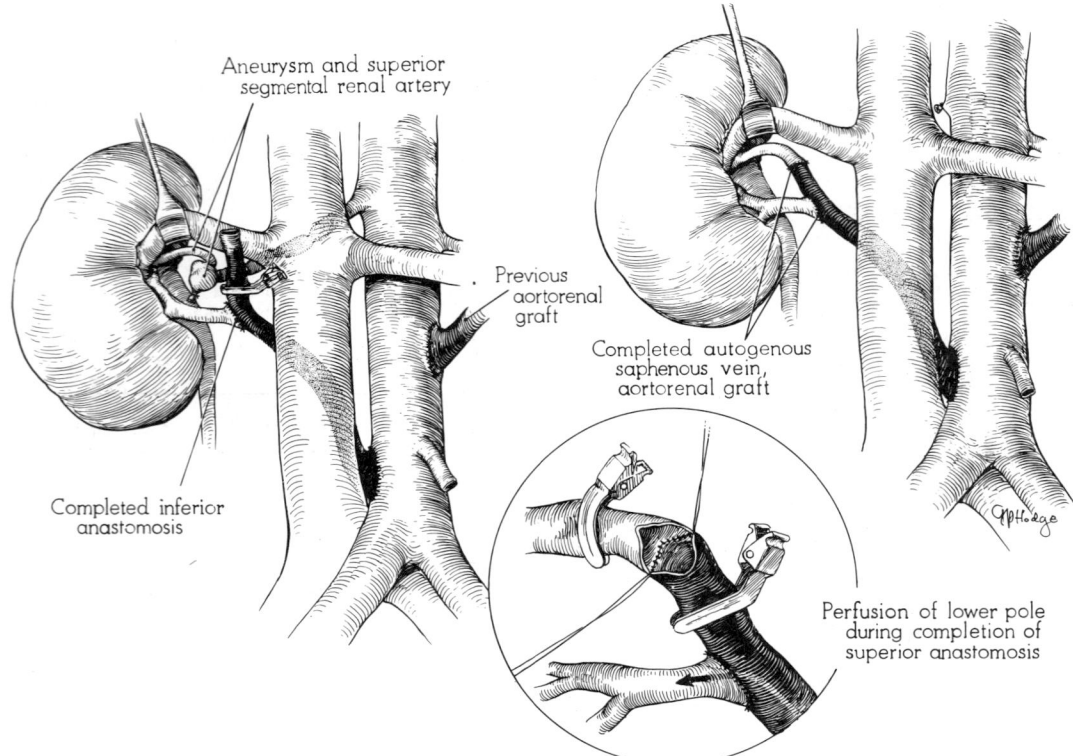

Figure 1 Autogenous saphenous vein aortorenal bypass for fibromuscular dysplasia and an associated aneurysm involving renal arterial bifurcation. A spatulated end-to-end anastomosis between the vein graft and one branch of the renal artery is constructed with 6-0 monofilament suture *(insert)*. The other branch is anastomosed to the side of the vein graft. (From Ernst CB, Stanley JC, Fry WJ. Multiple primary and segmental renal artery revascularization utilizing autogenous saphenous vein. Surg Gynecol Obstet 1973; 137:1023–1026, with permission.)

larization.[1] However, any patient with severe hypertension who would be a candidate for operation if a correctable renal arterial lesion is found merits study. For optimal results, patients must be properly selected, which frequently requires renal venous renin assays to document the functional significance of a renal arterial stenosis and detailed arteriography to document the hemodynamic significance of the lesion. Functional significance is suggested by lateralizing renal venous renin ratios of 1.4:1 or greater or a renal-systemic renin index (RSRI) of greater than 0.48. The RSRI is calculated by subtracting systemic renin activity (inferior vena cava blood renin) from individual kidney renal venous renin activity and dividing the remainder by systemic renin activity. A RSRI greater than 0.48 from an individual kidney reflects renin production that exceeds hepatic clearance and suggests hyperreninemia that should respond favorably to renal revascularization. Among patients with bilateral renal arterial stenoses, however, renal venous renin assays are not indicated because such studies seldom lateralize. Hemodynamic significance is best confirmed by arteriographic documentation of collateral vessels bypassing the stenosis. Noninvasive vascular laboratories that perform highly reliable renal duplex imaging studies are effectively able to exclude hemodynamically significant renal arterial stenotic lesions as a cause of renovascular hypertension or ischemic nephropathy.[6] It must be cautioned, however, that renal duplex imaging is applicable for only main renal artery disease; branch stenotic lesions responsible for renovascular hypertension cannot be consistently and accurately imaged.

Ischemic Nephropathy

Patients over 50 years of age with any level of hypertension who have recent onset of severe renal failure or accelerated renal dysfunction with serum creatinine levels of 2 mg/dl or greater are candidates for evaluation to identify a renovascular cause for the renal failure. The best candidates for renal revascularization for ischemic nephropathy are patients who have severe (80% or greater diameter stenosis) bilateral lesions (usually atherosclerotic but occasionally FMD) and patients with critically stenotic lesions involving solitary kidneys. Approximately 60% of such patients respond favorably to renal revascularization with improvement in renal function.[1,7] However, only 33% of patients with two kidneys and a significant unilateral lesion respond favorably to renal revascularization. Nonetheless, in a good-risk patient with unilateral disease in whom renal revascularization can be performed with an acceptable operative mortality, renal arterial reconstruction appears justified.

Renal Revascularization with Aortic Reconstruction

Aortorenal bypass adjunctive to aortic reconstruction may be required in 24% to 32% of patients.[1,2] In the author's opinion, adjunctive renal revascularization appears justified for all symptomatic renal arterial stenoses and for asymptomatic preocclusive lesions of approximately 80% diameter stenosis.[5] Although repair of an asymptomatic preocclusive lesion remains controversial, intuitively it seems that preservation of renal parenchymal tissue is beneficial, even though it is unclear what effect an unrepaired unilateral renal arterial stenosis that progresses to occlusion may have on patient survival or global renal function. Because the opportunity to revascularize a kidney after the renal artery becomes occluded may be limited, because the renal arterial stenoses are progressive, and because preocclusive lesions may jeopardize the kidney, prophylactic aortorenal bypass adjunctive to aortic reconstruction seems justified, provided such procedures can be performed in centers of excellence and with operative mortality rates of less than 3%.[5-8]

PREOPERATIVE EVALUATION

All candidates for aortorenal bypass should undergo thorough preoperative cardiac evaluation because many have significant left ventricular hypertrophy as a result of the long-standing hypertension. In addition, patients with atherosclerotic renal arterial lesions frequently have significant coronary artery disease, which is the leading cause of death following renal revascularization.

Beyond evaluation of the renal arterial stenosis for functional significance by determination of renal venous renin assays, all patients require detailed arteriographic studies to plan the operation. Duplex imaging has not yet evolved to the point that it can substitute for detailed contrast studies.

If the patient is to undergo prosthetic aortorenal bypass, prophylactic antibiotics are employed in the perioperative period. Patients undergoing autogenous tissue aortorenal bypasses are not given prophylactic antibiotics.

OPERATIVE APPROACHES

The operative approach to the aorta and renal arteries depends upon the indications for aortorenal bypass. If unilateral renal revascularization is indicated for a stenosis caused by either FMD or atherosclerosis and the aorta is not significantly diseased, then exposure is obtained transperitoneally through a supraumbilical transverse incision with right or left medial visceral rotation to expose the respective renal artery and aorta (Fig. 2). If, however, aortic reconstruction is required for

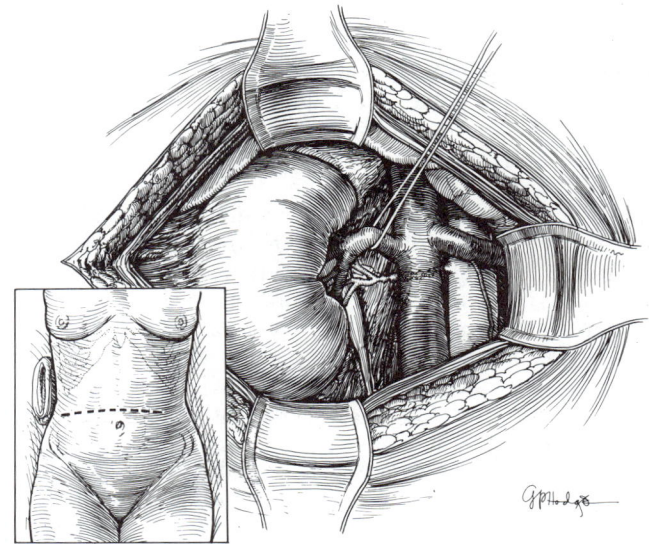

Figure 2 Exposure of the right renal artery through a supraumbilical transverse transperitoneal incision. Right medial visceral rotation provides excellent exposure of the renal artery and aorta. (From Ernst CB, Fry WJ, Stanley JC. Surgical treatment of renovascular hypertension. In: Stanley JC, Ernst CB, Fry WJ, eds. Renovascular hypertension. Philadelphia: WB Saunders, 1984, with permission.)

aneurysmal or occlusive disease in addition to renal revascularization, then exposure of the aorta is obtained transperitoneally through either a transverse supraumbilical or a midline abdominal incision. Because such adjunctive renal revascularization procedures are almost always performed for proximal atherosclerotic lesions, only the proximal half of the renal artery must be mobilized. Adequate exposure of either renal artery is easily obtained through the infracolic posterior peritoneum, and medial visceral rotation is usually not required. If the supraceliac aorta is to serve as an inflow source, a subcostal chevron upper abdominal transverse incision is used. The supraceliac aorta is exposed through the lesser space, and either or both renal arteries are exposed by right or left medial visceral rotation.

Aortorenal Bypass with an Undiseased Aorta

When the aorta is not significantly diseased, the right renal artery and aorta are exposed by mobilizing the ascending colon and duodenum to the left, anterior to the kidney (Fig. 2). The renal artery is dissected lateral to the inferior vena cava and mobilized over a sufficient length to permit proximal ligation, division, and an end-to-end anastomosis to the graft. The infrarenal abdominal aorta is exposed by further mobilizing the right-sided viscera to the left, anterior to the vena cava. Enough aorta is mobilized to permit application of a side-biting clamp.

For left-sided lesions, the renal artery is exposed by mobilizing the descending colon and occasionally the spleen and tail of the pancreas to the right, anterior to the kidney. Because the left renal artery lies behind the left renal vein, the left renal vein must be mobilized over a sufficient length to allow adequate exposure of the artery for ligation, division, and anastomosis.

The author prefers autogenous saphenous vein as the bypass graft when managing FMD because vein is more pliable than a synthetic prosthesis and facilitates the renal anastomosis, particularly if the FMD process involves the renal artery bifurcation and anastomoses to the primary branches are required (Fig. 1). To bypass proximal atherosclerotic lesions where the mid-renal artery is suitable for anastomosis, either saphenous vein or a synthetic graft is used. Under these circumstances, the author prefer a thin-walled expanded polytetrafluoroethylene (ePTFE) conduit.

The aortic anastomosis is performed first, using 5-0 polypropylene suture for vein grafts and PTFE suture for ePTFE grafts. After the patient is given 50 to 100 units heparin sodium/kg and 25 g mannitol intravenously, the renal artery is ligated proximally, clamped distally with a serrefine bulldog clamp, and divided. The vein graft is placed either in front of or behind the inferior vena cava, wherever it lies most comfortably, and an end-to-end vein to renal artery anastomosis is constructed with 6-0 polypropylene suture (Fig. 1). If an ePTFE graft is used, it is placed in a retrocaval tunnel to separate it from the overlying duodenum after the abdominal viscera are returned to their normal anatomic positions. In the event the ePTFE graft must be placed anterior to the inferior vena cava, it is covered by a tongue of omentum to isolate it from the duodenum.

Left renal revascularization is similar to the right but is simpler because one does not have to contend with the inferior vena cava. Significant bilateral lesions are treated with bilateral aortorenal bypasses at the same operation and are not staged.

Aortorenal Bypass Adjunctive to Aortic Reconstruction

Aortic reconstruction is virtually never required to treat FMD lesions unless such lesions are identified late in life, when symptomatic aortic disease is the indication for operation. For practical purposes, aortorenal bypass adjunctive to aortic reconstruction is performed only for atherosclerotic renal artery disease, using such renal revascularization prophylactically for preocclusive lesions, for hypertension, or for ischemic nephropathy.

Using 5-0 PTFE suture a 6 to 8 mm ePTFE sidearm is anastomosed to an ePTFE aortic graft before implanting the aortic graft. Standard aortic reconstruction is performed with either a straight or bifurcation graft. Because atherosclerotic renal artery stenoses usually involve only the proximal vessel, a suitable segment of renal artery can be exposed through the midline retroperitoneum. On the right, the inferior vena cava must be mobilized and retracted both medially and laterally to expose the renal artery. On the left, the left

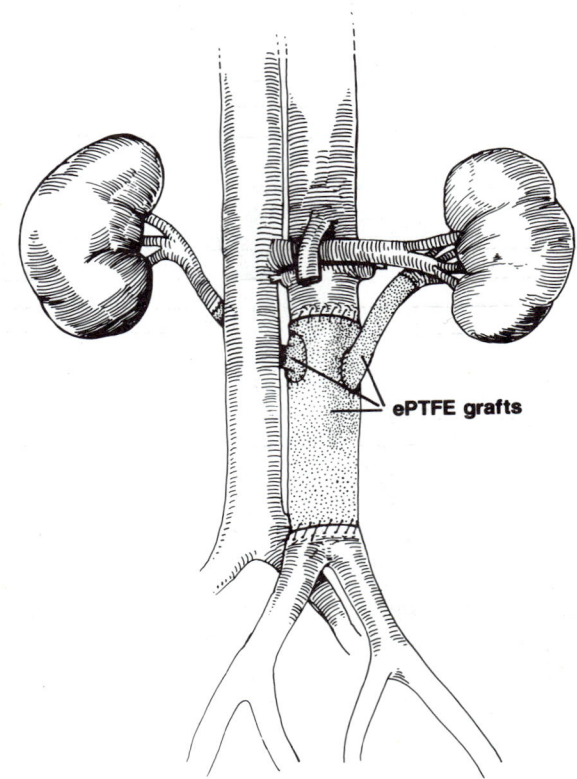

Figure 3 Bilateral aortorenal bypasses adjunctive to aortic reconstruction using ePTFE grafts. The right aortorenal graft lies behind the inferior vena cava.

renal vein must be adequately mobilized to expose the proximal half of the renal artery.

After reconstructing the aorta, the previously mobilized renal artery is ligated proximally, occluded distally with a serrefine vascular clamp, and divided. Using 5-0 PTFE suture, an end-to-end anastomosis is constructed between the ePTFE sidearm and the renal artery. On the right, if possible, the prosthesis is placed behind the inferior vena cava. During the anastomosis, the vena cava must be retracted; hence, the vena cava and left renal vein must be adequately mobilized. If bilateral renal revascularization is required, two sidearms are sutured to the aortic prosthesis and both renal arteries are repaired (Fig. 3). Contemporary practice dictates that such bilateral repairs are performed at the same operation and not staged. If, for some reason, suitable middle or distal right renal artery cannot be exposed through the midline, then right medial visceral rotation is required. For left renal arterial bypasses, left medial visceral rotation rarely, if ever, is required.

Use of the Supraceliac Aorta

If the infrarenal aorta does not require reconstruction and yet is unsuitable for clamp application, the undiseased supraceliac aorta provides a valuable inflow source for aortorenal bypass. Either autogenous saphenous vein or ePTFE may be used for the bypass graft. If

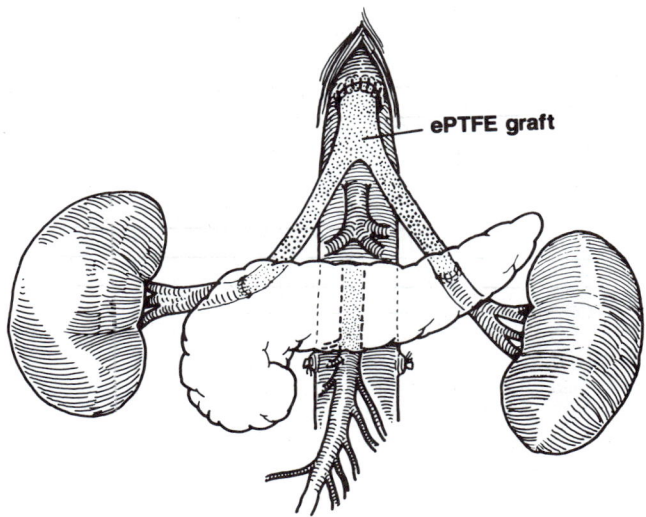

Figure 4 Supraceliac aortorenal bilateral bypass using an ePTFE bifurcation graft. The grafts reside behind the retroperitoneal viscera.

bilateral renal revascularization is required, a 14 by 7 mm ePTFE graft is used. Alternatively, two saphenous vein segments are sutured together to construct a bifurcation graft.[9]

The supraceliac aorta must be mobilized enough so that a partially occluding side-biting clamp can be applied proximal to the celiac axis. With blood flow maintained through the celiac and superior mesenteric arteries, the ePTFE graft is anastomosed to the anterior surface of the aorta using 5-0 PTFE suture. Occasionally, the aorta must be occluded with two clamps to allow an adequate aortotomy. After the end-to-side graft to aorta anastomosis is completed, the origin of the graft is clamped and the aorta is unclamped. Before renal anastomosis, 50 to 100 units of heparin sodium kg and 25 g of mannitol are given intravenously.

When using the supraceliac aorta, medial visceral rotation is required to expose either or both the renal arteries. On the right, the graft is tunneled behind the gastroduodenal ligament through the foramen of Winslow and behind the head of the pancreas. On the left, it is placed behind the stomach and pancreas (Fig. 4). End-to-end graft to renal arterial anastomoses are constructed after the respective renal arteries are ligated and divided.

RESULTS

Contemporary results clearly justify aortorenal bypass for renovascular hypertension as well as for ischemic nephropathy.[1] In properly selected patients with atherosclerotic renal arterial disease, a salutary effect on hypertension can be expected in 90% of patients, and renal function may be improved in almost 50%. Whereas two to three decades ago, aortorenal bypass along with aortic reconstruction had an operative mortality rate approaching 10%, contemporary anesthetic and surgical techniques have significantly improved results. Depending on the extent of generalized atherosclerosis, operative mortality rates approximate 3% for both solitary and adjunctive aortorenal bypass procedures.[1,2]

Among properly selected patients with FMD, results are even better, with no operative mortality and a salutary effect on hypertension of approximately 95%. Five-year patency rates for both prosthetic and autogenous tissue grafts are approximately 95%.[1,4]

REFERENCES

1. Hansen KJ, Starr SM, Sands E, et al. Contemporary surgical management of renovascular disease. J Vasc Surg 1992; 16:319–331.
2. Bredenberg CE, Sampson LN, Ray FS, et al. Changing patterns in surgery for chronic renal artery occlusive diseases. J Vasc Surg 1992; 15:1018–1024.
3. Moncure AC, Brewster DC, Darling RC, et al. Use of the splenic and hepatic arteries for renal revascularization. J Vasc Surg 1986; 3:196–203.
4. Cambria RP, Brewster DC, L'Italien GM, et al. The durability of different reconstructive techniques for atherosclerotic renal artery disease. J Vasc Surg 1994; 20:76–87.
5. Tollefson DFJ, Ernst CB. Natural history of atherosclerotic renal artery stenosis associated with aortic disease. J Vasc Surg 1991; 14:327–331.
6. Zierler RE, Bergelin RO, Isaacson JA, Strandness DE. Natural history of atherosclerotic renal artery stenosis: A prospective study with duplex ultrasound. J Vasc Surg 1994; 19:250–258.
7. Dean RH, Tribble RW, Hansen KJ, et al. Evolution of renal insufficiency in ischemic nephropathy. Ann Surg 1991; 213:446–456.
8. Chaikof EL, Smith RB III, Salam AA, et al. Ischemic nephropathy and concomitant aortic disease: A 10 year experience. J Vasc Surg 1994; 19:135–148.
9. Fry RE, Fry WJ. Supraceliac aortorenal bypass with saphenous vein for renovascular hypertension. Surg Gynecol Obstet 1989; 168:180–182.

EX VIVO ARTERIAL REPAIR FOR RENOVASCULAR HYPERTENSION SECONDARY TO FIBRODYSPLASIA

FOLKERT O. BELZER, M.D.
CHARLES W. ACHER, M.D.

Occasionally, fibromuscular dysplasia extends into the branches of the renal artery and dilation or operative reconstruction may be difficult, hazardous, or impossible. If the disease in the branch artery is minimal, dilation might be possible.[1] However, this method might not be applicable if the disease is extensive. In these complex cases, temporary nephrectomy and ex vivo repair utilizing microvascular techniques followed by autotransplantation allow precise repair of these lesions.

Renal autotransplantation for a ureter injury was first described by Hardy in 1963[2] and was first successfully performed for renal vascular hypertension by Woodruff and colleagues in 1964.[3] Ota and co-workers first reported nephrectomy and ex vivo microvascular reconstruction and successful autotransplantation in 1967. In 1970, we described a technique of reconstruction of renal artery branches in dogs using continuous extracorporeal hypothermic perfusion.[5] Corman and associates were the first to report the clinical use of this technique.[6] Subsequently, many case reports of nephrectomy and ex vivo repair using either hypothermic perfusion or hypothermia alone have been published.[7,8]

Ex vivo reconstruction should be considered only when in situ repair is deemed impossible. Extension of the disease to the primary renal artery branches does not necessarily preclude in situ repair. If the branches are 3 mm or more in diameter, in situ reconstruction can usually be performed with relative ease. Minimal stenosis of branch arteries can be successfully dilated, especially if there is no associated aneurysm.

In the past 20 years, we have used ex vivo reconstruction in 36 patients. The results of our first ten consecutive patients documented that all patients became normotensive without antihypertensive medication.[9] There was no mortality or morbidity in these ten patients and, although this series was relatively small, the uniform good results in these patients with extensive disease suggested that ex vivo renal artery construction was a safe and effective method of treatment. Arterial autografts were used exclusively for renal vascular reconstruction. These autografts included the hypogastric artery, splenic artery, common iliac artery, and external iliac artery. Although saphenous vein is used for most in situ renal vascular reconstruction, the long-term fate of autologous saphenous vein has shown an alarming 40% to 60% incidence of graft abnormalities, including thrombosis, expansion, dilation, aneurysm formation, and stenosis.[10] The hypogastric artery has been used in thousands of renal transplant procedures and only suture-line stenoses have been observed.

Since 1975, we have performed an additional ex vivo repair in 26 patients. The youngest patient was a 9-month-old weighing 16 pounds. The oldest patient was 63 years old. Arterial autografts were used in all patients. The indications were extensive fibromuscular dysplasia or complex large renal artery aneurysms, including multiple renal artery branches. There was one death, a 26-year-old man who died from a ruptured intracranial berry aneurysm 7 days after successful renal artery reconstruction. Morbidity has been minimal, with only one renal artery thrombosis. Long-term follow-up (mean 108 months) in these patients documented excellent results of blood pressure control (systolic of 140 mm Hg or less, diastolic less than 90 mm Hg) in 60% of the patients, and good blood pressure control (systolic less than 155 mm Hg, diastolic less than 95 mm Hg) in 36% of the patients. At follow-up, 40% (10/25) of patients remained normotensive off medications, and only 8% (2/25) required more than one medication for blood pressure control. Renal function was also maintained in these patients. The mean creatinine difference (preoperative creatinine minus follow-up creatinine) was 0.053 mg/dl with only two patients having any deterioration in renal function. In three patients who had high serum creatinine levels prior to revascularization, renal function returned to normal postoperatively and remained in the normal range at follow-up.

Several examples illustrate our experience. A 45-year-old man was found to be severely hypertensive. Aortography documented a normal left renal artery and a normal lower polar right renal artery. An upper polar artery was faintly visualized (Fig. 1A). Selective arteriography documented two high-grade stenoses, one in the main upper polar artery and the other in a branch vessel (Fig. 1B). Reconstruction involved the hypogastric artery. The anterior and posterior division of the artery was sutured end to end to the branch vessels of the upper renal artery. The normal renal artery was then inserted end to site into the hypogastric artery and the kidney autotransplanted (Fig. 1C).

In a 35-year-old woman found to be hypertensive, an arteriogram documented a complex, moderate-sized renal artery aneurysm involving multiple renal arteries (Fig. 2A). At the time of ex vivo repair, the kidney was supplied with two renal arteries, with the complex aneurysm arising from the upper renal artery. Arterial reconstruction, again using the hypogastric artery, was performed (Fig. 2B).

In a 28-year-old woman who was found to be severely hypertensive, arteriography documented a high-grade stenosis of the left renal artery, with a distal aneurysm supplying four arterial branches (Fig. 3A). Repair of the stenosis alone would have left the aneurysm unprotected from subsequent normal blood pressure. For this reason, the entire aneurysm was

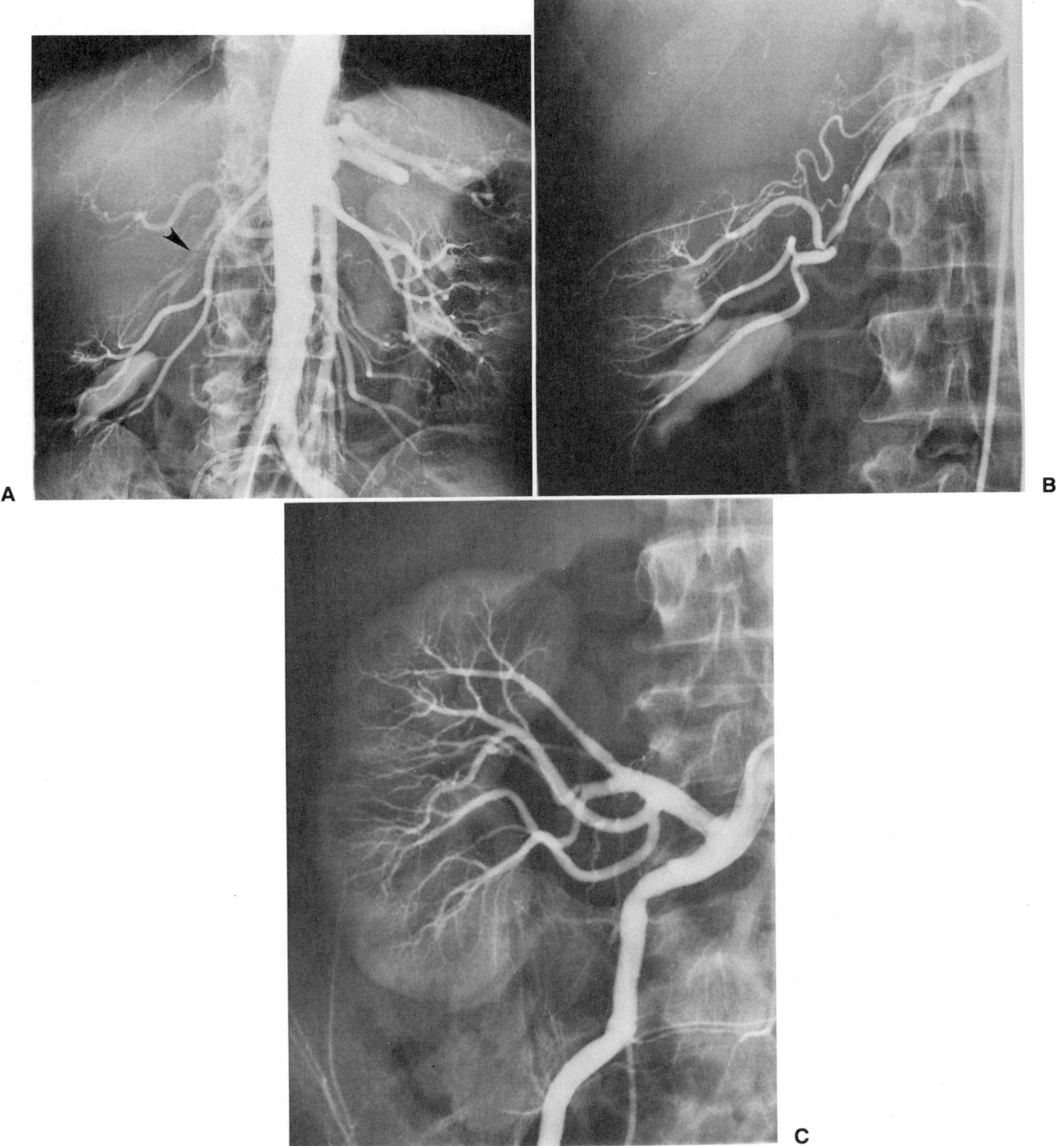

Figure 1 *A,* Aortogram in a 45-year-old, severely hypertensive man shows normal left renal and lower polar right renal arteries. An upper polar artery is faintly visualized *(arrow). B,* Selective arteriography shows high-grade stenoses in the main upper polar artery and in a branch vessel. *C,* During reconstruction, the anterior and posterior division of the hypogastric artery was sutured end to end to the branch vessels of the upper renal artery, and the normal renal artery was inserted end to side into the hypogastric artery; the kidney was then autotransplanted.

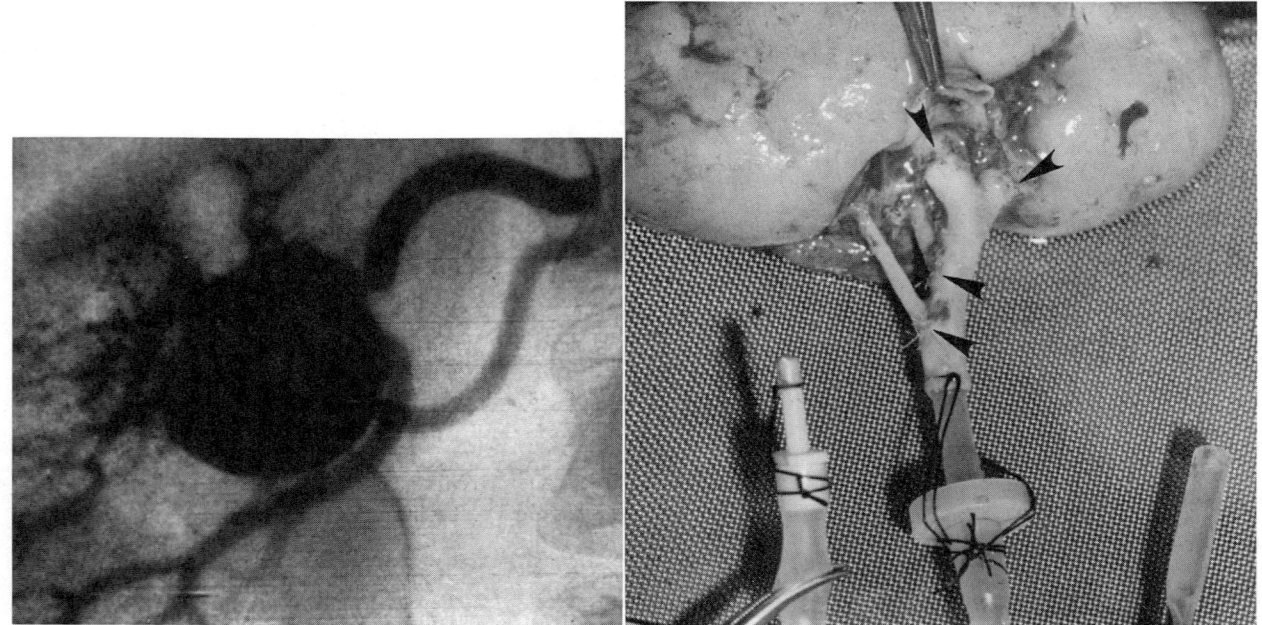

Figure 2 *A,* Complex aneurysm involving multiple renal arteries in a 35-year-old woman. *B,* Arterial reconstruction using the hypogastric artery; arrowheads indicate anastomoses.

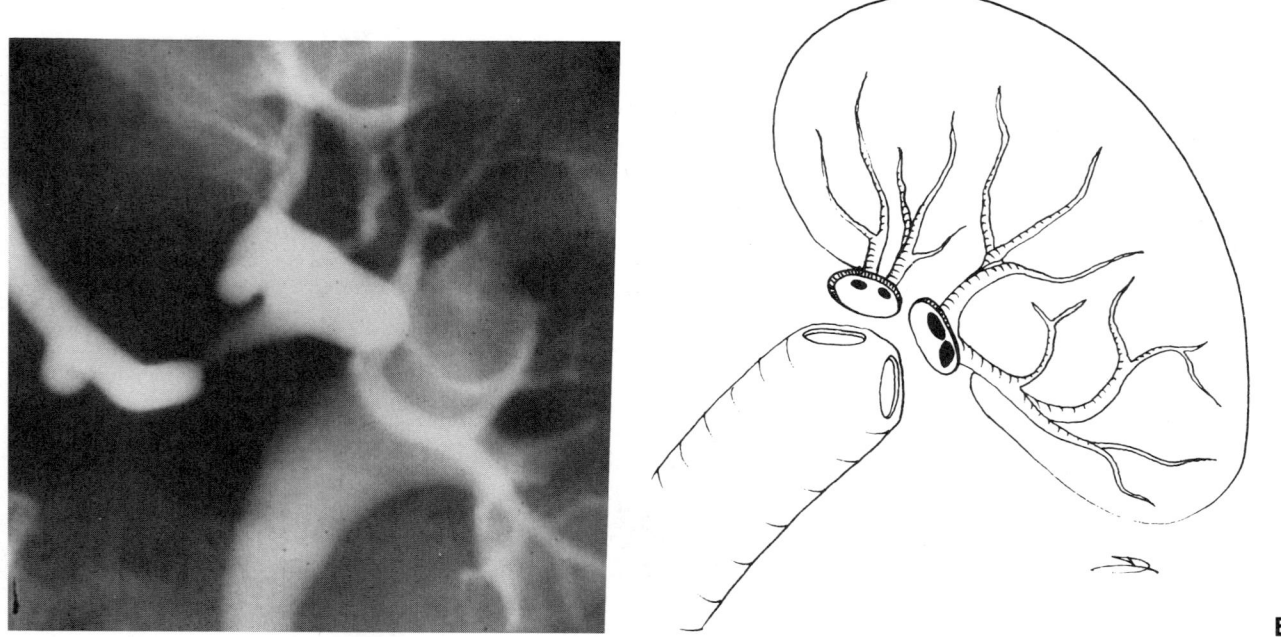

Figure 3 *A,* High-grade stenosis of the left renal artery with a distal aneurysm supplying four arterial branches in a severely hypertensive 28-year-old woman. *B,* The entire aneurysm was excised ex vivo, leaving two small Carrell patches, which were then anastomosed to the hypogastric artery bifurcation.

excised ex vivo, leaving two small Carrell patches that were then anastomosed to the hypogastric artery bifurcation (Fig. 3B).

In the early series, hypothermic, continuous perfusion was used during the ex vivo repairs. In the later series, simple hypothermic cooling appeared to be adequate. The kidney was flushed with a cold preservation fluid, and hypothermic conditions were maintained by placing ice packs around the kidney during the repair.

Initially, the ureter was divided prior to the surgical repair and reimplanted into the bladder at the time of autotransplantation. Later in this series, the ureter was mobilized, but not divided, and the surgical repair was performed on the patient's abdomen. No ureteral complications occurred with either approach.

Ex vivo arterial reconstructions provide for excellent results in the surgical management of renovascular hypertension secondary to arterial fibrodysplasia in patients in whom in situ revascularizations are not appropriately undertaken.

REFERENCES

1. Fry WJ, Brink BE, Thompson NW. New techniques in the treatment of extensive fibromuscular disease involving the renal arteries. Surgery 1970; 68:959–957.
2. Hardy JD. High ureteral injury: Management by autotransplantation of the kidney. JAMA 1963; 184:97–101.
3. Woodruff MFA, Doig A, Donalds KW, Nolan B. Renal autotransplantation. Lancet 1966; 1:433.
4. Ota K, Mori S, Awane Y, Ueno A. Ex situ repair of renal artery for renal vascular hypertension. Arch Surg 1967; 94:370–373.
5. Belzer FO, Reed TW, Pryor JP. A new method for renal artery reconstruction. Surgery 1970; 68:619–624.
6. Corman JL, Anderson JT, Taubman J, et al. Ex vivo perfusion, arteriography and autotransplantation procedures for kidney salvage. Surg Gynecol Obstet 1973; 137:659–665.
7. Belzer FO, Salvatierra O, Perloff D, Graus H. Surgical correction of advanced fibromuscular dysplasia of the renal arteries. Surgery 1974; 75:31–37.
8. Dean RH, Meacham PW, Weaver FA. Ex vivo renal artery reconstructions: Indications and techniques. J Vasc Surg 1986; 4:546–552.
9. Belzer FO, Salvatierra O, Palubinskas A, Stoney, RJ. Ex vivo renal artery reconstruction. Ann Surg 1975; 182:456–463.
10. Stanley JC, Ernst CB, Fry WJ. Fate of 100 aorto-renal vein grafts: Characteristics of late graft expansion and aneurysmal dilatation and stenosis. Surgery 1973; 74:931–944.

AORTORENAL ENDARTERECTOMY FOR TREATMENT OF RENAL ARTERY ATHEROSCLEROSIS

THOMAS S. HUBER, M.D., Ph.D.
JAMES C. STANLEY, M.D.

Renal revascularization is indicated for both renin-mediated hypertension and for progressive renal insufficiency secondary to renal artery stenotic disease. Renal artery atherosclerotic lesions account for 90% of all renal artery stenoses and are most often a manifestation of generalized atherosclerosis. Three specific patterns of atherosclerotic disease are relevant to renal endarterectomy procedures.

The most common atherosclerotic renal artery stenosis results from a "spillover" of aortic plaque. This type accounts for 65% of the stenoses and is bilateral in up to 75% of patients. An additional 30% of atherosclerotic renal artery stenoses present as focal eccentric or concentric narrowings within the proximal 1.5 cm of the artery. These stenoses are usually unilateral. These first two types of atherosclerosis are easily treated by endarterectomy. The remaining 5% of atherosclerotic renal artery stenoses occur as isolated lesions in the segmental branches. This form of renal atherosclerosis is rarely treated by endarterectomy.

Atherosclerotic renal artery stenoses have been reported to be progressive, causing approximately a 20% reduction in the vessel's cross-sectional area per year. Furthermore, nearly 10% of all lesions initially causing greater than a 60% reduction of the cross-sectional area progress to occlusion.[1] These facts must be considered in the decision to perform a bilateral endarterectomy in a patient whose disease appears primarily unilateral but in whom the contralateral artery is modestly narrowed.

Renal artery endarterectomy was one of the earliest forms of renal revascularization, first reported more than 40 years ago.[2] Renal artery occlusive lesions secondary to atherosclerosis are amenable to four principal means of endarterectomy: (1) aortorenal endarterectomy through an axial aortotomy, (2) aortorenal endarterectomy through the transected infrarenal aorta, (3) direct renal artery endarterectomy, and (4) eversion renal artery endarterectomy with subsequent reimplantation of the artery. The specific intervention undertaken depends upon the extent of aortic and renal artery disease, as well as the necessity to perform a simultaneous aortic reconstructive procedure.

OPERATIVE TECHNIQUE

Exposure

The usual approach to the renal arteries is an anterior one through the base of the mesocolon and root of the mesentery for all endarterectomy types, except for a unilateral direct renal artery endarterectomy, in which case an extraperitoneal approach after medial visceral rotation is favored.[3] The patient is placed supine on the operating table, and a rolled blanket is placed transversely under the lower back so as to accentuate the lumbar lordosis. A supraumbilical, transverse abdominal incision is preferred; it is extended from the contralateral anterior axillary line to the ipsilateral posterior axillary line. The small bowel is displaced from the abdominal cavity in a bowel bag, and the transverse colon is retracted into the upper abdomen with the aid of fixed retractor. The ligament of Treitz is divided and the duodenum is then mobilized, being retracted to the right. The retroperitoneum over the aorta is incised and dissection is advanced cephalad to the level of the left renal vein. The left renal vein is mobilized by transecting and ligating contributory adrenal, gonadal, and lumbar veins.

In the case of transaortic endarterectomy, the renal arteries are skeletonized from their aortic origin to a point well beyond the obvious distal extent of atherosclerotic plaque. Small nonparenchymal branches, such as those to the adrenal gland, must be transected and ligated close to the renal artery. This extensive mobilization is time consuming but is needed to facilitate easy eversion of the renal artery during the endarterectomy.

The aorta is dissected about its circumference to above the superior mesenteric artery. This requires incision of dense surrounding neural and fibrous tissues and division of the periaortic diaphragmatic crus. The crus is transected perpendicular to its fibers and the aorta with the electrocautery so as to prevent troublesome muscular bleeding. Ligation and transection of lumbar arteries may also be necessary to free the aorta completely from surrounding tissue, although these vessels are usually temporarily occluded with microvascular clamps.

Exposure of the renal artery for a direct unilateral endarterectomy is best provided with an extraperitoneal approach similar to the conventional medial visceral rotation used for aortorenal bypass. Patient positioning and the surgical incisions are the same as for other revascularizations. The renal arteries are approached by medial reflection of the colon and foregut structures to the contralateral side. The renal vein is dissected from the vena cava to the renal pelvis; it is extensively mobilized by transecting its small contributory venous branches. The renal artery is then dissected from its aortic origin to a point well beyond the obvious atherosclerotic plaque, usually just beyond the first branching of the main renal artery.

Systemic anticoagulation is achieved with intravenous administration of 150 units/kg of heparin sodium prior to aortic and renal artery clamping. Mannitol (12.5 g in an average adult) is administered intravenously at the same time to establish a diuresis. The four forms of endarterectomy differ in their performance.

Axial Aortorenal Endarterectomy

This is the most common direct method of restoring renal blood flow in cases of aortic spillover plaque (Fig. 1).[3,4] Clamping of the proximal superior mesenteric artery and distal renal arteries prior to aortic occlusion is done to prevent embolization of atheromatous debris from the aorta. Control of these vessels is achieved using low-pressure (30 to 70 g) microvascular clamps. Aortic control is obtained proximally just above the superior mesenteric artery and 3 to 4 cm below the level of the renal arteries. Aortic occlusion is occasionally required above the level of the celiac artery when little distance for clamping exists between the superior mesenteric and renal arteries.

An axial aortotomy is then made, beginning lateral to the superior mesenteric artery (Fig. 1). It is extended anteriorly in a curvilinear fashion to the midline of the aorta at the level of the renal arteries, where it is continued approximately 2 cm. The aortotomy must be sufficiently long to allow easy access to the renal artery orifices. An endarterectomy plane is developed between the diseased and normal aortic media and then extended circumferentially. The proximal extent of the plaque is transected immediately beneath the superior mesenteric artery orifice. Caution must be taken in the region of the superior mesenteric artery because it is not easily amenable to eversion endarterectomy through this exposure. The distal aortic plaque is transected approximately 1 cm below the renal artery orifices. Aortic tacking sutures are rarely necessary.

The endarterectomy is then accomplished by maintaining gentle traction on the aortic plaque extension into the renal artery while simultaneously pushing the everted arterial wall away from the lesion. The eversion is facilitated by the assistant's forceful advance of the distal artery into the more proximal vessel, which is often easier if the aortic plaque is transected anteriorly and posteriorly into two halves. A well-defined renal artery end point is usually established, with feathering of the plaque onto the distal artery. The aortotomy is closed with a continuous 4-0 polypropylene suture after vigorous irrigation of the endarterectomized aorta and renal arteries. Prior to the completion of the arterial closure, the superior mesenteric and renal arteries are backbled to remove any accumulations of intraluminal debris. Once the aortotomy has been closed, the aortic and renal artery clamps are removed, and antegrade flow to the kidneys is re-established. Intraoperative duplex scanning or directional Doppler examination

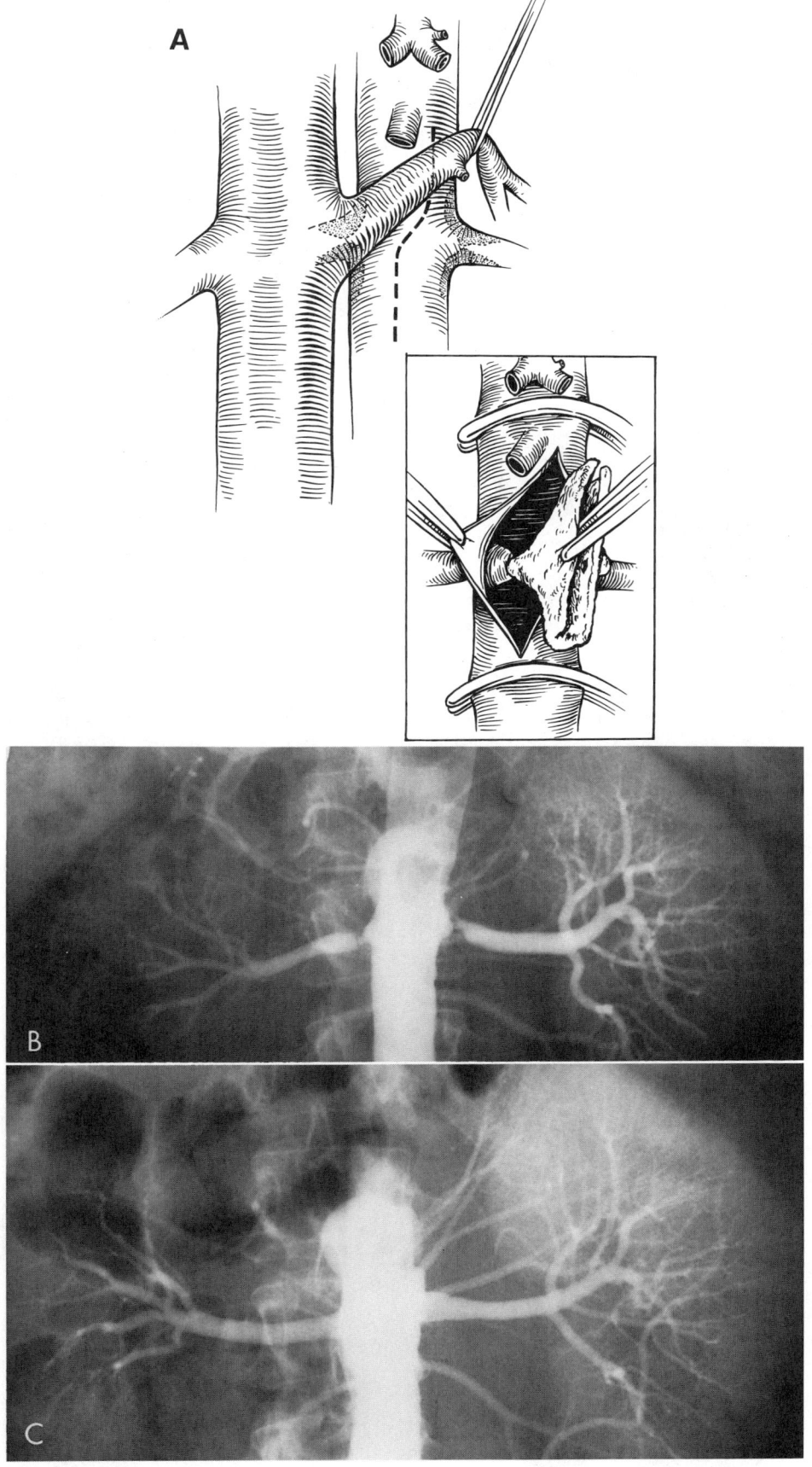

Figure 1 Technique of transaortic bilateral renal artery endarterectomy (*A*). Preoperative (*B*) and postoperative (*C*) aortography. (From Stanley JC, Messina LM, Wakefield TW, Zelenock GB. Renal artery reconstruction. In: Bergan JJ, Yao JST, eds. Techniques in arterial surgery. Philadelphia: WB Saunders, 1990:247; with permission.)

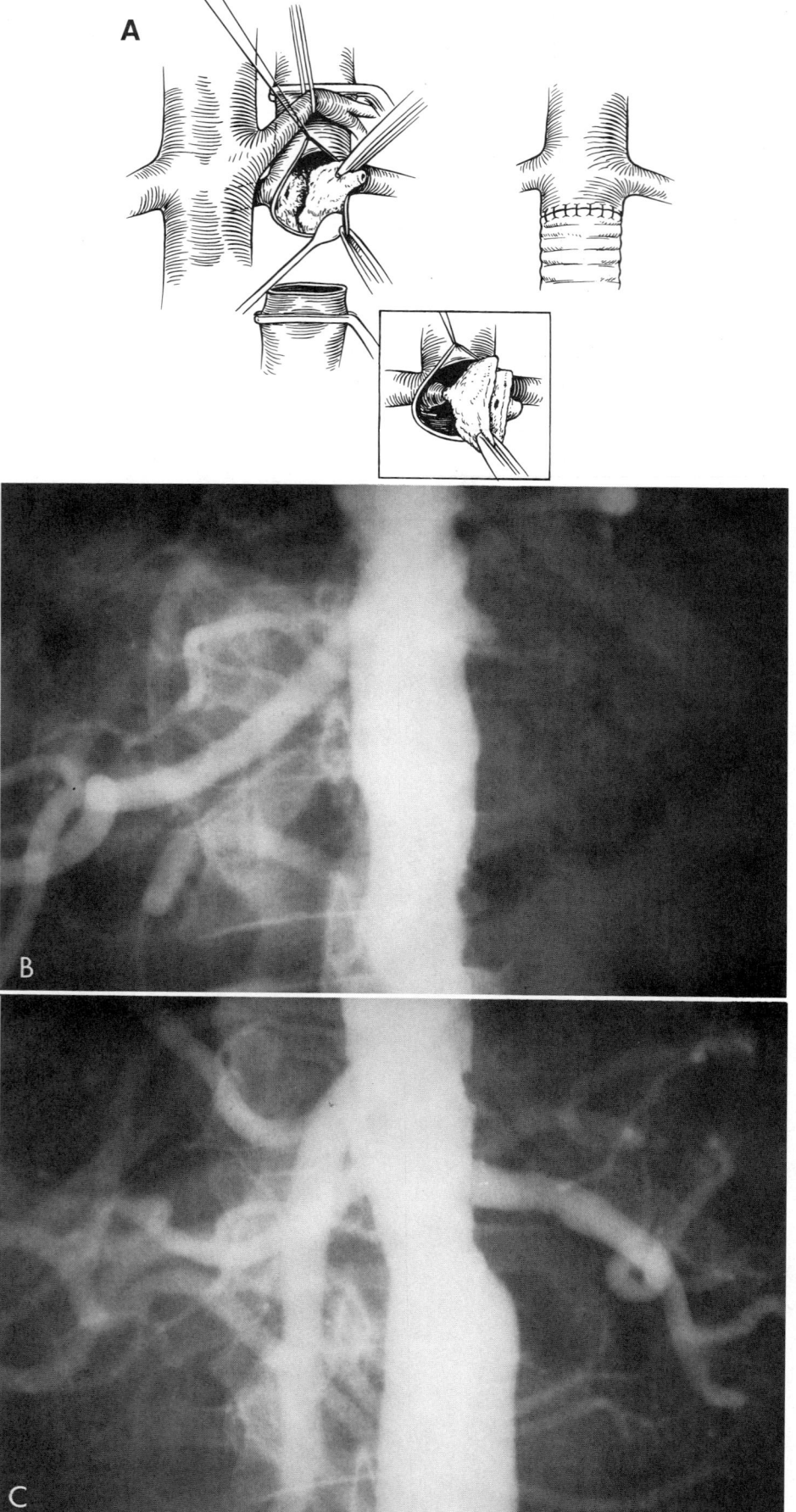

Figure 2 Technique of transaortic renal artery endarterectomy through a transected aorta undertaken in association with aortic reconstruction for aneurysmal or occlusive disease (*A*). Preoperative aortography documenting occluded left renal artery (*B*) and postoperative study revealing patent vessel (*C*). (From Stanley JC, Messina LM, Wakefield TW, Zelenock GB. Renal artery reconstruction. In: Bergan JJ, Yao JST, eds. Techniques in arterial surgery. Philadelphia: WB Saunders, 1990: 247; with permission.)

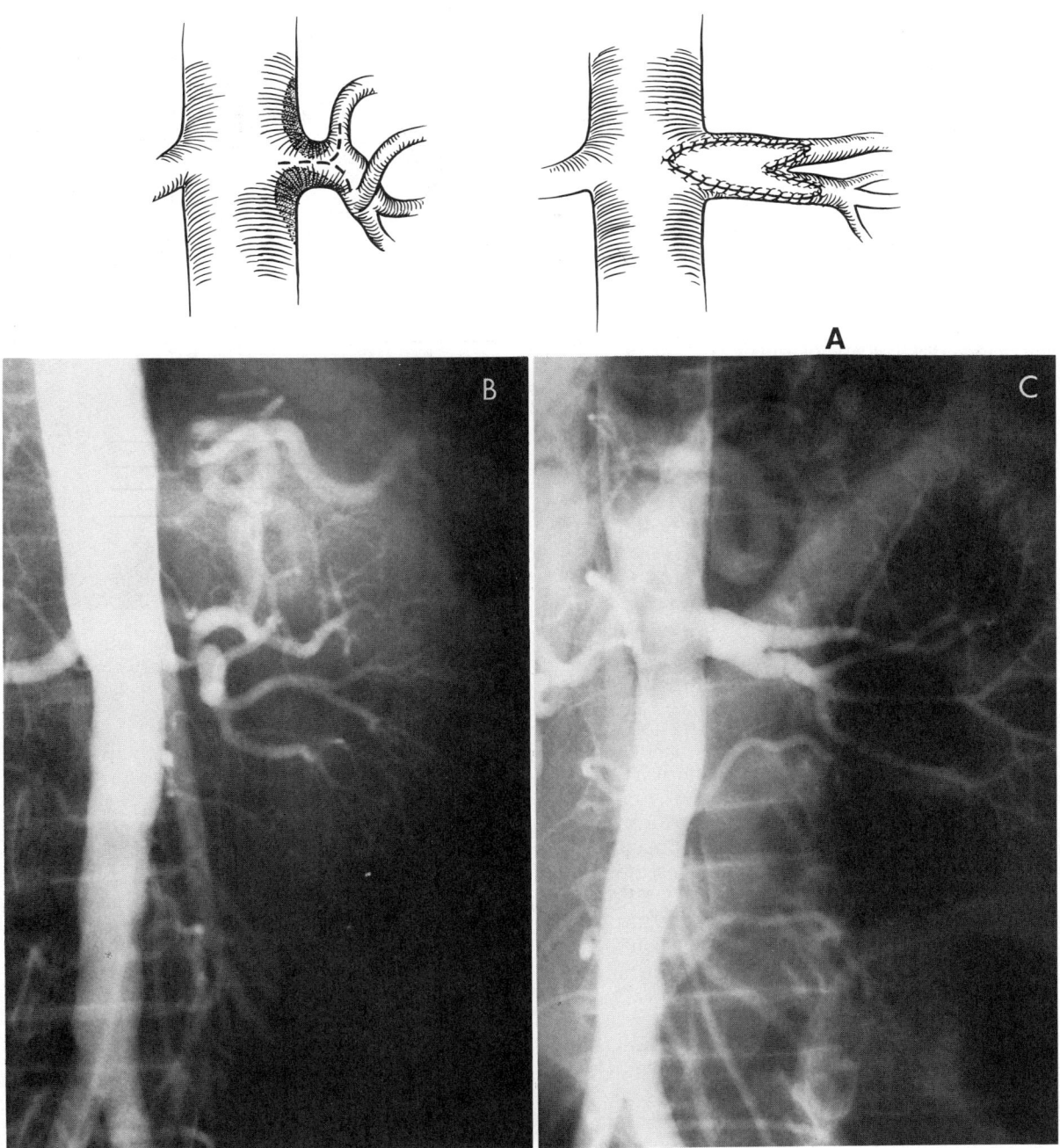

Figure 3 Technique of direct renal artery endarterectomy with patch graft arterial closure (*A*). Preoperative (*B*) and postoperative (*C*) arteriographic studies. (From Stanley JC, Messina LM, Wakefield TW, Zelenock GB. Renal artery reconstruction. In: Bergan JJ, Yao JST, eds. Techniques in arterial surgery. Philadelphia: WB Saunders, 1990: 247; with permission.)

establishes the adequacy of the endarterectomy.[3,5] If an intimal flap is suspected, a separate transverse renal artery incision should be made beyond the plaque's end point; after the plaque is removed or tacked down, the arteriotomy is closed. The heparin sodium effect is reversed with slow intravenous administration of protamine sulfate (1.5 mg/100 units heparin sodium). Just prior to re-establishment of renal blood flow, an additional 12.5 g of mannitol is administered.

This form of axial endarterectomy is particularly suited for arteriosclerotic stenoses limited to the proximal renal arteries (Fig. 1). The presence of a poststenotic dilation usually portends a good endarterectomy end point. This revascularization technique is the favored means of treating patients with multiple renal arteries in whom complex reconstruction would otherwise be required if conventional bypass procedures were undertaken.

Transaortic Renal Artery Endarterectomy

This technique is often performed in patients requiring concomitant renal artery and infrarenal aortic reconstructions[6] (Fig. 2). Vascular control is obtained in the same way as with the axial approach, except that placement of the distal clamp depends on the type and extent of aortic disease.

The aorta is transected approximately 5 mm below the renal arteries, and the endarterectomy is then performed through the open aorta. The endarterectomy plane is extended to approximately 1 cm above the renal artery orifices, and the plaque is transected transversely. Individual renal endarterectomies are often done after dividing the cylindrical aortic plaque in both the anterior and posterior midline. Endarterectomies are facilitated by everting each renal artery while maintaining gentle traction on the plaque. This form of endarterectomy is often made easier by transposing the transected aorta anterior to the left renal vein.[7] In these circumstances, following the endarterectomy and aortic graft anastomosis, the graft is repositioned beneath the left renal vein. A soft jaw clamp is placed on the graft, and early restoration of renal blood flow occurs with removal of the proximal aortic clamp. The remainder of the aortic reconstruction then proceeds in a standard manner.

Direct Renal Artery Endarterectomy

Renal artery reconstruction alone may be undertaken in certain patients without extensive aortic atherosclerosis. This is especially useful in treating complex proximal lesions (Fig. 3).[3] Once vascular control is achieved, an anterior renal arteriotomy is performed and extended distally beyond the atherosclerotic plaque and proximally onto the aorta. A direct endarterectomy of the focal renal artery lesion is then undertaken. Closure of the arteriotomy may occasionally be performed with a simple continuous suture, although a vein patch graft closure of the arteriotomy is more commonly undertaken. A patch of polytetrafluoroethylene or Dacron may suffice in managing large-caliber vessels. This direct renal artery endarterectomy technique is also applicable to treatment of bilateral disease. However, bilateral reconstructions are quite time consuming with this technique and offer no advantage over an axial aortorenal endarterectomy.

Renal Artery Eversion Endarterectomy and Aortic Reimplantation

A small subset of patients may benefit from reimplantation of a transected renal artery that has undergone eversion endarterectomy for proximal disease. This technique is well suited for revascularization of stenotic renal arteries arising from suprarenal or pararenal aortic aneurysms. The stenotic renal arteries arising from the diseased segment of aorta are usually transected along with a small cuff of aorta. An eversion endarterectomy is then performed in a conventional manner, and the endarterectomized arteries are then reimplanted onto

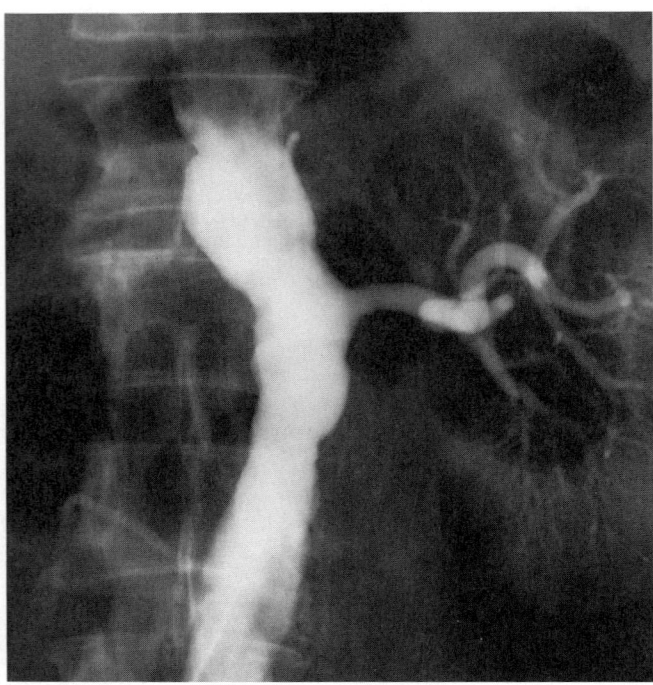

Figure 4 Renal artery reimplantation into the native infrarenal aorta following an eversion endarterectomy. Postoperative arteriographic study.

the prosthetic graft. This technique may occasionally be used with reimplantations into the native aorta (Fig. 4).

POSTOPERATIVE CARE

The primary objectives in the immediate postoperative period are to maintain blood pressure control and renal function. All patients are cared for 24 to 48 hours in the intensive care unit with continuous monitoring of pulmonary and systemic arterial pressures. Most patients are maintained on renal doses of dopamine (3 to 5 μg/kg/minute) for the first 24 hours. Preoperative antihypertensives are withheld during the immediate postoperative period, with the exception of agents such as clonidine (Catapres) that need to be discontinued slowly.

Severe hypertension in the postoperative period suggests renal artery occlusion and mandates evaluation. Conventional arteriography has been the standard diagnostic technique in this setting. However, its use is limited by potential nephrotoxicity of contrast agents. Renal perfusion scans may provide indirect evidence that the renal arteries are patent if a rapid uptake of the tracer is seen. A delay in tracer excretion may suggest acute tubular injury to explain the hypertension or renal dysfunction. Magnetic resonance angiography with gadolinium has overcome the limitations of both traditional contrast arteriography and renal perfusions scans. It is presently the study of choice at centers where it is available in this clinical setting.

The efficacy of aortorenal endarterectomy appears well established. However, no prospective, randomized trial has compared aortorenal endarterectomy to aortorenal bypass, percutaneous balloon angioplasty, or medical management alone. Nevertheless, aortorenal endarterectomy appears to be a durable and effective means of treating arteriosclerotic renovascular hypertension.

REFERENCES

1. Tollefson DFJ, Ernst CB. Natural history of atherosclerotic renal artery stenosis associated with aortic disease. J Vasc Surg 1991; 14:327–331.
2. Freeman NE, Leeds FH, Elliott WG, Roland SI. Thromboendarterectomy for hypertension due to renal artery occlusion. JAMA 1954; 156:1077–1079.
3. Stanley JC, Messina LM, Wakefield TW, Zelenock GB. Renal artery reconstruction. In: Bergan JJ, Yao JST, eds. Techniques in arterial surgery. Philadelphia: WB Saunders, 1990:247.
4. Wylie EJ, Perloff DL, Stoney RJ. Autogenous tissue revascularization techniques in surgery for renovascular hypertension. Ann Surg 1969; 170:416–428.
5. Hansen KJ, O'Neil EA, Reavis SW, et al. Intraoperative duplex sonography during renal artery reconstruction. J Vasc Surg 1991; 14:364–374.
6. Stoney RJ, Messina LM, Goldstone J, Reilly LM. Renal endarterectomy through the transected aorta: A new technique for combined aortorenal atherosclerosis. A preliminary report. J Vasc Surg 1989; 9:224–233.
7. Ernst CB, Fry WJ. Temporary aorto–left renal vein transposition: A simplified approach to the management of the aortic cuff in high aortic occlusions. Surgery 1971; 69:314–316.

ALTERNATIVE RENAL ARTERY RECONSTRUCTIVE TECHNIQUES: HEPATORENAL, SPLENORENAL, AND OTHER BYPASS PROCEDURES

ANDREW C. NOVICK, M.D.

A variety of surgical revascularization techniques are available for treating patients with hypertension or renal insufficiency due to renal artery disease.[1] In older patients with renal artery disease, involvement of the abdominal aorta with severe atherosclerosis, aneurysmal disease, or dense fibrosis from a prior operation may render a conventional aortorenal bypass or endarterectomy technically difficult and potentially hazardous. Simultaneous aortic replacement and renal revascularization have been associated with high operative mortality rates and should be considered only in patients with a significant aortic aneurysm or symptomatic aortoiliac occlusive disease. Alternate surgical approaches that allow safe and effective renal revascularization while avoiding operation on a badly diseased aorta are preferable in such individuals.[2]

Many patients with atherosclerosis present with bilateral renal artery stenoses. Bilateral simultaneous renal revascularization increases the risk of operation and is seldom necessary. In patients with bilateral renal artery disease, unilateral revascularization is safer and generally provides satisfactory treatment for associated hypertension or azotemia. The decision regarding which kidney to repair is based on the predominant indication for intervention. In patients with severe renovascular hypertension, the more ischemic kidney is repaired. If vascular reconstruction is being done primarily to preserve renal function, then the larger kidney is repaired.

SPLENORENAL BYPASS

Splenorenal bypass is the preferred vascular reconstructive technique for patients with a troublesome aorta who require left renal revascularization.[3] Transposition of the splenic artery by retroduodenal passage for right renal revascularization has been unsatisfactory and is not recommended. A requisite for performing splenorenal bypass is documentation by preoperative aortography, with both anteroposterior and lateral views, of widely patent celiac and splenic arteries. The splenic artery must also be carefully examined operatively for intramural atheromatous disease, which may be minimally occlusive and therefore not apparent on arteriography, but significant nonetheless. This problem, which is more commonly observed in women than in men, also mitigates against use of the splenic artery for renal revascularization.

The anatomic relationships of the splenic and renal vessels are relevant to these reconstructions (Fig. 1). To perform splenorenal bypass, an extended left subcostal transperitoneal incision is made, and the left colon and duodenum are reflected medially. The plane between Gerota's fascia and the pancreas is developed by blunt dissection, and the pancreas and spleen are gently retracted cephalad. The left renal vein is mobilized and retracted inferiorly to expose the main left renal artery. The pancreas is gently retracted upward to permit access to the splenic vessels. The splenic artery may be palpated posterior and superior to the splenic vein, and that portion lying closest to the distal aspect of the renal

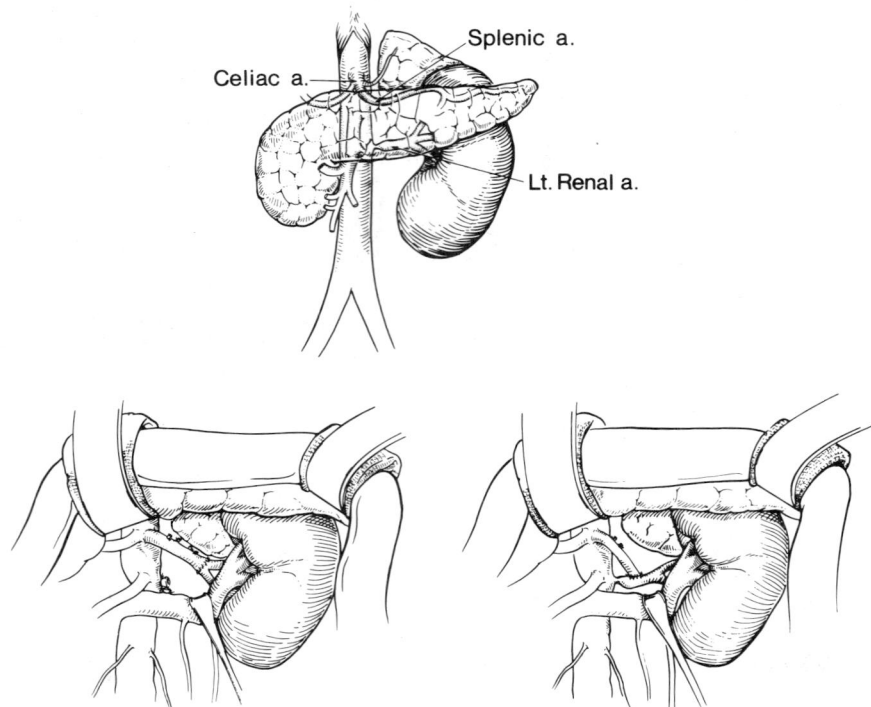

Figure 1 Normal anatomic relationship of the splenic and left renal arteries (*above*). Splenorenal bypass can be done with end-to-end (*bottom left*) or end-to-side (*bottom right*) anastomosis of splenic and left renal arteries.

artery is chosen for mobilization. Small pancreatic arterial branches are divided and secured with fine silk sutures. The splenic artery may be quite tortuous and should be mobilized proximally as close to the celiac artery as possible, where the vessel wall is thicker and the luminal diameter larger.

After its mobilization, the splenic artery is occluded proximally with a bulldog clamp, ligated distally with a 2-0 silk suture, and transsected. It is not necessary to remove the spleen, which receives adequate collateral supply from the short gastric and gastric epiploic vessels. After transection, the splenic artery is often observed to be in spasm with a considerably reduced luminal size. After irrigation of the lumen with dilute heparin sodium solution, this spasm can be relieved by gentle dilation of the splenic artery with graduated sounds. In general, there is no significant disparity in the caliber of the splenic and renal arteries, and a direct end-to-end anastomosis is performed. This type of anastomosis is preferred because it provides better flow, is easier to perform, and allows removal of the diseased arterial segment for pathologic study. An alternative method for performing splenorenal bypass involves end-to-side anastomosis of the splenic artery to the distal disease-free renal artery. This technique has been employed only in the unusual event of a significant disparity in the caliber of the splenic and renal arteries (Fig. 1).

Advantages of the splenorenal bypass technique are that the operation is done well away from the aorta, that only a single vascular anastomosis is necessary, and that revascularization is accomplished with an autogenous vascular graft.

HEPATORENAL BYPASS

Hepatorenal bypass is the preferred vascular reconstructive technique for patients with a troublesome aorta who require right renal revascularization. The hepatic circulation is ideally suited for a visceral right renal arterial bypass operation. The liver receives 28% of the cardiac output in resting adults and is unique in having a dual circulation from the portal vein and hepatic artery, which contribute 80% and 20% of hepatic blood flow, respectively. Hepatic oxygenation is equally derived from these two circulations. It has been documented that hepatic artery blood flow can be safely interrupted. When this occurs, hepatic function and morphology are maintained by increased extraction of oxygen from portal venous blood and by the rapid development of extensive collaterals to the liver.[4]

The hepatic artery arises from the celiac axis and runs anterior to the portal vein and to the left of the common bile duct. The first major branch is the gastroduodenal artery; thereafter, the hepatic artery divides into its right and left branches (Fig. 2A). In considering a hepatorenal bypass operation, one of the more clinically significant anatomic variations is origi-

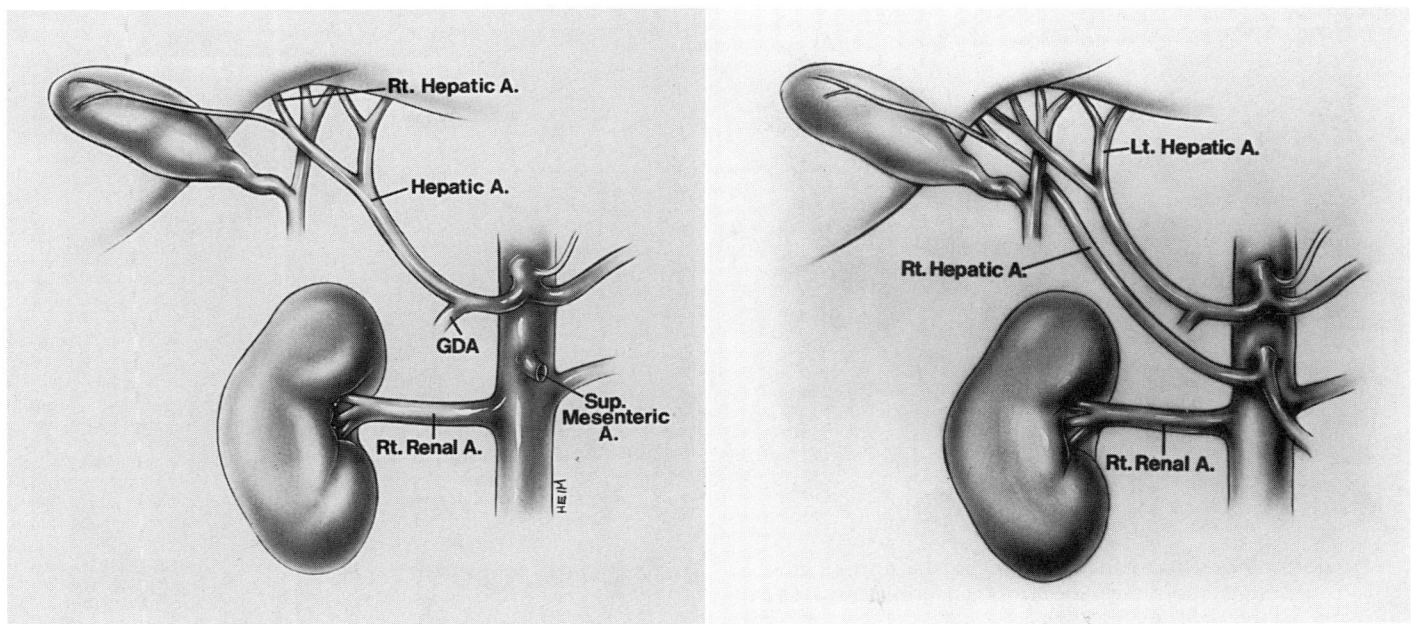

Figure 2 *A*, Normal course of the main hepatic artery and its various branches. *B*, Separate origins of the left and right hepatic arteries from the celiac and superior mesenteric arteries, respectively.

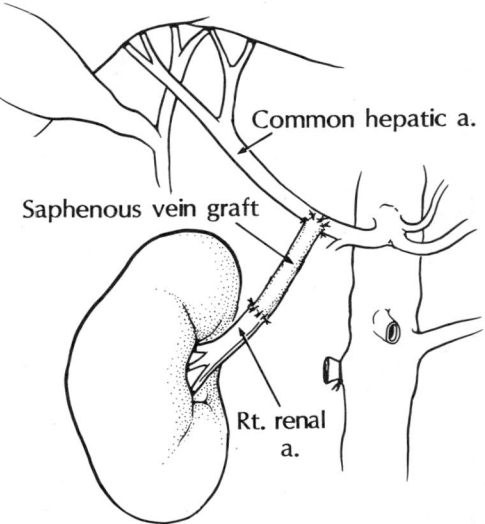

Figure 3 The most common method of performing hepatorenal bypass with an interposition saphenous vein graft anastomosed end to side to the common hepatic artery and end to end to the right renal artery.

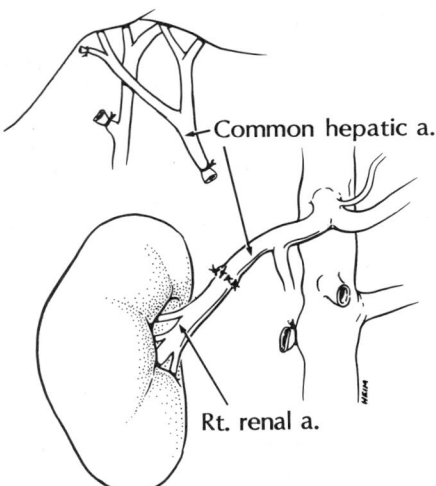

Figure 4 Performance of hepatorenal bypass by direct end-to-end anastomosis of the common hepatic artery to the right renal artery.

nation of the right hepatic artery from the superior mesenteric artery, which occurs in about 12% of patients (Fig. 2*B*). The left hepatic artery arises from the left gastric artery in approximately 11.5% of patients.

In patients considered for a hepatorenal bypass, preoperative aortography with lateral views must document patent celiac and hepatic arteries. In the author's experience, the hepatic artery is rarely involved with atherosclerosis and, certainly, less often than the splenic artery. Hepatorenal bypass should also only be undertaken when preoperative biochemical screening reveals normal liver function. The most common method of performing hepatorenal bypass is with an interposition saphenous vein graft anastomosed end to side to the common hepatic artery, just beyond the gastroduodenal origin, and then end to end to the right renal artery

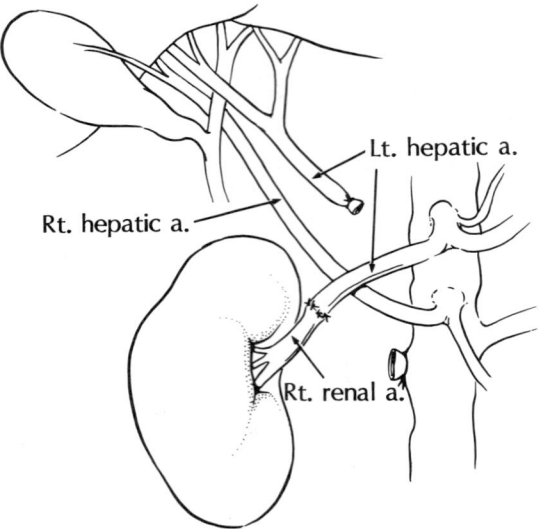

Figure 5 When the right and left hepatic arteries have a separate origin, the left hepatic artery can be anastomosed end to end to the right renal artery.

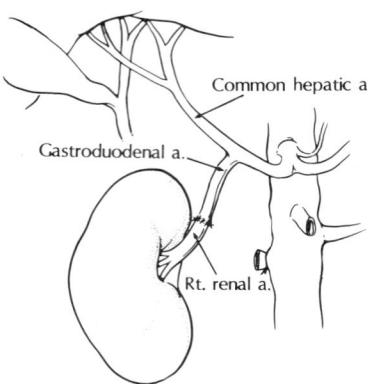

Figure 6 Use of the gastroduodenal artery to perform hepatorenal revascularization.

(Fig. 3). This technique preserves distal hepatic arterial blood flow and thereby reduces the risk of ischemic liver damage.[5]

In some patients, the common hepatic artery cannot be employed for vein graft hepatorenal revascularization either because it is smaller than the renal artery or because of an anatomic variation in which the right and left hepatic arterial branches each have separate origins. In these situations, the available major hepatic arteries are generally all of insufficient caliber to maintain adequate blood flow to both the liver and the right kidney. It is then preferable to perform end-to-end anastomosis of either the common, right, or left hepatic arteries to the right renal artery.[6] In some patients, a direct, tension-free anastomosis of these vessels can be performed (Fig. 4); otherwise, an interposition saphenous vein graft is needed. Despite the resulting total or segmental hepatic dearterialization in these patients, postoperative liver function studies have remained normal. However, the gallbladder is more susceptible to ischemic damage and may undergo necrosis when its blood supply from the right hepatic artery is interrupted.

There are three available strategies to avoid complications of gallbladder ischemia in patients undergoing end-to-end hepatorenal revascularization. First, when separate right and left hepatic arteries are present, the left hepatic artery should be used preferentially for anastomosis with the renal artery (Fig. 5). Second, if it is necessary to use the common or right hepatic arteries in this manner, cholecystectomy should be performed. A third option is to perform end-to-end anastomosis of the gastroduodenal and renal arteries, with an interposition saphenous vein graft, if necessary (Fig. 6). However, the origin and course of the gastroduodenal artery must be

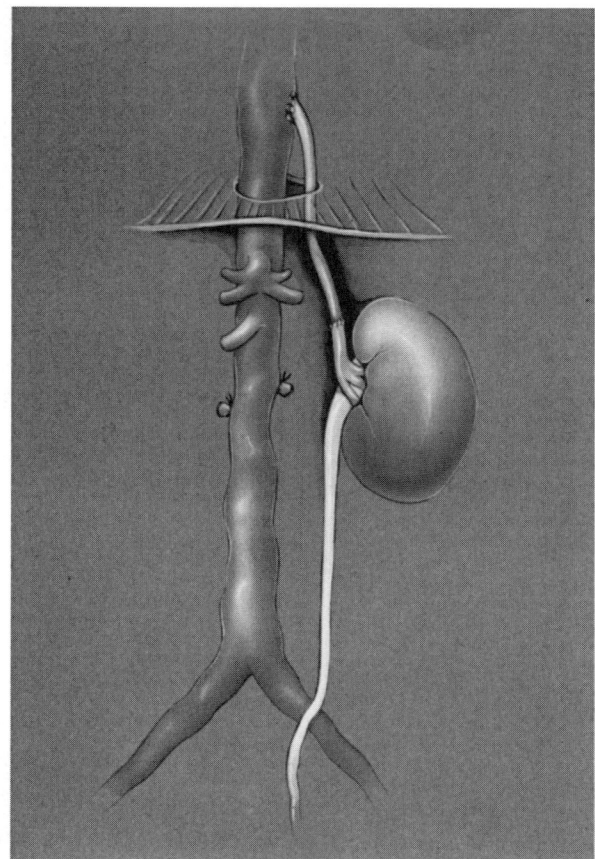

Figure 7 Thoracic aortorenal revascularization with an interposition saphenous vein graft.

such that proximal kinking does not occur when this vessel is rotated toward the right kidney. It is also somewhat more difficult to mobilize an adequate length of this artery, and care must be taken to avoid damage to the duodenum or pancreas. This technique is not as widely applicable as other methods of hepatorenal revascularization, but it does offer the advantage of preserving hepatic arterial flow.

The results of hepatorenal bypass for right renal arterial occlusive disease have been excellent and indicate that it is a safe and effective operative approach in patients with a diseased abdominal aorta.[5,6]

THORACIC AORTORENAL BYPASS

Use of the thoracic aorta for renal revascularization is a new surgical alternative for patients with significant abdominal aortic atherosclerosis, celiac artery stenosis, and no primary indication to replace the abdominal aorta. The subdiaphragmatic supraceliac and descending thoracic aorta are often relatively free of disease in such patients and can be used to achieve renal vascular reconstruction with an interposition saphenous vein graft (Fig. 7). Preoperative aortographic evaluation should include views of the supraceliac and thoracic aorta to verify their disease-free status.

For left renal revascularization, the descending thoracic aorta is used as a donor site because it is more readily accessible than the subdiaphragmatic supraceliac aorta. A left thoracoabdominal incision is made below the eighth rib and extended medially across the midline. This incision provides excellent simultaneous exposure of the thoracic aorta and renal artery with no need for extensive abdominal visceral mobilization. The left colon is reflected medially to expose the kidney and renal artery. The descending thoracic aorta is exposed above the diaphragm and is partially occluded laterally with a DeBakey clamp. A small aortotomy is made, a reversed saphenous vein graft is anastomosed end to side to the aorta, and the aortic clamp is then removed. During performance of the proximal anastomosis, distal aortic flow is preserved and systemic heparinization is not employed. A 2 cm incision is then made in the diaphragm just lateral to the aorta to enlarge the hiatus. The vein graft is passed alongside the aorta, through the diaphragmatic hiatus, posterior to the pancreas, and into the left retroperitoneum. End-to-end anastomosis of the vein graft and distal left renal artery are performed to complete the operation. On the right side, the subdiaphragmatic supraceliac or lower thoracic aorta are equally accessible through an anterior bilateral subcostal incision. The technique of thoracic aortorenal bypass is otherwise analogous to that described on the left side.

The initial results with thoracic aortorenal bypass in 23 patients with hypertension, abdominal aortic atherosclerosis, and celiac artery stenosis were: in 21 patients, renal artery stenosis was present bilaterally or in a solitary kidney.[7] There was one operative death due to a myocardial infarction. Postoperatively, among the remaining 22 patients, hypertension was cured or improved in 19 (86%), and renal function was stable or improved in 21 (95%).

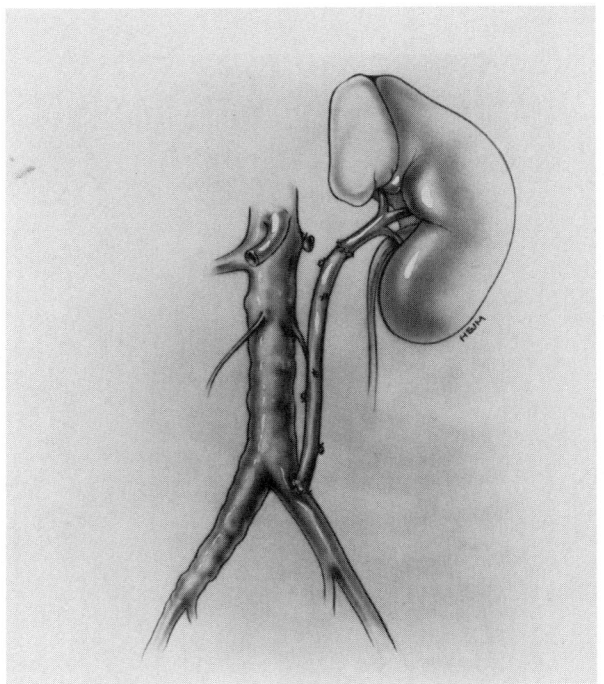

Figure 8 Iliorenal bypass with a saphenous vein graft.

Thoracic aortorenal revascularization is an attractive approach for several reasons. The thoracic aorta provides an excellent inflow source and the proximal end-to-side vein graft anastomosis yields an antegrade acute angle that is hemodynamically advantageous. Because the thoracic aorta is only partially occluded during performance of the proximal anastomosis, distal aortic blood flow is preserved, and systemic heparinization is unnecessary. The potential morbidity of aortic cross-clamping, which includes the risk of spinal cord ischemia, is avoided. The period of renal ischemia is also minimal and is limited to the time required for completion of the distal anastomosis, which is 15 to 20 minutes.

ILIORENAL BYPASS

Iliorenal bypass is an occasionally useful technique for revascularization in patients with severe aortic atherosclerosis, provided there is satisfactory blood flow through the diseased aorta and absence of significant iliac arterial occlusive disease (Fig. 8).[8] The author considers this operation only when a splenorenal, hepatorenal, or thoracic aortorenal bypass cannot be performed. This preference is based on the fact that aortic atherosclerosis may continue to progress in these patients, and, if so, this process is most likely to involve the infrarenal aorta. Such a development might then compromise flow to a revascularized kidney whose blood supply is derived exclusively from one of the iliac arteries.

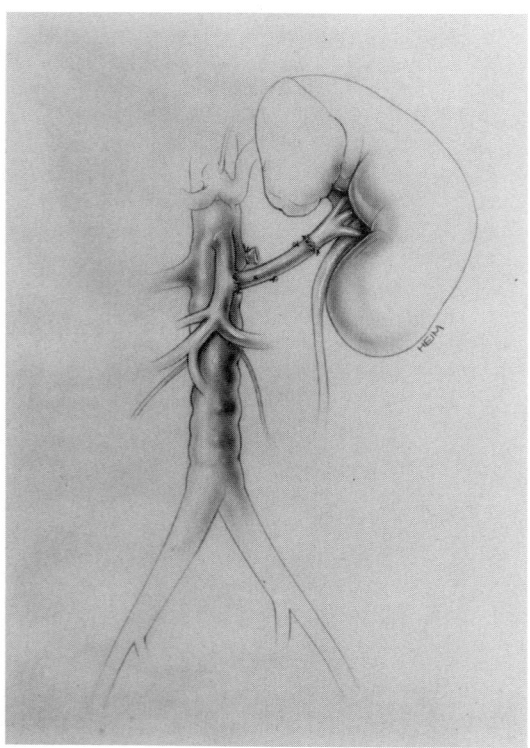

Figure 9 Superior mesenterorenal bypass with an interposition saphenous vein graft.

MESENTERORENAL BYPASS

Superior mesenterorenal saphenous vein bypass has limited and specific indications as a method of renal revascularization.[9] This technique has been used in the occasional patient with a surgically difficult aorta and a large superior mesenteric artery (SMA) in whom other alternative bypass procedures were not possible (Fig. 9). An enlarged and widely patent SMA is most often found in patients with occlusion of the infrarenal aorta. In such patients, the SMA has a wider caliber than normal because it is supplying collateral vessels to areas ordinarily supplied by the infrarenal aorta, including the large bowel, the pelvis, and lower extremities. Use of such an enlarged SMA for performance of a mesenterorenal bypass has been well tolerated with no compromise of intestinal blood flow. The author has not employed this approach in patients with a normal-sized SMA.

REFERENCES

1. Novick AC. Surgical correction of renovascular hypertension. Surg Clin North Am 1988; 68:7–25.
2. Novick AC, Ziegelbaum M, Vidt DG, et al. Trends in surgical revascularization for renal artery disease: Ten years' experience. JAMA 1987; 257:498–501.
3. Khauli R, Novick AC, Ziegelbaum W. Splenorenal bypass in the treatment of renal artery stenosis: Experience with 69 cases. J Vasc Surg 1985; 2:547–551.
4. Novick AC, Palleschi J, Straffon RA, Beven E. Experimental and clinical hepatorenal bypass as a means of revascularization of the right renal artery. Surg Gynecol Obstet, 1979; 148:557–562.
5. Chibaro EA, Libertino JA, Novick AC. Use of hepatic circulation for renal revascularization. Ann Surg 1984; 199:406–411.
6. Novick AC, McElroy J. Renal revascularization by end-to-end anastomosis of the hepatic and renal arteries. J Urol 1985; 134:1089–1093.
7. Novick AC. Use of the thoracic aorta for renal arterial reconstruction. J Vasc Surg 1994; 19:605–610.
8. Novick AC. Iliorenal and mesenterorenal bypass. In: Novick AC, Streem SB, Pontes J, eds. Stewart's operative urology. Baltimore: Williams & Wilkins, 1989:279.
9. Khauli RB, Novick AC, Coseriu GV, et al. Superior mesenterorenal bypass for renal revascularization with infrarenal aortic occlusion. J Urol 1985; 133:188–190.

OPERATIVE ASSESSMENT OF RENAL AND VISCERAL ARTERIAL RECONSTRUCTION USING DUPLEX SONOGRAPHY

KIMBERLEY J. HANSEN, M.D.
R. BRADLEY THOMASON, M.D.
RICHARD H. DEAN, M.D.

Renal and mesenteric artery reconstructions, whether performed as isolated procedures or combined with aortic reconstruction, pose challenges in anatomic exposure and vascular repair. Despite numerous refinements in surgical technique and advances in surgical materials, persistent or recurrent stenoses and occlusions affecting these repairs continue to occur. Serial arteriographic studies have documented persistent critical stenosis in 3% to 14% and thrombosis in 1% to 7% of aortorenal reconstructions. Likewise, up to 40% of retrograde aortomesenteric bypasses may fail during follow-up. In the elderly, atherosclerotic patient, the cost of these failures is potentially high. For renovascular repairs, postoperative failure may equate to unrelieved hypertension and loss of functioning renal mass in a group at high risk for major cardiovascular events and renal insufficiency. For visceral repairs, failure may lead to continued inanition associated with chronic visceral ischemia or frank intestinal infarction and death.

After completion of most peripheral artery reconstructions, technical errors have been defined by operative arteriography. This method has serious limitations, however, when applied to upper abdominal aortic branch reconstructions. At these locations, operative arteriography requires supraceliac or suprarenal aortic occlusion. The study obtained provides static images in the absence of pulsatile blood flow, and anatomic information is provided in only one projection. In addition, branch mesenteric and renal artery arteriolar vasospasm in response to cross-clamp ischemia and contrast injection may falsely suggest distal vascular occlusion. Finally, coexisting renal insufficiency is frequently present in patients undergoing either mesenteric or renovascular reconstruction, increasing the risk of postoperative contrast nephropathy.

These risks and the inherent limitations of arteriography are not shared by operative duplex sonography.[1-4] Because the ultrasound probe can be placed immediately adjacent to the vascular repair, high frequencies may be used that provide excellent B-scan detail sensitive to approximately 1 mm anatomic defects. Once imaged, defects can be viewed in a multitude of projections during pulsatile blood flow. Intimal flaps unapparent under static conditions are easily imaged while the adverse effects of additional mesenteric and renal ischemia are eliminated. In addition to superior anatomic detail, important hemodynamic information is obtained from the spectral analysis of the Doppler-

Table 1 Doppler Velocity Criteria for Renal and Mesenteric Artery Stenosis

Stenosis	Renal Criteria	Mesenteric Criteria
Less than 60% diameter-reducing stenosis	Peak systolic velocity (PSV) from entire artery < 2 m/sec	PSV from entire artery < 2.8 m/sec
60% or greater diameter-reducing stenosis	Focal PSV ≥ 2 m/sec *and* distal turbulent waveform	Focal PSV ≥ 2.8 m/sec *and* distal turbulent waveform
Occlusion	No Doppler-shifted signal from artery B-scan image	No Doppler-shifted signal from artery B-scan image
Inadequate study	Failure to obtain Doppler samples from entire arterial repair	Failure to obtain Doppler samples from entire arterial repair

PSV, Peak systolic velocity.

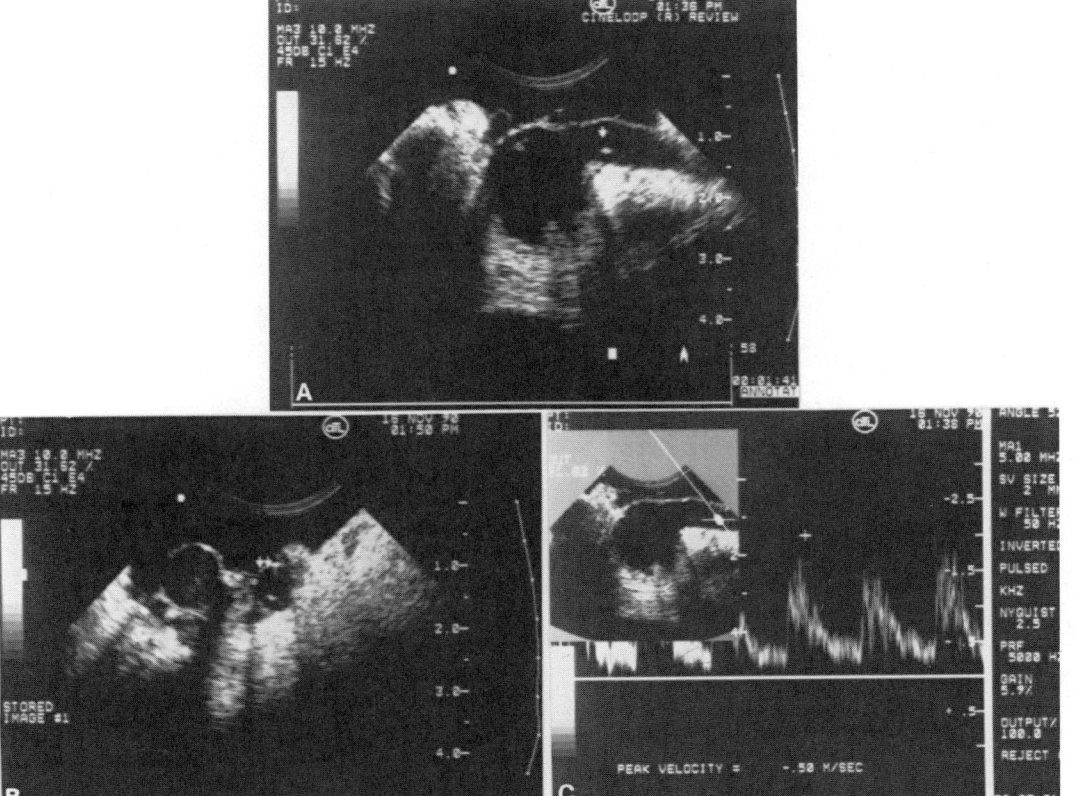

Figure 1 Sagittal *(A)* and transverse *(B)* B-scan images of intimal flap within the endarterectomy segment *(heavy arrows)* had normal spectral analysis of Doppler-shifted signal *(C)*. This minor defect was not revised. (From Hansen KJ, O'Neil EA, Reavis SW, et al. Intraoperative duplex sonography during renal artery repair. J Vasc Surg 1991; 14:364–374; with permission.)

shifted signal proximal and distal to the imaged defect. We believe freedom from limited static projections, the absence of nephrotoxic contrast material or additional ischemia, and the hemodynamic data provided by Doppler spectral analysis make duplex sonography the operative method of choice to assess both mesenteric and renovascular repairs.

As in surface duplex sonography, close cooperation between the vascular surgeon and the vascular technologist is required for accurate intraoperative assessment. Although the surgeon is responsible for manipulating the probe head to acquire optimal B-scan images of the vascular repair, proper power and time gain adjustments of the equipment are made best by an experienced technologist. Close cooperation is likewise required to obtain complete pulse-Doppler sampling associated with B-scan defects. While the surgeon images areas of interest at the optimal insonating angle, the technologist sets the Doppler sample depth and sample volume and determines blood flow velocities from the Doppler spectrum analyzer. Finally, participation in operative assessment enhances the vascular technologist's ability to obtain satisfactory surface duplex studies during follow-up. Our technique of operative assessment and the routine participation of a vascular technologist have yielded a 5 minute mean scan time and a 98% study completion rate.

We perform operative studies after renal and mesenteric reconstruction with either a 10 mHz mechanical probe with 5 mHz Doppler or a 5 mHz linear array probe with Doppler color flow. The probe head is placed in a sterile plastic sheath containing acoustic gel. Although plastic caps are available and designed to increase gel coupling to the mechanical scan head, we have found that they add an undesirable acoustic artifact. The operative field is flooded with warm saline, and B-scan images are obtained first in the longitudinal projection. Care is taken to image the entire upper abdominal aorta and renal or mesenteric artery origins along the entire length of the repair. All defects seen in longitudinal projection are imaged in transverse projection to confirm their anatomic presence and contribution to luminal narrowing. Doppler samples are then obtained just proximal and distal to imaged lesions in longitudinal projection to determine their potential contribution to blood flow disturbance.

Criteria used for hemodynamic defects, representing 60% or more diameter reductions, are similar to surface duplex studies (Table 1). These criteria have been found valid in our laboratory with a canine model

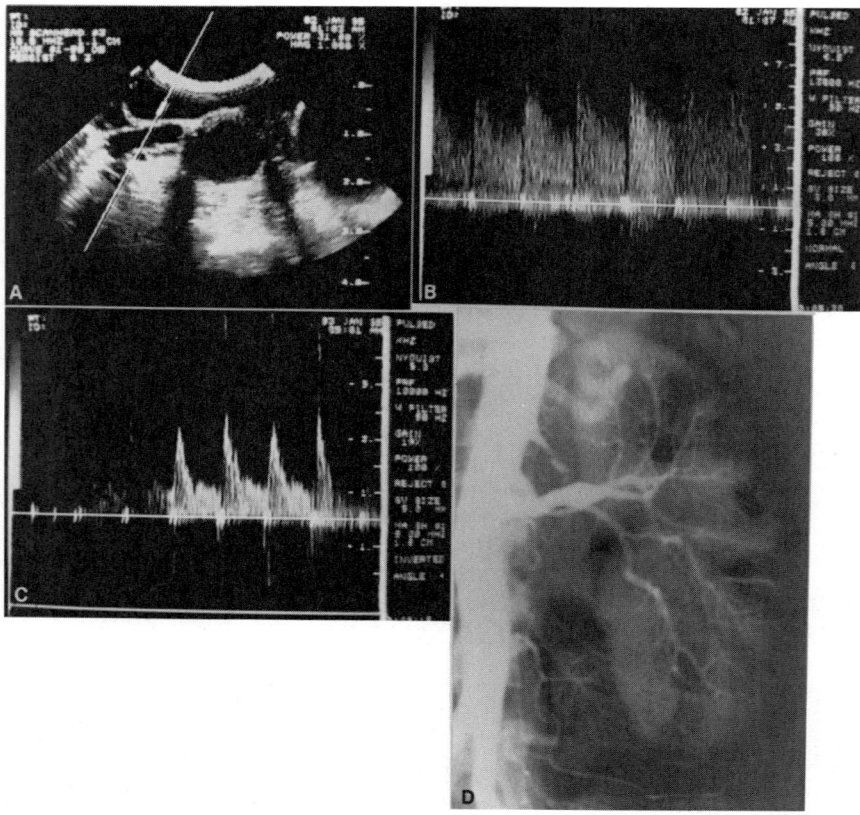

Figure 2 Sagittal image *(A)* of a major B-scan defect. This intimal flap at the proximal anastomosis *(B)* demonstrated a focal increase in renal artery peak systolic velocity (RA-PSV) (3.1 m/s). After revision, RA-PSV *(C)* was decreased (1.1 m/s), and follow-up angiogram *(D)* demonstrated a widely patent anastomosis. This patient was cured of hypertension. (From Hansen KJ, O'Neil EA, Reavis SW, et al. Intraoperative duplex sonography during renal artery repair. J Vasc Surg 1991; 14:364–374.)

of graded mesenteric and renal artery stenoses. They have also proved valid in a retrospective comparison with preoperative cut film arteriography in 19 patients and 34 renal arteries when radiographic studies were compared to operative prerepair duplex studies. Unlike surface duplex sonography in which the Doppler sample volume is large relative to the mesenteric and renal artery diameter, a small Doppler sample volume can be accurately positioned within mid-center stream blood flow. At this location, our laboratory and clinical experience suggests that spectral broadening and increased peak systolic and end-diastolic velocities relate to luminal narrowing in a fashion similar to that recognized in the carotid system. After mesenteric and renal artery repairs, however, at least moderate spectral broadening seems inherent to the Doppler signal and unassociated with anatomic defects.

In our first validity analysis of operative duplex sonography, we assessed 57 renovascular reconstructions in 35 patients who underwent unilateral (13 patients) or bilateral (22 patients) repair. Methods of reconstruction included aortorenal bypass in 29 patients (20 saphenous vein, 5 polytetrafluoroethylene [PTFE], 4 Dacron), reimplantation in 7 repairs, transrenal thromboendarterectomy (TEA) with PTFE patch angioplasty in 13 repairs, and transaortic TEA in 8 repairs. The group included branch renal artery repairs in 6 patients (5 in vivo, 1 ex vivo); 14 had combined aortic replacement.

Average time for operative duplex sonography was 4.5 minutes, and studies provided complete B-scan and Doppler information in 56 of 57 repairs (98%). Duplex sonography was considered normal in 44 repairs (77%), whereas B-scan defects were present in 13 (23%) (Fig. 1). Six of these B-scan defects (11%) had Doppler spectra with focal increases in peak systolic velocity of 2 m/sec or more with poststenotic turbulence. These defects were defined as major, and each underwent immediate operative revision (Fig. 2). In each of these revisions, a significant defect was discovered and corrected. Seven B-scan defects without Doppler spectral abnormality were defined as minor and not repaired. At a mean follow-up of 12.4 months, the status of 55 renal artery reconstructions in 34 patients was determined by either surface renal duplex sonography or renal arteriography. Forty-two of 43 renal artery repairs with normal operative duplex and 6 of 6 repairs with minor B-scan defects were patent and free of critical stenosis. Of the 6 revisions prompted by abnormal B-scan, with Doppler criteria for a major defect, 4 were patent without stenosis, 1 restenosed, and 1 occluded. For these criteria, operative duplex was 86% sensitive and 100% specific for technical defects associated with postoperative stenosis and occlusion. These anatomic results were supported by the clinical response to operation. Of hypertensive patients, 96% had a favorable blood pressure response, and 80% of patients with renal insufficiency had improved renal function. Similar results have been obtained for visceral reconstruction at the celiac and superior mesenteric artery positions (Fig. 3). As in the case of renal artery reconstructions, immediate revision of these repairs is reserved for B-scan defects defined as major by Doppler velocity criteria (Table 1). Among patients having normal or minor B-scan defects or major B-scan defects immediately revised, there have been no postoperative failures of mesenteric artery repairs.

Designation of B-scan defects according to Doppler velocity criteria provides accurate information to guide decisions regarding revision. However, there are special circumstances that deserve comment. Infrequently, an operative duplex study of either renal or mesenteric reconstruction documents peak systolic velocities that exceed criteria for critical stenosis when no anatomic defect exists. Under these circumstances, the peak systolic velocities are elevated uniformly throughout the repair, there is no focal velocity change, and there is no distal turbulent waveform. This scenario is most commonly encountered after renal artery reconstruction for nonatherosclerotic renovascular disease. Similarly, an increase in peak systolic velocity is observed in transition

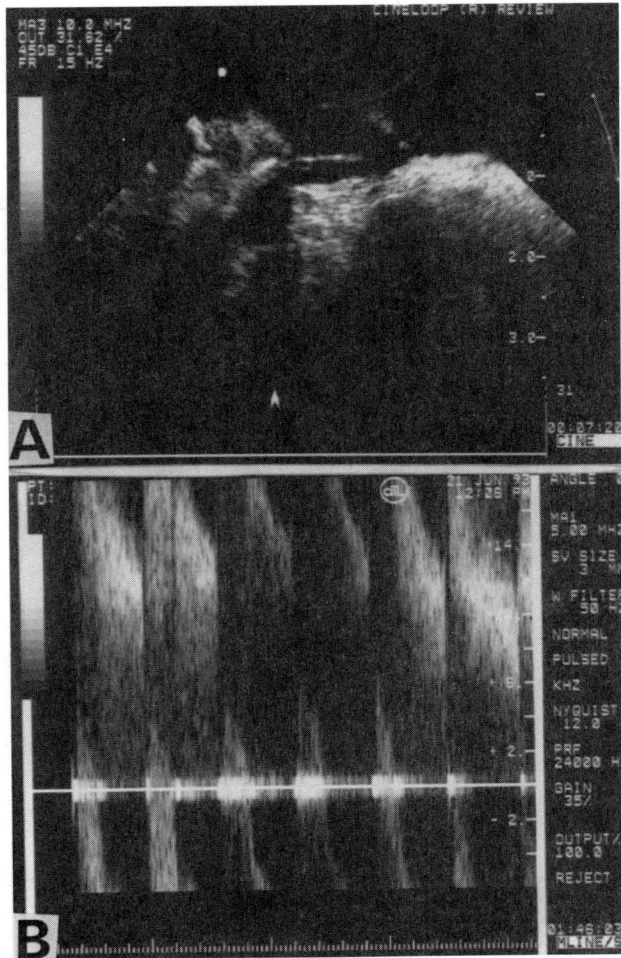

Figure 3 Operative duplex study during superior mesenteric artery reconstruction. The B-scan defect *(A)* was confirmed as major by Doppler spectral analysis *(B)*. A flow-limiting defect was confirmed during revision.

from the main renal artery to the segmental renal vessels after branch renal artery repair; however, no distal turbulent waveform will be observed. In addition, a renovascular repair to a solitary kidney frequently has increased velocities throughout. Similar to renal artery repairs of this variety, single-vessel mesenteric repairs that collateralize adjacent visceral circulation have a uniform increase in flow velocities.

In addition to these systolic spectral abnormalities, changes may be observed in the diastolic features of the spectra in the absence of technical error. A superior mesenteric artery repair with an unreconstructible but collateralized adjacent visceral circulation has the loss of a diastolic flow reversal characteristic of a fasting superior mesenteric artery signal. Likewise, abnormal diastolic spectra may be observed after revascularization of chronic renal and mesenteric ischemia. Reflecting increased vascular resistance in response to reperfusion, these spectra represent abbreviated systolic flow, short systolic acceleration times, and virtually no diastolic flow. This picture can mimic a distal embolic catastrophe. However, it may be distinguished by spectral changes observed after administration of vasodilator. This reactive vasospasm is relieved by intra-arterial administration, at the site of repair, of papaverine, 30 to 60 mg. The Doppler spectral signature characteristic for the renal or mesenteric artery reconstructed usually normalizes within 5 minutes.

Despite these infrequent spectral abnormalities in the absence of an anatomic defect, we believe our experience with operative duplex sonography as a completion study following mesenteric and renal reconstruction supports the technique as the operative method of choice to assess the repair objectively. Of reconstructions with normal operative duplex studies, 97% have remained patent and free of stenosis on follow-up. The B-scan image defects that are not associated with significant pressure-flow disturbance by Doppler velocity criteria do not seem to predispose to restenosis or occlusion and do not require treatment. However, B-scan defects associated with focal increases in peak systolic velocities exceeding 2 m/sec or 2.8 m/sec in renal or mesenteric artery repairs, respectively, should be considered for immediate revision.

REFERENCES

1. Okuhn SP, Reilly LM, Bennett JR, et al. Intraoperative assessment of renal and visceral artery reconstruction: The role of duplex scanning and spectral analysis. J Vasc Surg 1987; 5:137–147.
2. Goldstone J. Intraoperative assessment of renal and visceral arterial reconstruction using Doppler and duplex imaging. In: Ernst CB, Stanley JC, eds. Current therapy in vascular surgery. 2nd ed. Philadelphia: BC Decker, 1991:872.
3. Hansen KJ, Tribble RW, Reavis SW, et al. Renal duplex sonography: Evaluation of clinical utility. J Vasc Surg 1990; 12:227–236.
4. Hansen KJ, O'Neil EA, Reavis SW, et al. Intraoperative duplex sonography during renal artery reconstruction. J Vasc Surg 1991; 14:364–374.

SURGICAL TREATMENT OF RENOVASCULAR HYPERTENSION IN CHILDREN

HENRY D. BERKOWITZ, M.D.

Renal artery occlusive disease is second in frequency only to coarctation of the thoracic aorta as the most common form of surgically correctable hypertension in the pediatric population. Corrective operations in these children are technically challenging because they must correct the current problem and yet provide sufficient capacity for future growth and function over a normal lifespan.

The clinical presentation of renovascular hypertension in children is different than that in adults. Infants and young children frequently manifest failure to thrive and have seizure disorders secondary to hypertensive encephalopathy, which affects as many as 10% of these patients. In adolescents, the hypertension is usually silent and, once detected, usually resistant to control with conventional drug therapy.[1] Use of angiotensin converting enzyme (ACE) inhibitors in recent years has provided a salutary response regarding blood pressure. However, these agents can precipitate renal failure and must be monitored carefully.[2]

ARTERIAL LESIONS

The pediatric renovascular patient rarely presents with simple, unilateral renal artery disease. There is usually a complex spectrum of lesions involving renal and visceral arteries as well as the abdominal aorta.

The aortic lesions characteristically have a typical hourglass appearance on aortograms. They produce stenoses of the perirenal abdominal aorta and may obstruct orifices of renal and visceral arteries, the suprarenal aorta, and visceral arteries. This complex of lesions is referred to as the midaortic syndrome.

The aortic lesions most likely are not present at birth, but develop and progress with a variable time course. The median age of patients with this syndrome ranges from 12 to 17 years,[2-4] but it has been diagnosed in patients 4 to 5 years old. These aortic lesions may develop in an apparently previously normal aorta in as little as 2 months, but more commonly develop over several years. During this time the suprarenal aorta and, ultimately, the origin of the superior mesenteric artery (SMA) and celiac arteries may become constricted. The inferior mesenteric artery (IMA) is usually spared. This allows large collaterals to develop between the SMA, celiac, and the IMA, which perfuse the uninvolved distal aorta and iliac arteries. The relentless progression of aortic stenosis apparently is self-limited and may become quiescent after puberty.

PATHOLOGY

The chief differential diagnoses are Takayasu arteritis and neurofibromatosis. In Takayasu arteritis, the patient is generally older and has clinical signs of arteritis, including an increased erythrocyte sedimentation rate, malaise, fever, night sweats, anorexia, and weight loss. In addition, the frequent involvement of the pulmonary arteries may lead to dyspnea, which is not seen in patients with midaortic syndrome. Finally, the midaortic syndrome exclusively involves the midabdominal aorta, whereas Takayasu arteritis most frequently shows a mixed type of involvement including the branch vessels from the aortic arch and the pulmonary arteries. Histologic examination of involved regions of Takayasu arteritis shows inflammatory change, a finding not seen in patients with the midaortic syndrome. Patients with neurofibromatosis do not have clinical signs of inflammatory disease, and they also have the clinical stigmata of neurofibromatosis in addition to midaortic stenoses.

Typically, portions of the aorta and renal arteries obtained from patients with midaortic syndrome have intimal thickening, intimal fibrosis, and medial hyperplasia, singly or in combination. No evidence of round cell or granulomatous infiltration typical of periaortic inflammatory disease such as Takayasu arteritis is usually seen, and cells typical of giant cell arteritis are not present.[5] The usual pathologic diagnosis is a nonspecific arteriopathy.

DIAGNOSIS

Arteriography is the key to diagnosis. In addition to documenting the renal arterial lesions, it should document the origins of all abdominal visceral branches, as well as the abdominal aorta, aortic bifurcation, and iliac arteries. Biplane examinations with rapid-sequence imaging followed by delayed imaging are necessary for the depiction of early filling and collateral arterial flow.

PATIENT POPULATION

Few pediatric patients with renovascular hypertension have been reported. The total number of cases summarized from the literature is 145 as of 1989 (Table1). The most recent study from the University of Pennsylvania evaluated the results of 17 patients with renovascular hypertension. The ages ranged from 2 to 16 years. Bilateral renal artery lesions affected 71% (12/17) of the patients. Midaortic stenoses were present in 71% (12/17), and 47% (8/17) required surgical repair. Coexisting celiac or SMA disease was present in 59% (10/17). All of these lesions must be carefully documented preoperatively to effectively plan operation, which is usually performed in a one-stage procedure. In addition to operating on the renal artery lesions, the midaortic stenosis must be repaired in order to provide blood flow

Table 1 Pediatric Renovascular Hypertension: Comparative Results of Surgical Treatment

| Medical Center | Patients | Primary Procedures | | Secondary Procedures | Postoperative Status* | | | Operative Mortality (%) |
		Arterial Reconstruction	Nephrectomy		Cured (%)	Improved (%)	Failure (%)	
University of Michigan,† 1963–1980[1]	40	49	2	6	85	12.5	2.5	0
Cleveland Clinic, 1955–1977[7,8]	27	22	11	5	59	18.5	18.5	4
University of California, Los Angeles, 1967–1977[9]	26	19	11	7	84.5	7.5	4	4
Vanderbilt University, ‡ 1962–1977[10]	21	15	8	4	68	24	8	0
University of Pennsylvania, 1974–1987[2]	17	30	0	1§	76.5	23.5	0	0
University of California, San Francisco, 1960–1974[11]	14	10	4	2	86	7	0	7

*Criteria for blood pressure response defined in cited publications. Operative mortality not included in failure category. Data expressed to nearest 0.5%.
†Includes 34 cases from University of Michigan and 6 cases from University of Texas, Southwestern.
‡Results included data from four patients with parenchymal disease treated by nephrectomy.
§Two revascularized kidneys considered to have become infarcted postoperatively were not removed in this series.
From Stanley JC, Brothers TE. Surgical treatment of renovascular hypertension in children. In: Ernst CB, Stanley JC, eds. Current therapy in vascular surgery. 2nd ed. Philadelphia: BC Decker, 1991:880.

to the distal aorta between the IMA and aortic bifurcation, as well as the iliac arteries and pelvic viscera.

PREOPERATIVE EVALUATION

Renal venous plasma renin activity has not been an important preoperative study because the incidence of bilateral renal artery lesions is so high and these studies often fail to predict a beneficial response to surgery. In the Michigan experience, renal vein renin measurements expressed as a renal systemic renin index were felt to be useful prognostic studies.[6] However, renin measurements are not part of the preoperative evaluation in most reports because operation is not performed unless the renal artery obstructions are so severe that preservation of functioning renal parenchymal tissue becomes as important as controlling malignant hypertension.

ALTERNATIVE THERAPY

Percutaneous balloon angioplasty has not been successful in managing either the renal or aortic lesions. Unlike adult fibromuscular dysplasia, which affects the midportion of the renal arteries, the majority of lesions in the pediatric population are stenoses involving the proximal renal artery and represent true hypoplastic vessels characterized predominantly by adventitial elastic tissue. These particular lesions simply stretch with balloon inflation and return to their original contour with balloon deflation without remodeling the stenotic segment. Two patients in the University of Pennsylvania series were failures of balloon angioplasty (Fig. 1).[5] Some stenotic lesions limited to the midportion of the main renal arteries represent true arterial dysplasia and benefit from balloon angioplasty. Nonetheless, surgical therapy remains the primary treatment and is the most durable for restoration of renal blood flow and preservation of renal tissue in children.

SURGICAL REPAIR

Operation is usually performed in one stage, even when bilateral renal artery lesions and a concomitant midaortic stenosis must be repaired. Although waiting until the child is fully grown is desirable, this is often impossible because of the seriousness of the hypertension.

Surgical exposure is obtained through a midline or chevron incision. Medial rotation of the viscera gives excellent exposure of the proximal aorta up to the diaphragmatic hiatus and the visceral vessels. Thoracoabdominal incisions are rarely required. This approach is relatively easy in children, who usually do not have abundant retroperitoneal fat. The major technical considerations are the type of graft material to be used for the aortorenal bypass, the type of repair for the aortic stenosis, and whether the origin of the renal bypass grafts should come from native aorta or aortic graft.

The favored graft for renal artery reconstruction in children is the internal iliac artery.[4] Saphenous vein grafts undergo aneurysmal dilation (Fig. 1G and are generally not felt to be acceptable. However, external support of vein grafts with a Dacron mesh effectively prevented aneurysmal dilation in grafts observed up to 11 years postoperatively (Fig. 2).[2] This is an attractive technique because it allows the use of saphenous vein, which is easier to acquire than the internal iliac artery, especially when bilateral aortorenal bypasses are needed.

The midaortic stenosis is usually bypassed with a 12 to 14 mm Dacron graft inserted with enough redundancy to allow for future growth (Fig. 1F In an initial aortogram, the graft may appear to be too long, with a large redundant loop in it. Following the normal postpubertal growth spurt, however, the graft elongates and becomes straighter (Fig. 1G). There have been no late complications related to inadequate graft length or diameter. The graft is anastomosed in an end-to-side fashion to the proximal supraceliac aorta, and the distal end is placed just above the aortic bifurcation and below the IMA. This segment of aorta rarely becomes stenotic and is an excellent site for the proximal anastomosis of the aortorenal grafts. Alternatively, the grafts can be taken directly from the aortic graft. An alternative repair of the midaortic lesion is to use a primary patch aortoplasty with polytetrafluoroethylene graft or Dacron. This has been preferred for reconstructions in very young children.

Visceral artery stenoses are repaired along with the aortic and renal lesions if preoperative visceral ischemic symptoms are present. It is unclear that all of these lesions should be repaired in the absence of symptoms. However, one benefit of doing so would be to provide a potential for hepatorenal or splenorenal bypass in the future, if the primary renal bypass grafts failed.

The preferred technique for the renal artery anastomosis is an end-to-end anastomosis using interrupted sutures with widely spatulated ends to ensure a wide suture line and to allow for eventual circumferential growth. Interrupted suture technique is also used for part of the aortic anastomosis. In patients followed with postoperative arteriograms obtained more than 5 years after operation, there has been no evidence of stenosis in the aortic graft and only three stenoses observed in the 28 renal bypass grafts.[2]

RESULTS

The cumulative surgical experience with pediatric renovascular hypertensive patients reveals excellent results with respect to control of hypertension and preservation of renal function (Table 1). Although differences exist between institutions regarding primary arterial reconstructions versus primary nephrectomies, improved vascular surgical techniques have increased the likelihood of success for renal revascularization. The

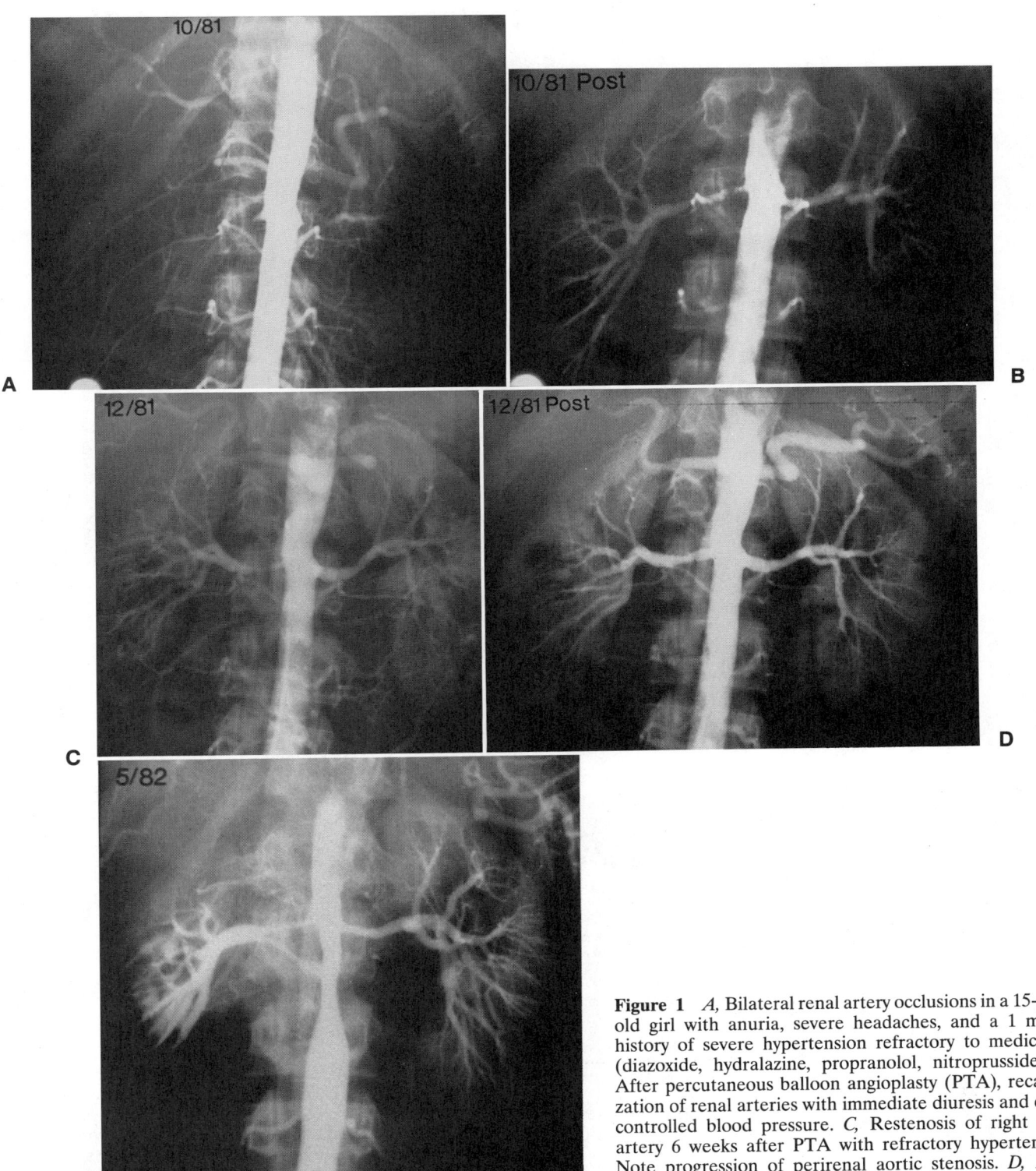

Figure 1 *A*, Bilateral renal artery occlusions in a 15-year-old girl with anuria, severe headaches, and a 1 month history of severe hypertension refractory to medication (diazoxide, hydralazine, propranolol, nitroprusside). *B*, After percutaneous balloon angioplasty (PTA), recanalization of renal arteries with immediate diuresis and easily controlled blood pressure. *C*, Restenosis of right renal artery 6 weeks after PTA with refractory hypertension. Note progression of perirenal aortic stenosis. *D*, After second PTA of right renal artery, hypertension easily controlled with propranolol. *E*, Five months later, both renal arteries are again narrowed (R greater than L), and severe infrarenal aortic stenosis is present with extension to origin of the superior mesenteric artery (SMA).

Continued.

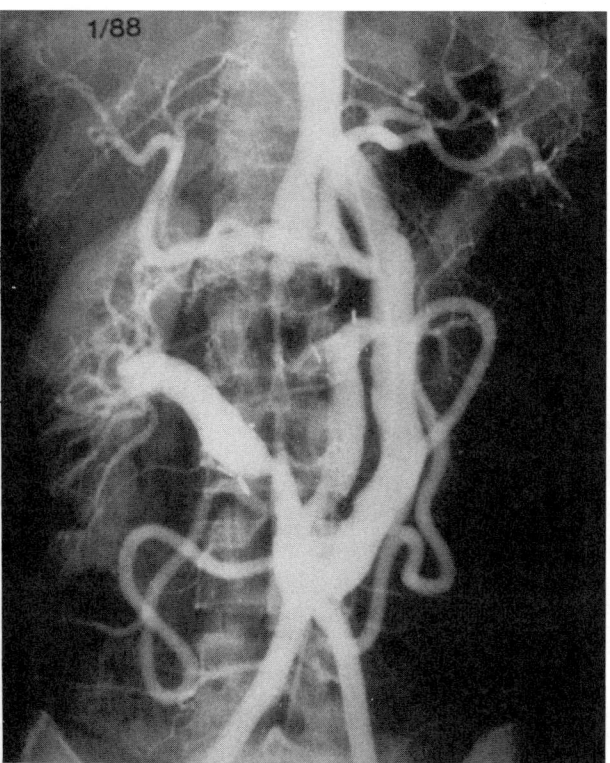
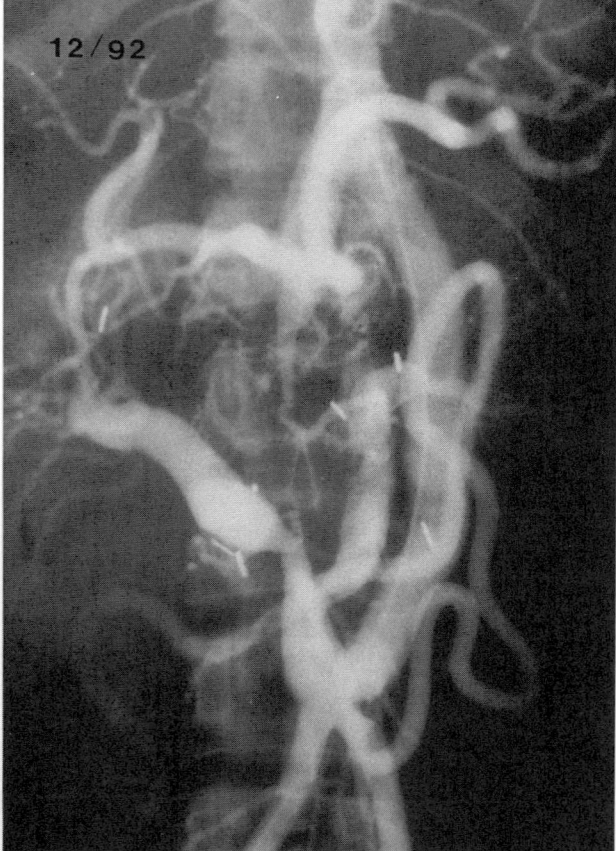

Figure 1, cont'd. *F,* Postoperative arteriogram 1 month after insertion of aortic graft and bilateral aortorenal bypasses. The catheter has been passed through the residual lumen of the narrowed native aorta. Note redundancy of aortic graft to allow for longitudinal growth. *G,* Follow-up after 5½ years. Patient normotensive with normal renal function. Both aortorenal vein grafts dilated (not supported with Dacron mesh). Note loss of previous aortic graft redundancy because of patient's growth and large meandering mesenteric artery collateral with flow from inferior to superior mesenteric artery due to proximal SMA stenosis. *H,* Follow-up after 10½ years. Patient normotensive with normal renal function. Vein graft dilation has not changed since previous study.

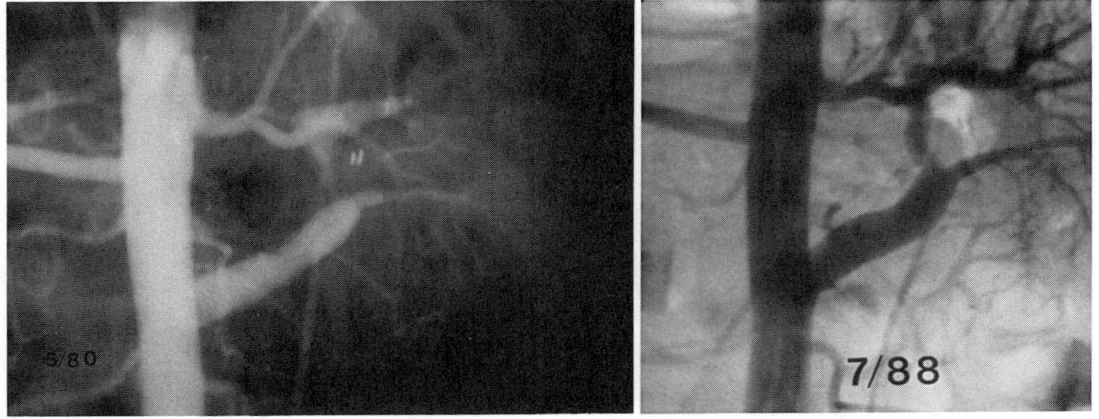

Figure 2 *A,* Postoperative aortogram of left aortorenal bypass for branch renal artery stenosis in 12-year-old boy. Saphenous vein graft was reinforced with Dacron mesh. *B,* Eight-year follow-up. No significant increase in vein graft diameter with Dacron mesh reinforced graft.

long-term results indicate that the repairs are durable and continue to function even after significant growth. Operative mortality for these extensive procedures was 0% in three reports and ranged from 4% to 7% in the remaining three. These excellent results support an aggressive surgical approach for pediatric renovascular hypertension.

REFERENCES

1. Stanley JC, Fry WJ. Pediatric renal artery occlusive disease and renovascular hypertension: Etiology, diagnosis and operative treatment. Arch Surg 1981; 116:669–676.
2. Berkowitz HD, O'Neill JA. Renovascular hypertension in children: Surgical repair with special reference to the use of reinforced vein grafts. J Vasc Surg 1989; 9:46–55.
3. Stanley JC, Graham LM, Whitehouse WM, et al. Developmental occlusive disease of the abdominal aorta, splanchnic and renal arteries. Am J Surg 1981; 142:190–196.
4. Messina LM, Goldstone J, Ferrell LD, et al. Middle aortic syndrome: Effectiveness and durability of complex arterial revascularization techniques. Ann Surg 1986; 204:331–339.
5. Lewis VD, Meranze SG, McLean GK. The midaortic syndrome: Diagnosis and treatment. Radiology 1988; 167:111–113.
6. Stanley JC, Gwertz BC, Fry WJ. Renal:systemic renin indices and renal vein renin ratios as prognostic indicators in remedial renovascular hypertension. J Surg Res 1976; 20:149–155.
7. Novick AC, Straffon RA, Stewart BH, et al. Surgical treatment of renovascular hypertension in the pediatric patient. J Urol 1978; 119:794–805.
8. Benjamin SP, Dustan HP, Gifford RW Jr, et al. Stenosing renal artery disease in children: Clinicopathological correlation in 20 surgically treated cases. Cleve Clin Q 1976; 43:197–206.
9. Stanley P, Gyepes MT, Olson DL, et al. Renovascular hypertension in children and adolescents. Radiology 1978; 129:123–131.
10. Lawson JD, Boerth R, Foster JH, et al. Diagnosis and management of renovascular hypertension in children. Arch Surg 1977; 122:1307–1316.
11. Stoney RJ, Cooke PA, String ST. Surgical treatment of renovascular hypertension in children. J Pediatr Surg 1975; 10:631–639.

RENAL ARTERY ANEURYSM

JAMES C. STANLEY, M.D.

Renal artery aneurysms occur in approximately 0.1% of the general population (Fig. 1).[1] Earlier reports suggested a higher incidence, but such is unlikely. The problem with many selective retrospective studies is evidenced by the greater frequency of complications and symptomatic aneurysms in surgical series, the nearly sevenfold increase of these aneurysms among hypertensive patients, and more than a ninetyfold increase in patients exhibiting renal artery fibrodysplasia.[1] Dysplastic renal artery disease undoubtedly accounts for the slightly greater occurrence of renal artery aneurysms in women. This gender difference may also account for the more frequent involvement of the right renal artery, which is known to exhibit medial fibrodysplasia more often than the left renal artery (Fig. 2).[2]

Few reports of renal artery aneurysms encompass more than 25 patients. Nevertheless, certain generalities regarding these aneurysms are widely accepted. Most aneurysms are saccular, and 90% occur in the extrarenal vessels. The remaining 10% affect intrarenal arteries. More than 75% of all renal artery aneurysms occur at branchings of the renal artery. Their mean diameter is 1.3 cm.

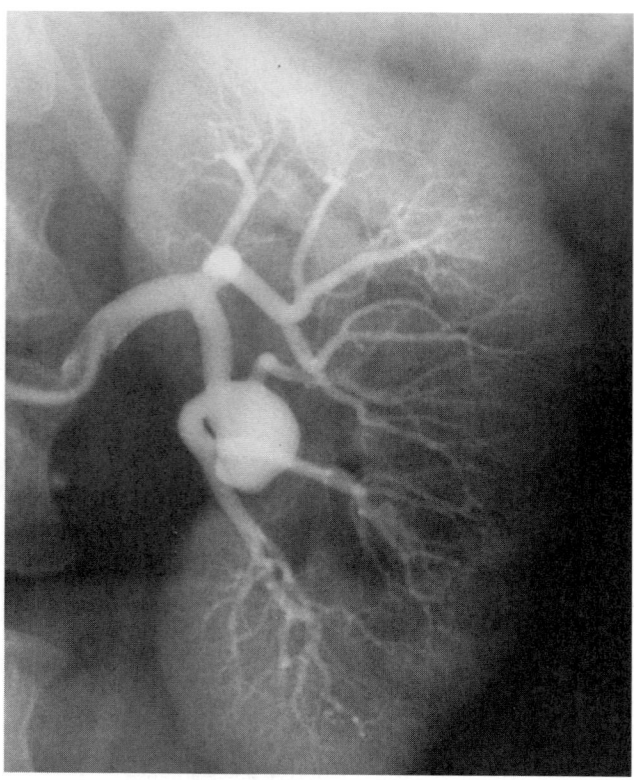

Figure 1 Renal artery aneurysm at a second-order branch. (From Stanley JC, Whitehouse WM Jr. Renal artery macroaneurysms. In Bergan JJ, Yao JST, eds. Aneurysms. New York: Grune & Stratton, 1982:417; with permission.)

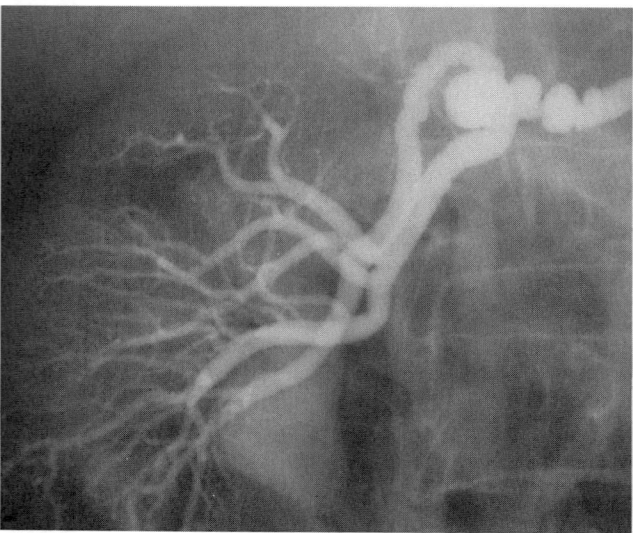

Figure 2 Saccular renal artery aneurysm occurring at the primary bifurcation of renal artery exhibiting medial fibroplasia. (From Stanley JC, Whitehouse WM Jr. Renal artery macroaneurysms. In Bergan JJ, Yao JST, eds. Aneurysms. New York: Grune & Stratton, 1982:417; with permission.)

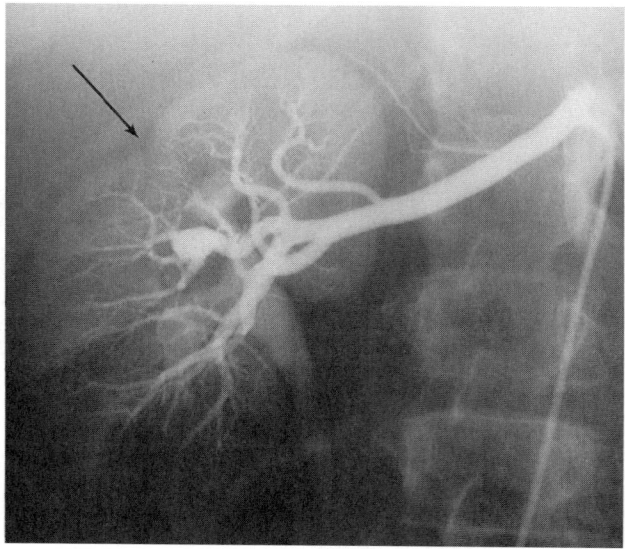

Figure 3 Small, nonatherosclerotic intraparenchymal aneurysm associated with segmental thromboembolic renal ischemia and cortical infarct (*arrow*). (From Stanley JC, Whitehouse WM Jr. Renal artery macroaneurysms. In Bergan JJ, Yao JST, eds. Aneurysms. New York: Grune & Stratton, 1982:417; with permission.)

PATHOGENESIS

The etiology of renal artery aneurysms appears related to both medial degeneration and an accompanying deficiency of the internal elastic lamina.[1] These changes are more pronounced in the presence of arterial fibrodysplasia. Hypertension affects nearly 80% of patients having renal artery aneurysms and is considered an additional risk factor for the development of mural changes leading to these aneurysms. Most large renal artery aneurysms are composed of acellular fibrous tissue. Areas of complicated atherosclerotic plaque with deposition of cholesterol crystals, mural necrosis, and calcification may be seen in certain aneurysms. The atherosclerotic process in most of these aneurysms is considered a secondary event rather than a primary etiologic process. This tenet is supported by the presence of calcific atherosclerosis in some but not all aneurysms of many patients with multiple aneurysms.[1]

CLINICAL MANIFESTATIONS

Very few renal artery aneurysms are symptomatic. In fact, serious complications of these lesions are relatively uncommon.[2,3] Nevertheless, not all of these aneurysms are innocuous. Approximately 2% are associated with occluded intraparenchymal arteries, thought to be due to embolization of aneurysmal thrombus (Fig. 3).[1] Severe secondary hypertension, rather than a small segmental renal infarction, may be the consequence of this complication.

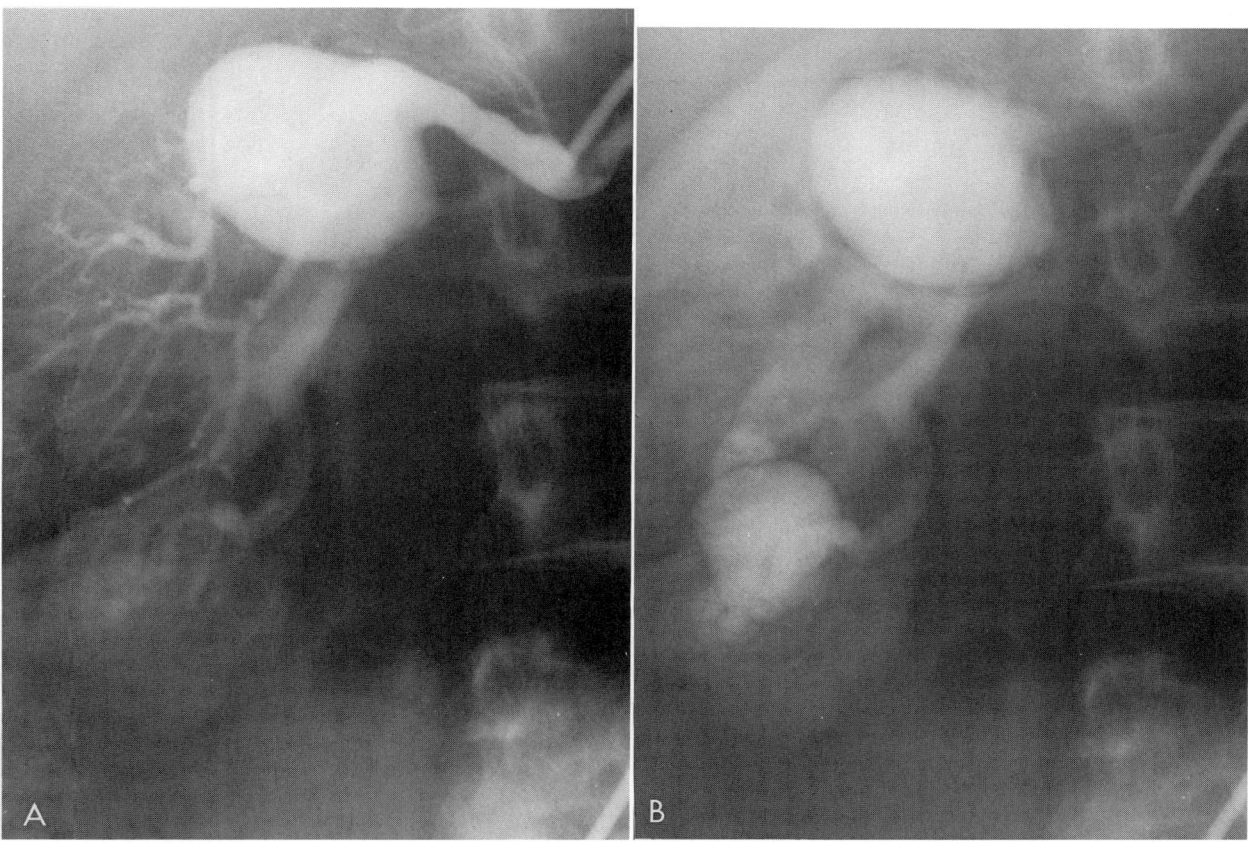

Figure 4 Large arteriovenous fistula associated with (A) covert inferior pole renal artery aneurysm rupture and with (B) ectatic interlobar artery and dilated vein. Superior pole aneurysm is intact. (From Stanley JC, Whitehouse WM Jr. Renal artery macroaneurysms. In Bergan JJ, Yao JST, eds. Aneurysms. New York: Grune & Stratton, 1982:417; with permission.)

Aneurysmal compression or torsion of adjacent renal arteries may reduce renal blood flow and result in secondary renovascular hypertension. However, this is very uncommon. In fact, the cause of blood pressure elevations in most patients with renal artery aneurysms is due to coexisting intrinsic renal artery occlusive disease, such as medial fibrodysplasia, rather than the aneurysm's effect on neighboring vessels.[1]

Rupture of a renal artery aneurysm represents the most serious complication attending these lesions, occurring in 3% of reported cases.[1] The actual frequency of rupture is undoubtedly less because select populations are represented by most reported series. Rupture may be covert into an adjacent vein (Fig. 4) or overt with initial bleeding into the perirenal extraperitoneal tissues. These two types of rupture occur with near equal frequencies.[1]

Renal artery rupture usually causes severe abdominal or flank pain. Bleeding may be contained initially within the retroperitoneum for a brief period before life-threatening free rupture occurs into the peritoneal cavity. Approximately 10% of reported patients with ruptured renal artery aneurysms have succumbed from this complication. In survivors, loss of the kidney occurs in all but the rarest case.[4] The belief is unfounded that renal artery aneurysm rupture is less likely in aneurysms that are smaller than 1.5 cm in diameter, are calcified, or are present in normotensive patients.

Renal artery aneurysms in pregnant women represent a unique problem.[5] Rupture of these lesions was responsible for the reported death of the mother and fetus in 55% and 85% of cases, respectively.[5] No obvious relation of repeated pregnancies to the evolution of renal artery aneurysms has been noted. However, many of these renal artery lesions undoubtedly evolve in young women who complete pregnancies without complications. Thus, most published rupture and mortality figures during pregnancy may be overstated. Nevertheless, renal artery aneurysms must be considered a serious health hazard in pregnant women or those likely to conceive.

SURGICAL THERAPY

Operative intervention for renal artery aneurysms is justified for (1) all symptomatic aneurysms, (2) aneurysms with coexistent renovascular hypertension due to stenotic disease of the renal artery, (3) patients manifesting embolization of thrombus from the aneurysm itself, (4) women of childbearing age, and (5) bland

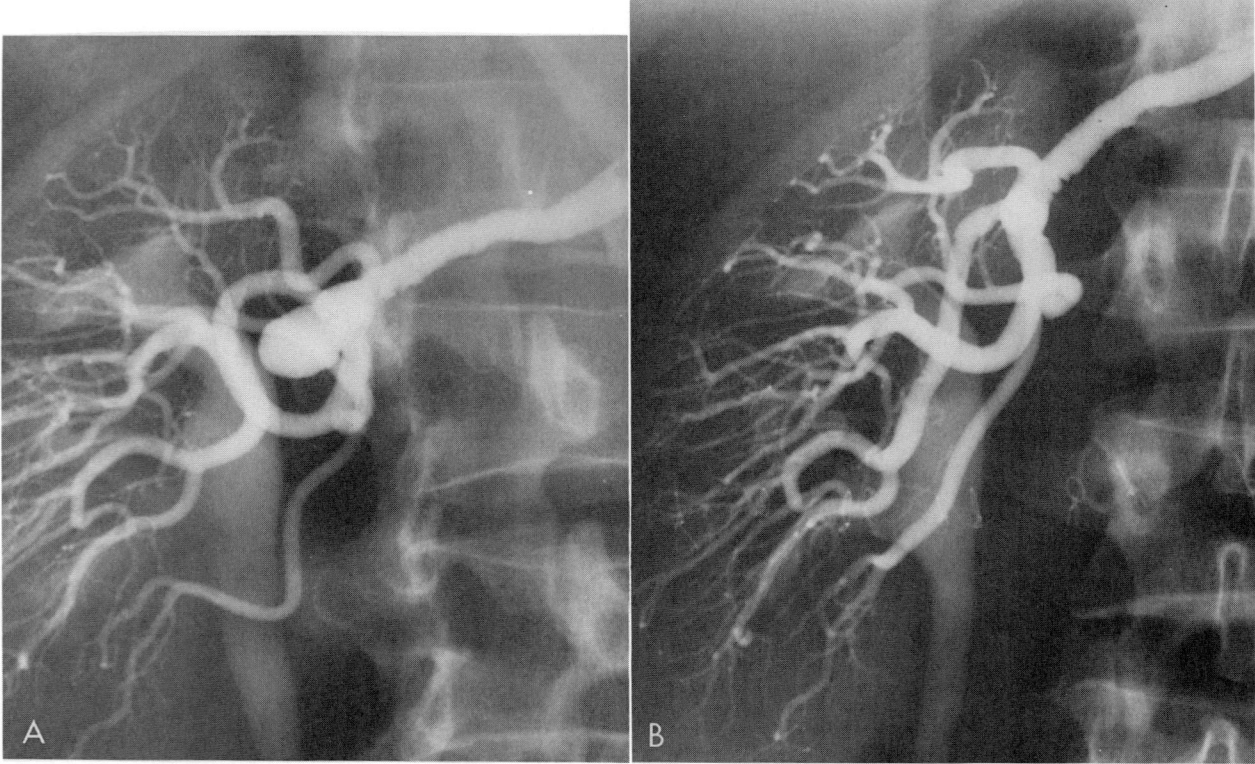

Figure 5 *A,* Renal artery aneurysm located at bifurcation of main renal artery. *B,* Surgical treatment included aneurysmectomy and vein patch graft closure of arterial defect. (From Stanley JC. Renal artery aneurysms and dissections. In: Veith FJ, ed. Current critical problems in vascular surgery, Vol 3. St Louis: Quality Medical, 1991:311; with permission.)

aneurysms whose diameter is greater than 2 cm. The justification for surgical therapy of bland aneurysms is relative and must be pursued only by those experienced in renal vascular reconstructive operations. The attendant risk of nephrectomy is considerable with operative treatment of these lesions by less experienced surgeons.

Bland aneurysms less than 2 cm in diameter may be followed with serial ultrasonography, computed tomography, or magnetic resonance imaging to assess the aneurysm's stability when surgical therapy is not pursued. In certain patients, such as those who become hypertensive, conventional arteriographic assessments may be necessary for the clinician to render an opinion as to the appropriateness of operative versus nonoperative therapy.

Surgical management of renal artery aneurysms is frequently complex.[1,4,6-8] Exposure is critical to successful operation. Supraumbilical transverse abdominal incisions are favored for these procedures, with medial visceral rotations of the colon and foregut structures to the opposite side. This provides generous extraperitoneal exposure of the renal artery and great vessels and facilitates performance of arterial reconstructive procedures in situ. Most moderate-sized aneurysms displace adjacent veins; because of this, the operative dissection of vessels in the region of the aneurysm is usually easier than dissections for comparable occlusive disease. Certain aneurysms are better approached posteriorly by elevating the kidney from its bed and reflecting it medially. Because the renal artery resides behind the renal vein, the posterior approach may obviate the sometimes tedious anterior dissection of certain aneurysms located deep within renal hilum.

The most commonly performed operation for a renal artery aneurysm is an aneurysmectomy and primary arterioplasty. This is performed with or without a vein patch closure, depending upon the size of involved vessels and the extent of adjacent vessel involvement (Fig. 5).[1,9] Use of magnification and fine monofilament cardiovascular suture, such as 6-0 polypropylene, with exacting technique allows most of these procedures to be completed in situ without difficulty.

The second most common means of treating renal artery aneurysms involves simple aneurysmectomy combined with an aortorenal bypass.[1,8,9] This is usually undertaken in patients with associated fibrodysplasia of the proximal renal artery. In some centers ex vivo repairs are commonly used in treating such aneurysms.[10]

The most recently introduced means of managing renal artery aneurysms is aneurysmectomy with reimplantation of the involved vessel into a normal adjacent or proximal renal artery (Fig. 6).[9] This is usually accomplished in situ, although some surgeons prefer ex vivo reconstructions in these circumstances. Lastly, very

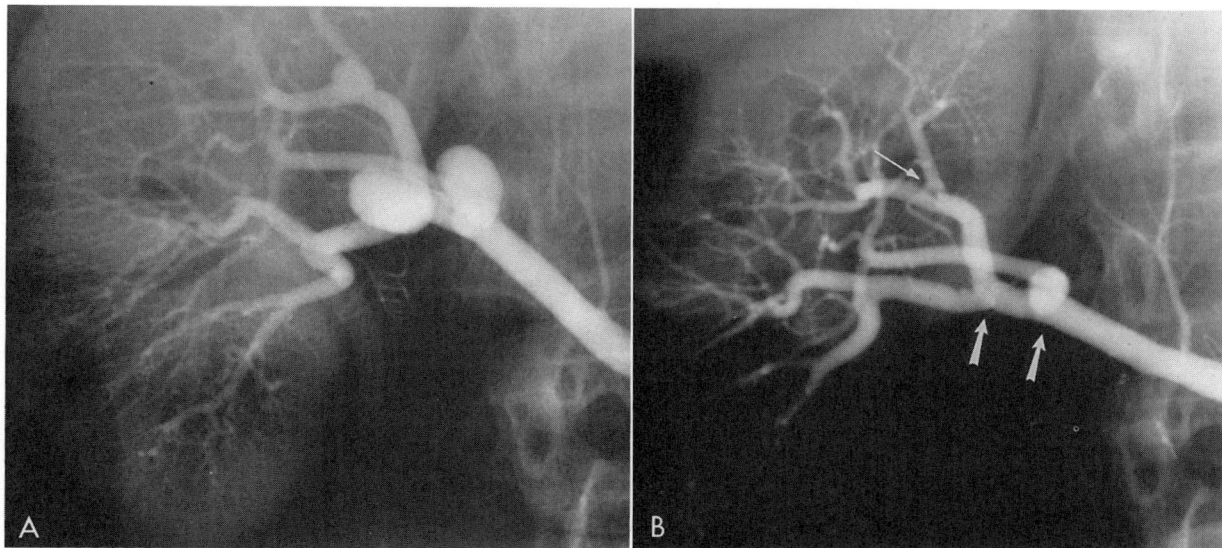

Figure 6 *A*, Renal artery aneurysm involving multiple segmental artery branchings. *B*, Surgical treatment included aneurysmectomy and end-to-side reimplantation (*large arrows*) of segmental vessels into adjacent artery, and closed aneurysmorrhaphy (*small arrow*). (From Stanley JC. Renal artery aneurysms and dissections. In: Veith FJ, ed. Current critical problems in vascular surgery, Vol 3. St Louis: Quality Medical, 1991:311; with permission.)

small aneurysms in the range of 2 to 3 mm may be treated by closed aneurysmorrhaphy, using a fine, continuous cardiovascular suture, such as 7-0 polypropylene, to plicate them.

Aneurysmectomy can be successfully performed in more than 95% of patients exhibiting extraparenchymal renal artery aneurysms. Treatment of certain intraparenchymal aneurysms may entail partial nephrectomy or transcatheter embolization with segmental infarction of the kidney.

REFERENCES

1. Stanley JC, Rhodes EL, Gewertz BL, et al. Renal artery aneurysms: Significance of macroaneurysms exclusive of dissections and fibrodysplastic mural dilations. Arch Surg 1975; 110:1327–1333.
2. Tham G, Ekelund L, Herrlin K, et al. Renal artery aneurysms: Natural history and prognosis. Ann Surg 1983; 197:348–352.
3. Henriksson C, Bjorkerud S, Nilson AE, Pettersson S. Natural history of renal artery aneurysm elucidated by repeated angiography and pathoanatomical studies. Eur Urol 1985; 11:244–248.
4. Mercier C, Piquet P, Piligian F, Ferdani M. Aneurysms of the renal artery and its branches. Ann Vasc Surg 1986; 1:321–327.
5. Cohen JR, Shamash FS. Ruptured renal artery aneurysms during pregnancy. J Vasc Surg 1987; 6:51–59.
6. Hubert JP Jr, Pairolero PC, Kazmier FJ. Solitary renal artery aneurysm. Surgery 1980; 88:557–565.
7. Martin RS III, Meacham PW, Ditesheim JA, et al. Renal artery aneurysm: Selective treatment for hypertension and prevention of rupture. J Vasc Surg 1989; 9:26–34.
8. Ortenberg J, Novick AC, Straffon RA, Stewart BH. Surgical treatment of renal artery aneurysms. Br J Urol 1983; 55:341–346.
9. Stanley JC, Messina LM, Wakefield TW, Zelenock GB. Renal artery reconstruction. In: Bergan JJ, Yao JST, eds. Techniques in arterial surgery. Philadelphia: WB Saunders, 1990:247.
10. Dubernard JM, Martin X, Gelet A, Mongin D. Aneurysms of the renal artery: Surgical management with special reference to extracorporeal surgery and autotransplantation. Eur Urol 1985; 11:26–30.

RENAL ARTERY DISSECTION

LINDA M. REILLY, M.D.

Renal artery dissection is most commonly associated with dissection of the aorta. Less than one-fourth of all dissections involving the renal vessels are isolated lesions.[1] Nonetheless, the renal artery is the most frequent site of isolated dissection of an aortic branch vessel. The causes of isolated renal artery dissection fall into two distinct categories, those that are primary and associated with underlying renal artery diseases such as fibromuscular dysplasia or atherosclerosis, and those that are secondary and a consequence of blunt trauma or percutaneous interventional procedures, such as selective renal arteriography or percutaneous renal artery angioplasty. The clinical sequelae of isolated renal artery dissection depend upon the degree of reduction of renal blood flow resulting from the compromised true lumen. They range from silent events, to hypertension due to renal ischemia, to frank renal infarction. The approach to treatment depends upon the clinical setting and the extent of the anatomic defect in the renal artery.

TRANSLUMINAL CATHETER-INDUCED DISSECTION

Subintimal renal artery dissection is a potential complication of catheter instrumentation of the renal artery. Selective renal catheterization carries a greater risk of this complication than does flush aortography. It is likely that many small, limited, catheter-induced dissections are clinically silent, and it is, therefore, difficult to establish the true incidence of this complication. Nevertheless, this type of dissection is certainly rare, as is supported by the report of Gewertz and colleagues, who recorded only 4 instances among 11,000 abdominal arteriographic studies, including approximately 2,200 selective renal artery studies.[2] The incidence of dissection following transluminal renal artery angioplasty is clearly greater; it occurred in 5 of 104 renal angioplasties in the series reported by Sos and associates.[3]

The occurrence of catheter-induced dissection is related to the presence of underlying disease in the renal artery. Dissection is more likely to occur in arteries with advanced atherosclerosis but relatively unlikely to occur in arteries involved by fibromuscular dysplasia (FMD). In reviewing 22 reported cases of catheter-induced renal artery dissections, Smith and co-workers noted associated atherosclerosis in 44% and FMD in only 18%.[4] These dissections are almost uniformly unilateral, involve renal artery branches in about one-quarter of patients, and have an equal gender distribution. Almost a third of the recognized catheter-related renal artery dissections were asymptomatic. Pain and hypertension occurred in about half of the patients, which is a much lower rate than that seen in primary dissections. Hematuria occurred in about 20% of patients.

In half the reported cases, the patients underwent renal artery reconstruction, usually involving renal artery bypass. About 15% of patients required nephrectomy, and the remainder were observed. An additional treatment option, which was not available at the time of published review articles, is deployment of a stent to correct the dissection and obliterate the false channel. This modality can be expected to ultimately reduce the number of patients requiring emergent renal artery reconstruction for serious clinical sequelae of catheter-induced renal artery dissection.

BLUNT TRAUMA–RELATED DISSECTION

Blunt injury to the renal pedicle commonly produces thrombosis of the renal artery. The underlying cause of the occlusion was not defined until careful histologic analysis of the removed kidneys was undertaken. It was then recognized that many of these thrombotic occlusions occur in the setting of intimal disruption and dissection. The exact mechanism for the dissection is unknown but has been attributed to either a deceleration injury or direct compression against the vertebral column.[5] Blunt trauma–induced dissection does not always produce occlusion, as was evident in the report by Gewertz and associates of seven nonocclusive post-trauma dissections.[2] It is likely that the exact incidence of this type of renal artery dissection will also be difficult to establish because dissection is not the only cause of an occluded renal artery following trauma.

Hematuria and flank pain are commonly present in patients with this injury. Although some authors feel that the hematuria is related to renal parenchymal injury, Stables and colleagues found accompanying renal parenchymal laceration to be rare.[6] In contrast, injuries to other organs are common. Often the patient is hypotensive because of the other associated injuries. However, if there are no other major injuries, hypertension is often present.

When the injury has led to occlusion of the renal artery, the prognosis is not good. There are several reasons for this. First, there is often a delay in diagnosis. Second, other major injuries may take treatment precedence, resulting in further delay before the renal artery thrombosis can be addressed or precluding any complex and lengthy renal artery repair. Third, the extent of the injury to the renal pedicle may make the repair difficult and less likely to be successful. In Stables and associates' study, only 2 of 26 trauma-related renal artery injuries were successfully reconstructed. Ultimately, complete loss of renal function occurred in 23 of the 26 kidneys with post-trauma renal artery occlusion, and 11 nephrectomies were required. The prognosis is better if the injury does not produce occlusion. Among Gewertz and co-workers' seven patients, only two nephrectomies and one partial nephrectomy were required. One patient underwent arterial reconstruction, and the other patients were followed. No patient lost renal function permanently (one needed transient dialysis), and all patients were normotensive (one required medication).

The technique of reconstruction is dictated by the extent of the arterial injury. Although some have recommended resection and primary reanastomosis, the injury is unlikely to be limited enough to allow such an approach. More commonly, the reconstruction requires bypass grafting, autotransplantation, or ex vivo repair. This last technique is especially suited to extensive injuries involving the renal artery branches, but can be performed only in an otherwise stable patient. The injury needs to be repaired very expeditiously, particularly if there is associated occlusion, if there is to be any expectation of success.

SPONTANEOUS DISSECTION

Spontaneous dissection of the renal artery is a rare phenomenon, representing less than one-fourth of all renal artery dissections.[1] It occurs in the absence of trauma and commonly in the presence of mural disease, such as FMD, atherosclerosis, or aneurysmal degeneration. The natural history of spontaneous renal artery dissection is unknown. However, the most consistent clinical sequence has been the abrupt onset of severe, poorly controlled, persistent hypertension in previously normotensive young men. Among the approximately 90 reported cases of spontaneous renal artery dissection (not including autopsy reports), in only 8 documented instances did reversion to normal blood pressure occur after varying intervals (2 to 45 months).[7] This clinical improvement was accompanied by the conversion of abnormal renin studies to normal in some patients and by an improved arteriographic appearance in others. Re-entry of the dissection is postulated as the mechanism for this resolution of hypertension. Additionally, in that silent dissections are occasionally discovered incidentally on arteriography, it has been suggested that resolution of dissection may be more frequent than implied by these examples. However, only one instance of a completely silent, isolated renal artery dissection has been reported so far. Therefore, it seems that the overall incidence of spontaneous cure of the hypertension associated with primary renal artery dissection may be about 10% at most. Importantly, there has been no report of spontaneous normalization of the renal artery anatomy following dissection. Although dramatic improvement has been documented in one patient by interval angiography, in general the anatomic defect remains.

In contrast to a clinical course characterized by improvement, worsening of blood pressure during diagnostic evaluation or initial attempts at medical therapy has been reported almost as frequently.[8] Additionally, at least nine patients, including one of our patients, had clinical histories notable for repeated episodes of the symptoms associated with the renal artery dissection, sometimes extending over many months. In one patient, distal progression of the dissection and increased aneurysmal dilation of the false channel were documented over a 3 month period after the patient initially declined operative intervention. The combined incidence of clinical deterioration and multiple symptomatic episodes suggesting extension of the dissection is at least equal to if not slightly greater than the incidence of spontaneous return to normal blood pressure. In summary, most of the patients with spontaneous renal artery dissection face a future of long-term, multidrug therapy to control their hypertension, a situation that is unlikely to improve and may actually worsen. In view of the young patient age at the onset of this disease, another approach would seem warranted.[7]

The most frequent operative approach to renal artery dissection has been nephrectomy or partial nephrectomy, which has been required in 38 of the 85 reported cases (44.7%). Although removing the ischemic renal tissue is very effective in curing hypertension, the significant incidence of bilateral FMD (30% to 50%), as well as of dissection (20% to 25%), makes this approach less attractive.[7] Many of these patients were explored with the intention of revascularization and renal salvage. The most common finding necessitating a change to nephrectomy was irreversible renal ischemia or extension of the dissection into renal artery branches, rendering reconstruction impossible.

Arterial reconstruction has been attempted in 28 patients (32 arteries) with spontaneous renal artery dissection, including the seven patients in our own series. Overall, 29 of 32 repairs (90.6%) were anatomically successful; that is, a new conduit was successfully constructed. However, clinical success has been less consistent (Table 1). Among the completed reconstructions reported, only eight patients (38.1%) were subsequently normotensive, one of whom required antihypertensive medication and one of whom was, in fact, normotensive preoperatively.[7,8] Three additional patients (14.3%) had improved blood pressure control. In contrast, all of the patients undergoing successful reconstruction in our series returned to their predissection blood pressure levels, without requiring additional medication. Undoubtedly, the key determinants of such a successful outcome are identification of correctable anatomic lesions, selection of the optimal operative technique, and intraoperative assessment of the status of the reconstruction.

It is evident from reviewing the reported cases of spontaneous renal artery dissection that at the time of initial presentation a substantial proportion of these patients are not candidates for renal salvage. Successful treatment of this disease requires restoration of normal arterial anatomy and normal renal perfusion. Identification of a reconstruction candidate, therefore, requires precise and accurate assessment of the extent of the dissection and the extent of parenchymal infarction. High-quality selective renal arteriography is the cornerstone of this assessment. Dissections extending into intraparenchymal arterial branches or producing multiple branch occlusions cannot be repaired. Isotope

Table 1 Spontaneous Renal Artery Dissection Outcome of Operative Repair

Outcome	UCSF* N (%)	Literature N (%)	Overall N (%)
Success—clinical	5 (71.5)	11 (52.4)	16 (57.1)
Failure—overall	2 (28.6)	7 (33.3)	9 (32.1)
Clinical		6 (28.6)	6 (21.4)
Anatomic	2 (28.6)	1 (4.8)	3 (10.7)
No follow-up		3 (14.3)	3 (10.7)

*University of California, San Francisco.

renography is also helpful in determining the extent and distribution of renal infarction.

Once a patient has been determined to have reconstructible anatomy, the appropriate operative technique must be selected. This, too, depends mainly upon the extent of the dissection. For the most part, main renal artery involvement—out to and including the first branch point—can usually be repaired in situ. If primary or secondary branches are involved, as long as the dissection remains extraparenchymal the ex vivo technique allows uncompromised exposure to get beyond the disease, as well as adequate time to perform a meticulous repair without unduly compromising renal function. One might also select the ex vivo technique for main renal artery repair if the exposure is particularly poor, if it is a redo operation, or if there is a solitary kidney. Among the reported repairs, the ex vivo technique has been utilized seven times in five patients, with a successful outcome in six reconstructions (four patients).[8] The only failure resulted from the inability to reverse parenchymal damage from long-standing ischemia, not from an inability to reconstruct the conduit.

In view of the young age of these patients and the frequent necessity for branch repair, we feel that autologous artery is the optimal conduit. The experience using other conduits would support this approach because 4 of 10 saphenous vein and Dacron conduits reported in the literature have failed clinically. Two additional venous conduits showed aneurysmal dilation only 4 years after implantation and have not been further studied. In contrast, among the 11 cases of renal artery dissection treated with some form of autologous arterial reconstruction (hypogastric artery graft in 5, excision and primary reanastomosis in 3, splenorenal bypass in 1, autotransplantation in 1, autotransplantation plus ex vivo repair in 1), 8 have been successful and only 1 has failed. Including the primary branches in harvesting the hypogastric artery facilitates size-matched branch repair, and using autogenous tissue seems to correlate with a durable reconstruction with minimal risk of late stenosis or occlusion.

Once the repair has been completed, it is mandatory to determine if it has been successful. It is essential to recognize that a successful repair must reverse renal ischemia as well as establish a normal conduit. Intraoperative duplex scanning of the reconstruction has become an important tool in assessing the functional status of the repair. If the intraoperative assessment documents poor blood flow through the new conduit, there is evidence of high resistance to blood flow through the kidney, or the appearance of the kidney has persistent areas of ischemia or infarction, then partial or complete nephrectomy should be undertaken. It is almost certain that the high clinical failure rate of the attempted reconstructions reported in the literature reflects failure to recognize persistent ischemic renal parenchyma.

Using the approach summarized here has allowed us to identify when repair is not possible or not successful. Consequently, we have been able to perform successful revascularization frequently (5 of 7, 71.4%), with restoration of predissection blood pressure (5 of 5, 100%), consistent preservation of renal function as indicated by the serum creatinine (5 of 5, 100%), yielding sustained and durable clinical benefit (14.5 year follow-up) (see Table 1).

Successful reconstruction is clearly facilitated by early treatment, before the dissection has extended into multiple branches and before significant infarction has occurred. Because extension of dissection is a continued threat that may have irreversible consequences, and because spontaneous reversion to normotension is uncommon, patients should not be uniformly treated medically. If the patient is a good candidate for operation, arterial reconstruction should be considered at the outset. Ultimately, a successful, durable repair may be more cost-effective and provide a better quality of life than three or four decades of multiagent antihypertensive therapy and continued risk of kidney loss.

REFERENCES

1. Foord AG, Lewis RD. Primary dissecting aneurysms of peripheral and pulmonary arteries: Dissecting hemorrhage of media. Arch Pathol 1959; 68:553–557.
2. Gewertz BL, Stanley JC, Fry WJ. Renal artery dissections. Arch Surg 1977; 112:409–414.
3. Sos TA, Pickering TG, Sniderman K, et al. Percutaneous transluminal renal angioplasty in renovascular hypertension due to atheroma or fibromuscular dysplasia. N Engl J Med 1983; 309:274–279.
4. Smith BM, Holcomb GW, Richie RE, Dean RH. Renal artery dissection. Ann Surg 1984; 200:134–146.
5. Slavis SA, Hodge EE, Novick AC, Maatman T. Surgical treatment for isolated dissection of the renal artery. J Urol 1990; 144:233–237.
6. Stables DP, Fouche RF, Van Niekerk JPde V, et al. Traumatic renal artery occlusion: 21 cases. J Urol 1976; 115:229–233.
7. Edwards BS, Stanson AW, Holley KE, Sheps SG. Isolated renal artery dissection: Presentation, evaluation, management, and pathology. Mayo Clin Proc 1982; 57:564–571.
8. Reilly LM, Cunningham CG, Maggisano R, et al. The role of arterial reconstruction in spontaneous renal artery dissection. J Vasc Surg 1991; 14:468–479.

RENAL ARTERY EMBOLISM

KENNETH OURIEL, M.D.

Embolism to the renal artery is associated with a characteristic spectrum of signs and symptoms, yet diagnosis is frequently delayed because of the relative rarity of the disorder and the failure to consider it. The primary sequelae of renal arterial emboli are renal insufficiency and hyperreninemic hypertension. Irreversible ischemia develops rapidly in the absence of a developed collateral circulation; thus, a renal artery embolus is frequently associated with infarction of the kidney by the time the diagnosis has been made.[1] Nevertheless, prompt diagnosis allows the institution of therapy directed at the preservation of functional renal parenchyma in those kidneys with sufficient residual blood flow to maintain viability, even in an anuric state.[2] In addition, the institution of adequate anticoagulation prevents subsequent embolic events to other organs.[3]

PATHOPHYSIOLOGY

Renal artery emboli are almost always of cardiac origin, associated with atrial arrhythmias, valvular disease, or acute myocardial infarction (Table 1). Less common sources include artificial heart valves and suprarenal aortic aneurysms. Emboli to a solitary kidney or simultaneously to both kidneys comprise a surprisingly high proportion of the cases reported, probably as a result of the difficulty in diagnosing a unilateral embolus in the presence of a normal contralateral kidney.

Morris and colleagues emphasized the importance of subfiltration arterial pressure on the development of irreversible renal ischemic injury.[4] Deterioration of renal function did not develop in canine kidneys subjected to suprarenal aortic occlusion and mean perfusion pressures of 24 mm Hg for up to 2 hours. By contrast, kidneys with negligible renal perfusion pressures suffered irretrievable damage within 60 minutes of onset. These laboratory studies suggest that renal salvage is unlikely in patients with complete renal artery obstruction and the absence of pre-existent collateral arterial channels. Indeed, most reports of renal arterial occlusions document poor rates of salvage in embolic disease and satisfactory rates of salvage in thrombotic disease.[5] Moreover, the timing of renal revascularization is poorly correlated with successful restoration of function. These observations are likely explained by the adequacy of collateral circulation in renal artery thrombosis and the absence of significant collaterals in most embolized kidneys. Not all renal arterial emboli, however, are totally obstructing, and occasional patients may have flow around the embolus or adequate pre-existing collateral circulation to maintain perfusion at a level insufficient to provide renal excretory function, yet adequate to preserve viability. Thus, an accurate and timely diagnosis of embolic renal artery occlusion remains the only means of effecting renal salvage and reducing the risk of subsequent embolic episodes.

DIAGNOSIS

Patients with renal emboli most often present with flank, back, or abdominal pain (Table 2). Nausea and vomiting may occur, and patients may note gross hematuria. A low-grade fever is common, as is new-onset hypertension. On examination, patients typically manifest flank tenderness to deep palpation. Laboratory findings consist of leukocytosis, and elevation in the lactate dehydrogenase level is common. The presence of erythrocytes, leukocytes, and protein is almost uniform on urinalysis.

When performed, an intravenous pyelogram documents absent function in complete renal artery obstruction and poor function when the obstruction is partial. Renal nuclear medicine studies mirror these findings, but renal arteriography is necessary and diagnostic in all patients (Figs. 1 and 2). The differentiation between a

Table 1 Etiology and Location of Renal Artery Emboli in Combined Series in the Literature

	Frequency
Etiology[1,3]	
Atrial fibrillation	53%
Valvular vegetation	12%
Acute myocardial infarction	23%
Aortic aneurysm	7%
Other	5%
Kidney affected[5,7]	
Right	55%
Left	45%
Solitary (left or right)	26%
Bilateral	10%

Table 2 Clinical and Laboratory Presentation in Renal Artery Embolism[3,5,8]

Parameter	Frequency (%)
Pain	
Abdominal	41%
Chest	24%
Flank	77%
Back	12%
Fever ($>38°$ C)	69%
Hypertension ($>170/100$)	85%
Creatinine elevation (>2 mg/dl)	46%
Leukocytosis ($>12,000/mm^3$)	94%
Urinalysis	
Protein	93%
Leukocytes (>10/hpf)	59%
Erythrocytes (>10/hpf)	71%
Lactase dehydrogenase elevation ($>2\times$ normal)	88%

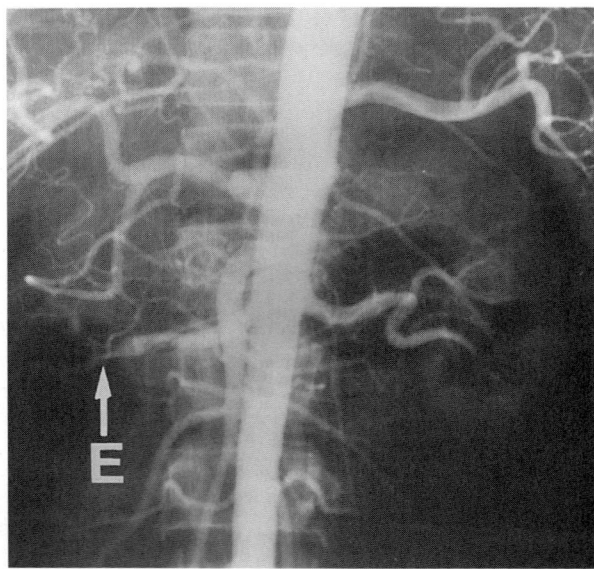

Figure 1 Embolic occlusion of the renal arteries bilaterally, with near complete obstruction of the right main renal artery *(E)* and the left superior pole branch.

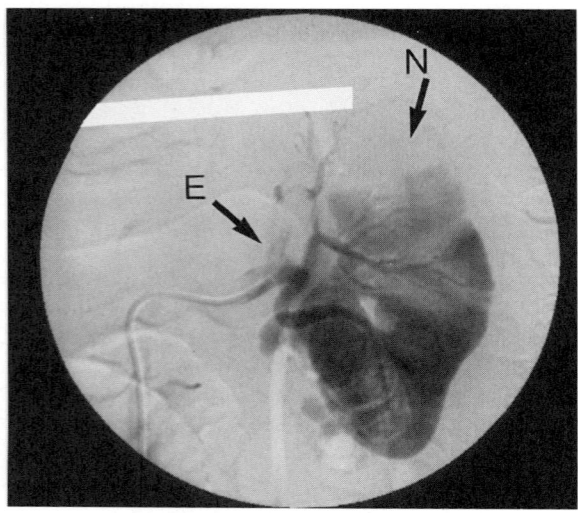

Figure 2 A selective left renal artery injection of the same patient, demonstrating occlusion of the superior pole branch vessel *(E)* and absence of a nephrogram *(N)* in the portion of the left kidney supplied by that branch.

renal artery embolus and renal artery thrombosis is sometimes difficult on arteriography. A meniscus may be seen in cases of embolism, whereas a smooth, tapering lesion is common in thrombotic occlusion. An aorta relatively free of atherosclerotic change is most unusual in cases of atherosclerotic renal artery thrombosis, and such a disease-free aorta suggests embolic occlusion. In a similar manner, the presence of abundant collateral channels feeding the distal renal artery implies a pre-existent, hemodynamically significant renal artery stenosis and a thrombotic rather than embolic etiology. Disease entities that mimic renal arterial embolism include renal artery thrombosis, aortic dissection, and pyelonephritis. These diseases can usually be excluded on the basis of an accurate history, physical examination, and arteriographic study.

TREATMENT

There are three options in the management of renal artery embolism: revascularization, nephrectomy, and observation with anticoagulation. Therapeutic decisions must be predicated on a determination of renal viability and the potential for salvage of functional parenchyma.

The renal perfusion scan and late phase of an aortogram have both been found to be predictive of renal viability.[5] Any degree of perfusion or the visualization of a nephrogram are indicative of adequate residual perfusion, and an attempt at revascularization is appropriate. In the absence of either criterion, renal salvage is so unlikely that attempts at revascularization are warranted only when the loss of the involved kidney would render the patient dialysis dependent.[1,3] Observation is indicated in the absence of prospects for salvage of significant renal mass, but the presence of concurrent factors such as persistent hypertension, pain, or infection mandate early nephrectomy.

The two general methods of restoring renal arterial perfusion are operative embolectomy and catheter-directed thrombolytic therapy. A number of anecdotal reports of renal arterial thrombolysis have appeared in the literature, but the relative merits of this procedure remain to be defined.[6] A variety of operative techniques are suitable for renal arterial exposure. Either an anterior or retroperitoneal approach may be undertaken. Using an anterior transperitoneal approach, either renal artery may be exposed after reflecting the right or left colon medially. The renal vein is usually identified first, and the artery is encountered with mobilization and gentle retraction of the vein. Alternatively, the left renal artery may be identified through a lesser sac exposure and the right renal artery after performing a generous Kocher maneuver. A third technique involves retraction of the transverse colon cephalad, following the infrarenal aorta proximally to the renal origins. This method provides adequate exposure of the proximal renal arteries, but distal exposure is difficult.

Balloon catheter thromboembolectomy is attempted after adequate renal artery exposure. Balloon catheters are passed proximally and distally in an attempt to clear all thromboembolic debris. Intraoperative arteriography, angioscopy, or duplex ultrasound may help to assure the complete removal of thrombus. Backflow is almost always poor and not generally indicative of subsequent outcome. Diuretics and mannitol may be useful after revascularization, as may be dopamine in doses of 3 to 5 µg/kg/minute. A period of acute tubular necrosis is expected, with renal function returning slowly over a period of several weeks.

RESULTS

Early studies of renal artery emboli reported successful renal salvage in more than 50% of patients.[7] However, these studies included partially occluding emboli, emboli to branch renal vessels, and patients with poorly documented embolic events that may have represented renal artery thrombosis in some. Unfortunately, most patients who experience complete embolic obstruction of a main renal artery do not have sufficient pre-existent collateral arterial blood flow to maintain viability until revascularization can be effected. Literature reports comprising patients with occluding main renal artery emboli document an extremely poor rate of salvage. We were unable to save any of 13 embolized kidneys, despite successful restoration of arterial flow in three-fourths of the patients who underwent operative revascularization.[5]

A review of reported series suggests that renal infarction has already occurred by the time the diagnosis is entertained and when the embolus occludes the main renal artery.[1,5] Operative or thrombolytic therapy is appropriate only in patients with partial renal artery occlusion or in the rare instance of embolization to a kidney with ample pre-existent collateral channels. These patients can be identified by the presence of a nephrogram on the late phase of an arteriogram or when the renal perfusion scan documents persistence of renal blood flow. Otherwise, revascularization is inappropriate and therapeutic strategies are directed at the prevention of recurrent embolization with prompt institution of systemic anticoagulation.

REFERENCES

1. Schoenbaum S, Goldman MA, Siegelman SS. Renal arterial embolization. Angiology 1971; 22:332–343.
2. Moyer JH, Heider C, Morris GC Jr, Handley C. Renal failure. I. The effect of complete renal artery occlusion for variable periods of time as compared to exposure to sub-filtration arterial pressures below 30 mm Hg for similar periods. Ann Surg 1957; 145:41–58.
3. Lessman RK, Johnson SF, Coburn JW, Kaufman JJ. Renal artery embolism. Clinical features and long-term follow-up of 17 cases. Ann Intern Med 1978; 89:477–482.
4. Morris GC Jr, Heider CF, Moyer JH. The protective effect of subfiltration arterial pressure in the kidney. Surg Forum 1956; 6:623–627.
5. Ouriel K, Andrus CH, Ricotta JJ, et al. Acute renal artery occlusion: When is revascularization justified? J Vasc Surg 1987; 5:348–355.
6. Campieri C, Raimondi C, Ratone F, et al. Normalization of renal function and blood pressure after dissolution with intra-arterial fibrinolytics of a massive renal artery embolism to a solitary functioning kidney. Nephron 1989; 51:399–401.
7. Lacombe M. Surgical versus medical treatment of renal artery embolism. J Cardiovasc Surg 1977; 18:281–290.
8. Winzelberg GG, Hull JD, Agar JWM, et al. Elevation of serum lactate dehydrogenase levels in renal infarction. JAMA 1979; 242:268–269.

RENAL VEIN THROMBOSIS

TIMOTHY J. NYPAVER, M.D.

Renal vein thrombosis is an uncommon clinical condition that, in general, responds to administration of anticoagulants and rarely requires operative intervention. Although renal vein thrombosis is considered a nonsurgical disease that is primarily within the domain of pediatricians, neonatologists, and nephrologists, the vascular surgeon should be familiar with this entity because of the instances in which operative intervention is necessary and because of its association with vena cava thrombosis and pulmonary embolism. The spectrum of renal vein thrombosis encompasses two discrete patient groups: (1) the neonatal-pediatric population, most commonly in association with severe dehydration; and (2) an adult population in association with renal disease, primarily nephrotic syndrome.

Approximately 0.26% to 0.7% of all autopsies in the neonatal-pediatric population and 0.4% of adult autopsies document renal vein thrombosis. Among patients with nephrotic syndrome, 20% ultimately develop renal vein thrombosis, although a substantial proportion remain occult.[1]

Historically, an accepted treatment for renal vein thrombosis was immediate nephrectomy. However, with improvements in diagnostic techniques, it became apparent that this condition was often unrecognized and that many patients responded to anticoagulation alone. The realization that the morbidity of renal vein thrombosis was related not to its existence but to the severity of the underlying predisposing systemic illness has served as the foundation for the present treatment guidelines.

PATHOPHYSIOLOGY

As with other venous thrombotic conditions, Virchow's triad of endothelial disruption, stasis, and hypercoagulability is also applicable to renal vein thrombosis. In the neonatal-pediatric population, venous stasis secondary to hemoconcentration, as well as low renal perfusion blood pressure as a consequence of two consecutive intrarenal capillary beds, predisposes to thrombus formation within the renal venous system.

The most common systemic disease associated with renal vein thrombosis in adults is the nephrotic syndrome. The nephrotic syndrome secondary to membranous or membranoproliferative nephropathy is associated with the highest risk of renal vein thrombosis. The nephrotic condition imposes a hypercoagulable state with susceptibility to multiple thrombotic complications. Specifically, changes in glomerular permeability lead to urinary loss of small-molecular-weight plasma proteins, including antithrombin III, producing a relative antithrombin III deficiency. In addition, thrombocytosis; increases in the levels of fibrinogen and factors V, VIII, and X; accelerated fibroblast degeneration; and increased activation of Hageman factor occur in the nephrotic state and contribute to this thrombotic tendency.[1-3] Last, patients with the nephrotic syndrome often have a contracted intravascular volume secondary to a low oncotic pressure and diuretic use, causing hemoconcentration, decreased renal vascular perfusion, and renal venous stasis. Although the nephrotic syndrome remains the most common etiologic factor, other conditions associated with adult renal vein thrombosis include pregnancy, ingestion of oral contraceptives, renal cell carcinoma, trauma, and retroperitoneal adenopathy or fibrosis.[2]

The thrombotic process is initiated in arcuate and intralobular venules with subsequent propagation into larger venous outflow vessels, proceeding centripetally to involve the renal vein. This has implications on operative thrombectomy in which, although patency of the major venous structures is established, the intralobular venules often remain occluded. Only with trauma, extrinsic compression, and renal cell carcinoma does the process begin in the major venous tributaries or renal vein.

CLINICAL PRESENTATION

In neonates, renal vein thrombosis most often occurs in association with hypoxia, sepsis, hypotension, dehydration, diarrhea, hypoglycemia, seizure disorders, or toxemia. Other predisposing conditions include maternal diabetes, congenital heart disease, polycythemia vera, sickle cell disease, congenital hypercoagulable conditions, and adrenal hemorrhage.[4,5] The clinical presentation is usually that of sudden onset of abdominal distention, a flank mass, hematuria, and proteinuria in a newborn less than 72 hours old. Bilateral renal vein involvement is heralded by the onset of progressive renal insufficiency. The condition may remain asymptomatic only to be detected later in life by the presence of an atrophic kidney.

Infants and neonates are more likely than adults to have hematologic evidence of intravascular consumptive coagulation, including thrombocytopenia, decreased fibrinogen concentration, and an increase in fibrin split products. Renal vein thrombosis may manifest itself by thrombus propagation into the inferior vena cava (IVC) with pulmonary artery embolization.

The clinical presentation in the adult can be divided into acute symptoms and chronic symptoms. Acute renal vein thrombosis typically presents with the sudden onset of flank pain, hematuria, proteinuria, or a deterioration in renal function. The obstruction of renal venous outflow causes congestion, edema, and later hemorrhagic infarction of the kidney. If venous outflow cannot be established through venous collaterals, the kidney is susceptible to rupture and potentially fatal retroperitoneal hemorrhage. Major retroperitoneal hemorrhage can also occur in neonates or children and, as with adults, requires immediate nephrectomy.

Chronic renal vein thrombosis may remain asymptomatic, demonstrate an extrarenal manifestation such as pulmonary embolus or remote thrombosis, or present with gradual decline in renal function, new onset of renal tubular dysfunction, or progressive proteinuria.[6]

For unilateral renal vein thrombosis, the outcome for the involved kidney depends on the acuity of the thrombotic process, the collateral venous circulation, and the rapidity and extent of recanalization. The involved kidney may follow one of three outcomes: (1) with adequate collateral venous circulation, the kidney may recover normal function; (2) circulatory compromise leading to increased renin production and hypertension; and (3) circulatory compromise progressing to an atrophic nonfunctioning kidney without hypertension.

DIAGNOSIS

The initial diagnostic procedure of choice for renal vein thrombosis is ultrasound, the accuracy of which can be enhanced by duplex imaging capability. The B-mode diagnostic criteria include renal enlargement without hydronephrosis, renal vein dilation, disruption and/or distortion of the normal renal internal echo pattern, and imaging of thrombus within the renal vein or IVC. The absence of a Doppler flow signal provides additional confirmatory evidence. With these diagnostic criteria, 93% accuracy can be achieved,[4] although as with any ultrasonographic technique, the test and its interpretation are subject to technologist expertise.

Computed tomography (CT) can establish the diagnosis of renal vein thrombosis. It is advantageous in that it documents both renal anatomy and function. However, CT does require the administration of potentially harmful intravenous contrast medium. The diagnosis may be established by imaging of thrombus within the renal vein or IVC. Indirect evidence for renal vein thrombosis includes renal enlargement, prolonged corticomedullary nephrogram, perirenal subcapsular fluid collection, and perirenal "cobwebs," which are serpiginous densities in the perinephric space caused by edema and enlarged venous collaterals and lymphatics (Fig. 1).[7] Magnetic resonance imaging avoids contrast administration, has superior soft tissue density imaging, and, although extensive experience is lacking, appears to be a useful accurate test for renal vein thrombosis.[8]

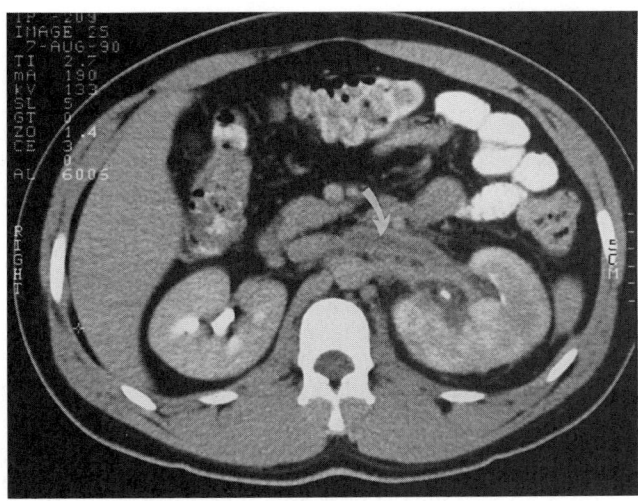

Figure 1 Computed tomography scan image demonstrating left renal vein thrombosis. Curved arrow points to thrombus in dilated left renal vein. Note enlargement of left kidney with increased enhancement of cortex, indicative of delayed excretion. Some "cobwebbing" is present in the left perirenal space.

Intravenous pyelography and renal arteriography are nonspecific and generally not first-line diagnostic tests. However, they are often performed because of the clinical suspicion of genitourinary pathology. The findings of unilateral renal enlargement, poor or absent contrast excretion, thinning of the infundibulum, and notching of the ureters should alert one to the diagnosis of renal vein thrombosis. The pelvicalyceal abnormalities develop as a result of parenchymal edema; ureteral notching may result from dilated collateral venous channels. Radionuclide renal scans, although nonspecific, may be useful in determining the degree of renal functional impairment and its progression with treatment.[2,6]

Inferior vena cavography, although generally accepted as the gold standard, is invasive, requires use of contrast medium, and may aggravate the thrombotic process. A persistent filling defect, the loss of streaming effect at the entry site of the renal vein into the IVC, and documentation of venous collaterals are diagnostic for renal vein thrombosis. The left renal vein, most likely related to its increased length, is involved three times more commonly than the right.

TREATMENT

In both the pediatric and adult populations, the mainstay for treatment of acute renal vein thrombosis is supportive and involves correction of fluid, electrolyte, and acid-base abnormalities and any underlying cause or hypercoagulable condition. Systemic anticoagulation with intravenous heparin sodium followed by conversion to oral anticoagulants, unless otherwise contraindicated, is the standard therapeutic regimen. Operative thrombectomy or thrombolytic therapy is limited to certain selected indications.

Acute life-threatening hemorrhage as a result of capsular rupture demands immediate nephrectomy. Long-term sequelae of renal vein thrombosis such as hypertension and infection occur infrequently but, when present, may require nephrectomy. Patients with a contraindication to anticoagulation, those who develop a complication as a result of anticoagulation, or those with recurrent pulmonary emboli despite anticoagulation are candidates for suprarenal IVC filter placement.

Neonatal-Pediatric Population

In all infants with suspected or documented renal vein thrombosis, attention is focused initially on treatment of the underlying condition. Anticoagulation with heparin sodium in infants, although controversial, is advocated in most instances. If the sonogram and Doppler studies indicate involvement of only one kidney and if renal function is stable, good recovery can be expected with conservative therapy.[4,9] However, if there is evidence of ongoing consumptive coagulation or bilateral renal involvement, anticoagulation is indicated. Cessation of thrombus propagation and prevention of pulmonary embolus are the primary goals of anticoagulation. By preventing further thrombus formation, one theoretically maintains patency of important venous collateral channels, thereby preserving renal function and allowing the patient's thrombolytic system the opportunity to recanalize the affected vein. Once renal function has stabilized or improved and the precipitating condition has been adequately treated with no further active thrombus formation, anticoagulation can be discontinued. Anticoagulation is generally continued for 5 to 10 days. Chronic long-term anticoagulation should be considered in infants with an underlying hypercoagulable condition or a history of multiple thromboembolic events.

Consideration for thrombolytic therapy or operative thrombectomy should be reserved for infants with renal failure who have bilateral renal vein thrombosis or renal vein thrombosis in a solitary kidney. Additionally, those with significant IVC involvement are also candidates for operation or thrombolytic therapy. Generally, thrombolytic therapy should be attempted prior to operative thrombectomy. Alternate administration techniques include systemic or regional with direct renal arterial or venous delivery systems. Selective regional infusion of urokinase (1,000 to 3,000 units/kg/hour) or streptokinase (50 to 100 units/kg/hour) through a catheter advanced into the region of the thrombus appears most effective while reducing the risks associated with the thrombolytic state. Nevertheless, it should be emphasized that experience with thrombolytic therapy in infants is limited, and it is further complicated by the difficulty of obtaining vascular access and the potential for pericatheter thrombosis, allergic reactions, and major hemorrhagic complications. These considerations warrant a cautious approach to the use of thrombolytic agents in neonates and children with renal vein thrombosis.[9,10] Operative thrombectomy in neonates and infants is associated with high mortality and should be reserved for patients with extensive IVC involvement and/or renal failure who fail thrombolytic therapy.

A recent study of renal vein thrombosis in infants and children reported a survival rate of 85.7%.[4] Most deaths occur secondary to the associated systemic disease and are rarely related to direct sequelae of the renal venous thrombosis.

Adults: Nephrotic Syndrome

The treatment protocol for adults depends primarily on the acuity of thrombosis and the presence or absence of any hypercoagulable condition. Regardless of the etiology, anticoagulation with heparin sodium is the mainstay of treatment for acute renal vein thrombosis. The duration of anticoagulation depends on whether an irreversible underlying hypercoagulable condition exists. Patients with a potentially reversible condition should be treated with a standard regimen of intravenous heparin sodium with conversion to oral sodium warfarin to be maintained for 3 to 6 months. Patients with a documented hypercoagulable condition, those with a history of previous thromboembolic complications, and those with severe nephrotic syndrome are candidates for long-term or lifetime anticoagulation. The risks of repetitive thromboembolic complications must be weighed against the susceptibility to hemorrhagic complications, a serious risk in patients with underlying renal insufficiency.

Thrombolytic therapy, with directed renal venous or renal arterial administration, offers an attractive alternative for selected patients with acute renal vein thrombosis. Although renal venous infusion of thrombolytic agents is preferable, arterial infusion may be beneficial in dissolving residual thrombosis within the intralobar venules and smaller branches of the renal venous system. Prompt institution of thrombolytic therapy and rapid recanalization may alleviate the deleterious effect of prolonged elevated renal venous pressure and ensure improved preservation of renal function. Thrombolytic therapy should be considered only in patients with acute onset of symptoms and renal dysfunction in whom no contraindication to a systemic lytic state exists. With the catheter embedded in the thrombus, an infusion of urokinase at 4,000 IU/minute is instituted. Heparin sodium is administered concurrently to maintain the partial thromboplastin time at 1.5 times the baseline value. Repeat phlebography is performed 3 to 4 hours after initiation of the infusion. If there is evidence of ongoing thrombolysis but residual thrombus remains, the urokinase infusion is reduced to 1,000 to 2,000 IU/minute and phlebography repeated at 8 to 12 hour intervals until complete dissolution occurs. As with the pediatric age group, regional thrombolysis is also recommended to patients with bilateral involvement, unilateral involvement of a single kidney, or significant IVC involvement. Operative thrombectomy for acute renal vein thrombosis is rarely indicated and is reserved for patients with renal failure in whom thrombolytic therapy is contraindicated or unsuccessful.

Chronic renal vein thrombosis often goes unrecognized and is the more common presentation in adults. There is no role for thrombolytic therapy in this setting. Long-term anticoagulation is indicated in the patient presenting with progressive renal dysfunction and to prevent further thromboembolic complications. In the adult, the ultimate prognosis depends on any complicating thrombotic events and the natural course of the inherent renal disease.

REFERENCES

1. Llach F. Hypercoagulability, renal vein thrombosis, and other thrombotic complications of nephrotic syndrome. Kidney Int 1985; 28:429–439.
2. Keating MA, Althausen AF. The clinical spectrum of renal vein thrombosis. J Urol 1985; 133:938–945.
3. Bernard DB, Cohen JJ, Harrington JT, et al. Extrarenal complications of the nephrotic syndrome. Kidney Int 1988; 33:1184–1202.
4. Ricci MA, Lloyd DA. Renal venous thrombosis in infants and children. Arch Surg 1990; 125:1195–1199.
5. Mocan L, Beattie TJ, Murphy AV. Renal venous thrombosis in infancy: Long-term follow-up. Pediatr Nephrol 1991; 5:45–49.
6. Llach F, Papper S, Massry SG. The clinical spectrum of renal vein thrombosis: Acute and chronic. Am J Med 1980; 69:819–827.
7. Glazer GM, Francis IR, Gross BH, Amendola MA. Computed tomography of renal vein thrombosis. J Comput Assist Tomogr 1984; 8:288–293.
8. Dietrich RB, Kangarloo H. Kidneys in infants and children: Evaluation with MR. Radiology 1986; 159:215–221.
9. Bromberg WD, Firlit CF. Fibrinolytic therapy for renal vein thrombosis in the child. J Urol 1990; 143:86–88.
10. Vogelzang RL, Moel DI, Cohn RA, et al. Acute renal vein thrombosis: Successful treatment with intraarterial urokinase. Radiology 1988; 169:681–682.

RENAL ARTERY OCCLUSIVE DISEASE IN CHRONIC RENAL FAILURE

RICHARD H. DEAN, M.D.

Traditional management of the sequelae of renovascular occlusive disease has centered on the resultant hypertension. Recent reports, however, have emphasized the potential for simultaneous retrieval of excretory function in some patients with combined hypertension and renal insufficiency.[1-3] These observations have renewed awareness of the functional consequence of renal ischemia and have resulted in the term ischemic nephropathy. By definition, ischemic nephropathy reflects the presence of anatomically severe occlusive disease of the extraparenchymal renal artery in a patient with excretory renal insufficiency.

Available information, frequently circumstantial, suggests that ischemic nephropathy may be a more common cause of progressive renal failure in the atherosclerotic age group than previously recognized. In a 1986 survey, 73% of end-stage renal disease (ESRD) patients were in the atherosclerotic age range (more than 40 years old), and the median age was older than 60 years.[4] Likewise, more than 50% of nondiabetic patients with ESRD have hypertensive nephropathy as their presumed diagnosis.[5] In a report by Mailoux and colleagues,[6] a presumed renal vascular cause of ESRD increased in frequency from 6.7% for the period 1978 to 1981 to a frequency of 16.5% for the period 1982 to 1985. The median age at onset of ESRD for that group was the oldest of all groups, falling in the seventh decade of life. Each of these clinical characteristics is in agreement with the demographic data of our patients with proved ischemic nephropathy. In our patients, all have had at least moderate hypertension, the mean age was 63 years, and only 14% had diabetes mellitus. These data argue that renovascular disease may be either the primary cause or a superimposed secondary accelerant of renal insufficiency in a larger proportion of patients with renal insufficiency than commonly acknowledged. Using this premise as a guide, we currently screen all adult patients over the age of 50 years who have newly recognized renal insufficiency when hypertension of any level coexists.

DIAGNOSTIC EVALUATION

Renal duplex sonography is the preferred method for preliminary screening. In a review of its use we found renal duplex sonography to have an overall accuracy of 96% for establishing the presence or absence of main renal artery occlusive disease.[7] Through this preliminary screening with renal duplex sonography, we limit the use of arteriography in renal insufficiency patients to those with either a positive renal duplex sonogram or severe hypertension. The results of arteriography in a group of 58 consecutive patients presenting for evaluation of ischemic nephropathy at our center are summarized in Table 1.

Evaluation with renal vein renin ratios is useless in this patient population because most patients have bilateral disease. Nevertheless, when a unilateral lesion is present, decisions regarding management should be based on both anatomic and functional assessments, including renal venous renin assays.

Table 1 Anatomic Variety of Disease in 58 Consecutive Patients with Ischemic Nephropathy

Location or Type of Disease	No. of Patients	No. of Lesions	%
Atherosclerotic	55	96	97
Fibromuscular dysplasia	3	3	3
Unilateral			
Occlusion		6	
Osteal stenosis		12	90
Nonosteal stenosis		2	
Bilateral	38		
Occlusion		31	
Osteal stenosis		44	99
Nonosteal stenosis		1	

OPTIONS FOR MANAGEMENT

Three options are available for treatment of patients with ischemic nephropathy: medical management, revascularization by percutaneous transluminal renal angioplasty (PTRA), and revascularization by operative intervention.

Medical Management

The merits of medical management center on the absence of the risks of diagnostic evaluation and interventional procedures. Although there is no randomized trial comparing the survival of medically managed patients to that of interventionally managed patients, the data we and others have collected suggest that dialysis-free survival is limited in patients treated only by medical management. In a retrospective analysis of the rate of decline in estimated glomerular filtration rate (EGFR) of patients prior to operative intervention, we found the rate of decline to be a 3.25% drop in EGFR per week during the 6 months prior to intervention.[8]

Although the rate of change of EGFR before intervention is probably affected by selection bias, it has been extremely rapid in our evaluated patients. It is even more pronounced if compared to the rate of decline of EGFR from other causes of renal insufficiency. In the preliminary data used to make sample size calculations for the initiation or the modification of diet in renal disease,[9] the decline in the glomerular filtration rate

(GFR) was estimated to be approximately 0.5 ml/minute/month for renal insufficiency patients on a standard diet. Noteworthy is that patients with known renovascular occlusive disease were excluded from entry into that data base. With the rate of deterioration suggested in the pilot data, it would require approximately 40 months for the GFR to drop from 40 ml/minute to 20 ml/minute. In contrast, using the rate of decline in our entire group for comparison, less than 5 months would be required for a patient with ischemic nephropathy to experience a similar level of deterioration.

The second theoretical benefit of medical management is the perceived prevention of morbidity and mortality associated with interventional procedures. If one accepts the data suggesting that the natural history of ischemic nephropathy under medical management is characterized by a rapid progression to end-stage renal failure, one must consider the morbidity and mortality that occur without interventional management.

In the study of the duration of survival after institution of dialysis, Mailoux and associates found that ESRD caused by uncorrected renovascular disease was associated with the most rapid rate of death during follow-up.[6] In their study, patients with renovascular disease had a median survival after initiation of dialysis of only 27 months and a 5 year survival of only 12%. This equates to a death rate in excess of 20%/year. Our conviction is that this risk associated with medical management is significant and justifies an aggressive attitude toward evaluation and intervention in these patients.

Percutaneous Transluminal Renal Angioplasty

The minimal invasion associated with PTRA is widely publicized and appreciated. The value of renal revascularization without the morbidity and mortality associated with operative intervention cannot be disputed. Nevertheless, one must examine the probability of successful revascularization by PTRA and the consequence of failed PTRA prior to adopting the philosophy of simply performing PTRA before submitting the patient to operation.

Unfortunately, our data argue that 97% of renal artery lesions associated with ischemic nephropathy are either orificial stenoses or occlusions. These anatomic varieties of disease have been associated with infrequent success (less than 20%) when treated by PTRA.[10] Furthermore, 29% of patients with ischemic nephropathy treated by operation in our experience had associated aortic disease that independently required correction. Therefore, we believe that PTRA is rarely a viable alternative to operative intervention for management of this variety of clinical presentation of renovascular disease.

Operative Renal Revascularization

The potential role of operative correction of ischemic nephropathy remains controversial, yet recent data argue for its preferential use in selected patients. Most pertinent to a discussion of this controversy is the risk of operative management and the associated anticipated benefit to dialysis-free survival. In this regard, review of our recently reported experience underscores both the risks and benefits of this approach.[8] This report reviewed the data collected during a recent 42 month period from 58 consecutive patients with ischemic nephropathy who were operated upon. Based on serum creatinine values, immediate preoperative EGFR ranged from 0 to 46 ml/minute (mean, 23.85 ± 9.76 ml/minute). Eight patients were dialysis-dependent or anuric at the time of operation. Patients with at least three sequential measurements for calculations of EGFR changes during the 6 months before operation ($n = 50$) and the first 12 months after operation ($n = 32$) were used to describe the preoperative rate of decline in EGFR and the impact of operation on this decrease in survivors. In addition, comparative analyses were performed of data from patients with unilateral versus bilateral lesions and patients classified as having improvement in EGFR versus no improvement after operation.

The operative mortality in this group was 9%. Included, however, were patients requiring both renal and aortic procedures. Patients with ischemic nephropathy are at increased risk for any major operative procedure. Nevertheless, one must place this risk and rate of survival into context with the probability of survival without operation.

The life table survival curve of our group of patients with ischemic nephropathy suggests that the patient who survives operation and the early follow-up period is afforded an improved probability of survival. Even when operative deaths are included, the probability for 2 and 3 year survival appears to be significantly better than that in patients who had not undergone operation and had progressed to the point of dialysis dependence.

There was significant improvement both in EGFR immediately after operation and in the amount of its subsequent deterioration (Fig. 1). Comparison of the rate of deterioration in EGFR before operation for the group who received immediate improvement in EGFR by operation versus those who received no benefit suggests that the rate of decline in GFR may have value in predicting the probability of retrieval of GFR by operation. Unfortunately, the heterogeneity of individual slopes of change in EGFR prevent comment on a critical rate of decline that would predict retrieval of renal function by operation. Nevertheless, a rapidly deteriorating GFR should alert the physician to the potential presence of ischemic nephropathy and should argue for the likelihood of retrieval of function by operation when ischemic nephropathy is identified.

The likelihood of benefit to renal function by correction of unilateral versus bilateral disease in our patients warrants special comment. The impact of revascularization on EGFR in these two subgroups reasserts our earlier observations regarding predictors of retrieval of renal function (Table 2).[11] We found significant improvement of EGFR after operation in an important minority (33%) of patients treated for unilat-

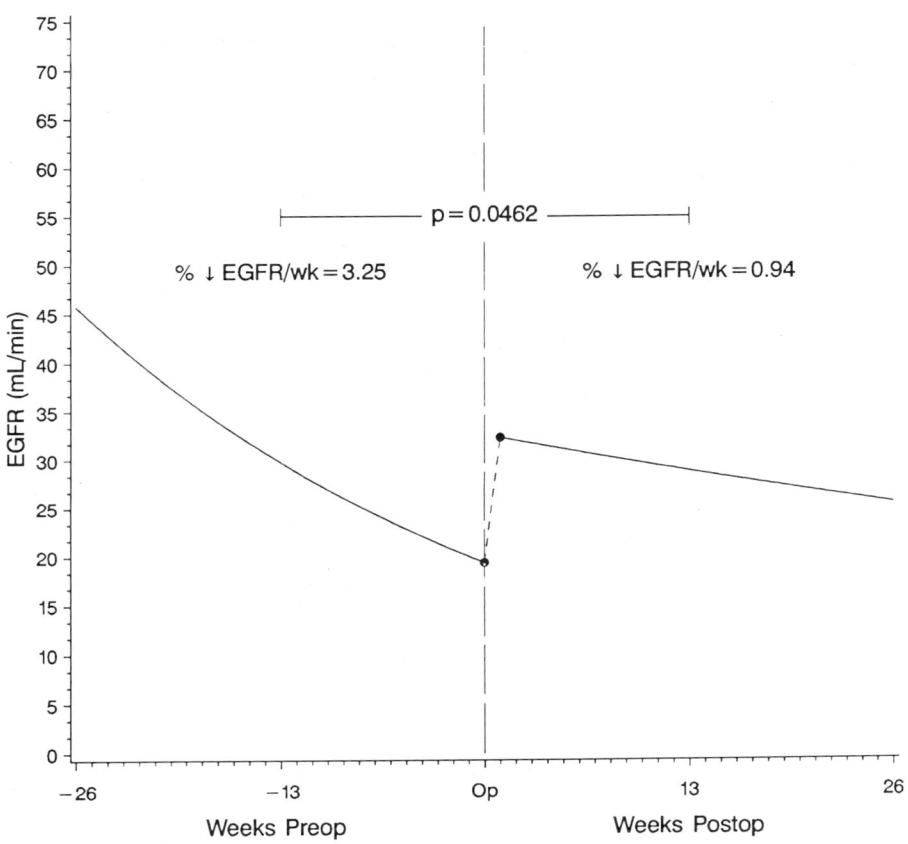

Figure 1 Graphic depiction of the percentage deterioration of estimated glomerular filtration rate (EGFR) per week for 5% patients with ischemic nephropathy during the 6 months before ($n = 50$) and after ($n = 32$) operation. The immediate effect of operation on EGFR is depicted. The p values for differences are determined using Student's t-test for unpaired data. Note the improvement in the slope of decline in EGFR after operation. (From Dean RH, Tribble RW, Hansen KJ, et al. Evolution of renal insufficiency in ischemic nephropathy. Ann Surg 1991; 213:446–456; with permission.)

Table 2 Change in EGFR Versus Site of Disease

	Unilateral		Bilateral	
Change	No.	%	No.	%
Improved ($\geq 20\%$ increase)	4	33	27	66
No change ($\pm 19\%$ change)	7	58	9	22
Worse ($\geq 20\%$ decrease)	1	9	5	12
	12		41	

From Dean RH, Tribble RW, Hansen KJ, et al. Evolution of renal insufficiency in ischemic nephropathy. Ann Surg 1991; 213:446–456; with permission.

Table 3 Predictors of Retrieval of Global Renal Function in Patients with Ischemic Nephropathy

Bilaterally of renal artery occlusions
Normal distal vessels documented on arteriogram
Renal length greater than 8 cm
History of rapidly declining renal function and severe hypertension

eral lesions. Because uncontrolled hypertension can be both an important independent cause of progressive renal insufficiency and an accelerator of cardiovascular morbid and mortal events, we believe that operative treatment of such patients with unilateral lesions who have secondary hypertension is justified, even without regard to the issue of retrieval of renal function.

Finally, we have found several factors of value as predictors of renal function retrieval by operation (Table 3). No single factor alone has high predictive value. In contrast, as a constellation of factors, we have enthusiasm for the probability of functional benefit from operative renal revascularization in these patients.

REFERENCES

1. Scobie JE, Maher ER, Hamilton G, et al. Atherosclerotic renovascular disease causing renal impairment: A case for treatment. Clin Nephrol 1989; 31:119–122.

2. Bengtsson U, Bergentz S-E, Norback B. Surgical treatment of renal artery stenosis with impending uremia. Clin Nephrol 1974; 2:222–229.
3. Novick AC, Pohl MA, Schreiber M, et al. Revascularization for preservation of renal function in patients with atherosclerotic renovascular disease. J Urol 1983; 129:907–911.
4. North Carolina Kidney Council. Annual report. Raleigh NC: North Carolina Kidney Council, 1986.
5. Eggers PW. Effect of transplantation on the Medicare end-stage renal disease program. N Engl J Med 1988; 318:223–229.
6. Mailoux LU, Bellucci AG, Mossey RT, et al. Predictors of survival in patients undergoing dialysis. Am J Med 1988; 84:855–862.
7. Hansen KJ, Tribble RW, Reavis SW, et al. Renal duplex sonography: Evaluation of clinical utility. J Vasc Surg 1990; 12:227–236.
8. Dean RH, Tribble RW, Hansen KJ, et al. Evolution of renal insufficiency in ischemic nephropathy. Ann Surg 1991; 213: 446–456.
9. Levey AS, Gassman JJ, Hall PM, Walker WG. Assessing the progression of renal disease in clinical studies: Effects of duration of follow-up and regression to the mean. J Am Soc Nephrol 1991; 1:1087–1094.
10. Sos TA, Pickering TG, Sniderman K, et al. Percutaneous transluminal renal angioplasty in renovascular hypertension due to atheroma or fibromuscular dysplasia. N Engl J Med 1983; 309:274–279.
11. Dean RH, Englund R, DuPont WD, et al. Retrieval of renal function by revascularization: Study of preoperative outcome predictors. Ann Surg 1985; 202:367–375.

RENAL ARTERIOVENOUS MALFORMATION AND ARTERIOVENOUS FISTULA

JOHN D. BENNETT, M.D., C.M.
SAADOON KADIR, M.D.

Abnormal renal arteriovenous communications are broadly classified as congenital, spontaneous, or acquired. Although duplex color Doppler sonography can identify such lesions, renal arteriography remains the mainstay in diagnosing and delineating these lesions. Transcatheter management has emerged as the treatment of choice for many patients with such lesions. With appropriate patient selection and meticulous technique, success rates exceeding 90% can be achieved.[1-10]

ARTERIOVENOUS MALFORMATION

Renal arteriovenous malformations (AVMs) are rare congenital lesions with an estimated incidence of 0.04% at arteriography.[8] They appear as a tangle of coiled, communicating vascular channels, usually associated with multiple, slightly enlarged feeding arteries and draining veins at the segmental or interlobar level. The degree of arteriovenous (AV) shunting is variable but usually not massive. They can be diffuse but are more commonly focal and are usually found in the renal medulla. The most common type of lesion is a small, hemangioma-like cirsoid malformation. It occurs more frequently in women than men and has a predilection for the right kidney.[8] A localized AVM can occasionally be mistaken for a vascular neoplasm; however, computed tomography or renal ultrasound confirms absence of a mass in the region of angiographic abnormality in the case of an AVM.

ARTERIOVENOUS FISTULA

Renal arteriovenous fistula (AVF) may be spontaneous or acquired. On arteriography, it is characterized by a single feeding artery and an early draining vein. The feeding artery may be enlarged, depending on the chronicity of the lesion and the size of the AVF. Frequently, a pseudoaneurysm is present. An acquired AVF occurs more frequently than a spontaneous lesion and is usually secondary to renal trauma. Whereas blunt trauma accounts for two-thirds of renal injuries, penetrating trauma is far more likely to be associated with AVF formation. The most common cause is renal biopsy. The incidence of renal biopsy AVF is estimated at approximately 16%[5,8] and occurs more commonly in patients with hypertension and nephrosclerosis. Most of these lesions heal spontaneously; however, 4% persist and necessitate treatment. Other causes of acquired AVF include stab wounds, antegrade pyelography, percutaneous nephrostomy tube insertion, and percutaneous stone manipulation. The most frequent site of the fistulous communication is at the interlobar or arcuate arterial level. An AVF between the main renal vessels can occur after penetrating injury or as a complication of operation and results from securing the renal artery and vein in the same ligature.

Spontaneous renal AVF is usually a complication of some other renal vascular abnormality. It has been described in association with renal arterial dissection and aneurysms and occurs as a result of arterial rupture into an adjacent vein. Spontaneous AVF may occur in association with arterial fibromuscular dysplasia even in the absence of an aneurysm. The etiology may be the rupture of arteriographically inapparent renal parenchymal microaneurysms.[8] Vasculitic, mycotic, postinflammatory, and congenital aneurysms are rare causes of renal AVF.

CLINICAL PRESENTATION

Nontraumatic renal AVMs and AVFs may remain clinically silent for years. When symptoms develop, the most common presentation is hematuria, which may be episodic, ongoing and mild, or massive and life-threatening. Patients may also present with perinephric or retroperitoneal hemorrhage. Systemic hypertension occurs occasionally as a result of focal renal ischemia. A bruit auscultated over the involved kidney is a characteristic sign. Large fistulas with a high degree of AV shunting can produce cardiac decompensation.

INDICATIONS FOR ARTERIOGRAPHY AND EMBOLIZATION

The indications for arteriography and therapeutic embolization in patients with suspected renal trauma include increasing hematuria, persisting or episodic hypotension, flank bruits, or ancillary studies suggesting significant renovascular injury. Indications for therapeutic embolization of nontraumatic renal AVM and AVF include hematuria, perinephric or retroperitoneal hemorrhage, hypertension, and cardiac decompensation.

PATIENT PREPARATION AND INTRAPROCEDURAL MONITORING

The procedure, risks, benefits, and alternatives are explained to the patient and informed consent is obtained, preferably the evening prior to elective procedures. In the emergency setting, the patient is clinically assessed and hemodynamic stabilization measures must be initiated before undertaking arteriography. Under these circumstances, the possibility of transcatheter embolization is discussed with the patient so that appropriate consent is obtained before the patient is sedated. Laboratory data and previous studies are reviewed, with particular attention to indicators of renal function. The patient is placed on a clear fluid diet beginning at midnight. Adequate hydration is of importance to avoid contrast media–induced nephropathy. Collaboration with a nephrologist may be helpful when dealing with situations of precarious fluid balance. Preprocedural sedation using 50 to 75 mg meperidine and 25 mg promethazine may be given intramuscularly 1 hour prior to the procedure. Alternatively, 5 mg morphine and 5 mg diazepam are given intravenously upon arrival in the angiography suite. Additional intravenous sedation is administered as required during the procedure. When extensive embolization is anticipated, broad-spectrum antibiotics are started the day before the embolization and are continued for about 3 days after the embolization.

During the procedure, the electrocardiogram and blood pressure are monitored. Embolization of renal parenchyma can be associated with considerable postprocedural pain and fever, necessitating ongoing analgesia and antipyretic therapy.

TECHNIQUE

Because the renal vascular bed is devoid of significant parenchymal anastomoses, interruption of an arterial branch causes tissue infarction beyond the point of occlusion. The amount of infarcted tissue corresponds to the size and number of vessels occluded. Embolization must, therefore, be highly selective in order to preserve the uninvolved branches.

A 5 or 6 Fr hemostatic sheath is inserted from the femoral approach. If the site of the lesion is known, the contralateral femoral approach is used, as it facilitates catheterization of the renal artery. If the pertinent arterial anatomy or location of the lesion is unknown, an abdominal aortogram is performed first to determine the number and location of the renal arteries. In the presence of penetrating flank injuries or if the lesion has previously been studied, selective arteriography of the affected kidney is performed as the initial procedure.

The affected branch is catheterized by using the 5 Fr visceral catheter or by using a coaxial system, such as an open-ended guide wire and 3 Fr Teflon or Tracker catheters. Catheter position in the appropriate branch is confirmed by digital subtraction angiography (DSA) before embolization.

The embolic agent is selected with consideration to the lesion type, feeding vessel size, degree of AV shunting, and whether temporary or permanent occlusion is desired. The most frequently used embolic agents are Gelfoam, Ivalon, and stainless steel coils. The size of the embolic agent is matched to the target vessel. For example, too small an embolic agent in the presence of a large AV shunt may pass into the venous system and result in pulmonary embolism. An oversized coil does not conform properly and may protrude proximally and even dislodge. Undersized coils may traverse the fistula and embolize to the lungs.

Trauma

For injuries to segmental and distal arterial branches, a temporary occluding agent is usually sufficient. We use absorbable gelatin (Gelfoam) cut into 2 to 4 mm pledgets soaked in cefamandole to enhance thrombogenicity. Pledgets of this size are injected through a 5 Fr catheter. Smaller pledgets (1 to 2 mm) are used with coaxial catheters or injectable guide wires. During the embolization, catheter position and flow within the vessel are repeatedly assessed by contrast injection. Once vessel occlusion occurs, embolization is concluded.

Table 1 Published Results for Renal Embolization in a Nonneoplastic Setting

Author	Embolic Agent	Clinical Success No. Patients	Complications
Kantor et al[1]	Gelfoam 12 Coils 8	19/20	Low-grade fever in "several"
Fisher et al[2]	Gelfoam 9 Coils 3 Both 3	15/15	Transient fever with low-grade hypertension in 1/15; resolved in 2 weeks
Uflacker et al[3]	Gelfoam 10 Coils 6 Clot 1	14/17	Transient fever in 1/17
Kadir et al[4]	Detachable balloons 9 (+ clot in 1 patient)	9/9	Mild pain, fever, and leukocytosis observed in most patients
Clark et al[5]	Gelfoam 11 Gelfoam + coil + cyanoacrylate 1	12/12	None reported
Nakamura et al[6]	Gelfoam 3	2/3	Transient hypertension in 2/3
White et al[7]	Detachable balloons 2	2/2	None reported
Cho et al[8]	Gelfoam 4 Clot 2	6/6	2/6 developed transient hypertension requiring medical therapy in 1 case
Chuang et al[9]	Clot 4 Amicar clot 1 Amicar clot + Gelfoam 1 Clot + Oxycel 1	6/7	2/6 had transient flank pain
Bookstein et al[10]	Clot 3	3/3	None reported
Overall success:		88/94 (94%)	
Transient hypertension		5/94 (5%)	

Arteriovenous Fistulas

Flow-directed detachable balloons provide a highly precise method of occluding AVF. Unfortunately, the silicone Mini Balloon is no longer on the market. Other balloon types are presently undergoing clinical trials.

Small AVFs, less than 3 mm in size, are managed by using Gelfoam or Ivalon pledgets, stainless steel coils, or the platinum minicoils alone or in combination. Fistulas up to 7 mm in size can be managed with stainless steel coils. However, in large AVFs, blood flow through the fistula is very rapid, and occlusion with coils is not always possible. In such patients, or if the patient's condition requires urgent operative intervention, a nondetachable occlusion balloon inflated in the proximal renal artery rapidly reduces blood flow and can stabilize the patient until operation can be performed.

Arteriovenous Malformations

Successful transcatheter treatment of congenital AVMs requires permanent occluding agents. Because of the paucity of parenchymal collaterals, embolotherapy of congenital renal AVMs is more successful than for those in the extremities where recurrence is a frequent problem. Ivalon pledgets or spheres soaked in cefamandole are injected through selectively placed 5 or 3 Fr catheters, open-ended guide wires, or Tracker catheters. We typically intersperse them with similar-sized particles of Gelfoam. The embolization technique is the same as described for traumatic lesions. Tissue adhesives and absolute alcohol have also been used for such lesions.

RESULTS

With meticulous technique, transcatheter treatment of renal AVFs and AVMs is successful, defined as complete resolution of clinical symptoms and signs attributable to the lesion, in more than 90% of patients (Table 1).[1-10] This requires careful delineation of the abnormal vascular anatomy and accurate placement of the embolic material (Fig. 1).

POSTEMBOLIZATION SYNDROME AND COMPLICATIONS

Following renal embolotherapy, most patients experience flank pain that varies directly with the amount of renal tissue embolized. It may be severe enough to require ongoing parenteral analgesia but is usually transient and resolves over 24 to 72 hours. Fever, associated with leukocytosis, occurs commonly but is self-limited. Transient hypertension occurs in 5% of patients.

The most serious potential complication of embolotherapy is inadvertent embolization of a nontarget vessel. Migration of the embolic agent through a fistula can result in pulmonary embolization. The most com-

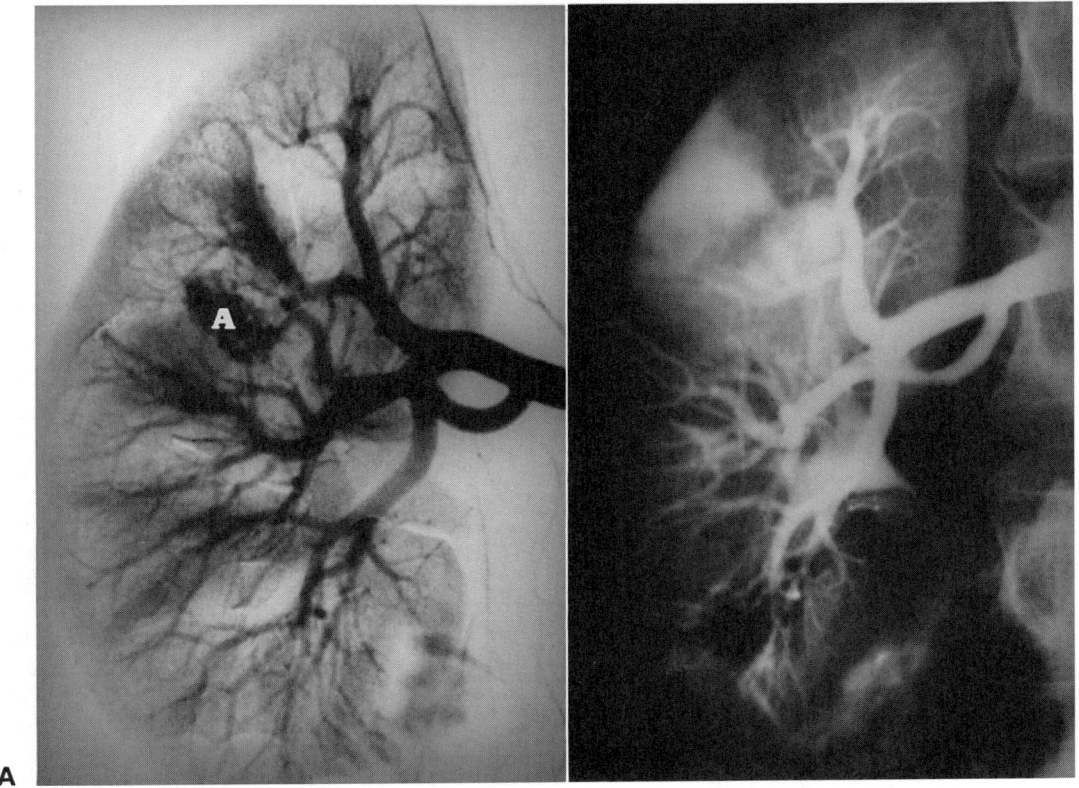

Figure 1 *A*, Subtraction film from a right renal arteriogram in a 34-year-old woman who presented with massive, episodic hematuria demonstrates a cirsoid vascular malformation. *B*, Arteriogram obtained following embolization with polyvinyl alcohol (Ivalon) pledgets soaked in cefamandole. The malformation is occluded.

mon cause of misplaced embolic material is catheter dislodgment or inadvertent reflux of the embolic material during the procedure. This complication is avoided if meticulous technique is used with subselective catheter placement and angiographic monitoring of the progress of the embolization.

REFERENCES

1. Kantor A, Sclafani SJA, Scalea T, et al. The role of interventional radiology in the management of genitourinary trauma. Urol Clin North Am 1989; 16:255–265.
2. Fisher RG, Ben-Menachem Y, Whigham C. Stab wounds of the renal artery branches: Angiographic diagnosis and treatment by embolization. Am J Roentgenol 1989; 152:1231–1235.
3. Uflacker R, Paolini RM, Lima S. Management of traumatic hematuria by selective renal artery embolization. J Urol 1984; 132:662–667.
4. Kadir S, Marshall FF, White RI, et al. Therapeutic embolization of the kidneys with detachable silicone balloons. J Urol 1983; 129:11–13.
5. Clark RA, Gallant TE, Alexander ES. Angiographic management of traumatic arteriovenous fistulas: Clinical results. Radiology 1983; 147:9–13.
6. Nakamura H, Uchida H, Kuroda C, et al. Renal arteriovenous malformations: Transcatheter embolization and follow-up. Am J Roentgenol 1981; 137:113–116.
7. White RI, Kaufman SL, Barth KH, et al. Embolotherapy with detachable silicone balloons: Technique and clinical results. Radiology 1979; 131:619–627.
8. Cho KJ, Stanley JC. Non-neoplastic congenital and acquired renal arteriovenous malformations and fistulas. Radiology 1978; 129:333–343.
9. Chuang VP, Reuter SR, Walter J, et al. Control of renal hemorrhage by selective arterial embolization. Am J Roentgenol 1975; 125:300–306.
10. Bookstein JJ, Goldstein HM. Successful management of post biopsy arteriovenous fistula with selective arterial embolization. Radiology 1973; 109:535–536.

ARTERIOVENOUS FISTULAS AND ARTERIOVENOUS MALFORMATIONS

CLASSIFICATION OF PERIPHERAL CONGENITAL VASCULAR MALFORMATIONS

ROBERT B. RUTHERFORD, M.D.

As a group, congenital vascular malformations (CVMs) are a complex mixture of malformed vessels. In earlier times, before their true nature was apparent, they were either labeled by descriptive terms such as hemangioma simplex, nevus angiectoides, cirsoid aneurysm, and venous angiodysplasia or by eponyms such as the Klippel-Trenaunay and Parkes-Weber syndromes. Both of the latter applied to the triad of a birthmark or vascular nevus, varicose veins, and an enlarged or elongated extremity. Convention has assigned these two eponyms to signify that the triad was caused by purely venous defects on the one hand, or by multiple arteriovenous fistulas (AVFs) on the other, respectively. The understandable confusion over the true nature or type of a CVM has been perpetuated by the relative rarity of these conditions in any single physician's practice, so that few have ever gained a large enough personal experience with them to analyze them.

However, the advent of angiography made possible studying the underlying vascular anatomy and making attempts at classification. Malan,[1] Degni,[2] and their colleagues proposed classification schemes, later modified by others, but their proposals, although with considerable merit, never gained wide acceptance. Some were too complex although inclusive, and others did not cover the full breadth of CVMs in a comprehensive, yet easily understood scheme.

Even agreement on a simple inclusive term under which to group these congenital vascular lesions has not been achieved. Currently, most are comfortable with the term congenital vascular malformations, but both congenital vascular anomalies and congenital vascular defects have their proponents. Disagreement has persisted as to whether to include all congenital defects, such as missing venous valves, which commonly lead to varicose veins, and whether to include the true cutaneous hemangiomas of infancy, which, although they are proliferating endothelial tumors and not CVMs, are important to distinguish from the cutaneous capillary or cavernous malformations seen in childhood, particularly in that these "birthmarks" are generally seen and treated by the same group of vascular specialists.

The importance of developing a classification system that was simple yet inclusive enough to gain acceptance is apparent from the failure of previous attempts and has been widely recognized. The frequent existence of mixed elements in these CVMs has been dealt with by assigning the primary categorization on the basis of the predominant component, as, for example, predominantly arterial, predominantly venous, or predominantly arteriovenous. In some CVMs major elements are significantly admixed. These have been labeled as combined CVMs by some, whereas others have felt that lesions should be designated by the single most important element. For example, if a patient presenting with varicosities had an anomalous vein, such as the so-called marginal vein that runs laterally up the leg, but it was fed by multiple microscopic AVFs, there might be disagreement as to whether this CVM was predominantly arteriovenous or venous.

Presuming ultimate agreement on criteria for assigning these lesions to basic categories such as arteriovenous, venous, capillary, lymphatic, and the like, there is still a major need for further differentiation within these categories if the classification scheme is to have any clinical impact, that is, to allow outcome assessment of the treatment of similar lesions and to be used as a framework for management decisions. Mulliken and Glowacki have suggested that these lesions be divided into high or low flow groups and that they be designated by an identifying alphabetical letter, such as CM, capillary malformation; VM, venous malformation; and LM, lymphatic malformation, which are all slow blood flow lesions; and AM, arterial malformation; AVM, arteriovenous malformation; and AVF, arteriovenous fistulas, which are all fast blood flow lesions.[3] In their system, combined malformations are dealt with by placing the predominant element first, such as CLM, capillary-lymphatic malformation; CVM, capillary-venous malformation; and LVM, lymphatic venous malformation. Because many of the complex CVMs present with distorted neuroectodermal and mesoder-

Table 1 Classification of Vascular Malformations

Slow flow
  Capillary (CM)
  Lymphatic (LM)
  Venous (VM)
Fast flow
  Arterial (AM): aneurysm, coarctation, ectasia
  Arteriovenous fistulas (AVF)
  Arteriovenous (AVM)
Complex-combined (often with associated skeletal overgrowth)
  Regional syndromes

Sturge-Weber:	Facial CM, intracranial CM, VM, AVM
Klippel-Trenaunay:	Limb-truncal CLVM
Parkes-Weber:	Limb CLVM with AVF

  Diffuse syndromes

Maffucci:	LVM, enchondromas
Solomon:	CM, VM, intracranial AVM, epidermal nevi, etc.
Proteus:	CM, VM, macrodactyly, hemihypertrophy, lipomas, pigmented nevi, scoliosis, etc.

From Mulliken JB. Cutaneous vascular anomalies. Semin in Vasc Surg 1993; 6:204–218; with permission.

---

mal elements, often with osseous overgrowth, these are included in Mulliken and Glowacki's system under named syndromes (Table 1).

Most European specialists in this field have preferred to subdivide these broad categories of venous, arteriovenous, and so on along lines that relate to their embryologic development. Based on the classic works of Woolard[4] and Rienhoff,[5] it has been generally accepted that the form a CVM takes depends on the stage of embryologic development at which the growth disturbance occurs. The vascular elements in a developing limb bud begin as a syncytial network of small undifferentiated channels (Fig. 1A). This is the undifferentiated or capillary network stage. Then, as an initial attempt at organization, some central main channels develop. At this, the retiform stage, there are still no recognizable mature elements; that is, the axial or truncal arteries and veins have not yet appeared (Fig. 1B). Their appearance marks the transition into the maturational or gross differentiation stage, as recognizable, named axial and other main truncal arteries and veins of the extremity develop (Fig. 1C). Capillary malformations (CMs, e.g., most birthmarks, port wine stains, or cutaneous vascular nevi) represent an arrest or disturbance in development at the earliest stage. Lesions with larger channels or lakes have been called cavernous hemangiomas or, more correctly, cavernous malformations, and mixed capillary-cavernous lesions are not uncommon. Clusters of venous angiomata, which are immature, thin-walled venous lakes, tangentially and often remotely connected to the main deep venous system, represent an inborn error during an intermediate stage of development. Aplasia or hypoplasia of the main deep venous trunks are maturational stage defects. They may be associated with persistence of the embryonal vein or other large embryonic venous channels as well as enlargement of recognized collateral pathways, such as the marginal vein. However, embryonal and marginal veins can occur with what appears to be a normally formed deep venous system.

Arterial defects tend to occur at later stages of development, usually in the form of aplasia or dilation. The former, occurring in a key segment, may be responsible for persistence of other primitive arterial segments, as is the case with a persistent sciatic artery. Arteriovenous fistulas represent a persistence of primitive connections between future arteries and veins. When this occurs early, during the retiform stage, microfistulas may result, whereas later, macrofistulas result, and occasionally only one or two major AVFs, without a surrounding network of small clustered vessels, are found. Lymphatic hypoplasia-aplasia, which involves the major lymphatics during the maturational phase, may occur alone as in lymphedema praecox, but some degree of hypoplasia also occurs in three-quarters of patients with venous dysplasias or multiple venous angiomata.[6] In contrast, secondary hyperplasia of lymphatics develops in all patients with significant numbers of AVFs. More primitive aberrations of the lymphatic system may be found as lymphatic cysts or multiloculated lymphoceles.

With this background in mind, the Hamburg Classification, which a group of European specialists in CVMs led by Belov[7] devised at an international workshop on CVMs held in Hamburg in 1988, can be considered. Although not universally accepted, even in Europe, it represents the latest, most popular classification system (Table 2). Most of the major categories are divided into truncular and extratruncular forms, which refers to involvement of the more mature, main vessels or trunks, on the one hand, or involvement of more immature, primitive vessels, typically located to the side of the main truncal vessels, on the other. Of the truncular forms, the arterial and venous defects are further divided according to whether they are dilated (aneurysmal) or obstructed/narrowed (hypoplasia, aplasia). Arteriovenous shunting defects are divided into deep and superficial forms, and "combined" defects combine either arterial and venous elements or blood and lymph vessels (hemolymphatic CVMs). All the extratruncular forms are subgrouped into infiltrating (diffuse) or limited (discrete) subtypes, according to whether they diffusely infiltrate the surrounding tissues or are anatomically localized or limited in extent. This approach not only does not acknowledge hemangiomas, which is understandable in that they are not CVMs, but also does not include capillary malformations, which may be the most common, albeit least significant, CVM. The reason given for this decision is that, as isolated findings, capillary malformations are of only cosmetic significance and not the concern of vascular specialists, whereas capillary lesions or nevi that are part of a more complex CVM, as the "birthmark" in the Klippel-Trenaunay or Parkes-Weber syndromes, are covered, as extratruncal elements, in their scheme.

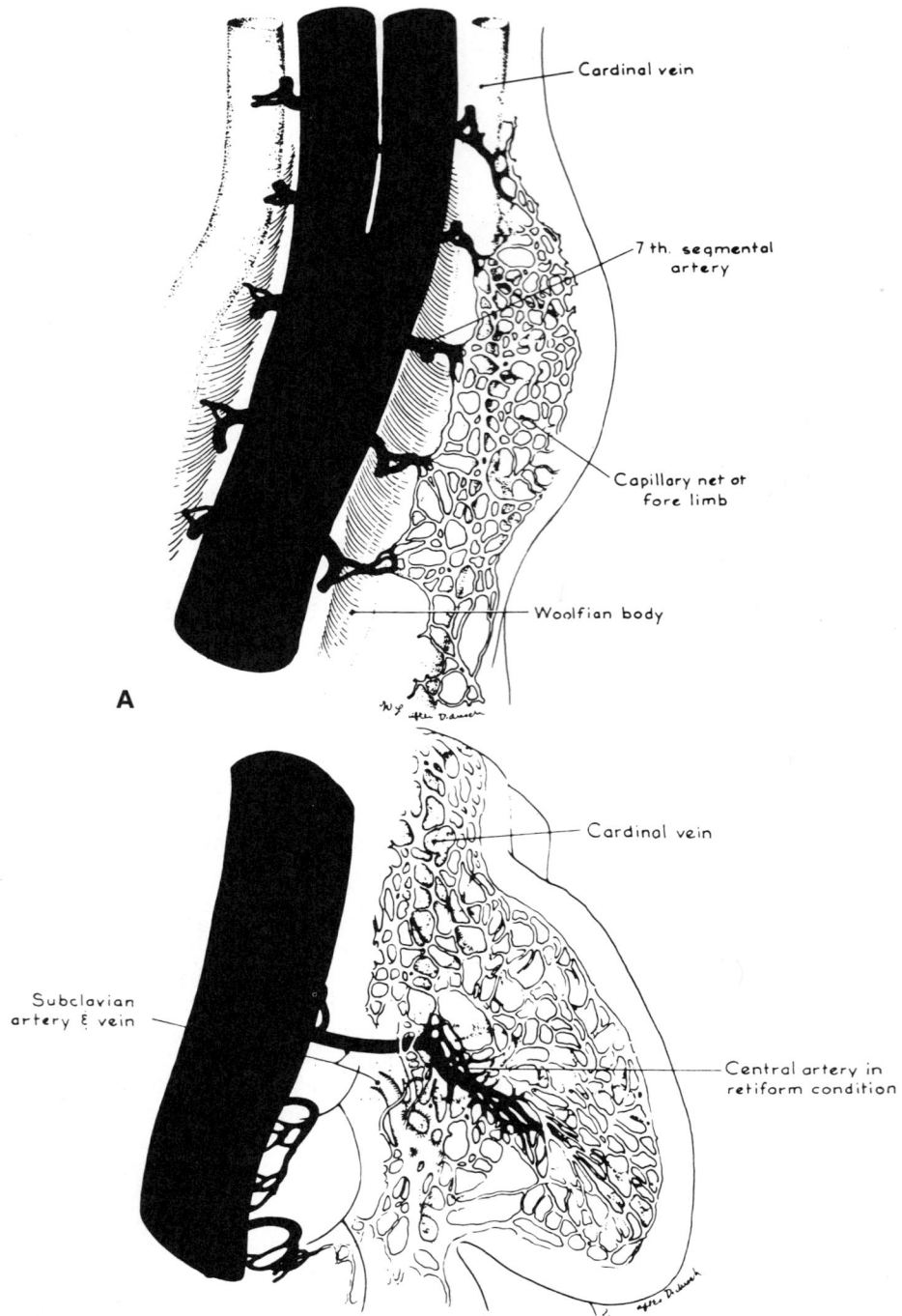

Figure 1 *A*, Capillary network stage of the developing vascular system in the forelimb bud of the 17-day-pig embryo. *B*, Retiform stage of development (20-day pig embryo).
Continued.

Truncular defects represent embryonic dysplasias of differentiated vascular trunks, whereas extratruncular defects are vascular defects derived from remnants of the primitive system. For example, one common truncular form of predominantly venous defects involves hypoplasia of segments of the deep venous system with compensatory persistence and enlargement of superficial pathways, such as a large marginal vein, or of parts of the primitive venous system, such as a persistent embryonal vein. By contrast, clusters of phlebectasias or so-called venous angiomas are often found in the remote backwaters of an otherwise normal venous system. These latter extratruncular forms are venous lagoons or lakes, which are remnants of the intermediate (retiform) stage of the primitive vascular bed. They often infiltrate through muscular compartments and appear in superfi-

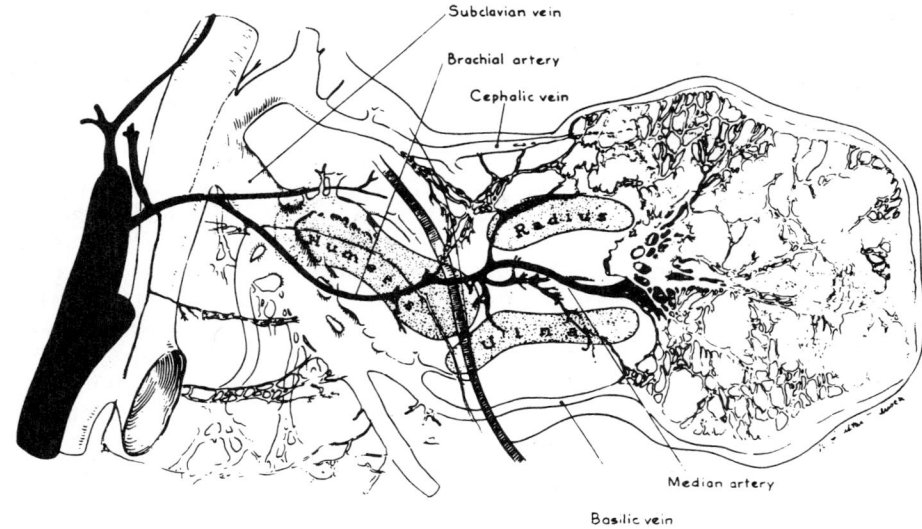

Figure 1, cont'd. *C,* Stage of gross differentiation (27-day pig embryo). Solid structures represent arterial elements; stippled structures, venous elements. (Adapted from Woolard HH: The development of the principal arterial stems in the forelimb of the pig. Contr to Embryology Carnegie Inst 1922; 4:141–154.)

Table 2 Classification of the Congenital Vascular Defects According to Their Species and Anatomical Form: Hamburg Classification 1988

Species		Anatomical Form
Predominantly arterial defects		
	Truncular forms	Aplasia or obstruction / Dilation
	Extratruncular forms	Infiltrating / Limited
Predominantly venous defects		
	Truncular forms	Aplasia or obstruction / Dilation
	Extratruncular forms	Infiltrating / Limited
Predominantly arteriovenous shunting defects		
	Truncular forms	Deep AV fistulas / Superficial AV fistulas
	Extratruncular forms	Infiltrating / Limited
Combined vascular defects		
	Truncular forms	Arterial and venous / Hemolymphatic
	Extratruncular forms	Infiltrating hemolymphatic / Limited hemolymphatic

From Belov ST: Classification, terminology and nosology of congenital vascular defects. In: Belov ST, Loose DA, Weber J, eds. Vascular malformations. Hamburg: Periodica Angiologica 16 Einhorn Presse, 1989:25.

cial tissues. Because they do not usually visualize on routine ascending phlebography, their true extent may be delineated only by direct puncture phlebography or closed-space phlebography, a technique in which injection of contrast is made after exsanguination by tourniquet and Esmark bandaging.

Predominantly venous defects are the most common CVM, comprising close to half of the total, and the extratruncular form is somewhat more common (close to 60%) than the truncular form.[8] In truncular defects of the arterial system, one can find hypoplasia or aplasia of segments of the differentiated arterial tree. Hypoplasia may stimulate collateral development but still result in slow bone growth. In severe cases with aplasia, parts of the primitive system persist in order to provide alternative arterial inflow pathways. The persistent sciatic artery is a classic example. However, predominantly arterial defects are rare, constituting less than 1% of CVMs.[8]

Lesions in which arteriovenous shunting predominates are second only to venous defects in frequency, constituting a little more than one-third of CVMs.[8] The Hamburg Classification arbitrarily divides them into superficial and deep subgroups. There may be good reason for this, but the author prefers to think in terms of macrofistulous and microfistulous lesions. The macrofistulous lesions create a hyperdynamic circulation, can be visualized angiographically, and may be treatable by embolotherapy, surgical excision, or a combination of the two. Such intervention may be required because of their major hemodynamic effects and the symptoms they cause. By contrast, microfistulous AV shunts are often not visualized, have minor or negligible hemodynamic impact, and intervention, which would be difficult in diffuse lesions, is not usually required. Furthermore, the microfistulous type is likely to be diffuse and infiltrative, whereas the macrofistulous type is more likely to be confined to a more circumscribed area, often to the branches of a particular segment or subsegment of the arterial tree. Although these larger congenital AVFs may present difficult challenges and significant risks with attempted surgical excision unless they are relatively well localized, they do respond well to embolotherapy or sclerotherapy applied either sequentially as needed for palliative control of symptoms or as a prelude to surgical excision that allows the latter to be performed more safely and thoroughly. Calling macrofistulous lesions truncular and microfistulous lesions extratruncular might be stretching things a bit, but doing so would make the Hamburg Classification more uniform. Another suggested modification would be to change the terms truncular and extratruncular to mature and primitive, in that the former terms are not as descriptive or familiar to English-speaking physicians.

Finally, combined vascular defects are common. Close to 15% of all CVMs had to be so categorized by the Hamburg system.[8] It would be desirable to limit, if not eliminate, this category by assigning these lesions to one or another of the other categories, arbitrarily classifying them, as suggested by Mulliken and Glowacki,[3] according to the most dominant or important component, for example, the one producing the most serious clinical problems. In this regard, one might be better off assigning these lesions according to the most serious component rather than the one with the largest anatomic contribution.

OVERVIEW

Whereas the Hamburg Classification system has made great strides in putting together a classification scheme that makes a great deal of sense from an anatomic, embryologic, and clinical point of view, a few aspects could be modified to make it even more universally acceptable. As suggested by Mulliken and Glowacki, the scheme could be represented by alphabetic letters and stratified in order of clinical importance, such as AV, A, V, L, and C.[3] Combinations could be used for mixed or combined forms, with the dominant component first and the secondary component second after a hyphen; for example, a venolymphatic malformation would be V-LM. Also as suggested by Mulliken and others, cutaneous lesions should be included. Some terminology other than truncular and extratruncular, which are not comfortable terms in the English language, could be applied, such as mature or primitive or some terms that would also allow AVMs to be divided into macrofistulous and microfistulous types. The final suggested subgrouping would be into diffuse and localized, which is similar to the infiltrating and limited terminology used in the Hamburg system. Finally, common, well-described syndromes could still be applied where useful, such as Klippel-Trenaunay, Parkes-Weber, Sturge-Weber (facial CM with intercranial CVM), Maffucci (LVMs associated with enchondromas), Soloman (CM, VM, intercranial AVM, epidermal nevus), and Proteus (CM, VM, macrodactylia, hemihypertrophy, lipomas, pigmented nevi, scoliosis). Eponyms that have stood the test of time still have some value, but the CVMs they represent could still be classified according to the system. It is anticipated that, at the next meeting of the International Society for Congenital Vascular Malformations, to be held in Budapest in 1994, suggested modifications such as these will be entertained and, hopefully, a universal classification scheme will finally be adopted that will satisfy the many complexities of CVMs but be a little more user-friendly.

REFERENCES

1. Malan E, Puglionisi A. Congenital angiodysplasias of the extremities (Note I: Generalities and classification; venous dysplasias). J Cardiovasc Surg (Torino) 1964; 5:87–130.
2. Degni M, Gerson L, Ishikawa K, et al. Classification of the vascular diseases of the limbs. J Cardiovasc Surg (Torino) 1973; 14:109–116.
3. Mulliken JB, Glowacki J. Hemangiomas and vascular malformations in infants and children: A classification based on endothelial characteristics. Plast Reconstr Surg 1982; 69:412–422.
4. Woolard HH: The development of the principal arterial stems in the forelimb of the pig. Contr to Embryology Carnegie Inst 1922; 4:141–154.
5. Rienhoff WF. Congenital arteriovenous fistula. Bull Johns Hopkins Hosp 1924; 35:271–284.
6. O'Donnell TFJ, Edwards JM, Kinmonth JB. Lymphography in congenital mixed vascular deformities of the lower extremities. J Cardiovasc Surg (Torino) 1976; 17:535–540.
7. Belov ST: Classification of congenital vascular defects. Int Angiol 1990; 9:141–146.
8. Tasnadi G. Clinical investigations in epidemiology of congenital vascular defects. In: P. Balas, ed. Progress in angiology. Torino: Edizioni Minerva Medica, 1992:391.

EVALUATION OF CONGENITAL VASCULAR MALFORMATIONS OF THE EXTREMITIES BY NONANGIOGRAPHIC METHODS

WILLIAM H. PEARCE, M.D.
ROBERT L. VOGELZANG, M.D.

Congenital vascular malformations represent the failure of the orderly development of the vascular system. As a result, these complex lesions may contain all components of the circulatory system. To fully evaluate these lesions, it is necessary to define, first, the dominant abnormality—arterial, venous, capillary, or lymphatic—and, second, the exact anatomic location. To obtain this information, a combination of direct imaging—computed tomography (CT) or magnetic resonance imaging (MRI)—and noninvasive hemodynamic testing is necessary. CT or MRI provides anatomic detail that is not possible with either arteriography or noninvasive testing. These imaging modalities accurately define the involvement of adjacent musculoskeletal elements. With present technology, however, CT and MRI do not provide arterial or venous hemodynamics. Computed tomography angiography (CTA) and magnetic resonance angiography (MRA) are emerging technologies that may add this information. At present, however, the duplex scan is used to estimate total limb blood flow and to define the characteristics of the lesion. Doppler studies are also useful to estimate cardiac output in patients with high output cardiac failure from arteriovenous fistulas (AVFs). Thus, no single test is able to supply all information necessary to accurately assess the abnormal anatomy and physiology of major vascular malformations. Arteriography and phlebography remain essential for many patients, particularly those for whom operation is contemplated.

PATHOGENESIS

Vascular malformations occur as an inborn error in normal embryologic development. The circulatory system is formed during three distinct embryologic stages: undifferentiated capillary network, retiform plexus, and formation of mature vessels. In the earliest phases of embryologic development, undifferentiated mesenchymal cells form cords with the development of angioblasts. These early capillary cells spontaneously form tubelike structures that are biologically similar to cells derived from capillary hemangiomas. During the retiform plexus stage, these structures coalesce to form recognizable blood vessels. The growth and development of these primitive blood vessels are then dependent on the establishment of normal hemodynamics. A failure in the early stages of embryologic development produces a congenital AVF with secondary venous and arterial enlargement. Large venous lakes and persistent fetal arteries are the manifestations of later embryologic events. Although many systems of classification and descriptive terms have been used to characterize congenital vascular malformations, the system described by Mulliken is perhaps the most useful and understandable.[1] In this system, vascular birthmarks are divided into either hemangiomas or malformations. Hemangiomas are well-circumscribed lesions that rapidly proliferate after birth, followed by a period of slow involution. Vascular malformations, although present at birth, are slow to expand and are not generally noticed until adolescence or later. Vascular malformations are complex lesions with a variety of manifestations and findings, depending on the dominant lesion—arterial, venous, lymphatic, or capillary.

ANATOMY

Computed Tomography Scan

Dynamic CT scanning with contrast enhancement identifies the location of the vascular malformation and documents associated musculoskeletal abnormalities.[2,3] For best results, a rapid bolus injection of contrast material is given with serial CT imaging. Deep intramuscular lesions give a muddled appearance, depending on the degree of cellularity and arteriovenous shunting. Contrast enhancement of a lesion is greater in high-flow fistulas with little cellularity and lower in lesions with low flow and a high degree of cellularity. Highly cellular vascular malformations may not enhance and, therefore, are underestimated by CT. In addition, associated bony involvement is easily detected by CT. Osseus erosion and calcified phleboliths are typical findings of some vascular malformations. Contrast-enhanced CT scanning also documents secondary arterial or venous enlargement resulting from increased arterial blood flow. Late aneurysm formation of the feeding artery is common. As with atherosclerotic aneurysms, the arterial wall is calcified. However, intraluminal thrombus is rare because of the high flow. The CT image is reconstructed in the transverse plane. A three-dimensional image is possible with special software and is best derived from spiral CT. Both three-dimensional reconstruction and CTA are possible with the new generation of spiral and ultrafast CT scanners. This new generation of CT scanners provides high-resolution, thin slices in rapid sequence. This technology has been untested in peripheral arteriovenous malformations (AVMs).

Magnetic Resonance Imaging

Yet another method of assessing congenital vascular malformations is MRI. The MRI is particularly suited for this purpose because of its tissue differentiation and ability to detect flow patterns.[4] Muscle groups are clearly defined by MRI, and invasion by an adjoining AVM is detected. Depending on the cellularity and blood content of the lesion, the vascular malformation appears as a bright image. The blood may be pulsed prior to entering the field of interest using the principle of time of flight. Here blood appears bright on subsequent images. On standard MRI, high-flow feeding vessels are identified as black holes that signify the passage of blood through the field.

Hemodynamic Studies

In a broad sense, vascular malformations may be grouped into three categories: high-flow AVMs and the low-flow malformations, venous and lymphatic. These categories are distinguished on the basis of noninvasive testing. The abnormal hemodynamics associated with arteriovenous arterial blood pressure are characterized by decreased resistance, decreased mean arterial blood pressure, increased venous blood pressure, and venous pulsatility.[5,6] Depending on the magnitude of shunting, these characteristics may vary. In large AVFs, arterial blood flow is high. Arterial blood flow is normal or only slightly elevated with microfistulas and venous and lymphatic malformations.

Segmental limb blood pressures are useful only when shunting through the fistula is sufficient to decrease distal arterial blood pressure. Digital blood pressures are more valuable because they may be reduced despite normal proximal blood pressures. Pulse volume recordings document similar findings, including increased pulsatility proximal to the fistulas and diminishment of pulsatility distal to the fistulas. Perhaps the simplest of all techniques is the handheld Doppler. Analysis of the waveform proximal to the fistulas documents increased forward flow and loss of reversal flow due to diminished resistance. In the artery distal to the fistulas, there is reversal flow that is continuous throughout the cardiac cycle. Also, in the veins draining the fistulas, there is continuous forward blood flow and pulsatility. With a discrete arteriovenous communication, it may be possible to occlude the arteriovenous communication and ablate the venous pulsatility. In patients with primary venous and lymphatic abnormalities, limb arterial hemodynamics are not altered.

The duplex scan with the color flow Doppler is currently our noninvasive diagnostic modality of choice. The duplex scan provides both an anatomic evaluation and hemodynamic evaluation of peripheral arteriovenous arteries and veins. However, current literature regarding the use of the duplex scan in congenital AVFs deals predominantly with intracranial vascular malformations in infants.[7] With the duplex scan, feeding vessels and draining veins are visualized intracranially. Further, changes in carotid artery blood flow are detected in large intracranial AVMs. Noninvasive assessment of cardiac output is also useful in infants with congestive heart failure secondary to high-output heart failure. In adolescents and adults, the duplex scan provides important information in patients with suspected high-flow AVMs. In the affected extremity, the major axial artery, femoral or subclavian, is visualized and the diameter determined. The diameter of the artery on the side of the vascular malformation is often larger than the contralateral extremity because of the adaptive enlargement with high blood flow. In addition, the arterial waveform documents a loss of resistance with increased velocity. A resistance index has been calculated for intracranial vascular malformations. (Peak systolic velocity − End-diastolic velocity / Peak systolic velocity). However, this formula has not been applied to other vascular malformations. An estimate of total blood flow is made when both the diameter of the vessel and the velocity of blood flow are known. If the arterial blood flow is not different on the affected side, the venous system is studied in detail. Major venous abnormalities often have incomplete deep systems with large lateral veins and aneurysm formation. Careful characterization of the deep venous system is most useful in diagnosing Klippel-Trenaunay syndrome.

IMAGING RESULTS

The results of the surgical treatment of congenital vascular malformations have, in general, been poor. The diffuse nature of these lesions and the inability to completely excise the arteriovenous communications have led to a high recurrence. These poor results reflect the limitations of our ability to accurately analyze such lesions. Previous clinical studies relied upon arteriography and to a lesser extent phlebography for diagnosis. In only the past several years have we gained a clear appreciation of the anatomic and physiologic complexities of these lesions by using ultrasound and newer imaging techniques. By using a multimodality approach, we are better able to select patients to undergo operation than in previous years. A comparison of commonly performed noninvasive tests in the evaluation of congenital vascular malformations is useful (Table 1). Arteriography and phlebography remain essential for patients in whom therapeutic interventions are being contemplated. Noninvasive testing and other imaging techniques provide additional information on the anatomy and physiology of the lesion. The hemodynamic data provided by the duplex scan estimate total limb flow, which is useful not only in diagnosing the vascular malformation but also in monitoring the success or failure of the surgical or radiologic intervention. If, for example, limb blood flow is unchanged after embolization, prognosis for cure is poor. We have had experience with patients who have undergone embolization with dramatic reduction of arterial blood flow in the affected limb. However, there has been a gradual recurrence of high flow. This finding is not unexpected, as new vessels are recruited to the low-resistance AVM.

The MRI is our imaging technique of choice for many patients with congenital vascular malformations. The ability to manipulate the image, both in tissue

Table 1 · Imaging of Vascular Malformations

	Arterial	Venous Malformation	Lymphatic Malformation
Computed tomography	Enhancing vascular mass Enlarged arteries and veins	Enhancing vascular mass Enlarged draining veins	Mass +/− enhancement No enlarged vessels
Magnetic resonance imaging	Flow voids in mass and draining vessels	*Signal brightness* *T1*: fat greater than malformation muscle (fat is the brightest tissue in the field) *T2*: malformation greater than fat muscle (malformation is the brightest tissue in the field)	*Signal brightness* Same as venous malformation
Ultrasound	Resistance index = 0 Increased flow velocity and volume flow	Resistance index: normal Dilated veins Normal flow	Resistance index: normal Normal flows

characterization and in reconstruction, makes it ideal. With the improvement in technology, it will be possible to quantify the blood flow in the feeding artery and draining vein. Similar to the duplex scan, these parameters may be used to follow therapy in a serial fashion and to determine the success or failure of treatment.

REFERENCES

1. Mulliken JB. Classification of vascular birthmarks. In: Mulliken JB, Young AE, eds. Vascular birthmarks. Philadelphia: WB Saunders, 1988:24–37.
2. Rauch RF, Silverman PM, Korobkin M, et al. Computed tomography of benign angiomatous lesions of the extremities. J Comput Assist Tomogr 1984; 8:1143–1146.
3. Bernardino ME, Jing BS, Thomas JL, et al. The extremity soft-tissue lesion: A comparative study of ultrasound, computed tomography and xeroradiography. Radiology 1981; 189:53–59.
4. Pearce WH, Rutherford RB, Whitehill TA, et al. Nuclear magnetic resonance imaging: Its diagnostic value in patients with congenital vascular malformations. J Vasc Surg 1988; 8:64–70.
5. Rutherford RB. Noninvasive testing in the diagnosis and assessment of arteriovenous fistulae. In: Bernstein E, ed. Vascular diagnosis. 4th ed. St. Louis: Mosby–Year Book, 1993:549–555.
6. Barnes RW. Noninvasive assessment of arteriovenous fistulae. Angiology 1978; 29:691–703.
7. Westra SJ, Curran JG, Duckwiler GR, et al. Pediatric intracranial vascular malformations: Evaluation of treatment results with color Doppler US. Radiology 1993; 186:775–783.

ACQUIRED ARTERIOVENOUS FISTULA

S. MARTIN LINDENAUER, M.D.

Acquired arteriovenous fistulas (AVFs) are almost exclusively the result of penetrating trauma caused by a knife, bullet, or other missile with simultaneous injury to an adjacent artery and vein (Fig. 1). Because traumatic vascular injuries occur most often to the extremities, the arms and legs are frequent sites for AVF. They also may occur when a similar injury takes place after suture ligation (Fig. 2) or percutaneous puncture for diagnostic study and, rarely, due to erosion of an adjacent vein by an atherosclerotic aneurysm, periarterial abscess, or neoplasm. Aortic aneurysm erosion most often occurs into the infrarenal vena cava, less often into a common iliac vein, and rarely into the left renal vein. With the advent of the in situ vein bypass technique, an overlooked branch of the vein bypass can result in an AVF.

Because most acquired AVFs are due to traumatic penetrating wounds, a concentrated experience in their management was reported in World War II, the Korean Conflict, and the Vietnam War. A less concentrated but continuing experience has been reported over the last three decades as the result of civilian violence in most large American urban regions. A steadily growing number of iatrogenic AVFs is a reflection of increasing percutaneous procedures performed in the groin for a multitude of diagnostic and therapeutic cardiac and radiographic procedures,[1] as well as percutaneous tissue biopsy for diagnosis of solid organ disease and for the assessment of transplanted organs.

William Hunter's early description included follow-up information on two patients over 5 years and 14 years and led him to comment that an AVF, "if not disturbed, produces no mischief.... I presume it will be best to do nothing." Despite this admonition, many attempts were made in subsequent years to define the most appropriate operative therapy. Historical surgical treatment techniques include proximal artery ligation, proximal and distal arterial ligation, proximal and distal artery and vein ligation (four-vessel ligation), and

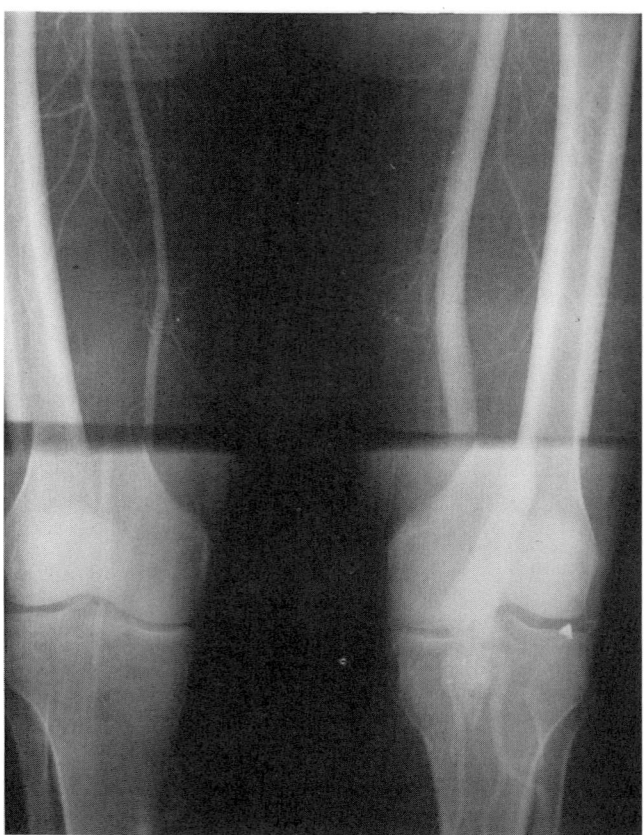

Figure 1 Arteriogram of lower extremities demonstrating a popliteal arteriovenous fistula in left leg. Note metallic projectile at lateral joint line and dilation of popliteal and superficial femoral artery.

nonsurgical intervention. Delay in definitive repair was recommended as recently as 1946 because of the lack of uniformly successful results. Delayed repair allows time for collateral circulation to develop and provide distal perfusion if direct arterial repair is not achieved. Although the presence of an acquired AVF in an extremity usually allows easy vascular exposure and control, the occurrence of a similar fistula in the head, neck, or trunk can be a demanding challenge in regard to exposure and control for even the most skilled and experienced surgeon.

PATHOPHYSIOLOGY

In a significant number of instances, a small AVF associated with in situ vein bypass grafts closes spontaneously. The reason is unclear but may relate to the volume flow through such connections and the capacity of the venous outflow bed.

In patients with an acquired AVF secondary to femoral catheterization, many such lesions resolved spontaneously.[1] Duplex scanning allows these lesions to be properly identified and to be followed and evaluated serially in a noninvasive fashion. Patients who undergo coronary balloon angioplasty are more likely to develop a femoral vascular complication that is less likely to resolve spontaneously than patients with lesions due to diagnostic catheterization. Femoral artery lesions that persist beyond 3 months should be repaired electively to avoid further complications.

The AVF that persists for several years has dilation and ectasia of the proximal artery, and the corresponding vein becomes thick-walled and dilated. These vessels are

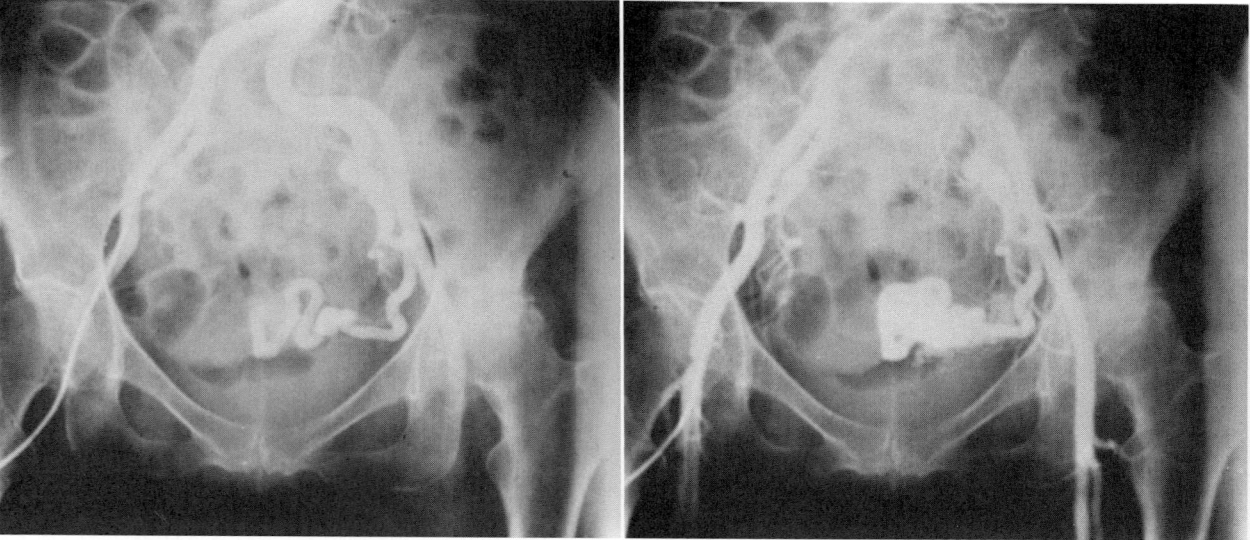

Figure 2 *A*, Early phase of pelvic arteriogram in a patient who has had a hysterectomy. Note dilated hypogastric and uterine artery on left. *B*, Later phase of pelvic arteriogram. Note uterine arteriovenous aneurysm with early venous fill and simultaneous visualization of hypogastric artery and vein (From Morley GW, Lindenauer SM. Arteriovenous fistula following pelvic operations. Obstet Gynecol 1968; 31:722; with permission.)

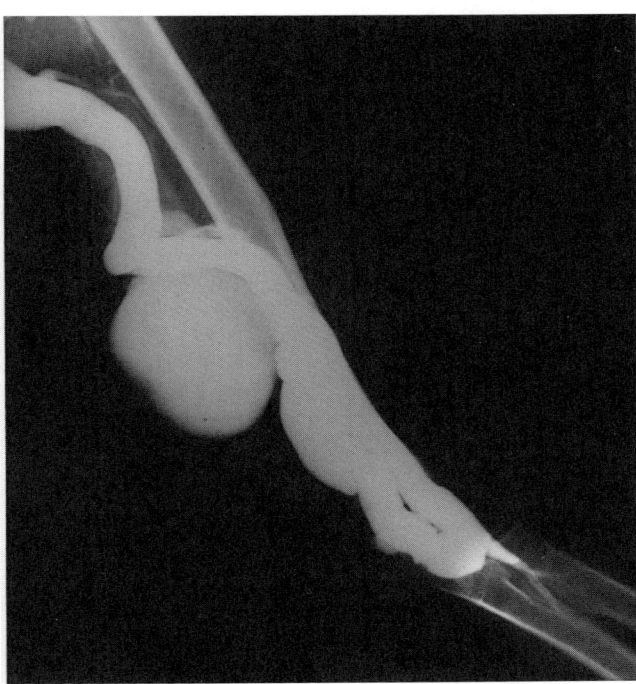

Figure 3 Arteriogram of chronic brachial artery arteriovenous fistula. Note arterial dilation early venous fill, venous dilation, and venous aneurysm (From Thompson NW, Lindenauer SM. Central venous aneurysm and arteriovenous fistulas. Ann Surg 1969; 170:852; with permission.)

unduly fragile and difficult to handle and may present problems when sutured. The intimal damage that occurs at the site of an AVF places this area at increased risk for infection, and bacterial endarteritis may occur. Depending upon the size of the fistula and its location, a significant amount of blood may be diverted through the fistula and result in symptoms of peripheral arterial insufficiency, venous congestion, venous valvular insufficiency, and edema formation. Venous stasis changes may occur and cause permanent damage to the skin and subcutaneous tissues. Varicosities may appear, and there may be an increase in limb girth. In young children, extremity AVF can lead to limb length inequality if the AVF is present before epiphyseal fusion.

Patients with large fistulas may have tachycardia, an increase in pulse pressure, and a decrease in diastolic blood pressure, as well as increased blood volume, cardiac output, stroke volume, heart rate, and central venous pressures. There may be cardiomegaly and signs of high-output congestive failure. Temporary compression of the fistula sometimes elicits a Branham-Nicoladoni sign with a rise in diastolic blood pressure and a fall in heart rate. This reflex is mediated by the vagus nerve and abolished by atropine.

The venous changes and possible venous aneurysm formation (Fig. 3) are usually not reversed by closure of the fistula, whereas the high-output congestive heart failure usually returns to normal promptly after fistula closure.

Arteriovenous fistulas between major abdominal arteries and veins are uncommon but can produce dramatic major hemodynamic alterations. Aortocaval fistula occurs most often from aneurysmal rupture into the inferior vena cava, whereas trauma and iatrogenic causes occur only rarely. Most aortocaval fistulas present with dramatic symptoms compatible with aortic rupture. There is a widened pulse pressure, a continuous abdominal bruit, dyspnea, cardiomegaly, extremity edema and mottling, and congestive heart failure. Gross hematuria is a common finding. The hematuria may originate from the kidneys or from dilated bladder veins with subsequent mucosal hemorrhage. The kidney may be a source of hematuria, probably as a result of renal injury caused by high retrograde renal vein pressure and an alteration in the pulse contour of the renal arterial blood flow.

DIAGNOSIS

Before one embarks upon operative repair of an AVF, it is mandatory to obtain precise arteriographic documentation of the relevant vascular anatomy. Arteriography is the preferred diagnostic procedure to document an AVF.[2] The fistula is readily identified by the presence of a dilated afferent artery with early venous filling and simultaneous visualization of arteries and veins. The increased vascularity may make it difficult to ascertain the precise site of communication. In selected instances, magnetic resonance imaging[3] and computed tomography[4] may be helpful in displaying the relevant arteriovenous anatomy and the exact site of the fistulous connection. Color flow duplex scanning has been used with success for noninvasive imaging of AVFs in the groin after catheterization injury.[5] It is occasionally useful in other locations as well. Aside from color flow duplex scanning in the groin, arteriography remains the mainstay of diagnosis in AVF.

TREATMENT

The technical aspects of the operative treatment of an AVF are similar to well-established standard vascular surgical techniques and require no elaboration. However, the difficulty of repairing such injuries should never be underestimated, and the importance of proximal and distal arterial and venous control cannot be overemphasized. When proximal and distal control have been obtained, the procedure is often facilitated by directly incising the arteriovenous connection or the connecting arteriovenous aneurysm, if present. Liberal use of the balloon embolectomy catheter is helpful to exclude and remove thrombi that may have been present or formed in the process of dissection. However, the balloon catheter must be used with caution in the venous segments so that injury to adjacent valves is avoided. Repair of veins the size of the popliteal or larger is feasible. Tibial veins most often are appropriately ligated because long-term patency is unlikely unless the vein is unusually dilated or there has been concomitant destruction of the remainder of the deep venous circulation. Preservation of the venous circulation may enhance the probability of successful arterial repair, and such efforts are appropriate if there has been concomitant unreconstructible loss of other main vessels. Operative completion arteriography is helpful and can document correctable technical errors.

Experience over the past 40 years has clearly defined optimal operative treatment: obliteration of the arteriovenous connection and restoration of normal arterial and venous blood flow.[2] It is occasionally facilitated by interposition of a vein autograft or prosthetic material in the arterial repair and the occasional requirement for a venous autograft for repair of the residual vein defect. Most often the venous defect can be managed by lateral suture.

If an arterial graft is required, an autogenous vein is preferred when the repair is in an extremity, whereas prosthetic materials serve equally well in larger vessels of the pelvis, trunk, and root of the neck.

If a venous autograft is required, it should be obtained from an unaffected extremity because of the significant potential for failure of the venous reconstruction. Furthermore, a large (1 cm) AVF in a vessel such as the superficial femoral or popliteal artery results in valvular incompetence of the deep venous circulation. Therefore, venous return should not be compromised further by interruption of the superficial venous circulation, which might occur if a vein autograft is required and it is obtained from the ipsilateral extremity.

Although successful restoration of arterial and venous blood flow can almost always be accomplished, on rare occasions four-vessel ligation may be required in a desperate circumstance as a lifesaving measure. Occasionally, following such a maneuver, the collateral circulation is sufficient to preserve viability of the distal extremity and allow time for a subsequent bypass procedure to be performed.

It is not appropriate to await the development of collateral circulation. In reality, the presence of multiple collateral channels in the area of a fistula adds an unnecessary measure of technical difficulty. Delay in repair only provides an opportunity for complications, such as bacterial endarteritis at the site of the fistula, cardiomegaly, and occasionally high-output congestive heart failure. Within days after formation of an AVF, proximal arterial dilation and proximal and distal venous dilation occur. If the fistula is present for a number of years and is large, the arterial wall degenerates. Structural weakening may manifest itself in unexpected and striking friability of the artery wall and sometimes result in technical difficulty in suture repair of the artery.

Certain fistulas may present technical difficulty in surgical closure. Such lesions can be safely eliminated by arterial embolization with wire coils, woolen tufts, autologous clot, gelatin sponge soaked in diatrizoate sodium, and detachable balloons[6] (Fig. 4). Embolization may be useful when extremity wounds are complex, such as those caused by shotgun blasts with multiple injuries to the femoral arterial system. Embolic occlusion of the profunda femoris artery is readily tolerated when the

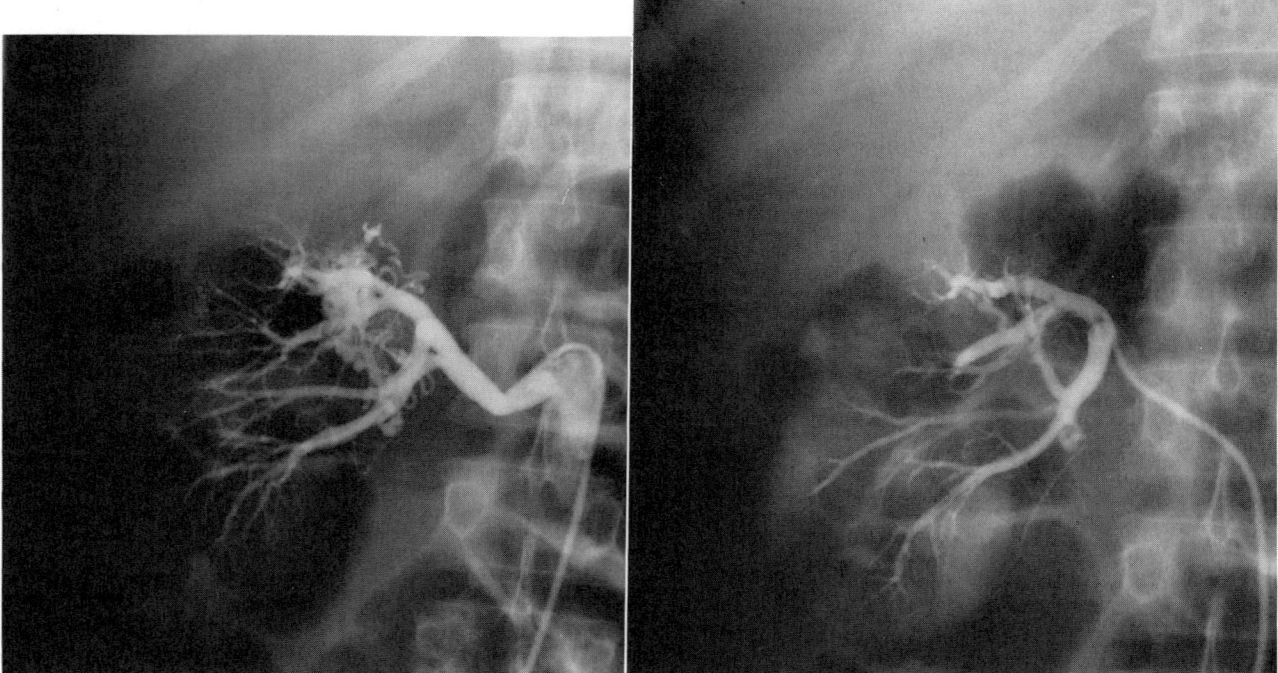

Figure 4 *A*, Arteriogram of renal arteriovenous fistula. Note early venous fill. *B*, Renal arteriogram following intra-arterial embolization. Note absence of early venous fill.

superficial femoral system is intact. Fistulas between the hypogastric artery and vein may also be difficult to control and can be successfully managed by embolization.

Embolization is not without complications. Distal ischemia, infarction, embolization to an undesired artery, and transvenous migration with pulmonary embolism have been reported. Embolization should be reserved for selected instances in which surgical exposure would be hazardous.

Hepatic artery to portal vein fistulas may occur as the result of both penetrating and blunt trauma. Although resection of the involved liver segment is possible, embolization of the involved artery is more easily accomplished.

Detachable balloons, although widely used as embolization material in neurovascular AVFs, are rarely used outside the head.[7] Detachable balloons offer a safe and precise method of embolization because they can be sited accurately, deflated, and repositioned if appropriate occlusion is not initially obtained. The balloons are advanced to the desired location and inflated with contrast material for evaluation of the balloon position. When the balloon is optimally positioned, it is filled with a silicone monomer that solidifies at body temperature, and the balloon is then detached. The two most common problems with the use of detachable balloons are early deflation and premature detachment.

A groin fistula can be treated by manual compression of the AVF track with the ultrasound transducer, and the real-time imaging allows precise localization and occlusion of the fistula. The amount of compression needed for occlusion can be determined by noting the disappearance of blood flow on the Doppler image. After 30 minutes of compression, Doppler imaging usually documents occlusion of the fistula.[8] Among the factors that increase the possibility of successful compression therapy are the age of the fistulous track (tracks more than 1 month old that have endothelialized are more difficult to thrombose than newer fistulas) and the anatomic characteristic of the track (long, thin tracks are easier to compress than short, broad tracks).

A recent report describes repair of a femoral AVF by endovascular placement of an intraluminal graft covered stent. The balloon expandable stented graft was used to obliterate an AVF due to a bullet injury to the superficial femoral artery and vein.[9]

Successful repair should be associated with the presence of easily palpable peripheral pulses. The absence of palpable pulses upon completion of the procedure should alert the surgeon to the possibility of technical error requiring further investigation and revision. Postoperative use of heparin sodium is not usually required for maintenance of the arterial repair; however, its cautious use may be considered to maintain the patency of the venous repair. Low-molecular-weight dextran (molecular weight 40,000) given for several days postoperatively (500 ml/day) may be of value and is associated with minimal risk of bleeding. Similarly, extremity elevation and external elastic compression may be useful to help maintain patency of the venous repair. Presence of a thrill or bruit postoperatively or the characteristic signal obtained from a Doppler ultrasonic velocity detector indicates failure of obliteration of the fistula or an overlooked second fistulous connection, which should be investigated, delineated, and repaired after a suitable interval. Successful long-term repair and normal function are expected in the vast majority of patients except those in whom there has been loss of venous valvular competence or when definitive repair has been long delayed.

When an AVF has been present for several years prior to repair, following repair long-term surveillance is required because of the risk of degeneration of the proximal artery with late aneurysm formation.[10]

REFERENCES

1. Kent KC, McArdle CR, Kennedy B, et al. A prospective study of the clinical outcome of femoral pseudoaneurysms and arteriovenous fistulas induced by arterial puncture. J Vasc Surg 1993; 17:125–133.
2. Osmundson PJ. Arteriovenous communications. Cardiovasc Clin 1992; 22:127–134.
3. Hatch WD, Pentecost MJ, Colletti PM, Weaver FA. Magnetic resonance imaging of a post-traumatic arteriovenous fistula in the lower extremity. Magn Reson Imaging 1991; 9:459–462.
4. Nakayama T, Hiyama Y, Ohnishi K, et al. Arterioportal shunts on dynamic computed tomography. Am J Roentgenol 1983; 140:953–957.
5. Roubidoux MA, Hertzberg BS, Carroll BA, Hedgepeth CA. Color flow and image-directed Doppler ultrasound evaluation of iatrogenic arteriovenous fistulas in the groin. JCU 1990; 18:463–489.
6. Ricketts RR, Finck E, Yellin AE. Management of major arteriovenous fistulas by arteriographic techniques. Arch Surg 1978; 113:1153–1159.
7. DeSouza NM, Reidy JF. Embolization with detachable balloons—applications outside the head. Clin Radiol 1992; 46:170–175.
8. Fellmeth BD, Roberts AC, Booksein JJ, et al. Postangiographic femoral artery injuries: Nonsurgical repair with US-guided compression. Radiology 1991; 178:671–675.
9. Marin ML, Veith FJ, Panetta TF, et al. Percutaneous transfemoral insertion of a stented graft to repair a traumatic femoral arteriovenous fistula. J Vasc Surg 1993; 18:299–302.
10. Lindenauer SM, Thompson NW, Kraft RD, Fry WJ. Late complications of traumatic arteriovenous fistula. Surg Gynecol Obstet 1969; 129:525–532.

CONGENITAL VASCULAR LESIONS IN INFANCY AND CHILDHOOD

STEVEN R. BUCHMAN, M.D.
DAVID J. SMITH, M.D.

Vascular anomalies in children are a frequent source of anxiety and concern to patients and their families, often requiring surgical evaluation and treatment. Perhaps the most important approach to managing the protean manifestations of vascular malformations is to classify them in a logical and orderly way (Fig. 1). An accurate classification method guided by an understanding of pathogenesis aids in arriving at a proper diagnosis, allows a realistic prognosis, and provides the basis for an effective treatment strategy.

The most sensible first step to take in evaluating a congenital vascular lesion is to separate the hemangiomas from all other vascular malformations. A congenital hemangioma displays histologic behavior and a clinical course that distinguishes it from other vascular lesions. These differences present a distinct set of problems and complications, calling for judicious management options in light of the unique natural history of the disease.

HEMANGIOMA

The hemangioma may be the most common tumor in the neonate. The incidence in the first week of life has been reported to be up to 2.6%. Most of these vascular lesions, however, manifest themselves clinically by 1 year of age, translating into a published frequency of between 10% and 12% for white infants. Females are affected more often than males at a ratio of about 3:1. Eighty percent of hemangiomas arise as an isolated finding; 60% are found in the head and neck, 25% in the trunk, and 15% in the extremities. These vascular anomalies may also be present in visceral organs; however, they frequently have simultaneous manifestations of the skin.

Histologically, these malformations exhibit endothelial hyperplasia concurrent with neovascularization and the formation of dilated vascular channels. The rapid neonatal proliferation of cells often appears as a syncytial mass interspersed with convoluted vascular lumina.

A complete and careful history from the parents is the most important determinant in the diagnosis of a hemangioma. The overwhelming majority of hemangiomas are not apparent at birth, but rather present in the first to fourth week of life. The sine qua non of the hemangioma is rapid proliferation, often commencing the first week after birth. The exuberant growth of the lesion is disproportionate to the growth of the child. Enlargement can proceed at an alarming rate during the first few months of life, often prompting overwhelming parental concern.

Physical examination as well as serial evaluation helps to corroborate clinical suspicions. These lesions most commonly appear as a flat red mark or a blotchy telangiectasia. Hemangiomas usually involve the superficial dermis and, as they grow, take on a coarse and stippled appearance with a darker, more intense scarlet color. Initially, the small, proliferating hemangioma was described as looking like a strawberry, hence the name strawberry hemangioma. These clinical descriptions, however, are unreliable and predispose to oversimplification and misdiagnoses. Deep lesions confined to the subcutaneous tissue exhibit the same proliferative growth phase common to all hemangiomas but may be

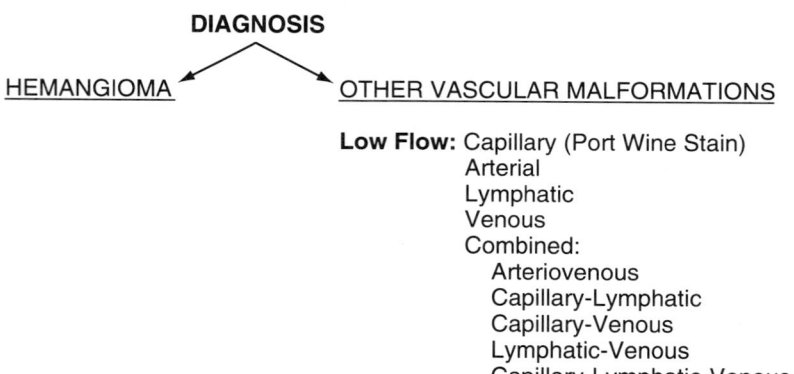

Figure 1 Classification of vascular malformations. (Adapted from Mulliken JB, Glowacki J. Hemangiomas and vascular malformations in infants and children: A classification based on endothelial characteristics. Plast Reconstr Surg 1982; 69:412; with permission.)

more difficult to diagnose (Fig. 2). These lesions may have normal-looking overlying skin or may transmit a faint bluish hue. Palpation reveals a noncompressible, rubbery, firm mass.

Extensive testing is not usually indicated in the evaluation of a hemangioma. However, complicated problems may require imaging the lesion using computed tomographic (CT) scan, magnetic resonance imaging (MRI), ultrasound, or even angiography. A deep hemangioma presenting as a firm, rapidly growing mass may need to be differentiated from a sarcoma. In these patients, radiographic evaluation and even biopsies may be necessary.

The angiographic appearance of a hemangioma is that of a homogeneous, well-circumscribed mass with a lobular pattern, prolonged tissue staining, and occasional feeding arteries. Computerized tomography with contrast as well as MRI with weighted imaging can provide a less invasive way to differentiate deep hemangiomas from other vascular malformations as well as from soft tissue tumors. Ultrasound can be helpful in characterizing a deep lesion as cystic or solid.

The natural history of these vascular anomalies is characterized by involution, regression, and resolution. Therefore, immediate treatment of uncomplicated hemangiomas is not necessary because virtually all will involute with time. Disproportionate growth usually slows within the first 6 months of life and finally ceases. Involution often starts by 6 to 10 months of age. A distinct phase of regression cannot usually be seen; instead, these lesions often exhibit a hybrid behavior of concurrent proliferation and involution. As regression continues, the hemangioma flattens, the color fades, and the mass shrinks in size. The skin texture may return to normal, exhibit areas of redundancy and wrinkling, or leave small atrophic patches. Complete resolution of hemangiomas can be documented in 50% of children by 5 years of age and in 70% of children by age 7. The final 30% of patients have continued regression of their lesions until the age of 12.

The goal of expectant care is to allow involution to progress to the point that excision is either not necessary or requires a much smaller procedure minimizing any long-term deformity. The benefits of this therapeutic plan must be balanced with the often severe psychosocial impact that, for example, a disfiguring facial hemangioma can have on a school-age child. When it is obvious that surgical intervention will ultimately be required, a procedure to improve shape and contour before the child starts school may be warranted. The balance of reconstructive efforts should be reserved for early adolescence when regression is complete.

The most challenging aspect in following the proper conservative course of serial inspection and expectant care is to console the overwhelming sense of anguish felt by the parents. Frequently, the child looks essentially normal at birth and the rapid progression of the often gruesome deformity may incite demands for action. Fear and frustration must be addressed with reassurance and empathy. Close consultation and family education can engender confidence and support during times of seemingly callous inaction.

Steroids are effective for patients requiring early intervention. The use of systemic steroids should be approached with caution in a growing child; however, their palliative effect in emergent situations can not be overstated. Treatment should be based on the sensitivity and response of the lesion. A trial of systemic therapy should be started using 2 to 3 mg/kg/day with a response evident by 10 days. Lesions responding to treatment should lighten in color and decrease in their rate of growth. If no change is observed, therapy should be discontinued. If a positive reaction is seen, the dose should be adjusted to a lower effective level. A cycle of 4 to 6 weeks of treatment at the lower steroid dose should be instituted. Additional treatment cycles can be tried on an individual basis, if rebound occurs. Once the entire lesion is in a stage of regression, there is no need to continue steroids. The goal of treatment should be the lowest effective steroid dose over the shortest duration to effect regression. Side effects of short-term systemic steroids in children include facial edema, decreased growth and appetite, and an increase in the rate of infection.

Flash lamp pulsed tuneable dye laser therapy for cutaneous proliferative lesions is controversial. Proponents claim that laser ablation of small lesions can be pre-emptive and forestall proliferative sequelae of a hemangioma. In practical terms many of these lesions do not present until proliferation is underway. Critics of the laser techniques note that too many treatments are required for too little effect and that the associated scarring may leave more of a deformity than involution and regression.

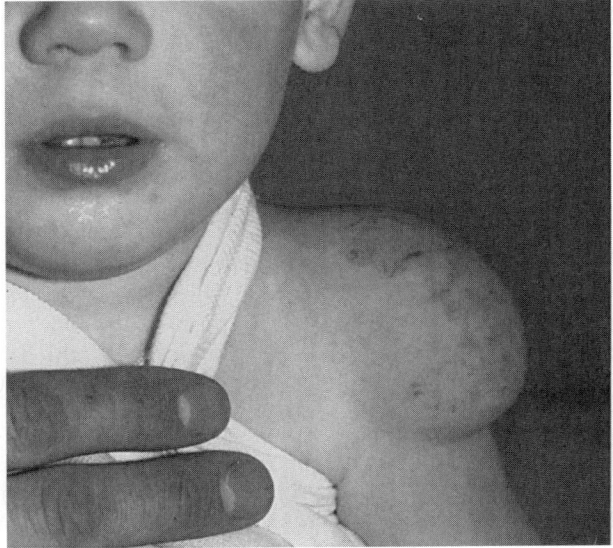

Figure 2 This 13-month-old child presented with a deep hemangioma predominantly in the subcutaneous tissue. A careful history and physical examination was the most important factor in confirming the diagnosis.

PROBLEMS ASSOCIATED WITH HEMANGIOMAS

Obstruction

Specific circumstances, such as a lesion adjacent to the eyelids, can affect normal functional development and necessitate more aggressive treatment. A hemangioma close to the eye may have enormous impact on ophthalmologic growth and performance. Visual field obstruction can induce deprivation amblyopia, which, unless quickly treated, can lead to a failure to develop binocular vision. A mass effect from an enlarging lesion can place pressure on the globe and distort the growing cornea, resulting in permanent refractive errors. In addition, infiltration of the extraocular muscles can cause strabismus. The severe consequences of ocular disturbances in infancy should prompt early ophthalmologic evaluation for any periorbital hemangioma. Therapy often is a collaborative decision based on the various clinical sequelae of the disease process for each individual patient. Treatment options include patching the unaffected eye, local or systemic steroids, laser ablation, and excision with direct closure or grafting.

If patching is not adequate for periorbital hemangioma, steroid therapy is the treatment of choice for lesions adversely affecting the eye. Steroids hasten the onset and rate of involution in from 30% to 90% of patients. A proliferating hemangioma is more responsive to treatment than one undergoing regression.

Intralesional steroids can give the benefits of treatment without the systemic drawbacks. Brief mask general anesthesia may be required to perform multiple injections and distribute the steroid well throughout the lesion. A response rate of up to 80% has been reported. A second treatment may be required 1 to 2 months after the first. Retrobulbar hemorrhage, occlusion of the retinal artery, and intraocular injection are all possible complications of local therapy. Posteriorly extending invasive ocular lesions should preferentially receive systemic treatment to avoid these complications.

Any child with cervicofacial hemangiomas and respiratory stridor should be evaluated for laryngeal involvement. Half of all subglottic hemangiomas are associated with cutaneous lesions. Endoscopy can confirm the diagnosis and define the size and extent of the obstruction. Treatment is determined by the endoscopic findings and clinical circumstances. Older children with minimal airway obstruction can undergo careful observation. A young child with minimal obstruction may be a candidate for systemic steroids, but higher grade obstructions may require more aggressive treatment. Carbon dioxide laser therapy can be efficacious in the treatment of laryngeal lesions that cause subglottic airway obstruction. Because of the risks for subglottic stenosis, laser therapy is not indicated for diffuse or circumferential lesions of the trachea. A tracheostomy may be necessary in certain patients to bypass the problem until regression occurs. Airway compromise can also result from blockade of the nose

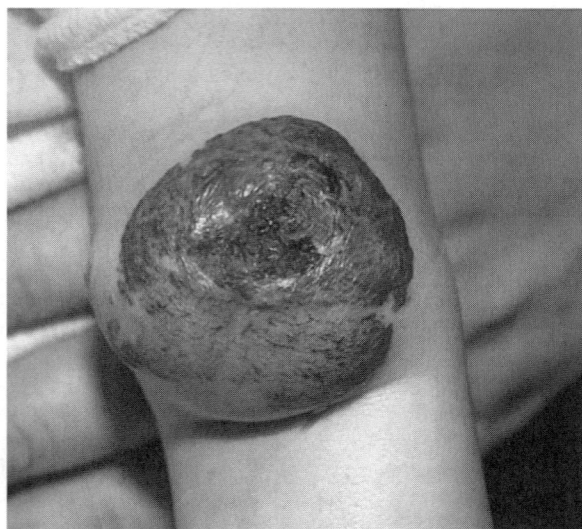

Figure 3 This 5-month-old child presented with a hemangioma complicated by a superficial ulceration. Local treatment was not adequate in this case, and surgical resection was required.

in early infancy when the neonate is an obligatory nose breather.

Ulceration

Ulceration as a complication in the proliferative phase of a hemangioma occurs in less than 5% of patients (Fig. 3). Skin breakdown is more common near an orifice such as the lips or anus and can be a significant source of morbidity. Secondary infection of an ulceration is also commonplace and can lead to destruction of local soft tissues and severe permanent deformity. Ulceration should be treated locally with cleansing, topical preparations, and dressing changes. Systemic antibiotics should be prescribed when indicated to help resolve a local cellulitis.

Bleeding

Parents should be advised on appropriate measures to be taken at home, such as using direct pressure and elevation of the affected part, if spontaneous bleeding occurs. Persistent or episodic hemorrhage should spur evaluation for the possibility of a generalized bleeding disorder.

Kasabach-Merritt syndrome is a bleeding diathesis secondary to thrombocytopenia in patients with expansive hemangiomas. This platelet-trapping coagulopathy results from decreased platelet survival and sequestration as well as increased consumption. Early signs of this disease include petechiae and bruising during the rapid proliferation of a neonatal hemangioma. A sudden tense enlargement of the hemangioma could signal intralesional hemorrhage. The most dangerous aspect of the disorder is the possible onset of acute systemic bleeding, which can be fatal, if uncontrolled.

Infants with multiple cutaneous and visceral lesions or lesions greater than 5 cm in diameter are at greater risk for the development of Kasabach-Merritt syndrome. Associated anemia and signs of bleeding tendencies should prompt further investigation. Helpful screening studies include complete blood and platelet counts as well as an examination of a peripheral blood smear for signs of microangiopathy. Evidence of thrombocytopenia may require searching for clues of consumptive coagulopathy. Neonates can often tolerate a decreased platelet count without complication, and mild cases are usually self-limited, with rebound in the platelet count after involution of the hemangioma.

Patients who develop Kasabach-Merritt syndrome require close observation and systemic treatment. Blood transfusions may be necessary, but platelet transfusions are not usually beneficial. The attendant clinical risk should dictate the necessity for a trial of systemic steroids, as the coagulopathy usually abates with regression of the hemangioma. Unresponsive or life-threatening lesions have been treated with cyclophosphamide or interferon. If the lesion is localized, embolization or excision may be efficacious. The success of antiplatelet treatment for Kasabach-Merritt syndrome is dubious.

CUTANEOUS-VISCERAL HEMANGIOMATOSIS

Neonates with multiple hemangiomas need to be closely monitored. Symptoms of congestive heart failure in an otherwise normal heart should signal danger. Subsequent evaluation of the liver is necessary to assess hepatomegaly. A systolic bruit heard over the liver or enlargement out of proportion to the degree of heart failure may help corroborate suspicion of a concurrent hemangioma in the liver. Although visceral lesions can also affect the lungs or the gastrointestinal tract, the liver is most commonly involved. This potentially lethal condition is associated with a high morbidity secondary to hemorrhage or cardiac complications.

A battery of tests, such as ultrasound, CT, and radionuclide scanning, help to confirm the diagnosis of visceral hemangiomatosis and often are sufficient evidence for institution of treatment. Arteriography in preparation for interventional therapy can characterize the lesion and define the blood supply to the affected area. The natural history of these proliferative vascular malformations should be one of involution and complete resolution over time; however, intercurrent complications contribute to a reported mortality of over 50%.

The high mortality associated with cutaneous visceral hemangiomatosis complicated by congestive heart failure usually mandates treatment. Patient management includes intensive care monitoring, fluid restriction, as well as the use of digoxin and diuretics. A trial of systemic steroids is warranted. Clinically, success of treatment can be evaluated by following differences of associated cutaneous lesions or documenting decrease in the size of visceral lesions on CT scan or ultrasound. Seventy percent of patients respond to these maneuvers. Treatment failures can undergo embolization or surgical resection, and radiation therapy can be tried as a last-ditch effort.

REFERENCES

1. Mulliken JB. Cutaneous vascular anomalies. In: McCarthy JG, ed. Plastic surgery. Vol 5. Philadelphia: WB Saunders, 1990:3191.
2. Achauer BM, Vanderkam VM. Vascular lesions. Clin Plast Surg 1993; 20:43–51.
3. Edgerton MT. The treatment of hemangiomas: With special reference to the role of steroid therapy. Ann Surg 1976; 183:517–532.
4. Esterly NB. Kasabach-Merritt syndrome in infants. J Am Acad Dermatol 1983; 8:504–513.
5. Mulliken JB. Diagnosis and natural history of hemangiomas. In: Mulliken JB, Young AE, eds. Vascular birthmarks: Hemangiomas and malformations. Philadelphia: WB Saunders, 1988:41.
6. Zak TA, Morin DJ. Early local steroid therapy of infantile eyelid hemangiomas. J Pediatr Ophthalmol Strabismus 1981; 18:25–27.
7. Mulliken JB, Glowacki J. Hemangiomas and vascular malformations in infants and children: A classification based on endothelial characteristics. Plast Reconstr Surg 1982; 69:412–422.
8. Kasabach HH, Merritt KK. Capillary hemangioma with extensive purpura: Report of a case. Am J Dis Child 1940; 59:1063.
9. Berman B, Lin HWP. Concurrent cutaneous and hepatic hemangiomata in infancy: Report of a case and review of the literature. J Dermatol Surg Oncol 1978; 4:869–873.

MANAGEMENT OF CONGENITAL ARTERIOVENOUS FISTULAS AND MALFORMATIONS IN ADULTS

THOMAS S. RILES, M.D.
MARK A. ADELMAN, M.D.

Congenital vascular lesions can occur in any part of the human body and may be associated with a wide spectrum of local and systemic signs and symptoms. These lesions are sufficiently rare that few clinicians encounter more than a handful in a lifetime of practice. Either from uncertainty as to how to manage complications or from unease about counseling a patient with an asymptomatic lesion, these patients are often referred to the vascular surgeon.

During the first three-quarters of this century, the treatment of congenital arteriovenous communications in the adult was limited to the closure or resection of congenital fistulas and the occasional resection of a small arteriovenous malformation (AVM). Although few reports describe radical resections,[1,2] large AVMs involving the abdomen, chest, or craniofacial region were seldom treated until the onset of life-threatening complications, such as bleeding, ulceration, or congestive heart failure. At that point, proximal ligation of the main feeding artery might have been attempted, often with only temporary improvement. Eventually, collateral circulation would develop, with return of the symptoms and the demise of the individual. Intravascular embolization of malformations was occasionally performed. These procedures were limited, however, by the need to repeatedly access the feeding arteries by surgical exposure and by the lack of appropriate embolic material to reach the center of the malformation.

Over the past decade and a half, major advances in the field of radiology have led to many new techniques for the diagnosis and treatment of congenital vascular communications. Patients heretofore considered untreatable are now routinely managed by the use of embolic materials, coils, glues, and detachable balloons.[3-6] Surgical resections that would have previously been associated with prohibitive risk are now made possible by preoperative embolization by the interventional radiologist. What has emerged is a better understanding and renewed hope for patients with congenital arteriovenous communications. Essential to successful treatment, however, is close cooperation among radiologists, surgeons, and hospital support groups and a careful premanagement plan with defined goals and realistic expectations.

ARTERIOVENOUS FISTULAS

Except for the anomalies of the great vessels, the patent ductus arterious, and the septal defects, congenital arteriovenous fistulas (AVFs), defined as single abnormal communications between the arterial and venous systems, are extremely rare. Most peripheral AVFs in adults are acquired from trauma, infection, neoplasms, or aneurysmal disease. When a fistula is identified in the peripheral vessels without an obvious etiology, remote trauma often is presumed. Congenital fistulas can occur, however. They may result from the anomalies during the very last stages of the embryology of the vascular system, when differentiation of the arterial and venous structures is in the final stage. Fistulas may occasionally be seen during routine arteriography for other conditions. Some congenital vascular syndromes such as the Klippel-Trenaunay syndrome may have associated AVFs.

Very small fistulas with no clinical manifestations, such as those seen unexpectedly on an arteriogram, may require no treatment. Even though fistulas in general increase in size over time, our experience with acquired lesions and surgically created AVFs has shown that this process may be extremely slow. As long as there are no symptoms, these small fistulas are irrelevant.

Larger fistulas may cause local symptoms such as ischemia due to a steal of arterial blood from the distal tissues and/or venous insufficiency from venous hypertension, and venous valvular incompetence. Either of these conditions may result in ulceration and tissue loss. If a fistula is very large, as measured by a shunt of 20% to 40% of the cardiac output, then myocardial hypertrophy, tachycardia, and congestive heart failure may occur. Fistulas that produce local or systemic symptoms or those that have the potential for causing problems during the life of the individual should be considered for closure, either by surgical or angiographic techniques.

The single AVF is relatively simple to manage. The choice of treatment is often determined by the location of the fistula and the need to maintain the arterial circulation through the feeding vessels. Those AVFs arising from vessels that can be sacrificed can generally be treated either by surgical ligation or percutaneous occlusion of the artery by a detachable balloon. The choice between these two methods may be dictated by the surgical or angiographic accessibility of the lesion. If the feeding vessel is essential to maintain viability of the distal tissues, management may require direct closure of the fistula while preserving the artery, or even an arterial reconstruction. By one method or another, closure can usually be performed.

ARTERIOVENOUS MALFORMATIONS

It is important to distinguish the congenital arteriovenous malformation (AVM) from the childhood hemangioma. The latter is actually a neoplasm characterized by rapid endothelial proliferation during infancy, followed by spontaneous resolution in early childhood. The AVM, in contrast, has no cellular growth component. These are nests of abnormal arteries and veins, being anomalies from the embryonic development, that increase in size because of the shunting of blood from one system to the other. Although periods of stability may occur, the general pattern is one of continuous growth. Although AVMs generally are isolated lesions in otherwise healthy individuals, associated anomalies may occur, either as coexistent anomalies or as the result of abnormal blood flow. The communication between the arterial and venous system is multifistulous. The actual sizes of the communications may vary widely.

The congenital AVM presents a much more difficult problem with respect to management. Although the indications for treatment are essentially the same as those for arteriovenous fistulas, the propensity for growth and ultimately troublesome complications behooves consideration of all available treatment options once the diagnosis is confirmed. By the time patients reach the vascular surgeon or interventional radiologist, many have undergone futile attempts at resection or proximal arterial ligation, creating an even more difficult management problem.

A thorough assessment of the patient is essential before any plan of management is proposed. It begins with a careful history and physical examination, in which the duration and severity of all signs and symptoms are noted. Depending on the location, the size, and the duration of the AVM, the presentation may be varied. Extremity AVMs may be associated with varicosities and signs of venous insufficiency, distal ischemia, and ulcerations. Those of long duration may have evidence of bone lengthening and hypertrophy. Malformations of the abdomen or pubis may produce pain or sexual dysfunction or may present with hematuria, gastrointestinal bleeding, or vaginal bleeding. Disfigurement may be the earliest sign of a craniofacial AVM, but bleeding from the gums, the nose, or from a dental extraction may also be the presenting symptom. Auscultation over the AVM characteristically reveals a loud, continuous murmur, and a thrill is often palpated. With large malformations, cardiomegaly, tachycardia, and symptoms of congestive heart failure may be present.

Among the many useful and innovative diagnostic tests to assess congenital AVMs, the two most important are arteriography and magnetic resonance imaging (MRI). Selective arteriograms are essential to document all feeding vessels and the exact location of the center of the lesion. To assess the involvement of adjacent bone and muscle and the overall extent of the lesion, both computed tomography (CT) and MRI are of value. The MRI is of particular value in distinguishing between high and low flow components. If the lesion involves the craniofacial structures of the gastrointestinal tract, endoscopy is usually indicated. Cardiac function tests are important for patients with large AVMs of long standing.

Once the AVM has been thoroughly evaluated, we have found it best to have a multidisciplinary conference to consider the advisability of treatment and the therapeutic options. These options, along with the possible risks and contingency plans, should be carefully explained to the patient. In many cases cure is not possible. It is important that the goals be realistic and well defined before treatment begins.

Patients with superficial AVMs of the trunk, face, scalp, and extremities and some lesions of the pelvis are preferably treated by surgical excision because complete removal offers the best opportunity for cure. Surgeons should be aware, however, that often the AVM involves more tissue than externally apparent. The MRI has greatly facilitated the presurgical planning for these lesions. Meticulous dissection and ligation of all branches feeding the AVM are essential. As resection of large lesions may be associated with considerable blood loss, tourniquet control and autotransfusion should be used when possible. Preoperative embolization can facilitate surgical resection and reduce operative blood loss. In such cases, embolization is best performed just prior to surgical resection. If there is a delay between embolization and operation, enlargement of collateral vessels may occur.

For AVMs that cannot be easily excised, percutaneous transcatheter embolization is generally the treatment of choice. As catheter technology has rapidly improved, superselective catheterization of small feeding vessels has become routine. Embolic materials have progressed from autologous clot, muscle, and Gelfoam to the embolic agents currently used, including polyvinyl alcohol, liquid silicone, and acrylic tissue adhesives. These newer agents that penetrate and obliterate the nidus of the malformation have significantly improved management. Many lesions heretofore deemed untreatable due to their extent or anatomic position are now controlled, if not cured, by embolization therapy.

The embolization procedure must be carefully planned in advance. The selective angiographic examinations are studied to determine the major arterial feeding vessels and collateral pathways, as well as the pathways for venous drainage. General anesthesia is frequently used to minimize patient discomfort. In many patients the embolization must be performed in multiple staged procedures to minimize the risk of tissue necrosis, contrast medium toxicity, and prolonged anesthesia. In addition to tissue necrosis, potential complications of transcatheter embolization include pulmonary embolization of embolic material and embolization of normal tissue from escaping particulate matter into adjacent arterial branches. In the extremities, compartment syndromes may also occur as a result of tissue necrosis and swelling. Little is known about the long-term risks of embolic materials since their clinical use began in the 1980s. Although the complications have been less than 5%, in each patient the risks and benefits must be carefully weighed and explained before treatment.

We cannot emphasize strongly enough that proximal arterial occlusion, whether by surgical ligation or transcatheter embolization, must be avoided. Although this was acceptable for life-threatening emergencies in the decades before embolization therapy, it has always been acknowledged that the benefits are short-lived. Revascularization of the AVM through collateral circulation and the return of symptoms soon follows. Now that embolization therapy is available, proximal arterial ligation or obliteration only inhibits catheter access to the malformation and in many patients precludes the chance for successful treatment.

Emphasizing the challenges is a series of patients we have encountered with craniofacial AVMs and prior external carotid ligations. Each of these patients presented with a unique problem and each required a different therapy.[7] Essential to their management, however, was close cooperation among the vascular surgeons, otolaryngologists, plastic surgeons, and the interventional radiologist. In these patients reconstruction of the ligated external carotid artery was the first step with the anticipation of subsequent embolization therapy.

VENOUS MALFORMATIONS

Purely venous malformations, sometimes called venous dysplasias or cavernous venous malformations, characteristically have no significant arteriovenous shunting. The network of abnormal veins is therefore under low pressure. Symptoms may result from venous distention and reflux, particularly in the lower extremity, from bleeding and ulceration, and from thrombosis. Many venous malformations require no treatment. Those of the extremities can often be managed by compression stockings or gauntlets. In some patients, excision of dilated veins may be indicated. This procedure may be more hazardous and associated with greater blood loss than that encountered during conventional varicose vein procedures. Sclerosing therapy by injection of absolute ethanol has also been used to manage symptomatic veins or those causing cosmetic problems.

REFERENCES

1. Szilagyi PE, Elliott JP, DeRusso FJ, et al. Peripheral congenital arteriovenous fistulas. Surgery 1965; 57:61–81.
2. Szilagyi DE, Smith RF, Elliott, et al. Congenital arteriovenous anomalies of the limbs. Arch Surg 1976; III:423–429.
3. Kaufman SL, Kumar AAJ, Roland JA, et al. Transcatheter embolization in the management of congenital arteriovenous malformations. Radiology 1980; 137:21–29.
4. Palmaz JC, Newton TH, Reuter SR, et al. Particulate intra-arterial embolization in pelvic arteriovenous malformations. Am J Roentgenol 1981; 137:117–122.
5. Berenstein A, Krucheff II. Catheter and material selection for transarterial embolization: Materials. Radiology 1979; 132:631–639.
6. Rosen RJ. Embolization in the treatment of arteriovenous malformations. In: Goldberg HI, Higgins CB, Ring EJ, eds. Contemporary Imaging. San Francisco: University of California Press, 1985:153.
7. Riles TS, Berenstein A, Fisher FS, et al. Reconstruction of the ligated external carotid artery for embolization of cervicofacial arteriovenous malformations. J Vasc Surg 1993; 17:491–498.
8. Rosen RJ, Riles TS, Berenstein A. Congenital vascular malformations. In: Rutherford RB, ed. Vascular surgery. 3rd ed. Philadelphia: WB Saunders, 1989:1049–1061.

ANGIOACCESS SURGERY

EXTERNAL METHODS OF ANGIOACCESS

JEFFREY D. PUNCH, M.D.
ROBERT M. MERION, M.D.

Establishing and maintaining hemodialysis access is a cornerstone of long-term renal replacement therapy. Hemodialysis techniques have improved sufficiently to allow many patients to survive for as long as dialysis access can be maintained. In order to achieve long-term dialysis access, an overall strategy planned by an experienced dialysis access surgeon is required. There is little debate that the best long-term access is a primary fistula between autologous artery and vein, followed by a prosthetic graft between artery and vein. In several situations, however, external methods of angioaccess are required for either temporary or permanent vascular access.

Temporary access is often needed for emergent hemodialysis in patients with reversible causes of renal failure who are expected to regain renal function in days to weeks. External angioaccess can usually be accomplished under local anesthesia at the bedside and can be used immediately for hemodialysis. Additionally, temporary access may be required for patients with sudden-onset renal failure to allow a primary arteriovenous fistula (AVF) or prosthetic graft to mature. External angioaccess methods are ideally suited to temporary use because they can easily be completely removed when they are no longer needed, they do not leave indwelling prosthetic material, and scarring and disfigurement associated with AVFs and prosthetic grafts are avoided.

External angioaccess is also the method of choice for infants who cannot undergo peritoneal dialysis. Children who weigh less than 25 to 30 kg usually do not have adequately developed vessels to maintain a patent upper extremity AVF regardless of whether prosthetic graft material is used. Because we aggressively pursue early living related renal transplantation as long-term renal replacement therapy in these patients, temporary access is frequently sufficient.

Finally, some patients are not candidates for an internal AVF. The sequential construction of multiple fistulas and prosthetic bridge grafts may result in utilization of virtually all anatomic locations for further fistula or graft construction, and occlusion or stenosis of the major central veins may complicate the intercurrent placement of temporary central venous cannulas. The latter may be suspected when extremity venous hypertension and swelling follow attempts at placement of a distal arteriovenous fistula. Peripheral vascular occlusive disease, particularly in patients with diabetes mellitus, may limit the quality of arterial inflow resulting in steal syndromes, if blood is diverted from the hand or foot directly across the fistula. A third group of patients that cannot tolerate AVFs are those with limited cardiac reserve. These patients may develop high-output congestive heart failure after an AVF with sufficient flow for hemodialysis is established.

CENTRAL VENOUS CANNULATION

The simplest method of external angioaccess involves cannulation of a central vein with a single- or double-lumen catheter. It is usually possible to cannulate the central venous system percutaneously with the Seldinger guide wire technique, and this method generally requires only a few minutes. This technique has largely replaced external connection of the radial artery to the cephalic vein using a Scribner shunt. The latter is placed operatively and may be problematic in the elderly and in small children. The use of a central dialysis access catheter also preserves the radial artery and cephalic vein for construction of a permanent Brescia-Cimino fistula, the optimal form of access for long-term hemodialysis. Blood flow is more reliable through a central vein catheter than a Scribner shunt, particularly when the patient is relatively hypotensive or peripherally vasoconstricted.

Several different sites are available for central vein cannulation, and the choice is largely one of personal preference and experience. The right subclavian vein is our preferred site for initial percutaneous placement of a dialysis catheter. The anatomy of the central veins on the right allows the catheter to take a more direct path to the superior vena cava without resting against the wall of the vessel and obstructing flow through the catheter. The right internal jugular vein is usually easy to cannulate but the catheter is more obtrusive to the patient and the dressing is less comfortable on the neck than on the chest. Use of the right side for access to the central venous system has the added advantage of preserving the patient's left side for a permanent dialysis access fistula. The left arm is more commonly nondominant and therefore the preferable side for a forearm fistula, especially for patients who will be maintained on home hemodialysis and perform their own fistula cannulation. Ideally, the temporary access is not placed on the same side as the permanent access in case a subclavian or brachiocephalic vein stenosis develops from the catheter. Also, removing a large-bore central venous cannula from the side of a high-flow arterialized vein could potentially result in significant bleeding.

For central venous catheters large enough for hemodialysis in infants or small children, it is often advisable to use an open cut-down technique on the cephalic vein, external jugular vein, or common facial vein. Cut-down technique is also advisable in patients with an uncorrectable bleeding diathesis due to hepatic dysfunction, systemic anticoagulation, thrombocytopenia, or disseminated intravascular coagulation. The qualitative platelet dysfunction associated with uremia can generally be corrected with desmopressin acetate (0.3 µg/kg IV over 30 minutes) and should not preclude a percutaneous attempt at central vein cannulation.

Femoral vein cannulation can also be used if necessary for urgent dialysis access, but has several distinct disadvantages. The catheter severely limits patient mobility and is uncomfortable. Also, the infection rate is high because of proximity to the urogenital region, necessitating frequent catheter changes. Finally, femoral venous cannulation is associated with venous thrombosis and the risk of pulmonary embolism originating from the lower extremities and pelvis. The practice of using the femoral site in patients with bleeding tendencies is similarly unsound because retroperitoneal hemorrhage can be as problematic as a hemothorax secondary to upper extremity or cervical venous access.

The choice of cannula depends on a number of factors. Satisfactory dialysis is possible using either a single-lumen or double-lumen catheter. The trend in recent years has been toward the latter. To avoid confusion, it should be noted that the dual-lumen catheter uses different halves of the same cannula, whereas the double-lumen cannula is essentially an inner venous cannula surrounded by an outer arterial cannula. Both use the same principle of simultaneous two-way flow. Dialysis using a single-lumen catheter, first described by Uldall in 1979, involves alternating inward and outward blood flow through the same cannula. Many observers believe that the phenomenon of recirculation—re-entry of the dialyzed blood back into the dialysis machine—is higher with the single-lumen catheter, although there is controversy about this point. Recirculation significantly reduces the effectiveness of dialysis. Using the dual-lumen cannula, inflow into the dialyzer is provided through access holes 3 to 4 cm from the tip of the cannula, with blood flowing through one of two D-shaped channels. Venous return to the patient is provided through the other channel, with outflow through the catheter tip. Dialyzer inflow and blood return to the patient are thus separated in the vascular system by 3 to 4 cm. The choice of technique depends upon the dialysis unit's capabilities because the single-lumen technique cannot be accomplished with the standard dialysis machine. So-called to-and-fro dialysis has been discontinued at our center, and dual-lumen catheters are exclusively utilized.

The composition of the catheter is another important consideration. Catheters for dialysis are made of polytetrafluoroethylene (PTFE), polyurethane, or Silastic. Catheters made of PTFE are stiffer and somewhat easier to insert but are believed to be more reactive to the vessel wall and are not suited for long-term external dialysis. Polyurethane catheters are initially stiff but soften at body temperature and thus combine relative ease of insertion with the advantage of subsequent pliability and lessened risk of venous perforation. The Silastic catheter is very soft and nonreactive and is the material used most commonly for long-term external cannulation. A popular catheter is the dual-lumen PermaCath, which comes with a Dacron cuff meant to be tunneled under the skin. Some surgeons believe the tunneled cuff reduces the incidence of infection. The PermaCath can be placed percutaneously with a split-sheath introducer or operatively through a cut-down incision. Patency rates for central venous cannulas used for dialysis access have been recently reported at 74% at 1 year and 43% at 2 years.[1]

ALTERNATIVE TYPES OF EXTERNAL ANGIOACCESS

Scribner Shunt

The Scribner shunt played a critical role in the evolution of hemodialysis but is now mostly of historical interest. The PTFE vessel tips are typically placed in the radial artery and cephalic vein at the wrist or into the dorsalis pedis artery and saphenous vein in the foot. The two vessel tips are then connected to two pieces of Silastic tubing that exit the skin and are connected in turn to the inflow and outflow of the hemodialysis machine. Between dialysis sessions the tubing from the arterial and venous sides are connected to each other to maintain the external AVF. Scribner shunts can also be used in patients who require continuous arteriovenous hemofiltration or long-term plasmapheresis. The Scribner shunt does have the advantage of requiring only superficial vessels and can therefore be placed safely at the bedside, even in patients with severe coagulopathy. Unfortunately, thrombosis is common, and the flow through the shunt may be variable enough to hinder effective hemodialysis. Flow through thrombosed Scribner shunts can sometimes be restored with the use of balloon embolectomy catheters, but results are generally temporary.

Thomas Shunt

The Thomas shunt consists of two Silastic tubes, each with a Dacron velour cuff. The cuffed ends are anastomosed to the common or superficial femoral artery and vein. The Silastic tubes are brought out through the skin separately and connected in the mid-portion. This shunt is most often used as the access of last resort when other vessels are unavailable. For its first 9 cm, the catheter is surrounded by a Dacron velour material, which is meant to encourage incorporation into a fibrous capsule with resistance to infection. Despite this feature, the Thomas shunt is susceptible to infection, with potentially catastrophic results. In one series, eight of ten shunts were ultimately removed secondary to infection.[2] Thomas recommended 6 weeks of prophylactic antibiotics to reduce the risk of infection. In our experience, a subcutaneous PTFE graft between the superficial femoral artery and the saphenous vein is a satisfactory alternative for patients who have no access sites available in their upper extremities; it has eliminated the need to ever place a Thomas shunt.

Hemasite External Angioaccess

The Hemasite implantable access system consists of a titanium T-piece, the two lateral ends of which are connected to PTFE prosthetic graft material. The vertical limb of the device contains an internal silicone rubber septum that protrudes through the skin to be available for connection to the dialysis machine. This system has the advantage of avoiding repeated painful needle punctures and for this reason was held in high regard by patients. Unfortunately, there was a high incidence of infection and thrombosis, and the device is no longer available. The high rate of infection was related to bacterial colonization that invariably developed in the excoriated skin adjacent to the site where the device protruded through the skin.

COMPLICATIONS OF EXTERNAL ANGIOACCESS DEVICES

Complications of external angioaccess devices fall into three broad categories: those related to catheter insertion, mechanical complications caused by the presence of a catheter in the vascular system, and infectious complications.

Complications at the Time of Catheter Insertion

The Seldinger guide wire technique has markedly decreased the rate of complications related to central venous cannulation from the old "catheter-through-the-needle" method, but significant risks remain. Several large studies have concluded that physician expertise is the dominant factor that determines the risk associated with these procedures. Experienced physicians have a complication rate of less than 2%, whereas inexperienced physicians have complication rates as high as 12%.[3]

The most common complication is pneumothorax, which occurs when the needle used to cannulate the vein initially traverses the pleura. The withdrawal of air into the syringe during attempted cannulation of the vein with the needle is not a reliable arbiter of whether a pneumothorax is likely to develop. Puncture of the visceral pleura does not necessarily result in a gush of air during the insertion of the needle and the development of a pneumothorax may be delayed for minutes to hours after catheter insertion. Pneumothorax may be precipitated by subsequent positive-pressure mechanical ventilation if, for example, the patient is placed under general anesthesia. A chest x-ray should always be obtained after any attempt at central venous cannulation, regardless of whether the attempt was successful. Also, if the patient develops shortness of breath or hypoxemia even hours later, the diagnosis of delayed pneumothorax must be entertained and a chest x-ray obtained. A small pneumothorax can be observed if the patient is asymptomatic. If the pneumothorax is stable over 12 hours, it is likely to be gradually resorbed. Symptomatic or larger pneumothorax should be treated with tube thoracostomy. Excellent success has been achieved using a small-diameter tube with a one-way valve if no significant air leak is present. These tubes are much less painful than a full-sized chest tube.

Other potentially serious complications of central venous catheter insertion include inadvertent cannulation of the subclavian or common carotid arteries and puncture of the superior vena cava or right atrium by the guide wire. If arterial cannulation is recognized before the guide wire is passed through the needle, the needle can be safely withdrawn and pressure held on the site for 15 minutes in most cases without the development of a hematoma or hemothorax. If arterial cannulation is unrecognized until the large-bore cannula has been inserted into the vessel, it is wise to remove the catheter only if one is prepared to explore the patient immediately should hemorrhage or hematoma result. However, catheters as large as 13 Fr can often be safely removed if pressure is held for 30 to 45 minutes. Perforation of the superior vena cava or right atrium is rare and less likely if the soft end of the guide wire is used to pass through the needle into the vein. No guide wire should ever be forced inward against resistance because caval perforation may result. This complication is manifested by sudden chest pain or hemodynamic collapse. Chest x-ray may document an abnormal catheter position, a widened mediastinum, or a new pleural effusion. Prompt recognition and treatment, which may include operation through a median sternotomy, are essential for the patient to survive this potentially lethal event.

Mechanical Complications

Inadequate flow through the catheter is usually related to positioning against the vessel wall, kinking of the catheter in the subcutaneous tunnel, or deposition of fibrin or thrombus within the lumen of the catheter itself. Repositioning of the catheter usually corrects the problem, although occasionally the catheter must be placed in a different site. Catheter thrombosis can often be successfully treated with infusion of streptokinase or urokinase into the catheter. Schwab and colleagues reported 95% successful salvage of central venous dialysis catheters using urokinase.[4] Although urokinase is not approved for use in children, Kellam and co-workers reported safe and successful treatment of thrombosed dialysis catheters with urokinase in 14 pediatric patients.[5] Due to the prevalence of thrombosis in catheters used for long-term hemodialysis access, some surgeons and nephrologists advocate long-term low-dose anticoagulation with either aspirin or sodium warfarin, although the utility of this practice has not been substantiated. Although there were early reports that recombinant human erythropoietin therapy predisposes patients to thrombosis of dialysis access sites, multiple studies have shown no decreased patency rates for AVFs or central venous dialysis catheters in patients receiving erythropoietin.

Subclavian vein stenosis or thrombosis secondary to indwelling central catheters is also a frequent occurrence in dialysis patients. When looked for carefully, sleeve thrombi have been noted in 42% of patients with subclavian catheters, and subclavian vein occlusion is reported in 8% of these patients. These complications often develop asymptomatically. The stenosis or occlusion rapidly become apparent if an AVF is placed in the ipsilateral distal extremity with resulting venous hypertension and massive edema. Fistula ligation relieves the edema but renders the extremity useless for further access procedures. Because the stenosis or occlusion may be silent, it is prudent to obtain a venous duplex scan of the subclavian veins prior to attempting percutaneous subclavian vein cannulation in patients who have had multiple subclavian catheters in the past. This practice can help to avoid useless attempts to cannulate a thrombosed or tightly stenotic vessel. Although subclavian vein occlusion is usually permanent, balloon angioplasty can successfully dilate proximal stenoses. Schwab and associates reported 100% successful restoration of normal flow in 12 patients using this technique.[6] Our experience, however, has been that this treatment is only temporary, and the stenosis often recurs. Interventional radiologists are currently exploring the use of intravascular prosthetic stents to maintain patency of fibrotic vessels that develop recurrent stenoses.

Occasionally, a subclavian vein stenosis secondary to a central catheter results in symptomatic venous hypertension. It may be correctable by an axillary or subclavian vein to internal jugular vein bypass using externally reinforced PTFE graft either under the clavicle or through the clavicular bed after claviculectomy.[7]

Rarely, long-term indwelling catheters can result in late perforation of the superior vena cava, causing hemothorax or perforation of the right atrium that results in cardiac tamponade. The contraction of the right atrium may predispose to cardiac perforation. Thus, the catheter tip should never be more than 3 cm below the junction of the sternal body and manubrium on the postinsertion chest x-ray. Chest pain and hypotension at the initiation of dialysis without electrocardiographic changes should make one suspicious of a perforation. A chest x-ray or echocardiogram may be diagnostic. Prompt recognition and operative repair are essential for the patient to survive.

Infectious Complications

Infections are the leading cause of morbidity and the second leading cause of death in hemodialysis patients. Patients with chronic renal failure are at increased risk of infection because of underlying disease, uremia, and protein malnutrition. The placement of percutaneous catheters, therefore, places the patient at risk for life-threatening sepsis. Central venous catheters become colonized with bacteria in 20% of patients, and bacteremia develops in about 10%.[8] The incidence of infection is even higher than that among patients with central hyperalimentation lines and is related to several factors. The larger size of central hemodialysis catheters creates more tissue trauma at the time of insertion. Catheter stiffness predisposes to dislodgement, increasing the difficulty of keeping an occlusive dressing over the puncture site and allowing skin contamination. Most importantly, the frequent manipulations necessary for hemodialysis predispose to contamination and emphasize the need for careful aseptic technique in handling the catheter. Nursing experience and patient education greatly influence the rate of infection.

In 70% of hemodialysis patients, the anterior nares are colonized with *Staphylococcus aureus,* the most common organism causing catheter sepsis. Colonization can be reduced with a combination of rifampin and topical bacitracin, but quickly recurs after cessation of antibiotic treatment. Recent reports of strains of *S. aureus* resistant to vancomycin are an ominous development because this antibiotic has been used broadly in dialysis patients. Its long half-life in patients with renal failure and its nearly universal efficacy as a bactericidal agent to combat most organisms that commonly infect intravascular catheters and grafts have made vancomycin a nearly ideal antibiotic in this setting. Attempts at binding antibiotics to the catheter have been tried but are not yet routinely available. Periodically changing the catheter over a guide wire has not been shown to reduce the incidence of catheter sepsis. It is critically important, therefore, that catheter manipulation be kept to a minimum and performed only by experienced personnel. Any patient with an indwelling central catheter who is febrile and in whom another source of fever cannot be identified should undergo drawback blood cultures from the catheter and, if these cultures grow any pathogenic organisms, prompt removal of the catheter. Although long-term antibiotic therapy to sterilize an infected catheter has been used with some success, catheter removal followed by a course of intravenous antibiotics remains the standard therapy for catheter infection. This removes the fibrin sheath surrounding the intravascular portion of the catheter, which may be the nidus of infection.

REFERENCES

1. Mosquera D, Gibson S, Goldman M. Vascular access surgery: A 2-year study and comparison with the Permcath. Nephrol Dial Transplant 1992; 7:1111–1115.
2. Beberide J, Miguel J, Sanz A. Experience with use of the Thomas prosthesis as vascular access for chronic hemodialysis. Dial Transplant 1982; 2:906–907.
3. Lockwood A. Percutaneous subclavian vein catheterization: Too much of a good thing? Arch Intern Med 1984; 144:1407–1408.
4. Schwab S, Buller G, McCann R, et al. Prospective evaluation of a Dacron cuffed hemodialysis catheter for prolonged use. Am J Kidney Dis 1988; 111:166–169.
5. Kellam B, Fraze D, Kanarek K. Clot lysis for thrombosed central venous catheters in pediatric patients. J Perinatol 1987; 7:242–244.
6. Schwab S, Quarles L, Middleton J, et al. Hemodialysis-associated subclavian vein stenosis. Kidney Int 1988; 33:1156–1159.
7. Currier C, Widder S, Ali A, et al. Surgical management of subclavian and axillary vein thrombosis in patients with a functioning arteriovenous fistula. Surgery 1986; 100:25–28.
8. Dahlberg P, Yutec W, Newcomer K. Subclavian hemodialysis catheter infections. Am J Kidney Dis 1986; 8:421–427.

DIRECT ARTERIOVENOUS ANASTOMOSIS FOR ANGIOACCESS

JEFFREY L. BUEHRER, M.D.
BLAIR A. KEAGY, M.D.

The radiocephalic arteriovenous fistula (AVF) remains the preferred access for chronic hemodialysis since its introduction in 1966. Developed initially as an alternative to the external Silastic arteriovenous shunt, its most common modern competitor is the polytetrafluoroethylene (PTFE) arteriovenous shunt. Advantages of the radiocephalic fistula over PTFE include superior primary patency, reduced risk of infection, and technical ease of construction. Unfortunately, many patients have had multiple peripheral venous procedures prior to referral for dialysis access. Consequently, the cephalic vein may be inadequate for construction of a radiocephalic fistula.

Several alternatives to the classic radiocephalic fistula have been described to extend the benefits of autologous dialysis access. Options include basilic vein to ulnar artery fistula at the wrist, brachiocephalic fistula above or below the elbow, reverse antecubital fistula at the elbow, and transposed basilic vein to brachial artery above the elbow. When it becomes clear that a patient will require hemodialysis, early referral improves the chance for constructing an autologous access. Early referral allows adequate time to fistula maturation prior to first access and avoids repeated percutaneous venipuncture or indwelling central venous catheter placement.

PREOPERATIVE EVALUATION

Cardiac risk factors and any history of vascular disease are documented. Careful history of previous access is essential. Although the nondominant hand is preferred, the limb with the most favorable anatomy should be used for initial access. Blood pressure is measured in both arms. A gradient of more than 20 mm Hg between sides suggests proximal arterial occlusive disease, which may cause fistula failure due to inadequate inflow. Brachial, radial, and ulnar pulses are palpated bilaterally. Previous surgical incisions are noted. Pre-existing sensorimotor deficits secondary to stroke or diabetes should be documented. Allen's test is helpful to assure a complete palmar arch but may be difficult in patients with dark skin or severe anemia. A continuous-wave Doppler increases the sensitivity of the test. A radiocephalic fistula may lead to digital ischemia in a patient with an incomplete deep palmar arch or an atretic ulnar artery. Preoperative arteriography is used when significant arterial occlusive disease is suspected.

The cephalic vein begins as the radial continuation of the dorsal venous arch of the hand at the anatomic snuffbox. It courses parallel to the anterior border of the brachioradialis muscle. At the antecubital fossa, it frequently communicates with the basilic vein via the median cubital vein, then continues upward in the lateral bicipital groove. It empties into the axillary vein deep in the deltopectoral triangle. If the examiner taps on the cephalic vein near the wrist, the impulse should be easily felt by an examining finger farther along the vein. An obstruction in the vein blocks transmission of the impulse. This simple tap test commonly identifies defects in the vein that may lead to fistula failure.

The basilic vein begins as the ulnar continuation of the dorsal venous arch of the hand. It continues along the ulnar border of the forearm and enters the antecubital fossa in front of the medial epicondyle of the humerus. It receives the median cubital vein and then continues in the medial bicipital groove. Near the middle of the arm, it pierces the brachial fascia to enter the neurovascular bundle and continues until it joins the paired brachial veins to form the axillary vein. The basilic vein is less conveniently located for dialysis access than the cephalic vein. However, it can be transposed to an easily accessible subcutaneous position in either the arm or forearm.

We perform a radiocephalic fistula as the first access for all patients with adequate vein who do not require urgent dialysis. The transposed ulnar vein in the forearm makes an equally acceptable conduit but is rarely available in our experience. If the cephalic vein in the forearm is unusable but sufficient in the upper arm, a primary brachiocephalic fistula is appropriate. In patients without a usable superficial vein and those who require immediate dialysis, we generally perform a PTFE forearm loop graft. If necessary, these grafts may be punctured immediately, although we prefer to wait 2 weeks. We make every effort to avoid indwelling central venous catheter placement. Apart from their immediate complications, the late incidence of subclavian vein stenosis or thrombosis from central venous catheters makes future dialysis access more difficult.

When a secondary site is required, we favor a brachiocephalic fistula if the forearm access has promoted arterialization of the cephalic vein in the upper arm. Transposed basilic vein to brachial artery fistula is the next choice if the vein is adequate. When these options are not available, we place an upper arm brachiobasilic PTFE bridge graft.

TECHNIQUE

The radiocephalic fistula is easily performed with local anesthesia. A longitudinal or transverse incision may be used. We prefer the transverse incision, which provides adequate exposure of both artery and vein. The incision is generally placed just cephalad to the radial styloid process, but may be moved proximally if the vein is inadequate at the wrist. The radial artery is identified between the brachioradialis and the flexor carpi radialis tendons. The superficial branch of the radial nerve lies lateral to and is separated from the radial artery by the brachioradialis muscle. The nerve is sensory at this level and should be preserved. After adequate mobilization, the vessels may be controlled with vessel loops or atraumatic aneurysm clips. Anastomosis may be performed in a side-to-side, end-to-end, or end-to-side fashion. All provide adequate flow. We prefer an end of vein to side of artery anastomosis using a continuous 6-0 or 7-0 monofilament suture. The side-to-side anastomosis has the highest flow rate but may lead to development of venous hypertension in the hand. The end-to-end anastomosis sacrifices the radial artery and has the lowest flow. Loupe magnification is helpful. Prior to anastomosis, the vein is gently dilated with heparin saline. Any resistance to flushing during this maneuver suggests venous obstruction, which may lead to fistula failure. The artery may be flushed with heparinized saline proximally and distally, but systemic heparinization is not required.

Upon completion of the anastomosis, a thrill should be palpable in the distal vein. Absence of a thrill indicates a probable technical or anatomic defect. Causes for immediate failure include inadequate vein, inadequate arterial inflow, technical anastomotic failure, kinking of the vein, or hypotension. Webs and thickened valve leaflets are common in upper extremity veins and may be the cause of poor outflow and fistula failure. The point of obstruction is occasionally palpable or may be localized with a coronary dilator. The continuous-wave Doppler study is occasionally helpful. Intraoperative arteriography is obtained if noninvasive procedures do not identify the cause of poor fistula blood flow. Focal lesions may be corrected with a vein patch, short segment interposition graft, or resection and primary anastomosis. Occasionally, the fistula must be revised to a more proximal segment of the vein.

We generally allow 4 to 6 weeks for adequate arterialization of the vein prior to use. Earlier vein puncture may result in intramural hematoma and fistula thrombosis. Veins previously exposed to arterial pressure by an earlier access may be used sooner, however. Hand exercise has been advocated to encourage fistula maturation, but it does not appear to increase fistula blood flow. Some surgeons encourage venous maturation by having patients occasionally occlude the cephalic vein in the forearm with gentle hand pressure.

The cephalic vein in the upper arm may be used in a similar fashion by constructing an end of vein to side of brachial artery anastomosis above or below the antecubital fossa. It may be performed as a primary access procedure or as a secondary procedure after a failed forearm access. Prior ipsilateral access in the forearm may cause dilation and maturation of the upper arm cephalic vein, allowing early use of the new fistula.

A transposed brachiobasilic fistula is another good choice to maintain autogenous access. This procedure is more extensive than other fistula procedures because complete mobilization of the entire vein is required. General or regional anesthesia is preferred. With a longitudinal continuous incision along the medial aspect of the arm, venous side branches are ligated and the basilic vein is mobilized up to the axilla. The upper extremity veins not uncommonly contain webs and areas of fibrosis that may render the conduit unacceptable. One method of assessment prior to complete mobilization of the vein is angioscopy, performed after exposure of the vein at the elbow. Preoperative duplex examination may also be useful. Gentle dilation of the vein with heparin saline may reveal intrinsic defects. The vein is marked to maintain orientation, and a blunt tunneler is used to transpose the mobilized vein into a subcutaneous position in the upper arm for easy venipuncture.

RESULTS

The 1 year cumulative patency of a native AVF ranges from 65% to 80%. Excluding those that fail immediately, the 1 year patency approaches 90%. Patency rates at 3 years are 57% to 65%.[1-3] Although many studies report essentially equivalent cumulative patency rates for PTFE grafts and native fistulas, these data invariably include a high immediate failure rate for the native fistulas. In addition, despite similar cumulative patency rates, PTFE grafts require more procedures per graft.[3]

Early postoperative fistula failure is most commonly due to inadequate venous outflow and is treated with thrombectomy if the fistula is salvageable. Occasionally, these grafts achieve long-term function. The best results are obtained when the defect responsible for graft failure is identified and corrected. Late failure is most commonly caused by intimal hyperplasia either in the outflow vein or at the anastomosis. Additional causes of late failure include subclavian vein stenosis or thrombosis, injury at sites of repeated puncture, subcutaneous hematoma, overly vigorous compression, or hypotension.

Salvage of a failing fistula is easier than resurrecting one that has thrombosed. Unfortunately, no standard method of surveillance is currently in widespread use to detect the failing access. Reported modalities include calculation of urea recirculation, venous dialysis pressure, and duplex scanning. Venous pressure during dialysis is simple to obtain and is commonly reported as abnormal when greater than 150 mm Hg at 200 to 225 ml/minute blood flow using a 16 gauge needle. At this level of venous pressure, 86% of patients studied with fistulography have a significant stenosis. Further, correction of these stenoses results in prolonged graft survival compared to grafts with uncorrected stenoses.[4] In high-efficiency dialysis systems with blood flows of 400 to 500 ml/minute, venous resistance is not a reliable indicator of graft stenosis.

Extent of urea recirculation appears to be indicative of graft stenosis even with high-flux dialysis.[5] Values greater than 15% have traditionally been reported as abnormal; however, recent work suggests that this may change depending on access site, dialysis flow rate, and time into the dialysis run. As the percentage urea recirculation increases, however, the positive predictive value for stenosis rises.[5]

Duplex and color flow Doppler technology are capable of detecting stenoses. Dialysis grafts are particularly suited for ultrasound examination because of their superficial location. Unfortunately, established standards for velocity waveform analysis do not yet exist to grade the degree of stenosis. One study found peak systolic frequency to be the most reliable indicator of anastomotic and outflow vein stenosis. Using a 5 mHz probe, a peak systolic frequency of 12 kHz was 81% accurate in identifying anastomotic stenoses. Using a cutoff of 8 kHz, this technique was 96% accurate in identifying stenoses in the efferent vein.[6] Color flow imaging has also been used to examine native fistulas. Criteria for stenoses using this technology include narrowing of the anastomosis or outflow vein with increased velocities and turbulent flow across the stenosis. This technique tends to overestimate the degree of stenosis more than arteriography.[7]

When a stenosis is suspected by one of these modalities, arteriography is indicated. Intervention is warranted for significant stenoses to reduce the incidence of access thrombosis. Similar to findings with peripheral vascular bypasses, patency rates of electively revised grafts are similar to grafts that never require intervention.[3] No one procedure is adequate for the treatment of all graft problems; rather, the procedure should be tailored to the offending lesion. Short stenoses respond favorably to percutaneous angioplasty. The initial success of this procedure is high, and 1 year patency ranges from 50% to 91%. Significant complications are unusual. Recurrences are common, and repeated dilations are often required. Stents have been used when lesions become refractory to angioplasty, but their exact role is presently undefined. Use of thrombolysis has further extended the role of interventional radiologists in the management of these problems. Operation is generally chosen when angioplasty fails or sequential or long-segment stenoses or occlusions are identified. Surgical options include resection of the area with primary anastomosis, patch angioplasty, short-segment vein interposition, or revision of the fistula to a more proximal vein segment. Only when no further radiologic or surgical interventions are deemed possible is the site abandoned.

Pseudoaneurysms or true aneurysms are occasional complications of native AVFs. When small, they are observed, but they may be excised if they are symptomatic, continue to increase in size, or threaten to erode through the skin. When possible, the fistula is salvaged by use of an interposition graft or by revision to a more proximal portion of the vein.

Ischemic steal syndromes in the hand occasionally occur. Symptoms may not be manifest immediately after construction of the fistula, but develop as it matures and blood flow increases. Complaints include pain and paresthesias, which may be constant or present only on dialysis. Intermittent mild paresthesias that develop early after fistula formation occasionally resolve. When significant symptoms of steal develop, however, delay in intervention may result in tissue loss. This complication is more common with upper arm AVFs because of higher flow rates. Although the fistula may be ligated in this situation, an attempt is generally made to salvage both the limb and the access. In the absence of an identifiable arterial occlusive lesion, the fistula is usually banded to reduce flow. The goal is to reduce fistula blood flow without resultant thrombosis. Technical adjuncts to assist with this problem include operative digital pulse volume or pressure recordings and also angiodynography.[8,9]

Subclavian vein stenosis or thrombosis, usually secondary to previous central venous access, may cause significant limb swelling or failure of an ipsilateral dialysis fistula. Although surgical correction of these lesions is possible, the ease and high success rate of angioplasty makes it the first choice for treatment of this problem. Multiple procedures may be required to obtain lasting results. The role of intravascular stents in treating venous stenoses remains undefined.[10,11]

REFERENCES

1. Cantelmo NL, LoGerfo FW, Menzoian JO. Brachiobasilic and brachiocephalic fistulas as secondary angioaccess routes. Surg Gynecol Obstet 1992; 155:545–548.
2. Wedgewood KR, Wiggins PA, Guillon PJ. A prospective study of end to side vs side to side arteriovenous fistulas for haemodialysis. Br J Surg 1984; 71:640–642.
3. Palder SB, Kirkman RL, Whittemore AD, et al. Vascular access for hemodialysis: Patency rates and results of revision. Ann Surg 1985; 202:235–239.
4. Schwab SJ, Raymond JR, Saeed M, et al. Prevention of hemodialysis fistula thrombosis. Early detection of venous stenoses. Kidney Int 1989; 36:707–711.
5. Collins DM, Lambert MB, Middleton JP, et al. Fistula dysfunction: Effect on rapid hemodialysis. Kidney Int 1992; 41:1292–1296.
6. Tordoir JHM, deBruin HG, Hoeneveld H, et al. Duplex ultrasound scanning in the assessment of arteriovenous fistulas created for hemodialysis access: Comparison with digital subtraction angiography. J Vasc Surg 1989; 10:122–128.
7. Dousset V, Grenier N, Douws C, et al. Hemodialysis grafts: Color Doppler flow imaging correlated with digital subtraction angiography and functional status. Radiology 1991; 181:89–94.
8. Rivers SP, Scher LA, Veith FJ. Correction of steal syndrome secondary to hemodialysis access fistulas: A simplified quantitative technique. Surgery 1992; 112:593–597.
9. Jain KM, Simoni EJ, Munn JS. A new technique to correct vascular steal secondary to hemodialysis grafts. Surg Gynecol Obstet 1992; 175:183–184.
10. Newman GE, Saeed M, Himmelstein S, et al. Total central vein obstruction: Resolution with angioplasty and fibrinolysis. Kidney Int 1991; 39:761–764.
11. Wisselink W, Money SR, Becker MO, et al. Comparison of operative reconstruction and percutaneous balloon dilatation for central venous obstruction. Am J Surg 1993; 166:200–205.

BRIDGE GRAFTS FOR ANGIOACCESS

RICHARD W. DOW, M.D.
SHELDON A. SCHWARTZ, M.D.

Two basic methods to provide access for hemodialysis are in current general use. One uses catheter access to the central venous blood pool, and the other uses an arteriovenous (AV) connection. Ordinarily, simple venous access is reserved for the short-term management of acute problems or for long-term use if AV access is inappropriate. Catheter-related sepsis, central venous stenosis or occlusion, catheter malfunction, thromboembolic phenomena, and insertion-related events are frequent complications of central venous devices.

Long-term access for most patients requiring hemodialysis involves intermittent needle cannulation of a surgically constructed AV fistula. There are only two fundamental types of AV fistulas. The first type uses an in situ autogenous vein, and the second uses a prosthetic conduit to make the AV connection.

Over the past several decades, numerous nonrandomized studies have evaluated the clinical performance of the autogenous fistula and the alternative of a prosthetic bridge graft. These studies support the conclusion that the long-term performance of autogenous tissues is superior to the long-term performance of prosthetic conduits.[1] The combined weight of these clinical studies has persuaded most experienced access surgeons that options for autogenous tissue construction in the upper extremity should be pursued before resorting to the use of prosthetic conduits in adult patients.

For patients who have an immediate need for dialysis, the interval required between the operative construction of fistula and its use is a problem. An average of 6 weeks is required for an autogenous fistula to develop sufficiently to permit reliable use for dialysis. With prosthetic conduits, this "maturation" time is substantially shorter. We prefer to construct autogenous fistulas in favorable candidates despite the longer maturation time required for development and clinical use. In our urban practice, about 80% of patients who present for the construction of their first AV dialysis access require urgent dialysis with a temporary venous device. Even in these circumstances, an autogenous fistula can be successfully constructed in about 60% of patients. In the increasingly common HIV-positive patient, the greater risk of infection of a prosthetic site provides additional motivation to explore all reasonable autogenous options before resorting to the use of prosthetic materials.

We proceed with bridge graft placement in most patients without obtaining specialized preoperative cardiac studies. Patients who demonstrate reasonable exercise tolerance by being able to climb a flight of stairs, have no current cardiac symptoms, give no history of cardiac disease, and maintain a normal cardiac rhythm do not undergo special preoperative cardiac evaluation. When decreased exercise tolerance, cardiac symptoms, history, or findings on examination suggest that cardiac reserve is compromised in spite of optimal medical support, formal preoperative cardiac evaluation is undertaken. Because of the wide array of variables, a reliable and simple decision algorithm relating AV site construction to cardiac status is not in general use. In questionable cases, we prefer an alternative peritoneal or long-term venous approach to dialysis.

Our practice is to evaluate the vascular anatomy and status of an extremity and select a site for bridge graft construction in most patients without obtaining contrast x-ray or noninvasive vascular laboratory studies. A difference in systolic pressure of greater than 10 to 15 mm Hg between arms is veiwed as presumptive evidence of a proximal occlusive lesion and prompts additional studies. The peripheral pulses and their quality are evaluated and recorded. Of particular importance is the evaluation of the radial artery in diabetic patients. Radial arteries with palpable thickening or calcification are poor for the construction of a bridge graft. Normal digital pulses are regularly palpable and should be sought. Their presence, especially in a diabetic patient, provides some reassurance that digital vessel disease will not complicate the construction of a proximal bridge graft. In 10% to 15% of the population, the brachial artery divides into radial and ulnar trunks proximal to the antecubital fossa. Our clinical impression is that this anomaly is associated with increased failure rates of standard bridge grafts in the forearm and the arm. Additionally, the anomaly appears to involve the venous side of the circulation, as the deep venous system is usually made up of multiple small communicating veins instead of the single or double venous channel normally encountered. When the anomaly is suspected clinically, the location of the brachial artery bifurcation is confirmed by ultrasound, and special care in planning an appropriate site is required. The final clinical maneuver in evaluating the arterial status is an estimation of the patency and adequacy of the palmar arches. When a lower extremity is being considered for dialysis site construction, noninvasive testing is advised, and evidence of significant occlusive disease contraindicates site construction at this location.

After we evaluate the arterial anatomy, we assess the venous anatomy. Because the presence of patent, visible or palpable, sizable, superficial, and straight veins ordinarily qualifies the patient for autogenous access construction, it is virtually axiomatic that examination does not reveal good superficial veins in candidates for bridge grafts. Because we regularly use the deep venous system as the outflow tract for bridge grafts, ultrasound evaluation is advocated to confirm the presence of adequate deep venous outflow in patients with no clinically evident superficial veins. Specific attention to axillary or subclavian venous stenosis or occlusion is necessary. Axillary or subclavian venous stenosis or occlusion is a major consequence of use of large-caliber central venous dialysis catheters.[2] These catheter-related occlusions and stenoses are ordinarily clinically silent. Although this feature makes preoperative detection difficult, the significant symptoms of venous hypertension and edema that follow the construction of a bridge graft make preoperative detection important. Additionally, bridge grafts that use these stenotic or obstructed outflow tracts are prone to thrombosis. Consequently, the liberal use of preoperative noninvasive or contrast imaging in patients with evidence of previous ipsilateral dialysis catheter use is suggested.

SELECTING THE SITE AND CONFIGURATION FOR THE BRIDGE GRAFT

Upper extremity sites are favored over lower extremity sites in adults, sites in nondominant extremities are favored over sites in dominant extremities, and sites distal in the extremity are favored over proximal sites. In the forearm, the graft is placed in either a straight or a looped configuration with the radial or brachial artery, respectively, as an inflow source and a superficial or deep vein in the antecubital fossa as the outflow. In the arm, the graft is placed in a gently curved configuration from the brachial artery above the elbow to the high brachial or axillary vein. In the leg, a looped configuration between the common femoral artery and the saphenofemoral junction is favored. Although a variety of prosthetic conduits have been used for dialysis site construction, most access surgeons now use a polytetrafluoroethylene (PTFE) conduit that tapers from 4 mm in diameter at the arterial end to 7 mm in diameter at the venous end.

Because both straight and looped forearm configurations use the same venous outflow at the elbow, the choice between straight and looped configurations is made on the basis of the size and quality of the radial artery. A straight configuration is advocated only in the presence of a normal radial artery at least 2.5 to 3 mm in diameter. If exposure of the distal radial artery reveals a small vessel or significant plaque, then a straight forearm graft is abandoned in favor of a looped configuration. When the looped configuration is selected, the arterial origin is selected on the basis of the quality of the arteries. Whereas the radial artery just distal to its origin from the brachial artery is preferred, the brachial artery itself is used if a diminutive or diseased radial arterial origin is encountered.

CONSTRUCTING THE ACCESS

The surgical manipulations used in the construction of bridge grafts are standard vascular techniques.[3] Loupe magnification is used. Perioperative antibiotics are advocated. Regional nerve block is preferred over general anesthesia or local infiltration techniques. For exposure and control of appropriate arteries and veins in the extremities, we favor axial incisions because they may be extended. Liberal regional use of heparin sodium is preferred to systemic heparinization. With the exception of the radial artery at the wrist, where a somewhat smaller normal artery can be used, an artery of at least 3 mm internal diameter and without significant proximal flow-restricting lesions is required to provide reliable inflow to a prosthetic dialysis site. A vein of 3.5 to 4 mm is required to provide adequate outflow, and there should be no flow-restricting lesions in the vein between the access site and the central venous structures. Tortuous collateral veins, even though they may have achieved a 4 mm diameter, are not used. Careful attention to tunneling and positioning of the graft minimizes the frequency of complications related to the tunnel or to the configuration of the prosthetic. A special effort is made to place the graft in a uniform subcutaneous position so that needle access to the full useful length of the graft is facilitated.

After the fistula is constructed and functioning, careful operative assessment is made. Blood flow should be easily detected by palpation of a continuous thrill. Operative imaging with contrast or ultrasound may provide useful information, but these imaging modalities are not routinely used in the absence of a clinical indication.

The postoperative care plan is simple. Patients are advised to position the extremity for comfort. Elevation is advised only if edema is a problem. A breathable adhesive polymer dressing is used to avoid the compression that may result when bulky dressings are used around mobile joints. Exercises are not advised.

Although others have punctured bridge grafts for dialysis within days of construction, we prefer to allow development of firm adherence between the graft and tissues of the tunnel before using the site. In the usual circumstances, 1 month of healing is preferred, but grafts are punctured 2 weeks after construction in pressing circumstances. The major risk of early utilization is the development of a perigraft hematoma with its attendant risks of infection and thrombosis. As the graft enters routine service, a follow-up program of surveillance to detect impending problems is advocated.

RESTORING FLOW IN NONFUNCTIONING BRIDGE GRAFTS

Unfortunately, bridge grafts constructed to provide access for hemodialysis have a limited duration of function and a high rate of complications.[4,5] Common complications of prosthetic access grafts include a range of problems associated with the arterial perfusion of the extremity, infection, aneurysms of the body of the prosthetic or the anastomosis, venous hypertension, and problems associated with high or low blood flow through the fistula. Thrombosis is the most frequent complication, and it can be expected about once every 12 months. In selected circumstances, a "crossed-catheter" technique of thrombolytic perfusion has been effective for restoring blood flow, but in most cases we favor a direct operative approach.

The evaluation of a patient with a thrombosed graft begins with a review of the performance history of the graft. Consultation with the dialysis technicians who had been using the site often provides valuable information.

A history of elevated venous pressures within the dialysis circuit, inadequate arterial flow, excessive bleeding from cannulation sites, prolonged external pressure on the site, episodes of hypotension during or after dialysis, or data suggesting excessive recirculation should be sought.

Assessment of Inflow

When the access is thrombosed, standard cuff blood pressures can be safely measured in that extremity. Systolic blood pressure differences of greater than 15 mm Hg between corresponding extremities suggest the presence of a proximal flow-restricting lesion.

A strong pulse in the "hood" of the thrombosed graft can usually be identified. When present, this pulse within the "hood" provides some assurance that adequate inflow for the site is readily available.

Evaluation of pulses is of special importance when the extremity has carried previous access sites because occlusion of the native vessels may have occurred with a previous failure. Collateral circulation through the palmar arch is evaluated by an Allen test or its equivalent, but the absence of adequate collateral circulation does not necessarily exclude reoperation at this site. An increased risk of hand ischemia accompanies operations in patients with inadequate distal pulses or poor palmar collaterals, and operations at such sites are not recommended if safer alternatives are feasible.

Examination of the arterial anastomosis may reveal a pulsatile mass representing a fibrin collection, a seroma, a hematoma, or a pseudoaneurysm. Anastomotic pseudoaneurysms may be difficult to distinguish from perianastomotic collections of serum or fibrin. Ultrasound or contrast examination ordinarily identifies these problems in functioning sites but may not conclusively differentiate them when the graft is clotted. Formal exposure, diagnosis, and repair of these lesions is advised.

Assessment of Outflow

Edema (which may have abated with shunt thrombosis), collateral veins around the shoulder or groin, and scars from previous central lines may indicate occlusion or stenosis of the central veins. Such physical findings should prompt consideration of preoperative imaging of the suspected venous segment. Re-establishment of flow into veins with inadequate central connections is not advised as it usually results in disabling venous hypertension, edema, or recurrent graft thrombosis.

The presence of large, pliable, low-pressure veins at the outflow end of the site suggests that adequate outflow options are available. Conversely, the presence of fibrotic, clotted, tense, undetectable, or small outflow veins may prompt a preoperative decision to change the location of the site.

Evaluation of the Prosthetic Graft

The condition of the prosthetic graft should be carefully assessed to determine if it has reached the end of its useful life. A prosthesis that is too deep or too tortuous, is palpably thickened to suggest extensive intraluminal fibrosis, has palpable defects in areas of multiple needle punctures, or exhibits significant pseudoaneurysms should be replaced.

The entire site should not be abandoned if only a segment of the prosthetic requires replacement. Preservation of a substantial segment of incorporated prosthetic is advantageous as the preserved segment may be used immediately following operation, and the need for a temporary venous catheter is eliminated.

Selecting the Site for the Initial Incision

Unless preoperative findings indicate a different approach, the incision is made at the venous anastomosis, the most common site of a lesion precipitating the thrombosis or requiring correction to re-establish long-term patency. Additionally, the graft in this area has not been subjected to repetitive needle cannulation. When a graft is exposed in the area of previous needle punctures, injury of the graft is more likely, subsequent closure of the graft may be difficult because the wall of the graft is honeycombed by the needle punctures, and needle puncture sites become a source of troublesome bleeding when flow is re-established.

Vascular Control

The prosthetic graft is mobilized near the venous anastomosis. Exposure of the anastomotic sutures is often the first clue to the precise location of the anastomosis. The decision to gain early control of the outflow vein is individualized. When control of the venous outflow is not obtained initially, an adequate breadth of exposure should be developed to allow easy control of the impending graftotomy site because venous back bleeding can be brisk.

Formal exposure or control of the arterial origin of the prosthesis is not obtained at this stage.

Graft Exploration

The graftotomy is made transversely within 1 or 2 mm of the suture line of the venous anastomosis. It is not uncommon to encounter the suture line of a previous graftotomy. If that suture line is in an appropriate position, it is reused.

When opening the graft adjacent to the venous anastomosis, it is often necessary to deepen the incision through a layer of tissue adherent to the inner surface of the prosthetic before gaining access to the lumen. This gray-white layer of hyperplastic myoendothelial cells is often 1 or 2 mm thick, and the flow lumen is subsequently recognized when frank clot is encountered. Intimal hyperplasia at the venous end of access grafts usually causes maximal narrowing within the graft very close to the anastomosis. This observation may be contrary to the general notion that the point of maximum narrowing is within the vein.

Structural Problems

Identification

External examination of the outflow vein by palpation and direct visual inspection often provides important clues about the status of the vein. If the vein is significantly thickened, contains adherent thrombus, or is small, revision to a new venous outflow site is usually appropriate.

Using suction and forceps, the clot is removed to permit direct inspection of the anastomotic area. Appreciating the extent of the hyperplasia may be difficult. We have found it helpful to calibrate, not dilate, the size of the venous anastomosis with a coronary artery dilator.

After calibration, the dilator is carefully advanced into the outflow vein to identify a more proximal area of stenosis. If a stenotic area is identified, we advise contrast imaging. Blind dilation of a proximal stenotic area is not advised, and simple dilation of an anastomotic stenosis is usually insufficient to obtain a longlasting result.

Another important observation involves the propagation of clot into the outflow vein. Anything more than a small tail of propagated clot into the outflow vein may indicate the presence of problems more proximally within the outflow vein. We consider the presence of thrombus in the outflow vein as an indication for operative phlebography.

Evaluation of the status of the outflow veins by assessing the backflow is unreliable. A widely patent venous outflow with low venous pressure and competent valves may have little backflow. Conversely, veins with proximal obstruction may produce a torrent of backflow. After evaluating and calibrating the outflow, regional heparinization of the venous segment is accomplished, and the adequacy of the outflow is additionally estimated by the ease of "flushing" the segment.

Before correcting any problems detected at the venous anastomotic site, we examine the body of the graft. A 4 Fr Fogarty catheter is used to progressively evacuate the clot from short segments of the graft. Ease of passage of the catheter, resistance to withdrawal of the catheter as it relates to the degree of inflation of the balloon, and the appearance of the site from the skin aspect as the balloon is withdrawn are evaluated. Areas of resistance to passage of the balloon are marked for attention at a later stage.

In these maneuvers, care is taken to avoid passage of the Fogarty catheter into the region of the arterial anastomosis. By careful measurement, palpation of the catheter as it is passed, and direct observation of the skin over the graft, it is possible to monitor the depth of insertion of the Fogarty catheter quite accurately. If a 0.5 to 1 cm area around the arterial anastomosis is not violated, premature arterial flow within the site is usually avoided. This strategy permits correction of structural problems in the body or outflow region of the site and without concern about reclotting in the body of the graft.

Correction

Over the past few years, we have become more aggressive about formal revision of the perianastomotic area in thrombosed sites where intimal hyperplasia or structural flow-disturbing-lesions of any severity are identified. Previously, only those sites where the perianastomotic lumen was smaller than 3.5 to 4 mm had been formally revised. Currently, we favor short-segment interposition procedures over both patching or direct operative "debridement" of the hyperplastic tissue at the venous anastomosis. If the previously utilized outflow vessel is no longer suitable for use, another vessel or the same vessel at a more proximal level is exposed and an interposition graft is fashioned of PTFE of the appropriate size. When joints are crossed, an externally supported prosthetic is often used.

When segmental declotting of the body of the graft reveals areas of narrowing, we have used a variety of instruments to remove the fibrous material that produces these areas of narrowing. This fibrous plaque is densely adherent to the prosthetic wall and is not ordinarily removed by even the most vigorous efforts with the Fogarty catheter. A uterine currette, intraluminal endarterectomy instrument, extraluminal vein strippers, and suction are all used with varying success in this effort. Judicious force must be used with these instruments, as perforation of the graft is a potential complication which usually requires major revision.

When dealing with a graft in a loop configuration from a single exposure at the venous end, the far side of the loop cannot be adequately "scraped" with any of these instruments. Careful individual judgment must be used in deciding whether independent exposure and currettage of this limb is required.

The degree of luminal fibrosis that is too extensive to be treated by these techniques is a point of judgment. If the body of the prosthesis is extensively fibrosed, a new prosthesis is interposed in a new subcutaneous tunnel adjacent to the old site. A new arterial anastomosis is usually not required, as the new prosthesis may be sutured end to end to the original graft close to the previous arterial anastomosis. A similar technique can be used at the venous end, but more often construction of a new venous anastomosis is required because of anastomotic narrowing.

Clearance of the Arterial Anastomotic Area

After the venous perianastomotic area and the body of the graft have been opened, No. 4 Fogarty catheter is used to remove the remaining thrombus from the arterial anastomosis. It is important to examine the thrombotic debris obtained. The bit of thrombus that forms the exact interface between flowing blood and luminal clot within the graft—"the bullet"—is characteristic. Inadvertent retention of this bullet usually leads to prompt rethrombosis of the site. Astonishingly vigorous arterial flow may be encountered even before this final bit of thrombus is cleared from the anastomotic area.

After retrieval of the bullet, the adequacy of arterial blood flow is assessed. We have no objective criteria to judge the adequacy of arterial inflow. In practice, when inflow is judged to be suspicious or inadequate, formal exposure with repair of any flow-reducing lesions is undertaken. If blood flow appears inadequate, contrast imaging directs further plans, which might include an extension of the operative procedure or arrangements for transluminal dilation of occlusive lesions of the proximal vessels.

After clearing the entire graft and reaching a decision about the adequacy of inflow, we fill the graft with heparinized saline while closing the graftotomy. The closure of the graftotomy is then accomplished expeditiously as the graft frequently clots even with heparin sodium instillation if more than 10 or 15 minutes of stasis is allowed to occur.

Final Intraoperative Evaluation

After the graftotomy is closed, the clamps are removed and flow in the site is assessed. A vigorous thrill should be palpable over the graft, and expansile pulsations should be minimal to absent. It is common for the intensity of the thrill to initially diminish somewhat from the arterial to the venous end of the graft. The thrill should be present throughout the cardiac cycle. Expansile pulsation of the graft reflects restriction of outflow from the site and strongly suggests poor venous outflow.

Wound Closure and Dressing

After satisfactory flow has been restored to the site, meticulous hemostasis must be obtained before the surgical incision is closed because a wound hematoma can have serious consequences. Graft compression by the hematoma may lead to thrombosis, and impaired wound healing or evacuation of the hematoma through the incision may lead to infection of the graft.

A plastic dressing is used to cover the incision. Gauze dressings are avoided as even a loosely applied gauze dressing may compress the access site when the elbow is flexed.

Same day use of the site for dialysis is permitted when the area of the graft to be punctured has not been mobilized from its surrounding tissue bed.

REFERENCES

1. Kherlakian GM, Roedersheimer LR, Arbaugh JJ, et al. Comparison of autogenous fistula versus expanded polytetrafluoroethylene graft fistula for angioaccess in hemodialysis. Am J Surg 1986; 152: 238–243.
2. Barrett N, Spencer S, McIvor J, et al. Subclavian stenosis: A major complication of subclavian dialysis catheters. Nephrol Dial Transplant 1988; 3:423–425.
3. Raju S. PTFE grafts for hemodialysis access. Ann Surg 1987; 206:666–673.
4. Zibari GB, Rohr MS, Landreneau MD, et al. Complications from permanent hemodialysis vascular access. Surgery 1988; 104: 681–686.
5. Munda R, First MR, Alexander JW, et al. Polytetrafluoroethylene graft survival in hemodialysis. JAMA 1983; 249:219–222.

SURVEILLANCE OF ANGIOACCESS GRAFT FUNCTION

ARMEN VARTANY, M.D.
MARTIN J. WINKLER, M.D.
SAMUEL E. WILSON, M.D.

The 115,000 patients in the United States who have end-stage renal disease require repetitive access to the vascular system for maintenance hemodialysis. Standard techniques for establishing angioaccess for hemodialysis are either construction of an autogenous arteriovenous fistula (AVF) or implantation of an arteriovenous conduit that can sustain at least 300 ml/minute of blood flow without thrombosis. Prosthetic vascular conduits have a high rate of thrombosis, often caused by stenosis of the venous outflow tract. Maintenance of adequate vascular access and the secondary complications of access sites are the most frequent causes of hospitalization in chronic hemodialysis. A program of regular surveillance of hemodialysis access function promises early detection of stenosis or recent thrombosis and extension of the patency of the shunt by prompt intervention.[1]

AUTOGENOUS ARTERIOVENOUS FISTULA

The optimal form of hemodialysis access is the autologous AVF. The fistula is usually constructed by anastomosis of the proximal end of the divided cephalic vein to the side of the radial artery in the distal forearm. Other sites for fistula formation include the ulnar artery and the basilic vein, the brachial artery and the cephalic or basilic veins, and distal placement of the fistula in the snuffbox. These autogenous fistulas have a relatively high rate of initial nonfunction (10% to 15%), usually due to inadequate dilation of the vein or lack of arterialization of the vein wall, which allows it to withstand multiple punctures. Their long-term patency rate, however, is higher than any other form of hemodialysis access, approaching 78% in 3 years.[2] Late failure is caused by fibrosis of the vein due to repeated puncture trauma with large-bore needles or aneurysm formation. Evaluation of blood flow and function, as well as imaging, have important roles in assessment of early fistula development and diagnosis of late failure. Identification of areas of stenosis along the vein can facilitate local correction by relatively simple techniques such as excision and anastomosis or interposition of a short prosthetic segment.

PROSTHETIC GRAFT ARTERIOVENOUS FISTULAS

In patients who do not have adequate native vessels for AVFs or have failed prior fistulas, prosthetic shunts are placed for hemodialysis. Currently, these shunts are the most common form of dialysis access. The standard prosthetic material used is expanded polytetrafluoroethylene (PTFE) graft. Prosthetic arteriovenous grafts may be placed between almost any artery and vein but are preferentially used in the upper extremity because of the lower risk of infection and hemodynamic complications than occurs with grafts placed in the lower extremity. The PTFE grafts are typically placed as straight 6 mm diameter segments or as loops in the forearm or brachium.

A lower incidence of early thrombosis is encountered with PTFE grafts than with arteriovenous fistulas because grafts have higher flow rates in the immediate postoperative period. However, their late thrombosis rate is higher, with the 2 year primary patency rates for grafts usually between 50% and 60%. In addition, grafts have a higher rate of infection, approximately 8%, and are subject to pseudoaneurysm formation, venous hypertension, and arterial steal more frequently than AVFs.[3]

GRAFT THROMBOSIS

The most common cause of late thrombosis of both AVFs and PTFE grafts is stenosis at, or just distal to, the venous anastomosis. Swedberg and colleagues found that the average time to failure due to venous stenosis occurred at 22.3 ± 13.1 months in AVFs, and at 16 ± 15 months in PTFE grafts.[4] The histology of the intimal hyperplasia that causes the venous stenosis includes both cellular and extracellular components. The cellular components are almost exclusively composed of smooth muscle cells, and the extracellular matrix is constituted by collagen, elastin, and proteoglycan. The release of platelet-derived growth factor from the blood-graft interface and the localized venous intimal injury caused by highly turbulent blood flow at the graft to vein anastomosis have been postulated as the causes of intimal hyperplasia. This compliance mismatch between the relatively rigid graft and elastic vein wall is also postulated as a cause of intimal hyperplasia. This aggressive form of intimal hyperplasia or venous runoff stenosis accounts for PTFE angioaccess graft thrombosis in more than three-quarters of patients. Other causes of thrombosis such as arterial inflow narrowing, sometimes seen in diabetic patients, or accumulating cellular and fibrin blood components on the interior graft wall are distinctly less common. Thus, early detection of the predictable development of venous runoff stenosis, before thrombosis occurs, would potentially reduce the failed graft rate, prolong life of existing grafts, and reduce hospitalization rates and cost of treatment of dialysis patients.

DIAGNOSIS OF GRAFT FAILURE

Detection of a failing graft on clinical grounds alone is difficult. A decrease in the palpable anastomotic thrill and a bruit audible with a stethoscope are subjective suggestions of decreased blood flow. Also, loss of the augmentation of graft pulsation on compression of the venous end suggests inflow or outflow obstruction. On occasion, one may feel a palpable cord in the region of the venous anastomosis, suggesting fibrosis of the venous outflow tract.

Elevated venous return pressure during hemodialysis is a more reliable indicator of venous stenosis. Schwab and colleagues measured venous dialysis blood pressures at extracorporeal blood flows of 200 to 225 ml/minute through an 18 gauge needle and considered pressures greater than 150 mm Hg as abnormal. This value detected venous stenosis with a specificity of 93% and sensitivity of 86%.[5] Elevated venous return dialysis blood pressures can be used for early detection of venous stenosis and elective treatment before thrombosis occurs.

Recirculation during hemodialysis is another indication of a failing graft. Recirculation is defined as a percentage of blood flow that is recirculated from the venous line into the dialyzer inflow by retrograde blood flow through the fistula. It is calculated as a percentage that equals $100 \times (P - A \div P - V)$ where P is the blood urea nitrogen (BUN) value in the vein of the nonfistula arm and V and A are BUN values in the venous and arterial dialysis lines, respectively. Recirculation values exceeding 15% are considered abnormal and can be used as screening tests for detection of a significant stenosis with a specificity of 82%.

Color Flow Doppler (CFD) imaging of vascular access grafts and fistulas has proven to be the most reliable, noninvasive method of evaluating function. Partial or complete obstruction is detected by identifying turbulent blood flow and outlining dimensions of the graft and vein lumina. The CFD is safer and cheaper than arteriography and is considered by some surgeons and nephrologists as the procedure of choice for evaluating a hemodialysis access prosthesis. It also detects graft occlusion, false aneurysms, and low blood flow velocity. Identification of a narrowing of greater than 50% is thought to predict the thrombosis of PTFE grafts. Thus, CFD may be used to identify patients at high risk for thrombosis and possibly allow intervention before acute thrombosis occurs.

The role of CFD for dialysis access surveillance is evolving. Middleton and co-workers reported a 94% accuracy rate for CFD in 17 patients with PTFE grafts who had stenoses greater than or equal to 50% when compared to the standard of digital subtraction fistulography. The CFD accuracy in six Brescia-Cimino fistulas was 67%.[6] Tordoir and associates reported similar accuracies for CFD versus fistulography in 36 patients with Brescia-Cimino fistulas and 28 patients with PTFE grafts.[7] Strauch and colleagues related CFD-diagnosed stenosis to subsequent graft occlusion. Patients were studied with CFD once and when graft failure was recorded over 6 months. Eight of 14 patients (57%) with stenoses greater than 50% had graft thrombosis within the 6 month study. In patients with lesser degrees of stenosis, only 14% of the patients developed graft thrombosis.[8]

The clinical utility of elective CFD graft surveillance was reported by Bay in 1992.[9] One hundred patients were studied, of whom 49% were female and 40% diabetic. The access sites were Brescia-Cimino fistulas in 31% and PTFE grafts in 69%. The CFD imaging was performed four times between October 1990 and April 1992. At each of the screenings, approximately 7% of the patients had stenoses of greater than 50%. Over the course of the study, CFD suggested a stenosis of greater than 50% in three patients with Brescia-Cimino fistulas, and this was confirmed by contrast fistulogram in two patients (66% accuracy). CFD suggested stenosis in 29 patients who had PTFE grafts. Fistulography confirmed stenosis in 28 patients (96% accuracy). Bay notes that these data are encouraging but acknowledges that it does not prove what clinicians hope to be true, that CFD surveillance at regular intervals will improve the long-term patency of hemodialysis access patients. Walker and Jones reported diagnostic utility of CFD in 50 patients who had failing grafts based on the following: increased venous return blood pressure, recirculation volume of 15%, access thrombosis, upper extremities edema, and expanding perigraft mass. This study illustrated the accuracy of CFD in detecting conditions other than stenosis that cause graft failure, such as false aneurysms, graft infection, and proximal venous outflow obstruction.[10]

Strauch and associates analyzed the relationship between blood flow velocities in PTFE dialysis grafts and thrombosis over a 6 month follow-up period.[8] In eight patients with blood flow velocities of less than 300 ml per minute, six (65%) patients developed graft thrombosis. This measurement is readily available from CFD imaging and may prove to be as valuable as stenosis in predicting the failure of grafts.

As a technique for graft surveillance, CFD imaging is promising. No controlled studies are available that document that overall outcome is improved with routine graft surveillance. It is probable that outcome is improved when CFD imaging is used to evaluate a graft that is felt to be failing based on other findings. Further, a cost analysis comparing overall graft patency in patients who have routine CFD surveillance with patients followed on clinical findings alone must be made. To be useful, such a trial should be randomized and prospective, with several centers contributing patients to achieve statistically significant results.

Clinicians have two options for graft surveillance: fistulography or CFD. CFD, although noninvasive, has the following disadvantages. Expensive equipment is required, and vascular laboratory technicians require extensive training to accurately identify stenotic lesions and to calculate blood flow volumes. The test requires 30 to 60 minutes to perform, and third-party payors are inconsistent in reimbursement for this study.

Advantages of fistulography include a hard copy study for the surgeon revising the fistula and the option to perform elective balloon angioplasty at the time of fistulogram. Fistulography can be performed at the completion of dialysis via cannula needles. Actual costs for fistulography are less than for an arteriogram.

Arteriography remains a highly accurate method for assessing graft or fistula morphology. Visualization of both the arterial and venous anastomoses of an autogenous fistula is possible by temporary occlusion of the arterial inflow at the brachium and filling the main venous channel with contrast that outlines the veins as well as both anastomotic sites. If arterial inflow is compromised, injection of contrast medium through the brachial artery is necessary, but if outflow is suspected to be the problem, contrast may be injected directly into the graft.

SALVAGE OF THE FAILING OR FAILED GRAFT

The principal role of surveillance in hemodialysis access function is to detect and treat stenoses prior to acute thrombosis. When a stenosis is suspected, prophylactic treatment has been shown to decrease the incidence of graft thrombosis. Schwab and colleagues investigated the value of prophylactic angioplasty and surgical revision in PTFE grafts with elevated venous blood pressures.[5] They documented a threefold decrease of graft thrombosis and a three and a half fold decrease in graft replacement.

The traditional management of a thrombosed hemodialysis access has been surgical thrombectomy and revision of the access, usually by reconstruction of the venous anastomosis as indicated. The principal alternative to operative management of acute graft thrombosis is thrombolysis and percutaneous transluminal angioplasty of the stenosis. Earlier reports describe administration of streptokinase at relatively low infusion rates of 1000 U/hour, but urokinase, which has a shorter half-life than streptokinase and is not antigenic, is commonly used today. After lysis of the clot, any hemodynamically significant vascular stenoses should be dilated to prevent rethrombosis.

Pulse-spray thrombolysis has been recently described as an improvement in delivery of the lytic agent over standard thrombolysis.[11] High concentrations of urokinase mixed with heparin sodium are administered in pulsatile fashion via two catheters that are threaded through the thrombus. Using this method in combination with angioplasty, a 93% success rate was reported in restoration of blood flow in thrombosed PTFE grafts. Experience with the use of thrombolytic therapy in thrombosis of autogenous AVFs is limited. Data on the long-term patency of grafts following thrombolysis are being accumulated, but early reports indicate that most access sites are patent after 3 months and that the average duration of patency is approximately 6 months.

The use of intravascular stents in PTFE grafts and fistulas has not yet been convincingly shown to be beneficial. They are useful in overcoming acute problems after angioplasty to prevent restenosis and may find a role in the correction of venous outflow stenosis. Stents placed in the subclavian vein have been shown in several case reports to correct stenoses proximal to an ipsilateral arm AVF and have decreased arm swelling and improved longevity of the access site.

REFERENCES

1. Kumpe DA, Cohen MAH. Angioplasty/thrombolytic treatment of failing and failed hemodialysis access sites: Comparison with surgical treatment. Prog Cardiovasc Dis 1992; 34:263–279.
2. Palder SB, Kirkman RL, Whittemore AD, et al. Vascular access for hemodialysis. Patency rates and results of revision. Ann Surg 1985; 202:235–239.
3. Ballard JL, Bunt TJ, Malone JM. Major complications of angioaccess surgery. Am J Surg 1992; 164:316–319.
4. Swedberg SH, Brown BG, Sigley R, et al. Intimal fibromuscular hyperplasia at the venous anastomosis of PTFE grafts in hemodialysis patients. Circulation 1989; 80:1726–1736.
5. Schwab SJ, Raymond RJ, Saeed M, et al. Prevention of hemodialysis fistula thrombosis. Early detection of venous stenoses. Kidney Int 1989; 36:707–711.
6. Middleton W, Picus D, Marx MV, Melson GL. Color Doppler sonography of hemodialysis vascular access: Comparison with angiography. Am J Radiol 1989; 152:633–639.
7. Tordoir JHM, de Bruin HG, Hoeneveld H, et al. Duplex ultrasound scanning in the assessment of arteriovenous fistulas created for hemodialysis access: Comparison with digital subtraction angiography. J Vasc Surg 1989; 10:122–128.
8. Strauch BS, Geoly KL, Yakub YN, et al. Clinical use of color flow Doppler. In: Henry ML and Ferguson RM, eds. Vascular access for hemodialysis. Hong Kong: WL Gore; Precept Press, 1993:102.
9. Bay W. Correlation of color flow Doppler and angiography. In: Vascular access for hemodialysis. Hong Kong: WL Gore; Precept Press, 1993:95.
10. Walker GK, Jones C. Color duplex evaluation of potential hemodialysis graft failure. J Vasc Tech 1992; 16:140–145.
11. Robert AC, Valji K, Bookstein JJ, Hye RJ. Pulse-spray pharmacomechanical thrombolysis for treatment of thrombosed dialysis access grafts. Am J Surg 1993; 166:221–225.

VENOUS DISEASE

COAGULATION CASCADE AND THROMBOEMBOLISM

THOMAS W. WAKEFIELD, M.D.

MECHANISMS OF COAGULATION

Initiating events in hemostasis involve collagen and tissue factor. Tissue factor released from injured cells activates the extrinsic pathway of coagulation while disruption of the endothelium exposes collagen to platelets. In blood, tissue factor complexes with activated factor VII (VIIa), activating factor X to factor Xa.[1] The enzyme responsible for the initial activation of factor VII is unknown. However, factors Xa and VIIa both catalyze activation of factor VII, so there is an amplification for formation of factor VIIa. At the same time, activated platelets change shape to allow their procoagulant phospholipid surface to become externalized. Coagulation cascade proteins assemble on the surface of platelets and form complexes that accelerate the rate of thrombus formation (Fig. 1).[1] Activated factor X (Xa), activated factor V (Va), ionized calcium, and factor II (prothrombin) form the prothrombinase complex, which markedly catalyzes the formation of thrombin (Fig. 2).[1]

Thrombin formation is central to all of coagulation. Among the many functions of thrombin, fibrinopeptide A (FPA) from the alpha-chain and fibrinopeptide B (FPB) from the beta-chain are removed to form a fibrin monomer.[1] This monomer then polymerizes with other fibrin monomers to form a clot. Thrombin activates factor XIII catalyzing the cross-linking of fibrin to make the clot firm, activates platelets leading to platelet aggregation, and activates factors V and factors VIII, two nonenzymatic cofactors, to Va and VIIIa.[1] This is important as it is the active factors, Va and VIIIa, not the inactive precursors, that are used in the coagulation complexes.

Tissue factor–factor VIIa complex can also activate factor IX to IXa. Factor IXa, X, ionized calcium, and thrombin-activated factor VIII (VIIIa) then assemble on the platelet surface (the Xase complex) to catalyze conversion of factor X to activated factor X (Xa) (Fig. 2).[1] This factor Xa can then enter into the prothrombinase complex for further thrombin formation. In addition, coagulation may be initiated through the contact activation system involving factor XII activation. High-molecular-weight kininogen, prekallikrein, and factor XI then interact with factor XIIa to initiate thrombosis through this pathway.[1] The contact pathway physiologically is most likely of less importance than the tissue factor–factor VIIa pathway and may be more important in thrombolysis than thrombosis.

At the same time that thrombus formation proceeds, natural anticoagulant mechanisms that oppose further thrombus formation are at work. Because thrombin generation is the key element in coagulation, antithrombin III is the first line of defense of natural anticoagulant proteins. This is a glycoprotein of approximate MW 70,000 that binds to thrombin to prevent the removal of FPA and FPB from fibrinogen, prevent the activation of factors V and VIII to Va and VIIIa, and inhibit activation and aggregation of platelets.[1] In addition, antithrombin III inhibits other serine proteases. Another natural anticoagulant is the serine protease-activated protein C (protein Ca) that inactivates factors Va and VIIIa. This inactivation reduces the ability of the Xase complex and prothrombinase complex to accelerate thrombin formation. A central role of thrombin for protein C activation is also evident. In the circulation, protein C is activated to protein Ca on endothelial cell surfaces by thrombin complexed with one of its receptors, thrombomodulin (Fig. 3).[1] The formation of this thrombin-thrombomodulin complex greatly accelerates the activation of protein C as compared to thrombin alone.[1] Protein S is a cofactor for protein Ca. Another natural anticoagulant is heparin cofactor II. Its concentration in plasma is estimated to be lower than antithrombin III, and its action is primarily in the regulation of thrombin formation in extravascular tissues. Finally, thrombin is inactivated after being incorporated into the clot itself.

The extrinsic pathway is short-lived because of the presence of another inhibitor, tissue factor pathway inhibitor (also known as lipoprotein-associated coagulation inhibitor, LACI, or extrinsic pathway inhibitor). This protein inactivates the tissue factor–factor VIIa

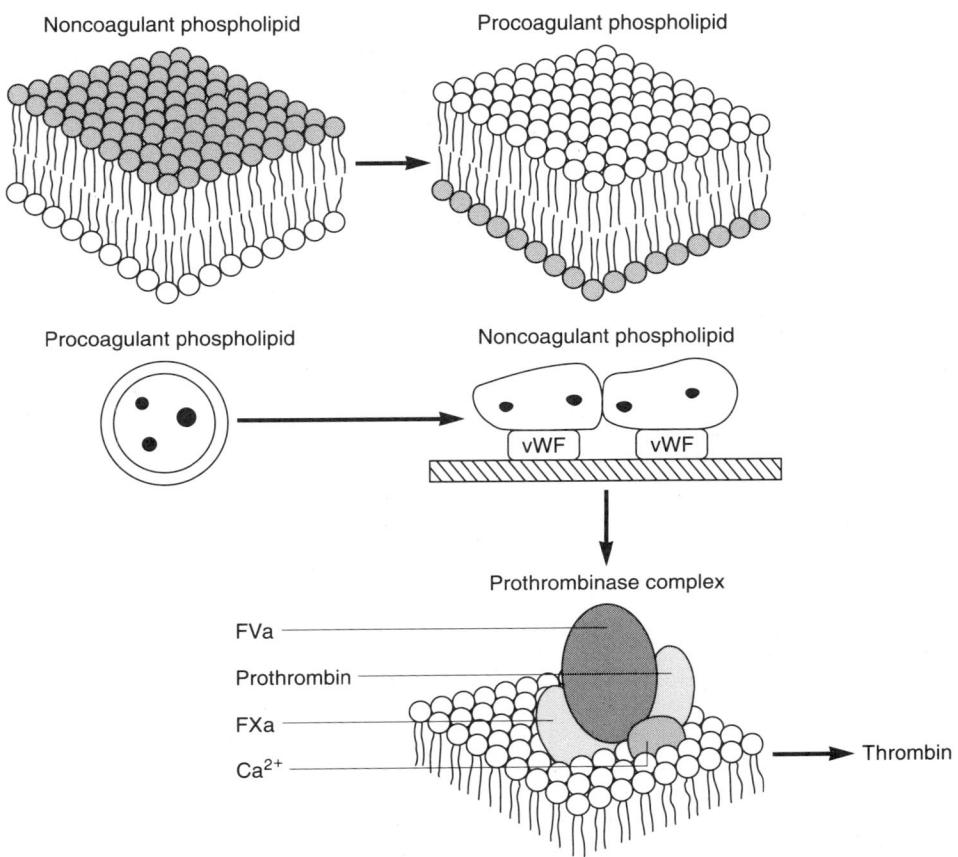

Figure 1 Formation of coagulation cascade assembly on the platelet phospholipid surface. (Adapted from Wakefield TW. Hemostasis. In: Greenfield LJ, Mulholland MW, Oldham KT, Zelenock GB, eds. Surgery: Scientific principles and practice. Philadelphia: JB Lippincott, 1993:103 and Hassouna HI. Laboratory evaluation of hemostatic disorders. In: Penner JA, Hassouna HI, eds. Coagulation Disorders II. Hematology/Oncology Clinics of North America, Dec, 1993, 1188.)

complex activation of factor X to Xa, but not of factor IX to IXa, thus shifting much of the coagulation cascade to the intrinsic system.

During thrombus formation, a constant process of thrombolysis prevents thrombus formation from leading to massive intravascular thrombosis. Plasminogen, tissue plasminogen activator (tPA), and alpha-2-antiplasmin (α-2-AP) are incorporated into the fibrin clot as it forms.[1] Thrombin promotes the release of tPA from endothelial cells. Tissue plasminogen activator catalyzes the conversion of plasminogen to plasmin, the main fibrinolytic enzyme in the body. This is a serine protease whose main substrates include fibrin, fibrinogen, and various other factors. Fibrin, when digested by plasmin, yields one molecule of fragment E and two molecules of fragment D. In physiologic clot formation, fragment D is released in dimeric form (D-dimer).[1] The D-dimer fragment is a marker for ongoing thrombosis and fibrinolysis. Alpha-2-antiplasmin is also secreted by endothelial cells. In physiologic fibrinolysis, these substances are bound to fibrin, and plasmin is inactivated.

In fibrinolytic states and during treatment with fibrinolytic agents (termed fibrinogenolysis), circulating fibrinogen, in addition to clot-bound fibrin, is digested by circulating plasmin, and circulating plasmin is less able to be inactivated. Fibrinogen is digested by removal of FPB and the carboxyl terminal portion of the alpha-chain, yielding fragment X, which is further converted to one molecule of fragment D and a fragment Y. After further degradation, two molecules of fragment D and one molecule of fragment E result.[1] In these fibrinolytic states, the fragments D are not cross-linked and D-dimer is not formed. The use of the D-dimer test, thus, can differentiate a process such as dissemination intravascular coagulation (DIC) with microvascular thrombosis and lysis from conditions with primary lysis alone.

The total inhibitory capacity opposing plasmin is less than the level of circulating plasmin.[1] Other sources of fibrinolytic enzymes in addition to endothelial cells include white blood cells, malignant tumor cells, and trophoblastic tissues.[1] The endothelial cell itself appears to have three systems for the promotion of a nonthrombotic surface: thrombin-thrombomodulin interaction, heparin-antithrombin III binding, and a recently described membrane-bound fibrinolytic system. The major categories of plasminogen activators include exogenous (streptokinase), endogenous (tPA and urokinase), and intrinsic (factors of the contact activation system).[1]

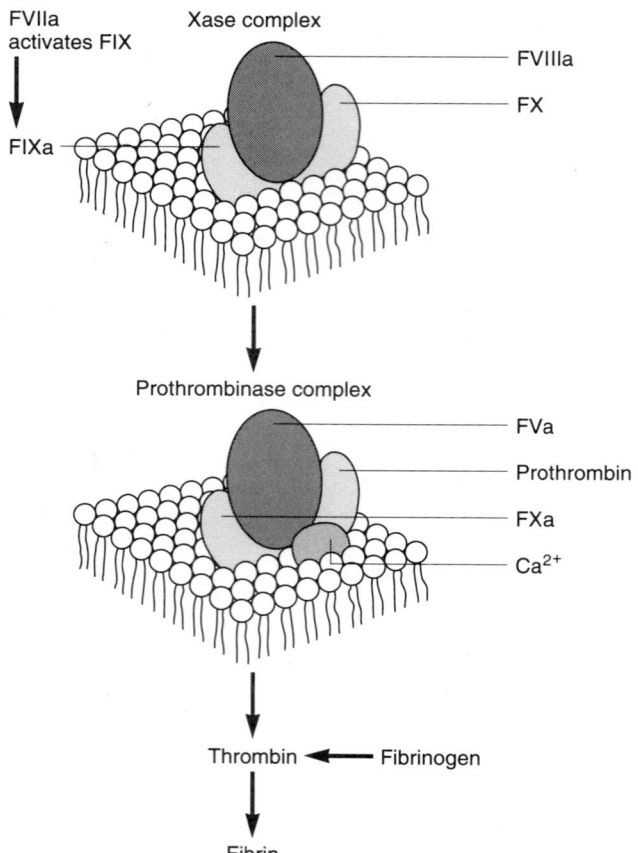

Figure 2 Formation of the Xase complex and prothrombinase complex with amplification of thrombin and fibrin formation. (Adapted from Wakefield TW. Hemostasis. In: Greenfield LJ, Mulholland MW, Oldham KT, Zelenock GB, eds. Surgery: Scientific principles and practice. Philadelphia: JB Lippincott, 1993:104 and Hassouna HI. Laboratory evaluation of hemostatic disorders. In: Penner JA, Hassouna HI, eds. Coagulation Disorders II. Hematology/Oncology Clinics of North America, Dec, 1993, 1177.)

These contact factors can independently convert plasminogen to plasmin. Finally, activated protein C (factor Ca) has been found to proteolytically inactivate tPA inhibitor, thus promoting fibrinolysis.

In summary, coagulation is an ongoing process of thrombus formation and thrombus dissolution with activation complexes speeding the process. The central mediator of coagulation is thrombin.[1] Abnormalities in coagulation occur when one process—thrombus formation, thrombus inhibition, or fibrinolysis—overcomes the others.

THROMBOEMBOLISM

Venous thrombosis and pulmonary embolism are associated with a number of risk factors encompassing Virchow's triad for thrombus formation including changes in the vein wall, stasis, and a procoagulant

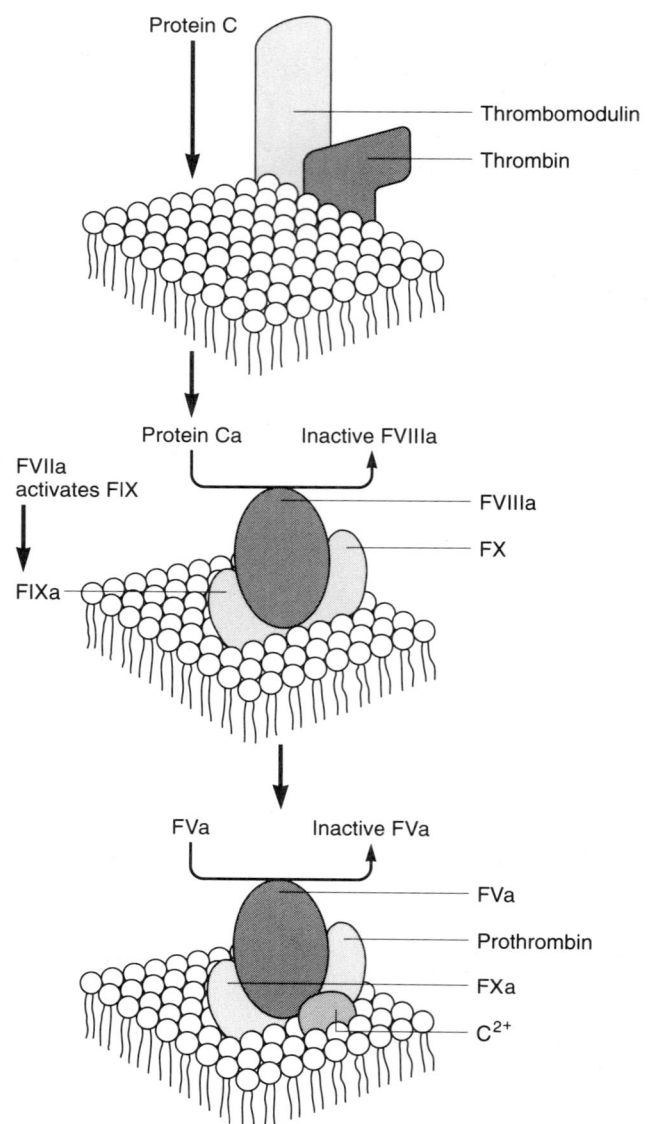

Figure 3 Activation of protein C by thrombin-thrombomodulin interaction. (Adapted from Wakefield TW. Hemostasis. In: Greenfield LJ, Mulholland MW, Oldham KT, Zelenock GB, eds. Surgery: Scientific principles and practice. Philadelphia: JB Lippincott, 1993:104 and Hassouna HI. Laboratory evaluation of hemostatic disorders. In: Penner JA, Hassouna HI, eds. Coagulation Disorders II. Hematology/Oncology Clinics of North America, Dec, 1993, 1175.)

tendency in the blood.[2] Other risk factors include age greater than 40, female sex, obesity, malignancy (especially pancreatic, genitourinary, stomach, lung, colon, and breast), previous history of venous thrombosis or pulmonary embolism, operative procedures, pregnancy and the puerperium, oral contraceptive use in premenopausal women, the nephrotic syndrome, blood group A, and a host of procoagulant syndromes including heparin sodium–associated thrombocytopenia, antithrombin III deficiency, protein C and S deficiency, dysfibrinogenemia, lupus anticoagulant and the presence of antiphospholipid antibodies, and abnormalities of fibrinolysis. Patients with heart disease, ulcerative colitis, and prolonged immobility also have an increased frequency of thromboembolism. The scope of the problem is significant. Approximately 500,000 cases of deep venous thrombosis annually result in approximately 50,000 deaths by pulmonary embolism in the United States.[2]

The constitution of a thrombus depends partly on the local hemodynamics at the site of thrombus formation. If flow remains active, as in the arterial circulation at the site of a developing thrombus, the thrombus is made up primarily of platelets, with limited amounts of fibrin and relatively few trapped red blood cells. Thrombi forming in areas of retarded flow, such as in the venous circulation, tend to be larger, occlusive, with more of a mixed pattern of blood elements not dominated by platelets. Under conditions of severe stasis, thrombi are dark red with fibrin and trapped red blood cells and relatively few platelets.

The clinical diagnosis of these thrombi in the venous circulation is unreliable and will be in error 50% of the time. A number of noninvasive tests are available for making the diagnosis of venous thrombosis, including Doppler probe examination, impedance plethysmography (IPG), phleborheography (PRG), radiolabeled fibrinogen scanning, magnetic resonance imaging (MRI), duplex imaging, and phlebography. Doppler probe, IPG, and PRG are all tests inferring the presence of thrombus based upon changes in flow or volume impedance and, as such, are observer dependent or not sensitive for small, nonocclusive thrombi or calf vein thrombi. Fibrinogen scanning is performed in only a few centers, and MRI, although a test with excellent sensitivity and specificity, involves equipment not readily available in most outpatient settings.

Duplex imaging, compared to phlebography, has a sensitivity between 88% and 100%, a specificity between 78% and 95%, a positive predictive value between 83% and 95%, and a negative predictive value between 88% and 100%.[3] In a study of 110 extremities in 103 patients evaluated with venous duplex imaging, PRG, and ascending phlebography within the same 24 hour period, patients were categorized into a diagnostic or surveillance group.[4] Duplex imaging had a sensitivity of 96% (98% diagnostic, 89% surveillance), specificity of 93% (86% diagnostic, 100% surveillance), positive predictive value of 96% (96% diagnostic, 100% surveillance), and a negative predictive value of 96% (96% diagnostic, 97% surveillance). Importantly, duplex imaging had reasonable sensitivity at both the above-knee and below-knee levels (100% and 78%, respectively). These results suggest that duplex imaging has similar diagnostic capability for patients in both diagnostic and surveillance groups, has a high diagnostic sensitivity for both above-knee and below-knee thrombi, and appears reasonable for diagnosing isolated infrapopliteal thrombi. The best variable(s) on the duplex image for diagnosing thrombus appear to be the absence of phasicity of flow with respiration or the combination of absence of spontaneous flow by Doppler ultrasonography and the absence of phasicity of flow with respiration. The addition of color flow imaging may greatly facilitate the ability to refine the diagnostic capability of venous duplex imaging and modify these ideal parameters.

Diagnostic approaches for pulmonary embolism include ventilation/perfusion (V/Q) scanning and pulmonary arteriography. In a recent multicenter study, the value of V/Q scanning was determined.[5] The V/Q scans were categorized as high probability, intermediate probability, and low probability for pulmonary embolism, based primarily on the size and number of perfusion defects. The sensitivity of a high-probability scan was only 41%, of a high- or intermediate-probability scan 82%, and of a high- intermediate- or low-probability scan 96%. However, the specificity of a high-probability scan was excellent at 97%, which decreased to 10% when all V/Q scans were considered together. When V/Q scans were combined with clinical assessments, the sensitivity improved, for example, up to 96% for high-probability studies. High-probability V/Q scans, thus, usually indicate pulmonary embolism, but only a minority of patients with pulmonary embolism have a high-probability V/Q scan. The most valuable V/Q scan would seem to be in patients with high-probability scans and a clinical suspicion of pulmonary embolism or in those with near-normal or normal scans. Management of acute massive pulmonary embolism depends on an accurate diagnosis that documents the presence and location of the embolus and in the situation of indeterminate V/Q scanning, pulmonary arteriography remains the gold standard. Additionally, pulmonary arteriography is indicated in patients in whom permanent interruption of the inferior vena cava is considered due to recurrent pulmonary embolism and in patients in whom catheter pulmonary embolectomy or open pulmonary embolectomy is performed.

PHARMACOLOGIC INTERVENTIONS

Heparin sodium, first discovered in 1916 by Jay McLean while working under William H. Howell, is a heterogeneous mixture of sulfated polysaccharide molecules of varying molecular weights. Heparin sodium accelerates the reaction between thrombin and antithrombin III. Thus, it accelerates the inhibition of thrombin and other serine proteases by antithrombin III. Additionally, heparin sodium directly inhibits coagulation proteases and is important for another selective inhibitor of thrombin, heparin cofactor II. After an intravenous bolus, heparin sodium has a half-life of approximately 90 to 120 minutes, although the half-life tends to correlate with the amount injected. Activated factors X and II are the clotting factors most sensitive to the heparin–antithrombin III complex. Heparin is not excreted through the kidney or liver, does not cross the placenta, and is cleared through the reticuloendothelial system. Commercial heparin sodium is obtained from pork or beef lung or intestine. Clinical use of heparin sodium in venous thrombosis and pulmonary embolism and as a prophylactic agent has been established.[6] In monitoring heparin effect, an activated partial thromboplastin time (aPTT) of 1.5 times control or a thrombin clotting time (TCT) of 2 times control reflects adequate anticoagulation; whole blood activated clotting times in a range of 150 to 250 seconds also suggest adequate anticoagulation. Higher levels are required for cardiovascular surgical procedures involving cardiopulmonary bypass. It has been documented that in many situations direct measurement of heparin levels does not correlate with the level of anticoagulation as measured by the aPTT. Although heparin sodium may decrease platelet aggregability while enhancing the generation of thromboxane from platelets, noncoagulant high-molecular-weight heparin fragments may also cause platelet aggregation, and heparin sodium–associated thrombocytopenia from an immune mechanism is a potential complication of heparin use. Patients receiving heparin sodium should have a platelet count measured every other day after the fourth day of therapy or earlier, if they are known to have been exposed to heparin sodium in the past. The most common complication of heparin sodium is bleeding. The risk of hemorrhage is increased in the elderly, postmenopausal women, and patients with pre-existing abnormalities of coagulation, thrombocytopenia, or uremia. Long-term therapy may be associated with alopecia and osteoporosis. Osteoporosis has been noted in patients receiving greater than 10,000 units/day for 6 months or longer.

Heparin sodium as used in venous thrombosis prophylaxis has received considerable attention. Low-dose heparin therapy is thought to protect against venous thrombosis through three different mechanisms. First, antithrombin III activity is enhanced by trace amounts of heparin sodium; second, there may be a decrease in thrombin availability that prevents its activation and its fibrin stabilizing effect; and third, small doses of heparin sodium may inhibit the second wave of platelet aggregation and the subsequent platelet release reaction. However, low-dose heparin therapy does carry an increased risk of wound hematoma; therefore, only appropriate patients at high risk for deep venous thrombosis (DVT) should be treated with this drug. The sodium and calcium salts of heparin seem to be equally effective for prophylaxis, and wound hematoma formation does not appear to be related to the type of salt in the heparin. In addition, there is only a slight advantage to giving 5,000 units three times a day rather than twice a day.

The use of low-dose heparin therapy has been endorsed for a number of applications by the National Institutes of Health Consensus Conference on venous thrombosis prophylaxis and in a recent meta-analysis of 70 randomized trials in 16,000 patients. The odds of developing DVT with low-dose heparin prophylaxis decreased 67% ± 4%; for pulmonary embolism (both fatal and nonfatal), the odds decreased 47% ± 10%.[7] For fatal pulmonary embolism, the odds reduction was even greater (64% ± 15%). No increase in mortality from other causes was found in patients treated with low-dose heparin therapy. Importantly, these reductions were noted not only in patients undergoing general surgical procedures but also in urologic, elective orthopaedic, and traumatic orthopaedic procedures.

Due to the bleeding complications related to low-dose heparin therapy, a number of investigations evaluating the role of low-molecular-weight heparin for venous thrombosis prophylaxis have commenced. Standard heparin sodium is a mixture of polysaccharide molecules that vary in molecular weight from 2,000 to 40,000 Daltons, with the anticoagulant effect centered over the lower end of the molecular-weight spectrum. Maximal heparin effect requires a three-way complex between heparin sodium, antithrombin III, and thrombin. However, a two-way complex between antithrombin III and thrombin with heparin sodium binding to antithrombin III but not thrombin (due to its small size in low-molecular-weight form) allows primarily anti-Xa activity with less anti-IIa activity and, theoretically, a decrease in systemic bleeding complications. Thrombin inhibition is felt to be responsible for much of the bleeding associated with heparin therapy. Additionally, with molecular weights below 5,000 to 8,000 Daltons, heparin sodium cannot simultaneously bind to both antithrombin III and platelets, thus decreasing the antiplatelet effect of the drug and the potential bleeding complications associated with platelet abnormalities. Although many variants of low-molecular-weight heparin are available, in general they are eliminated from the bloodstream more slowly than standard heparin sodium, have a half-life approximately twice as long as standard heparin sodium, have a rate of disappearance from the bloodstream that is not dose-dependent, and their reversal by protamine sulfate is not complete as measured by anti-Xa activity. In addition, low-molecular-weight heparins are readily absorbed from the subcutaneous injection sites and do not cross the placental barrier. Although promising studies on the use of low-molecular-weight heparins have been reported, bleeding complications still have been noted and in the aggregate are not appreciably different than with standard heparin prophylaxis. Clearly, more work with low-molecular-weight heparin is necessary, not only for venous thrombosis prophylaxis but also in its routine use in other cardiovascular applications, such as during extracorporeal bypass and cardiovascular operations. Low-molecular-weight heparins will invariably become very important in various applications in this country, as they have in Europe and Canada.

Oral anticoagulant therapy is recommended for chronic treatment of venous thromboembolism. Sodium warfarin interferes with the vitamin K–dependent factors II, VII, IX, and X, protein C, and protein S. In the liver, these factors are translated in an inactive form. At the level of the hepatocyte endoplasmic reticulum, the precursor factors are delivered to a membrane-bound carboxylase. This enzyme's cofactor is reduced vitamin K, and it converts a number of glutamic acid residues to gamma carboxy-glutamic acid residues (Fig. 4).[1] When

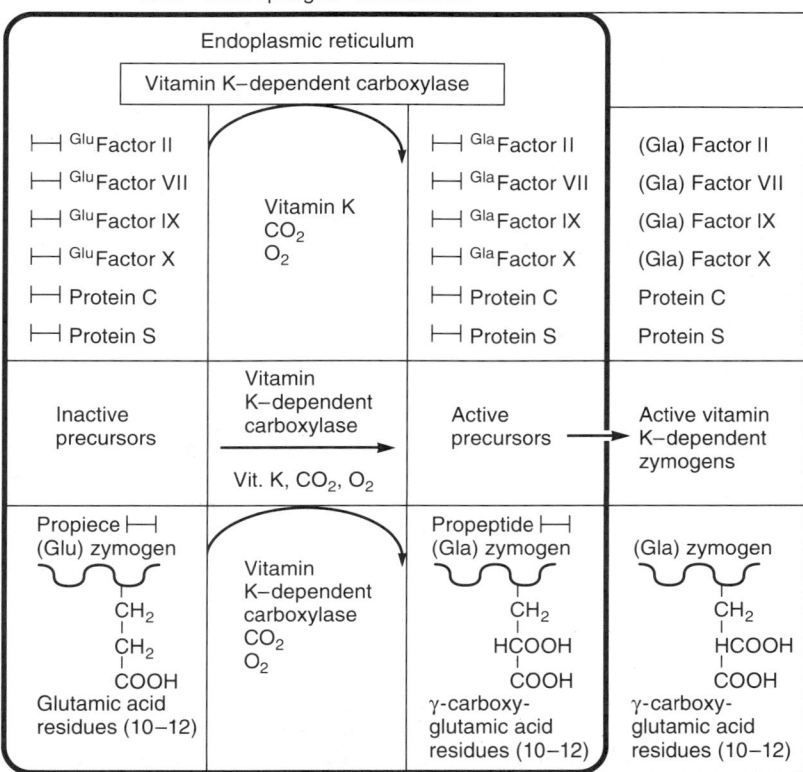

Figure 4 Conversion of glutamic acid residues to gamma carboxy-glutamic acid residues by vitamin K–dependent carboxylase for factors II, VII, IX, X, protein C and protein S. (Adapted from Wakefield TW. Hemostasis. In: Greenfield LJ, Mulholland MW, Oldham KT, Zelenock GB, eds. Surgery: Scientific principles and practice. Philadelphia: J.B. Lippincott, 1993:116 and Hassouna HI. Laboratory evaluation of hemostatic disorders. In: Penner JA, Hassouna HI, eds. Coagulation Disorders II. Hematology/Oncology Clinics of North America, Dec, 1993, 1219.)

these factors are released from the liver, they are secreted as active proteins. The carboxy-glutamic acid residues allow the binding of these proteins to phospholipid membranes, especially important for the formation of the Xase and prothrombinase complexes on the surface of activated platelets. Sodium warfarin blocks the reduction of vitamin K, resulting in the synthesis of inactive proteins. Two classes of compounds possess anticoagulant effects: 4-hydroxycoumarins (of which crystalline sodium warfarin [Coumadin] is the most common) and the 2-substituted 1,3-indandiones.[1] Using the prothrombin time measurement, effective anticoagulation occurs at a level of 1.3 to 1.4 times control. At higher levels, there is nearly a fivefold increase in bleeding complications.

Due to variations in the thromboplastins used for the prothrombin time determinations in different countries, a new system has been developed, the international normalized ratio (INR), in which the sensitivity of thromboplastins can be standardized and prothrombin times thus compared accurately.[8] Using this system, the proper INR for treatment of venous thrombosis by sodium warfarin is 2 to 3. Two major complications of sodium warfarin therapy include recurrent thrombosis and bleeding. It is recommended that sodium warfarin be continued 4 to 6 months after an initial episode of deep venous thrombosis. Between 10 weeks and 4 months after deep vein thrombosis, the recurrent thrombosis rate is approximately twice that between 4 months and 3 years after thrombosis. At 4 months, the risk of bleeding matches and exceeds the benefit from anticoagulant therapy and is the basis for discontinuing sodium warfarin administration at this time. However, with recurrent venous thrombosis, the thrombotic risk is greater, and sustained anticoagulation is appropriate. Further thrombosis has been found in up to 20% of patients with recurrent venous thrombosis who are treated with only a 6 month course of sodium warfarin.[9] Patients at highest risk for bleeding during sodium warfarin therapy include the elderly, those with gynecologic or urologic disorders, women after childbirth, and patients given large loading doses of sodium warfarin. A final important complication of sodium warfarin is skin necrosis in patients with protein C deficiency. This usually involves full-thickness skin sloughing over fatty areas and occurs because of inhibition of protein C and S before factors II, IX, and X, rendering the circulation procoagulant for a short period of time.

REFERENCES

1. Hassouna HI. The laboratory evaluation of hemostatic disorders. Hematol Oncol Clin North Am, 1993; 7:1161–1249.
2. Coon WW. Epidemiology of venous thromboembolism. Ann Surg 1977; 186:149–164.
3. Patterson RB, Fowl RJ, Keller JD, et al. The limitations of impedance plethsymography in the diagnosis of deep venous thrombosis. J Vasc Surg 1989; 9:725–730.
4. Comerota AJ, Katz ML, Greenwald LL, et al. Venous duplex imaging: Should it replace hemodynamic tests for deep venous thrombosis? J Vasc Surg 1990; 11:53–61.
5. Pioped Investigators. Value of the ventilation/perfusion scan in acute pulmonary embolism. Results of the prospective investigation of pulmonary embolus diagnosis (Pioped). JAMA 1990; 263: 2753–2759.
6. Hirsh J. Heparin. N Engl J Med 1991; 324:1565–1574.
7. Consensus conference. Prevention of venous thrombosis and pulmonary embolism. JAMA 1986; 256:744–757.
8. Hirsh J. Oral anticoagulation drugs. N Engl J Med 1991; 324: 1865–1875.
9. Hull R, Carter C, Jay R, et al. The diagnosis of acute, recurrent, deep-vein thrombosis: A diagnostic challenge. Circulation 1983; 67:901–906.

PATHOPHYSIOLOGY OF VENOUS THROMBOSIS

SESHADRI RAJU, M.D.

The well-known triad of stasis, hypercoagulability, and intimal injury was described by Virchow more than 150 years ago. The relative importance of the components of the triad and how they interact with each other are still subjects of continuing study and research.

"Stasis" is generally considered to be an important mechanism in the surgical patient. The velocity of venous blood flow and venous circulatory time in the lower limbs are decreased in the anesthetized recumbent patient. Blood in the soleal sinusoids may remain stagnant for hours in a patient who is undergoing operation because of the absence of muscular contractions and the dependent orientation of the sinusoids.[1]

Trauma, including surgical trauma, activates procoagulant factors and increased levels of these agents, including fibrinogen, platelets, and factors II, V, VII, and XIII, can be documented in the postoperative patient. Attempts to find a predictive correlation between increased levels of such procoagulant factors and venous thrombosis, however, have not been rewarding.

Evidence linking venous thrombosis with isolated deficiencies of certain coagulation-inhibiting and fibrinolytic proteins is more suggestive. As many as 13% of patients who present with venous thrombosis may be deficient in isolated proteins such as antithrombin-III, protein C, protein S, and plasminogen.[2] The incidence of these deficiencies may be even higher in patients who have familial, juvenile, or recurrent venous thrombosis. Some patients may harbor abnormal procoagulant factors such as lupus anticoagulant and cardiolipin antibody. These factors may be present transiently in some patients after pregnancy or viral illness.

The venous endothelium is a source of inhibitors of thromboplastin activation and promoters of plasminogen activity. Endothelial production of these factors may be deranged after anesthesia, operation, and prolonged bed rest. The relationship of endothelial factors to venous thrombosis remains to be elucidated. The role of intimal injury in the genesis of venous thrombosis is unclear. Pharmacologic and anesthetic agents, as well as intravenously administered fluids whose pH and osmolality differ from those of blood, may cause intimal injury and suppress fibrinolytic mechanisms. On the basis of experimental models, it has been suggested that stasis-induced white blood cell trapping by the endothelium in the anesthetized patient can mediate intimal injury.[3] Other possible mechanisms of intimal injury include mild anoxia due to stasis and intimal fracture due to hyperdilatation of the venous wall, especially in the region of the valve sinuses. High-resolution ultrasonography has been utilized to document such intimal fractures, but scanning electron microscopic inspection of the endothelium underlying a thrombus has failed to clearly document intimal injury.[3] Thus, the role of intimal injury in the triad remains controversial and unresolved.

PREDISPOSING FACTORS

On the basis of clinical observations, a number of factors have been identified that increase the risk of venous thrombosis (Table 1). Clinical experience suggests that a combination of such risk factors is additive. A previous history of deep venous thrombosis (DVT) is probably the most important risk factor. The risk for the occurrence of venous thrombosis is said to be increased fivefold with pregnancy and puerperium and threefold in the presence of varicose veins.[4] Approximately 30% of patients presenting with venous thrombosis in a hospital population are found to have intra-abdominal, intracranial, or other forms of malignancy. Intracranial tumors rich in factors that activate thromboplastin may gain entry into the circulation through breakdown of the blood-brain barrier. A variety of malignant and nonmalignant hematologic conditions associated with increased blood viscosity, including polycythemia, leukemia, multiple myeloma, and macroglobulinemia, predispose to venous thrombosis. Oral contraceptives reduce

Table 1 Conditions Predisposing to Venous Thrombosis

Previous venous thrombosis
Advanced age
Prolonged bed rest
Multiple systemic illnesses
Stroke and/or paraplegia
Pregnancy and puerperium
Cardiopulmonary disease
Birth control pills
Polycythemia
Obesity
Isolated deficiencies of antithrombotic proteins
Trauma, including surgical trauma
Malignancy
Varicose veins
Administration of procoagulant concentrates
Epsilon aminocaproic acid
Vasculitis (e.g., Buerger's disease)
Venous malformation (e.g., Klippel-Trenaunay syndrome)

antithrombin III levels and are recognized as a risk factor for thromboembolism.[3,4] It has been suggested that primary venous valvular reflux may predispose to venous thrombosis because of reflux stasis.[5] In a recent study,[6] 14% of patients with DVT were found to have venous valvular reflux at the time of presentation, suggestive of a pre-existing condition. Hemiplegic and paraplegic patients are prone to venous thrombosis.

VENOUS THROMBOSIS

Origin

Autopsy studies[1] that focused on pelvic veins as the primary origin of DVT have been supplanted by detailed autopsy studies documenting the frequent origination of thrombus in the calf veins, particularly the soleal sinusoids. Iodine-125 fibrinogen uptake studies and high-resolution phlebographic techniques[1] support the view that the calf and crural veins are the primary sites of thrombus formation. The initial thrombus is a platelet fibrin laminated clot (lines of Zahn) with extension occurring through propagation of red clot consisting predominantly of red blood cells and fibrin attached to the initial nidus. When the thrombus grows to become occlusive, flow is impeded and thus stasis is increased further. This results in rapid propagation of the clot proximally to the level of the next tributary. If the tributary blood flow is sluggish and the tributary itself becomes occluded by the thrombus, further propagation may occur. Because of relative stasis of blood flow, venous valve sinuses have been proposed as a favored site for initial nidus formation (Fig. 1). Although soleal sinusoids are devoid of venous valves, they are undoubtedly a primary site for thrombus formation also. The prevailing view is that venous thrombosis originates in the calf veins, probably initially in the soleal sinusoids, and propagates proximally. Four distinct patterns of venous thrombosis can be recognized on the basis of phlebographic appearance (Fig. 2). The pattern of calf

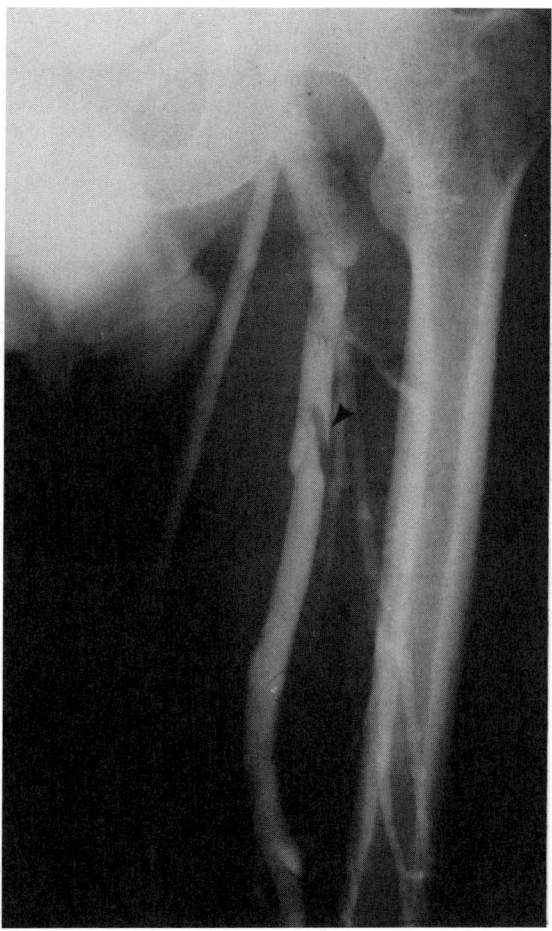

Figure 1 Thrombus in a venous valve sinus (*arrow*). Relative stasis of flow in the valve pockets has been proposed as a factor in such thrombus formation.

venous origin with or without proximal propagation (Fig. 2A and 2B) was identified in 92% of patients by careful phlebographic studies. Thrombosis involving proximal veins without calf/crural involvement (Fig. 2C) is much less frequent (6%) and can occur after orthopedic or pelvic operations that may cause direct or indirect local injury to the proximal veins in the vicinity. Infrequently (2%), thrombosis may occur at multiple independent sites (Fig. 2D).

Superficial venous thrombosis has traditionally been viewed as nonthreatening; therefore, systemic therapy was considered unnecessary. Recent duplex studies indicate that approximately 20% of patients with superficial venous thrombosis also have associated concurrent DVT.

The upper limbs and trunk are relatively rare sites for spontaneous venous thrombosis, accounting for less than 10% of total cases. With the increasing use of indwelling intravenous catheters and devices for dialysis, chemotherapy, hyperalimentation, and cardiac pacing, a higher relative incidence has been reported in recent years.[7] An incidence of up to 30% of venous thrombosis may be associated with such catheters and devices in the subclavian vein. Curiously, the incidence appears to be lower (10%) with indwelling devices introduced through the jugular vein. For the most part, however, these thrombi in the upper limb and trunk remain asymptomatic and nonthreatening, even though pulmonary emboli and significant symptomatic venous obstruction have been documented in several instances.

Bilaterality

Early autopsy studies documented that venous thrombi in the lower limb are bilateral in most patients.[3] More recent studies with duplex imaging, iodine-125 fibrinogen uptake, and phlebography, however, suggest that the incidence of bilaterality ranges from 20% to 40%.[1,3,4,6]

Incidence and Time Course

Careful epidemiologic studies from multiple sources[4] have documented an incidence of venous thrombosis of approximately 30% after major abdominal operations. The incidence may be even higher after certain types of procedures such as open prostatectomy (38%), elective orthopedic operations (52%), and emergency orthopedic operations for hip fracture (70%). The incidence appears to be particularly low after peripheral vascular procedures (7%) and cardiothoracic operations (3%), probably owing to frequent use of intraoperative heparin sodium. A 70% incidence was noted among medical intensive care unit patients who were seriously ill from a variety of life-threatening nonsurgical illnesses. Fibrinogen uptake studies have now established that 85% of postoperative venous thrombosis occurred during the first 96 hours postoperatively.[8] Fifty percent occurred during the first 24 hours, the majority probably during the operation. This information has important implications for optimal timing of appropriate prophylactic measures.

Embolization

It is estimated that about 78% of thrombi that originate in the calf veins lyse without sequelae or remain confined to the calf.[8] The remaining 22% propagate to involve the popliteal or proximal veins as indicated by serial iodine-125 fibrinogen uptake studies. The risk of embolization from thrombi confined to the calf is estimated to be about 20%. The risk of life-threatening emboli is negligible owing to the small size of the thrombi. The risk of embolization from thrombi

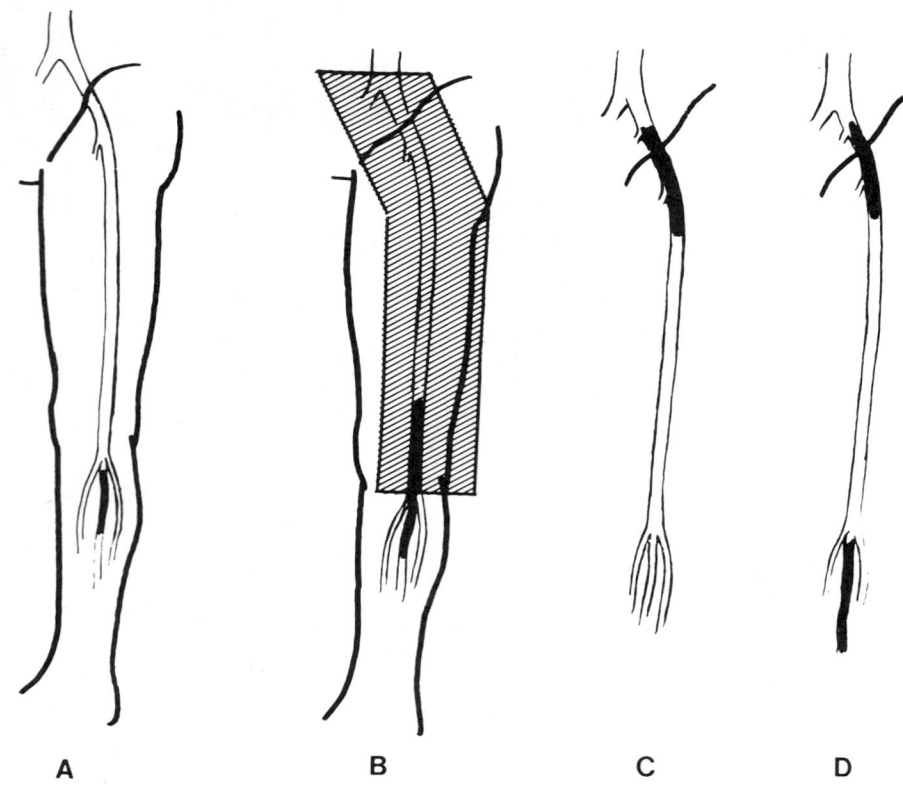

Figure 2 Four phlebographic patterns of venous thrombosis in the lower limb can frequently be recognized. *A*, Thrombus confined to the calf or crural veins in the leg. *B*, Calf/crural vein thrombus extending in continuity to a more proximal axial vein. Proximal extent of the thrombus may be variable (*shaded area*). *C*, Isolated continuous or discontinuous thrombus of variable length involving only the proximal axial veins with no calf or crural involvement. *D*, Combined calf-crural and proximal axial vein thrombus with intervening "skip" areas free of thrombus.

that have originated or extended into the popliteal vein is estimated at 50%. Because of the larger size of the thrombi, the incidence of life-threatening embolization is also higher. The incidence and mortality from pulmonary embolization are progressively higher from thromboses involving progressively larger, more proximal veins. A free-floating thrombus or one with a free tail may pose a particularly high risk of life-threatening embolus. Phlebographic appearance can be deceptive, however, as a thrombus that appears free floating may, in fact, be attached to the vein wall through part of its circumference.

Hemodynamic Changes and Symptoms

Thrombi confined to the calf veins seldom cause significant hemodynamic abnormality. High-grade venous obstruction is probably present in no more than 5% of such patients and only when there is extensive thrombosis involving the calf and crural veins.[9] With proximal involvement, the incidence of significant venous obstruction progressively increases. From retrospective studies, it is estimated that more than 50% of iliac vein thrombosis may present with high-grade venous obstruction. Because of rapid collateralization and clot lysis, even high-grade hemodynamic obstruction rapidly regresses in most patients. The dreaded conditions of phlegmasia cerulea dolens and venous gangrene, while dramatic when encountered, probably account for less than 1% of all cases of venous thrombosis.

The prominent symptoms of acute venous thrombosis—pain, swelling, and discoloration—are probably related to a combination of the degree of obstruction present and the inflammatory reaction elicited by the thrombus. The inflammatory response is variable. In some patients even major thrombi may sometimes be silent. Conversely, in some patients the degree of pain and local swelling may be severe and out of proportion to the small extent of thrombosis, presumably owing to the presence of a vigorous local inflammatory response. Most thrombotic inflammation is sterile and not septic. Consequently, the old distinction between thrombophlebitis and phlebothrombosis should be abandoned.

Swelling may be a prominent feature in thrombosis involving the proximal axial veins owing to hemodynamic obstruction. Swelling that occurs later with clot lysis is related to venous reflux rather than obstruction.[10] Stasis skin changes and skin ulceration are distinctly uncommon in acute venous thrombosis, even though localized dark skin patches may be present. Stasis skin changes follow the development of venous reflux with clot lysis. Patients followed sequentially after deep venous thrombosis may be observed to progress from early painful leg swelling to later stasis skin changes and ulceration with the development of recanalization and reflux.

Collateral Formation

Collateral development may be surprisingly rapid after the onset of venous thrombosis. Such collaterals develop from a variety of sources (Fig. 3). The vaso vasora may dilate around a segment of venous obstruction, presenting the interesting phlebographic appearance of outlining the occluded segment by contrast in the small collaterals. Axial collaterals form by dilatation and arborization of side branches of the axial vein itself around the occluded segment. More frequently, large collateral connections develop between the occluded axial vein and an adjoining important tributary such as the profunda or the hypogastric veins. The large size of such collaterals suggests putative connections that may have an embryologic basis.[9]

Clot Retraction, Lysis, and Recanalization

The process of thrombus resolution involves a variety of mechanisms including (1) endogenous fibrin-

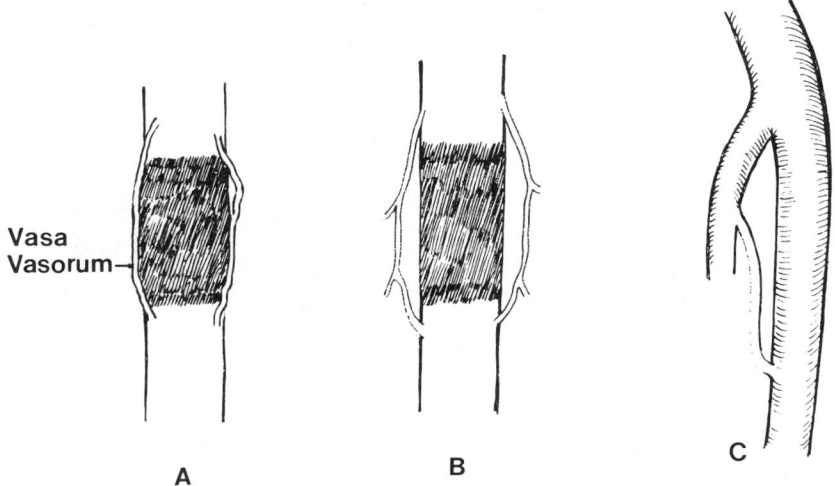

Figure 3 Collateral development following venous thrombosis. *A*, Vasovasora. *B*, Axial. *C*, Tributary.

olysis, which is particularly active during the first few days and for up to 3 weeks after the onset of the thrombosis, especially if aggressive anticoagulation is pursued; (2) retraction of the fibrin clot, which shrinks and re-establishes part of the venous lumen, a process that is due to polymerization of fibrin and that is active up to 12 weeks after thrombosis; and (3) organization of the thrombus, which is invaded by granulation tissue and within which numerous small channels develop, a process that may continue for 6 months or longer after initial onset.[3]

Important information about the incidence and time course of thrombus resolution has become available from sequential duplex studies[6,10] in patients followed from the time of onset of venous thrombosis. Evolution of thrombus appears to take one of three pathways: group 1, early lysis; group 2, early extension at 7 days after initial clot lysis; and group 3, late extension at 30 to 180 days after initial clot lysis. Both early and late extensions occurred despite anticoagulation therapy. Early clot lysis was the rule and occurred in 61% of patients studied. The other two groups accounted for 17% and 22% of patients, respectively. By 1 week after venous thrombosis, 17% of the initially thrombosed segments had recanalized with clot lysis. By 30 days 56% of the thrombosed segments had become patent, and by 90 days 86% of thrombosed segments had recanalized. The process appeared to slow and remained stable thereafter. Thus, 14% of venous segments remained occluded after 90 days. Clot lysis although prevalent was frequently incomplete and recanalization did not always lead to venous valve reflux. At 180 days after thrombosis, 25% of patent venous segments had developed reflux as documented by quantitative duplex examination.[10] By 1 year, more than two-thirds of patients had reflux in one or more segments initially affected by thrombus.[6] Some venous segments that were not initially involved in the thrombosis developed reflux after a lapse of 2 years. The mechanism for this late development of reflux in the absence of initial thrombosis is unknown. Observations of the post-thrombotic valve during valve reconstruction suggest that valve damage can be variable and clot lysis can occur without functional damage to the valve structure (Fig. 4). A redundant refluxive valve, indistinguishable in appearance from "primary" valve reflux, is frequently seen in post-thrombotic patients during valve reconstruction. It is presumed that these represent instances of primary reflux complicated by venous thrombosis from reflux stasis.

POSTPHLEBITIC SYNDROME

Incidence and Time Course

Early studies documented that 80% or more of patients ultimately develop venous stasis ulceration after venous thrombosis. These observations, undertaken at a time when anticoagulation was not widely used, are probably not relevant today. Recent studies document that approximately one-third of patients, when examined 5 to 10 years after onset of venous thrombosis,[3] escaped bad sequelae and remain symptom-free; another one-third have minor complaints of discomfort, aches, and pains but retain a nearly normal functioning extremity; the remaining one-third have severe and disabling symptoms with significant swelling, pain, and stasis skin changes. The precise incidence of skin ulceration is unknown but probably in the range of 5% to 10%. These data may underestimate the true incidence of postphlebitic syndrome as it evolves over many years and even decades. It is common to encounter patients who give a

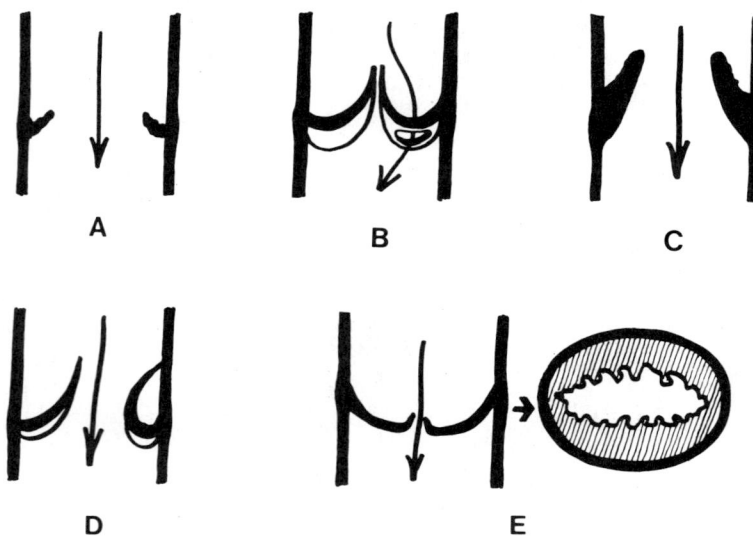

Figure 4 Pathology of post-thrombotic valve reflux. The degree of valve damage is variable. *A*, Destroyed valve cusp. *B*, Perforated cusp. *C*, "Frozen" and thickened valve cusp. *D*, Adherent valve cusp with some thickening. *E*, Redundant refluxive valve indistinguishable in appearance from "primary valve reflux."

history of previous venous thrombosis who remained asymptomatic for 10 or more years until a second or recurrent bout of venous thrombosis, after which more severe symptoms developed.

Pathophysiology

Patients with postphlebitic syndrome may have obstruction, reflux, or often a combination of the two. In addition, abnormalities of calf venous pump function are present. Venous capacitance may be reduced owing to the presence of organized thrombi in calf veins. In addition, compliance changes in the venous wall occur because of post-thrombotic thickening and fibrosis. As a result, calf pump ejection fraction may be reduced, and postejection recovery time may be very short. The compliance changes may further contribute to ambulatory venous hypertension, which is frequently present owing to the accompanying obstructive or refluxive abnormality. Even though symptoms of venous claudication, including increasing pain with ambulation, are present, elevation of ambulatory venous pressure to supranormal levels is seldom seen. In retrospective studies of post-thrombotic patients, 10% to 30% are found to have obstruction when examined 7 or more years after onset of thrombosis. In patients with venous obstruction, the site of obstruction was as follows: iliac-vena cava 58%, femoral 25%, and crural 27%;[9] 74% had multiple sites of obstruction. The pattern of reflux that develops in the post-thrombotic patient is variable. The most frequent site of reflux is the popliteal vein. Patients with severe reflux symptoms usually have multilevel reflux in the axial vein or multisystem involvement; that is, reflux in the profunda, superficial femoral, and popliteal veins. There is a significant association between post-thrombotic skin changes and reflux in the posterior tibial vein.[6] The profunda femoral vein is an important source of reflux in a patient whose axial vein was partially or totally obstructed by post-thrombotic changes.[9] Severe and symptomatic axial vein reflux at a lower level may be present even when the axial vein is partially or totally obstructed at a higher level. Massive collateral reflux may be present in addition to reflux present through the recanalized post-thrombotic axial vein. Large collateral axial vein connections, such as the profunda popliteal collateral connection, are a particularly relevant source of reflux.

REFERENCES

1. Nicolaides AN. Diagnosis of venous thrombosis by phlebography. In: Bergan JJ, Yao JST, eds. Venous problems. Chicago: Year Book, 1978:23.
2. Heijboer H, Brandjes DPM, Buller H, et al. Deficiencies of coagulation-inhibiting and fibrinolytic proteins in outpatients with deep-vein thrombosis. N Engl J Med 1990; 323:1512–1516.
3. Browse NL, Burnand KG, Thomas ML. Disease of the veins: Pathology, diagnosis and treatment. London: Edward Arnold, 1988.
4. Bergquist D. Post-operative thrombo-embolism: Frequency, etiology, prophylaxis. New York: Springer-Verlag, 1983.
5. Raju S. Venous insufficiency of the lower limb and stasis ulceration: Changing concepts and management. Ann Surg 1983; 198:688–697.
6. Markel A, Manzo RA, Bergelin RO, Strandness DE. Valvular reflux after deep vein thrombosis: Incidence and time of occurrence. J Vasc Surg 1992; 15:377–384.
7. McCarthy WJ, Vogelzang RL, Bergan JJ. Changing concepts and present-day etiology of upper extremity venous thrombosis. In: Bergan JJ, Yao JST, eds. Venous disorders. Philadelphia: WB Saunders, 1991:407.
8. Kakkar VV, Howe CT, Flanc C, et al. Natural history of postoperative deep vein thrombosis. Lancet 1969; 2:230–232.
9. Raju S, Fredericks R. Venous obstruction: An analysis of 137 cases with hemodynamic, venographic and clinical correlations. J Vasc Surg 1991; 14:305–313.
10. Killewich LA, Bedford GR, Beach KW, Strandness DE. Spontaneous lysis of deep venous thrombi: Rate and outcome. J Vasc Surg 1989; 9:89–97.

NONINVASIVE METHODS OF DIAGNOSING VENOUS DISEASE

ENRIQUE CRIADO, M.D.
GEORGE JOHNSON Jr., M.D.

The effective use of noninvasive testing for the diagnosis of venous disorders requires knowledge of both the disease process and the capabilities and limitations of the different diagnostic tests available.[1-8] Currently used noninvasive testing provides qualitative and quantitative information regarding the anatomy and function of the venous system. Noninvasive testing offers anatomic detail regarding size, location, and number of main venous trunks, intraluminal contents, possible extraluminal sources of venous compression, and position and integrity of venous valves.

Functional testing offers information about the presence of venous obstruction or valvular incompetence in a particular venous segment or in the limb as a whole. Diagnostic methods based on ultrasound technology can document venous anatomy and examine blood flow velocity patterns in individual veins. Physiologic methods of diagnosis generally rely on the assessment of extremity volume changes using different plethysmographic techniques and give information about extremity venous outflow or venous refill time patterns. Direct ultrasonic imaging methods have the advantage over physiologic tests of eliminating the uncertainty regarding the location and extent of the disease process in most instances, offering anatomic detail; when used in combination with pulsed Doppler ultrasound, they can also provide data regarding venous blood flow characteristics.

NONINVASIVE DIAGNOSIS OF DEEP VEIN THROMBOSIS

The diagnosis of deep vein thrombosis (DVT) is based on the documentation of the presence of intraluminal thrombus in the deep veins. Sound therapeutic decisions require, however, additional information regarding the location and extent of the thrombotic process, adherence of the thrombus to the vessel wall, and the interval propagation or regression of the thrombus spontaneously or in response to treatment. This information can be obtained noninvasively with the use of B-mode ultrasonography, which documents intraluminal thrombus by showing lack of venous compressibility when direct pressure is applied to the vein in question with the ultrasound probe. The presence of increased intraluminal echogenicity further strengthens the diagnosis of DVT. Ultrasound examination can provide a rough estimate of the age of the thrombus. Acute fresh thrombi have low echogenicity, are homogeneous, have a smooth surface and contour, are soft when compressed, occasionally are partially attached to the wall with free-floating ends, and do not have venous collaterals surrounding the thrombosed area. Old thrombi, on the contrary, display marked echogenicity and heterogeneous density, have irregular surfaces, are firm when compressed and well attached to the venous wall, and, when obstructive, have abundant collaterals surrounding the obstruction.

The combination of pulsed-wave Doppler ultrasound with B-mode imaging in duplex scanning further allows interrogating a specific venous segment for the absence of venous blood flow compatible with the presence of intraluminal thrombus. This function can be expedited with the use of color-coded flow scanning, which displays real-time flow images in long segments of the vein. Color flow scanning readily distinguishes arteries from veins, eases longitudinal vein tracking by the constant display of the flow pattern, documents partially occluding thrombi by narrowing of the flow image, and confirms venous occlusion when flow is absent. Although the use of color-coded flow duplex scanning for the diagnosis of DVT has not been shown to be more accurate than conventional duplex scanning in expert hands, it expedites the diagnostic study. It appears that color duplex scanning may be more sensitive in detecting calf vein thrombi, which are difficult to identify, than conventional duplex scanning.

There are limitations and potential sources of error, however, in the use of duplex scanning for the diagnosis of DVT. Visualization of the iliac veins is difficult, if not impossible, because of the presence of overlying intestinal gas. In those instances, indirect evidence of iliocaval vein patency can be obtained by showing spontaneous flow, phasic with respirations in the common femoral vein, whereas the finding of continuous, nonphasic flow suggests outflow obstruction. The femoral vein segment located in the region of the adductor canal is difficult to visualize and cannot be externally compressed because of the overlying musculotendinous structures. The presence of phasic flow in the femoral vein proximal to the adductor canal, which augments with distal calf compression, is compatible with patency of the more distal vein. However, absent or poor augmentation with distal compression implies intervening obstruction. A thrombus can be missed in patients with double femoral or popliteal veins when a single vein is thrombosed and only the patent one is identified. Nonocclusive fresh thrombi with low acoustic density are difficult to detect with duplex scanning and may be overlooked. Occasionally, patient obesity, lack of cooperation, limb pain or edema, the presence of multiple venous collaterals, surgical wounds, dressings, or casts can make the duplex examination technically difficult, if not impossible, thereby limiting its diagnostic value.

The sensitivity and specificity of duplex scanning in detecting DVT in the femoropopliteal veins in symptomatic patients are over 90% in most large series. The specificity remains high regardless of the location of the thrombus in the limb and whether the patient has symptoms or not. It is important to remember that the sensitivity of this test is much lower when used for the diagnosis of DVT in patients without symptoms or when the thrombi are confined to the tibioperoneal veins. Therefore, the diagnosis of DVT with duplex scanning is most accurate in patients who have symptoms suggestive of DVT and who have thrombi located in the popliteal or femoral veins. Color flow scanning may be better in detecting thrombi in the tibioperoneal veins; however, it still carries a low sensitivity and a substantial number of false-positive diagnoses. Fortunately, duplex scanning is most accurate in the diagnosis of popliteal and iliofemoral DVT, where treatment is most important because of the risk of pulmonary embolism and subsequent chronic venous insufficiency. The natural history of thrombosis of the tibioperoneal veins without popliteal involvement is benign in general and does not need to be treated in patients without an ongoing major risk factor for DVT. Therefore, it appears that the low sensitivity of duplex scanning in detecting calf vein thrombosis is of relatively little relevance and may only require surveillance in those patients with continued risks for thrombus propagation. A strategy exists for the diagnosis of DVT using duplex scanning (Fig. 1).

The diagnosis of recurrent DVT is particularly difficult regardless of the tests utilized. Phlebography and physiologic studies are of little help in discerning between old and new thrombosis. Evidence of acute thrombosis can be gained with radiolabeled fibrinogen injection, with high sensitivity for calf thrombi but low sensitivity for iliofemoral thrombosis. Unfortunately, AIDS has made this test impractical because it uses

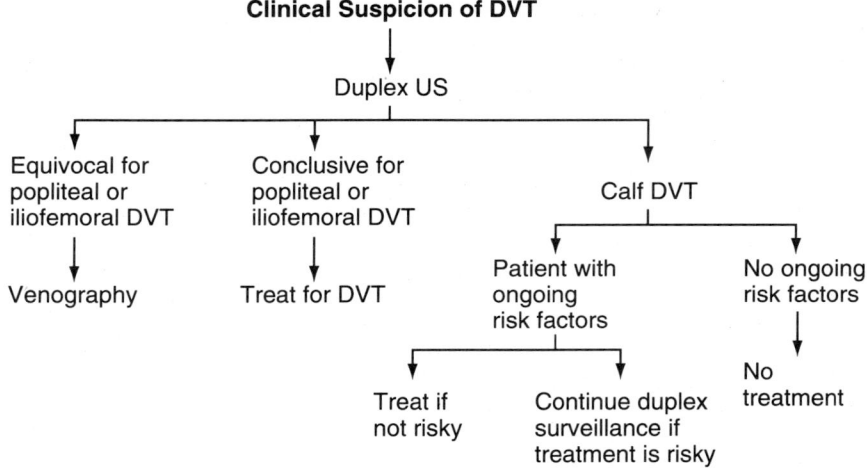

Figure 1 Algorithm for the diagnosis of deep venous thrombosis (DVT) using duplex ultrasound (US) scanning.

pooled plasma products, but if needed it can be done using autologous patient fibrinogen. Blood testing for fibrinogen degradation products, although still of experimental use, appears to be sensitive for detecting acute DVT, but its use is hampered by its large number of false-positive studies. In the absence of a study preceding the suspected recurrent DVT that can document an interval change in the extent of the thrombus, the clinician is forced to decide on an individual basis whether to treat a patient, based on the symptoms and the risks of embolization.

It is important to remember that the information gained with a duplex scanner is only as valid as the knowledge and skill of the sonographer who performs the study. At this time, it is unrealistic to expect that any laboratory can reproduce the accuracy in the diagnosis of DVT reported from centers with extensive experience in this area.

Physiologic tests for the diagnosis of DVT are based on the assumption that intraluminal thrombi produce obstruction to venous flow. Some of these tests have been widely used and rely on plethysmographic techniques (impedance plethysmography, strain gauge plethysmography, phleborrheography) that measure the rate of venous emptying of the leg after transient venous occlusion or a change in venous wave propagation. The sensitivity of physiologic testing in detecting proximal thrombosis is comparable to that of duplex scanning in some reports. Major limitations of plethysmographic testing, however, are poor sensitivity in detecting nonocclusive thrombi or those confined to the calf veins and an inability to differentiate between intraluminal and extraluminal sources of venous obstruction. Furthermore, physiologic tests do not provide any information regarding the location or extent of the thrombi and cannot identify free-floating thrombi or detect interval change in the extent of the thrombi over time, as can be done with duplex scanning.

The overall sensitivity and specificity of duplex scanning in the diagnosis of DVT is higher than that of physiologic tests using plethysmographic techniques. Because the duplex scanner has become the centerpiece of all modern vascular laboratories, where it is also used for arterial and visceral vascular testing, the argument of its higher cost than plethysmographic instruments is not sustainable. The use of hand-held continuous wave Doppler devices for the diagnosis of DVT has the advantage of portability and low cost, and in expert hands it can provide information regarding popliteal and femoral vein thrombosis. Then again, it is subjective, cannot detect nonocclusive thrombi, has little value in interrogating the iliac or calf veins, and is difficult to master. Therefore, a diagnosis of DVT based on a continuous wave Doppler survey should be confirmed with additional testing, if at all possible, and its use should be restricted to those situations in which duplex scanning or reliable physiologic testing is not available.

NONINVASIVE DIAGNOSIS OF CHRONIC VENOUS INSUFFICIENCY

Chronic venous insufficiency (CVI) results from poor emptying of the lower extremity venous system, leading to sustained venous hypertension. Measurement of the ambulatory venous pressure (AVP) has been considered the hemodynamic standard for the evaluation of patients with CVI. Unfortunately, measurement of the AVP is of limited value because it provides poor separation between patients with different clinical degrees of venous disease and has little correlation with clinical changes following surgical intervention. These limitations emphasize our partial understanding of the pathophysiology of CVI and suggest that the elevation in venous pressure is just one factor in its pathogenesis. Regardless of the etiology, the underlying pathology in most patients with CVI is venous obstruction, valvular incompetence, or both. Therefore, our diagnostic efforts are currently focused on the identification and quantitation of venous obstruction and reflux.

The three main questions to be answered in the diagnosis of CVI are what kind of venous problem is present (reflux or obstruction), where it is located, and how severe it is. In most patients, a combination of noninvasive tests can provide information regarding these three questions.

Duplex scanning is the single most valuable instrument for the diagnosis of CVI. It provides anatomic and functional information. From an anatomic standpoint it can document the diameter, number, and location of main venous trunks, document the presence of complete or partial obstruction in those vein segments in which adequate insonation is obtained, document luminal trabeculation suggestive of old DVT, and allow real-time visualization of valves. From a functional standpoint, duplex scanning is most useful in documenting valvular reflux. Color flow scanning has a clear advantage in this regard because it images forward and reverse flow in real time without the need to switch back and forth between B-mode imaging and pulsed wave Doppler insonation, as required in conventional scanning, thereby permitting the survey of the deep and superficial system in a relatively short time. To obtain reliable and comparable information regarding the magnitude of reflux in individual veins, it is essential to use a reproducible and standardized method for eliciting reflux. It has been shown that manual distal compression and release in the supine position generate extremely variable reverse venous blood flow velocities. A reproducible method of eliciting venous reflux, currently under study, can be achieved with the use of rapid inflation-deflation cuffs placed on the legs of a patient in the standing position. With this method, the major veins can be individually interrogated, and the peak and mean reverse blood flow velocities and duration of reflux can be measured accurately during the reversed flow phase generated upon cuff deflation. This information combined with vein diameter measurements yields data regarding the mean and peak reflux blood flow in volume units per second. This method provides objective quantitative measurement of reflux in individual veins and is best for documenting functional changes following deep valvular reconstruction. The use of this information is promising, but its wide clinical applicability is still being investigated.

Air plethysmography (APG) is based on the measurement of calf venous volume changes in response to a sequence of passive and active leg maneuvers in the supine and erect positions. It is currently the most valuable test for the evaluation of global limb venous function. It employs relatively inexpensive instrumentation and provides quantitative information regarding different aspects of venous function. From a practical standpoint, the most valuable parameters measured with APG are the venous filling index (VFI), calf ejection fraction (EF), and the residual volume fraction (RVF). The VFI measures, in milliliters per second, the volume of blood refluxing into the calf and is a reproducible index of overall limb valvular incompetence. The EF measures the volume of blood ejected from the calf with a single tiptoe exercise and assesses the effectiveness of the calf muscle pump mechanism. Finally, the RVF measures the blood volume remaining in the calf at the completion of ten consecutive tiptoe exercises. It has some correlation with the ambulatory venous pressure. The role of APG in the diagnosis of CVI is not yet well defined, but at present it appears to be the most useful and reproducible measure of global limb reflux and calf ejection capacity and best assessment of hemodynamic changes following venous operations.

Because most patients with CVI have valvular reflux, rather than obstruction, as their main problem, it is reasonable to start the evaluation of these patients with an assessment of valvular competence. The diagnostic approach varies, depending on the clinical presentation of the patient. In patients with varicose veins, assessment of reflux in the superficial system is the priority. The greater and lesser saphenous veins should be interrogated with duplex ultrasound in their entirety to delineate the incompetent segments. This is important in that about one-third of patients with varicose veins have reflux confined to a single segment of the greater saphenous vein, and only the incompetent segment needs to be stripped if operation is indicated. When operation is being considered, one should also survey the deep system to be sure that there is no deep obstruction or reflux. The VFI obtained with APG provides an estimate of the degree of reflux; when it corrects with the application of a thigh venous tourniquet, it suggests isolated superficial venous disease. Therefore, patients with varicose veins with reflux confined to the superficial system based on duplex examination, who have an increased venous filling index that corrects with an above-the-knee tourniquet are the best candidates for superficial venous operations and will have a predictably good result. In patients with varicose veins and severe forms of venous insufficiency (skin induration, hyperpigmentation, and ulceration), additional problems in the perforator or deep systems should be suspected and investigated. A rationale exists for the use of duplex scanning and air plethysmography in the management of patients with CVI (Fig. 2).

The assumption that patients with skin ulceration from chronic venous insufficiency always have underlying deep venous reflux or obstruction is wrong. One-third to one-half of patients with venous ulceration have reflux confined to the superficial veins, perforating veins, or both as the single problem. This is particularly important because these patients can benefit from a fairly simple operation with predictably good results. Therefore, patients with skin ulceration deserve an extensive evaluation. Once again, a complete duplex evaluation is done, investigating the presence of obstruction or reflux in the superficial, deep, and perforating veins. The identification of incompetent medial calf perforators requires color flow scanning and ascending phlebography in most patients. However, the sensitivity of either test in identifying perforator incompetence is

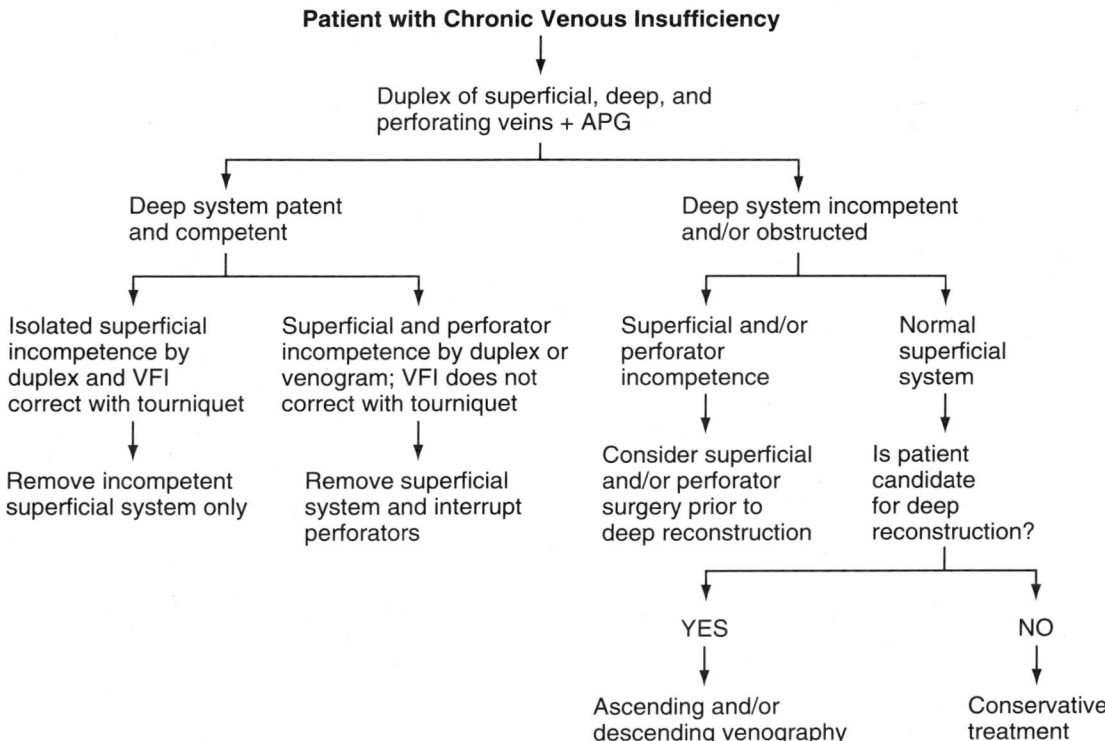

Figure 2 Algorithm for the management of chronic venous insufficiency using air plethysmography (APG) and duplex scanning. VFI, Venous filling index.

low, and the diagnosis has to be occasionally based on the physical examination and clinical suspicion. An APG aids in the evaluation of these patients by quantitating the severity of reflux and their overall venous hemodynamics, and it can be used to document objective changes following venous operations. Additionally, patients in whom deep venous reconstruction is being considered warrant descending or ascending phlebography or both to ascertain the presence of valves amenable to valvuloplasty or the exact extent of obstructed segments. In the future, higher-resolution instruments with three-dimensional imaging capability may obviate the need for phlebography.

Venous outflow obstruction is responsible for a minority of cases of venous ulceration. Its presence can be suspected on clinical grounds and confirmed with ultrasonography in most patients. When the venous occlusion is located in the iliac veins or inferior vena cava, ascending phlebography and cavography may be necessary to confirm the diagnosis and to delineate the proximal and distal extent of the obstruction for possible surgical reconstruction. Alternatively, cross-sectional imaging with computed tomography or magnetic resonance imaging are helpful in the diagnosis of caval or iliac vein obstruction. Quantitation of venous outflow obstruction can be done noninvasively by measuring the maximal venous outflow (MVO) with impedance or air plethysmography. Unfortunately, there is little correlation between the MVO and the clinical severity of disease. Therefore, when the evaluation of venous outflow obstruction is essential, measurement of the arm/foot venous pressure differential, although invasive, is a more reliable method.

REFERENCES

1. Hanrahan LM, Araki CT, Fisher JB, et al. Evaluation of the perforating veins of the lower extremity using high resolution duplex imaging. J Cardiovasc Surg 1991; 32:87–97.
2. Hanrahan LM, Araki CT, Rodriguez AA, et al. Distribution of valvular incompetence in patients with venous stasis ulceration. J Vasc Surg 1991; 13:805–812.
3. McEnroe CS, O'Donnell TF, Mackey WC. Correlation of clinical finding with venous hemodynamics in 386 patients with chronic venous insufficiency. Am J Surg 1988; 156:148–152.
4. Nicolaides AN, Sumner DS. Investigation of patients with deep vein thrombosis and chronic venous insufficiency. London: Med-Orion, 1991.
5. Van Bemmelen PS, Beach K, Bedford G, Strandness DE Jr. The mechanism of venous valve closure. Arch Surg 1990; 125:617–619.
6. Van Bemmelen PS, Bedford G, Beach K, Strandness DE. Quantitative segmental evaluation of venous valvular reflux with duplex ultrasound scanning. J Vasc Surg 1989; 10:425–431.
7. Van Bemmelen PS, Bergan JJ. Quantitative measurement of venous incompetence. Austin, Tex: RG Landes, 1992.
8. Vasdekis SN, Clarke GH, Nicolaides AN. Quantification of venous reflux by means of duplex scanning. J Vasc Surg 1989; 10:670–677.

INVASIVE METHODS OF DIAGNOSING VENOUS DISEASE

ANDREW N. NICOLAIDES, M.D.

DEEP VENOUS THROMBOSIS

Clinical Features

In the early stages of deep vein thrombosis (DVT), symptoms and signs may be absent and in 50% of patients thrombi never become clinically manifest. In some patients, thrombosis may be suspected by the occurrence of clinical pulmonary embolism or by a persistent swelling in the lower limbs. The patient experiences mild pain of gradual onset in the calf, with a sense of fullness, tightness, or actual swelling. The severity of these symptoms depends on the extent of the thrombosis and whether the patient is ambulant or not. Extensive thrombosis involving the popliteal vein may produce ankle edema, but thrombosis extending into the calf, popliteal vein, and superficial femoral vein, terminating just below the saphenofemoral junction, without any edema has been seen often in patients confined to bed. However, sometimes swelling may be the only sign. Extensive iliofemoral thrombosis results in a typically swollen white leg (phlegmasia alba dolens). Massive iliofemoral thrombosis involving the collateral vessels results in a very tender, tense, dusky blue leg with distended veins (phlegmasia cerulea dolens).

Although the clinical signs are notoriously unreliable because they can be elicited in the presence of other conditions, the most useful are deep induration at the site of tenderness and edema proximal to the calf. Homans' sign (i.e., calf pain produced by gentle dorsiflexion of the foot when the knee is flexed) is unreliable because it is present whenever there is calf tenderness irrespective of cause. Ideally, therefore, because of the inaccuracy of clinical signs, the first step in the management of DVT is to confirm the diagnosis with an objective test.

Ascending Phlebography

Until recently phlebography has been the method of choice, but the development of a number of accurate noninvasive tests has made phlebography unnecessary in most patients. Nevertheless, it remains the gold standard, and it is used to determine the accuracy of new tests. Because of this and because of some clinical indications, it is described briefly.

Methods

Contrast is injected in a vein on the dorsum of the foot and directed into the deep veins by an ankle tourniquet. Its ascent is slowed by a second mid-thigh cuff or by having the patient in a semierect position. It is possible to demonstrate the deep veins consistently from the muscular veins in the calf up to the inferior vena cava (IVC), but not the internal iliac and profunda veins.[1]

In a very small proportion of patients, it is not possible to obtain good visualization of the iliac veins and IVC with ascending phlebography, and yet in certain patients it is essential to do so. A good example is the patient with gross edema and iliofemoral vein occlusion in whom anticoagulants are contraindicated and an interruption procedure of the IVC is contemplated. A cavogram through a percutaneous injection of contrast material into the contralateral common femoral vein is indicated prior to cava interruption. Intraosseous phlebography has been used to study the venous collaterals in iliac vein obstruction but is not used routinely because it requires a general anesthetic and there is the possibility of producing osteomyelitis and fat embolism.

The phlebographic criteria for the diagnosis of DVT were established by De Weese and Rogoff as (1) the presence of well-defined filling defects in opacified veins, and (2) the demonstration of these defects on at least two radiographs.[2] Nonvisualization of one or more calf veins is not considered diagnostic of thrombosis because, in normal extremities, these veins are frequently not all visualized. Nonvisualization of the femoral vein with good opacification of the proximal and distal veins and the presence of collaterals is considered evidence of thrombotic obstruction.

Loose thrombus appears as a cylindrical filling defect surrounded by a thin white adherence to the wall. Using the image intensifier and obtaining several views of the same vein just before and after a Valsalva maneuver help distinguish most artifacts from thrombosis. Fresh thrombus fills most of the venous lumen but is not adherent to the wall. Old thrombus is partly adherent to the wall and partly lysed so that it produces the appearance of a recanalized vein.

Complications

The complications of ascending phlebography are pain, extravasation of contrast medium, and venous thrombosis. Pain may be alleviated by giving the patient an analgesic and injecting the contrast slowly during the early part of the examination. Minimal pain, tenderness, or swelling on the day after phlebography has been observed in a small number of patients. These symptoms are rarely severe and clear within 3 days of heparin sodium therapy. Thrombosis due to the contrast medium is another serious complication. In 50% of patients who had phlebography on the day before operation or varicose veins associated with recurrent leg ulcers, thrombi were found not only in the superficial but also in the subfascial veins at operation. These thrombi occurred despite routine flushing of the veins with heparinized saline.[3] Because thrombosis may be caused by phlebography, it is now recommended to be done under heparin therapy administered for 24 hours. Nonionic contrast medium, now available, should be used to minimize these complications.

CHRONIC VENOUS INSUFFICIENCY

Varicose veins, aches, pain, ankle or leg edema, skin irritation, pigmentation, and ulceration are the usual complaints of patients with chronic venous disease. The investigation aims to elucidate the underlying abnormalities (obstruction or reflux) in the venous system and determine their severity by quantitative measurements to enable the clinician to form a rational plan of management.

The symptoms of chronic venous insufficiency are produced by venous hypertension, which is itself the result of obstruction, reflux, or a combination of both. Venous hypertension results in dilation of the capillaries with an increased leakage of plasma, plasma proteins, and even red cells. Pericapillary fibrin deposits impair oxygen transport with eventual hypoxia, ischemia, fat necrosis, skin pigmentation, and ulceration.[4]

Outflow obstruction is found in patients who have had DVT without adequate subsequent recanalization and poor development of a collateral circulation. Less frequently it is the result of extramural venous compression. Reflux in the deep veins is often the result of venous thrombosis and recanalization with destruction of the venous valves but, more rarely, it may be idiopathic. In recent years routine descending phlebography performed in limbs with deep venous reflux has documented that in approximately 30% of such limbs there is no evidence of previous DVT, the reflux being the result of floppy valve cusps.

Two compensatory physiologic mechanisms tend to ameliorate the effects of venous hypertension. They are lymphatic drainage and the body's natural fibrinolytic activity. It has been documented that the rate of lymphatic drainage in post-thrombotic limbs may be increased up to 10 times, and the fibrinolytic activity that removes the pericapillary fibrin markedly varies between individuals. It is now believed that the development of edema, skin changes, and ulceration is the result of a delicate balance between the severity of venous hypertension and the compensatory mechanisms.

Clinical examination with the classic Trendelenburg's test and Perthes' tourniquet test can be misleading or impossible when varicose veins are not prominent, and it may offer relatively little information about the state of the deep veins (obstruction or reflux). However, in extreme conditions with a history of venous claudication, severe swelling, and prominent veins over the lower abdominal wall, the diagnosis is obvious. The author has seen patients whose symptoms became worse after operations on varicose veins that were acting as collaterals in the presence of undiagnosed and unsuspected deep venous obstruction, often in the superficial femoral vein. Also, many recurrent varicose veins are the result of failure to deal with unsuspected incompetent short saphenous veins. For this reason a number of diagnostic studies have been developed. They provide qualitative and quantitative information and can offer answers to most questions posed in a clinical practice. The difficulty is in deciding when to use these methods and how to interpret the results.

Ascending Phlebography

Ascending phlebography defines the anatomy and can give an indication of the basic abnormality. Unfortunately, it cannot provide quantitative measurements of any abnormality. The main reason for doing phlebograms is to confirm the presence and extent of outflow obstruction with documentation of the extent of collateral circulation and sites of reflux.

Until recently, phlebography was considered the gold standard for anatomic documentation. However, the development of high-resolution real-time ultrasonic imaging equipment, combined with Doppler ultrasound, is now producing a new, noninvasive gold standard. The availability of noninvasive techniques that provide quantitative measurements of the severity of obstruction and reflux and that can be used in combination with duplex scanning to answer almost all the questions posed has led to phlebography being performed less frequently. In the author's practice, it is performed in only 3% to 4% of all patients with venous problems.

Method

The technique of phlebography varies, depending on what one is trying to demonstrate or what questions have been posed by the clinician. When the aim is to confirm the diagnosis of outflow obstruction, it differs little from the standard techniques used for the detection of DVT.[1,5] Briefly, contrast is injected into a vein on the dorsum of the foot with a 21 gauge butterfly needle and directed into the deep veins by a narrow (2.5 cm wide) cuff at the ankle. It can be done with the patient horizontal, with an additional pneumatic cuff at the thigh or with the table tilted 60° to the horizontal (head up) to delay the disappearance of contrast proximally. With both cuffs deflated and further injection of contrast, opacification of the iliofemoral segment and inferior vena cava can be obtained. The use of a modern nonionic contrast medium makes the examination virtually painless and reduces the risk of contrast-induced thrombosis.

The detection of deep to superficial reflux requires a slightly different technique, ascending functional phlebography. In this instance, the table is tilted 60° to the horizontal (head up), and the patient's weight is on the opposite limb, which has a 6 cm wooden block under the foot. The latter allows the voluntary plantar flexion of the foot of the limb under examination. Contrast medium is injected and directed into the deep veins as previously described. When contrast medium is seen on the image intensifier to reach the popliteal vein, the patient is asked to plantar flex the foot once or twice. The result is movement of blood and contrast medium proximally in the deep veins during plantar flexion, but retrogradely (from deep to superficial) at incompetent sites during muscular relaxation.

Descending Phlebography

Method

The aim of descending phlebography is to assess the extent of reflux and by inference the degree of valvular damage in the deep veins of the lower limb. The patient is placed in the 60° semi-upright position.[6] An 18 gauge end-hole venous catheter is positioned in the common femoral vein at the level of the public bone. Repeated boluses of iso-osmolar contrast medium are injected. The competence of the common femoral, superficial femoral, profunda femoris, and popliteal veins, as well as the saphenofemoral junction, is assessed by determining the extent of distal reflux of the contrast material. Initially the examiner looks for spontaneous reflux and subsequently asks the patient to do a Valsalva maneuver while plantar flexing the foot as described for ascending functional phlebography.

Grades of Reflux

Five grades of reflux (0-4) have been described:[6,7] grade 0, no reflux below the confluence of the superficial and profunda femoris veins; grade 1, reflux into the superficial femoral vein but not below the middle of the thigh; grade 2, reflux into the superficial femoral vein but not through the popliteal vein (competent popliteal valves); grade 3, reflux to level just below the knee (incompetent popliteal valves, but competent valves in the axial calf veins); and grade 4, reflux through the axial veins (femoral, popliteal, and calf) to the level of the ankle. Although pathologic reflux through the popliteal vein has been shown to be associated with symptoms, the association is not clear. In one study, reflux through the popliteal vein was found in one of five limbs with skin changes or ulceration and in only 31% of postthrombotic limbs.[7]

The poor association between popliteal reflux and symptoms is probably because of the following two reasons, in addition to technical errors. It is now well established that skin changes and ulceration can often occur in the presence of reflux in the superficial veins only, provided the retrograde flow at peak reflux exceeds 7 ml/second.[8] It has also been documented that competent popliteal valves do not exclude postphlebitic changes, which may be the result of reflux in the tibial veins and incompetent calf perforating veins.[9] Unfortunately, the technique of descending phlebography fails to document reflux in the tibial veins in the presence of competent popliteal or more proximal valves.

Ambulatory Venous Pressure Measurements

The original observation made in the 1940s of decrease in venous pressure in the foot during walking and its gradual recovery to the resting value when walking stopped became the basis of ambulatory venous pressure (AVP) measurements used to supplement the anatomic information provided by phlebography. In recent years, AVP measurements became the hemodynamic gold standard used in the development of noninvasive methods for screening and diagnostic evaluation.[10]

Venous pressure is measured by inserting a 21 gauge butterfly needle into a vein on the dorsum of the foot. The needle is connected through a pressure transducer and an amplifier to a potentiometric pen recorder. The patient is supported in the standing position by holding onto an orthopedic frame so that the resting pressure is recorded. Holding onto a frame is important because it prevents contractions of the calf muscle that could produce artifacts during the resting period before and immediately after the end of exercise. The patient then performs a standard exercise of 10 tiptoe movements at the rate of one per second, synchronous to a metronome. At the end of exercise, the patient remains still as the recovery in pressure is recorded (refilling time in seconds). The exercise is then repeated after a 2.5 cm wide pneumatic cuff is inflated at the ankle to occlude the superficial veins. By applying the cuff at higher levels (upper thigh, lower thigh, and just below the knee) and repeating the exercise, the site or sites of deep to superficial reflux can be determined.[10]

Interpretation of Results

The mean AVP during the steady state (toward the end of the 10 tiptoe movements) (P) and the refilling time (90% RT) are the most useful measurements. The values of P based on 500 patients studied are shown in Table 1. This is perhaps the most useful single index of the overall efficacy of the calf muscle pump. Its correlation with the incidence of ulceration is shown in Table 2. Because of the exponential character of the refilling curve, it is much easier and more accurate to

Table 1 Values of Ambulatory Venous Pressure P (mm Hg) (95% Range)

Type of Limbs	No Ankle Cuff	Ankle Cuff Inflated
Normal	15 to 30	15 to 30
Primary varicose veins and competent perforators	25 to 40	13 to 30
Varicose veins and incompetent perforators	40 to 70	25 to 60
Deep venous valve incompetence and proximal occlusion	55 to 85	50 to 80
Proximal occlusion and competent popliteal valves	25 to 60	50 to 80

define 90% RT rather than 100% RT. The values of 90% RT are shown in Table 3.

In the presence of severe outflow obstruction and deep venous reflux (including reflux in the popliteal vein), the value of P may actually increase during exercise because of the increased blood flow as a result of the exercise hyperemia. This group of patients complain of "bursting" pain on walking despite the presence of competent popliteal valves.

Because the measurement of ambulatory venous pressure is invasive, it cannot be repeated frequently or used as a screening test. For this reason plethysmography, foot volumetry, and duplex scanning have been developed. Nevertheless, venous pressure movements remain the gold standard of overall hemodynamic function. They are useful for the validation of the noninvasive tests. Although they are no longer needed for the routine screening of patients, they are essential if the beneficial hemodynamic effect of surgical reconstructive procedures in the deep veins is to be convincingly documented. Venous pressure measurements should be part of the criteria used not only for the assessment of the results of such surgical reconstructions but also for the selection of patients.

OUTFLOW OBSTRUCTION

Outflow obstruction should be suspected when swelling is the predominant symptom. It may be associated with a history of DVT and the development of prominent collateral venous channels in the groin above the pubis or the anterior abdominal wall. It should be suspected and investigated in patients with postthrombotic limbs.

Arm/Foot Pressure Differential

The arm/foot pressure differential has been used by Raju as another method of assessing the severity of outflow obstruction.[11] This method consists of recording the venous pressure in the veins of the foot and hand simultaneously, with the patient in the supine position at rest. The measurements are repeated after inducing reactive hyperemia. In normal limbs the arm/foot pressure differential is less than 5 mm Hg; a rise of up to 16 mm Hg is observed during reactive hyperemia. Patients with phlebographic evidence of obstruction and P less than 5 mm Hg at rest and an increment of less than 6 mm Hg during reactive hyperemia are considered to be fully compensated (grade I). Using such measurements, Raju has classified limbs with outflow obstruction into four grades (Table 4).

Venous Outflow Resistance

Venous outflow resistance can be calculated from the outflow curves of volume and pressures obtained simultaneously. Pressure is measured by inserting a 21 gauge butterfly needle in a vein in the foot, and volume by placing the air chamber of the air plethysmograph around the leg. The foot is elevated 15 cm from the horizontal. A thigh cuff is inflated to 70 mm Hg for 2 minutes and then deflated suddenly. The flow Q can be calculated at any point on the volume outflow curve from the tangent at that point. The resistance R is calculated by dividing the corresponding pressure P from the pressure outflow curve with the flow Q ($R = P/Q$). The units are mm Hg/ml per minute. By calculating R at several points along the outflow curve and plotting it against pressure, it is possible to document how the

Table 2 Incidence of Leg Ulceration (Active or Healed) in Relation to Ambulatory Venous Pressure P in 251 Limbs

Number of Limbs	P (mm Hg)	Incidence of Ulceration (%)
34	<30	0
44	31 to 40	12
51	41 to 50	22
45	51 to 60	38
34	61 to 70	57
28	71 to 80	68
15	>80	73

Table 3 Values of 90% RT (sec) (96% Range)

Type of Limbs	No Ankle Cuff	Ankle Cuff Inflated
Normal	18 to 40	18 to 40
Primary varicose veins and competent perforators	10 to 18	18 to 35
Varicose veins and incompetent perforators	5 to 15	8 to 30
Deep venous valve incompetence	3 to 15	5 to 15

Table 4 Arm/Foot Pressure Differential (AP mm Hg) in Limbs with Outflow Obstruction

Grade	AP at Rest	Pressure Increment During Hyperemia
I: Fully compensated	<5	<6
II: Partially compensated	<5	>6
III: Partially decompensated	>5	>6 (often 10 to 15)
IV: Fully decompensated	>5 (often 15 to 20)	No further increase

resistance changes with different pressures. At high pressure when the veins and collateral channels are distended, the resistance is low. As the pressure decreases and the veins "collapse," the resistance decreases also.

By measuring the outflow resistance in a large number of patients without and with various grades of obstruction (Raju test grades I to IV), the relationship between the two methods has been found. The resistance has now become the gold standard to which noninvasive methods should be compared.

REFERENCES

1. Nicolaides AN, Kakkar VV, Field ES, Renney JTG. Origin of deep vein thrombosis: A venographic study. Br J Radiol 1971; 44:653.
2. De Weese JA, Rogoff SM. Plethysmographic diagnosis of deep venous thrombosis of leg. Aeta Chir Scand (Suppl) 1968; 398:33.
3. Cranley JJ. Vascular surgery, vol 2, Peripheral venous diseases. New York: Harper & Row, 1975:70.
4. Burnand KG, Browse NL. The post phlebitic leg and venous ulceration. In: Russel RCG, ed. Recent advances in surgery, 11th ed. New York: Churchill Livingstone, 1982:225.
5. Lea Thomas K. Phlebography of lower limb. Scotland: Churchill Livingston, 1982.
6. Herman RJ, Neiman HL, Yao JST, et al. Descending venography: A method of evaluating lower extremity valvular function. Radiology 1980; 137:63.
7. Ackroyd JS, Lea Thomas M, Browse NL. Deep vein reflux: An assessment by descending venography. Br J Surg 1986; 73:31.
8. Christopoulous D, Nicolaides AN. Noninvasive diagnosis and quantitation of popliteal reflux in the swollen and ulcerated leg. J Cardiovasc Surg (Torino) 1988; 29:535.
9. Moore DJ, Himmel PD, Summer DS. Distribution of venous valvular incompetence in patients with post-phlebitic syndrome. J Vasc Surg 1986; 3:49.
10. Nicolaides AN, Zukowski AJ. The value of dynamic venous pressure measurements. World J Surg 1986; 10:919.
11. Raju S. New approaches in the diagnoses and treatment of venous obstruction. J Vasc Surg 1986; 4:42.

NONOPERATIVE TREATMENT OF ACUTE SUPERFICIAL THROMBOPHLEBITIS AND DEEP FEMORAL VENOUS THROMBOSIS

MICHAEL J. VITTI, M.D.
ROBERT W. BARNES, M.D.

ACUTE SUPERFICIAL THROMBOPHLEBITIS

Acute superficial thrombophlebitis is a noninfectious inflammatory process caused by thrombosis of the greater or lesser saphenous veins of the lower extremity or of the superficial veins of the upper extremity. It has been estimated to occur in more than 125,000 patients annually in the United States. It is particularly common among elderly patients. Women are affected three times more commonly than men, as acute superficial thrombophlebitis commonly occurs during pregnancy.[1]

In the upper extremity, trauma to the superficial venous system from prolonged intravenous cannulation is the predominant causative factor. Acute superficial thrombophlebitis of the lower extremity is typically precipitated by trauma in the setting of pre-existing varicose veins. Lower extremity superficial thrombophlebitis, in the absence of varicose veins, has been associated with intra-abdominal carcinomas in a small percentage of patients.

Prevention

Prophylactic measures consist of elevation of the foot when seated or recumbent and the use of graduated compression stockings when the legs are dependent. Knee-length hose with pressure gradients of 20 to 30 mm Hg usually suffice. Such measures are recommended for patients at increased risk for superficial thrombophlebitis. These include pregnant women, and elderly or postoperative patients with varicose veins. Surgical extirpation of varicose veins as a means of prophylaxis is recommended only in patients with severe symptoms or venous stasis skin changes that cannot be controlled by compression stockings.[1]

Diagnosis

Acute superficial thrombophlebitis is characterized clinically by localized pain and tenderness, erythema or increased heat, and a palpable induration over the course of a superficial vein. Edema is not characteristic of superficial phlebitis but may indicate involvement of the deep venous system. In lower extremity superficial thrombophlebitis, these findings typically occur over pre-existing varicosities of the greater or lesser saphenous veins. In such patients, the clinical diagnosis of superficial thrombophlebitis can be made with certainty.

Superficial inflammation of the leg in the absence of varicose veins may also be caused by lymphangitis, cellulitis, subcutaneous fat necrosis, and vasculitis. Therefore, in the absence of predisposing varicose veins, superficial inflammation in the leg should be studied by duplex ultrasonography to assess the patency and flow characteristics of the saphenous system. If the saphenous vein in the inflamed area is patent with normal venous flow signals, lymphangitis or cellulitis is the most probable diagnosis, and the patient is treated with antibiotics. If venous thrombosis is indicated by duplex ultrasound, the diagnosis of superficial thrombophlebitis is confirmed. If thrombus extends near the saphenofemoral junction, the duplex examination is used to clarify the status of the deep venous system as well.[2]

Once acute superficial thrombophlebitis is diagnosed, patients should be monitored for clinical signs of thrombus propagation into the proximal thigh and into the deep venous system at the saphenofemoral junction. Venous duplex examination is recommended for any patient in whom proximal progression of superficial thrombophlebitis is suspected. Recent reports have cited a 23% to 28% prevalence of deep vein thrombosis (DVT) in patients with acute superficial thrombophlebitis when routine venous duplex examination was performed. In the vast majority of instances, deep venous involvement was clinically occult. This presence of associated DVT has been implicated as an explanation for the occurrence of pulmonary embolism in up to 10% of hospitalized patients with acute superficial thrombophlebitis of the lower extremity. In an effort to detect these clinically occult DVTs, some authors now advocate routine venous duplex examination for acute superficial thrombophlebitis of the saphenous veins.[3,4]

In addition to proximal extension of thrombus, infectious complications may also occur. Spiking fevers, leukocytosis, increased tenderness, and erythema over the course of a phlebitic vein may indicate the onset of septic phlebitis, a suppurative process involving the venous wall.

Treatment

Treatment of acute superficial thrombophlebitis depends upon the location of the thrombosis. When limited to the lower leg, conservative measures consisting of leg elevation, application of local heat, ambulation with graduated compression stockings, and nonsteroidal anti-inflammatory agents are employed. The vast majority of patients follow a benign, self-limited course with such therapy, although a 15% recurrence rate has been cited with medical management.

If thrombosis has progressed into the mid-thigh or in proximity to the saphenofemoral junction, duplex ultrasound is indicated to assess the deep venous system. If the deep veins are patent, bed rest and anticoagulation are instituted for thrombophlebitis that has progressed to the mid-thigh despite conservative treatment. If involvement is near the saphenofemoral junction, ligation is recommended to prevent propagation into the deep venous system. If the deep veins are already thrombosed, systemic anticoagulation is begun for treatment of DVT.[2]

In the case of septic thrombophlebitis, operative excision of the involved vein is the treatment of choice.

DEEP FEMORAL VENOUS THROMBOSIS

Acute DVT of the lower extremities and its major complication, pulmonary embolism (PE), have been estimated to cause the death of at least 100,000 hospitalized patients each year in the United States. Ninety percent of PEs originate in DVT of the lower extremities. Both DVT and PE manifest few specific symptoms and are, most often, clinically silent. Not uncommonly, the first manifestation of lower extremity DVT is a fatal PE. The clinical diagnosis of both entities is both insensitive and nonspecific.[5]

Most patients who die from PE do so within 30 minutes of the acute event. This deterioration is too rapid for anticoagulation to be effective. Unrecognized DVT may also lead to long-term morbidity from the postphlebitic syndrome as well as a predisposition to future episodes of recurrent venous thromboembolism. As a result, the prevention of DVT in hospitalized patients remains the focus of clinical research.[6]

Effective prophylaxis depends upon the knowledge of clinical risk factors, as defined by epidemiologic studies, that predispose to the development of DVT. These clinical risk factors include advanced age, prolonged immobility, prior DVT or PE, malignancy, operations (especially involving the pelvis or lower extremities), obesity, congestive heart failure, and oral contraceptive use. Hypercoagulable states such as antithrombin III deficiency, protein S deficiency, or protein C deficiency also predispose to DVT. In the presence of multiple risk factors, the risk for DVT development is cumulative. Because multiple risk factors are involved in the pathogenesis of DVT, no single prophylactic method is effective in all patients. The approach must be individualized to accommodate the patient's surgical situation and particular risk factors.[6]

Prevention

Most surgical patients are at risk for DVT, and prophylactic measures are essential components of their overall care. Low-risk patients are those under age 40, without additional risk factors, undergoing uncomplicated abdominal or thoracic operations. These patients have a less than 1% risk of femoral DVT and are the only surgical group in which prophylaxis may be excluded. In patients over age 40 who are undergoing major abdominal operations, the risk of femoral DVT is 7% and of PE is 1.6%. In patients undergoing elective hip replacement, the risk of DVT without prophylaxis is 45% to 50%, while PE occurs in 1.6%. After emergency hip operations, DVT occurs in 60% to 80% of patients and PE in 4% to 7% without prophylaxis.[6]

Two approaches can be taken to preventing PE. Primary prophylaxis utilizes either drugs or physical methods to prevent DVT development. Secondary prophylaxis relies on early detection and treatment of subclinical DVT by screening patients with noninvasive testing. Primary prophylaxis is more effective, less expensive, and the preferred method of DVT prevention. Secondary prophylaxis is reserved for patients in whom primary prevention is contraindicated or is used as a complement to primary prophylaxis in very high-risk patients.[6]

Mechanical methods of DVT prophylaxis are intended to increase blood flow in the proximal femoral vein, thereby reducing the potential for stasis and DVT development. These methods include graduated compression stockings and intermittent pneumatic compression devices. Graduated compression stockings apply a graded degree of compression to the ankle and calf with greater pressure applied more distally in the limb and an overall gradient of 20 mm Hg. Typically, stockings are applied preoperatively and are worn postoperatively until the patient is fully ambulatory. No difference exists in the effectiveness of the above-knee as opposed to below-knee stockings in reducing the occurrence of DVT. Graduated compression stockings reduce the incidence of postoperative DVT by only 5% to 10% when used as the only means of prophylaxis in moderate- and high-risk surgical patients. For this reason, they are considered only an adjuvant prophylactic measure.[5]

Intermittent pneumatic compression devices are inflatable sleeves placed around the lower leg and intermittently inflated to a pressure of 35 to 40 mm Hg for 10 seconds each minute. These devices not only inhibit venous stasis but also increase blood fibrinolytic activity. They are effective in reducing leg DVT in moderate- and high-risk general surgery patients. In trials comparing them to low-dose heparin (LDH) therapy, both agents were equivalent in the general surgery population. In orthopedic patients, intermittent pneumatic compression is highly effective in preventing DVT after knee operations but is less effective in preventing femoral DVT after hip operations.[6]

Antithrombotic drug prophylaxis is the most widely used method of DVT prevention. Among general surgery patients, subcutaneous LDH and low-molecular-weight heparin (LMWH) are the most effective agents in reducing the incidence of DVT. The pharmacologic effect of heparin sodium is as an antithrombin III agonist. Heparin sodium bonds to antithrombin III and forms a complex that binds and neutralizes thrombin. Circulating heparin sodium also neutralizes clotting factors VII, IX, and X.

The LDH subcutaneous regimen consists of 5,000 units given 2 hours before operation and continues every 12 hours after operation for 7 days (every 8 hours in high-risk patients). The LDH reduces the overall incidence of DVT in general surgery patients from 25% to 8% while also reducing the incidence of proximal femoral DVTs and clinically diagnosed PEs. It does not increase the incidence of major hemorrhagic complications, but the rate of wound hematomas is increased. Caution is, therefore, warranted for use of this regimen in patients with impaired hemostasis, prosthetic implants, and impaired wound healing. Among orthopedic patients, LDH is considerably less effective in preventing DVT, reducing the rate from 50% to 35%. As a result, LDH is the preferred regimen for DVT prophylaxis in moderate- and high-risk general surgery patients but not in the orthopedic population.[6]

Low-molecular-weight heparin is produced from conventional heparin by depolymerization into molecules of 2,000 to 7,000 daltons molecular weight. Their clinical usefulness is derived from their high bioavailability and longer half-life than conventional heparin sodium. In addition, LMWH loses its ability to inhibit Factor Xa, which results in an equivalent antithrombotic effect but less bleeding potential than conventional heparin sodium.[7] In the majority of trials in general surgery patients, LMWH was superior to LDH in preventing DVT (4% versus 8%). In orthopedic patients, LMWH is associated with a DVT incidence of 16%, compared to the LDH rate of 34%. Thus, LMWH appears to be superior to LDH in the orthopedic patient population.[6]

Another prophylactic regimen utilizes dextran, a branched polysaccharide of 40,000 or 70,000 daltons. Its antithrombotic properties have been attributed to decreased blood viscosity, reduced platelet interactions with the damaged vessel wall, and enhanced fibrinolytic activity. Dextran is given intravenously in a volume of 500 ml over 4 to 6 hours, starting at operation and then daily for 2 to 5 days postoperatively. It is not as efficacious in preventing leg DVT as are LDH and LMWH in general surgical patients. Dextran does, however, reduce the incidence of PE to the same extent as LDH. Although dextran does not prevent DVT, it does halt the growth and extension of thrombi so that PE is prevented. Dextran is somewhat more effective after hip operation but remains a second-line choice for DVT prophylaxis. Fluid overload and hypersensitivity reactions have been observed as side effects.[6]

Oral anticoagulation with sodium warfarin prevents DVT by inhibiting synthesis of vitamin K–dependent coagulation factors II, VII, IX, and X. When used at a fixed low dose of 2 mg/day or adjusted to mildly prolong the prothrombin time, sodium warfarin is effective in reducing the incidence of leg DVT. In general surgery patients, LDH is more effective and easier to use, but in orthopedic patients, sodium warfarin is the most satisfactory agent for the prevention of DVT after elective hip procedures. The need for preoperative treatment, the slow lag time prior to the onset of the antithrombotic effect, and its slow reversal in the setting of bleeding complications are all factors preventing wider acceptance of oral anticoagulation as DVT prophylaxis.[6]

Therefore, current recommendations for DVT prophylaxis are:

1. Low-risk general surgery patients (age under 40 years, no risk factors) require no prophylaxis other than early ambulation.
2. Moderate-risk general surgery patients (age older than 40 years, no risk factors, major operations) may receive graduated elastic compression stockings, intermittent pneumatic compression (IPC) devices, or LDH for effective prophylaxis.
3. High-risk general surgery patients (age older than 40 years, major operations, additional risk factors) require LDH or LMWH. In those prone to wound hematomas or infection, dextran and IPC are acceptable alternative treatments.

4. Very high-risk general surgery patients with multiple risk factors require LDH or LMWH in combination with IPC.
5. For orthopedic patients with hip fractures or hip replacement, sodium warfarin and LMWH are the most effective prophylactic agents. LDH, IPC, dextran, and elastic compression stockings all reduce the incidence of DVT but are considerably less effective.
6. Orthopedic patients undergoing knee surgery are recommended to have IPC.

Diagnosis

Despite the use of prophylaxis, a high index of suspicion for DVT must be maintained, as it often appears insidiously in critically ill patients. Calf pain is a frequently overlooked early symptom. The classic signs of DVT—edema of the extremity, calf tenderness, and Homan's sign (pain on passive dorsiflexion of the ankle)—are usually associated with an advancing process. Bedside signs and symptoms lead to detection of only 50% of affected patients, and diagnoses made on clinical grounds alone are in error in 30% of patients.[5]

Ascending contrast phlebography had been considered the gold standard for DVT diagnosis. However, phlebography is invasive, expensive, and associated with risks. Over the past 25 years, several noninvasive diagnostic modalities have been developed to diagnose DVT. Venous duplex examination has probably had the greatest impact. In many institutions, the use of venous duplex imaging has largely replaced phlebography for the diagnosis of acute DVT.

In the initial clinical and noninvasive assessment of a patient with suspected DVT, it is important to ascertain the anatomic site, chronicity, and extent of thrombosis. These factors may influence the treatment selected and the prognosis for a successful outcome. In femoropopliteal DVT, heparin sodium anticoagulation is recommended; more extensive common femoral and iliac vein thromboses of less than 5 days' duration may be considered for thrombolytic therapy.[5]

Five different clinical presentations of lower extremity DVT are recognized.

1. Distal DVT: thrombus localized to deep veins of the calf.
2. Proximal DVT: thrombus in popliteal and superficial femoral veins.
3. Phlegmasia alba dolens: unilateral edema of the entire leg without cyanotic discoloration due to thrombus in the common femoral vein with possible extension into the iliac veins.
4. Phlegmasia cerulea dolens: massive swelling of the entire leg with violaceous discoloration due to near total obstruction of the deep venous system including the femoral and iliac veins. Bilateral leg involvement may indicate thrombosis of the inferior vena cava.
5. Venous gangrene: areas of bleb formation and full-thickness skin necrosis due to rapidly progressive phlegmasia cerulea dolens. The necrosis is believed to be due to increasing venous outflow obstruction causing arterial insufficiency in the cutaneous microcirculation. Venous gangrene is the primary indication for venous thrombectomy and requires aggressive surgical management because it may lead to loss of the extremity if treatment is delayed.[1]

Treatment

Anticoagulants

Once acute DVT is diagnosed, the mainstay of medical treatment consists of heparin sodium followed by sodium warfarin anticoagulation. Ancillary supportive measures consist of bed rest for the first 4 to 5 days or until extremity pain abates. When discomfort and edema have subsided, the patient should be measured for below-knee graduated compression stockings providing a 30 to 40 mm Hg pressure at the ankle. After the initial period of bed rest, progressive exercise and ambulation are advised.[1]

Heparin sodium may be administered by two different methods: intermittent subcutaneous injection or continuous intravenous infusion. Heparin sodium does not cause dissolution of a thrombus but prevents the formation of new thrombi and permits the body's fibrinolytic system to function more effectively. Prior to beginning heparin sodium therapy, a baseline activated partial thromboplastin time (aPTT), prothrombin time (PT), and platelet count are obtained. If the continuous infusion protocol is selected, treatment is initiated with an intravenous dose of 5,000 units of heparin sodium. A solution of 20,000 to 40,000 units of heparin sodium in 500 ml of 0.9 normal saline is prepared and delivered via a continuous infusion pump at 1,500 units/hour initially. The level of anticoagulation is monitored by the aPTT done every 6 hours, and the heparin rate is adjusted to keep the aPTT between 1.5 and 2.5 times the control value. Platelet counts are also checked daily to monitor for the onset of heparin-induced thrombocytopenia.[1]

A minimum level of anticoagulation must be maintained to achieve an effective antithrombotic state. Inadequate anticoagulation results in unacceptably high rates of DVT and PE. Recurrent DVT is rare if the aPTT is kept greater than 1.5 times control. Failure to achieve this level of anticoagulation results in a 20% to 25% risk of recurrent DVT or PE. When the aPTT is less than 1.5 times control, the blood level of heparin sodium can be raised quickly and more reliably by giving another bolus and increasing the infusion rate simultaneously. When the aPTT is too prolonged, the heparin sodium infusion can be stopped for a short time, not to exceed 1 hour. Heparin requirements are usually greatest in the first few days after the acute thrombotic event. As stabilization of the aPTT occurs, laboratory monitoring can be changed from every 6 hours to daily.[8]

The intermittent subcutaneous heparin sodium regimen utilizes the abdominal panniculus as the preferred site of repeated subcutaneous injections. The initial heparin sodium dose should begin at 17,500 units every 12 hours with subsequent adjustments to maintain the aPTT at 1.5 times control. The aPTT must be drawn 1 hour before the next scheduled dose. Dosage requirements usually necessitate more frequent adjustments than with the continuous infusion method.[8]

After initial anticoagulation has been achieved and stabilized by heparin sodium, adequate long-term anticoagulation is maintained with sodium warfarin. Multiple randomized clinical trials of proximal DVT treatment have shown that when intravenous heparin sodium is given for 7 to 10 days, followed by long-term anticoagulation, the frequency of recurrent DVT or PE is less than 5%. The currently accepted approach is to begin heparin sodium and sodium warfarin therapy together at the time of diagnosis and to discontinue the heparin sodium on about the fifth day after the PT is in the therapeutic range.[8]

Sodium warfarin, which acts by inhibiting the synthesis of vitamin K–dependent coagulation factors II, VII, IX, and X and anticoagulation proteins C and S, does not act immediately. Time is required for the normal anticoagulation factors already present in the plasma to be cleared. This lag period depends on the plasma clearance rates of the vitamin K–dependent clotting factors. Clearance is fastest for factor VII and protein C, slowest for factor II. A large loading dose might prolong the PT within the first 24 hours, but in the presence of normal levels of factors II, IX, and X with low levels of protein C, a hypercoagulable state may be induced during the first 24 hours of therapy. This consideration supports the need for a period of overlap of heparin and warfarin therapy in the treatment of acute DVT.[8]

Sodium warfarin therapy is monitored by daily PTs. Multiple studies document that adequate anticoagulation is indicated by a PT prolongation by an international normalized ratio (INR) of 2 to 3. Monthly laboratory testing usually suffices during the more chronic phases of management. The duration of long-term sodium warfarin therapy must be tailored to the individual patient. Patients with slowly resolving risk factors such as prolonged immobilization should be treated for at least 3 months. Patients with malignancies, hypercoagulable states, or recurrent DVT or PE should be treated indefinitely.

Recently, the use of LMWH has been reported by Hull and associates to be as effective and safe as continuous intravenous heparin sodium in the treatment of proximal vein DVT. Patients who received LMWH had recurrent DVT or PE in 2.6% compared to 7% for intravenous heparin therapy. The LMWH was given subcutaneously once daily without laboratory monitoring. This report raised the possibility of caring for uncomplicated proximal vein DVTs on an outpatient basis, thereby resulting in substantial savings of hospital costs.[9]

The most common complications of anticoagulation therapy are bleeding, allergic reactions, and heparin-induced thrombocytopenia. A 5% to 20% rate of hemorrhagic complications or an unexpected fall in the hematocrit can be expected during heparin sodium therapy. The risk of bleeding also increases with the extent of anticoagulation. If the aPTT prolongation is two to three times control, complications increased threefold. When prolongation was greater than three times control, bleeding complications increased by a factor of eight.[8] Most bleeding episodes can be controlled by discontinuing the drug due to its half-life of 1 hour. If hemorrhage continues, blood transfusions are started and protamine sulfate can be given slowly over 10 to 15 minutes in a dose of 15 mg/1,000 units of estimated circulating heparin sodium. The maximum safe dose of protamine is 50 mg. If this is exceeded or if the drug is given too rapidly, acute hypotension or transient thrombocytopenia may occur.[1]

Heparin sodium therapy may also induce thrombocytopenia due to antibody-mediated injury to platelets and endothelium. Heparin-induced thrombocytopenia should be suspected in the setting of increased resistance to heparin sodium and a falling platelet count. If the platelet count falls below 100,000, platelet aggregation testing should be done on the patient's plasma to establish the diagnosis. If testing is positive, heparin sodium is stopped, and alternate means of anticoagulation are sought. If untreated, this syndrome may give rise to arterial thromboembolism and extension or recurrence of the existing DVT.[1]

Hemorrhage during sodium warfarin therapy is more difficult to manage due to its longer half-life of 2.5 days. The drug is discontinued and parenteral vitamin K up to a maximum dose of 50 mg is given to reverse the anticoagulation within 24 hours. If bleeding requires more prompt control, 5 to 25 mg of vitamin K are given intravenously with 500 ml of fresh frozen plasma.

Another complication seen with sodium warfarin is a vascular purpura that causes skin necrosis and occurs occasionally in the first weeks of therapy. It has been associated with protein C deficiency and malignancy. Sodium warfarin also crosses the placenta and may cause spontaneous abortion or embryopathies if given in the first trimester of pregnancy. All women of childbearing age taking sodium warfarin must avoid pregnancy. Subcutaneous heparin sodium dosed to maintain the aPTT beyond 1.5 times control is the therapy of choice in pregnant women.

Thrombolytic Agents

Thrombolytic therapy in the treatment of DVT is based on studies suggesting that early thrombolysis can decrease subsequent leg pain, swelling, loss of venous valves, and the incidence of postphlebitic syndrome. The use of thrombolytic therapy rather than heparin sodium is reserved for cases of acute massive DVT of the lower extremities in which symptoms have been present for less than 5 days. Fibrinolytic agents are used only when thrombosis extends to the origin of the deep femoral vein. Patients whose deep femoral vein can function as a collateral pathway are recommended for heparin anticoagulation.[5,8]

Thrombolytic agents dissolve thrombi by activating plasminogen to plasmin, which, in proximity to thrombus, degrades fibrin into soluble peptides. Streptokinase (SK), a protein derived from group C beta-hemolytic streptococci, is the agent of choice. It appears equally effective yet is less expensive than urokinase. The SK combines with plasminogen to form a complex that activates adjacent plasminogen to plasmin. It is antigenic and not recommended for repeated use within 6 months. The incidence of PE during thrombolytic therapy is similar to that during therapy with heparin sodium, 5%.

The major obstacle to the use of SK is the risk of bleeding. The SK treatment for acute DVT is designed to activate systemic fibrinolysis; therefore, it has the potential to lyse a fresh platelet-fibrin plug anywhere and cause bleeding at that site. Nonlethal bleeding has been reported to occur in 11.5% and lethal bleeding in 0.73% of patients on lytic therapy as compared to 7.3% and 0.3% respectively for heparin sodium anticoagulation.[8] This increased frequency of bleeding has led to the delineation of strict contraindications to lytic therapy, which include operation or major trauma within 1 month, active or recent hemorrhage, any intracerebral disease, pregnancy, and bleeding diatheses. A recent study of 209 patients with lower extremity DVT documented that contraindications to thrombolytic therapy were present in 93%. Recent operation was the most common factor precluding therapy. As a result, thrombolytic therapy for acute DVT is feasible in only a small proportion of patients.[10]

Currently, only patients with phlegmasia alba or cerulea dolens are considered acceptable candidates for thrombolytic therapy. Once the precise anatomic extent is defined with phlebography or duplex examinations, a pretreatment coagulation profile, which includes fibrinogen level and aPTT, is obtained. A loading dose of 250,000 units of SK is given intravenously over 20 minutes, followed by maintenance therapy with 100,000 units/hour delivered by a constant infusion pump. The extent of systemic fibrinolysis is monitored by the fibrinogen level and aPTT obtained 4 to 5 hours after initiation of treatment. Prolongation of aPTT by 10 seconds or more and fibrinogen less than 100 mg/dl indicates activation of fibrinolysis.[1]

For acute DVT, SK therapy is recommended for a total duration of 48 to 72 hours and, depending on the clinical response, is discontinued after that time. After lytic therapy is stopped, intravenous heparin sodium should be restarted once the aPTT is less than 1.5 times control. Heparin sodium and SK have a synergistic action, and the risk of bleeding is accentuated if both are used concomitantly. Heparin sodium is usually continued for 7 to 10 days after cessation of lytic therapy with sodium warfarin introduced at the midpoint of this time span. Heparin sodium is discontinued once the PT is within therapeutic range for 3 to 5 days. Sodium warfarin is usually continued for 3 to 6 months with PTs maintained at an INR of 2 to 3.[8]

If bleeding does occur with thrombolytic therapy, blood loss should be replaced with transfusions, and depleted fibrinogen levels are replaced by cryoprecipitate or fresh frozen plasma. Epsilon aminocaproic acid also may be helpful but is usually reserved for intracranial or other life-threatening hemorrhagic complications not being controlled by other measures.

Most surgeons today prefer the use of heparin sodium for patients with DVT confined to tibial, popliteal, and superficial femoral veins. The SK is reserved for DVT involving the common femoral or iliac veins of less than 5 days' duration. Both treatment methods have reduced the mortality rates due to PE from 18% to 33% in untreated patients to 8% in treated patients.[8]

As a result of newer therapeutic agents, the mortality and morbidity associated with DVT have improved significantly over the past several decades. Further clinical trials of such agents as LMWH and thrombolytic drugs may yet alter the nonoperative treatment of acute femoral DVT.

REFERENCES

1. DeWeese MS. Nonoperative treatment of acute superficial thrombophlebitis and deep femoral vein thrombosis. In: Ernst CB, Stanley JC, eds. Current therapy in vascular surgery. Toronto: BC Decker, 1991:952.
2. Barnes RW, Wu KW, Hoak JC. Differentiation of superficial thrombophlebitis from lympghangitis by Doppler ultrasound. Surg Gynecol Obstet 1976; 43:23–25.
3. Jorgensen JO, Hanel KC, Morgan AM, Hunt JM. The incidence of deep vein thrombosis in patients with superficial thrombophlebitis of the lower limbs. J Vasc Surg 1993; 18:70–73.
4. Lutter KS, Kerr TM, Roedersheimer R, et al. Superficial thrombophlebitis diagnosed by duplex scanning. Surgery 1991; 110:42–46.
5. Persson AV, Davis RJ, Villavicencio JL. Deep vein thrombosis and pulmonary embolism. Surg Clin North Am 1991; 71:1195–1209.
6. Clagett GP, Anderson FA, Levine MN, et al. Prevention of venous thromboembolism. Chest 1992; 102(suppl):391–407.
7. Hirsh J. Rationale for development of low molecular weight heparins and their clinical potential in prevention of venous thrombosis. Am J Surg 1991; 161:512–517.
8. Hyers TM, Hull RD, Weg JG. Antithrombotic therapy for venous thromboembolic disease. Chest 1992; 102(suppl):408–425.
9. Hull RG, Raskob GE, Pineo GF, et al. Subcutaneous low molecular weight heparin compared with continuous intravenous heparin in the treatment of proximal vein thrombosis. N Engl J Med 1992; 326:975–982.
10. Markel A, Manzo RA, Strandness E. The potential role of thrombolytic therapy in venous thrombosis. Arch Intern Med 1992; 152:1265–1267.

INJECTION COMPRESSION SCLEROTHERAPY OF SPIDER TELANGIECTASIA AND VARICOSE VEINS

JOHN R. PFEIFER, M.D.

Although many surgeons inject bulging varicose veins, we believe large, bulging varicose veins are best treated surgically, using small incisions and sparing the great saphenous vein when possible.[1] Although injection of cutaneous spider veins or telangiectasia of the lower extremity is often done for cosmetic reasons, most such lesions produce symptoms ranging from numbness or paresthesia to pain, either aching or burning. The procedure is tedious and time-consuming, with a significant incidence of recurrence. However, because of the unattractive appearance of telangiectasia and the associated symptoms, there is a high patient demand for this form of therapy.

We recently compared injection sclerotherapy using 22% hypertonic saline solution with carbon dioxide laser ablation of cutaneous spider veins of the lower extremities. Patients preferred injection sclerotherapy because laser treatment left small white scars, was more painful, and had a higher recurrence rate.

Laser treatment has now been abandoned for this reason, and we use only saline injection sclerotherapy.[2] Our current cumulative experience includes a total of 77,624 injections in 1,601 patients between January 1982 and August 31, 1993. Most of these patients presented with lower extremity lesions, with a limited number in the face, chest wall, and breast.

PATIENT EVALUATION

Our current practice is to perform a complete preliminary history and physical examination, with special attention to the arterial and venous system. The patient may have one or two noninvasive laboratory studies to complete the assessment of the venous system.

The patient is examined in the erect position, after 5 to 10 minutes of standing to allow for maximum inflation of bulging varicosities. Bulging varicosities and spider veins are accurately marked on leg diagrams at the time of initial examination. A copy of this diagram is on the chart at the time of each injection treatment to facilitate an accurate record of injection locations.

The patient is then measured for custom-fitted support hose by the office staff. A variety of brands are available. Over-the-counter hose are to be discouraged because the patient needs a stocking specific to his or her measurements. The stockings are available at the time of the first injection visit.

LABORATORY STUDIES

Initially, photoplethysmography (PPG) is used to evaluate venous valve function and the degree of venous insufficiency. With proper technique, superficial and deep venous insufficiency can be identified and managed prior to injection therapy. We now use Doppler examination and duplex scan to determine points of reflux. Tourniquet testing is no longer utilized.

If there is any question of deep vein thrombosis, phleborrheography (PRG) is used as a screening study for recent venous occlusion. Positive PRG studies are then confirmed by duplex scan. Duplex scanning is the best method of precisely assessing deep venous occlusion, either acute or chronic, as well as locations of major venous reflux. The presence of chronic deep vein occlusion is not a contraindication to sclerotherapy. However, the presence of acute deep vein thrombosis (DVT) is an absolute contraindication to sclerotherapy. If acute DVT is detected, sclerotherapy should be postponed for 6 months.

PATIENT PREPARATION

It is important to realize that although sclerotherapy is done for symptoms, most patients are treated for cosmetic concerns. Therefore, results are not based on the usual physician parameters of clinical improvement. Here, the patient's own assessment of results is important. In fact, the patient's decision to proceed with treatment depends on his or her reaction to the degree of pain during the procedure and assessment of the result. In sclerotherapy, patient comfort and patient satisfaction become critical factors in determining whether treatment is continued. The physician's preinjection preparation of the patient becomes an important component of treatment. A supportive physician is important, but supportive and kind office personnel are equally important as they handle the many questions posed by these patients.

EXPLANATION OF RISK

Before injection sclerotherapy is performed, a comprehensive explanation of the procedure with its attendant risks is given to the patient (Table 1).

PRESCLEROTHERAPY PHOTOGRAPHY

Evaluation of results in sclerotherapy is highly subjective. Frequently, as the series of treatments progresses, patients forget how extensive their veins were prior to injection. Therefore, it is important to photograph all areas of planned injection before beginning sclerotherapy.

We use a Minolta-7000 35 mm camera with a Macro 35-70 zoom lens. A data-back on the camera allows us to

Table 1 Injection Therapy for Spider Veins

As you begin a program of sclerotherapy for your spider veins, there are some things we would like you to remember.

1. Certain veins require 3 or 4 treatments before they disappear. The principle of injection therapy for small skin veins is to inject a sclerosing (scarring) agent into the vein, which causes the vein wall to become inflamed and seal together. When the vein can no longer carry blood, it is no longer visible through the skin.
2. There is occasional skin pigmentation (brown spots). When the tiny needle is inserted into the vein for injection purposes, occasionally as the salt solution is injected, the vein ruptures, allowing this solution to leak into the surrounding tissue. This may result in a brown pigmented spot in the skin that occasionally is permanent but usually disappears with time. It is usually small and no more obvious than the vein that was initially treated. However, you should be aware that this is a complication of injection of veins, although it only occurs in approximately 10% of the cases.
3. There is a rare occurrence of small skin ulcers forming after an injection. Very rarely, an injection is irritating enough to cause a small area of skin loss (or ulcer). In more than 70,000 injections, this complication has occurred 37 times. The size of a pencil eraser, these ulcers have healed without incident, leaving a small white scar.
4. You will be required to support your legs after treatment. After injection, your legs will be compressed with small gauze pads and a compression stocking (either calf high or a pantyhose). This compression support stays in place for 3 days and 2 nights, during which time you will not be able to shower or have a complete bath. Then the stocking alone is used, while you resume daily showers, for an additional 2 weeks.
5. During the injection treatments, your daily activities are not restricted. You may continue to work and perform your daily activities. However, aggressive exercising such as jogging, tennis, or high-impact aerobics should be avoided during a period of 1 to 3 weeks following treatment.
6. New spider veins may form, requiring subsequent treatment. Because we function and work in the erect position, there is extra pressure on the veins of the leg. Thus, there is a tendency for new spider veins to form. Even after the majority of your veins have been removed by sclerotherapy, be aware that *new spider veins can develop*. We ask all our patients to return for periodic re-evaluation so that any new veins can be injected before they become too large or too numerous.
7. Occasionally, immediately following injection, a new cluster of veins—a flare formation—may form in close proximity to the vein just injected. This has the appearance of a "blush" in the skin. (These can usually be controlled by repeat injection.)

protect the identity of the patient by assigning a code number to each patient. Prints are kept in the patient file and are periodically reviewed with the patient. This photographic record also allows the treating physician to objectively evaluate improvement as treatment progresses.

SCLEROTHERAPY (OPERATIVE) PERMIT

A signed permit is obtained, even though this is an office procedure. Written permission to photograph the patient is also included in a single consent to treatment form that covers both injection and photography (Fig. 1).

COMPRESSION STOCKINGS

Faria and Morales have noted that most spider telangiectasia are related to venous insufficiency and that there is direct communication between telangiectatic channels and the deep venous system.[3] Our observations have supported this finding. A leg that is not supported with a compression stocking after injection has a more rapid rate of recurrence of spider veins. Goldman and colleagues noted improvement in sclerotherapy results when compression was used.[4] The use of an adequate compression stocking is recommended[5] and in our experience has reduced recurrence by approximately 50%. Therefore, we maintain a full-time compression therapist on staff in our clinic, and we fit all patients for compression stockings at the time of preliminary evaluation.

If only below-knee injections are carried out, 30 to 40 mm Hg below-knee stockings can be used. If thigh injections are performed, a 20 to 30 mm Hg pantyhose is fitted. If large, bulging veins are injected, 4 or 6 inch Ace bandages are snugly applied to the leg, and the compression stocking is worn over the Ace bandages for the first 3 days.

The patient is required to wear the compression stocking for 3 days and 2 nights after treatment and is asked to avoid strenuous exercise. For the first 3 days, the injection sites are padded with gauze compression pads under the compression hose. After the first 3 days, the patient may take daily showers but must wear the support stocking during the day for 2 weeks, removing it only at night. When breast lesions are treated, they are compressed with elastic bandages overnight only.

On a long-term basis, we recommend that patients wear compression stockings for most of their standing activities. For women patients who are concerned about the appearance of compression stockings, several companies provide relatively sheer hose.

INDICATIONS FOR SCLEROTHERAPY

Vein Size

1. Small, bulging branch varicose veins, 3 to 6 mm
2. Dilated venules (reticular veins) 1 to 3 mm
3. Telangiectasia (spider veins), under 1 mm

Although controversial, many sclerotherapists inject larger veins. We believe that larger varicose veins should be surgically excised with quarter-inch phlebectomy

CONSENT TO TREATMENT

I have been informed by the doctor of the nature of injection treatment of varicose veins. I understand the possible side effects, which include recurrence, skin pigmentation, skin ulcers, and localized clotted veins.

I authorize the doctor to take photographs of me before and after treatment, and to permit such photographs to be used at the doctor's discretion for purposes of medical lecturing, research, or scientific publication, with the provision that I will not be identified.

FEES AND PAYMENT

Injections are billed individually at $_____ each. Most treatments will not exceed 20 injections per appointment.

Due to the costs of providing this treatment, payment is expected at the time this service is rendered.

A deposit of $100.00 is required no later than (10) days prior to your scheduled appointment. This deposit confirms your appointment time and will be credited to your balance on your treatment day. All future scheduled appointments will also require a deposit in advance.

The balance at the time of treatment will then be that which exceeds the $100.00 deposit.

For your convenience, we do accept payment by cash, check, Visa, or Mastercard.

I understand all terms as written above, and I authorize the doctor to administer such treatment to me.

_____
PATIENT'S SIGNATURE

_____
DATE

Due to the cost of providing these treatments, fees will be subject to change on an annual basis.

Figure 1 Form for consent to treatment, to be signed by patient before injection sclerotherapy.

---

incisions. The results are cosmetic, and the recurrence rate is low with operation. Large veins, when injected, often are complicated by skin pigmentation, which can be distressing to the patients.

Patient Symptoms

Weiss and Weiss have noted that most spider veins are symptomatic with numbness, paresthesia, aching and burning, or pain.[6] Injection of veins usually reduces or eliminates cutaneous symptoms, although the generalized aching of incompetent deep valves may persist.

CONTRAINDICATIONS TO SCLEROTHERAPY

The ongoing multicenter Food and Drug Administration trial on sotradecol/aethoxyscklerol has established excellent exclusion criteria for the study. A partial list of these exclusion criteria serves as a reference of relative and absolute contraindications to injection (Table 2).

Table 2 Contraindications to Sclerotherapy

Large varicose veins (above 6 mm in diameter) are best treated with operation because they are often in communication with a source of venous reflux
Pregnancy
Advanced age and sedentary lifestyle (older than 65 years of age)
Generalized systemic disease (cardiac, renal, hepatic, pulmonary, collagen diseases, and malignancies)
Advanced rheumatic disease, osteoarthritis, or any disease that interferes with patients' mobility
Arterial insufficiency of lower extremities
Bronchial asthma or demonstrated allergies
Acute superficial or deep thrombophlebitis
Acute febrile illness
Obesity
Patients on anticoagulants

INSTRUCTIONS FOR SCLEROTHERAPY

Occasionally, patients are injected on the day of preliminary evaluation. However, most are scheduled for a separate sclerotherapy appointment on another day. Instructions on what to do to prepare for injection are

Table 3 Preparation for Injection Treatment

On the day of your injections, bring your compression stockings.
Do not use bath oil or lotion on your legs the night before or the day of your injection treatment.
Dress in loose slacks, sweat pants, a dress, or skirt and comfortable, loose shoes to accommodate the dressing.
If possible, bring loose-fitting shorts to wear during the injection procedure.
Please call your insurance company if our office cannot advise you what your benefits are for this procedure.

---

given to the patients so they are adequately prepared for the injection procedure (Table 3).

SCLEROSANTS

A variety of solutions are available for injection.[7] Hypertonic saline is recommended because of the low risk of complications and generally excellent outcome.

INJECTION TECHNIQUE

1. Accuracy of intraluminal injection is enhanced by the use of 3-power loupes and a variable-intensity headlamp.
2. Patient lies flat in horizontal position on treatment table, either supine or prone, depending on location of venous lesion. A high-intensity light, preferably a headlamp, is an absolute necessity. Trendelenburg position and tourniquets are not necessary.
3. Legs are photographed and recorded in logbook. Photos may be in standing or horizontal position.
4. A copy of the initial venous mapping diagram is placed at the patient's bedside to allow accurate charting of all injections.
5. The leg area is prepped with aqueous Zephiran or similar colorless antiseptic solution. Infection after sclerotherapy is rare. One of the principal reasons for prepping the site is to render the skin more transparent so the veins are easier to see.
6. We use an injection solution of 23.4% saline (0.4 cc) plus 2% plain lidocaine (0.1 cc) mixed in a 1 cc tuberculin syringe. This solution is prepared in advance by injecting 2 cc of 2% plain lidocaine into a 30 cc multiple-dose vial of 23.4% saline. This dilutes the saline to 22%.
7. Each injection is limited to 0.5 cc of solution to minimize the risk of injectant traversing the communicating vein and reaching the deep venous system.
8. A 30 gauge needle is used to enter the vein. A 3-power ocular loupe facilitates accurate entry of the vein. Injection must be intraluminal.

Table 4 Instructions to Follow after Injection Treatment

Days 1-3: The stockings should remain in place for 3 days (including wearing them at night). The compression stockings are an important part of the treatment as they minimize the blood re-entering the injected vein. Elevate your legs as much as possible. Do no jogging or high-impact aerobics at this time. At the end of the 3 days, you may remove the stockings and discard the gauze pads. (You may find standing in the shower a convenient way to loosen the tape holding the gauze pads to avoid blistering sensitive skin.) Do not be surprised if injected areas appear bruised at this time; that is normal with many skin types.
Days 4-14: Continue to wear the compression stockings daily. Remove them at night to sleep. You may resume daily showers. Avoid jogging or high-impact aerobics during this time.
Day 15 on: Continue to wear the compression stockings whenever you can, as they reduce the rate of recurrence of spider varicose veins.

Perivenous injection leads to pigmentation and skin necrosis. We bend the needle to 30° to allow easier entry into the vein.
9. The injection should be made slowly. Watch the tip of the needle as the injection begins. The appearance of a small bubble suggesting extravasation means that individual injection should be terminated. If the physician stops the injection immediately when extravasation occurs, these small bubbles subside without leaving a blemish. It is not necessary—and may in fact be harmful—to attempt to dilute small extravasation bubbles.
10. Proper injection results in blanching along the course of the injected vein. Erythema around the injected vein appears immediately after injection and indicates that the saline solution has been injected correctly throughout the distribution of the vein.
11. After injection, withdraw the needle and apply a pressure pad of three 4 by 4 inch gauze squares folded once. Use paper tape to hold the gauze pad in place.
12. Our sessions average 15 injections, and the usual patient has three sessions. We have injected as many as 80 sites in a single session if the patient has constraints of travel distance or time.

IMMEDIATE POSTSCLEROTHERAPY PROCEDURES

During the course of the sclerotherapy treatment, the injection sites are compressed with gauze pressure pads secured with paper tape. The compression hose are applied before the patient is allowed to get off the treatment table. Thus, the patient's legs are not permitted in the dependent position until the compression stocking is in place. The office nurse, compression therapist, or a trained office assistant should put the stocking on the patients and instruct them in proper application and removal of the hose.

Patients are then given a list of instructions to follow for the first 2 weeks after treatment (Table 4).

COMPLICATIONS OF SCLEROTHERAPY

Although not a complication of sclerotherapy, patients view recurrence as a complication. Remember, this is a gravity-related disorder, and all varicose veins and spider veins tend to recur. Patients who are warned prior to injection are less concerned about recurrence and the need for repeat injections.

Pigmentation develops in 3% to 5% of patients. It usually disappears in a few months but may last as long as a year.

Telangiectatic matting or flare formation occurs in 1% to 3% of patients. These small venous blush formations near the site of injection are very distressing to patients. They can effectively be eliminated by subsequent injection of dominant veins within the blush formation.

Ulceration is very rare, occurring in 40 of 77,624 injections (1 per 1,900 injections). After hypertonic saline injection, these are usually small, full-thickness ulcers under 1 cm in diameter. They all heal in 1 to 3 months with minimal scarring. With some undiluted sclerosants, ulcers may be much larger.

Superficial phlebitis occasionally develops in veins adjacent to the injection site. In our series DVT has occurred in only two patients. Both were treated with anticoagulants and hospitalized; they experienced no long-term sequelae. If the patient experiences unusual pain, fullness, or edema in the first few weeks after injection, noninvasive studies to diagnose DVT should be performed.

REFERENCES

1. Hobbs JT. The treatment of varicose veins: A random trial of injection compression therapy versus surgery. Br J Surg 1968; 55:777.
2. Pfeifer JR, Hawtof GD. Injection sclerotherapy and CO_2 laser sclerotherapy in the ablation of cutaneous spider veins of the lower extremity. Phlebology 1989; 4:231–240.
3. Faria JL, Morales IN. Histopathology of the telangiectasia associated with varicose veins. Dermatologica 1963; 127:321–329.
4. Goldman MP, Beaudoing D, Marley W, et al. Compression in the treatment of leg telangiectasia: A preliminary report. J Dermatol Surg Oncol 1990; 16:4.
5. Fegan WG. Continuous compression technique of injecting varicose veins. Lancet 1963; 2:109.
6. Weiss RA, Weiss MA. Resolution of pain associated with varicose and telangiectatic leg veins after compression sclerotherapy. J Dermatol Surg Oncol 1990; 16:333–336.
7. Goldman, Ml P. Sclerotherapy. St Louis: Mosby–Year book, 1991.

EXCISION OF VARICOSE VEINS

JOSEPH P. ELLIOTT Jr., M.D.

Patients have struggled with the disfiguring, discomforting, and, at times, disabling affliction of varicose veins of the lower extremities since ancient times. A large percentage of adults (more females than males) have varying degrees of this problem. Methods of management include external support, ligation, sclerotherapy, and removal. The principles of treatment by excision were elucidated in the 1950s. Modifications, including the use of very small incisions for subcutaneous removal of clusters of varicosities along with the superficial ends of perforating veins, as well as the use of limited stripping, have resulted in a modern surgical approach that accomplishes very acceptable cosmetic results without sacrificing physiologic goals.

ANATOMY AND PHYSIOLOGY OF LOWER LIMB VEINS

Surgical treatment of varicose veins is based on a thorough knowledge of anatomy and physiology. Veins of the lower extremities consist of two systems: the deep and the superficial (Fig. 1). The deep veins follow named arteries deep to the deep fascia, and the superficial system lies between the skin and deep fascia. The two

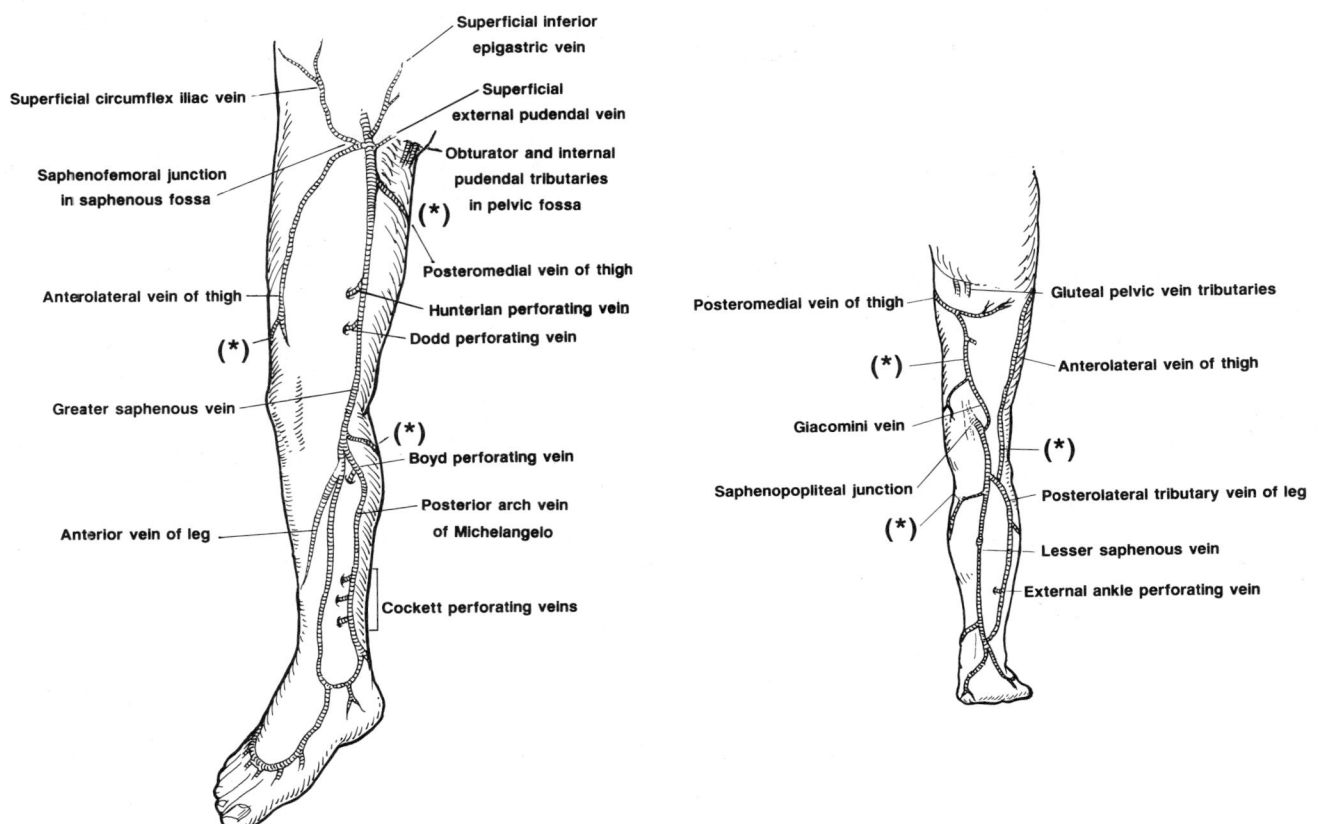

Figure 1 *A,* Anteromedial view of lower limb superficial veins with greater saphenous vein, saphenofemoral junction, greater saphenous tributaries, perforating veins, and veins communicating with lesser saphenous vein (*). (From Dodd H, Cockett FB. The pathology and surgery of the veins of the lower limb. Edinburgh: Churchill Livingstone, 1976:1–55; with permission.) *B,* Posterior view lower limb superficial veins with lesser saphenous vein, saphenopopliteal junction (at variable level), lesser saphenous tributaries, perforating veins, and veins communicating with greater saphenous vein (*). (From Bergan JJ. Common anatomic patterns of varicose veins. In: Bergan JJ, Goldman MP, eds. Varicose veins and telangiectasias: diagnosis and treatment. St Louis: Quality Medical, 1993:58–83; with permission.)

systems are connected by the saphenofemoral juncture, saphenopopliteal juncture, and the perforating veins.

The superficial system consists of the greater and lesser saphenous trunks and their tributaries (Fig. 1). The tributaries include veins that communicate between the greater and lesser systems. The posteromedial superficial thigh vein connecting with the vein of Giacomini is an important example of such a communicating vein. There are perforating veins traversing the deep fascia that separates the superficial and deep systems. Thin, translucent venous valves of low mass are located in the deep, superficial, and perforating veins. They are distributed more frequently in the caudal areas, where resting pressures are greater. Competent valves allow blood to flow only toward the heart and from the superficial to the deep veins via the perforators and the two superficial-deep junctions. In the erect human, these valves are subject to resting static venous pressures of up to 100 mm Hg. This venous pressure is greatly reduced in the foot after several steps because of calf muscle compression of the deep veins. Consequently, the calf muscles, deep veins, and valves combine to form the calf pump. The greater saphenous vein courses between the superficial membranous fascia and the inelastic deep fascia.

Below the knee, the greater saphenous vein receives the posterior arch vein of Michelangelo, as well as the anterior vein of the leg. These tributaries can be the origin of the Boyd perforator, which extends to the popliteal veins below the knee. The three Cockett perforating veins originate from the posterior arch vein above the ankle medially and enter the posterior tibial vein. Near the groin the saphenous vein receives variable combinations of five superficial vein tributaries, including the superficial circumflex iliac, the anterolateral thigh tributary, the posteromedial thigh tributary, the superficial external pudendal vein, and the superficial inferior epigastric vein. Unlike other perforators, the Dodd perforating vein above the knee and the Hunterian perforating vein in mid-thigh originate directly from the greater saphenous vein. Of the long saphenous veins, 90% have one or more perforators originating in the thigh. There are also potential interconnections with the gonadal vein through the pelvic veins via the internal obturator veins, the internal pudendal veins, and gluteal vein tributaries. Incompetent valves in these veins allow leaking into varicosities in the vulva, as well as the areas medial to the adductor muscles and inferior to the gluteal muscles. In the lower thigh, the saphenous nerve becomes superficial to accompany the greater saphenous vein to the foot.

The lesser saphenous vein starts at the lateral end of the dorsal venous arch of the foot, passes behind the lateral malleolus, and ascends in the midline of the calf. The lesser saphenous vein penetrates the deep fascia along its course and joins the deep system at or above the popliteal vein. The deep location of the proximal portion of the lesser saphenous vein along with the proximity of the sural, medial, and lateral popliteal nerves requires caution during surgical approach.

The lesser saphenous vein may communicate with the greater system in several ways. The lesser saphenous vein may have a posterolateral tributary vein. Superiorly, this lateral tributary may communicate with an anterolateral thigh vein. Frequently, the vein of Giacomini, a tributary of the lesser saphenous vein, becomes superficial to communicate medially high in the thigh with the greater saphenous vein via its posteromedial tributary. Also, the medial arch vein of the leg often communicates with the lesser saphenous vein. Unlike the main, thick-walled saphenous trunk, its thin-walled tributaries lie superficial to the membranous fascia. Thus, they are subject to dilatation sooner than the main saphenous vein. Frequently, the clusters of dilated tributary veins are situated over the external ends of perforating veins.

The two major saphenous veins are variable in size and location. Each segment can be duplicated, looped, branched, or absent. Also, their tributaries, as well as the perforating veins, vary in location, number, and size.

CLINICAL FINDINGS

Patients with primary varicosities complain of heaviness, aching, burning, fatigue, throbbing, or pain that may be relieved by walking, leg elevation, or external compression. Edema develops by evening but is resolved by morning. Delay in treatment can result in discoloration of the skin of the lower leg, dermatitis, cellulitis, ulceration, thrombosis within the varices, or hemorrhage through attenuated skin. Patients with postphlebitic syndrome or deep vein obstruction may have the same problems to a greater degree. In addition, these patients may develop venous claudication if venous hypertension is increased by walking or external compression.

In order to determine the anatomic distribution of varicosities, the veins of the lower limb are inspected in the recumbent and standing positions. The location of incompetent valves can be detected by first draining the blood from the elevated limb. Then rubber tourniquets or areas of finger pressure are applied at the level of the groin, above and below the knee, and at other levels as needed before having the patient stand. One then observes the effect of the location of the tourniquets and their release with the patient in the erect position.

The use of continuous wave Doppler or duplex examination defines further the extent of the pathology. Duplex examination can also confirm suspected deep vein obstruction. We have used light reflective rheography (LRR), an easy and rapid test, to separate gross valvular incompetence of the superficial versus the deep systems.[1]

In evaluating a patient with varicosities, coexisting problems that may mimic the symptoms of varicosities or affect the choice of treatment should be considered. It is important to exclude musculoskeletal and neurologic problems, arterial occlusive diseases, traumatic arteriovenous fistulas, or congenital arteriovenous malformations. In addition, severe venous obstruction, changes due to illicit drug abuse, malnutrition, cellulitis, and congestive heart failure must also be excluded. Selective use of roentgenograms, computed tomography, magnetic resonance imaging, ankle blood pressure indices, and arteriography, as well as Doppler and duplex evaluation, may be helpful.

The surgeon should also be alert for patients who have recently adopted a healthy lifestyle. Their new exercise regimen may cause musculoskeletal symptoms. Their use of nicotine patches in order to stop smoking can be a severe risk for anesthesia. In addition, patients on a strict weight reduction program may have unrealistic expectations concerning the treatment of their newly exposed varicosities.

TREATMENT ALTERNATIVES

Patients present with a wide variety of varicose veins and treatment expectations. Some need only reassurance and mild gradient pressure support stockings. Others need or desire definitive treatment. Many patients require extensive education about the pathophysiology of varicosities before they can make an informed choice about treatment. Before embarking on interventional treatment, patients need careful evaluation of their expectations and their general state of health. Their age, cardiopulmonary and renal status, or a history suggestive of coagulopathy or hypercoagulable state may limit alternatives or require investigation. For instance, evidence of arterial occlusive disease or atherosclerotic heart disease cautions against the sacrifice of a relatively normal saphenous vein that is potentially useful for a reconstructive arterial operation, even though the vein is incompetent.

The surgical treatment of uncomplicated varicose veins is rarely urgent, and well-fitted elastic gradient support stockings can be used effectively for prolonged periods. Patients may use waist-high leotards or knee-high stockings, depending on the distribution of the varicosities. Their use is recommended as an alternative until an operation is desired or until the patient's preoperative condition is optimized. Postoperatively, they are recommended to minimize recurrence of varicosities.

Varicose veins can be definitively managed by surgical methods alone, by operation in combination with sclerotherapy, or by sclerotherapy alone. In general, the excision of varicose veins has several advantages over sclerotherapy: (1) It avoids the risk of recanalization and recurrent symptoms from the same veins; (2) it allows precise removal of the tributaries that are potential collateral vessels, especially those close to the saphenofemoral junctions; and (3) it allows flush ligation of the greater saphenous vein just at the saphenofemoral junction without the risk of narrowing the common femoral vein or extension of thrombus caused by sclerosants into the common femoral vein. Objective reviews suggest that the long-term results of surgical treatment are significantly better (90%) than combined ligation and sclerotherapy (65%), whereas combined therapy had significantly better results than sclerotherapy alone (37%).[2,3] Therefore, for major varicosities, excision is recommended, especially if the saphenous veins are incompetent. However, excision is not suitable for the treatment of very small or superficial telangiectatic veins or for patients who are at high risk for anesthesia.

PREOPERATIVE MANAGEMENT

In the outpatient surgery area, while the patient is standing and before preoperative medication is administered, two important activities occur. First, the varicose veins are clearly outlined with an indelible, felt-tipped marking pen, with the patient and surgeon agreeing on the areas to be treated. Second, the anesthesiologist again reviews the anesthetic choices.

After induction of anesthesia, the patient is positioned depending upon the distribution of the varicose veins. The limb is prepared in a sterile field; the outlines of the varicose veins on the skin are carefully preserved. The table is then placed in a Trendelenburg position, or the limb can be elevated on a rack to empty the superficial veins. This maneuver minimizes bleeding and helps to maintain a clear surgical field to allow precise technique.

TECHNIQUE OF EXCISION OF VARICOSE VEINS

In recent years the treatment goals have been to remove all varicosities, to interrupt perforators, and to limit or delay recurrences. These goals have been accomplished while achieving an excellent cosmetic result by the judicious use of flush ligation, limited axial stripping of saphenous vein trunks, and extensive stab avulsion of varicose vein clusters. The technical aspects of surgical removal are considered under several anatomic locations: (1) flush ligation of the greater saphenous vein, (2) stripping of the greater saphenous vein while interrupting the perforating veins in the thigh, (3) stab avulsion of clusters of varicose veins and interruption of perforating veins of the leg, (4) removal of the lesser saphenous veins, and (5) management of pelvic leak.

Flush Ligation of the Long Saphenous Vein

If ligation of the saphenofemoral junction is elected, the junction can be located medial to the femoral arterial pulsation. The incision can be made obliquely or transversely, in or above the inguinal crease. The length of the incision depends on the amount of subcutaneous fat but should be adequate to allow clear visualization of the venous structures. The five tributaries of the greater saphenous vein should be carefully ligated and then gently mobilized to allow ligation and division of secondary tributaries as well, in order to forestall the development of varicosities in and through collateral veins. The tensile strength of the saphenous vein allows it to be skeletonized and controlled for 5 cm. The saphenous vein should be ligated under direct visualization flush with, but avoiding, narrowing of the common femoral vein.

Stripping of the Greater Saphenous Veins and Interruption of Perforating Veins of the Thigh

If the valves of the greater saphenous vein are incompetent and the vein itself is dilated and tortuous, there is clear indication for its removal. If the greater saphenous vein appears relatively normal in spite of documented incompetent valves, an argument can be made for its preservation, especially if it seems to be diminutive and, therefore, technically unsuitable for use of an intraluminal stripper.

In order to strip the greater saphenous vein, the intraluminal stripper is inserted into the greater saphenous vein, which is exposed in the groin incision. If the incompetent valves allow, the stripper is passed distally (Fig. 2). If necessary, the stripper is passed proximally, starting at a small incision over the greater saphenous vein either above or below the knee. The rounded acorn head of the stripper should be continually palpated while it courses through the vein to avoid injury of the deep structures by inadvertent passage of the stripper into a perforating vein. Once the distal greater saphenous vein is divided and ligated, the saphenous vein can be stripped with slow, steady traction on the stripper in a distal direction. To avoid making an offensively large, distal incision to accommodate the stripper head and the accordion-like mass of vein, the vein actually is removed in a proximal direction. A heavy, long suture tied to the saphenous vein and the head of the stripper assists with removal of the vein through the tunnel created by the stripping. Hemostasis throughout the procedure is maintained, using pressure on a folded towel over the wounds. Unless the greater saphenous vein below the knee is grossly abnormal, it is preserved. This restraint

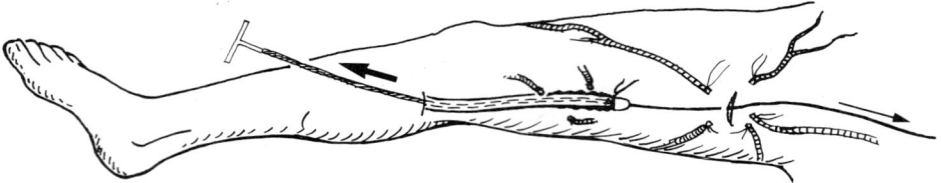

Figure 2 Stripping of greater saphenous vein between saphenofemoral junction and location above or below the knee. Rope silk used to withdraw stripper and mass of vein through larger groin incision.

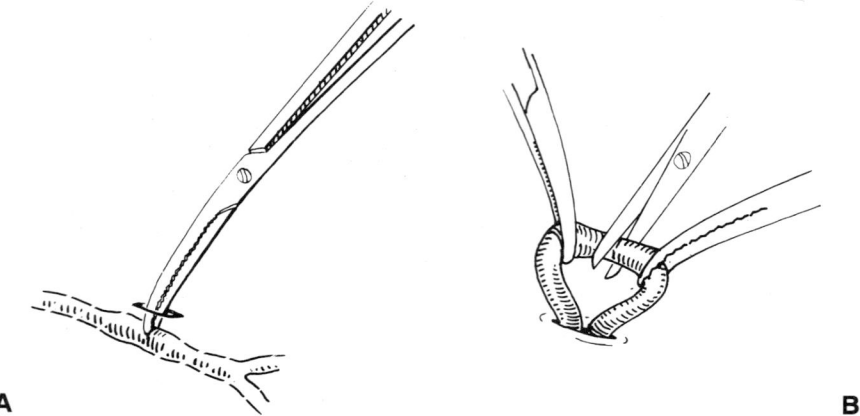

Figure 3 Stab avulsion of varicosity under the incision. *A*, Hemostat used to gently spread small incision and coax vein to surface. *B*, Varicose vein skeletonized and divided for maximum proximal and distal avulsion.

minimizes the chance of injuring the saphenous nerve. The several veins that perforate the deep fascia in the thigh and enter the deep system in the thigh originate directly from the greater saphenous vein. These perforators are interrupted in the process of stripping the greater saphenous vein from the level of the groin to just above or below the knee.

If there are large groups or clusters of varicosities in the tributaries of the leg or thigh veins, it may be advisable to delay actual clamping, division, and stripping of the greater saphenous vein until after the clusters have been removed because clamping often increases the venous pressure in the clusters.

Stab Avulsion of Clusters of Varicose Veins and Interruption of Perforating Veins of the Leg

Perforating veins in the legs do not originate directly from the saphenous veins; instead, they derive from tributaries, often the posterior arcuate vein of Michelangelo. It is not advisable to make prolonged searches through extensive incisions to ligate incompetent perforating veins. It is preferable to remove all of the detectable clusters of varicosities by the stab avulsion method. A secondary effect of extensive stab avulsion is to avulse the outer ends of the incompetent perforators and, therefore, to interrupt them. Thus, the clusters and the pathologic changes due to venous hypertension are eliminated at the same time. The clusters are removed by using the ink marks on the skin as guides. Multiple small incisions a few millimeters long are made over the clusters of varicose veins so that they can be removed by avulsion without ligation. Gentle spreading of the skin with a small hemostat temporarily increases the size of the wound. Occasionally, in large men with long-standing varicosities, the bulk of the vein requires a slightly larger incision. If a varicose vein is directly under the incision, it or the surrounding fibrous tissue can be grasped with a hemostat and the vein coaxed to the surface, where it is clamped and divided (Fig. 3). Mobility of the vein is increased by separating it entirely from surrounding subcutaneous tissues. By teasing the vein, rolling it on a hemostat, and gently pulling it in various directions while using digital skin retraction, the surgeon can often avulse long segments of vein through one small incision. However, the size and strength of the vein, as well as the degree of surrounding inflammation, determine the ease with which the vein can be removed and, therefore, the number of incisions required. As an alternative, veins near but not directly under the incision can be hooked with special instruments passed under the skin for 1 or 2 inches. By trapping the vein against the skin, it can be drawn into the wound (Fig. 4). Additional small incisions are made as needed, and the procedure is repeated until a maximum effort has been made to remove all of the marked varicosities. Several hooks ingeniously designed

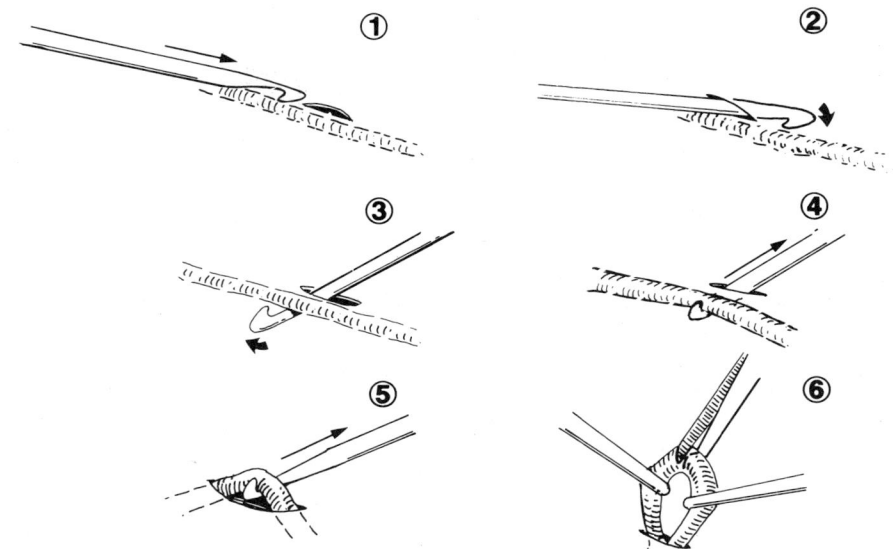

Figure 4 Stab avulsion of varicosity near incision. Hook used to turn under vein and capture it against the skin to coax it through the small incision (1–5); varicose vein skeletonized and divided for maximum proximal and distal avulsion (6).

specifically for vein avulsion are available commercially. In addition, various sizes of inexpensive crochet hooks are also very helpful.

Removal of the Lesser Saphenous Vein

Varicosities of the lesser saphenous veins are relatively infrequent, and they can be excised or stripped in a manner similar to that used for the greater saphenous vein. However, the distal end of the lesser saphenous vein is found posterior to the lateral malleolus; therefore, it must be carefully separated from the sural nerve. A distinguishing feature of the lesser saphenous vein is that it can dip below the deep fascia anywhere along its course toward the popliteal fossa. In addition, it may extend high in the thigh in the subcutaneous tissue and perforate to anastomose with the deep venous system at any level in the back of the thigh. If it is not obvious from observation and palpation, it is helpful to locate the termination of the lesser saphenous vein by duplex scanning.

The transverse popliteal incision used for flush ligation of the lesser saphenous vein should be adequate to allow close inspection of the popliteal veins, nerves, and geniculate tributaries, if necessary.

The patient should be warned about larger incisions in the groin, the popliteal spaces, and possibly in the mid-thigh. These larger incisions may be necessary to ligate large tributaries or to remove stripped vein.

Management of Pelvic Leak

This infrequent problem usually can be handled by excising the varicose vein on the medial and posterior aspects of the upper thigh. Rarely is it necessary to perform gonadal or pelvic phlebography or laparoscopy and ligation of intrapelvic gonadal veins.

Cosmetic Considerations

Frequently, cosmetic considerations are part of patients' motivation for having varicose veins removed. Therefore, details of surgical technique assume added importance. For example, should a large tributary or perforator vein need ligation, the ligature must be tied cleanly without dimpling the skin. In addition, closure of the wounds deserves careful attention. Subcutaneous and subcuticular closure of the wounds with absorbable sutures is desirable, but usually only groin or popliteal incisions are long enough or deep enough to allow the use of sutures. The remaining incisions are closed by meticulous use of short segments of paper adhesive strips applied parallel to the direction of the incision. If long strips are applied perpendicular to the incision, swelling and consequent increased tension on the skin can cause blisters to develop as the epidermal tissues slip. These blisters can cause blemishes that are more noticeable than the scars from the incisions. Also, removal of subcutaneous tissue should be minimized in order to avoid dimpling.

POSTOPERATIVE MANAGEMENT

Immediately after wound closure, gauze pads are placed on the wounds and secured with a layer of soft, pliable gauze bandage. Then, mild to moderate pressure is applied with an elastic bandage. Following anesthetic recovery, the patient may go home the same day with help. The limb is elevated above heart level to avoid swelling and minimize ecchymosis. The patient should be encouraged to walk increasing amounts starting with at least 5 minutes an hour for the first several days. On the third day the wounds are inspected, and on the tenth postoperative day the adhesive strips are removed. Sunscreen is advised until scars have matured.

COMPLICATIONS

Care in passing subcutaneous hooks and knowledge of the course of the saphenous nerve help to minimize the incidence of postoperative cutaneous anesthesia or dysesthesia. The frequency of this problem, as well as of hematoma, hemorrhage, infection, and deep phlebitis, is surprisingly low. We have had several episodes of troublesome thrombosis extending proximally in an interrupted but unresected greater saphenous vein. Treatment consisted of either systemic heparinization or a second operation to perform flush ligation and to excise remaining involved segment.

REFERENCES

1. Shepard AD, Mackey WC, O'Donnell TF Jr, et al. Light reflection rheography (LRR): A new noninvasive test of venous function. Bruit 1984; 8:266–270.
2. Jakobsen BH. The value of different forms of treatment for varicose veins. Br J Surg 1979; 66:182–184.
3. Hobbs JT. Surgery and sclerotherapy in the treatment of varicose veins. Arch Surg 1974; 109:793–796.

SURGICAL TREATMENT OF ACUTE SAPHENOUS AND DEEP FEMORAL VENOUS THROMBOSIS

ROBERT L. KISTNER, M.D.
BO EKLÖF, M.D., Ph.D.

Surgical treatment of acute venous thrombosis in the saphenous and femoropopliteal venous segments has a limited but important role. Considerations for the superficial and deep veins are quite different and are discussed separately.

ACUTE SUPERFICIAL VENOUS THROMBOSIS

The symptoms of saphenous thrombophlebitis are pain, swelling, and redness due to the inflammatory reaction. These are managed with anti-inflammatory medications and supportive therapy on an ambulatory basis with or without elastic support when the phlebitis is limited to the calf. When the pain and swelling are more dramatic, patients may require bed rest and elevation of the extremity. Because the process is inflammatory and not infectious, antibiotics are not indicated.

The important surgical consideration in saphenous thrombophlebitis is its potential for extension through the saphenofemoral junction into the common femoral vein with potential occlusion of the common femoral vein leading to iliofemoral thrombophlebitis with all of its sequelae, including pulmonary embolism (PE). This can also occur at the saphenopopliteal junction. This dangerous complication of saphenous thrombophlebitis can be prevented by awareness of its occurrence and careful diagnosis of the proximal extent of any saphenous thrombosis above the lower third of the thigh. In order to prevent this problem, saphenous thrombosis in the thigh should always be studied by duplex scan or, if this is not available, phlebography to be certain that the thrombosis that clinically extends into the lower thigh does not have a silent extension up through the saphenofemoral junction and into the common femoral vein.[1,2] If clinical examination alone is used to manage superficial thrombophlebitis, surgical interruption of the saphenofemoral junction should be done whenever the thrombosis ascends higher than the lower third of the thigh because the silent extension of the clot frequently is higher than the clinical symptoms suggest. In these patients clinical examination, including Doppler interrogation, may miss a thrombus extending into the common femoral vein.

It has been shown that 12% to 30% of patients with saphenous thrombophlebitis have accompanying deep vein involvement, usually in the same extremity and less frequently in the opposite extremity.[1-4] This reflects the tendency for thrombophlebitis to be of multicentric, concurrent origin. Not infrequently, the saphenous thrombosis is symptomatic while the deep vein thrombosis (DVT) is asymptomatic. In these patients, the saphenous thrombophlebitis can be thought of as a marker for the presence of silent DVT. Involvement of the deep system can occur by extension of the thrombus through the perforating veins into the tibial veins or by entirely separate multicentric origin of the thrombotic process in the deep and superficial veins.[1] Because of the multicentric origin with involvement of the deep veins, it is good practice that every patient with established saphenous thrombophlebitis have duplex scan of the deep veins in the involved extremity and, ideally, in both lower extremities. When the deep system is involved along with the saphenous system, the management changes from ambulant outpatient treatment to inpatient anticoagulation.

Since airplane travel is conducive to extension of an established thrombophlebitis and may represent a significant threat to the individual,[2] the patient with possible thrombophlebitis who intends to travel in the immediate future should undergo duplex scan of the involved extremity and, ideally, of both extremities before air travel. When thrombophlebitis of the saphenous system is found in an individual who must continue with air travel, the least that should be done is surgical interruption of the greater saphenous vein at the saphenofemoral junction prior to air travel, and anticoagulants should be considered for protection during travel.

The surgical treatment of greater saphenous thrombophlebitis is proximal ligation of the saphenous vein at the saphenofemoral junction, which may be accompanied by stripping of the saphenous vein as in a conventional high ligation and stripping procedure (Table 1). High ligation alone prevents the thrombotic process from extending into the deep veins as a DVT and leads to resolution of the inflammatory process in most patients. Because the superficial saphenous thrombophlebitis is an inflammatory process, one need not be concerned about infection and may complete the conventional vein stripping operation with the expectation of normal wound healing. These patients undergo a rapid resolution of the inflammatory process with a favorable postoperative course.

When thrombophlebitis is found at the time of ligation to have extended into the common femoral vein (CFV), a definitive procedure must be performed to remove all clot from the CFV itself. This is usually accomplished by simply withdrawing the clot from the CFV through the saphenofemoral junction at the time of proximal ligation. However, when there is more extensive involvement of the CFV, a formal iliofemoral venous thrombectomy should be performed. This requires exposure of the CFV with proximal and distal control and a venotomy extending into the CFV to be certain that all of the clot was removed from the CFV.

Table 1 Surgical Procedures in Acute Superficial and Deep Venous Thrombosis

Ligation of greater or lesser saphenous vein to prevent extension of DVT into deep veins with or without stripping of greater saphenous vein
Ligation of saphenous vein prior to airplane travel
Thrombectomy of common femoral vein with or without ligation of superficial femoral vein
Ligation of superficial femoral vein
   To control embolism from distal veins
   To prevent post-thrombotic reflux in superficial femoral-popliteal veins

ACUTE THROMBOPHLEBITIS OF THE FEMOROPOPLITEAL VEINS

The conventional and most appropriate treatment for acute DVT of the femoropopliteal veins is anticoagulation with heparin sodium, followed by conversion to sodium warfarin and continuation of the warfarin therapy for a minimum of 3 months. Because PE is well controlled with heparin sodium anticoagulation, surgical treatment is not indicated to decrease PE. The same, however, cannot be said for subsequent chronic venous insufficiency, which remains a significant late complication of acute DVT in the femoropopliteal segment.

The natural history of late sequelae following femoropopliteal thrombophlebitis remains undefined because diagnosis and follow-up of acute DVT have primarily been by noninvasive laboratory tests and clinical examination rather than objective definitive testing by phlebography or duplex scanning. Duplex scanning is available in almost all institutions and should be the minimum standard for diagnosing thrombophlebitis of the deep veins and outlining the specific segments involved.

Prior to the use of anticoagulants, the incidence of severe post-thrombotic sequelae could be expected to be 80% to 100% after an episode of extensive DVT.[5] The incidence of sequelae fell to 15% to 25% after the widespread introduction of heparin sodium therapy.[5] By duplex scan, it has been documented that much of the original thrombus is lysed during the first 3 months after thrombophlebitis,[6] and up to half of the patients have incompetent recanalized segments while the other half have patent vein segments without incompetence. Whether this is due to the retention of competent valves or to some other post-thrombotic blood flow mechanism has not been determined.

It is now well established that most of the post-thrombotic sequelae in the lower extremity are due to venous reflux rather than obstruction. The challenge is to discover ways to control the degree of reflux in the post-thrombotic patient, whether by ligation and interruption of involved venous segments, by lytic therapy to preserve valvular function, or by thrombectomy of the femoropopliteal veins. Before any of these treatments can be adopted, more complete knowledge about the natural course of events following DVT is necessary.

There are two potential areas where operative treatment of the deep veins may be used. One is the occurrence of PE where the source of embolism is below the inguinal ligament. In this instance, the potential for PE can be controlled by ligation of the superficial femoral vein (SFV). In some instances, this can be an alternative to the placement of an inferior vena cava filter. It has been found that patients who have competent profunda femoris veins (PFV), or patent and competent greater saphenous veins (GSV) have very few sequelae after ligation of the SFV.[7] The basic requirements for ligation of the SFV to prevent further PE are that the source of emboli is localized to a point distal to the ligation by duplex scan or phlebography and that the patient does not have huge collaterals between the popliteal vein and the PFV through which emboli could pass. When these conditions are met, we have found that the SFV can be ligated using local anesthesia and that this provides effective prevention of subsequent PE.

Another indication for operation in the femoropopliteal segment is during thrombectomy for iliofemoral DVT. The conventional operative method of treating iliofemoral DVT is to perform a transverse venotomy in the CFV and to aspirate clots proximally and distally until the segments are as clean as they can be made. The purpose of operation above the common femoral segment is to retain a patent iliofemoral vein and a patent inferior vena cava. Below the common femoral segment, the purpose is to prevent post-thrombotic reflux. When a catheter, such as a Fogarty catheter, is passed distally against the normal valves of the lower extremity, the possibility of injuring these valves is significant. Perhaps a more important threat to the valves is the presence of clot in the superficial femoral and popliteal venous segments with subsequent scarring of the valves that would render them incompetent after endogenous lysis of the thrombus. The late result in either case is a patent but incompetent superficial femoral-popliteal segment that sets the stage for the post-thrombotic syndrome due to late reflux.

To prevent postoperative reflux, a series of patients were operated upon by iliofemoral venous thrombectomy utilizing an approach designed to prevent post-thrombotic reflux in the SFV segment.[8] In this study, the common femoral vein was dissected in its entirety to gain control of each branch from the GSV proximally to the SFV and PFV distally. The vein was opened by a longitudinal venotomy, the clot removed from the CFV, and each branch of the CFV separately inspected (Fig. 1). Local thrombectomy of each branch was done with a balloon catheter, taking care to preserve valves as much as possible. Massage of the tissue was used to express deep clots. In some patients, the clot layers across the orifice of the branch and is readily removed, leaving a patent branch with intact valves. This is often the case in the PFV. If the SFV is involved with extensive clot that is not readily removed by gentle catheter and forceful massage, including an Esmarch bandage, the SFV is ligated and divided rather than left in continuity with the CFV. The purpose of this ligation is to minimize late axial reflux in the SFV-popliteal segment. This approach to iliofemoral venous thrombectomy was utilized in a series of 72 patients reported in 1979.[8] These patients were followed carefully postoperatively, and 11 were analyzed for late sequelae in a recent report of long-term 15 year sequelae of SFV interruption.[7] Late sequelae are minimal after this management, even though some element of physiologic obstruction may be demonstrable. The extremity appears to tolerate partial obstruction better than extensive reflux over the long term.

The ideal treatment for acute DVT limited to the femoral and popliteal veins remains to be proven. The minimal accepted treatment is heparin sodium for 5 to

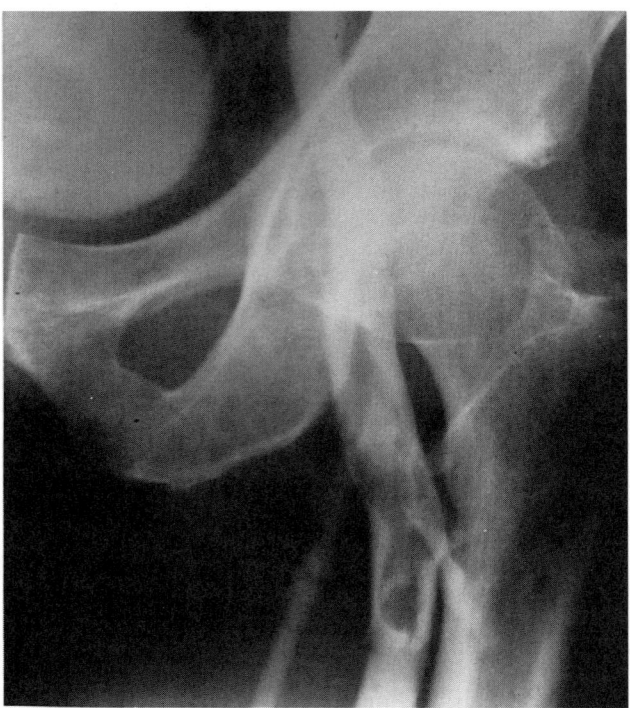

Figure 1 Common femoral vein thrombosis that is ideal for thrombectomy. This thrombus extended out of profunda femoris vein after hip reconstruction. It is similar to thrombosis from greater saphenous vein.

7 days, followed by sodium warfarin for 3 months. This provides 97% protection against subsequent pulmonary embolism but only 65% to 85% protection against late significant chronic venous insufficiency and ulceration. The natural history of the femoral-popliteal-tibial segments after DVT is still under scrutiny and needs to be determined to provide a baseline for comparison for other studies.

Surgical thrombectomy has been used in the SFV segment as part of the treatment of iliofemoral DVT but not as a stand-alone treatment of SFV-popliteal DVT. It is conceivable that there is a role for thrombectomy in DVT below the CFV level. It is more conceivable that surgical ligation of the completely thrombosed SFV will prevent late recanalization with reflux and subsequent chronic venous insufficiency in the leg. Evidence to support this concept is contained in the previously mentioned long-term 15 year study following SFV ligation, that documented minimal late clinical sequelae when the PFV or GSV was patent and competent.

REFERENCES

1. Lutter KS, Kerr TM, Roedersheimer R, et al. Superficial thrombophlebitis diagnosed by duplex scanning. Surgery 1991; 110:42–46.
2. Kistner RL, Ball JJ, Nordyke RA, Freeman GC. Incidence of pulmonary embolism in the course of thrombophlebitis of the lower extremities. Am J Surg 1972; 124:169–176.

3. Plate G, Eklof B, Jensen R, Ohlin P. Deep venous thrombosis, pulmonary embolism and acute surgery in thrombophlebitis of the long saphenous vein. Acta Chir Scand 1985; 151:241–244.
4. Skillman JJ, Kent KC, Porter DH, Kim D. Simultaneous occurrence of superficial and deep thrombophlebitis in the lower extremity. J Vasc Surg 1990; 11:818–824.
5. Bauer G. A roentgenological and clinical study of the sequels of thrombosis. Acta Chir Scand 1942; 86 (suppl 74):1–101.
6. Markel A, Manzo RA, Bergelin RO, Strandness DE Jr. Valvular reflux following deep vein thrombosis: Incidence and time of occurrence. J Vasc Surg 1992; 15:377–384.
7. Masuda EM, Kistner RL, Ferris EB. Long-term effects of superficial femoral vein ligation: Thirteen-year follow-up. J Vasc Surg 1992; 16:741–749.
8. Kistner RL, Sparkuhl MD. Surgery in acute and chronic venous disease. Surgery 1979; 85:31–43.

DEEP VENOUS THROMBOSIS IN PREGNANCY

ALI F. ABURAHMA, M.D.

Deep venous thrombosis (DVT) of the lower extremities is an infrequent complication of pregnancy. If proper treatment is not instituted, however, significant morbidity or mortality can occur in both the patient and the fetus.

INCIDENCE

The incidence of antepartum DVT has been reported to be no greater than 0.36% of deliveries.[1] Acute iliofemoral venous thrombosis is six times more frequent in pregnant women than in nonpregnant women.[1] Deep venous thrombosis is 3 to 5 times more common postpartum than antepartum, and 3 to 16 times more common in women delivered by cesarean section than in those delivered vaginally. Approximately 1 in 2,000 pregnancies is complicated by a pulmonary embolus (PE), which remains an important cause of maternal mortality, second only to abortion. Of particular importance is that PE occurs in 15% to 24% of patients with untreated DVT, resulting in a 12% to 15% mortality rate. With appropriate therapy, the incidence of PE declines to 4.5% with an overall mortality rate of 0.7%.

PATHOPHYSIOLOGY

Virchow's triad of vessel wall injury, stasis, and hypercoagulability remains the basis of venous thrombosis. Each element of Virchow's triad is present at some time during pregnancy. An increase in venous capacitance produces stasis. In the early part of the second trimester, the femoral venous pressure rises and continues to do so until term, when it falls rapidly after delivery. This increase in venous pressure appears to be secondary to mechanical venous obstruction. In general, there is no firm evidence that vascular injury plays a role in causing venous thrombosis in pregnancy; however, significant vascular damage can occur at delivery. Pregnancy has been described as an acquired hypercoaguable state. Factor I, V, VII, VIII, IX, X, and XII levels increase during pregnancy. Fibrinogen undergoes the most marked increase, with the total circulating amount almost doubling in preparation for the formation of a hemostatic endometrial fibrin mesh upon placental separation. In addition, plasma fibrinolytic activity is decreased, perhaps secondary to an increase in fibrinolysis inhibitors that may return to normal within an hour of delivery of the placenta. This change is most marked at term and immediate puerperium and helps to control blood loss after placental separation. A deficiency of antithrombin III, protein C, and protein S has also been implicated.[2]

DIAGNOSIS

The most common symptoms and signs are pain, tenderness, swelling, Homan's sign, change in limb color, and a palpable cord. When venous thrombosis is accompanied by massive swelling, discoloration, pain, and fever (phlegmasia cerulea dolens and phlegmasia alba dolens), a diagnosis can be confidently made based on the physical examination. However, because therapy entails significant risk, treatment of thromboembolic disease should never be initiated solely on the basis of a clinical diagnosis.

Several diagnostic tests have been used including phlebography and noninvasive testing. Diagnosis of venous thrombus requires identification of a well-defined filling defect in more than one radiologic view on phlebography. Unfortunately, the pelvic veins cannot be evaluated adequately. Consequently, nonobstructive thrombi in the common femoral vein may be missed. Because the clinical findings associated with DVT are common in pregnancy, the clinician may be reluctant to use ascending phlebography because of concerns about unnecessarily exposing the fetus to ionizing radiation. The use of pelvic shielding may also invalidate the results of ascending phlebography. Because of the time, expense, and potential risks involved with phlebography, a number of noninvasive tests have been developed.

The most commonly used noninvasive tests include impedance plethysmography (IPG), Doppler ultrasound, and standard and color duplex ultrasound.

Although the physiologic noninvasive tests are usually reliable, their accuracy may be affected by physiologic alterations associated with pregnancy.

Duplex Ultrasonography

Compression ultrasonography or color duplex imaging has been shown to have an accuracy of better than 90% for the diagnosis of venous thrombi located within the femoral and popliteal venous segments.[3] The imaging protocol consisted of using distention of the common femoral vein in response to the Valsalva maneuver to exclude obstructing thrombus in the iliac veins. The remainder of the femoral popliteal venous system is surveyed with color Doppler flow imaging with flow augmentation in the femoral and popliteal veins to exclude nonobstructing thrombosis. Compression ultrasonography is also performed along the course of the femoral and popliteal veins with a transducer held transverse to the vein. A normal vein has a spontaneous phasic augmented signal; DVT is diagnosed when a venous segment is noncompressible and does not show any flow signal.

TREATMENT

The choice of appropriate therapy is not well defined and has been widely debated. Sodium warfarin passes through the placenta and may cause fetal complications or death. Heparin sodium, in contrast, does not cross the placenta and is considered more effective therapy for DVT,[2] but long-term intravenous administration during pregnancy may be impractical and increases the risk of osteoporosis, alopecia, and neurologic complications.[4] The rationale of heparin sodium therapy is to prevent further thrombosis and PE and possibly to minimize the effect of post-thrombotic changes in the lower extremity. A review of published reports in which heparin sodium was administered documents conflicting results, with some showing significant fetal and maternal morbidity and mortality[5] and others concluding that heparin sodium can be safely used in the treatment of DVT in pregnancy.[6] It has also been reported that 36% to 90% of patients have chronic venous insufficiency after receiving conventional anticoagulation.[7]

In a comprehensive review of heparin sodium therapy for treatment of DVT in pregnancy, Hall and colleagues noted that only two-thirds of pregnancies in women treated with heparin sodium resulted in normal births.[5] Moreover, this did not differ from those treated with sodium warfarin. The complications associated with heparin sodium included stillbirths, spontaneous abortions, and a high incidence of prematurity. This report has been criticized by Weiner, who noted that pregnancy loss in the sodium warfarin group was usually related to placental abruption, fetal anomalies, or fetal/neonatal intracranial hemorrhage, each sodium warfarin related.[1] In contrast, pregnancy loss in the heparin sodium group was predominantly secondary to preterm delivery. A recent review of 22 children of mothers who took sodium warfarin during pregnancy revealed no significant difference from controls. This suggests that the incidence of significant abnormalities may be lower than previously reported.[8] However, the report by Hall and co-workers cannot be ignored.

Once the diagnosis of DVT has been confirmed, a sufficient quantity of heparin sodium should be administered to prolong the partial thromboplastin time (PTT) to 1.5 to 2 times baseline. Heparin sodium may be administered either subcutaneously or by continuous intravenous infusion with similar results.[9] If the intravenous route is selected, a loading dose of 110 units/kg is given, followed by a continuous infusion of 1,000 units/hour. The PTT should be monitored every 2 hours and adjustments made in the infusion rate until a stable prolongation is achieved. If the subcutaneous route is selected, a loading dose of 150 units/kg is given intravenously, followed by 20,000 units every 12 hours. The PTT is checked at mid-intervals until the plasma heparin activity level achieved with subcutaneous injection is stable. The duration of intravenous heparin sodium infusion is quite variable, but should be continued for a minimum of 2 days with DVT and 5 days for PE, depending on the severity of the disease. Although many authors recommended intravenous heparin sodium therapy for 7 to 10 days, adequate therapeutic responses may be achieved by the use of subcutaneous heparin sodium.[9] The period of continuous intravenous infusion is followed by therapeutic subcutaneous injection for the duration of the pregnancy. Postpartum thromboembolism should be treated with therapeutic anticoagulation for a minimum of 6 weeks for DVT and 3 to 6 months for PE.

There are three treatment options regarding peripartum management. One approach is continuation of therapeutic heparinization, which is recommended for high-risk patients, such as those with recent PE, iliofemoral thrombosis, or heart valve prosthesis. As a more uniform low therapeutic heparin activity level is desired, the patient may be changed from subcutaneous injection to continuous intravenous infusion, aiming for a heparin level of 0.1 to 0.2 units/ml or a low therapeutic PTT (1.5 of normal). Except for episiotomy hematomas, after vaginal delivery, patients have similar blood losses whether or not they are therapeutically anticoagulated. However, cesarean section patients receiving therapeutic heparin sodium have a significantly greater blood loss than usual. The second approach is to reduce the subcutaneous dose of heparin sodium to 5,000 units every 12 hours, which is suggested for patients with recent thromboembolism. The third approach is to stop intravenous heparin sodium administration 4 hours before delivery. If the heparin sodium therapy is subcutaneous, consider giving the last injection 6 hours before delivery. If the PTT is greater than 60 seconds, protamine sulfate reversal may be considered for minimization of bleeding from lacerations. As soon after delivery as possible, the patient should receive her next subcutaneous injection because it will take 2 to 4 hours before a therapeutic plasma level of heparin sodium can be obtained. Heparin sodium therapy (5,000 units subcutaneously every 12 hours) should be continued for 6 to 8 weeks postpartum. Sodium warfarin can be initiated after 4 to 7 days of heparin sodium therapy for nonlactating women, and the dose should be adjusted to keep the prothrombin time to 15 to 20 seconds. A progestational contraceptive should be considered for the anticoagulated ovulating woman to reduce the risk of hemorrhagic corpus luteum and menorrhagia. Postpartum suppression of lactation with estrogen is associated with a high incidence of thromboembolism and is contraindicated. Many physicians advocate either calf- or thigh-high compression stockings for prophylaxis.

Other Treatment Alternatives

The role of anticoagulation in the treatment of DVT in general is to prevent PE and to minimize the long-term sequelae of the post-thrombotic syndrome. Heparin sodium anticoagulation has been effective in achieving the former, but ineffective in preventing valvular damage and the postphlebitic syndrome.[7] In addition, bleeding from heparin sodium probably occurs in approximately 5% to 10% of patients but may affect as many as one-third.[2] Because of these concerns and because two pregnant patients in our medical center in 1 year had major complications while on heparin sodium therapy—one with significant retroperitoneal bleeding and one with PE—other therapeutic alternatives were explored.

A protocol was begun of inserting a Greenfield filter for the prevention of PE in patients with iliofemoral DVT, who are at high risk for this complication, and utilizing a lower dose of heparin sodium to prevent further thrombotic processes and as prophylaxis for DVT during the course of pregnancy. With the introduction of the percutaneous Greenfield filter, use became less invasive and more attractive. Fluoroscopy needs to be used briefly when the filter is placed. It has been estimated that 2 minutes of fluoroscopy to the abdomen exposes the area to 0.5 rads of irradiation. None of the patients needed more than 2 minutes of fluoroscopy.

The indications for inferior vera cava interruption in the treatment of DVT during pregnancy are similar to the indications in a nonpregnant state. Another indication is proposed, primarily for prevention of PE in pregnant patients with iliofemoral DVT in the third trimester in combination with lower dose heparin sodium for preventing further venous thrombosis.

Another alternative for iliofemoral venous thrombosis during pregnancy is thrombectomy and temporary arteriovenous fistula combined with heparin sodium therapy as proposed by Mogensen and associates who reported favorable results with such.[10]

THROMBOEMBOLIC PROPHYLAXIS DURING PREGNANCY

Patients at high risk for thromboembolic disease in pregnancy should be considered for anticoagulant prophylaxis during pregnancy. Such patients include those with a prior history of thromboembolic disease during or prior to pregnancy, operative delivery, concurrent malignant disease, pre-eclampsia, eclampsia, artificial heart valves, and primary hypercoagulable disorders such as antithrombin III, protein S, or protein C deficiencies. Patients with other risk factors such as age, higher parity, or obesity may also require prophylaxis. A patient with a thromboembolic event during an earlier pregnancy may receive prophylaxis throughout a later pregnancy. If thromboembolism was not associated with pregnancy, authors' opinions vary as to the need for prophylaxis during pregnancy, but all agree that prophylaxis is important during the puerperium. A protocol for prophylaxis has not yet been clearly established, but low-dose heparin sodium therapy is reasonable, with close clinical follow-up essential. Increasing uteroplacental coagulation and platelet activity as pregnancy progresses leads to progressive neutralization of heparin sodium. Heparin doses must, therefore, be increased from 5,000 units to 7,500 units, and possibly 10,000 units every 12 hours in the third trimester. A dose of 8,000 units is suggested for the puerperal period.

CLINICAL EXPERIENCE

Nineteen patients of 21,943 deliveries during a 6 year period (1987–1992) at our medical center were diagnosed as having DVT of the lower extremity with or without a PE during pregnancy. Two treatment protocols were used. Conventional therapy included continuous intravenous heparin sodium therapy for 7 to 10 days (5,000 to 10,000 units intravenous bolus; then the dosage was adjusted by a PTT of 2 to 2.5 of the control), followed by 5,000 units of subcutaneous heparin sodium every 12 hours until 6 to 8 weeks after delivery. Nonconventional therapy included lower dose subcutaneous heparin sodium for 7 to 10 days with or without Greenfield filter insertion (5,000 to 10,000 units intravenous bolus; then 5,000 to 10,000 units every 8 to 12 hours subcutaneously with the dosage adjusted for a PTT of 1.5 of the control), followed by 5,000 units of subcutaneous heparin sodium every 12 hours until 6 to 8 weeks after delivery. In both groups, subcutaneous heparin sodium therapy was stopped when active labor commenced and restarted as soon as possible after delivery. Three patients in the conventional group and two in the nonconventional group, who were not lactating, were maintained on 5 mg sodium warfarin daily for 6 to 8 weeks after delivery instead of subcutaneous heparin sodium. Patients in the nonconventional therapy group with iliofemoral DVT had a Greenfield filter inserted, some for therapeutic and others for prophylactic indications.

Fourteen of 19 patients were diagnosed with DVT in the third trimester, 4 in the second trimester, and 1 in the first trimester. The clinical diagnosis of DVT was confirmed in each patient by a duplex ultrasound study (15 patients) or phlebography (4 patients). There were 12 patients in the conventional group. Two of these were given full-dose intravenous heparin sodium for 24 hours and, because of complications (one bleeding and one PE), were converted to a lower dose subcutaneous heparin sodium regimen. Nine patients were in the nonconventional therapy group. Follow-up ranged from 6 to 72 months, with a mean of 29.5 months. Both groups were comparable in age and risk factors for DVT.

Eight patients in the nonconventional therapy group had Greenfield filters inserted; one for PE and one for bleeding, both of which occurred while on full-dose intravenous continuous heparin sodium therapy for 24 hours (after filter insertion, heparin sodium was changed to subcutaneous low-dose regimen); two for free-floating iliofemoral DVT; and four for PE prevention in patients with iliofemoral DVT, which was diagnosed less than 30 days prior to labor.

There were three major complications (two PE, one of which was fatal, and one case of significant retroperitoneal bleeding, which necessitated a blood transfusion) in the conventional therapy group (3 of 12 patients, 25%), but none in the nonconventional therapy group (none of nine). In long-term follow-up, three of seven patients in the conventional therapy group (43%) had significant leg swelling. By contrast, three of nine (33%) in the nonconventional group had leg swelling. There were no complications related to the insertion of the Greenfield filter in the nonconventional therapy group. There was no fetal morbidity or mortality in either group.

It was concluded that patients who received low-dose subcutaneous heparin sodium and Greenfield filter insertion tended to do better than those who received full-dose continuous intravenous heparin sodium treatment. However, the number of patients in this study is small, and further verification is needed.

REFERENCES

1. Weiner CP, Diagnosis and management of thromboembolic disease during pregnancy. Clin Obstet Gynecol 1985; 28:107–118.
2. Rutherford SE, Phelan JP. Thromboembolic disease in pregnancy. Clin Perinatol 1986; 13:719–739.
3. Polak JF, Wilkinson DL. Ultrasonographic diagnosis of symptomatic deep venous thrombosis in pregnancy. Am J Obstet Gynecol 1991; 165:625–629.
4. Hull RD, Raskob GE, Pineo GF, et al. Subcutaneous low-molecular-weight heparin compared with continuous intravenous heparin in the treatment of proximal-vein thrombosis. N Engl J Med 1992; 326:975–982.
5. Hall JG, Pauli RM, Wilson KM. Maternal and fetal sequelae of anticoagulation during pregnancy. Am J Med 1980; 68:122–140.
6. Rosenfeld JC, Estrada FP, Orr RM. Management of deep venous thrombosis in the pregnant female. J Cardiovasc Surg (Torino) 1990; 31:678–682.
7. Comerota AJ. An overview of thrombolytic therapy for venous thromboembolism. In: Comerota AJ, ed, Thrombolytic therapy. New York: Grune & Stratton, 1988:76.
8. Chang MKB, Harvey D, DeSwiet M. Follow-up study of children whose mothers were treated with warfarin during pregnancy. Br J Obstet Gynaecol 1984; 91:70–73.
9. Hommes DW, Bura A, Mazzolai L, et al. Subcutaneous heparin compared with continuous intravenous heparin administration in the initial treatment of deep vein thrombosis. Ann Intern Med 1992; 116:279–284.
10. Mogensen K, Skibsted L, Wadt J, Nissen F. Thromboectomy of acute iliofemoral venous thrombosis during pregnancy. Surg Gynecol Obstet 1989; 169:50–54.

NONOPERATIVE MANAGEMENT OF CHRONIC VENOUS INSUFFICIENCY

MARK C. RUMMEL, M.D.
MORRIS D. KERSTEIN, M.D.

Chronic venous insufficiency (CVI) is a common problem affecting approximately 6% of the population. An estimated 500,000 patients suffer from cutaneous ulceration, the most severe form of this disease. CVI has a spectrum of manifestations ranging from asymptomatic patients who may have some superficial varicosities to patients with severe insufficiency who suffer from cutaneous ulceration. The economic cost is staggering.

An estimated 2 million workdays are lost each year secondary to the sequela of stasis ulcers. The British National Health System estimates that it spends 100 million pounds per year on the treatment of cutaneous stasis ulcers.[1]

CLASSIFICATION

Venous stasis ulcers are classified according to their clinical severity. Asymptomatic patients may complain of no difficulties other than the dilatation of their superficial veins. These varicosities are a cosmetic problem that can be addressed after other more serious diagnosis are eliminated. Grade I or mild CVI is associated with mild to moderate ankle edema. Often the patient complains of a feeling of heaviness or pain in the legs. There may be some localized or generalized varicocele dilatation. This mild form of insufficiency is limited to the superficial venous system. Moderate CVI, class II, is manifest by hyperpigmentation of the skin, moderate brawny edema, and subcutaneous fibrosis all without ulceration. Often this is accompanied by prominent local or regional dilatation of the subcutaneous veins. Severe CVI, class III, is associated with ulceration and eczematoid changes, or severe edema. Extensive involvement of the deep venous system and diffuse loss of venous valvular function is seen.

ANATOMY

Venous anatomy in the lower extremity is divided into the deep and superficial systems. The deep system is composed of veins which usually follow the course of the major arteries of the leg. In many instances there are duplicate veins following the artery. The superficial system is composed of the series of veins superficial to the deep fascia. This series of veins has a high variability in its anatomic course. Two veins, the greater saphenous and the lesser saphenous, tend to have consistent anatomy. The greater saphenous vein is found anterior to the medial malleolus and courses along the medial aspect of the leg until it reaches the sapheno-femoral junction at the medial aspect of the groin. The lessor saphenous vein is located posterior to the lateral malleolus and courses along the posteriolateral aspect of the leg to the area of the popliteal fossa. Connecting the superficial and deep systems are a series of perforator veins.

The perforator veins are variable in their location. The most notable set of perforators is on the medial aspect of the lower leg. These perforators, called Cockett's perforators, are most typically affected in patients with severe chronic venous insufficiency and venous stasis ulceration. A second set of perforators arise between the greater saphenous trunk that drains into the posterior tibial vein known as Boyd's perforators. Finally, there are several communicating branches between the greater saphenous vein and the superficial femoral vein known as the Hunterian perforators or Dodd's Group.

Venous valves are present throughout the venous system. The central veins have few if any valves. There is a steady increase in the number of valves as the periphery is approached. Venous valves have been noted in veins of all sizes down to the postcapillary venous level where the vessel diameters are 80 to 200 μm.[2] Venous valves are a thin collagen matrix lined with endothelium and are usually bicuspid. A small sinus proximal to the valve prevents apposition of the valve leaflets to the vessel wall and helps facilitates valvular closure. The valves are opened during flow toward the heart and close with reversal of venous flow.

The calf muscle pump is crucial in the movement of blood toward the heart. The calf muscle pump is composed of the gastrocnemius and soleal sinusoids and the deep and superficial venous systems. The contraction of the calf muscles creates a high compartmental pressure propelling blood toward the heart through the popliteal vein. The blood flow in the lower leg is from the superficial to the deep system via the perforators. Blood is then propelled to the heart by the calf muscle pump. Failure of any of the venous valves, the perforators, or the calf muscle pump will create a situation where the lower leg is exposed to the pressure created by a column of blood extending from the foot to the heart. The sustained venous hypertension secondary to venous valvular failure, calf muscle pump failure, or rarely to venous obstruction, is felt to be the underlying cause of CVI.

Venous hypertension is believed to cause a series of events that eventually leads to sequelae associated with CVI. The chronically elevated pressure is transmitted to the skin resulting in dermal proliferation. Eventually, lymphatic destruction takes place with subsequent accumulation of colloid materials. The resultant edema and deposition of fibrin causes cellular damage and ulceration.

The theories concerning the origin of venous ulceration all assume that an increase of venous pressure results in damage to the microcirculation. No theory fully explains the etiology of the cellular damage. The hypothesis in the past was that cellular damage was secondary to cellular hypoxia. Multiple studies, however, have documented that the oxygen content of venous blood in ulcerated extremities is higher than normal. Two current theories attempt to explain the initiation of venous ulceration. The fibrin cuff theory asserts that increased venous pressure results in an enlargement of the pores between endothelial cells.[3] Fibrinogen traverses these pores into the interstitium. There it polymerizes and forms a pericapillary cuff. The cuff acts as a barrier to the diffusion of oxygen and other nutrients from reaching the skin. The white cell trapping theory postulates that white cells move slowly through the lower extremities when there is venous hypertension, marginate in the post capillary venules secondary to their slow rate of progression, plug the capillaries, and result in areas of ischemia. The trapped white cells become activated, release free radicals, proteolytic enzymes, and chemotactic substances. They also activate the surrounding endothelial cells which become more permeable and allow the deposition of fibrinogen, ultimately resulting in fibrin cuff formation. There is no evidence to support the hypoxic initiation of white cells, but there is evidence that supports the use of oxygen free radical scavengers in the treatment of venous stasis ulcers.

NONINVASIVE STUDIES

Non-invasive vascular studies have replaced ambulatory venous pressure measurements in most centers except in those rare occasions when non-invasive studies are indeterminate. The goal of non-invasive testing is to determine if proximal obstruction is the underlying cause of the venous insufficiency and to determine the level of incompetence, either the superficial, deep, or a combination of the two. The study should give some assessment of the severity of the insufficiency. Three tests are used for non-invasive assessment of venous insufficiency, Doppler assessment of venous reflux, plethysmography, and duplex scanning using a color-flow Doppler. These three tests provide answers to the different components of the venous insufficiency problem.

Venous reflux assessment using a Doppler is easily accomplished. The patient is positioned upright with the leg that is being assessed flexed, relaxed, and non-weight bearing. The upright position is necessary to assure that the flow reversal required to achieve valve closure is attained, and flexing the leg prevents the possible occlusion of the popliteal vein that occurs in 20% of the patients with hyperextension. The instrument can provide information about reflux at the saphenofemoral and saphenopopliteal junctions. Manual calf compression will produce cephalad flow. Reflux will occur when calf compression is released. If reflux is noted, the superficial vessels are compressed with a tourniquet and the leg reexamined. If reflux is abolished this is indicative of superficial venous valvular incompetence. A Doppler examination can provide an accurate assessment of venous reflux at the saphenofemoral or saphenopopliteal junction in 90% of the patients in experienced hands. Abnormal anatomy in the popliteal area is responsible for most of the errors with this test. The Doppler is unable to provide an assessment of the perforating vessels.

Photoplethysmography is able to provide information about the venous refill time and able to document superficial and deep venous insufficiency. A photodetector is applied to the ankle of the test leg. The patient is placed in a sitting position with the feet dangling. The patient is instructed to dorsiflex the foot ten times. This exercise drives the blood out of the lower leg by the calf pump mechanism. The blood is then allowed to return into the resting leg. A refill time of greater than 18 to 20 seconds is considered normal. Patients who have refill times less than 20 seconds are considered to have venous insufficiency. To differentiate between deep and superficial system incompetence, a tourniquet is applied to the upper thigh and the test is repeated. The tourniquet occludes the superficial system, and a recurrence of rapid refill with it in place would signify deep venous incompetence.

Duplex technology is able to document reflux in specific veins which can be individually identified and tested. Color has made duplex technology more accurate in identifying flow patterns and reflux. The femoral, popliteal, deep calf veins and perforating veins may be individually evaluated. A non-weight bearing limb is evaluated with a 5 or 7.5 MHz probe. The calf is compressed either manually or with a compression cuff. Compression with rapid release allows identification of the valves and an ability to assess their competence. The addition of color technology has permitted the identification and assessment of the perforator valves. Duplex technology may be used to quantify the reflux in the individual veins, however, acceptable reproducibility and accuracy are highly technician dependent and are more easily obtained with other testing methods.

NONOPERATIVE TREATMENT

The non-operative management of CVI has consisted of skin care, limb elevation, leg exercise, and compression therapy. Patient education and compliance are important aspects of non-operative therapy that can not be over emphasized. The benefit of non-operative measures is limited and inversely related to the severity of the insufficiency.

Skin care is an important and often ignored aspect of the treatment of CVI. Patients must be educated to wash their legs daily with neutral soaps and avoid rubbing their skin. The skin must be kept well hydrated and moist to prevent drying and the development of fissures. The poor healing ability of the lower leg makes even the smallest skin break the possible initial point for ulceration. Itching on the medial aspect of the leg is a recurrent complaint. Topical corticosteroids are used to decrease the topical dermatitis and pruritus associated with CVI. Inhibiting pruritus is an important aspect of treatment since recurrent itching may result in skin breaks and secondary infection. Topical corticosteroids, such as 1% hydrocortisone or 0.1% triamacinolone, are used to relieve pruritus.

Cellulitis is common and is associated with regional lymphadenopathy, leukocytosis, pain, chills, or fever. Secondary infection with *Staphylococcus aureus, Pseudomonas aeruginosa, Streptococcus, Proteus,* enterobacteria and *Klebsiella* is described and will significantly delay healing. The role of antibiotics in the treatment of venous stasis ulcers is not clearly defined. Often the ulcers are chronically contaminated with multiple bacteria. There are a number of different studies that have addressed the issue of the use of both topical and systemic antibiotics, and there is no definitive opinion on the issue. Our feeling is that topical and oral antibiotics should be used when specific cultures indicate their effectiveness. Intravenous antibiotics are reserved for the management of cellulitis.

Since prolonged exposure to a hydrostatic column of blood is the underlying etiology of cutaneous venous stasis manifestations, it is important to emphasize that patients avoid prolonged standing or sitting with their legs dependent. Patients should develop a routine to elevate the legs above the level of the heart several times a day. Additionally, since the calf muscle pump is instrumental in the return of blood to the heart, a program of exercise while wearing a gradient fitted elastic stocking should be instituted.

Compression therapy has been the mainstay of non-operative treatment of venous insufficiency since the time of Galen. Compression therapy is used in patients with skin changes, ulceration, or leg edema as prophylaxis for the development of the sequela of CVI or in patients who are not amenable to other forms of treatment. Typically, compression therapy is represented by Unna's boot or graduated pressure elastic stockings. Unna's boot has changed little since its original description in 1883. It delivers a constant volume while varying the amount of pressure applied to the leg. The paste bandage may be impregnated with a variety of substances including calamine, zinc oxide, and glycerin. Unna's boot provides excellent compression and allows drainage of the exudate produced by open ulcers. The warm moist environment provided by the boot promotes reepithelialization and cellular proliferation. The boot can be changed twice a week or worn for a week at a time. This helps to promote patient compliance. Drawbacks of Unna's boot include occasional poor tolerance from skin irritation, discomfort, odor, and unsightliness. The effectiveness of Unna's boots in the treatment of venous stasis ulceration is remarkable. Healing rates of 70% are reported.[4]

Some studies have attempted to use new materials for the treatment of venous stasis ulcers. Menzoian documented in a prospective, randomized trial of Unna's boot versus Duoderm plus compression therapy, that the latter was able to provide significantly quicker healing in the short term. Duoderm and compression therapy for 12 weeks appeared to promote healing more rapidly than the Unna's boot control group.[5] Further studies suggest that hydrocolloid dressings are easy to change and well tolerated by the patient. A decrease in pain and a small, but not statistically significant, improvement in healing was also documented.[6]

Graduated elastic stockings are integral to the treatment of CVI. They operate by varying the volume of the stocking while providing a constant pressure gradient. It is felt that the elastic stockings induce a significant reduction in ambulatory venous pressure by reducing the venous reflux and improving the calf muscle ejection capacity during usage.[7] Stockings are divided into classes dependent upon the pressure gradient delivered. Class I delivers 18 to 21 mm Hg of pressure and are indicated for "tired or heavy" legs, mild varices with edema, and as a probable anti-embolism prophylaxis. Class II delivers 25 to 32 mm Hg of pressure. They are used in patients with moderate edema, marked varices, after sclerotherapy or operations for varicose veins. Class III hose delivers 36 to 46 mm Hg of pressure. Patients suffering from the sequelae of deep venous thrombosis, marked edema, or healing venous stasis ulcers should be fitted with these stockings. Finally, Class IV stockings provide over 59 mm Hg of pressure. They are used in patients with severe sequelae of deep venous thrombosis or lymphedema.[8]

Patients with CVI should have Class III or Class IV graduated elastic stockings prescribed. Stockings come in a number of lengths and materials. The benefit of the stockings depends on the stocking being precisely matched to the leg. It is essential that the patient be individually fitted to obtain the optimal pressure gradient for effective therapy. Although stockings come in different lengths, there is no apparent hemodynamic benefit from either the thigh length or panty-hose length stockings. Patient compliance is imperative for the successful treatment of CVI and prevention of recurrent venous stasis ulcers and is often the limiting factor in patient therapy. Applying the stockings is especially hard for elderly, obese, or otherwise compromised patients. There are devices, such as the Medi-Butler, that can assist the patient in the application of their gradient stockings.

Other treatment modalities include the use of sequential gradient pneumatic compression systems. These systems provide compression through a series of bladders contained within a sleeve that is applied to the lower extremity. Treatment regimens require the application of the sleeve at home on a daily basis. Smith, in a randomized trial of a sequential pneumatic system and gradient elastic stockings versus gradient elastic stockings alone, documented a significant improvement in the sequential pneumatic system/gradient elastic stocking therapy group.[9] Although the patients in this study had difficulty with wearing the sleeve for the prescribed 4 hours daily, the pneumatic system was generally preferred to compressive bandages.

REFERENCES

1. Shami SK, Shields DA, Scurr JH, Coleridge-Smith PD. Leg ulceration in venous disease. Postgrad Med J 1992; 68:779–785.
2. Criado E, Johnson G. Venous disease. Curr Prob Surg 1991; 28:337–400.
3. Browse NL, Burnand KG. The cause of venous ulceration. Lancet 1982; 2:243–245.
4. Kikta MJ, Schuler JJ, Meyer JP, et al. A prospective, randomized trial of Unna's boots versus hydroactive dressing in the treatment of venous stasis ulcers. J Vasc Surg 1988; 7:478–486.
5. Cordts PR, Hanrahan LM, Menzoian JO, et al. A prospective, randomized trial of of Unna's boot versus Duoderm CGF Hydroactive dressing plus compression in the management of venous leg ulcers. J Vasc Surg 1992; 15:480–486.
6. Arnold TE, Stanley JC, Kerstein MD, et al. Prospective, multicenter study of managing lower-extremity venous ulcers. Ann Vasc Surg (accepted).
7. Noyes LD, Rice JC, Kerstein MD. Hemodynamic assessment of high-compression hosiery in chronic venous disease. Surgery 1987; 102:813–815.
8. Hohlbaum GG, Milde L, Schmitz R, et al. The Medical Compression Stocking. Stuttgart: Schattauer, 1989.
9. Smith PC, Sarin S, Hasty J, et al. Sequential gradient pneumatic compression enhances venous ulcer healing: a randomized trial. Surgery 1990; 108:871–875.

SURGICAL MANAGEMENT OF CHRONIC VENOUS INSUFFICIENCY

AGUSTIN A. RODRIGUEZ, M.D.
THOMAS F. O'DONNELL JR., M.D.

Conventional management of advanced (stage II/III) chronic venous insufficiency (CVI) has been the use of compressive bandages and a variety of ointments, none of which has been shown to be superior to the original compressive bandage developed by Unna more than 100 years ago. The lack of alternative therapy as well as ulcer recurrence despite aggressive conventional therapy led to the development of surgical approaches to this problem. Most procedures were performed on the superficial venous system, without regard to which system (superficial or deep) and level of system (proximal or distal) were involved. The majority of these operations were directed at the perforating or communicating veins, without regard to the status of the deep system. Ulcer recurrence was the rule in the latter situation, whereas wound morbidity complicated 20% to 30% of these operations.

Development of new noninvasive techniques, together with refinements in phlebography, has resulted in a better understanding of the anatomy and pathophysiology of CVI. Better evaluation of the disease process has also allowed a more rational approach to the surgical management of these patients. Patients can now be classified into two groups: venous outflow obstruction and valvular incompetence. Patients with valvular incompetence can be further subclassified as primary valvular incompetence (PVI) or post-thrombotic syndrome (PTS). These two entities can exist independent of one another or can coexist. Characterization of patients preoperatively will result in performance of the procedure that is best suited to the pathology present, and both patient and surgeon should be rewarded with better long-term results.

The modern era of venous reconstruction began with Kistner's original description of a direct approach to the repair of valves in patients with deep venous involvement.[1] Since this pioneering work, several other authors have described their modifications of both direct and indirect, as well as open and closed, approaches to deep valvular reconstruction.[2-4] Other techniques have also been described, such as popliteal vein valve transplantation,[5] femorofemoral cross-over graft,[6] venous bypass,[7] vein transposition,[8] external venous support,[9] and, more recently, even angioscopic approaches that allow direct repair of venous valves without the need for venotomy.[4]

Several reviews have documented that valvular incompetence is the cause of deep venous insufficiency in more than 70% of patients. Although this was initially thought to be due to the sequelae of the PTS, Kistner has observed that approximately 40% to 50% of limbs with deep venous reflux on descending phlebography or duplex scanning had PVI.[1] Primary valvular incompetence appears to be due to a fibroelastic tissue defect rather than thrombotic injury.[1] Therefore, different techniques are needed to repair PVI and post-traumatic valvular damage, and there are significant differences in long-term results.[10]

PREOPERATIVE EVALUATION

The clinical presentation of patients with valvular insufficiency differs somewhat from that of deep venous obstruction. With reflux due to valve incompetence, there is pain and a sensation of heaviness; with obstruction, there is the sensation of intense bursting pain on exercise. Patients with valvular reflux experience calf pain and heaviness when they become upright, irrespective of ambulation, in contrast to patients with deep venous obstruction. Edema is also a significant component in patients with valvular reflux.

Despite these clinical differences, only objective evaluation can reliably distinguish these two entities, and it is essential to guide proper therapy. Initially, the presence of valvular reflux should be documented with photoplethysmography (PPG). This technique is fast, operator-independent, and inexpensive, and it gives an idea of the magnitude of reflux. Once reflux is documented, more anatomic and physiologic data can be obtained with the use of the duplex scan and air plethysmograph.

All patients who are deemed candidates for operation undergo ascending and descending phlebography.

Table 1 Surgical Management of Chronic Venous Insufficiency

Valvular Reflux
  Primary venous insufficiency
    Valvuloplasty
      Open
      Closed (angioscopic)
    External venous support
      Diameter reduction of vein by interrupted sutures
      Psathakis external sling
      Dacron "cuff"
  Post-thrombotic syndrome
    Valve autotransplantation
    Vein segment transposition
Venous Outflow Obstruction
  Iliac vein obstruction
    Autogenous femorofemoral cross-over graft
    Prosthetic femorofemoral cross-over graft
  Femoral vein obstruction
    Autogenous saphenopopliteal bypass
    Prosthetic saphenopopliteal bypass
Superficial Venous Insufficiency
  Ligation and stripping
    Greater saphenous and/or tributaries
    Lesser saphenous and/or tributaries
  Interruption of perforating veins

For descending phlebography, the patient undergoes fluoroscopy on a 75° tilt table. The contralateral femoral vein is punctured, and the catheter is directed to the common femoral vein on the affected leg. Contrast is hand-injected, and the patient is asked to perform a Valsalva maneuver. The reflux of contrast is followed with fluoroscopy, and cut films are taken. Ascending phlebograms are also performed on a tilt table with the aid of fluoroscopy. Tourniquets are placed on the leg at ankle, below-knee, low-thigh, and high-thigh locations to aid in the identification of incompetent perforators.

Patients undergoing corrective venous procedures should have clinically class 2 or 3 disease, and should have grade 3 or 4 reflux on descending phlebography or incapacitating symptoms secondary to venous outflow obstruction. We recently compared the ability of the various noninvasive techniques, including PPG, duplex scanning, and air plethysmography, to select patients for descending phlebography. Duplex-derived valve closure time for the femoral-popliteal segment (superficial femoral vein valve closure time plus popliteal valve closure time) of 4 seconds or more had a sensitivity of 80% and specificity of 90%.[11] By contrast, venous filling index by air plethysmography and venous refill time were insensitive and nonspecific.

Based on the results of the noninvasive hemody-

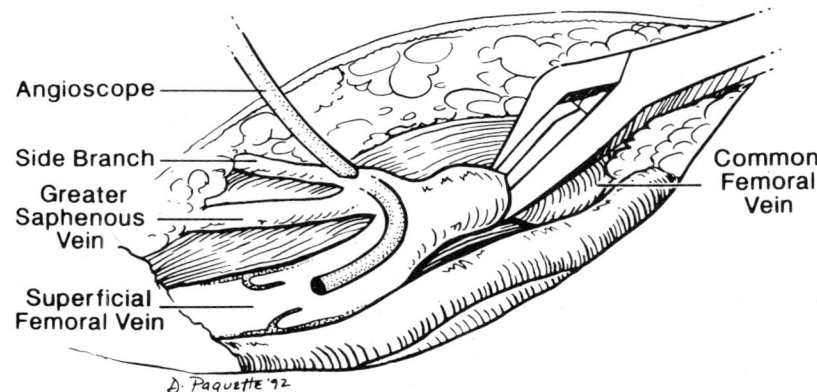

Figure 1 Technique of angioscopic valvuloplasty. Angioscope is inserted through tributary or stump of previously ligated greater saphenous vein into superficial femoral vein. Diagnosis of valvular incompetence is made, valve is repaired, and competency of repair is assessed under direct visualization with the angioscope. (From Welch HJ, McLaughlin RL, O'Donnell TF. Femoral vein valvuloplasty: Intraoperative angioscopic evaluation and hemodynamic improvement. J Vasc Surg 1992; 16:694; with permission.)

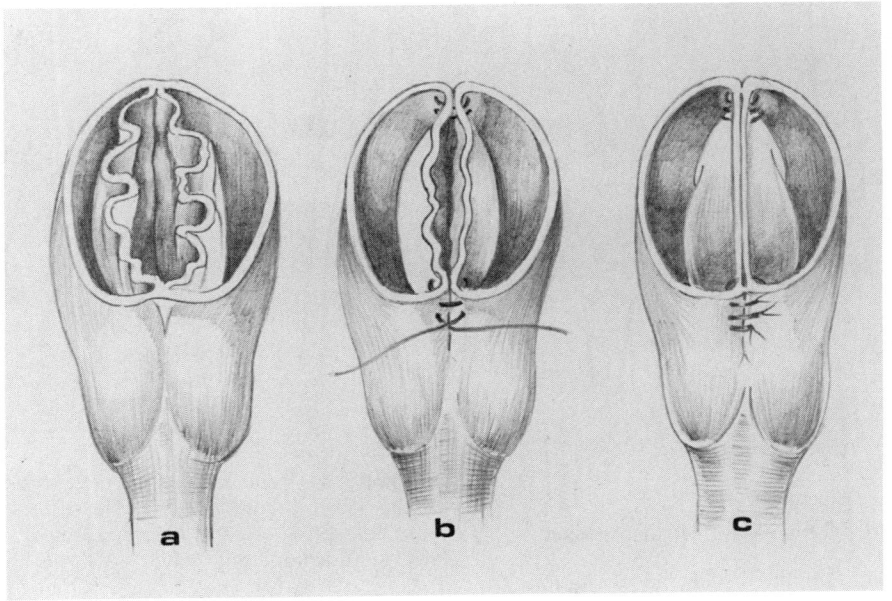

Figure 2 Valvuloplasty by the open technique. *A,* A venotomy has been made above the valve; the valve is seen to be incompetent and floppy. *B,* One suture has been placed at either side. *C,* The valve cusps have been reefed with three interrupted 7-0 prolene sutures and competence has been achieved. (Modified from Bergan JJ, Kistner RL. Atlas of venous surgery. Philadelphia: WB Saunders, 1992; with permission.)

namic and phlebographic studies, the patients can be classified into one of three groups:

Superficial Venous Insufficiency. Venous refill time (VRT) normalizes with above-knee or below-knee tourniquet. There is no evidence of deep venous obstruction or valvular incompetence by duplex or phlebography.

Deep Venous Valvular Incompetence. Abnormally shortened VRT; no evidence of occlusion on ascending phlebography, and abnormal descending phlebography with valvular reflux.

Deep Venous Obstruction. Abnormally shortened VRT; obstruction on ascending phlebography.

SURGICAL THERAPY (TABLE 1)

Superficial Venous Insufficiency

These patients should undergo ligation and stripping of the greater or lesser saphenous system with or without subfascial ligation of incompetent perforating veins. The incompetent perforating veins can be identified with the duplex scan or on ascending phlebography. Ligation has traditionally been done with the use of a medial subfascial incision or through a "stocking seam" incision. Duplex scanning can identify the specific site of perforator veins so that selective small incisions can be made over the site of the incompetent perforating vein. Alternatively, the laparoscopic superficial approach can be applied. Both lower the significant morbidity with the conventional approaches.

Valvular Reflux

Patients with isolated PVI are the best candidates for valvuloplasty. The valve most accessible for repair is located in the proximal superficial femoral vein near the junction of the superficial and profunda femoris veins. The repair can be undertaken according to the open techniques described by Kistner,[1] Raju and Fredericks,[2] and Sottiurai;[3] closed as described by Kistner, or closed under angioscopic guidance as described by our group[4] (Fig. 1). In the open technique, a venotomy is made and the valve cusps are then reefed with 7-0 prolene sutures until competence is achieved (Fig. 2). When the closed technique is employed, 7-0 prolene sutures are used to

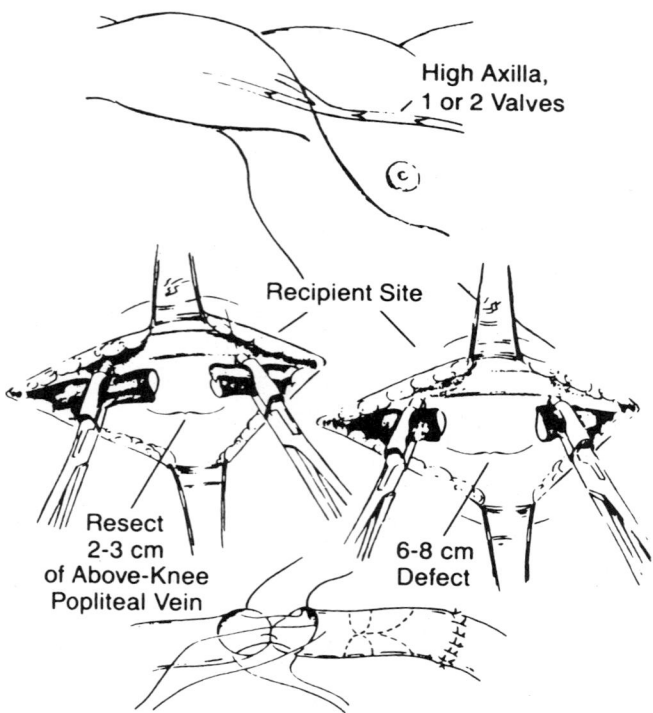

Figure 3 Axillary vein to popliteal vein transplantation. The surgical steps involved in axillary vein to popliteal vein transplantation are schematically shown. (From O'Donnell TF Jr, Mackey WC, Shepard AD, Callow AD. Clinical, hemodynamic, and anatomic follow-up of direct venous reconstruction. Arch Surg 1987; 122:474–482; with permission.)

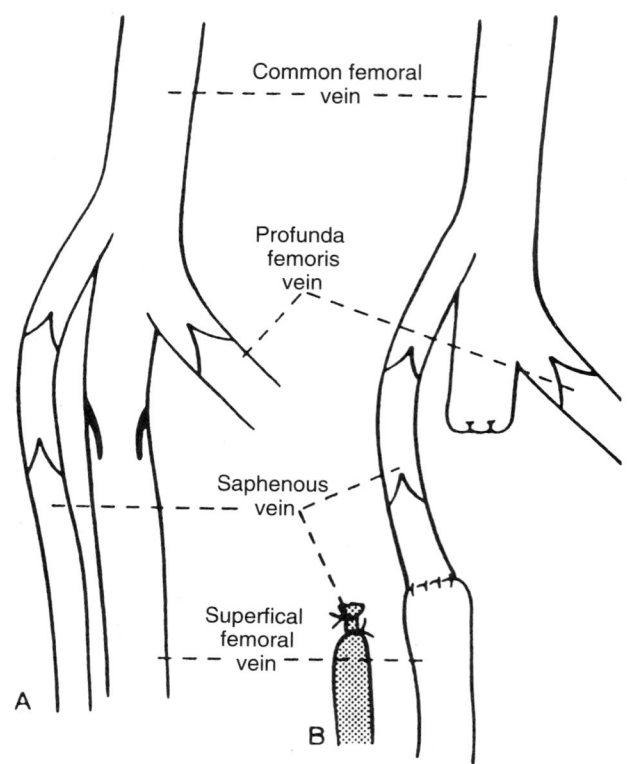

Figure 4 Venous segment transposition. *A*, Proximal valve of the SFV is incompetent. *B*, The distal superficial femoral vein is transposed to the greater saphenous vein to provide the latter's competent valves. Alternatively, the SFV may be anastomosed end to side, thus utilizing the competent valves of the PFV. SFV, superficial femoris vein; PFV, profunda femoris vein. (From O'Donnell TF Jr, Shepard AD. Chronic venous insufficiency. In: Jarrett F, Hirsch SA, eds. Vascular surgery of the lower extremity. St Louis: CV Mosby, 1985; with permission.)

Table 2 Reported Results of Surgical Therapy for Chronic Venous Insufficiency

Series (Author)	No. of Limbs	Percent Ulcer* (Preop)	Percent Ulcer Healing† (Short)	(Long)
Valvuloplasty				
Kistner	51	57	?	57%
Raju	107	78	85%	63%
Perrin	52	40	?	?
Eriksson	22	?	64%	62%
Sottiurai	20	100	?	80%
Simkin	7	100	?	50%
O'Donnell	9	100	100%	100%
Venous Transposition				
Ferris	14	?	80%	?
Queral	12	33%	100%	?
Johnson	12	33%	?	67%
O'Donnell	9	100%	100%	78%
Vein Valve Transplant				
Taheri	43	40%	?	94%
Raju	24	80%	79%	42%
O'Donnell	12	100%	100%	92%
External Venous Support				
Psathakis	44	23%	100%	100%

*Percentage of limbs studied preoperatively that had intractable ulcer.
†Percentage of limbs that healed completely after short (6 month) or long (>2 year) follow-up.
?, Information not reported.

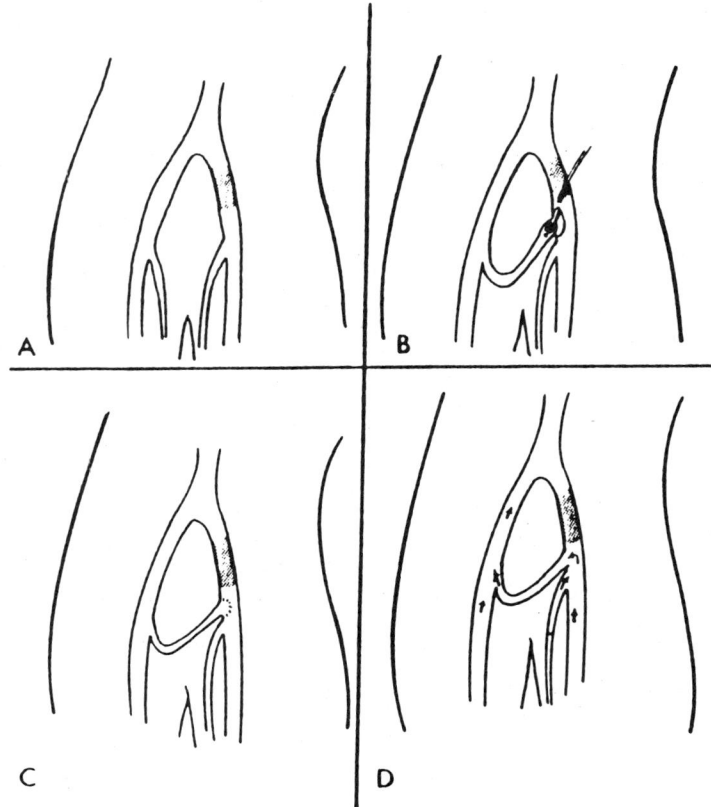

Figure 5 Saphenofemoral cross-over graft. *A,* Obstructed left ileofemoral segment. *B,* The contralateral saphenous vein is subcutaneously tunneled across the pubis to the left groin. *C,* End-to-side anastomosis. *D,* Venous return from the left leg now flows through the graft to the right iliac system. (Modified from Dale WA. Chronic ileofemoral venous occlusion including 7 cases of cross-over vein grafting. Surgery 1966; 59:127; with permission.)

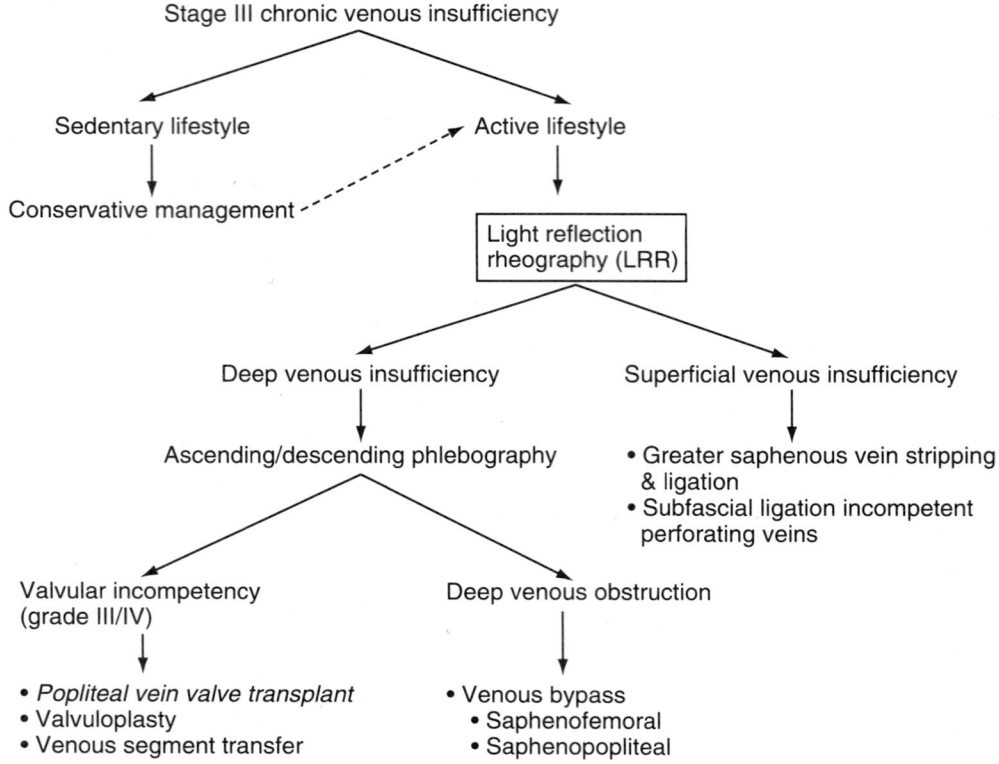

Figure 6 Algorithm for management of stage III chronic venous insufficiency (CVI). Patients with active lifestyles and disabling CVI should undergo initial assessment by noninvasive means (e.g., duplex scan, air plethysmography). Subsequent management is dictated by phlebography. We prefer angioscopic guided valvuloplasty for grade III/IV primary valvular incompetence, and popliteal vein valve transplantation for post-thrombotic syndrome; venous segment transfer or bypass is dictated by the nature of the obstructed segment.

bring the valve cusps together at the commissure until competence is assessed angioscopically (see Fig. 1). Incompetent perforating veins should be interrupted when present. If stripping is performed, it should not be done concomitantly with this procedure in order to avoid bleeding due to perioperative heparinization. With proper selection, good results can be expected in 60% to 90% of cases.[1-4]

Other options for these patients include the Psathakis external sling[12] and the Dacron cuff.[9] These procedures are indicated only when the valve is noted to become competent during the operation as a result of vasospasm and when it had been clearly shown to be incompetent in preoperative descending phlebography. Results so far are not as good as with the direct approach.

Patients with the PTS are candidates for vein valve transplant. A valve-bearing segment of axillary vein is interposed into the incompetent popliteal vein, or surperficial or profunda femoris veins. We have advocated that the popliteal vein is the logical choice—and is invariably incompetent in patients with advanced CVI—because it serves as the "gatekeeper" to the calf venous pump mechanism (Fig. 3). Another option would be venous segment transfer or transposition, which involves division of the incompetent superficial femoral vein close to its junction with the profunda femoris vein and anastomosing it to the greater saphenous vein below a competent venous valve (Fig. 4). Usually this vein is absent in patients with advanced CVI so that anastomosing the superficial femoral vein to the profunda femoris vein end to side is a better option.

Unfortunately, the reported results so far for segment transfer performed for PTS are not as encouraging as those reported for valvuloplasty performed for PVI (Table 2). This difference may be related to the very nature of the pathologic process.

Venous Outflow Obstruction

The first operations performed to relieve venous outflow obstruction were described by Palma and Esperon.[7] Their operation was a femorofemoral crosspubic graft to bypass iliac vein obstruction. Since then, a number of other operations have been described, using both autogenous and prosthetic materials. Some surgeons favor performing an arteriovenous fistula to increase flow through the graft and thereby prolong patency. Some of these operations also include the saphenopopliteal bypass, saphenofemoral bypass, and direct reconstruction of obstructed venous segments (Fig. 5). The optimal results are achieved when the obstruction is due to extraluminal pathology, with concomitant sparing of the intrinsic venous architecture.

Extirpation of secondary varicose veins and ligation of incompetent perforating veins appear to improve the results. Some advocates of the saphenopopliteal bypass suggest that failure does not worsen a patient's condition. The addition of an arteriovenous fistula distally appears to improve flow through the graft and may help prolong patency. This may be of greater importance when prosthetic materials, such as externally supported polytetrafluoroethylene are used for cross-pubic bypasses.

FOLLOW-UP EVALUATION

Patients should undergo some form of imaging either by duplex scan or by ascending phlebography alone, in the sapheno-cross-femoral bypass group, or both ascending and descending phlebography, in the valve transplant or valvuloplasty groups. Patients are then subsequently followed with duplex ultrasound examinations and air plethysmography. If the patient had an ulcer preoperatively, its size should be measured at each office visit. The goal should be the prevention of ulcer recurrence rather than just promoting ulcer healing, as most ulcers heal initially after most procedures only to recur later. The results of venous reconstructive operations can be evaluated only after 12 months of follow-up. A thorough evaluation and adherence to the principles outlined should reward both patient and surgeon with lasting results (Fig. 6).

REFERENCES

1. Kistner RL. Surgical repair of the incompetent femoral vein valve. Arch Surg 1975; 110:1336–1342.
2. Raju S, Fredericks R. Valve reconstruction procedures for non-obstructive venous insufficiency: Rationale, techniques, and results in 107 procedures with two- to eight-year follow-up. J Vasc Surg 1988; 7:301–310.
3. Sottiurai VS. Technique in direct venous valvuloplasty. J Vasc Surg 1988; 8:646–649.
4. Welch HJ, McLaughlin RL, O'Donnell TF. Femoral vein valvuloplasty: Intraoperative angioscopic evaluation and hemodynamic improvement. J Vasc Surg 1992; 16:694–700.
5. Waddell WG, Vogelfanger IJ, Prudhomme P, et al: Venous valve transplantation. Arch Surg 1964; 88:5–15.
6. Dale WA. Crossover vein grafts for iliac and femoral venous occlusion. Res Staff Phys 1983; 58–64.
7. Palma EC, Esperon R. Vein transplants and grafts in the surgical treatment of the post-phlebitic syndrome. J Cardiovasc Surg (Torino) 1960; 1:94–107.
8. Ferris EB, Kistner RL. Femoral vein reconstruction in the management of chronic venous insufficiency. A 14 year experience. Arch Surg 1982; 117:1571–1579.
9. Jessup G, Lane RJ. Repair of incompetent venous valves: A new technique. J Vasc Surg 1988; 8:569–575.
10. O'Donnell TF, McEnroe CS, Mackey WC, et al. Correlation of clinical findings with venous hemodynamics in 386 patients with chronic venous insufficiency. Am J Surg 1986; 156:148–156.
11. Iafrati MD, Welch H, Belkin M, O'Donnell TF. Correlation of venous non-invasive tests with the SVS/ISCVS clinical classification of chronic venous insufficiency. J Vasc Surg 1994; 19: 1001–1007.
12. Psathakis ND. The substitute "valve" operation by technique II in patients with post-thrombotic syndrome. Surgery 1984; 95: 542–548.

WARFARIN-INDUCED SKIN NECROSIS

DONALD P. SPADONE, M.D.
DONALD SILVER, M.D.

Oral anticoagulants are widely used for the prophylaxis and management of arterial and venous thromboembolism. The most commonly used oral anticoagulant in the United States is sodium warfarin (Coumadin). Approximately 1.8 million new sodium warfarin prescriptions are dispensed in the United States each year.[1] The most serious nonhemorrhagic complication of oral anticoagulant use is warfarin-induced skin necrosis.

Bishydroxycoumarin was introduced for clinical use in 1940. The first report of skin necrosis associated with use of this drug was published in 1943.[2] Soft tissue necrosis was first related to sodium warfarin by Verhagen in 1952.[3] There are now more than 300 publications documenting the manifestations of this condition,[1] which occurs in 0.01% to 0.1% of patients receiving sodium warfarin.[4] Warfarin-induced skin necrosis is manifested by thrombosis and hemorrhage of venules and capillaries within the subcutaneous fat and overlying skin. The thrombosis and hemorrhage frequently produce necrosis of the involved subcutaneous tissue and skin.

Patients who have previously tolerated oral anticoagulation may develop warfarin-induced skin necrosis during subsequent exposure to sodium warfarin. Most cases of warfarin-induced skin necrosis have occurred in patients being treated for deep venous thrombosis (DVT) or pulmonary embolism. The condition is rarely seen in patients being treated for arterial or cardiac embolism. The syndrome has occurred in orthopedic patients receiving low-dose warfarin prophylaxis for DVT and in patients with vitamin K deficiency.

The association between warfarin-induced skin necrosis and venous thrombosis suggests a predisposing hypercoagulable defect for both conditions. The presence of an anticardiolipin antibody (the lupus anticoagulant) and hereditary or acquired deficiencies of protein S, protein C, or antithrombin III have been associated with warfarin-induced skin necrosis.[1,4-8] Ischemic skin lesions similar to those of warfarin-induced skin necrosis have been described in end-stage renal failure patients who develop calciphylaxis, a rare, idiopathic syndrome of progressive soft tissue calcification and skin necrosis. In a series of five patients, protein C antigen levels were normal, but protein C serum activity was lower than that in control patients.[9] Although the exact mechanism for warfarin-induced skin necrosis is unknown, protein C deficiency seems to have an important role in the pathogenesis.

PATHOPHYSIOLOGY

Oral sodium warfarin is rapidly absorbed and competitively inhibits the action of vitamin K in the hepatocyte. Reduction of the level of active vitamin K reduces the gamma-carboxylation of glutamic acid residues of factors II (prothrombin), VII, IX, and X and proteins C and S. Coagulant activity is disrupted because the partially decarboxylated clotting factors lose their ability to interact with calcium or bind to phospholipid membranes. Protein C, a vitamin K–dependent 62 kD glycoprotein produced by the liver, is an important inhibitor of the rate-limiting steps in the coagulation cascade.[5] Protein C rapidly degrades factors Va and VIIIa, thereby limiting the progression of the thrombotic process. Protein C is activated by thrombin, and the reaction is catalyzed by binding of thrombin to thrombomodulin on the endothelial membrane. Lysis of activated factors Va and VIIIa by protein C is accelerated tenfold to twentyfold by protein S, which is a 75 kD vitamin K–dependent cofactor. Protein S has no anticoagulant effect of its own; it serves only as a cofactor for protein C. Protein C may also enhance fibrinolytic activity by inactivation of plasminogen activator inhibitor type I (PAI-1).

Deficiencies of proteins C and S may be genetic or acquired. The penetrance of genetic protein C deficiencies is highly variable. Heterozygotes may be asymptomatic or may begin to develop recurrent deep venous thrombosis in early adulthood.[5] Individuals with heterozygote protein C deficiencies have eight times more thrombotic events than individuals with normal protein C plasma levels.[7] Homozygotes have severe thrombotic complications and frequently develop purpura fulminans in the neonatal period. The overwhelming thrombotic process that occurs in these infants is secondary to the hypercoagulable state from the lack of protein C. The incidence of homozygous protein C deficiency is about 1 in 250,000 to 500,000 births. The frequency of heterozygous deficiency is 1 in 200 to 300 individuals.[7] The most common cause of protein C deficiency is depletion of vitamin K reserves from malnutrition, infection, cancer, operations, long-term antibiotic usage, or sodium warfarin use. Functional protein S deficiencies may result from the nephrotic syndrome, systemic lupus erythematosus, diabetes mellitus, sickle cell anemia, liver disease, and oral contraceptive use.

Plasma concentrations of factor VII and protein C rapidly decline after the initiation of warfarin therapy because the half-life of these factors is about 6 hours. The early changes in the prothrombin time (PT) that are induced by warfarin therapy reflect, predominantly, the reduced levels of factor VII. The other procoagulant vitamin K–dependent factors have significantly longer half-lives. Systemic therapeutic anticoagulation with sodium warfarin requires 3 to 4 days for the depletion of factor X (half-life 36 hours) and factor II (half-life 72 hours). The early induced deficiency of protein C in relation to the other clotting factors, especially in patients with pre-existing genetic or acquired protein C and protein S deficiency, induces a hypercoagulable state for the first 1 to 3 days of warfarin therapy. An unknown stimulus precipitates warfarin-induced skin necrosis in a small group of these hypercoagulable patients. The half-life of protein S is 3 to 4 days; thus, its reduction by sodium warfarin administration has little contribution to the hypercoagulable state caused by warfarin-induced protein C deficiency.[10]

PREVENTION

It is postulated that an imbalance between procoagulant and anticoagulant activity causes warfarin-induced skin necrosis, but it is not known why only a small fraction of patients receiving sodium warfarin actually develop the syndrome. Warfarin-induced skin necrosis occurs in approximately 3% of protein C–deficient patients beginning oral anticoagulation.[8] The rarity of this syndrome and the poor correlation between depressed activity of protein C, protein S, and antithrombin III and the development of warfarin-induced skin necrosis make screening of patients for these abnormalities impractical. A more realistic approach to prevent warfarin-induced skin necrosis is to limit the induction of a hypercoagulable state during the early stages of warfarin-induced anticoagulation. The use of large loading doses of sodium warfarin (15 to 20 mg or more per day) is discouraged. Patients receiving heparin sodium, either by continuous intravenous infusion or by subcutaneous injection, should be less coagulable and therefore less prone to develop warfarin-induced skin necrosis. However, clinical confirmation that heparin sodium will reduce the incidence of this syndrome is lacking. The authors recommend that all patients receive heparin sodium for the first 3 to 5 days during the initiation of warfarin therapy. Patients with known deficiency of protein C, protein S, antithrombin III, or vitamin K stores are considered to be at increased risk for warfarin-induced skin necrosis.

CLINICAL PRESENTATION

Warfarin-induced skin necrosis occurs most frequently in middle-aged or elderly females, with more than 75% of reported cases occurring in women. The areas of skin necrosis develop typically over areas with increased subcutaneous fat. The breasts are most frequently involved, with the thighs, buttocks, and legs the next most common areas affected. The preference of warfarin-induced skin necrosis for areas with increased amounts of subcutaneous fat has not been explained.

Warfarin-induced skin necrosis usually presents on the third to sixth day of warfarin therapy. The patient initially develops intense pain in areas that become erythematous with subsequent development of petechial hemorrhages and edema. Within 3 days, sharply demarcated hemorrhagic bullae and cutaneous cyanosis may develop and progress to infarctions extending into the subcutaneous tissues. Biopsy specimens of early lesions document dilation of the capillaries and fibrin deposition in the postcapillary venules.[6] Later, biopsy specimens document microvascular hemorrhage and necrotic changes. The soft tissue necrosis frequently becomes extensive and requires resection with split-thickness skin grafting in more than 50% of patients.[4] Recognition may be delayed because of confusion of the lesions secondary to warfarin-induced skin necrosis with ecchymoses from subdermal bleeding. The differential diagnosis of purpuric lesions associated with dermal vascular thrombosis is summarized in Table 1.

MANAGEMENT

Warfarin-induced skin necrosis must be recognized promptly to minimize the progression of this major complication. Physicians must be aware that the soft tissue necrosis may occur early during warfarin therapy, especially when the patient is being treated for venous thrombosis. The development of a painful, sharply defined erythematous lesion that progresses to petechiae, hemorrhage, and cyanosis should alert the physician to stop warfarin therapy and intervene to limit the skin necrosis. There are no controlled studies for the treatment of warfarin-induced skin necrosis. Reinitiation or continuation of heparin sodium therapy and reversal of sodium warfarin with intervenous vitamin K has been advocated. The infusion of fresh frozen plasma may reverse the imbalance between procoagulant and anticoagulant factors in individuals with protein C deficiency. Low-molecular-weight dextran infusion may improve the soft tissue microcirculation and prevent small vessel thrombosis. Corticosteroids are no longer advocated for treatment.[8] The skin necrosis that develops in these patients should be managed by routine methods, including serial debridements, split-thickness skin grafting, or amputation, depending upon the severity of the necrosis.

Treatment of patients requiring long-term anticoagulation who develop warfarin-induced skin necrosis is problematic. Long-term heparin sodium anticoagulation, usually by subcutaneous injection, is used most often. There are reports of successful reintroduction of sodium warfarin therapy after resolution of the skin necrosis and deep venous thrombosis.[1,4] Patients who require oral anticoagulation and who have had previous warfarin-induced skin necrosis, as well as those who have known deficiencies of protein C and protein S, should receive therapeutic doses of heparin sodium for at least the first 4 to 6 days of sodium warfarin therapy, and the sodium warfarin should be introduced at low doses (initial doses of 1 to 2 mg/day).

Table 1 Differential Diagnosis of Purpuric Lesions Associated with Dermal Vascular Thrombosis

Warfarin-induced skin necrosis
Protein C deficiency
Protein S deficiency
Calciphylaxis
Heparin-induced skin necrosis
Disseminated intravascular coagulation
Antiphospholipid antibody (lupus anticoagulant) medicated skin necrosis
Purpura fulminans
   Idiopathic
   Infectious
Thrombotic thrombocytopenic purpura
Paroxysmal nocturnal hemoglobinuria
Cryoglobulinemia
Myeloblastemia

Adapted from Adcock DM, Hicks MJ. Dermatopathology of skin necrosis associated with purpura fulminans. Semin Thromb Hemost 1990; 16:283–292; with permission.

REFERENCES

1. Comp PC, Elrod JP, Karzenski S. Warfarin-induced skin necrosis. Semin Thromb Hemost 1990; 16:293–298.
2. Flood EP, Redish MH, Bociek SJ, Shapiro S. Thrombophlebitis migrans disseminata: Report of a case in which gangrene of breast occurred. N Y State J Med 1943; 43:1121–1124.
3. Verhagen H. Local haemorrhage and necrosis of skin and underlying tissue, during anticoagulant therapy with dicumarol or dicumacyl. Acta Med Scand 1954; 148:453–467.
4. Cole MS, Minifee PK, Wolma FJ. Coumarin necrosis: A review of the literature. Surgery 1988; 103:271–277.
5. Marlar RA, Neumann A. Neonatal purpura fulminans due to homozygous protein C or protein S deficiencies. Semin Thromb Hemost 1990; 16:299–309.
6. Adcock DM, Hicks MJ. Dermatopathology of skin necrosis associated with purpura fulminans. Semin Thromb Hemost 1990; 16:283–292.
7. Locht H, Lindstrom FD. Severe skin necrosis following warfarin therapy in a patient with protein C deficiency. J Intern Med 1993; 233:287–289.
8. Pescatore P, Horellow HM, Conard J, et al. Problems of oral anticoagulation in an adult with homozygous protein C deficiency and late onset of thrombosis. Thromb Haemost 1993; 69:311–315.
9. Mehta RL, Scott G, Sloand JA, Francis CW. Skin necrosis associated with acquired protein C deficiency in patients with renal failure and calciphylaxis. Am J Med 1990; 88:252–257.
10. Berkompas DC. Coumadin skin necrosis in a patient with a free protein S deficiency: Case report and literature review. Indiana Med 1991; 84:788–791.

PATHOGENESIS OF CUTANEOUS VENOUS ULCERS

ARNOST FRONEK, M.D., PH.D.

Although changes in the microvasculature are still not clarified, there is now a consensus that venous hypertension is the underlying macrohemodynamic cause that ultimately leads to the development of cutaneous trophic changes. Specifically, it is the inability to significantly lower venous pressure during exercise. The location of these changes seems to be decisive because an increased venous pressure above the knee very rarely results in venous ulceration, whereas the same hemodynamic change below the knee often leads to the development of venous ulceration.

MACROHEMODYNAMICS

Deep venous thrombosis (DVT) and venous valvular insufficiency are the causes of increased venous pressure. This increase has to take place below the popliteal vein in order to trigger trophic changes in the ankle region. It should be pointed out that venous valvular insufficiency, even when limited to the superficial venous system, can lead to the development of venous ulceration.[1] However, often there is a coexistence of venous valvular insufficiency of the deep and superficial venous system, accompanied by an insufficiency of the communicating veins. This valvular incompetence can be primary or it can develop secondary to DVT. In the past, insufficient noninvasive diagnostic methods made it difficult to determine the cause of venous hypertension, and it can be expected that this question will be satisfactorily answered in the future. Although the original reports emphasized the importance of valvular intactness of the communicating veins in the genesis of venous ulceration, some recent publications also emphasize the importance of the competency of the superficial venous system.[2]

The circumstance of the combination of two factors, venous hypertension and ankle level, may underline the importance of photoplethysmographic methods in evaluating local venous hemodynamics. The most effective application of this method is at the ankle level, and the method itself is very sensitive to changes in valvular insufficiency of the deep, superficial, and communicating veins.

MICROHEMODYNAMICS

Changes in the Microvasculature

Only in recent years, with the advent of noninvasive microcirculatory clinical methods, have old theories been challenged and re-evaluated.

Homans's original hypothesis, in which venous ulceration is the end stage of venostasis and tissue hypoxia, quickly gained wide acceptance because it seemed to be in accord with general clinical experience, as well as with a report documenting decreased blood oxygenation in the effluent blood from ulcerated areas. Studies and results have now been refocused with the introduction of transcutaneous Po_2 ($tcPo_2$) measurements. Partsch found decreased Po_2 values in patients with venous ulceration.[3]

Micromorphologic Changes

Tortuous capillaries that are specific for venous hypertension have been described. These changes go hand in hand with increased permeability as documented by sodium fluorescence studies and with an increased pericapillary space (pericapillary "halo"). The question remains to be answered as to whether increased venous pressure directly leads to the described changes or if substances released from the endothelial cells are responsible, especially in view of the increased permeability. It should be noted, however, that capillary tortuosity per se is not accompanied by a reduced $tcPo_2$ as long as there is no reduction in the number of capillaries. Nevertheless, a very low $tcPo_2$ can always be found in the presence of significant changes in cutaneous vascularization, for instance, in atrophie blanche.

Arteriovenous Shunting

Occasional reports of increased oxygen tension in blood samples obtained from varicose veins focused attention on the possibility of the opening of arteriovenous anastomoses as a mechanism that ultimately leads to increased venous pressure. These studies were seriously challenged by Partsch's group, who utilized isotopically labeled macroaggregates of albumin and found no evidence of shunting in the vicinity of venous ulcers.[4] It can be concluded that current results do not support the hypothesis of arteriovenous shunts playing a significant role in venous hypertension or ulceration.

Impairment of Microlymphatics

Morphologic changes in microlymphatics have been described by several groups. Morphologic changes were identified especially in the lymphatic channels, but it remains to be seen whether this is a primary phenomenon or a reaction to the increase in venous pressure and permeability.

Pericapillary Fibrin Cuff Theory

Browse and Burnand proposed a mechanism that explained the pathogenesis of trophic changes in the skin accompanying chronic venous disease by the presence of fibrin around the capillaries, thus impeding oxygen diffusion.[5] This hypothesis originated with the observation that fibrin deposits were found around capillaries in biopsy specimens from areas close to the ulcer. It was postulated that the persistently increased capillary pressure led to increased permeability, which favors passing of fibrinogen into the extravascular space.

This hypothesis quickly gained wide acceptance despite reports of nonspecific deposits of fibrin in nonvenous ulceration. The results of a subsequent study documenting minimal therapeutic results from a drug (stanozolol) with some fibrinolytic effect did not support this hypothesis. Serious theoretical objections published by Michel indicated that the observed thickness of fibrin cuffs (around 50 μm) could not significantly influence oxygen diffusion.[6]

Ulcus Mixtum (Venous and Arterial)

Recent observations documented that a not-insignificant percentage of venous ulcers include a component of arterial occlusive disease (AOD). The additional presence of AOD can easily be overlooked, especially if the ulcus itself prevents measurement of ankle pressure. In this case, toe pressure measurement may help in arriving at a more complete diagnosis.

Leukocyte Trapping

Moyses and associates reported a retention of leukocytes in the legs of normal subjects after sitting for 30 minutes.[7] Retention of white blood cells, probably by adhesion, can have a deleterious effect on microhemodynamics in view of their larger size and higher stiffness compared to red blood cells. Based on these considerations, Coleridge-Smith and colleagues submitted a new hypothesis explaining the development of venous ulceration.[8] They assume that the reduced shear rate favors the adhesion of white blood cells to endothelial cells, which, in turn, activates the trapped leukocytes. This is followed by a release of lysosomal enzymes and different, yet unknown, chemotactic substances and proteolytic enzymes.

This hypothesis is indirectly supported by a recent study that concludes that patients with lipodermatosclerosis retain a significantly higher percentage of white blood cells than normal controls after 60 minutes of leg dependency.[9] The positive therapeutic results of pentoxifylline, which has some leukocyte deactivation effect, lend additional credence to the hypothesis of white cell trapping.

However, it should be pointed out that the assumed reduced shear rate may not be the primum movens for leukocyte adhesion. We postulate that the chronically increased venular pressure may lead to the expression of chemotactic substances by the endothelial cells, which attract the leukocytes, thereby initiating the vicious cycle of leukocyte-endothelium interaction. In vitro increased pressure, acting on isolated endothelial cells, caused a highly significant increase in cell adhesion forces.[10] Although this represents only a preliminary in vitro observation, it may elucidate the mechanism of leukocyte trapping in view of the fact that chronically increased venous pressure is most often a precursor of venous ulceration.

THERAPY-RELATED CONCLUSIONS

Although the last decade brought a renewed interest in the pathogenesis of venous ulceration, it can be concluded that many essential pathogenetic pathways are still unclear. The "venostatic" pathogenesis, as postulated by Homans and Linton, became the target of criticism with the advent of the fibrin cuff hypothesis. Considering, however, the compromised microhemodynamics induced by leukocyte trapping and reduced $tcPo_2$ findings, venostasis should, at least, be considered as one of the pathogenetic pathways.

Positive preliminary therapeutic results obtained with intermittent compression, accelerating the healing process, and the encouraging effect of leukocyte deactivating drugs are not only important from a therapeutic point of view but also may expand, if confirmed, an understanding of pathogenetic pathways underlying the development of venous ulceration.

REFERENCES

1. Cornwall JV, Doce C, Lewis JD. Leg ulcers: Epidemiology and aetiology. Br J Surg 1986; 73:693–696.
2. Sethia KK, Darke SG. Long saphenous incompetence as a cause of venous ulceration. Br J Surg 1984; 71:54–55.
3. Partsch H. Hyperemic hypoxia in venous ulceration. Br J Dermatol 1984; 110:249–251.
4. Lindemayr W, Löfferer O, Mostbeck A, Partsch H. Arteriovenous shunts in primary varicosis? A critical assay. Vasc Surg 1972; 6:9–13.
5. Browse NL, Burnand KG. The cause of venous ulceration. Lancet 1982; 2:243–245.
6. Michel CC. Oxygen diffusion in oedematous tissue and through pericapillary cuffs. Phlebology 1990; 5:223–230.
7. Moyses C, Cederholm-Williams SA, Michel CC. Haemoconcentration and accumulation of white cells in the feet during venous stasis. Int J Microcirc Clin Exp 1987; 5:311–329.
8. Coleridge-Smith PD, Thomas P, Scurr JH, Dormandy JA. Causes of venous ulceration: A new hypothesis. Br Med J 1988; 296:1726–2727.
9. Thomas PRS, Nash GB, Dormandy JA. White cell accumulation in dependent legs of patients with venous hypertension: A possible mechanism for trophic changes in the skin. Br Med J 1988; 296:1693–1695.
10. Sung P, Fronek A, Lee L. The effect of hydrostatic pressure on endothelial cell expression (unpublished data).

NONOPERATIVE TREATMENT OF VENOUS ULCERS

JAMES O. MENZOIAN, M.D.
WAYNE W. LaMORTE, M.D., PH.D.
JONATHAN WOODSON, M.D.

Despite the long history of attempts to treat venous ulcers effectively, it often remains a difficult and frustrating clinical problem for both physicians and patients. However, a sound understanding of the pathophysiology of venous ulcer disease can guide the development of effective treatment strategies for patients with this disorder.

EPIDEMIOLOGY

Venous leg ulceration occurs in about 1.5% of the adult general population or approximately 500,000 persons in the United States.[1] Venous leg ulcers are a chronic indolent and recurrent problem. In a recent survey the mean duration of venous ulcers was 95 months.[2] Whereas varicose veins appear to be more prevalent in females, venous ulcers occur with a greater frequency in males. In a recent survey comparing patients with chronic venous insufficiency (CVI) to patients with varicose veins, age, male gender, history of significant leg injury, and increased body mass index were consistently associated with a greater risk of CVI. These data further suggest that hypertension and smoking duration may also be risk factors for CVI. There is a high 5-year recurrence rate of venous leg ulcers ranging from 15% to 48%.

ETIOLOGY AND PATHOPHYSIOLOGY

Although it is generally accepted that ambulatory venous hypertension is the basis for stasis ulceration, the fact has always been perplexing that many patients with prominent varicose veins for many years have no skin changes and never develop ulceration, whereas other patients with no visible varicosities have extensive lipodermatosclerosis and venous ulceration.

Simply viewed, the normal individual with competent venous valves in the lower extremities maintains ambulatory pressures under 30 mm Hg through the action of the soleus muscle pump. Patients with incompetent valves are exposed to chronic ambulatory venous hypertension, but predicting which patients will develop ulcers is difficult. The factors involved in the pathogenesis of venous ulceration may be varied and could include abnormal venous hemodynamics, the formation of pericapillary fibrin cuffs, neutrophil trapping and activation, and increased plasma viscosity.

In a recent study of extremities in healthy volunteers, patients with primary varicose veins, and patients with CVI, the authors found abnormal hemodynamics in patients with CVI as well as in patients with varicose veins. The hemodynamic abnormalities in these two patient groups were quite similar, despite the vastly different clinical picture associated with these two conditions. Therefore, the pathophysiology of CVI is likely to involve not only hemodynamic abnormalities but also other factors that have not yet been clearly identified.[3]

The source of venous valve incompetence is often unknown. The previously held belief that most patients with valve incompetence and ulcers were postphlebitic has not been substantiated.[4,5] Additional factors, such as genetics, local trauma, and infection, are likely contributors. Furthermore, the extent of valvular incompetence is probably important, although up to 30% of patients with venous ulcers may have isolated superficial valvular incompetence.[6]

EVALUATION

The first step in effective treatment of venous ulcers is accurate diagnosis (Table 1). The relevant considerations are whether there is a history of previous ulceration, phlebitis, extremity trauma, or family history of venous problems. On physical examination the location, size, and depth of the ulcer are noted, along with the presence of lipodermatosclerosis, stasis pigmentation, edema, and palpable pulses. If pulses are not palpable, an adequate noninvasive evaluation is indicated to rule out coexisting arterial disease. All patients are evaluated by means of a standard, high-resolution duplex imager. The superficial, deep, and perforating venous systems are evaluated for the presence of acute or chronic thrombus and valvular competency.[7] Following this, all extremities are evaluated by air plethysmography,[8] which gives additional physiologic quantification of the degree of reflux present. We feel that a complete

Table 1 Differential Diagnosis of Leg Ulcers

Venous ulcers
Infections
    Tropical ulcers
    Tuberculous
    Bacterial
Ischemic
Mixed arterial-venous
Trauma
    Insect bites
    Pressure
Sickle cell disease
Diabetic
Lymphedema
Neoplasm
    Squamous cell carcinoma
    Karposi's sarcoma
Allergic dermatitis
Rheumatoid
Steroid

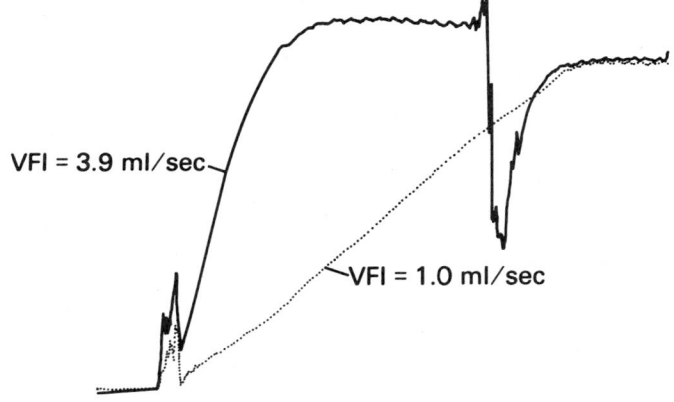

Figure 1 A portion of an air plethysmography study showing the venous filling index (VFI) prior to greater saphenous ligation and stripping *(solid line)* and following operation *(dotted line)* with a return of the VFI to normal.

Table 2 Organism Found in Leg Ulcers (Single or Multiple)

Staphylococcus
Pseudomonas
Streptococcus faecalis
Diphtheroids
Beta-hemolytic streptococci
Escherichia coli
Streptococcus viridans
Anaerobes*

*May be present in 44% of chronically infected wounds.

noninvasive evaluation is essential because some apparent venous ulcers have no evidence of venous insufficiency and, thus, the underlying etiology of these ulcers needs to be further evaluated by a skin biopsy and a dermatologist. In addition, if patients undergo subsequent operative intervention for the correction of venous insufficiency, these studies provide an anatomic road map for the operation and a baseline to compare the effects of operative intervention (Fig. 1).

It is important to realize that infection may be the primary source of nonvenous leg ulcers or may contribute to the persistence of the venous ulcer (Table 2). Biopsy of particularly indolent or painful ulcers for the purpose of deep tissue culture can be an important adjunct that allows tailoring appropriate antibiotic therapy. Surface cultures are not as helpful because all chronic ulcers are colonized. Additionally, in patients who have persistent or recurrent ulcers for years, there is a small possibility of developing squamous cell carcinoma. Biopsy allows accurate diagnosis of this problem.

TREATMENT

Local Wound Care

All wounds must be adequately measured because without accurate measurements it is impossible to assess whether therapy is having a positive effect on wound healing. Our practice is to place a plastic wrap directly over the wound, trace it with a felt-tipped pen, and then retrace on a clear acetate sheet that can be kept in the patient's record. Any obvious cellulitis needs to be treated with the appropriate antibiotics, generally first-generation cephalosporins. Any superficial necrosis can often be removed with a short course of saline wet to dry dressing changes. Extensive necrosis is uncommon but, if present, is best debrided in the operating room. In those patients with severe edema, measures should be undertaken to reduce the edema, in that wound healing is significantly impaired in the presence of edema.

In patients with significant lower extremity edema, sequential graded compression (SGC) may be an important adjunctive procedure that aids in the healing of chronic ulceration. Certain patients with primary venous ulcers, especially when they have had recurrent infections, may develop lymphatic scarring and worsening edema. The SGC aids in reducing edema and has been shown in small series to accelerate healing.[9] These findings have been substantiated in several patients with this problem that we have treated with SGC. Persistent use of graded sequential compression, plus appropriately fitted compression stockings, is usually necessary to maintain healing. The SGC device can be rented, and patients at home can use it on top of already applied compression wraps.

We do not make it a practice to use topical ointments on these ulcers. There is no evidence that they are beneficial, and many patients become sensitized to these ointments and can develop a dermatitis. We believe in the principle of moist wound healing and recently reported our results with Duoderm CGF hydrocolloid dressing. Treatment with the hydrocolloid dressing with compression resulted in ulcer healing rates that were faster than Unna's boot during the initial 4 weeks of therapy and may be faster over a 12 week treatment period.[2]

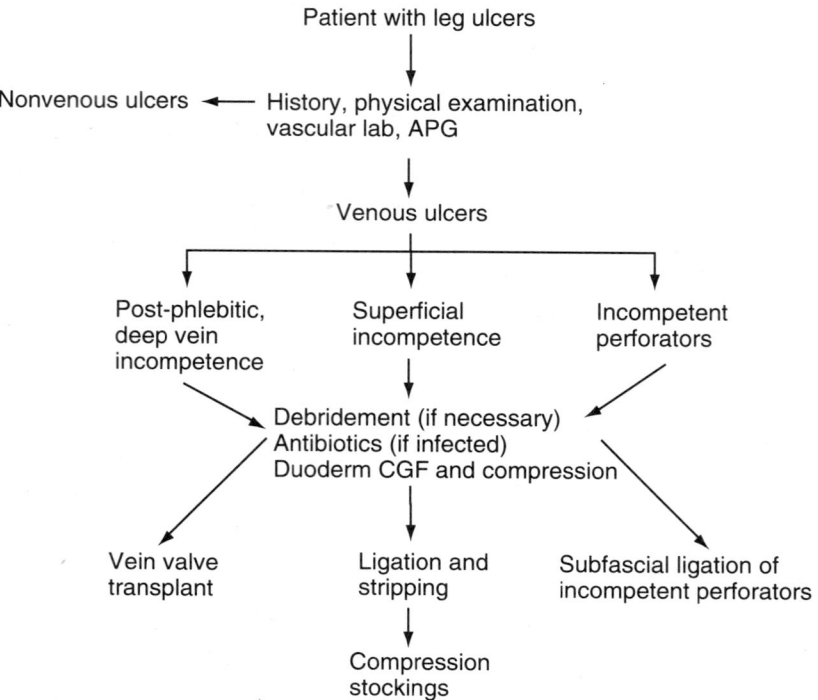

Figure 2 Algorithm for the approach to nonoperative management of venous ulcers. APG, Air plethysmography.

Compression

The mainstay of the treatment of patients with venous insufficiency is compression. It is not clear why compression therapy is beneficial, but venous ulcers unquestionably heal more slowly without compression. Although some feel that compression acts to correct the venous insufficiency, others feel that compression promotes wound healing by reducing edema.

A variety of agents can be used to apply compression therapy, including Unna's boot, Ace wraps, elastic compression stockings, Circaid Velcro wraps, Coban self-adhering wraps, and mechanical pumps. In an ambulatory setting, we feel that a composite dressing consisting of Duoderm CGF hydrocolloid, followed by a properly applied Unna's boot from the foot to just below the knee and an external Coban wrap, provides optimum treatment in the ambulatory patient. The dressings are left on for 1 week. They can be changed more frequently if there is excessive wound drainage, which is often seen with significant edema, prolonged leg dependency, or wound infection. The dressings can be applied by a visiting nurse or a family member with physician supervision every 2 to 3 weeks. In the presence of cellulitis, we temporarily remove compression therapy due to patient discomfort and immediately reapply compression once the cellulitis is resolved.

Routine use of topical or systemic antibiotics is not indicated. Antibiotics should be used only for established cellulitis or invasive wound infection. When infection is suspected, biopsy of the wound is the preferred method of assessment. Because infected ulcers often contain multiple organisms, broad-spectrum antibiotics are employed for treatment of infected ulcers. We have found newer broad-spectrum oral antibiotics (ciprofloxacin) to be useful in the treatment of outpatients with mild to moderate infections. Employment of these antibiotics in a timely fashion can prevent costly hospitalization for more rigorous intravenous therapy. A flow chart summarizes our approach to the nonoperative management of venous ulcers (Fig. 2).

There is some evidence from Great Britain that pentoxifylline may be beneficial in treating patients with venous ulceration. A randomized trial is currently underway in the United States. The routine use of antiplatelet agents or anticoagulants does not have a role in the treatment of venous ulcers.

Patient Education

Patient education plays a key role in the treatment of venous ulceration. The patient must be made to understand the basic principles of venous insufficiency so that they are more compliant with their wraps, periodic leg elevation, and periodic intermittent pneumatic compression, if indicated. Because most venous ulcers are treated on an ambulatory basis, treatment modalities are unsuccessful without active patient involvement and cooperation. Moreover, treatment of venous ulcers can be a prolonged affair, and the use of special assistants, such as a vascular nurse specialist, can be a valuable adjunct to reinforce educational and treatment concepts to patients, as well as monitor their progress.

PREVENTION OF RECURRENCE

Once a venous ulcer is healed, the likelihood of recurrence is great unless the underlying problem is corrected. At a minimum, patients need to be encouraged to wear compression support for the rest of their lives. Any patient who has significant venous disease resulting in a venous ulcer must be made to understand that without continued compression the chance of recurrence is very high. In addition, attention should be directed to any anatomic abnormalities that exist. For example, if the patient has a venous ulcer and has been shown to have an incompetent greater saphenous vein, the saphenous vein should be stripped. Many of these patients have defects at multiple levels, and the policy should be to first correct any abnormalities that exist in the saphenous venous system. If a recurrence develops, attention should be directed to ligation of incompetent perforating veins, repair of deep valvular incompetence, or repair of venous obstruction. We prefer to offer surgical intervention once the ulcer is healed to minimize the risk of wound infection. In selected patients where the wound appears clean, surgical venous correction may be combined with a skin graft procedure.

REFERENCES

1. Schultz LS, Joseph LG. Management of chronic venous insufficiency. Surgery Alert 1992; 12:65–66.
2. Cordts PR, Hanrahan LM, Rodriguez AA, et al. A prospective randomized trial of Unna's boot versus Duoderm CGF hydroactive dressing plus compression in the management of venous leg ulcers. J Vasc Surg 1992; 15:480–486.
3. Cordts PR, Hartono C, LaMorte WW, Menzoian JO. Physiologic similarities between extremities with varicose veins and with chronic venous insufficiency utilizing air plethysmography. Am J Surg 1992; 164:260–264.
4. Negus D, Freidgood A. The effective management of venous ulceration. Br J Surg 1983; 70:623–625.
5. Raju S. Venous insufficiency of the lower limb and stasis ulceration: Changing concepts and management. Ann Surg 1983; 197:688–697.
6. Cranley JJ. Non-operative management of the postphlebitic syndrome and other forms of chronic deep venous insufficiency. In: Rutherford RB, ed. Vascular surgery. 3rd ed. Philadelphia: WB Saunders, 1989:1604.
7. Hanrahan LM, Araki CT, Rodriguez AA, et al. Distribution of valvular incompetence in patients with venous stasis ulceration. J Vasc Surg 1991; 13:805–812.
8. Christopolus D, Nicolaides AN, Szendrog G. Airplethysmography and the effect of elastic compression on venous hemodynamics of the leg. J Vasc Surg 1987; 5:148–159.
9. Penkanmaki K, Kolari P, Kiistala U. Intermittent pneumatic compression treatment for post-thrombotic leg ulcers. Clin Exp Dermatol 1987; 12:350–353.

OPERATIVE TREATMENT OF VENOUS ULCERS

J. LEONEL VILLAVICENCIO, M.D.
JAMES A. COFFEY, M.D.
CHRISTOPHER CUNNINGHAM, M.D.

In most patients with venous ulcers of the legs and normal arterial circulation, the lesions heal when subjected to a program that includes elevation, pressure gradient external compression, daily ulcer washing with normal saline, and skin lubrication. Lymphatic dysfunction contributing to edema has been documented in patients with chronic venous insufficiency and must be controlled in order to achieve ulcer healing.[1] The importance of adequate compression and patient compliance in obtaining and maintaining ulcer healing has been recognized by every practitioner dealing with the problem. One-third of ulcers subjected to this form of treatment recur despite adequate supervision.[2]

Even though some unclear issues remain surrounding the pathophysiology of venous ulceration, evidence links a good number of venous ulcers to well-defined anatomic and pathophysiologic abnormalities that are surgically correctable.[3,4]

It does not make sense to submit an otherwise healthy, active individual to the expense, time, and discomfort of a prolonged conservative treatment if a permanent cure may be achieved through a relatively simple surgical procedure. This is particularly applicable to patients with severe superficial venous reflux or large incompetent perforators.

INVESTIGATION: IMPORTANCE OF AN ACCURATE DIAGNOSIS

Functional and anatomic tests should be used to obtain a complete picture of the venous abnormality. Various diagnostic tests are available for the assessment of venous ulcer patients. The most commonly used (Table 1) have quite different ratings with reference to accuracy, portability, training period, cost, quantitative results, and test type. Among the most useful studies for establishing the crucial diagnosis between primary and secondary venous insufficiency and to clarify the degree of obstruction or reflux present in an extremity are bidirectional Doppler, air plethysmography (APG), strain gauge plethysmography (SPG), duplex scanning, and photoplethysmography (PPG). Ascending and de-

Table 1 Comparison of Noninvasive Tests of the Venous System and Phlebography

| | Accuracy | | | | | | | | Quantitative | |
| | Thigh | | Calf | | | | | | | |
Test	Obstruction	Insufficiency	Obstruction	Insufficiency	Portability	Training Period	Cost	Results	Type
Doppler (CW)	1	4	1	4	5	Long	Low	1	Functional
Duplex ultrasound	5	5	4	5	3	Long	High	3	Anatomic and functional
Plethysmography									
Air (segmental, whole limb)	4	4	3	4	3	Short	Medium	5	Functional
Photo (standard)	1	4	1	4	4	Short	Medium	3	Functional
Photo (calibrated)	3	4	2	4	4	Short	Medium	5	Functional
Strain gauge	4	2	2	1	3	Short	Medium	4	Functional
Phlebography	5	4	4	4	0	Long	High*	2	Anatomic

Scale of 0–5, with 5 as best.
*Invasive.
Modified from The Alexander House Group. Consensus Paper on Venous Leg Ulcers. Phlebologie 1992; 7:48–58.

scending phlebography are utilized to identify anatomy, valve configuration, and reflux or obstruction in patients with venous insufficiency. Obstruction needs to be further investigated and graded using arm-foot venous pressure differential and foot venous pressure elevation induced by hyperemia, as well as direct determination of pressure gradient when applicable.

Ulcers that do not heal despite adequate treatment or that exhibit unusual appearance should be investigated by histologic examination to rule out malignancy.

Once the etiology of the ulcer has been identified by the judicious utilization of noninvasive and invasive methods of diagnosis, a decision must be made on the best form of treatment for the particular patient. All patients must be submitted to an intensive nonoperative treatment of the ulcer in order to improve the skin condition, alleviate the edema, and improve the ulcer as much as possible. The sequelae of venous hypertension, eczema, cellulitis, and liposclerosis, whether they are postphlebitic or due to primary venous insufficiency, improve rapidly with two simple measures: (1) bed rest in the Trendelenburg position and (2) firm elastic compression.

Conservative management is the treatment of choice in elderly, sedentary patients who have ulcers with relatively good subcutaneous tissue and who have shown a tendency to heal promptly. This form of treatment should be recommended also for patients who have severe chronic illnesses such as renal, hepatic, or cardiac disease or malignant tumors; and for patients with obesity, arthritis, achilles tendon fibrosis, or any other rheumatic type of disease. These patients do not use the calf pump mechanism effectively and could not comply appropriately with recommended postoperative measures.

After 6 to 12 weeks of conservative treatment, most ulcers either heal or show marked improvement. If the ulcer is of relatively short duration and the soft tissues

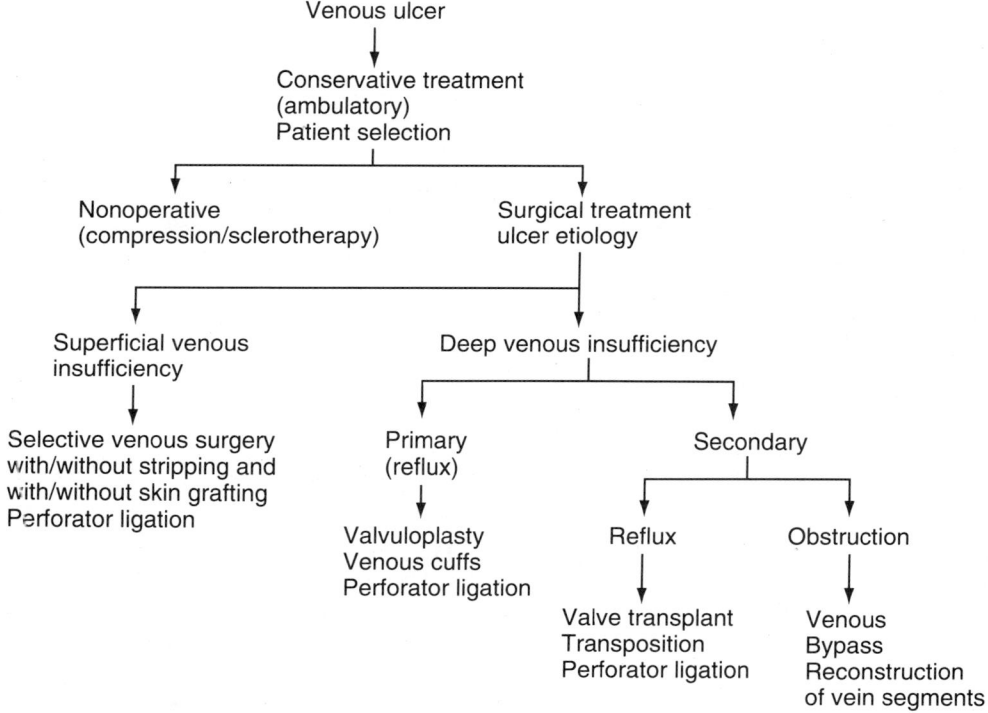

Figure 1 Guidelines for surgical management of patients with venous ulcers. Surgical management may be considered in active, relatively young individuals with recurrent ulceration, severe lipodermatosclerosis and lifestyle-impairing symptoms. Selective venous surgery with or without skin grafting is the procedure of choice in patients with primary superficial venous insufficiency. This type of varicose veins usually have a normal deep venous system. Skin grafting may be considered to accelerate healing in very large ulcers. After successful skin grafting, the surgical treatment of the underlying venous problem should be undertaken. By contrast, there are patients whose problem is deep venous insufficiency, which can be either primary or secondary to deep venous thrombosis. The group with primary deep valve incompetence responds well to valvuloplasty of the incompetent valve(s). There is documentation of long-term competence in studies extending 15 years and beyond. In primary incompetence, the hemodynamic problem is purely reflux. This is in sharp contrast with the pathology observed in secondary or post-thrombotic venous incompetence, in which valves are scarred, weakened, and deformed and often there is a combination of obstruction and reflux as sequelae of deep venous thrombosis and erratic recanalization. This type of disease can be corrected only by valve transplantation or transposition techniques. Typically, recurrences in this group are higher than in primary venous insufficiency. Severe obstruction of major venous trunks is treated with bypass, using either prosthesis or autogenous conduits, with or without a temporary arteriovenous fistula.

around it are fairly normal, external compression while the patient is ambulatory usually results in healing. Once optimal healing has been achieved, the decision of continuing indefinitely with conservative treatment or having the patient undergo operation should be made.

SURGICAL MANAGEMENT

Surgical management should be considered in active, compliant, and relatively young individuals who use their calf pump mechanism and have impaired lifestyles. Particularly suited for this type of treatment are individuals with saphenous venous insufficiency. There is a group of relatively young, active individuals in whom the tissue surrounding the ulcer is the site of chronic induration and calcification. The degree of induration in these ulcers may be very severe. The ulcer area is transformed into a firm plaque, and no known compression system can obliterate the large venous channels going through it. Operation in these patients offers the best possibility for long-term healing. These type of lesions are usually found among the patients with post-thrombotic sequelae.

Certain factors should be taken into consideration and steps followed in selecting a surgical procedure (Fig. 1).

Primary Superficial Venous Insufficiency

This group comprises patients with incompetence of the greater or lesser saphenous systems and large incompetent perforators. If reflux at the greater or lesser saphenous systems is identified, and the duplex scanning or phlebography documents an abnormal, dilated, tortuous, and damaged venous trunk, the greater or lesser saphenous veins must be stripped and all the large, incompetent perforators ligated. Such veins must be identified preoperatively by carefully marking the location of incompetent perforators, as well as the areas of varicose vein clusters. If stripping is considered, it should be done from the saphenofemoral junction to a point just below the knee. This technique has decreased the incidence of saphenous neuritis and does not increase the recurrence rate.

The ulcer area should be considered separately. If the ulcer area is transformed into a firm plaque and there is severe lipodermatosclerosis, en bloc resection of the ulcer, including fascia and subfascial ligation of incompetent perforator veins, must be performed (Fig. 2). The clean surgical wound can be treated as a noninfected ulcer on an ambulatory basis. Six to 8 weeks later, skin grafting should be performed. Cosmetic results are far superior with delayed skin grafting than with immediate intraoperative grafting.

The long-term results of operation for venous ulcers secondary to primary superficial venous incompetence are excellent. Healing in 90% of the patients at 5 years has been reported.

Primary Deep Venous Insufficiency: Interruption of Incompetent Perforating Veins

Incompetent perforator veins may be localized by using the color duplex scanner, ascending phlebography, and bidirectional Doppler. Incompetent perforators are carefully marked with an indelible marker. A 12 cm incision is carried out 3 cm parallel to the medial border of the tibia beginning behind the internal malleolus and extending to the junction of the medial and lower thirds of the leg. Whenever possible, the incision should be posterior to the ulcer area (Fig. 3). The incision is carried down to the fascia. Using three-pronged blunt retractors, the medial and posterior flaps are elevated and dissected, searching for perforators (Fig. 4). If the subcutaneous tissue is in good condition and the induration of

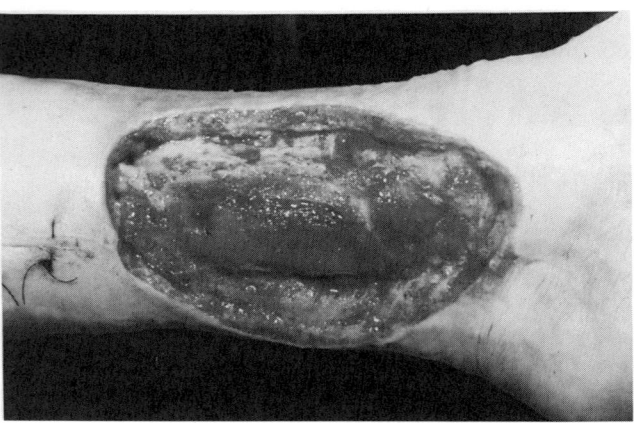

Figure 2 Clean ulcer bed after en bloc resection of infected ulcer and ligation of perforators under the ulcer bed. Healthy granulating tissue fills the defect in 4 to 6 weeks. Skin grafting completes the treatment.

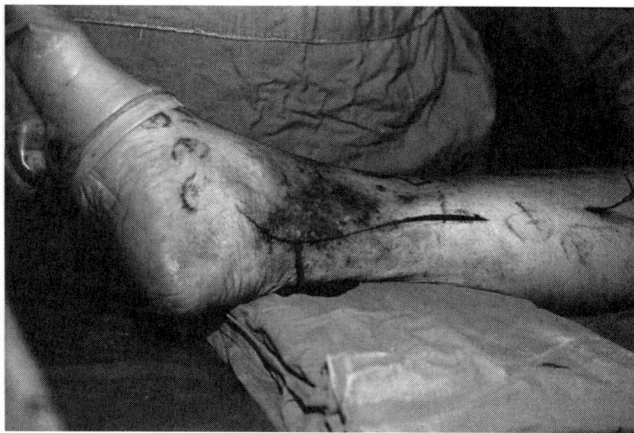

Figure 3 Cockett incision. Incision along the Cockett line utilized for ligation of incompetent perforators localized under the ulcer bed. To reach the large perforators located behind the medial malleolus and proximal third of the foot (*circles*), the incision needs to be curved around the malleolus and extended toward the foot.

the skin is not severe, perforator dissection and identification should be done extrafascially. If this approach is selected, care should be taken to avoid extensive flap undermining, which may lead to flap necrosis. This is the most common mistake by inexperienced operators. There are usually one to three large perforator veins in this area; they are especially large under the ulcer bed (see Fig. 4). The perforators are divided and ligated with absorbable material.

In patients with severe lipodermatosclerosis, the operation must be done subfascially. In this approach, the flaps are elevated, including fascia, and the dissection is carried out toward the posterior edge of the tibia medially and to the lesser saphenous vein, posteriorly. Once the perforators have been ligated, the skin edges should be approximated using a nonpinching technique, and the wound closed with interrupted 3-0 monofilament sutures. Good apposition of the skin edges is essential, and for this reason stapling is not recommended. In patients in whom the ulcerated area is severely scarred, sclerosed, and woody, the entire damaged area should be resected en bloc, including fascia. The procedure of perforator division and ligation is carried out at the same time that the flap containing the ulcer is elevated and excised. The ulcer bed is left open, covered only with a thin layer of Vaseline gauze. Skin grafting is performed 4 to 6 weeks later on a healthy granulating ulcer bed.

The long-term results of subfascial ligation of perforators are quite reasonable (Table 2). The recurrence rate of the subfascial procedures varies from 9.5% to 55% at 5 years. However, in none of the reported series, including our own, has an analysis of the hemodynamic problem leading to the ulcers been made. In our experience, ulcers in patients with hemodynamic manifestations of obstruction are more difficult to heal than in patients who have reflux as their predominant problem. Some patients have a combination of perforator incompetence and deep venous valvular insufficiency. In this group, a careful assessment of the magnitude and severity of the valvular reflux, as well as the size and relative importance of the role of the incompetent perforators, should be made. If the analysis of the clinical and hemodynamic data suggest that both factors are significant, then the surgical procedure must include correction of both hemodynamic problems. There are reports in the literature indicating that the ulcer may recur after subfascial procedures if severe valvular reflux was not recognized and if a successful

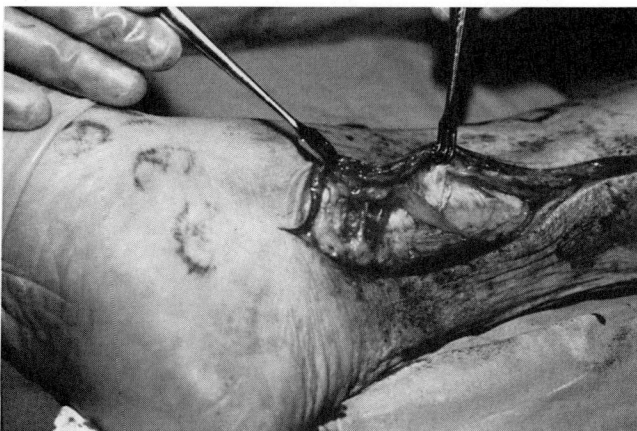

Figure 4 Same patient as Figure 3. Skin and fascia have been elevated with three-prong blunt retractors. Two large (greater than 3.5 mm), previously identified incompetent perforators connecting with the posterior tibial veins can be observed under the ulcer bed near the distal end of the incision. Three smaller perforators were interrupted at the upper third of the incision. This patient healed uneventfully and has been ulcer-free for more than 10 years.

Table 2 Long-Term* Results after Subfascial Perforator Ligation for Venous Ulceration

Author (Reference)	Year	Number	Healed (%)	Wound Complications (%)	Recurrence (%)
Silver, et al	1971	28	100	14	10
Thurston and Williams	1973	89	100	12	13
Bowen	1975	55	56	44	32
Burnand, et al	1976	41	100	NR	55†
DePalma	1979	53	100	2	6
Hyde, et al	1981	109	100	15	24
Negus and Friedgood	1983	77	100	22	13
Johnson, et al	1985	37	100	14	41 (3 yr)‡
					51 (5 yr)‡
Cikrit, et al	1988	27	100	26	22

*Mean of 3 years or greater.
†Length of follow-up not given.
‡Life-table recurrence.
NR, not reported.
Modified from: Mayberry JC, Moneta GL, Taylor LM, Porter JM. Nonoperative Treatment of Venous Stasis Ulcer. In: Bergan JJ, Yao JST, eds. Venous disorders. Philadelphia: WB Saunders, 1991:381.

valvuloplasty is followed by ulcer recurrence secondary to perforator incompetence that was not corrected during the first operation.

Current concepts on utilization of skin grafts in venous ulcers have been summarized in the Consensus Paper on Venous Leg Ulcers:[6] "Success in healing leg ulcers can be achieved both by split-skin grafting and by pinch-grafting. Skin grafting is seldom required for small ulcers, but for larger ulcers the technique may be cost effective as a mean of achieving shorter healing times. The recurrence rate following skin grafting is not high provided that the procedure is integrated into the general plan for managing the patient's venous disease and is accompanied by appropriate venous surgery and compression therapy."

REFERENCES

1. Hammond SL, Gomez ER, Collins PS, et al. Involvement of the lymphatic system in chronic venous insufficiency. In: Bergan JJ, Yao JST, eds. Venous disorders. Philadelphia: WB Saunders, 1991:333.
2. Mayberry JC, Moneta GL, Taylor LM, Porter JM. Non-operative treatment of venous stasis ulcer. In: Bergan JJ, Kistner RL, eds. Atlas of venous surgery. Philadelphia: WB Saunders, 1992:81.
3. Negus D, Friedgood A. The effective management of venous ulceration. Br J Surg 1983; 70:623–627.
4. Sethia KK, Darke S. Long saphenous incompetence as a cause of venous ulceration. Br J Surg 1984; 71:754–755.
5. Villavicencio JL, Rich NM, Salander JM, et al. Leg ulcers of venous origin. In: Cameron JL, ed. Current surgical therapy. 3rd ed. Philadelphia: BC Decker, 1989:610.
6. The Alexander House Group. Consensus paper on venous leg ulcers. Phlebologie 1992; 7:48–58.

SURGICAL TREATMENT OF ACUTE ILIOFEMORAL THROMBOSIS

BO EKLÖF, M.D., Ph.D.
ROBERT L. KISTNER, M.D.

The objectives of treatment of acute iliofemoral venous thrombosis (IFVT) are to prevent fatal pulmonary embolism (PE); to prevent further swelling of the leg with development of an acute compartment syndrome, which can lead to phlegmasia cerulea dolens, venous gangrene, and loss of limb; and to prevent the post-thrombotic syndrome. Based on our combined experience of more than 300 patients with acute IFVT treated surgically, thrombectomy is the treatment of choice if the history of swelling of the thigh indicating iliac vein obstruction is less than 7 days and the activity expectancy of the patient is more than 10 years.[1,2]

SURGICAL TREATMENT

Diagnosis and Preoperative Preparation

Evaluation must detect the proximal extension of the iliofemoral thrombus. Duplex scanning verifies the presence of the thrombus with a high degree of accuracy but can rarely determine the central extent of the thrombus. A femoral phlebogram from the contralateral side is usually required to achieve this purpose. Ventilation-perfusion ($\dot{V}/\dot{Q}$) lung scanning is routinely performed preoperatively to be used as baseline information. When the diagnosis is established, heparin sodium infusion is started. Two units of blood are ordered for routine femoral thrombectomy, 6 units if the caval approach is considered. The cell-saver autotransfusion device is used during the procedure. Prophylactic antibiotics are given to reduce the incidence of wound infection in the groin.

Technique

The operation is performed using general endotracheal anesthesia.[3] A longitudinal incision is made in the groin to expose the long saphenous vein, which is followed to its confluence with the common femoral vein, which is dissected up to the inguinal ligament. The superficial femoral artery 3 to 4 cm below the femoral bifurcation is prepared for construction of the arteriovenous fistula (AVF). Further dissection depends upon the etiology of the IFVT.

In primary IFVT with subsequent distal progression of the thrombus, a transverse venotomy is made in the common femoral vein, and a venous Fogarty thrombectomy catheter is passed through the thrombus into the inferior vena cava (IVC). The balloon is inflated, and repeated passages with the Fogarty catheter are performed until no more thrombotic material is extracted. With the balloon inflated in the common iliac vein, a suction catheter is introduced to the level of the internal iliac vein to evacuate thrombi from the internal iliac vein. Backflow is not a reliable sign of clot clearance because a proximal valve in the external iliac vein may be present in 25% of patients, preventing retrograde flow in a cleared vein. Then again, backflow can be excellent from the internal iliac vein and its tributaries, despite a remaining occlusion of the common iliac vein. Therefore, an operative completion phlebogram is mandatory. An alternative is the use of an angioscope, which enables removal of residual thrombus material under direct vision.

The distal thrombus in the leg is removed by manual massage of the leg starting at the foot. The Fogarty catheter can sometimes be gently advanced in retrograde fashion. The aim is to remove all fresh thrombi from the leg. In IFVT secondary to ascending thrombosis from the calf, the thrombus in the superficial femoral vein (SFV) is often adherent to the vein wall and the valves are damaged. The objective is to restore patency and preserve valvular function. If iliac patency is established but the thrombus in the SFV is too old to remove, it is preferable to ligate the SFV. Recanalization otherwise leads to valvular incompetence and subsequent reflux. In a 13 year follow-up after SFV ligation, we found excellent clinical and physiologic results without the post-thrombotic syndrome.[4]

If blood flow in the SFV cannot be re-established, distal extension of the incision is recommended to explore the orifices of the deep femoral branches. These are isolated and venous blood flow is restored with a small Fogarty catheter. The SFV is ligated. The distinction between primary and secondary IFVT can be made by duplex scanning or ascending phlebography documenting persistent blood flow around the thrombus in the femoropopliteal vein in primary IFVT.

The venotomy is closed with continuous polypropylene suture and an AVF is constructed by anastomosing the long saphenous vein end-to-side to the superficial femoral artery. An operative phlebogram is performed through a catheter inserted in a branch of the AVF. After a satisfactory completion phlebogram, the wound is closed in layers without drainage.

If phlegmasia cerulea dolens or venous gangrene is present, the operation is started with fasciotomy of the calf compartments. If there is extension of the thrombus into the IVC, it is approached transperitoneally through a subcostal incision. The IVC is exposed by reflecting the duodenum and ascending colon medially. Depending upon the phlebographic findings relative to the central extension of the thrombus, the IVC is controlled, usually just below the renal veins. The IVC is opened and the thrombus is removed by massage, especially of the iliac venous system. If the iliofemoral segment is involved, the operation is continued in the groin as described previously. When celiotomy is contraindicated in patients in poor condition, a caval filter of the Greenfield type can be introduced before the thrombectomy to protect against fatal PE.

Heparin sodium therapy is continued at least for 5 days postoperatively, and sodium warfarin is started the first postoperative day and continued for 6 months. The patient is ambulant the day after the operation and wearing a compression stocking.

If there is immediate reocclusion of the iliac vein resulting in a compromised outflow from the leg, previously uninvolved or cleared distal veins, and a picture of phlegmasia cerulea dolens, reconstruction with a synthetic femorofemoral cross-over bypass graft is considered to prevent retrograde formation of thrombus and subsequent valve destruction. The patient is usually discharged on the tenth postoperative day to return after 6 weeks for closure of the AVF.

Role and Closure of Temporary AVF

The objectives of a temporary AVF are to increase blood flow in the thrombectomized segment to prevent rethrombosis, to allow time for healing of the endothelium, and to promote development of collaterals in case of incomplete clearance or immediate rethrombosis of the iliac segment. Closure of the AVF is performed after 6 weeks. In the early years of our practice, fistulas were closed using local anesthesia by ligation and division. We sometimes had more problems with the closure of the AVF than the original operation. With the new percutaneous technique developed by Endrys and associates these problems have almost vanished.[5] Through a puncture of the contralateral femoral artery, a catheter is positioned at the fistula level, through which the AVF is occluded by a detachable balloon or coil. Prior to inflation and release of the balloon or coil, an arteriophlebogram can be performed to evaluate the patency of the iliac veins (Fig. 1). The arteriophlebogram is of prognostic value because more than 10% of patients may have a significant stenosis of the iliac vein despite initial successful operation. A transvenous percutaneous angioplasty with stenting can be performed under the protection of the AVF, which is closed 4 weeks later after repeat arteriophlebogram.

Mortality

In our series of more than 300 patients, 2 died. One patient died of acute respiratory failure due to chronic pulmonary fibrosis. Autopsy did not document any fresh PE. The other patient had undetected cirrhosis of the liver. He also had IVC extension of the thrombus. This patient died of multiorgan failure 32 days postoperatively following intra-abdominal hemorrhage due to overanticoagulation.

Pulmonary Embolism

Our study identified no fatal PE in the perioperative period. To avoid this problem, it is important to exclude extension of the thrombus into the IVC, which can be fractured during manipulation with the Fogarty catheter. Instead of using a separate balloon catheter to occlude the IVC, we routinely ask the anesthetist to apply positive endotracheal pressure (PEEP) during the operative manipulation of the thrombotic vein. In a retrospective study using V̇/Q̇ lung scan in 79 patients preoperatively, 50 positive scans (63%) were found, 20 of which showed large defects. In 18 of the 50, the PE was the presenting symptom; in 23 the PE was silent. New emboli occurred during the course of treatment in 8%.[6] In a prospective randomized study, positive perfusion scans were found at admission in 45% of patients, with additional defects detected after 1 and 4 weeks in the conservatively treated group in 11% and 12%, respectively, and in the thrombectomized group in 20% and none, respectively.[7] No additional perfusion defects developed after

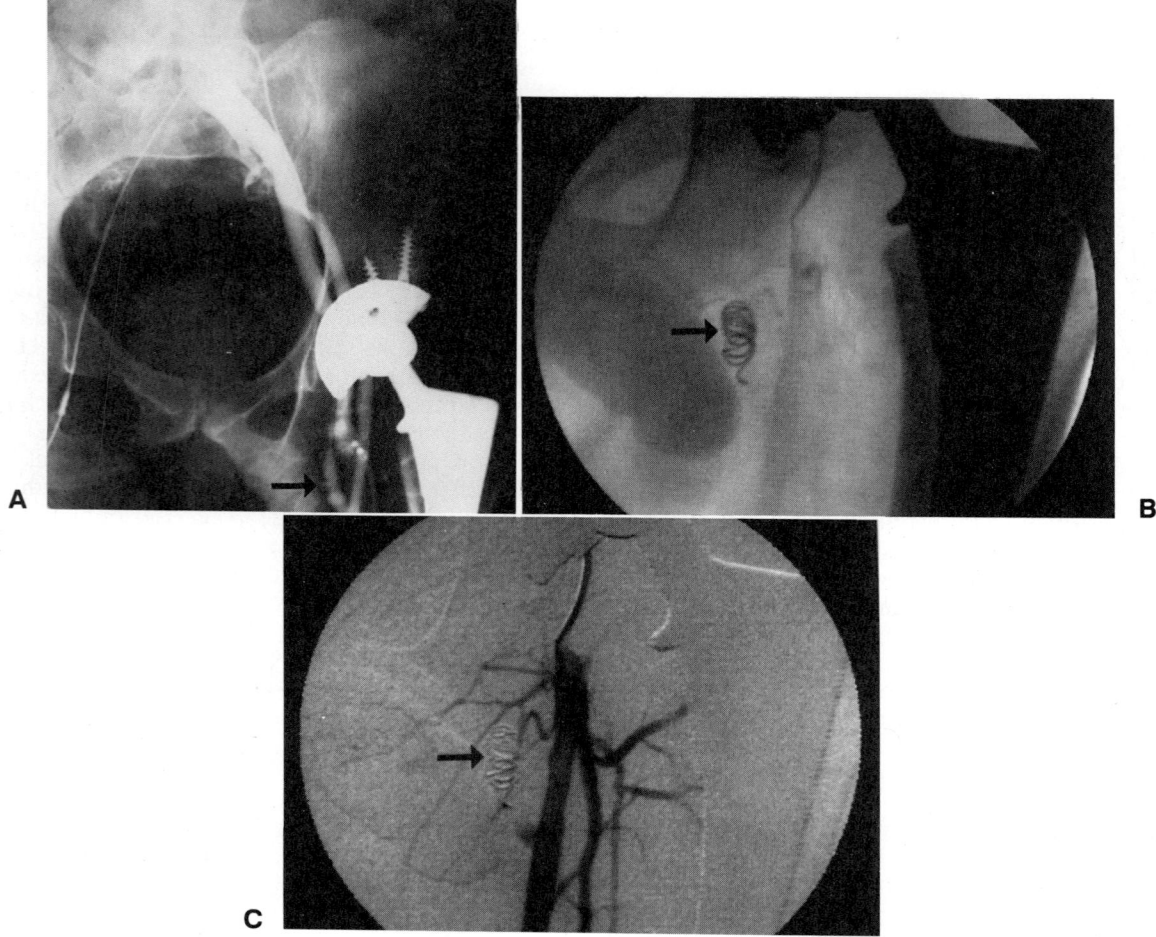

Figure 1 *A,* Arteriophlebography of the left external iliac artery with catheter introduced from the right femoral artery 8 weeks after thrombectomy showing well-functioning arteriovenous fistula (AVF, *arrow*) with normal common femoral vein, external and common iliac vein, and distal inferior vena cava. *B,* A coil is deposited in the AVF *(arrow). C,* Repeat arteriogram shows the arterial stump and the occluded AVF *(arrow).*

the first postoperative week following thrombectomy with AVF. Because the AVF effectively prevented rethrombosis, it was assumed that the fistula was one reason for the low incidence of postoperative PE.

Earlier reports of high mortality due to fatal PE have not been borne out in our experience. Possible reasons for the decreased risk of significant symptomatic and fatal PE with the present technique are (1) careful selection of patients; (2) preoperative documentation by phlebography of the central extension of the thrombus, requiring an extended surgical approach if the IVC is involved; (3) use of PEEP during operation to decrease the risk of perioperative PE; (4) operative phlebography or venoscopy to prove clearance of the iliac vein; and (5) utilization of an AVF to decrease risk of immediate rethrombosis and subsequent PE.

Early Morbidity after Thrombectomy

The rate of early rethrombosis of the iliac vein varies. In our retrospective study, it was 34% in primary IFVT (8 of 24) and 18% in secondary IFVT (27 of 33) without use of temporary AVF.[1] In the prospective randomized study using an AVF, 13% had early rethrombosis of the iliac vein.[8] This low rate of early rethrombosis using a temporary AVF was confirmed by a collected series of 421 patients documenting 15% rethrombosis.[2] Important factors to avoid early rethrombosis are (1) rarely operating if the symptoms of iliac obstruction are beyond 7 days; (2) use of the Fogarty catheter to clear the external and common iliac veins with special consideration of the internal iliac vein; (3) direct approach when the IVC is involved; (4) intraoperative phlebography or venoscopy to document clearance of the iliac vein; (5) liberal and early use of decompressive leg fasciotomy in patients with phlegmasia cerulea dolens; (6) use of a temporary AVF; (7) early ambulation wearing compression stockings; and (8) carefully monitored postoperative anticoagulant therapy.

Postoperative bleeding with hematoma formation in the groin was not uncommon, despite drainage of the wound, as all patients were anticoagulated with heparin sodium. Groin infection was very common until preoperative hygiene was improved and prophylactic antibiotics started. Still, lymphatic drainage is seen, which usually ceases after 2 to 3 weeks.

In two patients, the AVF did cause high-output cardiac failure, which subsided after closure of the fistula. Both operations were performed in elderly patients with previously known compromised cardiac function. One objection to the fistula has been the assumption of increased venous pressure leading to swelling of the lower limb. No increase of the iliac vein pressure was found if the outflow was normal. If there was a stenosis of the vein central to the fistula, the pressure was higher. This stresses the importance of clearing the proximal vein.

LATE RESULTS

Follow-up after an average 4 years of 77 patients, of whom 33 patients with primary IFVT had thrombectomy and 44 patients with secondary IFVT had thrombectomy and interruption of the SFV, documented good or excellent clinical results in 86%.[1] A strong relationship between phlebographic patency and good or excellent clinical result was noted in 57 patients. There was a 75% overall patency of the iliac vein, with 66% in primary IFVT and 82% in secondary IFVT. In nonadherent clots, a 92% iliac patency was documented, compared to 45% patency in patients with adherent clots. This study also suggested that patients with early, nonadherent clots can expect a 70% to 75% chance of having a good or excellent, functional extremity after 4 years and only a 2% chance of developing the post-thrombotic syndrome. The development of a post-thrombotic syndrome takes many years, so the final clinical outcome is unclear in most reports. In the prospective randomized study from Sweden, a highly significant difference in asymptomatic patients was found in the group undergoing thrombectomy (42%) versus 7% in the conservative group.[8] At 5 years follow-up 37% of the patients undergoing operation were free of symptoms, compared to 18% in the conservative group.[9] The 6 month iliac patency in the randomized study was 76% in the group undergoing operation, compared to 35% in the conservative group. After 5 years, radionucleotide phlebography documented a patency of 77% in the surgical group. The iliac vein was normal in 71% of patients in the surgical group, compared to 30% in the conservative group.

Very few reports contain information on postoperative valvular competence. It is vital to preserve the valves and retain a normal calf muscle pump function in order to prevent the development of the post-thrombotic syndrome. In the randomized study, after 6 months we found patent and competent valves in the femoropopliteal segment in 52% of the surgical group compared to 26% in the conservatively treated group, using phlebography with Valsalva, which correlated with Doppler ultrasound. After 5 years there was a decreased risk for developing severe post-thrombotic syndrome after operation and more pronounced venous hypertension among patients treated with anticoagulants only. The surgical patients had a significant reduction in ambulatory venous pressure, improved venous emptying as shown by plethysmography, and a better calf pump function with less reflux as measured by foot volumetry. Taking the results of all functional tests, at the 5 year follow-up 36% of surgical patients had a normal venous function, compared to 11% of those conservatively treated.

Of 52 patients with extension of IFVT into the IVC that were treated from 1983 to 1989, 27 underwent surgical removal of the thrombus combined with anticoagulation, and 25 were treated with anticoagulation only.[5] At follow-up after a mean of 23 months, the surgical group was substantially better, with asymptomatic legs in 56% versus 25%, venous ulcers in none versus 15%, and secondary varicose veins in 6% versus 30%. These clinical findings were confirmed by functional tests using photoplethysmography and Doppler ultrasound. The most striking finding was that all patients without surgical removal of the caval thrombosis developed venous thrombosis in the opposite leg during follow-up. This suggested that venous thrombectomy may better preserve valve function and prevent contralateral retrograde thrombus formation by removal of the caval outflow obstruction.[10]

REFERENCES

1. Kistner RL, Sparkuhl MD. Surgery in acute and chronic venous disease. Surgery 1979; 85:31–43.
2. Eklöf B, Juhan C. Revival of thrombectomy in the management of acute iliofemoral venous thrombosis. Contemp Surg 1992; 40: 21–30.
3. Eklöf B, Juhan C, Neglén P. Iliofemoral thrombectomy and temporary arteriovenous fistula. In: Bergan JJ, Kistner RL, eds. Atlas of venous surgery. Philadelphia: WB Saunders, 1992:223.
4. Masuda EM, Kistner RL, Ferris EB. Long-term effects of superficial femoral vein ligation: Thirteen-year follow-up. J Vasc Surg 1992; 16:741–749.
5. Endrys J, Eklöf B, Neglén P, et al. Percutaneous balloon occlusion of surgical arteriovenous fistulae following venous thrombectomy. Cardiovasc Intervent Radiol 1989; 12:226–229.
6. Kistner RL, Ball JJ, Nordyke RA, Freeman GC. Incidence of pulmonary embolism in the course of thrombophlebitits of the lower extremities. Am J Surg 1972; 124:169–176.
7. Plate G, Ohlin P, Eklöf B. Pulmonary embolism in acute iliofemoral venous thrombosis. Br J Surg 1985; 72:912–915.
8. Plate G, Einarsson E, Ohlin P, et al. Thrombectomy with temporary arteriovenous fistula: The treatment of choice in acute iliofemoral venous thrombosis. J Vasc Surg 1984; 1:867–876.
9. Plate G, Akesson H, Einarsson E, et al. Long-term results of venous thrombectomy combined with a temporary arterio-venous fistula. Eur J Vasc Surg 1990; 4:483–489.
10. Neglén P, Nazzal M, al-Hassan H, et al. Surgical removal of an inferior vena cava thrombus. Eur J Vasc Surg 1992; 6:78–82.

NONOPERATIVE TREATMENT OF ACUTE ILIOFEMORAL AND CAVAL THROMBOSIS

MICHAEL J. KIKTA, M.D.
DONALD SILVER, M.D.

Thromboses of the iliofemoral veins and inferior vena cava (IVC), if untreated, are associated with a 40% incidence of pulmonary embolism (PE), of which 20% may be fatal.[1] Patients who recover from the thrombotic episodes are at risk for developing lower extremity venous insufficiency. Nearly 90% of patients with iliofemoral thromboses treated with anticoagulation develop venous ulcerations within 5 years.[2] The goal of therapy is to prevent PE, re-establish venous patency, and preserve venous valvular function. Nonoperative management includes aggressive anticoagulation or, with increasing frequency, a combination of thrombolytic and anticoagulation therapy.

CLINICAL FEATURES

Iliofemoral and caval thromboses occur in 15% to 20% of patients with deep venous thrombosis.[3,4] Most of the thromboses arise from proximal extension of distal deep vein thromboses (DVT), although up to 20% may occur as isolated iliac or caval thromboses.[1] Trauma, major operations, compression of the IVC or iliac veins by tumor or other masses, indwelling catheters for venous access, and intracaval filter devices are known causes of thrombosis. Right-heart catheterization is frequently associated with thrombosis in infants. The venous stasis that occurs after myocardial infarction, stroke, serious illness, and malignancy predisposes these patients to venous thromboembolism. Iliac vein thrombosis occurs more commonly on the left than on the right. The right iliac artery crosses anterior to the left iliac vein, occasionally compressing it against the pelvic brim and causing stasis and thrombosis, as the May-Thurner syndrome. Other conditions associated with iliofemoral and caval thrombosis include collagen vascular diseases, retroperitoneal fibrosis, radiation therapy, and hypercoagulable states.

Patients with iliofemoral and caval thromboses may present with hypovolemic shock due to the loss of fluid from the intravascular compartment that occurs with the formation of massive edema. The edema can cause lower extremity compartmental hypertension, which may lead to a decreased arterial flow with ischemia and tissue loss. A temporary anemia may occur from the sequestration of red blood cells into the thrombus. Lower extremity pain and swelling are present in 70% of patients with acute iliofemoral and caval thrombosis. Back pain, probably due to venous distention or accompanying inflammation, may be a sign of caval thrombosis. Caval thrombosis extending into the renal veins may cause renal failure. More proximal extension may cause hepatic vein thrombosis, with ascites and hepatomegaly, as the Budd-Chiari syndrome.

DIAGNOSIS

Impedance plethysmography is highly accurate for the diagnosis of iliofemoral venous and caval thromboses, but its use has largely been supplanted by venous color flow duplex scanning. Venous duplex scanning is both sensitive (90% to 95%) and specific (90% to 100%) for the diagnosis of iliofemoral and popliteal DVT. Duplex scanning is also useful for the detection of major pelvic and intra-abdominal venous thromboses, although visualization of the iliac veins and the IVC may be hindered by overlying bowel gas and obesity. Nonadherent thromboses can generally be discerned from adherent ones, but sometimes a moving thrombus is difficult to differentiate from flowing blood.

Phlebography remains the gold standard for the diagnosis of iliofemoral and caval thromboses. Complete visualization of extensive iliofemoral and caval thromboses may require contrast injections from the ipsilateral foot, ipsilateral femoral vein, contralateral femoral vein, and the proximal IVC catheterized through the internal jugular vein. Catheters placed into or adjacent to the thrombus may be used for administration of thrombolytic agents. If appropriate, percutaneous placement of a vena cava filter can also be done following phlebography. Computed tomography and magnetic resonance imaging also effectively document large iliofemoral and caval thromboses. The accuracy of these modalities has not been determined and their expense does not justify their use in preference to duplex scanning or phlebography for the diagnosis of iliofemoral and IVC thrombosis.

NONOPERATIVE THERAPY

Patients presenting with hypovolemia should be resuscitated while specific therapy for the iliofemoral or caval thrombosis is instituted. Pulmonary embolism must also be ruled out in patients presenting with cardiorespiratory compromise.

Anticoagulation

The standard specific treatment for iliofemoral and caval thrombosis is anticoagulation with heparin sodium. Heparin sodium is given, unless contraindicated by bleeding diatheses, heparin sensitivity, or the presence of antibodies to heparin. Heparin sodium accelerates the action of antithrombin III (AT III), which inhibits activated clotting factors II, IX, X, XI, and XII. Large doses of heparin sodium are necessary initially to stop the ongoing thrombosis. Patients usually receive an initial intravenous bolus of 150 to 200 units/kg of heparin sodium, which is followed by a continuous infusion at a rate of 15 to 20 units/kg/hour. The activated partial thromboplastin time (aPTT) should be maintained at 1.5 to 1.8 times the normal value. This may require early repeat boluses of heparin sodium or infusions at rates substantially higher than initially estimated. The aPTT should initially be repeated at 4 to 6 hour intervals until the desired level of anticoagulation is achieved. When a stable heparin sodium dose is determined, the aPTT is determined at least twice daily.

Adjusted dose subcutaneous heparin sodium has been found to be as effective as intravenous heparin sodium therapy for the treatment of DVT.[5] The initial dose of subcutaneous heparin is 250 units/kg, given twice daily. This dose is adjusted to maintain the aPTT measured approximately 30 minutes prior to the next dose of heparin sodium at 1.5 to 2 times normal. We prefer intravenous heparin sodium administration, as do most surgeons, because its effect is more easily titrated than subcutaneous heparin sodium and bleeding complications are more easily avoided. Heparin sodium therapy should be maintained until active thrombosis has stopped and adequate oral anticoagulation is established, usually 5 to 10 days.

Despite the high initial doses required to stop ongoing thrombosis, complications from heparin sodium administration are relatively infrequent. Major bleeding episodes occur in fewer than 5% of patients. They are more common in elderly women, in postoperative patients, and in patients with underlying hemostatic defects. Most major bleeding episodes occur after the first 48 to 72 hours of heparin sodium administration, when heparin requirements are decreasing as the thrombosis is controlled. The heparin sodium dose must be decreased accordingly to prevent bleeding. Bleeding is uncommon unless the aPTT exceeds 3 times normal for several hours.

If the thrombosis continues despite the usual dose of heparin sodium, the aPTT remains low, and the platelet count is normal, then the patient is likely to have an AT III deficiency. Many AT III–deficient patients can be successfully anticoagulated with high doses of heparin sodium. If this is ineffective, AT III supplements with AT III concentrate or fresh frozen plasma, 2 units every 12 hours, should be given. Patients with AT III deficiency who develop recurrent DVT should be anticoagulated with sodium warfarin for life.

Heparin-induced thrombocytopenia develops in 4% to 5% (range 0.9% to 31%) of patients. Thromboembolic complications occur in 18% to 61% of patients with heparin-induced thrombocytopenia, and hemorrhagic complications occur in less than 5% of patients. Patients receiving heparin sodium should have platelet counts monitored daily. A platelet count of less than 100,000/mm^3, a greater than 50% decrease in platelet count, the development of resistance to anticoagulation, or the development of new thromboembolic or, rarely, bleeding episodes while the patient is receiving heparin sodium suggests that the patient has developed heparin-induced thrombocytopenia. The administration of heparin sodium should be stopped and the plasma assayed for heparin-associated antiplatelet antibodies. Aspirin (325 mg twice daily) and dextran (10 to 40 ml/hour of 10% dextran-40) should be given until anticoagulation can be established with sodium warfarin. The platelet count usually returns to normal in 2 to 4 days. Hypersensitivity reactions (urticaria, bronchospasm, and anaphylaxis) occur in fewer than 2% of patients who receive heparin sodium. They should be treated with antihistamines and discontinuation of heparin sodium therapy.

Ancrod has been used for anticoagulation in patients in whom heparin sodium cannot be given.[6] Ancrod enzymatically cleaves fibrinogen to form a product that cannot form a stable clot. Blood viscosity is lowered. Other proteins of the coagulation and fibrinolytic systems are unaltered. A 70 unit bolus given intravenously over 2 to 4 hours causes the fibrinogen level to fall into the therapeutic range, between 20 and 50 mg/dl, for ancrod anticoagulation. A continuous infusion of ancrod, 70 units every 24 to 36 hours, is given to maintain anticoagulation. Ancrod is excreted in urine. Its dose must be reduced in patients with renal insufficiency. Bleeding complications occur in 12% of patients treated with ancrod. If the severity of bleeding requires reversal of anticoagulation, cryoprecipitate and, rarely, an antivenom specific for ancrod can be given. Minor allergic reactions and the development of resistance are rare with intravenous ancrod administration.

Low-molecular-weight heparins (LMWH) and heparinoids have also been used successfully to treat DVT. Compared to unfractionated heparins, LMWH and heparinoids have a longer half-life when given subcutaneously and may have a lower incidence of heparin-induced thrombocytopenia and heparin sensitivity. The theoretic advantage of a decreased incidence of bleeding complications with LMWH and heparinoids has not been realized in clinical use. Heparinoids and LMWH have also been used as heparin substitutes in patients with heparin-induced thrombocytopenia. Due to a 20% to 61% likelihood that plasma from patients with heparin-induced thrombocytopenia will cause continued platelet aggregation with LMWH and heparinoids, LMWH and heparinoids should not be used as heparin substitutes for patients with heparin-induced thrombocytopenia unless platelet aggregation testing with the patient's plasma and the LMWH or heparinoid intended for use is negative.[7]

Sodium warfarin anticoagulation should be initiated after heparin sodium administration has begun, usually on the first or second day of heparin therapy. A vitamin K antagonist, sodium warfarin inhibits formation of the functional forms of clotting factors II, VII, IX, and X. Sodium warfarin doses of 5 ot 10 mg/day are usually given for the first few days of therapy. Maintenance doses are usually 2.5 to 5 mg/day. Lower doses are usually effective in the elderly and in patients with hepatic insufficiency. Sufficient sodium warfarin is given to prolong the prothrombin time (PT) to 1.5 to 1.7 times normal (international normalized ratio of 2 to 3).

Plasma concentrations of protein C, a vitamin K–dependent natural anticoagulant, are also decreased by sodium warfarin administration. Because protein C's half-life of 6 hours is significantly shorter than the half-lives of most of the vitamin K–dependent coagulation factors, a transient hypercoagulable state is present during the first days of sodium wafarin administration. For this reason, heparin sodium should be given during the first 3 to 5 days of sodium warfarin administration.

Bleeding complications develop in about 4% of patients on well-controlled sodium warfarin anticoagulation.[8] If a major bleeding episode occurs while a patient is appropriately anticoagulated, the sodium warfarin should be withheld. Vitamin K (5 to 10 mg intravenously) usually reverses the warfarin effect within 24 hours. Fresh-frozen plasma can be given if faster reversal is required. When the bleeding has been controlled, sodium warfarin may cautiously be resumed. Consideration should be given to placement of a vena cava filter in patients who cannot be reanticoagulated.

Anticoagulation with sodium warfarin or subcutaneous heparin sodium should be continued for a minimum of 3 months. At this time, the risk of recurrence decreases and the anticoagulant may be stopped in patients who have had only one episode of DVT. Patients with recurrent DVT should be anticoagulated for 6 to 12 months after their second DVT and indefinitely after their third DVT. Long-term or lifelong warfarin anticoagulation should also be considered for patients with continuing risks for DVT and pulmonary embolism, such as malignancy and hypercoagulable states.

Anticoagulation effectively prevents PE in patients with these extensive thromboses. In three recent studies including a total of 76 patients with iliofemoral and IVC thrombosis, no new PE occurred once anticoagulation was established.[1,3,4] This result compares favorably to the 2% PE rate previously reported for patients with lower extremity venous thromboses treated with anticoagulation.[8]

Thrombolytic Therapy

Thrombolytic therapy is used to restore venous patency and, potentially, prevent the development of the post-phlebitic syndrome by relieving venous outflow obstruction and preserving valve function. Fresh or nonocclusive thrombi are most amenable to lysis. The thrombolytic agents are usually given through a distal peripheral vein. Drug properties, typical doses, and relative cost data are listed in Table 1. Streptokinase (SK) and urokinase (UK) have been used more often than recombinant tissue plasminogen activator (rtPA) for venous thrombolysis. The incidence of bleeding complications with UK may be lower than with SK, although both are equally effective lytic agents.[9] Urokinase is free of sensitivity reactions, whereas up to 53% of patients receiving SK have sensitivity reactions.[9] Heparin sodium is usually given concurrently with the thrombolytic agent to prevent additional thrombosis from occurring during thrombolysis. The current choice of agents for thrombolysis is UK and heparin sodium.

During thrombolysis, the PT, aPTT, thrombin time, and fibrinogen level are monitored two to four times daily. None of these tests are predictors of success or bleeding, but they can be used to guide therapy if bleeding occurs. The amount of residual thrombus should be monitored every 12 hours with duplex scanning or phlebography. Thrombolytic therapy is stopped when the thrombus is completely lysed or when no further thrombolysis has occurred. Several days of infusion may be required to achieve complete lysis. After lytic therapy, anticoagulation with heparin sodium and sodium warfarin is continued as previously described.

Although thrombolytic therapy would seem to have particular benefit for patients with phlegmasia cerulea dolens and those with extensive proximal venous obstruction, this group has the poorest rate of successful lysis. The literature contains only a few case reports of inferior vena cava thrombosis successfully treated with lytic therapy. The success rate for lytic management of iliofemoral thrombosis is only 28%.[10] This low likelihood of restoration of venous patency probably exists because limited flow prevents the thrombolytic agent from coming in contact with the massive amounts of thrombus present in these patients. In an effort to solve this problem, clot lacing and intrathrombus administration techniques have been used.[11] Intra-arterial administration has also been recommended for phlegmasia cerulea dolens. Successful restoration of venous patency has been reported in a small number of patients in whom these techniques have been used.[11,12]

The likelihood that thrombolysis of a DVT will cause PE is low. However, because of these concerns it has been recommended that an IVC filter be placed prior to initiating lytic therapy in patients with iliofemo-

Table 1 Thrombolytic Agent Doses for Treatment of DVT

Thrombolytic Agent	Fibrin Specificity	Antigenicity	Relative Cost*	Dose
Streptokinase	+	Yes	1	250,000 unit bolus + 100,000 units/hour infusion
Urokinase	+ +	No	16	4,400 units/kg/hour bolus + 4,400 units/kg/hour infusion
Tissue plasminogen activator (rtPA)	+ + +	No	24	0.6 mg/kg/hour

*Based upon University of Missouri Hospital Pharmacy costs, June 1993.

ral and caval thrombosis who have already had a PE.[11] If PE were to occur during thrombolytic therapy, these emboli would likely be quickly lysed with continued administration of the thrombolytic agent. We have rarely recommended filter placement to patients receiving lytic therapy.

Bleeding risks comprise the major contraindications and complications from thrombolytic therapy. Thrombolytic therapy is contraindicated in patients with recent (less than 10 days earlier) operations, obstetric delivery, gastrointestinal bleeding, and major trauma. Bleeding diatheses, intracranial pathology, and recent (less than 2 months earlier) stroke and intracranial and spinal operations are also contraindications to lytic therapy. Bleeding complications occur in 0% to 17% of patients having lytic therapy for DVT.[9]

Reports of long-term preservation of venous valvular function and prevention of the post-thrombotic syndrome are favorable but very limited in number and length of follow-up.[11] Because long-term advantages over heparin sodium have not yet been shown in a large series, thrombolytic therapy for DVT cannot be routinely recommended at this time. However, given the potential advantages that lytic therapy offers, its use in selected patients with iliofemoral and caval thrombosis is often considered.

ADJUNCTIVE MEASURES

Adjunctive measures for the management of patients with iliofemoral and caval thrombosis include leg elevation and bed rest. For elevation to be effective, the legs must be higher than the heart. Patients are kept at bed rest until the pain and swelling resolve. They are then allowed to ambulate while wearing a compression stocking. When the edema subsides, the patient should be fitted for graduated compression stockings. If pain and swelling return when ambulation is begun, bed rest is again prescribed and heparin sodium is continued until the patient can ambulate without pain. Aspirin, 325 mg daily, is given to suppress platelet function. Bleeding due to concomitant administration of aspirin and anticoagulants, including sodium warfarin, is not increased when the anticoagulation is properly controlled.

At the time of hospital discharge, patients should be instructed on ways to avoid recurrent DVT, including performance of calf muscle exercises when sedentary and avoidance of positions of stasis. They should wear graduated compression stockings when not supine. Unless contraindicated, enteric-coated aspirin is recommended indefinitely.

REFERENCES

1. Farber SP, O'Donnell TF, Deterling RA, et al. The clinical implications of acute thrombosis of the inferior vena cava. Surg Gynecol Obstet 1984; 158:141–144.
2. O'Donnell TF, Browse NL, Burnand KG, Thomas ML. The socioeconomic effects of an iliofemoral venous thrombosis. J Surg Res 1977; 22:483–488.
3. Menzoian JO, Sequeira JC, Doyle JE, et al. Therapeutic and clinical course of deep vein thrombosis. Am J Surg 1983; 146:581–585.
4. Girard P, Hauuy MP, Musset D, et al. Acute inferior vena cava thrombosis: Early results of heparin therapy. Chest 1989; 95:284–291.
5. Andersson G, Fagrell B, Holmgren K, et al. Subcutaneous administration of heparin: A randomized comparison with intravenous administration of heparin to patients with deep venous thrombosis. Thromb Res 1982; 27:631–639.
6. Cole CW, Bormanis J. Ancrod: A practical alternative to heparin. J Vasc Surg 1988; 8:59–63.
7. Kikta MJ, Keller MP, Humphrey PW, Silver D. Can low molecular weight heparins and heparinoids be safely given to patients with the heparin-induced thrombocytopenia syndrome? Surgery 1993; 114:705–710.
8. Hull R, Hirsh J, Jay R, et al. Different intensities of oral anticoagulant therapy in the treatment of proximal-vein thrombosis. N Engl J Med 1982; 307:1676–1681.
9. Graor RA, Young JR, Risius B, Ruschhaupt WF. Comparison of cost-effectiveness of streptokinase and urokinase in the treatment of deep vein thrombosis. Ann Vasc Surg 1987; 1:524–528.
10. Hill SL, Martin D, Evans P. Massive venous thrombosis of the extremities. Am J Surg 1989; 158:131–135.
11. Comerota AJ, Aldridge SC. Thrombolytic therapy for acute deep vein thrombosis. Semin Vasc Surg 1992; 5:76–81.
12. Robinson DL, Teitelbaum GP. Phlegmasia cerulea dolens: Treatment by pulse-spray and infusion thrombolysis. Am J Roentgenol 1993; 160:1288–1290.

NONOPERATIVE TREATMENT OF ACUTE PULMONARY EMBOLISM

DOUGLAS W. HARRINGTON, D.O.
JOHN POPOVICH JR., M.D.

The diagnosis of pulmonary embolism (PE) is often clinically challenging and elusive, yet nonoperative treatment for this disorder is relatively straightforward. The cornerstone of therapy for venothromboembolic disease after 50 years of clinical use remains anticoagulation. Other aspects of nonoperative therapy for PE are predicated on the severity of the cardiopulmonary embarrassment resulting from the event and the likelihood of recurrent embolism.

GENERAL APPROACH

Evaluation of patients with suspected PE should include the assessment of hemodynamic stability and adequacy of oxygenation with pulse oximetry or arterial blood gases. Patients should remain at bed rest. Pain and anxiety should be treated with a narcotic analgesic, such as morphine sulfate, and a low-dose anxiolytic agent. Frequent clinical assessment of respiratory condition, volume status, and peripheral perfusion is necessary. Baseline laboratory studies, including complete blood count, platelet count, prothrombin time (PT), activated partial thromboplastin time (aPTT) or thrombin clotting time, and stool for occult blood, should be obtained.

Most patients with PE do not need to be admitted to a critical care unit unless they are experiencing some cardiorespiratory aberration requiring anticipatory monitoring or active treatment. The one exception may be where adequate infusion of heparin sodium and monitoring of anticoagulant effects cannot be performed on general nursing units. Critically ill patients with PE should be monitored with continuous electrocardiogram, noninvasive measurement of blood pressure, and pulse oximetry. Arterial catheterization should be considered in patients with significant hemodynamic compromise, such as persistent systolic blood pressure less than 90 mm Hg. More invasive procedures, such as central venous catheterization, repetitive intravenous (IV) or intra-arterial blood sampling, or needle diagnostic procedures, should be carefully considered in the anticipated event of thrombolytic therapy. Supplemental oxygen should be delivered to achieve an arterial oxygen saturation of at least 90%, arterial Po_2 of greater than 60 mm Hg. Cardiac dysrhythmias require correction. Hypotensive patients with PE should receive a challenge of volume expansion in the absence of cardiogenic pulmonary edema. Excessive volume loading of patients with acute PE may result in a worsening of right ventricular performance and must carefully be assessed. If hypotension is unresponsive to fluid challenge, vasoactive drugs, such as norepinephrine, should be considered to support the patient.[1]

ANTICOAGULATION

The principal acute therapy for PE is anticoagulation with IV heparin sodium (Table 1). Therapy with anticoagulants has been documented to reduce mortality from PE from 33% to 8%.[2] Heparin sodium acts by accelerating the effect of a plasma inhibitor, antithrombin III, which inactivates a number of clotting factors. Neither hepatic nor renal dysfunction interferes with clearance of heparin sodium.

With a strong clinical suspicion for PE and/or deep venous thrombosis (DVT), heparin sodium therapy should be initiated unless there is a contraindication, such as active or recent hemorrhage (Fig. 1). This should be done prior to confirmation of the diagnosis with further studies. Initially, a bolus of 5,000 units of heparin sodium is given. There is some rationale to give an initial larger bolus of heparin sodium, such as 10,000 to 20,000 units. This large bolus has two principal effects: platelet aggregation to the fresh embolus is diminished, and pulmonary vasoconstriction from vasoactive amines is blocked. Once the diagnosis of PE or DVT is confirmed, the patient should be rebolused with 5,000 to 10,000 units of heparin sodium and started on a continuous infusion of IV heparin sodium at 1,300 units per hour (Fig. 2).

The most critical factor in heparin therapy is achieving early and adequate levels of anticoagulation. Subtherapeutic anticoagulation within the first 24 hours has been shown to result in a fifteenfold increase in recurrence of thromboembolic disease and is generally felt to contribute to possible mortality from this disor-

Table 1 Guidelines for Anticoagulation

Disease	Guideline
Suspected	Give heparin sodium 5,000 U IV and order imaging study
Confirmed	Rebolus with heparin sodium 5,000 to 10,000 U IV and start maintenance infusion at 1,300 U/hour (heparin sodium 20,000 U in 500 ml D5W, 40 U/ml infused at 33 ml/hour)
	Check aPTT at 6 hours to keep aPTT between 1.5 and 2.5 times control
	Check platelet count daily
	Start sodium warfarin therapy on day 1 at 5 to 10 mg daily for first 2 days, then adjust warfarin daily
	Stop heparin sodium therapy after 5 to 7 days of joint therapy with sodium warfarin when INR is 2 to 3
	Anticoagulate with sodium warfarin for 3 months at an INR of 2 to 3

From Hyers TM, Hull RD, Weg JG. Antithrombotic therapy for venous thromboembolic disease. Chest 1992; 102:411S; with permission.

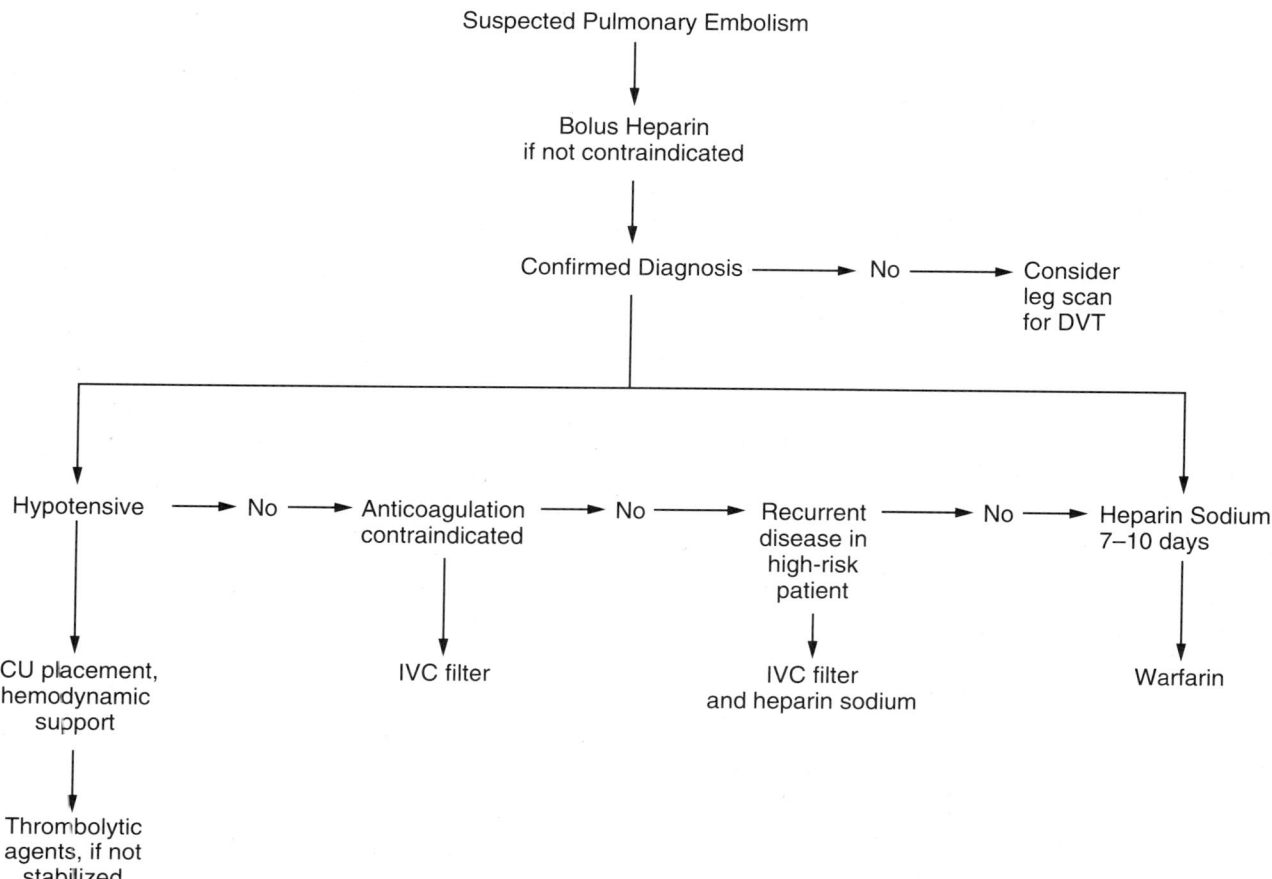

Figure 1 Algorithm for treatment of a patient with suspected pulmonary embolism.

der.[3,4] Heparin sodium therapy based on intuitive ordering results in inadequate therapy. The adequacy of anticoagulation should be assessed by measurement of aPTT or thrombin clotting time every 6 hours for the first several days of therapy, with the heparin sodium infusion adjusted to keep the level between 1.5 and 2.5 times control values (Table 2).[5,6] Heparin sodium requirements are usually largest in the first few days. After 48 to 72 hours, aPTT can be measured daily for the duration of therapy.

Heparin sodium has certain side effects that require clinical scrutiny. Heparin sodium–induced thrombocytopenia occurs in up to 15% of treated individuals, more commonly with bovine than with porcine preparations.[7] Most episodes are asymptomatic and occur after 3 to 15 days of treatment. This syndrome has been associated with arterial thromboembolism and extension of existing venous thromboembolism. Due to the risk of heparin sodium–induced thrombocytopenia, platelet counts should be checked at the time of initiation of therapy and daily thereafter. If the platelet count falls below 100,000/cm^3, heparin sodium should be discontinued, at which point other forms of management, including sodium warfarin or inferior vena cava filters, should be considered. Platelet counts return to normal after heparin sodium discontinuation. Heparin sodium is also associated with other side effects, including hypokalemia and elevated liver function studies. Hypokalemia occurs uncommonly, attributed to heparin sodium–induced hypoaldosteronism. Asymptomatic transient elevation in liver function studies occurs in most individuals taking heparin sodium after 5 to 10 days of treatment.

Bleeding risk with heparin sodium anticoagulation ranges from 5% to 20%, with major hemorrhage occurring in 3.8%. There is little evidence that heparin sodium anticoagulation producing aPTT levels of greater than 2.5 times control in the first few days of treatment increases the risk of significant bleeding. Independent factors associated with an increased risk for bleeding include acute myocardial infarct, hypotension, bilirubin greater than 1 mg/dl, creatinine greater than 1.5 mg/dl or an increase of 50%, hematocrit less than 30%, serious illness, and advancing age.[5]

Sodium warfarin (Coumadin) therapy is generally started on the first day of heparin sodium therapy in patients with uncomplicated PE, although it may be prudent to delay this for 1 to 2 days in critically ill patients due to the uncertainty of their clinical course. Traditionally, heparin sodium was continued for 7 to 10 days with overlapping Coumadin begun toward the end

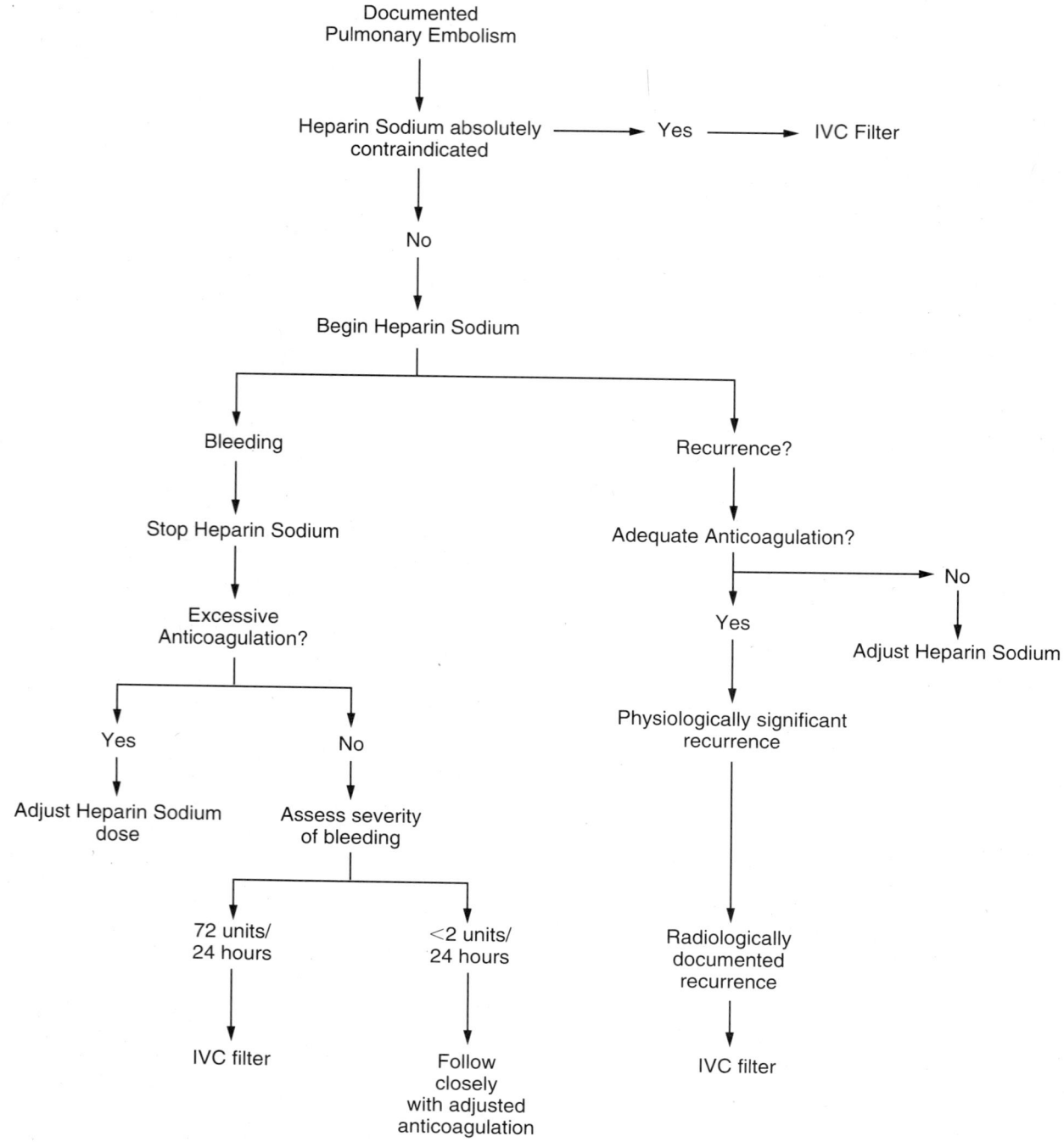

Figure 2 Algorithm for treatment of a patient with documented pulmonary embolism.

of heparin sodium therapy. Recently, studies have documented equally effective anticoagulation and low venothrombotic recurrence rates when heparin sodium is given for 4 to 5 days and Coumadin is begun on day 1 or 2.[8] Heparin sodium should be continued for at least 5 to 7 days, with longer duration of therapy considered in patients with larger clot burdens, as seen with massive PE or iliofemoral venous thrombosis.[8] Coumadin is used for long-term maintenance anticoagulation, which is continued for 3 months in most patients with PE. Coumadin should be considered for more prolonged treatment if there is an ongoing high risk for venothrombosis. Coumadin therapy should be monitored using the INR (international normalized ratio) with a target of 2 to 3. The INR is a mathematical correction derived from the patient's PT and control PT by using the international sensitivity index to avoid variations in PT testing.

Heparin sodium anticoagulation may also be administered subcutaneously, starting with 17,500 units every 12 hours and adjusting the dose to achieve an aPTT

Table 2 Intravenous Heparin: Monitoring and Adjusting Dosage*

aPTT†	Rate Change ml/hour	Dose Change U/24 hours	Additional Action	Next aPTT
≤45	+6	+5,760	Rebolus with 5,000 U	4 to 6 hours
46-54	+3	+2,880	None	4 to 6 hours
55-85‡	0	0	None	Next morning§
86-110	−3	−2,880	Stop infusion 1 hour	4 to 6 hours after restart
>110	−6	−5,760	Stop infusion 1 hour	4 to 6 hours after restart

*A starting bolus of 5,000 to 10,000 U is given IV, followed by IV infusion of 1,300 U/hour.
† Normal aPTT range with Dade-Actin FS reagent of 27 to 35 seconds.
‡The therapeutic range of 55 to 85 seconds is roughly equivalent to a plasma heparin sodium concentration range of 0.2 to 0.4 U/ml by protamine titration or to 0.35 to 0.7 U/ml by inhibition of factor Xa. The therapeutic range varies with different aPTT reagents and coagulation machines.
§During the first 24 hours, repeat aPTT in 4 to 6 hours. Thereafter, monitor aPTT daily unless it is subtherapeutic.
From Hyers TM, Hull RD, Weg JG. Antithrombotic therapy for venous thromboembolic disease. Chest 1992; 102:412S; with permission.

greater than 1.5 times control 1 hour before the next dose, although this method is more commonly employed in the treatment of DVT that has not been complicated by PE.

LOW-MOLECULAR-WEIGHT HEPARIN

Heparin sodium is not a homogeneous substance but is a mixture of polysaccharide molecules that varies in molecular weight from 5,000 to 40,000 daltons; the anticoagulant effect is only a small part of heparin sodium. Low-molecular-weight heparin (LMWH) is a homogeneous polysaccharide with an average molecular weight of 5,000 daltons. It binds to antithrombin III and can inactivate factor X to produce anticoagulation. The anticoagulation response is correlated with body weight; therefore, it is possible that LMWH may be effective when given in standard dose (unit/kg) without stringent laboratory monitoring. Coupled with its longer half-life, LMWH can be administered subcutaneously 1 to 2 times per day. Several studies have documented that LMWH is as effective as continuous heparin sodium in thromboembolic disease.[9] Presently, LMWH has Food and Drug Administration approval only for DVT prophylaxis, but it is likely to add another therapeutic option in treating patients with pulmonary thromboembolism.

THROMBOLYTIC THERAPY

Despite years of investigation, the specific role of thrombolytic agents in the treatment of PE is still debated and requires individualization. Thrombolytic therapy rapidly clears clots from the deep venous and pulmonary arterial vasculature. Thrombolytic agents are superior to heparin sodium in the rapidity of resolution of PE, as assessed by pulmonary arteriography, lung scan, or hemodynamic derangements improvement. One study noted a small improvement in carbon monoxide diffusing capacity at 2 weeks and 1 year in patients treated with thrombolytic therapy in comparison to conventional anticoagulation. Nevertheless, mortality improvement and other meaningful outcome parameters have not been documented. Although careful selection of patients has diminished hemorrhagic complications of thrombolytics, the risk of significant hemorrhage with this therapy is greater than in patients treated with conventional anticoagulant therapy. This is especially so in the critically ill patient, who may be harboring clinically unrecognized bleeding sites, such as upper gastrointestinal abnormalities, that have previously clotted. These "good" clots are indiscriminately lysed through systemic thrombolysis, leading to hemorrhagic complications. Multiple invasive lines in critical care patients also serve as additional bleeding sites for complications with thrombolytic agents. Furthermore, most patients who are in the hospital at the time of diagnosis of PE have contraindications to the use of thrombolytics.

The principal clinical indication for thrombolytic agents is persistent hypotension or refractory hypoxemia, despite optimal medical therapy, for which rapid reduction in the clot volume occluding the pulmonary vasculature may be hemodynamically beneficial. Patients with hemodynamic instability and PE should be considered for thrombolytic therapy if there are no bleeding tendencies or absolute contraindications. Some authors have suggested a widened role for thrombolytic agents, although outcome studies have not supported this approach to date in the broad spectrum of patients with pulmonary thromboembolism.

Three thrombolytic agents are available for use: streptokinase, urokinase, and tissue plasminogen activator (Table 3). Although tissue plasminogen activator is more fibrin specific than streptokinase or urokinase, bleeding complications appear to occur equally with each agent. Modification of dosing schedules of available thrombolytic agents, including the combined use of heparin sodium with thrombolytic agents at lower than conventional doses, have been used, but these regimens have not documented advantages in lowering bleeding complications. Intrapulmonary arterial infusion of thrombolytic agents has also not been convincingly demonstrated to improve clot lysis or reduce hemorrhagic complications. The thrombolytic capacity of all three agents is not discernibly different.

Table 3 Thrombolytic Agents in Venous Thromboembolism

Stop heparin infusion. Start thrombolytic infusion when aPTT or thrombin time (TT) is 1.5 times control or less.

Streptokinase*	250,000 IU loading dose
	100,000 IU/hour maintenance
Urokinase*	4,400 IU/lb loading dose
	4,400 IU/lb/hour maintenance
Tissue plasminogen activator*	100 mg (56 million IU) over 2 hours

After terminating thrombolytic infusion, restart heparin sodium infusion without a loading dose or with a small loading dose when aPTT or TT is 1.5 times control or less.

*Duration of therapy: Streptokinase is recommended for 24 hour infusion in pulmonary embolism 48 to 72 hours of infusion in deep venous thrombosis. Urokinase is recommended for 12 hour infusion in pulmonary embolism, 24 to 48 hours in deep venous thrombosis. Tissue plasminogen activator is recommended for a 2 hour infusion in pulmonary embolism at a total dose of 100 mg.
From Hyers TM, Hull RD, Weg JG. Antithrombotic therapy for venous thromboembolic disease. Chest 1992; 102:417S; with permission.

VENA CAVA FILTERS

Most patients can be successfully managed with anticoagulation. Patients who cannot be anticoagulated require inferior vena caval (IVC) interruption for mechanical protection against recurrent embolism (Fig. 2). Indications for IVC filters include (1) a contraindication to anticoagulation (absolute contraindications include active or recent hemorrhage, history of hemorrhagic stroke, or postoperative ocular, spinal, or neurosurgery within 2 weeks; relative contraindications include recent operation, major trauma, intracranial neoplasm, recent gastrointestinal hemorrhage), (2) a complication of anticoagulation, (3) significant recurrent PE with adequate anticoagulation, (4) large free-floating iliofemoral thrombosis, (5) chronic recurrent PE with associated pulmonary hypertension, (6) postoperative pulmonary embolectomy, and (7) history of significant PE with marginal cardiopulmonary reserve.

The Greenfield filter is the most thoroughly studied and accepted IVC filter available. It has excellent efficacy and safety. Recurrent PE after filter placement is 2.4%, and its occlusion rate is 3.1%, with most occurring within 1 month of placement.[10]

Anticoagulation should be continued after placement of IVC filters if no absolute contraindication exists. The filters protect against only recurrent PE and do not address the present PE and DVT. Animal studies have documented in situ progression of PE when not treated with anticoagulation.

Newer developments with IVC filters include the introduction of a new titanium Greenfield filter and increasing data to support the use of suprarenal placement with no risk to renal function.

REFERENCES

1. Molloy WD, Lee KY, Girling L, et al. Treatment of shock in a canine model of pulmonary embolism. Am Rev Respir Dis 1984; 130:870–874.
2. Barritt DW, Jordan SC. Anticoagulant drugs in treatment of pulmonary embolism. Lancet 1960; 1:1309–1312.
3. Hull RD, Raskob GE, Harsh J, et al. Continuous intravenous heparin compared with intermittent subcutaneous heparin in initial treatment of proximal vein thrombosis. N Engl J Med 1986; 315:1109–1114.
4. Hull RD, Raskob GE, Rosenbloom, et al. Optimal therapeutic level of heparin therapy in patients with venous thrombosis. Arch Intern Med 1992; 152:1589–1595.
5. Cruickshank MK, Levine MN, Harsh J, et al. A standard heparin nomogram for the management of heparin therapy. Arch Intern Med 1991; 151:333–337.
6. Hyers TM, Hull RD, Weg JG. Antithrombotic therapy for venous thromboembolic disease. Chest 1992; 102:408S–425S.
7. Warkenten TE, Kelton JG. Heparin induced thrombocytopenia. Prog Hemost Thromb 1991; 10:1–34.
8. Hull RD, Raskob GE, Rosenbloom D, et al. Heparin 5 day vs 10 day in the initial treatment of proximal venous thrombosis. N Engl J Med 1990; 322:1260–1264.
9. Hull RD, Pineo GF. Treatment of venous thromboembolism with low molecular weight heparin. Hematol Oncol Clin North Am 1992; 6:1095–1103.
10. Kanter B, Moser KM. The Greenfield vena cava filter. Chest 1988; 93:170–175.

PERCUTANEOUS DEVICES FOR VENA CAVA FILTRATION

DANIEL B. WALSH, M.D.
MICHAEL BETTMANN, M.D.

Patients with deep venous thrombosis or pulmonary emboli (PE) who cannot be anticoagulated and patients with PE that occurs during anticoagulation may be treated by placement of a filtration device in the inferior vena cava (IVC). Percutaneous placement of these devices is becoming commonplace. This technique avoids the perceived costs in time, discomfort, and resources associated with operating room placement. Eight different filters have been described for percutaneous placement in the IVC (Table 1). All are placed using the Seldinger technique. The right femoral vein is the site most commonly selected for venous access. The internal jugular vein is preferred when the iliac veins or the IVC is involved with thrombus. This approach generally remains the second choice due to its associated risk of air embolism. The left femoral approach is possible but is often avoided due to increased difficulty in correct placement caused by the greater angle of entry of the iliac vein into the IVC. External jugular and arm veins have been used successfully but are usually avoided due to their smaller size, greater distance, and less direct access to the infrarenal IVC. Inferior vena cavography is routinely performed prior to filter placement, for the size and orientation of the vena cava can significantly affect the function of filter devices.

STAINLESS STEEL GREENFIELD FILTER

The stainless steel Greenfield filter (Fig. 1) consists of a central hub from which six stainless steel legs extend

Table 1 Physical Characteristics of Eight Vena Cava Filters

Filter	Material	Length (mm)	Diameter (mm)	Diameter of Delivery System (Fr)	
				Carrier	Sheath
Steel Greenfield	Stainless steel	41	30	24	29.5
Bird's Nest	Stainless steel	70	54	11	14.0
Vena Tech	Eligiloy	46	30	10	12.0
Titanium Greenfield	Beta-3 titanium	47	38	12	14.3
Nitinol	Nickel titanium	38	28	7	9.0
Gunther	Stainless steel	75	22–30	10	12.0
Amplatz	Stainless steel	25	36	12	14.3
Prothia	Stainless steel	75	25 or 30	7	

After Dorfman GS. Percutaneous inferior vena caval filters. Radiology 1990; 174:987–992; with permission.

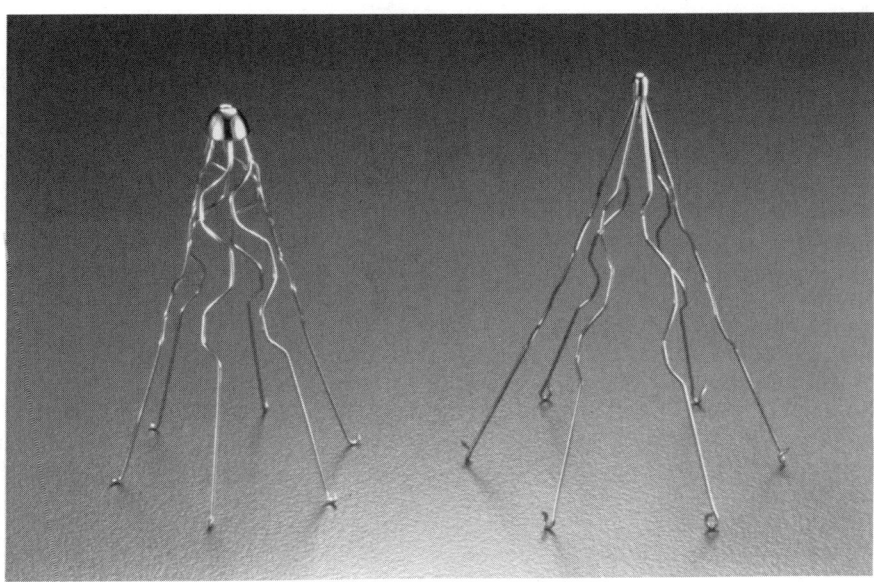

Figure 1 Stainless steel Greenfield filter on right; titanium Greenfield filter on left.

in a slightly bent fashion to create a cone. Each leg ends in a finely curved hook that anchors the device in the caval wall. The hub contains a central hole to allow passage of a guide wire to aid correct alignment during placement. This filter, which for so long was placed most frequently via an internal jugular vein cut-down, can now be placed percutaneously and offers the longest, most extensively published experience among contemporary filtration devices.

Percutaneous placement of the stainless steel Greenfield filter was first performed and reported in 1983. This device has performed well, regardless of placement technique, with an incidence of complications—including caval thrombosis, penetration of the caval wall, filter migration, PE, and lower extremity symptoms—after placement in less than 5% of patients.[1] However, percutaneous placement of this relatively large device (24 Fr) has been associated with a relatively high incidence of thrombosis of the access vein (19% to 41%).[2] Although most authors state that this venous thrombosis infrequently leads to symptoms, long-term follow-up is lacking, and deep venous thrombosis of the femoral vein from other causes is associated with significant long-term morbidity. The fear of significant sequelae secondary to femoral venous thrombosis has led to the development of other devices.

TITANIUM GREENFIELD FILTER

The titanium Greenfield filter (Fig. 1) is similar in shape to the stainless steel Greenfield filter but is 8 mm wider at its base and 5 mm taller. It is less than half the weight of the stainless steel Greenfield and more compressible, but lacks a central hole, so that it cannot be placed via a guide wire. After some initial difficulties with migration and alignment, which forced redesign of the anchoring struts, this filter placed via a 14 Fr sheath has been widely utilized.

The published experience with the modified hook titanium filter is limited only by length of follow-up (30 days).[3] This filter was successfully placed in 97% of 186 patients, most commonly (70%) via the right femoral vein. Over this 30 day period, 3% of patients suffered recurrent PE. Venous thrombosis at the site of insertion occurred in 8.7% of patients, a significantly lower rate than reported with the stainless steel Greenfield filter. New lower extremity edema occurred in 9.7% of patients. Patency of the IVC was documented only by the presence or absence of these symptoms.

Advantages of this particular filter appear to be ease of insertion from femoral and jugular sites, combined with function likely similar to the well-tested stainless steel model. This filter cannot be used in the relatively unusual circumstance of a vena cava larger than 28 mm diameter. Accurate alignment of this filter requires careful attention. When the IVC is tortuous or a left femoral vein insertion is required, placement of the filter without some angulation is difficult. This angulation, particularly if it is greater than 30° from the vertical axis of the IVC, may compromise filter function.

BIRD'S NEST FILTER

The Bird's Nest filter is a device constructed of four stainless steel wires each 25 cm long, preshaped with nonmatching bends (Fig. 2). Each wire is attached to a strut with a hook at its end for attachment to the IVC. The Bird's Nest filter can be placed by either the jugular or femoral approach. The introducing mechanism has a 14 Fr outer diameter. Its method of delivery, although somewhat complex, is readily mastered. The Bird's Nest filter has the advantage of being large enough to be effectively used in any size vena cava. The major disadvantage of the Bird's Nest filter is its length. If the infrarenal portion of the IVC is short or if suprarenal placement is required, the placement of this filter becomes problematic. An additional problem, at least theoretically, is prolapse of portions of the small wires connecting the major components. The incidence or importance of this phenomenon is unknown.

The largest and most recently published experienced with the Bird's Nest filter consists of 568 patients, only 37 of whom underwent follow-up vena cavography or ultrasound examination to determine IVC patency.[4] The authors report a clinical patency rate of the IVC of 97% with a possible recurrent PE rate of 3%. Dorfman reports (personal communication) that the second generation Bird's Nest filter has a caval occlusion rate of 1.4% and recurrent PE in 0.5% of 211 patients, although these data are otherwise unpublished.[5] If only the "scattered and random" 37 patients with the first-generation filters studied radiographically are considered, the IVC thrombosis rate is 19% and PE recurred in at least one and possibly two of the three patients studied.[4]

VENA TECH FILTER

In 1986 another percutaneous cone-shaped filter was introduced from France as the LGM filter, now named after the marketing company in the United States as the Vena Tech filter. This device is made from Phynox, the same substance as temporary cardiac pacing wires. It is inserted through a 12 Fr introducer via either the jugular or femoral approach. The filter has six arms with hooks attached to each arm. Like the Greenfield filter, placement of the Vena Tech filter in a vena cava larger than 28 mm in diameter is contraindicated.

Significant experience with this filter has been reported only by two groups, the most recent of which offers no follow-up. Among the original 100 patients with this filter followed for 1 year, there was an 8% caval thrombosis rate, 32% experienced lower extremity swelling, and two patients suffered PE.[6] Because it is less self-centering and less self-aligning than other filters, proximal migration, incomplete opening, and misplace-

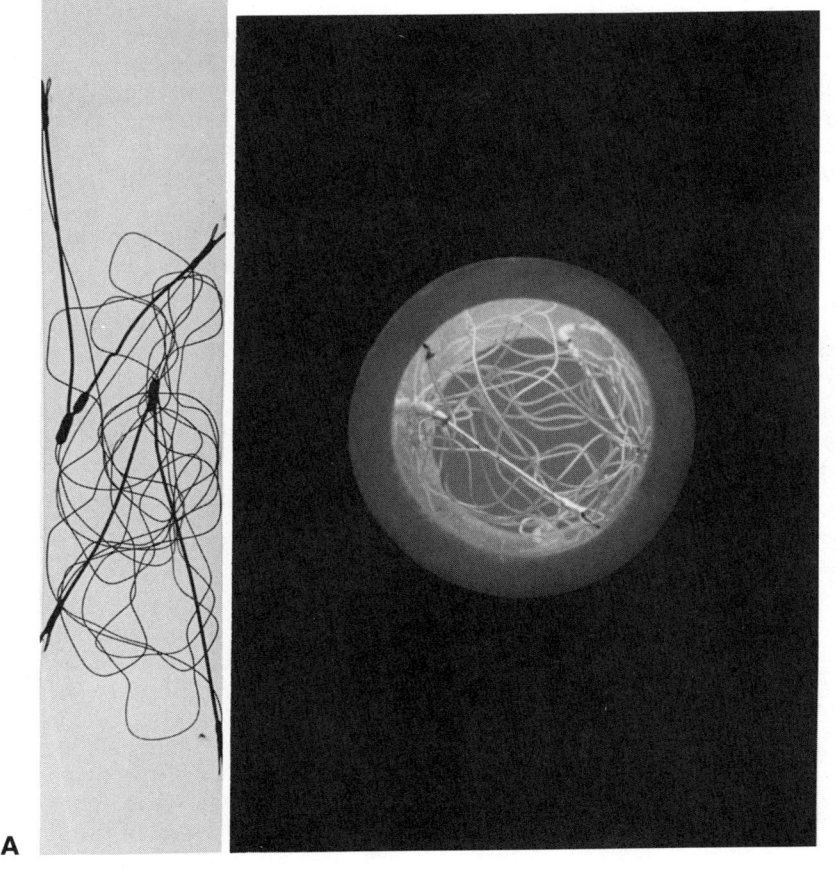

Figure 2 *A,* The Bird's Nest filter deployed in anterior-posterior view. *B,* Luminal views of the Bird's Nest filter.

ment were significant problems in this experience, although there is some indication that complications from placement decreased measurably with experience.

AMPLATZ

This filter is cone-shaped, made of stainless steel, and placed through a 14 Fr introducer. It is inserted in the IVC in an "inverted" position, with the top of the cone farthest from the diaphragm. This filter is also meant to be retrievable, although how easily this may be accomplished after a prolonged period of time in place remains to be demonstrated. This design characteristic, however, may facilitate realignment if misplacement occurs.

In the two published trials, involving a total of 82 patients, the caval occlusion rate appears prohibitively high (23% in one study; 21% in the other).[7,8] Recurrent PE also occurred in 2% to 7% of patients. Thrombosis at the insertion site occurred in 3% of patients in both studies. There is also a concern that thrombi might propagate through this device. Unless further experience improves these results, it seems unlikely this filter would or should achieve broad use.

NITINOL FILTER

This filter is made of nitinol (Fig. 3), a nickel titanium alloy, which is a pliable straight wire when cool but, when warmed, rapidly transforms into a previously imprinted rigid shape. It is inserted using a 9 Fr introducer via femoral, jugular, or brachial approaches. The thermal memory feature requires iced saline running through the introducer at the time of placement. Due to its 28 mm size, placement in vena cavas larger than this is contraindicated. Vigorous abdominal contraction has been thought to lead to strut fracture in these filters. Thus, placement in quadriplegics is also contraindicated.

In the only large published experience, 103 of these filters have been placed and followed at 11 centers.[9] Twelve patients are thought to have suffered IVC thrombosis. Two patients likely experienced recurrent PE. Five of 18 (28%) patients examined had evidence of insertion site thrombosis. The dome of the filter was frequently observed to tilt 20° to 25° toward the vein wall. This was felt to be secondary to the dome geometry in a small vena cava. This tilt was not felt to threaten filter function as such a tilt might with a Greenfield filter.

GUNTHER FILTER

The Gunther filter was developed to be readily retractable. The original design was a stainless steel combination of a basket attached to an inverted cone. It can be placed via the jugular or femoral veins using a 10 Fr introducer. Due to its design, tilting was not a problem. Experience with the filter has been reported only from Europe. Initially planned clinical trials have not been undertaken in the United States.

Only one PE has been reported after placement of this filter in 93 patients, although in one anecdotal report, 2 of 9 patients developed recurrent PE.[10-12] Caudal migration of the filter has been observed in as many as 70% of patients, with caval thrombosis occurring in 7%. There has been very little follow-up reported with these filters and little quantitative data comparable to that available for other devices. The filter was 7.5 cm in length and thus likely not suitable for use in the suprarenal position or in patients with short IVC segments. Due to metal fatigue and fractures, this device has been redesigned to a tulip-shaped configuration (Fig. 4). This design has obviated the problem of strut fracture and is currently in initial clinical studies in Germany.

PROTHIA REMOVABLE FILTER

The Prothia filter is a stainless steel basket inserted via the femoral or jugular approach using a long catheter that remains in place while the basket is in use. Once the basket is retracted into the catheter, the entire device is removed. The filter is 7.5 cm in length and is available in two diameters, 25 mm and 30 mm. This device is meant to be used during thrombolytic therapy or in other circumstances when the risk of PE is felt to be high. The theoretical advantage of the device is easy removal, thus avoiding long periods with permanent devices that expose patients to the risk of the device with minimal benefit.

Use of the device has been reported in 65 patients.[13] No patient suffered PE during the use of or within 7 months of the use of this device. Nearly a quarter of the filters had thrombus seen in the filters at removal. Thirty-eight percent of patients bled sufficiently around the catheter to require blood transfusion. Fifteen percent of patients experienced bacteremia documented by positive blood cultures. Thrombosis around the

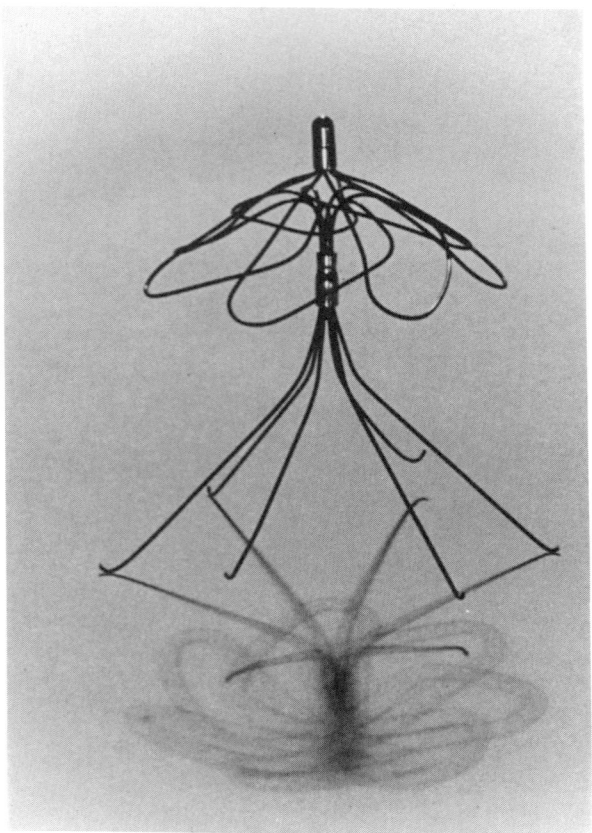

Figure 3 Anterior-posterior view of the Nitinol filter.

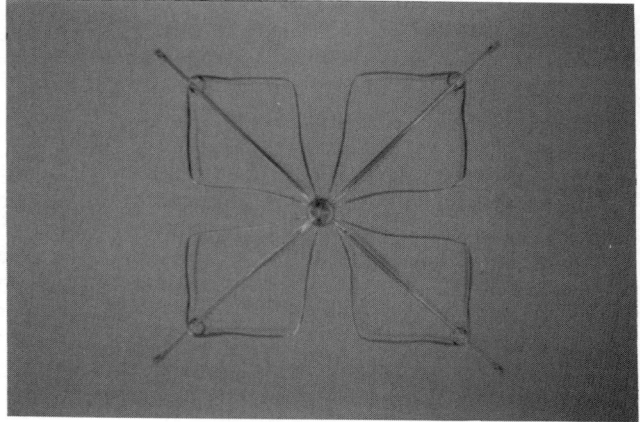
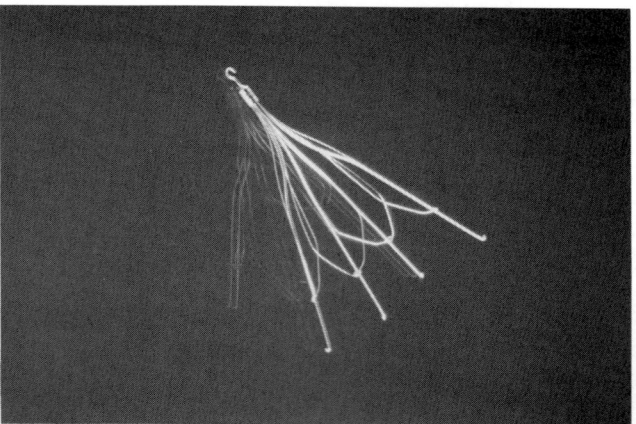

Figure 4 *A*, End-on view of the Gunther filter. *B*, Anterior-posterior view of the redesigned Gunther filter.

catheter or in the insertion site during or after the device was removed was not studied.

Overall Results

The two Greenfield filters, the Vena Tech filter, and the Bird's Nest filter are the devices most commonly used for vena caval filtration in the United States. The published experience with each device is minimal compared with their actual usage. Unfortunately, the few published reports available do not often examine experience with a view toward unbiased and accurate comparison of results. Clearly, the search for the perfect device to prevent PE should continue. None of the available devices can be placed without some incidence of failure, misalignment, or caval thrombosis, and none has a 0% incidence of PE or insertion site thrombosis. Comparison of published results for each filter has been further complicated by the lack of standard, quantitative follow-up of patients over a period long enough for possible venous complications to be observed. Detailed and comparable examination of IVC filter results is becoming more important as the usage of these devices increases.

REFERENCES

1. Becker DM, Philbrick JT, Selby JB. Inferior vena cava filters. Indications, safety, effectiveness. Arch Intern Med 1992; 152:1985-1994.
2. Pais SO, Tobin KD. Percutaneous insertion of the Greenfield filter. AJR Am J Roentgenol 1989; 152:933-938.
3. Greenfield LJ, Cho KJ, Proctor M, et al. Results of a multicenter study of the modified hook-titanium Greenfield filter. J Vasc Surg 1991; 14:253-257.
4. Roehm JOF Jr, Johnsrude IS, Barth MH, Gianturco C. The Bird's nest inferior vena cava filter: Progress report. Radiology 1988; 168:745-749.
5. Dorfman GS. Percutaneous inferior vena cava filters. Radiology 1990; 174:987-992.
6. Ricco JB, Crochet D, Sebilotte P, et al. Percutaneous transvenous caval interruption with the "LGM" filter: Early results of a multicenter trial. Ann Vasc Surg 1988; 2:242-247.
7. Epstein DH, Darcy MD, Hunter DW, et al. Experience with the amplatz retrievable vena cava filter. Radiology 1989; 172:105-110.
8. McCowan TC, Ferris EJ, Carver DK, Baker ML. Amplatz vena caval filter: Clinical experience in 30 patients. Am J Roentgenol 1990; 155:177-181.
9. Simon M, Athanasoulis CA, Kim D, et al. Simon nitinol inferior vena cava filter: Initial clinical experience. Work in progress. Radiology 1989; 172:99-103.
10. Fobbe F, Dietzel M, Korth R, et al. Günther vena caval filter: Results of long-term follow-up. Am J Roentgenol 1988; 151:1031-1034.
11. Schneider PA, Geissbühler P, Piguet JC, Bounameaux H. Follow-up after partial interruption of the vena cava with the Günther filter. Cardiovasc Intervent Radiol 1990; 13:378-380.
12. Lofaso F, Messadi AA, Anglade MC, Huet Y. Failure of the intracaval filter of Günther to prevent recurrence of pulmonary embolism: Report of two cases. Intensive Care Med 1990; 16:457-459.
13. Thery C, Asseman P, Amrouni N, et al. Use of a new removable vena cava filter in order to prevent pulmonary embolism is patients submitted to thrombolysis. Eur Heart J 1990; 11:334-341.

OPERATIVE INFERIOR VENA CAVA INTERRUPTION

HOLT A. McDOWELL Jr., M.D.
ERNESTO ANAYA, M.D.

The most serious complication of venous thrombosis is pulmonary embolism (PE), a problem under increasing consideration that unfortunately has not resulted in a decreased mortality rate. It is estimated that deep venous thrombosis (DVT) and PE are associated with 300,000 to 600,000 hospitalizations a year and that as many as 50,000 individuals die each year as a result of PE.[1] Because some groups of patients at high risk for the development of venous thromboembolism can be identified, it is reasonable and desirable to consider ways of prevention. A particular group of patients of interest in vascular surgery practice, in which prophylaxis for PE is of consideration, are those submitted to aortoiliac reconstruction. Even though the incidence of this complication is less than 1%, due to the use of heparin sodium during the surgical procedure, if this event occurs, the use of postoperative anticoagulants carries increased hemorrhagic risk.[2,3]

Even though heparin sodium has proven to be useful in the prevention of DVT, the risk of bleeding and hematoma formation has been reported when this prophylactic agent is used.[4] More severe complications or death due to bleeding are not as frequent. Another complication of the use of heparin sodium for anticoagulation is heparin-induced thrombotic thrombocytopenia, which through antibody-mediated induction of platelet aggregation may cause a drop in platelet count with a paradoxic hypercoagulable state. A past history of this event is an absolute contraindication for heparin sodium therapy. Other absolute contraindications to systemic anticoagulation are malignant hypertension, recent central nervous system or eye operations, subarachnoid or cerebral hemorrhage, and major, active bleeding.

Ligation of the inferior vena cava (IVC) to prevent progression and embolization of infected thrombi in patients with puerperal sepsis was first recommended by Trendelenburg in 1910. Homans suggested ligation of the femoral vein for prevention of PE but later revised his recommendation to include ligation of the IVC when the source of emboli was supposed to be above the inguinal ligament. This procedure is associated with both early and late morbidity.

PARTIAL INTERRUPTION OF THE VENA CAVA

As a result of the morbidity that ligation of the IVC carries, a variety of surgical methods were developed to reduce the chance of large emboli to generate PE. These alternatives can be divided in two groups, those that require intimal penetration and those that do not. The first group has a high incidence of subsequent thrombophlebitis that can be explained by the combination of intimal injury in a slow flow system. Procedures in this group include the suture filtration described by DeWeese and Hunter, Spencer's suture plication, and the staple compartmentation introduced by Ravitch. In the second group are the clips developed by Miles, Adams-DeWeese, Moretz, and the Abdu clip.

Venous interruption is indicated in patients with contraindication to or failure of anticoagulant therapy (38%), recurrent PE (27%), complication of anticoagulation (17%), and prophylaxis (17%).[5]

Vena caval interruption does not prevent the development of lower extremity DVT or its propagation. Vena caval interruption only decreases the incidence of fatal PE.

TECHNIQUE OF VENA CAVAL LIGATION

A transperitoneal or an extraperitoneal approach can be performed, always using general anesthesia. When the extraperitoneal approach is chosen, a transverse muscle-splitting incision is used, displacing the peritoneal sac medially. The limitation of the retroperitoneal approach is that it does not provide the best exposure of the vena cava at the level of the renal veins. Ligation should be done using nonabsorbable suture. Division of the IVC could be cumbersome and does not offer any benefit.

Ligation of the IVC in humans can produce hazardous hemodynamic alterations.[6] These alterations were thought to result from diminished venous return and blood sequestration. The mortality rate after IVC ligation is higher in patients with cardiac disease because they are less capable of tolerating the fall in the preload. Another problem detected after IVC ligation is the development of retroperitoneal venous collaterals. These vessels are, in many instances, the cause of recurrent embolization, sometimes fatal, as the size of these collateral veins is quite adequate to allow thrombi of considerable size to pass.[7] These large collateral vessels, and in some instances thrombus extending above the level of the ligature, are responsible for the rate of recurrent PE, which is 6.4% after this procedure. In cases of septic emboli, multiple small PE that have resulted in the development of pulmonary hypertension or cor pulmonale, and recurrent emboli following caval plication, ligation has not been replaced by partial interruption. In septic pelvic thrombophlebitis, ligation of ovarian veins should be included.

One of the major objections to caval ligation is the risk of chronic venous stasis in the lower limbs, estimated to be 20%. Sequelae of this range from mild ankle edema to phlegmasia cerulea dolens.

TECHNIQUE OF VENA CAVAL PLICATION

The procedure can be performed through a right retroperitoneal approach or a transperitoneal approach, both using general anesthesia. The transperitoneal approach provides a better exposure of the IVC, and the left ovarian or spermatic vein can easily be identified entering the left renal vein. The IVC is dissected over a distance of 5 cm below the renal veins, and the clip should be placed just below them, trying to avoid the formation of a cul-de-sac above the plicated area. The preferred clip is the one described by Moretz, made of polytetrafluoroethylene and nonserrated, because it is very easy to apply. In some cases a Silastic tubing may guide an atraumatic passage if necessary. The Moretz clip is available in aperture range between 3 and 3.5 mm.[8] An effort should be made for the clip to lay flat.

In the setting of abdominal aortic reconstruction, it seems that the best therapy would be prophylaxis. During such operations the retroperitoneal exposure needed for aortic reconstruction also provides exposure of the IVC, which can easily be plicated without increasing the operative risk.

In an unpublished series of our patients who have undergone IVC plication performed simultaneously with a major abdominal vascular operation since July 1985, 125 patients were identified in whom a Moretz clip was placed. At the time of review, 29 patients had died of various causes, none from pulmonary thromboembolism. Ninety-four patients were available for follow-up study; of these, 29 had symptoms of lower extremity venous hypertension, 19 of whom had had the symptoms before the plication. Sixty-four patients underwent one or more studies to evaluate the patency of the IVC and, in all, patency was confirmed.

CURRENT APPROACH

These results document that prophylactic plication of the IVC can be done safely, expeditiously, and without the concern of mortality and late morbidity. Our current criteria for prophylactic plication are less liberal than in the past. We are restricting its application to patients who are in the classic high-risk groups for developing DVT, including prior episodes of DVT or pulmonary thromboembolism, chronic venous stasis, leg edema, malignancy, expectation of prolonged bed rest, and varicose veins.

The availability of transvenous intracaval devices has made caval interruption a less frequently used method for prophylaxis against PE. However, considering the comparable patency rates with the ease and safety of application, clip plication is a reasonable alternative to intraluminal filters for high-risk patients undergoing abdominal operations. Additional advantages are the avoidance of a second procedure in the operating room or radiographic suite with Greenfield filter insertion and avoidance of the need for systemic heparin sodium therapy in the postoperative patient who develops DVT.

REFERENCES

1. Moser KM. Pulmonary thromboembolism. In: Braunwald E, Isselbacher KJ, Petersdorf RG, et al, eds. Harrison's principles of internal medicine. 11th ed. New York: McGraw-Hill, 1987:1105.
2. Reilly MK, McCabe CJ, Abbott WM, et al. Deep venous thrombophlebitis following aortoiliac reconstructive surgery. Arch Surg 1982; 117:1210–1211.
3. Ariyan S, Stansel HC. Further hazards of heparin therapy in vascular surgery. Arch Surg 1976; 111:120–121.
4. Persson AV, Davis RJ, Villavicencio JL. Deep venous thrombosis and pulmonary embolism. Surg Clin North Am 1991; 71:1195–1209.
5. Greenfield LJ, Peyton R, et al. Greenfield vena cava filter experience. Late results in 156 patients. Arch Surg 1981; 116:1451–1456.
6. McDowell HA. Prophylactic Teflon clip plication of the inferior vena cava for prevention of pulmonary embolism. South Med J 1973; 66:356–358.
7. Piccone VA, Vidal E, Yarnoz M, et al. The late results of caval ligation. Surgery 1970; 68:980–998.
8. Moretz WH, Still JM, Griffin LH, et al. Partial occlusion of the inferior vena cava with a smooth Teflon clip: Analysis of long-term results. Surgery 1972; 71:710–719.

TRANSVENOUS CATHETER PULMONARY EMBOLECTOMY

E. JOHN HARRIS Jr., M.D.
THOMAS J. FOGARTY, M.D.
CHRISTOPHER K. ZARINS, M.D.

Massive pulmonary embolus (PE), defined as at least 50% obstruction of the total pulmonary vasculature with associated hemodynamic instability, continues to be a leading cause of sudden death in hospitalized patients. Many patients who suffer massive PE die within the first several hours despite prompt medical intervention, and up to 85% die within 6 hours. Of patients who survive the initial insult of a massive PE, one-third eventually succumb to the hemodynamic sequelae.

Postmortem studies document that massive PE account for 2% to 14% of hospital deaths; however, the diagnosis of PE is established premortem in only 30% of these patients. Unlike most patients, those with massive PE usually do not respond to heparin sodium anticoagulation alone. Dalen and co-workers documented that in patients with angiographically proved bilateral PE, heparin sodium therapy alone resulted in minimal resolution of pulmonary vascular obstruction during the first few days after embolization. Complete resolution, with normal arteriograms and hemodynamics, was not realized for weeks.[1]

Therapies for massive PE have been largely unsuccessful in patients suffering from shock or cardiac arrest. Thrombolytic therapy, combined with heparin sodium anticoagulation and vena caval filtration for massive PE, has shown encouraging improvements in pulmonary hemodynamics, yet these improvements require hours to days for realization. Thrombolytic therapy is inadequate in patients with massive PE who are in shock or who have impending cardiac arrest. Pulmonary embolectomy offers the promise of removing the obstructing thrombi and instantly improving pulmonary hemodynamics. However, this requires thoracotomy, and open pulmonary embolectomy is not a simple procedure; intraoperative hemorrhage can be problematic, and there is a high operative mortality rate. The development of extracorporeal cardiopulmonary support devices allowed more aggressive approaches to PE. Currently, open pulmonary embolectomy is indicated for patients with arteriographically documented massive PE who are in shock and (1) have an absolute contraindication to thrombolytic therapy, (2) have no response or have deterioration with thrombolytic therapy, (3) are in a hemodynamic state suggesting impending cardiac arrest, or (4) have echocardiographic documentation of right atrial emboli that may be "in transit." Results for operative pulmonary embolectomy have improved over the last 10 years, yet operative mortality remains high.[2]

The limitations of thrombolytic therapy and the poor results for open pulmonary embolectomy have led to the development of alternative methods for the treatment of massive PE. One such method is transvenous catheter pulmonary embolectomy. Because the time to successful intervention appears critical in determining outcome in massive PE, methods for the removal of obstructing pulmonary arterial thrombi, using transvenous catheter retrieval without thoracotomy or general anesthesia, have been developed for rapid means of pulmonary embolectomy.

The initial work to evaluate the feasibility of removal of PE with a transvenous large-bore catheter was

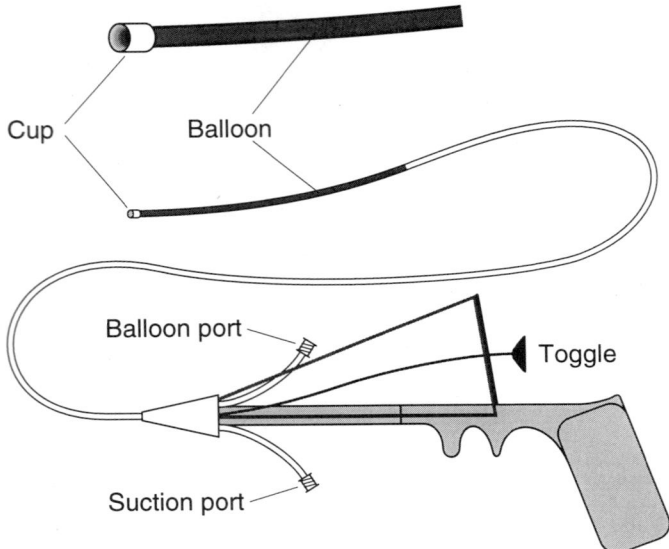

Figure 1 The current iteration of the pulmonary embolectomy catheter. A guide wire can be passed through the suction port, which can also be used for arteriography. The distal tip is steerable by the toggle switch.

performed by Fisher, Fogarty, and Nolan in 1968.[3] In a dog model of PE, a Teflon-reinforced Silastic catheter was manipulated transvenously under fluoroscopic guidance into the pulmonary arteries, and, with gentle suctioning and flushing, PE were successfully removed. Passage of the large catheter did not significantly alter pulmonary arterial (PA) pressure, ventricular pressure, cardiac output, or systemic arterial pressure in normal control animals. Greenfield and colleagues subsequently described a technique of transvenous catheter pulmonary embolectomy, with a special vacuum-cup catheter tip.[4] They also used a dog model of PE to develop their catheter and reported similar results in animal studies. The Fogarty group employed large-bore catheters, 5 to 8 mm internal diameter (I.D.), whereas the Greenfield group used a smaller catheter with an enlarged, 7 mm I.D., conical vacuum-cup at its tip. The clinical application of transvenous pulmonary embolectomy has been performed using the catheter system developed by Greenfield.

PULMONARY EMBOLECTOMY CATHETER

The current catheter is steerable, with a radiopaque cup at its tip that may be passed intravenously with or without a guide wire. A joystick apparatus on the handle of the catheter provides steering control. Contrast material may be injected through the lumen of the catheter, and PA pressures may be measured through an external port. Suction is applied to the plastic cup at the tip of the catheter by a syringe on the external port (Fig. 1).

Either the femoral or jugular venous route can be used for access (Fig. 2, left). The femoral vein is preferred because manipulation of the catheter is somewhat easier, a venotomy is easily performed for retrieval of the embolus, and the head and thorax are available for cardiopulmonary resuscitative efforts, if needed, during the procedure. The catheter is passed under fluoroscopic guidance. Difficulty in passage may be encountered at the tricuspid and pulmonic valves, especially in unstable patients with low cardiac outputs. A guide wire is then passed into the pulmonary artery, and the embolectomy catheter is then passed over the guide wire.

Once the catheter is in the pulmonary artery, a baseline PA pressure is measured. The cup is then positioned adjacent to the embolus, and position is confirmed with a small injection of nonionic contrast material. Suction is then applied to the distal catheter port with a 30 ml syringe. If the embolus becomes lodged in the cup, there is no return of blood. Embolectomy is then performed by withdrawal of the catheter while an assistant maintains suction (Fig. 2, right). A venotomy, with proximal and distal control of the vein, facilitates removal of the catheter and trailing embolus. Free flow of blood into the syringe at any time suggests noncapture or dislodgment of the embolus from the plastic cup during withdrawal of the catheter.

After removal of an embolus, the patient's physiologic response is evaluated by measuring Pao_2, PA pressure, and cardiac output. If the embolus has been causing significant hemodynamic alterations, its removal should lead to immediate increases in Pao_2 and cardiac output. The PA pressures should diminish, and, in the presence of adequate fluid resuscitation, the mean PA pressure should decrease to 20 mm Hg or less. Once this response has been realized, inotropic and pressor support may be successfully weaned. Further attempts at embolectomy for residual emboli are not necessary and may, in fact, be harmful. The goal of catheter embolec-

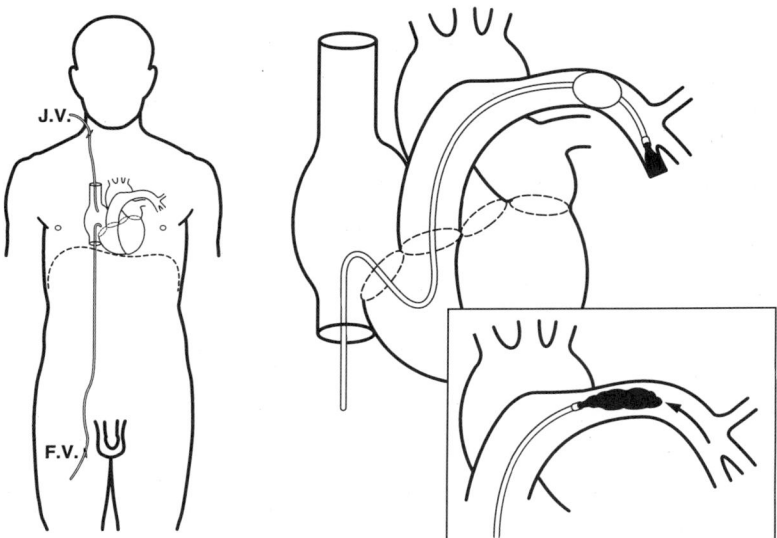

Figure 2 Left, Access sites for passage of the pulmonary embolectomy catheter. J.V., jugular vein; F.V., femoral vein. Passage of a guide wire under fluoroscopic control is the first procedure, with the embolectomy catheter then passed over the wire into the pulmonary artery. In the upper panel on the right, the catheter has been positioned adjacent to the embolus, and the balloon is inflated. Once the balloon is occluding the artery, suction is applied to the catheter, and the embolus becomes impacted in the cup. With suction maintained, the balloon is deflated and the catheter is withdrawn.

tomy is improvement of hemodynamic status; therefore, completion pulmonary arteriography is not needed.

Early experience with catheter embolectomy was hampered by recurrent emboli. Subsequent development of vena cava filtering devices has considerably reduced the risk of recurrent embolism. Current recommendations are for the placement of a vena cava filter at the completion of the transvenous catheter embolectomy, with the location dictated by the extent of iliofemoral and gonadal venous thrombosis. The patient also should receive standard anticoagulation with heparin sodium followed by long-term sodium warfarin therapy after successful catheter embolectomy.

Pulmonary emboli begin to adhere to the pulmonary artery within 48 to 72 hours after embolization. Transvenous catheter removal of these emboli usually results in fragmentation of the clot and removal of only small fragments rather than the removal of the entire embolus. Thus, there usually is little or no improvement in the patient's hemodynamic condition. Similarly, in patients with chronic recurrent thromboembolism, most of the pulmonary vascular bed has been converted to fibrous scar tissue, and removal of only the most recent emboli does not improve the associated pulmonary hypertension.

TREATMENT OPTIONS

All patients with confirmed PE and those with suspected massive PE should receive immediate intravenous heparin sodium. A bolus dose of 150 to 200 units/kg is then followed by a continuous heparin sodium infusion. The natural history of PE treated with heparin sodium therapy alone has been reported, showing substantial resolution of the emboli within 1 week. The heparin sodium retards further venous thrombosis, and resolution of the emboli is mediated by natural plasminogen activation. Continued resolution of PE is observed for 2 to 3 more weeks but is not complete at that stage. Intravascular webs and synechiae may persist indefinitely, with numerous webs causing chronic pulmonary artery obstruction and secondary pulmonary hypertension.

Several controlled, randomized clinical trials have documented that thrombolytic therapy combined with intravenous heparin sodium can accelerate the resolution of PE compared to heparin sodium therapy alone. These same studies have failed to document a clear survival benefit for thrombolytic therapy over heparin sodium therapy alone. Thrombolytic therapy would seem indicated in a patient with submassive PE and hemodynamic instability, in whom rapid thrombus resolution might be beneficial.

For massive PE, there is no clear consensus of recommended indications for pulmonary embolectomy. Most often, patients with massive PE, with or without shock, are treated with thrombolytic therapy. For patients not responding to thrombolytic therapy or those in profound shock, pulmonary embolectomy may be considered. Since the first reports of successful open pulmonary embolectomy with the assistance of cardiopulmonary bypass (CPB), most successfully treated patients have been associated with CPB. Pulmonary embolectomy performed with CPB allows bilateral embolectomy through the main pulmonary artery. Recent advances in CPB equipment have made these support systems potentially mobile. The early institution of partial CPB for circulatory support is now possible in the angiography suite or in the intensive care unit, with increased potential for salvage of patients with massive PE and cardiorespiratory arrest. Alternatively, others have chosen to perform pulmonary embolectomy without CPB, but rather with venous inflow occlusion or unilateral pulmonary artery occlusion. In spite of the preponderance of support for pulmonary embolectomy using CPB, recent studies report similar success rates for pulmonary embolectomy without CPB.[5]

RESULTS

The largest experience with the transvenous pulmonary embolectomy catheter has been reported by Greenfield.[6] The series now includes 46 patients treated over a 22 year period. Pulmonary emboli were classified as massive in 72%, major in 9%, and chronic in 19% of patients. Access to the pulmonary arterial tree was by way of the femoral vein in 61% and the right internal jugular vein in 39% of patients. Emboli were successfully extracted in 35 of 46 patients (76%), with a 30 day mortality of 30%. Successful extraction of emboli was more likely in major or massive emboli (84%) than in chronic emboli (56%). Hemodynamic data before and after embolectomy revealed an average reduction in mean PA pressure of 8 mm Hg and a significant increase in mean cardiac output from 2.59 L/minute to 4.47 L/minute.

A recent study from France described the use of the embolectomy catheter through a percutaneously placed sheath. The reported results were similar to those of Greenfield, with successful removal of thrombus and hemodynamic improvement in 13 of 18 patients (72%) and a mortality rate of 28%.[7] Catheter embolectomy was attempted in some patients who may have had chronic PE, and this may explain the high failure rate. Greenfield cautioned against the use of the percutaneous flexible sheath when performing embolectomy.[8] The catheter sheath is not necessary to control hemorrhage at the insertion site, it may shear off thrombus from the embolus attached to the vacuum cup, and it has the potential to allow air embolism to occur. The only other experience with transvenous catheter pulmonary embolectomy has been limited to case reports.

Another approach to transvenous catheter intervention for PE has been suggested. A conventional 8 Fr diagnostic catheter is advanced into the pulmonary artery in standard fashion and then used to mechanically fragment the embolus. The fragments then disperse into the distal pulmonary arterial tree. The rationale of this approach is that the volume of the embolus is large relative to the size of the main pulmonary arteries but small compared to the total volume of the smaller distal pulmonary arterial tree. Thus, dispersing the emboli into the distal branches theoretically increases total pulmonary blood flow.[9] The success of this approach is limited to case reports in three patients, and more experience and investigation with this technique are necessary.

Complications with transvenous catheter embolectomy have been numerous, with wound hematoma from anticoagulation the most frequently reported. In the early experience with this technique, bolus contrast injections through the embolectomy catheter were used, and several patients suffered cardiac arrest during angiography. With modification of the technique to small, selective contrast injections, this complication no longer occurs. Other reported complications have included pulmonary infarction, myocardial infarction, hemorrhagic pleural effusion, ventricular perforation, rupture of the pulmonary artery (from Swan-Ganz catheter placement after embolectomy), recurrent PE, pneumonia, empyema, and wound infection.[6]

Although the transcatheter pulmonary embolectomy technique has appeal due to its ability to be rapidly initiated in the arteriography suite, it has not been widely employed. The technique is complex and requires a venous cut-down. Manipulation of the catheter through the heart into the involved pulmonary artery can be difficult and requires fluoroscopy. Cardiac arrest precludes the use of fluoroscopy, as one needs access to the upper body to initiate resuscitative efforts. The role of suction embolectomy in the treatment of acute PE is limited and uncertain.

CURRENT TREATMENT RECOMMENDATIONS

Symptoms of PE may range from very mild alterations in respiratory patterns to severe dyspnea, hypoxia, and hemodynamic collapse. A classification of pulmonary thromboembolism based on observed physiologic effects has been previously reported by Greenfield.[6] This classification has been used to help stratify patients into treatment groups for accurate comparisons of therapeutic options and to allow more uniform predictions of prognosis. Class I, with 20% to 30% occlusion of the pulmonary vasculature, is considered minor. Signs and symptoms consist of anxiety and hyperventilation. Hypoxemia is typically mild with a Pao_2 greater than 80 mm Hg and $Paco_2$ less than 35 mm Hg. Hemodynamics remain stable in class I, with a tachycardia frequently observed. Class II, with 30% to 50% occlusion of the pulmonary vasculature, is considered major. Signs and symptoms include dyspnea and perhaps cardiorespiratory collapse. Hypoxemia is more pronounced, with a Pao_2 less than 65 mm Hg and a $Paco_2$ less than 35 mm Hg, reflecting a more pronounced tachypnea. Hemodynamic instability is observed with elevated central filling blood pressures and hypotension, yet this level of hemodynamic instability responds to resuscitation. Class III, with more than 50% occlusion of the pulmonary vasculature, is considered massive PE. Signs and symptoms are severe dyspnea and often shock. Hypoxemia is severe, with Pao_2 less than 50 mm Hg. Hemodynamic instability is frequent, with elevated filling pressures; the mean PA pressure is 25 mm Hg or more. These patients often require inotropes and vasopressors in order to maintain blood pressure. Class IV is referred to as chronic pulmonary embolism. The pulmonary vasculature is more than 50% occluded, and these patients often experience dyspnea and syncope. Hemodynamically, there is a fixed low cardiac output with mean PA pressure above 40 mm Hg. Hypoxemia is less severe with PaO_2 less than 70 mm Hg. One must also keep in mind that significant pre-existing cardiac or pulmonary insufficiency may reduce substantially the degree of PA occlusion necessary to produce severe symptoms.

Sumner has proposed a useful diagnostic algorithm for a patient with suspected PE.[10] A patient presenting with symptoms suggestive of massive PE should undergo immediate pulmonary arteriography. All others with suspected submassive PE should receive a ventilation-perfusion lung scan if the chest radiograph is normal. If the scan is normal, no further diagnostic efforts need be performed, and another diagnosis should be sought. If the perfusion scan shows multiple segmental or lobar defects and there is a clear ventilation-perfusion mismatch, it can be assumed that the patient has PE. All other patients should undergo noninvasive or phlebographic studies of the lower extremities. When the lower extremity studies are positive, the patient may be treated as one who has PE. If the lower extremity studies are negative, a pulmonary arteriogram should be performed. Examination of the leg veins may also be indicated if the diagnosis of PE has been firmly established and one is considering vena caval interruption.

Once the diagnosis of massive PE is made, a clinical decision should be made to either initiate adjunctive therapy in addition to the administration of systemic anticoagulation with intravenous heparin sodium or to treat the patient with systemic anticoagulation alone. Thrombolytic therapy is indicated for patients with massive PE, without shock, and without contraindications to lytic agents. For patients with massive PE with shock or cardiac arrest, open pulmonary embolectomy should be employed. Transvenous catheter pulmonary embolectomy remains an experimental device with insufficient experience to allow objective evaluation of its efficacy. The device, although innovative and well conceived, remains bulky and difficult to manipulate without experience. In Greenfield's own experience at the University of Michigan, only five procedures have been performed in 4 years.[7]

REFERENCES

1. Dalen JE, Banas JS Jr, Brooks HL, et al. Resolution rate of acute pulmonary embolism in man. N Engl J Med 1969; 280:1194–1199.
2. Daily PO. Embolectomy for acute pulmonary embolism. In: Bergan JJ, Yao JST, eds. Venous disorders, Philadelphia: WB Saunders, 1991:531–541.
3. Fisher RD, Fogarty TJ, Nolan SP. A catheter technique for the removal of pulmonary emboli without cardiopulmonary bypass. Surg Forum 1968; 19:247–249.
4. Greenfield LJ, Kimmell GO, McCurdy WC III. Transvenous removal of pulmonary emboli by vacuum-cup catheter technique. J Surg Res 1969; 9:347–352.
5. Clarke DB, Abrams LD. Pulmonary embolectomy: A 25 year experience. J Thorac Cardiovasc Surg 1986; 92:442–445.
6. Greenfield LJ, Proctor MC, Williams DM, et al. Long-term experience with transvenous catheter pulmonary embolectomy. J Vasc Surg 1993; 18:450–458.
7. Timsit JF, Reynaud P, Meyer G, Sors H. Pulmonary embolectomy by catheter device in massive pulmonary embolism. Chest 1991; 100:655–658.
8. Greenfield LJ. Catheter pulmonary embolectomy. Chest 1991; 100:593–594.
9. Brady AJB, Crake T, Oakley CM. Percutaneous fragmentation and dispersion versus pulmonary embolectomy by catheter device in massive pulmonary embolism. Chest 1992; 102:1305–1306.
10. Sumner DS. Diagnosis of deep vein thrombosis. In: Rutherford RB, ed. Vascular surgery. 3rd ed. Philadelphia: WB Saunders, 1989; 2:1520.

SURGICAL TREATMENT OF ACUTE AND CHRONIC PULMONARY EMBOLI

MARK IANNETTONI, M.D.
MARVIN KIRSH, M.D.

Approximately 600,000 episodes of pulmonary embolism (PE) occur annually in the United States alone.[1] The true mortality associated with PE is unknown, but it is estimated that 50,00 to 200,000 people die per year. Approximately 10% of these patients die within the first hour. However, of the 90% who survive, the diagnosis is frequently established late in the clinical course or not established at all. Coon showed that in only 27% of the patients who survived the initial event was the correct diagnosis ever established.[1] The mortality in patients in whom the correct diagnosis was established was only 8% but was 30% in those in whom the diagnosis was never established. Rubinstein in 1988 reported similar results in that in only a third of fatal cases of PE was the correct diagnosis ever established ante mortem.[1]

ACUTE PULMONARY EMBOLI

Pathophysiology

The adverse hemodynamic effects of acute PE result from a combination of mechanical obstruction of the pulmonary vasculature with the reflex and hormonal responses secondary to the emboli. The abrupt increase in pulmonary artery pressure places an undue strain on the normal right ventricle. When the pulmonary artery blood pressure exceeds 30 to 40 mm Hg, right ventricular dysfunction occurs because the normal right ventricle can acutely generate a pressure of only up to 40 mm Hg. Cardiovascular collapse occurs when the right ventricle is unable to compensate for the abrupt increase in pulmonary artery pressure. Various hormonal factors such as serotonin or thromboxane A_2 and other vasoactive amines have been documented to cause severe vasoconstriction of the muscular pulmonary arteries in acute PE.[2] These vasoactive amines are released from the platelet aggregation portion of the thrombus causing the embolus. Another source of pulmonary artery hypertension may be secondary to the baroreceptors in the pulmonary arteries, which may respond with intense vasoconstriction when obstruction, regardless of its size, occurs within the pulmonary artery. This, in association with the hormonal factors, may account for the cardiovascular collapse that may occur in patients with a relatively small PE.

Hypoxia is a cardinal finding in patients with acute PE. The pulmonary artery obstruction results in an increase in alveolar dead space because there are areas of ventilation without perfusion. The resultant hypoxia produces compensatory hyperventilation with hypocarbia. Additional hypoxia results from the decreased perfusion secondary to the right ventricular dysfunction, which leads to additional increases in alveolar dead space. Serotonin causes bronchoconstriction, which leads to additional hypoxia.

In addition, the vasoactive amines have been documented to cause a reduction in pulmonary surfactant distal to the embolus, producing atelectasis, further increasing the alveolar dead space ratio and causing more hypoxia. Consequently, a vicious cycle is created, with hypoxia leading to more hypoxia, that, if uninterrupted, results in death.

Management

Any patient suspected of sustaining a PE should be begun immediately on heparin sodium therapy while awaiting the establishment of the diagnosis. Ventilation perfusion ($\dot{V}/\dot{Q}$) scanning is useful as a screening procedure in stable patients. It is especially helpful when normal because a normal $\dot{V}/\dot{Q}$ scan is almost never associated with a major PE. We believe that pulmonary angiography is the optimal method of establishing the diagnosis. Not only does it confirm the diagnosis especially in those patients with an abnormal $\dot{V}/\dot{Q}$ scan but also it establishes the size and location of the embolus.

The role of pulmonary embolectomy for acute PE has been the subject of continuing controversy despite the fact that only a small percentage (2% to 6%) of patients with an acute PE require surgical pulmonary embolectomy.

The indications for operation are (1) severe hemodynamic compromise unresponsive to inotropic support and (2) progressive hypoxemia, with or without hemodynamic compromise, not responding to aggressive medical therapy, including intubation and mechanical ventilatory support.[3,4]

Pulmonary embolectomy can be performed with either inflow occlusion or cardiopulmonary bypass (CPB). The authors prefer the latter because the former is associated with a prohibitive mortality (40%) and the time constraints associated with inflow occlusion limit the amount of thrombus that can be removed.

Technique

A median sternotomy provides optimal exposure of the main pulmonary artery and its major branches. Prior to the sternotomy, the patient is placed on CPB via the femoral artery and vein and converted to total CPB after the sternotomy by cannulating the superior vena cava via the right atrial appendage. Transesophageal echocardiography is carried out at the time the patient is on partial CPB in an attempt to visualize the location of the PE. Both the superior and inferior vena cava are occluded with tourniquets. The main pulmonary artery and its right and left branches are circumferentially exposed. A longitudinal incision is made in the main pulmonary artery and extended onto the left pulmonary artery. All visible thrombus is removed. The thrombus is best grasped with either ring forceps or a sponge stick. Following removal of all visible thrombi, a Fogarty catheter is placed distally into the pulmonary artery branches to extract any distal clot. If there is distal clot that cannot be removed with the Fogarty catheter, the lungs are manually massaged in an attempt to remove the remaining thrombi. After all the clot is removed, the pulmonary artery is closed with a running 5-0 polypropylene suture. After cessation of CPB, a Greenfield filter is inserted via either the femoral vein or the right atrial appendage.

Results

The operative mortality for pulmonary embolectomy ranges from 16% to 38%. The mortality is directly related to the preoperative condition of the patient. In the study of Gray and associates, patients who sustained a cardiac arrest and required external cardiac massage had a 36% survival, whereas those who did not sustain a cardiac arrest had an 89% survival.[3,4] In a study by Kieny and colleagues, the mortality was directly related to the preoperative systolic blood pressure. In those who had a blood pressure lower than 60 mm Hg but did not sustain a cardiac arrest, the mortality rate was 12%. It was 10% for those with a blood pressure between 60 and 100 mm Hg, and only 5% with those with a blood pressure greater than 100 mm Hg.[5]

Complications

Because many patients are hypotensive before initiation of CPB, approximately 25% of those undergoing a pulmonary embolectomy have some central nervous dysfunction postoperatively. This is especially true in patients who sustained a cardiac arrest prior to operation. The other major complication unique to this operation is pulmonary edema and/or hemorrhage. It has been reported to occur to some extent in all patients who undergo pulmonary embolectomy.[4] The etiology is unknown but is felt by most to be a reperfusion injury that is exacerbated by the release of vasoactive amines. Kieny and co-workers believe it is secondary to manipulation of the lungs or the technique of reversed perfusion that is used to express the distal thrombus. In their study, in which these maneuvers were not performed, the incidence was only 1 in 134 patients.[5] Although, as a rule, this complication is self-limiting, it may be fatal if severe enough to produce profound hypoxemia. If there is no contraindication, patients with severe hypoxemia should be supported by extracorporeal membrane oxygenation until the process revolves.

Long-Term Management

Even though a vena cava filter has been inserted, it is our opinion that these patients should be placed on lifelong anticoagulant therapy with sodium warfarin, which should be closely monitored.

CHRONIC PULMONARY EMBOLI

If the patient survives the acute episode and appropriate measures are taken to prevent recurrence, the thrombus usually resolves completely. However, in 0.1% to 0.2% of patients surviving the acute embolism, the emboli fail to resolve and consequently chronic pulmonary hypertension develops.[6] The exact etiology of the chronic pulmonary hypertension is unknown, but it is felt by Moser and associates to result from hypertensive changes in the nonelastic arteries in the "open" vascular bed.[7] The true prevalence is unknown because the symptoms and physical findings are subtle until right ventricular failure occurs.[2]

The major symptoms of these patients are dyspnea on exertion and fatigue. The respiratory insufficiency, at first mild, becomes progressive and incapacitating. A history of deep venous thrombosis is obtained only in approximately 40% of patients, and only 50% give a history of PE. The initial physical examination may be completely normal. However, with passage of time there is an increased second heart sound, a systolic murmur associated with tricuspid regurgitation, an additional high-pitched continuous murmur over the chest wall, hepatomegaly, ascites, and peripheral edema. Also late in the course of the disease, the patient becomes hypoxic, develops clubbing, and becomes cyanotic with exercise. The chest roentgenogram usually documents right ventricular enlargement, prominent main pulmonary arteries, and decreased pulmonary vasculature. A $\dot{V}/\dot{Q}$ scan documents areas of poor perfusion in areas of normal ventilation ($\dot{V}/\dot{Q}$ mismatch). Pulmonary angiography is diagnostic of chronic PE. In patients who are severely symptomatic, the emboli obstruct 50% to 75% of the pulmonary vasculature.

Medical treatment with chronic anticoagulants and vasodilator therapy has not been demonstrated to affect the prognosis in patients with chronic PE. The mortality in these patients is directly correlated with their pulmonary artery blood pressures. If the pulmonary artery blood pressure varies between 30 and 50 mm Hg, the 5 year survival with medical therapy was 30%, whereas it was only 10% when the pulmonary artery blood pressures were greater then 50 mm Hg.

Although surgical therapy has been documented to be beneficial, fewer than 300 cases have been reported. Criteria for thromboendarectomy in those severely symptomatic included (1) thrombi that are readily accessible, (2) pulmonary artery blood pressure of at least 30 mm Hg, and (3) pulmonary vascular resistance greater than 4 Wood units. Contraindications to thromboendarectomy include (1) small peripheral emboli, (2) comorbid diseases such as renal or coronary artery disease, (3) small pulmonary arteries not amenable to patch reconstruction, and (4) irreversible right heart failure.[8]

Technique

The operation involves a median sternotomy, use of CPB, and brief periods of circulatory arrest. The circulatory arrest allows the excellent visualization that is needed for distal dissection without interference from bronchial artery backbleeding. Additional exposure of the right pulmonary artery can be obtained by circumferential mobilization of the superior vena cava, allowing either medial or lateral retraction. Incisions are made from the main pulmonary artery and onto both lower lobe branches. The thrombi in these patients become incorporated into the vascular wall over time with a resultant densely adherent thrombus. An endarterectomy plane, similar to that for a carotid endarterectomy, is established. The thrombus and intimal layer are removed as a unit. The clot is retrieved as far distally as possible, leaving a well-tapered end. The pulmonary arteriotomy is closed, primarily with a running suture of 5-0 polypropylene. At times, it may be necessary to utilize a pericardial patch to reconstruct the pulmonary arteries. The right atrium should be routinely explored for an atrial septal defect or the presence of additional thrombi. After cessation of CPB, a Greenfield filter is inserted via the femoral vein or the right atrial appendage, if not previously placed.[9]

Recently, Jamieson and co-workers recommended the use of preoperative angioscopy as an aid to planning the surgical approach by more accurately identifying the most proximal location of chronic thrombus. This practice would amplify the information gained by the pulmonary arteriogram.[10] Intraoperative transesophageal echocardiography enables one to evaluate left and right ventricular function and aid in the selection of inotropic support in the immediate postoperative period.

Tricuspid annuloplasty as a rule has been avoided.

Although severe tricuspid regurgitation may be present prior to endartectomy, relief of the elevated pulmonary artery blood pressures and decrease in pulmonary vascular resistance result in improved right heart hemodynamics and obviate the need for tricuspid annuloplasty.

In an attempt to decrease the occurrence of postperfusion vasoconstriction and its sequelae, as well as the potential for postprocedure in situ rethrombosis, intravenous prostaglandin E should be begun just prior to cessation of CPB and continued for at least 72 hours. If the patient develops postembolectomy reperfusion injury, prostaglandin should be continued until the process resolves.

The operative mortality ranges from 9% to 22%, depending upon the experience of the surgeon.[8-10] This operation is technically demanding and requires superb clinical judgment. Therefore, this procedure should only be performed by experienced surgeons at centers familiar with the difficult perioperative management of these patients.

The most common cause of death is right ventricular failure secondary to high residual pulmonary artery blood pressures and unremitting severe reperfusion edema. Elevated pressures are likely to occur in patients in whom there is little, if any, backbleeding from the bronchial arteries during the thromboendarectomy and in patients with inaccessible thrombi. Excellent hemodynamic improvement is usually obtained in those who survive operation. In the studies of Moser and associates, this symptomatic improvement was maintained long term. In their report, more than 95% of the survivors were the New York Heart Association (NYHA) class I.[7] This is a stark contrast to their preoperative conditions, when more than 95% of the patients were either NYHA class III or IV. The patients should remain on lifelong anticoagulation, which should be carefully regulated.[7]

REFERENCES

1. Greenfield LJ. Pulmonary emboism: Pathophysiology and treatment. In: Baue AE, ed. Glenn's thoracic and cardiovascular surgery. Englewood Cliffs, NJ: Appleton & Lange, 1991:2:1561.
2. Elliott CG. Pulmonary physiology during pulmonary embolism. Chest 1992; 101 (suppl):163–71.
3. Gray HH, Morgan JM, Paneth M, Miller GA. Pulmonary embolectomy for acute massive pulmonary embolism: An analysis of 71 cases. Br Heart J 1988; 60:196–200.
4. Meyer G, Tamisier D, Sors H, et al. Pulmonary embolectomy: A 20-year experience at one center. Ann Thorac Surg 1991; 51:232–236.
5. Kieny R, Charpentier A, Kieny MT. What is the place of pulmonary embolectomy today? J Cardiovasc Surg (Torino) 1991; 32:549–554.
6. Ridel M, Stanek V, Widimsky J, Prerovsky I. Long term follow-up of patients with pulmonary embolism: Late prognosis and evolution of hemodynamic and respiratory data. Chest 1982; 81: 151–158.
7. Moser KM, Auger WR, Fedullo PF, Jamieson SW. Chronic thromboembolic pulmonary hypertension: Clinical picture and surgical treatment. Eur Respir J 1992; 5:334–342.
8. Lyerly HK, Sabiston DC. Surgical treatment of chronic pulmonary embolism. Annu Rev Med 1991; 42:501–517.
9. Daily PO, Dembitsky WP, Iversen S. Technique of pulmonary thromboendarterectomy for chronic pulmonary embolism. J Cardiovasc Surg (Torino) 1989; 4:10–24.
10. Jamieson SW, Auger WR, Fedullo PF, et al. Experience and results with 150 pulmonary thromboendarterectomy operations over a 29-month period. J Thorac Cardiovasc Surg 1993; 106:116–127.

UPPER EXTREMITY VENOUS OCCLUSION

HERBERT I. MACHLEDER, M.D.

After 100 years of sporadic reports in the medical literature on spontaneous thrombosis of the axillary-subclavian vein, Hughes undertook the first real analysis of the subject in 1949.[1] He wrote, "The association of a more or less acute venous obstruction in the upper extremity of an otherwise perfectly healthy person constitutes a syndrome which, in the absence of accurate knowledge of the etiology and pathology, can be called the 'Paget-Schroetter syndrome,' after the first two to describe it as a clinical entity." For the next 40 years, a patchwork of surgical and medical approaches were directed to the treatment of this problem, all encumbered by poor understanding of the pathophysiology and characterized by a very high incidence of failure.

In 1985 a structured, comprehensive management strategy for the treatment of patients with Paget-Schroetter's syndrome was initiated at UCLA. This approach was based on improved understanding of the underlying pathophysiology as well as advances in thrombolytic and vascular interventional techniques. In 1993 the results were reported for 50 consecutive patients entered prospectively into what was termed a "staged, mutidisciplinary approach."

NATURAL HISTORY

Untreated patients with Paget-Schroetter's syndrome can be expected to have varying degrees of disability as a consequence of chronic venous hypertension and/or recurrent episodes of venous thrombosis. This disability incidence ranges from a low of 25% reported by Linblad from Sweden, to 40% reported by

Gloviczki from the Mayo Clinic, 47% reported by Donayre, and 74% by Tilney. In addition to the upper extremity morbidity, there is a persistent, although small, incidence of pulmonary embolism.

MANAGEMENT

The algorithm for management contains several stages that incorporate specific treatment steps, based on our own experience as well as published results of others[2,3] (Fig. 1). At the outset, verification by venography is essential for proper diagnosis, as duplex ultrasound scanning is relatively inaccurate for venous assessment in the area of the retroclavicular space.

Thrombolytic and Anticoagulant Therapy

Immediately after verification of the diagnosis, patients should be treated by catheter-directed fibrinolytic therapy into the thrombus. Heparin sodium is administered concomitantly and continued until therapeutic anticoagulation with warfarin sodium is accomplished.[4] Although streptokinase had been used successfully in axillosubclavian vein thrombosis, much of the reported experience suggests the superiority of urokinase for this disorder. To avoid rethrombosis, surgical therapy is delayed for 1 to 3 months after successful thrombolysis. This delay is imposed with the recognition that the vein remains highly thrombogenic for a variable period of time following an acute thrombotic episode. Laboratory and clinical research have identified high levels of cytokines in the vein wall for at least 1 month and reduced fibrinolytic activity of the endothelium for at least 3 months.

Surgery

The rationale for operative treatment derives from an understanding of the pathologic anatomy and recognition of the natural history. In untreated patients or those treated only with thrombolytic or anticoagulant therapy, there is a high incidence of repetitive thrombosis. In the UCLA series, of 50 patients followed prospectively, there was a 34% incidence of repeat (venographically documented) thrombosis prior to sur-

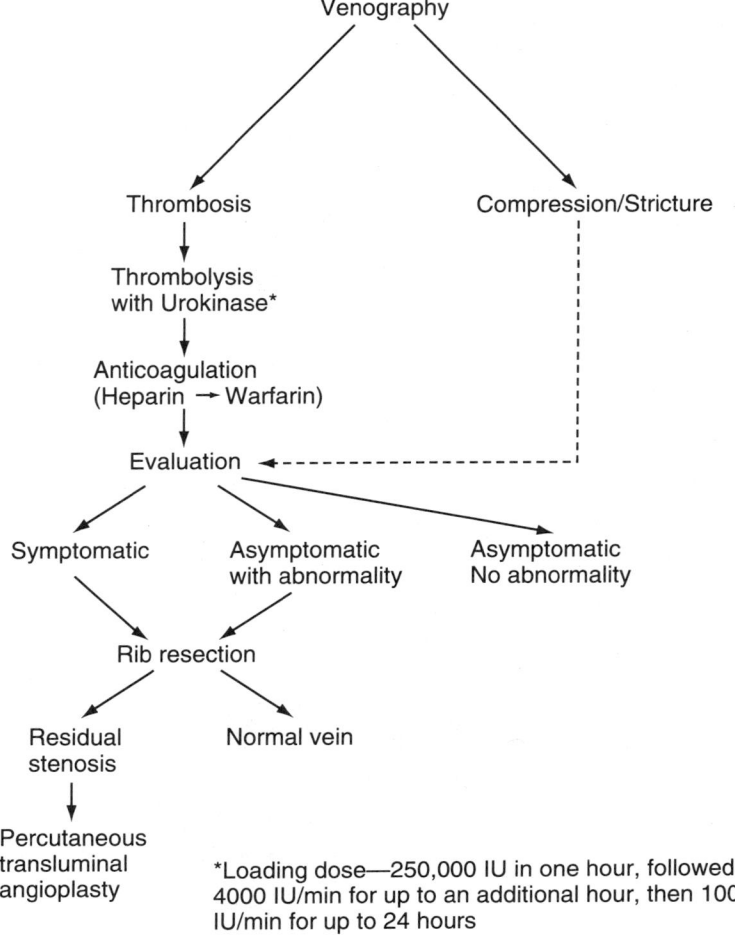

Figure 1 Algorithm for the management of suspected axillosubclavian vein thrombosis.

gical correction of the underlying abnormality (Figs. 2 and 3).

Surgical treatment is recommended in two settings: (1) if, following restoration of vein patency, there remains an underlying compressive abnormality, or (2) if symptomatic patients with an occluded vein demonstrate obstruction of the venous collaterals with abduction of the arm. Venography is performed in two supine positions: with the arm at the patient's side and with the humerus at right angles to the chest wall. Transaxillary first rib resection is the procedure of choice, based on the extensive literature documenting long-term results, effectiveness, and the excellent anatomic visualization of the area.

Transluminal Balloon Venoplasty

Postoperative transluminal angioplasty can be employed when the subclavian vein does not return to a normal configuration, with a residual stricture demonstrated on postoperative venogram. The continued presence of collateral venous channels after operation is

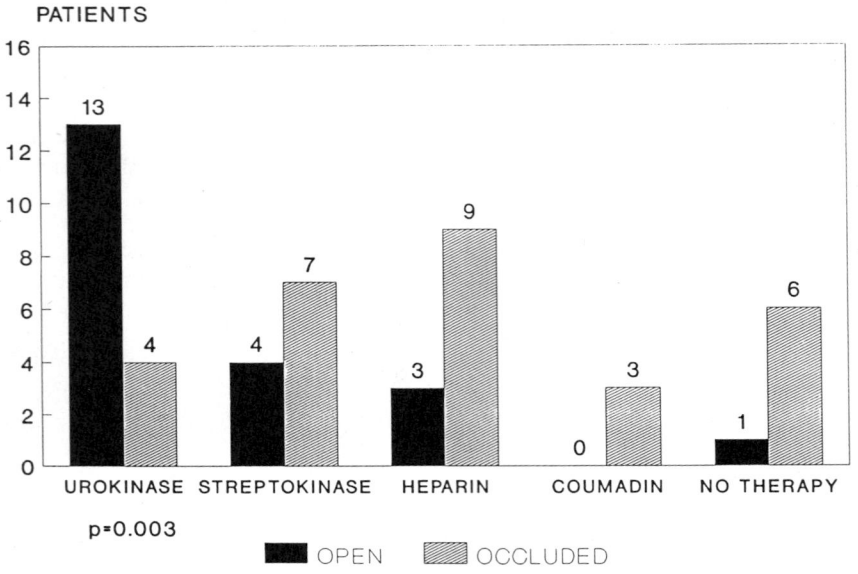

Figure 2 Venous patency after various types of initial medical management (studied in 50 consecutive patients).

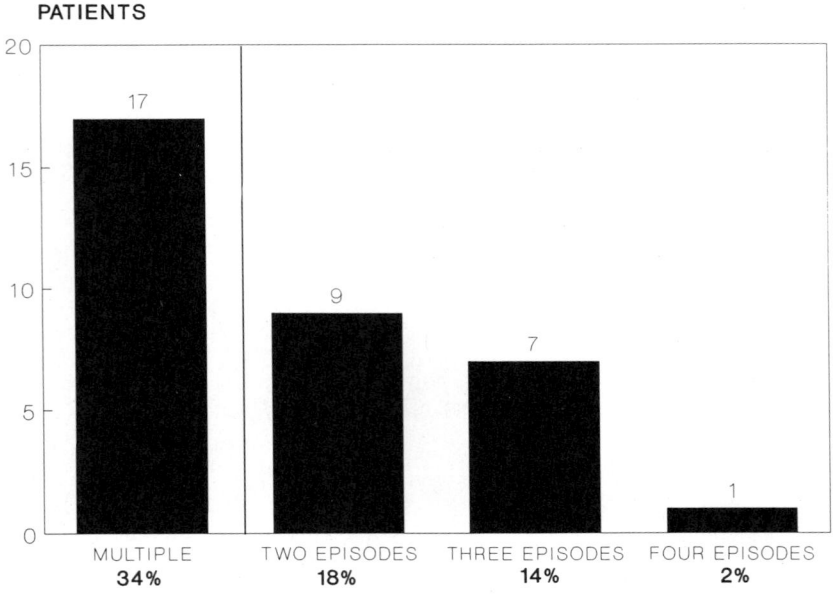

Figure 3 Episodes of venographically documented recurrent thrombosis (after initial successful restoration of patency) prior to definitive surgical correction of the compressive abnormality.

interpreted as indicating that a stricture is hemodynamically significant. When this modality is used preoperatively, it often leads to rethrombosis and, in our experience, a serious compromise of ultimate patency (Fig. 4). Seven of 12 balloon angioplasties performed after successful thrombolytic therapy but before operation resulted in immediate rethrombosis of the vein. Seven of nine balloon angioplasties performed for residual stricture after surgical decompression were patent at long-term venographic follow-up evaluation. In two patients, the stricture could not be crossed with a guide wire.

BASIS FOR THE STAGED MULTIDISCIPLINARY ALGORITHM

The concept of a definitive multidisciplinary treatment strategy derives from improved understanding of the role of operative treatment as well as the development of endovascular techniques for angioplasty and the delivery of thrombolytic agents.

The underlying cause of Paget-Schroetter's syndrome is a mechanical abnormality at the costoclavicular portion of the axillosubclavian vein, with superimposed thrombosis resulting in the complexity of the clinical manifestations (Figs. 5 and 6). A treatment strategy that deals with the thrombotic process and then corrects the underlying mechanical abnormality can relieve the acute as well as the chronic manifestations of this disorder.

ALTERNATIVE APPROACHES

Despite the rationale of the staged approach, there have been proponents of other treatment strategies for this problem. Although initial thrombolytic therapy has been gaining wider acceptance, there remain surgeons committed to early surgical thrombectomy as well as initial surgical repair. We believe that this initial surgical approach should be abandoned.

Several authors have suggested treating the throm-

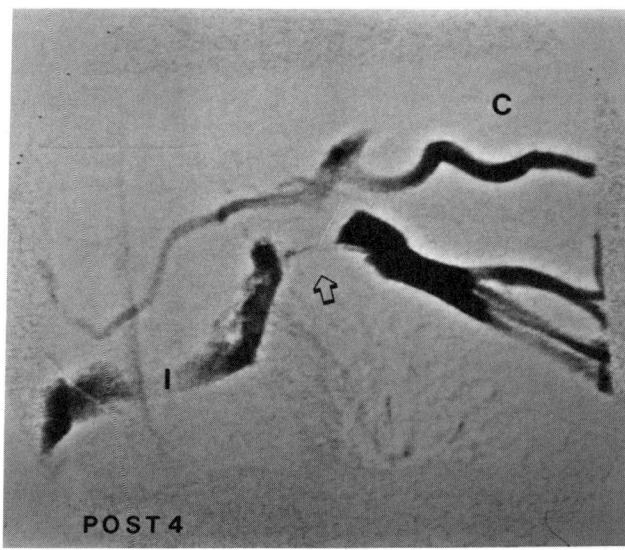

Figure 4 Status of subclavian vein after four attempts to balloon dilate the stricture. (This was done immediately after successful thrombolytic therapy but prior to surgical correction.)

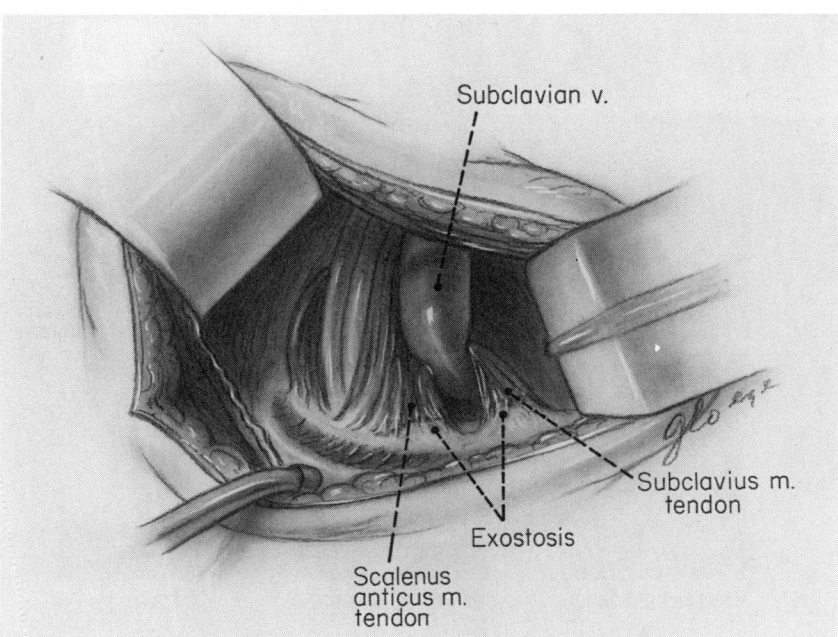

Figure 5 Anatomic deformity (seen from the transaxillary exposure) in a typical patient with the Paget-Schroetter syndrome.

botic process alone without addressing the underlying anatomic abnormality. The rationale for this approach is supported by neither these authors' published data nor by our own experience.[5] Some authors have accepted the concept of initial thrombolytic therapy and suggest that surgical correction can be undertaken immediately in the postlytic period.[6,7] This is a deceptively appealing concept that seems to be encumbered by the same problems complicating surgical thrombectomy, specifically, that of attempting definitive repair at a time when the vein is in its most thrombogenic condition and that of potentially increasing the risk of adequate followup anticoagulant therapy.

At this phase, the staged approach is justified by the excellent postoperative patency rates achieved. The recommendation for immediate surgical intervention has yet to be validated by any objective followup studies.

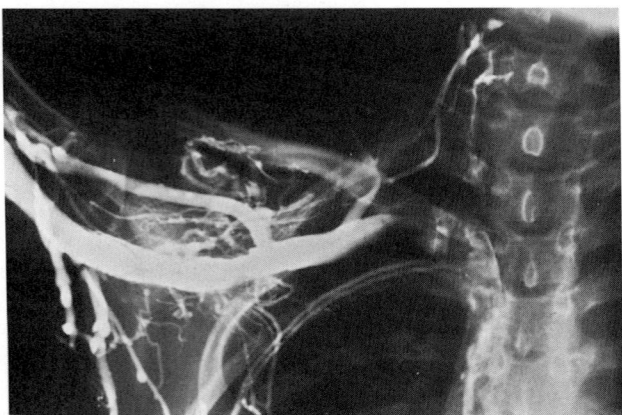

Figure 6 Phlebogram of the compressive abnormality at the thoracic outlet. Often described as a beaklike deformity.

In patients in whom recognition of the problem has been prompt and the lytic program carried out expeditiously, revealing a relatively normal vein with typical external compressive abnormality, the interval to operation has been shortened to 4 weeks without adversely affecting long-term patency.

It has additionally been suggested that the vein can be decompressed by an anterior infraclavicular resection of the parasternal portion of the first rib. As noted by Urschel, this procedure places the brachial plexus at particular risk.[8] Authors reporting extensive experience with first rib resection uniformly document the hazards of leaving a posterior segment of first rib and scalenus medius muscle abutting the inferior trunk of the brachial plexus. The resultant fibrous scar is a frequent and serious cause of later neuropathic symptoms from the brachial plexus.[9]

The protocol described by Kunkle appears safe as well as effective, with infrequent complications of generally minimal and transient consequence.[2] Thrombolytic therapy was efficacious in these young patients, who, in general, have no contraindications to the use of lytic agents. In the group of patients studied at UCLA, there were few minor bleeding episodes, no cerebral complications, and, in the case of urokinase, no allergic reactions.

When a decision is made for aggressive therapy, the staged multimodal algorithm for management appears to be effective in restoring patients to normal function, maintaining venous patency, and preventing recurrent thrombosis (Fig. 7).

REFERENCES

1. Hughes ESR. Venous obstruction in the upper extremity. Int Abst Surg 1949; 88:89.

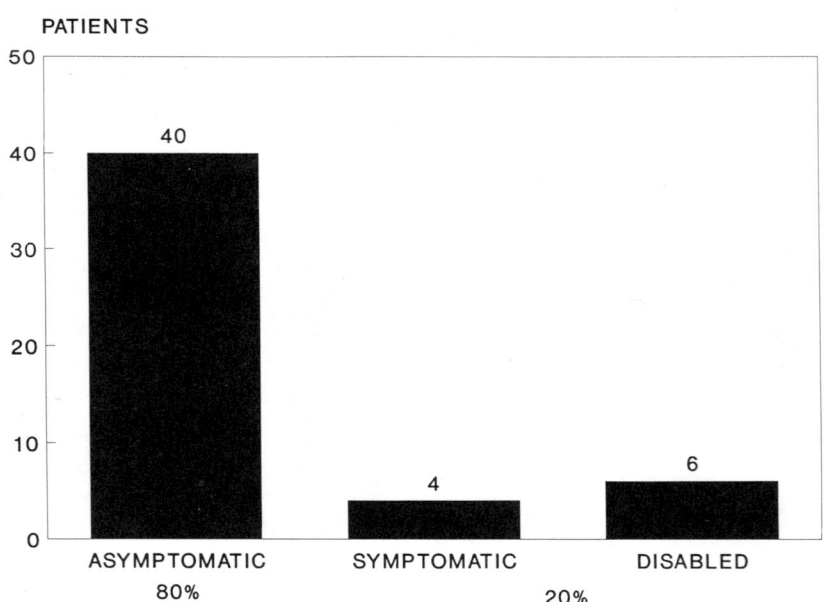

Figure 7 Final clinical result in 50 consecutive patients, after 3 years of follow-up evaluation.

2. Kunkel JM, Machleder HI. Treatment of Paget-Schroetter syndrome: A staged, multidisciplinary approach. Arch Surg 1989; 124:1153–1158.
3. Machleder HI. Evaluation of a new treatment strategy for Paget-Schroetter syndrome: Spontaneous thrombosis of the axillary-subclavian vein. J Vasc Surg 1993; 17:305–317.
4. Machleder HI. Upper extremity venous thrombosis. Semin Vasc Surg 1990; 3:219–226.
5. Wilson JJ, Zahn CA, Newman H. Fibrinolytic therapy for idiopathic subclavian-axillary vein thrombosis. Am J Surg 1990; 159:208–211.
6. Molina JE. Surgery for effort thrombosis of the subclavian vein. J Thorac Cardiovasc Surg 1992; 103:341–346.
7. Urschel HC, Razzuk MA. Improved management of the Paget-Schroetter syndrome secondary to thoracic outlet compression. Ann Thorac Surg 1991; 52:1217–1221.
8. Urschel HC. In discussion of, Surgery for effort thrombosis of the subclavian vein, by Molina JE. J Thorac Cardiovasc Surg 1992; 103:346.
9. Roos DB. Recurrent thoracic outlet syndrome after first rib resection. Acta Chir Belg 1980; 5:363–371.

SEPTIC THROMBOPHLEBITIS

MARK REYNOLDS, M.D.
J. DAVID RICHARDSON, M.D.

Septic or suppurative thrombophlebitis is an intense local inflammatory response to infiltration of the venous wall by invasive micro-organisms. Perivascular and intravascular suppuration, thrombosis, and systemic septicemia are frequent findings. This is the surgical manifestation of a spectrum of disorders, including bland venous thrombophlebitis, aseptic phlebitis, catheter contamination and colonization, and catheter-associated sepsis. This disease that often begins so simply may have protean manifestations dependent upon its location, extent, and severity. The systemic sequelae of intravascular sepsis, including pneumonia, multiple and recurrent episodes of bacteremia, systemic septic physiology, and metastatic abscess, may hide the relatively modest signs of local infection. It may be easily neglected in a cursory examination of a septic patient. However, it is not a diagnosis that one can afford to overlook. Septic thrombophlebitis is a condition with a high associated mortality when it is not treated in a timely and aggressive fashion.[1] Even when promptly treated, it may significantly lengthen hospital stay and cause increased morbidity.

Septic thrombophlebitis occurs as several distinct clinicopathologic entities. These may be distinguished on the basis of the anatomic location of the primary lesion: (1) superficial, (2) central pelvic, (3) portal, (4) intracranial, or (5) cervical. The last three forms have become rare since the advent of effective antimicrobial chemotherapy. By contrast, superficial and central septic thrombophlebitis have become relatively more prevalent in recent decades. This rise in incidence is a result of the increasingly invasive nature of modern medicine.

Superficial or central venous suppurative thrombophlebitis is usually a consequence of chronic, indwelling, intravenous catheters in the patient with a prolonged critical illness.[1] Pelvic thrombophlebitis is a disease of women of childbearing age. It is associated with pregnancy, parturition, abortion, pelvic infection, and gynecologic surgery. Portal or mesenteric suppurative thrombophlebitis (pylephlebitis) is a complication of neglected intra-abdominal infection, most commonly appendiceal, diverticular, or biliary sepsis. Suppurative thrombophlebitis of the internal jugular (Lemierre syndrome or postanginal septicemia) occurs now as a rare complication of acute oropharyngeal infection. Intracranial suppurative thrombophlebitis (septic cavernous sinus or lateral sinus thrombophlebitis) is a dreaded and highly lethal complication of superficial facial, otitic, and sinus infections.

EPIDEMIOLOGY

Prior to the widespread use of intravenous (IV) therapy, superficial thrombophlebitis was associated with local skin and soft tissue infections.[2] Now, with a large proportion of all hospitalized patients receiving IV therapy, the major cause of superficial suppurative thrombophlebitis is the presence of long-term venous catheters.[3] Suppurative thrombophlebitis is the most extreme and uncommon form of catheter-associated phlebitis and catheter-associated sepsis.

Phlebitis is an inflammation of the vessel that is usually not associated with infection. In the majority of infusion-associated phlebitic episodes, there is no evidence of sepsis or bacteremia, and there is only a slightly enhanced risk of catheter colonization and infection. Phlebitis is a common iatrogenic disease. About 25% of all hospitalized patients suffer an iatrogenic complication during their hospital course; of these, catheter-related phlebitis represents approximately 75%.[4] Overall, bland phlebitis occurs in 13.7% to 20% of general medical patients who have intravenous catheters placed.[4]

A Centers for Disease Control study of patients with intravenous catheters found that the incidence of catheter colonization and catheter-associated sepsis was 34.5% and 3.6%, respectively. The incidence of bacteremia due to intravenous catheters is approximately 0.1% to 6.5% of all those receiving intravenous therapy.[5] Catheter-associated sepsis is defined clinically by the improvement in the septic patient after catheter re-

Table 1 Risk Factors for Septic Thrombophlebitis

Emergency catheter placement
Venous cut-downs
Lower extremity placement
Plastic catheter use
Prolonged catheter use
Burns
Multiple use of intravenous needle
Intravenous drug abuse
Immunosuppressed state (cancer and steroid therapy)

moval. Confirmation is provided by growth from the catheter tip of greater than 15 CFU of the same organism isolated from the blood. The course of catheter-associated sepsis is complicated in 33% of patients. Suppurative thrombophlebitis accounts for 21% of the complications that occur in 7% of all episodes of catheter-assocated sepsis.[6]

Suppurative thrombophlebitis is the most severe complication of IV catheter use. The overall incidence of suppurative thrombophlebitis is 88 per 100,000 hospital discharges (0.08%), and it may account for 7% to 12% of all nosocomial infections.[7] Multiple adverse risk factors have been identified[8] (Table 1). It is 40 times more likely to occur in patients with a plastic cannula in place than in those with a steel needle. It is associated with lines that are placed under emergency conditions and with the infusion of sclerosing solutions, such as potassium chloride. It occurs with greater frequency and virulence in burn patients. It has been reported to be one of the most common causes of septic death in the burn patient, occurring in 4% to 8% of all those who develop infectious complications.[9] Patients with a history of IV drug abuse or cancer and those receiving steroids are also at increased risk. Suppurative thrombophlebitis is among the many complications of IV drug use, and its incidence as a non-nosocomial finding parallels the incidence of IV drug abuse in the community.[10]

Catheter-associated septic central venous thrombosis is the simultaneous occurence of two uncommon entities: central venous catheter–associated sepsis and catheter-associated central venous thrombosis. Central venous catheter–associated sepsis complicates an average of 2% to 10% of all episodes of central venous catheterization. Clinically apparent or hemodynamically significant catheter-associated central venous thrombosis necessitating catheter removal occurs in approximately 4% to 10% of all insertions. The simultaneous occurrence of these two complications is extremely rare. In 1986 Kaufman and colleagues reported on a series of five patients with this complication accrued over the course of 2 years. At that time they were able to find only 37 confirmed or probable cases reported in the literature. The rapidity with which they accrued their series and the difficulty of making the diagnosis argue that this complication is significantly underreported.[11] Twenty-five cases have been reported in the literature since that time.

PATHOPHYSIOLOGY

Suppurative thrombophlebitis can be conceptualized as a subset of venous thrombosis, and Virchow's triad is relevant to an understanding of the etiology of this disease. Damage to the vessel wall and intima can occur through direct mechanical abrasion from a venous cannula, from the chronic presence of high concentrations of hyperosmotic and cytotoxic solutions, or from extrinsic compression and trauma caused by the presence of a nearby expanding abscess or gravid uterus. Relative low flow states may exist in many of these patients. This may be due to hypovolemia and hemoconcentration secondary to dehydration or hypoperfusion, or to local compromise of venous drainage secondary to extrinsic masses or chronic venous disease. Hypercoagulable states are probably contributory in some patients, including cancer patients and pregnant women in particular.

The thrombus becomes a nidus for the development of infection. The micro-organisms that colonize the thrombus may reach it from many distant or local sites. There are three major routes of dissemination: Local spread is the traditional route by which suppurative thrombophlebitis results from otitis media, oropharyngeal infections, diverticulitis, endometritis, and suppurative lymphadenitis. In suppurative thrombophlebitis associated with indwelling IV catheters, local spread may occur from the skin down the tract of the catheter or from contamination of the catheter, with seeding at the time of insertion. Hematogenous spread from distant foci of infection is possibly the most common route of colonization of the organizing thrombus. In catheter-associated disease, contaminated infusate is another potential source of infection. The association of catheter-related sepsis with an increasing number of ports available for infusion is indicative of the potential importance of this source of contamination. The degree to which these three routes of dissemination contribute to the pathogenesis of suppurative thrombophlebitis is dependent upon the patient population involved.

The resultant nidus of intravascular infection gives rise to the lethal sequelae. Suppurative thrombophlebitis is a progressive disease. It invades tributary veins and spreads centrally. The pulmonary circulation may be showered with multiple septic emboli, resulting in a diffuse pneumonitis, pneumonia, and the adult respiratory distress syndrome. The entire circulatory system is subjected to a chronic intermittent bacteremia. The source may not be apparent, but the systemic sequelae may be dramatic, and frequently these secondary effects are all that is apparent of the underlying disease.

CLINICAL MANIFESTATIONS

The local signs of suppurative thrombophlebitis include erythema, tenderness, swelling, lymphangitis, or a palpable venous cord, usually in close proximity to the site of IV catheter insertion. The reported incidence of these local findings varies from 33%[7] to 62%[10] to 94%,[3] depending upon the patient population involved.

The disease is more common and more difficult to diagnose in the burn patient. Formerly, suppurative thrombophlebitis occurred in approximately 7% of all burn patients suffering more than 20% total body surface area burns. The site of the infection was in the lower extremity in 76%, upper extremity in 24%, and elsewhere in 8%. The duration of cannulation prior to the onset of infection was 4 to 5 days, but suppuration at the site of catheterization may occur up to 10 days after removal. Fever occurs in 70%. Local signs of infection were present in only 32%, but 84% had symptomatic bacteremia, and 44% developed pneumonia secondary to septic pulmonary emboli.[8] The most common presenting signs are positive blood cultures in the setting of clinical sepsis. In this setting, suppurative thrombophlebitis is associated with high mortality.

When suppurative thrombophlebitis supervenes in the typical medical or surgical patient, it is usually less catastrophic and easier to diagnose. These patients tend to be mostly over the age of 50, hospitalized with severe, debilitating diseases, and frequently on intravenous antibiotics for the treatment of sepsis. The veins of the upper extremity are involved in two-thirds of patients, and the lower extremity is rarely involved. Signs of local infection have been reported to be present in over 90% in some series[3] and are said to be a rare finding in others.[1,8] Swelling and erythema are present in approximately a third to a half, and purulent fluid may be expressed from the catheter site in 50% to 70%. Pain at the site occurs frequently. Fever of greater than 102°F is present in about half of these patients, and a third have fevers of between 104 and 106°F.[1,10] Leukocytosis is a frequent finding, but it is usually moderate. Bacteremia is present in approximately 70% to 80% of patients, and in 80% the isolate from the blood cultures is identical or similar to the organisms isolated from the thrombus.[3] About two-thirds of the infected cannulas were in place for greater than 5 days.

Suppurative thrombophlebitis of the central venous system is a rare complication. There is rarely any clinical evidence of venous occlusion or thrombosis. The clinical findings are consistent with sepsis. This syndrome is differentiated clinically from central venous catheter-associated sepsis by the persistence of the septic state after removal of an infected catheter. The febrile course is characterized by a hectic pattern. Evidence of a phlegmonous mass involving the central venous system may be found on computed tomographic (CT) examination of the chest.

MICROBIOLOGY

The microbiology of suppurative thrombophlebitis has changed considerably over the decades. In the sentinel report from the preantibiotic era,[2] beta-hemolytic *Streptococcus* (44%) and *Staphylococcus aureus* (24%) were the most prevalent bacteria isolated. Less commonly, *Escherichia coli,* Friedländer's bacillus, *Streptococcus viridans,* and *Enterococcus* were cultured. O'Neill and co-workers have reported on the incidence and bacteriology of this disease in the burn patient over the course of the past 30 years.[7] In the experience of this group, the bacteriology of suppurative thrombophlebitis has changed with the changing microbiology of the burn unit. During the period from 1960 through 1966 staphylococci were the causative organisms in 77% of the positive cultures, alone in 40%, with Gram-negative rods in 41%, and with *Candida* in 5.7%. Forty-three percent of cultures were polymicrobial. During 1967 through 1974, Gram-negative organisms were ascendent, in particular, *Pseudomonas aeruginosa* and *Providencia stuartii.* From 1975 to the present, *Staphylococcus aureus* has once again emerged as the predominant organism, isolated in nearly three-quarters of the patients.[9] In the past decade there has been increasing involvement of nonbacterial species, in particular, *C. albicans* and *Aspergillus*.[12]

TREATMENT

Treatment depends on the site and the severity of the infection. For infection in a location that is amenable to excision, this is the most effective and efficient therapy. For inaccessible infection, prolonged therapy with parenteral antibiotics with or without thrombolytic or anticoagulant therapy is reasonably effective.

In the retrospective review of superficial suppurative thrombophlebitis by Baker and co-workers, 17% of the patients with superficial suppurative thrombophlebitis were treated successfully with nonoperative therapy.[10] Treatment in these patients consisted of heat, elevation, and parenteral antibiotics. Operative therapy combined with antibiotic therapy was pursued in the remaining patients by a variety of means. Excision of the involved vein, with incision and drainage of associated abscesses as needed, was performed in most of the patients. In a few patients, incision and drainage were also performed alone. Simple ligation of the vein was performed in 9%. The length of hospital stay was not affected by the mode of treatment.

Most authors advise complete excision of the infected vein. The margins of the excision should include all thickened, phlegmonous tissue and all thrombus. The vein should appear normal where it is transected, and free-flowing blood should be seen. The wound should be left open and packed with saline or antibiotic-soaked gauze. After 3 or 4 days, if the wound appears to be clean, a delayed primary closure may be performed. Most of these procedures may be performed under local or regional anesthesia.

Clearly, when purulence is present, the vein must be completely excised and all areas of thrombus must be excised. We have encountered instances where excision was performed including only the grossly infected vein, leaving thrombus in the unresected portion of the vein.

These patients have generally failed to improve unless the entire vein is re-excised.

One of the difficult decisions in treatment is distinguishing between chemical phlebitis and septic thrombophlebitis. Both may be erythematous, locally warm, associated with some degree of systemic fever, and showing signs of local tenderness. The sicker the patient, the greater the index of suspicion should be for septic thrombophlebitis. The puncture site should be frequently inspected and may require local incision to detect purulence. Chemical phlebitis usually responds to local measures such as heat and elevation, whereas septic phlebitis does not. If adverse risk factors are also present, the index of suspicion favoring infection should increase.

If total excision of the involved segment is impossible, proximal ligation of the venous trunk should performed. This is frequently all that is necessary to forestall the systemic consequences of the disease.

If the infection is centrally located, eradication by surgical excision is frequently impossible. In this situation Neuhof and Seley advocated the use of incision and drainage of any localized collections in combination with prolonged parenteral antibiotics.[2] The thrombus represents a privileged endovascular environment that is resistant to the penetration of antbiotics, a situation analogous to bacterial endocarditis. For this reason, parenteral antibiotics should be administered in a dose and for a duration similar to those for endocarditis. The addition of anticoagulant or thrombolytic therapy has been advocated in order to improve response. The rationale for the use of anticoagulant therapy is that it prevents further central spread of the infected thrombus. This therapy fails in approximately 30%. It is most likely to fail in patients with a discrete abscess collection adjacent to the vein. In this situation, surgical intervention becomes a necessity.

We have excised the subclavian vein on three occasions when septic clots were present due to prolonged subclavian catheterization. The patients appeared to be showering the lungs with septic emboli. These procedures were difficult to perform and were generally unsatisfactory, although two of the three patients survived. In this situation, long-term anticoagulants and specific antibiotics are probably the best therapy.

PREVENTION

The incidence of this disease can be limited by the institution of strict precautions and surveillance of all IV catheter sites. Pruitt and McManus reported a decrease in the incidence of this complication in burn patients from 6.9% during 1969–70 to 1.4% during 1977–78 to 0.71% during the 8 years from 1982 to 1990.[12] This decrease in incidence was a result of recognition of the problem and strict adherence to improved standards of catheter care, the technique of catheter insertion, routine replacement of lines every 48 to 72 hours, and avoidance of lower extremity IV lines.[12] The use of dedicated IV teams who place, care for, and monitor the condition of IV catheters and the catheter sites has reduced the incidence of this disease. Catheters that have any evidence of phlebitis should be removed immediately. Intravenous lines placed in the field or in any emergency setting should be replaced within 24 hours. Intravenous boluses of potassium are also associated with an increased incidence of thrombophlebitis and should be avoided. Institution and strict enforcement of these practices have served to reduce significantly the incidence of suppurative thrombophlebitis.

REFERENCES

1. Hammond JS, Varas R, Ward CG. Suppurative thrombophlebitis: A new look at a continuing problem. South Med J 1988; 81:969–971.
2. Neuhof H, Seley GP. Acute suppurative phlebitis complicated by septicemia. Surgery 1947; 21:831.
3. Garrison RN, Richardson JD, Fry DE. Catheter-associated septic thrombophlebitis. South Med J 1982; 75:917–919.
4. De la Sierra A, Cardellach F, Cobo E, et al. Iatrogenic illness in a department of general internal medicine: A prospective study. Mt Sinai J Med 1989; 56:267–271.
5. Tager IB, Ginsberg MB, Ellis SE, et al. An epidemiologic study of the risks associated with peripheral intravenous catheters. Am J Epidemiol 1983; 118:839–851.
6. Arnow PM, Quimosing EM, Beach M. Consequences of intravascular catheter sepsis. Clin Infect Dis 1993; 16:778–784.
7. O'Neill JA, Pruitt BA, Foley FD, et al. Suppurative thrombophlebitis: A lethal complication of intravenous therapy. J Trauma 1968; 8:256.
8. Stein JM, Pruitt BA. Suppurative thrombophlebitis: A lethal iatrogenic disease. N Engl J Med 1970; 282:1452.
9. Pruitt BA, McManus WF, Kim SH, et al. Diagnosis and treatment of cannula related intravenous sepsis in burn patients. Ann Surg 1980; 191:546.
10. Baker CC, Peterson SR, Sheldon GF. Septic phlebitis: A neglected disease. Am J Surg 1979; 138:97–103.
11. Kaufman J, Demas C, Stark K, et al. Catheter-related septic central venous thrombosis: Current therapeutic options. West J Med 1986; 145:200–203.
12. Pruitt BA Jr, McManus AT. The changing epidemiology of infection in burn patients. World J Surg 1992; 16:57–67.

PRIMARY AND SECONDARY VENA CAVAL TUMORS

THOMAS F. DODSON, M.D.
ROBERT B. SMITH III, M.D.

Primary tumors of the vena cava are rare, on the one hand, with a recent review identifying 141 patients from 1871 to 1989.[1] Secondary vena caval tumors are, on the other hand, quite common, given the fact that 23,000 patients in the United States were expected to be diagnosed with renal cell carcinoma in 1993 and that approximately 5% to 10% of those patients will have tumor extension into the inferior vena cava (IVC).[2,3] Other nonrenal tumors, including adrenal and colon tumors, may also involve the IVC, but they are rare occurrences. Because the relationships of gender, presentation, and outcome are different in the two types of IVC involvement, it is useful to consider each separately (Table 1).

PRIMARY IVC TUMORS

As noted by Dzsinich and colleagues from the Mayo Clinic, vascular leiomyosarcomas constitute only 2% of all leiomyosarcomas, and they are found in five times as many veins as arteries.[4] In addition, there is a female preponderance among patients with IVC tumors such that seven of eight patients in their report and about 80% of patients previously described were women. All three patients added to the literature by Mingoli and associates were women as well.[1] In their review of 144 patients with leiomyosarcoma of the IVC, the mean age at the time of admission was 54 years. Only four patients in this series were asymptomatic, and they were diagnosed during radiologic procedures or unrelated operations. Abdominal pain was present in 66% of patients, and an abdominal mass was palpable in nearly 50%. Lower limb edema was noted in only a minority of patients (38.9%), and it was surmised that this was due to the probable slow growth of the tumor and the corresponding development of venous collateral circulation.

Plain x-ray films of the abdomen are seldom helpful. The examination of choice is either computed tomography (CT) or magnetic resonance imaging (MRI). In a personal series involving 7 primary tumors that were all leiomyosarcomas and 11 secondary tumors, 10 arising from renal carcinomas and 1 from an adrenal carcinoma, Kieffer and co-workers performed retrograde cavography in all patients with partial or complete obstruction of the IVC.[5] A clear delineation of the limits of tumor extension was made possible by this examination, together with an assessment of the potential for hepatic venous involvement.

In the 144 patients reported by Mingoli and colleagues, the tumor arose from the infrarenal portion of the IVC in 34% of patients, from the middle segment (origin of the renal veins and retrohepatic portion) in 42%, and from the upper segment (origin of the hepatic veins and suprahepatic portion) in 24%.[1] Most patients (24/35) with tumor in the upper segment had symptoms of Budd-Chiari syndrome. One-third of the total patients in the series were inoperable due to either poor condition or metastatic disease. Of the 96 patients who underwent operations, radical resection of the tumor was accomplished in 82 patients (57%), and palliative resection was performed in 14 patients (10%). Only two early postoperative deaths were recorded among the patients who had a complete tumor resection, a postoperative mortality of 2.4% in that subgroup. Of the 82 patients who underwent radical resection, 11 were readmitted with local recurrence at a median time of 12 months. By 36 months, 26 patients had died of recurrent disease, and 4 patients had died of unrelated causes. At the time of the report, 12 of the total 82 patients were alive without signs of recurrence and 7 others were alive with known recurrent disease. Unfortunately, 31 patients were lost to follow-up. The 5 and 10 year survival rates for patients undergoing curative operations were 27.9% and 14.2%, respectively. Two factors were predictive of high risk: tumor involvement of the upper segment of the IVC and a poorly differentiated tumor. In patients whose tumor was in the upper segment and who were found to be inoperable, the median survival was 1 month. Only three patients with upper segment tumors underwent radical resection, with one death due to metastatic disease at 48 months. Factors associated with a good outcome were radical tumor resection, the presence of abdominal pain, and the absence of a palpable abdominal mass.

In our operative approach to patients with primary IVC tumors, if the tumor involves only the infrarenal portion of the IVC, the tumor and surrounding structures as well as the involved segment of the IVC are removed. No attempt at reconstruction of the IVC is made in these patients. In patients found to have involvement at the level of the renal veins or the retrohepatic portion of the IVC, replacement of the IVC by an externally supported polytetrafluoroethylene (PTFE) graft is preferred. If a simple venous patch is needed to replace a portion of the IVC in this location, the internal jugular vein may be utilized. Patients with tumor involving the IVC from the origin of the hepatic veins or the suprahepatic portion are often inoperable. In those rare instances in which radical resection is possible, externally supported PTFE is the graft replacement of choice.

SECONDARY IVC TUMORS

Whereas few surgeons are faced with the need to care for a primary tumor of the IVC, most vascular surgeons are called upon to assist with the treatment of

Table 1 Primary and Secondary Vena Caval Tumors

	Mean Age at Presentation (Years)	Gender	Common Presentation	Operative Mortality	Poor Prognostic Factors	Prognosis (Survival)	Chemo/Radiation
Primary (leiomyosarcomas), Mingoli, et al	54.4	80% F 20% M	Abdominal pain (66%) Mass (48%)	2.4%	Involvement of upper IVC; poorly differentiated tumor	27.9% (5 years) 14.2% (10 years)	No consistent protocol
Secondary (renal cell carcinomas), Boring, et al; Suggs, et al	56	60% M 40% F	Hematuria (42%) Mass (26%) Flank pain (23%)	3.4%	Presence of distant metastases; involvement of perinephric fat or regional nodes	57% (5 years; actuarial in patients without known metastatic disease)	Alpha-interferon and immunotherapy are under investigation

secondary tumors of the IVC. Most of these tumors are renal cell carcinomas. Approximately 1,000 to 2,000 such patients are diagnosed with extension of tumor thrombus into the IVC each year. In 1991, the Cleveland Clinic reported on 68 patients with renal cell carcinoma involving the IVC over 21 years.[6] That same year, Emory published results of a series of 31 patients over the previous 13 years.[7]

An aggressive approach to renal cell carcinoma with extension into the IVC followed from the report by Skinner and associates in 1972 that a 55% 5 year survival occurred in 11 patients who had undergone radical nephrectomy with concomitant removal of intracaval tumor.[8] Most patients with this type of tumor are men, with nearly a 2:1 male to female ratio. The average age at presentation is between the fifth and seventh decades, but the tumor has been reported in neonates and adolescents. Hematuria, a common form of presentation, affected 42% of our patients. Whereas a mass was palpable in nearly 50% of patients with a primary IVC tumor, it was palpable in only a quarter of patients with renal cell carcinoma.

Both CT and MRI are used to define the anatomic limits of the tumor, and it is rare that contrast angiography or echocardiography is needed (Figs. 1 to 3). The operative approach is dictated by the extent of tumor thrombus. If the tumor is limited to the infrahepatic IVC, only an abdominal incision is required. If the tumor extends to the retrohepatic cava but below the diaphragm and atrium, either a right thoracoabdominal incision or a bilateral subcostal incision is utilized to allow control of the suprahepatic IVC. Tumor extension into the right atrium mandates a median sternotomy along with a midline abdominal extension. Cardiopulmonary bypass is generally used in this situation and was performed in three of the five patients in our series who appeared to have tumor extension above the diaphragm. We have no experience with total circulatory arrest, but Shahian and associates in 1990 described successful use of that technique in seven patients with no postoperative deaths, myocardial infarctions, or strokes.[9] It is not clear, however, whether the advantages of a bloodless field are sufficient to warrant the potential complexities of this procedure.

One of the operative goals is to gain venous control both above and below the tumor. Therefore, it is necessary to encircle the contralateral renal vein as well as the IVC below the tumor. Similarly, the IVC above the tumor must be controlled, either at the inferior border of the liver or between the liver and the diaphragm. Sturdy mechanical retraction devices are helpful in elevating the costal margins and allowing the surgeon to work almost directly over the suprahepatic IVC when

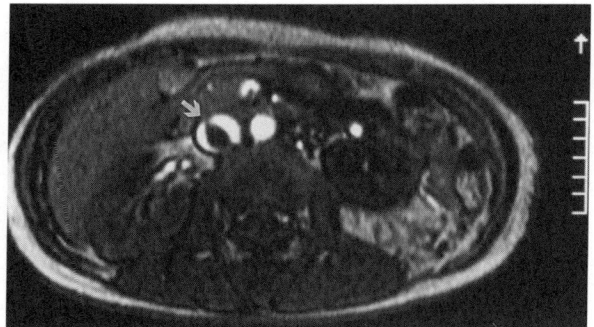

Figure 1 Tumor thrombus (*arrow*) in infrahepatic vena cava.

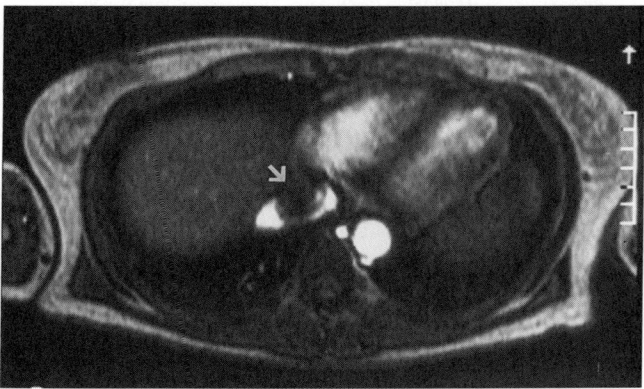

Figure 2 Tumor thrombus (*arrow*) at level of diaphragm.

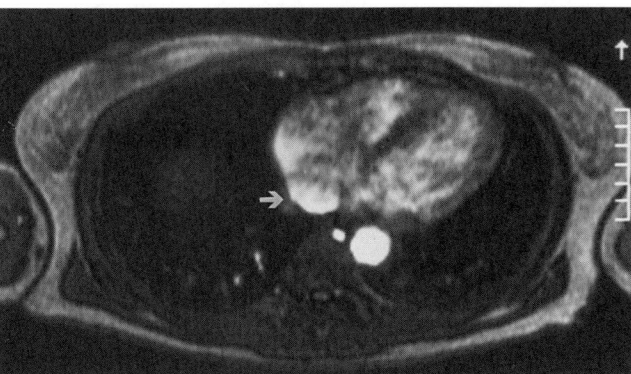

Figure 3 Tumor thrombus *absent* (*arrow*) at level of right atrium.

this exposure is necessary. Any lumbar veins that can be identified prior to cavotomy should be clipped to reduce blood loss. If the tumor extends behind the liver such that it is necessary to clamp the suprahepatic IVC, a Pringle maneuver is performed to occlude hepatic blood flow temporarily. Montie and colleagues also suggest clamping both the superior mesenteric and inferior mesenteric arteries to help maintain intravascular volume.[6] We have not employed this extra maneuver.

Given the magnitude of the operation and the considerable blood loss attendant on operations on the IVC, the operative mortality is quite low, 3.4% in the Emory series and 7% in the Cleveland Clinic report. Operative blood loss in our series was related to the complexity of the procedure. Patients with tumor confined to the infrahepatic IVC averaged 990 ml, patients with tumor into the retrohepatic IVC averaged 3,675 ml, and patients with tumor extending to the level of the atrium averaged 4,600 ml. Postoperative morbidity, however, is not inconsequential, as 9 of our 29 patients suffered major complications, resulting in a complication rate of 31%.

Distant metastasis or tumor involvement of the perinephric fat or regional lymph nodes is associated with a poor prognosis. Most patients with metastatic disease do poorly and die within a year of operation. Our 5 year actuarial survival rate in the 21 patients without known preoperative metastatic disease was 57%. In patients with perinephric fat or regional lymph node involvement, that survival declines to 12% to 25%.[3] Given that renal cell carcinoma involving the IVC is diagnosed in 1,000 to 2,000 patients yearly, and that this involvement is associated with detectable metastatic disease in 30% to 40% of patients, 600 to 1,200 patients each year are candidates for radical resection of the tumor. At present, surgical extirpation is the only effective treatment. New developments in immunotherapy may make it possible in the future to offer resectional therapy to even those patients with metastatic disease.[10]

REFERENCES

1. Mingoli A, Feldhaus RJ, Cavallaro A, Stipa S. Leiomyosarcoma of the inferior vena cava: Analysis and search of world literature on 141 patients and report of three new cases. J Vasc Surg 1991; 14:688–699.
2. Boring CC, Squires TS, Tong T. Cancer statistics, 1993. 1993; 43:7–26.
3. Richie JP. Neoplasms of the genitourinary tract. In: Holland JF, Frei E, Bast RC, et al, eds. Cancer medicine. 3rd ed. Philadelphia: Lea & Febiger, 1993:1529.
4. Dzsinich C, Gloviczki P, van Heerden JA, et al. Primary venous leiomyosarcoma: A rare but lethal disease. J Vasc Surg 1992; 15:595–603.
5. Kieffer E, Bahnini A, Koskas F. Nonthrombotic disease of the inferior vena cava: Surgical management of 24 patients. In: Bergan JJ, Yao JST, eds. Venous disorders, Philadelphia: WB Saunders, 1991:501.
6. Montie JE, El Ammar R, Pontes JE, et al. Renal cell carcinoma with inferior vena cava thrombi. Surg Gynecol Obstet 1991; 173:107–115.
7. Suggs WD, Smith RB III, Dodson TF, et al. Renal cell carcinoma with vena caval involvement. J Vasc Surg 1991; 14:413–418.
8. Skinner DG, Pfister RF, Colvin R. Extension of renal cell carcinoma into the vena cava: The rationale for aggressive surgical management. J Urol 1972; 107:711–716.
9. Shahian DM, Libertino JA, Zinman LN, et al. Resection of cavoatrial renal cell carcinoma employing total circulatory arrest. Arch Surg 1990; 125:727–732.
10. Sella A, Swanson DA, Ro JY, et al. Surgery following response to interferon-α-based therapy for residual renal cell carcinoma. J Urol 1993; 149:19–22.

VENOUS ANEURYSMS

BRUCE A. PERLER, M.D.

Venous aneurysms are exceedingly uncommon and have received scant attention in most surgical textbooks. The first venous aneurysm was recognized clinically and reported by Sir William Osler in 1913,[1] but because it was associated with an arteriovenous fistula, it would probably not be considered a true venous aneurysm by contemporary criteria. Subsequently, multiple case reports and small clinical series have appeared, although venous aneurysm, as a specific clinical entity, was not established until publication of a comprehensive review in 1964.[2]

It is difficult to characterize the true incidence of this peculiar entity for two reasons. First, there has been confusion with respect to the definition of a true venous aneurysm. Currently, a venous aneurysm is defined as a solitary area of venous dilation that communicates with the main venous structure by a single channel.[2] A venous aneurysm is not a lesion normally associated with varicosities. Second, there should be no evidence of an arteriovenous communication. Similarly, although several venous aneurysms have been identified in patients with a history of antecedent trauma, a true venous aneurysm is not a contained hematoma, analogous to an arterial false aneurysm.

There has been less than complete agreement on the histologic findings characteristic of a true venous aneurysm. In some cases, for example, there is a paucity of smooth muscle cells and a considerable concentration of fibrous connective tissue within the vein wall.[3] Others have reported a thinning of the wall with either an increase or decrease in the amount of connective tissue, as well as an increase or decrease in the concentration of elastic fibers present.[4] In part, these discrepancies may reflect differences in the location or the chronicity of the lesions examined.

ETIOLOGY

In view of the relatively small number of patients reported, confusion with respect to the true definition, and discrepancies in reported histologic findings, it is not surprising that the etiology of venous aneurysms remains speculative and unsettled. Traumatic, inflammatory, and congenital etiologies have been suggested.[4] Some have proposed that endophlebosclerosis or endophlebohypertrophy, a degenerative process in the vein wall, is responsible.[3,5] It has been postulated that these changes, resulting in aneurysm formation, develop as a result of physical stress secondary to the pressure exerted by adjacent continuous arterial pulsations.[3] Others have questioned whether abnormalities of connective tissue metabolism may underlie the development of at least some venous aneurysms.[3] Because most patients have solitary lesions, it seems reasonable to assume that some local factors must contribute to the development of these lesions, even if a more generalized systemic abnormality exists.

ANATOMIC DISTRIBUTION AND CLINICAL PRESENTATION

Venous aneurysms have been identified in both superficial and deep veins of the neck, chest, abdomen, and the extremities (Table 1).[2,3,6] Although it appears that venous aneurysms may occur almost anywhere in the body, there does appear to be a predilection of certain veins to develop these lesions. For example, at least 17 aneurysms of the superior vena cava (SVC), both saccular and fusiform, have been reported, whereas only 3 have been identified in the inferior vena cava (IVC).[7,8] Within the peripheral circulation, aneurysms have been reported most frequently in the popliteal vein and its branches. At least 12 popliteal vein aneurysms have been reported.[3]

Venous aneurysms have been identified in individuals of all ages. Although most lesions have been reported in adults, several aneurysms have been diagnosed in children, involving the internal jugular, common femoral, greater saphenous, and lesser saphenous veins. There does not appear to be a gender predilection.

The clinical presentation of these aneurysms depends upon their anatomic location. Aneurysms involving the neck and upper extremity typically present as painless soft tissue masses, although in some patients there may be tenderness to palpation. The differential diagnosis includes most subcutaneous tumors and cysts.[5] Intra-abdominal and intrathoracic venous aneurysms, typically involving the IVC or SVC, are almost always asymptomatic and detected as "masses" during radiologic evaluation for other causes. Compression of adjacent structures and spontaneous rupture of a venous aneurysm are almost unheard of, although there has been one report of a ruptured persistent left SVC aneurysm, presumably secondary to thrombosis of the draining veins.[3] In addition, at least one thrombosed inferior vena cava aneurysm has been identified in association with deep venous thrombosis.[7]

The most serious clinical presentation associated with venous aneurysms is pulmonary embolism (PE). This complication has been reported almost exclusively in patients with popliteal vein aneurysms. Among 12 patients with popliteal venous aneurysms, 9 (75%) had PE.[3] It has been suggested that PE in the absence of deep venous thrombosis may be a sign of popliteal venous aneurysm, and it should stimulate further evaluation to rule out this entity.[3] Then again, PE has not been associated with aneurysms of the saphenous or upper extremity venous systems.

Table 1 Venous Aneurysms: Reported Locations

Neck
   Internal jugular
   External jugular
   Facial
Chest
   Superior vena cava
Abdomen
   Inferior vena cava
   Portal
   Splenic
Upper extremity
   Subclavian
   Axillary
   Cephalic
Lower extremity
   Common femoral
   Popliteal
   Greater saphenous
   Lesser saphenous

DIAGNOSIS

Most aneurysms involving superficially located veins present as nonpulsatile soft tissue masses. The location of the mass, usually along the course of the vein, and its easy compressibility suggest the diagnosis, although in several reports the correct diagnosis was not made until operative exploration. Provocative or positional maneuvers are also helpful in making the correct diagnosis. For example, venous aneurysms in the neck enlarge as the patient performs a Valsalva maneuver. Venous aneurysms in the upper or lower extremities increase in size with dependency and usually during a Valsalva maneuver, and they decrease in size with elevation of the extremity. The diagnosis can be confirmed by phlebography (Fig. 1) or in most patients by venous duplex evaluation. Duplex examination is particularly helpful in evaluating the patient with a suspected popliteal venous aneurysm because it may document mural thrombus or complete thrombosis of the lesion that may not be apparent on conventional phlebography. Impedance

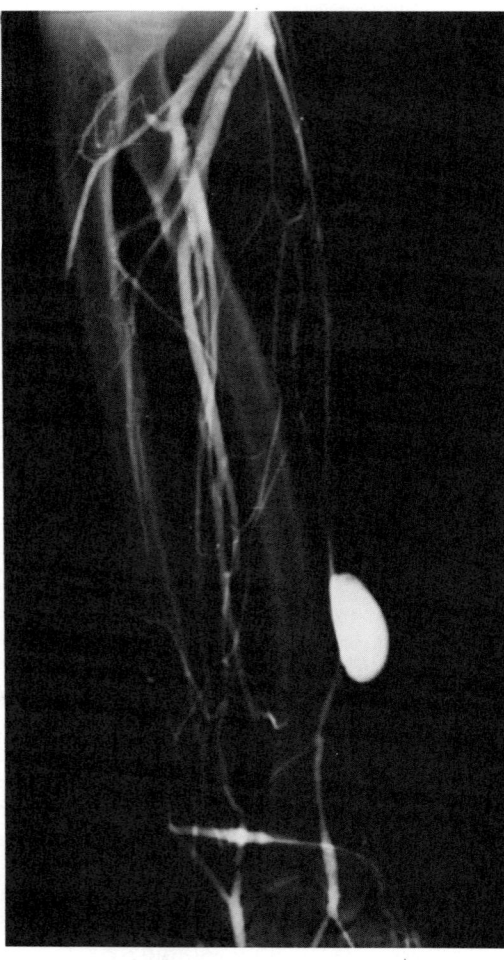

Figure 1 Phlebogram demonstrating large upper extremity superficial venous aneurysm. (From Perler BA, Venous aneurysm—an upper extremity mass. Arch Surg 1990; 125:124; with permission.)

plethysmography and conventional Doppler examination with venous augmentation maneuvers have not been found helpful in establishing the diagnosis.[9]

Aneurysms involving abdominal or thoracic venous structures are difficult to diagnose accurately. In fact several intrathoracic venous aneurysms have been diagnosed only at thoracotomy performed to establish a tissue diagnosis in the patient with a mass lesion of unknown etiology. In evaluating the patient with a mediastinal mass, supine and upright as well as inspiratory and expiratory chest x-rays are invaluable. One should observe a change in the size of the lesion with these maneuvers, if one is dealing with a venous aneurysm. In most patients, computed tomography or magnetic resonance imaging is very helpful in diagnosing intrathoracic or intra-abdominal venous aneurysms. If not completely thrombosed, the diagnosis may be confirmed by phlebography.

TREATMENT

Indications for treatment of a venous aneurysm include local discomfort or cosmetic reasons, usually in the neck or extremities; to establish a tissue diagnosis, typically of lesions in the chest or abdomen; and to prevent PE, particularly originating in popliteal venous aneurysms. Venous aneurysms in the neck and superficial veins in the extremities can usually be excised after ligating the segment communicating with the main venous channel, often with local anesthesia. No serious sequelae have been reported after such treatment. By contrast, up to 50% of patients undergoing excision or ligation of a popliteal venous aneurysm have developed postoperative deep venous thrombosis.[9] It might be reasonable, therefore, to anticoagulate patients perioperatively, although there are few objective clinical data to address this issue. Finally, intra-abdominal or intrathoracic venous aneurysms have in most patients been resected after exploration to establish the diagnosis of a mass lesion detected radiographically. Most experience has been reported in excising aneurysms of the SVC. Saccular aneurysms can usually be easily excised after ligating the base of the aneurysm. Fusiform lesions may require primary aneurysmorraphy, or vein patching, after excision of the lesion.[10] Because these lesions are not believed to have a significant risk of PE or rupture, if the diagnosis of a caval aneurysm is made by phlebography or by some other noninvasive examination, one could make a case for expectant treatment rather than surgical excision.

REFERENCES

1. Osler W. An arteriovenous aneurysm of the axillary vessels of 30 years duration. Lancet 1913; 2:1248.
2. Abbott OA, Leigh TF. Aneurysmal dilatations of the superior vena caval system. Ann Sug 1964; 159:858–872.
3. Friedman SG, Krishnasastry KV, Doscher W, Deckoff SL. Primary venous aneurysms. Surgery 1990; 108:92–95.
4. Spiro SA, Coccaro SF, Bogucki E. Aneurysms of the internal jugular vein manifesting after prolonged positive pressure ventilation. Head Neck 1991; 13:450–452.
5. Schatz IJ, Fine G. Venous aneurysms. N Engl J Med 1962; 266:1310–1312.
6. Perler BA. Venous aneurysm: An unusual upper extremity mass. Arch Surg 1990; 125:124.
7. Sweeny JP, Turner K, Harris KA. Aneurysm of the inferior vena cava. J Vasc Surg 1990; 12:25–27.
8. Itoh S, Ohe H, Tokuyana N, et al. Congenital saccular aneurysm of the superior vena cava. Jpn J Surg 1988; 18:588–591.
9. Ross GJ, Violi L, Barber LW, Vujic I. Popliteal venous aneurysm. Radiology 1988; 168:721–722.
10. Modry DL, Hidvegi RS, LaFleche LR. Congenital saccular aneurysm of the superior vena cava. Ann Thorac Surg 1980; 29:258–262.

LYMPHATIC DISEASE

PRIMARY LYMPHEDEMA

GEORGE H. RUDKIN, M.D.
TIMOTHY A. MILLER, M.D.

Lymphedema is the accumulation of protein-rich interstitial fluid in the skin and subcutaneous tissues due to abnormal lymphatic function. The deep muscle compartments remain uninvolved. This process results in swelling of the affected region and predisposes to lymphangitis and cellulitis. Lymphedema may result from congenital lymphatic dysfunction or from acquired disease. Those cases in which the etiology is congenital or unknown comprise *primary* lymphedema. Most cases of primary lymphedema are thought to be the result of in utero vascular dysplasia. Those resulting from known causes, including infection, operations, and radiation therapy are termed *secondary* lymphedema. No cure for lymphedema exists, although medical and surgical treatment may greatly ameliorate the condition and the resulting disability.

PATHOPHYSIOLOGY

The lymphatic system may be described as having three components: initial or terminal lymphatics, collecting ducts, and lymph nodes. Initial lymphatics are analogous to capillaries but have a poorly defined basement membrane, allowing absorption of lymph fluid from the interstitium. As the lymphatics progress in size, they become valved collecting ducts, which parallel the venous drainage in the extremities. Separate deep and superficial systems drain to common regional lymph nodes and ultimately to the thoracic duct or cisterna chyli. Skeletal muscle contractions, lymphatic valves, and an intrinsic lymphatic contractile mechanism result in proximal lymph flow.

The lymphatic system functions to transport interstitial fluid and macromolecular protein lost from the capillary system, as well as foreign material and infectious agents, back into the circulation. The accumulation of protein-rich lymphatic fluid results when fluid formation exceeds lymphatic transport capacity. Normal lymphatics have a substantial reserve capacity and may increase their flow rate by a factor of 10. An increase in interstitial fluid formation alone does not produce lymphedema. Lymphatic dysfunction is required to produce the accumulation of protein-rich fluid. In the early stages of lymphedema, accumulation of interstitial fluid results in a soft, pitting edema. With time, protein concentrations in the interstitium rise and result in subcutaneous fibrosis, which may in turn cause additional lymphatic dysfunction. Recurrent lymphangitis, which occurs in roughly 15% to 25% of patients, may further damage the lymphatic system.

CLASSIFICATION

Primary lymphedema may be classified by age of onset or lymphangiographic findings. Congenital lymphedema is present at birth, representing 10% to 15% of primary lymphedema cases. One form, Milroy's disease, presents with extremity lymphedema at birth and is a familial sex-linked form of lymphatic aplasia. Lymphedema precox presents in adolescence and represents 70% to 80% of primary lymphedema cases. Those patients whose lymphedema presents after the age of 35 years are classified as having lymphedema tarda.

Lymphedema may be classified by lymphangiography into hypoplastic and hyperplastic forms. In the hypoplastic forms, which represent the majority, lymphatics are narrowed and reduced in number. Distal and proximal forms of hypoplasia have been described. In the hyperplastic forms, which represent fewer than 10% of cases, lymphatics are dilated and increased in number due to obstruction or incompetent lymphatic valves. Because lymphangiograms may produce lymphatic damage and cause the edema to progress, we do not routinely use this classification system for patients with primary lymphedema.

DIAGNOSIS

In most patients with lymphedema, the diagnosis can be made by history and physical examination alone.

Table 1 Treatment of Lymphedema

Medical	Surgical-physiologic	Surgical-excisional
Skin care	Lymphangioplasty	Total skin and subcutaneous excision (Charles procedure)
Elevation	Omental transposition	Buried dermal flap (Thompson procedure)
Compressive garments	Enteromesenteric bridge	Subcutaneous excision underneath flaps (modified Homans procedure)
Pneumatic compression pumps	Lymphovenous anastomoses	
Manual lymph drainage/bandaging	Lympholymphatic anastomoses	
Benzopyrones		
Treatment of infection		

Primary lymphedema is more common in females and most commonly first presents around the time of menarche. In most patients the edema begins distally and progresses proximally over months or years. In lower extremity lymphedema, the left leg is more commonly affected than the right. Involvement of the forefoot may produce a characteristic "buffalo hump" appearance. Involvement of the digits produces Stemmer's sign, in which the skin of the dorsum of the digit cannot be easily tented up. At first, the edema is soft and pits easily, but, as fibrosis occurs, the edema gradually becomes nonpitting, and the tissue may become indurated or spongy. In later stages, skin changes including lichenification and hyperkeratosis may occur, but ulceration is infrequent. As the edema progresses, patients may complain of fatigue or pressure in the extremity, but pain is unusual and suggests an alternative cause for the swelling. A history of recurrent infection of the affected extremity is not infrequent. A family history of lymphedema is atypical.

Lymphedema can be differentiated from edema of other etiologies on clinical grounds. Cardiac, renal, and hepatic insufficiency are distinguished from lymphedema on the basis of history and physical examination. Venous stasis disease is a common cause of lower extremity edema, but the characteristic skin changes and pigmentation assist in the differential diagnosis. *Lipedema* causes the enlargement of the lower extremities and may be confused with lymphedema. This lipodystrophy characteristically affects females with symmetric enlargement of the lower extremities and is often associated with obesity. A history of infection is rarely, if ever, obtained, whereas a family history of the condition is not uncommon. Combined forms of lymphedema and lipedema have been described.

It is important to note that lymphangiosarcoma may arise in any patient with chronic lymphedema, although it occurs more frequently in acquired, or secondary, cases. This malignant endothelial cell tumor is characterized by bluish, papular lesions of the extremity. Early radical resection remains the treatment of choice. Radiation therapy and chemotherapy may be used as palliative or adjuvant therapy.

Laboratory studies are obtained as needed to rule out other sources of edema. Venous studies are ordered if a component of venous insufficiency is suspected. A variety of radiologic tests may be employed in the study of lymphedema. Computed tomography (CT) is useful early in the diagnosis of lymphedema to rule out malignancy. Lymphangiography, although used frequently in the past, is now rarely indicated. It seldom influences therapy and may further damage lymphatics. Lymphoscintigraphy using radiolabeled albumin, gold colloid, and technetium colloid has been successfully used to study lymphatic function and largely replaced lymphangiography. Lymphoscintigraphy is useful in planning physiologic forms of surgical therapy and in studying the effects of treatment on the lymphedematous extremity.[1] It may also have a diagnostic role when the etiology of edema is unclear.

TREATMENTS

Lymphedema is a chronic disease process, and no treatment option is completely and permanently curative. A variety of medical and surgical therapies are available and may significantly alter the course of the disease (Table 1). The primary goals in the treatment of lymphedema are to reduce limb volume, which provides improved function and cosmesis, and to prevent recurrent infections.

Medical

Most patients with lymphedema can be effectively managed with nonsurgical forms of treatment, consisting of skin care, treatment of infection, pharmacologic therapy, and mechanical compression with elevation to reduce limb volume.

Skin Care

Basic skin care is vital in the prevention of infection and may assist in preventing the secondary skin changes. The daily use of a low-pH, water-based skin lotion is recommended. Fungal infections of the web spaces may predispose to secondary infection and can be prevented by careful drying of the digits and web spaces after washing, together with the use of an antifungal powder. Localized fungal infections can be treated with antifungal creams, but invasive infection requires treatment with oral griseofulvin.

Treatment of Infection

Recurrent lymphangitis or cellulitis occurs in 15% to 25% of patients with lymphedema. Beta-hemolytic streptococci are the most common etiologic agent. *Staphylococcus aureus* and gram-negative organisms have been implicated as well. When infection occurs, it must be treated promptly and aggressively, as it may pursue a fulminant course to sepsis. The patient should receive a systemic antistaphylococcal and antistreptococcal agent for 5 to 7 days and should be restricted to bed rest with the affected limb elevated. Occasionally, it may be necessary to place a patient with recurrent infections on long-term prophylactic antibiotic therapy, typically penicillin. Cephalexin or erythromycin may also be used.

Pharmacologic Therapies

Diuretics have been widely used in the treatment of lymphedema. Although they may reduce limb volume in some patients, the effects are short-lived. By reducing the limb water content, diuretics may increase the concentration of interstitial fluid protein, and some authors have suggested that this process may accelerate the formation of subcutaneous fibrosis. We do not routinely use diuretic therapy in the treatment of lymphedema.

Benzopyrones, including sodium warfarin, have been used in the treatment of lymphedema abroad. Clinical trials in Europe and Australia have documented moderate improvement in limb volume and skin softness. Theoretically, these compounds act by increasing protein lysis by macrophages in the interstitium. We have not used sodium warfarin in the treatment of lymphedema because of the potential for bleeding complications.

Reduction of Limb Volumes

Reduction of limb volume is essential in improving limb function and cosmesis. Limb size should be assessed objectively at the initial visit and at regular intervals so that the clinician may accurately determine a patient's response to therapy. Measurements of limb circumference have been employed by many clinicians, but they are prone to error in reproducibility. The measuring tapes used for fitting compressive stockings, which consist of a series of tapes at specific intervals, assist in reducing this error. Limb volume measurements by water displacement are more precise but do not identify changes in a specific region of the limb. Photography is also important in following these patients.

Limb elevation is most effective in the early stages of lymphedema. Patients should be advised to elevate the affected extremity at night to prevent the accumulation of dependent edema. This may be accomplished by elevating the foot of the bed on 4 to 6 inch blocks for lower extremity edema or through the use of a sling for upper extremity edema. During the day, custom-fit compressive garments (sleeves or stockings) are often necessary to maintain limb volume. Measurements should be made after a period of bed rest so that compression can be maintained at lower limb volumes, and the length of the stocking or sleeve should match the extent of the disease. Typically, these should have a 40 to 50 mm Hg gradient, although some patients cannot tolerate this level of compression initially. A comfortable fit is essential to assure patient compliance.

Compressive pump therapy has proven very effective in the reduction of limb volume[2] and is most effective if initiated early, before the onset of significant subcutaneous fibrosis. In compressive pump therapy, an inflatable sleeve is placed over the affected limb and intermittently inflated to a specified pressure, forcing edema out of the extremity. The most advanced pneumatic pumping devices are the gradient sequential pumps (Lymphapress, Biocompression Systems). These devices use multiple compression chambers, which inflate sequentially along the limb to create a milking action. The pressure is adjustable and delivers higher pressures distally, creating a pressure gradient along the extremity. Several studies have documented compressive pump therapy to be effective in reducing limb volume. Therapy must be continued at regular intervals in order to maintain its benefits, however, and compressive garments should be worn between treatments. Deep venous thrombosis, active infection, and cardiac failure are considered contraindications to pump therapy.

Manual lymph drainage (MLD) and compressive bandaging therapy have been utilized effectively in Europe for the treatment of lymphedema[3] and have recently been introduced to several centers in the United States. A massage technique, MLD is designed to stimulate lymph flow in the diseased extremity and in adjacent tissues. A variety of theories have been advanced regarding its mechanism of action. It is often combined with compressive bandaging therapy, in which the extremity is wrapped with a nonelastic bandage. We have recently used these treatments in a select group of patients with promising results.

Surgical

If optimal medical therapy is ineffective in controlling lymphedema, surgical intervention may be considered. The primary goals in lymphedema operations are reduction in limb bulk with improvement in function and cosmesis and the prevention of recurrent infections. A cosmetically perfect result is not possible, and we consider functional impairment to be the primary indication for operation. The patient must understand that operation for lymphedema is palliative only and does not cure the disease or obviate the need for continued medical therapy, including the use of compressive stockings postoperatively.

Numerous operations for the treatment of lymphedema have been described. These procedures may be categorized as either physiologic or excisional. The physiologic procedures attempt to re-establish lymphatic drainage. The excisional procedures debulk the limb by removing skin and subcutaneous tissue. Some procedures, such as Thompson's buried dermal flap, may have both physiologic and excisional components.

Physiologic procedures

Physiologic procedures are most appealing theoretically in instances where a localized obstruction to lymphatic drainage is identified, as in obstructive forms of primary lymphedema or in postsurgical secondary lymphedema.

In lymphangioplasty, described by Handley in 1908, silk threads were placed subcutaneously in the affected limb(s), with the hope that fibrous channels would form around the implants and transport lymph from the extremity by capillary action. No patients had a sustained benefit from this procedure. Lymphangioplasty has been tried with multifilament Teflon implants.[4] Despite a short-term reduction in extremity size, edema had reaccumulated or progressed in all patients by 5 years postoperatively.

In the omental transposition of Goldsmith, a portion of omentum was transposed into the affected limb, based on a gastroepiploic vascular pedicle. Although the omentum is rich in lymphatic vessels, anastomoses between the lymphatics of the omentum and those of the diseased limb have never been documented. This procedure failed to produce long-term benefits and may produce serious complications including hernia and intestinal obstruction. Hurst and colleagues have described a similar procedure, the enteromesenteric bridge, in which a segment of ileum is denuded of its mucosa and apposed to transected iliac or inguinal lymph nodes. This procedure may prove useful in select patients with primary lymphedema due to proximal obstruction. Sustained results may be obtained with this procedure, and persistent patency of the anastomosis has been documented by lymphangiography.[5]

Lymphovenous shunts, which include lymphonodalvenous and lymphovenous procedures, have been performed since the 1960s. In these procedures, an anastomosis is performed between a lymph node or lymphatic vessel and a neighboring vein. Sustained reduction in limb size has been documented in obstructive secondary lymphedema.[6] Although some have suggested that primary lymphedema is an absolute contraindication to these procedures, lymphovenous shunts have been used effectively in selected patients with hyperplastic lymphedema.[7] These procedures are ineffective in hypoplastic lymphedema, which represents most cases of primary disease.

Lympholymphatic shunts were developed in the 1970s. In these procedures, autologous lymphatic vessels are harvested from a nondiseased extremity and transposed or transplanted to the affected limb. There they are used to bypass a region of lymphatic obstruction with microsurgical anastomoses to native lymphatics. Long-term anastomotic patency has been documented by lymphoscintigraphy, with sustained reduction in extremity volume. As is true with lymphovenous shunts, these procedures are ineffective for most patients with primary lymphedema but may be used successfully in select patients.[8]

Excisional Procedures

The Charles procedure, or total skin and subcutaneous excision, was described in 1912. In this operation, virtually all skin, subcutaneous tissue, and fascia are resected from the tibial tuberosity to the malleoli. Wound coverage is provided by split-thickness or full-thickness skin grafts taken from the resected specimen or by split-thickness skin grafts from an alternate donor site. Severe secondary skin changes including hyperkeratosis, keloid formation, hyperpigmentation, and weeping dermatitis may occur in the skin graft postoperatively; they are more common if split-thickness grafts are used.[9] This procedure remains an option only for those patients with severe edema and skin changes. It should not be used routinely because of the risk of severe postoperative skin changes and poor cosmetic results.

Thompson's buried dermal flap is an excisional procedure that may have a physiologic component. In this operation, subcutaneous tissue is resected through a medial leg incision, and skin flaps are raised anteriorly and posteriorly. The posterior flap is shaved with a dermatome and buried within the underlying muscle after fascial excision. A lateral procedure may also be performed at a later date. Theoretically, this operation improves lymphatic drainage by establishing lymphatic connections between the subdermal lymphatic plexus and the deep lymphatics of the muscle compartment. Such connections have never been documented, however, and the success of this operation may be attributable to its excisional component alone.

Suction curettage has been utilized in the treatment of both primary and secondary lymphedema.[10] We have found suction curettage to be a useful adjunct to excisional procedures in some patients and most helpful in the thigh. In our experience, the use of this technique for the treatment of lymphedema is limited, however. The suction cannula retrieves very little tissue, most likely because of the subcutaneous fibrosis found in chronic lymphedema.

Sistrunk described a staged subcutaneous excision underneath flaps for the treatment of lymphedema in 1918. This procedure was later popularized by Homans, and it is our preferred approach to the surgical treatment of lymphedema. The degree of debulking obtained is directly related to the quantity of skin and subcutaneous tissue removed. Results are comparable to those obtained with the buried dermal flap, and the complication rate is lower. Additionally, the severe postoperative skin changes that may occur after the Charles procedure are avoided.

Staged Subcutaneous Excision. Patients are admitted 24 to 72 hours prior to the procedure, depending on the severity of the edema, and kept at bed rest with the affected extremity elevated by a Thomas orthopedic

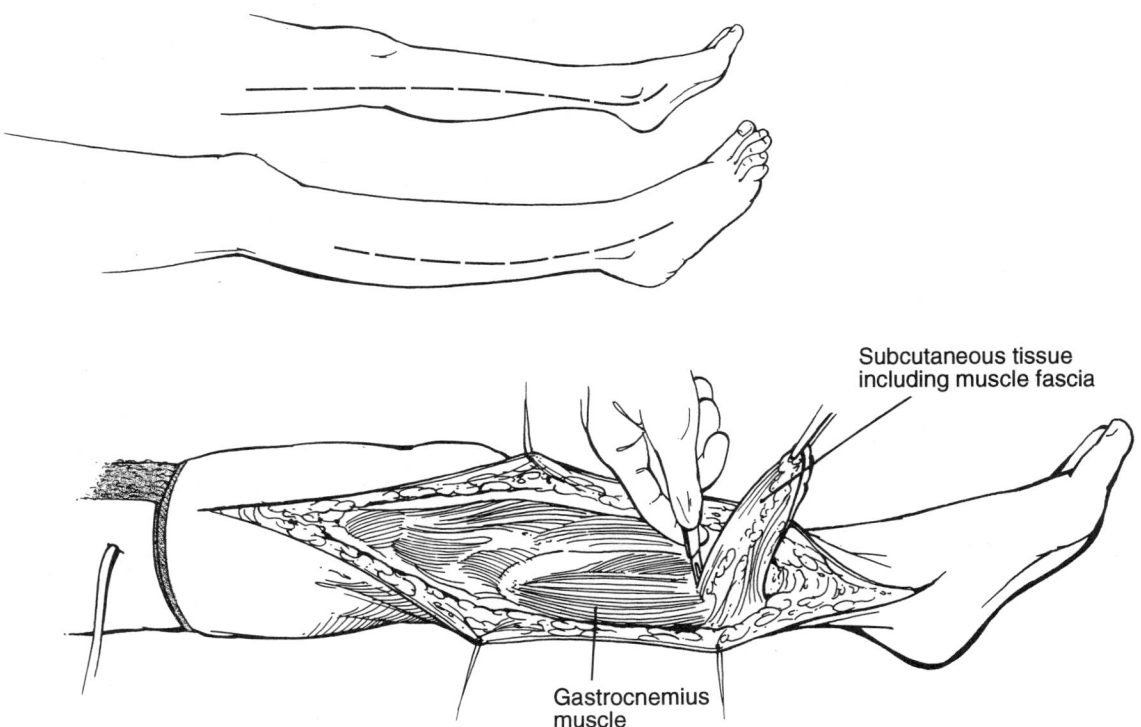

Figure 1 Subcutaneous excision on the medial aspect of the leg. Medial and lateral incisions are shown. (From Abdou MS, Ashby ER, Miller TA. Lymphedema. In Ritchie WP Jr., Steele G Jr., Dean RH eds. General Surgery. Philadelphia: JB Lippincott, 1995;761.)

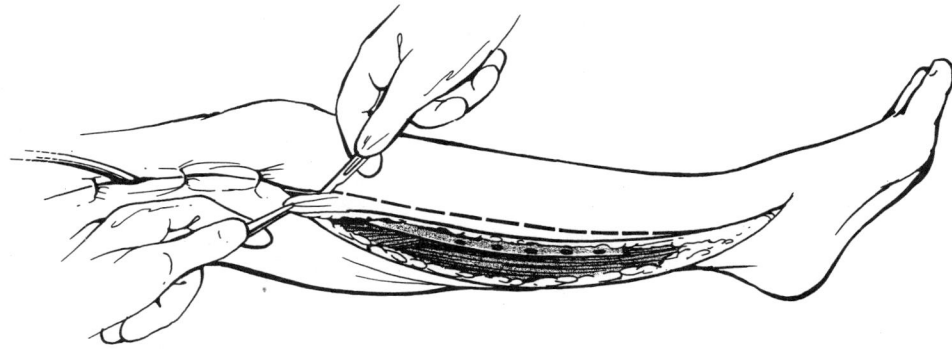

Figure 2 Closure after excision of redundant skin. (From Abdou MS, Ashby ER, Miller TA. Lymphedema. In Ritchie WP Jr., Steele G Jr., Dean RH eds. General Surgery. Philadelphia: JB Lippincott, 1995;761.)

splint. We have added pneumatic compression pump therapy to this regimen for some patients with severe edema. The extremity is washed daily in the preoperative period. A single dose of preoperative antibiotics is administered.

Typically, we perform this procedure in two stages. A medial resection is performed first, as this requires the larger tissue resection in most patients. A lateral procedure is performed 3 months after the initial procedure, as necessary. In patients with bilateral disease, the operation may be performed serially on both involved limbs during the initial operation, except as massive edema makes this prohibitive because of prolonged operative time or excessive blood loss.

After skin preparation, a pneumatic tourniquet is placed proximally on the affected leg. A medial incision is made 1 cm posterior to the tibial border in the leg and extended proximally into the thigh (Fig. 1). Flaps of 1.5 cm thickness are elevated anteriorly and posteriorly to the midsagittal plane in the calf, with less extensive dissection in the thigh and ankle. The subcutaneous tissue underneath the flaps is then removed, with care taken to preserve the sural nerve. The deep fascia of the calf is incised over the tibia and resected, sparing the fascia about the knee and ankle in order to preserve joint integrity. Redundant skin is then resected, and the wound is closed in a single layer with 4-0 nylon (Fig. 2). Prior to closure, a suction catheter is placed in a dependent position under the posterior flap and left in place for 5 days. The extremity is immobilized with a posterior splint, and the patient is placed at bed rest with the extremity elevated. Sutures can usually be removed by the eighth postoperative day. Prior to allowing dependency of the limb, the patient should be measured for compressive stockings, after which the patient may be allowed to sit in a chair for brief intervals. Ambulation can be started, with the legs wrapped, by the eleventh postoperative day. The lateral procedure is performed 3 months later, if necessary. The procedure is essentially the same, except that the deep fascia is left intact. Care must be taken to avoid the peroneal nerve during the dissection.

The arm is prepared as described for the leg. A medial incision is started at the distal ulna and extended proximally across the medial epicondyle of the humerus and into the posterior aspect of the upper arm. One cm flaps are elevated anteriorly and posteriorly to the midsagittal plane in the forearm and tapered both distally and proximally. The deep fascia is spared. Care is taken to identify and preserve the ulnar nerve at the medial epicondyle. If necessary, the tourniquet may be removed in order to carry the dissection into the axilla. After excising redundant skin, the wound is closed over a suction catheter. The postoperative care is similar to that described for the leg. Lateral procedures are seldom necessary.

Results. Of 82 lower extremity operations in 49 patients, 65% experienced a significant reduction in extremity size that was maintained during 2 years of follow-up. An additional 10% had modest improvement. In the remaining patients, the edema had returned to preoperative levels or progressed. The prognosis was worse for males than for females. There were three postoperative complications of partial flap necrosis. All three wounds closed by secondary intention, and none required an additional procedure. Several patients experienced decreased sensation at the incision site, but this has not been a source of complaint. In our experience, skin and subcutaneous excision represents the most reliable and uncomplicated method of managing lymphedema.

REFERENCES

1. Gloviczki P, Calcagno D, Schirger A, et al. Noninvasive evaluation of the swollen extremity: Experiences with 190 lymphoscintigraphic examinations. J Vasc Surg 1989; 9:683–689.
2. Pappas CJ, O'Donnell TF Jr. Long-term results of compression treatment for lymphedema. J Vasc Surg 1992; 16:555–562.
3. Hutzschenreuter P, et al. Post-mastectomy arm lymphedema: Treated by manual lymph drainage and compressive bandage therapy. Eur J Phys Med Rehabil 1991; 1:161.
4. Silver D, Puckett CL. Lymphangioplasty: A ten year evaluation. Surgery 1976; 80:748–755.
5. Hurst PA, Stewart G, Kinmonth JB, Browse NL. Long term results of the enteromesenteric bridge operation in the treatment of primary lymphoedema. Br J Surg 1985; 72:272–274.
6. O'Brien BMcC, Mellow CG, Khazanch RK, et al. Long-term results after microlymphaticovenous anastomoses for the treatment of obstructive lymphedema. Plast Reconstr Surg 1990; 85:562–572.
7. Olszewski WL. The treatment of lymphedema of the extremities with microsurgical lymphovenous anatomoses. Int Angiol 1988; 7:312–321.
8. Baumeister RG, Siuda S. Treatment of lymphedemas by microsurgical lymphatic grafting: What is proved? Plast Reconstr Surg 1990; 85:64–74.
9. Miller TA. Charles procedure for lymphedema: A warning. Am J Surg 1980; 139:290–292.
10. O'Brien BM, Khazanchi RK, Kumar AK, et al. Liposuction in the treatment of lymphoedema: A preliminary report. Br J Plast Surg 1989; 42:530–533.

SECONDARY LYMPHEDEMA

HARRY S. GOLDSMITH, M.D.
WILLIAM HOLMES, M.D.

Long-standing obstruction of lymphatic channels caused by either interruption or pressure can result in secondary lymphedema. Diverse views regarding the management of this disorder exist.[1-8] The physiologic basis of the disease is better understood. When lymph fluid is unable to pass through obstructed lymphatic vessels, there is an increase in intralymphatic pressure distal to the obstruction, resulting in increasing losses of lymph fluid through the wall of the lymphatics into the surrounding interstitial space. This causes an increase in osmotic pressure within the interstitial space as a result of an increased volume of protein-rich lymph. This elevated osmotic pressure further attracts additional lymph fluid into the region. As the interstitial fluid compartment expands, because of the increased lymph fluid accumulation, connective tissue fibers attached to lymphatic vessels within the interstitial space become taut. When these fibers are put on tension, they prevent the valves within the lymphatics from coapting, thereby further hindering lymph flow. As the process progresses and interstitial pressure continues to rise, the lymph fluid compression upon lymphatics, in association with the inability of lymphatic valves to close, makes lymph drainage increasingly ineffectual. This situation in which there is a continuing cycle of lymphstasis, interstitial fluid overload, and lymphatic valve incompetence eventually results in the chronic condition of secondary lymphedema.

The most common cause of secondary lymphedema worldwide is parasitic infection within the lymphatic

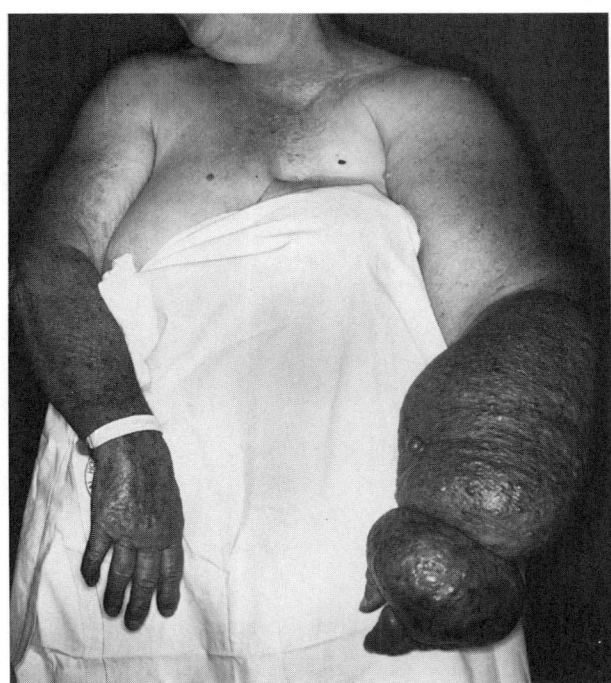

Figure 1 Massive lymphedema following radical mastectomy and radiation therapy 18 years earlier.

system caused by a mosquito-borne nematode, *Wuchereria bancrofti*. Mosquitoes, mainly in the developing countries, deposit these filariae subcutaneously, which then multiply and eventually disseminate throughout the body by way of the lymphatic and hematogenous systems. The greater the degree of parasitic infestation within the lymphatic system, the greater the subsequent degree of lymphedema.

In developed countries, secondary lymphedema usually does not occur from infection, but from surgical interruption and/or excision of lymphatic vessels, malignant disease, or radiation therapy. The surgical procedure that most commonly caused secondary lymphedema in the past was radical mastectomy for cancer of the breast (Fig. 1). It was estimated that up to a quarter of all women who had this operation developed some degree of secondary lymphedema of the arm on the side of the excised breast. With the recent de-emphasis on the need for radical mastectomy for breast cancer, the number of patients with lymphedema of the arm has diminished.

The surgical procedure that continues to result in a high incidence of postoperative lymphedema is a radical groin dissection. Any surgical procedure, such as a groin dissection, where lymphatics are interrupted in an area that is highly susceptible to wound contamination greatly increases the chance for developing infection and subsequent secondary postoperative lymphedema. It was Halsted who first showed the connection between infection and the development of lymphedema. Because of this relationship, every effort should be made to minimize the possibility of wound infection, especially during and after an axillary or radical groin dissection.

CONSERVATIVE TREATMENT

The treatment of patients with secondary lymphedema may prove to be a major problem for both the patient and the doctor. Patients can often be helped by conservative methods. Such measures allow most patients to lead a relatively normal life without any surgical procedure. Many patients with secondary lymphedema are overweight. If significant weight reduction can be accomplished, the lymphedematous extremity may decrease in size. Another simple measure that is helpful, but must be carefully explained to the patient, is frequent elevation of the lymphedematous extremity. This requires that the involved limb be elevated for at least 5 to 10 minutes, every 1 to 2 hours during the day. If it is a lower limb, it is essential that the foot of the patient's bed be raised at night at least one foot above the floor. It is sometimes necessary for the patient to move from a shared bed because the partner may be uncomfortable with bed elevation. The patient must understand that putting pillows under the legs or the mattress does not maintain leg elevation and is unacceptable. When a patient reports little or no reduction in the size of a lymphedematous extremity in spite of leg elevation throughout the night, this usually indicates severe and long-standing secondary lymphedema. This situation results from extensive fibrotic reaction within and around lymphedematous tissue within the leg, which hinders lymph drainage even when the limb is elevated for a prolonged period.

Another conservative measure that can help to some degree is restriction of sodium intake. Elevated sodium levels lead to increased fluid retention, with the propensity for excess fluid to accumulate in the lymphedematous extremity. It is especially important that women observe strict salt restriction during their premenstrual period. The attempt to reduce retained fluid volume in a limb by curtailing fluid intake has never been a reasonable way to treat lymphedema. Even though diuretics can lead to the temporary loss of fluid, the fluid loss is quickly replaced after ingestion of liquids.

Well-fitted elastic compression garments benefit patients with lymphedema, especially if the condition is minimal to moderate in degree. The principal use of these compressive devices is to maintain the size of the lymphedematous limb. It is therefore necessary that measurements for these elastic garments be made when the limb is at its smallest. More aggressive therapy using a pneumatic compression garment can help some patients with lymphedema, but they must spend many hours a day using a mechanical device.

Acute lymphangitis is particularly threatening to patients with, or predisposed to, secondary lymphedema. Even a minor abrasion or infection can lead to severe systemic manifestations such as chills, high fever, and septicemia. Recurrent episodes of lymphangitis frequently are associated with progressive lymphedema. Because secondary lymphedema is a chronic condition that becomes increasingly difficult to treat, any patient who has had more than one bout of severe lymphangitis should be placed on long-term antibiotic prophylaxis. Fortunately, such therapy prevents further attacks of lymphangitis in 80% of patients. It is important that patients who must take antibiotics for occasional lymphangitic attacks do so as early as possible in the episode of lymphangitis.

SURGICAL THERAPY

The majority of patients who suffer from secondary lymphedema can be treated medically. However, approximately 10% to 20% of patients with this chronic form of lymphedema may eventually require operation. Indications for such operation are (1) an increase in size of an involved extremity, despite aggressive medical treatment; (2) significant functional impairment, especially in the young patient; (3) serious cutaneous changes resulting from vesicular formation on the skin that become sources for recurrent infections despite prophylactic antibiotic treatment; and (4) severe emotional disturbances resulting from the appearance of the lymphedematous extremity. Many surgical procedures have been proposed for treating patients with secondary lymphedema. The large number of operations that have been performed indicates that no surgical procedure is

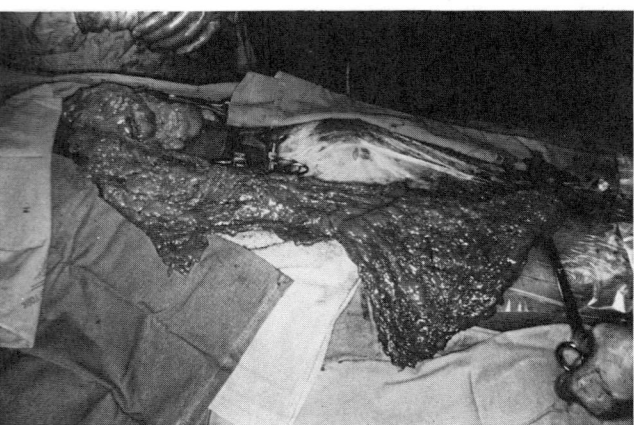

Figure 2 Omentum being lengthened and transposed. Upper left shows colon; lower right demonstrates omentum being positioned at the level of the patella (indicated by surgical instrument). Further omental division will allow mobilization to the level of the lower leg.

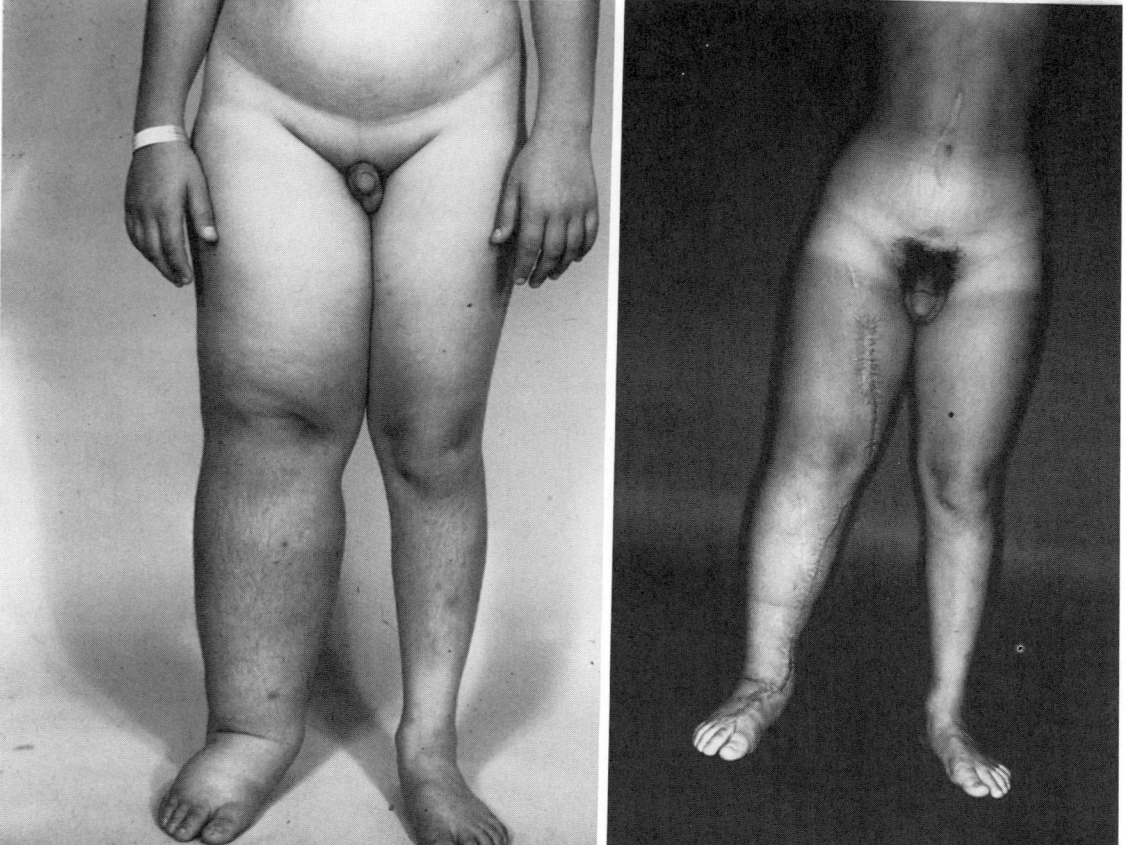

Figure 3 *A*, A patient before omental transposition to the right leg and foot. *B*, Same patient 4 years after operation.

successful on a routine basis. The operations that have been devised for treating a lymphedematous extremity are based on three procedures: (1) the attempt to stimulate the formation of neolymphatic channels within the lymphedematous extremity, (2) the removal of large segments of lymphedematous tissue from the involved limb, and (3) the transfer of normally functioning lymphatics into a lymphedematous limb.

Formation of Neolymphatic Vessels

Surgical operations in this category involve the subcutaneous implantation of threads of foreign material into a lymphedematous limb. The reasoning behind these procedures is that fine fibrotic tubes will develop around the implanted threads and that these new fibrotic tubes will function as lymphatic vessels. Even though fibrotic channels can form around the implanted threads, there appears to be no way for lymph fluid to be propelled along the course of these valveless fibrotic tubes. Insertion of foreign material to develop lymphatics has been generally discarded.

Excision of Lymphedematous Tissue

Another group of surgical procedures is based on the reduction of the size of an enlarged limb by excising large amounts of lymphedematous tissue. The various operations devised for this purpose can improve the appearance of a lymphedematous limb by decreasing its circumference, but this is due solely to excision of tissue. The theory as to why the operation might be effective over a long period of time is based on the idea that lymphatic connections will develop between subcutaneous lymphatics and lymphatics deep to the excised tissue. Operations based on this concept frequently fail to prevent the slow return of lymphedema to the extremity. Excisional procedures for lymphedema are still carried out, however, when indicated. There has been interest more recently in removing lymphedematous material from an involved extremity by liposuction.[10] This procedure, which simply removes material resulting from lymphatic obstruction, would not be expected to have long-standing effects.

Transfer of Normal Lymphatics into a Lymphedematous Limb

Surgical techniques have been designed to transfer normally functioning lymphatic vessels within a lymphedematous limb. One such procedure involves the burial of an intact dermal flap deep into the limb to improve lymph drainage.[11] This is accomplished by excising skin and subcutaneous tissue in a longitudinal plane along the edematous extremity, leaving an inch-wide dermal flap. This long dermal flap is then tucked into the deep tissues of the leg and sutured in place. The theory behind this operation is that the intact lymphatics within the buried dermal flap will function as more effective conduits for lymphatic drainage within the limb.

Another operation to develop lymphatic flow from a lymphedematous extremity into the core of the body is the transposition of the pedicled omentum into the involved limb (Fig. 2). When such a lengthened omentum is placed in the swollen extremity, omental lymphatics have been documented by lymphangiography to connect to deep lymphatics within the lymphedematous limb, with subsequent lymph drainage into lymphatics and lymph nodes within the peritoneal cavity and retroperitoneum. The senior author has been involved in omental transposition to lymphedematous extremities over a number of years, and the operation has been found to be effective in approximately 25% of patients (Fig. 3). The operation is especially effective in the control of persistent lymphangitis associated with secondary lymphedema.

A late complication associated with omental transposition is a 10% to 15% chance of postoperative abdominal hernia formation. This is not unexpected in that the procedure itself is a controlled herniation of the omentum into the extremity. Fortunately, most of these postoperative hernial defects do not require surgical repair (Fig. 4).

There has been recent interest in the use of microvascular techniques to treat secondary lymphedema. This involves an anastomosis between the end of a normally functioning lymphatic vessel to a lymph node,

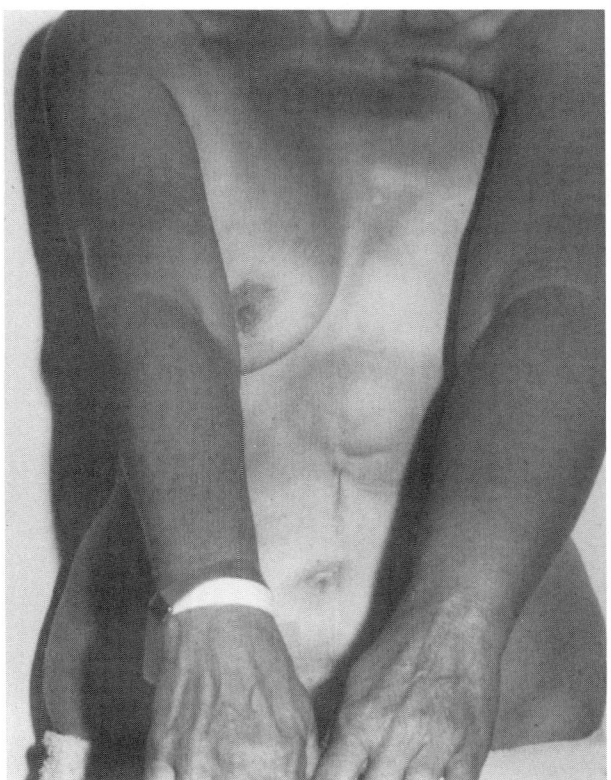

Figure 4 Asymptomatic hernial defect at upper pole of abdominal incision in a patient after omental transposition (15 years earlier) to a markedly lymphedematous left arm following a radical mastectomy.

a vein, or another lymphatic vessel. The most impressive results with this highly technical surgical treatment have been in patients with early secondary lymphedema who are free from massive swelling of the involved limb and without fibrotic changes within the leg—the same type of patients with secondary lymphedema who might be expected to do well with conservative therapy. A basic problem with microsurgical procedures is that the area of the lymphatic anastomosis becomes involved in a fibrotic reaction as the result of the normal healing process. Such scarring in the region of the microvascular anastomosis would be expected to decrease long-term success.

At this time it is difficult to draw a conclusion from available published data as to which operation is best for the individual patient with secondary lymphedema.

REFERENCES

1. Baumeister R, Siuda S. Treatment of lymphedema by microsurgical lymphatic grafting: What is proved? Plast Reconstr Surg 1990; 85:64–74.
2. Foldi E, Foldi M, Clodius L. The lymphedema chaos: A lancet. Ann Plast Surg 1989; 22:505–515.
3. Gloviczki P, Fisher J, Hollier LH, et al. Microsurgical lymphovenous anastomosis for treatment of lymphedema: A critical review. J Vasc Surg 1988; 7:647–652.
4. Goldsmith HS. Long-term evaluation of omental transposition for chronic lymphedema. Ann Surg 1974; 180:847–849.
5. Kinmonth JB. The lymphatics, surgery, lymphography and diseases of the chyle and lymph systems. 2nd ed. London: Edward Arnold, 1982.
6. Miller TA. A surgical approach to lymphedema. Am J Surg 1977; 134:191–195.
7. O'Brien BM, Shafroff BB. Microlymphaticovenous and resectional surgery in obstructive lymphedema. World J Surg 1979; 3:3–15.
8. Pappas C, O'Donnell T. Long-term results of compression treatment for lymphedema. J Vasc Surg 1992; 16:555–562.
9. Puckett CL, Jacobs GR, Hurvitz JS, et al. Evaluation of lymphovenous anastomoses in obstructive lymphedema. Plast Reconstr Surg 1980; 66:116–120.
10. Sando WC, Nahi F. Suction lipectomy in the management of limb lymphedema. Clin Plast Surg 1989; 16:369–373.
11. Thompson N. Buried dermal flap operation for chronic lymphoedema of extremities: Ten year survey of results in 79 cases. Plast Reconstr Surg 1970; 45:541–548.

INDEX

A

Abdomen
  angina in, 702
  duplex ultrasound of, 711-712
  plain film of, 707
  vascular injury in, 619-625
Abdominal aorta
  coarctation and hypoplasia of, 359-363
  percutaneous transluminal angioplasty of, 367
  in radiation-induced arteritis, 134, 136
Abdominal aortic aneurysm
  arteriography in, 210-213
  coronary artery disease in, 345-350
  endovascular grafting of, 265-268
  genetics of, 198-200
  iliac aneurysm after, 296-297
  imaging of, 214-218
  infected, 232-235
  inferior vena cava fistula and, 261-262
  inflammatory, 204-205, 229-231
  intra-abdominal disease and, 235-238
  in intravascular ultrasound, 528, 530
  retroperitoneal approach to, 238-241
  rupture of, 224-226
  small, 227-229
  visceral and renal artery disease with, 242-245
ABI; *see* Ankle-brachial index
Above-elbow amputation, 684
Above-knee amputation, 677-680
  below-knee versus, 669-671
Above-knee grafts, 481
Abscess
  infected femoral artery pseudoaneurysm versus, 319
  in intravenous drug abuse, 638
  in obturator foramen bypass grafts, 322-325
Abuse, drug
  infected femoral artery pseudoaneurysm and, 319-321
  vascular injury secondary to, 637-644
Acrocyanosis, 154
Activated partial thromboplastin time, 554-555

Adamkiewicz, artery of; *see* Radicular artery
Additives in intravenous drug abuse, 637
Adult
  congenital arteriovenous fistulas and malformations in, 850-852
  renal vein thrombosis in, 824, 826
Adventitial cystic disease, 509-512
Air plethysmography
  in aortoiliac occlusive disease, 351
  in chronic venous insufficiency, 882
Airway
  hemangioma obstruction of, 848
  in penetrating carotid trauma, 599
Alcohol
  in atherosclerotic disease prevention, 532
  in stroke and transient ischemic attacks, 26
Algorithm
  for asymptomatic carotid artery stenosis, 32, 33
  for axillosubclavian vein thrombosis, 959
  for bleeding varices, 733
  for cardiac risk in aortic reconstruction, 346, 347
  for carotid and coronary artery disease, 101
  for carotid endarterectomy neurologic deficit, 74
  for chronic venous insufficiency, 883, 918
  for chyloperitoneum treatment, 428
  for chylothorax treatment, 429, 430
  for deep vein thrombosis diagnosis, 881
  for extracranial carotid occlusive disease, 22, 23
  for extremity arterial injury, 594, 595
  for femoral artery embolectomy, 579
  for graft revision, 498
  for groin graft infection, 566
  for hemodynamic vertebrobasilar insufficiency, 86, 87
  for nonocclusive mesenteric ischemia, 708
  for pulmonary embolism, 941, 942, 955
  for upper extremity vasospastic disease, 149, 150

  for venous ulcers, 926, 929, 930
  for vertebral artery injury, 604, 605
Alopecia, 557
Ambulation in below-knee amputation, 674
Ambulatory venous pressure, 886-887
Amplatz, 947
Amputation, 669-685
  above-knee, 677-679
  below-knee, 674-677
  in Buerger's disease, 158
  guillotine, 563
  limb salvage versus, 632-633
  noninvasive assessment of, 669-672
  profundaplasty in, 459
  of toe and foot, 672-674
  of upper extremity, 680-685
Analgesia in arteriography, 441
Anastomosis
  in aortic reconstruction, 272
  of arm veins, 478-480
  arteriovenous, 857-860
  axillary, 387
  in bridge graft, 863, 864
  in carotid body tumor embolization, 122-123, 124
  femoral, 385-386
  between prosthetic and vein, 474
Anastomotic aneurysm, 415-419
Ancrod, 937
Anesthesia
  in balloon catheter embolectomy, 577
  for carotid endarterectomy, 44-45
  cerebral ischemia and, 54-55
  for nonruptured infrarenal aortic aneurysm, 221
Aneurysm
  abdominal aortic
    arteriography in, 210-213
    coronary artery disease in, 345-350
    endovascular grafting of, 265-268
    genetics of, 198-200
    iliac aneurysm after, 296-297
    imaging of, 214-218
    infected, 232-235
    inferior vena cava fistula and, 261-262
    inflammatory, 229-231
    intra-abdominal disease and, 235-238
    in intravascular ultrasound, 528, 530

Aneurysm—cont'd
    retroperitoneal approach to, 238-241
    rupture of, 224-226
    small, 227-229
    visceral and renal artery disease with, 242-245
  anastomotic, 415-419
  aortic, 198-314
    aneurysmosis and, 292-296
    arteriomegaly and, 292-296
    definition of, 218
    inflammatory, 204-205
    pathogenesis of, 200-203
    thoracoabdominal, 255-261
    visceral and renal artery disease with, 242-245
  of axillary artery, 188-194
  of celiac artery, 714-715
  definition of, 293
  in direct arteriovenous anastomosis, 859
  extracranial carotid artery, 105-109
  of femoral artery, 315-318
  of hepatic artery, 715-716
  iliac, 211, 296-302
  infrarenal aortic
    ruptured, 224-226
    unruptured, 218-223
  intracranial, 66-67
  mycotic, 639-640
  pararenal, 218
  of popliteal artery, 325-327
    in arteriography, 445, 446
  of popliteal vein, 971
  in renal artery, 813-817
  of splenic artery, 716-718
  of subclavian artery, 188-194
  of ulnar artery, 195
  in umbilical vein grafts, 485
  of upper extremity, 188-194
  venous, 970-972
Aneurysmectomy
  elective, 238-241
  intra-abdominal disease and, 235-238
  of renal artery aneurysm, 816-817
Aneurysmosis, 292-296
Angina, abdominal, 702
Angioaccess surgery, 853-867
  bridge grafts for, 860-864
  direct arteriovenous anastomosis for, 857-860
  external methods of, 853-857
  surveillance in, 865-867
Angiodysplasia, 718-720
Angiography
  of carotid artery, 13-15
  of carotid artery dissection, 111-112
  in cutaneous foot ulcers, 562
  in ergotism, 160
  in fibromuscular dysplasia, 116
  in giant cell arteritis, 131-132
  of infrainguinal occlusive disease, 443, 444, 447-453
Angioplasty
  in angioaccess graft failure, 867

  in atherosclerotic aortoiliac occlusive disease, 365-373
  in axillosubclavian vein thrombosis, 960-961
  in bilateral renal artery stenosis, 775
  for carotid endarterectomy, 61-63
  of carotid kinks, 120-121
  in chronic renal failure, 828
  in failing bypass grafts, 521-523
  in femorofemoral bypass, 393-394
  in fibromuscular dysplasia, 118
  in iliac artery occlusion, 369
  in intravascular ultrasound, 529-530
  for lower extremity occlusive disease, 512-517
  pediatric renovascular hypertension and, 810, 811-812
  percutaneous transluminal, 689-690
  for renovascular hypertension, 780-785
  in Takayasu's arteritis, 127-128
  of visceral ischemia, 692
Angioscopy
  in infrainguinal occlusive disease, 524-526
  intravascular ultrasound versus, 527
Angiotensin, 776
Ankle pressure
  in cutaneous foot ulcers, 560
  in infrainguinal occlusive disease, 432-433
Ankle-brachial index
  in aortoiliac occlusive disease, 331-332
  in graft surveillance, 494
  in infrainguinal occlusive disease, 433
  in penetrating injury, 598
  in popliteal vascular entrapment syndrome, 504, 505
Ankle-brachial systolic pressure ratio, 513, 514
Annuloplasty, 957-958
Antecubital fossa, 640
Antibiotics
  in cutaneous foot ulcers, 563
  in femoral anastomotic aneurysm, 416
  in graft coating, 566
  in infected abdominal aortic aneurysm, 233, 234-235
  in septic thrombophlebitis, 965
  in thoracic great vessel injury, 610
  in venous ulcer treatment, 926
Antibodies
  antiphospholipid, 550-551
  antiplatelet, 556-557
  monoclonal, 585
Anticoagulants
  for arterial macroembolism, 572-573
  in axillosubclavian vein thrombosis, 959
  in cerebral hyperfusion syndrome, 70
  in deep femoral venous thrombosis, 891-892
  in femoropopliteal thrombophlebitis, 905

  in graft patency, 548-549
  in intravenous drug abuse, 638
  in septic thrombophlebitis, 966
  for transient ischemic attacks, 27-28
Anticoagulation
  in acute graft thrombosis, 539
  in acute iliofemoral and caval thrombosis, 936-938
  in acute pulmonary embolism, 940-943
  in carotid artery dissection, 112-113
  in concomitant venous repair, 654
  in occluded extracranial carotid artery, 48
  in paradoxical embolism, 590-591
  in renal vein thrombosis, 825, 826
  in reperfusion syndrome, 650, 652
  in umbilical artery injury, 661
Antidepressants, 163
Antigen, proliferating cell nuclear, 2, 3
Antihypertensive therapy, 342
Antiphospholipid antibodies, 550-551
Antiplatelet agents
  in graft patency, 546-548
  for lower extremity occlusive disease, 536
  for transient ischemic attacks, 26-27
Antiplatelet antibodies, 556-557
Antithrombin III
  in coagulation, 868, 870
  deficiency
    in aortic reconstruction, 273
    as heparin therapy complication, 556
    as prothrombotic state, 551
Antithrombotic therapy
  for deep femoral venous thrombosis prophylaxis, 890
  in graft patency, 544-550
  in graft thrombosis, 545
  for ischemic stroke, 26-28
  for transient ischemic attacks, 26-28
Aorta
  abdominal
    percutaneous transluminal angioplasty of, 367
    in radiation-induced arteritis, 134, 136
  acute occlusion of, 378-380
  aortorenal bypass with, 787-788
  coarctation and hypoplasia of, 359-363
  cross-clamping of, 620-621
  developmental narrowing of, 361
  dissection of, 206-209
    medical management of, 305-308
    surgical treatment of, 309-314
  graft infection in
    diagnosis of, 400-405
    treatment of, 405-411
  graft of
    enteric fistula and, 411-413
    limb occlusion in, 419-426
  infrarenal, 367, 368, 369-370
  pediatric lesions of, 808-809
  penetrating injury of, 608-613

reconstruction of
  acute limb ischemia and, 271-274
  autotransfusion in, 287-289
  intestinal ischemia and, 274-277
  neurologic complications in, 278-282
  renal ectopia and renal fusion with, 246-249
  renal transplants and, 250-251
  spinal cord ischemia in, 282-286
  venous anomalies and, 252-255
  stump closure of, 408-409
  surgical risk assessment in, 349-350
  thoracic to femoral bypass, 381-383
  in thoracotomy, 612
Aortic aneurysm, 198-314
  abdominal
    arteriography in, 210-213
    coronary artery disease in, 345-350
    endovascular grafting of, 265-268
    genetics of, 198-200
    iliac aneurysm after, 296-297
    imaging of, 214-218
    infected, 232-235
    inferior vena cava fistula and, 261-262
    inflammatory, 229-231
    intra-abdominal disease and, 235-238
    in intravascular ultrasound, 528, 530
    retroperitoneal approach to, 238-241
    small, 227-229
  aneurysmosis and, 292-296
  arterial prostheses deterioration in, 289-292
  arteriomegaly and, 292-296
  definition of, 218
  femoral artery aneurysm and, 315
  inflammatory, 204-205
  infrarenal
    nonruptured, 218-223
    ruptured, 224-226
  pathogenesis of, 200-203
  thoracoabdominal, 255-261
  visceral and renal artery disease with, 242-245
Aortic dissection; see Aorta, dissection of
Aortoduodenal fistula, 226
Aortoenteric fistula, 262-264
Aortofemoral graft
  in acute aortic occlusion, 379-380
  for atherosclerotic aortoiliac occlusive disease, 355-359
  infection of, 408, 409
  in infrarenal aortoiliac hypoplasia, 362-363
  limb occlusion in, 419, 420
Aortography
  arteriography and, 210, 211
  of infrainguinal occlusive disease, 44
  in innominate artery atherosclerosis, 96

  in nonruptured infrarenal aortic aneurysm, 220
  in subclavian to carotid transposition, 89-92
  in thoracic aorta dissection, 310
Aortoiliac endarterectomy, 356, 363-364
Aortoiliac occlusive disease, 328-431
  acute aortic occlusion in, 378-380
  anastomotic aneurysm in, 415-419
  aortic graft infection in, 400-411
    diagnosis of, 400-405
    treatment of, 405-411
  aortic graft limb occlusion in, 419-426
  aortic graft-enteric fistula in, 411-413
  atherosclerosis in
    anatomic distribution of, 328-332
    endarterectomy for, 363-364
    percutaneous arterial dilation for, 365-373
  bypass in
    aortofemoral, 355-359
    axillofemoral, 384-390
    femorofemoral, 393-396
    retroperitoneal iliofemoral, 391-392
    thoracic to femoral, 381-383
  chyloperitoneum and chylothorax in, 426-431
  coarctation in, 359-363
  coronary artery disease in, 345-350
  groin lymphocele in, 413-415
  hyperlipidemia in, 336-339
  hypertension in, 340-345
  hypoplasia in, 359-363
  lymph fistula in, 413-415
  physiologic studies of, 350-354
  smoking and, 333-335
  transabdominal medial visceral rotation in, 373-377
  vasculogenic impotence in, 397-400
Aortoiliac reconstruction, 399
Aortoplasty, 362
Aortorenal bypass
  for renovascular hypertension, 785-789
  thoracic, 802, 803
Aortorenal endarterectomy, 793-799
Appendicitis, 236
Arm
  bridge graft in, 861
  elevated stress test of, 176
  hyperabduction of, 614
  pressure differential of, 887
  veins of, 476-480
Arteria radicularis magna, 278, 279
Arterial thoracic outlet syndrome, 176
Arteriography
  in abdominal aortic aneurysm, 210-213
  in acute graft thrombosis, 538
  in angioaccess graft failure, 867
  in aortic graft infection, 404
  in blunt arterial injury of shoulder, 614

  in carotid artery fibrodysplasia, 6
  cost of, 593
  in cutaneous foot ulcers, 561, 562
  emergency, 632
  in fibromuscular dysplasia, 115-116
  of graft infection, 565
  in infected femoral artery pseudoaneurysm, 319-320
  of infrainguinal occlusive disease, 441-447
    versus duplex mapping, 440
    versus magnetic resonance angiography, 447, 450-452
  in intra-arterial injection, 641
  intravascular ultrasound versus, 527
  mesenteric, 711
  in nonocclusive mesenteric ischemia, 707-709
  in pediatric renovascular hypertension, 809
  in penetrating trauma, 596-598
    carotid, 599-600
    vertebral, 604-606
  in popliteal artery adventitial cystic disease, 510
  renal duplex sonography versus, 773
  of renovascular hypertension, 779-780
  in reversed autogenous vein grafts, 466
  in spontaneous atheroembolism, 570
  in vasculogenic impotence, 398
Arteriomegaly, 292-296
Arteriopathy
  in carotid artery fibrodysplasia, 4-6
  in upper extremity arterial disease, 141
Arteriosclerosis, 315-318
Arteriotomy
  in balloon catheter embolectomy, 577
  in carotid endarterectomy, 42
Arteriovenous anastomosis, 857-860
Arteriovenous fistula
  acquired, 841-845
  in acute iliofemoral thrombosis, 932-933
  autogenous, 865
  congenital, 850-852
  in percutaneous arterial puncture, 630-631
  portal, 721-724
  prosthetic graft, 865
  renal, 830-833
  splanchnic, 721-724
Arteriovenous malformation, 718-720
  congenital, 850-852
  transcranial Doppler ultrasound and, 18
Arteriovenous shunting
  in congenital vascular malformations, 838
  venous ulcers and, 922
Arteritis
  giant cell, 130-133
  microbial, 232
  radiation-induced, 133-137

Arteritis—cont'd
    Takayasu's, 125-129
        pediatric renovascular hypertension versus, 809
    in upper extremity arterial disease, 140-141
Artery
    in arteriographic puncture, 441-442
    in bridge grafts, 861
    cannulation of, 855
    congenital vascular malformations of, 835
    deterioration of prostheses for, 289-292
    diseased
        intravascular ultrasound of, 527-531
        venous ulcers in, 923
    enlargement of, 202
    macroembolism in, 572-576
    pressure index of, 594
Arthritis, 139
Ascending phlebography
    of chronic venous insufficiency, 885-886
    of deep vein thrombosis, 884-885
Ascites
    in chyloperitoneum, 428-429
    in portal hypertension, 761, 763
Aspiration of perigraft fluid, 565
Aspiration thromboembolectomy, 580-582
Aspirin
    in graft patency, 546-547
    for lower extremity occlusive disease, 536
    in stroke and transient ischemic attacks, 26-27
Atherectomy devices, 517-520
Atheroembolism, spontaneous, 568-571
Atheroma, 517
Atherosclerosis
    in aortic aneurysm, 201, 202-203
    aortoiliac occlusive disease
        anatomic distribution of, 328-332
        endarterectomy for, 363-364
        percutaneous arterial dilation for, 365-373
    in arteriography, 444, 445-446
    in cardiovascular disease, 340-345
    carotid artery, 1-4
        aneurysm of, 105-106
        evolving stroke and, 34-38
        fixed stroke and, 38-40
        transient ischemic attack and stroke secondary to, 80-84
    dry gangrene in, 672
    endarterectomy in
        aortorenal, 793-799
        carotid, 40-43
        superficial femoral artery, 453-457
    in graft failure, 545-546
    of innominate artery, 96-99
    prevention of, 531-533
    renal artery, 764-765
        occlusive disease of, 774

in renovascular hypertension, 782
sequential bypass for, 473-475
upper extremity
    aneurysms of, 189, 190
    arterial disease of, 139-140
    in vasculogenic impotence, 398-399
Atrial fibrillation, 586
Atriocaval shunt, 624
Atropine sulfate, 441
Auth Rotablator, 519-520
Autogenous arteriovenous fistula, 865
Autogenous reversed vein graft, 465-469
Autologous preoperative blood deposit, 287
Autologous vein, 480-482
Autotransfusion, 287-289
Autotransplantation of kidney, 234
Avulsion of varicose vein clusters, 902-903
Axillary artery
    aneurysm of, 188-194
    blunt injury of, 614
    iatrogenic catheter injury to, 626
Axillary-subclavian lesions, 134, 135
Axilloaxillary bypass, 94-95
Axillofemoral bypass, 384-390
Axillosubclavian vein thrombosis, 958-963
Azotemic arteriopathy, 141

B

Bacteria
    in cutaneous foot ulcers, 563
    in septic thrombophlebitis, 965
Balloon angioplasty; see Angioplasty
Balloon catheter
    embolectomy
        in acute aortic occlusion, 379
        for macroembolism, 576-580
    thromboembolectomy, 822-823
Balloon occlusion, 54
Balloon tamponade, 734
Basilic vein, 857-858
Below-elbow amputation, 683
Below-knee amputation, 674-677
    above-knee versus, 669-671
Below-knee grafts, 481
Benzopyrones, 975
Beta-blocker
    in blood pressure instability, 73
    cardiovascular risk and, 342
Bifurcated graft, 267-268
Biliary atresia, 760
Biliary tract disease, 237
Biofilm
    culture of, 407
    infection of, 409-410
Biopsy
    abdominal aortic aneurysm and, 237
    in giant cell arteritis, 131
    of venous ulcers, 925
Biplane arteriography, 695
Bird's nest filter, 946, 947

Bleeding
    in abdominal vascular injury, 619
    in aortic graft-enteric fistula, 411
    in hemangioma, 848-849
    in varices, 733
Blindness in giant cell arteritis, 130
Block, stellate ganglion, 166
Blood
    autotransfusion of, 287-289
    lipids in, 26
    salvage of, 288
Blood flow
    in amputation assessment, 670
    in aortic aneurysm, 202
    cerebral
        in carotid artery reconstruction, 55
        in carotid endarterectomy shunting, 57
    in lumbar sympathectomy, 462
    in sequential bypass, 475
    velocity of
        in graft surveillance, 493-494
        transcranial Doppler ultrasound and, 15-16
Blood pressure
    ankle-brachial ratio of, 513, 514
    carotid endarterectomy and, 71-73
    of finger, 147-148
    gradients of, 352-354
    in hypertension
        diastolic, 340, 341
        systolic, 343, 344
    measurements of, 354
    penile, 397-398
    segmental Doppler measurement of
        in amputation assessment, 669
        in aortoiliac occlusive disease, 351
        in infrainguinal occlusive disease, 433-434
    of stump
        in carotid artery reconstruction, 55
        in carotid endarterectomy shunting, 57
Blood supply
    to spinal cord, 285
    in abdominal aortic reconstruction, 278-282
    in vasculogenic impotence, 397
Blue toe syndrome, 568-571
    lumbar sympathectomy in, 463
Blunt injury
    abdominal, 619-625
    of elbow arteries, 615-616
    of extracranial carotid artery, 601-603
    to knee, 634-636
    renal, 657-659
    in renal artery dissection, 818-819
    of shoulder arteries, 614-615
    of vertebral artery, 606-608
B-mode ultrasonography
    of abdominal aortic aneurysm, 214
    in duplex scanning, 8-9
Body tumors of carotid artery, 121-125
Boot, Unna's, 913

Bowel viability, 696
Brachial artery, 625
Brachial plexus, 614
Brachiobasilic fistula, 858
Brain infarction, 19-20
Bridge grafts, 860-864
Bruit
    in asymptomatic carotid artery stenosis, 29
    in neck, 11
    in thoracic great vessel injury, 609
Budd-Chiari syndrome, 748-751
    in children, 760
    hepatic vein thrombosis in, 727
Buerger's disease, 154-159
    lumbar sympathectomy in, 463
    in upper extremity arterial disease, 140
Bulbocavernous reflex latency, 398
Burn patient, 965
Bypass; see also Graft
    aortofemoral
        for aortoiliac occlusive disease, 355-359
        in infrarenal aortoiliac hypoplasia, 362-363
    aortorenal, 785-789
    axilloaxillary, 94-95
    axillofemoral, 384-390
    cardiopulmonary, 953-954
    carotid-subclavian, 93-95
    for chronic mesenteric ischemia, 701-703
    extracranial-intracranial, 53
    femorofemoral
        in aortic graft limb occlusion, 424
        for aortoiliac occlusive disease, 393-396
    femoropopliteal, 480-482
    femorotibial, 480-482
    hepatorenal, 800-803
    iliofemoral, 391-392
    iliorenal, 803
    of lower extremity, 465
    mesenterorenal, 804
    in profundaplasty, 459
    in radiation-induced arteritis, 135
    saphenous vein, 454-455
    sequential, 473-475
    as spinal cord protection, 285
    splenorenal, 799-800
    in spontaneous atheroembolism, 571
    thoracic aortorenal, 802, 803
    thoracic to femoral, 381-383
    thoracoabdominal, 361-362
    in upper extremity revascularization, 144
    in vasculogenic impotence, 400
Bypass graft
    acute thrombosis of, 537-539
    of coronary artery, 102-104
    failing infrainguinal, 521-523
    in innominate artery repair, 612
    of obturator foramen, 322-325
    in radiation-induced arteritis, 135
    surveillance of, 492-499

C

Calcium channel antagonists, 306, 307
Calf muscle pump, 911
Calf veins, 875, 876
Cancer
    colonic, 236-237
    in inferior vena cava, 969
Cannulation
    central venous, 853-854
    in iatrogenic catheter injury, 625-626
Capillaries
    in amputation assessment, 671
    congenital vascular malformations of, 835, 836
Captopril renography, 777-778
Cardiac emboli, 586-589
    in renal artery, 821
Cardiac risk
    assessment of, 346-348
    in carotid endarterectomy, 100-102
Cardiology reservoir of salvaged blood, 288-298
Cardiomyopathy, 586-587
Cardiopulmonary bypass, 953-954
Cardiovascular disease, 340-345
L-carnitine, 536
Carotid artery
    angiography of, 13-15
    atherosclerosis of, 1-4
        collagen gene expression in, 3-4
        evolving stroke secondary to, 34-38
        fixed stroke secondary to, 38-40
        growth factors in, 2-3
        hemodynamic factors in, 2
        plaque composition in, 1-2
        transient ischemic attack and stroke secondary to, 80-84
    body tumors of, 121-125
    computed tomography of, 20
    concomitant occlusive disease of, 100-104
    dissection of, 109-114
    duplex scanning of, 8-13
    extracranial
        aneurysm of, 105-109
        blunt injury of, 601-603
        embolus of, 16
        occlusive disease of, 22, 23
        penetrating injury of, 598-601
    fibrodysplasia of, 4-7
    fibromuscular disease of, 114-118
    kinks and coils of, 118-121
    occluded extracranial, 45-53
        contralateral carotid endarterectomy in, 50
        extracranial-intracranial bypass of, 53
        thrombectomy of, 50-52
        thromboendarterectomy of, 52-53
    in radiation-induced arteritis, 135
    reconstruction of, 54-56
    stenosis of
        asymptomatic, 29-34
        duplex scanning and, 12
        in fibroplasia, 4-5
        recurrent, 76-80
        transcranial Doppler ultrasound in, 16
    stump blood pressure in, 55
    transcranial Doppler ultrasound in, 16-17
    transposition to subclavian artery, 89-92
Carotid endarterectomy
    anesthesia for, 44-45
    atherosclerotic disease and, 40-43, 82, 83
    blood pressure instability and, 71-73
    in carotid artery atherosclerosis, 82, 83
    carotid artery stenosis and
        asymptomatic, 30-31
        recurrent, 78-80
    cerebral hyperfusion syndrome and, 68-71
    cerebral steal syndrome and, 94
    computed tomography of, 20
    contralateral, 50
    coronary artery disease and, 100-102
    duplex scanning and, 12
    intracranial aneurysms and, 66-67
    intracranial occlusive disease and, 65-66, 67
    patch graft closure for, 60-64
    pseudoaneurysm after, 109
    in radiation-induced arteritis, 135
    restenosis in, 334
    shunting in, 57-60
    stroke and, 73-75
        evolving, 35
        fixed, 38-40
    transcranial Doppler ultrasound monitoring in, 17
Carotid-subclavian bypass, 93-95
Catheter
    central venous cannulation, 854
    embolectomy
        pulmonary, 952-953
        retrograde balloon, 379
    Fogarty adherent clot, 577, 579
    Fogarty graft thrombectomy, 423, 424
    iatrogenic injury with, 625-627
    in infrainguinal occlusive disease
        arteriography, 441-442
        atherectomy, 517-520
    in intravascular ultrasound, 527-528
    for macroembolism, 576-580
    in renal artery dissection, 818
    in septic thrombophlebitis, 963-964
    in thrombolytic therapy, 573
    in umbilical artery injury, 661-662
    in variceal embolization, 735
Causalgia, 162-165
    sympathectomy in, 166
Caval filter, 592
Caval thrombosis, 936-939
Cavernosography, 398
Cavotomy, 969-970
CEA; see Carotid endarterectomy

Celiac artery, 703
  aneurysm of, 714-715
Celiac compression syndrome, 703-706
Celiotomy, 619-620
Cell proliferation in plaque, 2-3
Cellulitis, 638
Central nervous system, 663
Central splenorenal shunt, 745
Central venous cannulation, 853-854
Cephalic vein
  in direct arteriovenous anastomosis, 857
  in lower extremity revascularization, 476
Cerebral blood flow
  in carotid artery reconstruction, 55
  in carotid endarterectomy shunting, 57
  collateral, 80, 81
Cerebral embolus, 18
Cerebral hyperfusion syndrome, 68-71
Cerebral ischemia, 54-56
Cerebral perfusion, 16-17
Cerebral steal syndrome, 93-95
Cerebrospinal fluid, 283-284
Cerebrovascular disease, 1-137
  arteritis in
    giant cell, 130-133
    radiation-induced, 133-137
    Takayasu's, 125-129
  carotid artery atherosclerosis in, 1-4
    evolving stroke secondary to, 34-38
    fixed stroke secondary to, 38-40
    transient ischemic attack and stroke secondary to, 80-84
  carotid artery in
    angiography of, 13-15
    asymptomatic stenosis of, 29-34
    body tumors of, 121-125
    concomitant occlusive disease of, 100-104
    dissection of, 109-114
    duplex scanning of, 8-13
    extracranial aneurysm of, 105-109
    fibrodysplasia of, 4-7
    fibromuscular disease of, 114-118
    kinks and coils of, 118-121
    occluded extracranial, 45-53
    recurrent stenosis of, 76-80
  carotid endarterectomy in
    anesthesia for, 44-45
    atherosclerotic disease and, 40-43
    blood pressure instability and, 71-73
    cerebral hyperfusion syndrome and, 68-71
    cerebral ischemia and, 54-56
    intracranial aneurysms and, 66-67
    intracranial occlusive disease and, 65-66, 67
    patch graft closure for, 60-64
    shunting during, 57-60
    stroke and, 73-75
  computed tomography evaluation of, 19-21
  innominate artery atherosclerosis in, 96-99
  ischemic stroke in, 24-29
  magnetic resonance imaging of, 21-24
  subclavian artery in
    carotid transposition with, 89-92
    cerebral steal syndrome and, 93-95
    transcranial Doppler evaluation of, 15-19
    transient ischemic attacks in, 24-29
    vertebral artery reconstruction in, 84-89
Cervical lesions, 134, 135
Cervical rib anomalies, 171, 172
Cervical sympathectomy, 163, 164
Cervico-dorsal sympathectomy, 166-167
Charcot foot, 558, 559
Charles procedure, 976
Chelation therapy, 536
Chemical phlebitis, 966
Chest tube, 609-610
Chilblains, 665-666
Child
  aortoplasty in, 362
  biliary atresia in, 760
  Budd-Chiari syndrome in, 760
  congenital hepatic fibrosis in, 760
  congenital vascular lesions in, 846-849
  iatrogenic vascular injury in, 659-662
  portal hypertension in, 759-763
  portal vein thrombosis in, 760
  renal artery stenosis in, 782-783
  renal vein thrombosis in, 824, 825-826
  renovascular hypertension in, 808-813
  stroke in, 25
Cholecystectomy, 237
Cholesterol
  in atherosclerotic disease prevention, 531-532
  in hyperlipidemia, 336
Chopart amputation, 673
Chronic venous insufficiency
  invasive diagnosis of, 885-887
  noninvasive diagnosis of, 881-883
  nonoperative management of, 910-913
  surgical management of, 914-919
Chyloperitoneum, 426-431
Chylothorax, 426-431
Cigarette smoking
  in atherosclerotic disease prevention, 532-533
  in stroke and transient ischemic attacks, 26
  and vascular disease, 333-335
Circulation
  in aortic reconstruction, 274-275
collateral
  in abdominal aortic reconstruction, 279-280, 281
  in acquired arteriovenous fistula, 844
  in carotid artery atherosclerosis, 80, 81
  in iatrogenic pediatric vascular injury, 659
  in occluded extracranial carotid artery, 46
  in portal hypertension, 726
  portosystemic, 728
  profunda femoris artery in, 457-458
  stimulation of, 533-534
  transcranial Doppler ultrasound in, 16
  in venous thrombosis, 877
Cirrhosis, 727
Cisterna chyli, 426
Claudication
  intermittent
    in collateral circulation stimulation, 533
    reversed autogenous vein grafts in, 465
    smoking and, 333
  in popliteal artery adventitial cystic disease, 509-510
Clip, Moretz, 950
Clot
  one-handed aspiration of, 581-582
  removal of, 863-864
  retraction of, 877-878
Coagulase-negative staphylococci, 406
Coagulation
  disorders of, 555
  in graft thrombosis, 544, 545
  of plasma, 552
  in ruptured infrarenal aortic aneurysm, 225
Coagulation cascade, 868-874
Coarctation of subisthmic thoracic aorta, 359-363
Coils of carotid artery, 118-121
Colapinto needle, 752
Cold in Raynaud's phenomenon, 145-146
Cold injury, 663-668
Colitis, 275
Collateral circulation
  in abdominal aortic reconstruction, 279-280, 281
  in acquired arteriovenous fistula, 844
  cerebral
    in carotid artery atherosclerosis, 80, 81
    transcranial Doppler ultrasound in, 16
  in iatrogenic pediatric vascular injury, 659
  in occluded extracranial carotid artery, 46
  in portal hypertension, 726
  portosystemic, 728

profunda femoris artery in, 457-458
stimulation of, 533-534
in venous thrombosis, 877
Colon
  abdominal aortic aneurysm and, 236-237
  blood flow of, 686
  ischemia
    in aortic reconstruction, 276
    in visceral revascularization, 243
Colonoscopy, 719
Color flow scanning
  in angioaccess graft failure, 866
  in chronic venous insufficiency, 882
  of deep vein thrombosis, 880
  in duplex scanning, 9-10
  in infrainguinal occlusive disease, 437-440
Coma, 600
Compartment syndrome, 644-648
  in blunt knee trauma, 636
  popliteal vascular entrapment syndrome versus, 505-506
Compression
  in chronic venous insufficiency, 912-913
  intermittent pneumatic, 890
  in lymphedema, 975
  in percutaneous arterial puncture hemorrhage, 628
  in venous ulcer treatment, 926
Compression garments, 975, 979
Compression stockings; see also Stockings
  for deep femoral venous thrombosis, 890
  in injection compression sclerotherapy, 895
Computed tomography
  of abdominal aortic aneurysm, 214-215, 216
  in aortic graft infection, 403-404
  in aortic graft-enteric fistula, 411
  for cardiac macroemboli, 587-588
  of carotid body tumors, 122
  in cerebrovascular disease, 19-21
  of congenital vascular malformations, 839
  of graft infection, 565
  in groin lymphocele, 414
  in inflammatory abdominal aortic aneurysm, 230
  in mesenteric venous thrombosis, 711-712
  in popliteal artery adventitial cystic disease, 510, 511
  in renal vascular injury, 657
  in renal vein thrombosis, 824, 825
  in ruptured infrarenal aortic aneurysm, 225
  of venous anomalies, 252, 254
Congenital arteriovenous fistulas, 850-852
Congenital arteriovenous malformations, 850-852
Congenital hepatic fibrosis, 760
Congenital vascular lesions, 846-849

Congenital vascular malformations
  classification of, 834-838
  nonangiographic evaluation of, 839-841
Congenital wall defects, 141
Conjugated diene, 584
Connective tissue disorders, 139
Contraceptives, oral, 26
Contrast
  in arteriography, 442-444
  in computed tomography monitoring, 19-20
Coral reef syndrome, 329, 330
Coronary artery
  bypass grafting of, 102-104
  concomitant occlusive disease of, 100-104
Coronary artery disease
  in abdominal aortic aneurysms, 345-350
  antithrombotic drugs in, 549
  nonruptured infrarenal aortic aneurysm and, 219
  reversed autogenous vein grafts and, 465-466
Coronary caval shunt, 731
Coronary heart disease
  blood pressure and
    diastolic, 340, 341
    systolic, 343, 344
  in hyperlipidemia, 337
Corticosteroids
  in giant cell arteritis, 132
  in inflammatory abdominal aortic aneurysm, 230
  Takayasu's arteritis and, 127
Cosmetics in varicose vein excision, 903
Cost
  of abdominal aortic aneurysm arteriography, 212
  of arteriography, 593
  in below-knee amputation, 674
Cotinine in smoking, 333
Coumadin; see Warfarin
Creeping amputation, 669
Cross-clamping
  of aorta, 620-621
  in spinal cord protection, 283
Cross-over graft, 917, 918-919
Crural vein, 875, 876
Crutches, 189, 190-191
Crystallization in frostbite, 666
CT; See Computed tomography
Culture of biofilm, 407
Cure, defined, 781
Curettage, 976
Cutaneous ischemic ulcers, 462-465
Cutaneous-visceral hemangiomatosis, 849
Cystic disease, 509-512
Cystic medial necrosis, 208-209

D

Dacron graft
  antibiotic-coated, 566
  in aortofemoral bypass, 355-359
  aspirin in, 546
  in axillofemoral bypass, 384-385
  dilation of, 290-291
  in innominate artery repair of, 612
  in pediatric renal artery reconstruction, 810
  in ruptured infrarenal aortic aneurysm, 226
  structure of, 289-290
  in upper extremity aneurysms, 194
Debridement
  of cutaneous foot ulcers, 563
  in graft infection, 565
  of infected femoral artery pseudoaneurysm, 321
Decompression
  in celiac compression syndrome, 705
  in reperfusion syndrome, 585
  for variceal hemorrhage, 744-748
Deep vein thrombosis
  femoral, 889-893
  in intravenous drug abuse, 638
  invasive diagnosis of, 884-885
  noninvasive diagnosis of, 880-881
  in paradoxical embolism, 590
  in pregnancy, 907-910
  as risk factor, 874-875
  saphenous thrombophlebitis and, 904
Defibrillation, 664
Defibrotide, 536
Deficiency
  of antithrombin III
    as heparin therapy complication, 556
    as prothrombotic state, 551
  of protein C, 551
  of protein S, 551
Dermal flap, Thompson's buried, 976
Descending phlebography, 886-887, 915
Devascularization, 740-744
Development
  of renal artery stenosis, 767-768
  in thoracic outlet syndrome, 170-174
Dexamethasone, 641-642
Dextran
  for deep femoral venous thrombosis prophylaxis, 890
  in graft patency, 548
  low-molecular-weight
    in ergotism, 161
    in intravenous drug abuse, 641-642
Diabetes
  in aortoiliac atherosclerosis, 328, 329
  cutaneous foot ulcers in, 558-564
  percutaneous transluminal angioplasty and, 515
  in stroke and transient ischemic attacks, 26
  wet gangrene in, 672
Dialysis, 853
Diastolic blood pressure, 340, 341
Diene, conjugated, 584

Diet
  in atherosclerotic disease prevention, 531-532
  in chyloperitoneum treatment, 428
  in hyperlipidemia, 337-338
Diffuse medial fibroplasia, 766
Digit pulse amplitude, 463
Digital amputation, 681
Digital plethysmography, 148
Digital subtraction angiography, 443, 444
Dilatation
  in aortic anomalies, 361
  in graft failure, 291
Dilation, graduated intraluminal, 117-118
Dipyridamole
  in graft failure, 546-547
  stroke and transient ischemic attacks and, 26-27
Dipyridamole-thallium scintigraphy, 346-348
Disarticulation
  of elbow, 683
  of hip, 677-680
  of wrist, 682-683
Dislocation
  of elbow, 615-616
  of knee, 632
  of shoulder, 614
Dissection
  aortic, 206-209
    medical management of, 305-308
    surgical treatment of, 309-314
  of carotid artery, 109-114
    by finger, 382, 383
  of renal artery, 818-820
Diuretics
  cardiovascular risk and, 342
  in lymphedema, 975
Diverticulitis, 237
Diverticulum, Kommerell's, 191, 192
Doppler ultrasound
  in aortoiliac occlusive disease, 351
  in duplex scanning, 8
  pressure measurement
    in amputation assessment, 669
    in aortoiliac occlusive disease, 351
    of infrainguinal occlusive disease, 432-435
    in penetrating injury, 594
  transcranial
    in carotid artery reconstruction, 55
    in carotid endarterectomy shunting, 57-58
    in cerebrovascular disease, 15-19
  in vascular laboratory, 148-149
  in vasculogenic impotence, 397-398
  velocity
    in infrainguinal occlusive disease, 432, 433
    for renal arterial stenosis, 805, 806-807
Drainage
  of cerebrospinal fluid, 283-284
  of lymph, 975

Dressing
  in Buerger's disease, 158
  Epigard, 649
Drug abuse
  infected femoral artery pseudoaneurysm and, 319-321
  vascular injury secondary to, 637-644
Drug therapy
  in hyperlipidemia, 338-339
  for lower extremity occlusive disease, 534-537
  in Raynaud's phenomenon, 152-153
  in thromboembolism, 871-873
  for variceal hemorrhage, 732-734
Dry gangrene, 672
Duoderm
  in chronic venous insufficiency, 913
  in venous ulcer treatment, 925, 926
Duplex scanning
  and angiography, 14
  B-mode imaging in, 8-9
  of carotid artery occlusive disease, 8-13
  in chronic renal failure, 827
  in chronic venous insufficiency, 882, 912
  color-flow imaging in, 9-10
  of congenital vascular malformations, 840
  of deep vein thrombosis, 880-881
    in pregnancy, 908
  duplex concept in, 8
  in graft surveillance, 493, 495-498
  of infrainguinal occlusive disease, 436-440
  instrumentation and technique in, 10-11
  operative assessment with, 804-808
  in penetrating injury, 594-595, 598
  for renal arterial occlusive disease, 768-774
  spectral waveform analysis in, 9-10
  in splanchnic artery occlusive disease, 686-689
  in thromboembolism, 871
  in vascular laboratory, 148-149
  in vasculogenic impotence, 397-398
DVT; see Deep vein thrombosis
Dye in groin lymphocele surgery, 414
Dynamic infusion cavernosography, 398
Dysplasia
  fibromuscular, 4-7
    of carotid artery, 114-118
    in renal arterial occlusive disease, 774
    in renal artery aneurysm, 813, 814
    in renovascular hypertension, 781
  renovascular hypertension secondary to, 790-793
  in upper extremity arterial disease, 140
  of vertebral artery, 5-6
  perimedial, 766-767
Dystrophy, reflex sympathetic, 162-165

E

Echocardiography
  for cardiac macroemboli, 587
  in paradoxical embolism, 590
  in thoracic aorta dissection, 310
Ectasia
  of arm veins, 478
  vascular, 718-720
Ectopic kidney, 246-249
Edema
  in intra-arterial injection, 641
  pulmonary, 777
Education in venous ulcer treatment, 926-927
Edwards procedure, 453-454
Ehlers-Danlos syndrome
  abdominal aortic aneurysm and, 199
  in upper extremity arterial disease, 141
  vascular complications of, 302-303
Ejaculation mechanism, 399
Elastic stockings, 913; see also Stockings
Elbow
  blunt arterial injury of, 615-616
  disarticulation of, 683
Electroencephalography
  in carotid artery reconstruction, 55-56
  in carotid endarterectomy, 42
Elevated arm stress test, 176
Elevation
  of limb, 975
  in secondary lymphedema, 979
Embolectomy
  in acute aortic occlusion, 379
  in acute pulmonary embolism, 956
  for arterial macroembolism, 575
  balloon catheter, 576-580
  of renal artery embolism, 822
  transvenous catheter pulmonary, 951-955
Embolic disease, of extremities, 568-592; see also Extremity, embolic disease of
Embolism
  in arteriography, 444, 446
  ischemia of, in mesenteric vascular disease, 693-697
  paradoxical, 589-592
  in percutaneous arterial puncture, 630
  pulmonary
    in acute iliofemoral thrombosis, 933-934
    in deep femoral venous thrombosis, 889
    nonoperative treatment of, 940-944
    in pregnancy, 909
    in thromboembolism, 871
  of renal artery, 821-823
Embolization
  in acquired arteriovenous fistula, 844-845
  after aortic reconstruction, 272
  in arteriovenous malformation, 851

of carotid body tumors, 122-123, 124
of variceal hemorrhage, 735
in venous thrombosis, 876-877
Embolus
  in acute aortic occlusion, 378
  cerebral, 18
  extracranial carotid, 16
  infarction of, 20
  in stroke and transient ischemic attacks, 24, 25
  in thromboembolic vertebrobasilar insufficiency, 84
Emergency department
  arteriography in, 632
  thoracic great vessel injury in, 609-610
Endarterectomy
  aortoiliac, 356, 363-364
  aortorenal, 793-799
  carotid
    anesthesia for, 44-45
    in asymptomatic carotid artery stenosis, 30-31
    atherosclerotic disease and, 40-43
    blood pressure instability and, 71-73
    in carotid artery atherosclerosis, 82, 83
    carotid artery stenosis and
      asymptomatic, 30-31
      recurrent, 78-80
    cerebral hyperfusion syndrome and, 68-71
    cerebral steal syndrome and, 94
    computed tomography of, 20
    contralateral, 50
    coronary artery disease and, 100-102
    duplex scanning and, 12
    intracranial aneurysms and, 66-67
    intracranial occlusive disease and, 65-66, 67
    patch graft closure for, 60-64
    pseudoaneurysm after, 109
    in radiation-induced arteritis, 135
    restenosis in, 334
    shunting in, 57-60
    stroke and, 73-75
      evolving, 35
      fixed, 38-40
    transcranial Doppler ultrasound monitoring in, 17
  in chronic pulmonary embolism, 957
  in innominate artery atherosclerosis, 97
  mesenteric, 695-696
  splanchnic, 699-701
  stripper for, 423
  of superficial femoral artery, 453-457
Endoscopy
  in aortic graft-enteric fistula, 411
  in esophageal varices sclerotherapy, 736-738
  in variceal hemorrhage, 761-762
Endothelial disorders, 553

Endothelium-derived relaxing factor, 333
Endovascular surgery
  of abdominal aortic aneurysm, 265-268
  of infrainguinal occlusive disease, 439-440
Enhancement in computed tomography monitoring, 19-20
Enteric fistula, 411-413
Entrapment syndrome, popliteal vascular, 446-447
Environment in hypertension, 343-344
Enzyme, proteolytic, 201-202
Epigard dressing, 649
Ergotamine, 159, 160-161
Ergotism, 159-162
Erythrocyte sedimentation rate
  in giant cell arteritis, 132
  in inflammatory abdominal aortic aneurysm, 230
  in Takayasu's arteritis, 127
Esmolol
  in acute aortic dissection, 306, 307
  in blood pressure instability, 73
Esophagus
  thoracic great vessel injury and, 613
  transection of, 741-742
  varices in, ligation of, 738-739
  varices of, 725
    in children, 760-761
    sclerotherapy of, 735-738
Estrogen replacement therapy, 339
Estrogens, 552
Evoked potentials, 285-286
  somatosensory
    in carotid artery reconstruction, 55-56
    in carotid endarterectomy shunting, 58
    in spinal cord ischemia, 285
Ex vivo arterial repair, 790-793
Excision
  in graft infection, 565
  aortic, 407-408
  in hypothenar hammer syndrome, 197
  in lymphedema
    secondary, 981
    staged subcutaneous, 976-978
  in septic thrombophlebitis, 965-966
  of varicose veins, 898-904
Exercise
  in collateral circulation stimulation, 533-534
  in infrainguinal occlusive disease, 434-435
Extracorporeal membrane oxygenation, 661
Extracranial aneurysm, 105-109
Extracranial carotid artery
  blunt injury of, 601-603
  penetrating injury of, 598-601
Extracranial cervical lesions, 134, 135
Extremity
  causalgia and mimocausalgia of, 162-165

  concomitant venous repair in, 652-656
  congenital vascular malformations of, 839-841
  embolic disease of, 568-592
    anticoagulant therapy in, 572-573
    balloon catheter embolectomy in, 576-580
    cardiac macroemboli in, 586-589
    lytic therapy in, 573-576
    oxygen free radical scavengers in, 582-585
    paradoxical embolism in, 589-592
    percutaneous aspiration thromboembolectomy, 580-582
    reperfusion syndrome in, 582-585
    spontaneous atheroembolism in, 568-571
  ischemia of, 128
  lower; see also Lower extremity
    aneurysm of, 315-327
    occlusive disease of, 432-567
  upper, 138-197; see also Upper extremity
    amputation of, 680-685
Eye, hemangioma and, 848

F

Failure
  defined, 781
  graft
    in angioaccess, 865-867
    antithrombotic drugs in, 544-549
    balloon angioplasty in, 521-523
    hemodynamics in, 492-494, 495
Fasciotomy, 644-649
  in blunt arterial injury of elbow, 616
  in concomitant venous repair, 656
  in extremities penetrating injury, 618
  in iatrogenic catheter injury, 627
  in reperfusion syndrome, 585
Fat in atherosclerotic disease prevention, 531
Femoral artery
  aneurysm of
    anastomotic, 415-419
    arteriosclerotic, 315-318
    aortic graft limb occlusion of, 419-420
  atherosclerosis in, 328
  embolectomy of, 579
  iatrogenic pediatric injury of, 660-661
  infected pseudoaneurysm of, 319-321
  percutaneous transluminal angioplasty in, 512-516
  stenosis of, 212
  superficial
    endarterectomy of, 453-457
    short vein grafts in, 488-491
  thoracic aorta bypass to, 381-383

Femoral vein
   acute thrombophlebitis of, 905-906
   cannulation in, 854
   deep venous thrombosis of, 889-893
Femorofemoral bypass
   in aortic graft limb occlusion, 424
   for aortoiliac occlusive disease, 393-396
Femoropopliteal bypass, 480-482
Femorotibial bypass, 480-482
Fentanyl, 441
Fibric acid, 338-339
Fibrillation, atrial, 586
Fibrin cuff theory, 922-923
Fibrinogen, 880-881
Fibrinolysis
   for acute lower extremity thrombosis, 540-544
   in coagulation, 869
   thrombosis and, 553
Fibrocartilaginous band anomalies, 172-173
Fibrodysplasia; see also Fibromuscular dysplasia
   of carotid artery, 4-7
   in renal artery aneurysm, 813, 814
   of vertebral artery, 5-6
Fibromuscular disease of renal artery, 765-767
Fibromuscular dysplasia
   of carotid artery, 114-118
   in renal arterial occlusive disease, 774
   in renovascular hypertension, 781
   renovascular hypertension secondary to, 790-793
   in upper extremity arterial disease, 140
Filter
   bird's nest, 946, 947
   Greenfield
      in acute pulmonary embolism, 944
      for deep vein thrombosis, in pregnancy, 909
      stainless steel, 945-946
      titanium, 945, 946
   Gunther, 948
   nitinol, 947, 948
   in paradoxical embolism, 592
   Prothia, 948-949
   vena cava, 945-949
      in acute pulmonary embolism, 944
      transvenous catheter pulmonary embolectomy and, 953
   Vena Tech, 946-947
Finger
   blood pressure of, 147-148
   dissection by, 382, 383
   vibratory white, 139
Finger plethysmography, 196
Finger-brachial pressure index, 147-148
First rib
   anomalies of, 171, 172
   transaxillary resection of, 182-184

Fistula
   aortic graft-enteric, 411-413
   aortoduodenal, 226
   aortoenteric, 262-264
   arteriovenous
      acquired, 841-845
      in acute iliofemoral thrombosis, 932-933
      autogenous, 865
      congenital, 850-852
      in percutaneous arterial puncture, 630-631
      portal, 721-724
      prosthetic graft, 865
      renal, 830-833
      splanchnic, 721-724
   brachiobasilic, 858
   in groin, 845
   hepatic, 723-724
   inferior vena cava, 261-262
   lymph, 413-415
   radiocephalic, 857
   splenic, 723
Fistulography, 866-867
Flap
   pedicle, 566
   Thompson's buried dermal, 976
Fluoroscopy, 591
Fogarty catheter
   adherent clot, 577, 579
   graft thrombectomy, 423, 424
Foot
   amputation of, 672-674
   Charcot, 558, 559
   diabetic cutaneous ulcers of, 558-564
   pressure differential of, 887
   protection of, 534
Foramen ovale, 589
Forearm
   compartmental anatomy of, 647
   fasciotomy of, 616
Forequarter amputation, 684
Fossa, antecubital, 640
Fracture
   arterial injury and, 631-634
   in blunt arterial injury of shoulder, 614
Frostbite, 665-667
Frostnip, 665
Functional popliteal entrapment, 506-508
Fungal infection, 974
Fusion, renal, 246-249

G

Gallbladder ischemia, 802-803
Gallium-67, 401
Ganglia in lumbar sympathectomy, 462
Gangrene, 672
Gastric disease, 236
Gastric zone in portal hypertension, 725
Gastrocnemius muscle, 504, 505

Gastroesophageal devascularization, 740-744
Gelfoam, 831-832
Gemifibrozil, 338-339
Genetics
   of aortic aneurysm, 198-200, 201
   of hypertension, 341
Giant cell arteritis, 130-133, 141
Glomerular filtration rate, 827-829
Glucocorticosteroids, 132
Gradient sequential pumps, 975
Graduated compression stockings
   in chronic venous insufficiency, 913
   for deep femoral venous thrombosis, 890
Graduated intraluminal dilation, 117-118
Graft; see also Bypass
   above-knee, 481
   in acquired arteriovenous fistula, 844
   antithrombotic drugs in, 544-550
   aortic
      infection of, 400-411
      limb occlusion in, 419-426
   aortofemoral; see Aortofemoral graft
   below-knee, 481
   bridge, 860-864
   bypass
      acute thrombosis of, 537-539
      of coronary artery, 102-104
      failing infrainguinal, 521-523
      in innominate artery repair, 612
      of obturator foramen, 322-325
      in radiation-induced arteritis, 135
      reversed vein, 525-526
      surveillance of, 492-499
   in carotid artery dissection, 113
   cross-over, 917, 918-919
   Dacron; see Dacron graft
   endovascular, 265-268
   failure of
      in angioaccess, 865-867
      antithrombotic drugs in, 544-549
      balloon angioplasty in, 521-523
      hemodynamics in, 492-494, 495
   fibrinolytic therapy for, 542-543
   infection of
      in axillofemoral bypass, 390
      groin in, 564-567
   in infrarenal aortic aneurysm
      nonruptured, 220-222
      ruptured, 226
   in innominate artery atherosclerosis, 97, 98-99
   interposition, 316-317
   patch closure, 60-64
   perfusion of, 250-251
   removal of, 408-409
   reversed vein, 525-526
      autogenous, 465-469
   revision of, 498
   saphenous vein, 334, 335
      in situ, 469-472
   selection of, 384-385
   in sequential bypass, 473-474

short vein, 488-491
skin, 932
tension of, 386-387
thrombosis of, 865
umbilical vein, 484-487
in upper extremity aneurysms, 193
Graftotomy, 863
Gram staining, 233
Greenfield filter
  in acute pulmonary embolism, 944
  in paradoxical embolism, 592
  in pregnancy, 909
  stainless steel, 945-946
  titanium, 945, 946
Groin
  dissection of, 979
  fistula in, 845
  infected grafts in, 564-567
  lymphocele of, 413-415
  sepsis of, 322-325
Growth factors
  in cutaneous foot ulcers, 563
  in plaque, 2-3
Guillotine amputation, 563
Gunshot wounds, 604, 606
Gunther filter, 948

H

Hamburg classification of congenital vascular malformations, 835-838
Hand-held continuous wave Doppler device, 881
Headache in cerebral hyperfusion syndrome, 70
Heart
  in hypothermia, 663
  in renal artery embolism, 821
  valve vegetations in, 639
Heart disease
  in hypertension, 340, 341
  in stroke and transient ischemic attacks, 24, 25
Hemangioma, 846-849
  in vascular malformation, 720
Hemangiomatosis, 849
Hemasite external angioaccess, 855
Hematoma
  in abdominal vascular injury, 622-623
  in aortic dissection, 206
  in penetrating carotid trauma, 599
  in percutaneous arterial puncture, 628-630
Hemodialysis, 853
Hemodilution, 535-536
Hemodynamic vertebrobasilar insufficiency, 85-86
Hemodynamics
  in aortic aneurysm, 202
  of congenital vascular malformations, 840
  of graft failure, 492-494, 495
  in plaque, atherosclerosis in, 2
  of renin-angiotensin system, 775-776

in venous thrombosis, 877
of venous ulcers, 922-923
Hemorrhage
  as heparin therapy complication, 554-555
  intracerebral, 71
  in percutaneous arterial puncture, 628-630
  in renal vascular injury, 658
  variceal, 732-735
    decompressive shunts for, 744-748
    gastroesophageal devascularization for, 740-744
  in portal hypertension, 761
Hemorrhagic infarction, 20
Heparin sodium
  in acute aortic occlusion, 378
  in acute iliofemoral and caval thrombosis, 936-937
  in acute pulmonary embolism, 940-941, 943, 956
  in aortic reconstruction, 273
  for arterial macroembolism, 572-573
  in axillosubclavian vein thrombosis, 959
  in carotid endarterectomy stroke, 75
  complications of, 554-557
  in deep femoral venous thrombosis, 891-892
  in ergotism, 161
  evolving stroke and, 34-35
  in graft patency, 548
  in intra-arterial injection, 641-642
  in intravenous drug abuse, 638
  low-dose, 890
  and papaverine, 709
  in pregnancy, 908
  in stroke and transient ischemic attacks, 26, 27-28
  in thromboembolism, 871-872
  in transvenous catheter pulmonary embolectomy, 953
Heparin-induced thrombocytopenia
  in acute iliofemoral and caval thrombosis, 937
  in aortic reconstruction, 273
  in deep femoral venous thrombosis, 892
  thrombosis and, 551-552
Hepatic artery
  aneurysm of, 715-716
  in hepatorenal bypass, 800-803
Hepatic fibrosis, 760
Hepatic fistula, 723-724
Hepatic vein thrombosis, 727
Hepatorenal bypass, 800-803
Heredity in abdominal aortic aneurysm, 198-200
Hernia, 236
H-graft interposition mesocaval shunt, 744-745
Hindbrain, 85-86
Hip disarticulation, 677-680
Hirudin, 547
Horner's syndrome, 169
Horseshoe kidney, 246, 248

Hyperabduction of arm, 614
Hypercholesterolemia, 337
Hypercoagulable states, 550
  in aortic reconstruction, 273
  laboratory assessment of, 553
  in venous thrombosis, 874
Hyperemia, reactive, 69
Hyperhidrosis
  in acrocyanosis, 154
  sympathectomy in, 166
Hyperlipidemia, 336-339
Hyperplasia
  intimal
    in angioaccess graft thrombosis, 865
    in graft failure, 545
  medial, 765
  myointimal
    in graft surveillance, 493
    in recurrent carotid artery stenosis, 78-79
    in in situ saphenous vein graft, 470
Hypersplenism, 761, 763
Hypertension
  in aortic anomalies, 361
  in aortic dissection, 206
  atherosclerotic cardiovascular disease in, 340-341
  carotid endarterectomy and, 72
  in carotid endarterectomy patch angioplasty, 63
  in elderly, 342-343
  genetics of, 341
  in occluded extracranial carotid artery, 48-50
  portal, 725-763; *see also* Portal hypertension
  renovascular
    aortorenal bypass for, 785-789
    arteriographic diagnosis of, 779-780
    ex vivo arterial repair for, 790-793
    pediatric surgery for, 808-813
    percutaneous arterial dilation for, 780-785
    renin-angiotensin system in, 774, 775-778
    secondary, 815
  in stroke and transient ischemic attacks, 25-26
  in Takayasu's arteritis, 128
  in thoracoabdominal aortic reconstruction, 283-284
Hypertrophy, left ventricular, 341-342
Hypogastric artery, 790-793
Hypoperfusion, 275
Hypoplasia of subisthmic thoracic aorta, 359-363
Hypotension, 72
Hypothenar hammer syndrome, 139, 195-197
Hypothermia, 663-665
  as spinal cord protection, 284
Hypovolemia, 599
Hypoxia, 956

I

IADSA; see Intra-arterial digital subtraction angiography
Iatrogenic trauma
    pediatric, 659-662
    in renal vascular injury, 658-659
Iliac aneurysm, 296-302
    abdominal aortic aneurysm and, 211
Iliac artery
    in abdominal vascular injury, 622, 623
    in femorofemoral bypass, 393
    in pediatric renal artery reconstruction, 810
    percutaneous transluminal angioplasty of, 366, 367-369
    stenosis of, 212
    stent placement in, 370-372
Iliofemoral bypass, 391-392
Iliofemoral thrombosis
    nonoperative treatment of, 936-939
    surgical treatment of, 932-935
Iliorenal bypass, 803
Imaging sequence in arteriography, 442-443, 444-445
Impedance plethysmography, 881
Impotence, 397-400
Improvement, defined, 781
In situ replacement, 566
In situ saphenous vein graft, 469-472
In situ vein bypass, 468-469
Incompetent valves, 900
Index
    ankle-brachial
        in aortoiliac occlusive disease, 331-332
        in graft surveillance, 494
        in infrainguinal occlusive disease, 433
        in penetrating injury, 598
        in popliteal vascular entrapment syndrome, 504, 505
    arterial pressure, 594
    finger-brachial pressure, 147-148
    profunda-popliteal collateral, 459
    renal-systemic renin, 786
    thigh ankle gradient, 459
Indium-111
    in aortic graft infection diagnosis, 401-402
    in graft infection, 565
Infant
    central venous cannulation in, 854
    congenital vascular lesions in, 846-849
    iatrogenic vascular injury in, 659-662
    renal vein thrombosis in, 824, 825-826
Infarction
    brain, 19-20
    embolic, 20
    hemorrhagic, 20
    myocardial
        antithrombotic drugs in, 549
        cardiac macroemboli in, 586
    of skin, 569
    of spinal cord, 280
Infection
    in abdominal aortic aneurysm, 232-235
    of aortic graft
        diagnosis of, 400-405
        treatment of, 405-411
    of arterial prosthesis, 322-325
    in axillofemoral bypass, 390
    in below-knee amputation, 674
    in cutaneous foot ulcers, 558-559
    as external angioaccess complication, 856
    in femoral anastomotic aneurysm, 415
    of femoral artery pseudoaneurysm, 319-321
    of groin vascular grafts, 564-567
    in lymphedema, 975
    parasitic, 978-979
    in septic thrombophlebitis, 964
    of soft tissue, 637-638
Inferior vena cava; see Vena cava
Inflammatory aortic aneurysm, 204-205
    abdominal, 229-231
Inflammatory process
    in intravenous drug abuse, 637
    in reperfusion syndrome, 651
Inflow
    in aortic graft limb occlusion, 422-424
    in bridge graft, 862
    in unilateral retroperitoneal iliofemoral bypass, 391
Infrageniculate arterial reconstruction, 477
Infrainguinal atherosclerosis, 328-332
Infrainguinal occlusive disease
    angioscopy in, 524-526
    in aortoiliac occlusive disease, 330
    atherectomy devices in, 517-520
    conventional arteriography of, 441-447
    Doppler pressure assessment of, 432-435
    duplex imaging of, 436-440
    failing bypass grafts in, 521-523
    magnetic resonance angiography of, 447-453
Infrainguinal reconstruction
    in aneurysmosis, 295
    arterial, 480-482
    bypass graft in
        acute thrombosis of, 537-539
        surveillance of, 492-499
    short vein grafts in, 488
Infrapopliteal artery, 488-491
Infrarenal aorta
    aneurysm of
        nonruptured, 218-223
        ruptured, 224-226
    stent placement in, 367, 368, 369-370
Injection
    arteriographic parameters of, 442-444
    intra-arterial, 640-644
Injection compression sclerotherapy, 894-898
Injury; see also Trauma
    blunt
        abdominal, 619-625
        of elbow arteries, 615-616
        of extracranial carotid artery, 601-603
        to knee, 634-636
        renal, 657-659
        in renal artery dissection, 818-819
        of shoulder arteries, 614-615
        of vertebral artery, 606-608
    cold, 663-668
    intestinal ischemic, 693-694
    intimal, 874
    occupational, 139
    penetrating
        abdominal, 619-625
        in acquired arteriovenous fistula, 841, 842
        arteriography of, 596-598
        of extracranial carotid artery, 598-601
        of extremities, 617-619
        nonarteriographic assessment of, 593-595
        renal, 657-659
        of thoracic great vessels, 608-613
        of vertebral artery, 604-608
    radiation, 140
Innominate artery
    atherosclerosis of, 96-99
    penetrating injury of, 608-613
    repair of, 612
Inokuchi shunt, 731
Insufficiency, chronic venous
    nonoperative management of, 910-913
    surgical management of, 914-919
Insulin resistance, 340
Intercostal arteries, 284-285
Intermittent claudication
    in collateral circulation stimulation, 533
    reversed autogenous vein grafts in, 465
    smoking and, 333
Intermittent pneumatic compression, 890
International normalized ratio in prothrombin time, 873
Interposition graft, 316-317
Intestinal ischemia
    in aortic reconstruction, 274-277
    mesenteric vasospasm and, 693-694
Intima
    of persistent sciatic artery, 500, 501, 502
    in venous thrombosis, 874
Intimal fibroplasia, 765
Intimal hyperplasia
    in angioaccess graft thrombosis, 865
    in graft failure, 545
Intra-abdominal disease, 235-238

Intra-arterial digital subtraction angiography, 13-14
   in cutaneous foot ulcers, 562
Intra-arterial injection, 640-644
Intra-arterial pressure gradients, 440
Intracerebral hemorrhage, 71
Intracranial occlusive disease
   in carotid endarterectomy, 65-66, 67
   transcranial Doppler ultrasound in, 17-18
Intrahepatic veno-occlusive disease, 727
Intraluminal stripper, 901-902
Intramural hematoma, 206
Intravascular stents, 783-785
Intravascular ultrasound, 527-531
Intravenous pylogram, 657
Irrigation
   in graft infection, 565-566
   in infrainguinal occlusive disease angioscopy, 524
Ischemia
   in acute graft thrombosis, 538
   after aortic reconstruction, 271-274
   cerebral, 54-56
   in diabetic foot, 558-564
   of gallbladder, 802-803
   intestinal
      in aortic reconstruction, 274-277
      mesenteric vasospasm and, 693-694
   mesenteric
      acute embolic, 694
      acute thrombotic, 694-695
      chronic, 697-703
      nonocclusive, 706-709
      in visceral revascularization, 242, 243
   oxygen free radicals in, 582-585
   profundaplasty in, 459
   in renal fibromuscular disease, 767
   spinal cord
      in abdominal aortic reconstruction, 278-282
      in thoracoabdominal aortic reconstruction, 282-286
   in Takayasu's arteritis, 128
   of upper extremity, 142
   vertebrobasilar
      computed tomography and, 20-21
      insufficiency in, 86-87
   visceral, 689-693
Ischemic colitis
   in aortic reconstruction, 277
   percutaneous transcatheter therapy for, 691
Ischemic nephropathy, 827
   aortorenal bypass for, 786-787
   in renal arterial occlusive disease, 777
Ischemic stroke
   antithrombotic therapy for, 26-28
   medical therapy for, 24-29
Ischemic ulcers, 462-465
Isosulphan blue dye, 414
Isoxsuprine, 535

J
Juxtarenal aortic aneurysm, 218-223
Juxtarenal aortoiliac occlusive disease, 373-377

K
Kasbach-Merritt syndrome, 848-849
Kidney
   angiotensin in, 776
   autotransplantation of, 234
   ectopic, 246-249
   horseshoe, 246, 248
   in hypothermia, 664
   renal duplex sonography of, 770
Kinks of carotid artery, 118-121
Knee
   amputation above, 677-679
   amputation below, 674-677
   blunt arterial injury to, 634-636
   dislocation of, 632
Knee joint, 473
Knit fabric
   in aortofemoral bypass, 355-359
   in arterial grafts, 290
Kommerell's diverticulum, 191, 192

L
Labetalol, 73
Laboratory, vascular, 147-149
Landmark in elective aneurysmectomy, 239, 241
Laser ablation, 847
L-carnitine, 536
Leg
   blood pressure of, 433-434
   bridge graft in, 861
   compartmental anatomy of, 646, 647
   perforating veins of, 902-903
   protection of, 534
Leiomyosarcoma, 967
Leukocytes, 923
Ligation
   in carotid artery dissection, 113-114
   in chyloperitoneum, 429
   in chylothorax treatment, 431
   in concomitant venous repair, 652-653
   of esophageal varices, 738-739
   of extracranial carotid artery aneurysm, 108
   in femoropopliteal thrombophlebitis, 905-906
   of infected femoral artery pseudoaneurysm, 320-321
   of inferior vena cava, 950
   in penetrating carotid trauma, 600
   of perforating veins, 930-932
   of persistent sciatic artery, 502-503
   in saphenous thrombophlebitis, 905
   in superficial venous insufficiency, 916
   in upper extremity aneurysms, 193
   of variceal hemorrhage, 740-741
   of varicose veins, 901
   in vertebral artery injury, 607
Limb
   aortic graft occlusion of, 419-426
   elevation of, 975, 979
   ischemia of, 271-274
   salvage of
      amputation versus, 632-633
      short vein grafts in, 488-491
Lipedema, 974
Lipids
   in hyperlipidemia, 336-337
   peroxidation of, 584
   in stroke and transient ischemic attacks, 26
Lipoproteins
   in atherosclerotic disease prevention, 532
   in hyperlipidemia, 336
Lisfranc amputation, 673
Livedo reticularis, 153-154
Liver
   hemangioma in, 849
   transplantation
      in Budd-Chiari syndrome, 750-751
      in portal hypertension, 755-759
Local anesthesia
   for carotid endarterectomy, 44-45
   cerebral ischemia and, 54-55
Long vein bypass, 489-490
Lovastatin, 338, 339
Low-dose heparin, 890
Lower extremity
   aneurysm of, 315-327
      arteriosclerotic femoral artery, 315-318
      infected femoral artery, 319-321
      obturator foramen bypass grafts in, 322-325
      popliteal artery, 325-327
   concomitant venous repair in, 655-656
   occlusive disease of, 432-567
      acute graft thrombosis in, 537-539
      angioscopy in, 524-526
      antithrombotic drugs in, 544-550
      arm veins in, 476-480
      atherectomy devices in, 517-520
      bypass graft surveillance in, 492-499
      conventional arteriography in, 441-447
      cutaneous foot ulcers in, 558-564
      Doppler pressure assessment in, 432-435
      duplex imaging in, 436-440
      expanded polytetrafluoroethylene graft for, 480-484
      failing grafts in, 521-523
      fibrinolytic therapy in, 540-544
      heparin therapy complications in, 554-557
      intravascular ultrasound in, 527-531

Lower extremity—cont'd
  occlusive disease of—cont'd
    lumbar sympathectomy in, 462-465
    magnetic resonance angiography in, 447-453
    nonoperative, nonpharmacologic management of, 531-534
    percutaneous arterial dilatation for, 512-517
    persistent sciatic artery in, 499-504
    pharmacologic treatment of, 534-537
    popliteal artery adventitial cystic disease in, 509-512
    popliteal vascular entrapment syndrome in, 504-508
    profundaplasty in, 457-461
    prothrombotic states and thromboses in, 550-554
    reversed autogenous vein grafts in, 465-469
    sequential bypass for, 473-475
    short vein grafts in, 488-491
    in situ saphenous vein graft in, 469-472
    superficial femoral artery endarterectomy in, 453-457
    umbilical vein grafts for, 484-487
    vascular graft infection in, 564-567
  percutaneous arterial puncture in, 628-631
  trauma to, 631-634
  vein anatomy in, 898-900
Low-molecular-weight dextran
  in ergotism, 161
  in intra-arterial injection, 641-642
Low-molecular-weight heparin
  in acute iliofemoral and caval thrombosis, 937
  in acute pulmonary embolism, 943
  for deep femoral venous thrombosis prophylaxis, 890
  in thromboembolism, 872
L-propionylcarnitine, 536
Lumbar sympathectomy
  for cutaneous ischemic ulcers, 462-465
  livedo reticularis, 153
Lymph fistula, 413-415
Lymphangioplasty, 976
Lymphangiosarcoma, 974
Lymphangitis, 979-980
Lymphatics in venous ulcers, 922
Lymphedema
  primary, 973-978
  secondary, 978-982
Lymphocele of groin, 413-415
Lympholymphatic shunt, 976
Lymphorrhea, 413
Lymphoscintigraphy, 974
Lymphovenous shunt, 976
Lysis
  for arterial macroembolism, 573-576
  of clot, 877-878
  of valve, 525

M

Macroembolism
  balloon catheter embolectomy for, 576-580
  cardiac sources of, 586-589
  therapy for, 572-576
Magnetic resonance angiography
  in atherosclerotic aortoiliac occlusive disease, 355-356
  of carotid artery dissection, 111-112
  of infrainguinal occlusive disease, 447-453
Magnetic resonance imaging
  of abdominal aortic aneurysm, 215-217
  in aortic graft infection, 404
  for cardiac macroemboli, 587-588
  of carotid artery dissection, 111-112
  of cerebrovascular disease, 21-24
  of congenital vascular malformations, 839-840
  in cutaneous foot ulcers, 559-560, 562
  of graft infection, 565
  in mesenteric venous thrombosis, 711-712
  in popliteal vascular entrapment syndrome, 506, 507
Mal perforans ulcers, 558, 559
Malformation
  arteriovenous, 718-720
    congenital, 850-852
    renal, 830-833
    transcranial Doppler ultrasound and, 18
  congenital vascular
    classification of, 834-838
    nonangiographic evaluation of, 839-841
  of splanchnic circulation, 718-720
Malignancy in thrombosis, 552
Mandibular subluxation, 41
Mannitol, 652
Manual lymph drainage, 975
Marfan syndrome
  abdominal aortic aneurysm and, 199
  vascular complications of, 303-305
Markers
  of coronary artery disease, 349
  of smoking, 333
Mastectomy, 979
Media
  in aortic aneurysm, 202-203
  of persistent sciatic artery, 500, 501, 502
Medial arcuate syndrome, 703-706
Medial fibrodysplasia, 813, 814
Medial fibroplasia, 765-766
Medial visceral rotation, 373-377
Median sternotomy
  in innominate artery atherosclerosis, 96-99
  in thoracic great vessel thoracotomy, 610
Mesenteric artery
  in abdominal vascular injury, 623-624
  anatomy of, 693
  in aortic reconstruction, 274-275
  thromboendarterectomy of, 695-696
  in visceral revascularization, 243
Mesenteric collateral circulation, 279-280, 281
Mesenteric vascular disease, 686-724
  aneurysms in, 714-718
  arteriovenous fistula in, 721-724
  celiac compression syndrome in, 703-706
  ischemia in
    bypass procedure for, 701-703
    embolic, 693-697
    nonocclusive, 706-709
    thrombotic, 693-697
    transaortic splanchnic endarterectomy for, 697-701
    visceral, 689-693
  splanchnic circulation in
    duplex scanning of, 686-689
    vascular malformation of, 718-721
  venous thrombosis in, 710-713
Mesenterorenal bypass, 804
Mesocaval shunt, 729
Metacarpal amputation, 682
Metastatic disease in vena caval tumors, 970
Metatarsal
  amputation, 673
  head resection, 563
Microbial arteritis, 232
Microbubbles in paradoxical embolism, 590
Microembolization, 568
Microscopy, capillary, 671
Microvasculature
  in diabetics, 558
  in venous ulcers, 922
Midazolam, 441
Mimocausalgia, 162-165
  sympathectomy in, 166
Moist dressing in Buerger's disease, 158
Monoclonal antibody, 585
Morbidity
  in acute aortic occlusion, 380
  in acute iliofemoral thrombosis, 934-935
  in in situ saphenous vein graft, 471
  transabdominal medial visceral rotation and, 376-377
Moretz clip, 950
Mortality
  in acute aortic occlusion, 380
  in acute iliofemoral thrombosis, 933
  in aortic graft infection, 409
  in pulmonary embolectomy, 956
  in ruptured infrarenal aortic aneurysm, 224
  in thoracic great vessel injury, 608, 609
  transabdominal medial visceral rotation and, 375-376
Motor evoked potentials, 285-286
MRA; see Magnetic resonance angiography

MRI; *See* Magnetic resonance imaging
Multisystem organ failure, 700-701
Muscle flap closure, 566
Mycotic aneurysm, 639-640
Myocardial infarction
    antithrombotic drugs in, 549
    cardiac macroemboli in, 586
Myoglobinuria, 650-652
Myointimal hyperplasia
    in graft surveillance, 493
    in recurrent carotid artery stenosis, 78-79
    in in situ saphenous vein graft, 470
Myonecrosis, 650-652

N

Naftidrofuryl, 536-537
Necrosis
    in reperfusion syndrome, 582
    warfarin-induced, 919-921
Needle biopsy, 237
Neolymphatic vessel formation, 981
Neonate
    hemangioma in, 846
    renal vein thrombosis in, 824, 825-826
Nephrectomy, 819
Nephropathy, ischemic
    aortorenal bypass for, 786-787
    in chronic renal failure, 827
    in renal arterial occlusive disease, 777
Nephrotic syndrome, 824, 826
Nervous system
    in hypothermia, 663
    thoracic great vessel injury and, 613
    in vasculogenic impotence, 397
Neuralgia in lumbar sympathectomy, 463
Neurogenic thoracic outlet syndrome, 177-178
    disputed, 179-180
Neurologic deficit, 599
Neurologic thoracic outlet syndrome, 182-183
Neuropathy, diabetic, 558
Nicotine supplements, 157-158
Nicotinic acid, 338, 339
Nifedipine, 152
Nitinol filter, 947, 948
Nitroglycerin
    in arteriography, 444
    in nonruptured infrarenal aortic aneurysm, 221
    in percutaneous transluminal renal angioplasty, 781
Nitroprusside
    in acute aortic dissection, 306, 307
    in blood pressure instability, 73
    in ergotism, 161
    in nonruptured infrarenal aortic aneurysm, 221
Nocturnal penile tumescence, 398
Nylidrin, 534-535

O

Obesity, 337
Obstruction of airway, 848
Obturator foramen, 322-325
Occlusion
    of internal carotid artery, 80-83
        stenosis versus, 513-515
    of transjugular portosystemic shunt, 754
Occlusive disease
    aortoiliac, 328-431; see also Aortoiliac occlusive disease
    of carotid and coronary artery, 100-104
    in carotid endarterectomy, 65-66, 67
    of lower extremity, 432-567; see also Lower extremity, occlusive disease of
    of renal artery, 764-768
    of splanchnic artery, 686-689
    of suprainguinal arteries, 391-392
    of visceral artery, 211-212
Occult infection, 415
Occupational injury, 139
Octreotide, 734
Omental transposition, 976, 980, 981
One-handed clot aspiration valve set system, 581-582
Open endarterectomy, 453-454
Oral contraceptives, 26
Orthopedics in blunt knee trauma, 636
Osteomyelitis, 559-560
Osteoporosis, 557
Outflow
    in aortic graft limb occlusion, 424-425
    in bridge graft, 862
    calculation of resistance in, 887-888
    in graft thrombosis, 545
    obstruction of, 887-888
        in chronic venous insufficiency, 917, 918-919
        in intra-arterial injection, 640-641
Overdosage of heparin, 554-555
Oxygen
    in extracorporeal membrane, 661
    transcutaneous pressure of
        in amputation assessment, 670-671
        in cutaneous foot ulcers, 561
Oxygen free radicals, 582-585

P

Paget-Schroetter's syndrome, 958-963
Pain
    in intra-arterial injection, 641
    in lumbar sympathectomy, 463
    in reflex sympathetic dystrophy, 163
    sympathectomy and, 165
Palmaz stent
    in atherosclerotic aortoiliac occlusive disease, 365-367
    studies of, 372
Palpable pulse, 669

Papaverine
    in blood pressure measurement, 354
    in nonocclusive mesenteric ischemia, 709
    in provocative testing, 398
    in spinal cord ischemia, 286
Paracentesis, 427
Paraclavicular operative approach, 187
Paradoxical embolism, 589-592
Paragangliomas, 121-125
Paraparesis, 282-283
Paraplegia
    in thoracoabdominal aortic aneurysm, 255
    in thoracoabdominal aortic reconstruction, 282-283
Pararenal aneurysm, 218
Pararenal aorta, 373-377
Parasitic infection, 978-979
Partial thromboplastin time, 554-555
Patch angioplasty, 120-121
Patch graft
    in aortic anomalies, 362
    for carotid endarterectomy, 60-64
    in profundaplasty, 460, 461
Patency
    antithrombotic drugs in, 544-550
    in axillofemoral bypass, 387-388, 389-390
    in balloon angioplasty, 521, 522
    of femorofemoral bypass, 396
    of infrageniculate arterial reconstruction, 477
    in reversed autogenous vein grafts, 467-469
    of runoff vessels, 450-452
    in short vein grafts, 488-490, 491
    of in situ saphenous vein graft, 471, 472
    smoking and, 334, 335
    of umbilical vein grafts, 484-487
Patent foramen ovale, 589
PCNA; *see* Proliferating cell nuclear antigen
Peak systolic velocity, 769-770
Pediatric; *see* Child
Pedicle
    in abdominal vascular injury, 623
    flaps, 566
Pelvic leak, 903
Pelvic steal syndrome, 398, 399-400
Penetrating injury
    abdominal, 619-625
    in acquired arteriovenous fistula, 841, 842
    arteriography of, 596-598
    of extracranial carotid artery, 598-601
    of extremities, 617-619
    nonarteriographic assessment of, 593-595
    renal, 657-659
    of thoracic great vessels, 608-613
    of vertebral artery, 604-608
Penile artery, 397
Pentoxifylline
    in intermittent claudication, 465

Pentoxifylline—cont'd
    for lower extremity occlusive disease, 535
Peptic ulcer disease, 236
Percutaneous arterial dilatation; see Percutaneous transluminal angioplasty
Percutaneous arterial puncture, 628-631
Percutaneous transluminal angioplasty, 689-690; see also Angioplasty
    in atherosclerotic aortoiliac occlusive disease, 365-373
    in femorofemoral bypass, 393-394
    in fibromuscular dysplasia, 118
    for lower extremity occlusive disease, 512-517
    renal
        in chronic renal failure, 828
        for renovascular hypertension, 780-785
Perforating veins
    in chronic venous insufficiency, 911
    interruption of, 901-902
        venous ulcers and, 930-932
    in vein anatomy, 899-900
Perfusion of renal graft, 250-251
Pericapillary fibrin cuff theory, 922-923
Perigraft fluid aspiration, 565
Perigraft seroma, 388
Perigraft tissue, 406-407
Peripheral arterial disease, 333, 334
Peripheral medial fibroplasia, 766
Peritoneovenous shunt, 429
Pernio, 665-666
Persistent sciatic artery, 499-504
PET; see Dacron
Phalangeal amputation, 673
Pharmacology
    in hyperlipidemia, 338-339
    in lower extremity occlusive disease, 534-537
    in Raynaud's phenomenon, 152-153
    in thromboembolism, 871-873
    for variceal hemorrhage, 732-734
Phenomenon, Raynaud's, 151-153
    diagnosis of, 145-151
    sympathectomy in, 166
Phlebitis, 963
    chemical, 966
    septic, 638
Phlebography
    ascending, 884-885
    of chronic venous insufficiency, 885-887
    descending, 915
    in thoracic outlet syndrome, 176-177
    of venous aneurysm, 971-972
    of venous anomalies, 252-254
Photography, 894-895
Photoplethysmography
    in chronic venous insufficiency, 912
    in lumbar sympathectomy, 463
    in vascular laboratory, 147-148
Physical examination
    in penetrating injury, 594
    in thoracic great vessel injury, 609

Physical therapy, 181
Pirogoff amputation, 673
Plaque
    in aortic aneurysm, 202, 203
    collagen gene expression in, 3-4
    composition of, 1-2
    growth factors in, 2-3
    hemodynamic factors in, 2
    intravascular ultrasound and, 527-528
Plasma coagulation, 552
Plasmin, 869
Platelets
    activation of, 552
    in graft thrombosis, 544, 545
Plethysmography
    air
        in aortoiliac occlusive disease, 351
        in chronic venous insufficiency, 882
        in cutaneous foot ulcers, 561
        for deep vein thrombosis diagnosis, 881
    digital
        in hypothenar hammer syndrome, 196
        in vascular laboratory, 148
Pleurocentesis, 427
Pleuroperitoneal shunt, 431
Plication of inferior vena cava, 950
Pneumatic compression, 890
Pneumothorax
    as external angioaccess complication, 855
    in thoracic outlet syndrome surgery, 187
Poiseuille's law, 432
Polar renal arteries, 771
Polyarteritis nodosa, 141
Polyethylene terephthalate; see Dacron
Polytetrafluoroethylene
    aneurysmal deterioration and, 289
    in aortic graft infection, 408, 409-410
    in aortic graft-enteric fistula, 412-413
    arm veins versus, 476-477
    aspirin and, 546
    in axillofemoral bypass, 384
    in bridge graft, 861
    for carotid endarterectomy patch graft, 61-62
    expanded
        in aortorenal bypass, 788
        in femoral anastomotic aneurysm, 416-418
        for lower extremity occlusive disease, 480-484
    in femorofemoral bypass, 395
    suture, 466-467
    in upper extremity aneurysms, 194
Popliteal artery
    adventitial cystic disease of, 509-512
    aneurysm of, 325-327
        arteriography in, 445, 446
        femoral artery aneurysm and, 315

        blunt injury to, 634-636
        percutaneous transluminal angioplasty in, 512-516
        short vein grafts in, 488-491
Popliteal vascular entrapment syndrome, 504-508
    in arteriography, 446-447
Popliteal vein
    acute thrombophlebitis of, 905-906
    aneurysm of, 971
Portacaval shunt, 744
Portal arteriovenous fistulas, 721-724
Portal hypertension, 725-763
    anatomic basis of, 725-731
    Budd-Chiari syndrome and, 748-751
    in children, 759-763
    classification of, 726-727
    esophageal varices in, 735-740
    liver transplantation in, 755-759
    transjugular portosystemic shunts in, 751-754
    variceal hemorrhage in
        decompressive shunts for, 744-748
        gastroesophageal devascularization for, 740-744
        pharmacologic intervention for, 732-735
Portal vein
    circulation of, 623-624
    occlusion of, 728-729
    presinusoidal obstruction of, 728-731
    thrombosis of
        in children, 760
        liver transplantation and, 757-758
Portosystemic collaterals, 728
Portosystemic decompression, 749
Portosystemic shunts
    in children, 762-763
    transjugular, 751-754
Postendarterectomy pseudoaneurysm, 109
Postphlebitic syndrome, 878-879
Post-traumatic pain, 163
Prazosin hydrochloride, 161-162
Prednisone, 132
Pregnancy
    deep vein thrombosis in, 907-910
    renal artery aneurysm in, 815
    thrombosis and, 552
Presinusoidal portal obstruction, 728-731
Pressure
    ambulatory venous, 886-887
    assessment
        in aortoiliac occlusive disease, 352-354
        in infrainguinal occlusive disease, 432-435
        in vascular laboratory, 147-148
    in compartment syndrome, 645-646
    in cutaneous foot ulcers, 560-561
    transcutaneous oxygen, 561
Pressure gradient
    equation for, 352-354
    intra-arterial, 440

percutaneous transluminal angioplasty and, 515
Prevention of hypertension, 343-345
Probucol, 338, 339
Profunda femoris artery, 457-461
Profundaplasty, 457-461
  in aortic graft limb occlusion, 424
Profunda-popliteal collateral index, 459
Proliferating cell nuclear antigen, 2, 3
Prophylaxis
  in angioaccess graft failure, 867
  for deep femoral venous thrombosis, 889-891
  in pregnancy, 909
L-propionylcarnitine, 536
Propranolol, 306, 307
Prostaglandins, 537
Prosthesis
  aneurysmal deterioration of, 289-292
  arteriovenous fistula, 865
  in bridge graft, 862-863
  cardiac macroemboli in, 586
  infected arterial, 322-325
  in sequential bypass, 473-474
  of upper extremity, 685
Protein C
  in coagulation, 868, 870
  deficiency
    as prothrombotic state, 551
    in warfarin-induced skin necrosis, 920
Protein S deficiency, 551
Proteolytic enzymes, 201-202
Prothia filter, 948-949
Prothrombotic states, 550-554
Provocative testing, 398
Pseudoaneurysm
  in direct arteriovenous anastomosis, 859
  of femoral artery, 319-321
  in percutaneous arterial puncture, 628-630
  postendarterectomy, 109
Pseudo-occlusion, 47-48
Pseudoxanthoma, 141
PTA; see Percutaneous transluminal angioplasty
PTFE; see Polytetrafluoroethylene
Pulmonary edema, 777
Pulmonary embolism
  acute
    nonoperative treatment of, 940-944
    surgical treatment of, 955-957
  in acute iliofemoral thrombosis, 933-934
  chronic, 957-958
  in deep femoral venous thrombosis, 889
  in paradoxical embolism, 590
  in pregnancy, 909
  in thromboembolism, 871
  transvenous catheter embolectomy of, 951-955
Pulmonary system in hypothermia, 663-664

Pulse
  in amputation assessment, 669
  in bridge graft, 862
  digital, 463
  in penetrating injury, 598
  in thoracic great vessel injury, 609
Pulse volume recorder
  in infrainguinal occlusive disease, 435
  in popliteal vascular entrapment syndrome, 504
Pump
  calf muscle, 911
  gradient sequential, 975
Puncture
  arterial
    in arteriography, 441-442
    in lower extremity, 628-631
  portal venous, 752-753

R

Radial artery
  in direct arteriovenous anastomosis, 858
  iatrogenic catheter injury to, 625
Radiation injury, 140
Radiation-induced arteritis, 133-137
Radical mastectomy, 979
Radicals, oxygen free, 582-585
Radicular artery, 278, 280
Radiocephalic fistula, 857
Radiography, 609
Radionuclides
  in aortic graft infection, 401-403
  in cutaneous foot ulcers, 561
Ray amputation
  of toe and foot, 673
  of upper extremity, 681-682
Raynaud's phenomenon, 151-153
  diagnosis of, 145-151
  sympathectomy in, 166
Reactive hyperemia, 69
Recanalization
  of iliac artery, 372
  in venous thrombosis, 877-878
Reconstruction
  aortoiliac, 399
  disease recurrence after, 334-335
  of infected femoral artery pseudoaneurysm, 321
  infrainguinal
    in aneurysmosis, 295
    short vein grafts in, 488
  in innominate artery atherosclerosis, 97, 98-99
  in renal artery dissection, 819-820
  in Takayasu's arteritis, 128, 129
  of vertebral artery, 84-89
Recovery room stroke, 74-75
Recurrence
  of cutaneous foot ulcers, 563-564
  of venous ulcers, 927
Red blood cells, 584
Reflex sympathetic dystrophy, 162-165
Reflux
  in chronic venous insufficiency, 886, 912

  in femoropopliteal thrombophlebitis, 906
  valvular, 915, 916-918
Regional anesthesia
  for carotid endarterectomy, 44-45
  cerebral ischemia and, 54-55
Rehabilitation, 674-675
Relaxing factor, 333
Renal artery
  abnormalities of, 211
  alternative reconstructive techniques for, 799-804
  aneurysm in, 813-817
  aortic aneurysm and, 242-245
  atherosclerosis of, 793-799
  dissection of, 818-820
  embolism of, 821-823
  injury to, 657-659
  occlusive disease of
    in chronic renal failure, 827-830
    duplex scanning for, 768-774
    functional significance of, 774-779
    pathology in, 764-768
  reconstruction of, 804-808
  stenosis of, 782-783
Renal cell carcinoma, 969
Renal duplex sonography, 768-769
Renal ectopia, 246-249
Renal failure
  chronic, 827-830
  in renal arterial occlusive disease, 777
  secondary, 650-652
Renal fusion, 246-249
Renal pedicle, 623
Renal transplants
  aortic reconstruction and, 250-251
  in renovascular hypertension, 782
Renal vein thrombosis, 823-826
Renal-systemic renin index, 786
Renin, 242
Renin-angiotensin system, 774, 775-778
Renography, captopril, 777-778
Renovascular disease, 764-833
  alternative reconstructive techniques for, 799-804
  aneurysm in, 813-817
  aortorenal endarterectomy for, 793-799
  arteriovenous malformation in, 830-833
  in chronic renal failure, 827-830
  duplex scanning in, 768-774
    operative assessment with, 804-808
  embolism in, 821-823
  functional significance of, 774-779
  hypertension in
    aortorenal bypass for, 785-789
    arteriographic diagnosis of, 779-780
    ex vivo arterial repair for, 790-793
    pediatric surgery for, 808-813
    percutaneous arterial dilation for, 780-785

Renovascular disease—cont'd
  hypertension in—cont'd
    renin-angiotensin system in, 774, 775-778
    secondary, 815
  pathology of, 764-768
  renal artery dissection in, 818-820
  renal vein thrombosis in, 823-826
Reperfusion in compartment syndrome, 646
Reperfusion injury, 636
Reperfusion syndrome, 650-652
  oxygen free radicals in, 582-585
Resection
  of carotid body tumor, 123-125
  in popliteal artery adventitial cystic disease, 511-512
  transaxillary first rib, 182-184
  in upper extremity aneurysms, 193
Reserpine, 306, 307
Reservoir of salvaged blood, 288-298
Resins in hyperlipidemia, 338, 339
Rest pain, 463
Restenosis, 783
Resuscitation, 609, 611
Retrograde balloon catheter embolectomy, 379
Retrohepatic inferior vena cava, 624-625
Retroperitoneal hematoma, 622-623
Retroperitoneal iliofemoral bypass, 391-392
Revascularization
  aortorenal bypass with, 787
  for cerebral steal syndrome, 93-95
  in chronic renal failure, 828-829
  of coronary artery, 102-104
  in cutaneous foot ulcers, 563
  of lower extremity, 476-480
  of renal artery, 242-243
  in Takayasu's arteritis, 128
  of upper extremity, 142-145
  of visceral artery, 242, 243
Reversed vein grafts
  autogenous, 465-469
  in infrainguinal occlusive disease, 525-526
Revision of graft, 498
Rewarming
  in frostbite, 666-667
  in hypothermia, 664
Rheological agents, 535-536
Rheumatoid arthritis, 139
Rib anomalies, 171, 172
Rifampin, 566
Right-to-left shunt, 590
Rosch-Uchida transjugular needle, 752
Runoff; *see also* Outflow
  in magnetic resonance angiography, 450-452
  percutaneous transluminal angioplasty and, 515
Rupture
  in aortic dissection, 207
  of iliac aneurysm, 300
  of renal artery aneurysm, 815

S

Salmonella, 232
Salvage
  in angioaccess graft failure, 867
  of blood, 288
  limb
    amputation versus, 632-633
    short vein grafts in, 488-491
Saphenous vein
  acute superficial thrombophlebitis in, 888-889
  acute superficial venous thrombosis of, 904-905
  in blunt arterial injury, 615
  bypass versus endarterectomy, 454-455
  for carotid endarterectomy patch angioplasty, 61-62, 63
  flush ligation of, 901
  patency of, 334, 335
  in reversed autogenous vein grafts, 466
  in situ graft of, 469-472
  in upper extremity aneurysms, 194
  in vein anatomy, 899-900
Sarcoma
  lymphedema and, 974
  vena caval, 967
Saturation in magnetic resonance angiography, 448
Scalene muscle
  anomalies of, 173-174
  ultrastructural studies of, 174-175
Schistosomiasis, 727
Sciatic artery, 499-504
Scimitar sign, 510
Scintigraphy, 346-348
Scleroderma, 139
Sclerosants, 897
Sclerotherapy
  of esophageal varices, 735-738
  injection compression, 894-898
  ligation versus, 739
  medical therapy versus, 738
  shunt versus, 738
Scribner shunt, 854-855
Sedation
  in arteriography, 441
  in renal arteriovenous embolization, 831
Segmental pressure
  in amputation assessment, 669
  color flow duplex scanning versus, 438-439
  in infrainguinal occlusive disease, 433-434
Seldinger percutaneous technique, 365
Semiclosed endarterectomy, 454
SEP; *see* Somatosensory evoked potentials
Sepsis
  catheter-associated, 963-964
  in groin, 322-325
  in phlebitis, 638
  in thrombophlebitis, 963-966

Sequential bypass, 473-475
Seroma, perigraft, 388
Sexual dysfunction, 397-398
Shivering, 663
Short vein grafts, 488-491
Shoulder, 614-615
Shunt
  atriocaval, 624
  central splenorenal, 745
  coronary caval, 731
  decompressive, 744-748
  direct mesocaval, 729
  in external angioaccess, 854-855
  H-graft interposition mesocaval, 744-745
  liver transplantation versus, 755-756
  lympholymphatic, 976
  lymphovenous, 976
  nonselective versus selective, 730-731
  peritoneovenous, 429
  pleuroperitoneal, 431
  portacaval, 744
  previous, 757
  right-to-left, 590
  selective, 745
  as spinal cord protection, 285
  splenorenal
    in portal hypertension, 728-729, 730
    in variceal hemorrhage, 745
  total, 744-745
  transjugular portosystemic, 751-754
  Warren, 730
Shunting
  arteriovenous
    in congenital vascular malformations, 838
    venous ulcers and, 922
  in carotid endarterectomy, 57-60
    for atherosclerotic disease, 42
    of fixed stroke, 39-40
Simpson Atherocath, 517-518, 519
Sinogram, 565
Siphon stenosis
  in intracranial occlusive disease, 65
  in occluded extracranial carotid artery, 46-47
Skin
  blood flow of, 670
  care of
    in chronic venous insufficiency, 912
    in lymphedema, 974
  grafting of, 932
  infarction of, 569
  ulceration of, 882-883
  warfarin-induced necrosis of, 919-921
Skull base aneurysm, 106-108
Small aorta syndrome, 328, 330
Small bowel disease, 236
Smoking
  in atherosclerotic disease prevention, 532-533
  in Buerger's disease, 155
  in stroke and transient ischemic attacks, 26
  and vascular disease, 333-335

Sodium intake, 979
Sodium warfarin
  in acute iliofemoral and caval thrombosis, 937-938
  in acute pulmonary embolism, 941-942
  for arterial macroembolism, 572-573
  in axillosubclavian vein thrombosis, 959
  in deep femoral venous thrombosis, 892
  for deep femoral venous thrombosis prophylaxis, 890
  in graft patency, 548-549
  pregnancy and, 908
  in stroke and transient ischemic attacks, 28
  in thromboembolism, 872-873
  thrombolytic therapy and, 573
Soft tissue
  arterial injury and, 631-634
  in intravenous drug abuse, 637-638
Solid-state transducer, 646
Somatosensory evoked potentials
  in carotid artery reconstruction, 55-56
  in carotid endarterectomy shunting, 58
  in spinal cord ischemia, 285
Somatostatin, 734
Sonography; *see* Duplex scanning
Spectral analysis
  of carotid artery occlusive disease, 8-13
  intravascular ultrasound versus, 527
Sphygmomanometer, 432
Spider telangiectasia, 894-898
Spinal cord
  blood supply to, 285
  ischemia
    in abdominal aortic reconstruction, 278-282
    in thoracoabdominal aortic reconstruction, 282-286
Spins in magnetic resonance angiography, 447-448
Splanchnic arteriovenous fistulas, 721-724
Splanchnic circulation
  occlusive disease of, 686-689
  vascular malformation of, 718-720
Splanchnic endarterectomy, 699-701
Splenectomy, 741
Splenic artery
  aneurysm of, 716-718
  in splenorenal bypass, 799-800
Splenic fistula, 723, 724
Splenic vein
  occlusion of, 728, 729
  thrombosis of, 729
Splenorenal bypass, 799-800
Splenorenal shunt
  in bilharzial portal hypertension, 747-748
  in portal hypertension, 728-729, 730
  in variceal hemorrhage, 745

Spontaneous atheroembolism, 568-571
Spontaneous dissection of renal artery, 819-820
Stab avulsion of varicose vein clusters, 902-903
Staged subcutaneous excision, 976-978
Staphylococci
  coagulase-negative, 406
  as external angioaccess complication, 856
  in graft infection, 565
    aortic, 400, 405
Stasis
  ulcers, 910-913
  in venous thrombosis, 874
Statin, 338, 339
Steal syndrome
  cerebral, 93-95
  in direct arteriovenous anastomosis, 859
  pelvic, 398, 399-400
  subclavian, 139-140
Stellate ganglion block, 166
Stenosis
  balloon angioplasty in, 521
  of carotid artery
    asymptomatic, 29-34
    duplex scanning and, 12
    in fibroplasia, 4-5
    transcranial Doppler ultrasound in, 16
  criteria defining, 437-438
  in direct arteriovenous anastomosis, 859
  of femoral artery, 212
  in graft surveillance, 494-495, 496
  of iliac artery, 212
  in magnetic resonance angiography, 452
  occlusion versus, 513-515
  of profunda femoris artery, 457
  of renal artery, 242, 767-768
    aortorenal endarterectomy for, 793-799
    in child, 782-783
    Doppler velocity criteria for, 805, 806-807
    unilateral versus bilateral, 774-775, 776
  in renal duplex sonography, 770
  short vein grafts and, 490
  siphon
    in intracranial occlusive disease, 65
    in occluded extracranial carotid artery, 46-47
  of subclavian artery, 93-95
  of subclavian vein, 856
  in transjugular portosystemic shunt, 754
Stent
  in iliac artery, 370-372
  in infrarenal aorta, 367, 368, 369-370
  renal artery angioplasty and, 783-785
  ureteral, 231

Sternotomy
  in innominate artery atherosclerosis, 96-99
  in thoracic great vessel thoracotomy, 610
Steroids in hemangioma, 847
Stockings
  in chronic venous insufficiency, 913
  for deep femoral venous thrombosis, 890
  in injection compression sclerotherapy, 894, 895
  for varicose veins, 900-901
Strecker stent, 372
Streptokinase
  for arterial macroembolism, 573
  in deep femoral venous thrombosis, 893
  in ergotism, 161
  in fibrinolytic therapy, 540
Stress test, elevated arm, 176
Stretch syncope, 606
Stripper, endarterectomy, 423
Stripping
  of varicose veins, 901-902
  in venous ulcers, 930
Stroke
  after carotid endarterectomy, 73-75
  cardiopulmonary bypass and, 103
  in carotid artery atherosclerosis, 80-84
  in carotid endarterectomy shunting, 58
  evolving, 34-38
  fixed, 38-40
  hypertension and, 342
  in intracranial occlusive disease, 65
  ischemic
    antithrombotic therapy for, 26-28
    medical therapy for, 24-29
  magnetic resonance imaging and, 23
  occluded extracranial carotid artery and, 50
  in recurrent carotid artery stenosis, 76
  in young patients, 25
Stump
  aortic, 408-409
  in below-knee amputation, 674
  blood pressure of
    in carotid artery reconstruction, 55
    in carotid endarterectomy shunting, 57
Subclavian artery
  aneurysm of, 188-194
  blunt injury of, 614
  to carotid transposition, 89-92
  penetrating injury of, 608-613
  repair of, 612
  stenosis of, 93-95
  thoracic outlet compression of, 138
Subclavian steal syndrome, 93-95
  in upper extremity arterial disease, 139-140

Subclavian vein
    central venous cannulation in, 853-854
    stenosis of, 856
    transluminal balloon angioplasty of, 960-961
Subclavian-axillary lesions, 134, 135
Subclavius muscle anomalies, 174
Suction curettage, 976
Sugiura procedure
    in portal vein occlusion, 729
    for variceal hemorrhage, 742-744
Sulcal arteries, 278
Sulfinpyrazone, 547
Supernumerary scalene muscles, 173
Support hose; see Stockings
Suppurative thrombophlebitis, 963-966
Supraceliac aorta, 788-789
Supraclavicular operative approach, 185-188
Suprainguinal arteries, 391-392
Suprarenal aorta, 373-377
Surgery
    of carotid body tumor, 123-125
    of small abdominal aortic aneurysm, 228
Suture
    in concomitant venous repair, 654
    polytetrafluoroethylene, 466-467
Syme's amputation
    of toe and foot, 673
    of upper extremity, 681
Sympathectomy, 165-169
    anterior transthoracic dorsal, 167-169
    cervical, 163, 164
    cervico-dorsal, 166-167
    lumbar
        for cutaneous ischemic ulcers, 462-465
        livedo reticularis, 153
    in Raynaud's phenomenon, 153
    stellate ganglion block in, 166
    thoracoscopic dorsal, 169
    transaxillary thoracic dorsal, 167, 168
Syncope, 606
Systemic lupus erythematosus, 139
Systolic blood pressure
    coronary heart disease and, 343, 344
    segmental Doppler measurement of, 669

T

Takayasu's arteritis, 125-129
    pediatric renovascular hypertension versus, 809
    in upper extremity arterial disease, 140
TCD; see Transcranial Doppler ultrasound
Teflon; see Polytetrafluoroethylene
Telangiectasia
    spider, 894-898
    in splanchnic circulation, 720

Temporal arteritis, 130-133
    in upper extremity arterial disease, 141
Temporal artery biopsy, 131
Terlipressin, 733-734
Terminal device in amputation, 685
Terminal Syme's amputation, 681
Theratek catheter, 518-519
Thermography, 671
Thigh
    blood pressure of, 433-434
    neuralgia of, 463
    perforating veins of, 901-902
Thigh ankle gradient index, 459
Thomas shunt, 855
Thompson's buried dermal flap, 976
Thoracentesis, 427-428
Thoracic aorta
    coarctation and hypoplasia of, 359-363
    dissection of, 309-314
    to femoral bypass, 381-383
Thoracic aortorenal bypass, 802, 803
Thoracic dorsal sympathectomy, 167, 168
Thoracic great vessels, 608-613
Thoracic outlet obstruction, 189, 190
Thoracic outlet syndrome, 169-188
    diagnosis of, 176-179
    etiology and anatomic pathology of, 169-175
    management of
        nonoperative, 179-181
        supraclavicular operative, 185-188
        transaxillary operative, 182-184
    as upper extremity arterial disease, 138
Thoracoabdominal aortic aneurysm, 255-261
Thoracoabdominal bypass, 361-362
Thoracoscopic dorsal sympathectomy, 169
Thoracostomy, 609-610
Thoracotomy, 610-613
Thrombectomy
    in acute aortic occlusion, 379
    in acute graft thrombosis, 539
    in acute iliofemoral thrombosis, 934-935
    in aortic graft limb occlusion, 422-424
    of expanded polytetrafluoroethylene graft, 483
    in femoropopliteal thrombophlebitis, 906
    of occluded extracranial carotid artery, 50-52
    in umbilical artery injury, 661
Thrombin, 868, 870
Thromboangiitis obliterans, 140
Thrombocytopenia
    as heparin therapy complication, 556-557
    heparin-induced
        in acute iliofemoral and caval thrombosis, 937

in aortic reconstruction, 273
    in deep femoral venous thrombosis, 892
    thrombosis and, 551-552
Thromboembolectomy
    balloon catheter, 822-823
    percutaneous aspiration, 580-582
Thromboembolic vertebrobasilar insufficiency, 84-85
Thromboembolism, 870-874
    after aortic reconstruction, 272
    in percutaneous arterial puncture, 630
    in pregnancy, 909
    in upper extremity aneurysms, 191
Thromboendarterectomy
    in chronic pulmonary embolism, 957
    of mesenteric artery, 695-696
    of occluded extracranial carotid artery, 52-53
Thrombolytic therapy
    in acute graft thrombosis, 538-539
    in acute iliofemoral and caval thrombosis, 938-939
    in acute pulmonary embolism, 943, 944
    in angioaccess graft failure, 867
    aortic graft limb occlusion and, 424
    for arterial macroembolism, 573-576
    in axillosubclavian vein thrombosis, 959
    in deep femoral venous thrombosis, 892-893
    evolving stroke and, 35-36
    iatrogenic pediatric vascular injury and, 662
    in paradoxical embolism, 591-592
    in popliteal artery aneurysm, 326
    in renal artery embolism, 822
    in renal vein thrombosis, 825-826
    transient ischemic attacks and, 28
    transvenous catheter pulmonary embolectomy and, 951
Thrombophlebitis
    acute superficial, 888-889
    of femoropopliteal veins, 905-906
    of saphenous vein, 904-905
    septic, 963-966
Thromboplastin time, 554-555
Thrombosis
    in angioaccess, 865
    in aortic occlusion
        acute, 378
        graft limb, 419
    in arteriosclerotic femoral artery aneurysm, 315
    axillosubclavian vein, 958-963
    in catheter, 856
    caval, 936-939
    deep vein
        femoral, 889-893
        in intravenous drug abuse, 638
        invasive diagnosis of, 884-885
        noninvasive diagnosis of, 880-881
        in paradoxical embolism, 590
        in pregnancy, 907-910
        as risk factor, 874-875

saphenous thrombophlebitis and, 904
fibrinolytic therapy for, 540-544
graft
    bridge, 862
    bypass, 537-539
    expanded polytetrafluoroethylene, 482
    failure of, 544-546
    surveillance of, 493
as heparin therapy complication, 555-557
in iatrogenic injury
    catheter, 625-626
    pediatric vascular, 660
iliofemoral
    nonoperative treatment of, 936-939
    surgical treatment of, 932-935
in mesenteric ischemia, 693-697
in occluded extracranial carotid artery, 45-46
in percutaneous arterial puncture, 630
prothrombotic states and, 550-554
of renal vein, 823-826
venous, 875-878
    acute, 904-906
    mesenteric, 710-713
    in septic thrombophlebitis, 964
warfarin-induced skin necrosis and, 919

Thrombus
    evolving stroke and, 35-36
    in thromboembolism, 871

TIA; see Transient ischemic attacks

Ticlopidine
    in graft patency, 547-548
    for lower extremity occlusive disease, 536
    in stroke and transient ischemic attacks, 26, 27

Time
    activated partial thromboplastin, 554-555
    of aortic cross-clamp, 283

Tissue
    in aortic graft infection, 406-407
    in coagulation, 868

Tissue ischemia score, 642-943
Tissue plasminogen activator, 573

Toe
    amputation of, 672-674
    blue toe syndrome of, 568-571
        lumbar sympathectomy in, 463
    in cutaneous foot ulcers, 560-561
    disarticulation of, 673

Tolazoline
    in arteriography, 444
    for lower extremity occlusive disease, 535

Tortuosity of carotid artery, 119
Tracheobronchial injury, 613
Transabdominal medial visceral rotation, 373-377
Transaortic splanchnic endarterectomy, 697-701

Transaxillary first rib resection, 182-184
Transaxillary thoracic dorsal sympathectomy, 167, 168
Transcatheter therapy
    in nonocclusive mesenteric ischemia, 692
    of visceral ischemia, 689-693
Transcranial Doppler ultrasound
    in carotid artery reconstruction, 55
    in carotid endarterectomy shunting, 57-58
    in cerebrovascular disease, 15-19
Transcutaneous oxygen pressure, 561
Transducer
    in duplex scanning, 446
    solid-state, 646
Transesophageal echocardiography, 587-588
Transfusion, 298
Transient ischemic attacks
    after carotid endarterectomy, 75
    antithrombotic therapy for, 26-28
    in carotid artery atherosclerosis, 80-84
    computed tomography and, 20
    definition of, 24
    evolving stroke and, 34
    mechanisms of, 24-25
    medical therapy for, 24-29
    risk reduction in, 25-26
    in thromboembolic vertebrobasilar insufficiency, 84-85
Transjugular portosystemic shunts, 751-754
Translumbar aortography, 44
Transluminal angioplasty; see Angioplasty
Transluminal catheter-induced dissection, 818-820
Transmetatarsal amputation, 673
Transmural intestinal ischemia, 277
Transplant
    liver
        in Budd-Chiari syndrome, 750-751
        in portal hypertension, 755-759
    renal
        aortic reconstruction and, 250-251
        in renovascular hypertension, 782
Transposition
    omental
        in lymphedema, 976
        in secondary lymphedema, 980, 981
    subclavian to carotid, 89-92
Transthoracic dorsal sympathectomy, 167-169
Transverse arteriotomy, 695
Trapdoor aortotomy, 698
Trauma, 593-668; see also Injury
    blunt injury in
        abdominal, 619-625
        elbow arterial, 615-616
        extracranial carotid artery, 601-603
        knee, 634-636
        renal, 657-659
        shoulder arterial, 614-615
        vertebral artery, 606-608
    cold injury in, 663-668
    compartment syndrome in, 644-648
    concomitant venous repair in, 652-656
    drug abuse in, 637-644
    fasciotomy in, 648-649
    fractures in, 631-634
    iatrogenic arterial catheter, 625-627
    iatrogenic pediatric, 659-662
    penetrating injury in
        abdominal, 619-625
        arteriography of, 596-598
        extracranial carotid artery, 598-601
        extremities, 617-619
        nonarteriographic assessment of, 593-595
        renal, 657-659
        thoracic great vessels, 608-613
        vertebral artery, 604-608
    percutaneous arterial puncture as, 628-631
    reperfusion syndrome in, 650-652
    soft tissue in, 631-634
Treadmill, 434-435
Trenchfoot, 666
Triad, Virchow's
    in mesenteric venous thrombosis, 710
    in venous thrombosis, 874
Tricuspid annuloplasty, 957-958
Tricyclics, 163
Tumescence, nocturnal penile, 398
Tumor
    body, 121-125
    gastric, 236
    vena caval, 967-970
Tunnel
    in axillounifemoral bypass, 385
    in descending thoracic aorta to femoral bypass, 382, 383

U

Ulcer
    in chronic venous insufficiency, 882-883
    diabetic foot, 558-564
    of esophageal varices, 737
    of hemangioma, 848
    lumbar sympathectomy for, 462-465
    stasis, 910-913
    venous
        nonoperative treatment of, 924-927
        operative treatment of, 927-932
        pathogenesis of, 922-923
Ulnar artery aneurysm, 195
Ultrasonography; see also Doppler ultrasound
    of abdominal aortic aneurysm, 214
    in groin lymphocele, 414
    in inflammatory abdominal aortic aneurysm, 230

Ultrasonography—cont'd
  in lower extremity occlusive disease, 527-531
  in renal vein thrombosis, 824
Umbilical artery, 661-662
Umbilical vein grafts, 484-487
Underdosage of heparin, 555-557
Unilateral retroperitoneal iliofemoral bypass, 391-392
Unna's boot, 913
Upper extremity, 138-197
  amputation of, 680-685
  aneurysms of, 188-194
  arterial disease pathology of, 138-141
  Buerger's disease of, 154-159
  causalgia and mimocausalgia in, 162-165
  concomitant venous repair in, 655
  ergotism in, 159-162
  hypothenar hammer syndrome in, 195-197
  iatrogenic arterial catheter injury to, 625-627
  revascularization of, 142-145
  sympathectomy of, 165-169
  thoracic outlet syndrome in, 169-188
    diagnosis of, 176-179
    etiology and anatomic pathology of, 169-175
    nonoperative management of, 179-181
    supraclavicular operative approach to, 185-188
    transaxillary operative management of, 182-184
  vasospastic disease in
    acrocyanosis as, 154
    diagnosis of, 145-151
    livedo reticularis as, 153-154
    Raynaud's phenomenon as, 151-153
    treatment of, 151-154
  venous occlusion in, 958-963
Ureteral stent, 231
Urokinase
  for arterial macroembolism, 573
  in axillosubclavian vein thrombosis, 959
  evolving stroke and, 35-36
  in fibrinolytic therapy, 540

V

Valve
  in chronic venous insufficiency, 911
  incompetent
    in chronic venous insufficiency, 914
    in varicose veins, 900
    in venous ulcers, 922
  lysis of, 525
  post-thrombotic, 878
  prosthetic, 586
  reflux, 915, 916-918
  in in situ saphenous vein graft, 470

vegetations
  cardiac macroemboli in, 586
  in intravenous drug abuse, 639
Valvuloplasty, 915, 916-918
Valvulotomy, 470
Vancomycin, 856
Variceal hemorrhage
  decompressive shunts for, 744-748
  gastroesophageal devascularization for, 740-744
  pharmacology in, 732-735
  in portal hypertension, 761
Varices
  bleeding, 733
  esophageal
    ligation of, 738-739
    sclerotherapy of, 735-738
  mesenteric, 720
Varicose veins
  acute superficial thrombophlebitis and, 888
  in chronic venous insufficiency, 885
  excision of, 898-904
  injection compression sclerotherapy of, 894-898
Vasa vasorum
  in aortic dissection, 206
  in renal fibromuscular disease, 767
  in venous thrombosis, 876
Vascular laboratory, 147-149
  digital plethysmography in, 148
  duplex and Doppler examinations in, 148-149
  pressure measurements in, 147-148
  vasospasm tests in, 149
Vascular trauma; see Trauma
Vasculitides, 446
Vasculogenic impotence, 397-400
Vasodilation, sympathectomy and, 165
Vasodilators
  in arteriography, 444
  for lower extremity occlusive disease, 534-535
Vasopressin, for treatment of variceal hemorrhage, 733
Vasospasm
  in iatrogenic pediatric vascular injury, 660
  mesenteric, 693-694
  transcranial Doppler ultrasound and, 18
  in vascular laboratory, 149
Vasospastic disease
  diagnosis of, 145-151
  treatment of, 151-154
Vegetations, valvular
  cardiac macroemboli in, 586
  in intravenous drug abuse, 639
Vein
  anomalies of, 252-255
  arm, 476-480
  in bridge grafts, 861
  concomitant repair of, 652-656
  congenital vascular malformations of, 837
  malformation of, 850-852

in thoracic great vessel injury, 613
thrombosis of, 710-713
Vein graft
  reversed, 525-526
    autogenous, 465-469
  in sequential bypass, 473-474
  short, 488-491
  in situ
    reversed autogenous vein grafts versus, 468-469
    saphenous, 469-472
Velocity
  of blood flow, 493-494
  detector of, 432, 433
  Doppler criteria of, 805, 806-807
  in duplex imaging, 437-438
Velour in arterial grafts, 290
Vena cava
  in abdominal vascular injury, 624-625
  aortic reconstruction and, 252-255
  filter in
    in acute pulmonary embolism, 944
    percutaneous devices for, 945-949
    transvenous catheter pulmonary embolectomy and, 953
  fistula of, abdominal aortic aneurysm and, 261-262
  operative interruption of, 949-951
  perforation of, 855
  thrombosis in, 936-939
  tumors of, 967-970
Vena Tech filter, 946-947
Venography; see Angiography
Veno-occlusive disease, 727
Venous disease, 868-972
  acute iliofemoral thrombosis in
    nonoperative treatment of, 936-939
    surgical treatment of, 932-935
  acute superficial thrombophlebitis in, 888-889
  acute thrombosis in, 904-906
  aneurysms in, 970-972
  chronic insufficiency in
    invasive diagnosis of, 885-887
    noninvasive diagnosis of, 881-883
    nonoperative management of, 910-913
    surgical management of, 914-919
  coagulation cascade in, 868-874
  deep femoral thrombosis in, 889-893
  injection compression sclerotherapy in, 894-898
  invasive diagnosis of, 884-888
  noninvasive diagnosis of, 879-883
  pathophysiology of, 874-879
  in pregnancy, 907-910
  pulmonary embolism in
    nonoperative treatment of, 940-944
    surgical treatment of, 955-958
    transvenous catheter embolectomy of, 951-955
  septic thrombophlebitis in, 963-966

thromboembolism in, 868-874
ulcers in
   nonoperative treatment of, 924-927
   operative treatment of, 927-932
   pathogenesis of, 922-923
   upper extremity occlusion in, 958-963
varicose vein excision in, 898-904
vena cava in
   filtration devices for, 945-949
   interruption of, 949-951
   thrombosis of, 936-939
   tumors of, 967-970
warfarin-induced skin necrosis in, 919-921

Venous thoracic outlet syndrome, 176-177
  transaxillary first rib resection in, 182
Venovenous bypass, 756-757
Ventilation/perfusion scanning
  in acute pulmonary embolism, 956
  in thromboembolism, 871
Ventricular hypertrophy, 341-342
Vertebral artery
  blunt injury of, 606-608
  fibrodysplasia of, 4-7
  penetrating injury of, 604-608
  reconstruction of, 84-89
Vertebrobasilar insufficiency, 84-89
Vertebrobasilar ischemia, 20-21
Vibratory white finger, 139
Virchow's triad
  in mesenteric venous thrombosis, 710
  in venous thrombosis, 874
Visceral artery
  aortic aneurysm and, 242-245
  occlusive disease of, 211-212
  reconstruction of, 804-808
Visceral ischemia, 689-693
Visceral rotation, transabdominal medial, 373-377

W

Walking, 533
Wallstent
  in atherosclerotic aortoiliac occlusive disease, 369-370
  studies of, 372
  in transjugular portosystemic shunts, 753
Warfarin
  in acute iliofemoral and caval thrombosis, 937-938
  in acute pulmonary embolism, 941-942
  for arterial macroembolism, 572-573
  in axillosubclavian vein thrombosis, 959
  for deep femoral venous thrombosis, 890, 892
  in expanded polytetrafluoroethylene graft, 482
  in graft patency, 548-549
  pregnancy and, 908
  in stroke and transient ischemic attacks, 28
  in thromboembolism, 872-873
  thrombolytic therapy and, 573
Warfarin-induced skin necrosis, 919-921
Warren shunt, 730
Waveform
  in aortoiliac occlusive disease, 351
  in graft surveillance, 494, 495
  in infrainguinal occlusive disease, 437-438
Wet gangrene, 672
White blood cells
  in graft infection, 565
  in reperfusion syndrome, 584
  in venous ulcers, 923
Wound care
  in graft infection, 565-566
  in venous ulcers, 925
Woven fabric in arterial grafts, 290
Wrist disarticulation, 682-683